Textbook of
MEDICINE

Textbook of
MEDICINE

Sixth Edition

Volume II

KV Krishna Das
BSc FRCP (E) FAMS DTM&H
Retired Director and Professor
Department of Medicine
Government Medical College
Thiruvananthapuram, Kerala, India

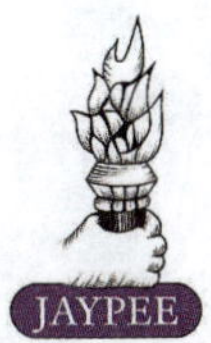

JAYPEE BROTHERS MEDICAL PUBLISHERS
The Health Sciences Publisher
New Delhi | London

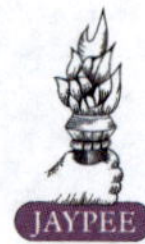

Jaypee Brothers Medical Publishers (P) Ltd

Headquarters
EMCA House
23/23-B, Ansari Road, Daryaganj
New Delhi 110 002, India
Landline: +91-11-23272143, +91-11-23272703
+91-11-23282021, +91-11-23245672
E-mail: jaypee@jaypeebrothers.com

Corporate Office
Jaypee Brothers Medical Publishers (P) Ltd.
4838/24, Ansari Road, Daryaganj
New Delhi 110 002, India
Phone: +91-11-43574357
Fax: +91-11-43574314
E-mail: jaypee@jaypeebrothers.com

Overseas Office
JP Medical Ltd.
83, Victoria Street, London
SW1H 0HW (UK)
Phone: +44-20 3170 8910
E-mail: info@jpmedpub.com

EU GPSR Authorised Representative
Logos Europe, 9 rue Nicolas Poussin
17000, La Rochelle, France
Phone: +33 (0) 6 67 93 73 78
E-mail: Contact@logoseurope.eu

Website: www.jaypeebrothers.com
Website: www.jaypeedigital.com

Inquiries for bulk sales may be solicited at: jaypee@jaypeebrothers.com

Textbook of Medicine (Sixth Edition, Volume II)

First Edition	:	1986
Second Edition	:	1990
Third Edition	:	1996
Fourth Edition	:	2002
Fifth Edition	:	2008
Reprint	:	2014
Sixth Edition	:	2017
Reprint	:	2023, 2024, **2025**

ISBN: 978-93-86056-10-8

Printed at: Samrat Offset Pvt. Ltd,

This book is dedicated to my alma mater
Medical College and Hospital, Thiruvananthapuram
*where I started learning the first principles of medicine and
thereafter; had the honor to serve as its staff and
continue my close association with the college
even several years after my retirement*

Contributors

A George Koshy MD (Med) DM Cardiology FACC FSCAI FRCP
Professor and Head
Department of Cardiology
Government Medical College
Thiruvananthapuram, Kerala, India

AG Unnikrishnan MD DM
Formerly, Professor of Endocrinology
Amrita Institute of Medical Sciences
Kochi, Kerala, India
Consultant in Diabetology
Chellaram Diabetes Institute
Bavdhan, Pune, Maharashtra, India

Anand Kumar MD DM
Professor and Head
Department of Neurology
Amrita Institute of Medical Sciences
Kochi, Kerala, India

Anjali Bhatt MD-Medicine Fellowship in Diabetology
Consultant in Diabetology
Chellaram Diabetes Institute
Bavdhan, Pune, Maharashtra, India

Arun N Babu MD DM
Assistant Professor
Department of Neurology
Amrita Institute of Medical Sciences
Kochi, Kerala, India

AS Girija MD DM
Retd Professor and Head
Department of Neurology
Government Medical College
Kozhikode, Kerala, India
Professor
Department of Neurology
Christian Medical College
Vellore, Tamil Nadu, India
Consultant Neurologist
Malabar Institute of Medical Sciences
Kozhikode, Kerala, India

Aswini Kumar MD
Professor and HOD of Medicine
Government Medical College
Parippally, Kollam, Kerala, India

B Jayakumar MBBS MD DM
Professor and Head of Department of General Medicine
Chief of Endocrinology and Diabetology
Government Medical College
Thiruvananthapuram, Kerala, India

B Krishna Swamy MD
Professor and Head
Department of Geriatric Medicine
Madras Medical College
Chennai, Tamil Nadu, India

Balu Vaidyanathan MD DNB DM FACC
Clinical Professor
Pediatric Cardiology
Fetal Cardiology Division
Amrita Institute of Medical Sciences
Kochi, Kerala, India

Binoy J Paul MD PhD DNB
Formerly Professor of Medicine
Government Medical College
Professor of Medicine and In-charge of Rheumatology
KMCT Medical College
Kozhikode, Kerala, India

C Sudheendra Ghosh MD (Med) MD (Resp) Dip NB MPH (USA)
Formerly Joint Director of Medical Education
Government Medical College
Professor of Respiratory Medicine
Sree Gokulam Medical College
Thiruvananthapuram, Kerala, India

CG Bahuleyan MBBS MD DM FRCP FSCAI
Formerly Professor and Head
Department of Cardiology
Government Medical College
Consultant Cardiologist
Ananthapuri Hospitals and Research Institute
Thiruvananthapuram, Kerala, India

CP Murali MD
Associate Professor of Chest Diseases
Government Medical College
Thrissur, Kerala, India

CV Soumya MD DM
Neurophysician
AKG Hospital
Kannur, Kerala, India

Davis Paul MD
Professor and HOD of Chest Diseases
Government Medical College
Thrissur, Kerala, India

George Kurian MD DM
Professor of Nephrology
Amrita Institute of Medical Sciences
Kochi, Kerala, India

Gomathy S MD DM
Additional Professor of Nephrology
Government TD Medical College
Vandanam, Alappuzha, Kerala, India

Jacob George MD DM FRCP (Glasgow) FICP (India)
Professor and Head
Department of Nephrology
Government Medical College
Thiruvananthapuram, Kerala, India

Jaisy Mathai MBBS Dip in Blood Transfusion
HOD-Transfusion Medicine
SCTIMST
Thiruvananthapuram, Kerala, India

Jayant Thomas Mathew MD DM
Professor of Nephrology
Amala Institute of Medical Sciences
Amalanagar, Thrissur, Kerala, India

Jigy Joseph MD DM
Associate Professor of Nephrology
Sree Gokulam Medical College
Thiruvananthapuram, Kerala, India

K Sreekanthan MD
Professor and Head
Department of Medicine
Azeezia Medical College
Meeyannoor, Kollam, Kerala, India

K Suresh MD DM
Formerly, Professor and Head
Department of Cardiology
Government Medical College
Consultant Cardiologist
KIMS Hospital
Thiruvananthapuram, Kerala, India

KA Kabeer MBBS MD DM
Additional Professor
Department of Neurology
Government TD Medical College
Alappuzha, Kerala, India

Kapilamoorthy MD DMR
Professor and Head
Department of Imageology
SCTIMST
Thiruvananthapuram, Kerala, India

Karru Venkata Ravi Teja MBBS PhD ICMR Fellowship
Senior Resident
NIMHANS
Bengaluru, Karnataka, India

Kasim Salim MD FRCP FRCP (Ed) FRCPath (Hematology)
Retd HOD–Medicine
Government Medical College
Consultant Hematologist
Kozhikode, Kerala, India

KE Elizabeth MD PhD
Professor and Head
Department of Pediatrics
Sree Mookambika Institute of Medical Sciences
Kulasekharam, Kanyakumari District, Tamil Nadu, India

KE Rajan MD
Professor–Respiratory Medicine
SUT Academy of Medical Sciences
Vattappara, Kerala, India

KP Poulose BSc MD FRCP
Retd Professor of Medicine
Government Medical College
Kottayam, Kerala, India
Consultant
Sree Uthradom Thirunal Group of Hospitals
Thiruvananthapuram, Kerala, India

KR Vinaya Kumar MD DM MRCP
Former Professor
Department of Gastroenterology
Government Medical College
Thiruvananthapuram, Kerala, India
Professor of Gastroenterology
Travancore Medical College Hospital
Kollam, Kerala, India

M Thomas Mathew MD DM
Formerly Professor
Government Medical College
Consultant-Nephrology
Baby Memorial Hospital
Kozhikode, Kerala, India

M Zulfikar Ahamed MD DM
Professor of Pediatric Cardiology
SAT Hospital
Government Medical College
Thiruvananthapuram, Kerala, India

Manu G Krishna MD DM
Assistant Professor
Pushpagiri Medical College
Thiruvalla, Kerala, India

Mathew John MD DM
Former Faculty
Department of Endocrinology
Christian Medical College
Vellore, Tamil Nadu, India
Chief Consultant
Providence Endocrine and Diabetes Specialty Centre
Murinjapalam, Thiruvananthapuram, Kerala, India

Mathew Thomas MD
Professor and Head
Department of Medicine
Dr Somervell Memorial CSI Hospital and Medical College
Karakonam, Thiruvananthapuram, Kerala, India

Mirza Masoom Abbas MBBS MD DM
Consultant in Neurology, currently in Singapore

N Krishnan Kutty MD (Psych)
Currently Consultant Psychiatrist
Formerly Professor and HOD–Psychiatry
Government Medical College
Thiruvananthapuram, Kerala, India

N Sudhaya Kumar MD DM
Consultant Cardiologist
Formerly HOD–Cardiology
Government Medical College
Kottayam, Kerala, India

Nethravathi M MD DM
Additional Professor
Department of Neurology
NIMHANS
Bengaluru, Karnataka, India

Noble Gracious MD DM
Associate Professor of Nephrology
Government Medical College
Thiruvananthapuram, Kerala, India

PK Jabbar MD DNB DM
Additional Director–Endocrinology
Indian Institute of Diabetes
Pulayanarkotta, Thiruvananthapuram, Kerala, India

PK Sasidharan MD
Ex-Professor and Head
Government Medical College
Consultant–Internal Medicine
PVS Hospital
Kozhikode, Kerala, India

R Jayachandran MBBS MD DM
Staff of NIMHANS on training in USA

R Kasi Visweswaran MD DM FRCP
Retd Professor and HOD
Department of Nephrology
Government Medical College
Consultant in Nephrology
Ananthapuri Hospital
Thiruvananthapuram, Kerala, India

R Sajith Kumar MD
Professor of Infecious Diseases
Government Medical College
Kottayam, Kerala, India

Ramdas Pisharody MBBS MD DM MSc (Clin. epidemiology)
Formerly Professor of Nephrology
Government Medical College
Hon Sr Consultant–Nephrology
KIMS Hospital, Thiruvananthapuram, Kerala, India

Ranjit Sanu Watson MD DNB (Neurology)
Additional Professor
Department of Neurology
Government Medical College
Thiruvananthapuram, Kerala, India

Reena Thomas MD DM
Associate Professor of Nephrology
Pushpagiri Medical College
Thiruvalla, Kerala, India

Rita Christopher MBBS MD
Professor and Head
Department of Neurochemistry
NIMHANS
Bengaluru, Karnataka, India

RK Shenoy MD
Retd Professor and Head
Government TD Medical College
Vandanam, Alappuzha, Kerala, India

RV Jayakumar MD DM FRCP MNAMS
Former HOD–Medicine
Government Medical College
Kottayam, Kerala, India
Professor of Endocrinology
Amrita Institute of Medical Sciences
Kochi, Kerala, India

S Bhasi MD
Professor–Medicine
Sree Gokulam Medical College
Thiruvananthapuram, Kerala, India

S Pradeep Nair MD
Professor and Head
Department of Dermatology and Venereology
Government Medical College
Thiruvananthapuram, Kerala, India

Sajan Z Ahmed MD
Resident
Department of Cardiology
Government Medical College
Thiruvananthapuram, Kerala, India

Salim Shafeek MD FRCP FRCP (Ed) FRCPath (Hematology)
Consultant Hematologist and
Clinical Director of Hemato-oncology
Worcestershire
Honorary Sr Lecturer in Clinical Hematology
University of Birmingham
United Kingdom

SR Chandra MD DM
Professor and Head
Department of Neurology
NIMHANS
Bengaluru, Karnataka, India

SR Srinivasa Kannan MD DM
Director
Vivek Laboratories
Nagercoil, Tamil Nadu, India

Sreelatha M MD DM
Professor of Nephrology
Government Medical College
Kozhikode, Kerala, India

Suhail Mohammed PT MBBS MD FCD DND (Cardiology)
ALMAS Hospital
Kottakkal, Malappuram, Kerala, India

Susan Uthup MD DM
Assistant Professor
Department of Nephrology (Pediatric)
SAT Hospital and Medical College
Thiruvananthapuram, Kerala, India

Swaraj Sathyan MD DM
Consultant Nephrologist
ALMAS Hospital
Kottakkal, Malappuram, Kerala, India

Thomas Gregor Issac MBBS MD PhD (Clinical neurology)
Resident
Department of Psychiatry
NIMHANS
Bengaluru, Karnataka, India

Thomas Iype MD DM
Professor and Head
Department of Neurology
Government Medical College
Thiruvananthapuram, Kerala, India

TK Suma MD
Professor of Medicine
Government TD Medical College
Vandanam, Alappuzha, Kerala, India

Usha Samuel MD DM
Professor of Nephrology
Government TD Medical College
Vandanam, Alappuzha, Kerala, India

Usha Vaidhyanathan MBBS DNB
Consultant in Dermatology and Cosmatology
KIMS Hospital
Anayara, Thiruvananthapuram, Kerala, India

Vidhya Annapoorni CS MBBS MS MCH
SAT Hospital
Government Medical College
Thiruvananthapuram, Kerala, India

Vimala A MBBS MD DM (Nephrology), FRCP (London)
Professor and Head–Nephrology
Dr Somervell Memorial CSI Hospital and Medical College
Karakonam, Thiruvananthapuram, Kerala, India

Vinu Thomas MD DM
Professor of Medicine
Government Medical College
Thrissur, Kerala, India

VN Unni MD DM
Consultant in Nephrology
Aster Medcity Hospital
Kochi, Kerala, India

VP Gopinathan MD MNAMS
Professor of Chest Diseases
Amala Institute of Medical Sciences
Amalanagar, Thrissur, Kerala, India

Preface to the Sixth Edition

During the past 6 years, the quantum and quality of a textbook in internal medicine to be used by a wide range of readership—undergraduates, primary care physicians, practitioners, teaching staff of medical colleges and first, second year postgraduate students in medicine and allied subjects in the Indian Universities and under the National Board of Exams, have grown enormously due to the results of studies under new scientific equipment, biologicals, genetic and molecular studies, and molecular tools employed in both research and treatment, especially monoclonal antibodies and others. This has made the volume grow in size, and subject has become more complex and difficult to comprehend by students and practitioners. I along with my contributors have taken all pains to make the subjects up-to-date, reader-friendly and authentic. Most of the contributors, particularly the section editors, are chosen among the best teachers and researchers with wide hands-on experience in the subject. They have made their contributions clear and understandable for the young students as well as postgraduates and practitioners.

All chapters have been thoroughly scrutinized with the addition of newer information and removal of redundant material. Tables, figures, flowcharts and other study aids have been introduced wherever necessary. Reference to the source has been included wherever new information has been added.

This volume mainly deals with the theoretical and clinical aspects of health and diseases. Its companion volume, (4th edition of clinical medicine) published by Jaypee Brothers Medical Publishers in 2013, edited by me, gives hands-on clinical information of examination of patients, planning the investigations and interpreting the results.

I hope these two volumes will serve to give the necessary information for learning the theory and practice of medicine needed by medical personnel in our country and abroad. I consider my mission fulfilled if my purpose is achieved.

The publishers, Jaypee Brothers Medical Publishers, headed by Shri Jitendar P Vij, has also encouraged us to bring out a full textbook which may evolve to be the flagship of the publishers.

The contributors have done their job. It is hoped that the 6th edition of *Textbook of Medicine* serves the purpose, it is intended to perform.

I would also like to thank Dr Archith Boloor, MBBS MD (Internal Medicine), Associate Professor of Medicine, Kasturba Medical College, Manipal University, Mangaluru, Karnataka, India for his contribution in the book.

KV Krishna Das

Preface to the First Edition

This book is written to fulfil a long-felt and widespread need among the undergraduate students. A questionnaire sent to several hundreds of clinical students revealed that majority of them rely on class notes and handbooks written on the subject by several authors. Many had no access to textbooks in the subject and the big volumes available were beyond their understanding. Comprehensive textbooks catering to the need of undergraduates written by Indian authors are only a few. Books published in other countries are quite freely available to our students, but naturally their emphasis is on conditions prevailing in their lands.

The medical problems of India are unique in that the disease-spectrum is a blend of what is seen in the affluent countries with what is seen in developing countries. This book has been written with this picture in mind. The section on 'tropical diseases' which usually gets a separate deal in most of the textbooks has been dovetailed into the other sections such as infections, physical agents, nutrition, etc. It is my feeling that with modern jet travel and the rapidly changing life-styles of Indian subjects, all diseases—the most modern and the most ancient are likely to be encountered by the clinical students in this country. Moreover, the so-called tropical diseases which used to be confined to the tropical belt, are now seen widely all over the world as a result of free and fast migration of population.

I consider my purpose fulfilled if the undergraduates in this country find this book useful.

KV Krishna Das

Acknowledgments

I acknowledge the support given to me by my wife Smt LN Kamalam, who stood with me and encouraged me to complete the task of editing the sixth edition, despite all her heavy domestic commitments and my strenuous schedule to complete this heavy task.

I thank to all my section editors and contributors who prepared the manuscript and periodically updated the material, due to the delay in bringing out the edition.

I thank Dr Archith Boloor, MBBS MD (Internal Medicine), Associate Professor of Medicine, Kasturba Medical College, Manipal University, Mangaluru, Karnataka, India, who was commissioned by the publishers for helping me to provide charts and tables which have made the material more reader-friendly.

I express my thanks to Shri Jitendar P Vij (Group Chairman), Mr Ankit Vij (Group President), Ms Chetna Malhotra Vohra (Associate Director–Content Strategy), Dr Madhu Choudhary (Content Strategist), Ms Payal Bharti (Project Manager), Ms Neelam Kakriya (Proofreader), Mr Akshay Thakur (DTP Operator) and staff of Jaypee Brothers Medical Publishers (P) Ltd, New Delhi for prompt execution of the work required for this rather voluminous textbook.

I express my humble *Pranam* to The Almighty, to have allowed me to complete this task of editing the sixth enlarged edition, with my section editors and contributors.

Editorial Committee

Section Editors	Sections	Titles	Chapters
KV Krishna Das	Section 1	General Topics	Ch 1–8
KV Krishna Das	Section 2	Diseases due to Arthropods, Marine Animals and Snakes	Ch 9–11
KV Krishna Das	Section 3	Disorders due to Physical Agents	Ch 12–21
KV Krishna Das	Section 4	Toxicology	Ch 22–26
KV Krishna Das	Section 5	Nutrition	Ch 27–33
S Bhasi Usha Vaidhyanathan	Section 6	Diseases caused by Infections	Ch 34–71
R Kasi Visweswaran	Section 7	Fluid and Electrolytes	Ch 72–74
KR Vinaya Kumar	Section 8	Gastroenterology	Ch 75–81
KR Vinaya Kumar	Section 9	Hepatobiliary System and Pancreas	Ch 82–90
AG Unnikrishnan	Section 10	Diabetes Mellitus, Other Metabolic Disorders and Inherited Disorders of Connective Tissue	Ch 91–95
KP Poulose	Section 11	Endocrinology	Ch 96–105
Binoy J Paul	Section 12	Rheumatology	Ch 106–118
K Suresh A George Koshy	Section 13	Cardiology	Ch 119–137
C Sudheendra Ghosh	Section 14	Respiratory System	Ch 138–157
Mathew Thomas KV Krishna Das	Section 15	Hematology	Ch 158–178
R Kasi Visweswaran	Section 16	Nephrology	Ch 179–192
SR Chandra	Section 17	Neurology	Ch 193–218
Usha Vaidhyanathan S Pradeep Nair	Section 18	Dermatology	Ch 219–234
N Krishnan Kutty	Section 19	Psychiatry	Ch 235–251
B Krishna Swamy KV Krishna Das	Section 20	Geriatrics	Ch 252–253

Contents

Volume I

SECTION 1 — GENERAL TOPICS

1. Introduction to Medicine — 1
KV Krishna Das

2. Medical Genetics — 5
KV Krishna Das

3. Defense Mechanisms of the Host and Clinical Immunology — 23
KV Krishna Das

4. Principles of Drug Administration — 40
KV Krishna Das

5. Antimicrobial Agents — 47
KV Krishna Das, S Bhasi

6. Therapeutics of Glucocorticoids — 63
S Bhasi

7. Principles of Oncology — 67
KV Krishna Das

8. Imaging Sciences and Interventional Radiology — 80
Kapilamoorthy

SECTION 2 — DISEASES DUE TO ARTHROPODS, MARINE ANIMALS AND SNAKES

9. Myiasis — 90
KV Krishna Das

10. Arthropod Bites and Stings, and Injuries due to Marine Animals — 91
KV Krishna Das

11. Snake Bite — 96
KV Krishna Das

SECTION 3 — DISORDERS DUE TO PHYSICAL AGENTS

12. Disorders caused by Heat — 102
KV Krishna Das, TK Suma

13. Injuries due to Cold — 107
TK Suma, KV Krishna Das

14. Disorders due to Alterations in Barometric Pressure — 109
TK Suma, KV Krishna Das

15. Diseases due to High Altitude — 111
TK Suma, KV Krishna Das

16. Drowning — 113
TK Suma, KV Krishna Das

17. Injuries due to Ionizing Radiations — 115
TK Suma, KV Krishna Das

18. Electrical Injuries and Lightning — 116
TK Suma, KV Krishna Das

19. Dangers of Nuclear Explosion — 118
TK Suma, KV Krishna Das

20. Adverse Effects due to Noise and Vibrations — 119
KV Krishna Das, TK Suma

21. Motion Sickness, Problems due to Air Travel and Road Accidents — 121
TK Suma, KV Krishna Das

SECTION 4 — TOXICOLOGY

22. Acute Poisoning: General Considerations — 124
KV Krishna Das, TK Suma

23. Common Poisons — 130
KV Krishna Das, TK Suma

24. Food Poisoning — 142
TK Suma, KV Krishna Das

25. Endemic Fluorosis — 147
TK Suma, KV Krishna Das

26. Therapy of Chronic Tobacco Addiction — 149
KV Krishna Das, KE Rajan, TK Suma

SECTION 5 — NUTRITION

27. Nutrition: General Considerations — 154
KV Krishna Das

28. Starvation — 162
KV Krishna Das, KE Elizabeth

29. Protein-energy Malnutrition — 163
KV Krishna Das, KE Elizabeth

30. Fat-soluble Vitamins — 167
KV Krishna Das

31. Water-soluble Vitamins — 174
KV Krishna Das

32. Minerals — 179
KV Krishna Das

33. Obesity — 186
KV Krishna Das

SECTION 6 — DISEASES CAUSED BY INFECTIONS

34. Infections: General Considerations — 192
S Bhasi

35. Fever of Unknown Origin — 197
S Bhasi

36. **Sepsis and Septic Shock** 202
S Bhasi

37. **Systemic Diseases caused by Cocci** 206
KV Krishna Das

38. **Common Bacterial Infections of Childhood** 223
KV Krishna Das

39. **Salmonella Infections** 228
S Bhasi, KV Krishna Das

40. **Gram-negative Bacterial Infections** 234
S Bhasi

41. **Anthrax, Plague, Brucellosis, Melioidosis** 239
S Bhasi, KV Krishna Das, R Sajith Kumar

42. **Diarrheal Diseases of Infective Origin** 245
KV Krishna Das, VP Gopinathan

43. **Bartonellosis, Legionellosis, Listeriosis, Yaws, Pinta, Relapsing Fevers, Lyme Borreliosis** 253
KV Krishna Das

44. **Leptospirosis** 260
R Sajith Kumar, KV Krishna Das

45. **Rickettsial Diseases, Q Fever, Human Ehrlichiosis and Anaplasmosis** 263
KV Krishna Das, VP Gopinathan

46. **Anaerobic Infections: Tetanus and Gas Gangrene** 268
KV Krishna Das

47. **Sexually Transmitted Diseases** 273
KV Krishna Das, Usha Vaidhyanathan

48. **Sexually Transmitted Viral Diseases** 284
KV Krishna Das, Usha Vaidhyanathan, R Sajith Kumar

49. **Mycobacterial Infections Tuberculosis, Nontuberculous Mycobacteria and Leprosy** 298
KV Krishna Das, Usha Vaidhyanathan

50. **Chlamydial Respiratory Infections: Psittacosis and Primary Atypical Pneumonia** 319
KV Krishna Das

51. **Viral Infections** 321
KV Krishna Das, R Sajith Kumar

52. **Viral Infections of the Respiratory Tract** 323
R Sajith Kumar, KV Krishna Das

53. **Exanthems and Enanthems** 328
KV Krishna Das

54. **Mumps** 338
KV Krishna Das

55. **Viral Hepatitis** 339
KV Krishna Das, KR Vinaya Kumar

56. **Enteroviruses** 352
KV Krishna Das

57. **Adenovirus Infections** 357
KV Krishna Das

58. **Arenavirus Infections, Filovirus Infections and Hemorrhagic Fevers** 358
KV Krishna Das, R Sajith Kumar

59. **Rabies** 361
KV Krishna Das, K Sreekanthan, Aswini Kumar

60. **Arboviruses** 365
K Sreekanthan, KV Krishna Das, R Sajith Kumar

61. **Other Viral Infections** 374
KV Krishna Das

62. **Systemic Fungal Infections** 377
KV Krishna Das, R Sajith Kumar

63. **Actinomyces and Nocardia** 382
KV Krishna Das, R Sajith Kumar

64. **Disease caused by Protozoa** 384
PK Sasidharan, KV Krishna Das, VP Gopinathan

65. **Amebiasis, Giardiasis, Balantidiasis, Toxoplasmosis and Cryptosporidiosis** 405
KV Krishna Das, VP Gopinathan

66. **Helminthiasis: General Considerations** 413
RK Shenoy, KV Krishna Das

67. **Intestinal Nematodes** 415
RK Shenoy, KV Krishna Das

68. **Cestodiasis** 423
RK Shenoy, KV Krishna Das

69. **Trematode (Fluke) Infections** 428
RK Shenoy, KV Krishna Das

70. **Tissue Nematodes** 432
RK Shenoy, KV Krishna Das

71. **Rare Helminthic Infestations** 441
KV Krishna Das, RK Shenoy

SECTION 7 FLUID AND ELECTROLYTES

72. **Abnormalities of Water and Electrolyte Balance** 442
R Kasi Visweswaran

73. **Abnormalities of Acid-base Balance** 452
R Kasi Visweswaran

74. **Disturbances of Osmotic Equilibrium** 464
KV Krishna Das, R Kasi Visweswaran

SECTION 8 GASTROENTEROLOGY

75. **Digestive Organs: General Considerations** 470
KR Vinaya Kumar, KV Krishna Das

76. **Diseases of the Mouth and Tongue** 480
KR Vinaya Kumar, KV Krishna Das

77. **Diseases of the Esophagus** 484
KR Vinaya Kumar, KV Krishna Das

78. **Diseases of the Stomach** 489
KR Vinaya Kumar, KV Krishna Das

79. **Diseases of the Small Intestine** 499
KR Vinaya Kumar, KV Krishna Das

80. **Diseases of the Colon** 511
KR Vinaya Kumar, KV Krishna Das

81. **Diseases of the Peritoneum** 518
KR Vinaya Kumar, KV Krishna Das

SECTION 9 — HEPATOBILIARY SYSTEM AND PANCREAS

82. **Hepatobiliary System: General Considerations** 521
KR Vinaya Kumar, KV Krishna Das

83. **Jaundice** 523
KR Vinaya Kumar, KV Krishna Das

84. **Cirrhosis of the Liver** 528
KR Vinaya Kumar, KV Krishna Das

85. **Hepatic Failure** 536
KR Vinaya Kumar, KV Krishna Das

86. **Liver Transplantation** 543
KR Vinaya Kumar

87. **Portal Hypertension** 545
KR Vinaya Kumar, KV Krishna Das

88. **Other Hepatic Disorders** 551
KR Vinaya Kumar, KV Krishna Das

89. **Diseases of the Gallbladder and the Major Bile Ducts** 562
KR Vinaya Kumar, KV Krishna Das

90. **Diseases of the Pancreas** 565
KR Vinaya Kumar, KV Krishna Das

SECTION 10 — DIABETES MELLITUS, OTHER METABOLIC DISORDERS AND INHERITED DISORDERS OF CONNECTIVE TISSUE

91. **Diabetes Mellitus** 577
AG Unnikrishnan, Anjali Bhatt

92. **Complications of Diabetes Mellitus** 601
AG Unnikrishnan, Anjali Bhatt

93. **Fibrocalcific Pancreatic Diabetes and Other Causes of Meliturias** 615
KV Krishna Das, KP Poulose, RV Jayakumar

94. **Other Metabolic Disorders** 618
KV Krishna Das, TK Suma

95. **Inherited Disorders of Connective Tissue** 628
KV Krishna Das

SECTION 11 — ENDOCRINOLOGY

96. **Endocrinology: General Considerations** 631
KP Poulose, B Jayakumar

97. **Hypothalamus, Pituitary and their Disorders** 641
KP Poulose, B Jayakumar

98. **Pineal Gland and its Disorders** 657
KP Poulose, B Jayakumar

99. **Thyroid and its Disorders** 658
KP Poulose, B Jayakumar

100. **Parathyroids and their Disorders** 676
KP Poulose, B Jayakumar

101. **Disorders of the Adrenal Cortex and Adrenal Medulla** 684
KP Poulose, Mathew John, AG Unnikrishnan

102. **Gonads and their Disorders** 696
Mathew John, KP Poulose, KV Krishna Das

103. **Miscellaneous Endocrine-related Conditions** 711
B Jayakumar, KP Poulose

104. **Multiple Endocrine Neoplasia** 715
PK Jabbar, KP Poulose

105. **Polyglandular Autoimmune Syndromes** 717
PK Jabbar, KP Poulose

SECTION 12 — RHEUMATOLOGY

106. **Disease of Locomotor System** 719
Binoy J Paul, KV Krishna Das

107. **Rheumatoid Arthritis and its Variants** 727
Binoy J Paul, KV Krishna Das

108. **Systemic Lupus Erythematosus and Antiphospholipid Antibody Syndrome** 739
Binoy J Paul, KV Krishna Das

109. **Progressive Systemic Sclerosis** 748
KV Krishna Das, Binoy J Paul

110. **Systemic Vasculitis** 752
Binoy J Paul, KV Krishna Das

111. **Polymyositis and Dermatomyositis** 760
Binoy J Paul, KV Krishna Das

112. **Miscellaneous Rheumatic Syndromes** 762
KV Krishna Das, Binoy J Paul

113. **Seronegative Spondyloarthropathies** 763
Binoy J Paul, KV Krishna Das

114. **Metabolic Arthropathies** 769
Binoy J Paul, KV Krishna Das

115. **Osteoarthritis** 777
Binoy J Paul, KV Krishna Das

116. **Other Bone Diseases** 780
KV Krishna Das, Binoy J Paul

117. **Rheumatological Manifestations of Systemic Diseases** 784
Binoy J Paul, KV Krishna Das

118. **Newer Diagnostic and Therapeutic Modalities in Rheumatology** 787
Binoy J Paul

Volume II

SECTION 13 — CARDIOLOGY

119. Cardiology: General Considerations — 791
K Suresh, CG Bahuleyan

120. Heart Failure (Cardiac Failure) — 803
CG Bahuleyan

121. Shock — 814
N Sudhaya Kumar

122. Congenital Heart Disease — 817
M Zulfikar Ahamed, Balu Vaidyanathan

123. Chronic Valvular Heart Disease — 838
N Sudhaya Kumar

124. Infective Endocarditis — 855
K Suresh, Suhail Mohammed PT

125. Cardiac Arrhythmias — 861
K Suresh

126. Systemic Hypertension — 881
K Suresh

127. Ischemic Heart Disease — 895
CG Bahuleyan

128. Diseases of the Myocardium — 916
K Suresh, CG Bahuleyan

129. Diseases of the Pericardium — 921
CG Bahuleyan, K Suresh

130. Pulmonary Embolism — 924
A George Koshy, K Suresh

131. Diseases of the Aorta — 928
N Sudhaya Kumar

132. Cardiac Manifestations of Systemic Diseases — 933
A George Koshy, Sajan Z Ahmed

133. Pregnancy and Heart Disease — 939
N Sudhaya Kumar, K Suresh

134. Cardiac Tumors — 942
A George Koshy, Sajan Z Ahmed

135. An Introduction to Interventional Cardiology — 945
A George Koshy, Sajan Z Ahmed

136. Cardiac Surgery — 948
A George Koshy, CG Bahuleyan

137. Preventive Cardiology — 951
K Suresh, CG Bahuleyan

SECTION 14 — RESPIRATORY SYSTEM

138. Respiratory System: General Considerations — 953
C Sudheendra Ghosh, CP Murali

139. Respiratory Failure — 968
C Sudheendra Ghosh, CP Murali

140. Diseases of the Upper Respiratory Tract — 973
KE Rajan

141. Pneumonias — 977
C Sudheendra Ghosh, CP Murali

142. Lung Abscess and Pleuropulmonary Amebiasis — 981
C Sudheendra Ghosh, Davis Paul

143. Allergic Disorders of the Lung — 984
KE Rajan

144. Diseases of the Lower Airways — 996
C Sudheendra Ghosh, Davis Paul

145. Occupational Lung Diseases — 1005
KE Rajan

146. Sarcoidosis — 1008
KV Krishna Das

147. Pulmonary Fibrosis — 1010
C Sudheendra Ghosh, Davis Paul

148. Circulatory Disturbances in Lungs — 1012
C Sudheendra Ghosh, Davis Paul

149. Obstructive Sleep Apnea Syndrome — 1015
C Sudheendra Ghosh, CP Murali

150. Neoplasms of the Lung — 1019
C Sudheendra Ghosh, CP Murali

151. Pulmonary Cysts — 1026
C Sudheendra Ghosh

152. Pulmonary Involvement in Systemic Diseases — 1027
C Sudheendra Ghosh, Davis Paul

153. Diseases of Pleura — 1028
C Sudheendra Ghosh, Davis Paul

154. Diseases of the Chest Wall — 1034
KE Rajan

155. Diseases of the Diaphragm — 1036
KE Rajan

156. Diseases of the Mediastinum — 1039
C Sudheendra Ghosh, Davis Paul

157. Pulmonary Rehabilitation and Respiratory Physiotherapy — 1041
KE Rajan

SECTION 15 — HEMATOLOGY

158. Hematology: General Considerations — 1044
KV Krishna Das

159. Anemias: General Considerations — 1057
KV Krishna Das

160. Nutritional and Other Anemias — 1063
KV Krishna Das

161. Hemolytic Anemias — 1072
KV Krishna Das

162. Anemias Characterized by Defective Erythrocyte Production — 1089
Mathew Thomas, KV Krishna Das

163. Blood Transfusion — 1096
KV Krishna Das, Mathew Thomas, Jaisy Mathai

164. Leukemias: General Considerations 1103
*Salim Shafeek, Kasim Salim,
KV Krishna Das, Mathew Thomas*

165. Acute Leukemias 1113
*Salim Shafeek, Kasim Salim,
KV Krishna Das, Mathew Thomas*

166. Chronic Leukemia 1122
Salim Shafeek, Kasim Salim, KV Krishna Das

167. Myelodysplastic Syndrome 1131
Mathew Thomas, KV Krishna Das

168. Agranulocytosis (Severe Neutropenia) 1135
PK Sasidharan, KV Krishna Das

169. Plasma Cell Dyscrasias 1137
*Salim Shafeek, Kasim Salim,
Mathew Thomas, KV Krishna Das*

170. Malignant Disorders of Lymphoid Cells 1147
*Salim Shafeek, Kasim Salim,
KV Krishna Das, Mathew Thomas*

171. Myeloproliferative Disorders 1160
PK Sasidharan, KV Krishna Das

172. Spleen and its Disorders 1167
KV Krishna Das, PK Sasidharan

173. Hemostasis: General Considerations 1169
Mathew Thomas, KV Krishna Das

174. Platelet and Vascular Disorders 1174
Mathew Thomas, KV Krishna Das

175. Defects of Coagulation 1185
Mathew Thomas, KV Krishna Das

176. Therapeutics of Anticoagulants 1194
Mathew Thomas, KV Krishna Das

177. Fragmentation Hemolysis 1199
Mathew Thomas, KV Krishna Das

178. Thrombophilia 1204
Mathew Thomas, KV Krishna Das

SECTION 16   NEPHROLOGY

**179. Structure and Function of the Kidneys
and Urinary Tract** 1207
R Kasi Visweswaran, Susan Uthup

**180. Clinical Approach:
Evaluation and Investigations** 1212
Jacob George

181. Glomerulonephritis 1220
Jacob George, Noble Gracious

182. Acute Kidney Injury 1230
Jigy Joseph, Vimala A

183. Chronic Kidney Disease 1236
Ramdas Pisharody, Gomathy S

**184. Diseases of Renal Tubules
and Interstitium** 1242
VN Unni, Manu G Krishna

185. Urinary Tract Infection 1250
Sreelatha M, Swaraj Sathyan

186. Nephrolithiasis 1256
Ramdas Pisharody, Vinu Thomas

187. Kidney in Systemic Diseases 1260
M Thomas Mathew

188. The Kidney and Hypertension 1266
R Kasi Visweswaran, Reena Thomas

**189. Renal Involvement in Systemic Diseases
with Special Reference to Pregnancy** 1270
Jacob George, Usha Samuel

190. Urinary Tract Obstruction 1274
Jayant Thomas Mathew, M Thomas Mathew

191. Renal Replacement Therapy 1276
VN Unni, George Kurian

192. Drugs and the Kidney 1284
Jacob George

SECTION 17   NEUROLOGY

193. Nervous System: General Considerations 1288
SR Chandra, Vidhya Annapoorni CS

**194. Neurological Examination
and Investigations** 1294
SR Chandra, SR Srinivasa Kannan

195. Cranial Nerves 1316
SR Chandra, Karru Venkata Ravi Teja

196. Coma and Brain Death 1333
SR Chandra, CV Soumya

197. Headache 1339
AS Girija

**198. Nutritional Disorders of the
Nervous System** 1344
Thomas Gregor Issac, SR Chandra

**199. Infections of the Central
Nervous System** 1351
*SR Chandra, Nethravathi M,
Thomas Gregor Issac*

200. Dementias and Metabolic Encephalopathy 1365
AS Girija

201. Prion Disease and Related Encephalitis 1373
SR Chandra, Thomas Gregor Issac

202. Epilepsies 1379
AS Girija

**203. Parkinson's Disease and
Related Disorders** 1391
SR Chandra, R Jayachandran

**204. Extrapyramidal Disorders other than
Parkinsonism and Related Syndromes** 1398
SR Chandra, Thomas Iype

205. Cerebrovascular Diseases 1406
SR Chandra, Ranjit Sanu Watson

206. Intracranial Space-Occupying Lesions 1417
Anand Kumar, Arun N Babu

**207. Multiple Sclerosis and other
Demyelinating Lesions** 1425
Anand Kumar, Arun N Babu

208. Motor Neuron Disease 1430
SR Chandra, KA Kabeer

209. Diseases of the Cerebellum 1435
Anand Kumar, Arun N Babu

**210. Diseases of Spinal Cord, Nerve
Roots and Plexuses** 1439
*SR Chandra, Vidhya Annapoorni CS,
Thomas Gregor Issac, KV Krishna Das*

xxii

211. Diseases of the Vertebral Column Causing Neurological Lesions 1448
Anand Kumar, KV Krishna Das

212. Diseases of the Peripheral Nervous System 1453
Anand Kumar, Arun N Babu

213. Disorders of the Autonomic Nervous System 1460
SR Chandra

214. Myasthenia Gravis 1466
SR Chandra, KA Kabeer

215. Diseases of Muscles 1472
SR Chandra

216. Rehabilitation in Neurology 1481
SR Chandra

217. Investigation of a Child with a Suspected Neurometabolic Disorder 1483
Rita Christopher

218. Central Nervous System Manifestations in Systemic Disorders 1489
SR Chandra, Mirza Masoom Abbas

SECTION 18 DERMATOLOGY

219. Skin: General Considerations 1496
Usha Vaidhyanathan

220. Infections of the Skin and Appendages 1500
Usha Vaidhyanathan

221. Skin Infestations 1507
Usha Vaidhyanathan

222. Acne and Rosacea 1509
Usha Vaidhyanathan

223. Papulosquamous Disorders 1511
Usha Vaidhyanathan

224. Eczema 1517
Usha Vaidhyanathan

225. Vesiculobullous Disorders 1523
S Pradeep Nair

226. Urticaria and Angioedema 1526
S Pradeep Nair

227. Cutaneous Drug Reactions 1528
S Pradeep Nair

228. Disorders of Blood Vessels and Lymphatics 1531
S Pradeep Nair

229. Disorders of Pigmentation 1533
S Pradeep Nair

230. Disorders of Hair and Nails 1534
S Pradeep Nair

231. Disorders of Elastin and Collagen Fibers 1537
S Pradeep Nair

232. Cutaneous Manifestations of Systemic Disorders 1539
S Pradeep Nair

233. Skin Tumors 1542
S Pradeep Nair

234. Pregnancy and Skin 1544
Usha Vaidhyanathan

SECTION 19 PSYCHIATRY

235. Basic Concepts 1546
N Krishnan Kutty

236. Organic Mental Disorders 1552
N Krishnan Kutty

237. Schizophrenia and Delusional Disorders 1554
N Krishnan Kutty

238. Mood Disorders: Mania, Depression, Dysthymia 1557
N Krishnan Kutty

239. Anxiety Disorders 1560
N Krishnan Kutty

240. Obsessive Compulsive Disorders 1562
N Krishnan Kutty

241. Conversion Disorders, Dissociative Disorders, Somatoform Disorders, Cultural Bond Syndromes, Reaction to Stress and Adjustment Disorders 1563
N Krishnan Kutty

242. Torture 1566
N Krishnan Kutty

243. Disorders of Adult Personality 1567
N Krishnan Kutty

244. Psychoactive Substance-use Disorders and Alcohol-related Disorders 1568
N Krishnan Kutty

245. Behavioral Syndromes Associated with Physiological Disturbances and Physical Factors 1571
N Krishnan Kutty

246. Psychological Factors Affecting Systemic Medical Disorders 1574
N Krishnan Kutty

247. Mental Retardation 1575
N Krishnan Kutty

248. Behavioral and Emotional Disorders Occurring in Childhood and Adolescence 1576
N Krishnan Kutty

249. Psychiatric Emergencies 1577
N Krishnan Kutty

250. General Principles of Management of Psychiatric Disorders 1579
N Krishnan Kutty

251. Psychological Methods of Treatment (Psychotherapy) 1583
N Krishnan Kutty

SECTION 20 GERIATRICS

252. Principles and Practice of Geriatric Medicine 1586
KV Krishna Das

253. Clinical Aspects of Geriatric Diseases 1590
B Krishna Swamy, KV Krishna Das

Index .... I-i

Volume II

Volume II

CHAPTER 119

Cardiology: General Considerations

K Suresh, CG Bahuleyan

Chapter Summary

- Cardiac Physiology
- Symptomatology in Cardiovascular Diseases
- Physical Examination
- Special Investigations

CARDIAC PHYSIOLOGY

The normal adult human heart weighs 250–350 g. The left ventricle (LV) is 2–3 times the thickness of the right ventricle (RV). The former constitutes 60% of the total weight. Histologically, the cardiac muscle forms a syncytium, though the myocardial cells are electrically isolated by high resistance membranes. Cardiac muscle possesses intrinsic properties such as excitability, contractility, rhythmicity, conductivity and distensibility. As the cardiac muscle gets stretched, within physiological limits, the force of contraction increases *(Starling's law)*. Though the sinoatrial (SA) node, atrioventricular (AV) node, the conducting tissues and cardiac muscle are all capable of impulse production, in health, the heart beat is initiated by impulses from the SA node. Vagal impulses depress the rate of the SA node and increase the refractory period of the cardiac muscle. Sympathetic fibers arising from the cervical and upper thoracic ganglia supply the heart and they accelerate the SA node and decrease the refractory period of the myocardium. Atrial contraction is followed by ventricular contraction. Atrial contraction helps in pumping blood remaining in the atria toward the end of diastole and this helps to augment ventricular filling, thus preparing the ventricles for more effective contraction. Atrial contraction gives rise to the A wave in the jugular veins. With the onset of ventricular systole, AV valves close and the AV valve apparatus bulges toward the atria giving rise to the C wave in the jugular veins. As the ventricular pressure increases rapidly, the semilunar valves open and blood is ejected into the aorta and the pulmonary artery. The ventricles eject 60–70% of their contents during each systole. Initial phase is one of rapid ejection. This is followed by the period of slowed ejection. During each cardiac cycle, the ventricles eject 70 mL of blood which is the stroke volume. The atrial filling continues during ventricular systole and the rise of pressure in the right atria gives rise to the V-wave of the jugular venous tracing. At the end of ejection, the semilunar valves close and the isometric relaxation follows. Though, in a broad sense, the ventricular contraction occurs synchronously on the right and left sides of the heart, closer examination will reveal that the right ventricular (RV) ejection starts earlier and is completed slightly later than left ventricular (LV) ejection. AV valves open when the ventricular pressure falls below that of the atria during diastole. Atrial blood flows into the ventricle rapidly in the early part of diastole and this may give rise to the third heart sound (S3). This is followed by the slow filling phase and the period of diastasis. The last phase of ventricular diastole is atrial systole. Atrial systole in a young person normally contributes to less than 20% of ventricular filling. Atrial contribution to ventricular filling is especially important in elderly persons with ventricular hypertrophy and stiff ventricles (diastolic dysfunction). Atrial systole can contribute much more to ventricular filling in such individuals, especially with faster heart rates.

Cardiac Cycle: Phases

The cardiac cycle can be divided into ventricular systole and ventricular diastole given in Table 119.1.

Heart Sounds

These are produced by deceleration of blood impinging on elastic structures in the heart, giving rise to vibration. More rapid deceleration gives rise to louder sounds and vice versa. The pitch of the sound (frequency) is determined by the relative contribution of the mass of blood and the elastic properties of the structures which are responsible for producing the sounds.

First heart sound (S1) occurs at the commencement of systole and coincides with the closure of the AV valves. *Second heart sound (S2)* marks the onset of diastole and indicates closure of the semilunar valves. *The third heart sound (S3)* occurs in the earlier part of diastole and it coincides with rapid ventricular filling. *The fourth heart*

Table 119.1: Phases of the cardiac cycle (ventricular systole and ventricular diastole)

Ventricular systole (0.3 s)	Ventricular diastole (0.5 s)
• Isovolumetric contraction (0.05 s)	• Protodiastole (0.04)
	• Isovolumetric relaxation (0.06 s)
• Rapid ejection (0.10 s)	• Rapid filling phase (0.10 s)
• Reduced ejection (0.15 s)	• Diastasis (0.2 s)
	• Atrial filling phase (0.10 s)

sound (S4) is produced by atrial contraction and this is a late diastolic sound.

Cardiac Output

This is the volume of blood pumped by the LV in 1 minute. Normal average is 5–6 L in healthy adults. It is also expressed as the cardiac index, when related to the surface area of the individual. **Normal cardiac index** is 2.8–4.2 $L/min/m^2$ (mean 3.4 $L/min/m^2$). Cardiac output is the product of heart rate and stroke volume (CO = HR × SV). It is controlled by several factors such as heart rate, effective filling pressures of the ventricles, compliance of the chambers, contractile force of the ventricles, neurohumoral factors and blood pressure (BP). Generally, an increase in cardiac output is achieved by increasing the heart rate and stroke volume. Exercise and emotion normally increase the cardiac output, whereas extreme tachycardia, extreme bradycardia, atrial fibrillation (AF), myocardial dysfunction and anatomical or functional obstruction to the outflow of blood, reduce it.

Heart receives its oxygen supply and nutrition from the coronary arterial blood flow, which is 72–85 mL/100 g of cardiac muscle per minute in the resting phase. The heart utilizes 8–10 mL of oxygen per 100 g every minute. The oxygen demand during systole is thrice that during diastole. Diastole is also an active energy-consuming process. Proper diastolic function is essential to accommodate the optimum quantity of blood before the onset of systole.

Right Ventricular Physiology

RV has the same output as the left. It has only one-sixth the muscle mass and performs only one-fourth the stroke work as the LV. This is due to the fact that the pulmonary vascular resistance is only one-tenth that of systemic resistance. The two ventricles differ in shape but their function is made interdependent through the mechanism of action of the interventricular septum and surrounding pericardium. The systolic pressure wave caused by LV septal contraction augments the systolic force of the RV and promotes pulmonary perfusion.

Arterial Blood Pressure

The arterial BP is influenced by several factors such as the cardiac output, peripheral resistance in the arterial system, blood volume in the arterial system, viscosity of blood and elasticity of the arteries. The control of BP is achieved mainly by alteration in the cardiac output and peripheral resistance. Normally, arterial BP fluctuates depending on exercise and emotional stress, time of the day and posture. The systolic BP falls by 15–30 mm Hg during sleep. In the erect posture, diastolic BP is greater than during recumbency.

Average systolic BP readings are as follows:

- **Neonates:** 40 mm Hg
- **Infants aged 2 weeks:** 70 mm Hg
- **Children up to 12 years:** 105 mm Hg
- **Above 17 years:** 120 mm Hg.

In adults, for a considerable period of life (up to the 6th or 7th decade), the BP remains more or less steady, but with old age, due to reduction in elasticity of the arterial wall, the systolic pressure may tend to rise.

SYMPTOMATOLOGY IN CARDIOVASCULAR DISEASES

Dyspnea is the most common symptom, which brings the patient to the doctor in most instances. This is the uncomfortable awareness of breathing. Several factors, notably pulmonary venous congestion and hypoxemia, contribute to dyspnea. The New York Heart Association (NYHA) has proposed, based on the restriction of activity produced by symptoms, a functional classification for patients with heart disease to assess the severity and for helping in follow-up. Although dyspnea, palpitation, fatigue and chest pain are all considered in this NYHA functional classification, dyspnea is the most commonly assessed symptom.

- **NYHA class I (slight):** Patients with cardiac disease, but no restriction of ordinary activity; symptoms are provoked only by more than ordinary activity like running, climbing uphill.
- **NYHA class II (moderate):** Patients with cardiac disease and slight symptoms; mild restriction of ordinary activity like walking briskly, going two flights of stairs.
- **NYHA class III (considerable):** Patients with cardiac disease and marked restriction of activity, with symptoms on less than ordinary activity like walking on level ground, light household work.
- **NYHA class IV (gross):** Patients with cardiac disease resulting in **inability** to carry on any physical activity without discomfort or with total incapacity and dyspnea at rest and recumbency.

Orthopnea: It is dyspnea on recumbency, which is relieved by sitting up and is common in left-sided heart failure. **Paroxysmal nocturnal dyspnea** (PND) is the occurrence of sudden onset of dyspnea, which abruptly wakes the patient up in the early hours of sleep. The patient jumps up for breath with cough and frothy sputum. Assuming the erect attitude relieves the distress in many cases. PND (also used to be known as **cardiac asthma**) is an early symptom of left-sided heart failure. Pulmonary congestion and edema account for this phenomenon. Cheyne-Stokes respiration (CSR) is the periodic alteration in the rate and depth of breathing. The respiratory rate waxes and wanes with apneic pauses in between. CSR occurs in several conditions, left-sided heart failure being a common cause.

In the presence of other evidences of heart disease, dyspnea is a strong pointer of cardiac failure.

Edema: Subcutaneous edema is demonstrated by the phenomenon of pitting on pressure. Considerable amount of fluid (>2 L) should accumulate in the body before manifesting as generalized edema. Abnormal increase in weight (0.5–1 kg/day) associated with oliguria occurs early. When edema is manifest, the skin is stretched and shiny and pitting can be demonstrated. The edema is **dependent**, i.e. it is more prominent in the most dependent parts of the body. In those who are ambulant, the edema is maximal on the feet and that too in the evening. In bedridden patients, the edema is localized to the back and sacral region. Edema is a manifestation of heart failure and the factors which contribute to the production of edema are:

- Increased hydrostatic venous pressure and transudation of fluid into the interstitium
- Reduction in the cardiac output leading to compensatory salt and water retention by overactivity of aldosterone and antidiuretic hormone.

Precordial pain: Among the several causes of precordial pain, cardiac disease is the most important. Pain sensitive structures in the heart are the pericardium, which gives rise to pain due to inflammation (pericarditis) or stretching as in pericardial effusion, and the myocardium in which severe pain may occur as a result of ischemia. Pain arising from the pericardium and myocardium are distinguishable in many cases, but sometimes they are identical. Endocardium is not pain sensitive.

Pain of myocardial ischemia is vague, felt over the precordium or retrosternal region and may be described as crushing, bursting, lancinating, burning or otherwise. Anginal pain usually is precipitated by exertion or emotional stress and is relieved with rest. In myocardial infarction (MI), the pain is of longer duration and is experienced usually at rest. The pain shows characteristic radiation. The classical sites of radiation are: (1) Along the inner aspect of the left arm to the little finger, (2) left or both sides of neck and jaw, (3) left scapular region, (4) right shoulder and arm, (5) epigastrium. Pericardial pain is usually superficial, sharp, retrosternal in location with radiation to the shoulder or back. It worsens with movements, respiration, coughing and swallowing. Patients with cardiac neurosis and hypochondriasis may also complain of chest pain. This pain is often localized to the cardiac apex and may be described as catching or pricking. Such pain may not have any organic basis.

Palpitation: This is awareness of the heartbeat. Though normal individuals can experience the heartbeat during exercise or emotional stress, under pathological states this symptom may be troublesome. Palpitation may be due to tachycardia, extreme bradycardia, irregularity of cardiac rhythm or increase in force of contraction due to increase in stroke volume. In anxious individuals, this is a common symptom.

Syncope (faint): Loss of consciousness occurs when the cardiac output is not sufficient to maintain cerebral blood flow. The patient loses consciousness rapidly over seconds, unlike epilepsy in which the loss of consciousness is more abrupt. As the patient sinks into the flat position, consciousness is regained. If cerebral ischemia continues the patient may develop convulsions ***(Stokes-Adams attacks)***. Syncope is a common symptom in obstructive lesions like Fallot's tetralogy, aortic, pulmonary and mitral stenosis and tumors like myxomas. It is also seen in arrhythmias such as intermittent heart block, sick sinus syndrome and at the onset of acute MI.

Other causes of syncope include pooling of blood in the lower limbs as seen in persons standing still for a long-time (e.g. parade or drill), sudden rise in intrathoracic pressure resulting in diminution of venous return to the heart (e.g. cough syncope) or hyper-reactivity of the carotid sinus in which sudden neck movements or pressure over the carotid sinus leads to severe bradycardia and syncope.

Apart from these specific symptoms, general symptoms such as extreme fatigue may be the result of low cardiac output states. Anemia and fever occur in infective endocarditis. Clubbing of fingers is a common symptom of cyanotic congenital heart disease (CHD) and infective endocarditis.

PHYSICAL EXAMINATION

Before proceeding to the examination of the cardiovascular system, a full general examination should be performed. Findings that may point to the disease of the cardiovascular system are cyanosis, digital clubbing and dependent edema. Other general findings like anemia, skin rashes, pyrexia and obesity may have relevance in the final analysis.

Cyanosis

CHD gives rise to central cyanosis due to mixing of arterial and venous blood within the heart or outside it. In central cyanosis due to cardiac causes, the extremities and tongue are all cyanosed, the periphery is warm and the cyanosis is not abolished by breathing 100% oxygen (Fig. 119.1).

Low cardiac output states may give rise to peripheral cyanosis in which there is stagnation of blood in the capillaries and overextraction of oxygen by tissues resulting in cyanosis. The limbs are cold to feel and only the periphery is affected, the central parts like tongue are not cyanosed.

Edema

Careful search for edema and its distribution is essential in all cases.

Temperature of the Limbs

This depends on the state of arterial circulation. In low cardiac output states, peripheral vasoconstriction gives rise to coldness of the palms and feet. In high cardiac output states (e.g. thyrotoxicosis), the limbs are warm and the arterial pulsations may become prominent.

Arterial Pulse

The radial artery is generally taken up for examining the pulse. The rate, rhythm, volume, character of the pulse and nature of the arterial wall are noted. The normal pulse rate is 60–100 beats/minute and rhythm is regular. Any increase or decrease in pulse rate and irregularity in rhythm should be noted. Pulse volume is the amplitude of excursion of the vessel wall during the passage of the pulse

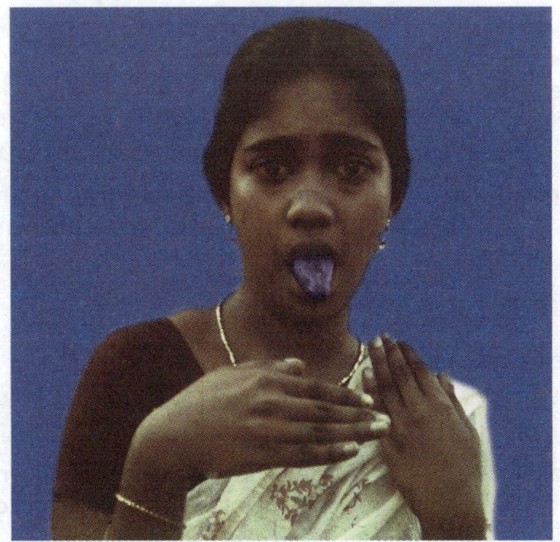

Fig. 119.1: Central cyanosis

wave. Pulse is of high volume in high cardiac output states, such as thyrotoxicosis and anemia, and in conditions where the stroke volume is high as in aortic incompetence. Low volume pulse (*pulsus parvus*) occurs in low cardiac output states such as mitral stenosis. When there is anatomical obstruction to the outward flow of blood as in aortic stenosis, the pulse is small in volume and slow rising (*slow-rising pulse* or *pulsus parvus et tardus*). The pulse is jerky in hypertrophic subaortic stenosis. When the stroke volume is large and there is vasodilatation, the pulse is of high volume and such a pulse is called **collapsing pulse** or **Corrigan's pulse**. This occurs classically in aortic incompetence and in some cases of patent ductus arteriosus (PDA). The term **bisferiens pulse** is used, when the pulse wave shows two upstrokes in systole. This is classically described in hypertrophic cardiomyopathy with obstruction. It is also seen in combined lesions of aortic stenosis and incompetence (when aortic incompetence is the dominant lesion) or sometimes even in pure aortic incompetence. Pulsus bisferiens may be more clearly identified over the carotid artery.

In normal subjects, during inspiration the pulse volume falls slightly, but this is often not noticeable. Marked fall of pulse volume and pulse pressure during inspiration is called *pulsus paradoxus* which is actually only an exaggeration of the normally observed inspiratory fall. This is classically seen in pericardial effusion with cardiac tamponade. It is also seen in one-third cases of constrictive pericarditis. *Pulsus alternans* is a condition in which alternate beats are weak. This difference may be palpable in most cases.

The difference between the stronger and weaker beats may be up to 40 mm Hg. Presence of pulsus alternans signifies gross impairment of LV function.

Examination of the arterial wall for thickening, nodularity and calcification reveals several abnormalities. When the medium-sized arteries like the radials are nodular and thickened, it suggests medial sclerosis (***Mönckeberg's sclerosis***), which is generally seen with advancing age.

All major arteries should be palpated to assess whether they are patent or occluded. Generally the carotid, axillary, brachial, radial, femoral, popliteal, dorsalis pedis and posterior tibial are examined. Simultaneous palpation of the radial and ipsilateral femoral artery helps to detect occlusion of the aorta. Normally, the femoral pulse precedes the radial pulse by about 15 ms. The femoral pulse is delayed in coarctation of the aorta and aortoarteritis. Auscultation over the arteries may reveal bruit. Bruit may be the result of narrowing of the lumen (e.g. carotid stenosis and renal artery stenosis) or may arise from increased blood flow through the artery (e.g. carotid artery opposite to the side of carotid occlusion, thyroid arteries in Graves' disease) (Table 119.2).

Jugular Venous Pulse

It is conventional to examine the internal jugular vein with the patient resting comfortably at an angle of 45°. The jugular vein closely reflects the pressure changes within the right atrium (RA). In health at 45° incline, the upper limit of the venous column lies just behind the right sternoclavicular

Table 119.2: Findings in the waveforms and their significance

Types	Waveforms	Significance
Catacrotic pulse	Percussion (p): Ejection of blood Tidal (t): Reflected waves Dicrotic: Elastic recoil of vessel	Normal
Anacrotic pulse	Slow rising	Aortic stenosis
Pulsus bisferiens	Rapid rising Twice beating Both waves felt in systole	Severe AR AR + AS with dominant AS HOCM
Dicrotic pulse	Twice beating First wave in systole, second wave in diastole Seen when pulse rate and diastolic pressure is low	Fever: Typhoid Severe LVF Dilated cardiomyopathy
Pulsus parvus et tardus	Slow rising late peaking	Severe AS
Collapsing pulse Corrigan's or water hammer pulse	High volume pulse Sharp rise Ill-sustained peak Sharp fall Pulse pressure is at least 60 mm Hg	Aortic regurgitation PDA, AP window, rupture of sinus valsalva, AV fistula Hyperdynamic circulation states
Pulsus paradoxus	Systolic BP falls more than 10 mm Hg during inspiration (exaggeration of normal phenomenon)	Cardiac tamponade Constrictive pericarditis Acute severe asthma or COPD Tension pneumothorax Massive pulmonary embolism
Reverse pulsus paradoxus		Positive pressure ventilation HOCM
Jerky pulse		HOCM
Pulsus alternans	Alternating weaker and stronger pulses, doubling rate of Korotkoff sound on lowering cuff pressures	LVF

Abbreviations: AR = Aortic regurgitation; AS = Aortic stenosis; HOCM = Hypertrophic obstructive cardiomyopathy; AV = Atrioventricular; AP = Anteroposterior; LVF = Left ventricular failure; COPD = Chronic obstructive pulmonary disease; PDA = Patent ductus arteriosus

joint, which is at the same horizontal level as the sternal angle. When right atrial pressure is increased as in right-sided heart failure, the venous column is seen above the right sternoclavicular joint and the vertical height of this column above the sternal angle is measured to express the increase in venous pressure. The waves a, c and v and the troughs x and y are studied. The jugular vein is a low pressure system and, therefore, the waves are occluded easily by palpation.

- A wave is caused by atrial contraction and is presystolic. It is more prominent when the RA is contracting against increased resistance. It disappears in AF.
- C wave is recordable but not usually visible as a separate wave. It reflects the bulging motion of the closed tricuspid valve during isovolumic systole.
- V wave is systolic and is due to passive filling of rheumatoid arthritis (RA) during systole when tricuspid valve is closed.
- X descent is the trough caused by atrial relaxation.
- Y descent is caused by opening of the tricuspid valve and rapid inflow of blood into the RV.
- The various events in the cardiac cycle and their relation to the arterial, venous, atrial and ventricular pressure tracings and the ECG can be understood from the diagram (Figs 119.2 and 119.3).

Usually it is easy to distinguish carotid artery pulse from jugular venous pulse, but sometimes when the former is very prominent or when both coexist, difficulty may arise (Table 119.3).

Hepatojugular Reflux

While observing the jugular vein, the abdominal wall is pressed. Rise in intra-abdominal pressure drives blood from the liver to the inferior vena cava (IVC), thus increasing the venous return to the heart. This results in rise of the jugular venous pressure (JVP). Release of abdominal pressure promptly brings back JVP also to the normal level. In early right-sided heart failure, abdominal

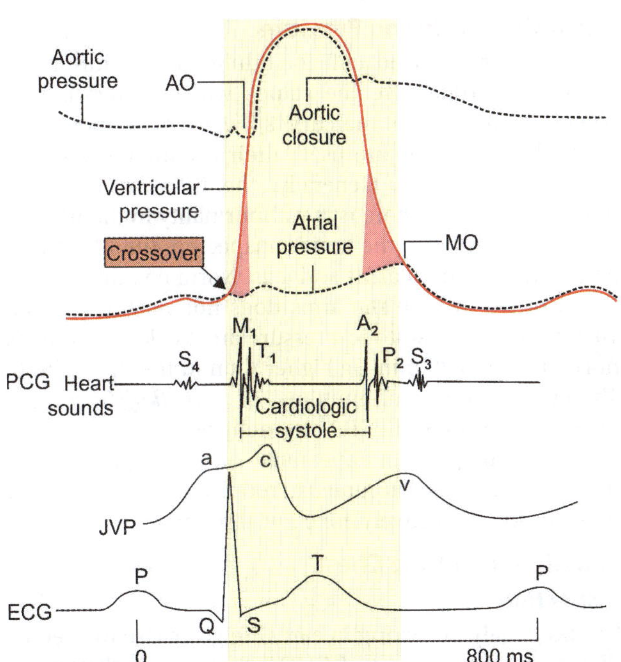

Fig. 119.3: Various events in the cardiac cycle and their relation to the arterial, venous, atrial and ventricular pressure tracings and electrocardiogram (ECG)

Abbreviations: JVP = Jugular venous pressure; PCG = Phonocardiogram

Table 119.3: Differences between jugular venous pulse and carotid artery pulse	
Jugular venous pulse	**Carotid artery pulse**
Better seen than felt	Seen and felt well
Wavy column with 2–3 waves	Jerky, only one wave
During inspiration the vein becomes empty	Not much change with phases of respiration
Hepatojugular reflux present	No change
Vein becomes more prominent when the patient lies flat	No change

pressure raises the JVP, but release of the pressure is not followed by prompt fall of the jugular venous column.

Proper examination of the jugular venous pulse is a simple and very reliable bedside method to assess the hemodynamic events in the RA and it is absolutely essential that the clinical student spends time to learn this technique fully.

JVP is increased in right-sided heart failure, in which this is the earliest sign. Hypervolemic states (overhydration) lead to engorgement of the jugular veins (e.g. acute nephritic syndrome). Study of the wave pattern helps in diagnosing arrhythmias such as AF and AV dissociation. In AF, A waves are absent in the JVP. ***Cannon waves*** are jugular venous waves occurring in conditions such as complete heart block or extrasystoles when the atrium contracts against a closed tricuspid valve. Regular cannon waves may occur in junctional rhythm and in ventricular rhythms with 1:1 retrograde conduction. Irregular cannon waves are more common and occur in complete heart block and ectopic beats (ventricular or junctional) and ventricular tachycardia without retrograde atrial activation.

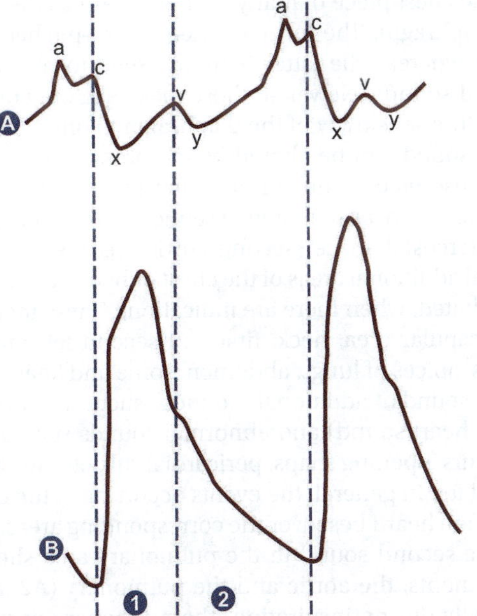

Fig. 119.2: Jugular venous tracing and arterial pulse: (A) Jugular venous pulse; (B) Carotid arterial pulse—(1) Systole; (2) Diastole

Recording the Blood Pressure

The appropriate sized cuff for adults and children has to be used, otherwise the values will be altered. It is conventional to use mercury sphygmomanometers. If aneroid instruments are used, their accuracy should be verified periodically. Generally, the BP is recorded in one of the arms. If there is any abnormality in the BP or if arterial occlusion in the arm is suspected, the BP should be recorded in both arms and legs. Normally, the systolic BP recorded in both the arms does not vary more than 10 mm Hg. The systolic pressure in the lower limb is normally up to 20 mm Hg higher than in the upper limb. Though the point of muffling of *Korotkoff's sounds* denotes the diastolic BP, to achieve consistency in recording, the point of appearance and disappearance of these sounds can be accepted to represent the systolic and diastolic BP, respectively, for clinical purposes.

Examination of the Chest

Inspection

Cardiomegaly occurring in early life gives rise to precordial bulge. This is true of CHD and juvenile rheumatic heart disease. In the majority of these cases, RV is enlarged. Displacement of the apex beat and abnormal pulsations occurring in ventricular aneurysm or aortic aneurysm can be made out. The epigastrium pulsates in RV hypertrophy. Liver pulsates in tricuspid incompetence.

Palpation

It is the method to locate the apical impulse. Other valuable information obtained by palpation are the presence of ventricular hypertrophy, expansile pulsation of aneurysms, abnormally loud heart sounds and thrills produced by loud murmurs.

Normal apex beat is palpable in thin and moderately built individuals. It just lifts the palpating finger, but not beyond the plane of the adjoining ribs and is sustained for less than half of systole. Normally the apex beat is felt in the fifth left intercostal space 1 cm inside the midclavicular line. It may be impalpable if the chest wall is thick or if it is behind a rib. Pathological causes include emphysema and pericardial effusion. When the apex beat is not located in the normal position, the right side should be palpated, so as not to miss dextrocardia. When there is volume overload of a ventricle, the palpating finger is lifted beyond the plane of the adjoining ribs but is not sustained. Such an apical impulse is called *forceful* or *hyperdynamic apex beat*. Pressure overload of the ventricles as in hypertension or outflow stenosis causes a forceful and sustained impulse (heaving apex beat). LV hypertrophy is manifested by heaving apex beat, whereas RV hypertrophy manifests as left parasternal heave. Normal pulmonary artery pulsation may be visible in the second and third left intercostal spaces in thin individuals. If this is prominent, it suggests abnormal pulsation and pulmonary hypertension.

Thrills are caused by vibrations imparted to the palpating hand by turbulent blood flow.

Percussion

The precordial dullness is increased in cardiomegaly due to various causes and in pericardial effusion. The

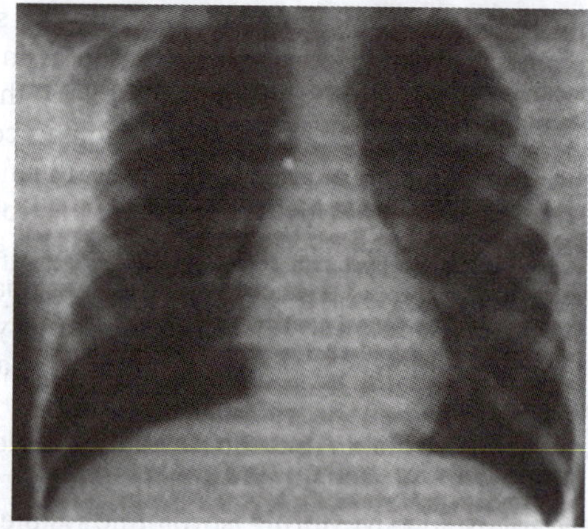

Fig. 119.4: Skiagram of normal chest. **Note:** Lungs are translucent and bronchial and vascular markings are traceable to the chest wall. The cardiothoracic ratio is less than 50%. The blood vessels at the hilum and major bronchi are visible

cardiac dullness is obliterated in emphysema and left-sided pneumothorax. Enlargement of the pulmonary artery, occurring in atrial septal defect or gross pulmonary hypertension can be detected by extension of the dullness outside the normal in the left second intercostal space. Normal pulmonary artery dullness does not extend more than 2 cm beyond the left sternal edge. Since assessment by percussion can at best be only approximate, more accurate estimation by radiography or ultrasonography has to be resorted to in all cases when facilities permit (Fig. 119.4).

Auscultation

René-Théophile-Hyacinthe Laennec (1781–1826 French Physician) invented the stethoscope between 1816 and 1819 AD and introduced auscultation in cardiology. The original instrument was made of cedar wood or ebony. It was 30 cm long, 3.7 cm thick and with a central lumen of 0.6 cm in diameter. He named it stethoscope (*stethos*—chest, *scopein*—to observe). The modern stethoscope has undergone many changes.

The chest piece of many stethoscopes has the bell and the diaphragm. The former picks up low-pitched sounds better, whereas the latter is more useful to receive high-pitched sounds. Newer stethoscopes have only one chest piece. The sensitivity of the diaphragm to different pitches of the sound can be altered by the pressure exerted with the chest piece. The mitral, tricuspid, pulmonary and aortic areas are auscultated in sequence and then the third left intercostal space (second aortic area) is auscultated. Several additional areas of the chest or body have also to be auscultated, when there are indications. These include the interscapular area, neck, first and second left intercostal spaces, apices of lungs, abdomen, spine and head. Normal heart sounds, additional sounds such as (third and fourth heart sound) and abnormal sounds such as clicks, murmurs, opening snaps, pericardial rub, etc. are specially looked for. In general, the events occurring at the different valves are heard best over the corresponding areas.

The second sound in the pulmonary area shows two components, the aortic and the pulmonary (A2 and P2). Normally during inspiration, the pulmonary component becomes delayed whereas the aortic component occurs slightly earlier and S2 becomes split. In expiration, both the components come closer and S2 becomes almost single. Wide but mobile splitting of the second sound can be appreciated in inspiration and expiration and occurs when the RV contraction is delayed or takes longer time. This occurs in conditions like right bundle branch block or pulmonary stenosis. Splitting of the second sound is called *fixed*, if it does not show a variation between inspiration and expiration. This happens in atrial septal defect and RV failure. In atrial septal defect, the phasic changes in venous return during respiration are associated with reciprocal changes in the volume of left to right shunt. Inability to vary its stroke volume by the failing RV accounts for the fixed splitting of S2 in RV failure. If the splitting of the second sound becomes narrow during inspiration, it is called *reversed split (paradoxical split)*. This occurs in aortic stenosis, left bundle branch block (LBBB) and left ventricular failure (LVF).

Gallops

They are diastolic events and appear to be related to filling of the ventricles. When S3 or S4 becomes pathologically accentuated giving rise to a characteristic cadence resembling the canter of a horse, it is termed *gallop rhythm*. The ventricular diastolic gallop also known as *protodiastolic gallop* is due to the third heart sound that occurs during the rapid filling phase. This is an early sign of ventricular dysfunction, although it can occur physiologically in normal children and young adults. The atrial gallop also known as *presystolic gallop* is due to the fourth heart sound that occurs during the presystolic filling phase due to atrial systole. It is abolished in AF. When the heart rate is fast and the diastolic interval is shortened, they may merge and such a phenomenon is called *summation gallop*.

Murmurs

These are produced by turbulence of blood flow at or near the valves or through abnormal communications. If a murmur occurs as a result of abnormally large amount of blood flowing through a normal valve or artery, this is termed flow *murmur* (previously known as functional murmurs). This disappears when the hemodynamic abnormality is corrected. On the other hand, organic murmurs are produced by structural abnormality in the heart or blood vessels and these murmurs tend to persist. In addition, murmurs may occur without intrinsic structural or functional abnormalities in the heart valves and blood vessels. These are generally benign, without any hemodynamic abnormality (Table 119.4). In addition to the location of the murmur several other characteristics help to identify its source. These are timing, duration, character (high-pitched or low-pitched), change with respiration and position of the patient, conduction and response to maneuvers like hand grip, valsalva and squatting. Additional sounds include cardiac sounds such as opening snaps, tumor polyps, endocardial, pericardial or pleuropericardial rubs and extracardiac sounds such as venous hum, bruit over arteries, soufflé, etc.

SPECIAL INVESTIGATIONS

Radiology

The size and shape of the heart can be assessed from chest radiographs. Posteroanterior views, lateral views and oblique views are used to assess abnormalities of the

Table 119.4: Eponyms of some classic murmurs

Name of murmur	Author	Nationality and date	Details
Austin Flint	Austin Flint	American—Early and mid 19th century	Mid-diastolic and presystolic mitral murmur in nonrheumatic aortic regurgitation
Barlow's syndrome	John Barlow	South African –1968	Mitral valve prolapse syndrome nonejection click, late systolic murmur changing with maneuvers
Cabot-Locke murmur	Richard Cabot Frank Locke	American–1912	Diastolic murmur that sounds like aortic incompetence without decrescendo—seen in anemia especially left sternal borders; disappears on clearance of anemia
Carey Coombs murmur	Carey Coomb	English–1924	Short mid diastolic murmur heard in acute rheumatic carditis affecting the mitral valve
Dock's murmur	William Dock	American –1967	Continuous diastolic murmur with early and late accentuation sharply localized 4 cm to the left of the sternum. Due to stenosis of the descending branch of left coronary artery
Gibson's murmur	George Gibson	London–1906	Continuous murmur due to persistent ductus arteriosus
Graham Steell murmur	Graham Steell	Scotish Horseman – 1873	Pulmonary incompetence murmur due to pulmonary hypertension in MS, best heard in the localized space in the left upper sternal border
Key-Hodgkin murmur	Charles Aston Key–19th century	London-Charles Aston Key and Thomas Hodgkin–1828	The diastolic murmur of syphilitic aortic incompetence
Roger's murmur	Henri-Louis Roger	French pediatrician mid-late 1800's	Pan systolic murmur of ventricular septal defect
Still's murmur	George Fredrick Still	English physician 1897–1902	Medium to long systolic ejection murmur of a musical nature quality heard at the lower sternal border and apex. Innocent murmur heard in children

Abbreviation: MS = Mitral stenosis

different chambers. Normally the cardiothoracic ratio is less than 50%. Enlargement of different chambers gives characteristic configuration in the X-ray. The contraction of the chambers can be seen by fluoroscopy. Pulsation of the aorta and pulmonary artery can be observed. Pulmonary congestion, pulmonary oligemia and pulmonary edema can be diagnosed. Serially taken chest radiographs also help in assessing the progress of cardiac disease (Figs 119.4 to 119.6). Chest radiographs taken in different views bring out the different chambers clearly.

Electrocardiography (ECG)

The electrical changes that take place in the heart during different phases of the cardiac cycle are recorded in the ECG. The standard 12-lead ECG consists of three standard bipolar limb leads (L1, L2 and L3), three augmented unipolar limb leads (aVR, aVL and aVF) and six precordial unipolar leads (V1–V6) (Fig. 119.7). When required, further additional leads such as right-sided chest leads, high anterior chest leads or posterior leads are also taken. Normal ECG shows the P-wave which is caused by electrical activation of the atria, QRS which represents ventricular depolarization and T-wave which is caused by ventricular repolarization. The amplitude of these waves, their configuration, their duration and the time interval between various deflections (PR, QRS and QT, PP and RR intervals) are all studied to derive diagnostic information (Fig. 119.8).

Clinical Applications

Following are the clinical applications of ECG:

- Determining the heart rate and rhythm
- To detect atrial or ventricular enlargement

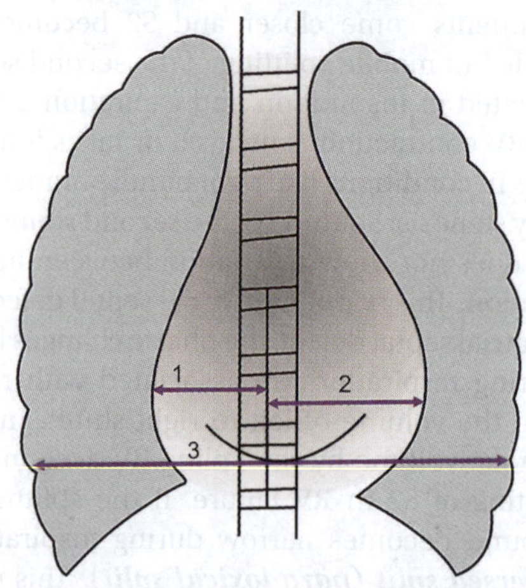

Fig. 119.5: Schematic representation of chest X-ray. **Note:** Transverse diameter of the heart is 1 + 2. Cardiothoracic ratio $\underline{(CTR)}$ is $\dfrac{1 + 2}{3}$

- Diagnosis of all arrhythmias and disorders of impulse production and conduction
- Detection, localization and semiquantitation of myocardial ischemia (reversible and irreversible)
- Diagnosis of myocardial diseases (myocarditis or cardiomyopathy)
- Diagnosis of pericardial diseases (pericarditis, effusion)
- Monitor toxicity of drugs like digoxin and other ingested toxins such as cerebra odollum
- Diagnosis of the cardiac involvement in metabolic diseases like myxedema, thyrotoxicosis and others
- Determining the cardiac effects of electrolyte disturbances, especially hyper and hypokalemia.

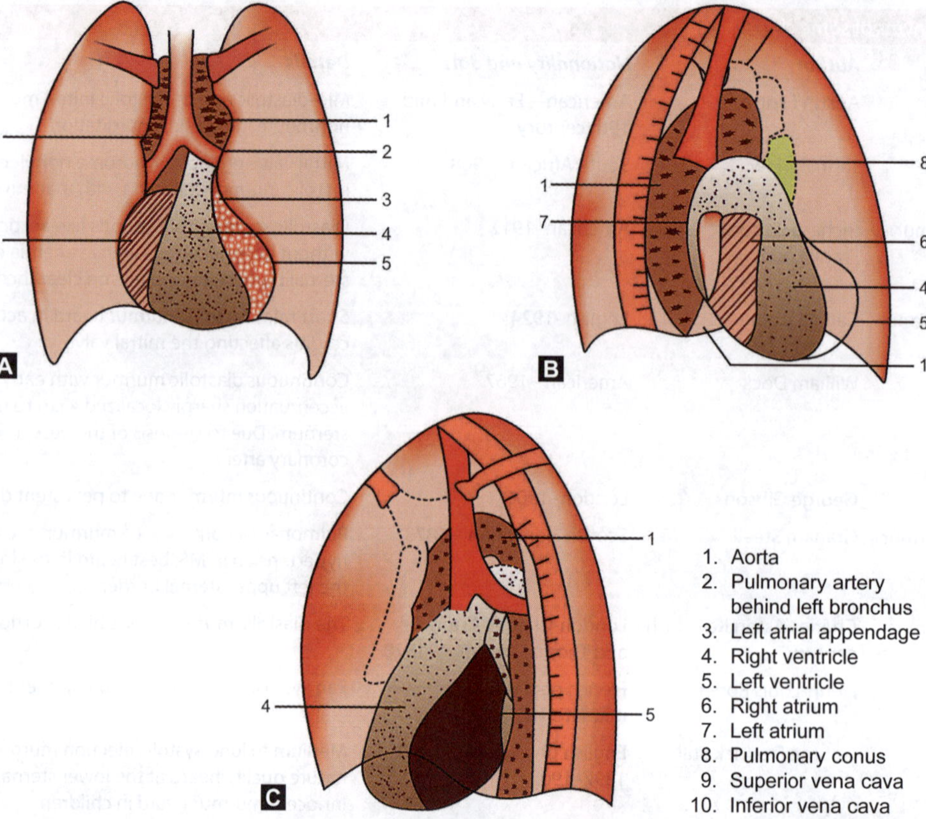

Figs 119.6A to C: X-ray: **A.** PA view of the chest; **B.** Right oblique view; **C.** Left oblique view

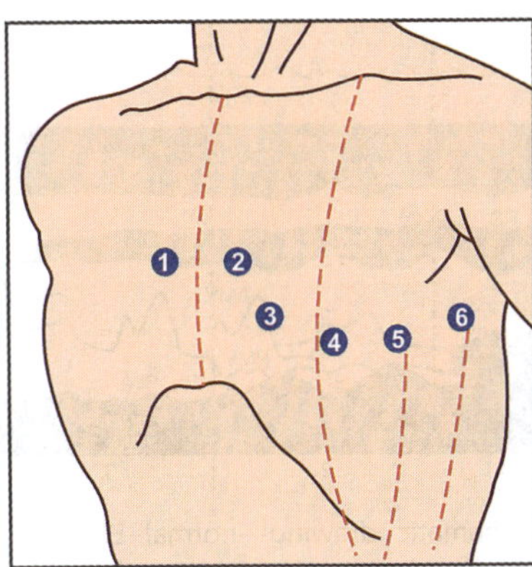

Fig. 119.7: Position of chest leads—V1–V6

Recording the ECG is a routine basal investigation to look for evidence of heart disease. The following modifications have been made over the conventional ECG.

- ***Stress test:*** Treadmill test is the most commonly used type of stress test. This can be used to assess the likelihood and extent of coronary artery disease (CAD), prognosis of CAD, functional capacity and effects of therapy. Stress test is positive for inducible ischemia when ECG shows more than or equal to 0.1 mV horizontal or downsloping ST depression or more than or equal to 0.15 mV slow upsloping ST depression or a ST segment elevation of more than or equal to 0.1 mV in a noninfarct territory. This is a highly reliable test. The commonly used method is the Bruce protocol for graded exercise testing on the treadmill.

- ***Holter monitoring:*** ECG is recorded continuously for long periods in ambulant subjects and is later analyzed. This is very useful for evaluation of paroxysmal arrhythmias and episodic silent or symptomatic ischemia.

- ***His bundle electrography:*** Electrical activity of the bundle of His may be recorded by an electrode catheter placed near the tricuspid valve under fluoroscopy. This technique known as His bundle electrography permits division of the PR interval into two subintervals, namely, the AH interval (an approximation of AV nodal conduction time) and HV interval (representing conduction time within the His-Purkinje system). Thus, more precise localization of the site of AV block and distinction between supraventricular and ventricular beats become possible.

- ***Signal averaged ECG (or) high resolution ECG:*** This technique is used to identify the different frequencies and voltage components that constitute the QRS complex. Late potentials (delayed low-voltage signals) detected by this technique serve as predictors for the development of ventricular arrhythmias especially in ischemic heart disease (IHD).

Echocardiography (ECHO)

In principle, this method records the reflection of pulsed ultrasound from various parts of the heart studied in different directions. Ultrasound of 1–7 MHz frequency is generally used. The earlier machines used time-motion mode display, but later versions permitted two-dimensional imaging. Color coding has also been introduced for specialized investigations. The ECHO can be visualized on a fluorescent screen, photographed or recorded for future analysis and interpretation. In the ECHO, the anterior RV wall, both sides of the interventricular septum, mitral valve, posterior LV wall, pericardium, walls of the aorta, aortic valve, pulmonary artery and valve, pulmonary veins, posterior left atrial wall, both atria and the tricuspid valve can be identified distinctly. Conventionally, M-mode ECHO at different levels and two-dimensional real time imaging from the different parasternal, apical and other windows form the cornerstone of a basic ECHO evaluation. Incorporation of Doppler into ECHO helps to assess normal blood flow and also abnormal flow of blood as occurring in septal defects and valvular stenosis

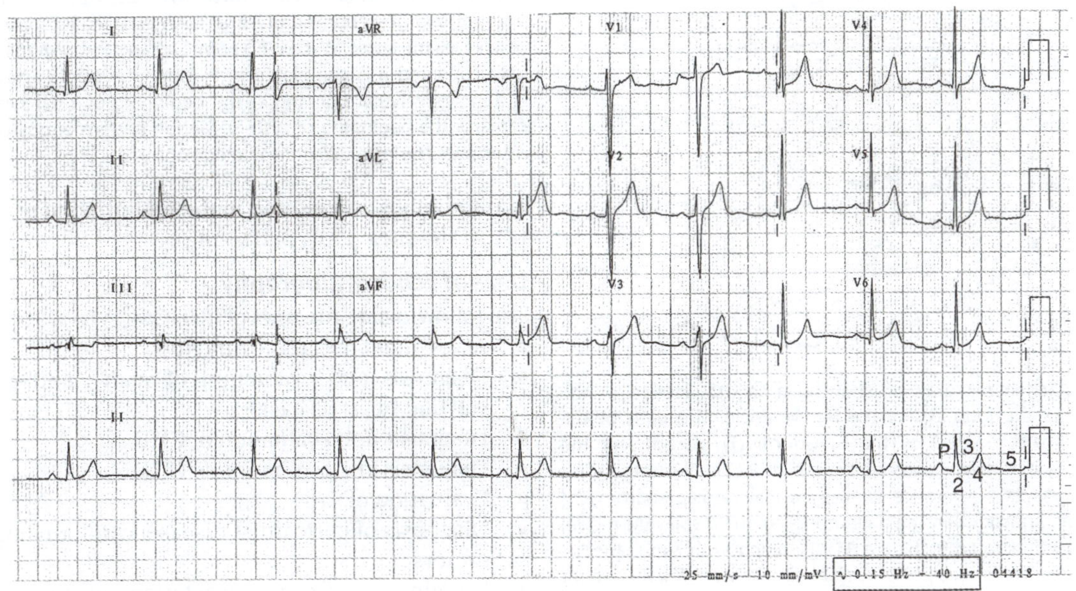

Fig. 119.8: Normal ECG shows sinus rhythm. Each QRS complex is preceded by a P wave. PR interval in this ECG is 0.16 sec (normal PR interval is up to 0.21 sec). QRS duration is also normal, i.e. 0.08 sec (normal up to 0.1 sec). No ST segment of T wave changes—I, II, III, limb leads; aVR, aVL, aVF augmented unipolar leads; V1–V6 unipolar chest leads; 2. QRS segment; 3. ST segment; 4. T wave; 5. Position of U wave

or incompetence and other lesions. Being a simple, easily available and noninvasive procedure, the use of ECHO has become an integral part of cardiac assessment. With its use, invasive and more expensive investigations such as catheterization and angiocardiography can be avoided in many cases (Figs 119.9 to 119.11).

One of the drawbacks of conventional transthoracic ECHO has been the difficulty to get proper images of the posterior aspect of the heart and finer details such as valvular vegetations and intra-atrial thrombi. This has been overcome by the introduction of *transesophageal ECHO* in which the probe is introduced into the esophagus and images are recorded. Better visualization of the intracardiac structures is possible, especially in the setting of prosthetic valves or suboptimal transthoracic views. Coupling this method with *Doppler imaging* and *color-coding* of the images helps to assess the dynamics of blood flow and its abnormalities. Another application is the intraoperative use of this method to get continuous recording of cardiac events during procedures such as mitral valve reconstructive surgery.

Stress ECHO is a very useful technique in the evaluation of CAD and valvular heart disease. This is done by evaluating the cardiac chambers, wall motion and hemodynamics by ECHO at rest, during and immediately after applying some forms of stress. Commonly used modalities of stress are exercise, atrial pacing and pharmacologic methods (dobutamine and adenosine).

Intravascular ultrasound uses crystals mounted on arterial catheter. This probe can be passed through small arteries, like the coronary arteries. This technique is employed in the assessment of arterial lesions such as atherosclerosis

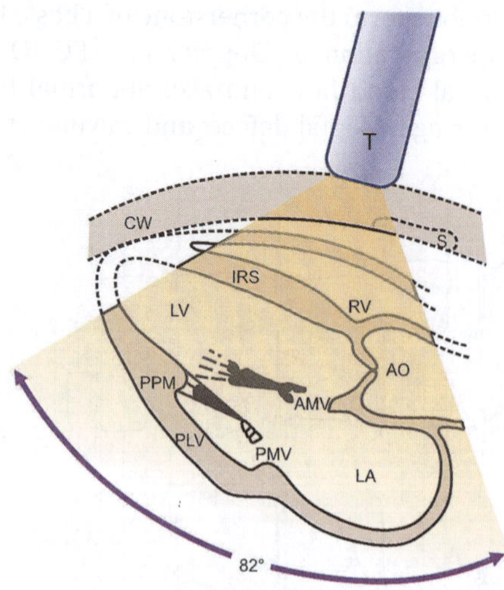

Fig. 119.9: Schematic drawing showing a sagittal section of the heart through the long-axis of the left ventricle. The path of the ultrasound beam emitted by the transducer (T) placed over the chest wall, as it is swept through an arc of 82° is illustrated. This diagram serves as a reference for the normal cardiac anatomy as visualized by ultrasound in the time motion mode display (M-mode) schematically illustrated in Figure 119.11 along with simultaneous ECG record. T—Transducer; CW—Chest wall; S—Sternum; RV—Right ventricle; IVS—Intraventricular septum; RV—Right ventricular wall; AMV—Anterior mitral valve leaflet; PMV—Posterior mitral valve leaflet; LV—Left ventricle; PPM—Posterior papillary muscle; PLV—Posterior left ventricular wall; AO—Aorta; LA— Left atrium

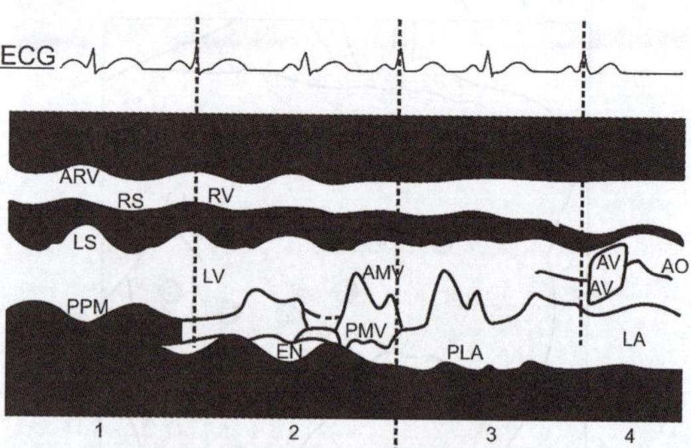

Fig. 119.10: Schematic drawing—normal ECHO. PLA—Posterior left atrial wall, Ao—Aorta, AV—Aortic valve, LA—Left atrium, ECG—Electrocardiogram, 1. At papillary muscle level, 2. At the level of chordae tendinae, 3 and 4-further up. The ventricular internal dimensions and ventricular and septal thickness are measured at this level. Slight superior angulation of the transducer brings into view the anterior and posterior leaflets of the mitral valve. The normal leaflet motion pattern has a characteristic appearance of M and W for the anterior and posterior leaflets respectively. The normal aortic valve (AV) echogram has a box like configuration in systole. The left atrium is immediately posterior to the aorta

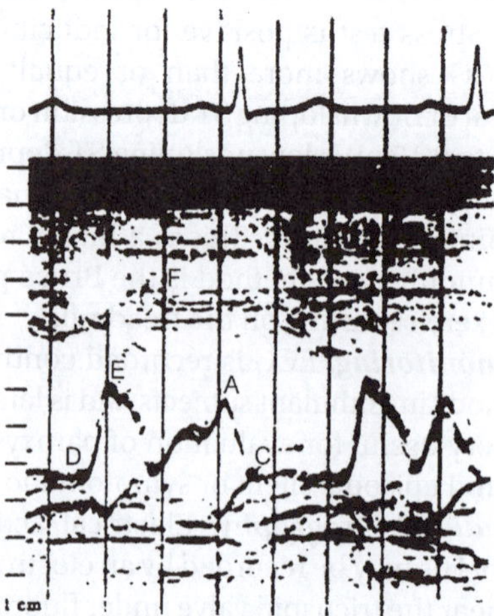

Fig. 119.11: Normal ECHO. *Note:* The pattern of motion of the anterior and posterior mitral leaflets. Anterior leaflet motion pattern resembles the letter 'M' (DEFAC) point D marks the beginning of mitral valve opening it is completed at E. F denotes mid-diastolic closure. A denotes valvular opening at the beginning of atrial systole. Point C marks the beginning of systole. Motion pattern of posterior leaflet resembles the letter 'W' (mirror image of M)

and thrombus and utilized in the optimization of treatment of CAD by angioplasty and stenting.

Uses of Echocardiography

The following are the uses of ECHO:

- Assessment of cardiac function
- Diagnosis and evaluation of native and prosthetic valvular heart disease
- Diagnosis and evaluation of CHD
- Diagnosis and evaluation of CHD
- Evaluation of CAD
- Diagnosis of pericardial disease, cardiomyopathy and tumors
- Demonstration of the vegetations of infective endocarditis.

From its original introduction, the ultrasound scanners and the techniques have undergone steady improvement in machine design, probe specifications and probe positioning. Whereas the early studies are conducted with the transducer probe positioned outside the body, at present, probes which can be attached to endoscopes and arterial or venous percutaneous catheters are available. These permit evaluation in real time of events inside the chambers and vascular lumen.

In many conditions such as valvular lesions, congenital heart disease, cardiac failure, IHD, cardiomyopathy, pericardial disease and others, accurate measurement of the structural and hemodynamic abnormalities is possible. Being noninvasive and repeatable, the ECHO has established its place in preoperative and postoperative assessment. In the follow-up of patients with diseases of the cardiac muscle, this investigation is invaluable.

Isotopic Investigations

Availability of radionuclides such as [99m]technetium (half-life 6 hours) and [201]thallium (half-life 73 hours) and sestamibi has enabled isotopic studies to assess blood flow and myocardial perfusion. Isotopic studies are also noninvasive.

Flow studies: [99m]Technetium compounds are used for dynamic flow studies. These include—delineation of the various cardiac chambers during systole and diastole (*nuclear angiocardiography*); calculation of ejection fraction; evaluation of congenital cyanotic heart disease; demonstration of akinetic segments of the ventricular wall following MI and quantitation of intracardiac shunts.

Myocardial scanning: For this purpose [201]thallium which is concentrated in the myocardium is employed. This isotope behaves similar to potassium and its concentration in the myocardium depends on the myocardial blood flow. Areas of diminished perfusion can be detected as **cold** areas in IHD. Appearance of cold areas during exercise is an indication of stress-induced ischemia. Sestamibi is another isotope used for myocardial imaging. It is not taken up by necrotic myocardium. Isotope studies are employed for the following conditions:

- For assessing myocardial perfusion during rest and exercise
- Studying the configuration of the myocardium, especially hypertrophy
- To detect the presence of myocardial infarct, its extent, and viability of the ischemic myocardium
- For the evaluation of postbypass surgery patients
- For the identification of hibernating myocardium
- For the assessment of the prognosis in MI.

Magnetic Resonance Imaging in Clinical Cardiology

Magnetic resonance imaging (MRI) has established its place in cardiology over the past 10 years. It is a useful investigation in various situations for the assessment of cardiac structure, function, perfusion and myocardial viability. MRI is accurate and reproducible. Images of cardiac chambers and the great vessels help to assess morphological and functional changes in these locations. MRI is being increasingly used for imaging the coronary circulation, myocardial perfusion, study of intravascular plaques and for the delineation of heart valves. Hypertrophic cardiomyopathy and cardiac tumors are well-demonstrated. Next to skiagram and ECHO, MRI is the investigation of choice in the study of pericardial lesions. More sophisticated and dedicated machines are being introduced into this branch of investigative cardiology. Cardiac MRI studies show promise as noninvasive investigative tools to assess coronary artery occlusions. Unlike the contrast agents used in conventional angiocardiography, gadolinium used in MRI is not nephrotoxic.

Multiparametric cardiovascular magnetic resonance (CMR) protocol has high diagnostic accuracy in CAD and it is superior to single-photon emission computed tomography (SPECT) study. CMR has a sensitivity of 86.5% and specificity of 83.4%. Positive predictive value is approximately 77% and negative predictive value is 90%. These are even superior to those in SPECT.

Single-photon emission computed tomography and *positron emission tomography* (*PET*) can be employed to study the myocardium in greater detail. These studies are available in India in several centers in all states. Studies employing these methods help to identify potentially salvageable myocardium in IHD. Using appropriate radiolabeled isotopes, the metabolic activity of the myocardium can be assessed.

Cardiac Catheterization

The right and left sides of the heart can be catheterized using special catheters. Pressures in the different chambers can be recorded during catheterization and this helps in identifying anatomical abnormalities.

Blood can be sampled from different locations for estimation of oxygen (*oximetry*) and this helps to quantitate left-to-right or right-to-left shunts. Cardiac output and cardiac index can be calculated by oximetric studies in the aortic and pulmonary arterial blood. Normal cardiac index is 2.8–4.2 L/min/m^2. Reduction below 2.4 indicates abnormality. Pressure tracing of the ventricles enables detection of obstruction to ventricular filling, outflow obstruction, intactness of interventricular septum and the presence of large septal defects, and also permits the calculation of the *systolic ejection time*. Systolic ejection time is the interval between the end of isometric contraction and the end of ejection.

A suitable catheter can be passed into the right side of the heart and manipulated into the pulmonary artery and advanced till it gets impacted in a small branch. Measurement of the pressure at this site (*pulmonary wedge pressure*) reflects the left atrial pressure.

Upper limit of normal pulmonary artery pressure is 30/14 mm Hg. Rise in RV end diastolic pressure above 8 mm Hg and LV end diastolic pressure above 12 mm Hg is indicative of ventricular failure or restriction to ventricular filling due to pericardial disease or myocardial fibrosis.

Selective Angiocardiography

It is the imaging of different cardiac chambers after injecting contrast material into them. This method helps to visualize the cardiac chambers and sequential flow of the dye during different phases of the cardiac cycle. Angiocardiography clearly demonstrates the anatomical and functional abnormalities in the heart. Mitral incompetence, mitral stenosis, aortic stenosis, aortic incompetence, tricuspid and pulmonary valve lesions, cardiac aneurysms and complex congenital malformations can be fully visualized.

Coronary Angiography

It is the method of demonstrating right and left coronary arteries after selective retrograde arterial catheterization from the radial, ulnar or femoral access using special catheters (Fig. 119.12).

Angiocardiographic studies provide invaluable information in several disorders where other noninvasive methods fail. Therefore, angiocardiography has to be resorted to particularly in the preoperative assessment of some of the cardiac lesions.

Interventional Cardiology: Catheterization Laboratory Procedures

This term is used for the therapeutic procedures done by an interventional cardiologist in a cardiac catheterization laboratory. This specialty has expanded rapidly during the last 3 decades. The procedures include primary angioplasty for acute MI, coronary angioplasty and stent for CAD, renal angioplasties, peripheral angioplasties, closure of PDA by coil or device, device closure of atrial septal defect (ASD) and ventricular septal defect (VSD) and balloon valvuloplasties for mitral stenosis, pulmonary valve stenosis and aortic stenosis in addition to other procedures for an expanding array of indications.

Coronary angioplasty is widely used for management of single vessel disease and two vessel disease. For three vessel disease with normal LV function and suitable lesions for angioplasty, the results are comparable to bypass surgery except for the greater need for repeat revascularization. However, complex three vessel disease, especially in diabetics, is traditionally considered for coronary artery bypass surgery. The details of angioplasty are determined beforehand by coronary angiography which is done by selective catheterization of the coronary arteries using special catheters (Fig. 119.13).

Routine stenting during angioplasty helps to keep vascular patency over long period. Conventional bare metal stents have given place to drug eluting stents. These stents are coated with drugs such as sirolimus, everolimus, tacrolimus, praclitaxel and others. The initial studies over a few years have shown that the rate of reocclusion of the coronary arteries is lower and the patency of the lumen is maintained for longer periods with drug-coated stents. Newer generation drug eluting stents, especially the bioabsorbable stents, are considerably more expensive than the plain stents.

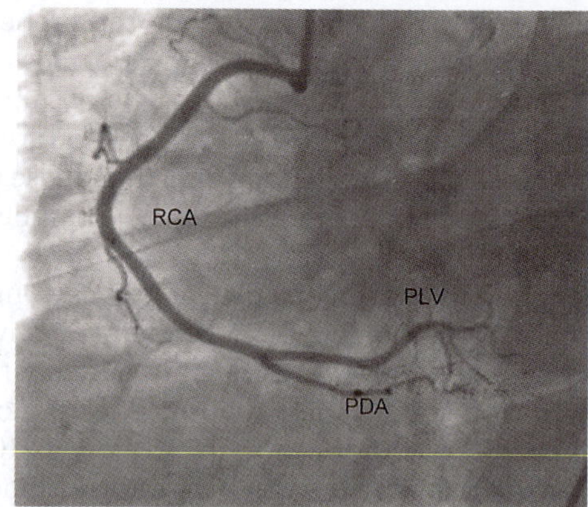

Fig. 119.12: Normal right coronary angiogram showing the right coronary artery (RCA), posterior descending artery (PDA) and posterior left ventricular branch (PLV)

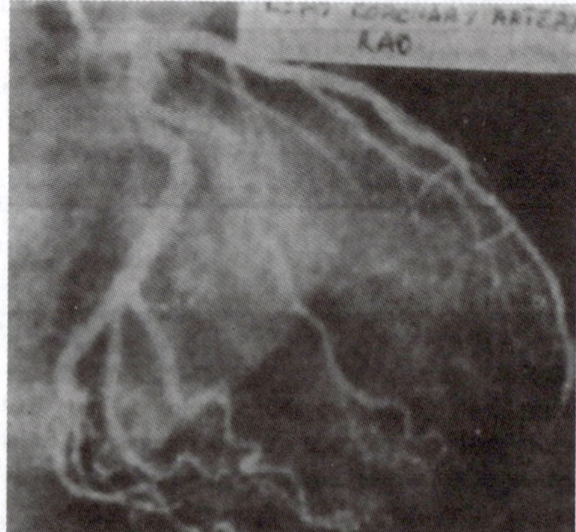

Fig. 119.13: Normal coronary angiogram showing the various branches filling normally

Balloon valvuloplasty is employed for definitive treatment of mitral stenosis and pulmonary valve stenosis. Balloon pulmonary valvuloplasty is the treatment of choice for pulmonary valve stenosis. Mitral stenosis with suitable valve morphology treated by balloon mitral valvuloplasty has excellent short-term and long-term outcome, which is comparable to open surgical commissurotomy. Balloon aortic valvuloplasty in adults still remains largely as a palliative measure.

Digital subtraction angiography: In this technique, the bony cage and soft tissue shadows are eliminated by computer-aided subtraction which makes the vascular anatomy stand out prominently. Enhancement of vascular image obtained by elimination of other shadows enables one to visualize lesions in the major arteries (cerebral, thoracic, visceral or peripheral) by venous injection of small doses of contrast media, thereby avoiding arterial puncture.

Heart Failure (Cardiac Failure)

CG Bahuleyan

Chapter Summary

- General Considerations
- Pathophysiology
- Hemodynamic Alterations
- Neurohumoral Alterations
- Cellular and Molecular Mechanisms
- Types of Heart Failure
- Clinical Features
- Management
- Ace Inhibitors
- Angiotensin Receptor Blockers
- Beta Blockers
- Mineralo Corticoid Receptor Antagonist
- Anticoagulants
- Hydralazine and Isosorbide Dinitrate
- Antiarrhythmics
- Positive Inotropes
- Selective Sinus Node if Channel Inhibitor (Ivabradine)
- Surgical Options
- Cardiac Transplantation
- Gene Therapy
- Refractory Cardiac Failure
- Emergency Treatment of Acute Pulmonary Edema

GENERAL CONSIDERATIONS

Definition: Heart failure is a pathophysiological state in which the heart is unable to pump at a rate commensurate with the requirement of the metabolizing tissues (systolic failure) or can do so only with elevated filling pressures (diastolic failure).

Heart failure manifests as a complex clinical syndrome characterized by circulatory congestion, impaired systolic function, impaired diastolic function or both, and progressive activation of the neuroendocrine system. ***In all forms of cardiac disease, if the abnormality is allowed to progress without treatment, heart failure sets in, invariably after varying periods of time***.

Though there have been significant advances in the treatment and prevention of heart failure, it is still increasing in incidence and prevalence. Approximately, 1.5–2% of the population has some form of cardiac failure and the prevalence increases to 6–10% in patients more than 65 years old. In India, the estimated prevalence of heart failure is 18.8 million (1.76% of the population) and the incidence of 1.57 million per year (0.15%).

The incidence of heart failure increases with the aging of the population, and in the elderly it is associated with several comorbidities like renal failure, anemia, diabetes mellitus, obstructive sleep apnea, all of which increase the morbidity and mortality.

Chronic heart failure is a dangerous debilitating and common disease. Prevalence of chronic heart failure in the population is 1%. Thirty two percent of patients with chronic heart disease die within 1 year of hospitalization. Incidence of chronic heart failure (CHF) in India has been estimated to be between 0.49 million and 1.8 million in 2020.

Source: On the horizon of heart failure. Lancet. 2011;378:637.

PATHOPHYSIOLOGY

During the past 4 decades there has been a progressive evolution in the concept and understanding of heart failure (Box 120.1).

In 1940–60s, heart failure was considered as a ***cardiorenal*** disorder where it was thought that impaired ventricular function leads to reduced cardiac output, and reduced renal perfusion leads to salt and water retention. Later on in 1960–80s, heart failure was considered as ***cardiocirculatory*** disorder where the ***hemodynamic abnormality*** was given more emphasis. Now it is known that heart failure cannot be simply defined in hemodynamic terms and the role of neurohumoral, cellular and molecular mechanisms are all important.

HEMODYNAMIC ALTERATIONS

In the early stages of heart failure, the hemodynamic abnormalities occur only during exercise. As the heart

---

Box 120.1: Pathophysiology of heart failure

- Hemodynamic alterations
  - Increased end diastolic pressure (EDP), end diastolic volume (EDV)
  - Reduced cardiac output
- Neurohumoral alterations
  - Alterations in autonomic nervous system
    - Increased norepinephrine
    - Altered baroreceptor control
  - Alterations in beta adrenergic receptors
    - Down regulation of beta receptors
    - Increased beta-adrenergic receptor kinase
  - Alterations in renin-angiotensin system
    - Increased renin
    - Increased angiotensin II
    - Increased aldosterone
    - Down regulation of angiotensin I and II receptors
  - Others
    - Elevated atrial/brain natriuretic peptide
    - Elevated endothelin
    - Role of cytokines
- Cellular and molecular alterations
  - Calcium kinetics
    - Reduced Ca^{++} cycling
    - Reduced sarcoendoplasmic reticulum calcium (SERCA) 2-enzyme level
    - Reduction in calcium release channels
  - Changes in contractile apparatus
    - Re-expression of genes
  - Free radicals and apoptosis

failure progresses, they occur at rest as well. Reduction in cardiac output is associated with a rise in end-diastolic pressures (EDP) in the ventricle and increased venous pressure. Increase in EDP is accompanied by increase in end-diastolic volume (EDV). Generally, the EDP and volume determine the extent to which myocardial fibers are stretched prior to acute active contraction and this is termed **preload**. The load that the ventricle has to move once it starts contracting is called **afterload**. As the preload and afterload increase, venous congestion develops behind the failing chamber to manifest as pulmonary or systemic venous congestion in right-sided and left-sided heart failure, respectively. Reduction in cardiac output leads to reduction in tissue perfusion. Blood flow to the vital organs like brain and heart is maintained by diverting the flow from less vital organs. Reduced cardiac output and reduced renal perfusion leads to salt and water retention.

NEUROHUMORAL ALTERATIONS

Consequent to the two principal hemodynamic alterations viz reduced cardiac output and elevated mean atrial pressure, a complex series of neurohumoral alterations occur. In early stages, these alterations act as compensatory mechanisms, but later on they lead to undesirable effects and injury.

Alterations in Autonomic Nervous System

These include increased sympathetic activity and elevation of plasma norepinephrine (NE) levels. Extent of elevation of plasma NE correlates directly with the severity of heart failure. Augmented, sympathetic activity and elevated NE causes vasoconstriction and arrhythmias which predisposes to sudden cardiac heart death. The increase in adrenergic activity is mainly due to altered control of adrenergic outflow from the central nervous system (CNS).

Alterations in the Beta-adrenergic Receptor Pathway

Increased levels of local NE concentration cause down regulation of beta-1 adrenergic receptors in the ventricles. In addition there is increase in beta-adrenergic receptor kinase (BARK) enzyme level, which leads to uncoupling of beta receptors. Down regulation of beta-receptors can be reversed by beta blockers.

Alteration in Renin Angiotensin System

Increased adrenergic activity stimulates the alpha-1 receptor in juxtaglomerular apparatus of the kidneys. Also, decreased blood flow to kidney activates the baroreceptors. Both these lead to release of renin. Renin acts on **angiotensinogen** to form **angiotensin I** which is acted upon by angiotensin converting enzyme (ACE) to form **angiotensin II**. Angiotensin II is a potent vasoconstrictor and leads to elevated systemic vascular resistance. Angiotensin II also stimulates production of aldosterone and NE.

Only 1–10% of ACE is found in circulation; 90–99% is present in tissues such as blood vessels, heart and kidneys. Angiotensin has two receptor subtypes angiotensin-type-1 (AT1) and angiotensin-type-2 (AT2). Angiotensin acts on these receptors and causes cell growth and altered gene expression. In patients with severe heart failure these receptors are down regulated.

Role of Arginine Vasopressin

In congestive heart failure (CHF), arginine vasopressin (AVP) is elevated. This leads to salt and water retention and systemic vasoconstriction.

Role of Natriuretic Peptides

Three natriuretic peptides, atrial natriuretic peptide (ANP), brain natriuretic peptide (BNP) and C-type natriuretic peptide (CNP) have been identified. ANP is stored mainly in the right atrium. BNP is stored mainly in the ventricles. They counteract the effects of adrenergic, renin angiotensin system (RAS) and AVP systems and cause vasodilatation, natriuresis and diuresis. CNP is located primarily in the vasculature and it is produced by vascular endothelium as a response to shear stress, primarily in the vasculature. In addition, these peptides inhibit myocytes and vascular smooth muscle hypertrophy. They improve functions of the failing myocardium. Circulating levels of ANP and BNP are increased in heart failure and they confer beneficial effects. Estimation of blood level of natriuretic peptides has been utilized in the diagnostic evaluation of cases of suspected heart failure. Levels of BNP and ANP have been utilized as diagnostic tests in ventricular failure. Normal level is < 100 pg/mL. In heart failure, the levels go above 675 ± 450 pg/mL. This estimation supports the diagnosis of heart failure in doubtful cases.

Estimation of both BNP and N-terminal pro-BNP (NT-pro-BNP) have been found useful in the diagnosis and determining the prognosis of heart failure. Plasma BNP values of less than 100 µg/mL and NT-pro-BNP values of more than 300 µg/mL are useful to exclude the diagnosis of heart failure.

Role of Endothelin

It is a potent vasoconstrictor released by endothelial cells. Three types of endothelins 1, 2 and 3; two subtypes of receptors A and B have been recognized in CHF. Circulating endothelin levels are increased.

Role of Cytokines

Cytokines implicated in the pathogenesis of CHF include tumor necrosis factor alpha, transforming growth factor beta, peptide growth factors and interleukin-1 (IL-1) beta. They have crucial roles in mediating the changes in myocardial structure and function in CHF.

CELLULAR AND MOLECULAR MECHANISMS

Role of Calcium

Calcium plays a central role in myocardial contraction and relaxation. In CHF, there is prolonged elevation of intracellular calcium during relaxation and calcium cycling is reduced by 50%. Calcium uptake is mediated by ATP-dependent enzyme, sarcoendoplasmic reticulum Ca^{2+}-ATPase (SERCA2). SERCA2 activity is inhibited by phospholamban. In CHF, SERCA2 activity is reduced.

Calcium release channel (CRC) located on the sarcoplasmic reticulum (SR) mediates release of Ca^{2+} from the

SR into the myoplasm during systole. In CHF, messenger RNA (mRNA) level for CRC is decreased.

Changes in the Contractile Apparatus

There occurs a qualitative and quantitative change of the contractile proteins. Myosin ATPase activity is reduced in CHF. Also there occurs a re-expression of genes coding for fetal and neonatal isoforms of myosin, rather than adult isoforms. In addition, there is alteration in the regulatory protein-expression of *troponin T.* In normal myocardium, 98% of the regulatory protein is *troponin T.* In CHF, there is a change to *troponin T2.*

Role of Free Radicals and Apoptosis

In CHF, altered mitochondrial oxygen metabolism results in formation of free radicals, i.e. molecules with unpaired electrons. These molecules cause cell damage.

Apoptosis is programmed cell death. Free radicals produced by various mechanisms have been shown to result in apoptosis of cardiac myocytes in CHF.

Diastolic Heart Dysfunction and Failure

Nearly 50% of patients with congestive heart failure have diastolic dysfunction—often referred to as diastolic heart–failure. The left ventricular (LV) function and ejection fraction may be normal. Diastolic heart dysfunction and failure is more common in older age groups, and in women. Hypertension is more common and ischemic heart disease less common in them. Some show impairment of active ventricular relaxation and compliance of the ventricles. Ventricular diastolic pressures rise. This results in increase in pulmonary venous pressure. Stroke volume does not increase with exercise. When effort intolerance, dyspnea, venous congestion and pulmonary edema develop, it is termed diastolic heart failure.

TYPES OF HEART FAILURE

Forward versus Backward Heart Failure

In backward failure hypothesis, when the ventricles fail to discharge the content, blood accumulates and pressure rises in the atria and venous systems proximal to them.

In forward failure hypothesis, manifestations of CHF are due to reduction in cardiac output. In most cases, both these mechanisms operate simultaneously.

Right-sided versus Left-sided Failure

In right-sided failure, systolic output of right ventricle and/or right atrium falls. Common causes include pulmonary artery hypertension (PAH) due to various causes, atrial septal defect, cor pulmonale, pericardial diseases, pulmonary stenosis, right sided cardiomyopathy, massive pulmonary embolism and tricuspid stenosis. This manifests as elevated right atrial pressure, elevated jugular venous pressure, and systemic venous congestion leading to edema and hepatomegaly.

Left-sided failure is caused by pulmonary venous congestion resulting from dysfunction of left ventricle and left atrium, chronic ischemic heart disease, systemic hypertension, and aortic or mitral valve disease. This manifests as dyspnea, orthopnea and paroxysmal nocturnal dyspnea. Persistent left heart failure gives rise to pulmonary hypertension which results in right heart failure as well.

Low Output versus High Output Failure

In the former, the cardiac output is reduced resulting in inadequate tissue perfusion, e.g. mitral stenosis, ischemic heart disease and hypertensive heart disease. In the latter, cardiac output is above the normal range, but it falls from the original levels as heart failure sets in, e.g. thyrotoxicosis, anemia, beriberi.

Acute versus Chronic Heart Failure

In acute heart failure, there is insufficient time for compensatory mechanisms to become operative and hence clinical manifestations are marked, e.g. acute myocardial infarctions (acute MI), tachyarrhythmias, acute pulmonary embolism.

In chronic heart failure, there is time for adaptive mechanisms to develop and hence patients are able to tolerate the reduction in cardiac output better.

Systolic Versus Diastolic Heart Failure

When the abnormality is in systolic function leading to defect in ejection of blood, it is systolic heart failure whereas, if the abnormality is in diastolic function leading to defect in ventricular filling, it is diastolic heart failure. More often both coexist, but in a third cases of heart failure, it may be purely diastolic.

Pathology: At autopsy, the heart may be dilated in cases of chronic congestive cardiac failure. The underlying cardiac lesions may be evident. The lungs are heavy, congested and edematous. In chronic cases the pulmonary vessels show medial hypertrophy and intimal hyperplasia. Liver is enlarged, firm and edematous. The central hepatic veins and sinusoids are congested. Cardiac cirrhosis is histologically characterized by centrilobular necrosis, atrophy and extensive fibrosis.

The spleen may be enlarged and congested. Pancreas may show venous congestion. Intestines may reveal infarction and hemorrhagic necrosis. Kidneys and brain show chronic venous congestion. Mechanism in heart failure and their common causes have been given in Table 120.1.

CLINICAL FEATURES

Symptoms: Most common symptom is dyspnea, which is more marked in left-sided heart disease. Orthopnea, paroxysmal nocturnal dyspnea and Cheyne-Stokes respiration (CSR) are seen in left-sided heart failure.

Weakness, fatigue, and apathy are suggestive of low cardiac output states. Oliguria and nocturia may develop even before dependent edema manifests. Nocturia occurs in the early stages of heart failure. During daytime when the patient is ambulant, cardiac function is impaired and fluid accumulates. At night, with recumbency edema fluid is reabsorbed into the circulation, cardiac function improves with rest, and the excess fluid is eliminated.

Edema is the most prominent symptom in right-sided heart failure. Initially, the edema is dependent, later it becomes generalized. In the early stages, the edema readily pits on pressure but in long-standing cases the part becomes indurated and pigmented. Hepatic

Table 120.1: Mechanism in heart failure and their common causes

• Myocardial causes which reduce the contractile force of the myocardium
  ▪ Myocarditis
  ▪ Coronary artery disease
  ▪ Cardiomyopathy
  ▪ Infiltrations
	• Infective (e.g. rheumatism, typhoid, coxsackie infection)
	• Toxins-diphtheria, scorpion stings, drugs like emetine, adriamycin
	• Nutritional causes—Beriberi
	• Dyscollagenosis—Lupus erythematosus
	• Other miscellaneous causes: Alcohol, diabetes, myxedema
	• Acute myocardial infarction

• Chronic pressure overload • Structural abnormalities in the heart or great vessels which reduce the cardiac output • Pericardial disease which leads to interference with diastolic filling of the ventricles especially the right ventricle • Arrhythmias	• Chronic ischemic myocardial damage • Primary and secondary • Amyloidosis, hemochromatosis, sarcodosis, leukemia, malignant deposits • Hypertension • Valvular heart disease (rheumatic, syphilitic, congenital and atherosclerotic)
• Tachycardias which lead to reduction in the diastolic interval, thereby reducing the end diastolic volume • Extreme bradycardia in which the ventricular rate goes below 30/min • Increased demand on cardiac output. Normal heart is able to cope up with even extremes of demand within physiological limits, since the reserve capacity is great In the majority of pathological states increased demand is associated with impairment of cardiac function as well. • Cor pulmonale • Increased resistance to ventricular emptying	• Infective endocarditis, traumatic lesions (injury or postsurgical) • Congenital heart diseases • Pericardial effusion, constrictive pericarditis • Paroxysmal tachycardias, atrial flutter and fibrillation • Heart block, cardiac poison, e.g. cerbera odollam • Pregnancy, fever, thyrotoxicosis, severe exercise, arteriovenous fistula, chronic respiratory failure, hepatic failure • Acute cor pulmonale as in pulmonary embolism or chronic cor pulmonale as in obstructive airway disease • Systemic arterial hypertension leads to left ventricular failure, and pulmonary hypertension leads to right ventricular failure

congestion manifests with upper abdominal pain and tender hepatomegaly. In long-standing CHF, weight loss and emaciation develop as a result of inadequate intake of food and wasting of tissues. This picture is termed *cardiac cachexia.* Alterations in the cytokine system, especially increase in levels of tumor necrosis factor (TNF), interferon gamma (IFN-gamma) and interleukin 3 (IL-3) also play a part in the production of cardiac cachexia (Fig. 120.1).

Physical Examination

Pulse and blood pressure (BP): The pulse becomes rapid as a result of compensatory adrenergic activity. ***Pulsus alternans*** is suggestive of LV failure. The blood pressure is not generally affected in mild and moderately severe cases. But in severe heart failure, the systolic pressure may fall due to reduction in cardiac output. The diastolic pressure is maintained by increase in the peripheral resistance.

Engorgement of the jugular vein: This is seen characteristically in right-sided and combined heart failure. Abnormality of the hepatojugular reflux can be demonstrated even before the jugular venous pressure is elevated.

Examination of the precordium: In the majority of cases, the heart is dilated, though in many cases (e.g. mitral stenosis, acute MI, myocarditis, and constrictive pericarditis) it may not be so. Evidence of the underlying heart disease may be found. In LV failure a protodiastolic gallop (S3) may be heard over the apex beat, and it is better heard during expiration. In right ventricular failure, S3 gallop is heard over the lower left sternal border and it is better heard during inspiration. Rise in pulmonary arterial pressure gives rise to accentuation of the pulmonary second sound. Dilatation of the ventricle gives rise to valvular incompetence. Functional pansystolic murmurs arising from the mitral or tricuspid valves may be audible, which disappear when the heart size returns to normal.

Abdomen: The liver is enlarged, soft and tender and this may be evident even before overt edema manifests. Hepatic enlargement persists for varying periods after edema clears up with treatment, but with intensive therapy it recedes completely. Mild jaundice and impairment of hepatic function may occur. In long-standing right-sided heart failure with ***cardiac cirrhosis,*** the liver is firm and nontender. It does not recede with treatment at this stage. Mild-to-moderate splenomegaly occurs in some cases initially due to passive venous congestion; later the organ may become fibrotic. Significant splenomegaly should suggest the possibility of infective endocarditis. Ascites may develop as a result of passive venous congestion. Prominent ascites occurs in organic tricuspid valve disease, constrictive pericarditis, and right ventricular endomyocardial fibrosis (Fig. 120.2).

Lungs: Physical signs in the lungs are more pronounced in left-sided heart failure. These are the presence of rales over the interscapular regions, bronchospasm, unilateral or bilateral hydrothorax, frequent respiratory infections

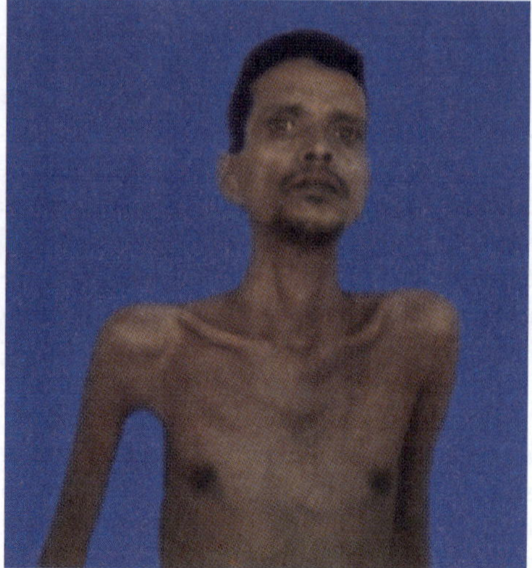

Fig. 120.1: Cardiac cachexia. ***Note:*** Feature of cardiac failure and emaciation

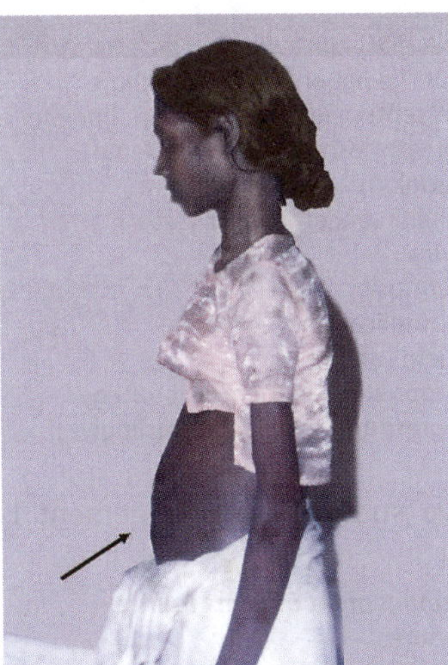

Fig. 120.2: Female 35 cardiac cirrhosis. **Note:** Cachexia and prominent abdomen (arrow)

(pneumonia, bronchopneumonia or bronchitis) and pulmonary infarcts.

Diagnosis

Framingham criteria for diagnosis of heart failure

Major criteria
- Paroxysmal nocturnal dyspnea
- Neck veins distension
- Rales (crackles) over the lower portions of the lung
- Cardiomegaly
- Acute pulmonary edema
- S3 gallop
- Increased venous pressure >16 mm Hg
- Circulation time >25 sec
- Hepatojugular reflux

Minor criteria
- Ankle edema
- Night cough
- Dyspnea on exertion
- Hepatomegaly
- Pleural effusion
- Decrease of vital capacity exceeding 1/3
- Tachycardia >120/mt

Major or minor criteria
- Weight loss >4.5 kg in 5 days in response to treatment
- Major +2 minor criteria if present concurrently establishes the diagnosis of congestive heart failure

Note: Framingham is a township in the USA where a cohort of persons have been followed up meticulously over a long period of time and several biological parameters have been recorded continuously. This study has become a classic prospective study, for several disorders, especially for cardiovascular disorders. The follow-up and observations are still continuing

Investigations

Based on the American College of Cardiology/American Heart Association Task Force Guidelines

Class I: Investigations (usually indicated and always acceptable)
- Blood counts—helpful to exclude infections
- Urinalysis—proteinuria may occur due to renal congestion
- Blood biochemistry:
    - Serum Na⁺, K⁺. In severe CHF, dilutional hyponatremia occurs. Diuretics may cause hypokalemia.
    - Blood urea nitrogen and creatinine are moderately elevated. Severe elevation indicates reduction in renal blood flow.
    - Blood glucose, phosphorus, magnesium, calcium and albumin levels are helpful in etiological diagnosis.
    - TSH levels help to point to thyroid function.
- **ECG:** Though not directly diagnostic of CHF, underlying diseases like ischemia, ventricular hypertrophy, arrhythmias and conduction defects can be diagnosed.
- **Chest X-ray:** This may show cardiomegaly, and features of pulmonary venous or arterial hypertension. Acute pulmonary edema gives characteristic butterfly-shaped opacity extending on both sides from the hilum (Fig. 120.3). A normal chest radiograph does not rule out systolic or diastolic dysfunction.
- **Echo-Doppler evaluation:** This is very useful in evaluating both RV and LV functions and identifying causes like ischemic heart disease, valvular abnormalities, ventricular hypertrophy, congenital heart disease, infiltrative myocardial and pericardial diseases and thrombi. Quantitative measurement of systolic function like ejection fraction, fractional shortening, stroke volume, cardiac output and rate of changes of ventricular pressure (dp/dt) can be obtained with accuracy. Doppler echocardiography is the corner stone for evaluation of diastolic heart failure. Measurements like isovolumic relaxation time (IVRT), mitral inflow pattern, declaration time; and pulmonary and hepatic venous flow patterns are very helpful in the diagnosis and quantification of diastolic dysfunction.
- **Non-invasive stress testing (treadmill test; stress echocardiography and nuclear perfusion studies):** These tests can detect ischemia in patients with and without angina, but with a high probability of coronary artery disease who could be candidates for revascularization and in patients with previous coronary artery disease.
- **Assessment of myocardial viability:** In patients with ischemic heart disease, it is necessary to determine the amount of viable myocardium which is the important determinant for assessing prognosis and formulating therapy. This can be done using dobutamine or dipyridamole stress echocardiography, myocardial contrast echocardiography, nuclear imaging using thallium or sestamibi and positron emission tomography.
- **Cardiac catheterization and coronary angiography:** This is indicated in patients with angina or large areas of ischemic viable myocardium and those at risk of coronary artery disease who require surgical coronary revascularization and those who have to undergo surgery for noncardiac conditions. Right and left heart catheterization can determine the cardiac output, filling pressures, pulmonary artery pressure, pulmonary and systemic vascular resistance, shunts and parameters of diastolic function.

Class II: Investigation (acceptable but of uncertain efficacy)
- **Serum iron and ferritin** to exclude iron overload states.
- **Endomyocardial biopsy:** This is indicated in patients with clinical indication of myocarditis and systemic disease with possible cardiac involvement such as hemochromatosis, amyloidosis, sarcoidosis, subendocardial fibroelastosis and those who have received adriamycin chemotherapy.

Abbreviation: TSH = Thyroid stimulating hormone

Complications of Cardiac Failure

Cardiac failure on its own can produce many complications. These include:
- Arrhythmias and sudden death
- Venous thrombosis and pulmonary embolism
- Intracardiac thrombi and related problems
- Pulmonary infections due to venous congestion
- Cardiac cirrhosis in long-standing cases
- Renal failure.

Course and Prognosis

The prognosis depends upon the type of heart failure and the nature of underlying disease. In the majority of cardiac disorders, cardiac failure is a major cause of death. Acute pulmonary edema occurring in MI, systemic hypertension, mitral stenosis and myocarditis may prove fatal, if emergency treatment is not instituted. In systemic hypertension, ischemic heart disease, aortic valvular disease and chronic cor pulmonale, onset of cardiac failure marks a steady downhill course and the majority die within two years, if not properly managed. On the other hand, in mitral stenosis, tricuspid valve disease, pericardial diseases and right ventricular endomyocardial fibrosis, chronic right-sided heart failure may become established and these cases progress to cardiac cirrhosis with ascites, or *cardiac cachexia* (*See* Fig. 120.1). They show waxing and waning of cardiac function from time to time.

In the Framingham heart study, the median survival was 3.2 years. The risk for death in mild CHF is 5–10% annually which increases to levels as high as 30–40% annually in patients with advanced CHF [New York Heart Association (NYHA) class II and IV]. Many factors affect the prognosis adversely (Box 120.2).

MANAGEMENT

The principles of management include: restoration of cardiac function; removal of the precipitating factors, and elective correction of all remediable lesions after controlling the heart failure.

Based on these guidelines, the broad principles of management may be considered as under and the

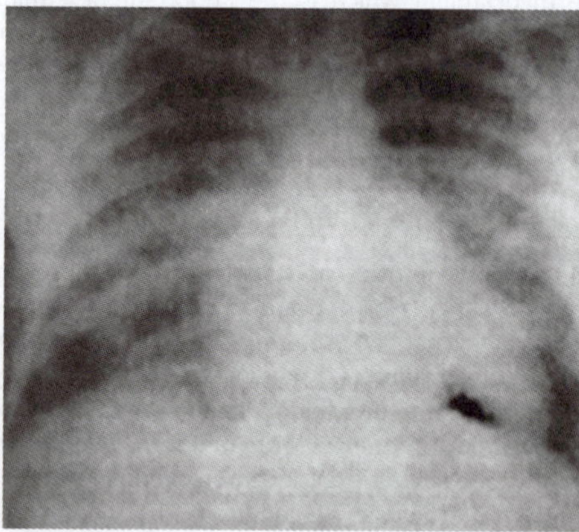

Fig. 120.3: Acute aortic regurgitation with pulmonary edema. *Note:* Cardiomegaly with left ventricular contour, filled up pulmonary artery segment, enlarged left atrium and 'bat-wing' type of pulmonary opacity

Box 120.2: Poor prognosis criteria of heart failure

- Diabetes mellitus
- Hypertension
- Tobacco use
- ECG abnormalities—left ventricular conduction abnormalities
- Ejection fraction < 25%
- Peak exercise capacity < 14 mL/kg/mt of oxygen consumption
- Pulmonary capillary wedge pressure >18 mm Hg
- Poor socioeconomic factors
- Age > 65 years and male gender
- Serum sodium < 135 mmol/L
- Arrhythmias—esp. ventricular
- Plasma norepinephrine levels > 400 microgram/dL

Abbreviations: ECG = Electrocardiogram; ESP = End-systolic pressure

Box 120.3: Management outline

- Establish that the patient has heart failure
- Ascertain presenting features, acute pulmonary edema, exertional breathlessness/fatigue, edema
- Determine etiology
- Identify relevant concomitant disease
- Assess severity
- Estimate prognosis
- Anticipate complications
- Counsel patients and relatives
- Choose appropriate management strategy
- Monitor progress and manage accordingly

comprehensive strategy of management is outlined in Box 120.3.

Principles of management of heart failure:
- General measures
- Pharmacologic therapy
- Devices
- Surgery
- Newer evolving therapies.

General Measures

- *Rest:* During periods of acute decompensation, bed rest is recommended. Since restriction of activity promotes physical deconditioning on prolonged immobilization, bed rest should not be prolonged indefinitely. Activities leading to exhaustion should not be undertaken. Aerobic training may improve symptoms and exercise capacity. Ambulation reduces the incidence of venous thrombosis and pulmonary embolism.
- Tobacco smoking should be stopped forthwith and alcohol discontinued. There are reports that tobacco produces systemic effects also when chewed. Therefore, it is better to stop this form of tobacco as well.
- Comorbidities like hypertension, dyslipidemia and diabetes should be controlled
- Weight reduction is advised in obese patients
- Factors aggravating or precipitating CHF such as anemia and systemic infections should be corrected
- Salt restriction like sodium intake should be limited to less than 2 g/day equivalent to 4 g sodium chloride
- Fluid restriction to 1–2 L/day is advisable in patients with dilutional hyponatremia
- Daily weight measurement helps to detect early occurrence of fluid retention
- Regular follow-up to monitor progress
- The patient and his family members should be informed regarding the disease, treatment and prognosis in order to enlist their cooperation
- Specific interventions for treatable causes, e.g. revascularization in patients with ischemic heart disease and correction of valvular heart disease.

Pharmacologic Therapy

Drugs used in treatment of heart failure

Indicated and acceptable drugs
- ACE inhibitors
- Angiotensin receptor blockers
- Beta blockers
- Mineralocorticoid receptor antagonist
- Diuretics
- Digoxin

- Anticoagulants
- Hydralazine and isosorbide dinitrate

Acceptable; as alternate drugs or add-on drugs
- Antiarrhythmica
- Positive inotropes
- Selective sinus node if channel inhibitor (ivabradine)

Ace Inhibitors

Angiotensin converting enzyme inhibitors (ACEI) have shown survival benefit in all classes of heart failure due to their actions on the heart as well as vasodilatory effect on blood vessels.

Indications

All patients with heart failure and systolic dysfunction benefit from ACEI; and these are indicated, unless otherwise contraindicated.

Mechanism of action

Angiotensin converting enzyme inhibitors act by reducing the formation of angiotensin II. In addition they block kininase II, which is responsible for degradation of kinin, thereby augmenting effects of kinins. By these actions, ACEI suppress the neurohumoral mechanisms, reduce the afterload and improve the hemodynamic parameters such as cardiac output.

Drugs: The ACEI approved for the CHF treatment include captopril, enalapril, lisinopril, quinapril, fosinopril and ramipril.

Adverse effects

- ***Hypotension:*** Patients with hyponatremia or on diuretics experience hypotension more frequently. This can be avoided by correcting hyponatremia, decreasing the dose and frequency of diuretics, and by initiating ACEI therapy with smaller doses.
- ***Renal failure:*** This is seen more in patients with concurrent use of diuretics, hyponatremia and in NYHA class 4 patients. Renal failure has been reported in 5–15% of patients.
- ***Hyperkalemia:*** This can be severe enough to cause cardiac arrhythmias. Patients at risk include those taking potassium supplements, potassium sparing diuretics or those having renal failure.
- ***Cough:*** This is characteristically a non-productive and irritating cough which can be very distressing. It is seen in 5–15% of patients and this is the most common reason for withdrawing ACEI.
- ***Angioedema:*** This is seen in 1% of patients and this can be life-threatening at times.

Benefits and contradictions of ACEI are given in Table 120.2.

Angiotensin Receptor Blockers

These drugs are also effective in reducing symptoms, rehospitalization and mortality of heart failure. These drugs include losartan, valsartan, irbesartan, candesartan and eprosartan. These are as effective as and others. They are not substitutes for ACEI in patients who are tolerating ACEI. They are useful in patients who are intolerant to ACEI, due to disturbing cough or angioedema. Like ACEI they can also cause hypotension, worsen renal failure and cause hyperkalemia. At present there is no indication to replace ACEI with these drugs in patients well controlled by the former. ACEIs and angiotensin receptor blockers (ARBs) can be combined for better results in resistant cases. ***Combining ACEI with ARB is better avoided in treating heart failure.***

Table 120.2: Benefits and contradictions of angiotensin converting enzyme inhibitors

Benefits of ACEI	Contraindications to ACEI

• Alleviation of symptoms
• Reduces mortality
  ▪ Improves ejection fraction
  ▪ Improves NYHA class
• Decreases need for hospitalization
	• Hypotension; SBP < 80 mm Hg
	• Serum creatinine > 3 mg/dL
	• Bilateral renal artery stenosis
	• Hyperkalemia (K^+ > 5.5 mmol/L)
	• History of angioedema

Abbreviations: ACEI = Angiotensin converting enzyme inhibitors; NYHA = New York Heart Association

Beta Blockers

Beta adrenergic blockers have shown survival benefit in heart failure basically due to their antiadrenergic activity.

Indications

All functional classes of heart failure unless otherwise contraindicated benefit by beta blockers.

Mechanism of action

The effects on sympathetic nervous system help to prevent progression of CHF. Risk of fatal arrhythmia is reduced. Ventricular volumes and peripheral vasoconstriction are reduced. Cardiac hypertrophy and apoptosis of cardiac muscle are reduced.

Initiation and maintenance

Beta blockers that have been found most beneficial in CHF include carvedilol, metoprolol and bisoprolol. Treatment is initiated with small doses such as carvedilol 3.125 mg twice daily; bisoprolol 1.25 mg once daily or metoprolol sustained release tablet 12.5 mg once daily. The dose is increased every 2–4 weeks till the target dose is achieved. In clinical trials optimal dose of carvedilol was 50–100 mg/day and that of metoprolol was up to 200 mg/day. The dose of bisoprolol was 5–10 mg/day.

Contraindications

- Progression of PR interval of ≥240 ms
- Acute decompensated heart failure (HF), severe pulmonary edema
- Bronchospasm, asthma
- Symptomatic bradycardia with heart rate below 60 minutes.
- Prolonged PR interval ≥ 240 ms
- Higher grades of blocks in patients who have no implanted pacemakers
- Patients on IV inotropic support
- Acute decompensated heart failure; severe pulmonary edema.

Benefits of beta blockers

- Reduction in mortality, especially by retarding progression of CHF and abolition of fatal arrhythmias.
- Reduces symptoms
- Retards progression of CHF

- Improves NYHA class
- Reduces the risks of hospitalization
- Improves ejection fraction
- The benefit offered by beta blockers are over and above that produced with the use of ACEI/ARB
- Beta blockers produce additive effects with ACEI or with ARB. However, triple combination of beta blockers, ACEI and ARB (triple blocker) should be avoided in the treatment of heart failure.

Risks of treatment with beta blockers:

- Hypotension
- Fluid retention and worsening of CHF
- Bradycardia and heart blocks.

Mineralocorticoid Receptor Antagonist

Aldosterone antagonists are considered in the treatment of heart failure because of the observation that despite the use of ACEI, the aldosterone concentration remains increased in heart failure and also that spironolactone prevents myocardial fibrosis in experimental animals with hypertension. Spironolactone and more selective aldosterone antagonist, eplerenone have been found useful in patients with NYHA class IV symptoms and LV ejection fraction less the 35% as well as in postmyocardial infarction patients with reduced LV systolic function. A dosage of 25–50 mg/day is recommended. Use of mineralocorticoid receptor antagonist (MRA) has been associated with survival benefit in heart failure. The main concern with the use of MRA is hyperkalemia especially in combination with ACEI/ARB. Close monitoring for hyperkalemia is required and when serum K^+ is more than 5.5 mmoL/L, the dose should be reduced and when more than 6 mmoL/L the drug should be stopped.

Aldosterone antagonists have gained importance in the management of heart failure. *Eplerenone* is a selective aldosterone receptor blocker which reduces the rate of death and hospitalization from cardiovascular causes by approximately 37%. These drugs act by inhibition of fibroblast proliferation and perivascular fibrosis which are promoted by chronic hyperaldosteronism and reversal of coronary and renal vascular remodelling caused by endothelial and baroreceptor dysfunction (EMPHASIS Heart Failure Trial). Aldosterone antagonists have pleotropic effects. These include prevention of K^+ and Mg^+ depletion which produces ventricular arrhythmias and sudden death. Eplerenone in a dose of 50 mg oral daily reduce the risk of death and hospitalization among patients with systolic heart failure and mild symptoms. Use of aldosterone antagonist in the treatment of heart failure has gained acceptance.

Source: Armstrong PW. Aldosterone antagonists—last man standing? New Engl J Med. 2011;364:79-80.

Diuretics

Diuretics inhibit the reabsorption of sodium and chloride at specific sites in the renal tubules and thereby prevent sodium retention. Commonly used agents include frusemide, torsemide and bumetanide which act at the loop of Henle (loop diuretics) and thiazides, metolazone and potassium sparing agents which act at the distal tubule. Loop diuretics are more powerful. They increase sodium excretion by 20–25% whereas thiazides increase sodium excretion only by 5–10% in moderately impaired renal function.

Indications

Diuretics should be prescribed for all patients with symptoms of heart failure who have fluid retention. Goal of diuretic therapy is to eliminate symptoms and signs of fluid retention. Diuretics produce symptomatic benefit more rapidly than any other drug. Appropriate use of diuretics is complementary for the successes of other drugs. Underdosing of diuretics may lead to fluid retention, and decrease the efficacy of ACEI. Overdosing can lead on to volume depletion, and increase the risk of hypotension and renal failure with ACEI.

Risks of diuretic therapy

Electrolyte depletion: Hypokalemia and hypomagnesemia can occur which may cause serious arrhythmias particularly those caused by digitalis therapy. Concomitant administration of ACEI or combination with potassium sparing agents such as spironolactone can prevent potassium depletion.

Neurohumoral activation: Diuretics increase the activation of endogenous neurohumoral systems particularly renin angiotensin system. In the long-term this can increase the risk of disease progression. Hence, neurohumoral antagonists are combined.

Hypotension and azotemia: Excessive use of diuretics can cause hypotension and azotemia. Other problems include allergic rashes and damage to the auditory nerves.

Dose: Therapy is initiated with low doses such as 20–40 mg frusemide/day. The dose is increased till the symptoms or signs of fluid retention are abolished. The dose is 20–120 mg/day. Wherever possible, the drug is given orally. The action starts within 2 hours and lasts for 6–8 hours or more. In emergencies such as acute pulmonary edema, frusemide is given IV as slow injection not exceeding 4 mg/minute, to a dose of 40 mg, increased if necessary up to 120 mg. Action starts within 15–30 minutes. Other diuretics such as thiazides and potassium sparing diuretics such as spironolactone or amiloride can be given as per indications, once the emergency is tided over. Some patients develop diuretic resistance, which can be overcome by use of diuretic combinations or by using IV diuretics.

Nonsteroidal anti-inflammatory drugs can inhibit the therapeutic effect of diuretics and may precipitate the development of azotemia.

Benefits of diuretics

- Alleviate symptoms and signs of CHF
- Improve cardiac function and NYHA class
- Improves effort tolerance.

Digoxin

This is the most commonly used digitalis glycoside and the most time-honored drug used in treatment of CHF. William Withering (British) published his treatise on the use of foxglove (**Digitalis purpurea**) in 1785. Digoxin improves exercise tolerance and quality of life in patients with heart failure. Survival benefit with long-term administration of digoxin has not been proven.

Indications

It is indicated in patients with congestive heart failure and atrial fibrillation with fast ventricular rate. It is also indicated in patients who continue to be symptomatic despite treatment with ACEI or beta blockers.

Mechanism of action

It inhibits Na^+, K^+-ATPase enzyme in the myocytes and increases the contractility. Digoxin also decreases the sympathetic outflow from CNS. Thus, it acts both as a positive inotropic agent and neurohumoral attenuator.

Clinical effects

It reduces the heart rate, relieves symptoms, enhances diuresis and brings about overall symptom benefit even though it does not affect the ultimate fatal outcome.

Adverse effects

Digoxin is a double-edged weapon since the difference between the therapeutic and toxic levels is narrow.

- **Arrhythmias:** Ventricular ectopics and bigeminy, paroxysmal atrial tachycardia with block; ventricular tachycardia (VT) especially bidirectional VT and ventricular fibrillation. These arrhythmias may be fatal unless proper care is taken. The therapeutic margin of digoxin is narrow and therefore in selected cases, estimation of serum digoxin levels should be done to guide therapy.
- Different grades of atriventricular (AV) blocks
- **Gastrointestinal symptoms:** Anorexia, nausea, vomiting
- **Central nervous system symptoms:** Disorientation, visual disturbances

Optimal therapeutic level of digoxin in serum is 1–1.5 ng/mL. Serum levels of more than 2.0 ng/mL are toxic. Those at particular risk include elderly patients with renal failure, hypokalemia, hypothyroidism and on concurrent medication with quinidine, verapamil, amiodarone, spironolactone and flecainide. Estimation of serum digoxin levels is helpful for optimal therapeutic benefit without the risk of toxicity.

Recently, the practice of digitalizing the patient with heart failure has been given up. Most often the therapy is started with the oral maintenance dose.

Dosage

Tablets are available in strengths of 0.0625 mg; 0.125 mg and 0.25 mg. Parenteral preparation containing 0.25 mg/mL is available for IV injection. Effect of oral dose of digoxin manifests in 30–45 minutes. **The drug is cumulative on repeated administration. The digitalizing dose is the total dose of digoxin required to produce optimum therapeutic effect.** Following the full digitalizing dose, maximal action is seen in 3–5 hours and some activity persists for 2–6 days. Rapid digitalization is done by giving 0.5–0.75 mg initially followed by 0.25–0.5 mg at 48 hours intervals. In the majority of patients the digitalizing dose is 2–2.5 mg. In slow digitalization 0.25 mg is given once or twice a day and the serum level reaches the desired maximum in 5–7 days. After initial digitalization, the serum level is kept up by maintenance therapy given in a dose of 0.125–0.25 mg daily for 5–6 days a week.

Intravenous digoxin is only rarely used. Dose is 0.5–1 mg slowly over 3–5 minutes. After a loading dose the clinical effect starts within minutes, and the full effect occurs in 2–3 hours. A lower maintenance dose of digoxin is advised in patients above 70 years and those with impaired renal function. In appropriate situations it is life saving.

Benefits of digoxin

- Improves symptoms, quality of life, functional capacity and effort tolerance
- Improves ejection fraction
- Withdrawal results in hemodynamic and clinical deterioration
- No significant reduction in mortality.

Contraindications to digoxin

- Atrioventricular (AV) blocks—second degree, complete heart block and unstable AV blocks
- Pure diastolic dysfunction
- Wolff-Parkinson-White syndrome
- Suspected digitoxicity
- Hypertrophic obstructive cardiomyopathy.

Treatment of digitoxicity: The remedial measures depend on the serum levels of the drug. Depending on the severity of toxicity and serum levels, the therapy has to be modified. Principles of therapy include the following:

- Withdrawal of digoxin
- Potassium supplementation—2–4 g orally once or twice a day
- Phenytoin, beta blockers or lignocaine for ventricular arrhythmias
- Temporary pacing for AV blocks or symptomatic sinus bradycardia
- Digoxin antibodies in severe grades of toxicity. These are available for use in critical situations.

Anticoagulants

Heart failure patients are at increased risk for thromboembolic complications. Incidence is 1–3% annually. Current recommendation is that warfarin is justified in patients with heart failure who have experienced a previous embolic episode or who are in atrial fibrillation and when echocardiography reveals mural thrombus in the cardiac chambers.

Hydralazine and Isosorbide Dinitrate

The combination acts as venodilator and arterial dilator agents. They reduce the preload and afterload and improve ejection fraction. This combination is recommended in patients who are intolerant to ACEI, or having renal insufficiency. There is no evidence to support the use of nitrates alone or hydralazine alone.

Antiarrhythmics

Patients with CHF have frequent complex arrhythmias and are at high risk for sudden death. Hence, there has been considerable interest in the use of antiarrhythmic intervention. Three groups of antiarrhythmics have been evaluated in patients with heart failure.

- **Class I agents (quinidine, procainamide, flecainide and encainide):** These drugs have shown increased mortality in clinical trials

- ***Class II agents:*** Beta blockers have shown definite benefit
- ***Class III agents (amiodarone, d-sotalol and dofetilide):*** Amiodarone may have benefit in nonischemic CHF patients and in those with supraventricular and ventricular arrhythmias.

Positive Inotropes

Though theoretically these drugs may be expected to produce benefit, in clinical trials their effects are disappointing, and hence drugs such as dobutamine, milrinone and vesnarinone are not routinely used in CHF.

Selective Sinus Node If Channel Inhibitor (Ivabradine)

If channel and ivabradine

If-ion channel (funny channel) is the principal channel determining the sinoatrial (SA) nodal pacemaker current and it decides the slope of spontaneous diastolic depolarization and consequently the sinus rate. Ivabradine is a specific and selective inhibitor of this channel without any effect on the other parts of the conducting system. It is useful as a pure sinus slowing drug. Normally, it does not influence hemodynamics, ventricular contractility or BP. Recent trials have shown that addition of ivabradine reduces the heart rate and improves LV function and symptoms of patients with low output heart failure. It can be combined with beta blockers in whom the resting heart rate continues to be above 70 beats per minute. Usual dose of Ivabradine is 5–7.5 mg twice daily.

In some patients with stable angina and LV dysfunction, ivabradine gives beneficial results. It is not useful in patients with atrial fibrillation.

Source: Swedberg K, Komajda M, Böhm M, et al. Ivabradine and outcomes in chronic heart failure (SHIFT) a randomized placebo controlled trial. Lancet. 2010;376:875-85.

Mechanical Devices

- Ventricular assist devices (VADs): Both left ventricular and dual chamber assist devices are available. These include:
  - Hemopumps: Indicated only for a short-term use
  - Centrifugal devices (BioMedicus BioPump)
  - Pulsatile devices (Abiomed BVS—5000)
  - Implantable devices, e.g. heart mate

These are used in many cases to tide over the waiting period before cardiac transplantation. Newer assist devices are being introduced.

- Extracorporeal membrane oxygenator (ECMO): This device has a centrifugal pump to drive blood from patient to a membrane for CO_2 and O_2 exchange.
- Implantable cardiovertor fefibrillator (ICD)
- Cardiovertor defibrillator implantation is done for delivering shock for ventricular tachyarrhythmias and prevention of sudden death (Fig. 120.4)
- Patients with CHF who had episodes of definite VT/VF are likely to benefit from ICD. These are capable of producing regular impulses for pacing to terminate the tachyarrhythmia and also defibrillate the heart in case of emergencies.
- Pacemakers in CHF.

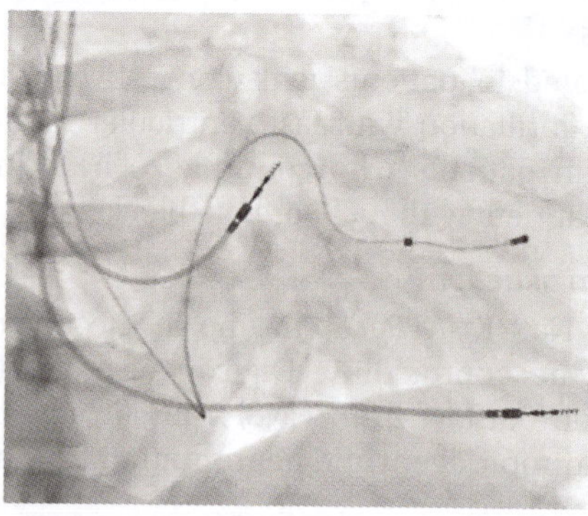

Fig. 120.4: Cardiac resynchronization therapy, three leads are shown: atrial (top), ventricular (lowermost) and left ventricular (LV) pacing lead in a tributary of the coronary sinus (middle)

Courtesy: George Koshy

There is growing evidence in support of hemodynamic benefits and long-term improvement in clinical status of patients with CHF after ventricular and dual chamber (DDD) pacing. The main mechanism is by resynchronization of LV activity. Among patients with NYHA class II or III heart failure, wide QRS complex with LBBB morphology and LV systolic dysfunction, addition of cardiac resynchronization therapy (CRT) with ICD reduces mortality and recurrent hospitalization. This is called CRT-D or combo device. CRT with only pacing function and no ability to deliver a shock to terminate VT/VF is called CRT-P.

Source: Tang AS, Wells GA, Talajic M, et al. New Engl J Med. 2010;363:2385-95.

Surgical Options

Dynamic cardiomyoplasty: In this procedure the latissimus dorsi muscle with its pedicle is wrapped around the cardiac apex and a myostimulator is implanted. Though there is improvement in the cardiac indices, long-term outcome is disappointing.

Mitral annuloplasty and mitral valve repair: Where there is associated secondary MR, these procedures are indicated.

Partial left ventriculectomy (Batista procedure): This procedure was introduced in 1994 by the Brazilian surgeon Batista. The principle is that return of the dilated ventricle to a more normal volume/mass/diameter relation reduces the wall stress and improves the function. Basic procedure involves resection of the lateral wall from apex to the atrioventricular groove. The results are good in experienced hands.

Aneurysmectomy: Left ventricular aneurysm causes paradoxical expansion and loss of effective contraction and it contributes to CHF. Aneurysmectomy improves the cardiac function.

Cardiac Transplantation

When the myocardium is damaged beyond repair, life cannot be sustained by the failing heart. Cardiac transplantation is indicated under such circumstances if a donor heart and technical expertise are available.

Indications

- Persistent cardiogenic shock requiring mechanical assistance
- Refractory CHF with continuous inotropic infusion

- NYHA class 3–4 with a poor 12 months prognosis
- Progressive symptoms despite maximal therapy
- Severe symptomatic hypertrophic cardiomyopathy (HCM) or restrictive cardiomyopathy
- Refractory angina with unsuitable anatomy for revascularization
- Life-threatening ventricular arrhythmias despite aggressive medical and device interventions
- Cardiac tumors with only low tendency for metastasis
- Hypoplastic left heart syndrome and complex congenital heart disease.

Prerequisites for Surgery

- Received maximal medical therapy
- Been considered for alternative surgical options
- Been addressed for all reversible causes
- Peak oxygen consumption (VO_2 max) falls below 14 mL/kg/min or it shows a marked and steady decline.

Gene Therapy

This is an evolving treatment strategy where attempt is made to increase the myocardial contractility at molecular level. This is accomplished by using nanoparticles as potential gene therapy carriers or vectors.

In this method, over expression of $\beta 2$ receptors in the myocardium is accomplished using adenovirus vector. Genes expressing SERCA2 are increased by using adenovirus transfection of myocytes. Preliminary studies have shown that this improves contraction and relaxation, but there was increased incidence of arrhythmias.

Cell based treatments are undergoing clinical trial approaches include both adult and embryonic stem cells and adult stem cells. Both erythroid precursor cells and mesenchymal cells are being assessed.

REFRACTORY CARDIAC FAILURE

Refractory CHF is defined as NYHA class III or IV CHF, in whom symptoms have not improved or have actually worsened following recent attempts to escalate therapy. Triple therapy with digoxin, diuretics and vasodilators should have been attempted prior to labeling the heart failure as refractory.

Management

- Take a fresh look to find out conditions causing recent deterioration in CHF like
  - Excessive diuretics
  - Digitoxicity
  - Electrolyte abnormalities
  - Renal failure
  - Untreated medical problems such as infections.
- Search for factors causing refractory CHF
  - Myocardial problems like ongoing or recurrent ischemia, mitral regurgitation, arrhythmia, hypertension
  - Compounding illnesses like renal failure, infections, pulmonary embolism, uncontrolled diabetes, hypothyroidism.
  - Patient factors: Dietary indiscretion, noncompliance, alcohol abuse
  - Iatrogenic problems: NSAIDs, antiarrhythmias
- Optimize the medical therapy
- Consider positive inotropic agents
- Consider devices
- Consider surgical options.

INTRACTABLE CARDIAC FAILURE

If patient fails to respond to the above measures and needs a mechanical assist device, heart failure is considered intractable and they are candidates for transplantation.

EMERGENCY TREATMENT OF ACUTE PULMONARY EDEMA

- Patient is hospitalized and put to rest with a back rest or cardiac table, in the position of maximum comfort
- The patient is given oxygen immediately at a flow rate of 7–10 L/minute.
- Morphine sulfate 3–5 mg is given intravenously over 3 minutes and repeated to a total dose of 15–20 mg, at 15 minute intervals. In less acute cases, the drug can be given intramuscularly in doses of 15–20 mg. Morphine abolishes anxiety, depresses the respiratory center, allays dyspnea, and reduces the adrenergic vasoconstrictor stimuli.
- ***Diuretic:*** Frusemide 40 mg should be given intravenously. If the effect is not evident in 30 min the dose may be repeated.
- Aminophylline in a dose of 5 mg/kg given IV slowly is very effective in increasing the cardiac output and relieving bronchospasm. Aminophylline has different actions such as improvement of cardiac output, stimulation of the respiratory center, bronchodilation and diuresis. Hypotension and anaphylaxis are potential complications. In many cases the effect of aminophylline is dramatic.
- ***Reduction of preload:*** Tourniquets are applied to the extremities proximally to reduce venous return and thus reduce preload. The venous return from three limbs is obstructed at a time and the tourniquets are rotated at 15 minute intervals. This method of physiological venesection is very effective. Rarely open venesection to remove 300–500 mL blood rapidly may be required. Venesection should not be done on hypotensive patients.
- ***Digitalization:*** Rapid digitalization is done by intravenous injection of 0.5–1 mg digoxin when there is clear indication.
- Vasodilators such as nitroglycerin and nitroprusside given IV may be required in many cases. Once the emergency is managed successfully, further elective management depends upon the underlying condition.
- In intractable cases, ventilatory support either noninvasive or invasive may have to be given.

N Sudhaya kumar

CHAPTER
121

Shock

Chapter Summary

- Pathophysiology
- Classification of Shock
- Organ Responses
- Clinical Features
- Complications
- Management

INTRODUCTION

Shock (acute circulatory failure) is a syndrome associated with an acute reduction in effective blood flow resulting in gross impairment of tissue perfusion with failure to maintain the transport and delivery of essential substances to sustain the function of vital organs. Hypotension with obtundation, cold and clammy extremities, rapid thready pulse and oliguria are the typical clinical features of acute circulatory shock.

A simple working model of circulation incorporating the following eight primary components is helpful to understand the hemodynamic mechanisms of shock:

- Intravascular volume (venous return or preload)
- Heart (pump)
- Resistance circuit (arteries and arterioles)
- Capillary exchange bed
- Venous resistance bed (postcapillary venules and small veins)
- Metarterioles (which connect the precapillary arteries and postcapillary veins–arteriovenous shunts)
- Medium-sized and major veins
- Obstruction to mainstream of blood flow.

PATHOPHYSIOLOGY

Based on the above-mentioned eight component model, shock can occur due to hypovolemia, pump failure (cardiogenic), increased vascular resistance, capillary leak, arteriovenous shunting, venous pooling or obstruction to circulation. Compensatory phenomena, such as sympathetic overactivity leading to vasoconstriction and reflex tachycardia, serve to maintain the blood pressure and systemic perfusion. These vascular responses are maximal in the vessels of the skin, kidneys, splanchnic areas and skeletal muscles. These vasomotor phenomena serve to redirect the available blood to the vital organs, like brain, heart and kidneys. If shock persists or becomes severe, the compensatory mechanisms fail and progressive tissue damage occurs.

CLASSIFICATION OF SHOCK

A classification of shock based on the following four hemodynamic defects has evolved (Fig. 121.1):

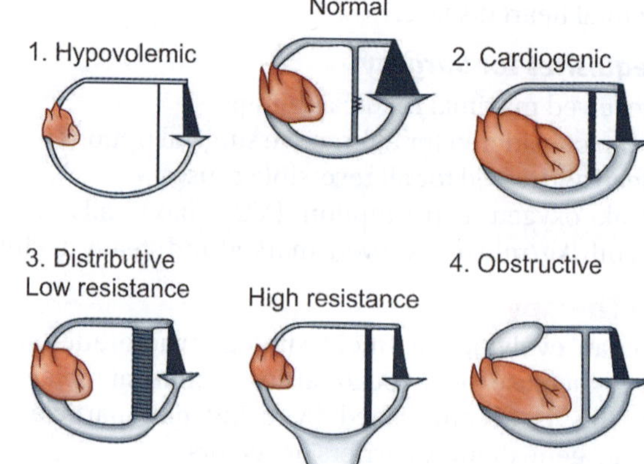

Fig. 121.1: Main pathophysiological mechanisms of various types of shock

- ***Hypovolemic shock:*** Due to volume loss which could be exogenic (hemorrhage, gastrointestinal loss, excessive diuresis, burns, inflammation, etc.) or endogenous (capillary leak due to inflammation, anaphylaxis, snake venom, etc.). Basic hemodynamic abnormality in this situation is reduction in central venous and pulmonary artery wedge pressures.
- ***Cardiogenic shock:*** Failure of the cardiac pump to maintain systemic blood flow at adequate filling pressures, e.g. MI, myocarditis, cardiomyopathies, valvular and other structural heart diseases, cardiac arrhythmias, etc.
- ***Obstructive shock:*** Due to obstruction to circulation, e.g. cardiac tamponade, pulmonary embolism, atrial myxomas, ball valve thrombi, etc.
- ***Distributive shock (vasomotor dysfunction):*** Due to abnormal distribution of blood flow. Abnormalities in distribution could be due to either low resistance (arteriovenous shunting as in sepsis) or high or normal resistance (expanded venous capacitance) and high arterial resistance as in advanced stages of septic shock, neurogenic shock, spinal shock, etc. The low resistance state results in hyperdynamic shock and high resistance in hypodynamic shock.

When the perfusion of tissues and delivery of oxygen are decreased, anaerobic metabolism supervenes. Hypoxia, hypercapnia and acidosis (both metabolic and lactic) ensue. Cellular injury created by inadequate delivery of oxygen and substrates also induces the production and release of inflammatory mediators that further compromise perfusion through functional and structural changes within the microvasculature. Integrity of the capillary wall is lost leading to extravasation of protein-rich fluid into the extravascular space. This leads to a vicious cycle in which impaired perfusion is responsible for cellular injury, which causes maldistribution of blood flow, further compromising cellular perfusion leading to multiorgan dysfunction. Intense ischemia damages the intestinal mucosa resulting in the entry of bacteria and toxins into the circulation. This leads to further aggravation of hypotension and shock. Release of histamine and histamine-like substances enhances vasodilation and capillary permeability. Disseminated intravascular coagulation (DIC) results from the release of thromboplastic substances and this further occludes the microcirculation of vital organs. This worsens the shock. Irrespective of the primary cause, persistence of shock leads to myocardial dysfunction and further reduction in cardiac output.

ORGAN RESPONSES

Neuroendocrine Response

Hypovolemia, hypotension and hypoxia are sensed by baro and chemoreceptors, which contribute to autonomic response resulting in increased adrenergic output and decreased vagal activity. This leads to peripheral and splanchnic vasoconstriction, increase in heart rate, systemic vascular resistance and cardiac output, and metabolic changes, like glycogenolysis, gluconeogenesis and reduced pancreatic insulin release. Severe pain and stress cause release of adrenocorticotropic hormone (ACTH) which stimulates cortisol secretion leading to elevated blood glucose levels. Renin release is increased in response to adrenergic discharge and reduced renal perfusion, which results in production of angiotensin II, aldosterone and vasopressin.

Pulmonary Response

Shock results in a relative increase in pulmonary vascular resistance as in the systemic circulation. Shock-related tachypnea reduces tidal volume, increases minute ventilation and dead space, and induces alkalosis. Shock, especially septic shock, is an important cause of acute lung injury leading to adult respiratory distress syndrome (ARDS).

Renal Response

Decreased renal blood flow and increased afferent arteriolar resistance lead to reduced glomerular filtration rate. The physiologic response of kidney to hypotension is salt and water retention. Acute tubular necrosis occurs as a result of interaction of shock, sepsis, nephrotoxic drugs and rhabdomyolysis. All these result in oliguria and acute renal failure.

CLINICAL FEATURES

Cardiogenic Shock

Clinically, shock is usually accompanied by hypotension, i.e. a mean arterial pressure less than 60 mm Hg in a previously normotensive person. Compensatory sympathetic stimulation produces tachycardia, cutaneous vasoconstriction and sweating, which results in rapid thready pulse and cold clammy skin (an important exception is the warm shock in low resistance hyper-

dynamic state of septic shock). Alterations in sensorium, obtundation, irritability, agitation, somnolence, confusion or coma are the manifestations of brain hypoperfusion. The urinary output falls below 20 mL/h with the urinary sodium falling below 30 mmol/L. Metabolic acidosis manifests with tachypnea and Kussmaul's respiration. Several complications leading to multiorgan failure syndrome (MOFS) contribute to the high mortality in severe cases.

Intrinsic Cardiogenic Shock

This form of shock is caused by failure of the heart to act as an effective pump. The onset is usually sudden. It occurs most commonly as a complication of acute myocardial infarction. It can also occur due to severe brady or tachyarrhythmias, valvular heart disease, or in the terminal stage of chronic heart failure of any cause, including ischemic heart disease and dilated cardiomyopathy. Cardiogenic shock is characterized by a low cardiac output, diminished peripheral perfusion, pulmonary congestion, and elevation of systemic vascular resistance and pulmonary vascular pressures. Acute right heart failure can arise as a result of right ventricular myocardial infarction or may complicate the acute respiratory distress syndrome (ARDS) and severe pulmonary hypertension of any etiology. As a consequence of right ventricular failure, left ventricular preload falls, and this in turn, reduces systemic perfusion. In contrast to other forms of shock, absolute or relative hypovolemia is usually not present in cardiogenic shock (Table 121.1).

Compressive Cardiogenic Shock

This is caused by extrinsic compression of the heart. The heart becomes less compliant, and therefore, normal filling pressures are inadequate to achieve proper diastolic filling. Blood or fluid collecting in the pericardial sac may cause tamponade since the pericardium is not distensible. Any cause of increased intrathoracic pressure such as tension pneumothorax, herniation of abdominal viscera through a diaphragmatic hernia or use of excessive positive pressure ventilation produces compressive cardiogenic shock. Acute right heart failure with sudden decline in cardiac output can be caused by pulmonary embolism obstructing right ventricular outflow tract and this impairs ventricular filling. Although initially this condi-

Parameters	Hypovolemic shock	Distributive shock	Cardiogenic shock	Obstructive shock
Heart rate	Increased	Increased (normal in neurogenic shock)	May be increased or decreased	Increased
Jugular venous pressure	Low	Low	High	High
Blood pressure	Low	Low	Low	Low
Skin temperature	Cold	Warm (cold in severe shock)	Cold	Cold
Capillary refill	Slow	Slow	Slow	Slow

Table 121.1: Clinical features of different forms of shock

tion responds to increased filling pressures produced therapeutically by volume expansion, as the compression increases, cardiogenic shock ensues.

COMPLICATIONS

Various complications as follows:

- *Pulmonary:* ARDS, characterized by tachypnea, diffuse bilateral rales and respiratory failure.
- *Cardiac:* Myocardial dysfunction and arrhythmias.
- *Renal:* Acute tubular necrosis and obstruction of tubules by casts.
- *Gastrointestinal:* Hepatocellular failure, mesenteric vasoconstriction, hemorrhagic necrosis of bowels.
- *Hematological:* DIC.

All these above-mentioned factors proceed unchecked, if the condition becomes nonresponsive to treatment and end up in multiorgan failure and death in the vast majority.

MANAGEMENT

A critical clinical assessment of the circulatory status, meticulous evaluation to detect the mechanism and cause of the entity, close monitoring of the patient supported by laboratory parameters are of prime importance in the final outcome. Blood gases, renal parameters and blood lactate levels have to be serially monitored. Quantitative estimation of blood lactate helps in predicting the prognosis; when lactate level increases from 2 to 8 mmol/L, survival progressively decreases from 90 to 10%.

General Principles

A useful guide to initial evaluation and management is the acronym VIPS.

- V: Ventilation; proper assessment and maintenance of adequate pulmonary gas exchange.
- I: Infusion; assess intravascular volume and infuse to obtain optimal central venous and pulmonary artery wedge pressures.
- P: Pump function; maintain cardiac competence by inotropes and optimizing preload and afterload.
- S: Specific and supportive measures; correct biochemical abnormalities and treat the underlying cause.

Shock should be diagnosed early. Survival is inversely related to the duration of the shock before starting treatment. Prompt institution of specific treatment reduces mortality. The patient is put to bed with foot-end of the bed elevated to increase the venous return to the heart. Patency of the airway is established by removing foreign bodies from the mouth and throat and by keeping the neck extended backward to prevent the tongue from falling back. Vital signs, like pulse, respiration, blood pressure and urine flow are to be continuously monitored. A venous cannula introduced into the jugular vein helps in monitoring the central venous pressure and also in administering fluids, if prolonged treatment becomes necessary. It is ideal to keep the central venous pressure at 10–14 cm of water. Metabolic acidosis is corrected by administration of 50–100 mmol of sodium bicarbonate given as a 7.5% solution.

Vasopressor Drugs

Sympathomimetic drugs are used to improve vascular tone. Dopamine is given intravenously (IV) at a rate of 3–15 µg/kg/min, depending upon the response of blood pressure and urine output. Other drugs in this group are isoprenaline (4–8 µg/min) and dobutamine (3–15 µg/kg/min) given as infusions. These drugs cause improvement in cardiac output and blood pressure, but cardiac arrhythmias may be precipitated.

Vasodilator drugs commonly used include:

- Sodium nitroprusside infusion given IV at a dose of 10–20 µg/min
- Nitroglycerine infusion given IV at a dose of 10–20 µg/min or
- Phentolamine infusion given IV at a dose of 0.5 µg/min.

Vasodilators have the following effects:

- Reduction of ventricular afterload due to dilation of systemic arterial bed
- Decrease in ventricular preload by dilating venous capacitance vessels and reducing pulmonary capillary, arterial and right ventricular pressures
- Decrease in myocardial oxygen demand and increase in the subendocardial flow of blood.

Vasodilators should be started in small dosage and the dose should be worked up, depending on the response. Combination of vasodilators with inotropic agents gives better results.

Apart from these general measures each type of shock demands appropriate specific management. For example, thrombolytic therapy and interventional or surgical revascularization for acute MI, antibiotics for septic shock and dialysis procedures for poisoning.

Hypovolemic Shock

Rapid replacement of the blood volume by administration of the appropriate fluid (depending on the fluid lost) is life-saving and this should be undertaken without delay. Blood, isotonic saline or plasma volume expanders such as 6% w/v dextran or other colloidal solutions should be used. The rate of infusion should match the rate of fluid loss. In severe cases of gastroenteritis up to 3–4 L of fluid may have to be infused in the first 1–2 hours. Fluid infusion is continued until the systolic blood pressure comes up to 100 mm Hg. Further, maintenance depends on rate of fluid loss. If the shock is unresponsive to replacement of conventional fluids, infusion of 7.5% saline (100–400 mL) may help to restore the blood pressure.

Cardiogenic Shock

Inotropic agents to improve cardiac contractility, vasodilators to reduce the afterload on the heart and correction of the cardiac abnormality are the main principles of treatment. If the cardiac output is persistently low, the circulation can be assisted by means of balloon counterpulsation in the aorta if facilities permit. The balloon is positioned in the upper part of descending aorta. It is inflated during diastole and deflated during systole. This helps to reduce afterload in systole and to increase the filling pressure of the ventricles and coronary arteries during diastole. By these mechanisms, balloon counter pulsation improves the cardiac output and coronary circulation. In conditions such as rupture of interventricular septum or acute damage to a valve, emergency surgery may have to be undertaken, if the shock remains unresponsive to medical treatment. In shock due to acute MI, thrombolytic therapy is beneficial, but results are less rewarding than in those without shock. Early revascularization procedures, such as percutaneous transluminal coronary angioplasty (PTCA) or coronary artery bypass surgery (CABG), bring about dramatic benefit and improve survival, and in many centers early revascularization is the method of choice.

Anaphylactic Shock

It is treated by intramuscular injection of 1 mL of 1/1,000 adrenaline, repeated if needed every 5–10 minute. Adrenaline corrects the hypotension and bronchospasm. If the bronchospasm is severe, 250 mg of aminophylline is given IV slowly. In severe cases, hydrocortisone in doses of 100 mg or its analogues (betamethasone or dexamethasone 8 mg) are given IV either by repeated injections or through an intravenous drip, until the condition improves. If laryngeal edema obstructs the airways, emergency tracheostomy has to be done to save life.

CHAPTER

122

Congenital Heart Disease

M Zulfikar Ahamed, Balu Vaidyanathan

Chapter Summary

- Epidemiology
- Burden of Congenital Heart Disease in India
- Etiopathogenesis
- Genetic Disorders and Congenital Heart Disease
- Basic Hemodynamics
- Acyanotic Congenital Heart Defects
  - Additional Lesions
    - Anomalous Origin of LCA From Pulmonary Artery
- Cyanotic Congenital Heart Disease
  - Algorithmic Approach to Cyanotic CHD
  - Tetralogy of Fallot
  - Dextro-Transposition of Great Arteries
  - Admixture Lesions
  - Anomalous Pulmonary Venous Connection
  - Tricuspid Atresia
- Eisenmenger Syndrome
- Other Congenital Cyanotic Heart Disease
- Prenatal Diagnosis of Congenital Heart Disease
- Newborn Screening for Critical Congenital Heart Disease

INTRODUCTION

Congenital heart disease (CHD) is defined as structural abnormality of heart and intrathoracic great vessels present at birth. This need not present itself at birth. Approximately, one out of hundred babies may have a CHD. This estimate usually excludes bicuspid aortic valve (BAV) present in 1%, persistent left superior vena cava (PLSVC) present in 2% and mitral valve prolapse (MVP) present in 3% of children.

EPIDEMIOLOGY

The prevalence of CHD ranges from 6/1,000 to 8/1,000 livebirths. One-third of CHD are critical which usually present in the newborn, one-third are trivial lesions and one-third are significant and yet noncritical CHD.

The incidence of CHD shows a slight increment, probably due to increasing number of preterm patent ductus arteriosus (PDA) and improved detection of small ventricular septal defects (VSD). This secular trend is evident in India also. Adult CHD is yet another significant entity, the number of which is increasing due to increased survival of CHD. The gender ratio in CHD is more or less equal. However, hypoplastic left heart syndrome (HLHS), aortic stenosis (AS), coarctation of aorta (CoA) and d-transposition of great arteries (d-TGA) are more common in males and atrial septal defect (ASD), PDA and atrioventricular septal defect (AVSD) are more common in females. White population may have a slightly increased prevalence of Ebstein anomaly and pulmonary atresia.

BURDEN OF CONGENITAL HEART DISEASE IN INDIA

We have no community-based data for the incidence of CHD in India. The published incidence of CHD in various studies across the globe has been fairly consistent at 6–8 per 1,000 livebirths. Serious CHD requiring treatment in infancy occurs in 2.5–3 per 1,000 livebirths. Extrapolating these statistics with the total number of livebirths in the country, it is assumed that nearly 180,000 children are born with CHD every year in India. Of these, nearly 60,000–90,000 suffer from critical CHD requiring early intervention. Only less than 10% of these are actually receiving specialized pediatric cardiac care. The remaining are either not diagnosed or referred or do not have access to pediatric cardiac care due to various logistic reasons. Thus, every year a large number of children are added to the total pool of cases with CHD. We also have a large number of adult patients with uncorrected CHD, primarily because of lack of healthcare awareness and inadequate healthcare facilities. With currently available treatment modalities, more than 75% of infants with CHD can survive beyond the first year of life and with many correctable lesions, can lead near normal lives thereafter. Delay in seeking definite care significantly increases mortality and morbidity due to CHD. Approximately, 10–15% of the present infant mortality in India may be accounted for by congenital heart defects alone. The four major questions regarding CHD, which parents are likely to pose to the clinician are:

1. Why did this happen? (Cause)
2. What will happen to the baby? (Outcome)
3. How can we treat it? (Remedy)
4. Will it happen again? (Prevention)

ETIOPATHOGENESIS

In 85% of the cases, CHD is multifactorial in origin, resulting from interplay between unknown genetic and environmental factors. In the rest, the causes may vary. They include:

- Chromosomal disorders
- Gene disorders (single gene)
- Intrauterine infection
- Maternal diseases
- Teratogens.

Genetic Disorders and CHD

Modes of inheritance of genetics
- Chromosomal
  - Number
  - Deletion
  - Duplication
- Single gene
  - Autosomal dominant
  - Autosomal recessive
- Presumed

Chromosomal disorders	Congenital heart disease	
	Incidence	Defects
Trisomy 21	40%	AVSD, VSD, TOF
Trisomy 18	99%	Septal defects
Trisomy 13	90%	Septal defects
Turner syndrome	30%	Coarctation, BAV
Klinefelter syndrome	30%	PDA

Abbreviations: AVSD = Atrioventricular septal defect; VSD = Ventricular septal defect; TOF = Tetralogy of Fallot; BAV = Bicuspid aortic valve; PDA = Patent ductus arteriosus

- Mendelian gene disorders could be autosomal dominant or recessive. In addition, microdeletion can also cause CHD, the prime example being DiGeorge syndrome which can have associated conotruncal defects like Tetralogy of Fallot (TOF) and truncus.
- Probably the only intrauterine infection capable of causing CHD is Rubella. The defects are PDA, pulmonary artery (PA) branch stenosis, VSD and TOF. Fetal mumps has been implicated in endocardial fibroelastosis (EFE) in the infant.
- Maternal diseases which can cause CHD include diabetes mellitus (DM), systemic lupus erythematosus (SLE), phenylketonuria (PKU) and ankylosing spondylitis. Recently, obesity in the mother, maternal viral infection and smoking also have been shown linked to CHD.
- Teratogenic influences lead to CHD. The most prominent among them are phenytoin (VSD), lithium (Ebstein), alcohol (VSD), vitamin A (VSD, TGA) valproate (CoA and VSD) and warfarin (PDA).
- There have been attempts to prevent or reduce incidence of CHD by folic acid administration and multivitamin pills. Prevention can also be facilitated by preventing teratogen exposure, rubella vaccination, controlling maternal diseases and regulating maternal medications.
- Recurrence risk in sibling is usually 2–4%. This can be higher in certain CHD like aortic stenosis or HLHS. The risk for offspring is 5%, if father has a CHD and 10%, if mother has a CHD.
- Isolated CHD occurs in 75–80%. Nearly, 25% will have additional problems. These could be either syndromic (8–10%) or nonsyndromic (15%). Syndromes can be genetic or nongenetic.

SYNDROMES OF CHD

Ellis-van Creveld	Single atrium
Holt-Oram	ASD
VATER anomaly	VSD, TOF
Rubinstein-Taybi	PDA
Noonan	PS, HCM
Carpenter	VSD
Alagille	PA branch stenosis
Cornelia de Lange	VSD
CHARGE (DiGeorge)	Truncus, TOF

Abbreviations: ASD = Atrial septal defects; VSD = Ventricular septal defect; TOF = Tetralogy of Fallot; PDA = Patent ductus arteriosus; HCM = Hypertrophic cardiomyopathy; PS = Pulmonary stenosis; VATER = Vertebral anomalies, anal atresia, tracheoesophageal fistula and renal agenesis; VSD = Ventricular septal defect; PA = Pulmonary artery

CLASSIFICATION

- ***Acyanotic CHD*** (arterial saturation >95%)
  - Left-to-right shunts (40%)
    - Pre-tricuspid—ASD, PAPVC (partial anomalous pulmonary venous connection)
    - Post-tricuspid—VSD, PDA, AVSD, APW (aorto-pulmonary window)
  - Obstructive lesions (20%)
    - Right sided: Pulmonary stenosis (PS)
    - Left sided: Aortic stenosis, CoA
  - Regurgitant lesions (< 5%)
    - Congenital mitral regurgitation (MR)
    - Congenital tricuspid regurgitation (TR)
  - Additional lesions
    - Anomalous origin of left coronary artery (LCA) from PA
    - Coronary arteriovenous fistula (CAVF)
    - Systemic arteriovenous fistula (SAVF)
    - Ruptured sinus of Valsalva (RSOV)
    - PA branch stenosis
- ***Cyanotic CHD:*** Arterial saturation < 95% (usually < 85%)
  - Reduced pulmonary blood flow ($\downarrow$PBF) (20%)
    - With PS and VSD
    - With PS alone
    - With pulmonary arterial hypertension (PAH)

Table 122.1: Basic hemodynamic

Superior vena cava	Carries 35–40% of all systemic venous return	Saturation of 65%
Inferior vena cava	Carries 65% of all venous return	Saturation of 65–70%
Coronary sinus	Drains into right atrium	Saturation of 60%
Pulmonary veins	Enter left atrium	Saturation of 99–100%
Right atrium	Has a mean pressure of 4 mm Hg. A wave is taller than V by 2 mm Hg	Saturation of 65–70%
Left atrium (LA), pulmonary artery wedge pressure (PAWP) is more or less same as LA pressure	Has a mean pressure of 6 mm Hg. In both LA and PAWP, V is taller than A	Saturation of 99%
Right ventricle	The pressure is usually 25/0 with an end-diastolic pressure (EDP) of 4–6 mm Hg	Saturation of 65–70%
Left ventricle	The pressure is 80-120/0 usually with EDP of 6–8 mm Hg	Saturation of 98%
Pulmonary artery	The pressure is usually 25/12 mm Hg	Saturation of 65–70%
Aorta	The pressure ranges from 80–120/60–/80 mm Hg.	Saturation of 98%

- Increased pulmonary blood flow ($\uparrow$PBF) (15%)
  - Parallel circulation
  - Admixture lesions
- Miscellaneous lesions (< 2%)
  - Ebstein, pulmonary arteriovenous fistula (PAVF)
- ***Malpositions***
  - Dextrocardia
  - Isomerism—right-sided, left-sided.

BASIC HEMODYNAMICS

Basic hemodynamics have been described in Table 122.1.

Right atrium (RA) to right ventricle (RV) gradient and left atrium (LA) to left ventricle (LV) gradient are normally zero. Ventricle to great vessel gradient is less than 5 mm Hg. Normal systemic vascular resistance (SVR) is 8–20 Wood units. Normal pulmonary vascular resistance (PVR) is 1–3 Wood units. Normal ejection fraction (EF) is 65 ± 5 %. Abnormal EF is—(adult) <50%; (child) <55%.

Step up in oxygen saturation on oxymetry indicates L ≥ R shunt. A significant step up is defined as more than 9% at the atrial level, more than 6% at the ventricle level and more than 6% at the great vessel level.

Step down in oxygen saturation on oxymetry by more than 3% indicates R-L shunt. Arterial saturation under 92% also usually indicates R-L shunt.

ACYANOTIC CONGENITAL HEART DEFECTS

OBSTRUCTIVE LESIONS

Congenital Aortic Stenosis (AS)

Obstruction to the left ventricular outflow tract (LVOT) may be valvar, subvalvar, or supravalvar, valvar being the most common (80%), accounting for 5% of CHD. Aortic stenosis is more common in males. It can have associated lesions like CoA, PDA and muscular VSD.

Pathology: The AS valve is most often bicuspid (75%), although tricuspid aortic valve may also become stenotic in the younger age group.

Hemodynamics: AS leads to a significant gradient between LV and aorta. It is graded as mild, moderate or severe, based on the pressure gradients across the aortic valve or LVOT. A peak systolic gradient of more than 75 mm Hg is often considered as severe, while values between 25–50 and 50–75 are classified as mild and moderate

stenosis respectively. Mean gradients of less than 25, 25–50 and more than 50 mm Hg, likewise are graded as mild, moderate and severe aortic stenosis. Significant stenosis leads to increase in afterload which in turn causes left ventricular hypertrophy (LVH) and elevated systolic and end-diastolic pressures of LV. Consequently, this will cause dyspnea, myocardial ischemia and later LV dysfunction.

Clinical evaluation: Mild cases are asymptomatic and are picked up during routine examination when a murmur is detected on clinical evaluation. Severe forms may present with exertional syncope, effort angina or cardiac failure. Critical AS produces congestive heart failure (CHF) in infancy. AS predisposes to infective endocarditis (IE). Bicuspid valve develops degenerative changes early and leads to stenosis on an average by 20–30 years of life.

In moderate and severe cases, the pulse is characteristically small in volume with slow rising ascending limb of the pulse wave (pulsus parvus et tardus) and pulse pressure is less than 20 mm Hg. The heart may not be enlarged, but the apex beat is heaving in nature. In most of the cases, there is a systolic thrill, best felt in the right upper sternal border as well as over the carotids. Auscultation reveals ejection systolic murmur preceded by a constant ejection click, best audible over the right upper sternal border and conducted to the carotids. In many cases, the murmur and click are very well audible over the cardiac apex also. An early diastolic murmur (EDM) of associated mild aortic regurgitation may also be heard in some cases. In mild cases of AS, the murmur may be present without any abnormality in the pulse or apex beat. The presence of a constant ejection click suggests that the stenosis is at valvar level. This is associated with post-stenotic dilatation of the ascending aorta. Both these features are absent in subvalvar stenosis. Features indicating severity of AS are:

- ***Symptoms:*** Dyspnea, chest pain and syncope
- ***Pulse:*** Pulsus parvus et tardus
- ***Blood pressure (BP):*** Narrow pulse pressure
- ***Apex beat:*** Heaving apex
- Suprasternal thrill
- Fourth heart sound heard at apex
- Long, loud murmur with late peaking.

Congenital subvalvar AS may take the form of a discrete membrane or a tunnel type of obstruction. Supravalvar AS may be familial, associated with a characteristic facies, hypercalcemia and mental retardation (Williams-Beuren syndrome). In supravalvar AS, the jet of blood flow may be directed towards the innominate artery resulting in a higher pulse volume and higher BP in the right arm than on the left (anisosphygmia).

Natural history: AS is a potentially progressive disease. Even mild AS can potentially progress to severe AS. The average increment in gradient may be 2–3 mm Hg annually.

Diagnostic evaluation: Chest X-ray findings include normal cardiac size with LV contour, dilated aorta and occasionally left arterial enlargement (LAE).

Electrocardiogram (ECG) will demonstrate LVH in severe AS in 75%, with or without strain pattern (Figs 122.1A and B). Echocardiogram is diagnostic, confirming AS, its severity and the level of obstruction. It will also confirm the presence of LVH and associated lesions. ***Catheterization*** is essentially done for therapeutic purpose.

Management protocol: Mild forms of AS do not require any treatment except follow-up and observation of IE prophylaxis. Some limitation of activity is prescribed in moderate and severe stenosis. Treatment is recommended in more severe forms based on clinical symptoms or assessment of pressure gradient.

Indications for interventions:

- Presence of LV dysfunction, irrespective of pressure gradient.
- Gradient of more than 80 mm Hg (peak systolic) or more than 50 mm Hg (mean) with normal LV function irrespective of symptoms.
- Moderate AS with symptoms or resting ECG changes.

Most cases of valvar AS in childhood are amenable to catheter based balloon aortic valvotomy. Subvalvar and supravalvar forms are treated by surgical techniques. Valve replacement is usually reserved for older patients with congenital AS or those with significant associated aortic regurgitation (AR). This can be done either using mechanical prosthesis or by substituting the pulmonary valve for the aortic valve (Ross procedure). Ross procedure is ideal for children, as it avoids a mechanical prosthesis and anticoagulation.

Coarctation of Aorta (CoA)

This condition is characterized by obstruction of the thoracic descending aorta in the region of the ductus arteriosus or ligamentum arteriosum just distal to the left subclavian artery (LSA). Very rarely, it may occur at a more proximal site in the arch or in abdominal aorta. It is more common in males (2:1) and is the most common CHD in Turner syndrome.

Pathology: In majority of cases, coarctation occurs as a discrete infolding of the dorsal aortic wall. In about 20% of cases, coarctation exists as the only abnormality, whereas the rest have some associated abnormalities like BAV, PDA, VSD, ASD, mitral stenosis, mitral regurgitation (MR) and transposition of great vessels. BAV is the most common associated anomaly, majority of them being hemodynamically insignificant. Shone's complex consists of coarctation with supramitral membrane and subaortic or aortic valve obstruction. When coarctation is severe, arterial blood from the proximal part is taken to the distal part through collateral circulation which develops from the intercostal arteries and the subclavian system. CoA is associated with the presence of berry aneurysms in the cerebral arterial tree, especially circle of Willis.

Hemodynamics: CoA produces elevated pressure in the proximal aorta and the branches (cephalobrachial hypertension). LVH ensues. Hypertension in CoA is multifactorial—due to distal mechanical obstruction, activation of renin-angiotensin mechanism, increased sympathetic discharge, resetting of baroreceptors and diffuse ***aortopathy***.

Clinical evaluation: Approximately 50% of coarctation presents in the neonatal period, many of them with varying degrees of heart failure. Those who present during adolescence and adulthood give history of intermittent claudication of legs, mild fatigue and dyspnea. In older individuals, it may present as CHF. The upper limb pulses, suprasternal pulse and carotid pulse are prominent, and the BP is high in the arms. The lower limb systolic BP is at least 10 mm Hg lower than upper limb BP. The femoral pulse is felt feebly and is delayed. The apex beat may be heaving in nature. Usually, there is an ejection systolic murmur with a constant ejection click, best heard over the right sternal border. This is caused by the associated BAV. Sometimes, there may be an EDM of aortic incompetence. The collaterals may be visible and palpable over the back of the chest, around the scapula and sometimes in front of the chest. Continuous murmur may be produced from the site of coarctation or from the collaterals. Rib erosion due to dilated chest collateral may occur in Figure 122.2. The diagnosis should be suspected by the finding of absence or delay of the femoral pulses, presence of high BP in the upper limbs, low BP in the lower limbs and the cardiac abnormalities.

Natural history: CoA can lead to major complications like CHF, intracranial hemorrhage due to berry aneurysm rupture, severe hypertension and IE. The longevity is significantly reduced in untreated CoA.

Diagnostic evaluation: Echocardiogram shows LVH. In newborn coarctation, in view of the associated PAH, the ECG typically shows right axis deviation (RAD) and right ventricular hypertrophy (RVH).

X-ray shows localized indentation of aorta at coarctation site with dilatation above and below (3 sign). X-ray also shows rib notching (Fig. 122.2). These findings are seen only after 4 years. On barium swallow, esophageal indentation due to aortic dilatation occurs (E sign, reverse 3 sign).

Echocardiogram: Suprasternal view shows narrowing of aorta just beyond LSA. Color flow localizes the site of narrowing. Continuous wave Doppler can assess gradient across coarctation. Gradient of more than 25 mm Hg defines the presence of coarctation. However, in the presence of an open ductus arteriosus, assessment of severity by gradients can be erroneous.

Catheterization: It can be avoided with a good echo study. However, it may be indicated for precise definition of anatomy of coarctation site, assessment of ductus and collaterals, and for assessment of other intracardiac

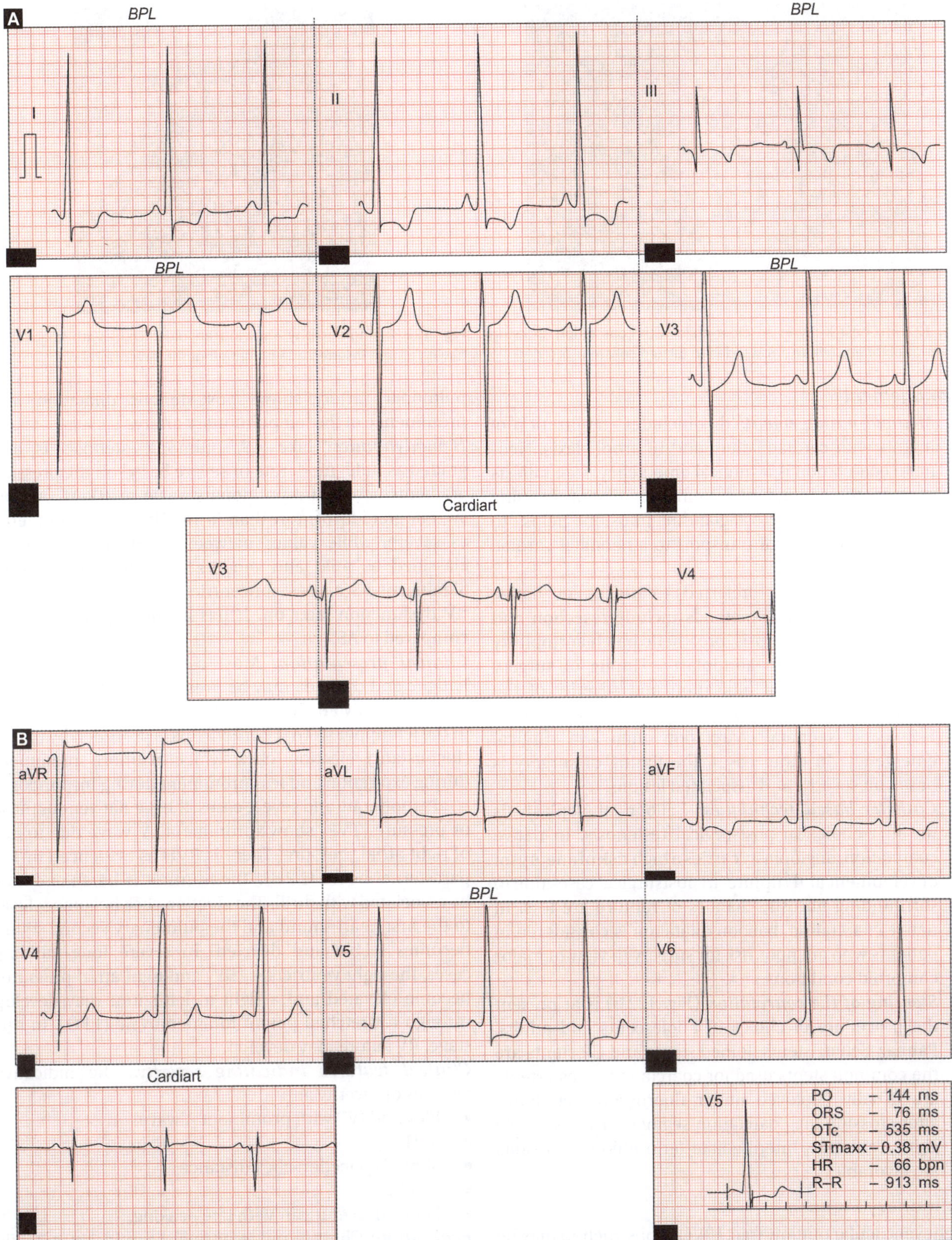

Figs 122.1A and B: ECG of a child with AS having left ventricular hypertrophy with strain

Abbreviations: aVR = Augmented vector right; aVL = Augmented vector left; aVF = Augmented vector foot

lesions. In the current era, the role of cardiac catheterization is mostly reserved for the purpose of catheter based interventions and in adults with coarctation.

Magnetic resonance imaging (MRI) is increasingly being used for evaluation of CoA, both native and postprocedure.

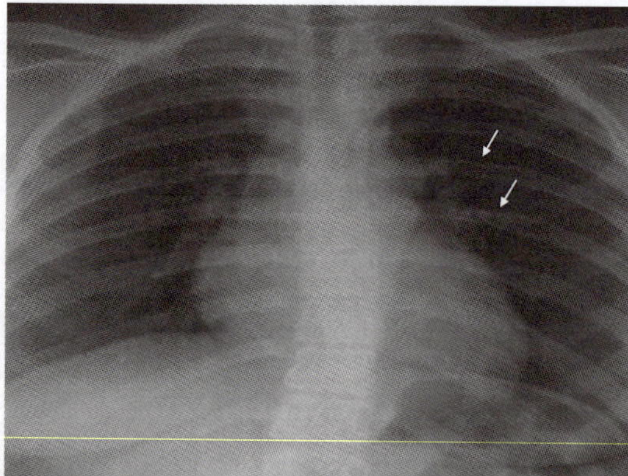

Fig. 122.2: Chest X-ray in an older child with coarctation showing indentation of ribs (white arrows) due to dilated collateral arteries

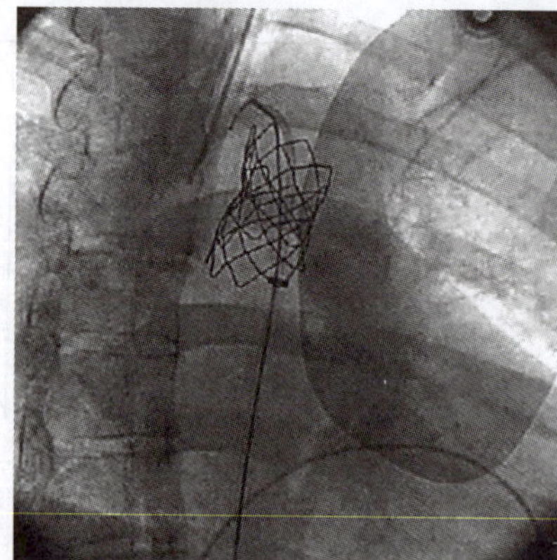

Fig. 122.3: Angiography showing an older child with coarctation having a stent inserted as a percutaneous intervention

Management

- ***Medical management:*** This includes stabilization of infants with cardiac failure and IE prophylaxis. Neonatal coarctation is a surgical emergency. It manifests as a ductus dependent systemic circulation keeping the PDA open. Prostaglandin infusion helps to stabilize the child for transport to a neonatal cardiac surgical unit.
- ***Surgery:*** It is the preferred treatment in native coarctation. Surgical methods include resection and end-to-end anastomosis, prosthetic patch aortoplasty and subclavian flap aortoplasty. Timing of surgery is based on clinical indication and severity of the coarctation. The optimal timing has come down to 1–2 years. Neonatal coarctation often is a surgical emergency. In other cases, the timing of surgery is based on severity and associated lesions.
- ***Catheter-based techniques:*** Balloon angioplasty is the first choice in postsurgical restenosis. In native coarctation, angioplasty carries a high risk of aneurysm development and rupture. In postsurgical cases due to surrounding fibrosis, chances of rupture are less. In native coarctation, balloon dilatation is considered in patients who are poor risk for surgery in view of major comorbid conditions.
- ***Stenting of the coarctation*** (Fig. 122.3) is at present the procedure of choice in adolescents and adults. Palmaz-Schatz stents, Jomed stents and CP stents are the common stents used for coarctation. These stents are usually deployed under fluoroscopic guidance after crossing the coarctation segment using suitable guide catheters. Intermediate term follow-up results are favorable.

Pulmonary Stenosis

Right ventricular outflow tract (RVOT) obstruction may be valvar, supravalvar or subvalvar. As an isolated anomaly, pulmonary valve stenosis (PVS) is the most common type of RVOT obstruction. It forms 5–7% of CHD and is classically associated with Noonan's syndrome.

Pathology: This is characterized by a thick valve with fused commissures and central or eccentric opening. The valve demonstrates characteristic doming with varying degrees of restriction of opening during systole. The main pulmonary artery shows post-stenotic dilatation with prominence of the left pulmonary artery.

Hemodynamics: Like AS, pulmonic stenosis is also graded as mild, moderate or severe based on the pressure gradients across the pulmonary valve or RVOT. A peak systolic gradient of more than 75 mm Hg is often considered as severe, while values between 25–50 and 50–75 are classified as mild and moderate stenosis respectively. Significant PS causes concentric RVH and it may cause RV dysfunction later on. It has a slower progression as compared to AS.

Clinical presentation: Most cases are asymptomatic. Fatigue and dyspnea may be present in some. Mild cases may show only an ejection systolic murmur, best audible in the left upper sternal border. This is preceded by phasic (inconstant) ejection click which is more prominent during expiration and less prominent during inspiration.

In moderate and severe cases, the jugular venous pulse or pressure (TVP) shows prominent 'A' wave due to rise of right atrial pressure. There is RVH as evidenced by left parasternal heave (LPH). The murmur is harsh and may be associated with thrill. The ejection click becomes closer to the first heart sound and the pulmonary second sound becomes feeble and delayed. In severe long-standing cases, the right ventricular (RV) and right atrial pressures become elevated and a right to left shunt may develop through a stretched patent foramen ovale (PFO). In this stage, RV failure may develop.

Clinical features indicating severity: The indicative features of severity are:

- Elevated JVP with prominent A wave
- LPH
- Short S1–ejection click distance
- Soft P2
- Long, loud murmur with late peaking.

Evaluation: Chest X-ray is normal in mild cases, while in severe cases enlargement of the right atrium and prominent main pulmonary artery segment maybe noted. Cardiomegaly is unusual. Lung vascularity is usually normal.

Echocardiography characteristically shows RAD and RVH. An estimate of the RV systolic pressures may be obtained from the height of the R wave in lead V1 (Fig. 122.4). Right atrial enlargement (RAE) and evidence of ischemic

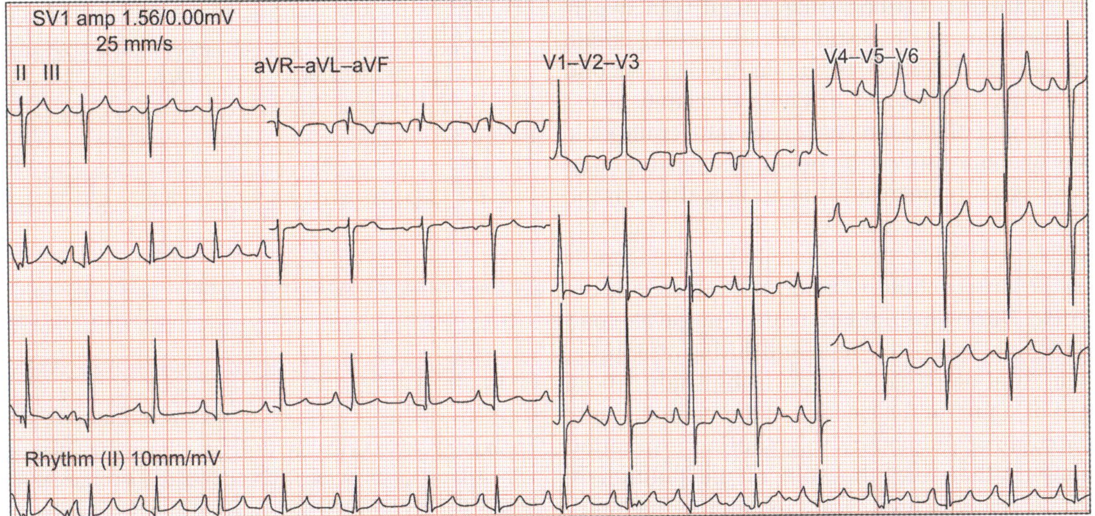

Fig. 122.4: ECG of a child with pulmonary stenosis having right ventricular hypertrophy

changes in RV herald onset of RV failure. In Noonan's syndrome, ECG may typically show left axis deviation (LAD) or right upper quadrant axis (RUQ).

Echocardiography confirms the diagnosis and it can be used to assess the RV function, degree of severity of stenosis and indication for treatment.

Management protocol: Mild cases usually do not progress further and require no intervention except follow-up and observation of endocarditis prophylaxis.

Indications for Treatment

- RV dysfunction, irrespective of gradient.
- Gradients of more than 60 mm Hg (peak systolic) or more than 40 mm Hg (mean) with normal RV function.

Balloon valvuloplasty has replaced surgical therapy as the first approach (Fig. 122.5). Balloon is inflated to about 20–40% greater size than the measured pulmonary annulus thus opening the valve. A dysplastic valve as in the case of Noonan's syndrome responds less favorably to balloon valvuloplasty. Pulmonary valve replacement or open surgical valvotomy are very rarely required in the pediatric age group.

LEFT-TO-RIGHT SHUNT LESIONS

Atrial Septal Defect (ASD)

This is the second most common CHD found in children (10%) and most common in adults (30%). There is a female predominance (2:1). Familial ostium secundum ASD is noted. ASD may occur as an isolated anomaly or in association with other intracardiac anomalies like PS or VSD. Syndromic association includes Ellis-van Creveld. Rheumatic mitral stenosis may coexist with ASD (Lutembacher's syndrome).

Pathology: ASD is characterized by the presence of one or more defects in the interatrial septum. Based on the developmental abnormality, ASD can be classified into mainly three types.

1. ***Ostium secundum (Fossa ovalis) defect (70%):*** Ostium secundum defect occurs in the region of the fossa ovalis and this is the most common type. It results from the maldevelopment of the septum secundum. The only abnormality is the presence of the ASD.

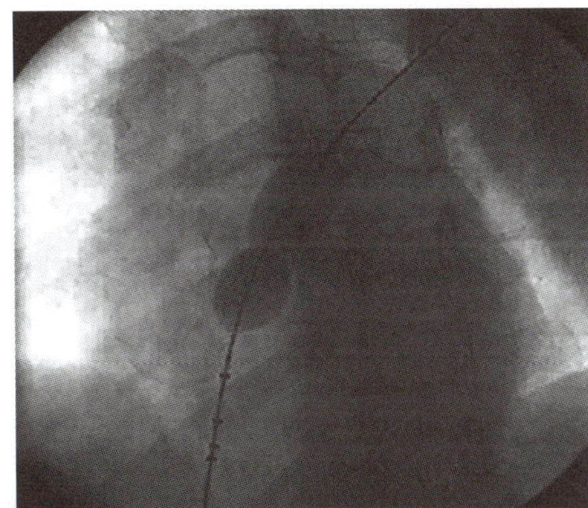

Fig. 122.5: Balloon dilatation of pulmonary valve in a child with pulmonary stenosis

2. ***Ostium primum defect (20%):*** It is the result of abnormal development of the endocardial cushion. The defect is in the lower portion of the interatrial septum. This is typically associated with defects in the mitral valve in the form of a cleft and sometimes MR.

3. ***Sinus venosus type of defect (10%):*** It occurs in the upper portion of the interatrial septum. It is due to the abnormality of development of the upper part of the interatrial septum and it is associated with anomalous connection of one or more pulmonary veins (typically right) to the SVC or RA.

Hemodynamics: In ASD, the blood is shunted from LA to RA and then to the highly compliant right ventricle. The right ventricle acts as a conduit, pumping this increases return into the pulmonary arteries. This leads to progressive enlargement of the RA, RV and pulmonary arteries. Even though pressures are equal, shunt occurs from LA to RA as the right ventricle is more compliant than LV. There is no pulmonary venous hypertension (PVH). PAH can develop late in the natural history.

Clinical presentation: Most ASDs are asymptomatic. Palpitation and recurrent respiratory infections are the usual symptoms. Effort intolerance usually develops in the third and fourth decades and thereafter features of CHF develop.

Clinically, there is cardiac enlargement with hyperactive precordium as a result of RV enlargement. Pulmonary artery pulsation is felt in the left second intercostal space. In rare cases, a systolic thrill may be felt over the upper part of the sternum, on the left. A pulmonic ejection systolic murmur will be heard. The murmur and thrill are produced by increased blood flow through the pulmonary valve. The second sound in the pulmonary area is widely split since the pulmonic valve closure is delayed by the larger volume of blood to be ejected by the right ventricle. During inspiration, more vena caval blood flows into the right side of the heart and during expiration, more of left atrial blood flows through the shunt. These phenomena account for the ejection of the same quantity of blood across the pulmonary valve during inspiration and expiration. Therefore, the split of the pulmonary second sound remains fixed. The auscultatory hallmark is wide fixed split of second heart sound. Increased flow across the tricuspid valve during diastole may produce a tricuspid mid-diastolic murmur (MDM), best heard along the left lower sternal border. This is sometimes preceded by a RV third heart sound. Severity of shunt is assessed by cardiomegaly, presence of RVS3 and tricuspid MDM. A thrill palpable in pulmonary area can occur in large shunt or with associated mitral stenosis or associated PS.

Natural history: Small ASDs may close and below 4 mm are common in infants up to 1 year. They are known to close spontaneously or remain as persistent foramen ovale. Defects more than 6 mm in infancy have been noted to become larger in natural history studies. When the shunt is large, the right-sided chambers progressively enlarge. Pulmonary hypertension develops in course of time. The pulmonary pressure may be elevated to high levels and same is reflected in the RV and RA. When right atrial pressure exceeds that of the LA, the blood flow is reversed and this leads to the development of central cyanosis. This phenomenon is called ***Eisenmenger syndrome***. Pulmonary hypertension and reversal of shunt occurs in less than 10% patients. Premium type of ASD carries a poorer prognosis than the secundum type. Other complications include paradoxical embolism, arrhythmias like atrial fibrillation and very rarely IE.

Diagnostic Evaluation

ECG: It shows RAE, rsR' pattern in lead V1, RVH and RAD (Fig. 122.6). LAD is seen in ***ostium primum ASD***. PR interval prolongation is seen in familial types of ASD and in ostium primum defects.

Chest X-ray: It shows cardiomegaly, enlargement of right atrium without the engorgement of the SVC, increased pulmonary vascularity as evidenced by multiple end on vessels and enlargement of main pulmonary artery, right pulmonary artery and left pulmonary artery, if the shunt is large (Fig. 122.7).

Echo with color Doppler: It can diagnose the type of ASD, measure the size of ASD, note the direction of shunt and quantify the shunt. The suitability for transcatheter closure can also be assessed by echo (Figs 122.8A to C). Pulmonary venous drainage can also be visualized and anomalous pulmonary venous drainage can be made out. Doppler

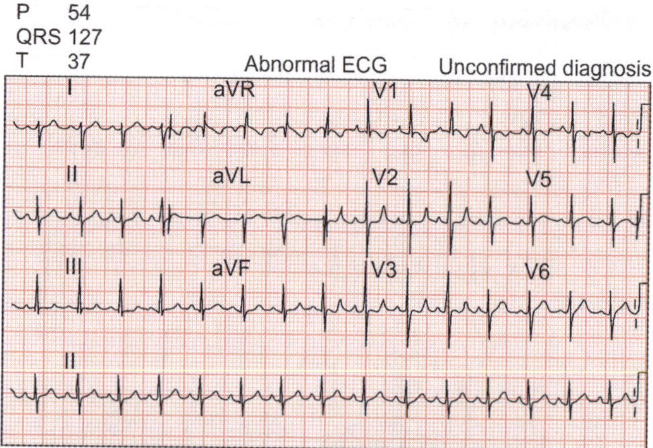

Fig. 122.6: ECG of a patient with large atrial septal defect. ***Note:*** The right axis deviation of the QRS complex and incomplete right bundle branch pattern in the lead V1

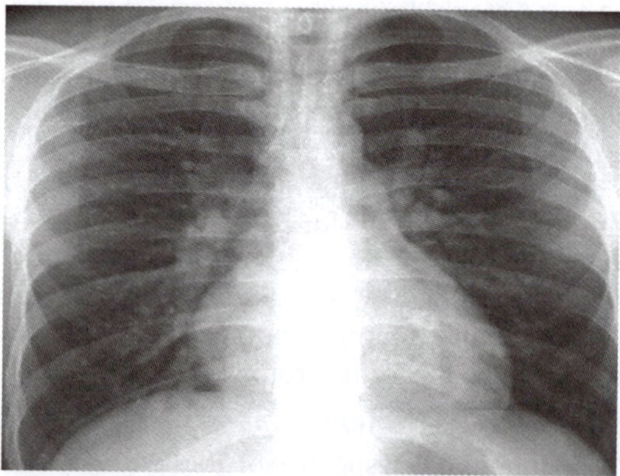

Fig. 122.7: Chest X-ray of a patient with a large ASD. ***Note:*** Cardiomegaly, right atrial enlargement and prominent pulmonary arteries

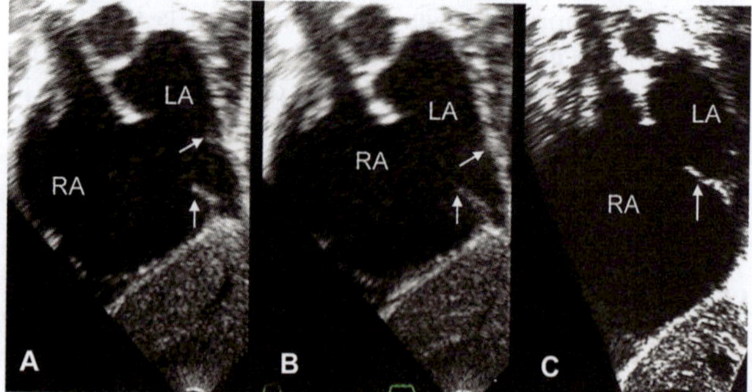

Figs 122.8A to C: Transthoracic echocardiography in ostium secundum atrial septal defect. **A.** A large defect with a thin inferior vena cava (IVC) rim (transparent arrow); **B.** A defect with absent IVC rim; **C.** A central defect with good rims, ideal for transcatheter closure

with color mapping is comparable with angiographic visualization of intracardiac shunting.

Cardiac catheterization: Generally, this is not required for preoperative diagnosis. It is indicated for the following reasons:

- In adults, to assess pulmonary vascular resistance and hence, to decide on surgery
- To assess coronary arteries in patients above the age of 40 years, when corrective surgery is contemplated
- If any disparity between clinical and echo quantification of shunt exists.

Catheterization will show increase in oxygen saturation from SVC to RA. LA can be entered from right atrium through the ASD and the pressures in the two chambers are equal can be measured.

Management Protocol

Medical: ASD by itself has a very low risk for IE. If associated MR is present, IE prophylaxis is advised. In late stages as the patient goes in for cardiac failure, digoxin and diuretics are to be used.

Indications and timing of intervention: Any hemodynamically significant ASD should be closed. The timing of intervention is as follows:

- *Asymptomatic child*—2–4 years of age (for sinus venosus ASD at around 4–5 years)
- *Symptomatic ASD* in infancy (seen in around 5–10% cases)—early closure recommended
- *Presentation in older children and adults:* Elective closure irrespective of age as long as the shunt is hemodynamically significant and pulmonary vascular resistance index (PVRI) is less than 5 Wood units.

Type of Intervention

Surgical: Surgery is the treatment of choice for all ostium primum and sinus venosus ASDs. In a very large secundum, ASDs with deficient margins, surgery is the first choice for closure of the ASD. Median sternotomy, left posterolateral or right thoracotomy or atrial wall approach can be used. ASD closure is done by suturing the edges of ASD directly or by using pericardial patch or prosthetic material.

Catheter-based techniques: This is applicable only for the ostium secundum type of ASD. About 80% of this type of ASDs can be treated by the catheter-based method in the current era. Presence of a very large ASD with deficient margins is a relative contraindication for transcatheter closure. Transcatheter closure is ideally done after the age of 3 years with the patient weight above 10 kg. Various types of devices have been used for transcatheter closure. Presently used devices are of the third generation and include Amplatzer device and CardioSEAL. The Amplatzer septal occluder is the most commonly used device and this is made of Nitinol, which imparts the property of in-built memory allowing the device to be deployed through smaller delivery systems. Complications rates with this procedure in carefully selected cases are very less and the long-term results are comparable to surgery (Figs 122.9A and B).

Ventricular Septal Defect (VSD)

This is the most common CHD in the pediatric age group (25%). This is characterized by one or more defects in the ventricular septum.

Types

- The most common are perimembranous with variable extension into the inlet, trabecular or outlet sections of muscular septum (80%)
- Subarterial defects/subpulmonic (5–7%)
- Inlet defects (5–8%)
- Muscular septum defects (20%).

VSD may occur as an isolated anomaly in the majority, or in association with other cardiac anomalies such as ASD, RVOT obstruction, CoA and transposition of great vessels. The blood flows from LV to the right and then to the pulmonary circulation. This leads to enlargement of left and right ventricles, pulmonary artery and the LA.

Hemodynamics: VSD results in a left-to-right shunt at the post-tricuspid level. In a large VSD, there is equalization of systolic pressures in both ventricles and this pressure is directly transmitted into the pulmonary arteries with significantly increased flow of blood into the pulmonary system (hyperkinetic PAH). This ↑PBF returns to the left side of the heart leading to enlargement of the left sided chambers and increased flow across the mitral valve in diastole. Small VSDs maintain a significant pressure gradient across the defect and the PBF is not significantly increased. Hence, there is no left heart enlargement either with the development of pulmonary vascular disease, the pulmonary compliance and blood flow reduces, the overall shunt across the defect gets obliterated and left heart enlargement comes down. When the pulmonary vascular resistance increases further, there will be reversal of shunt and cyanosis.

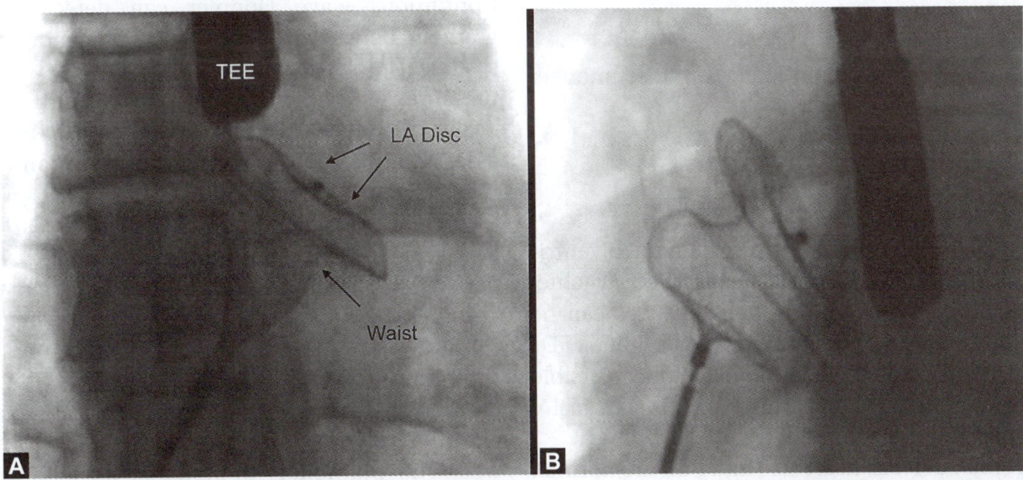

Figs 122.9A and B: Transcatheter closure of secundum atrial septal defect with the Amplatzer septal occluder. ***Note:*** The characteristic double disc feature of the device

Abbreviations: TEE = Transesophageal echocardiography; LA = Left atrium

Clinical presentation: Large VSDs can lead to congestive cardiac failure in infancy. Recurrent respiratory infection and failure to thrive (FTT) may also be noticed. Those who survive develop varying degrees of pulmonary hypertension. Moderate VSDs present with feeding difficulties and recurrent respiratory infections. Small VSDs are asymptomatic and they are detected on routine examination.

Small VSDs are characterized by a harsh pansystolic murmur associated with thrill, best heard in the left third and fourth intercostal spaces. Moderate VSDs produce pansystolic murmur and cardiac enlargement. Large VSDs are relatively silent, as there is no pressure gradient between the right and left ventricles. The apex beat is forceful with hyperactive precordium. Pulmonary artery pulsation may be felt. There may be LV third heart sound. Typically, large VSDs will cause a systolic flow murmur across the pulmonary valve due to increased blood flow into the lungs, and a MDM is heard over the cardiac apex suggestive of increased blood flow across the mitral valve.

Assessment of severity: LV third heart sound, MDM over mitral area and cardiomegaly indicate a large shunt. The presence of these findings indicates that the pulmonary hypertension is secondary to increased flow (hyperkinetic PAH) and hence, the patient will have benefit from closure of the defect. With the onset of irreversible PAH (Eisenmenger syndrome), the cardiomegaly comes down and the flow murmurs disappear.

The major complications due to a large VSD are heart failure, FTT and recurrent respiratory tract infections (RTIs) in infancy. Typically after 2 years, irreversible pulmonary hypertension and reversal of shunt (Eisenmenger syndrome) can develop. Other complications, typically with smaller defects include IE, development of RVOT obstruction, aortic valve prolapse and AR (typically with subpulmonic VSD).

Natural history: The natural history of VSD is variable.

- About 60% of small VSD close spontaneously, maximum closure occurring before 3 years. Moderate VSD can also close (10–20%). Large VSDs seldom close. Subpulmonic and inlet VSDs never close spontaneously
- VSDs can become small
- They can develop PAH and later on Eisenmenger syndrome
- A small proportion can develop AR
- VSD can develop RVOT obstruction.

Diagnostic Evaluation

ECG: Large VSDs cause RAD with prominent biventricular forces in the mid-precordial leads (Katz-Wachtel phenomenon) (Fig. 122.10). Prominent q waves can be seen in LV leads due to LV volume overload. Inlet VSDs typically cause LAD of the QRS. The onset of irreversible PAH is associated with disappearance of Q waves in LV leads and findings of predominant RV hypertrophy.

X-ray: With small defects, heart size and PBF are normal. With large defects, moderate to marked enlargement of heart, prominent main pulmonary artery and pulmonary plethora are seen (Fig. 122.11). Left atrial enlargement

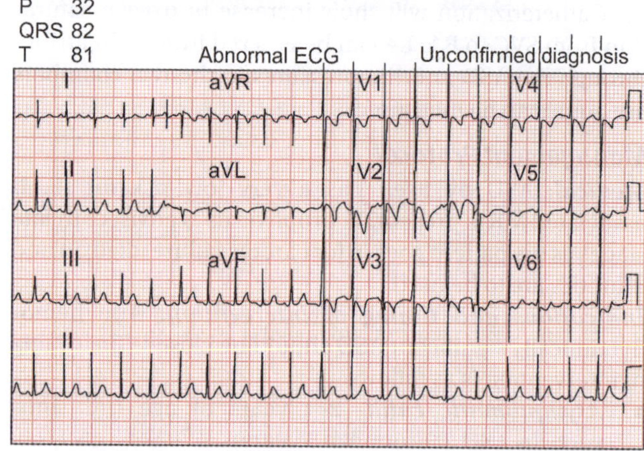

Fig. 122.10: ECG of a child with large ventricular septal defect. ***Note:*** The characteristic biventricular forces in precordial leads (Katz-Watchel phenomenon)

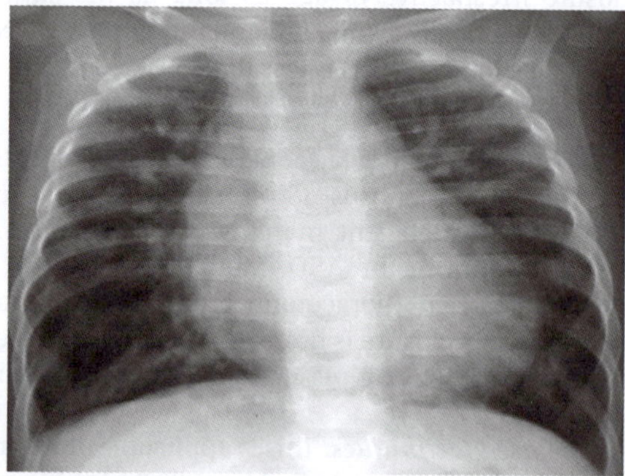

Fig. 122.11: Chest X-ray in a child with large ventricular septal defect. ***Note:*** The prominent cardiomegaly, left atrial enlargement and increased pulmonary vascular markings (plethora)

(LAE) is prominent. There is no RAE unlike ASD and unlike PDA, the aorta is not prominent.

Echocardiogram: Visualization of the site of VSD and size measurement is possible with 2D-echo which is very useful and noninvasive and is the initial investigation. Color flow mapping can identify small muscular defects. Continuous wave Doppler can detect the pressure gradient between the two ventricles and from this RV systolic pressure can be derived. This will assess PA pressures. Presence of associated features can also be evaluated. Echocardiogram can be used for hemodynamic assessment of significance of the shunt and operability (Fig. 122.12).

Catheterization: The only indication for cardiac catheterization in the current era is a large VSD in an older patient with doubtful operability on clinical assessment. The typical findings in a large VSD with significant left-to-right shunt will be a significant step-up in oxygen saturations on right heart oxymetry with significant elevation of pulmonary artery pressures. There will be elevation of pulmonary capillary wedge pressures as well. The pulmonary-to-systemic blood flow ratio will be elevated (> 2:1). PVRI of less than 8 Wood units is considered to be a feature of operability. In selected cases, vasodilator testing with various agents may be required to

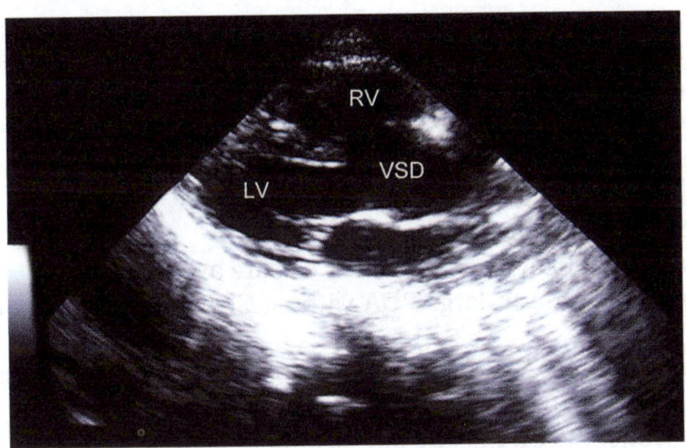

Fig. 122.12: Echocardiography in a child with large ventricular septal defect. **Note:** The subaortic location

assess operability and plan long-term medical therapy if the data is not favorable for closure of the defect.

Management Protocol

Medical: This includes IE prophylaxis and treatment of cardiac failure using diuretics, digoxin and ACE inhibitors.

Indications and timing of intervention: Closure is recommended in all hemodynamically significant VSDs. The timing and choice of intervention depends on the age of the patient and location of the VSD.

- Large VSD with uncontrolled heart failure: As early as possible
- Large VSD with severe hyperkinetic PAH: 3–6 months of age
- Moderate-large VSD with significant left-to-right shunt: 6–12 months of age
- Small VSD: Needs no intervention. Elective closure by 2–3 years of age if—
  - Aortic valve prolapse with regurgitation
  - Episode of IE
  - Development of RVOT obstruction.

Some clinicians recommend that all subpulmonic VSDs should be electively closed by 2–3 years in view of higher risk of aortic valve complications in future life.

Surgical: Surgery is the mainstay of treatment in patients with VSD. Transatrial and transventricular approaches are utilized for VSD closure. The long-term results of surgical closure of VSD are excellent and majority of patients can lead near normal lives.

Catheter-based techniques: Unlike ASD and PDA, the role of catheter-based therapy for VSD closure is restricted to a selected group of patients only. Typically, these are the older children (>15 kg) with muscular VSDs with a hemodynamically significant shunt. Several types of devices including the PDA devices and various VSD devices are used. The role of device closure for children with membranous VSDs is under development with selected older patients suitable for this technique. Careful follow-up of the aortic valve and cardiac rhythm is required when such procedures are considered.

Patent Ductus Arteriosus (PDA)

It accounts for 5–10% of all CHD. It is associated with prematurity, low birth weight (LBW), Rubella syndrome, Cornelia de Lange and Rubinstein Taybi syndrome. The female to male ratio is 2:1. It is more common in high altitude.

Pathology: Embryologically, the ductus arteriosus is the posterior part of the persistent left sixth aortic arch. In the fetus, it allows the egress of blood pumped from the RV into the pulmonary trunk to the descending aorta bypassing the lungs which are nonfunctional. Normally, as the lungs get aerated after birth, functional closure of the ductus occurs in 12–24 hours and anatomical closure within 2–3 weeks after delivery. Patency of the ductus after birth results in the flow of blood from the aorta to the pulmonary artery since the pulmonary artery pressure is lower. The aortic end of the ductus lies beyond the origin of the LSA, and the pulmonary end is located immediately to the left of the bifurcation of the pulmonary trunk. In the early stages of the disease, blood from the aorta flows to the pulmonary artery throughout systole and diastole. When pulmonary hypertension develops this blood flow diminishes the diastolic flow initially. The blood flow may be reversed when Eisenmenger syndrome develops.

Hemodynamics: PDA causes a left-to-right shunt at the level of the great arteries with consequent run-off from the aortic side to the pulmonary arteries. The hemodynamic assessment is similar to that of VSD. In large PDA, in view of a significant shunt occurring in both systole and diastole from aorta to pulmonary arteries, a continuous murmur is audible and due to the aortic run-off, the aortic diastolic pressures are often reduced leading to a wide pulse pressure. With the development of pulmonary vascular disease, the shunt and aortic run-off declines, leading to normalization of pulse pressures, disappearance of the diastolic segment of the continuous murmur and eventual reversal of shunt leading to differential cyanosis in the lower extremities.

Clinical presentation: Many cases remain asymptomatic, even though the mother would have detected the murmur and thrill in the child. Palpitation and exertional dyspnea set in if the ductus is large and pulmonary hypertension develops. Later, CHF supervenes. The pulse may be collapsing in character. There is LV type of cardiac enlargement. Cases with pulmonary hypertension may reveal LPH. In the vast majority of cases, a continuous thrill may be felt over the left second intercostal space outside the sternal border. The most characteristic auscultatory finding is the presence of a continuous machinery type of murmur, audible most loudly over the left upper sternal border. The murmur is louder during systole and less so during diastole. The systolic phase is interrupted by multiple systolic clicks. Less commonly, large shunts may be accompanied by LV third heart sound followed by a decrescendo mid-diastolic murmur best heard over the apex beat. This indicates large blood flow across the mitral valve. The second heart sound is usually immersed in the murmur. In cases with pulmonary hypertension, the pulmonic component becomes louder and well-heard.

Course and prognosis: Mild cases do not impair cardiac function and they may remain asymptomatic. Large ductus may present with CHF in infancy. Those cases which recover from heart failure may develop pulmonary hypertension later in life. Large left-to-right shunt leads to enlargement of LA, LV, aorta and pulmonary artery.

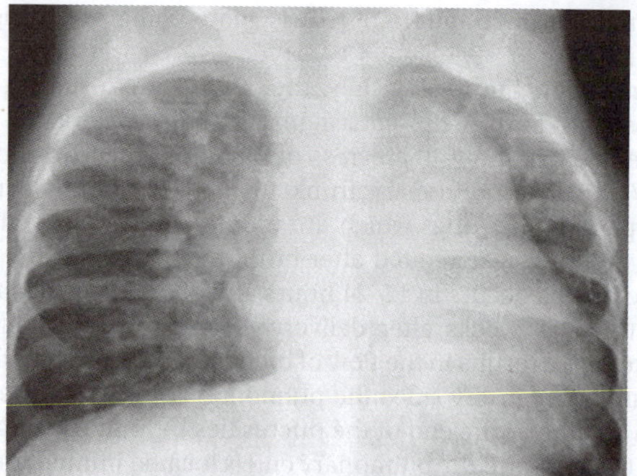

Fig. 122.13: Chest X-ray of a child with large PDA. **Note:** The cardiomegaly, dilated pulmonary artery and pulmonary plethora

Complications: Cardiac failure, IE, paradoxical embolism and Eisenmenger syndrome may complicate PDA.

Diagnostic Evaluation

ECG: LAE and LVH is noted with large shunts.

Chest X-ray: It shows cardiomegaly, pulmonary plethora, prominent aortic arch and sometimes ductal calcification (Fig. 122.13).

Echocardiogram: Color flow mapping shows shunt flow into left pulmonary artery. Using Doppler, the gradients in systole and diastole between aorta and pulmonary artery can be calculated and this may gives an idea regarding pulmonary artery pressures. The size and the anatomy of the PDA can be evaluated and suitability for transcatheter closure can be assessed comprehensively (Figs 122.14A and B).

Catheterization: This is mostly done as a predevice-closure procedure. In selected cases of older patients with large PDA and PAH, a diagnostic cardiac catheterization and test balloon occlusion of the PDA for hemodynamic assessment of operability maybe required.

Management Protocol

Closure of PDA is advised in all cases, except in those without a murmur (silent PDA) due to high risk of IE.

Medical: Indomethacin 0.1 mg/kg/bw can be given in the neonatal period 12 hourly (2 doses) for ductus closure in preterm PDA. It acts as by inhibiting prostaglandin. Alternatives to indomethacin include ibuprofen or paracetamol. Other medical measures include correction of cardiac failure and IE prophylaxis.

Indications and timing of intervention

- Large PDA with CHF: Early closure by 3–6 months
- Moderate-to-large PDA with no CHF: 6–12 months of age
- Small PDA with continuous or long systolic murmurs: By 12–18 months of age
- Silent PDA: Closure not recommended.

Surgical closure: In the current era, surgical ligation of PDA is recommended only in very large PDA in very small infants where transcatheter closure is not feasible. In preterm infants with large PDA needing closure, surgical ligation can often be done in the neonatal intensive care unit (NICU) by the bedside.

Catheter-based techniques: More than 95% of the PDAs can be closed by catheter-based techniques in the current era. In most cases, the transcatheter closure can be accomplished from the venous side without the need for arterial access. Smaller PDAs can be closed with **Gianturco coils** while larger ones are best occluded by the **duct occluder device**. Long-term results are comparable with surgical ligation, though follow-up of branch pulmonary artery and aortic flows are recommended, especially in smaller patients (Figs 122.15A to C).

Atrioventricular Septal Defects (AVSD)

These are also referred to as Endocardial Cushion defects. These lesions are characteristically more common in patients with trisomy 21.

Pathology: The embryological basis of these lesions is characterized by lack of fusion of the endocardial cushions during cardiac development leading to abnormalities of the atrioventricular valve and presence of atrial and ventricular level shunts.

Classification: Based on the features of the atrioventricular valve and location of the shunts, these defects are classified into:

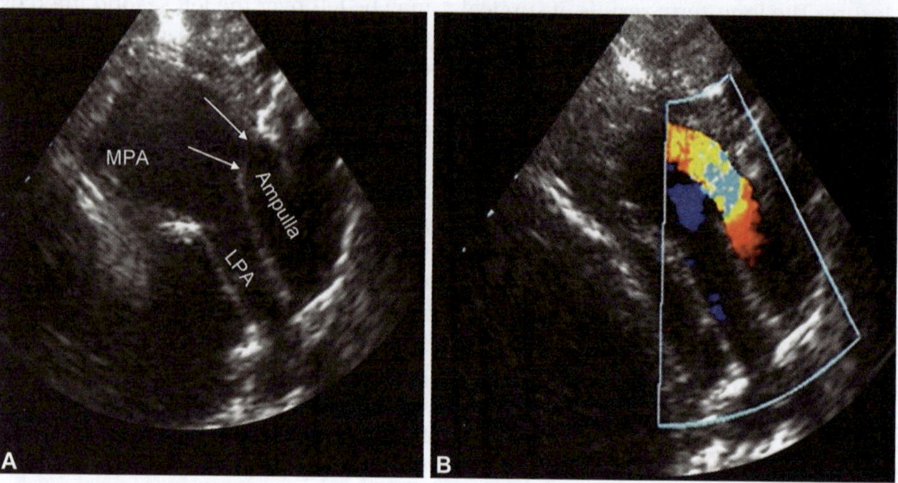

Figs 122.14A and B: Transthoracic echocardiogram of patent ductus arteriosus (PDA). **A.** The arrows indicate the pulmonary artery end of the PDA where the size is measured; **B.** Color flow confirms left-to-right shunt

Abbreviations: MPA = Main pulmonary artery; LPA = Left pulmonary artery

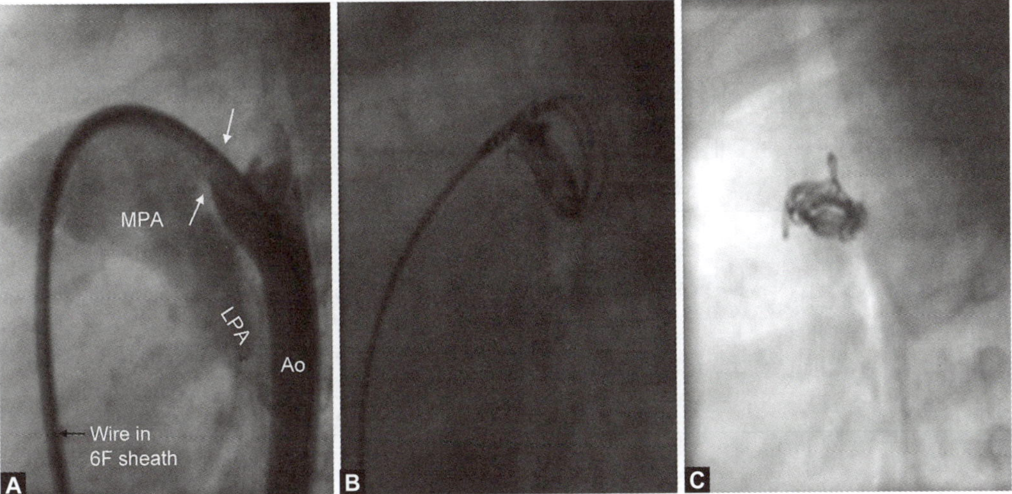

Figs 122.15A to C: Transcatheter closure of patent ductus arteriosus (PDA) using Gianturco coils. **A.** Aortic angiogram showing the PDA (arrows); **B.** Multiple coils being delivered using a bioptome; **C.** The coil mass after deployment

Abbreviations: MPA = Main pulmonary artery; LPA = Left pulmonary artery; Ao = Aorta; descending aorta.

- Partial AVSD (ostium primum ASD)
- Transitional AVSD: Ostium primum ASD with a restrictive VSD.
- Complete AVSD.

Some morphologists have characterized an intermediate form of AVSD based on the morphology of the common atrioventricular valve. The common anatomic features of these defects include the presence of a common atrioventricular valve, a typically unwedged and anteriorly displaced aortic valve, and abnormalities of the left-sided atrioventricular valve with cleft and abnormal orientation of conduction system. Various schemes of classification of the atrioventricular valve with implications for surgical repair have been described (Rastelli classification).

Hemodynamics: These are typically very similar to patients with ASD (for partial AVSD) or VSD (for complete AVSD). The development of pulmonary vascular disease and Eisenmenger syndrome is much more rapid in patients with complete AVSD. About 50% of patients with complete AVSD show phenotypic features of trisomy 21. The onset and severity of CHF is more rapid and severe compared to a large VSD. Patients with trisomy 21 in addition may have significant respiratory symptoms also, complicating the assessment of shunts and operability.

Diagnostic Evaluation

ECG: Typical finding in ECG is the presence of LAD of the QRS complexes (Fig. 122.16).

Additional findings depend on the presence of associated shunts like ASD or VSD. There may be RVH or biventricular hypertrophy (BVH). Biatrial enlargement is common in complete AVSD.

Chest X-ray: Cardiomegaly with biatrial and ventricular enlargement is found in complete AVSD along with pulmonary vascular congestion.

Echocardiography: Echo permits a comprehensive evaluation of the anatomy, presence of atrial or ventricular level shunts, valve regurgitation and hemodynamic assessment. Intraoperative echo in the operating room permits assessment of completeness of repair and residual issues.

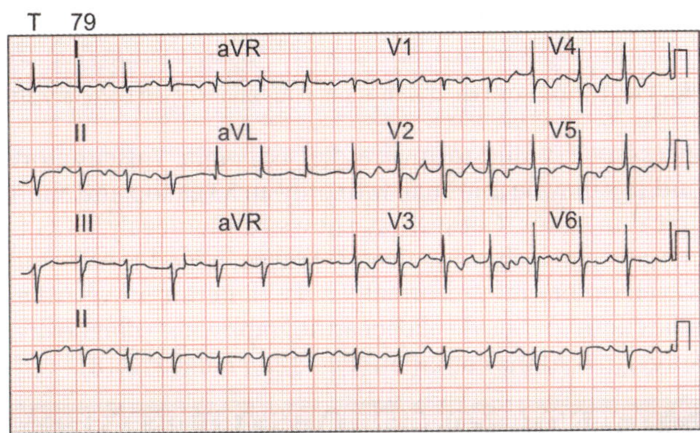

Fig. 122.16: ECG of a patient with atrioventricular septal defect showing characteristic left axis deviation of the QRS complex

Cardiac catheterization: This is reserved for the selected older patient with severe PAH and borderline operability.

Management Protocol

All forms of AVSD require intervention and the choice of intervention is surgical correction in all cases.

Timing of surgery

- Complete AVSD with uncontrolled heart failure: Surgery as soon as possible
- Complete AVSD with controlled heart failure: 3–6 months of age
- Partial AVSD: 2–3 years of age.

Surgery involves closure of the atrial and ventricular level shunts (using a single patch or two separate patches), repair of the atrioventricular valve and correction of any valvar regurgitation. Patients require long-term follow- up for residual issues like MR and LVOT obstruction. About 10–20% of patients require reoperation for these two reasons.

ADDITIONAL LESIONS

Anomalous Origin of LCA from Pulmonary Artery

This is a rare but a critical CHD where LCA arises from PA. This presents in infancy as severe CHF mimicking dilated cardiomyopathy (DCM). The babies may have episodes of

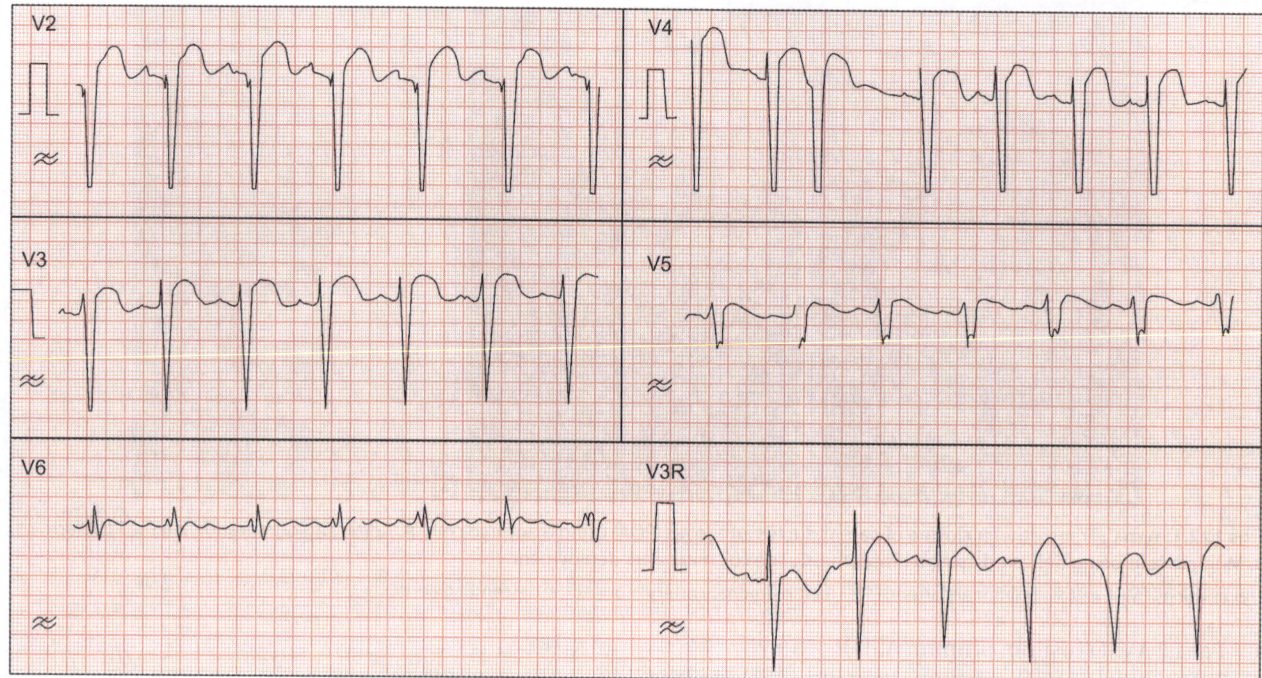

Fig. 122.17: ECG of a child with anomalous origin of left coronary artery from pulmonary artery. ***Note:*** The ST elevation in V1 to V3

incessant cry due to myocardial ischemia. Auscultatory findings may be minimal, with only an S3 gallop and short apical murmur. Chest X-ray shows cardiomegaly. ECG is characteristic, showing deep Q waves in lead I, AVL and ST elevation in precordial leads (anterior myocardial infarction pattern). Echocardiography is diagnostic. Surgery cures the condition (Figs 122.17 and 122.18).

CYANOTIC CONGENITAL HEART DISEASE

Cyanotic CHD characteristically has a right to left shunt causing arterial desaturation and ensuing hypoxemia. The shunt is usually at an intracardiac level. The saturation is below 95%. When arterial O_2 saturation drops to below 85%, clinical cyanosis results.

The subject of cyanotic CHD is very complex since several abnormalities involving the different chambers, blood vessels, valves, septa and functional derangements have been identified with the help of modern investigations such as echocardiography, cardiac catheterization, MR-angiography, CT-positron emission tomography (CT-PET) and isotopic studies. These may be present at birth producing life-threatening situations (incompatible with life unless urgently corrected) or less severe conditions which require elective correction during infancy or childhood. This branch has become a major subdivision of cardiology involving all branches from the cardiologists, electrophysiologists, imageologists, intervention cardiologist and cardiac surgeons. A brief indication of these conditions is added below for bringing home to the young student about the vastness and complicated nature of the problem. For further details, monographs on this subject have to be consulted. This is the domain of pediatric cardiologist.

ALGORITHMIC APPROACH TO CYANOTIC CHD

Cyanotic CHD reduced pulmonary blood flow (PBF)
- With pulmonary stenosis
  - VSD
  - No VSD
- With PAH/pulmonary venous obstructive disease (PVOD)

Group I
- Reduced PBF [↓PBF, PS, intact ventricular septum (IVS)]
- Severe PS will develop R-L shunt across PFO/ASD and will cause desaturation

Group II
- ↓PBF, PS, VSD
- TOF and its variants have this physiology

Group III
- ↓PBF, PAH/PVOD
- Eisenmenger syndrome is the example. It can be simple or complex

Cyanotic CHD with increased blood flow (↑PBF)
- Parallel circulation:
  - d-TGA
  - Taussig-Bing anomaly
- Admixture lesions:
  - Total anomalous pulmonary venous connection (TAPVC), single atrium (SA)

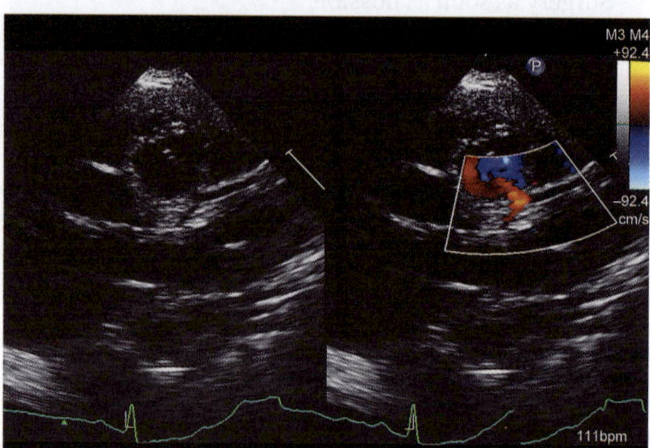

Fig. 122.18: Echocardiogram of a child with anomalous origin of left coronary artery from pulmonary artery. ***Note:*** The origin of left coronary artery from pulmonary artery and its bifurcation

- Single ventricle, double outlet right ventricle (DORV)
- Truncus

Miscellaneous: Ebstein, pulmonary A-V fistula (PAVF), persistent pulmonary hypertension in newborn (PPHN).

Abbreviations: VSD = Ventricular septal defect; PAH = Pulmonary arterial hypertension; PBF = Pulmonary blood flow; PS = Pulmonary stenosis; TOF = Tetralogy of Fallot; d-TGA = d-Transposition of the great arteries

TETRALOGY OF FALLOT (TOF)

It is the most common cyanotic CHD in children, accounting for 10% of all CHD. There is a slight male preponderance. Teratogens responsible for TOF include maternal PKU, diabetes and excess vitamin A ingestion. Syndromes associated with TOF are DiGeorge, Down, Alagille, Poland and Goldenhar.

Pathology

The four components of TOF are:

1. Large malaligned perimembranous VSD
2. Pulmonary stenosis—infundibular (always) and also valvar (occasionally)
3. RVH
4. Aortic over-ride (biventricular origin of aorta).

Additional defects may be present. These are PFO, ASD (pentalogy of Fallot), coronary artery anomalies, left SVC, PDA and right-sided aortic arch (25%).

Hemodynamics

In TOF, due to the presence of a large VSD, LV and RV systolic pressures are equal and the same as aortic pressure. PA pressure is normal or low. Because of obstruction at RV outflow, blood reaching the RV will shunt to aorta through the large subaortic VSD and will cause a right-to-left shunt and desaturation. The desaturation will depend on:

- Severity of RVOT obstruction
- Presence of PDA
- Other sources of supply to lung (collaterals).

Clinical Presentation

TOF seldom presents at birth. Usually, the baby presents with cyanosis on crying, progressing to cyanosis at rest around 3 months (deferred cyanosis). They can develop cyanotic spells, between 3 months and 6 months characterized by increasing cyanosis, fast and deep breathing and extreme irritability. Such episodes can be life-threatening. Older children often squat to get relief, when they become breathless. Dyspnea on exertion such as feeding and walking becomes evident in infancy and childhood.

Clinically, varying grades of cyanosis and clubbing occur. There is no CHF or cardiomegaly. There are no prominent LPH and precordial pulsations (quiet precordium). JVP is normal as well as pulse. On auscultation, S2 is single and well-heard. There will be an ejection systolic murmur of 2–3/6 intensity over mid left sternal border. The intensity of the murmur is inversely proportional to severity of TOF.

Classic Features

- Central cyanosis
- No CHF; normal JVP
- Normal cardiac size
- Quiet precordium; No LPH
- Single S2
- Ejection systolic murmur.

Additional findings include an ejection click over base of the heart and collateral murmur.

Features of Severity

- Early onset cyanosis
- Deep cyanosis
- Presence of ejection click (aortic)
- Short murmur
- Soft murmur
- Collateral murmur.

Complications of TOF include cyanotic spells and cerebral thrombosis, both of which are common before 2 years and cerebral abscess and IE in later years. Other complications include severe polycythemia, bleeding tendency and hyperuricemia. CHF is uncommon and when occurs may be due to iron deficiency anemia (IDA), IE, restrictive VSD (due to prolapse of tricuspid valve), AR or hypertension in the adult.

Natural History

Without intervention, survival of TOF at 1 year is 65% at 10 years survival is 25% and at 20 years survival is only 10%.

Diagnostic Evaluation

- ***Chest X-ray*** will show normal cardiac size, RV apex, no RAE, concave pulmonary bay and reduced lung vascularity. Right arch is seen in 25% (Fig. 122.19).
- ***ECG*** will show, RAD, RVH and early transition of R waves from V1 to V2 and no RAE (Fig. 122.20).

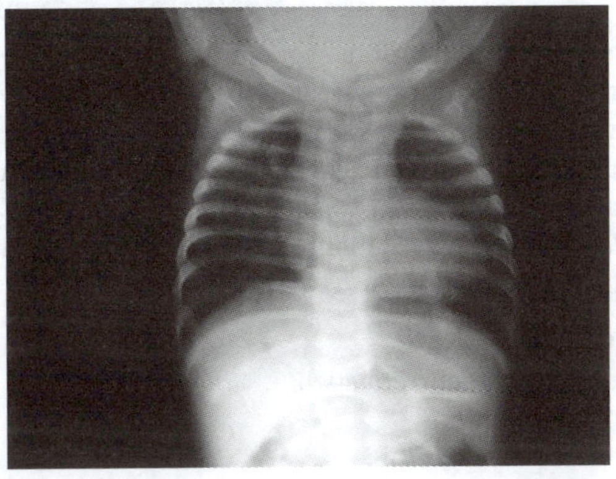

Fig. 122.19: Chest X-ray of a baby with TOF. ***Note:*** The right ventricular apex, concave pulmonary bay and pulmonary oligemia

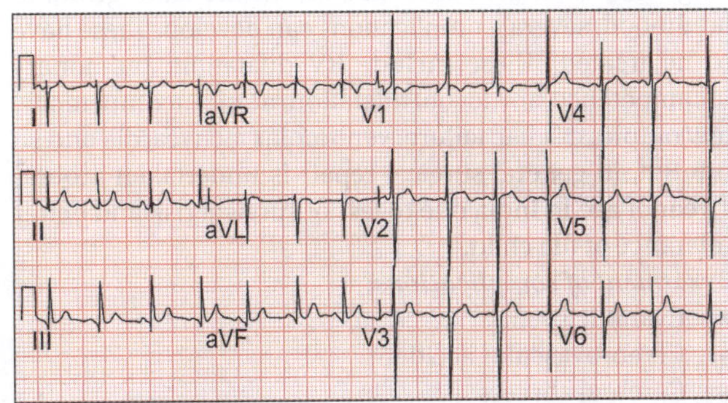

Fig. 122.20: ECG of a child with TOF. ***Note:*** The right axis deviation, right ventricular hypertrophy and early transition of QRS from V1 to V2

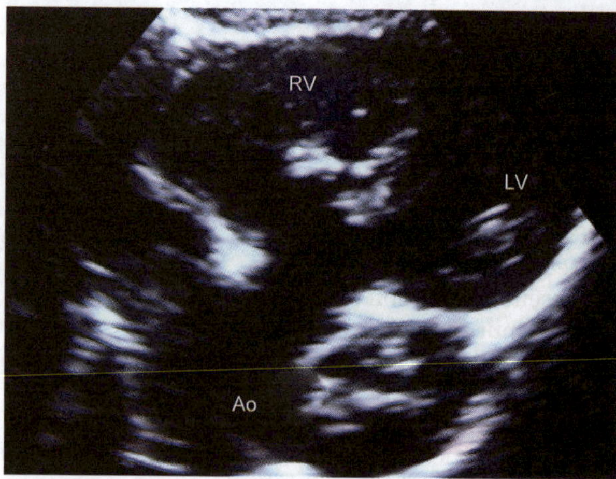

Fig. 122.21: Echocardiogram of a child with tetralogy of Fallot. **Note:** The over-riding of the aorta and large ventricular septal defect

Abbreviations: RV = Right ventricle; LV = Left ventricle; Ao = Descending aorta

- Echocardiography is confirmatory. It will also assess additional abnormalities and pulmonary artery size and confluence (PA anatomy) (Fig. 122.21).
- Catheterization is seldom done now. Cardiac MRI and CT could be useful in delineation of anatomy, especially in adult TOF.
- Other investigations include hemoglobin (Hb), packed cell volume (PCV), red cell indices and peripheral smear.

Management Protocol

Medical measures:

- IE prophylaxis
- Iron supplementation
- Prevent dehydration; treat dehydration
- Treating cyanotic spell (if it occurs)
- Preventing recurrence of spell—propranolol 3 mg/kg/day divided doses.

Surgical measures: Palliative: Blalock-Taussig-Thomas shunt (BTT shunt)

Indications

- Refractory/recurrent spell
- Poor PA anatomy
- Severe polycythemia
- Corrective: Intracardiac repair at around 1 year of age. Optimum age for repair is 3–6 months. Early surgery is generally successful, but as the child grows to adulthood, several complications can develop. These have to be treated. These include RV dilatation, pulmonary incompetence, aortic root dilatation, aortic incompetence, low output, cardiac failure, ventricular tachycardia and so on. But, in general surgical repair is undertaken around 1 year of age in India due to less of surgical risk and better tolerance of the child.

Treatment of complications:

- Cyanotic spell
- Cerebrovascular accident
- Cerebral abscess
- IE
- Severe polycythemia

- Treating cyanotic spell:
  - Putting the child in knee-chest position. It increases SVR and hence, reduces R-L flow; PBF is improved
  - Administration of oxygen (100%) improves saturation
  - Intravenous (IV) morphine (0.1 mg/kg) as two doses, 15 minutes apart. It causes sedation, allays anxiety and may improve infundibular spasm
  - IV fluids (normal saline/dextrose saline) will increase intravascular compartment and elevate SVR. Sodium bicarbonate (1 mL/kg) to combat metabolic acidosis
  - Beta blockers (IV propranolol or IV metoprolol). It will reduce dynamic infundibular obstruction and increase SVR
  - Vasopressors (noradrenaline/phenylephrine) to increase SVR
  - Additional measures like ventilation
  - If all measures fail, one has to do an emergency BTT shunt.

Blalock-Taussig-Thomas shunt:

- Classical
- Modified (using gore-textube)—standard
- Subclavian artery to ipsilateral pulmonary artery shunt

Intracardiac repair: Close the VSD, remove infundibular obstruction and do pulmonary valvotomy (if required). Mortality is below 1% with a 20 years survival of above 95%.

TOF Variants

Generally, cyanotic CHDs with a VSD and PS are called TOF variants. They are:

- DORV, VSD, PS can be clinically indistinguishable from TOF. ECG may show prolonged PR interval and extreme right axis deviation and may not show the early transition.
- d-TGA, VSD, PS presents very early with cyanosis and the murmur of PS may be prominent inspite of deep cyanosis. Chest X-ray will show egg on side appearance with pulmonary oligemia. ECG will have RAD and RVH with no early transition.
- L-transposition of great arteries (L-TGA), VSD, PS will behave more like TOF. It is a common CHD in dextrocardia. There could be an apical systolic murmur due to left AV valve regurgitation. Chest X-ray will show L-posed aorta and ECG shows the classical features of LAD, qR in V1 and no q in V6, with varying degrees of atrioventricular block.
- AVSD, PS could be found in Down syndrome. It can have an apical murmur of MR. ECG is quite characteristic with first degree AV block, LAD and RVH.
- Single ventricle with PS behaves more or less like TOF. The murmur need not become soft on deep cyanosis. ECG will show LAD, No q in V5 and V6 and may show monotonous r/S pattern from V1 to V6.
- Pulmonary atresia with VSD will have no PS murmur. Instead there will be a continuous murmur either due to PDA or collaterals. ECG will be similar to that of TOF.
- Truncus arteriosus with PS will have high volume pulse and also a short EDM due to truncal regurgitation.

- Tricuspid atresia (TA) also behaves more or like TOF, even though the VSD in TA is restrictive. TA will have early onset cyanosis, good murmur and a prominent JVP. Apex may be of LV type. ECG will show LAD, RAE, poor RV forces and good LV forces. Chest X-ray will have RAE.

DEXTRO-TRANSPOSITION OF GREAT ARTERIES (d-TGA)

It is the second most common cyanotic CHD in infants and children. More than 5% all CHD are due to d-TGA. It is the most common cyanotic CHD in newborn.

Epidemiology

Familial d-TGA has been reported. It may have an association with maternal diabetes and progesterone intake. It is more common in male babies (4:1).

Pathology

There are four subsets of d-TGA:
1. d-TGA with intact interventricular septum
2. d-TGA, large VSD, PAH
3. d-TGA, large VSD, PS
4. d-TGA, large VSD, PVOD.

Hemodynamics

It is the classical example of parallel circulation, where there is AV concordance with VA discordance. Blood reaches RA from systemic veins, travels to RV and reaches aorta and again comes back to RA. Blood reaches LA from pulmonary veins, travels to LV and reaches pulmonary artery and lungs. It again comes back to LA. This is a parallel circulation. Survival beyond birth is possible only if there is some intercirculatory mixing at atrial, ventricular and arterial levels (ASD/VSD/PDA).

Presentation and survival in d-TGA depends on:
- Adequacy and level of intercirculatory mixing
- Bronchopulmonary collaterals
- Pulmonary stenosis (LVOT) obstruction.

Clinical Presentation

d-TGA with intact IVS will present with progressive cyanosis and acidosis within 1 week of life. Clubbing will not be present. There could be mild CHF with a high volume pulse (PDA). S2 is single in almost all d-TGA. Murmurs are not prominent. Without intervention, 30% die within 1 week, 50% die within 1 month and 90% die by 1 year.

d-TGA with large VSD and PAH will present with significant cyanosis and CHF. CHF develops within 2 weeks. There will be significant cardiomegaly, single S2 and murmur of VSD with MDM at apex.

d-TGA with VSD and PS (LVOT obstruction) will behave like severe TOF. Spells can occur.

d-TGA, VSD and pulmonary vascular occlusive disease will present as Eisenmenger syndrome, but with intense central cyanosis.

Natural History

Without intervention, course is dismal. Survival at 1 year is only 10%.

Diagnostic Evaluation

Chest X-ray in d-TGA beyond 2 weeks of life will have an egg on side appearance, with cardiomegaly, RAE, RV apex, narrow pedicle and pulmonary plethora. d-TGA with VSD and PS will show pulmonary oligemia (Fig. 122.22).

ECG will show RAD, RAE and RVH. BVH is expected in the presence of large VSD or PDA.

Echocardiography is confirmatory. It detects AV concordance and VA discordance and categorizes all associated defects (VSD, ASD, PDA, coronary anomaly, LVOT obstruction, arch anomalies) (Fig. 122.23).

Protocol for d-TGA Management (Flowchart 122.1)

It is initially managed with taking care of acidosis, CHF and hypoxemia. Prostaglandin E_1 (PGE$_1$) is useful in maintaining ductal patency and improving saturation. Balloon atrial septostomy is done whereby the already existing ASD is made bigger to facilitate intercirculatory mixing and hence, improve saturation (Fig. 122.24). In d-TGA, VSD, PS, severe hypoxemia is tackled with a BTT.

ADMIXTURE LESIONS

Admixture lesions are those CHD, where there is a common mixing chamber, usually with increased ↑PBF. It can clinically as follows:
- At atrial level—SA and total anomalous pulmonary venous connection (TAPVC)
- At ventricular level—single ventricle and DORV
- At great vessel level—truncus.

They have usually significant CHF with mild cyanosis, presenting within 3 months of life. They will develop PAH early.

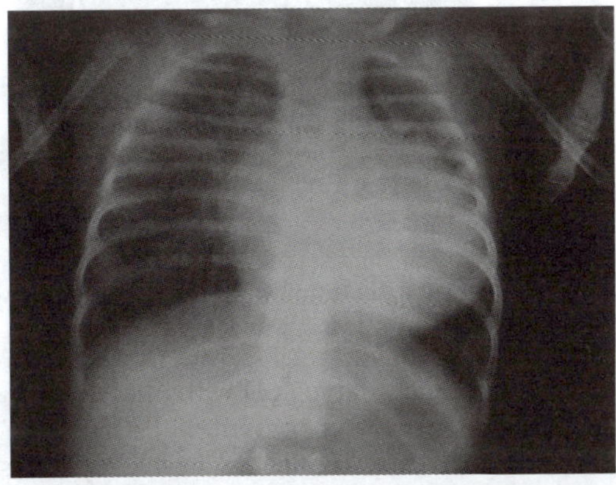

Fig. 122.22: Chest X-ray of a baby with transposition of great arteries. ***Note:*** The right ventricular apex, right atrial enlargement, narrow base and pulmonary plethora, ***egg on side*** appearance

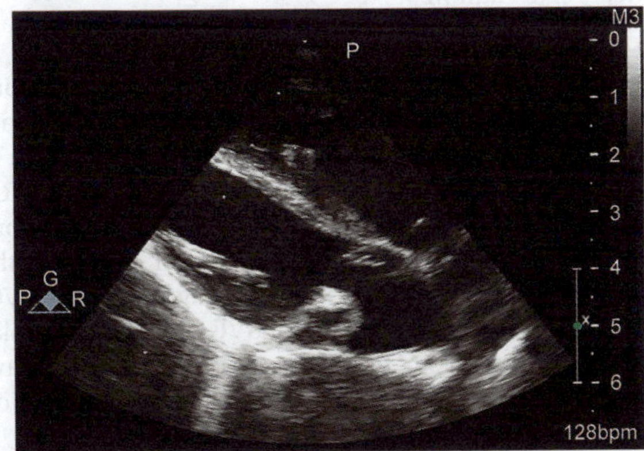

Fig. 122.23: Echocardiogram of transposition of great arteries. ***Note:*** The pulmonary artery arising from the posterior right ventricle

Flowchart 122.1: D-transposition of great arteries with IVS

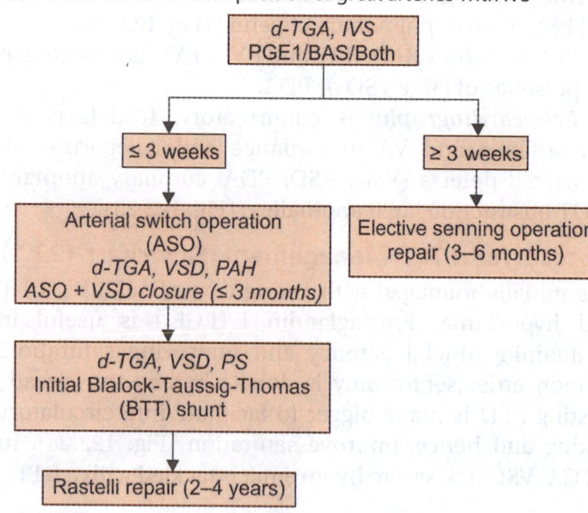

Abbreviations: d-TGA = D-transposition of great arteries; IVS = Intact ventricular septum; PGE1 = Prostaglandin E1; BAS = Balloon atrial septostomy; VSD = Ventricular septal defect; PAH = Pulmonary arterial hypertension; PS = Pulmonary stenosis

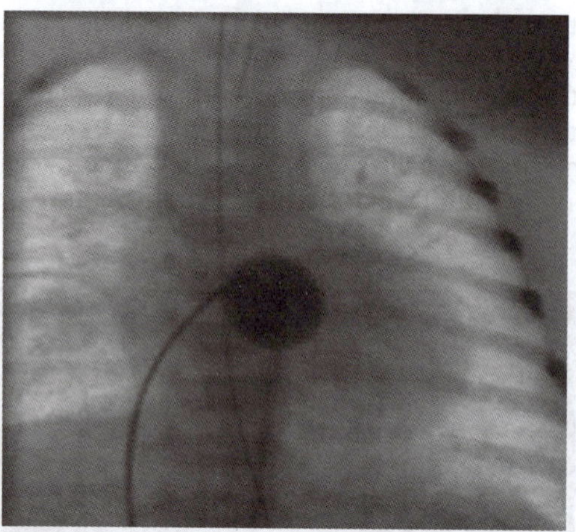

Figs 122.24: Balloon atrial septostomy and angiogram in a newborn with transposition of great arteries

SA will behave like a large ASD with mild desaturation and early PAH. TAPVC can present with CHF, FTT and tinge of cyanosis. The appearance on chest X-ray is classical in unobstructed TAPVC. Both single ventricle and DORV will present like a large VSD with mild cyanosis. Truncus will behave like a VSD. PAH with high volume pulse due to truncal regurgitation.

Anomalous Pulmonary Venous Connection

This is also known as total anomalous pulmonary venous drainage. It is the condition in which all the four pulmonary veins enter the RA, or vena cava or other systemic veins. In the partial variety, one or more of these veins enter the RA.

Often there is associated ASD. In total anomalous pulmonary venous drainage, the site of entry of the pulmonary veins may be supradiaphragmatic (left SVC, vertical vein, coronary sinus, right SVC or RA) or infradiaphragmatic portal vein, hepatic veins or inferior vena cava (IVC). Varying degrees of pulmonary venous obstruction may exist.

The clinical picture is variable. Some may be cyanotic, others present with CHF from early life, yet others present

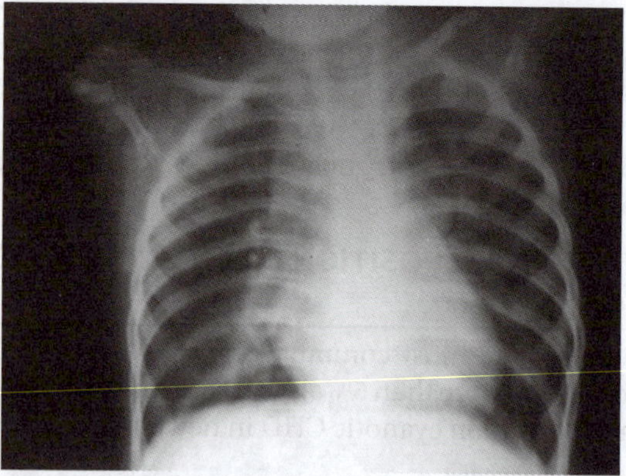

Fig. 122.25: Chest X-ray of a baby with total anomalous pulmonary venous connection. *Note:* The *figure of eight* appearance

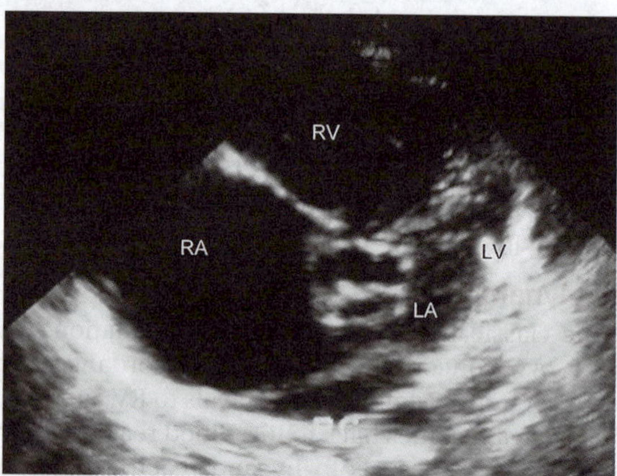

Fig. 122.26: Echocardiogram of a child with total anomalous pulmonary venous connection. *Note:* The large right atrium (RA) and right ventricle (RV) and a posterior chamber behind left atrium (LA)

a picture similar to ASD. Correction of the defects is by surgery.

X-ray shows normal sized heart with figure of 8 configuration (Fig. 122.25).

Echo will reveal the lesion clearly (Fig. 122.26).

Tricuspid Atresia (TA)

It is an important cyanotic CHD where there is no tricuspid valve opening, varying degrees of RV hypoplasia, VSD and PS. It accounts for 3% of all CHD. The most common variety of TA has a VSD and PS.

Systemic venous blood reaches RA and enters LA entirely through an ASD and reaches LV and then RV through the VSD. The PS will reduce the PBF further and it causes significant desaturation.

TA presents with early, deep cyanosis with a prominent JVP, minimal cardiomegaly and absence of any RV impulse. S2 is single and there is a long ejection murmur.

Chest X-ray will reveal minimal cardiomegaly, with a box like heart, RAE and oligemia (Fig. 122.27). ECG is quite characteristic (Fig. 122.28). Echocardiography is confirmatory.

TA is a univentricular physiology, where a Fontan type of surgery is the choice of treatment. If baby is deeply cyanotic, a Glenn (SVC to PA) or BTT shunt can be done in infancy (Flowchart 122.2). Fontan (RA-PA connection) or TCPC (connecting both SVC and IVC directly to PA) can be done between 2 and 4 years.

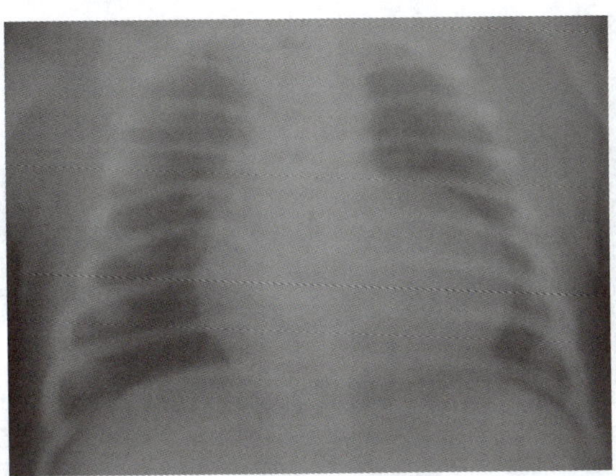

Fig. 122.27: Chest X-ray in baby with tricuspid atresia. **Note:** The box like heart with right atrial enlargement and pulmonary oligemia

EISENMENGER SYNDROME

PAH may develop at variable period of time in CHD with initial L–R shunt. When severe PAH develops it can diminish the L–R shunt and subsequently severe PVOD causes a reversal of flow.

Simple Eisenmenger	ASD, VSD, PDA, AP window AVSD
Complex Eisenmenger	Single ventricle, DORV d-TGA VSD, TAPVC truncus

VSD and PDA can lead to Eisenmenger in childhood itself whereas ASD develops PVOD by adulthood.

The history will be that of recurrent chest infections, FTT and CHF in infancy, which **improves** later on. The 'improvement' is essentially due to development of PVOD and curtailing of PBF. The clinical hallmark is the combination of cyanosis, clubbing and PAH. Differential cyanosis will be apparent in PDA Eisenmenger. Cardiomegaly is prominent in ASD with Eisenmenger. All the children with Eisenmenger syndrome will have features of PAH. The second sound is the key to diagnosis of the underlying shunt in Eisenmenger. ASD Eisenmenger will have a fixed split of S2, VSD has a single S2 and PDA a closely split S2.

Features of PAH

- RV apex, LPH, epigastric impulse, palpable P2
- Ejection click, loud P2, RVS4, RVS3.
- Ejection systolic murmur at PA. Pansystolic murmur (TR)
- EDM (PR).

X-ray shows normal sized heart, huge dilated pulmonary artery and pulmonary oligemia valve (Fig. 122.29).

Course and Prognosis

Once Eisenmenger syndrome develops, the symptoms related to left-to-right shunt disappear. At this stage, easy fatigability and tiredness dominate the clinical picture. Once, CHF sets in steady deterioration occurs culminating in death within 3–5 years.

Treatment

Supportive therapy includes home oxygen therapy, anticoagulation and digoxin for heart failure. Patients should be counseled to avoid heavy physical exertion and high altitudes. Female patients should be strongly counseled against pregnancy. Progesterone only contraceptives or other methods are recommended. Medical therapy with newer pulmonary vasodilators like phosphodiesterase inhibitors (sildenafil) and endothelin antagonists (bosentan, ambrisentan) has been shown to significantly improve symptoms and survival in these patients. In patients with advanced disease, IV prostacyclin infusion is the treatment of choice. Heart-lung transplantation or single-lung transplant are the treatment options available for advanced disease in selected centers.

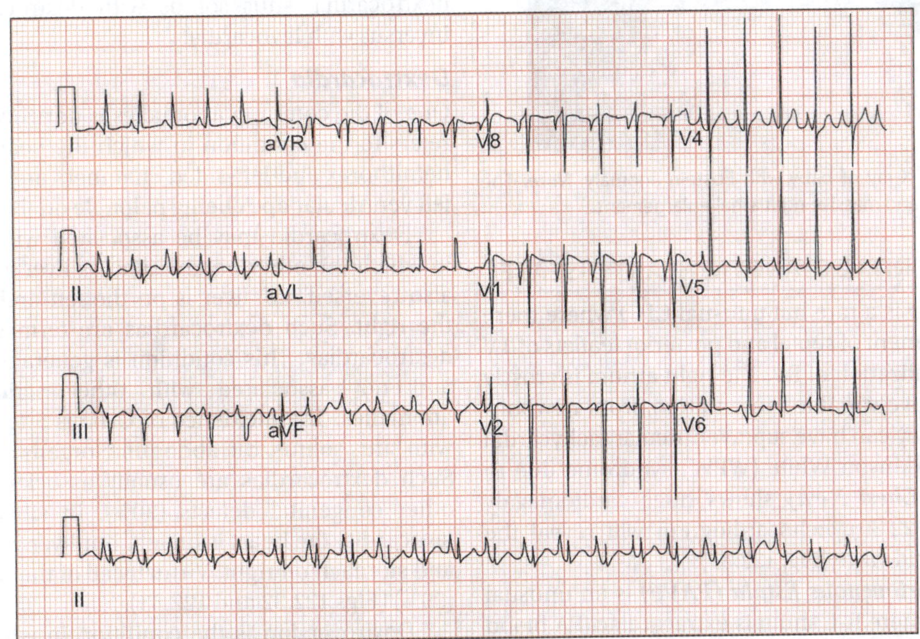

Fig. 122.28: ECG of a child with tricuspid atresia. **Note:** The left axis deviation, right atrial enlargement, poor right ventricle forces and good left ventricle forces

Flowchart 122.2: Management of tricuspid atresia: Blalock-Taussig-Thomas (BTT) shunt

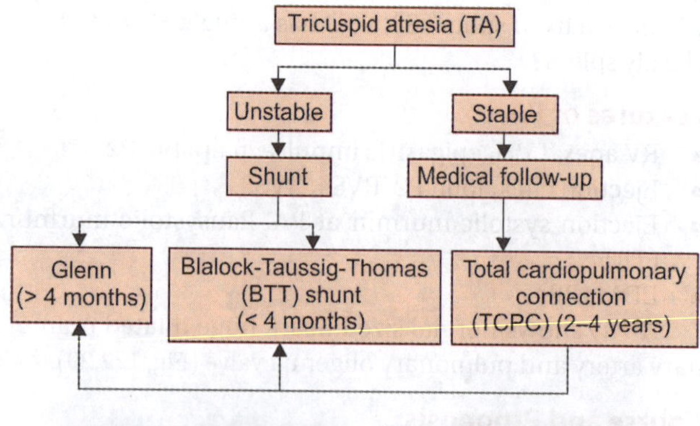

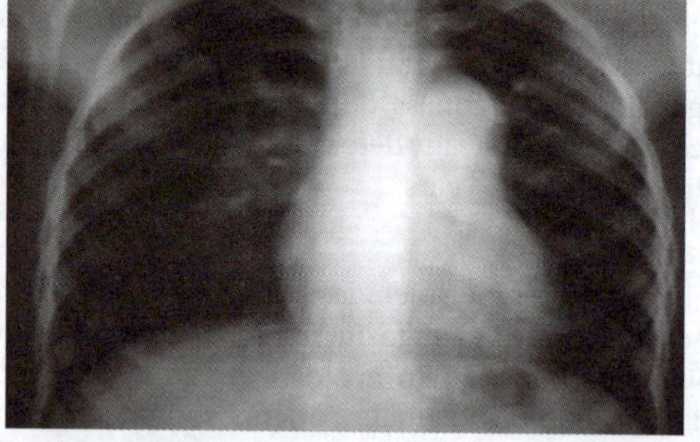

Fig. 122.29: Chest X-ray of a child with Eisenmenger syndrome. *Note:* The normal cardiac size, hugely dilated pulmonary artery and pulmonary oligemia

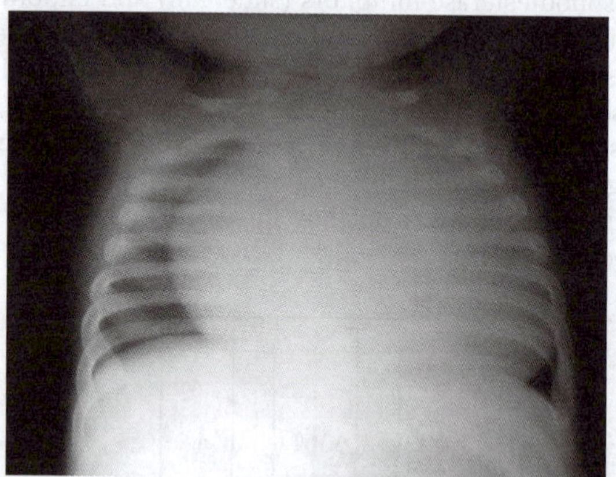

Fig. 122.30: Chest X-ray of baby with Ebstein anomaly. *Note:* The huge cardiomegaly and massive right atrial enlargement

OTHER CONGENITAL CYANOTIC HEART DISEASE

Ebstein anomaly is a rare but unusual CHD where there is distal displacement of septal and posterior leaflets of TV into RV and atrialization of RV. The right atrium is grossly dilated. It can have variable presentation, from newborn to adulthood. They can have supraventricular tachycardia due to Wolff-Parkinson White (WPW) syndrome due to a bypass tract. ***Chest X-ray*** shows huge cardiomegaly and RAE (Fig. 122.30). Echocardiogram will reveal the displaced tricuspid valve (Fig. 122.31).

Pulmonary arteriovenous fistula (PAVF) is an unusual cyanotic CHD, where R-L shunt is extracardiac. PA blood reaches PV and causes desaturation. Characteristically, children with PAVF will have central cyanosis and

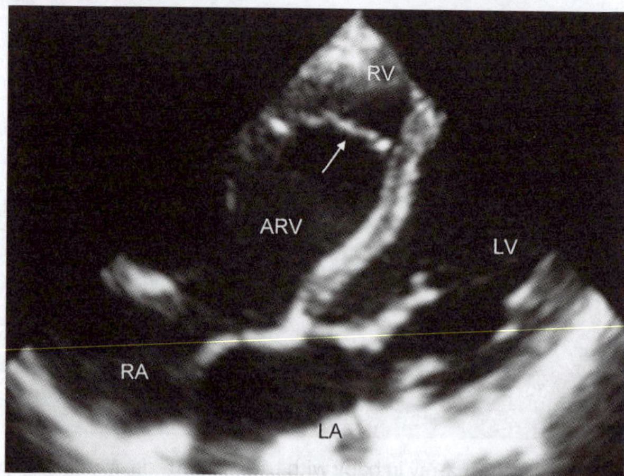

Fig. 122.31: Echocardiogram of a child with Ebstein anomaly. *Note:* The distal displacement of tricuspid valve

Abbreviations: ARV = Atrialized right ventricle; RA = Right atrium; LV = Left ventricle; LA = Left atrium

clubbing with no cardiac findings. Chest X-ray and ECG will be normal. A contrast echo will pick-up the possibility of PAVF in such situation.

MANAGEMENT FOR CYANOTIC CHD

Flowchart 122.3 shows the management for cyanotic CHD.

Malpositions of the Heart

The position of the heart and major blood vessels may be abnormal due to aberrations during embryonic development. Cardiac malpositions can be associated with or without visceral heterotaxy. The term heterotaxy refers to anomalous placement or location of viscera and vascular structures. In patients with visceral heterotaxy, the organ and vascular arrangements are not in an orderly concordant manner.

There are three basic cardiac malpositions in patients without visceral heterotaxy—situs inversus with dextrocardia, situs solitus with dextrocardia and situs inversus with levocardia.

Dextrocardia

One of the common anomalies is dextrocardia. This term refers to the condition in which the heart is in the right hemithorax and left-sided chambers are on the right, the left ventricular apex being palpable on the right side.

Dextrocardia may be associated with situs inversus in which the other organs such as liver and stomach are also reversed, i.e. liver is on the left and stomach is on the right. Such dextrocardias are termed mirror-image dextrocardias. This condition is generally asymptomatic and not associated with other serious congenital anomalies. The incidence of CHD is 5%. In dextrocardia with situs solitus, the abdominal organs are not reversed. Such dextrocardias are usually associated with several other congenital defects (90%). In situs inversus with levocardia, the heart is on left, but liver will be on the left and stomach on right. Virtually all of them will have CHD (99%) (Figs 122.32 and 122.33).

Dextroversion is the condition in which the viscera, atria and aortic arch are in the normal position, but the cardiac apex is on the right.

Flowchart 122.3: Management for cyanotic CHD

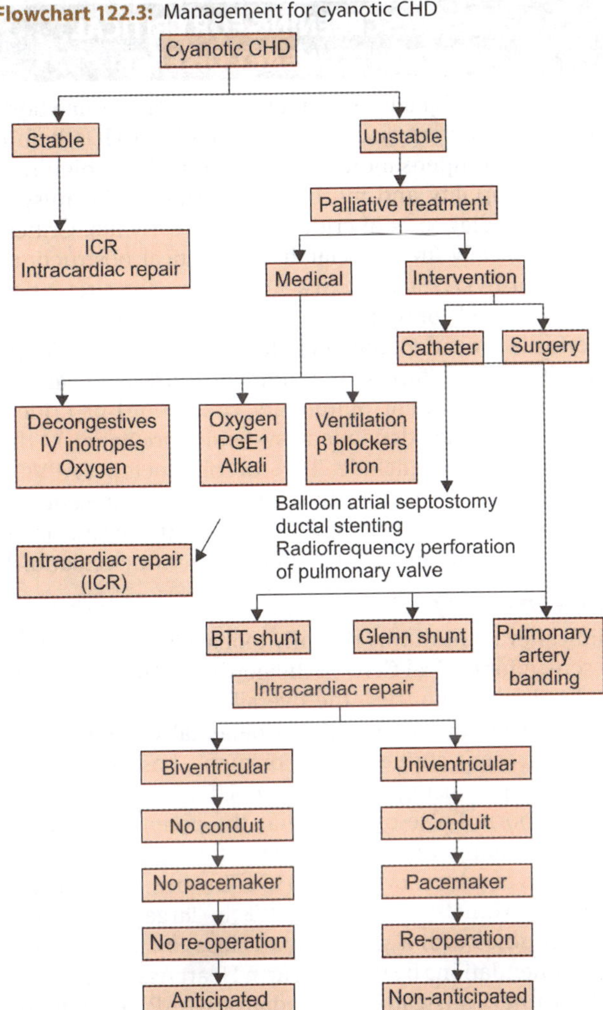

Dextrocardia gives rise to diagnostic findings in the skiagram and ECG. Dextrocardia has to be differentiated from dextroposition of the heart in which the heart is shifted to the right hemithorax due to lesions such as pulmonary fibrosis, pleural effusion or thoracic skeletal abnormalities.

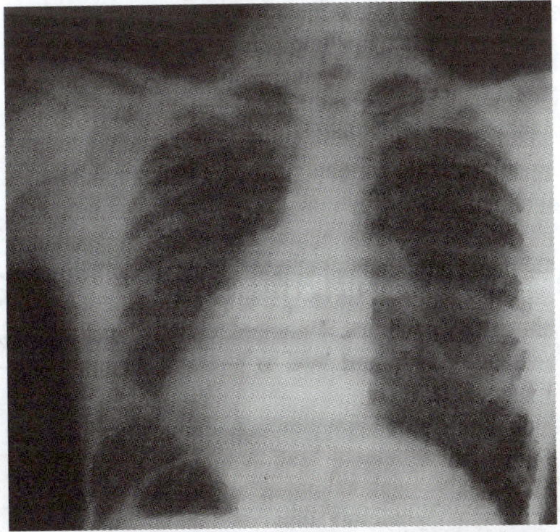

Fig. 122.32: Dextrocardia with situs inversus. ***Note:*** The heart is in the right hemithorax with apex to the right. The stomach (G) is under the right hemidiaphragm which is at the lower level than the left. The liver is on the left side (situs inversus). Associated anomalies are rare

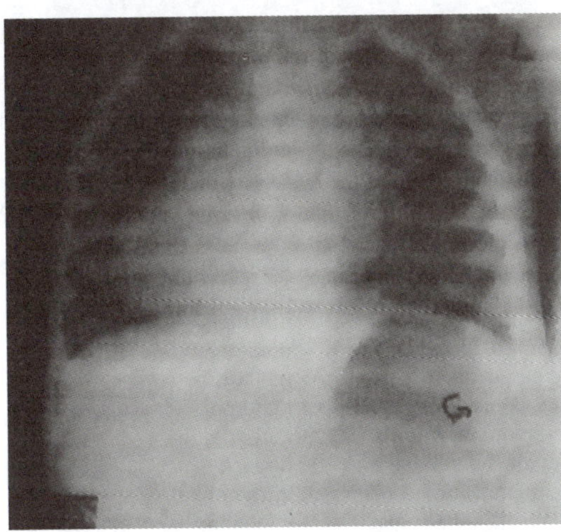

Fig. 122.33: Dextrocardia with situs solitus Heart is on the right with apex pointing to the right, stomach (G) is on the left, and liver is on the right. This anomaly is associated with complex malformations

Visceral heterotaxy can occur with right or left isomerism. The term isomerism refers to bilateral similarity, if not equivalence of structures.

Features of Right Isomerism

- Right isomerism:
  - Bilateral morphologic right bronchi
  - Bilateral morphologic right atrial appendages
- Visceral heterotaxy:
  - Liver: Transverse
  - Stomach: Left-sided, right-sided or rarely midline
  - Lungs: Trilobed
- Heart: Dextrocardia (common)
- Asplenia common but not invariable.

Features of Left Isomerism

- Left isomerism:
  - Bilateral morphologic left bronchi
  - Bilateral morphologic left atrial appendages
- Visceral heterotaxy:
  - Liver: Transverse
  - Stomach: Right-sided, occasionally left-sided, but not midline
  - Lungs bilobed
- Heart: Levocardia (common)
- Polysplenia.

PRENATAL DIAGNOSIS OF CONGENITAL HEART DISEASE

Fetal echocardiography enables a comprehensive evaluation of the fetal heart from as early as first trimester of pregnancy. A detailed fetal echocardiography is indicated in specific high-risk situations (Table 122.2), but basic screening views of the heart should be obtained as a part of the anomaly scan in all pregnancies. The ideal gestational age for performing fetal echocardiography is between 16 and 18 weeks gestation. A combination of four-chamber view with evaluation of the outflow tracts with a three-vessel view will enable detection of most critical forms of CHD. A basic cardiac rhythm assessment should also be performed to complete the study. Prenatal

Table 122.2: Indications for fetal echocardiography

Fetal	Maternal	Familial
• Abnormal four chamber view • Extracardiac anomalies—gastrointestinal tract, spina bifida • Chromosomal anomalies—VACTERL, trisomies, DiGeorge • Increased first trimester nuchal thickness • Nonimmune hydrops • Irregular heart beat—tachy/bradyarrhythmias • Abnormal cardiac axis • *In-vitro* fertilization	• Maternal congenital heart disease (CHD) • Teratogen exposure • Metabolic disorders—diabetes mellitus • Maternal autoimmune disease • Intrauterine infections	• Previous child with CHD • Paternal CHD • Mendelian syndromes—tuberous sclerosis, Noonan's, DiGeorge

Abbreviations: VACTERL = Vertebral anomalies, Anal atresia, Cardiac defects, Tracheooesophageal fistula, Renal and radial anomalies, Esophageal atresia, Limb defects

diagnosis of CHD offers more management options for the family depending on the complexity of the lesion, possibility of corrective intervention and the long-term outcomes after treatment. For very complex CHDs with suboptimal outcomes after treatment (e.g. HLHS, complex forms of univentricular heart) the option of medical termination of pregnancy maybe considered in accordance with the local rules and regulations of the region. For critical, but correctable lesions (e.g. transposition of great vessels, CoA, etc.), the option of planned delivery at or near a cardiac facility can result in a better planning of neonatal care leading to improved outcomes after corrective intervention. Fetal arrhythmias, especially tachyarrhythmias, are amenable to transplacental therapy. Several studies from the developed world have reported a significant positive impact of prenatal diagnosis on the outcomes of CHD, especially the critical forms. In the context of limited resource environments, prenatal diagnosis may facilitate a more optimal utilization of resources for CHD management by triaging those CHDs with better outcomes for a targeted postnatal cardiac care.

NEWBORN SCREENING FOR CRITICAL CONGENITAL HEART DISEASE

The principal objective of screening for CHD in newborn babies is to detect critical life-threatening CHDs before clinical decompensation. Several studies have highlighted the mortality and morbidity associated with missed or delayed diagnosis of critical CHD in early life. Critical CHDs typically are associated with critical obstructions to right or LVOTs leading to a state, where the circulation is maintained only in presence of an open ductus arteriosus (duct dependent circulation). These conditions include various forms of pulmonary atresia (cyanosis with duct dependent pulmonary circulation) or critical AS or CoA (duct dependent systemic circulation). The other conditions include TGA or obstructed TAPVCs. The hallmark of most of these lesions is the presence of cyanosis (uniform cyanosis or differential cyanosis in lower extremities in duct dependent systemic circulation).

Pulse Oximetry

Clinical evaluation was the only tool available in the past to screen for critical CHD in the newborn. However, even in developed countries, the overall sensitivity of careful clinical examination for critical neonatal CHD was only 50%. In recent studies, pulse oximetry has emerged as the most promising screening tool for critical CHD in the newborn. Pulse oximetry has the potential to detect clinically inapparent cyanosis and thus facilitates early diagnosis of critical cyanotic CHDs. The overall sensitivity of pulse oximetry is around 70% in large population-based studies with a specificity of close to 100%. Current recommendations by the American Heart Association and (AHA) American Academy of Pediatrics (AAP) recommend a single lower extremity screening 24 hours after birth for all babies and a repeat testing in case the initial screen is positive (oxygen saturation < 95%). The potential utility of this screening tool for larger populations of various ethnic backgrounds and healthcare infrastructures across the globe remains to be tested. As of now, a combination of antenatal screening, careful clinical examination after birth and pulse oxymetry offers the best possible method to screen for critical CHD in the newborn period.

Textbook of Medicine

CHAPTER
123

Chronic Valvular Heart Disease

N Sudhayakumar

Chapter Summary

- Mitral Valve Apparatus
  - Mitral Stenosis
  - Mitral Regurgitation
  - Mitral Valve Prolapse Syndrome
  - Aortic Stenosis

- Aortic Regurgitation
  - Acute Aortic Regurgitation
- Tricuspid Valve Lesions
  - Tricuspid Stenosis
  - Tricuspid Regurgitation
- Acquired Lesions of the Pulmonary Valve

INTRODUCTION

Valvular heart diseases are major contributors to cardiac morbidity and mortality all over the world; rheumatic fever being one of the common causes. Approximately 40% of patients with acute rheumatic carditis develop chronic valvular lesions as sequelae. The incidence of rheumatic heart disease (RHD) in India varies from 1.8 to 11.0 per 1,000 among school children as per the surveys conducted by Indian Council of Medical Research (ICMR) in different parts of India. Currently, there is a decrease in the incidence of rheumatic fever in India, especially, in states like Kerala. *Mitral, aortic, tricuspid* and *pulmonary valves* are affected in order of frequency; in many cases valvular lesions are multiple. Very rarely all the four valves are involved.

Common causes of chronic valvular heart disease

- Rheumatic fever
- Myxomatous degeneration as in mitral valve prolapse (MVP)
- Heritable disorders of connective tissue, e.g. Marfan syndrome
- Congenital
- Ischemic heart disease (IHD)
- Degenerative changes
- Infiltrative and storage diseases
- Collagen vascular diseases
- Rheumatoid disease
- Tumors of heart
- Infective causes
  - Infective endocarditis (IE)
  - Syphilis
  - Coxsackie B virus
- Miscellaneous causes
  - Drugs—fenfluramine, phentermine and dexfenfluramine (appetite suppressants)
  - Trauma
  - Anticardiolipin antibody
  - Hypereosinophilic syndrome (HES)

MITRAL VALVE APPARATUS

Mitral valve apparatus is a complex structure as shown in Figure 123.1. It includes—two leaflets, annulus, chordae tendineae, two papillary muscles, ventricular myocardium and the floor of left atrium (LA). Pathology involving any of these components can result in mitral stenosis (MS), regurgitation or both.

MITRAL STENOSIS (MS)

Rheumatic fever is the most common cause of narrowing of the mitral valve orifice and other causes, which are rare, include congenital lesions, storage disorders, connective tissue diseases (CTDs) and drugs. About 50% of patients with MS give history suggestive of antecedent rheumatic fever; others might have had subclinical episodes. In the developed countries, it takes about 5 years for stenosis to develop and another 5 years for it to become severe. However, in tropical countries like India and Africa where rheumatic fever prevalence is high, MS occurs at a younger age (juvenile MS), probably because of severe and multiple episodes of rheumatic fever.

Pathology and Pathophysiology

Rheumatic carditis results in inflammation followed by fibrosis resulting in commissural, cuspal and chordal fusion of the mitral valve apparatus resulting in narrowing of the mitral orifice. In long-standing cases, calcification develops. Normal mitral valve orifice is 4–6 cm^2 in adults (4 cm^2/m^2 body surface area). When it is reduced to 2.5 cm^2, auscultatory findings suggestive of MS appear. Based on the mitral valve area (MVA), stenosis is graded as mild, if aperture size is 2.5–1.6 cm^2; moderate, if orifice is 1.5–1.1 cm^2 and a valve area below 1 cm^2 is considered as severe.

Hemodynamically, MS means obstruction to flow of blood from LA to left ventricle (LV) resulting in transmitral diastolic pressure gradient, which is the hallmark of stenosis (Fig. 123.2). This leads to elevation of left atrial pressure that is reflected back to the pulmonary veins [pulmonary congestion and pulmonary venous hypertension (PVH)]. LA pressure in severe cases can rise to more than 25 mm Hg (normal being 4–12 mm Hg). To maintain the forward flow, pulmonary artery (PA) pressure has to rise, i.e. passive PA hypertension. Later, the PA pressure rises progressively due to reactive vasoconstriction (reactive pulmonary hypertension). Rarely, in long-standing cases, structural changes occur in the pulmonary vasculature resulting in the irreversible obliterative type of pulmonary arterial hypertension (PAH).

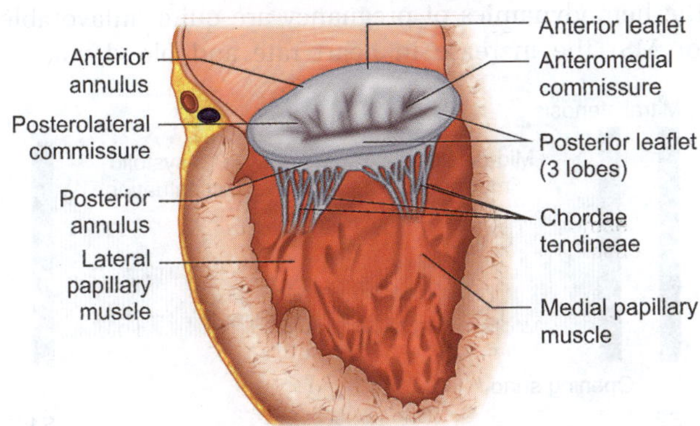

Fig. 123.1: Complex anatomy of the mitral valve apparatus

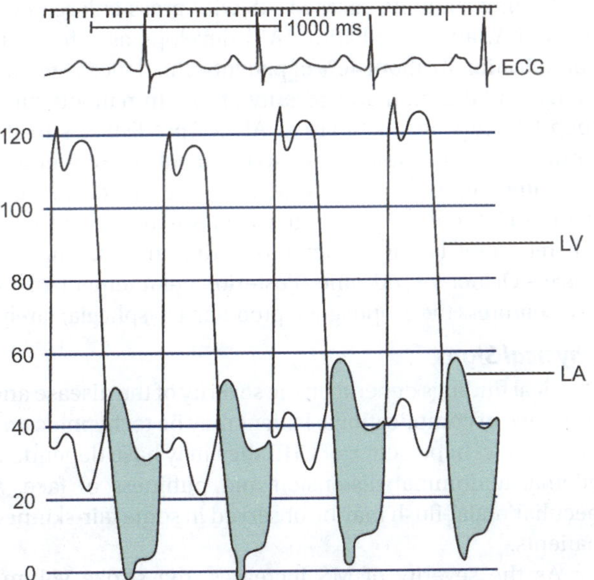

Fig. 123.2: Transmitral gradient (shaded green) in mitral stenosis; left atrium pressure is higher than left ventricle pressure in diastole

Abbreviations: ECG = Electrocardiogram; LV = Left ventricle; LA = Left atrium

Chronic pulmonary hypertension leads to right ventricular hypertrophy (RVH) and, eventually, tricuspid regurgitation (TR) and right ventricular (RV) failure.

Clinical Features

Symptoms

Mild-to-moderate MS may remain asymptomatic or may be only mildly symptomatic. Severe MS is mostly symptomatic. Initial symptoms are related to the elevated LA pressure being transmitted to the pulmonary veins and capillaries. Most common symptom is exertional dyspnea and its severity depends upon the degree of stenosis and, hence, the magnitude of the pulmonary capillary pressure. Exertion leads to tachycardia and increased venous return. During tachycardia, diastole gets shortened resulting in reduced left atrial emptying. Resultant stasis of blood in LA and the increased venous return during exercise leads to increased left atrial volume and pressure, producing the symptom of dyspnea. The rise in LA pressure causes pulmonary venous and capillary engorgement and when pulmonary capillary pressure goes above 25 mm Hg, transudation of fluid occurs into the interstitium and alveoli. As a result, compliance of the lung reduces which manifests as dyspnea, paroxysmal nocturnal dyspnea (PND), orthopnea and in acute cases as pulmonary edema. As the disease progresses, PAH ensues leading to TR and congestive heart failure (CHF), which manifest as edema, abdominal pain, puffiness of face, fatigue, loss of appetite, etc. Other common symptoms are palpitation, cough and hemoptysis.

> **Common causes of hemoptysis in mitral stenosis**
> - Recurrent bronchitis
> - During paroxysmal nocturnal dyspnea (PND)
> - During acute pulmonary edema
> - Pulmonary infarction
> - Rupture of bronchopulmonary veins due to rise in pulmonary venous pressure resulting in massive self-limiting hemoptysis (pulmonary apoplexy)

In long-standing cases of MS with gross enlargement of the LA, atrial fibrillation (AF) develops as a frequent complication in about 40% of patients. Incidence is related to age and duration and severity of MS. In patients more than 50 years age, 80% are in AF. AF predisposes to the formation of thrombi in the atria and subsequent embolization commonly manifesting as stroke. In severe cases with PAH, the dilated hypertensive PA may compress the left recurrent laryngeal nerve resulting in hoarseness of voice—Ortner's syndrome. Posterior enlargement of LA can compress the esophagus—producing dysphagia, rarely.

Physical Signs

Physical findings depend on the severity of the disease and presence of complications. Patient may be tachypneic and orthopneic. In presence of CHF, they may have dependent edema, abdominal distension and puffiness of face. A peculiar malar flush may be observed in some fair-skinned patients.

As the severity of MS increases, the stroke volume decreases, especially, when they develop pulmonary hypertension and cardiac failure. This results in a low-volume pulse (pulsus parvus). Totally irregular pulse should suggest the presence of AF. Jugular venous pulse during sinus rhythm may show prominent A wave in cases with PAH and prominent V wave in those with TR. The A wave will be absent when the rhythm is AF due to absence of atrial contraction. In patients with CHF, the mean jugular venous pressure (JVP) is elevated.

The apex beat is characteristically tapping and it is usually felt in the normal position. A diastolic thrill may be palpable over the apex beat. This can be made more prominent by palpating in the left lateral position. In severe cases when they develop PAH, systolic pulsation of the dilated PA and palpable shock of the loud second heart sound (S2) can be felt in the second left intercostal space (2LICS). The RVH can be felt as left parasternal heave and epigastric pulsation.

The characteristic auscultatory findings of MS include a loud sharp first heart sound (S1), rough rumbling mid diastolic murmur and the high-pitched *opening snap* (OS). The murmur is best heard over apex in left lateral position during expiration and is accentuated by increasing heart rate (exercise). During sinus rhythm, the atrial contraction increases the LA pressure and produces the presystolic accentuation of the murmur; this accentuation is often lost in presence of AF. The murmur starts with a sharp high-pitched sound—OS—which is widely transmitted and, hence, it can be heard along left sternal border also (Fig. 123.3). The OS may disappear, when the valve becomes nonpliable due to fibrosis or calcification. In presence of PAH, pulmonary component (P2) of second heart sound (S2) gets accentuated and split of S2 may get narrowed. The early diastolic murmur secondary to PAH (**Graham Steell murmur**) is usually localized to the pulmonary area [in contrast to aortic regurgitation (AR) murmur, which is widely transmitted along lower left sternal border] and may be preceded by an ejection click. In severe PAH, the pansystolic murmur of TR and a fourth sound may be audible along left sternal border. As RV failure sets in, third heart sound also becomes audible.

Severity of MS can be assessed with reasonable accuracy based on clinical features. Severe symptoms [New York Heart Association (NYHA class III/IV, orthopnea and PND)], PAH and CHF indicate severe MS. As the severity increases, the mid-diastolic murmur (MDM) becomes longer and the OS moves closer to S2 resulting in short S2-OS interval.

Pregnancy and Mitral Stenosis

The hemodynamics of pregnancy are quite unfavorable for MS. The increase in heart rate and blood volume

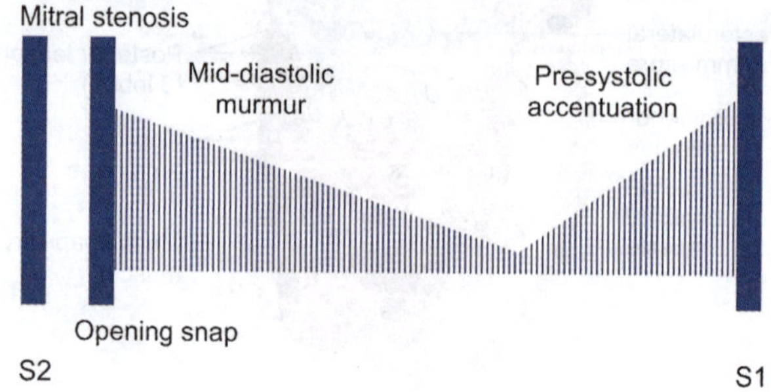

Fig. 123.3: Auscultatory signs of mitral stenosis

increases the LA pressure and, hence, the patients will become more symptomatic. They may develop pulmonary edema or CHF, especially, during mid-trimester and in the peripartum period when the hemodynamic load is maximum. Hence, proper evaluation and counseling have to be done before pregnancy; in severe cases, it is safer to have mitral valvotomy before they conceive. If, during pregnancy, the patient becomes symptomatic balloon mitral valvotomy (BMV) can be done safely in second trimester.

Investigations

Basic investigations, like 12-lead electrocardiogram (ECG) and skiagram of the chest provide valuable information; near complete data can be obtained by a meticulous echo-cardiographic study. Cardiac catheterization is seldom indicated.

Electrocardiogram

In addition to documenting the presence of AF (Fig. 123.4), ECG also provides information regarding chamber enlargements. When in sinus rhythm, left atrial enlargement produces a broad-notched P wave in lead II (P mitrale). In cases with PAH, there will be evidence of RVH manifesting as right axis deviation and tall R waves in lead V1. QRS axis correlates with severity of MS. When QRS axis is $0 \pm 60°$ the MVA is more than 1.3 cm^2 and if more than $+ 60°$, MVA is less than 1.3 cm^2. Axis more than $+ 150°$ indicates PA pressures at systemic levels.

Radiology

The characteristic X-ray findings include (Figs 123.5A to D):

- Straightening of the left border of the heart, which is often due to the small LV and the prominence of left atrial appendage below the PA
- Prominent main PA segment in cases with PAH
- ***Enlargement of the LA: Superiorly***—pushing up the left bronchus, which becomes more horizontal and manifesting as widening of carinal angle or splaying of the left bronchus; ***leftward***—causing a prominent left atrial appendage along left border; ***rightward***—giving rise to the double shadow along right border, a shadow with increased density having a convex border medial to right atrial (RA) border, ***posteriorly***—leading to compression of the lower part of the esophagus. The indentation caused by the enlarged LA can be demonstrated by a barium swallow picture taken in the right anterior oblique view.

- ***Pulmonary vasculature abnormalities:*** The earliest evidence of PVH is the redistribution of pulmonary blood flow from the normal lower zone dominance to the upper lobe, i.e. prominent upper lobe vessels. In severe cases when PAH develops, the main PA and its branches become prominent
- ***Evidence of fluid transudation:*** When the pulmonary capillary pressure exceeds the oncotic pressure, fluid transudes into the interstitium, alveoli and pleural spaces. Acute rise in LA pressure leads to pouring out of fluid into the alveoli producing the classical bat's wing appearance of pulmonary edema. Excess fluid drainage by the lymphatics results in dilated and fibrosed interlobular lymph channels producing the ***Kerley B lines (short horizontal lines seen near the costophrenic angles more on the right side)***
- RV and RA enlargement—when they develop TR and CHF
- Miliary mottling pattern in the lung field—seen in patients with recurrent hemoptysis due to deposition of hemosiderin pigments
- Occasionally, calcification of the mitral valve can also be picked up, especially, by fluoroscopy
- Radiology can be normal in mild cases.

Echocardiography (Fig. 123.6)

This is the most useful and reliable noninvasive method for evaluation of MS. Echocardiography can detect the structural details of the mitral valve including calcification, thickening, mobility and subvalvular pathology and also presence of clot in LA. MVA can be measured and severity can be graded. Presence of other valvular lesions and ventricular function can also be assessed. A scoring system by Abascal, et al. has been found useful in assessing the suitability of mitral valve for BMV. This score evaluates four factors—(1) Leaflet mobility, (2) leaflet thickening, (3) calcification and (4) degree of subvalvular fusion. A score of eight or less indicates excellent results with BMV and score more than 10 indicates suboptimal results. Transesophageal echocardiography (TEE) provides better images of the LA and mitral valve and this is more sensitive in detecting LA thrombi. Doppler echocardiogram gives additional information like gradient across mitral valve, PA pressure and associated mitral regurgitation (MR).

Complications

Major complications of MS include acute pulmonary edema, PAH, cardiac failure, AF and thromboembolism; infective endocarditis (IE) is relatively rare in MS. Acute

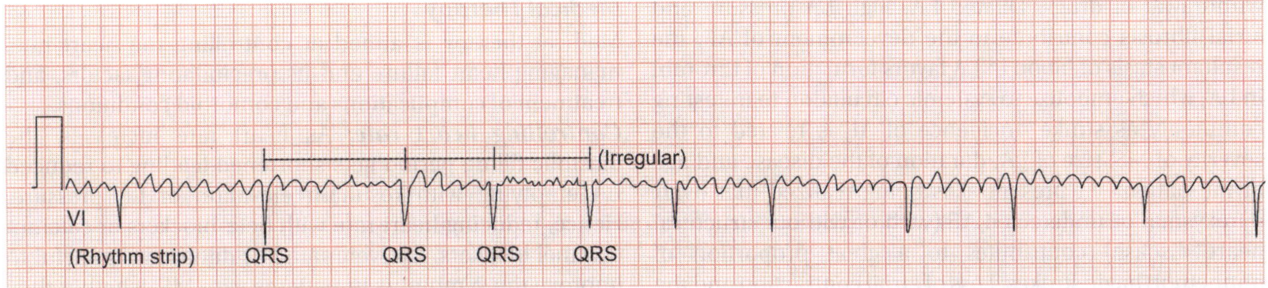

Fig. 123.4: Atrial fibrillation—ECG absence of P waves, which are replaced by fibrillary waves (irregular baseline) and irregular R-R interval

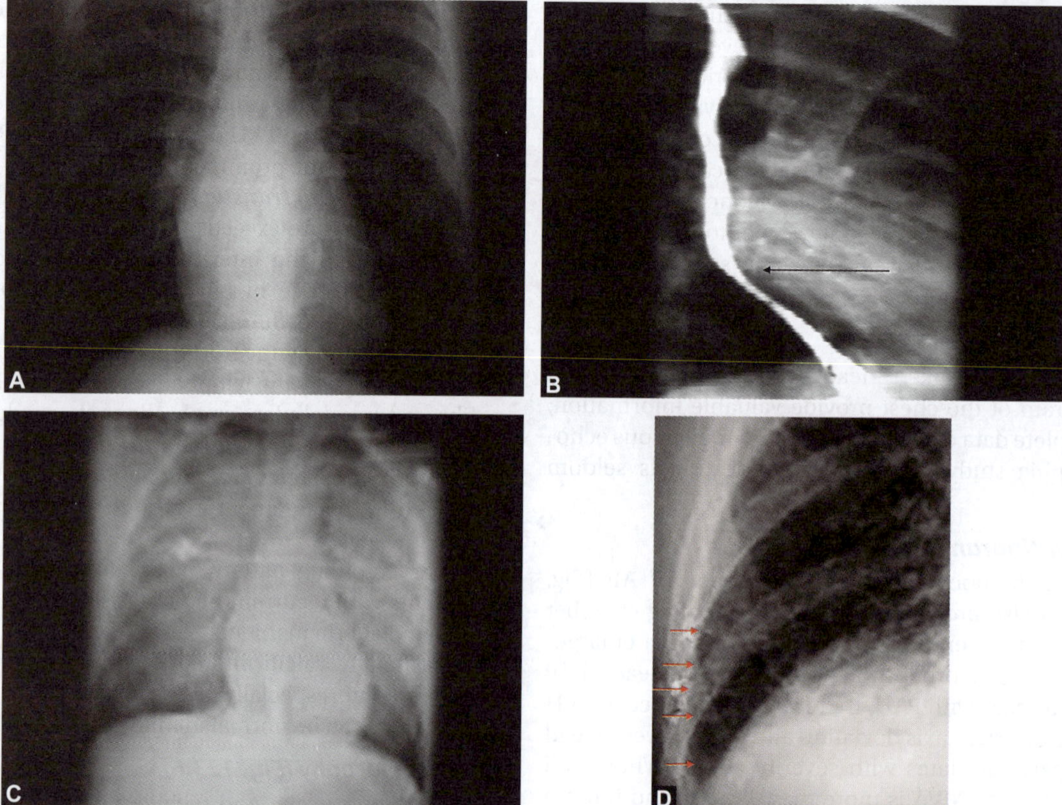

Figs 123.5A to D: Radiological findings in mitral stenosis: **A.** Straight left border, left atrium enlargement (double shadow along right border), left atrium appendage (below pulmonary artery) and prominent upper lobe vessels; **B.** Indentation of lower-third of esophagus by the dilated left atrium; **C.** Bat's wing appearance of pulmonary edema; **D.** Kerley B lines (arrows)

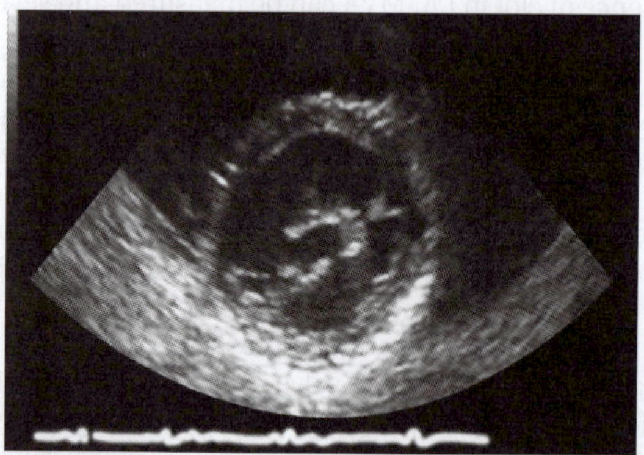

Fig. 123.6: Parasternal short-axis view showing the thickened mitral leaflets with narrow orifice in the center of the round left ventricle

pulmonary edema, a fatal complication unless treated promptly, is the sequelae of an acute elevation of LA pressure, which is precipitated by many factors like infection, AF, anemia, pregnancy undue exertion and withdrawal of drugs. Dilated LA, high LA pressure and atrial fibrosis contribute to the development of AF; the resultant stasis of blood in LA favors formation of thrombi in LA, which embolize to systemic circulation manifesting commonly as stroke. Incidence of AF is related to the severity of MS, size of LA, duration of the disease and age of the patient. At present, it is being realized that overt paroxysmal or undetected AF (with or without structural heart disease) contributes to a great proportion of nonhemorrhagic strokes. Loss of atrial contraction and the fast heart rate in AF elevates the LA pressure and lowers the cardiac output leading to acute pulmonary edema and cardiac failure.

Prognosis

Prognosis of patients with MS depends on the severity of stenosis, age, presence of PAH and most importantly, the functional status of patient. Ten years mortality in patients in NYHA class II is 85% while those in class IV seldom survive beyond 10 years. Majority of deaths are due to CHF (around 60%) and systemic embolism (around 20%).

Treatment

General Measures

As such, MS does not resolve with medical treatment. In a considerable proportion of cases, several coexistent remediable factors like anemia, systemic and pulmonary infections, thyrotoxicosis and pregnancy aggravate the disability. Proper management of these conditions will give considerable symptomatic relief.

Medical Therapy

Medical therapy is aimed at controlling the heart rate, managing heart failure and its precipitating factors, and treatment of complications and comorbid conditions.

Controlling heart rate: As heart rate increases, the diastolic filling period gets shortened leading to reduced LA emptying with resultant elevation of LA pressure. Hence, reducing heart rate with beta-blockers or calcium channel blockers, like verapamil or diltiazem, is useful to improve the symptoms in patients with MS, whether they are in sinus rhythm or in AF.

Treatment of cardiac failure: Rest, fluid and salt restriction and adequate doses of diuretics (furosemide, spironolactone alone or in combination) along with small dose of digoxin (especially in presence of AF) help to control the ***cardiac failure*** and stabilize the patient prior to valvotomy.

Atrial fibrillation (AF): In patients with MS-developing AF, the main aim is to control heart rate rather than aiming to restore sinus rhythm (as it is difficult to maintain sinus rhythm in view of large LA) and to prevent thromboembolism. Hence, these patients require long-term oral anticoagulation. Any episode of embolism is a definite indication for anticoagulation irrespective of the cardiac rhythm; older age and very large LA are also possible indications for anticoagulation even in the presence of sinus rhythm. Paroxysmal AF has been detected in many such cases before they develop persistent AF.

Rheumatic fever prophylaxis: Long-term antibiotic prophylaxis against rheumatic fever recurrence is essential, ideally with parenteral penicillin (benzathine penicillin 1.2 million units once in 3/4 weeks).

IE prophylaxis: Currently IE prophylaxis is not recommended for pure MS.

Definitive Treatment

Relief of the mitral valve obstruction (commissurotomy/valvotomy) is the definitive management for significant MS (symptomatic patients, severe MS, presence of PAH, etc.). Table 123.1 shows the echocardiographic criteria for grading the severity of MS. Valvotomy can be achieved by catheter intervention (percutaneous mitral commissurotomy—PMC/BMV) or by surgical approach. If the valve is heavily calcified or if there is associated significant MR, patient will require mitral valve replacement (MVR).

Balloon mitral valvotomy (BMV): Catheter with inflatable balloon (Inoue, Accura) is introduced via the femoral vein and manipulated to LA by puncturing interatrial septum under fluoroscopy; the balloon is positioned across the mitral valve and inflated to open up the valve (Figs 123.7A and B). This has now become the treatment of choice in patients with pliable valve and has replaced closed or open surgical valvotomy. Randomized clinical trials comparing BMV and surgical techniques, like open mitral valvotomy (OMV) and closed mitral valvotomy (CMV), have shown no significant differences in terms of acute results, rates, clinical improvement and exercise time at 1 year and 3 years.

Surgical correction: Surgery is indicated, if the valve is not pliable or if there is associated significant MR or LA thrombus:

- ***Closed mitral valvotomy:*** In this technique, surgical commissurotomy is performed on beating heart without cardiopulmonary bypass, using either transatrial or transventricular approach. Pliable noncalcified valves without subvalvular fusion achieve best results
- ***Open mitral valvotomy:*** In developed countries, OMV is preferred to CMV, if BMV is not feasible. OMV allows direct inspection of the valve under cardiopulmonary bypass so that commissures can be split under direct vision. Mortality in different centers varies from 1 to 3%
- ***Mitral valve replacement:*** MVR is the accepted procedure for patients who are not candidates for surgical commissurotomy or BMV. Mortality is less than 5%. However, postoperative problems of prosthetic valves, like risk of anticoagulation, IE, valve malfunction and embolic events, are of concern. Basically, there are two types of prosthetic valves: Metallic and bioprosthetic (Figs 123.8A and B). Bioprostheses are less durable, but have the advantage that they do not require anticoagulation; hence, preferred in those who have contraindications for long-term anticoagulation.

Mitral Restenosis

Rheumatic pathology is a progressive phenomenon and, hence, following valvotomy many patients develop restenosis after a variable period of follow-up. Diagnosis is made by serial clinical and echocardiographic evaluation. Murmur and OS may persist even after successful valvotomy; but murmur will be short and S2-OS interval will be longer. Recurrence of symptoms and clinical findings after successful valvotomy (as defined

Table 123.1: Echocardiographic grading of severity of mitral stenosis			
	Mild	*Moderate*	*Severe*
Mean gradient (mm Hg)	< 5	5–10	> 10
PA systolic pressure (mm Hg)	< 30	30–50	> 50
Valve area	> 1.5	1.0–1.5	< 1.0

Abbreviation: PA = Pulmonary artery

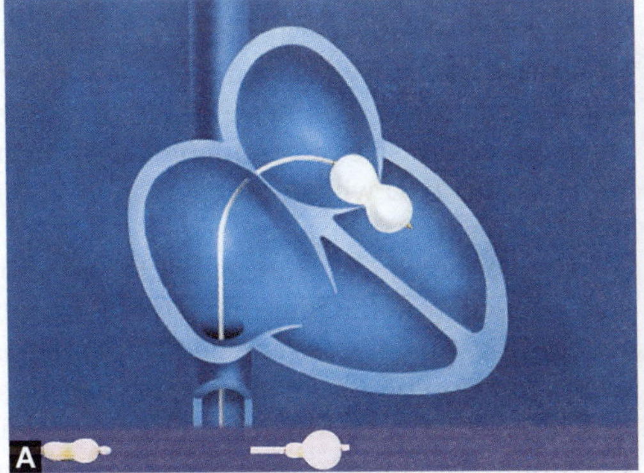
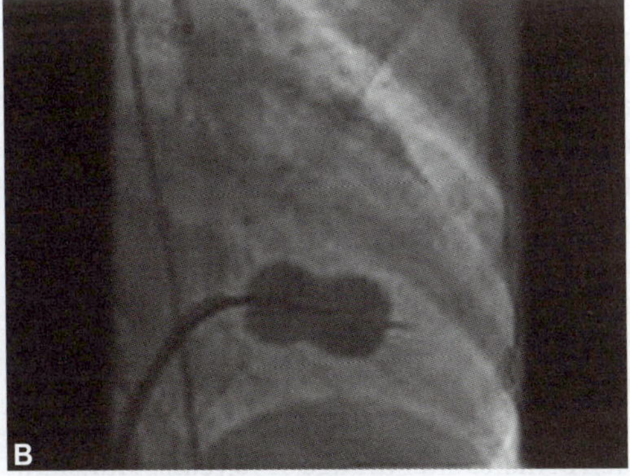

Figs 123.7A and B: Balloon mitral valvotomy: **A.** Illustration; **B.** X-ray of balloon mitral valvotomy

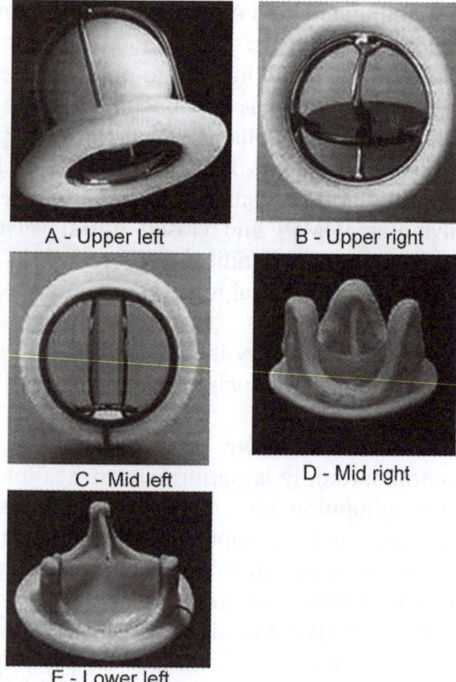

Figs 123.8A and B: A. Different types of prosthetic valves; **B.** X-ray chest lateral view showing metallic valves in mitral (inferior and posterior) and aortic positions

by sustained improvement in symptoms by at least two functional classes, achievement of MVA to more than 1.5 cm² or by more than 50% from prevalvotomy level) along with echocardiographic evidence of reduction in MVA are the clues for restenosis. True restenosis occurs in about 20% of patients by 10 years. Restenosis produces recurrence of symptoms similar to the original condition and may require evaluation and reintervention—re-BMV or surgical option.

MITRAL REGURGITATION (MITRAL INCOMPETENCE)

The complex anatomy of the mitral valve apparatus has already been illustrated in Figure 123.1. Coordinated functioning of all the components is essential for proper mitral valve closure, which is an active phenomenon requiring normal contraction of the myocardium and papillary muscles to maintain optimal coaptation of the leaflets [as the left ventricular pressure is much higher than the LA pressure in systole (LV)]. Defective function of one or more of these components may lead to inadequate coaptation of the mitral leaflets in systole giving rise to various degrees of mitral regurgitation (MR). The common etiological factors of isolated MR are listed in Box 123.1. As the incidence of rheumatic fever is coming down, nonrheumatic causes, especially mitral valve prolapse have become the common causes for MR.

In rheumatic MR, the valve leaflets are thickened, fibrosed and contracted; the chordae are also shortened and fused. This process causes inadequate closure of the mitral leaflets in systole and, hence, MR results.

Ischemic heart disease (IHD) leading to MR is commonly seen in males after the age of 40 years. Transient or permanent dysfunction of the papillary muscles leads

---

Box 123.1: Common cause of mitral regurgitation

Chronic MR
- ***Inflammatory:*** Rheumatic, lupus erythematosus and scleroderma
- ***Degenerative:*** Mitral valve prolapse, Marfan's syndrome and Ehlers-Danlos syndrome
- ***Congenital:*** Cleft mitral leaflet and parachute mitral valve
- ***Infective:*** IE
- IHD
- Cardiomyopathies
- Mitral annular calcification
- Trauma
- Postsurgical/intervention

Acute MR
- ***Mitral leaflet disorders:*** IE, acute rheumatic fever and trauma
- ***Rupture of chordae:*** Spontaneous, endocarditis, myxomatous valve (prolapse) and trauma
- ***Annulus disorders:*** Endocarditis, surgery and paravalvular leak
- ***Papillary muscle disorders:*** CAD and trauma
- Mitral valve prosthesis disorders.

Abbreviations: MR = Mitral regurgitation; IE = Infective endocarditis; IHD = Ischemic heart disease; CAD = Coronary artery disease

to MR, posterior papillary muscle being more commonly involved. Occasionally, rupture of the papillary muscles may complicate myocardial infarction (MI), which results in severe acute MR. Ischemia of the myocardium can result in transient dyskinesia of the portion of LV, where the papillary muscles are implanted and this may result in MR. Chronic IHD with ventricular aneurysm may also be associated with MR.

Cardiomyopathy involving the LV can produce MR. It may be seen in all the three main types of cardiomyopathy [endomyocardial fibrosis, dilated cardiomyopathy (DCM) and hypertrophic cardiomyopathy], mechanisms being different. Severity of MR varies widely in these cases. In IE, rupture of chordae may occur and this gives rise to acute MR. Annular dilatation as in Marfan's syndrome and mitral annular calcification seen in the elderly result in failure of coaptation of the leaflets causing MR.

Hemodynamic Changes

As the LV pressure exceeds the LA pressure in systole, if the valve does not coapt properly, blood regurgitates from LV into the LA during systole. This along with the normal pulmonary venous return to LA in systole increases the LA volume. The enhanced volume of blood in LA flows across the mitral valve in next diastole leading to diastolic overload of the LV. The forward systolic output into the aorta is maintained normal or near-normal for considerable periods, but the systolic ejection time is shortened and this gives the characteristic rapid upstroke for the pulse. LV function is well-compensated for quite long; in severe cases, left ventricular dilatation and hypertrophy develop. Ultimately, left ventricular failure (LVF) supervenes resulting in pulmonary hypertension and RV failure, as well. Fall in the ejection fraction (EF) below 60% and rise in the end systolic volume of LV are indicators of poor prognosis.

Clinical Features

Clinical picture depends on severity of MR, LV function, PA pressure and cardiac rhythm. Symptoms are similar to that in MS but quite delayed. Many patients with even severe MR may remain asymptomatic or minimally symptomatic for a long period till they develop LV dysfunction. The only abnormality in mild cases is the presence of a pansystolic murmur over the cardiac apex. In severe MR, pulse is described as pseudocollapsing (normal/low volume collapsing) due to the abrupt ejection of the forward stroke volume, which is not high. Left ventricular enlargement is evidenced by the forcible apex beat, which is shifted down and out. S1 is usually soft in severe MR, especially, if the etiology is rheumatic. Occasionally in MR due to nonrheumatic causes like mitral valve prolapse, S1 can be loud. Early closure of aortic valve due to the shortened LV ejection time can make S2 widely split; but as LV dysfunction sets in the split becomes closer. Loud P2 indicates development of PAH. The characteristic murmur of MR is a high-pitched soft blowing pansystolic murmur heard best over the apex beat. In nonrheumatic MR, like mitral valve prolapse or ischemic, the murmur may be mid or late systolic. In cases, where the anterior mitral leaflet is damaged, the murmur is conducted to the axilla because of the direction of the regurgitant stream from LV toward the body of LA. If posterior leaflet is involved, the murmur is conducted to the anterior chest and to the upper sternal border because the regurgitant stream impinges on the interatrial septum adjacent to the aortic root. In moderate and severe cases, the murmur occupies the whole of systole and is moderately loud in intensity. The enhanced flow of blood from LA to LV in diastole produces a left ventricular third heart sound and/or a decrescendo MDM over apex. In severe cases, evidence of PAH may be evident, which leads to TR and RV failure.

Acute Mitral Regurgitation

Acute onset of severe MR is a medical emergency, which manifests as acute pulmonary edema. LV systolic pressure is acutely transmitted to the noncompliant LA resulting in marked elevation of LA and pulmonary venous and capillary pressures. Common causes of acute severe MR are acute myocardial infarction (acute MI) with papillary muscle rupture, IE with leaflet destruction, chordal rupture as in myxomatous pathology, trauma and acute rheumatic fever.

Investigations

Electrocardiogram

ECG remains normal in mild cases. In moderate and severe cases, left ventricular hypertrophy (LVH) and LA enlargement are seen. In later stages, development of AF can be confirmed by ECG. As PAH develops, ECG may show features of biventricular hypertrophy. The ECG may also help in determining the etiology of MR as in the case of IHD or cardiomyopathy.

Chest X-ray

In mild to moderate cases, X-ray can be normal. In severe MR, cardiomegaly of left ventricular type and LA enlargement are seen (Fig. 123.9). Very large LA (giant LA) occurs in some of the severe cases. The pulmonary findings mimic those in MS.

Echocardiography

As in any other valvular lesions, echocardiography is the most useful noninvasive investigation to assess the etiology and severity of MR (Fig. 123.10). It is also useful to decide the timing and choice of surgery. With widespread use of Doppler and color Doppler echocardiography, severity of MR can be assessed accurately. Information on ventricular function and pulmonary hemodynamics are obtainable from echocardiographic studies obviating the need for invasive investigations. TEE provides better information regarding the nature of the pathology, presence of LA clots and choice of the procedure (surgery/intervention) needed. Newer imaging modality, like magnetic resonance imaging (MRI), may provide additional information. Cardiac catheterization is seldom indicated (in patients above 40 years to assess coronary artery status prior to surgery).

Complications

These are similar to those seen in MS; however, the risk of IE is relatively high. Development of PAH is relatively late compared to MS.

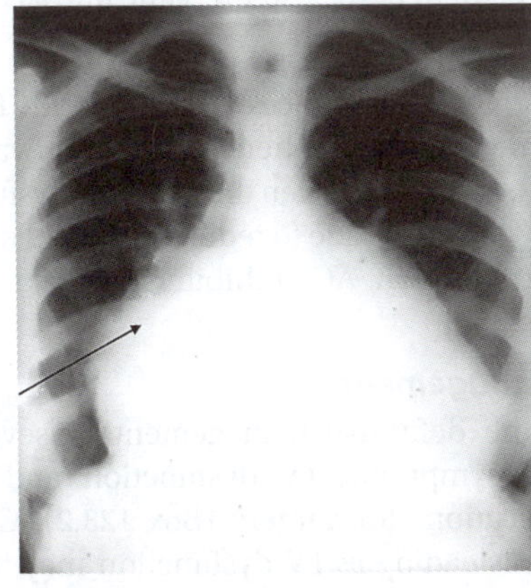

Fig. 123.9: X-ray findings in severe mitral regurgitation. **Note:** The cardiomegaly and aneurysmal left atrium (arrow)

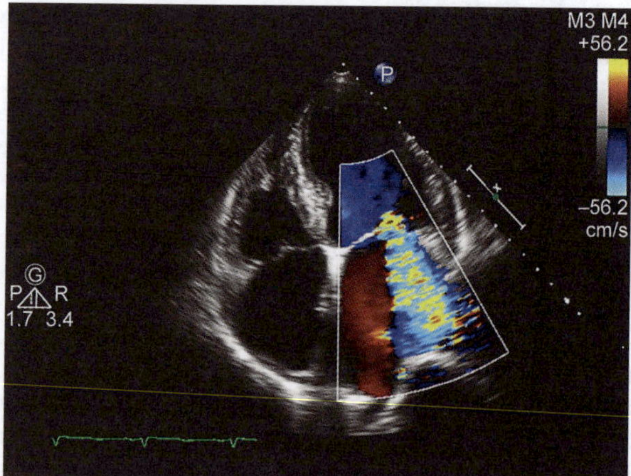

Fig. 123.10: Color Doppler echocardiography in mitral regurgitation (ventricles above and atria below); mosaic color pattern of the mitral regurgitation jet in left atrium during systole (atrioventricular valves are closed)

Course and Prognosis

Mild MR usually remains asymptomatic; progression to severe MR occurs in only a small percentage of these patients, usually following IE or chordal rupture. Moderate and severe cases become symptomatic in due course. Development of pulmonary hypertension is relatively slow in MR and the pulmonary pressure tends to be lower than that seen in MS. Severe MR usually progresses and results in CHF. AF leads to systemic thromboembolism, which contributes to morbidity and mortality. Five-year survival in symptomatic patients, who declined surgery, was reported to be only 30%. In contrast, the prognosis of patients with asymptomatic severe MR and normal LV function is good with an annual mortality of less than 1%.

Treatment

Management depends on the etiology and severity of MR and presence of complications, like AF, PAH, cardiac failure, etc. Mild MR requires only follow-up and endocarditis prophylaxis. If the etiology is rheumatic, rheumatic fever prophylaxis has to be given as in MS. Patients with severe MR presenting with symptoms of congestion require adequate dose of diuretics and vasodilators, like angiotensin-converting enzyme inhibitors (ACEI). In presence of CHF, digoxin is indicated especially, if they are in AF. Management of AF is in the same line as in MS.

Afterload Reduction

Reducing the aortic resistance can enhance the LV forward stroke volume to aorta and hence, the role of vasodilators in severe MR, especially, when they have LV dysfunction. In acute MR, IV nitroprusside to reduce afterload may be life-saving. In chronic MR, ACE inhibitors or oral hydralazine may be used.

Surgical Management

Surgery is the definitive management in severe cases. Presence of symptoms, LV dysfunction and PAH are definite indications for surgery (Box 123.2). Calculating EF can be misleading as LV dysfunction may be present even with normal EF (LV empties part of the stroke volume to the low-resistant LA). Mitral valve repair and MVR are the available options. Valve repair is preferred, whenever possible, especially in nonrheumatic MR. Rheumatic MR usually requires valve replacement as the leaflets are grossly damaged or calcified.

Optimal timing of surgery is important. Patients with asymptomatic MR should be followed-up periodically to decide the progression of MR as well as to detect onset of LV dysfunction. Aim is to give the corrective treatment before onset of LV dysfunction. Recently, the mortality of MVR has declined in good centers to 1–2%, so that surgical-corrective treatment can be advised more liberally. However, surgery in presence of severe LV dysfunction (EF < 30%) carries a high mortality and such patients may be followed-up with optimal medical management and restriction of physical activity.

Nonsurgical catheter interventions, like annular rings and mitral valve clipping, are also being done for selected nonrheumatic MR.

MITRAL VALVE PROLAPSE SYNDROME

Syn: Mid-systolic click syndrome, Floppy valve syndrome, Barlow's syndrome

Prolapse of the mitral valve into the left atrial cavity during systole may develop in 5–10% of apparently healthy young adults. Mitral valve prolapse syndrome (MVPS) is a heterogeneous condition. When strict echocardiographic criteria are applied, the frequency of this disorder is 3% in the general population. Most of the cases are sporadic; but autosomal-dominant familial incidence is noted in a few. In most of them, the abnormality remains asymptomatic till detected by routine medical examination or investigative procedures. In some, the valve cusps show myxomatous degeneration, which makes them redundant. MVP may be classified into three types:

1. MVPS—younger age, predominantly females, classical click, murmur and benign long-term course
2. Myxomatous mitral valve (MMV) disease—elderly males, high likelihood of progression
3. Secondary (MVP)—Marfan syndrome, Ehlers-Danlos syndrome, other CTDs, rheumatic fever, hypertrophic cardiomyopathy, atrial septal defect (ASD) and hyperthyroidism.

MVP may exist with or without MR. The mechanism of myxomatous degeneration of the valve leaflets is not clear. The middle spongiosa layer of the valve cusps is thickened due to accumulation of proteoglycans. The leaflets and chordae become abnormal. There are abnormalities in the distribution and architecture of fibrillin, elastin and

---

Box 123.2: Indications for surgery in chronic mitral regurgitation

- Symptomatic severe MR
- Moderate MR with class III/IV symptoms
- Asymptomatic severe MR, if:
  - LVEF is < 60%
  - LV end systolic diameter is > 40 mm
  - In AF
  - PAH develops

Abbreviations: MR = Mitral regurgitation; LVEF = Left ventricular ejection fraction; LV = Left ventricle; PAH = Pulmonary arterial hypertension; AF = Atrial fibrillation

collagen I and II. Chordal rupture may complicate the lesion resulting in acute severe MR.

Clinical Features

Majority of patients with MVP remain asymptomatic for a long period till they develop severe MR, which occurs only in a small percentage. Palpitation, vague chest pain, dyspnea and noncardiac symptoms such as vascular headache and anxiety state are not uncommon. In a few, there may be associated spasm of the coronary artery; undue stretch on the papillary muscles may also impair the blood flow in the branches of the coronary artery adjacent to them. These factors may lead to anginal pain. Palpitation may result from anxiety or arrhythmias such as ectopic beats or rarely paroxysmal tachycardias (both supraventricular and ventricular).

Apart from the features of associated clinical entities, MVP has typical auscultatory findings—a nonejection systolic click and a mid or late systolic murmur, best heard over the apex. Compared to aortic ejection click, the nonejection click of MVP is late (at least 0.14 seconds after S2) and is dynamic in timing.

As the LV size decreases (reduced venous return, reduced afterload, increased contractility and tachy-cardia), the prolapse occurs earlier resulting in early click and long murmur and vice-versa. This is the basis of dynamic auscultation in MVP. On standing and during the straining phase of Valsalva maneuver, the venous return decreases and heart rate increases resulting in early click and long murmur; the reverse occurs in supine position, on squatting, during release phase of Valsalva and expiration. In general, all murmurs increase on squatting and decrease on standing except the murmurs of MVP and hypertrophic obstructive cardiomyopathy (HOCM). As the severity of MR increases, the murmur becomes longer and may be even pansystolic, when the click may not be audible.

ECG and X-ray findings are similar to other cases of MR. Echocardiography is diagnostic for MVP. Thickening with classical billowing of the leaflet into LA is the characteristic finding of MVP (Fig. 123.11). Other findings are those of the associated MR. More than 2 mm billowing of one or

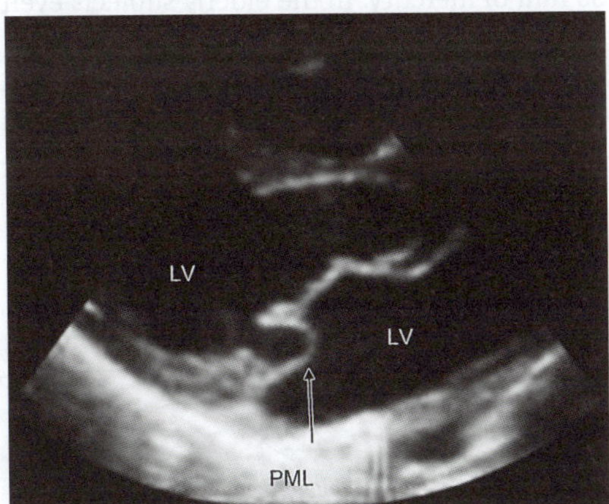

Fig. 123.11: Parasternal long-axis view showing the typical billowing of posterior mitral leaflet (arrow) in mitral valve prolapsed

Abbreviations: LV = Left ventricle; LA = Left atrium; PML = Posterior mitral leaflet

both leaflets in parasternal long-axis view as well as apical four chamber view is diagnostic.

Complications

Ninety percent of cases of MVP are hemodynamically normal. Ten percent develop significant MR; some may progress and become severe in which case the complications are similar to any other type of severe MR. Acute MR may result from chordal rupture. In presence of MR, the risk of endocarditis is high. Sudden cardiac death due to ventricular arrhythmias is rare.

Treatment

Management is in the same line as for any case of MR. However, patients who are anxious and having ventricular ectopics may benefit with beta-blockers.

AORTIC VALVE LESIONS

AORTIC STENOSIS

Obstruction to the LV outflow [aortic stenosis (AS)] can occur at different levels resulting in valvular, subvalvular and supravalvular stenosis. Unless specified, AS refers to valvular stenosis, which is discussed below.

Etiology

Valvular AS has three principal causes: (1) Congenital bicuspid aortic valve (BAV) with or without superimposed calcification, (2) rheumatic fever with fibrosis, commis-sural fusion and calcification, and (3) degenerative calcific AS of the elderly (Figs 123.12A to C). Current evidence is that stenosis developing in congenital BAV is the most common cause. Above the age of 70 years, degenerative calcification is frequent. In a series of 933 patients undergoing surgery for AS, bicuspid valve accounted for more than 50% (< 70 years—65% and >70 years—40%). Other rare causes include congenital unicuspid valve, athe-rosclerotic in severe hypercholesterolemia, ochronosis with alkaptonuria and rheumatoid arthritis (RA).

Congenital Aortic Stenosis

Rarely, children are born with critical AS due to unicuspid aortic valve. Such children are quite sick with high mortality rate. However, the most frequent congenital malformation, i.e. the BAV are functionally competent at birth and in childhood. As age advances due to hemodynamic trauma and calcification, they develop progressive stenosis with or without regurgitation.

Rheumatic Aortic Stenosis

Active rheumatic endocarditis of the aortic valve leads to thickening of the valve cusps with fusion of one or all commissures. This results in varying degrees of narrowing of the aortic valve orifice. Subsequently, hemodynamic stress on this abnormal valve produces further degene-rative changes and consequent calcification. However, calcification occurs much later than in the case of congenital BAV. Pure AS is rare to develop in RHD. In most cases, it is associated with aortic incompetence and many times with mitral valve disease. In a series reported from Christian Medical College (CMC) Vellore, MS was present in 11.8% of cases with aortic valve disease; 91.7% had associated AR.

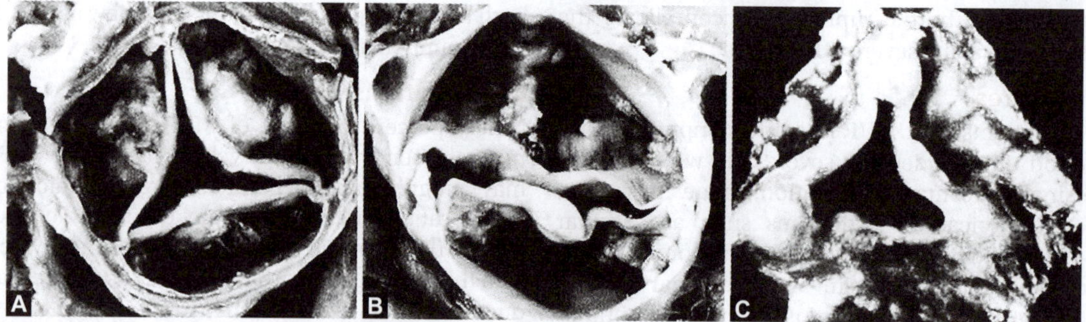

Figs 123.12A to C: Calcific aortic valves: **A.** Degenerative of elderly; **B.** Bicuspid aortic valve; **C.** Rheumatic

Degenerative Calcification of Aortic Valve

This results from the degeneration and calcification of the tricuspid aortic valve. The calcification is more toward the base of the aortic leaflets and the commissures are free. Hypertension and hypercholesterolemia accentuate the process.

Pathophysiology

The aperture of the normal valve is 3.0–4.0 cm². Clinically significant AS manifests when the valve narrows to less than 2.0 cm²; valve area 1.5–2.0 cm² is mild, 1.0–1.5 cm² is moderate and less than 1.0 cm² (valve area index—0.6 cm²/m² body surface area) is severe AS. Valve area of less than 0.75 cm² (index < 0.5 cm²/m² body surface area) is considered as critical AS. In view of the obstruction to the outflow, LV has to generate higher pressure in systole to empty its contents to aorta resulting in the pressure gradient across the aortic valve (Fig. 123.13). The LV consequently undergoes concentric hypertrophy. The hypertrophy is both adaptive—to increase the force of contraction and maladaptive in that the hypertrophied myocardium is less perfused even in the presence of normal coronary arteries. Finally, the LV dilates and fails. Heart failure may be the result of diastolic dysfunction, systolic dysfunction or both. The former is due to increased thickness of the LV, which impairs relaxation. Systolic dysfunction results from excessive afterload, decreased ventricular contractility, myocardial fibrosis and ischemia.

Hemodynamic consequences of LV outflow obstruction are low stroke volume and elevated LV systolic and diastolic pressure. With exercise, the LV will not be able to increase the cardiac output adequately and, hence, the LV diastolic pressure further rises. The high LV pressures, LV outflow gradient, LVH and fibrosis, low cardiac output, myocardial ischemia and ventricular arrhythmias are the basis of the clinical features in AS.

Low-flow Low Gradient Aortic Stenosis

In some patients with severe AS when they develop LV dysfunction, the cardiac output falls and, hence, the transvalvular gradient decreases mimicking DCM with mild AS, i.e. low-flow low gradient AS. It is defined as valve area less than 1.0 cm², left ventricular ejection fraction (LVEF) less than 40% and mean gradient less than 30 mm Hg; with dobutamine infusion the aortic velocity increases to more than 4 m/sec and the valve area remains less than 1.0 cm². These patients are benefited with surgery though at a higher risk.

Clinical Features

The three most important symptoms of significant AS are: (1) Exertional angina, (2) exertional syncope and (3) symptoms of LVF. Severe AS can remain asymptomatic for a long period; however, presence of these symptoms indicate severe AS, 50% of patients above the age of 40 years with angina are found to have associated significant coronary artery disease (CAD) on coronary angiogram. Other symptoms include palpitation, exertional fatigue and visual field defects probably secondary to minute calcific emboli from the aortic valves.

The pulse in severe AS is described as anacrotic pulse or pulsus parvus et tardus, i.e. low volume (parvus) slow rising (tardive) pulse, which is best felt over carotids (Fig. 123.14). The pulse pressure is usually narrow, less than 30 mm of mercury. In the elderly subjects even with

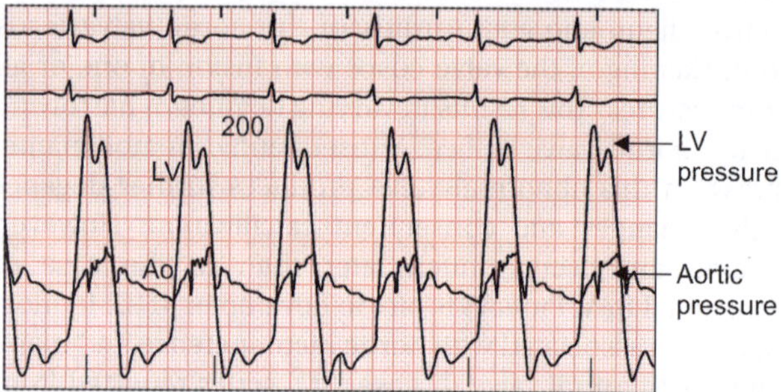

Fig. 123.13: Catheterization data in aortic stenosis. ***Note:*** The pressure difference between left ventricle and aorta (arrows)

Abbreviations: LV = Left ventricle; AO = Aorta

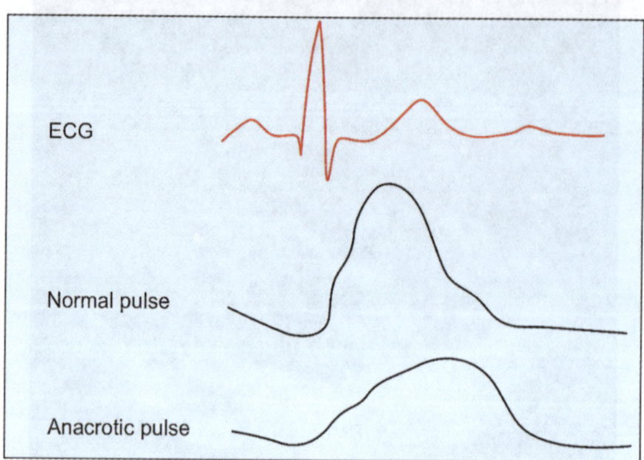

Fig. 123.14: Arterial pulse in aortic stenosis (top—ECG; middle—normal pulse; bottom—anacrotic pulse). ***Note:*** The low volume and slow rise

Abbreviation: ECG = Electrocardiogram

significant AS, the systolic pressure may occasionally reach 160 mm Hg or more due to inelasticity of the aorta. Consequently, in such patients, the severity of AS cannot be predicted from the amplitude of pulse pressure.

Apex beat is characteristically forceful and sustained (heaving). There may be a systolic thrill, best felt in the second right intercostal space, or along the left sternal border and very rarely over the apex also. S1 is usually normal; but can be soft in severe cases. As the LV ejection time is prolonged due to the obstruction, A2 is delayed resulting in single S2 or even paradoxical split of S2 in severe cases. LVH results in impaired relaxation affecting the rapid filling phase, which is compensated by a strong atrial kick producing a LV S4 over apex. As LV systolic dysfunction sets in LV, S3 appears. Noncalcified BAV generates a constant ejection click over the base, which may be well-audible over the apex also. Turbulent flow across the stenotic aortic valve produces a harsh grunting crescendo-decrescendo mid systolic murmur best heard in the aortic area and conducted to the carotids. The palpable harsh vibration in the carotids with the slow rising pulse produces the typical carotid shudder in severe AS. The murmur may be well-heard over the apex as well. The ejection systolic murmur corresponds to the period of ejection, i.e. it starts with the opening of the aortic valves and is over before the second sound. The murmur becomes louder with the phase of maximal ejection and comes down during the latter part of systole. In severe stenosis, the murmur is longer, louder and its peak is reached later in systole. In patients with calcified valves, high-frequency components of the murmur may be selectively radiated to the apex (Gallavardin phenomenon) mimicking MR murmur. When LV fails, cardiac output falls and the murmur becomes soft and may even disappear.

Investigations

Electrocardiogram

It is normal in mild cases. In significant AS, ECG shows LVH with strain (ST-segment depression and T-wave inversion) as well as left atrial overload pattern (Fig. 123.15). The ECG pattern of LVH generally correlates with the severity and prognosis of AS. AF is relatively rare and late in the course of the disease.

Radiological Findings

In pure AS, the heart is usually not enlarged until they develop LV dysfunction. Poststenotic dilation of the aorta may be seen in congenital AS (Fig. 123.16). This poststenotic dilation does not have any relation with the severity of AS. Calcification of the valve may be seen, better on fluoroscopy.

Echocardiography

It is the basic noninvasive technique for evaluating and following-up patients with AS and also planning the timing and nature of intervention. It allows the accurate definition of valve pathology, severity of stenosis, LVH and ventricular function. Doppler echocardiography helps to assess the transvalvular gradient and effective valve area, the accuracy of which correlates very well with hemodynamic data obtained by cardiac catheterization.

Cardiac Catheterization and Angiography

These are seldom indicated except for assessing the coronary status in patients with symptom of angina and before surgery.

Assessment of Severity of Aortic Stenosis

Table 123.2 shows the grading of severity of AS based on echocardiographic data.

Presence of the typical symptoms (exertional angina, exertional syncope and heart failure symptom), anacrotic pulse, heaving apex, LV S4, paradoxically split S2 and long murmur with late systolic peaking indicate severe AS. ECG evidence of LVH with strain pattern, left atrial overload,

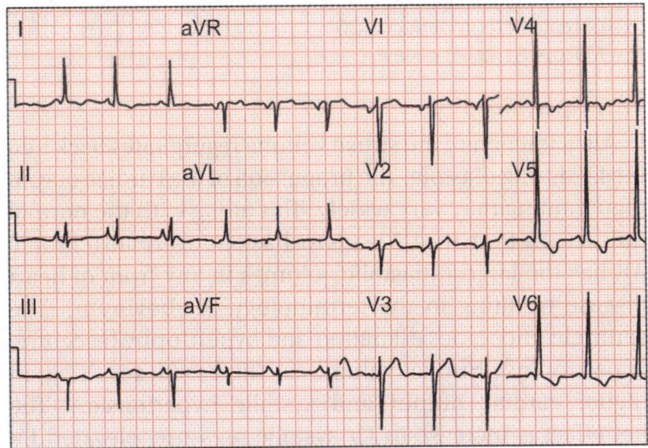

Fig. 123.15: Electrocardiogram in severe AS showing left ventricular hypertrophy with strain pattern

Abbreviations: aVF = Augmented vector foot; aVL = Augmented vector left; aVR = Augmented vector right.

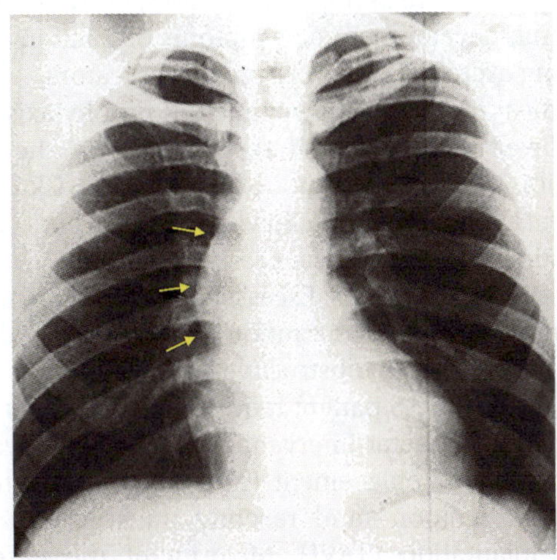

Fig. 123.16: Post-stenotic dilatation in valvular aortic stenosis (arrows)

Table 123.2: Echocardiographic grading of severity of aortic stenosis			
Parameter	**Mild AS**	**Moderate AS**	**Severe AS**
Doppler jet velocity (m/sec)	< 3.0	3.0–4.0	> 4.0
Mean gradient (mm Hg)	< 25	25–50	> 50
Valve area (cm²)	> 1.5	1.0–1.5	< 1.0
Valve area index (cm²/m²)	> 0.9	0.6–0.9	< 0.6

Abbreviation: AS = Aortic stenosis

LBBB and conduction abnormalities are also clues for severe lesion.

Course and Prognosis

Mild cases do not generally progress and may remain asymptomatic for long. However, the course of AS cannot be predicted with confidence because of the variability in its progression due to the deposition of calcium. In patients with mild thickening but no obstruction, only 2.5% will develop severe stenosis at an average follow-up of 8 years.

Even severe AS can remain asymptomatic for a long period. Once they become symptomatic with angina, syncope or LVF, the average survival is only 5, 3 and 2 years, respectively. Sudden cardiac death may occur in symptomatic patients; however, in asymptomatic patients it is rare (2% annually). Risk of IE is more moderate.

The strongest predictor of progression to symptoms is the Doppler aortic jet velocity. Survival, free of symptoms is 84% at 2 years when jet velocity is less than 3 m/sec compared with only 21% when it is more than 4 m/sec. Presence of valve calcification is also a positive predictor for rapid progression of stenosis. The average progression of AS is an annual decrease in valve area by 0.12 cm^2, increase in jet velocity by 0.32 m/sec/year and increase in mean gradient by 7 mm Hg/year.

Management

Basic principle in management is patient education in disease progression and recognition of symptoms of severity. Serial clinical and echocardiographic evaluation is the key point. Serial echocardiography has to be performed yearly in asymptomatic severe AS, every 1–2 years for moderate AS and every 3–5 years in mild cases. In moderate-to-severe asymptomatic cases, exercise test may be helpful; development of symptoms or a fall in systolic BP during exercise is poor prognostic indicators.

Medical management includes IE prophylaxis, rheumatic fever prophylaxis, if the etiology is rheumatic, evaluation and treatment of coronary risk factors and treatment of heart failure when it occurs. As the obstruction is a mechanical pressure load to LV, medical treatment has limitations. Excessive diuretics can produce hypotension and, hence, caution is needed. Vasodilators are contraindicated in obstructive lesions.

Symptomatic AS patient requires relief of obstruction by surgery or catheter intervention. Procedures available are aortic valve replacement (AVR), aortic valvotomy—surgical or balloon—and recently transcatheter aortic valve implantation (TAVI). Majority of the cases are handled by AVR; it is combined with coronary artery bypass grafting (CABG) for associated CAD. Young patients with noncalcified bicuspid valve stenosis without regurgitation can be considered for valvotomy; however, the restenosis rate is much higher compared to the restenosis rate after BMV for MS. Elderly patients with calcific AS who are at high-risk for surgery are recently being treated with TAVI.

Indications for surgery

- Symptomatic patients
- Asymptomatic moderate-to-severe AS undergoing CABG for active coronary atherosclerotic heart disease
- Asymptomatic severe AS with LVEF < 50 or exercise-induced hypotension
- Low-flow low gradient severe AS

Abbreviations: AS = Aortic stenosis; CABG = Coronary artery bypass grafting; LVEF = Left ventricular ejection fraction

Overall operative mortality for isolated AVR in patients with good LV function is 2–5% and 5.6%, when it is combined with CABG. Risk factors associated with high-operative mortality include a high NYHA class, LV dysfunction, advanced age and associated coronary atherosclerotic heart disease.

AORTIC REGURGITATION (AORTIC INCOMPETENCE)

Aortic regurgitation results when the aortic valve cusps are not able to close the aortic orifice completely during diastole, which could be due to abnormalities of the valve, dilatation of the aortic root or combination. Aortic root disease as a cause for AR is increasing over the last years accounting for more than 50% of the cases undergoing AVR for isolated AR. AR like MR could be acute or chronic.

Various causes of aortic regurgitation

Valvular causes
- Congenital—bicuspid, tricuspid, quadricuspid valves
- Rheumatic valvulitis
- Prolapse of aortic leaflet as in ventricular septal defect (VSD)
- Infective endocarditis (IE)
- Calcific valve

Root dilatation
- Ankylosing spondylitis
- Marfan's syndrome
- Aortic aneurysm
- Aortic dissection
- Annuloaortic ectasia
- Hypertension

Root dilatation + valve pathology
- Atherosclerosis
- Rheumatoid arthritis (RA)
- Aortoarteritis
- Systemic lupus erythematosus (SLE)
- Myxomatous degeneration
- Ehlers-Danlos syndrome
- Syphilis
- Trauma
- Reiter's syndrome
- Behcet's syndrome
- Osteogenesis imperfecta (OI)
- Mucopolysaccharidoses

Pathophysiology

In AR, a fraction of the stroke volume regurgitates back into the LV during diastole. The proportion of the cardiac output regurgitating may vary widely. This along with the normal inflow to LV from the LA leads to diastolic overload (chronic AR has the largest diastolic volumes in any from of heart disease resulting in the terminology cor bovinum). The ventricle undergoes dilatation and hypertrophy (eccentric hypertrophy). Stroke volume is increased resulting in higher cardiac output and systolic hypertension. The net effect is increase in LV systolic pressure, elevated LV diastolic volume, high LV end diastolic pressure (LVEDP) and LVH. All these contribute to increased wall tension (as per Laplace's law) and afterload. Thus AR is a unique lesion imposing both preload and afterload excess to LV (only preload in MR; only afterload in AS). To maintain forward flow and to reduce regurgitation, systemic vascular resistance decreases as a compensatory mechanism with considerable lowering of the diastolic pressure. This along with the high-stroke volume produces the wide pulse pressure in AR. Similar to reduction in systemic resistance, tachycardia is also favorable to the AR hemodynamics. As the heart rate increases, the diastolic time decreases and, hence, the fraction of regurgitation will come down. Both these hemodynamic factors are important in the medical management of AR.

Myocardial ischemia can occur in severe AR. Increase in wall tension and LVH increase the myocardial oxygen demand. As the diastolic blood pressure falls, coronary perfusion decreases as the flow to LV subendocardium occurs predominantly in diastole. The imbalance between oxygen supply and demand results in development of angina in AR, more during night as the heart rate drop during sleep accentuates AR. The impact of the vigorous aortic pulsation over the chest wall may produce nonanginal chest pain.

The heart compensates and maintains the cardiac output for considerable period by dilatation and hypertrophy, but ultimately LVF develops. In advanced stages of decompensation, LVEDP rises, which will be transmitted to LA, pulmonary capillaries and PA resulting in PAH, RV failure and reduction in cardiac output (still the cardiac output will be more than the normal range—high output failure).

Clinical Features

Mild, moderate and even severe cases remain asymptomatic for a long period. Chronic severe AR is associated with symptoms like palpitation (increased force of contraction due to volume overload), exertional dyspnea and chest pain. The symptoms are gradually progressive and when the compensatory mechanisms become inadequate, CHF ensues. Physical examination may reveal features of the underlying etiopathological disorders, like Marfan's syndrome. Pulse is characteristically collapsing or bisferiens in severe AR, which is better felt in brachials and femorals than in carotids (Figs 123.17 and 123.18). Pulse pressure is wide due to elevated systolic pressure and low diastolic pressure.

Investigations

Auscultation

First heart sound is usually normal till LVF develops when it becomes soft. Longer ejection time and low-systemic vascular resistance (with resultant long-aortic hangout interval) delay the aortic valve closure resulting in single or closely split S2. A2 is usually soft in severe valvular AR or, if the valve is calcified; but is loud in AR due to root dilatation. LV S3 may be heard in severe AR; it indicates an elevated end systolic volume, which may be a clue for LV dysfunction. BAV or aortic dilatation can produce a sharp sound (ejection click) at the onset of ejection, i.e. after S1.

The characteristic murmur of AR is a high-pitched soft blowing decrescendo early diastolic murmur best heard in the third left intercostal space (3 LICS) close to

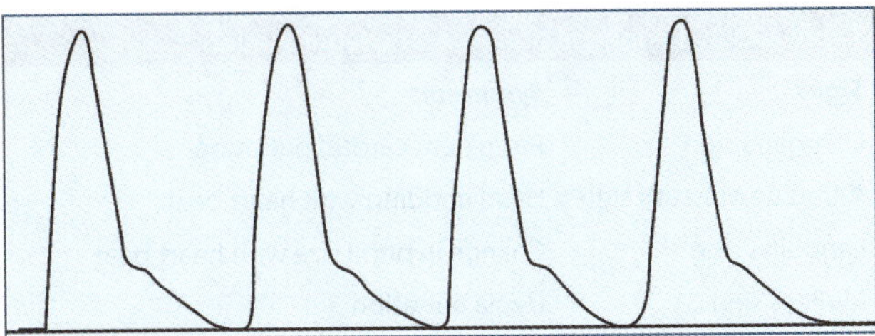

Fig. 123.17: Pulse tracing of aortic incompetence. **Note:** The wide pulse pressure with very low diastolic pressure (collapsing pulse)

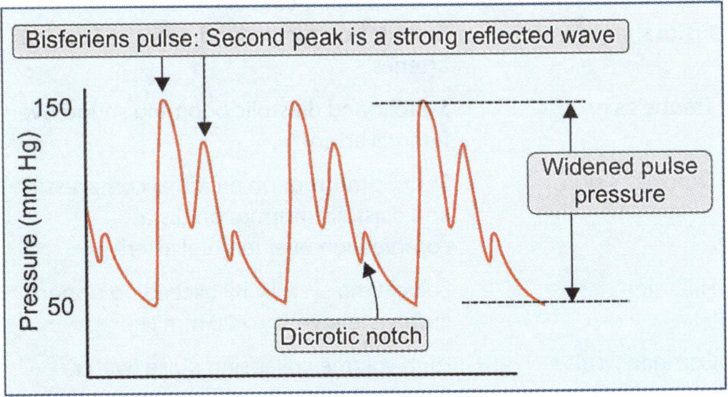

Fig. 123.18: Bisferiens pulse in aortic regurgitation. **Note:** The second peak, widen pulse pressure and dicrotic notch

sternum (second aortic area/Erb's area); it is conducted down along the left sternal edge and is better heard with diaphragm of stethoscope, patient sitting up, leaning forward and breath held in expiration. The vibration of the anterior mitral leaflet between the two diastolic flows into LV (AR jet and mitral inflow jet from LA) produces a mid and late diastolic rumble—Austin Flint murmur. Another explanation for this murmur is the functional mild MS related to premature partial closure of the mitral valve in diastole due to the elevation of LV diastolic pressure by the regurgitant pressure and volume (LV diastolic pressure may exceed the LA pressure producing even diastolic MR, especially in acute AR—Rytand's murmur). The ejection of enhanced stroke volume across the aortic valve produces a mid-systolic murmur in the aortic area.

AR due to aortic root dilatation can be differentiated from valvular AR by a few findings—murmur is better transmitted along right sternal border, A2 is loud and ejection click is common.

Wide pulse pressure produces a lot of peripheral signs as listed in Table 123.3.

Electrocardiogram

It is normal in mild cases. As severity of AR increases ECG findings of LVH appear.

Chest Radiograph

It shows LV enlargement in severe cases. The aorta in most of the cases appears dilated and on fluoroscopy it is hyperdynamic (Fig. 123.19).

Echocardiography

Two-dimensional ECG along with Doppler and color-flow mapping can provide anatomical information on the aortic valve and aortic root, etiology and severity of AR, LV function and presence of other valvular involvement

Table 123.3: Peripheral signs of aortic regurgitation

Signs	Symptoms
Corrigan's sign	Prominent carotid pulsation
Alfred de Musset's sign	Head nodding with heart beat
Landolfi's sign	Change in pupil size with heart beat
Muller's sign	Uvula pulsation
Rosenbach's sign	Liver pulsations
Gerhardt's sign	Spleen pulsations
Quincke's sign	Digital capillary pulsations
Pistol shot sound	Systolic booming sound over the femoral arteries
Traube's sign	Systolic and diastolic booming sound over femoral artery
Duroziez's sign	Systolic murmur on proximal compression and diastolic murmur on distal compression over femoral arteries
Hill's sign	Lower limb systolic BP exceeding upper limb systolic BP by > 20 mm Hg
Corrigan's pulse	High volume collapsing pulse (water-hammer pulse)
Becker's sign	Retinal artery pulsations

Note: Water-hammer—this term refers to the percussion made by water in the pipe when the flow is suddenly turned off.

Source: Concise Oxford Dictionary

Abbreviation: BP = Blood pressure

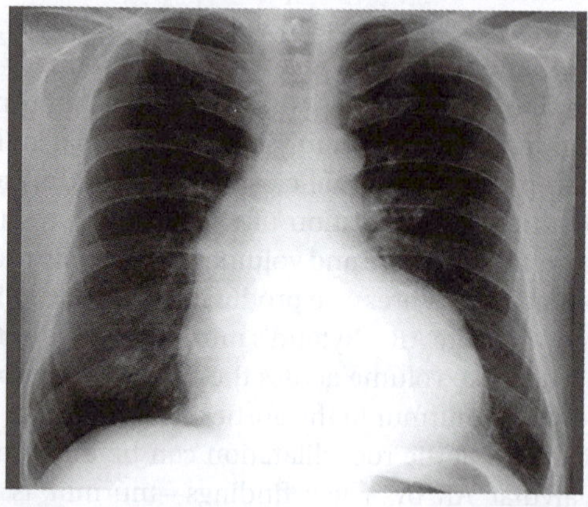

Fig. 123.19: Chest X-ray AR showing cardiac dilatation (LV type) and dilated aorta

(Fig. 123.20). ECG also helps in assessing the PA pressures and deciding the timing and type of surgery.

Cardiac catheterization and angiography and cardiac MRI can provide accurate assessment of the hemodynamic abnormality; however, these are indicated only in a few selected cases.

Course and Prognosis

Mild cases usually do not progress. If the regurgitant valve orifice is more than 0.3 cm² and the regurgitant volume is more than 60 mL/beat, it is severe AR. Moderate or even severe asymptomatic AR has a favorable long-term prognosis. Natural history is more favorable in younger patients compared to the older. In one series, among younger patients (mean age 39 years) with severe AR and normal LVEF, the annual mortality was less than 1%.

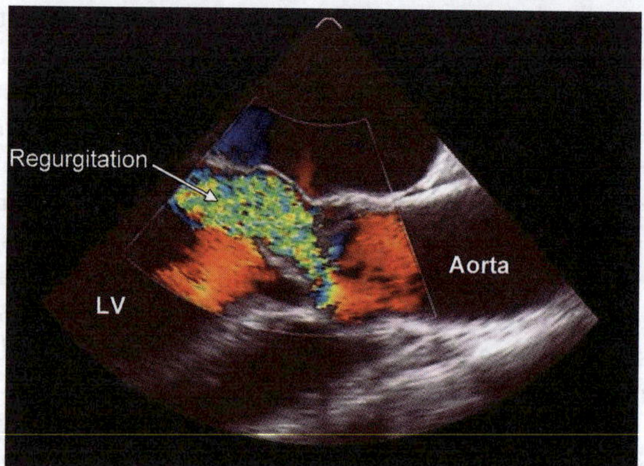

Fig. 123.20: Color Doppler echocardiography jet in aortic regurgitation—aorta and left ventricle (LV)

However, once the patient becomes symptomatic, the downhill course is rapid. Without surgical treatment, the average survival is 4 years once they develop angina and less than 2 years after the onset of heart failure. Patients with CHF, angina and those in NYHA class III and IV are at high-risk of mortality (25% per year), if untreated. Risk of aortic dissection is increased in those with annuloaortic ectasia and those with BAV and dilated aortic root.

Treatment

Medical

There is no definite specific therapy to prevent progression of AR. Serial clinical, radiologic and echocardiographic follow-up is essential in asymptomatic cases. Meticulous control of systemic arterial diastolic hypertension is needed to prevent worsening of the regurgitation. The role of vasodilators like nifedipine, hydralazine and ACE inhibitor to prevent the progression of AR is debatable. Patients with fast heart rate may benefit with small dose beta-blockers to maintain heart rate at around 80 per minute. LV dysfunction and heart failure should be treated with ACE inhibitor, diuretics and digoxin to stabilize them for surgery. IE and rheumatic fever prophylaxis should be considered, whenever indicated.

Surgical

Surgery should be deferred in asymptomatic cases with good LV function, in view of the good long-term prognosis in such groups. Serial echocardiographic evaluation to look into the LV size and EF helps in timing the surgery (Box 123.4).

Box 123.4: Indications for surgery

- Symptomatic patients with severe AR
- Asymptomatic patients with severe AR and depressed LV function—LVEF< 50%
- Asymptomatic severe AR with dilated LV end-diastolic dimension > 75 mm; end-systolic dimension > 55 mm
- AR due to aortic root dilatation > 55 mm (> 50 mm in presence of BAV)
- Asymptomatic severe AR undergoing other cardiac surgeries, like CABG, MVR
- Acute AR

Abbreviations: AR = Aortic regurgitation; LV = Left ventricle; LVEF = Left ventricular ejection fraction; CABG = Coronary artery bypass grafting; MVR = Mitral valve replacement; BAV = Bicuspid aortic valve

The standard surgical approach is valve replacement with or without aortic root surgery. The valve replacement may be prosthetic or biological valves (porcine or bovine). The former necessitates anticoagulant therapy, the latter may not require it. Cardiac prosthetic valves are manufactured in India, a popular one being Chitra valve developed at the Sree Chitra Thirunal Institute of Medical Sciences and Technology by MS Valiathan and associates. This valve is cheaper than imported valves and it is in active use for more than 20 years. Aortic valve repair may be done by experienced group in selected cases like perforation of leaflet, traumatic leaflet tear and aortic leaflet prolapse as in association with ventricular septal defect.

Acute Aortic Regurgitation

IE, trauma, aortic dissection and rheumatic fever are some of the causes of acute onset of severe AR, which in a normal-sized LV produces acute rise in LV diastolic pressure leading to acute onset of severe LVF (pulmonary edema). Transmission of the aortic diastolic pressure to LV results in marked elevation of LV pressure in early-to-mid diastole itself (exceeding LA pressure) leading to premature closure of mitral valve and even diastolic MR. In view of severe diastolic volume and pressure overload, LV fails and, hence, the cardiac output will not be increased, in contrast to chronic AR. In response to acute LVF, systemic vascular resistance increases (hence, diastolic BP may not fall) which will augment the regurgitation.

Patients with acute AR will be quite sick with severe dyspnea, orthopnea, peripheral cyanosis, cold extremities, tachypnea, tachycardia and acidosis. Pulse may not show the characteristic features of chronic severe AR and peripheral signs will be lacking. Pulse pressure may not be wide and even could be narrow. Marked elevation of left heart pressures can lead to PAH and RV failure with resultant elevation of JVP. Cardiomegaly is inconspicuous and apex is not hyperdynamic. S1 is soft or may be even absent; LV S3 is invariable but LV S4 does not occur in view of premature mitral valve closure. PAH produces accentuated P2 and audible RV S3 and S4. AR murmur will be short and unimpressive; Austin Flint murmur due to diastolic MR is usually short.

As early mortality is high despite aggressive medical management, emergency surgery is warranted. Till then, the patient has to be stabilized with diuretics, positive inotropes, vasodilators like nitroprusside and ventilatory assistance along with other supportive measures. Intra-aortic balloon pump (IABP) is contraindicated in acute AR in contrast to acute MR.

TRICUSPID VALVE LESIONS

TRICUSPID STENOSIS (TS)

Normal tricuspid orifice is larger than the mitral orifice (5–7 cm²). The tricuspid leaflets differ from the mitral leaflets in being thinner, more translucent and less clearly separated into well-defined leaflets. The three major leaflets are: (1) Anterior, (2) septal, and (3) posterior. The tricuspid valve may be stenotic, regurgitant or both. Tricuspid stenosis (TS) is clinically detectable in 3–5% of cases with multivalvular involvement, but tricuspid lesion can be demonstrated in a much higher proportion (up to 30%), during autopsy. Rheumatic TS is almost always associated with MS and most often with aortic valve disease also.

Etiology

- Rheumatic valvulitis
- Congenital tricuspid stenosis
- Carcinoid syndrome
- Endocardial fibroelastosis
- Endomyocardial fibrosis
- Systemic lupus erythematosus (SLE)

Rheumatic valvulitis causes fusion of the adjacent free edges of the leaflets. The valve cusps are also moderately thickened. The involvement of the subvalvular apparatus is less marked compared to the distortion in MS.

When the valve area falls below 1 cm², it leads to severe TS. If the valve area is between 1 cm² and 1.5 cm², it is designated as moderate stenosis. Transtricuspid gradient (mean gradient > 2 mm Hg) with elevation of RA pressure is the hemodynamic hallmark of TS.

Clinical Features

Presence of TS leads to reduction in the RV output, thereby decompressing the LA; hence, the pulmonary venous congestion and, therefore, the symptoms of associated MS such as PND, pulmonary edema and hemoptysis are considerably less. The most common symptoms attributable to TS are easy fatigability due to low cardiac output and systemic venous congestion symptoms (edema, abdominal distention and puffiness of face) due to high RA pressure. Physical examination reveals low volume pulse. The JVP is elevated with prominent A waves and slow Y descent (latter due to slow emptying of blood from RA to RV in early diastole). In the presence of AF, the A wave disappears but the slow Y descent persists. The characteristic auscultatory feature is the presence of a mid-diastolic or presystolic murmur, which is best heard at the lower-left sternal border. Though the murmur is also rumbling in character, its pitch is higher than the murmur of MS. It increases in intensity with inspiration (*Carvallo's sign*). The first sound is often split as a result of delay in tricuspid valve closure. Usually, there will be an associated TR murmur.

Investigations

The ECG shows evidence of RA enlargement in sinus rhythm; quite often the patients will be in AF. Chest X-ray shows disproportionate RA dilatation; the findings of MS will be attenuated. ECG clearly demonstrates the lesion in the valve. Cardiac catheterization is seldom required for tricuspid valve disease.

Course and Prognosis

Though the symptoms of PVH in patients with MS are ameliorated by the coexistence of TS, the cardiac output is considerably reduced and systemic venous hypertension (SVH) develops. In such cases, failure to identify TS preoperatively and correct it during surgery of the mitral and aortic valves, leads to poor postoperative results.

Treatment

Moderate or severe TS should be corrected by commissurotomy at the time of surgery for the mitral lesion.

Balloon valvotomy has also been found feasible in TS. However, if valvotomy is not feasible or if it does not give good results, tricuspid valve replacement is needed.

TRICUSPID REGURGITATION

It results from inadequate closure of the tricuspid orifice by the valve leaflets, which could be due to valve pathology, annular dilatation or both. The most frequent cause of TR is functional incompetence secondary to pulmonary hypertension with resultant high RV systolic pressure and annular dilatation (functional/hypertensive TR). Less commonly, TR occurs due to primary RV or tricuspid valve pathology without PAH (primary or nonhypertensive TR) (Box 123.5).

Regurgitation of blood from right ventricle (RV) to RA in systole leads to elevation of RA pressure and RA dilatation. Similar to the mechanism in MR, enhanced diastolic flow into RV in the next diastole results in RV dilatation and RV failure. Marked dilatation of RA leads to AF, which is very common in tricuspid valve disease (80–90%).

Clinical Features

Symptomatology is similar to that in TS. The most conspicuous finding is elevation of JVP with prominent V wave and exaggerated Y collapse. The characteristic murmur of TR is a high-pitched pansystolic murmur best heard in the lower-left sternal border. This murmur increases in intensity with inspiration and with passive leg raising. Inspiratory augmentation of the murmur may not be very conspicuous in cases with severe CHF. In primary TR, the murmur is medium-pitched and short; inspiratory augmentation is less conspicuous. When TR is severe, a third heart sound as well as a mid-diastolic flow murmur may be heard along the lower-left sternal border.

Investigations

Chest X-ray will show evidence of RA enlargement (Fig. 123.21). Echo delineates the lesion well. Using Doppler, ECG pulmonary pressures can be assessed and this may help in differentiating primary and secondary TR. Cardiac catheterization and angiography are seldom needed.

Treatment

Medical treatment is given for those cases with functional TR. Valvuloplasty or valve replacement may be necessary in cases with primary TR. Even in functional TR surgical correction may have to be done, if the lesion is severe.

ACQUIRED LESIONS OF THE PULMONARY VALVE

The pulmonary valve is only rarely involved by acquired heart disease. In carcinoid syndrome, the pulmonary

---

Box 123.5: Causes of primary tricuspid regurgitation

- Rheumatic valvulitis
- Congenital anomalies (Ebstein malformation, atrioventricular cushion defects)
- Carcinoid syndrome
- Infective endocarditis (IE)
- Trauma
- Right ventricular (RV) pacing
- RV endomyocardial fibrosis
- RV myocardial infarction
- Myxomatous valve—tricuspid valve prolapse (Marfan syndrome)

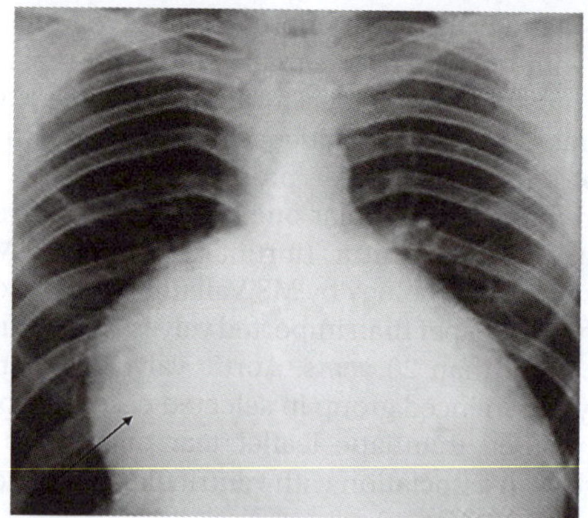

Fig. 123.21: Chest X-ray showing aneurysmal dilatation of RA in tricuspid valve disease (arrow)

valve shows fibrous scarring with retraction leading to pulmonary stenosis (PS) and regurgitation. In severe forms of RHD, the pulmonary valve also may be involved as part of the quadrivalvular affection. Bacterial endocarditis may affect congenitally abnormal or even normal pulmonary valve resulting in pulmonary regurgitation (PR). The pulmonary valve may be the seat of tumors such as myxoma or fibroma in rare cases. In Marfan's syndrome, the valve shows myxomatous degeneration. The valve may be damaged during surgery for tetralogy of Fallot (TOF) or PS. Severe pulmonary hypertension resulting from any cause may produce functional PR with pulmonary early diastolic murmur (Graham-Steell murmur). Very rarely pulmonary valve may be involved by tuberculosis and syphilis.

Clinical manifestations depend upon the severity of valve involvement and its cause. In quadrivalvular involvement, identification of the pulmonary lesion is difficult because the clinical features are those of the other lesions. Isolated pulmonary stenosis (which is usually congenital) is characterized by prominent a wave in JVP, wide split S2 with soft P2 and ejection click followed by loud ejection systolic murmur often associated with a thrill most prominent over the left upper sternal border. PR produces an early diastolic murmur along the left sternal border. Careful examination can distinguish it from AR murmur (Table 123.4).

Course and prognosis: In quadrivalvular disease, the hemodynamic abnormalities are largely determined by

Table 123.4: Differentiation of aortic regurgitation and pulmonary regurgitation diastolic murmurs

Features	AR	PR
Inspiratory increase	–	+
Murmur begins with A2	+	–
Murmur begins with P2	–	+
Site	Widely heard along LSB	Localized to PA
S2	Normal/loud A2	Usually loud P2
Murmur increases with phenylephrine and hand grip	+	–
Murmur decreases with amylnitrate	+	–

Abbreviations: AR = Aortic regurgitation; PR = Pulmonary regurgitation; A2 = Closure of the aortic valve; P2 = Pulmonic valve closure; LSB = Left sternal border; PA = Pulmonary area

the lesions of the proximal valves. Pulmonary valve disease may not alter the natural history significantly. However, recognition of pulmonary valve disease is important to decide the line of management. When PR is mild or moderate, RV accommodates the increased diastolic blood volume without considerable hemodynamic disturbance, but severe PR may cause progressive RV failure.

Treatment: Management largely depends on the status of the associated lesions. Pulmonary valve replacement may have to be considered under the following indications:

- Severe and progressive PR following surgical correction of TOF or PS
- Tumors involving the pulmonary valve
- IE, when medical treatment fails.

CHAPTER
124

Infective Endocarditis

K Suresh, PT Suhail

Chapter Summary

- Acute Infective Endocarditis
- Subacute Bacterial Endocarditis
- Indication for Surgery in Infective Endocarditis
- Recommendation for Endocarditis Prophylaxis

INTRODUCTION

Infective endocarditis (IE) is defined as microbial infection of the endothelial surfaces of heart and great vessels (infective endarteritis). Endocarditis may be acute or subacute.

ACUTE INFECTIVE ENDOCARDITIS

The heart valves and endocardium may be the seat of direct invasion by microbes. Virulent organisms such as *Staphylococcus aureus*, *Streptococcus hemolyticus* and *Pneumococci* produce acute ulcerative endocarditis during the course of a septicemia and these affect normal valves. Fortunately, this complication is rare.

Acute infective endocarditis and subacute bacterial endocarditis (SBE) differ in their etiology, microbial flora, pathology, clinical features and management. Whereas acute endocarditis presents as a part of more fulminant generalized infection, the subacute form often takes the picture of a stealthy superinfection on an already existing cardiovascular lesion by organisms which are of low virulence in normal individuals (Table 124.1).

Table 124.2 shows the degree of risk of IE in common cardiac lesions.

SUBACUTE BACTERIAL ENDOCARDITIS

Etiology

Predisposing Causes

Infection is predisposed by congenital heart disease (CHD) or rheumatic heart disease (RHD). Organisms may colonize on the endocardium, valves or arteries that are already damaged or subjected to hemodynamic abnormalities. Combined valvular lesions are more often the seat of vegetations than pure stenosis or incompetence. In immunodeficient individuals and intravenous (IV) drug users, even normal valves may become colonized by pathogens.

Microbial Flora

Common organisms are *Streptococcus viridans*, *Streptococcus mutans*, *Streptococcus faecalis* and other streptococci. Less common organisms include staphylococci, pneumococci, *Haemophilus influenzae*, gonococci, meningococci, *Salmonellae*, *Escherichia coli*, *Bacterium anitratum*, *Candida* species, *Aspergillus* species, anaerobes and *Coxiella burnetii*. Most of these organisms form commensals in the human body, particularly abundant in sites such as the mouth, upper respiratory tract, genitalia and urinary tract. Any infective illness or minor surgical procedures such as dental surgery, tonsillectomy, urinary instrumentation, parturition, abortion or medical termination of pregnancy (MTP) causes transient bacteremia which conveys the organisms to the abnormal cardiac tissues, where they settle and multiply.

Table 124.1: Primary cardiac lesion and the most common precipitating event	
Pre-existing heart disease	**Precipitating factors**
Congenital heart disease (CHD)	Dental procedures, abortion, procedures on lower urinary tract, intravenous (IV) drug use
Rheumatic valvular disease	Dental procedures, minor surgery, systemic infections
Atherosclerotic valve lesions and degenerative lesions	Urinary endoscopy and other manipulations
Prosthetic heart valves	Bacteremias
Cardiac surgery	IV cannulae and shunts, foreign materials
Normal valves in immunocompromised individuals	Emergency room procedures including IV catheter and injections
Drug addicts: Normal valves	Needle sharing, IV injections

Table 124.2: Degree of risk of infective endocarditis in common cardiac lesions

High-risk	Intermediate risk	Low/negligible risk
• Prosthetic valves • Aortic valve disease • Mitral regurgitation • PDA • AV fistula • VSD • Coarctation of aorta • Previous infective endocarditis • Marfan's syndrome	• Mitral valve prolapse • Mitral stenosis • Tircuspid valve disease • HOCM • Calcific aortic stenosis • TOF • Nonvalvular intracardiac prosthesis	• Degenerative heart disease • ASD • Luetic aortitis (syphilis) • CABG • Surgically corrected congenital lesions • Pacemakers

Abbreviations: ASD = Atrial septal defect; PDA = Patent ductus arteriosus; HOCM = Hypertrophic obstructive cardiomyopathy; CABG = Coronary artery bypass graft; AV = Arteriovenous; VSD = Ventricular septal defect; TOF = Tetralogy of Fallot

Pathology

On the endocardial surface, the organisms multiply and proliferate. Fibrin is deposited over the organisms and this gives a protective coat against the defense of the host. Further, growth of the organisms and fibrin deposition result in the formation of friable vegetations which show three layers—(1) the inner layer made up of erythrocytes, leukocytes and platelets, (2) the middle layer containing a heavy growth of the organisms and (3) an outer layer made up of fibrin. As fibrin gets deposited further, the vegetations grow and they get embolized from time to time. Organisms which reach the cardiac tissues adhere to the damaged valves and other parts within minutes. After adhesion to tissues they multiply and envelope themselves in fibrin and this may leads to the development of vegetations. Monocytes which adhere to these sites do not engulf the organisms. On the other hand, they produce procoagulant factors which favor the development of further fibrin and vegetations. Normally, adhesion of platelets tends to inhibit organisms, but in IE, this does not happen; but further growth of vegetations may occur. Tissue invasion and abscess formation follow (Figs 124.1A and B).

The vegetations are located differently on the different valves. Generally, vegetations are located at the downstream portions of a communication between high and low pressure areas.

- Mitral valve—atrial surface and line of apposition
- Aortic valve—ventricular surface
- Ventricular septal defect (VSD)—on the right ventricular endocardium where the abnormal jet impinges and around the defect
- Patent ductus—pulmonary artery and the ductus arteriosus.

Site of development of vegetations on the affected valves are listed in Table 124.3.

The chordae tendinae and papillary muscles may be affected. These may leads to rupture leading to acute valvular incompetence or they may undergo fibrosis when they heal.

Embolic Episodes

Embolic episodes form an integral clinical feature of IE. The emboli may be septic or sterile. Embolism leads to infarction of organs. Septic emboli reaching the vasa vasorum lead to weakness of the arterial wall and the formation of mycotic aneurysms especially in the intracranial vessels.

Repeated release of organisms into the circulation starts off immunological processes. Large amounts of antibodies are formed which give rise to the formation of immune complexes. Complement activation occurs. As a result, immunological lesions like glomerulonephritis (GN), perisplenitis and vasculitis develop. Septic emboli also lead to focal GN. Spleen enlarges due to reticuloendothelial hyperplasia and formation of microabscesses.

Untreated cases end fatally. Death is caused by massive embolism to vital organs (brain or heart), cardiac failure or renal failure.

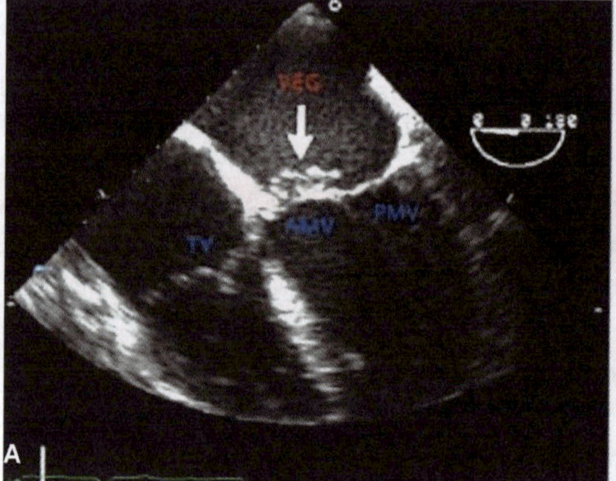

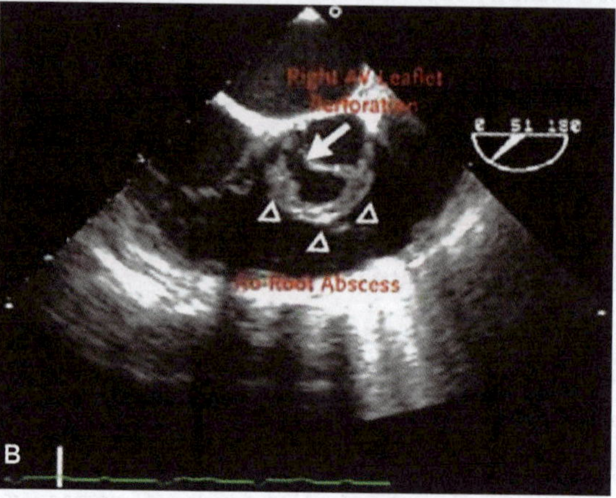

Figs 124.1A and B: Transesophageal echocardiogram (TEE). **A.** Vegetation attached to mitral valve (arrow); **B.** Aortic root abscess on right side (arrow)

Table 124.3: Site of development vegetations on the affected valves

Valve affected	Site of vegetation/complication
Mitral valve	Along chordae tendineae toward papillary muscle causing their rupture
Aortic valve	Develop ring abscess
VSD	Right ventricular wall, the site of jet impact
Regurgitant mitral lesion	Wall of left atrium in the area termed MacCallum's patch
Regurgitant aortic lesion	Chordae tendineae of anterior mitral leaflet
PDA	On the pulmonary artery and ductus

Abbreviations: VSD = Ventricular septal defect; PDA = Patent ductus arteriosus

Clinical Features

Symptomatology can be described under four groups:

1. ***Features of subacute infection:*** This manifests as low-grade or high-grade intermittent or continuous fever, often associated with chills and rigor. Digital clubbing may develop within weeks and this may be painful. In some cases, the symptoms may be nonspecific. Even unexplained fatigue, anemia or resistant cardiac failure should draw attention to endocarditis. Splenomegaly develops and the organ is well-palpable by the 2nd week. A brownish pigmentation develops over the face and limbs—cafe-au-lait pigmentation (meaning, coffee with milk) (Fig. 124.2).

2. ***Hemodynamic changes:*** Destruction of a valve may result in valve rupture leading to the development of fresh murmurs, aggravation of existing murmurs and sudden cardiac failure. In some cases, the vegetations obstruct the valves. The papillary muscles and the chordae tendineae may rupture giving rise to incompetence of the atrioventricular (AV) valves.

3. ***Embolic phenomena:*** The emboli are generally small though large fatal emboli may develop at times. Emboli produce several manifestations.
   - ***Cutaneous embolism:*** This may leads to painless, erythematous or hemorrhagic lesions on palms and soles called ***Janeway lesions***
   - ***Nails:*** Splinter hemorrhages occur as longitudinal streaks under the nails

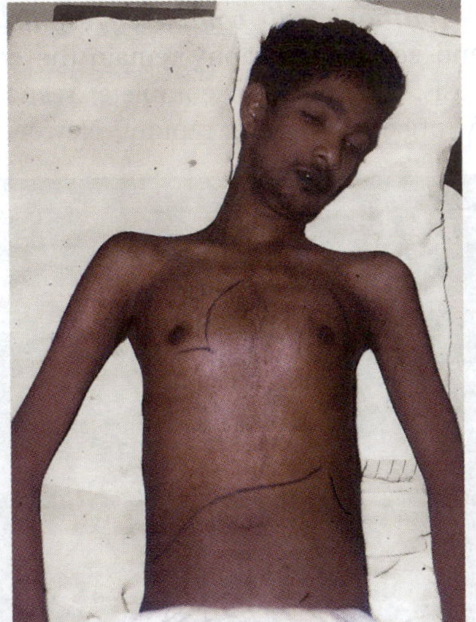

Fig. 124.2: 25-year-old (male), mitral valve disease with infective endocarditis. ***Note:*** Pallor, splenomegaly, cardiomegaly

- ***Spleen:*** Painful splenomegaly and splenic infarcts may develop
- ***Peripheral arteries:*** Occlusion of the arteries to the extremities gives rise to absence of peripheral pulses, claudication and distal gangrene
- ***Central nervous system (CNS):*** The carotid or vertebral system may be involved giving rise to paralysis, convulsions, visual loss, aphasia and cerebellar disturbances
- ***Renal infarction:*** This condition causes hematuria and renal failure
- ***Pulmonary embolism:*** Pulmonary embolism gives rise to pulmonary infarction, pleurisy and pleural effusion.

4. ***Immunological disturbances:*** These lead to vasculitis which manifests as ***Osler's nodes*** (raised tender nodules on the pulps of the fingers), ***Roth's spots*** (circular hemorrhages with central white spots) seen on the retina and ***GN***.

Diagnosis

A high index of clinical suspicion is very essential for early diagnosis. In persons with CHD, fever, anemia, clubbing, refractory cardiac failure, new murmurs, development of emboli or even vague ill health should suggest the possibility of IE. It should be differentiated from activation of rheumatic fever, disseminated lupus erythematosus, drug toxicity and other prolonged fevers. Development of normocytic-normochromic anemia, mild leukocytosis, elevation of erythrocyte sedimentation rate (ESR), proteinuria and microscopic or frank hematuria should strengthen the clinical diagnosis.

C-reactive protein (CRP) is elevated in 90% of cases but lacks specificity.

Procalcitonin, a circulating calcitonin precursor has been shown to be a marker of systemic bacterial infection including IE. A value exceeding 2.3 ng/mL among patients with suspected IE has a sensitivity of 81% and a specificity of 85% in diagnosing definite IE.

Criteria for diagnosis evolved from Duke University (Duke Criteria) in 1994. These criteria offer improved sensitivity and specificity for diagnosis of endocarditis.

Duke's Criteria for Diagnosis of IE

Definite IE

Pathologic criteria

- ***Pathologic lesions:*** Vegetation or intracardiac abscess present, confirmed by histology showing active endocarditis

Textbook of Medicine

- **Microorganisms:** They demonstrated by culture or histology in a vegetation or in a vegetation that has embolized or in an intracardiac abscess.

Clinical criteria

It is using specific definitions are listed below:
- Two major criteria
- One major and three minor criteria
- Five minor criteria.

Definitions of terms used in the Duke criteria for the diagnosis of IE:
- Major criteria
  - **Positive blood culture for IE:** Typical microorganism for IE from two separate blood cultures, or persistently positive blood culture defined as recovery of a microorganism consistent with IE from:
    - Blood cultures drawn more than 12 hours apart
    - All of three or a majority of four or more separate blood cultures, with first and last drawn at least 1 hour apart
    - Single positive blood culture for *Coxiella burnetii.*
  - **Evidence of endocardial involvement:** Positive echocardiogram for IE:
    - Oscillating intracardiac mass on valve or supporting structure, or in the path of regurgitant jet or on implanted material in the absence of an alternative anatomic explanation
    - Abscess
    - New partial dehiscence of prosthetic valve, or new valvular regurgitation (increase or change in pre-existing murmur not sufficient).
- Minor criteria
  - **Predisposition:** Predisposing heart condition or IV drug use
  - **Fever** > 38°C (100.4°F)
  - **Vascular phenomena:** Major arterial emboli, septic pulmonary infarcts, mycotic aneurysm, intracranial hemorrhage, conjunctival hemorrhage, Janeway lesions
  - **Immunologic phenomena:** GN, Osler's nodes, Roth's spots, rheumatoid factor (RF)
  - **Microbiologic evidence:** Positive blood culture but not meeting major criterion as previously defined or serologic evidence of active infection with organism consistent with IE
  - **Echocardiogram:** Consistent with IE but not meeting major criteria as previously defined.

Possible IE

Findings consistent with IE that fall short of definite but not rejected (one major criteria plus one minor criterion or three minor criteria).

Rejected

- Either a firm alternate diagnosis for manifestations of endocarditis, or
- Resolution of manifestations of endocarditis, with antibiotic therapy for 4 days or less, or
- No pathologic evidence of IE at surgery or autopsy after antibiotic therapy for 4 days or less.

To use bacteremia caused by coagulase-negative staphylococci or diphtheroids (organisms that may cause IE but more often contaminate blood cultures) to support the diagnosis of endocarditis, blood culture must be persistently positive or the organisms recovered in several sporadically positive cultures must be proved to represent a single clone.

Investigations

Echocardiogram

Vegetations above 0.5 cm can be detected easily. Smaller vegetations may escape detection and, therefore, a negative result should not be a reason for ruling out the diagnosis. In practice, demonstration of vegetations by echocardiogram is the most rapid and definite method to establish the diagnosis. Since demonstrable vegetations take days to weeks to develop, repetition of echocardiography is indicated if clinical suspicion is strong. Echocardiogram also helps to assess progress with treatment (Figs 124.1 and 124.3).

Blood Culture

Organisms can be cultured from blood and this should be attempted in all cases. Blood is collected before starting antimicrobial drugs. Three separate sets of blood culture; each from separate venipuncture, obtained over 24 hours are recommended to evaluate patients with suspected endocarditis. Each sample should be inoculated in aerobic and anaerobic medium. The organisms are slow growers and, therefore, the cultures should be continued for 2–3 weeks. In doubtful cases, they should be subcultured. In many cases mixed flora may be seen or with treatment, the microbial flora may change. Hence, repeat cultures should be done when treatment is prolonged or the progress is not fully satisfactory. Drug sensitivity of the organisms should be determined to assess the choice of antibiotics. The organisms vary considerably in their drug sensitivity and, therefore, prior assessment of the antibiotic sensitivity is of great value in ensuring successful therapy.

Other Investigations

Computed tomography-positron emission tomography (CT-PET) (pathological complete response): Blood cultures and echocardiography remain the cornerstone for diagnosis. Pathological complete response helps to identify organisms more rapidly. Newer diagnostic

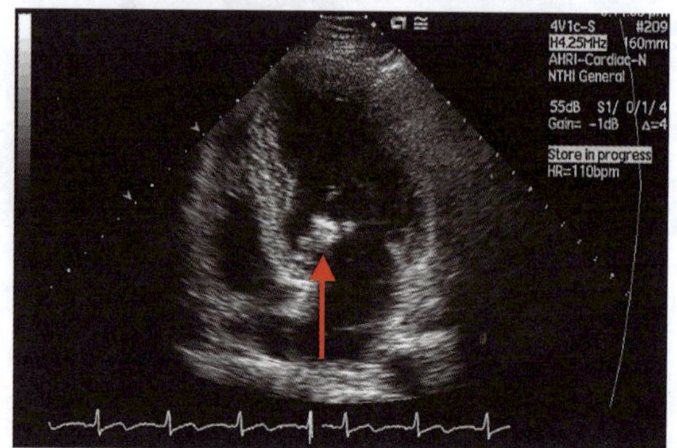

Fig. 124.3: Transthoracic echocardiogram shows vegetation attached to anterior mitral leaflet (arrow)

imaging modalities include 3D echocardiography, multi-slice, CT-PET, molecular imaging and magnetic resonance imaging (MRI). MRI can detect subclinical cerebro-vascular complications in about 50% of cases.

Prognosis

With the help of echocardiography and microbiological studies, the diagnosis can be confirmed in most cases if clinical suspicion is high. Prognosis depends on the timely institution and prolonged administration of appropriate antibiotic combination. Prognosis is best when the specific organism and its antibiotic sensitivity are known. ***Therefore, it is of utmost importance, that blood should be taken for microbiological studies before starting antibiotics empirically, even if treatment may be delayed slightly.***

It is important to prevent the onset of IE in all patients with anatomical lesions in the cardiovascular system (CVS).

Identification of high-risk patients: Heart failure, stroke, abnormal mental status, recurrent embolism, septic shock, fever persisting more than 7–10 days, large enlarging vegetation, perivascular extension of lesion (abscess, pseudoaneurysm, fistula), new heart block, severe left-sided regurgitation, severe prosthetic dysfunction, signs of alteration in left-sided cavity filling pressures, pulmonary hypertension, low left ventricular ejection fraction, pathogens other than *Staphylococcus viridans*, e.g. *S. aureus*, fungi and gram-negative bacilli, acute renal failure and comorbidity are all associated with higher risk for mortality and morbidity.

Treatment

Use of bactericidal antibiotics is the cornerstone of successful therapy.

Empirical Therapy

When the causative organism is not known, the choice of empirical therapy should depend on whether the patient has acute or subacute disease. Acute bacterial endocarditis (ABE) requires broad spectrum therapy that covers *S. aureus* as well as many species of streptococci and gram-negative bacilli. SBE requires a regimen that eradicates most streptococci, including *Enterococcus faecalis*.

- ***For ABE:*** Nafcillin 2.0 g IV q4h + ampicillin 2.0 g IV q4h + gentamicin 1.5 mg/kg IV q8h. If methicillin-resistant *Staphylococcus aureus* (MRSA) is a possibility, for example, in a hospital-acquired case, vancomycin, 1.0 g IV q12h should be substituted for nafcillin
- ***For SBE:*** Ampicillin 2.0 g IV q4h + gentamicin 1.5 mg/kg IV q8h.

Treatment should be appropriately modified when the etiologic organism is identified and antibiotic sensitivity established.

Standard Therapy

The standard treatment for endocarditis due to penicillin susceptible *Viridans streptococci* is aqueous penicillin G 12–18 million unit/24 hours either continuous or every 4 hours in six equally divided doses for 4 weeks and gentamicin 1 mg/kg IM/IV 8 hourly for first 2 weeks. Vancomycin is recommended for patients allergic to penicillin.

Treatment of *S. aureus* endocarditis, in the absence of prosthetic material includes nafcillin or cefazolin or vancomycin (for methicillin resistant 15–20 mg/kg/q12h). In the presence of prosthetic material, vancomycin plus rifampicin (300 mg PO 8th hourly) and gentamycin (1 mg/kg IM or IV 8th hourly) for 6 weeks is the preferred regimen (Table 124.4).

For *Haemophilus*, *Actinobacillus*, *Cardiobacterium*, *Eikenella* and *Kingella* (HACEK group organisms which are a group of gram-negative bacilli causing IE), ceftriaxone (2 g od) or ampicillin-sulbactam (2 g/q4h) for 4 weeks is recommended.

Indication for Surgery in IE

Although the mainstay of treatment in IE is medical, surgery has a role in certain specific situations when medical

Table 124.4: Effective antibiotics for common organisms causing infective endocarditis

Organism	Treatment
Infective endocarditis awaiting culture report	Benzylpenicillin plus gentamicin at the dose given below OR Amoxicillin/clavulanate 12 g/day in four divided doses plus gentamicin 1 mg/kg thrice a day for 4–6 weeks
Suspected staphylococcal endocarditis	Vancomycin 30 mg/kg/day in two divided doses (not to exceed 2 g/day) for 6 weeks and gentamicin 1 mg/kg three times a day for 1–2 weeks. Add rifampicin 20 mg/kg/day in two divided doses in prosthetic valve endocarditis
Streptococci highly sensitive to penicillin	Benzylpenicillin 2–3 million units IV 4 hourly for 4 weeks OR Ceftriaxone 2 g IV once a day for 4 weeks OR Benzylpenicillin or ceftriaxone for 2 weeks plus gentamicin 3 mg/kg once a day for 2 weeks Vancomycin 30 mg/kg/day in two divided doses (not to exceed 2 g/day) for 4 weeks in penicillin-sensitive patients
Streptococci less sensitive to penicillin	Benzylpenicillin (24 million units/day in six divided doses) or ceftriaxone for 4–6 weeks and gentamicin 3 mg/kg/day (as single infusion) for at least 2 weeks
Anaerobic streptococci	Benzylpenicillin, metronidazole
Staphylococcal endocarditis (methicillin-sensitive)	Cloxacillin 2 g 4 hourly or cefazolin 2 g 8 hourly for 6 weeks plus gentamicin 1 mg/kg three times a day for 3–5 days
Enterococcal endocarditis	Ampicillin 2 g 4 hourly or vancomycin plus gentamicin 1 mg/kg three times a day for 6 weeks
Candida	Amphotericin B 1 mg/kg qid 2 weeks maximum up to 4 weeks. Do not exceed 50 mg/day Flucytosine 150 mg/kg oral for 4 days

treatment fails to clear the infection, the underlying abnormality may have to be corrected surgically and this has to be done as a life-saving procedure. Other indications for surgery include acute valvular incompetence leading to cardiac failure, large friable vegetations which are likely to embolize, unstable prosthesis and perivalvular extension of infection.

Surgery in the presence of infection is more risky. Still in the case of intractable infection, not responding to medical therapy, the mortality will be high without surgery. Indications for surgery include conditions such as early prosthetic valve endocarditis (PVE), paravalvular leak (PVL), annular abscess, fungal endocarditis and persistence of fever for more than 2 weeks despite antibiotics in the absence of other evident causes of embolism. Surgical procedure includes thorough debridement, vegetectomy valve or appliance replacement and valve repair. The recurrence rate of postoperative endocarditis in the replaced valve is only below 2–3%. Surgical treatment of IE (valve surgery) results depends greatly on the surgeon's skills. Valvular repair is preferable if possible. After discharge from hospital, close monitoring of patients for 1 year is essential to detect complications.

RECOMMENDATION FOR ENDOCARDITIS PROPHYLAXIS

Revised guidelines on IE prophylaxis were aimed at simplifying recommendations and ensuring consistency with the published evidence over the past 2 decades. The target groups and the procedures for which prophylaxis is reasonable have been drastically reduced in number. Four primary reasons were cited to form the rationale for revising the guidelines:

1. IE is much more likely to result from frequent exposure to random bacteremias associated with daily activities than from bacteremia caused by a dental, gastrointestinal tract (GIT) or genitourinary (GU) tract procedure
2. Prophylaxis prevents an exceedingly small number of cases of IE, if any, in individuals who undergo a dental, GI tract or GU tract procedure
3. The risk of antibiotic-associated adverse events exceeds the benefit, if any, from prophylactic antibiotic therapy except in very high-risk situations
4. Maintenance of optimal oral health and hygiene may reduce the incidence of bacteremia from daily activities and thus the risk of IE, and is more important than the use of prophylactic antibiotics for dental procedures.

Prophylaxis

Prophylaxis indicated and not indicated for IE are shown in Table 124.5.

Prophylaxis against IE is not recommended in patients with valvular heart disease for nondental procedures [e.g. transesophageal echocardiography (TEE), esophagogastroduodenoscopy (EGD), colonoscopy or cystoscopy] in the absence of active infection.

The procedures for which prophylaxis is reasonable are as follows.

Table 124.5: Prophylaxis indicated and not indicated for infective endocarditis

Prophylaxis indicated	Prophylaxis not indicated
• Prosthetic cardiac valves • Previous infective endocarditis • Unrepaired cyanotic congenital heart disease, including palliative shunts and conduits • Completely repaired congenital heart defect with prosthetic material or device, during the first 6 months after the procedure • Repaired congenital heart disease with residual defects at the site or adjacent to the site of a prosthetic patch or prosthetic device (which inhibit endothelialization) • Cardiac transplant recipients with cardiac valvulopathy • Rheumatic heart disease if prosthetic valves or prosthetic material used in valve repair	• Atrial septal defects • Ventricular septal defects • Patent ductus arteriosus • Mitral valve prolapse • Previous Kawasaki disease • Hypertrophic cardiomyopathy • Previous coronary artery bypass graft surgery • Cardiac pacemakers (intravascular and epicardial) and implanted defibrillators • Bicuspid aortic valves • Coarctation of the aorta • Calcified aortic stenosis • Pulmonic stenosis

Dental Procedures

Recommended for procedures that involve manipulation of gingival tissue, periapical region of teeth or perforation of oral mucosa. The following procedures and events do not require prophylaxis—routine anesthetic injections through noninfected tissue, taking dental radiographs, placement of removable prosthodontic or orthodontic appliances, adjustment of orthodontic appliances, placement of orthodontic brackets, shedding of deciduous teeth and bleeding from trauma to the lips or oral mucosa.

Respiratory Tract Procedures

Recommended to individuals who undergo an invasive procedure of the respiratory tract that involves incision or biopsy of the respiratory mucosa, such as tonsillectomy and adenoidectomy. Prophylaxis is not required for bronchoscopy unless the procedure involves incision of the respiratory tract mucosa.

Gastrointestinal or Genitourinary Tract Procedures

Prophylaxis is no longer recommended for these patients. However, for high-risk patients who have an established GIT or GU tract infection, or for those who receive antibiotic therapy to prevent wound infection or sepsis associated with a GIT or GU tract procedure, the antibiotic regimen should include an agent active against enterococci, such as ampicillin or vancomycin.

Procedures on Infected Skin, Skin Structure or Musculoskeletal Tissue

The antibiotic regimen should include coverage against staphylococci and group A streptococci. Appropriate agents include an antistaphylococcal penicillin or cephalosporin. Vancomycin or clindamycin may be used in patients allergic to beta-lactams. If methicillin-resistant *S. aureus* is suspected, vancomycin is recommended.

Antibiotics Regimen for Prophylaxis

Antibiotics regimen for prophylaxis is shown in Table 124.6.

Table 124.6: Antibiotic regimens for dental procedures (single dose administered 30–60 minutes before the procedure

Situation	Agent	Adults*	Children**
Able to take oral medication	Amoxicillin	2 g	50 mg/kg
Unable to take oral medication	Ampicillin	2 g IM or IV	50 mg/kg IM or IV
	Cefazolin or ceftriaxone	1 g IM or IV	50 mg/kg IM or IV
Allergic to penicillin or ampicillin	Cephalexin***	2 g	50 mg/kg
	Clindamycin	600 mg	20 mg/kg
	Azithromycin or clarithromycin	500 mg	15 mg/kg
Allergic to penicillin or ampicillin and unable to take oral medication	Cefazolin or ceftriaxone	1 g IM or IV	50 mg/kg IM or IV
	Clindamycin	600 mg IM or IV	20 mg/kg IM or IV

* Vancomycin 20 mg/kg IV over 1–2 hours and gentamicin 1.5 mg/kg IV/IM

** Total children's dose should not exceed adult dose

***Cephalosporins should not be used in individuals with immediate type hypersensitivity reaction (urticaria, angioedema, or anaphylaxis) to penicillin.

Abbreviations: IM = Intramuscular; IV = Intravascular

CHAPTER
125

Cardiac Arrhythmias

K Suresh

Chapter Summary

- General Considerations
- Modern Developments in Cardiac Electrophysiology
- Sinus Arrhythmia
- Sinus Bradycardia
- Sinus Tachycardia
- Ectopic Beats
- Paroxysmal Tachycardias
- Supraventricular Arrhythmias
- Wolff-Parkinson-White Syndrome (WPW syndrome)
- Atrial Flutter
- Atrial Fibrillation
- Torsade-de-pointes
- Arrhythmogenic Right Ventricular Dysplasia
- Ventricular Tachycardia (VT)
- Ventricular Fibrillation (VF)
- Heart Blocks
- Pacemaker Implantation
- Ventricular Standstill (Ventricular Asystole)
- Cardiac Arrest and its Management
- Sick Sinus Syndrome (SSS)

GENERAL CONSIDERATIONS

The myocardial cells have the property of spontaneous excitability (automaticity). This is responsible for the pacemaking function of the heart. The sinoatrial (SA) node which has the fastest rate of excitability controls the heart rate. The SA node contains specialized electrically active cells known as P cells which are most excitable. The rate of impulse production and conduction is controlled by various physiological, pharmacological and pathological processes. In normal adults the heart rate varies between 60 and 100/min.

The Action Potential

The cardiac action potential is generated by movement of charged ions across the cell membrane through various channels. The action potential has five phases (phase 0, 1, 2, 3 and 4). However, the two major phases involved in depolarization are—spike (phase 0) and plateau (phase 2). A large fast inward movement of Na^+ through the fast sodium channel is responsible for the early spike. A slower steady influx of Ca^{++} through a separate set of slow channels accounts for the plateau phase. The SA node and the atrioventricular node (AV node) contain cells whose action potential is dominantly mediated by the slow calcium channels. In contrast, the Purkinje cells and the working myocardial cells have both fast and slow channels.

The Calcium Channel

The exact structural details of the calcium channels in the sarcolemmal membrane are not known. It is believed that each ionic channel is a specific protein that floats in a lipid bilayer matrix with a water filled central pore for ion movement. These channels have a selective filter which determines the nature of ions passing through them. In addition, the channels are also influenced by intracellular voltage variations, and hence they are also called *voltage-dependent channels*.

The slow response type of action potential seen mainly in the SA node and AV node is mediated by the slow channels. Although there are various types of slow channels, the calcium-mediated slow channel is most widely recognized. Compared to the fast channels, these channels are not only kinetically slower, but they also operate at a less negative to a more depolarized voltage range. A variety of agents block the slow channels. Local anesthetics, volatile general anesthetics and others produce a nonspecific blockade of both fast and slow channels. In contrast, drugs like verapamil, nifedipine and diltiazem produce a selective direct blocking action on the slow channels. The result is blockade of calcium entry into the cell. Calcium channel blockers are extensively used in the treatment of arrhythmias and hypertension.

The Conduction System

From the SA node, the impulse travels through the atria to the AV node. There are three functionally specialized pathways in the atria which conduct impulses from the sinus node to the AV node. These are the: (1) Anterior, (2) middle and (3) posterior internodal tracts. A branch of the anterior tract—the Bachmann's bundle connects the two atria also. From the AV node, the impulse travels through the bundle of His, bundle branches and the Purkinje system to reach the ventricular musculature.

In general, arrhythmias may be of two types—disorders of impulse production or disorders of impulse conduction and may be caused by abnormalities of automaticity, and/or abnormalities of conduction. When the main pacemaker is suppressed, the lower centers become active and take up the pacemaking function. This gives rise to escape rhythms such as junctional escape or ventricular escape. Enhanced automaticity of ectopic foci may occur and this leads to the development of ectopic rhythms and ectopic tachycardias (junctional ectopics and junctional tachycardia).

Abnormality in the conduction of impulses may give rise to *reentry phenomenon* which is considered as one of the common mechanisms of tachyarrhythmias. When the normal conducting pathway becomes refractory, an incoming impulse may take a different course and pass down. By the time it reaches lower down, the refractoriness of the distal end of the normal pathway would have passed off and it may become capable of conduction. Hence, the abnormal impulse gets into it and it is conducted in a retrograde direction. This is designated as reentry phenomenon and is responsible for genesis and perpetuation of ectopic tachycardias. In order for reentry to occur three conditions must be met: (1) Two functionally distinct conducting pathways, (2) Unidirectional conduction block in one of the pathways and (3) a differential in the conduction rates in the pathways, with slow conduction via one pathway and return of conduction via the second.

In some individuals, accessory pathways for conduction exist. These accessory pathways are anomalous extranodal connections which connect the epicardial surfaces of the atrium and ventricles along the AV groove. Accessory pathways may conduct impulses in both anterograde and retrograde directions—the former mostly silent. The accessory and normal pathways conduct impulses from the atria to the ventricles in various combinations resulting in the production of reentrant tachyarrhythmias, e.g. Wolff-Parkinson-White (WPW) syndrome.

MODERN DEVELOPMENTS IN CARDIAC ELECTROPHYSIOLOGY

Study of cardiac electrophysiology has reached a high degree of advancement starting from the classic electrocardiogram (ECG) studies, special leads to record the electrical variations from different parts of the heart, study of electrical activity of the His-Purkinje system from their trunks to their ultimate ramification, study of abnormal conducting pathways in and across the AV junctions, accessory conducting pathways, their exact localization, and total electrophysiological mapping of the heart and other studies. Several types of antiarrhythmic drugs have been made available with well-defined indications and contraindications.

Arrhythmias which are not amenable to medications can be traced back to their anatomical source such as mapping abnormal bundles (e.g. Kent bundle) which can be cured by radiofrequency ablation.

Heart blocks do not usually respond to drug therapy. They can be managed by electrical pacing of the heart which can be done on a short-term external pacing or long-term pacing using implanted pacemakers which have become very popular and common, though still expensive. Several newer models incorporating newer modalities in function and operations are available in the market.

Fatal arrhythmias such as cardiac standstill and ventricular fibrillation (VF) can be sensed by the defibrillator pacemaker devices and major cardiac events and death can be avoided.

Many patients who have abnormalities in cardiac electrophysiology are fitted with implanted pacemaker, defibrillators/pacemakers and their improved versions such as demand pacemakers and so on. In the earlier phase of their development, such devices were to be protected from high energy, electrical and magnetic influences. At present pacemakers compatible with MRI sources are available. Though all these developments are highly expensive by Indian standards many people are provided with such components by the help of governmental and charitable sources. The subspecialty of cardiac electrophysiology has developed as a major subdivision of cardiology and exciting developments are taking place. Many tertiary cardiac centers have these facilities.

A relatively recent innovation is the use of resynchronization of ventricular function in dysfunctional states of the ventricle using single ventricular or biventricular pacing (cardiac resynchronization therapy). This has resulted in considerable functional improvement and improvement in ventricular function.

SINUS ARRHYTHMIA

Even in normal subjects with sinus rhythm, slight beat to beat variation in time-interval occurs. When the difference between the longest and the shortest cycles exceeds 0.12 sec, it is termed as sinus arrhythmia. This is seen more often in children and young adults. In the vast majority of cases, this is a benign condition with no detectable underlying disorder of the heart.

Sinus arrhythmia may occur in two forms: (1) Phasic and (2) nonphasic. In the **phasic form**, which is more common, there is characteristic acceleration of the heart rate with inspiration and slowing with expiration. This is caused by the respiratory fluctuations in the vagal tone mediated through the **Bainbridge reflex**. The **nonphasic form** does not show any relation to the phases of respiration. The ECG shows a difference of at least 0.12 sec between the longest and the shortest PP intervals. The configuration of the P wave and the PQ intervals remain constant (Figs 125.1 and 125.2).

SINUS BRADYCARDIA

Sinus bradycardia implies a sinus rate below 60/min. Often this is seen normally in athletes and heavy manual laborers. Disease states such as hypothyroidism, obstructive jaundice, raised intracranial tension and acute inferior wall myocardial infarction (MI) may be associated with bradycardia. Drugs like digoxin, verapamil and propranolol may produce sinus bradycardia. Pathological processes affecting the SA node give rise to sick sinus syndrome (SSS) in which the patients may present with extreme sinus bradycardia, sinus arrest, sinus blocks and escape rhythms.

SINUS TACHYCARDIA

Sinus tachycardia implies a sinus rate of more than 100/min. It is seen normally during exercise and anxiety. Fever, thyrotoxicosis, infections, hypoxia, anemia, hemorrhage, hypotension, heart failure and shock are the common pathological causes. Drugs like atropine, adrenaline and ephedrine cause sinus tachycardia. Usually the heart rate does not exceed 150/min (Fig. 125.3).

ECTOPIC BEATS

Heartbeat produced prematurely as a result of impulse originating in areas other than the sinus node is designated as ectopic beat. It may be early or late in diastole. Following a premature beat the normal impulse reaching the AV node finds the ventricle refractory and so the subsequent normal beat is missed. This is the **compensatory pause**. If the RR interval in the ECG encompassing the ectopic is twice the normal it is called fully compensated, otherwise it is partial. Premature beat may be atrial, junctional or ventricular.

Atrial Premature Beats

These are premature beats arising from ectopic foci in the atria. Ectopic foci may be single or multiple. All age groups may be affected and in many cases, there is no detectable organic disease of the heart. **Common causes** include anxiety, excessive intake of coffee or tea and heavy tobacco smoking. However, in the presence of organic heart disease it can predispose to atrial tachyarrhythmias such as atrial tachycardia, flutter and fibrillation. Clinically, premature beats are appreciated as dropped beat. The compensatory pause is not full in atrial premature beat. The normal beat coming after the compensatory pause is more forceful on account of the longer diastolic filling and this may be felt as a thud by the patient. ECG shows the abnormally shaped ectopic P wave preceding the normal QRS complex. The compensatory pause is not full. The PQ interval is usually short though sometimes it may be prolonged (Fig. 125.4).

Junctional Premature Beats

These beats arise from the AV junction. These are less common than atrial and ventricular premature beats (VPBs). The physical findings resemble those of atrial premature beats. Sometimes cannon waves may be observed in the neck veins if the atria contract, while the AV valves remain closed. The conduction of impulse in the atrium is retrograde and so the P wave appears inverted in LII, LIII and aVF, but it is upright in lead aVR. They may precede the QRS with a shortened PQ interval, be immersed in the QRS or follow the QRS. The QRS of the junctional premature beat is usually normal. The compensatory pause is not full.

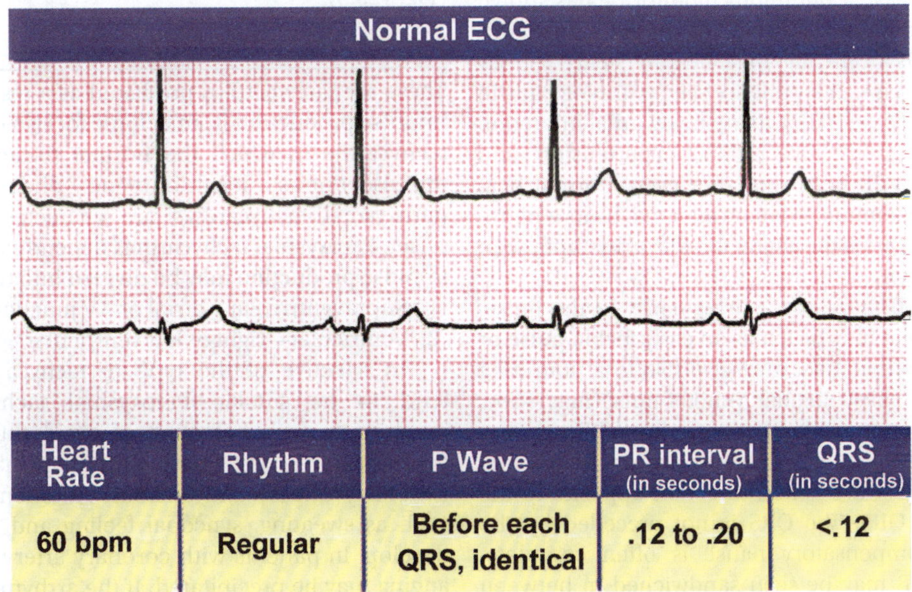

Heart Rate	Rhythm	P Wave	PR interval (in seconds)	QRS (in seconds)
60 bpm	Regular	Before each QRS, identical	.12 to .20	<.12

Fig. 125.1: Normal ECG with sinus bradycardia. **Note:** The QRS rate is around 60/minute. The rhythm is regular with normal P and other complexes. QRS duration is less than 0.12 seconds

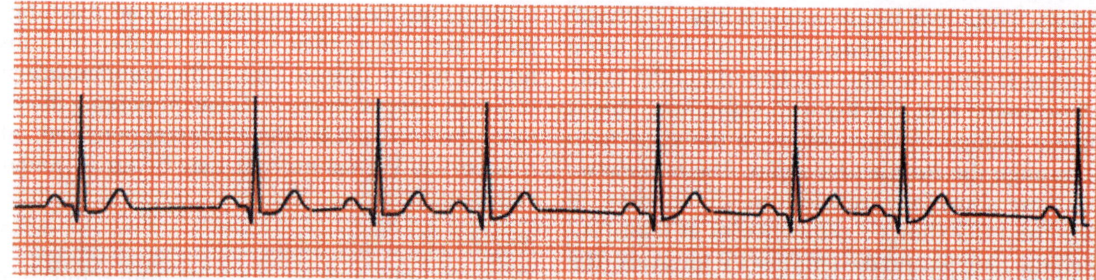

Fig. 125.2: *Sinus arrhythmia. Note:* The change in heart rate with inspiration and expiration—increase during inspiration with shorter RR intervals and decrease during expiration. This is a normal phenomenon

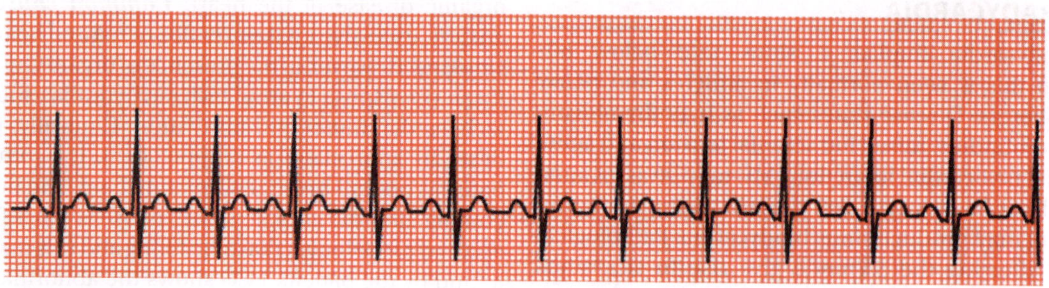

Fig. 125.3: **ECG sinus tachycardia.** *Note:* Heart rate is 150/minute. P waves precede all QRS complexes

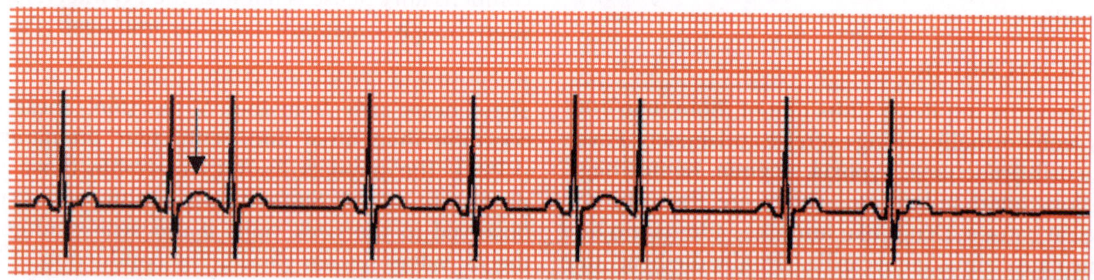

Fig. 125.4: *Atrial premature beats. Note:* 1. The 3rd and 7th beat of the rhythm are premature beats. 2. The QRS morphology of premature beat is same as the normal beat. 3. The premature beat is preceded by abnormal P wave (arrow)

Ventricular Premature Beats

An ectopic focus in any part of the ventricle can give rise to VPBs. This is the most common arrhythmia seen both in health and in disease. Continuous monitoring has shown that even apparently healthy individuals may show this arrhythmia. VPBs occurring in a healthy heart usually disappear on exercise. The VPBs are seen pathologically in ischemic heart disease (IHD), acute myocardial infarction (MI), cardiomyopathy, myocarditis, hypertension and digitalis toxicity. VPB occurring after every normal beat leads to pulsus bigeminus in which after two beats a pause occurs regularly. This is the characteristic arrhythmia seen in digitalis toxicity.

Clinically, VPB manifests as irregularity in the pulse. The premature beat may be felt as an early feeble pulse or the strong postectopic beat may give rise to a pounding sensation in the chest. Jugular venous pulse may show irregular cannon waves. In the ECG, the VPB appears as a widened QRS which is often bizarre in shape. The ST segment and T wave is in a direction opposite to the direction of the QRS. The QRS is not preceded by the P wave. The compensatory pause is often complete. Sometimes a VPB may be seen sandwiched in between two sinus beats. They are known as interpolated VPBs. The RR interval encompassing the VPB is equal to one cardiac cycle. The interval between the sinus beat and the VPB is known as coupling interval. Coupling interval is constant in case of unifocal VPB, but it is variable in multifocal VPBs (Fig. 125.5).

PAROXYSMAL TACHYCARDIAS

These are tachycardias produced as a result of enhanced impulse production from ectopic foci (in contrast to sinus tachycardia in which the normal pacemaker produces impulses) or as a result of reentry phenomenon. All the paroxysmal tachycardias are characterized by abrupt onset. Paroxysmal tachycardias depending on the focus of impulse production may be divided into two types:

1. Supraventricular—atrial or AV junctional
2. Ventricular—right or left ventricular.

Irrespective of the type of tachycardia, symptoms tend to be similar. Paroxysmal tachycardias usher in abruptly with a feeling of rapid thumping cardiac contractions in the chest. This may make the patient extremely uneasy and anxious. Autonomic phenomena such as sweating, syncopal feeling and tachypnea may develop. In patients with coronary artery disease (CAD), angina may be precipitated. If the arrhythmia tends to be prolonged beyond a few hours, signs of cardiac failure may develop especially if there are underlying abnormalities.

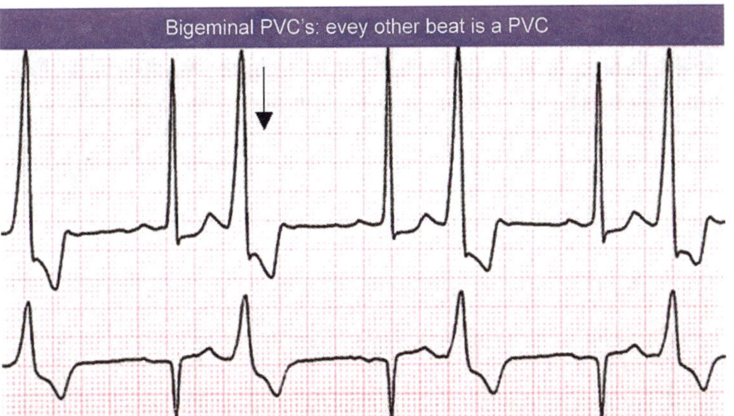

Fig. 125.5: *Premature ventricular beat (PVC). Note:* The bizarre ventricular ectopic beat. Compensatory pause (arrow)

Termination of the attack is also felt as an abrupt cessation of the tachycardia. This may be accompanied by diuresis, usually in supraventricular tachyarrhythmias.

In predisposed individuals, tachyarrhythmias are triggering factors to induce cardiac failure. In all forms of these arrhythmias, ECG is absolutely essential to arrive at the diagnosis.

SUPRAVENTRICULAR ARRHYTHMIAS

Paroxysmal Atrial Tachycardia (PAT)

Impulses arise in the atrium and the arrhythmia is usually produced as result of reentry phenomenon. The heart rate varies from 140 to 230/min and the rhythm is regular. The ECG shows normal QRS with a rate of 140–230/min. In some cases the P waves may be identifiable. Vagal stimulation (carotid pressure, dipping the face in or swallowing ice-cold water or pressure over eyeball) generally slows the rate and abolishes an attack. In the majority there is no underlying cardiac disease. Common causes are excess of caffeine or tobacco, alcohol, anxiety or thyrotoxicosis (Fig. 125.6).

Paroxysmal Atrial Tachycardia with Block

This is an ectopic atrial tachycardia due to enhanced automaticity. This is a special form of paroxysmal atrial tachycardia in which some of the atrial impulses are not conducted down to the ventricles. This gives rise to varying grades of AV block. Electrocardiographically P waves occur at a rate of 140–230/min, with an isoelectric shelf separating the P waves, and a slower QRS rate. This abnormality is characteristically seen in digitalis toxicity. It is an indication for withdrawing digitalis (Fig. 125.7).

Multifocal Atrial Tachycardia

This is characterized by an irregular rhythm and P waves with different morphology. It is seen in conditions such as bronchitis emphysema syndrome, cor pulmonale, hypoxia from any cause, IHD, diabetes mellitus and after cardiac surgery. It indicates a poor prognosis. Diagnosis of multifocal atrial tachycardia can be made only with ECG. The ECG criteria include the following (Fig. 125.8):

- Rate above 100/min
- At least three different forms of P waves in the same lead
- Variability of PP, PR and RR intervals.

Atrioventricular Junctional Tachycardia

Both paroxysmal (ventricular rate 130–240/min) and nonparoxysmal (ventricular rate 70–140/min) forms exist. The ECG shows normal QRS complexes, but the P wave usually follows the QRS.

Atrioventricular Nodal Reentrant Tachycardia

Atrioventricular nodal re-entrant tachycardia (AVNRT) is a tachycardia with a narrow QRS complex and a ventricular rate typically in the range of 150–250 beats/min. The mechanism in AVNRT appears to be a reentrant circuit composed of separate slow and fast pathways involving the AV node. The typical variety is the slow-fast pathway where the antegrade conduction is through the slow pathway and the retrograde conduction to the atria is through the fast pathway. It is generally seen in subjects without underlying heart disease. Palpitations are common presenting complaints. Angina, congestive heart failure and rarely shock may be seen in those with a history of underlying heart disease. Syncope occurs rarely.

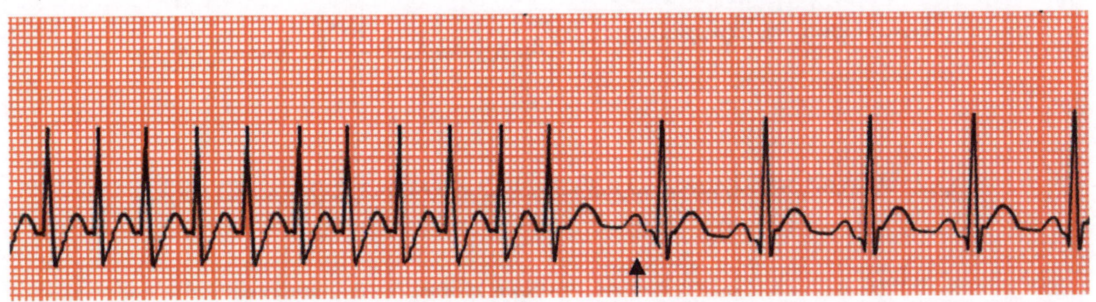

Fig. 125.6: Paroxysmal atrial tachycardia (PAT). *Note:* The first half of the rhythm strip shows rate of nearly 190/minute. The run of tachycardia terminates and is replaced by sinus rhythm in the latter part (arrow)

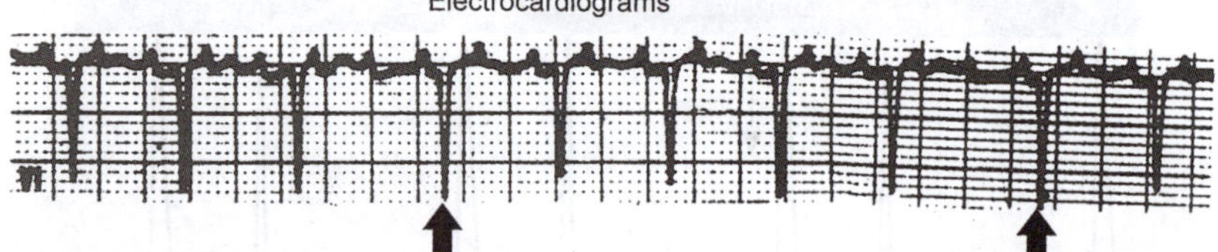

Fig. 125.7: Paroxysmal atrial tachycardia with block

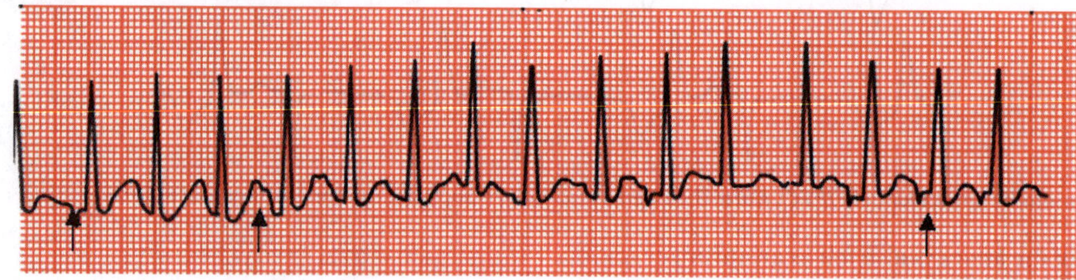

Fig. 125.8: *Multifocal atrial tachycardia (MAT). Note:* 1. The varying morphology of the P waves indicated by arrows. 2. Tachycardia with a rate of nearly 150/min

Clinical examination may reveal regular cannon waves in the neck and absence of variation in the intensity of first heart sound. The pulse and heart sounds are absolutely regular. ECG shows narrow QRS regular tachycardia with a rate of 150–250/min. Retrograde P waves are often seen deforming the terminal part of the QRS complex. This can lead to a pseudo-R in V1 and a terminal in V5 and V6 simulating an incomplete right bundle branch block (RBBB). After conversion to sinus rhythm, this terminal-R in V1 will no longer be seen indicating that it is produced by the retrograde P. In roughly half of the cases, the retrograde P waves may not be seen as they are hidden within the QRS complex (Fig. 125.9).

Management

- Carotid sinus massage in the recumbent posture may serve to abolish PAT. Only one side should be massaged at a time

- Intravenous (IV) administration of adenosine, verapamil, diltiazem or esmolol may terminate the episode
- Other antiarrhythmics that may be tried include amiodarone or the class I antiarrhythmics.

In resistant cases, direct current (DC) shock may be required. ***Investigation*** for the underlying condition and specific measures should be instituted to prevent recurrence.

Atrioventricular Reentrant Tachycardia

Atrioventricular reentrant tachycardia (AVRT) is another narrow QRS tachycardia with ventricular rates often greater than 200/min.

The clinical features are very similar to those of AVNRT but are distinct on an electrophysiological basis. The mechanism in AVRT relies on the presence of reentrant circuit comprising of an accessory pathway as one portion

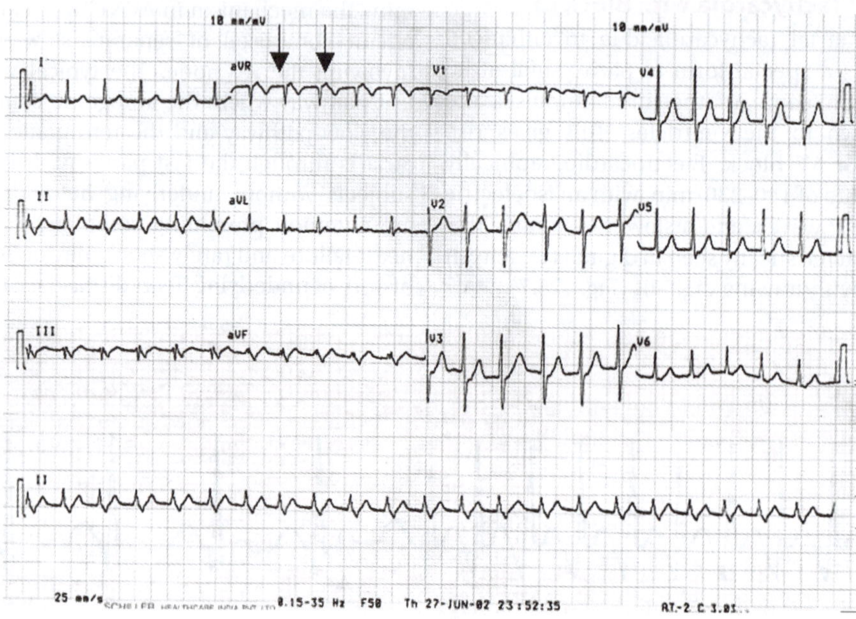

Fig. 125.9: *AVNRT. Note:* 1. AVNRT is a reentrant tachycardia which utilizes the fast and slow pathways in the AV node for its circuit. The uniform and narrow QRS complexes at a rate of nearly 180/min. 2. Short RP intervals and long PR intervals (marked by arrows in aVR) is a hallmark of AVNRT

of the circuit and the AV node as the other portion. Accessory pathways may be ***concealed*** (inapparent by ECG) due to having only retrograde conduction properties (V to A) or ***manifest*** (apparent on ECG as delta waves) due to variable degrees of antegrade conduction (e.g. WPW pattern as described below).

AV reentrant tachycardia may be orthodromic or antidromic. Orthodromic AVRT is a narrow-complex tachycardia that uses the AV node as the antegrade limb and the accessory pathway as the retrograde limb of the circuit. Antidromic AVRT is a wide QRS complex tachycardia that is the opposite such that the accessory pathway serves as the antegrade limb and the AV node as the retrograde limb of the circuit.

Orthodromic AVRT is the most common reentrant AVRT accounting for 95% of cases. It is a narrow QRS complex regular tachycardia and the P wave will be seen just after the QRS complex inscribed on the ST segment (unlike AVNRT where the P waves are hidden in the QRS).

WOLFF-PARKINSON-WHITE SYNDROME (PRE-EXCITATION SYNDROME)

Wolff-Parkinson-White syndrome is not an uncommon cause of tachyarrhythmia seen in both sexes. In this condition, an abnormal band of atrial tissue connects the atria and ventricles. In sinus rhythm this tissue conducts impulses faster bypassing the AV node. Conduction of impulse from atrium to ventricle occurs partly through the AV node and partly through the faster bypass tract. The ECG shows shortening of the PR interval and slurring of the ascending limb of the QRS complex, termed the delta wave, in addition to widening of the QRS complex (Fig. 125.10).

Since the AV node and the abnormal conducting tract have different conduction velocities, reentrant tachycardias occur frequently resulting in paroxysmal tachycardias. Depending upon the direction of passage of the impulse through the AV node and the abnormal conducting tissue, the reentry mechanisms vary giving rise to ECG patterns either resembling supraventricular tachycardia (SVT) or with broader QRS complexes resembling ventricular tachycardias (VTs). Usually the antegrade conduction during tachycardia is through the AV node and the retrograde conduction is through the accessory pathway and hence the QRS tends to be narrow. Atrial fibrillation (AF) can occur and is associated with a very fast ventricular response which can degenerate into VF and sudden cardiac death. The condition is disabling since it affects the quality of life of the patient.

Management of Supraventricular Tachycardia

This includes pharmacological therapy, radiofrequency ablation of the abnormal conduction pathway or surgical treatment. At present, catheter ablation is done for life-threatening arrhythmias (e.g. WPW syndrome, VT, incessant SVT, AF, atrial flutter, etc.) where accessory pathways are demonstrable. Electrophysiological studies and radiofrequency ablation of the accessory pathway is preferred to long-term medical management by many physicians and patients.

Pharmacological Therapy

Mainly three types of drugs are employed:
1. Those that prolong the conduction time or refractoriness in the AV node, e.g. adenosine, propranolol and digoxin
2. Those that prolong the conduction or refractoriness of the accessory pathway, e.g. class 1A and 1C drugs
3. Prolongation of conduction time and refractoriness of both pathways. Class III drugs, e.g. amiodarone, sotalol.

Digoxin, IV verapamil and lignocaine can be used, but with caution, and not if the patient presents with AF. In patients with anterograde conduction through the accessory pathway, use of digoxin, adenosine, calcium blockers and beta-blockers, etc. may be contraindicated since these drugs increase accessory pathway conduction and predispose to fast ventricular rates.

Amiodarone: This is a potent antiarrhythmic drug which is effective both in supraventricular and ventricular arrhythmias. It may be given both parenterally as well as orally. Peak levels occur within 4–5 hours after an oral loading dose. It has a long half-life in the body (more than 8 days). It is concentrated in the myocardium. Initial dose

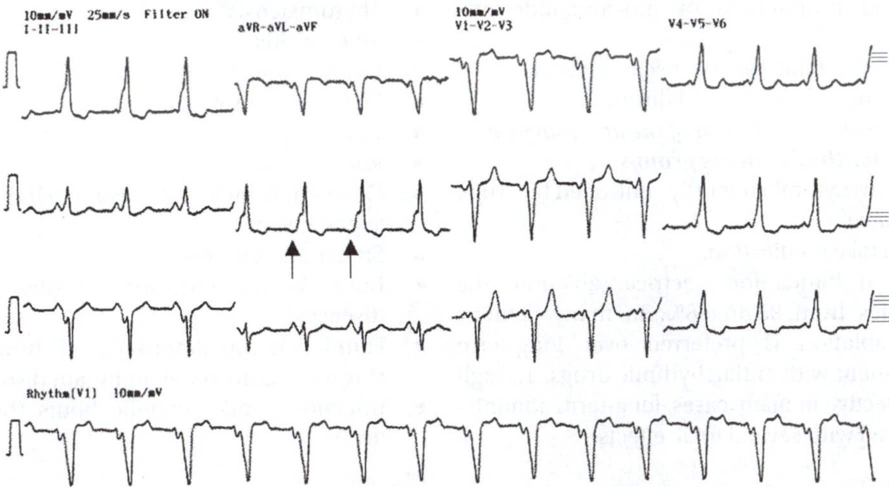

Fig. 125.10: *Wolff-Parkinson-White (WPW) syndrome. Note:* The classic triad of WPW syndrome include: 1. Short PR interval. 2. Delta wave (arrows) 3. QRS widening. The delta wave represents the conduction through the aberrant bypass tract

is 100–200 mg, 6–8 hourly orally for 5–7 days and then the dose is reduced gradually to reach a maintenance dose of 100–200 mg/day. Adverse side effects include antagonism to vitamin K dependent coagulation factors and photosensitivity. This drug is useful in the treatment of resistant supraventricular and ventricular arrhythmias and WPW syndrome. This drug can also be given IV as a bolus injection in a dose of 150 mg, followed by a continuous infusion of 1.0–1.2 g over 18–24 hours.

Calcium channel blockers: Verapamil and diltiazem have pronounced antiarrhythmic properties. They reduce the SA node activity and AV nodal conduction. Verapamil is very effective in the treatment of SVTs when given IV in a dose of 5 mg to be repeated 10 min later, if necessary. Diltiazem is also effective particularly when given parenterally and also in the more conventional mode orally. Both these drugs are contraindicated in the presence of left ventricular failure, shock and conduction defects. They are not effective in the treatment of VTs.

When drug therapy fails and the condition of the patient demands rapid termination of the arrhythmia, more aggressive methods have to be used. These include DC shock and catheter ablation of the abnormal conduction pathways. In the latter, radiofrequency energy is used to ablate the abnormal pathways.

Termination of an Acute Episode

If there is no hemodynamic compromise, vagal pressure can be applied initially to reduce the rate. This is followed up with IV adenosine (6–12 mg IV rapid bolus) and later IV verapamil or diltiazem. AF with fast heart rate may occur after drug administration, particularly adenosine. This should be treated with electrical cardioversion.

In those with very rapid ventricular rates or signs of hemodynamic impairment, electrical cardioversion is the treatment of choice.

For AF or fibrillation, drugs that prolong refractoriness in the accessory pathway often coupled with drugs prolonging AV nodal refractoriness such as procainamide and propranolol are used (Flowchart 125.1).

Prevention of Tachycardia

Drug combinations are usually employed:

- Quinidine and propranolol or procainamide and verapamil
- Amiodarone or sotalol can be used singly. Dose of solatol 80–320 mg/day in divided doses.

Radiofrequency catheter ablation of the accessory pathway is advisable for the following groups:

- Symptomatic arrhythmia not fully controlled by drugs
- Drug intolerance
- Reluctance to take medication.

In experienced hands for electrical ablation, the success rate varies from 95 to 98%. In many centers, radiofrequency ablation is preferred over long-term medical management with antiarrhythmic drugs. Though amiodarone is effective in many cases, long-term administration is associated with several toxic effects.

Surgical Ablation

Rarely surgical interruption of accessory pathway may be necessary.

ATRIAL FLUTTER

This is an uncommon arrhythmia in which the atria contract at the rate of 300/min. The mechanism is one of reentrant tachycardia affecting the atria. Since the AV node cannot conduct impulses at this rate, a physiological block develops and only half, a third or a fourth of the atrial impulses are transmitted to the ventricles. The ventricles contract at a lower rate, but regularly. Flutter waves are seen in the jugular vein. Carotid pressure increases the block and reduces the ventricular rate further (Figs 125.11 and 125.12).

Treatment

Generally atrial flutter is resistant to drug treatment, but it responds to DC shock readily, 50 joules may be sufficient. Digoxin either abolishes the arrhythmia or converts it into AF and reduces the ventricular rate. On withdrawing digoxin, normal rhythm may be restored. Quinidine is also effective in the treatment of atrial flutter. But it is less commonly due to its unpleasant side effects.

ATRIAL FIBRILLATION

This is the condition in which the coordinated contraction of the atrium is abolished and the atrial muscle fibrillates. Abnormality of atrial activation is caused by impulses arising from different foci at the rate of 400–600/min. Since coordinated contraction at this rate is not possible, fibrillation sets in. This is the most common sustained arrhythmia in clinical practice. Prevalence increases with age. Above the age of 65 years, AF occurs in 5% of persons and above 75 years it affects 10% or more. Five percent of persons with paroxysmal AF and 20% of those with persistent or permanent AF have no other demonstrable pathology.

Etiology

Atrial fibrillation may be due to different causes. In the order of frequency these are the following:

- Rheumatic mitral valvular disease, mixed mitral lesions (mitral stenosis and mitral regurgitation)
- IHD
- Hypertensive heart disease
- Thyrotoxicosis
- Myocarditis
- Cardiomyopathies
- Digoxin toxicity
- Chronic pericardial disease
- Pneumonia
- Congenital heart disease (CHD) especially atrial-septal defect
- Sick sinus syndrome
- Lone AF (AF without any obvious predisposing diseases)
- Familial AF (an abnormality of chromosome 16 occurring as an autosomal dominant disorder)
- Infections and alcoholic bouts (holiday heart syndrome).

Classification

- ***Paroxysmal atrial fibrillation:*** Transient, reverting to normal sinus rhythm spontaneously

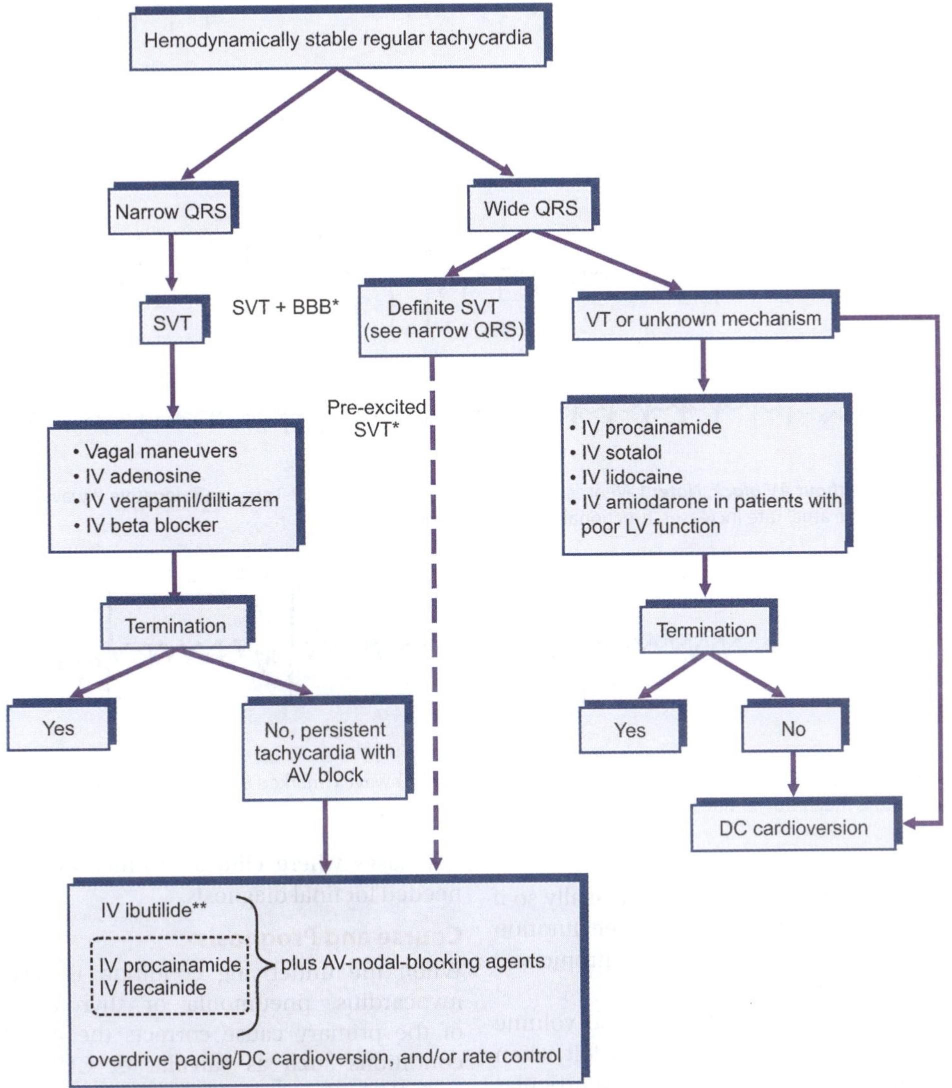

Source: Modified from ACC/AHA/ESC guidelines for the management of tachyarrhythmias. Circulation. 2003;108:1871-1909.
Abbreviations: AF = Atrial fibrillation; AV = Artrioventricular; BBB = Bundle-branch block; DC = Direct current; IV = Intravenous; LV = Left ventricular; QRS = ventricular activation on ECG; SVT = Supraventricular tachycardia; VT = Ventricular tachycardia; EF: Ejection fraction

- ***Persistent atrial fibrillation:*** It does not revert spontaneously, but does so with electrical or pharmacological intervention
- ***Permanent atrial fibrillation:*** It cannot be reverted to sinus rhythm by electrical or pharmacological intervention.

Pathophysiology

Ectopic impulses arise in the atria or pulmonary veins and their ostia at the rate of 400–600/min. They reach the AV node at irregular intervals. Many of them find the AV node totally or partially refractory and therefore, conduction to the ventricle is totally irregular. In AF the electrical activity produces multiple wavelets which circle round the atria. Some of these circles back themselves forming reentry loops. The conduction velocity and refractory periods of portions of the atrial wall vary so that wavelets follow altering courses. A few complete classic reentrant loops.

Atrial enlargement predisposes to AF by accommodating more wavelets.

Rheumatic valvular disease predisposes to AF since it leads to deranged hemodynamics, atrial inflammation, fibrosis and impaired propagation of the impulse.

Ventricular contraction occurs irregularly—both in rhythm as well as in force. The A wave in the jugular vein disappears since the atrium fails to contract as a whole. Loss of atrial contraction abolishes the augmented transit of atrial blood into the ventricle during end diastole, thereby abolishing the stretch to the ventricular muscle preceding systole (atrial booster effect). In normal hearts this may not be clinically significant, but in a diseased heart, AF precipitates cardiac failure because of the loss of atrial booster effect. Thrombi form in the atria as a result of stagnation. These embolize periodically resulting in systemic or pulmonary embolism.

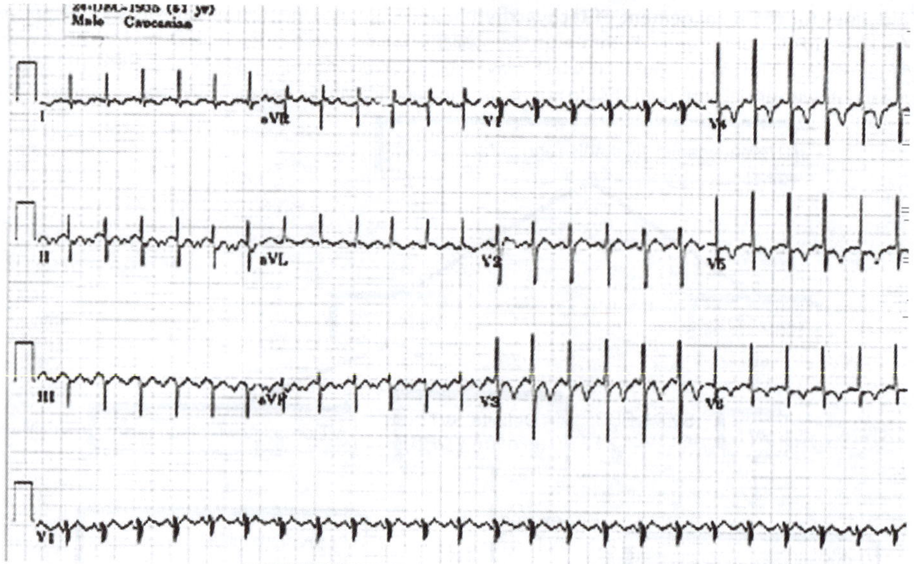

Fig. 125.11: *Atrial flutter without AV block. Note:* 1. Ventricular rate above 180/minutes. 2. Large and negative P waves in leads II, III and avF. Comment: Generally when the atrial rate increases, functional AV block develops

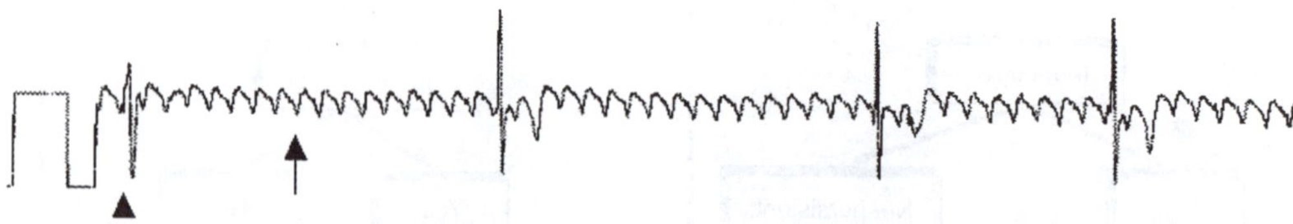

Fig. 125.12: **Atrial flutter:** Lead V1 to show the flutter waves. 1. The rapid flutter waves (marked by arrow) which are usually inverted in leads II, III and avF. 2. The QRS rate is much slower due to associated AV block (arrow head)

Clinical Features

The onset of AF may be felt as palpitation, especially so if the heart rate is high. AF is considered acute when duration is less than 48 hours. It may be paroxysmal or chronic and insidious in onset and course.

The pulse is totally irregular in rhythm and volume (irregularly irregular). The irregularity is best felt when the heart rate is rapid. In slow heart rates with ventricular contraction around 70/min, the arrhythmia may be more difficult to detect clinically at rest. Pulse deficit can be made out by simultaneous palpation of the pulse and auscultation of the heart rate (by two different observers). A difference of more than 10 beats/min is highly suggestive of AF. The irregularity increases with exertion. Auscultation reveals total irregularity and varying intensity of the first heart sound. The a-wave of the jugular venous pulse is abolished. The presystolic accentuation of the mid-diastolic murmur of mitral stenosis disappears in most cases. If the fourth heart sound was audible prior to the onset of AF, it disappears. Confirmation of the diagnosis is made by ECG which shows absence of P-waves and the presence of fibrillary waves instead. The QRS complexes are irregular in rhythm but may be normal in pattern (Fig. 125.13).

Differential Diagnosis

Frequently occurring irregular extrasystoles may be mistaken for AF, especially if the heart rate is slow. Exercise abolishes the extrasystoles whereas it aggravates AF. In a few cases where clinical distinction is difficult ECG is needed for final diagnosis.

Course and Prognosis

When the underlying condition is reversible such as myocarditis, pneumonia or thyrotoxicosis, treatment of the primary cause corrects the AF also. In chronic conditions such as valvular or CHD, cardiomyopathy and IHD, the arrhythmia tends to persist even after treatment of the primary disease. AF in the setting of acute MI tends to be transient. In the setting of right coronary artery involvement leading to inferior wall MI and right ventricular involvement, AF is usually associated with slow ventricular response. Sometimes, AF is associated with complete heart block, when pulse as well as RR interval in the ECG tends to be regular. AF in the setting of anterior wall MI very often is associated with fast ventricular rate and left ventricular dysfunction.

AF gives rise to thromboembolic episodes. The risk is much higher when there is obstruction to AV flow as in mitral stenosis. Risk of thromboembolism is increased considerably in all cases of AF, compared to sinus rhythm. Other abnormalities such as left ventricular function impairment, disturbances of hemostatic mechanism and hypercoagulability accentuate the risk. Presence of mitral stenosis increases this risk several fold further. People with history of previous thromboembolic episodes are at considerable risk for recurrent stroke. The thromboembolic risk is higher in those with history of hypertension, DM as well as in elderly. In patients with nonvalvular AF

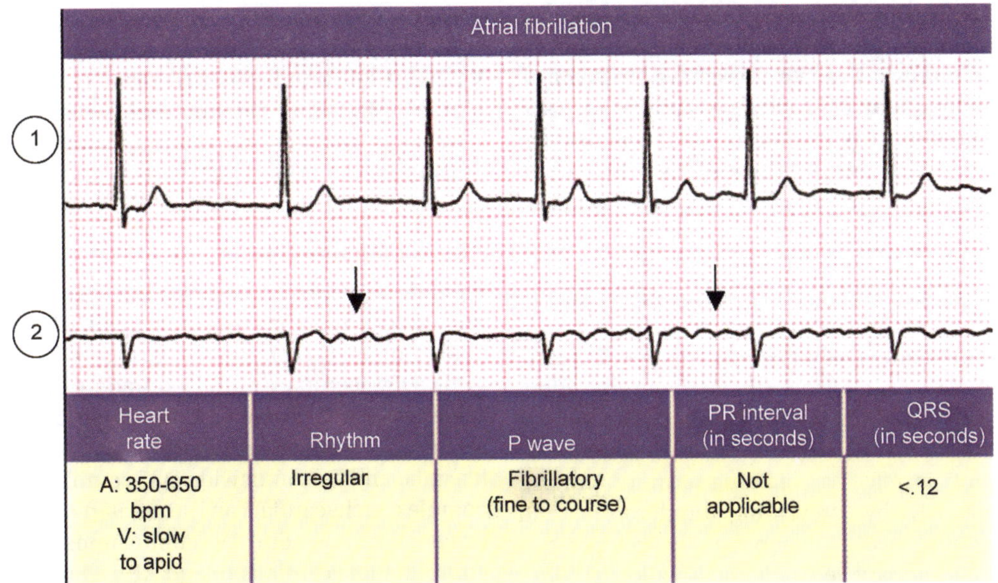

Fig. 125.13: ***Atrial fibrillation. Note:*** 1. Totally irregular RR intervals. 2. Absent negative P waves. 3. Fibrillary waves marked by arrows. Usually the QRS rate is fast in untreated atrial fibrillation. This record is made after starting treatment and slowing of the heart rate: (1) Upper tracing lead 2, (2) Lower tracing shows the fibrillary waves best brought out in lead V1

the average annual risk for arterial thromboembolism, including stroke is 5% and the risk is higher in patients older than 75 years. Stroke risk in AF increases from 1.5% at age 50–59 years to 23.5% at age 80–89 years. About 40% of AF patients in primary care may be at high risk of stroke. Several recent studies involving long-term (up to several months) monitoring using implanted devices have shown that paroxysmal AF has been the underlying cause for many cases of obscure nonhemorrhagic stroke. In paroxysmal AF usually embolization occurs on restoring sinus rhythm. In general 65% of emboli arise from the atrial appendage.

Occurrence of AF leads to deterioration in the cardiac status and a progressive downhill course in chronic rheumatic heart disease (RHD), cardiomyopathies and systemic hypertension. Total mortality is doubled by the presence of AF in all forms of serious underlying heart disease.

Table 125.1 shows the quantitation of risk of stroke in patients with cardiovascular disease.

Risk stratification of ischemic stroke in patients with nonvalvular AF is shown in Table 125.2.

Management

The aims of treatment are:
- To restore sinus rhythm if possible (rhythm control)
- If not, reduce the ventricular rate so as to improve the cardiac output (rate control)
- Prevent recurrences and maintain sinus rhythm
- Prevention of thromboembolism.

DC shock helps to convert AF to sinus rhythm in 70–80% of cases. If the AF is less than 2 days duration, electrical conversion can be attempted without anticoagulation. Flecainide is given to maintain sinus rhythm if the LV function is good. If it is compromised amiodarone is the drug of choice.

If the AF is more than 2 days duration, cardioversion should be attempted only after instituting anticoagulation with warfarin for 3 weeks. Warfarin has to be continued for 4 weeks after the procedure. The International Normalized Ratio (INR) has to be kept between 2 and 3.

Table 125.1: Quantitation of risk of stroke in patients with cardiovascular disease

Risk factors	Scores
C—congestive heart failure	1 point
H—hypertension	1 point
A—age >75 years	1 point
D—diabetes	1 point
S—prior stroke/TIA	2 point
CHADS$_2$ scores	**Stroke rate/100 patient years**
0	1.9
1	2.8
2	4.0
3	5.9
4	8.5
5	12.5
6	18.2

Abbreviation: TIA = Transient ischemic attack

Table 125.2: Risk stratification of ischemic stroke in patients with nonvalvular atrial fibrillation

Risk factors	Scores
C—congestive heart failure	1
H—hypertension	1
A—age ≥ 75 years	2
D—diabetes mellitus	1
S$_2$—prior stroke/TIA	2
V—vascular disease	1
A—age 65–74 years old	1
Sc—sex category (female)	1

- ***0 point:*** Low risk (1.2–3.0 strokes/100 patient years)
- ***1–2 points:*** Moderate risk (2.8–4.0 strokes/100 patient years)
- ***Greater than or equal to 3 points:*** High risk (5.9–18.2 strokes/100 patient years)

Abbreviation: TIA = Transient ischemic attack

Ventricular rate control in AF can be done with digoxin, beta-blockers, amiodarone and calcium channel blockers (verapamil or diltiazem). In acute cases these drugs can be given IV, but for long-term use oral route is preferred. Beta-blockers are the best drugs for controlling the ventricular response both at rest and during exercise. In certain cases, the AV blocking drugs may have to be combined for optimum rate control. Generally resting heart rate between 60 and 70 and a heart rate of approximately 100–120 can be considered reasonable in individuals with chronic AF.

Conversion to sinus rhythm can be achieved with drugs such as amiodarone (64%) also. AF less than 48 hours duration responds well. In AF more than 48 hours duration, drugs are less effective—dofetilide or amiodarone may be tried (success rate 25–40%).

Atrial pacing is effective on long-term to prevent recurrences of AF, by preventing bradycardia and suppressing ectopic beats. Ablation of the ectopic foci in the atria or pulmonary vein ostia or isolation of these foci from conducting to the rest of the heart can be done by either catheter based radiofrequency techniques or surgically. The maze procedure and the corridor procedure are such methods. The reentrant circuits perpetuating AF are disrupted.

The risk factors for stroke in AF include mitral valve disease, age more than 65 years, hypertension, left ventricular dysfunction and previous history of transient ischemic attack or stroke. In patients less than 65 years of age with no risk factors for stroke, only aspirin (150 mg/day) is required to prevent thromboembolic episodes, in all other patients with AF anticoagulation with warfarin is required, titrated to maintain INR (2–3) to prevent thromboembolic episodes.

TORSADE-DE-POINTES

This is an acquired or congenital polymorphic VT in the range of 180–250/min characterized by QRS complexes of progressively changing amplitude and contour that seem to revolve around the isoelectric line. Successive bursts of nonsustained VT occur. Sometimes these attacks may be prolonged and lead to syncope. The ECG shows prolonged QT interval VT (Fig. 125.14). QT prolongation in the ECG can be due to congenital or acquired causes.

ARRHYTHMOGENIC RIGHT VENTRICULAR DYSPLASIA

Arrhythmogenic right ventricular dysplasia is a cardiomyopathy in which the right ventricular muscle becomes increasingly replaced by adipose and fibrous tissue as the disease progresses. VT arising in the right ventricle is often an early manifestation of this disorder. VT has a left bundle branch block (LBBB) morphology, although in sinus rhythm there is often inversion of T waves in the anterior leads and a slurring of the terminal portion of the QRS complex known as an *epsilon wave*.

General Points in the Management of Acute Tachycardias

Paroxysmal tachycardias present as medical emergencies demanding acute care management. The ECG gives the clue to the nature of the tachycardia whether VT or SVT. Wide QRS complex with a duration of more than 140 millisec is suggestive of VT unless proved otherwise. Based on the ECG, the tachycardias may be classified as regular or irregular and narrow or wide QRS complex. Regular narrow complex tachycardia can be treated with adenosine or drugs that slow the AV conduction. Irregular narrow complex tachycardia is due to AF and warrants treatment with drugs to achieve rate control by AV nodal blocking action. Monomorphic wide QRS tachycardia should be presumed to be VT unless otherwise proved and procainamide, amiodarone or electrical cardioversion should be tried. Polymorphic wide complex irregular tachycardia should be classified into those with wide QT, those with normal QT and those with AF with WPW. Treatment of choice in these situations is magnesium, beta-blockers and procainamide or amiodarone respectively.

VENTRICULAR TACHYCARDIA

When three or more ventricular ectopic beats occur in succession, it is called VT. The common causes are IHD, myocarditis, digitalis toxicity, electrolyte disturbances and cardiomyopathies. Rarely this may occur in an otherwise normal heart. The ventricles beat regularly at the rate of 150–210/min, slight irregularity may occur. VT can be monomorphic or polymorphic. The blood pressure (BP) is low and the patient may go into shock. Carotid massage does not bring down the rate as in the case of SVT.

Ventricular tachycardia may be preceded by the occurrence of ventricular ectopics. Frequency of more than 6 ectopics/min, multifocal ectopics, ectopics occurring in succession and ectopics falling on the T wave of the preceding beat (R on T phenomenon) are features which are associated with a higher risk of developing VT. VT is common in the presence of structural heart disease (very often postmyocardial infarction left ventricular dysfunction and dilated cardiomyopathy) and can degenerate into VF and sudden cardiac death.

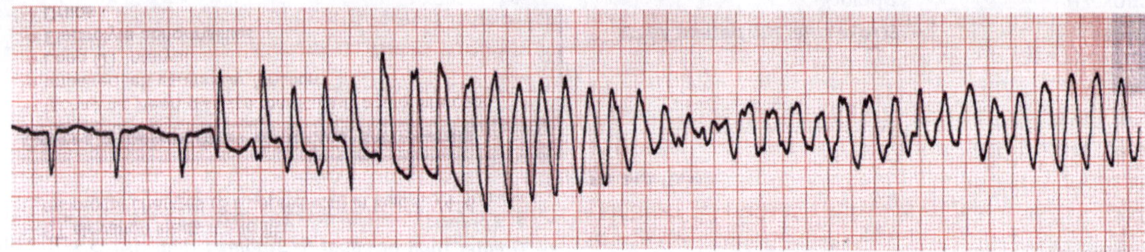

Fig. 125.14: *Torsade de pointes. Note:* 1. Torsade is a form of malignant ventricular tachycardia. 2. The QRS is polymorphic. 3. The axis of the QRS shifts across the baseline around a point. 4. Often this occurs in the setting of prolonged QT interval

Diagnosis

Ventricular tachycardia is confirmed by the ECG which shows wide, regular, QRS complexes with evidence of dissociation between P waves and QRS. Occasional sinus capture beats and fusion beats due to the inherent AV dissociation may be seen. VT needs to be distinguished from other wide QRS complex tachycardias like SVT with aberrant intraventricular conduction, pre-existing bundle branch block (BBB), antegrade conduction over an accessory pathway. Presence of AV dissociation is diagnostic of VT (Fig. 125.15).

Prognosis

Ventricular tachycardia is a grave arrhythmia associated with high mortality, since it usually indicates serious underlying heart disease. Death is due to shock or transition to VF.

Management

Patient presenting with shock and VT should be given synchronized DC shock of 100–150 joules to convert the rhythm to normal without delay. Antiarrhythmic drugs tend to take time for action and aggravate hypotension. Pressor agents such as dopamine may be required if the BP does not come up.

In uncomplicated cases, lidocaine can be tried. It is given as a 2% solution IV. Bolus doses of 50–100 mg are repeated (up to a total dose of 250 mg) till the tachycardia is arrested. Then a maintenance dose of 2–4 mg/min is given continuously as an IV drip, 1 g added to 500 mL 5% glucose and 1–2 mL given every minute. The drip is tapered off within 48–72 hours. If the VT recurs despite lignocaine, other antiarrhythmic drugs should be tried to control the arrhythmia. Drugs like procainamide disopyramide, mexiletine, propranolol or amiodarone are given IV for immediate control of VT. The dose of amiodarone is 150 mg IV bolus in 15 min followed by an infusion of 900 mg in 24 hours (1 mg/min for 6 hours and then 0.5 mg/min for 18 hours). IV amiodarone is gradually emerging as the preferred pharmacological agent for hemodynamically tolerated VT. Once the VT is controlled, oral maintenance therapy can be continued preferably with the same drugs. The following drugs are for oral use:

- Procainamide 1–3 g daily in divided doses
- Quinidine sulfate 0.8–2 g daily in divided doses
- Disopyramide 400–600 mg daily in divided doses
- Dilantin sodium 100 mg thrice daily
- Amiodarone 100–300 mg/day
- Mexiletine 200 mg thrice daily to start with and then continued at 100 mg thrice daily
- Sotalol dose 80–320 mg/day in divided doses.

In acute MI with a slow ventricular rate, transvenous pacing to increase the heart rate prevents the development of VT. The development of curative catheter based therapies especially in patients with normal heart and implantation of implantable cardioverter defibrillator (ICD) especially in postischemic VT have reduced the role of antiarrhythmic drugs in the prevention of recurrence.

VENTRICULAR FIBRILLATION

This is the most common fatal arrhythmia in IHD. VF is the underlying rhythm in 80% cases of sudden cardiac death. The myocardium of the ventricles contract asynchronously and fractionally to produce a fibrillary movement without any sustained synchronous beat. Pumping action of the heart is abolished, circulation comes to a standstill and death ensues if resuscitative measures are not instituted immediately. The physical signs are exactly those of cardiac asystole. The ECG distinguishes VF from asystole.

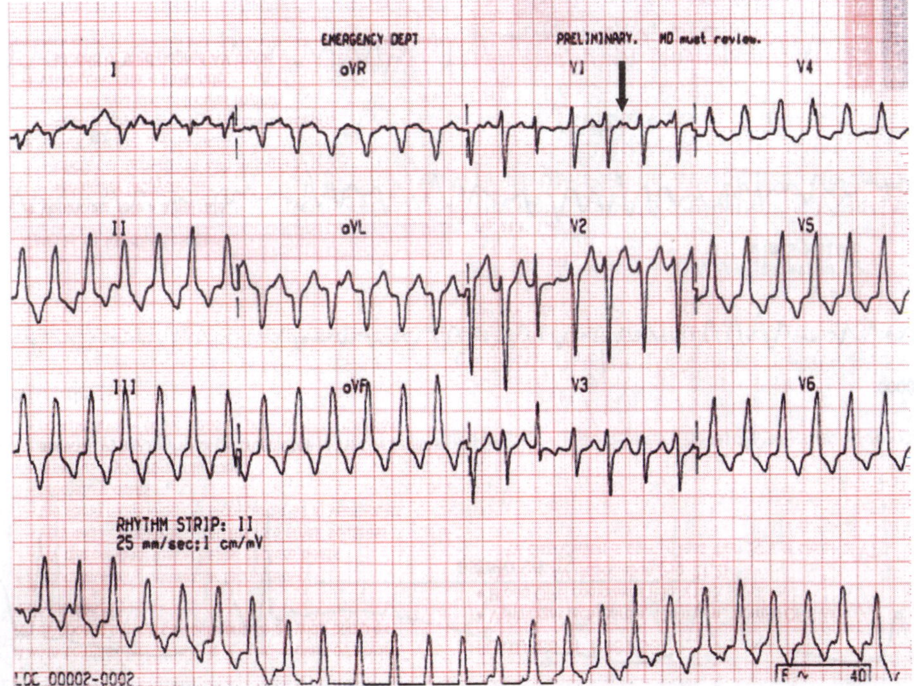

Fig. 125.15: *Ventricular tachycardia (VT)*. ***Note:*** The non-uniform QRS complexes. 1. Broad QRS complexes at rate of 150/minute. 2. Mild irregularity in RR intervals. 3. Mild variation in morphology of QRS complexes. 4. Evidence of AV dissociation. Marked by arrow in V1

Management

ECG is mandatory for diagnosis. VF is recognized on the ECG by the absence of QRS complexes and T waves and the presence of low amplitude baseline undulations which are quite variable both in amplitude and rhythm (Fig. 125.16). The heart is defibrillated by biphasic asynchronized DC shock of 150–200 joules. Management of VF is the same as that of sudden cardiac arrest.

Bretylium tosylate given IV in a dose of 5–10 mg/kg/bw is very effective in preventing the recurrence of VF. Implantable cardiac defibrillator (ICD) are used to detect the arrhythmia and delivers the shocks to terminate the same. Implantations of pacemakers defibrillators is commonly done at present. ICD have become available in recent years. These compact devices detect VT and fibrillation and automatically deliver shocks on to the myocardium, to terminate the arrhythmias.

Shock resistant VF is defined as VF persisting even after three attempts of electrical defibrillation.

Life Support Measures

In many developed countries, the public has been trained to give emergency cardiac support by external cardiac massage, mouth-to-mouth respiration and external cardiac defibrillation. In many of the public places, emergency defibrillators are also provided. If cardiac rhythm is restored within 3 min of onset of ventricular fibrillation or asystole the chance for recovery and brain function are good. Standardized practice guidelines have been laid down to assist physicians in clinical decision making in such emergencies. In many public places like airports, trade centers, pilgrim centers and the like, automated external defibrillator devices can be provided.

HEART BLOCKS

Delay or interruption of the conduction of impulses from the SA node along the normal pathway to the ventricular myocardium results in heart block. The SA node produces impulses at the rate of 70–80/min. Velocity of conduction in the atria is 1 millisec. It is 0.2 millisec in the AV nodal tissues and 4 millisec in the Purkinje system. The AV node being less conductive, there is a delay of 80–120 millisec, at this level. Heart block can be caused by abnormalities of impulse conduction at the SA node as in sinus blocks or conduction at the AV node, the bundle of His and its branches.

- *Sinus arrest:* In this condition the sinus node ceases to produce impulses (Fig. 125.17).
- *Sinoatrial block:* Impulses arising from the SA node are blocked at the junction of the SA node with the atrial musculature and hence the beat is missed. The ECG shows a pause with total absence of the PQRST complexes, corresponding to the missed impulses. Sometimes escape beats or escape rhythms may occur (Fig. 125.18).
- *AV block:* This is caused by abnormalities at the AV junction or along His-Purkinje system. Three forms may occur:

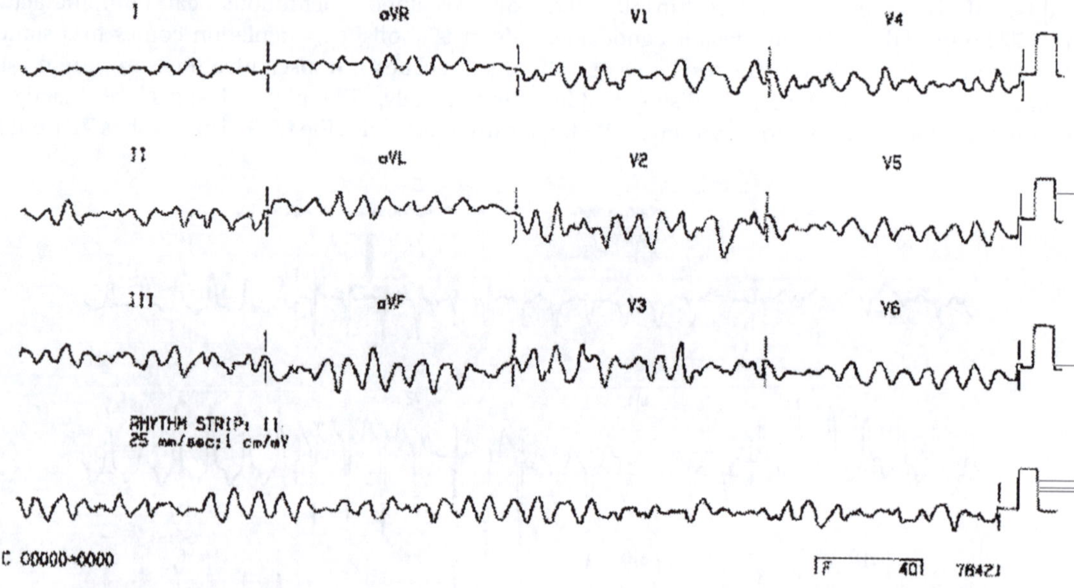

Fig. 125.16: *Ventricular fibrillation. Note:* 1. Totally irregular QRS activity with undulating base line. 2. Absence of normal QRS and T waves

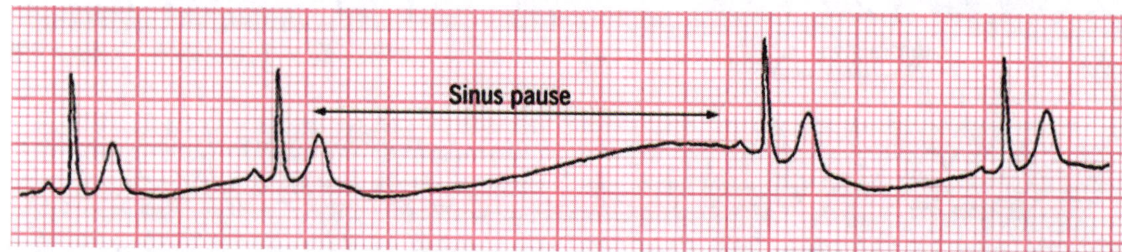

Fig. 125.17: *Sinus arrest. Note:* The absence of all complexes with long pause

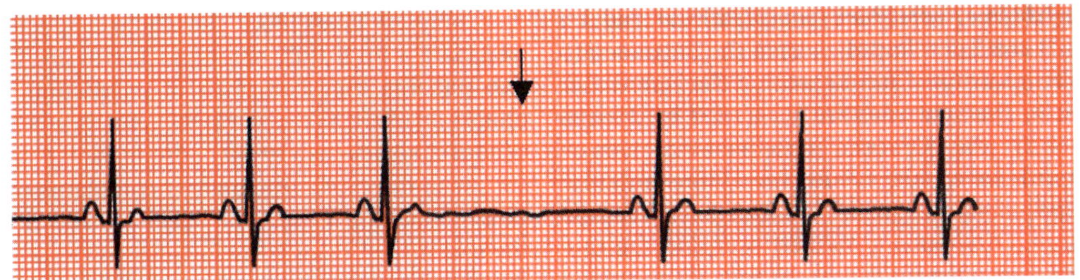

Fig. 125.18: SA block. The PR interval is normal. The sinus fails to produce impulse as is seen by the absence of P wave and the QRS (arrow)

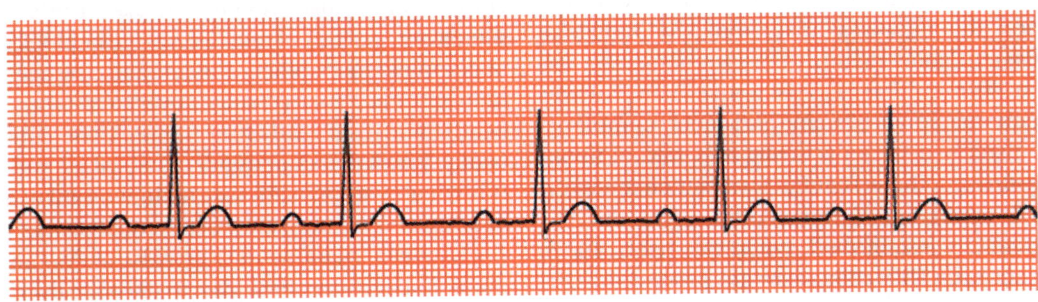

Fig. 125.19: *First degree A-V block. Note:* The prolonged PR interval beyond 0.2 second (i.e.) > 5 small divisions

1. ***First degree AV block:*** Clinical detection of this form may be difficult. The ECG shows prolongation of PR interval exceeding 0.20 sec (Fig. 125.19).
2. ***Second degree AV block:*** This block is of two types. In both the types some of the impulses from the SA node fail to reach the ventricles resulting in dropped beats.
   - ***Mobitz type I block (Wenckebach phenomenon):*** The PR interval increases progressively till a QRS is totally missed. This is clinically evident as a regular irregularity. Almost always this is caused by a block in the AV node (Fig. 125.20).
   - ***Mobitz type II block:*** This is a more serious arrhythmia than type I block. The PR interval of the conducted beats is fixed, but some of the P waves are not conducted to the ventricles and are not followed by QRS. The P waves outnumber the QRS complexes. Mostly this is due to a block in the His-Purkinje system and often the QRS may show some widening (Fig. 125.21).

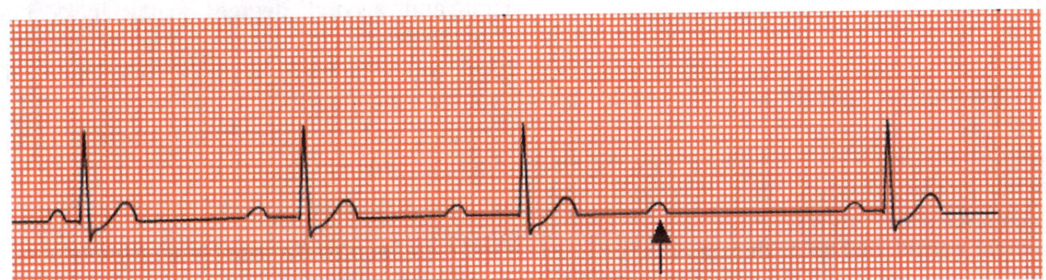

Fig. 125.20: *Second degree heart block Mobitz type 1. Note:* 1. Progressive prolongation of PR interval. 2. The fourth P wave is blocked and is not followed by a QRS (arrow) Wenckebach's phenomenon

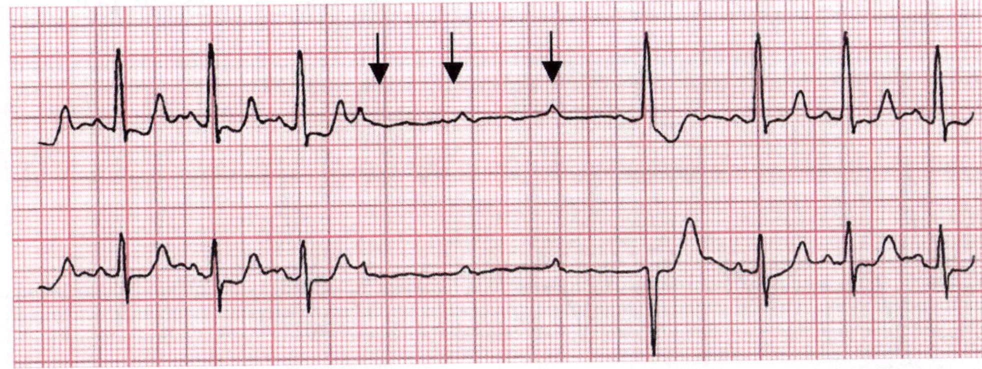

Fig. 125.21: *Second degree heart block Mobitz type 2: High grade AV block: Note:* The 4th, 5th and 6th P waves (marked by arrows) are not conducted to the ventricles indicating high grade A-V block 2. All the conducted beats show PR interval which remain constant

3. ***Third degree heart block (complete heart block):*** In this condition impulses from the SA node are totally interrupted from reaching the ventricular muscle. The ventricles are controlled by a focus either in the junction (idiojunctional escape rhythm) or in the ventricles (idioventricular escape rhythm). With idiojunctional escape rhythm, QRS tends to be narrower and the rate faster, very often more than 40/min. If the escape focus is idioventricular, the rate tends to be slower and the QRS complex will be usually wider. When the impulses arise from the ventricles (idioventricular rhythm) the rate is usually less than 40/min. The ECG shows regular P waves occurring at 70–80/min and QRS complexes are usually bizarre occurring at a rate of about 30–40/min. There is total dissociation between the P-waves and QRS complexes. The pulse is regular in established complete heart block because the QRS complexes are produced regularly (Fig. 125.22).

Clinical Features

First degree heart block is an abnormality usually detected by ECG. Second degree heart block causes regular missing of heart beats and the pulse. Unlike benign extrasystoles in which the irregularity disappears with exertion, the irregularity in heart block tends to persist. Mobitz type II is associated with more serious disorders such as acute MI in the background of anterior wall MI or degenerative disorders of the conduction system. It is considered a more serious block because often it progresses to complete AV block.

Etiology of Heart Block

- Primary degeneration of the conducting tissues (Lev's disease, Lenegre's disease)
- ***Diseases affecting the myocardium:*** MI, chronic CAD and myocarditis
- ***Drugs and toxins:*** Digoxin, quinidine, procainamide, β-adrenergic blocking drugs, *Cerbera thevetia*, *Cerbera odollam* and *Nerium oleander*
- Trauma to the conducting tissue during surgery
- Congenital abnormality of the conducting tissue (congenital heart block)
- ***Infections:*** Tertiary syphilis, south American trypanosomiasis (Chagas' disease) and cysticercosis
- Sick-sinus syndrome.

Complete heart block should be suspected when the heart rate is 30–40/min or less, not increasing with exercise. The patients may complain of palpitation or syncopal attacks on exertion or even at rest. Syncope is transient loss of consciousness as a result of diminution of arterial blood supply to the brain. The patient complains of dimness of vision, a sinking feeling and may become unconscious. In the majority of cases consciousness is regained on falling down due to resumption of cerebral circulation.

If the heart beats are not resumed, the patient develops convulsions—Stokes-Adams attacks. These attacks are seen when periods of asystole or transient VT or VF occur in complete heart block. This may also be seen when one idioventricular focus changes over to another. If the heart beat is not resumed within minutes, the condition ends fatally. When the lesion is fully established and the rhythm is regular even at a slow rate, compensatory mechanisms develop and the frequency of syncopal attacks diminishes.

Physical examination reveals slow, high volume pulse, forceful apex beat (due to diastolic overdistension), presence of irregular cannon waves in the jugular veins, widened pulse pressure (high systolic and normal or low diastolic) and varying intensity of the first heart sound. Independent atrial sounds may be heard.

The ECG shows the slow ventricular rate and complete dissociation of the P and QRS complexes.

Diagnosis

Complete heart block should be suspected when the heart rate is slow and regular. His-bundle electrography gives further information about the site of lesion (infra-Hisian or supra-Hisian).

Prognosis

First and second degree heart blocks may resolve completely with treatment or proceed to complete heart block when the lesion is progressive. During the stage of evolution the prognosis should be guarded. In the stage of evolution and when the lesion is unstable complete heart block can progress to cardiac arrest or VF.

Management

First and Second Degree Heart Blocks

Apart from close ECG monitoring and observation of the clinical state, no specific treatment may be indicated. Treatment of the primary condition may clear the conduction defect as well. Atropine 0.5 mg given IV abolishes vagal tone and improves the heart rate in AV

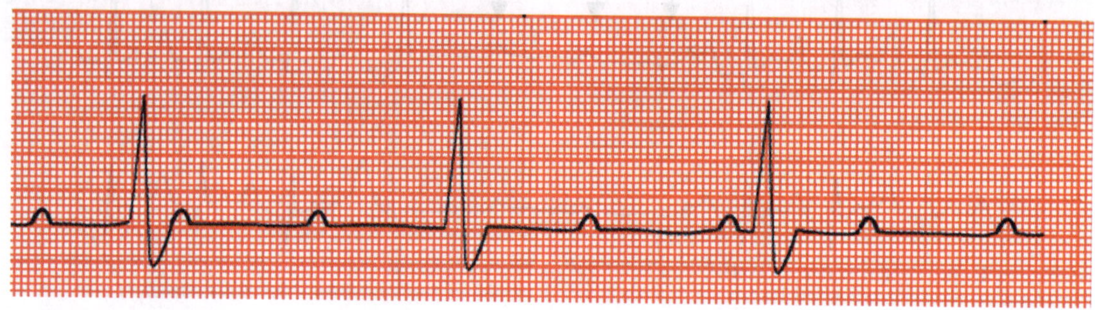

Fig. 125.22: ***Third degree A-V block.*** 1. P waves are regular and normal in rate. 2. QRS are also regular but much slower in rate and wider. 3. No relation between P and QRS

blocks. Isoprenaline or adrenaline given intravenously increases the heart rate and this is life-saving in an emergency. The heart rate can be maintained at a high level by giving orciprenaline 10 mg orally thrice daily. These sympathomimetic drugs have the risk of triggering off serious tachyarrhythmias and hence in acute MI these are not recommended.

When a patient with MI develops progressive heart block leading to complete heart block, it is an indication for transvenous pacing using an external pacemaker and electrode catheter introduced into the right ventricle.

PACEMAKER IMPLANTATION

In established *complete heart block*, long-term prognosis is poor and therefore, permanent pacemakers are implanted (Fig. 125.23). Pacemaker consists of two components. 1. Pulse generator which is made of various type of batteries and 2. The lead which can be connected to the heart. The pulse generator is implanted into the body by making a pocket in the subcutaneous tissue in the infraclavicular area or on the abdominal wall. The generator is connected to one end of the lead and the other end of the lead may be placed in the right ventricle transvenously (endocardial pacemaker) or over the left ventricular apex (epicardial pacemaker). Dual chamber pacemakers are available in which stimulation of the atrium is followed by stimulation of the ventricle so that the normal sequence of contraction is reproduced. These are also known as physiological pacemakers. Modern pacemakers are programmable regarding the rate, voltage output and refractory period by telemetry from outside. Sensors which recognize the level of activity of the patients are incorporated in the pacemakers so that the rate of pacing is automatically adjusted to the requirement.

Since the advantage of pacemakers in giving symptomatic relief and prolonging life has been established it should be the aim to provide pacemakers wherever indicated. The cost ranges from ₹ 40,000 to 60,000 for the basic models to higher prices for more advanced options. Majority of them have a trouble free life exceeding 10 years.

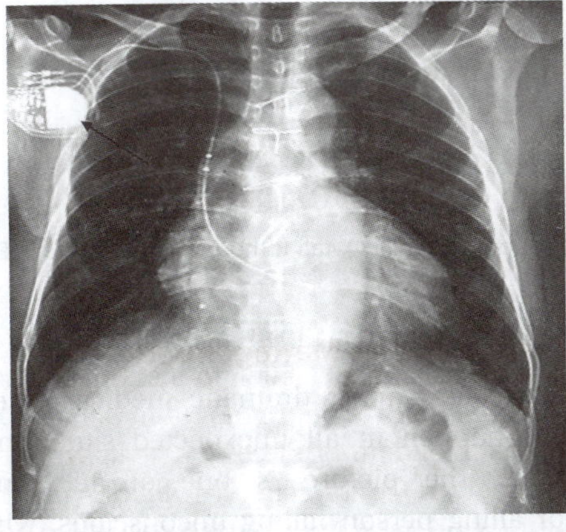

Fig. 125.23: A permanent pacemaker has been inserted for this patient with a postoperative complete heart block. **Note:** The pulse generator in the right infraclavicular area and the ventricular lead reaching the right ventricle (arrow) (via the right subclavian vein, superior vena cava, right atrium and into the right ventricle)

Dual chamber pacemakers probably are more effective with better hemodynamics and quality of life.

It is important that patients with implanted pacemaker should avoid strong magnetic fields such as MRI installations and metal detecting equipment. It is ideal to implant pacemakers early to avoid the development of Stokes-Adams attacks or sudden cardiac death. Once implanted, they require regular follow-up care. Now, MRI compatible leads and pacemakers are available.

Bundle Branch Block (BBB)

His bundle divides into right and left branches, the left further divides into the anterosuperior and posteroinferior fascicles. Conduction of impulse below His bundle occurs through these three fascicles (trifascicular conduction). Conduction disturbance occurring in the RBBB and LBBB. Blocks at the fascicles of the bundle are called fascicular blocks. These may be involving two or three fascicles (bifascicular or trifascicular blocks). BBB do not produce any arrhythmia by themselves.

Complete Left Bundle Branch Block

This involves the main stem of the left bundle. The anterosuperior or posteroinferior fascicle may be selectively affected at times. These are called left anterior hemiblock (LAHB) and left posterior hemiblock (LPHB) respectively. Sometimes the main left bundle may be affected, along with one or both of its branches (Fig. 125.24).

Complete Right Bundle Branch Block

Interruption of the right bundle may occur as the lone abnormality or along with block of one or both of the branches of the left bundle. The combination of RBBB with LAHB or LPHB is called bifascicular block. In trifascicular block, RBBB exists with alternating LAHB and LPHB. RBBB plus LAHB/LPHB with prolonged PR interval is also a form of trifascicular block (Fig. 125.25).

Partial Bundle Branch Blocks

Complete interruption of conduction of impulses in the bundle branch causes the QRS complex to prolong beyond 0.12 sec. When there is only delay without complete block of the impulse (partial BBB) the duration of the QRS is between 0.10 and 0.12 sec (normal 0.08 sec).

Bifascicular and trifascicular blocks give rise to characteristic ECG patterns. When the bundle branches are blocked, ventricular activation takes place through the remaining bundle or its fascicles (Fig. 125.26).

BBB may result from IHD, sclerodegenerative disorder of the conduction system of the heart, myocarditis, cardiomyopathy, drugs like quinidine and surgical trauma. In addition, RBBB may be seen in atrial septal defect, acute pulmonary embolism, right ventricular dilation and right ventricular failure. Congenital RBBB may occur rarely. Though RBBB can exist as an isolated ECG abnormality, LBBB is usually indicative of underlying structural heart disease.

In MI, presence of bifascicular or trifascicular block is considered an indication for temporary transvenous pacing of the heart, since complete heart block or the fatal arrhythmias are likely to develop in such patients.

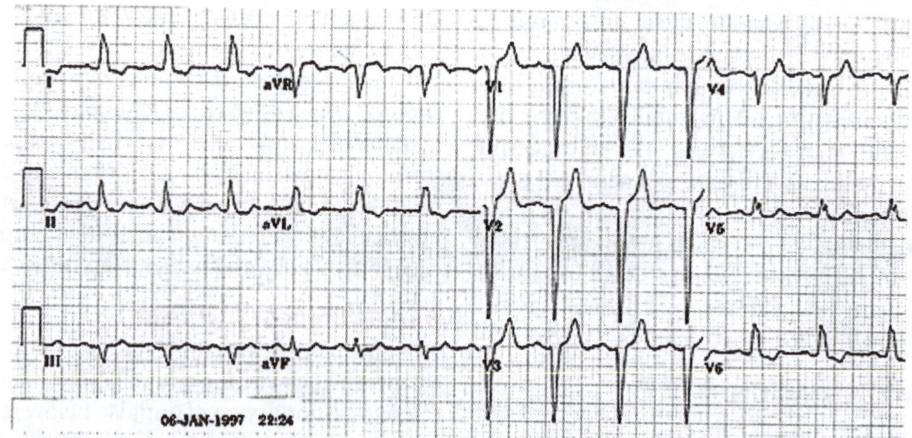

Fig. 125.24: *ECG left bundle branch block (LBBB). Note:* 1. Duration of QRS exceeds 0.12 seconds. 2. Widened, slurred and bizarre R waves in lead 1 aVL, V5 and V6 slurred S waves in V1 and V2

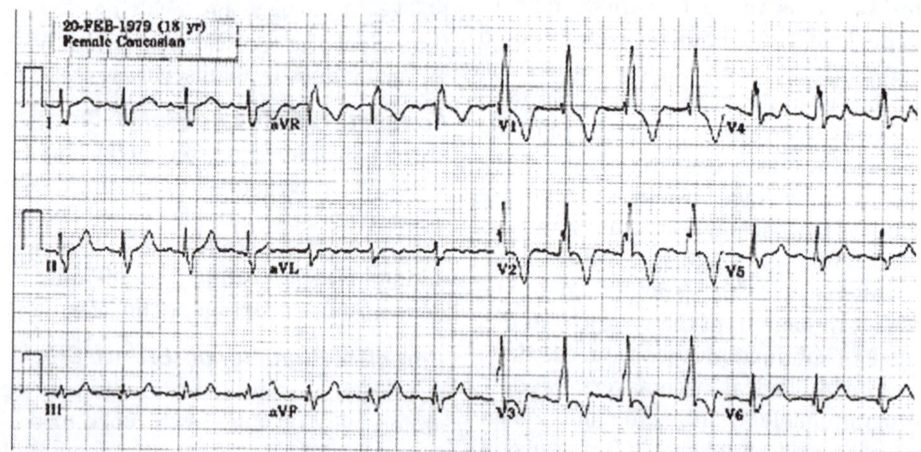

Fig. 125.25: *Complete right bundle branch block. Note:* 1. Prolongation of QRS duration above 0.12 seconds. 2. Slurred R'waves in V1 and V2. 3. Wide S waves in L1, aVL and V5 and V6

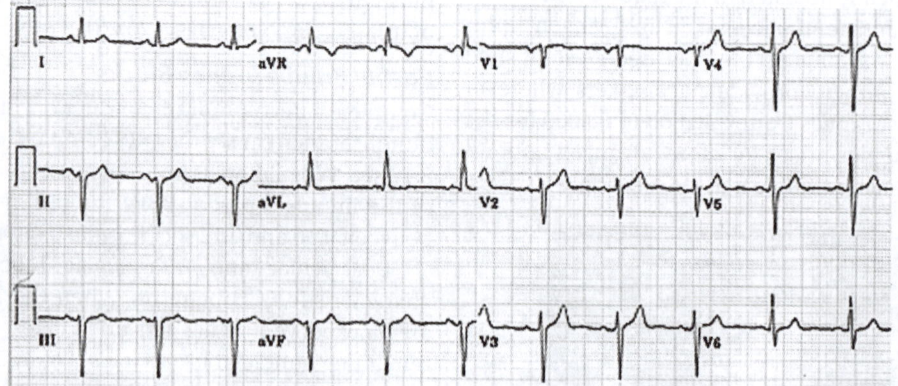

Fig. 125.26: *LAHB. Note:* 1. QRS axis is abnormally shifted to the left (left axis deviation). 2. Small Q, tall R morphology in aVL. 3. Persistent S waves in V5 and V6

VENTRICULAR STANDSTILL (VENTRICULAR ASYSTOLE)

When there is total cessation of stimuli reaching the ventricles, ventricular standstill develops. The ECG shows absence of QRS. Often the P wave may also be absent. Cardiac asystole may occur in MI and other forms of IHD or in complete heart block. Treatment involves external cardiac massage and instituting the procedure for cardiac resuscitation (Fig. 125.27).

Cardiac Arrest and its Management

Cardiac arrest is a most dramatic medical emergency which may happen in all unexpected situations from time-to-time. The picture is one of an apparently healthy or ailing person falling unconscious, with total loss of consciousness and cessation of heart beat and pulse. The most common causes are VF and ventricular asystole. If cardiac standstill is not corrected within 3–4 min, irreversible damage occurs to the brain and vital

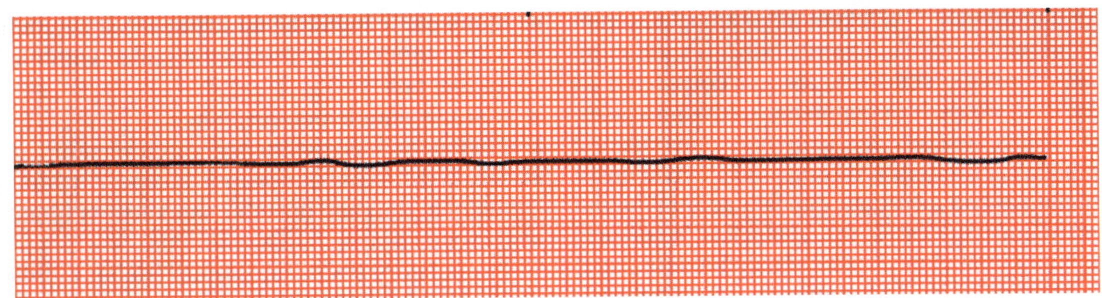

Fig. 125.27: *Asystole. Note:* Complete electrical silence (ventricular standstill)

centers. Resuscitation becomes futile thereafter or even if the cardiac rhythm is restored, full consciousness is not regained. Such a patient may continue to live a vegetative existence without regaining consciousness and other cerebral functions.

Other supportive evidences are:

- Dilation of the pupils
- Cessation of breathing or gasping respiration
- Cyanosis or pallor
- Loss of consciousness.

The ECG will confirm whether the heart is in asystole or VF.

A planned line of management is absolutely essential to avoid these catastrophes.

Resuscitative measures should be instituted if the main pulses are not palpable and heart sounds are not heard. Management of cardiac arrest is a teamwork. One person starts the procedure, the others soon join him for assistance. It is mandatory to distinguish between the ventricular asystole and the VF for specific management.

Steps to be followed:

- Put the patient on a firm nonresilient surface and clear the airway. Remove dentures and foreign bodies from the mouth and throat, loosen clothing, pull the chin up so that the tongue does not fall back to obstruct the throat and remove secretions from the air passages by proper positioning and suction. Introduce an airway, if available.
- Start external cardiac massage by pressing firmly over the sternum (so as to compress the precordium) and releasing it, at the rate of 50–60/min. If the maneuver is properly done, the carotid pulse will be felt.
- Start artificial ventilation simultaneously by mouth-to-mouth respiration or using an Ambu bag. If facilities are available, the trachea is intubated with a cuffed endotracheal tube and positive pressure respiration given with oxygen-enriched air at the rate of 10–12 L/min, without interference to the external cardiac massage.
- Start an IV line with 5% glucose, to act as a route of medication.
- If ECG shows VF, apply the electrodes and give a DC shock of 200 joules (100–400 joules). Often the fibrillation disappears and heart resumes normal beat. The DC shock can be repeated if conversion is not achieved with single shock. If ventricular asystole is detected, adrenaline 0.5 mg is given IV or intracardiac (0.5 mL of 1/1,000 solution) into the cavity of the right ventricle using a lumbar puncture needle inserted

through the third or fourth left intercostal space. Often this converts asystole into VF and this can be converted by DC shock. In many centers adrenaline is given by the IV route. This is adequate if external cardiac massage is performed effectively.

- ***Other drugs:*** Sodium bicarbonate is given IV in a dose of 100 mmol (100 mL of 7.4% solution) for an adult, rapidly to counteract metabolic acidosis.
- If the heart returns to activity, continue massage till the systolic BP is maintained at 70–80 mm Hg.
- If the heart is beating, but BP is low, dopamine may be started as an IV drip at the rate of 2–3 µg/kg/min.
- If the heart continues in asystole after adrenaline, and massage 20 mL of 5% solution of calcium chloride can be given IV, after repeating sodium bicarbonate and adrenaline.

External cardiac massage and resuscitatory measures are stopped if the heart fails to recover within 1 hour or the pupils remain dilated and fixed despite adequate massage.

As soon as the emergency team starts to give first aid, steps are taken to transport the patient to the hospital in a suitably equipped ambulance. Emergency first aid management of cardiac arrest is taught to several groups such as ambulance personnel, paramedical staff, porters, scouts and so on. Periodically, guidelines are published to simplify the procedure so that more persons can practice emergency resuscitation. Life-saving equipment such as defibrillators, ventilators and oxygen delivery systems are available in public places and in several aircraft. Emergency resuscitation helps to prevent death and permanent morbidity.

SICK SINUS SYNDROME

Normal sinus node produces impulses at the rate of 60–70/min under basal conditions. Depending on physiological demands it may increase the rate up to 180/min (exceptionally 200/min). During sleep, heart rate may go down to 50–60/min (exceptionally as low as 40/min). Persons with increased vagal tone achieved by physical training or otherwise have lower resting heart rates, then the rate of rise of heart rate with exercise is also lower. When the sinus node is diseased and consequently the impulse production becomes defective it may give rise to various electrophysiological abnormalities of the heart. The clinical spectrum resulting from these is termed SSS. In about 30% of cases AV node (AV junction) may also show abnormality.

Sick sinus syndrome is relatively common in clinical practice, particularly among the elderly. Although various drugs such as digitalis, β-blockers, verapamil, diltiazem and quinidine produce dysfunction of the sinus node, these functionally reversible situations are not considered as part of SSS. IHD, idiopathic sclerodegenerative processes, toxic myocarditis, various types of cardiomyopathies, Friedreich's ataxia, infiltrative disorders like amyloidosis, hemochromatosis and metastatic deposits account for the vast majority. In many cases, the etiological factor may not be apparent. The clinical picture may be dominated by bradyarrhythmias such as severe sinus bradycardia, SA block, intermittent sinus arrest or sinus pause singly or in combination. Because of this, patient may develop dizziness, mental confusion, syncope or near syncope. In patients with underlying heart disease progressive congestive heart failure may result.

The other group of manifestations results from atrial tachyarrhythmias, such as recurrent AF, flutter or reentrant tachycardia. Sudden onset AF with relatively slow ventricular response, especially in elderly subjects, should alert the possibility of SSS. Palpitation, confusion, syncope, near-syncope, angina pectoris and congestive heart failure may result from the tachyarrhythmia. SSS may produce extreme bradyarrhythmia associated with sudden change into tachyarrhythmia in the same patient. This is termed as bradytachyarrhythmia syndrome (BTS).

Diagnosis

Diagnosis can be suspected from the clinical manifestations. Routine 12 lead ECG is very useful in the diagnosis. ECG manifestations may include:

- Persistent, inappropriate and marked sinus brady-cardia
- SA block
- Sinus arrest

- Long pause following an atrial premature contraction
- Chronic atrial fibrillation or flutter with slow ventricular rate
- Carotid sinus hypersensitivity
- Unstable sinus rhythm after cardioversion
- Atrioventricular junctional escape rhythm with or without slow and unstable sinus activity (Fig. 125.28)
- Bradytachyarrhythmia syndrome.

Ambulatory electrocardiogram (Holter monitoring) is particularly useful for diagnosis and prognosis. Those with equivocal findings can be studied by treadmill exercise test or response to drugs like atropine or isoproterenol. Electrophysiological studies for determining the sinus node recovery time or sinoatrial (SA) conduction time and His bundle electrocardiogram (ECG) may be required in selected cases for diagnosis and management.

Prognosis

The abnormality of the sinus node tends to be chronic, progressive and permanent. In those who present with symptoms of recurrent syncope or near syncope, progressive angina and congestive heart failure especially with underlying heart disease, the prognosis is bad. Sudden death may occur in untreated cases.

Management

Once the diagnosis is established, in symptomatic patients, implantation of suitable permanent pacemaker is the treatment of choice, particularly in those with symptomatic bradycardias. It helps to relieve the symptoms and improve the quality of life. Tachyarrhythmias due to sick sinus syndrome (SSS) may be safely managed with antiarrhythmic drugs provided a pacemaker is also implanted.

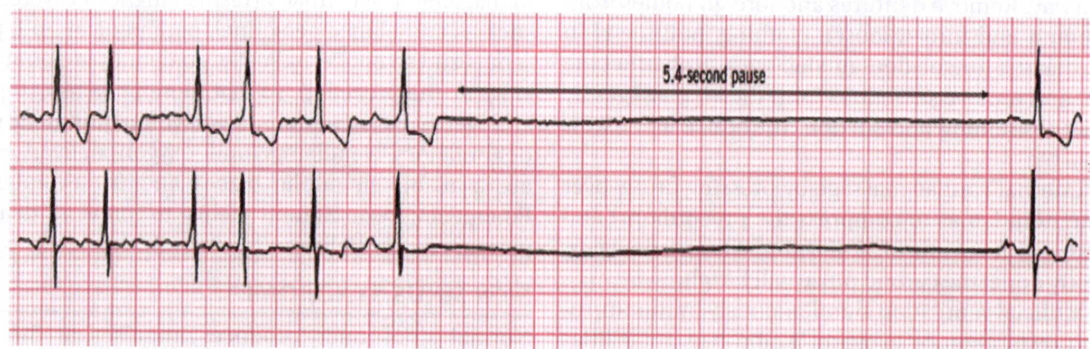

Fig. 125.28: *Sick sinus syndrome. Note:* The tachy and bradyarrhythmias. 1. The first half shows atrial fibrillation with fast heart rate. 2. The latter half shows a long pause

APPENDIX

Appendix 125.1: Antiarrhythmic drugs—dosage and indications

S. no.	Antiarrhythmic drugs	Dosage (oral)	Dosage (parenteral)	Indications
1.	Quinidine	200–400 mg three to four times a day (up to 600 mg q6h)	IM 600 mg followed by 400 mg every 2 hours or IV 800 mg in 50 mL 5% dextrose at the rate of 1 mL/min infusion	Atrial flutter, atrial fibrillation AVNRT
2.	Procainamide	2–4 g/day in three to four divided doses (maximum daily dose 6 g)	IM or IV 25–50 mg over 1 min to repeat at 5 min interval till arrhythmia controlled or IV infusion 2–6 mg/min	Atrial fibrillation SVT (AVNRT, AVRT)

Contd...

S. no.	Antiarrhythmic drugs	Dosage (oral)	Dosage (parenteral)	Indications
3.	Disopyramide	100–200 mg q6h maximum 1,200 mg/day	IV 1–2 mg/kg bolus followed by 1 mg/kg/hr	Atrial flutter, Atrial fibrillation SVT (AVNRT, AVRT) VT
4.	Lignocaine	NA	IV 1–2 mg/kg bolus maximum 5 mg/kg then infusion at 1–4 mg/min	Rapid termination of VT Refractory VT/VF
5.	Mexiletine hydrochloride	200 mg tid	100–250 mg IV bolus followed by 250 mg infusion over 1–2 hours	Ventricular tachycardia
6.	Phenytoin	1 g loading dose day 1 followed by 500 mg day 2 and day 3 and 300–400 mg daily thereafter	IV 100 mg, repeated up to maximum 1 g	Digoxin related atrial and ventricular arrhythmias
7.	Flecainide	100 mg every 12 hours, maximum 400 mg/day	IV 2 mg/kg then 100–200 mg q12h	Paroxysmal AF, SVT, VT
8.	Esmolol	NA	IV 500 µg/kg loading followed by 50–200 µg/kg/min	Rapid rate control in SVT
9.	Amiodarone	200 mg tid × 1 week then 200 mg bd for a week maintenance, 100–200 mg/day	150–300 mg IV bolus then 1 mg/kg/min for 6 hours and 0.5 mg/kg/min for 18 hours	Atrial flutter fibrillation AVNRT refractory VT/VF
10.	Sotalol	80 mg/day in one to two divided doses, maximum of 640 mg/day	IV 100 mg over 1–2 min	Atrial flutter atrial fibrillation, VT
11.	Bretylium	4 mg/kg/daily	IV 5–10 mg/kg bolus followed by 0.5–2 mg/min infusion	Refractory VT and VF
12.	Ibutilide	NA	IV 1 mg over 10 min to repeat if needed	Termination of a/c episode of atrial flutter/atrial fibrillation
13.	Dofetilide	0.1–0.5 mg bd	IV 2.5 µg/kg, to repeat if needed	Acute and chronic AF
14.	Verapamil	120–480 mg/day in three to four divided doses	IV 5–10 mg over 2–3 min	SVT
15.	Adenosine	NA	6–12 mg IV as rapid bolus	Termination of PSVT
16.	Digoxin	0.5–1 mg loading followed by 0.125 mg 0.25 mg daily	IV 0.5–1 mg	Control of heart rate in atrial flutter/fibrillation

Abbreviations: IV = Intravenous; IM = Intramuscular; NA = Not applicable; SVT = Supraventricular tachycardia; PSVT = Paroxysmal supraventricular tachycardia; VT = Ventricular tachycardia; AVNRT = Atrioventricular nodal reentrant tachycardia; VF = Ventricular fibrillation; AF = Atrial fibrillation; AVRT = Atrioventricular reentrant tachycardia

CHAPTER
126

Systemic Hypertension

K Suresh

Chapter Summary

- General Considerations
- Factors which Influence BP
- Systemic Hypertension
- Epidemiology
- Pathology
- Clinical Features
- Complications of Hypertension
- Management
- Risk Stratification
- General Guidelines
- Resistant Hypertension
- Hypertensive Urgencies and Emergencies
- Renal Hypertension
- Mineralocorticoid Hypertension
- Orthostatic Hypertension

GENERAL CONSIDERATIONS

Systemic arterial hypertension is one of the most common maladies of mankind, affecting 30–45% of the general population globally, with a steep increase with ageing. Though, it was considered to be a disease related to affluence, it is no longer so. All sections of the population in India suffer from the disease. Prevalence of hypertension has increased in both urban and rural subjects. It is presently 25% in urban adults and 10–15% among rural adults. Along with diabetes, ischemic heart disease and strokes, hypertension is another major public health problem for India. Diabetes and hypertension coexist in about 30–40% of cases, and the combination adversely affects the long-term prognosis of both. Hypertension leads to damage of the target organs–heart, brain, optic fundi, kidneys and blood vessels both acutely and on a long-term basis.

The damage to the target organs correlates generally with the values of elevated blood pressure (BP) (both systolic and diastolic). However, other factors such as hyperlipidemias and tobacco smoking may also influence the final outcome.

Measurement of BP

This is traditionally done using a mercury sphygmoma-nometer. The patient should be seated in a quiet room for 15 minutes before recording BP. BP may also be recorded in the supine and standing position. At all postures, the arm should be supported at heart level. Measurement of BP at the upper arm is preferred, cuff and bladder dimensions should be adapted to the arm circumference, and the arm with the higher BP values should be taken. A significant (>10 mm Hg) and consistent systolic BP differ-ence between arms has been shown to carry an increased cardiovascular risk. The BP cuff for adults should have a bladder 12–13 cm wide and 30–35 cm long, which is adequate for most of the average sized persons.

Larger cuffs are required for stout arms (arm circumference > 32 cm) and vice versa. Using a cuff of smaller size gives erroneously higher values. The cuff is rapidly inflated to 30–40 mm Hg above the level at which the pulse becomes impalpable and then deflated at the rate of 2 mm/sec. Auscultating over the cubital fossa, the onset of Korotkoff sounds (phase I) and their disappearance (phase V) are recorded. The former denotes the systolic and the latter, the diastolic BP. At least two measurements made 1–2 minutes apart are taken and the average values taken as the BP. The unit of BP is expressed as mm Hg or as kilo Pascals (KPa = 7.5 mm Hg). All other instruments used to record BP such as aneroid manometers, electronic devices and others should be periodically calibrated with the mercury instrument. Other modalities of measuring BP are automatic instruments preset to record at regular intervals, direct intra-arterial measurement, instruments that can be fitted to a finger with the patient lying supine and ambulatory recording. BP measurements should always be associated with measurement of heart rate, because in hypertensive patients increased resting heart rate values independently predict cardiovascular morbid or fatal events.

The BP values in a community follow a bimodal pattern lying within a broad range of normalcy. The rather arbitrary cut off points separating normal and abnormal BP, are based on statistical evidence of adverse consequences of raised systolic and diastolic pressure.

When measuring BP in the office, care should be taken

- To allow the patients to sit for 3–5 minutes before beginning BP measurements
- To take at least two BP measurements, in the sitting position, spaced 1–2 min apart, and additional measurements if the first two are quite different. Consider the average BP if deemed appropriate
- To take repeated measurements of BP to improve accuracy in patients with arrhythmias, such as atrial fibrillation
- To use a standard bladder (12–13 cm wide and 35 cm long), but have a larger and a smaller bladder available for large (arm circumference > 32 cm) and thin arms, respectively

- To have the cuff at the heart level, whatever the position of the patient
- When adopting the auscultatory method, use phase I and V (disappearance) Korotkoff sounds to identify systolic and diastolic BP respectively
- To measure BP in both arms at first visit to detect possible differences. In this instance, take the arm with the higher value as the reference
- To measure at the first visit, BP 1-3 min after assumption of the standing position in elderly subjects, diabetic patients, and in other conditions in which orthostatic hypotension may be frequent or suspected
- To measure, in case of conventional BP measurement, heart rate by pulse palpation (at least 30 seconds) after the second measurement in the sitting position

White-Coat (or Isolated Clinic) Hypertension and Masked (or Isolated Ambulatory) Hypertension

'White-coat' or 'isolated clinic hypertension' refers to condition in which BP is persistently elevated in the office and normal out of the clinic. The prevalence of white-coat hypertension is approximately 13%. Some of the factors related to increased prevalence of white-coat hypertension include age, female sex and anxiety. Some studies show that these patients have increased long-term risk of new-onset diabetes and progression to sustained hypertension.

Conversely, BP may be normal in the office and abnormally high out of the medical environment, which is termed 'masked' or 'isolated ambulatory hypertension'. The prevalence of masked hypertension also averages about 13% in the population. Several factors may raise out-of office BP relative to office BP, such as younger age, male gender, smoking, alcohol consumption, physical activity, exercise-induced hypertension, anxiety, job stress, obesity, diabetes, chronic kidney disease (CKD) and family history of hypertension. Both white-coat hypertension and masked hypertension are diagnosed by out of office BP monitoring; it is recommended that the diagnosis should be done within 6 months from the initial presentation.

The major advantage of out of office BP monitoring is that it provides a large number of BP measurements away from the medical environment, which represents a more reliable assessment of actual BP than office BP. Out of office BP is commonly assessed by ambulatory blood pressure monitoring (ABPM) or home blood pressure monitoring (HBPM). Office BP is usually higher than ambulatory and home BP (Table 126.1).

Ambulatory BP monitoring is performed with the patient wearing a portable BP measuring device, usually on the nondominant arm, for a 24 hours period. Subject

Table 126.1: Categories of hypertension by office and home BP levels

Category	Systolic BP (mm Hg)		Diastolic BP (mm Hg)
Office BP	≥ 140	and/or	≥ 90
Ambulatory BP			
• Daytime (or awake)	≥ 135	and/or	≥ 85
• Night-time (or asleep)	≥ 120	and/or	≥ 70
• 24-h	≥ 130	and/or	≥ 80
Home BP	≥ 135	and/or	≥ 85

is instructed to engage in normal activities, but to refrain from strenuous exercise, so that it gives information on BP during daily activities and at night during sleep. This can be undertaken in special cases. The test is expensive.

In more than two-third of cases of hypertension, both the systolic and diastolic BP levels (SBP and DBP) are elevated. In about a third, the SBP is greater than 140 mm Hg while the DBP is 90 mm Hg or less (isolated systolic hypertension). SBP appears to be a better predictor of events than DBP after the age of 50 years, is associated with higher risk of vascular occlusions in the coronary and cerebral vasculature. SBP and DBP together and also individually are associated with increased risk of complications. Systolic BP increases with age up to the 8th decade, whereas DBP increases only up to the age of 50 years. In the elderly, the DBP may actually fall and pulse pressure widens. In the Framingham study, SBP and widening of pulse pressure were found to be important predictors of risk in the elderly.

FACTORS WHICH INFLUENCE BP

Age: There is a positive relation between age and BP in most of the population groups.

Sex: Males have slightly higher values than females of the same age.

Ethnic groups: Some communities show higher prevalence of hypertension. In USA the BP in the black races is higher than that in the whites.

Risk Factors

Hereditary factors: Family history of hypertension is the strongest predictor for the development of hypertension.

Genetic factors: Several factors and genes have been studied. The inheritance seems to be polygenic.

- *Birth weight:* Low birth weights and adverse environment in early life are associated with higher prevalence of hypertension and diabetes.
- *Obesity:* In adults, obesity may confer a two-fold risk to develop hypertension. Central obesity is a stronger predictor of risk.
- *Dietary sodium:* The SBP and DBP are related directly with sodium intake and urinary sodium loss. Reduction to about 5 g/day has a modest (1–2 mm Hg) SBP-lowering effect in normotensive individuals and a somewhat more pronounced effect (4–5 mm Hg) in hypertensive individuals. Contrary to old concepts, recent studies show that neither increased potassium nor calcium diets improves hypertension and such diets are not recommended.

Other factors: Alcohol intake, tobacco smoking, sedentary lifestyle and noise pollution markedly elevate the BP level. Modification of lifestyle helps to lower the BP considerably.

In clinical practice, over 97% of hypertension belongs to idiopathic or primary variety and 3% may be secondary. Clinical features which should suggest the possibility of secondary hypertension include a positive history of hypertension and renal diseases in the family, history of intake of drugs, endocrinological disorders and resistance to the action of common antihypertensive drugs.

SYSTEMIC HYPERTENSION

Systemic hypertension is a major risk factor for coronary artery disease, heart failure, stroke and renal disease. So early detection and effective management of hypertension is important in reducing the morbidity and mortality attributed to it. The risk of cardiovascular diseases in a hypertensive patient is also determined by other coexisting cardiovascular risk factors in addition to the level of BP.

Hypertension is defined as systolic BP of 140 mm Hg or greater, and diastolic BP of 90 mm Hg or greater. Isolated systolic hypertension is defined as systolic BP of 140 mm Hg or greater and diastolic BP below 90 mm Hg (Tables 126.2 and 126.3).

When the BP is elevated without an evident organic cause, it is called *essential hypertension*. Hypertension produced by an identifiable cause is called *secondary hypertension*.

Essential hypertension far outnumbers secondary hypertension. It is necessary to detect the primary cause for secondary hypertension since correction of the cause leads to regression of the hypertension. In essential hypertension, since no underlying removable cause is detectable, treatment has to be, at best, palliative.

Causes of Secondary Hypertension

Renal
- Renal parenchymal disease
  - Acute glomerulonephritis
  - Chronic nephritis
  - Polycystic disease of kidney
  - Diabetic nephropathy
  - Hydronephrosis
  - Post-traumatic renal damage
- Renovascular
  - Renal artery stenosis
  - Intrarenal vasculitis
- Renin producing tumors
- Primary sodium retention

Table 126.2: Classification of BP

Category	Systolic		Diastolic
Optimal	< 120	and	< 80
Normal	120 –129	and/or	80–84
High normal	130 –139	and/or	85–89
Grade 1 hypertension	140 –159	and/or	90–99
Grade 2 hypertension	160 –179	and/or	100–109
Grade 3 hypertension	≥ 180	and/or	≥ 110
Isolated systolic hypertension	≥ 140	and	< 90

Note: 'Prehypertension' terminology has been removed in recent guidelines

---

Table 126.3: SBP and DBP in different age groups

Age	Normal	Significant hypertension
< 2 years	104–111 / 70–73	112–117 / 74–81
10–12 years	122–125 / 78–81	126–133 / 82–89

Note: BP in a one day old infant is ± 70 mm Hg. It rises to ± 85 mm Hg at 1 year. Boys have a slightly higher BP than girls

Endocrine
- Acromegaly
- Hypothyroidism and hyperthyroidism
- Hyperparathyroidism
- Adrenal
  - Cortical
    - Cushing's syndrome
    - Primary hyperaldosteronism (Conn's syndrome)
    - Congenital adrenal hyperplasia
  - Medullary—pheochromocytoma
- Exogenous hormones
  - Estrogen
  - Glucocorticoids
  - Mineralocorticoids
  - Sympathomimetic drugs
  - Tyramine containing foods and monoamine oxidase inhibitors

Vascular causes: Coarctation of aorta

Pregnancy induced hypertension

Neurological disorders
- Increased intracranial pressure
  - Brain tumors
  - Encephalitis
- Guillain-Barré syndrome
- Familial dysautonomia

Miscellaneous causes: Sleep apnea, acute stress, postoperative, hypoglycemia, burns, postresuscitation, alcohol withdrawal, etc.

EPIDEMIOLOGY

Overall prevalence of hypertension in India is about 26.2% in men and 23.6% in women. The prevalence is significantly more in urban subjects (30.9%) than in rural population (21.2%). A prospective study conducted at Chandigarh showed that the prevalence of hypertension rose from 26.9% in 1968 to 44.9 in 1996–97. A report from Chennai showed the crude prevalence rate of hypertension was 21.1% whereas the age standardized prevalence was 17%. The body mass index and waist-hip ratio were significantly higher in the hypertensive group. The prevalence of diabetes mellitus (DM), obesity and coronary artery disease were significantly higher in those with hypertension.

A recent study from Himachal Pradesh in rural communities showed that 35.89% were hypertensive (39.8% in males and 33.15% in females) in adults > 18 years age, 24.85% had prehypertension. Only 39.6% had normal BP levels, only 21.98% were aware of their hypertension. Among these only 20.23% has their BP under control.

Source: Bhardwaj R, Kandori A, Marwah R, et al. Prevalence, awareness and control of hypertension in rural communities of Himachal Pradesh. J Assoc Physicians India. 2010;58: 423-4, 429.

Longitudinal study of the population at Framingham (USA) revealed that the prevalence of hypertension was 29.7%. The BP showed a rise of 20 mm in SBP and 10 mm DBP when persons were followed up from 30–65 years. Systolic BP continued to rise in women up to 80 years and in men up to 70 years. There was strong genetic and familial predisposition to hypertension. Persons with DM and impaired glucose tolerance have a high prevalence of hypertension (even up to 50%), whereas hypertensive have a 15–18% chance of having associated abnormalities of glucose metabolism.

Contributory factors: Following factors contribute to the occurrence of this condition.

- ***Genetic factors:*** Essential hypertension shows a polygenic pattern of inheritance. Mutation in the MYH9 gene encoding nonmuscle myosin, strongly associated with end stage renal disease in hypertensive nephropathy, independent of the BP. Several rare, monogenic forms of hypertension have been described, such as glucocorticoid-remediable aldosteronism, Liddle's syndrome and others.
- ***Psychological stress:*** Persons who have to undergo mental stress during the course of their duties and those with tense personality are affected more.

Neural mechanisms:

- ***Sympathetic:*** Overactivity has been demonstrated in early primary hypertension and in hypertension associated with diabetes, CKD, obesity, sleep apnea and heart failure.
- ***Baroreceptors:*** In hypertension, the baroreceptor is reset to defend a higher level of BP. Partial baroreceptor dysfunction is common in elderly and is typically manifested with the triad of orthostatic hypotension, supine hypertension and symptomatic postprandial hypotension.
- ***Obesity:*** Weight gain and reflex sympathetic activation may be an important compensation to burn fat, but at the expense of sympathetic overactivity in kidney and vascular smooth muscle that produces hypertension.
- ***Obstructive sleep apnea:*** Patients with obstructive sleep apnea can have markedly elevated plasma and urine catecholamine levels, mimicking pheochromocytoma. Apnea produces sustained reflex sympathetic over activation and hypertension even during waking hours.

Salt and water intake: Communities with high salt intake have a higher prevalence of essential hypertension.

The renal hormones: The role of renin-angiotensin aldosterone system has been extensively studied. Renin is produced by the juxtaglomerular apparatus in response to various stimuli.

The control of renin release is complex. Several stimuli lead to renin release. These are:

- The impulses from pressor receptors in the afferent arterioles of the glomeruli
- Chemoreceptors of the macula densa which are stimulated by hyponatremia
- The sympathetic stimuli which lead to renin release on assuming the upright posture
- Chemical stimuli such as hypokalemia, etc.

Renin converts angiotensinogen to angiotensin I, which is further converted to angiotensin II, by the converting enzyme. Angiotensin II stimulates the production of aldosterone.

Angiotensin II causes vasoconstriction and aldosterone leads to retention of salt and water.

Among the hypertensives, 60% have normal, 30% have low and 10% have high values of plasma renin activity.

Low birth weight: Because of fetal undernutrition, low birth weight with reduced nephrogenesis increases the risk for development of adult salt dependent hypertension.

Other factors: Factors such as deficiency of prostaglandins and kinins which normally help in lowering the vascular tone have also been incriminated in the production of essential hypertension.

Atrial natriuretic hormone: Atrial tissue secretes a group of peptides, at least one of which is secreted as a regulatory hormone. In vivo experimental studies show that this peptide produces immediate marked increase in sodium loss, increase in glomerular filtration rate (without altering the total renal blood flow) and fall in arterial BP. The other effects include inhibition of renin secretion, aldosterone secretion and opposing the vasoconstrictor effect of angiotensin II.

Vascular factor: The endothelial lining of blood vessels is critical to vascular health and constitutes a major defense against hypertension. Oxidative stress, free radical injury deceases the bioavailability of nitric oxide—powerful vasodilator and thus leads to hypertension.

PATHOLOGY

Main pathological process occurs in the heart and several parts of the arterial tree as follows:

Cardiac Changes

The left ventricle hypertrophies in 20–50% of mild to moderate hypertensives. The muscle fibers hypertrophy and this process is reversible with antihypertensive therapy. At autopsy, left ventricular hypertrophy is diagnosed if it weighs above 131 g/m^2 body surface in men and 100 g/m^2 body surface in women. Unlike physiological hypertrophy occurring as a result of exercise, in hypertension left ventricular hypertrophy leads to diastolic dysfunction, arrhythmias, acceleration of coronary atherosclerosis and left ventricular failure. Cardiac failure is caused by degeneration and lysis of myofibrils. The extent of hypertrophy and levels of BP do not correlate in all cases but hypertrophy is more pronounced in those with early onset hypertension.

Arterial Changes

Arteries and arterioles show thickening (arteriolosclerosis). Arteriolar changes are well seen in the kidneys. Renal vessels show medial hypertrophy and intimal fibrosis. Progressive occlusion of arterial lumen leads to scarring of glomeruli and tubular atrophy.

In the coronary arteries there is accelerated progression of atherosclerosis. Cerebral arteries, renal arteries, aorta and its major branches show progressive atheromatous change. Hypertension is a major risk factor for aortic dissection, abdominal aortic aneurysm, and peripheral arterial disease. Small arteries of the brain show microaneurysms, known as Charcot-Bouchard aneurysms, which may rupture resulting in cerebral hemorrhage. Thrombotic and embolic occlusion of atheromatous arteries gives rise to infarction in the heart, brain and kidneys.

CLINICAL FEATURES

Essential Hypertension

The condition is asymptomatic and over 50% of the patients are unaware of the condition. Elevated BP is detected during a routine medical examination in such subjects. A few of them present for the first time with one of the major complications. Many develop symptoms after knowing that they are hypertensives. The symptoms are vague and nonspecific in such patients. These symptoms include fatigue, dizziness, palpitation, headache and anxiety. Though many types of headache have been described, throbbing headache, felt in suboccipital region on waking up after sleep is suggestive of hypertension.

Physical examination may reveal a heaving apex beat and loud aortic second sound in many cases. The pulse may show rise in tension (requiring more pressure to obliterate) in some. Further, physical signs develop as the target organs (heart, brain, kidneys and retinae) are involved.

Secondary Hypertension

In secondary hypertension, evidence of the primary disorder may be detectable in many cases. In others, hypertension may be the only evident abnormality and the diagnosis has to be established by investigation (Table 126.4).

Coarctation of the aorta has to be diagnosed by detection of weak or delayed femoral pulse and presence of hypertension in the upper limbs with lower pressure in the lower limbs. Renal artery bruit may be auscultated over the abdomen lateral to the umbilicus or over the renal angles and this finding is a clue to renovascular cause for hypertension. Palpability of the kidneys suggests polycystic disease, hydronephrosis or tumor.

COMPLICATIONS OF HYPERTENSION

Attributable to Hypertension

- Accelerated–malignant hypertension (grade III and IV retinopathy)
- Encephalopathy
- Cerebral hemorrhage
- Left ventricular hypertrophy
- Congestive heart failure
- Renal insufficiency
- Aortic dissection.

Atherosclerotic Complication

- Cerebral thrombosis
- Coronary artery disease
- Peripheral occlusive vascular disease.

Changes in the Cardiovascular System

- ***Left ventricular hypertrophy [LVH]:*** This is the most common cardiac abnormality in hypertension. LVH is a powerful predictor of serious cardiovascular sequelae. Electrocardiography can detect LVH only in 5–10% of hypertensives, whereas echocardiography LVH present in nearly 30% of patients. Cardiac MRI is most sensitive.
- ***Congestive heart failure [CHF]:*** The various alterations of LV systolic and diastolic function seen with LVH ultimately leads to the development of CHF. Hypertension remains as an important and major preventable factor leading to the development of CHF.

Table 126.4: Causes, clinical indications and diagnostic investigations in suspected secondary hypertension

	Clinical indications			Diagnostics	
Common causes	**Clinical history**	**Physical examination**	**Laboratory investigations**	**First-line test(s)**	**Additional/ confirmatory test(s)**
Renal parenchymal disease	History of urinary tract infection or obstruction, hematuria, analgesic abuse; family history of polycystic kidney disease	Abdominal masses (in case of polycystic kidney disease)	Presence of protein, erythrocytes, or leukocytes in the urine, decreased GFR	Renal ultrasound	Detailed work-up for kidney disease
Renal artery stenosis	Fibromuscular dysplasia: Early onset hypertension (especially in women)	Abdominal bruit	Difference of > 1.5 cm in length between the two kidneys (renal ultrasound), rapid deterioration in renal function (spontaneous or in response to RAA blockers)	Renal duplex doppler ultrasonography	Magnetic resonance angiography, spiral computed tomography, intra-arterial digital subtraction angiography
Primary aldosteronism	Muscle weakness; family history of early onset hypertension and cerebrovascular events at age < 40 years	Arrhythmias (in case of severe hypokalemia)	Hypokalaemia (spontaneous or diuretic-induced); incidental discovery of adrenal masses	Aldosterone-renin ration under standardized conditions (correction of hypokalemia and withdrawal of drugs affecting RAA system)	Confirmatory tests (oral sodium loading, saline infusion, fludrocortisone suppression, or captopril test); adrenal CT scan; adrenal vein sampling
Uncommon causes					
Pheochromocytoma	Paroxysmal hypertension or a crisis superimposed to sustained hypertension; headache, sweating, palpitations and pallor; positive family history of pheochromocytoma	Skin stigmata of neurofibromatosis (café-au-lait spots, neurofibromas)	Incidental discovery of adrenal (or in some cases, extra-adrenal) masses	Measurement of urinary fractionated metanephrines or plasma-free metanephrines	CT or MRI of the abdomen and pelvis; 123 I-labelled metaiodobenzyl-guanidine scanning; genetic screening for pathogenic mutations
Cushing's syndrome	Rapid weight gain, polyuria, polydipsia, psychological disturbances	Typical body habitus (central obesity, moon-face, buffalo hump, red striae, hirsutism)	Hyperglycaemia	24-hour urinary cortisol excretion	Dexamethasone-suppression tests

Abbreviations: GFR = Glomerular filtration rate; RAA = Renin-angiotensin aldosterone; CT scan = Computed tomgraphy scan; MRI = Magnetic resonance imaging

- ***Ischemic heart disease:*** It is more common in them. This may present as angina pectoris, silent ischemia, myocardial infarction or sudden death. Acute myocardial infarction may be unrecognized in 30–32%.
- ***Atherosclerosis:*** It is accelerated. Atherosclerosis of coronary, cerebral, renal and peripheral arteries lead to their progressive occlusion.
- ***Arrhythmias:*** Both supraventricular and ventricular are more common in hypertensives. Tobacco smoking worsens the cardiovascular complications.

Changes in the Central Nervous System

Stroke is among the most common complications in hypertension. The lesion may be an ischemic infarct resulting from thrombosis (80%) or a hemorrhage (20%) resulting from rupture of an artery. Hypertension is the most important single factor leading to all forms of strokes in the general population (50%). Hypertensive patients with asymptomatic carotid bruit should undergo Doppler

USG. The relationship between the incidence of stroke or coronary heart disease with BP is linear at all ages.

Hypertensive encephalopathy: It is a specific complication seen in hypertensives when there is a rapid rise of BP. The incidence is higher in acute glomerulonephritis, pheochromocytoma and malignant hypertension. The cerebral arteries go into spasm in response to a rapid rise in BP. Edema and ischemia of the brain develop.

Clinically, it is characterized by intense headache, visual disturbances, convulsions, loss of consciousness and varying degrees of focal neurological deficits. Prompt reduction of BP completely revert the attacks and restores the normal state. This feature distinguishes hypertensive encephalopathy from cerebral infarction or hemorrhage in which the neurological deficit persists.

Changes in the Kidneys

Atheroma of the renal arteries results in reduction of blood supply to the kidney and progressive loss of renal function.

In malignant hypertension renal function deteriorates rapidly, ending in renal failure.

Changes in Retina

The retinal arterioles undergo changes. These have been graded. The retinal changes give an indication of the progress of hypertension and help to determine the prognosis. Grades I and II are seen in the early phases of hypertension. Grade III is suggestive of the accelerated phase and grade IV indicates transition to the malignant phase.

Grade I: Arteriolar narrowing and increase in light reflex over the arterioles.

Grade II: Marked arteriolar narrowing and arteriovenous nicking.

Grade III: Grade II + flame-shaped hemorrhages and fluffy (soft) exudates.

Grade IV: Grade III + papilledema.

Malignant Hypertension and Accelerated Hypertension

Malignant hypertension is a hypertensive emergency, clinically defined as the presence of very high BP associated with papilledema and often ischemic organ dysfunction (retina, kidney, heart or brain). Secondary hypertension occurring in renal disease and pheochromocytoma shows a greater tendency to progress to the malignant phase. At this stage, there is widespread fibrinoid necrosis of arterioles. Retinopathy may lead to visual impairment. The diagnosis of malignant phase and accelerated phase depends on the evidence of vascular damage in a patient with severe hypertension. Malignant hypertension is characterized by papilledema whereas accelerated hypertension shows only grade III retinopathy. Once the malignant phase sets in, death occurs within two years as a result of cardiac failure, renal failure, or cerebral hemorrhage. Prompt treatment arrests the malignant phase and its complications. The retinal changes also regress and revert to Grade II (Fig. 126.1).

Prognosis

Hypertension leads to reduction of lifespan, and also considerable morbidity. Death is caused by ischemic heart disease, cardiac failure, cerebrovascular diseases or renal failure. Damage to the target organs worsens the prognosis considerably. Target organ damage (TOD)

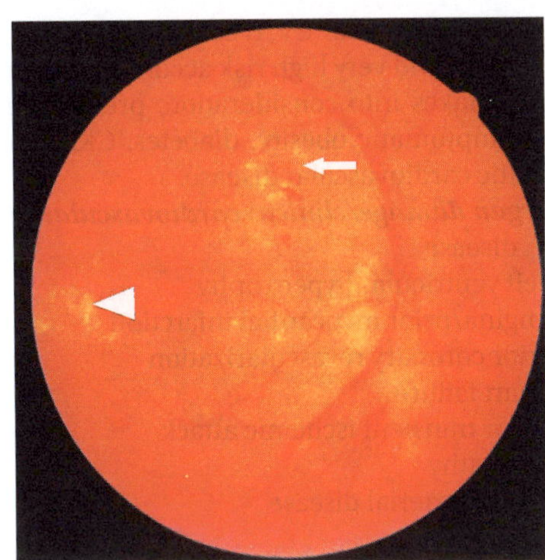

Fig. 126.1: Hypertensive retinopathy in malignant hypertension. ***Note:*** Papilledema, hemorrhages (arrow and soft exudates -arrowhead)

should be diagnosed if any one or more of the following abnormalities are detectable.

- Cardiac failure
- Signs and symptoms of atherosclerotic vascular disease
- ECG evidence of myocardial infarction, ischemia or left ventricular hypertrophy
- Evidence of previous stroke
- Renal insufficiency or proteinuria, and hypertensive changes on funduscopy
- Hypertension is associated with higher incidence of retinal venous and retinal arterial occlusions and visual loss.

ECG evidence of left atrial enlargement and presence of late diastolic gallop (S4 gallop) indicate the presence of diastolic dysfunction. Proper control of BP leads to reduction of the complications—reduction of strokes by 35–40%, coronary artery events by 20–30%, congestive heart failure by 50–60% and overall cardiovascular mortality by 20%.

Major Risk Factors (Table 126.5)

- Smoking
- Dyslipidemia
- Diabetes mellitus
- Age above 60 years
- Sex (men and postmenopausal women)
- Family history of cardiovascular disease.

Table 126.5: Major risk factors altering the BP

Other risk factors, asymptomatic organ damage or disease	Blood pressure (mm Hg)			
	High normal: SBP 130–139 or DBP 85–89	*Grade 1 HT: SBP 140–159 or DBP 90–99*	*Grade 2 HT: SBP 160–179 or DBP 100–109*	*Grade 3 HT: SBP ≥ 180 or DBP ≥ 110*
No other RF		Low risk	Moderate risk	High risk
1–2 RF	Low risk	Moderate risk	Moderate to high risk	High risk
≥ 3 RF	Low to moderate risk	Moderate to high risk	High risk	High risk
OD, CKD stage 3 or diabetes	Moderate to high risk	High risk	High risk	High to very high risk
Symptomatic CVD, CKD stage ≥ 4 or diabetes with OD/RFs	Very high risk	Very high risk	Very high risk	Very high risk

Abbreviations: BP = Blood pressure, CKD = Chronic kidney disease; CVD = Cardiovascular disease; DBP = Diastolic blood pressure; HT = Hypertension; OD = Organ damage; RF = Risk factor; SBP = Systolic blood pressure

Stratification of total CV risk into categories as low, moderate, high and very high risk according to sytolic and diastolic BP takes into consideration, prevalence of risk factors, asymptomatic obesity, diabetes, CKD stage, and symptomatic cardiovascular disease.

Target organ damage/clinical cardiovascular disease

- Heart disease
  - Left ventricular hypertrophy
  - Angina/prior myocardial infarction
  - Prior coronary revascularization
  - Heart failure
- Stroke or transient ischemic attack
- Nephropathy
- Peripheral arterial disease
- Retinopathy.

This empiric classification stratifies patients with hypertension into risk groups for making therapeutic decisions.

MANAGEMENT

The goal of management of hypertension is to reduce morbidity and mortality by the least invasive means as possible. This may be accomplished by achieving and maintaining SBP below 140 mm Hg and DBP below 90 mm Hg, while controlling other modifiable risk factors for cardiovascular disease. BP reduction therapy is required particularly to prevent stroke, to preserve renal function and prevent or slow heart failure progression. This goal may be achieved by lifestyle modification alone or with pharmacologic treatment.

RISK STRATIFICATION

Risk of cardiovascular disease in patients with hypertension is determined not only by the levels of BP but also by the presence or absence of target organ damage (TOD) or other risk factors. Hypertensive patients can be classified into high, moderate or low risk based on the presence or absence of major risk factors, TOD and clinical cardiovascular disease (CCD).

Lowering of BP provides similar relative protection at all levels of baseline cardiovascular risk. As the baseline risk increases, the risk reduction also increases. These results support the reduction of BP at all levels of cardiovascular risks. Meta-analysis of 67,475 individuals included in 37 studies supported these findings.

Source: Blood pressure lowering trailists collaboration. Blood pressure lowering treatment based on cardiovascular risks, a meta-analysis of individual patient data. The Lancet. 2014;384:(9943): 591-8.

Lifestyle Modifications

- Lose weight, if overweight. The mean SBP and DBP reductions associated with an average weight loss of 5.1 kg are 4.4 and 3.6 mm Hg, respectively. Maintenance of a healthy body weight [body mass index (BMI) of about 25 kg/m²] and waist circumference (102 cm for men and 88 cm for women) is recommended.
- Hypertensive men who drink alcohol should be advised to limit their consumption not more than 20–30 g, and hypertensive women not more than 10–20 g, of ethanol per day.

- At least 30 min of moderate-intensity dynamic aerobic exercise (walking, jogging, cycling or swimming) on 5–7 days per week. Isometric exercises are not recommended.
- Salt intake present recommendation is up to 4 g sodium chloride/day. The effect of sodium restriction is greater in older people and in individuals with diabetes, metabolic syndrome or CKD. Salt restriction may reduce the number and doses of antihypertensive drugs. Advice should be given to avoid added salt and high-salt food.
- Stop smoking and reduce intake of dietary saturated fat to below 7% of total calorie intake for overall cardiovascular health.
- Relaxation and biofeedback technique—transcendental meditation, yoga exercise such as *Savasana*.

Hypertensive patients should be advised to eat vegetables, low-fat dairy products, dietary and soluble fiber, whole grains and protein from plant sources, reduced in saturated fat and cholesterol. Fresh fruits are also recommended although with caution in overweight patients because sometimes their high carbohydrate content may promote weight gain. The Mediterranean type of diet, especially, has attracted interest in recent years. Patients with hypertension should be advised to eat fish at least twice a week and 300–400 g/day of fruit and vegetables. Soy milk appeared to lower BP when compared with skimmed cow's milk. Lifestyle modification brings down BP and also helps to reduce the dosage of drugs needed.

Pharmacological Treatment

Reduction of BP with drugs clearly decreases cardiovascular morbidity and mortality. Objective reduction of stroke, coronary events, heart failure, progression of renal disease, progression to more severe hypertension and all cause mortality has been demonstrated in several trials.

GENERAL GUIDELINES

Dosage and Follow-up

Therapy for most patients with uncomplicated hypertension (stages 1 and 2) should begin with the lowest dosage in order to avoid the adverse effects of abrupt reduction in BP. In hypertensive patients, abrupt lowering of BP produces signs of cerebral hypoperfusion. If BP remains uncontrolled after 1 or 2 weeks of drug therapy, the next dosage levels should be tried.

Optimal formulation should provide 24 hours efficacy with once daily dosage with at least 50% of peak effect remaining at the end of 24 hours.

JNC 8 Recommendations (Modified to Indian Conditions by the Editor)

- In the general population aged ≥ 60 years, initiate pharmacologic treatment to lower BP if SBP ≥ 150 mm Hg or DBP ≥ 90 mm Hg (goal < 150/90 mm Hg and goal < 90 mm Hg).
- In the general population < 60 years, initiate pharmacologic treatment to lower BP at SBP ≥ 140 mm Hg and DBP > 90 mm Hg and treat to a goal SBP < 140 mm Hg and DBP < 90 mm Hg.

- Same is the target in both CKD and diabetic patients.
- In the general population, including those with diabetes, initial anti-hypertensive treatment should include a thiazide-type diuretic, calcium channel blocker (CCB), angiotensin-converting enzyme inhibitor (ACEI), or angiotensin receptor blocker (ARB).
- In the population aged ≥ 18 years with CKD, initial (or add-on) anti-hypertensive treatment should include an ACEI or ARB to improve kidney outcomes. This applies to all CKD patients with hypertension regardless of race or diabetes status.

If BP goal is not reached within one month of treatment increase the dose or the drug or add second drug and if not reached with 2 drugs, add and titrate a third drug from the above mentioned class.

If the goal BP cannot be reached using only the drugs from class of thiazide-type diuretic, CCB, ACEI or ARB due to some contraindication or the need to use more than 3 drugs to reach goal BP, anti-hypertensive drugs from other classes can be added.

Drug Combinations

Combinations of low doses of two agents from different classes have been shown to provide additional antihypertensive efficacy, thereby minimizing the likelihood of dose dependent adverse effects. Very low dose of diuretics can potentiate the effects of other agents without producing adverse metabolic effects. Low dose combinations with ACE inhibitor and a nondihydropyridine calcium antagonist may reduce proteinuria more than either drug given singly. Combination of dihydropyridine calcium antagonist and ACE inhibitor reduce the incidence of pedal edema compared to calcium antagonist given alone. Although verapamil and diltiazem are sometimes used with a beta-blocker to improve ventricular rate control in permanent atrial fibrillation, only dihydropyridine calcium antagonists should normally be combined with beta-blocker for hypertension management (Fig. 126.2 and Table 126.6).

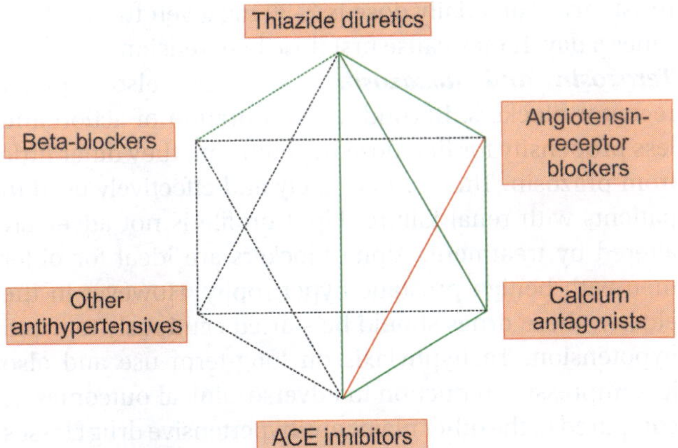

Fig. 126.2: Angiotensin converting enzyme—possible combinations of classes of antihypertensive drugs. Green continuous lines—preferred combinations; green dashed line—useful combination (with some limitations); black dashed lines—possible but less well-tested combinations; red continuous line—not recommended combination

Abbreviation: ACE = Angiotensin-converting enzyme

Table 126.6: Indications for specific drugs

Indications	Drugs
Asymptomatic organ damage	
LVH	ACE inhibitor, calcium antagonist, ARB
Asymptomatic atherosclerosis	Calcium antagonist, ACE inhibitor
Microalbuminuria	ACE inhibitor, ARB
Renal dysfunction	ACE inhibitor, ARB
Clinical CV event	
Previous stroke	Any agent effectively lowering BP
Previous myocardial infarction	BB, calcium antagonist
Angina pectoris	BB, calcium antagonist
Heart failure	Diuretic, BB, ACE inhibitor, ARB, mineralocorticoid receptor antagonists
Aortic aneurysm	BB, calcium antagonist
Atrial fibrillation, prevention	Consider ARB, ACE inhibitor, BB or mineralocorticoid receptor antagonist
Atrial fibrillation, ventricular rate control	BB, non-dihydropyridine calcium antagonist
ESRD/proteinuria	ACE inh ibitor, ARB
Peripheral artery disease	ACE inhibitor, calcium antagonist
Other	
ISH (elderly)	Diuretic, calcium antagonist
Metabolic syndrome	ACE inhibitor, ARB, calcium antagonist
Diabetes mellitus	ACE inhibitor, ARB
Pregnancy	Methyldopa, BB, calcium antagonist
Blacks	Diuretic, calcium antagonist

Abbreviations: LVH = Left ventricular hypertrophy; ACE = Angiotensin converting enzyme; CV = Cardiovascular; ISH = Isolated systolic hypertension; ARB = Angiotensin II receptor blockers; BP = Blood pressure; BB = Beta-blockers

Step-Down Therapy

An effort to decrease the dosage and number of antihypertensive drugs should be considered after hypertension has been controlled effectively for at least 1 year. Step-down therapy is often successful in patients who are also making lifestyle modifications. This may be possible in approximately 10–20% of patients.

Drugs Used in Hypertension and their Dosages

Diuretics

Diuretics initially lower BP by increasing urinary sodium excretion and by reducing plasma volume, extracellular fluid (ECF) volume and cardiac output. Within 6–8 weeks, the lowered plasma volume, ECF volume and cardiac output return to normal. On a long-term basis, antihypertensive effect is due to a fall in peripheral vascular resistance—the mechanism responsible for lowering peripheral vascular resistance is not clearly known.

Dosage and choice of agent

A thiazide diuretic is the usual initial choice often in combination with a potassium sparing agent. Loop diuretics should be reserved for those patients with renal insufficiency, resistant hypertension or hypertension associated with acute left ventricular failure or congestive cardiac failure. There is no guideline to suggest one diuretic is superior over others.

Hydrochlorothiazide : 6.25–50 mg/day (OD)
Chlorthalidone : 12.5–50 mg/day (OD)
Indapamide : 1.25–5 mg/day (OD)
Furosemide : 40–240 mg/day (2–3 times)
Amiloride : 5–10 mg/day (OD)
Spironolactone : 25–100 mg/day (OD)
Triamterine : 25–100 mg/day (OD)

Side effects

Hypokalemia, hypomagnesemia, hyperuricemia, hyperlipidemia, hyperglycemia, insulin resistance, hypercalcemia and impotence are the side effects.

The incidence of gynecomastia with spironolactone is dose-related whereas the exact incidence of menstrual disturbances in premenopausal women with spironolactone is unknown. A small dose of a thiazide diuretic, triamterene or amiloride, can be added to avoid a higher dose of spironolactone, which may cause side effects.

Eplerenone is a newer, selective mineralocorticoid receptor antagonist without antiandrogen and progesterone agonist effects, thus reducing the rate of side effects; it has 60% of the antagonist potency of spironolactone. Because of its shorter duration of action, multiple daily dosing is required (with a starting dose of 25 mg twice daily).

Spironolactone and eplerenone which have been found to have beneficial effects in heart failure, can be used as a third- or fourth-line drug in hypertension and help in effectively treating undetected cases of primary aldosteronism.

Inhibitors of Adrenergic System

- Peripheral neuronal inhibitors
  - Reserpine (seldom used now)
- Central adrenergic inhibitors
  - Methyldopa
  - Clonidine
- Alpha-receptor blockers
  - Alpha 1 and alpha 2 receptors
    - Phenoxybenzamine
    - Phentolamine
- Alpha 1 receptor
  - Prazosin
  - Doxazosin
  - Terazosin
- Beta receptor blockers
  - Nonselective
    - Propranolol, nadolol, timolol, pindolol
  - Cardioselective
    - Atenolol, acebutolol, metoprolol, bisoprolol
- Alpha and beta receptor blockers
  - Labetolol
- Newer-renin inhibitors-aliskerin

Note: Pindolol, acebutolol and bisoprolol also have intrinsic sympathomimetic activity (ISA). These do not lower the heart rate like the other beta blockers without ISA activity.

Reserpine: It acts by depleting the levels of norepinephrine in postganglionic adrenergic neurons by inhibiting the uptake of norepinephrine into storage vesicles. It depletes the central catecholamine levels. Daily dose is 0.1 to 5 mg. Adverse side effects include nasal congestion, mental depression and the development of parkinsonism. This drug is seldom used now. Initial studies on reserpine were conducted by Rustom Jal Vakil, the celebrated cardiologist from Bombay, in the 1950's. This drug has been superceded by newer drugs with less serious side effects.

Methyldopa: The primary site of action of methyldopa is central nervous system. It stimulates central alpha adrenergic receptors, thereby reducing the sympathetic outflow from the central nervous system. It is effective in a dose of 250–500 mg given orally 3–4 times a day. It does not reduce the renal blood flow and therefore can be given safely even in the presence of renal impairment. Adverse side effects include dryness of mouth, sedation, extrapyramidal features, fever, hepatitis and hemolytic anemia. Currently the role of methyl dopa is mainly in the management of resistant hypertension and also in pregnancy induced hypertension.

Clonidine: It acts centrally and is effective in an oral dose of 0.1 to 1 mg a day. Dryness of the mouth and drowsiness are the adverse side effects. Sudden withdrawal of the drug causes rebound hypertension.

Alpha-adrenergic Receptor Blocking Drugs

Nonselective (alpha 1 and alpha 2 blockers): Phenoxybenzamine and ***phentolamine*** belong to this class. Mainly they are used to control the excessive rise of BP in pheochromocytomas. The former is slow in action and the effect is sustained. The latter is quicker in action, but the effect is short lived. The dose of phentolamine is 2–5 mg IV slowly. Upto 5–30 mg given intravenously in a drip, the rate of flow is adjusted depending upon the response. Phentolamine is used to control the hypertensive crisis occurring in pheochromocytomas. It is also used as a diagnostic test.

Selective Alpha 1 Blockers

Prazosin: It is a selective antagonist of postsynaptic alpha-1 receptors. It acts by blocking alpha mediated vasoconstriction, thereby reducing peripheral vascular resistance. Total daily dose is 2–30 mg given two or three times a day. It may cause first dose hypotension.

Terazosin and doxazosin: These are also alpha-1 receptor blockers. Beyond longer duration of action and less propensity for first dose hypotension, they differ little from prazosin. They can be safely and effectively used in patients with renal failure. Lipid profile is not adversely altered by treatment. Alpha blockers are ideal for older men with benign prostatic hypertrophy. However in the elderly, these drugs should be started cautiously to avoid hypotension. Tachyphylaxis on long-term use and also less impressive reduction in adverse clinical outcomes as compared to the other major antihypertensive drug classes are the major limitations of most alpha blocking drugs.

Alpha blockers are not recommended as first-line therapy because in one study initial treatment with an alpha blocker resulted in worse cerebrovascular, heart failure, and combined cardiovascular outcomes than initial treatment with a diuretic.

Beta-adrenergic Blocking Drugs

Beta-adrenergic blocking drugs are the second most widely used antihypertensive drugs after diuretics. They reduce cardiac output, inhibit renin release and reduce sympathetic tone by central mechanisms. In cases with coexistent ischemic heart disease, beta blockers are found to be more useful. Long-term use of beta blockers in this context has been shown to reduce mortality by preventing major cardiac events such as myocardial infarction and fatal arrhythmias.

Although beta blockers were formerly thought to be contraindicated in patients with heart failure, they have now been found to be useful, especially metoprolol, carvedilol and bisoprolol. Atenolol is currently not preferred for management of hypertension as it has not been found to be less effective in reducing the risks of stroke and adverse cardiac effects.

Side effects: The most common side effect is fatigue. It may cause worsening of other concomitant problems like bronchospasm and peripheral vascular disease. In diabetics, warning signs of hypoglycemia may be masked. Other problems are insomnia, nightmares, depression, impotence and alteration of lipid metabolism leading to hyperlipidemia.

Cardioselective beta blockers are available for use. These are acebutalol 100–200 mg/day, metoprolol 100–400 mg/day, atenolol 100 mg/day and pindolol 10–40 mg/day. Of these atenolol and metoprolol have become the most popular drugs due to their effectiveness, ease of administration and freedom from major adverse effects.

Drug with both alpha and beta blocking action e.g. labetolol is given orally in doses of 100 mg twice daily orally.

A large meta-analysis has shown beta-blocker initiated therapy to be as equally effective as the other major classes of antihypertensive agents in preventing coronary outcomes. The vasodilating beta-blockers, such as celiprolol, carvedilol and nebivolol, which are more widely used today reduce central pulse pressure and aortic stiffness better than atenolol or metoprolol and affect insulin sensitivity less than metoprolol. Nebivolol has been shown not to worsen glucose tolerance. Some beta-blockers have also been reported not to increase, but even reduce, the risk of exacerbations and to reduce mortality in patients with chronic obstructive lung disease.

Vasodilators

These drugs cause vasodilation in various vascular compartments.

Hydralazine: This drug causes predominantly arteriolar dilation. It is effective in a dose of 20–50 mg thrice daily. This drug increases the renal, coronary and hepatic blood flow. Adverse side effects include angina induced by reflex tachycardia and lupus erythematosus, which regresses on withdrawing the drug. Though it is at present rare to start a patient on hydralazine as the first drug, many patients who are on this drug for a long-term, find it acceptable to continue with the same.

Sodium nitroprusside: This is an effective vasodilator which rapidly lowers BP and, therefore, it is used in hypertensive emergencies. It is given only as an intravenous drip, 50 mg being added to 500 mL 5% glucose and infused at the rate of 1–8 μg/kg/min, the response being monitored continuously. The drug is withdrawn when the emergency is controlled. Adverse side effects include severe hypotension, nausea, psychotic behavior and muscle spasms.

Diazoxide: This is a potent vasodilator with short action and therefore, it is used in hypertensive emergencies. When given in a dose of 100–300 mg intravenously, it lowers the BP rapidly.

Minoxidil: This is effective when given orally in doses up to 20–40 mg daily. It is effective in patients with severe hypertension associated with renal impairment. Side effects may be troublesome, but uncommon. These include hypertrichosis (increased hair growth), coarsening of facial appearance, salt and water retention, and tachycardia. Minoxidil should always be given along with diuretics.

Angiotensin Converting Enzyme Inhibitors (ACEI)

These drugs inhibit the ACE enzyme which converts angiotensin I to angiotensin II, thereby leading to the reduction in the production of angiotensin II and also aldosterone. In addition, this group of drugs has other beneficial effects in correcting impaired cellular metabolism and improving myocardial function. Drugs in this group are captopril, enalapril, lisinopril, ramipril, perindopril and others. The same enzyme, ACE is involved in the breakdown of bradykinin, and therefore ACEI also reduce the breakdown of bradykinin. Bradykinin is responsible for some of the adverse side effects such as cough, angioedema, renal dysfunction and hypotension. ACE inhibitors do not abolish the production of angiotensin II completely, since it may be formed by other pathways also.

Captopril: It is effective in oral doses of 150–400 mg daily. It is particularly effective in high renin hypertension. Captopril lowers peripheral resistance without altering the cardiac output and heart rate. It is effective in hypertension resistant to other drugs. It can be combined with other drugs. Side effects include fever, rashes, pruritus, distaste in the mouth, orthostatic hypotension, nephropathy, bronchospasm, hyperkalemia and leukopenia.

Enalapril: It is an analogue similar in action but with a longer half-life of 12–24 hours. It is given in a total dose of 5–40 mg per day in divided doses. Lisinopril is a lysine derivative of enalapril. It is absorbed and is effective when given orally. The action is prolonged and therefore the whole dose may be given together once a day. The initiating dose is 2.5–5 mg once or twice a day. This may be increased up to 20 mg daily. In patients with renal impairment the dose should be reduced. Ramipril is effective in a single oral dose of 1.25–10 mg daily. Perindopril is given in doses of 2–8 mg daily, starting at 2 mg and working up to 8 mg if needed.

Angiotensin II Receptor Blockers

Drugs in this class act by displacing angiotensin II from its specific receptor. They are at least as effective as ACE inhibitors. However, since they do not cause accumulation of bradykinin; cough as a side effect is infrequent. The major advantage is the minimal side effect profile for this class of antihypertensives. Moreover since they act on the final common pathway, viz. the receptor, alternate pathway production of angiotensin II does not blunt the effectiveness. There is total blockade of angiotensin II effects.

Currently available drugs in this class are ***losartan, valsartan, telmisartan, olmesartan candesartan*** and ***irbesartan***. Studies have found that they are at least as effective as ACEI in controlling BP. Dose: losartan—25–100 mg/day, valsartan—80–320 mg/day, telmisartan—40–80 mg/day, candesartan—8–16 mg/day and irbesartan—150–300 mg/day.

In USA, difference in the response to antihypertensive drugs (both efficacy and side effects) have been documented, but such studies are not widely done in India.

Aliskiren, a direct inhibitor of renin at the site of its activation, is available for treating hypertensive patients, both as monotherapy and when combined with other antihypertensive agents, but due to its adverse effects its regular use has not been recommended.

Calcium Channel Blocking Drugs

Calcium antagonists are commonly used in the treatment of hypertension. Dihydropyridine calcium antagonists (***nifedipine, amlodipine, cilnidipine*** and ***felodipine***) have the greatest peripheral vasodilator action with little effect on cardiac automaticity, conduction or contractility. Vasodilation leads to dependent edema.

The nondihydropyridine calcium antagonists (***diltiazem, verapamil***) cause less peripheral vasodilatation compared to dihydropyridines, but they have profound effects on cardiac contractility, automaticity and conduction. So they cause fewer side effects related to vasodilatation but may aggravate established cardiac failure or bradyarrhythmia.

Dosage: Amlodipine 2.5–10 mg/day once a day, felodipine 2.5–20 mg/day once a day, nifedipine extended release 30–120 mg once a day. These drugs may cause dependent edema in some patients due to peripheral vasodilatation. Withdrawal of the drug leads to prompt relief.

Dose of diltiazem is 30–90 mg and that of verapamil is 40–80 mg twice or thrice a day. Parenteral preparations are available for emergency. Verapamil 5–10 mg IV is given over 3 minutes.

Compared with diuretics, beta blockers and ACE inhibitors, calcium channel blockers (CCB) are inferior in heart failure. But calcium antagonists have shown a greater effectiveness than beta blockers in slowing down progression of carotid atherosclerosis and in reducing LV hypertrophy. Over all, dihydropyridine CCB (amlodipine) are preferred first line drugs for hypertension, especially in blacks.

Not recommended as first line drugs are:

- Central α2-adrenergic agonists (e.g. clonidine) Direct vasodilators (e.g. hydralazine)
- Aldosterone receptor antagonists (e.g. spironolactone)
- Peripherally acting adrenergic antagonists (e.g. reserpine)
- Loop diuretics (e.g. furosemide).

General Principles in Antihypertensive Therapy

Optimum benefit is obtained only if the BP is maintained at the desired levels throughout the day and night continuously. Proper adjustment of dosage, frequent consultation, and counseling to ensure drug compliance are all important to ensure success. Since adverse side effects may lead to loss of morale and discontinuation of therapy, all patients should be fully informed of the side effects (Table 126.7).

ACE inhibitors are preferable when there is left ventricular dysfunction with ejection fraction below 40% and in those with diabetes mellitus. In both groups, ACE inhibitors reduce mortality. In the latter, it also delays the onset of renal failure.

In patients with signs of prostatism, alpha blockers are useful as these reduce both hypertension and prostatic symptoms.

Failure to comply with therapy is the most frequent cause for failure of control of hypertension. Abrupt withdrawal of therapy may lead to rebound rise of BP and hypertensive complications such as hypertensive encephalopathy or cerebrovascular accidents. Self-monitoring of BP and adjusting the dose by the patient has being tried. Average of 4 days reading should be kept as 130/85 for otherwise normal people and 130/75 for diabetes.

Table 126.7: Side effects and contraindications to the most frequently used antihypertensives

Drug	Compelling	Possible
Diuretics (thiazides)	Gout	Metabolic syndrome Glucose intolerance Pregnancy Hypercalcemia Hypokalemia
Beta-blockers	Asthma A-V block (grade 2 or 3)	Metabolic syndrome Glucose intolerance Athletes and physically active patients Chronic obstructive pulmonary disease (except for vasodilator beta-blockers)
Calcium antagonists (dihydropyridines)		Tachyarrhythmia Heart failure
Calcium antagonists (verapamil, diltiazem)	A-V block (grade 2 or 3, trifascicular block) Severe LV dysfunction Heart failure	
ACE inhibitors	Pregnancy Angioneurotic edema Hyperkalemia Bilateral renal artery stenosis	Women with child bearing potential
Angiotensin receptor blockers	Pregnancy Angioneurotic edema Hyperkalaemia Bilateral renal artery stenosis	Women with child bearing potential
Mineralocorticoid receptor antagonists	Acute or severe renal failure (eGFR < 30 mL/min) Hyperkalemia	

Once established, essential hypertension tends to persist and, therefore, life-long therapy may be required in most cases, but it may be possible to reduce the dose in many or even withdraw drugs in a few.

RESISTANT HYPERTENSION

Hypertension is defined as resistant to treatment when a therapeutic strategy that includes appropriate lifestyle measures plus a diuretic and two other antihypertensive drugs belonging to different classes at adequate doses (but not necessarily including a mineralocorticoid receptor antagonist) fails to lower SBP and DBP values to, <140 and < 90 mm Hg, respectively. After excluding potential identifiable causes of hypertension, clinicians should carefully explore reasons why the patient is not at the goal BP. Particular attention should be paid to the type of diuretic and its dose in relation to renal function. Consultation with a hypertension specialist should be considered if goal BP cannot be achieved, but remember:

- Persistence of an alerting reaction to the BP-measuring procedure, with an elevation of office (although not of out-of-office) BP
- Use of small cuffs on large arms, with inadequate compression of the vessel
- Pseudohypertension, i.e. marked arterial stiffening, (more common in the elderly, especially with heavily calcified arteries), which prevents occlusion of the brachial artery—all these can result in false labeling of resistant hypertension.

Causes of Resistant Hypertension

- Improper BP measurement
- Volume overload and pseudotolerance
  - Excess sodium intake
  - Volume retention from kidney disease
  - Inadequate diuretic therapy
- Drug-induced or other causes
  - Nonadherence
  - Inadequate doses
  - Inappropriate combinations
  - Nonsteroidal anti-inflammatory drugs especially cyclooxygenase 2 inhibitors
  - Cocaine, amphetamine, other illicit drugs
  - Sympathomimetics (decongestants, anorectics)
  - Oral contraceptives
  - Adrenal steroids
  - Cyclosporine and tacrolimus
  - Erythropoietin
  - Licorice (including some chewing tobacco)
  - Selected over-the-counter dietary supplements and medicines (ephedrine)
- Associated conditions
  - Obesity
  - Excess alcohol intake, smoking tobacco
- Identifiable causes of hypertension (sleep apnea, renal diseases, endocrine causes, etc.)

A good response has been reported to the use of mineralocorticoid receptor antagonists, i.e. spironolactone, even at low doses (25–50 mg/day) or eplerenone, the α-1 blocker doxazosin and a further increase in diuretic dose, loop diuretic replacing thiazides or chlorthalidone

if renal function is impaired. At variance from an earlier report, endothelin antagonists have not been found to effectively reduce clinic BP in resistant hypertension and their use has also been associated with a considerable rate of side effects. New BP-lowering drugs (nitric oxide donors, vasopressin antagonists, neutral endopeptidase inhibitors, aldosterone synthase inhibitors, etc.) are all undergoing early stages of investigation. No other novel approach to drug treatment of resistant hypertensive patients is currently available. Avoidance of precipitating factors should be the first approach. Chronic field electrical stimulation of carotid sinus nerves (carotid baroreceptor stimulation) via implanted devices has recently been reported to reduce SBP and DBP in resistant hypertensive individuals.

Renal Denervation

This involves a bilateral destruction of the renal nerves travelling along the renal artery, by radiofrequency ablation. The rationale for renal denervation lays in the importance of sympathetic influences on renal vascular resistance, renin release and sodium reabsorption, the increased sympathetic tone to the kidney and other organs displayed by hypertensive patients, and the pressor effect of renal afferent fibers. Though it is promising theoretically, recent studies could not convincingly prove its efficacy.

HYPERTENSIVE URGENCIES AND EMERGENCIES

Hypertensive emergencies are defined as large elevations in SBP or DBP (>180 mm Hg or >120 mm Hg, respectively) associated with impending or progressive organ damage, such as major neurological changes, hypertensive encephalopathy, cerebral infarction, intracranial hemorrhage, acute LV failure, acute pulmonary edema, aortic dissection, renal failure, or eclampsia. Isolated large BP elevations without acute organ damage (hypertensive urgencies) are often associated with treatment discontinuation or reduction, as well as with anxiety—should not be considered an emergency but treated by reinstitution/intensification of drug therapy and treatment of anxiety.

Treatment of hypertensive emergencies depends on the type of associated organ damage and ranges from no lowering or extremely cautious lowering of BP in acute stroke to prompt and aggressive BP reduction in acute pulmonary edema or aortic dissection.

In most other cases, it is suggested that physicians induce a prompt but partial BP decrease, aiming at a less than 25% BP reduction during the first hours, and proceed cautiously thereafter. Drugs to be used, initially intravenously and subsequently orally, are those recommended for malignant hypertension.

Patients with markedly elevated BP but without acute target organ damage (urgency) usually do not require hospitalization, but they should receive immediate combination oral antihypertensive therapy. They should be carefully evaluated and monitored for hypertension-induced heart and kidney damage and for identifiable causes.

Emergency drugs for rapid control of BP in hypertensive emergencies:

Sodium nitroprusside	0.25–10 μg/kg IV infusion
Nitroglycerine	50–150 μg/min IV infusion
Diazoxide	50 mg IV bolus repeated or 15–30 mg/min infusion

Additional Considerations in Antihypertensive Drug Choices

Antihypertensive drugs can have favorable or unfavorable effects on other comorbidities.

Potential Favorable Effects

Thiazide-type diuretics are useful in slowing demineralization in osteoporosis. Beta-adrenergic blockers (BB) can be useful in the treatment of atrial tachyarrhythmias/fibrillation, migraine, thyrotoxicosis (short term), essential tremor, or perioperative hypertension. Calcium channel blockers (CCB) may be useful in Raynaud's syndrome and certain arrhythmias, and alpha-blockers may be useful in prostatism.

Potential Unfavorable Effects

Thiazide diuretics should be used cautiously in patients who have gout or who have a history of significant hyponatremia. BBs should generally be avoided in individuals who have severe asthma or severe reactive airway disease, or second or third degree heart block. ACEIs and ARBs support recommendations that these drugs should not be used in pregnancy or in women who are likely to become pregnant. ACEIs should not be used in individuals with a history of angioedema. Aldosterone antagonists and potassium-sparing diuretics can cause hyperkalemia and should generally be avoided in patients who have serum potassium values more than 5.0 mmol/L while not taking medications.

RENAL HYPERTENSION

See also Section 16, Ch 188

Renal parenchymal hypertension which results from primary glomerular and tubulointerstitial disease of the kidney is both volume dependent and renin-mediated. These account for about 70% of all cases of renal hypertension. In glomerular disease, renal symptoms and hypertension set in almost simultaneously, whereas in tubulointerstitial diseases, hypertension precedes the renal symptoms by several years. Renovascular hypertension (RVH) constitutes only around 1% of the total cases of hypertension but in children below 15 years without gross urinary abnormalities, RVH constitutes more than 60% of cases. Suitable medical regimens can include ACEI or ARBs blockers, except in bilateral renal artery stenosis or in unilateral artery stenosis with evidence of functional importance by ultrasound examinations or scintigraphy. Renal angioplasty is another option for the treatment of RVH, and it may result in good control of BP with fewer medications.

HYPERTENSION IN CHILDREN

BP in children correlates more with that of their mothers. Elevated BP in children may be a forerunner of essential hypertension in adults. The clinical features of elevated BP in neonates and young infants is failure to thrive, irritability, feeding problems including vomiting, cyanosis, respiratory distress, cardiac failure and seizures. Most common causes include renal artery thrombosis following umbilical artery catheterization, coarctation of the aorta, congenital renal diseases, renal artery stenosis, hypercalcemia, neurofibromatosis and endocrine disorders.

HYPERTENSION IN PREGNANCY

See also Section 16, Ch 189

MINERALOCORTICOID HYPERTENSION

This is caused mostly by increase in aldosterone production by the adrenal cortex, rarely it may be any other mineralocorticoid such as 11-deoxycorticosterone. Mineralocorticoid induced hypertension is associated with hypokalemia.

Normally, aldosterone production is regulated by angiotensin II levels, which in turn is controlled by renin levels. Increased aldosterone levels in turn suppress renin levels, and low renin levels are the hallmark of primary hyperaldosteronism.

Primary hyperaldosteronism may result from aldosterone producing adrenocortical adenoma, bilateral adrenocortical hyperplasia or rarely carcinoma. The first two conditions may form part of familial multiple endocrine neoplasia type one (MEN-1).

Clinical features: In the early stages, it may resemble other forms of hypertension, but when hypokalemia and alkalosis develop, additional features such as muscle weakness, tetany and cardiac arrhythmias may develop. Classic diagnostic markers are hypertension resistant to drug therapy and hypokalemia. Diagnosis is established by simultaneously estimating plasma levels of renin, aldosterone and potassium, in a patient who is seated for 5 minutes. The ratio of aldosterone to renin is very high in such cases. Further, confirmatory tests are available. The site of overproduction of the hormone can be identified by sampling the adrenal venous blood on either side. CT may reveal the tumor if it is of sufficient size.

Treatment: Dexamethasone given orally with a view to suppress corticotrophin also suppresses aldosterone levels in familial hyperaldosteronism type-1. Familial hyperaldosteronism type-2 is not suppressible by glucocorticoid.

Adenomas have to be removed surgically. In case of bilateral adrenal hyperplasia, medical treatment with spironolactone, amiloride or eplerenone (25–100 mg bd) is beneficial. Spironolactone may be required in small doses of 12.5–25 mg twice daily given orally. Dose of amiloride is 2.5 mg daily.

ORTHOSTATIC HYPOTENSION

See also Section 17, Ch 213

Sudden fall of BP may occur on adopting the erect posture leading to symptoms such as giddiness and syncope. Generally, this may result from several underlying diseases. The term postural hypertension is used when the SBP falls by 20 mm Hg or to below 100 mm Hg on standing for 5 minutes.

When a person stands, there is a tendency for 10–15% of blood to get sequestrated in the splanchnic circulation and the lower limbs. The consequent fall in BP is counteracted by counter-regulatory mechanisms which include sympathetic activity and discharge of hormones like catecholamine, renin, angiotensin and vasopressin. Peripheral vasoconstriction increase in heart rate and rise in plasma volume help to maintain the BP steady. When a normal person stands, it takes about a minute for circulatory adaptation. The heart rate and diastolic BP rise by 10%. The systolic BP is not affected. In postural syncope, the BP falls immediately after standing. Fainting occurs due to fall in cerebral perfusion.

Orthostatic hypertension may result from two groups of lesions:

- Lesions affecting the afferent pathways from the baroreceptors to the vasomotor center
- Lesions affecting the efferent pathways from the vasomotor center to the arterioles.

Various neurological disorders that can lead to orthostatic hypertension.

Afferent lesions	Neuropathies
Central lesions	Multiple system atrophy, Parkinson's disease
Spinal lesions	Lesions of cervical and dorsal regions of the spinal cord
Ganglionic lesions	Progressive autonomic failure
Postganglionic lesions	Neuropathies

Common Causes of Orthostatic Hypotension

- Polyneuropathy in diabetes, beriberi and amyloidosis
- Autonomic neuropathy in syringomyelia, tabes dorsalis and subacute combined degeneration
- Following surgical or medical sympathectomy
- Adverse reaction to drugs, especially antihypertensive drugs
- Idiopathic autonomic neuropathy (Shy-Drager syndrome)
- Dehydration, blood loss, fever, severe anemia, convalescence from debilitating illnesses, prolonged bed rest and starvation.

Clinical features: Dizziness or fainting on standing is the presenting symptom. Fainting from autonomic failure differs from other causes of fainting by the absence of sweating, pallor and cardiac slowing in the former.

Shy-Drager Syndrome

It is the condition where postural hypotension is associated with other autonomic phenomena such as sphincter disturbances, anhidrosis and impotency and other neurological disorders such as external ocular palsies, Parkinsonism and cerebellar disturbances.

Diagnosis: It is important to diagnose the condition and establish the cause since the outlook varies in the different types. In normal subjects, the BP falls during sleep and rises prior to waking up. This circadian rhythm of BP is reversed in patients with autonomic failure.

Management: Immediate management is to put the patient supine and elevate the legs or press the thighs against the abdomen to improve venous return. In many cases, the patient recovers. Stimulating drinks such as coffee or lime juice containing 20 g sugar and 6 g salt help to raise the BP within a short time. In more severe cases with syncope or sustained hypertension, an IV drip of 10% glucose saline should be started. Still, if the condition does not recover pressor agents such as ephedrine 30 mg oral or IV infusion of dopamine may be required. Fludrocortisone in doses of 0.01–0.02 mg/day is the best treatment on a long-term basis. The underlying causes should be detected and corrected.

Long-term management consists of dietary advice to take more salt, avoid hypotensive drugs and exercise programs to improve muscle tone, and treatment of the cause.

The term ***orthostatic intolerance*** is given to a syndrome characterized by adrenergic symptoms that occur when upright posture is assumed. The heart rate increases by at least 30 beats/min without developing orthostatic hypotension. Most subjects are women between the ages 20–50. These symptoms overlap with the clinical presentation of other functional disorders such as Da Costa's syndrome, Soldier's heart, neurocirculatory asthenia and also mitral valve prolapse.

CHAPTER
127

Ischemic Heart Disease

CG Bahuleyan

Chapter Summary

- General Considerations
- Acute Myocardial Infarction
- Coronary Artery Bypass Graft (CABG)
- Right Ventricular Infarction
- Stable Angina Pectoris
- Unstable Angina Pectoris
- Prinzmetal's Angina (Synonym: Variant Angina)
- Asymptomatic Coronary Artery Disease

GENERAL CONSIDERATIONS

A wide spectrum of clinical disorders is included under this term. All of these are caused by reduction in arterial blood supply to the myocardium. The lumen of the coronary arteries is narrowed leading to impairment of blood supply and in vast majority of cases, this results from atherosclerosis.

The right and left coronary arteries arise from the root of the aorta. The left coronary artery (LCA) divides into two major branches, the left anterior descending and left circumflex. Branches of the left descending branch supply the free wall of the left ventricle (LV) and a major portion of the interventricular septum (IVS). The left circumflex artery supplies the left atrium (LA) and parts of the posterior and lateral walls of the LV. In 45% of cases this artery supplies the sinoatrial (SA) node as well. The right coronary artery (RCA) supplies the right ventricle (RV), a major portion of the diaphragmatic surface of the LV, the atrioventricular (AV) node (in 90%) and the SA node (in 55%). Venous blood from the heart is drained into the right atrium (RA) through the coronary sinus, thebesian veins and the anterior cardiac veins.

Around 4–6% of the cardiac output flows into the coronary arteries in health. The coronary arteries run on the epicardial surface and their branches penetrate to supply the myocardium. The outer two-third portion is supplied by the epicardial branches and the inner one-third is supplied by perforating branches which form subendocardial ramifications. The left ventricular (LV) myocardium receives blood almost exclusively during diastole whereas the normal right ventricular (RV) myocardium receives blood during both phases of the cardiac cycle. In normal persons, myocardial blood flow is controlled by constriction and dilation of the microcirculation (vessels < 400 μm). The large coronary arteries offer no resistance to blood flow. When stenosis occurs, the arterial pressure drops distally. In health, coronary blood flow can increase 3.5–8.0 times the resting blood flow. When coronary obstruction occurs, the microcirculation dilates and compensates to maintain the blood flow. When arterial stenosis becomes severe, even this vasodilation will fail to maintain adequate blood flow. Such occlusions become functionally important.

Metabolism of cardiac muscle is aerobic. The myocardium extracts 70% of the oxygen supplied to it in arterial blood. If the oxygen supply is interrupted for over 2 minutes, the myocardium becomes ischemic and the mechanical activity ceases totally. Ischemia may result from atherosclerotic narrowing of the coronary arteries or spasm or both. In normal subjects, blood flow to the myocardium is maintained even when the coronary diameter is reduced to 50%, i.e. the cross-section is reduced by 75%. The resting blood flow is maintained till the arterial lumen is reduced by 90%. Factors, which further reduce coronary blood flow, are extreme tachycardias (due to reduction of diastolic interval), hypertension, elevation of intraventricular pressure as in aortic and pulmonary stenosis (PS), and cardiomegaly. Ischemia to the myocardium causes the characteristic pain.

ETIOLOGY

The etiology of ischemic heart disease (IHD) includes:

- *Coronary atherosclerosis:* This is the most common cause for myocardial ischemia.
- *Non-atheromatous coronary artery disease (CAD):*
  - *Arteritis:* Polyarteritis nodosa (PAN), Takayasu's disease, Kawasaki's syndrome, nonspecific arteritis, syphilitic aortitis, systemic lupus erythematosus (SLE), thromboangiitis obliterans (TAO) and others.

- *Thickening of coronary arteries:* Mucopolysaccharidoses, amyloidosis.
- *Spasm of coronary arteries:* Generally, spasm supervenes on diseased arteries but sometimes no other pathological lesion may be detectable. Under extreme conditions of stress, even normal arteries may undergo spasm. This can lead to myocardial ischemia and fatal arrhythmias.
- *Dissecting aneurysm of the aorta, dissection of the coronary arteries.*
- *Embolism:* Infective endocarditis (IE), emboli from the LA or LV, left atrial myxoma or paradoxical embolism may affect the coronary arteries.
- *Congenital anomalies:* Anomalous origin of the LCA from the pulmonary artery, single coronary artery, coronary arteriovenous fistula (CAVF), aneurysms of the coronary arteries, myocardial bridges.
- *Trauma to the coronary arteries*, penetrating wounds, injury during pericardiocentesis.
- *Thrombosis without underlying atherosclerotic plaque:* Polycythemia, thrombocytosis, hypercoagulability states.
- *Substance abuse:* Cocaine, amphetamines.
- *Imbalance between oxygen demand and blood supply:* Severe aortic stenosis, aortic regurgitation, prolonged hypotension, severe anemia, thyrotoxicosis and other conditions of ventricular hypertrophy.

EPIDEMIOLOGY

In all the developed countries where reliable statistics are available, IHD is one of the most common cause of death and cardiac morbidity in middle and elderly age groups. Till the early part of this decade, the incidence was rising, but there is a slight drop recently. Though complete statistics are not available in India, cardiovascular diseases account for 24% of total deaths of which coronary heart disease (CHD) appears to be the dominant form. IHD death rates are 3 times higher than stroke rates. Men suffer 9 times more frequently than premenopausal women, but after menopause the risk of coronary atherosclerosis rapidly increases to catch up with that of men over a period of several years. The disease is more common in the affluent classes of society, but the poor socioeconomic groups and manual laborers are not totally spared.

RISK FACTORS FOR ATHEROSCLEROSIS

Several risk factors have been identified as contributing to the development of coronary atherosclerosis. For purposes of management, they have been broadly divided into modifiable and nonmodifiable risk factors.

Nonmodifiable Risk Factors

- *Age:* As age advances, the prevalence of CHD increases. Increase in age is a strong predisposing factor for atherosclerosis. It is difficult to distinguish the specific influence of age in the causation of atherosclerosis and therefore in practical terms, 'higher the age, higher the prevalence of atherosclerosis' can be a general proposition, with a minority of exceptions. Now, that the aging population in India is increasing, a higher burden of IHD is to be expected if effective preventive interventions are not implemented.

- **Genetic predisposition** to atheroma is revealed by a positive family history of IHD [sudden deaths, myocardial infarction (MI), or angina] or cerebrovascular accidents occurring at relatively younger ages among close relatives. The higher prevalence of CAD in persons having diagonal crease in the earlobe has been found in many population groups including that in Kerala.
- **Personality factors:** High strung aggressive and competitive individuals (type A) are more prone to develop MI than the more relaxed type of personality (type B).
- **Sex:** The disease is considerably less prevalent in women during their reproductive periods of life. In the Framingham Study, the male-to-female ratio in the 35–44 years age group was 6.8:1 but in the age group 75–84 years, the prevalence equaled in both sexes. Despite the lower prevalence, once the disease manifests, it runs a more aggressive course in women.

Modifiable Risk Factors

- **Cigarette smoking:** Cigarette consumption is the single most important modifiable risk factor for CAD. Even among nonsmokers, passive exposure to cigarette smoke increases coronary risk. The offending agents are nicotine and carbon monoxide (CO) present in cigarette smoke.
- **Hyperlipidemia:** The risk of coronary atherosclerosis is directly related to elevation of serum cholesterol. Increase in levels above 250 mg/dL is associated with increasing risk. Lipids circulate in blood in the form of lipoproteins. Based on electrophoretic pattern and density gradient, they can be classified into α-lipoproteins [high-density lipoprotein (HDL)], β-lipoproteins [low-density lipoprotein (LDL)] and pre-β-lipoproteins [very-LDL (VLDL)]. An elevated LDL-cholesterol level appears to be the primary CHD risk factor, and the higher the total and LDL-cholesterol levels are, the greater is the risk of an atherosclerotic event. A low level of HDL-cholesterol is also a potent individual predictor for IHD. Many types of hyperlipidemias are genetically determined, but by proper dietary modification, exercise and drug therapy the serum levels can be lowered and this risk can be brought down to some extent (*See* also Section 10, Ch 93: Other metabolic disorders).
- **Hypertension:** Systemic arterial hypertension is a major independent risk factor for CHD, although it appears pathogenetically to be a cholesterol dependent accelerator of atherosclerosis. Raised blood pressure (BP) increases the rate of progression of atheroma, especially when present along with hyperlipidemia. It has been suggested that associated hormonal changes, including generation of angiotensin II by systemic and/or local renin-angiotensin systems (RAS), could also play a pathogenetic role.
- **Diabetes mellitus (DM):** It appears another pathogenetically cholesterol dependent, but statistically independent, major cardiovascular risk factor is DM. Diabetes and hypercholesterolemia interact strongly in the genesis of IHD. The precursor to type 2 diabetes, insulin resistance with impaired glucose tolerance (IGT) also carries a strongly increased risk for cardiovascular disease. The risk of developing coronary atherosclerosis is considerably increased.
- **Exercise:** Persons with sedentary jobs develop CAD more often than those having regular physical exercise.
- **Novel risk factors:** Increased levels of homocysteine, C-reactive protein (CRP), plasma fibrinogen and fibrin D-dimer, and lipoprotein-α have been implicated as independent risk factors for atherosclerosis and IHD.

Work done at Bangalore has shown that in resident Indians of South India, tobacco smoking, hypertension, diabetic state and central obesity were the more important risk factors seen in patients with the first attack of acute myocardial infarction (Acute MI). In western countries, the incidence of IHD is coming down in the richer groups due to modification of lifestyles whereas, it is increasing in the more poor groups.

C-reactive Protein and hs-CRP

It is a well-characterized marker of vascular inflammation. Epidemiologic studies have demonstrated that CRP when measured with high-sensitivity assays (hs-CRP) is more strongly and independently predictive of the risk of MI, stroke, peripheral arterial disease and sudden cardiac death in apparently healthy individuals even in the absence of conventional risk factors like elevated LDL-cholesterol. hs-CRP levels below 1 mg/L is associated with lower vascular risk whereas a level exceeding 3 mg/L is associated with high vascular risk. Values between 1 mg/L and 3 mg/L can be considered to represent moderate risk. Statins have been shown to reduce the hs-CRP levels by about one-third. Rosuvastatin has been studied in a major primary prevention trial and was shown to reduce MI and stroke in those with low LDL-cholesterol but elevated hs-CRP. Routine measurement of hs-CRP as a screening test in the general population is not recommended due to higher cost and lesser availability.

PATHOLOGY

Atheroma commonly affects the epicardial vessels. This may lead to single or multiple obstructions.

The location of infarct depends upon the vessel occluded. Occlusion of the left anterior descending branch causes infarction of the anterior and apical portions of LV. Occlusion of the left circumflex branch causes infarction of the lateral and inferoposterior walls of the LV. RCA occlusion causes infarction of the inferior portion of the IVS and inferoposterior wall.

In atherosclerosis, focal fibrofatty elevations (plaques) develop in the intimal and subintimal regions resulting in progressive narrowing of the lumen. Inflammation is an important component in the development of atheroma. It is associated with activation and proliferation of macrophages, endothelial cells and smooth muscle cells and generation of cytokines and growth factors. The lipid-rich atheromatous material itself is a potent inducer of inflammation. Oxidized LDL is taken up by macrophages to form subintimal foam cells. Oxidized LDL also acts as a chemotactic factor for macrophage accumulation.

The inflammatory changes have been the focus of intense research in recent years. Inflammation within the arterial wall starts with the entry of low-density lipoprotein (LDL) through the damaged intima. This attracts cellular components, such as monocytes, macrophages which are transformed monocytes and T lymphocytes. Several cytokines, such as interferon gamma (IFN-γ), tumor necrosis factor (TNF), interleukin-1 (IL-1) and others have been detected and incriminated in the process. Several microbial antigens have been detected. These include *Chlamydia pneumoniae*, herpesviridae, cytomegalovirus (CMV) and others. Several markers of inflammation, such as CRP, fibrinogen, IL-7, IL-8 and others have been detected. All these point to a strong possibility of inflammation playing a major role in atherothrombotic CAD.

Several Complications

Several complications may develop in the atheroma. These include hemorrhage into the atheroma, ulceration of the intimal surface with thrombosis over the atheroma, embolization of the atheromatous material and calcification. Progressive occlusion of the lumen of the coronary arteries may remain totally asymptomatic till the circulation is considerably diminished. In general, the development of complications gives rise to one of the clinically detectable syndromes.

Once a coronary artery is occluded and the myocardium is infarcted, gross changes are noticeable by 6 hours. The infarct appears pale, blue and edematous. Early histological features are interstitial edema, neutrophilic infiltration and clumping of muscle cells. Granulation tissue appears by the 10th day. The infarcted area is converted into a scar by the 6th week. An infarct may involve the total thickness of the ventricular myocardium (transmural infarcts) or may be confined to the subendocardial region.

Further changes may develop over the area of initial infarction. These are:

- Extension of the infarct leading to further loss of ventricular function
- Involvement of conducting tissues leading to disruption of impulse conduction

- Rupture of the infarct resulting in hemopericardium
- Inflammation of the overlying pericardium giving rise to pericarditis
- Formation of ventricular aneurysm.

The ischemic myocardium is electrically unstable and heterogeneous and this acts as a focus for re-entry, which gives rise to ventricular arrhythmias in the immediate postinfarction period.

CLINICAL PRESENTATIONS

The following distinct clinical syndromes have been recognized:

- Acute MI; with ST-segment elevation [ST-elevation myocardial infarction (STEMI)] without ST-segment elevation [non-STEMI (NSTEMI)]
- Unstable angina pectoris
- Stable angina pectoris
- Sudden cardiac death
- Arrhythmias and conduction defects
- Ischemic cardiomyopathy
- Asymptomatic CAD.

ACUTE MYOCARDIAL INFARCTION

Despite impressive strides in diagnosis and management over the past 3 decades, acute MI continues to be a major public health problem. Almost all MIs result from coronary atherosclerosis, generally with superimposed coronary thrombosis. Before the thrombolytic era, clinicians typically divided acute MI patients into those suffering a Q wave or non Q wave infarct, based on the evolution of the pattern on the electrocardiogram (ECG) over several days after acute MI. In the thrombolytic era, acute MI is classified based on the presence or absence of ST-segment elevation in the 12-lead ECG—into STEMI or NSTEMI (Figs 127.1 to 127.4).

Pathogenesis

Slowly developing high-grade stenoses of epicardial coronary arteries may progress to complete occlusion, but do not usually precipitate acute MI, probably because of the development of a rich collateral network. During the natural evolution of atherosclerotic plaques, especially those that are lipid laden, an abrupt and catastrophic transition may occur, characterized by plaque rupture. After plaque rupture, there is exposure of substances that promote platelet activation and aggregation, thrombin

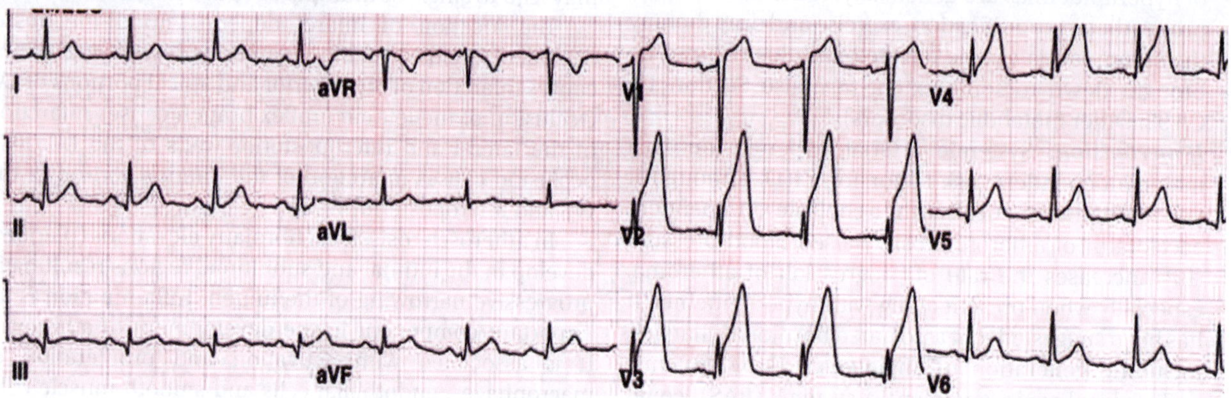

Fig. 127.1: ECG of anterior wall MI showing ST-elevation in leads V1-V5

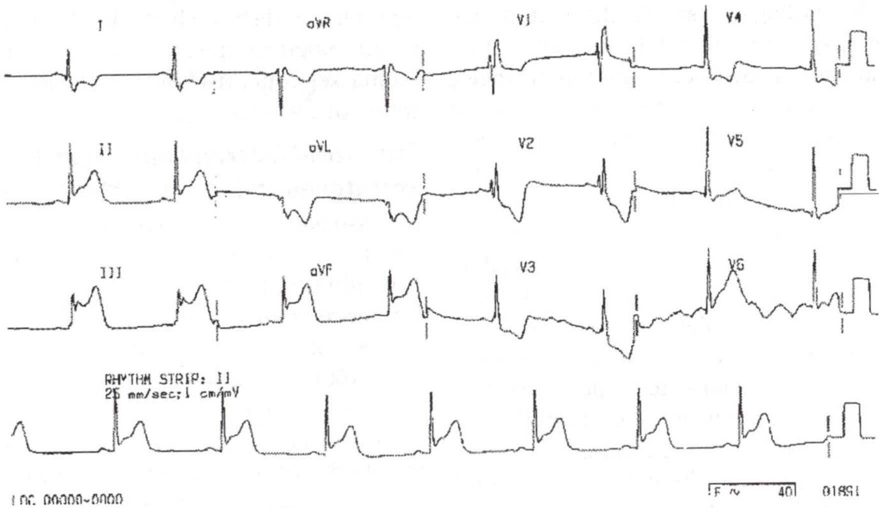

Fig. 127.2: ECG: Hyperacute inferior wall myocardial infarction. ***Note:*** (1) ST-elevation in inferior leads– viz lead II, III, and aVF (2) Reciprocal ST segment depression in V2-V4

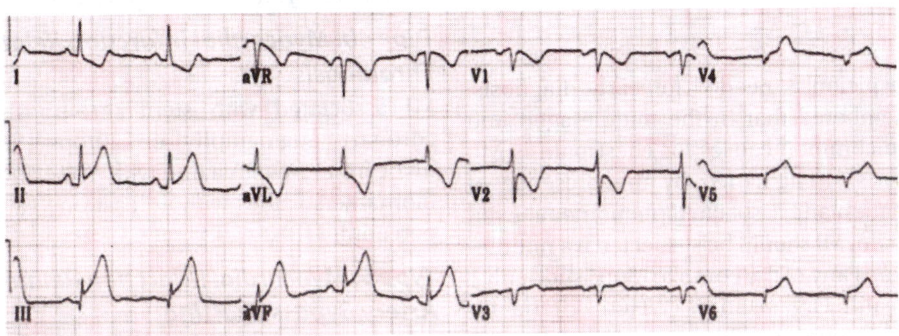

Fig. 127.3: ECG showing inferior and lateral MI. ***Note:*** ST-elevation in leads 2, 3, aVF, V5,V6 and ST depression in leads I, aVL, V1,V2

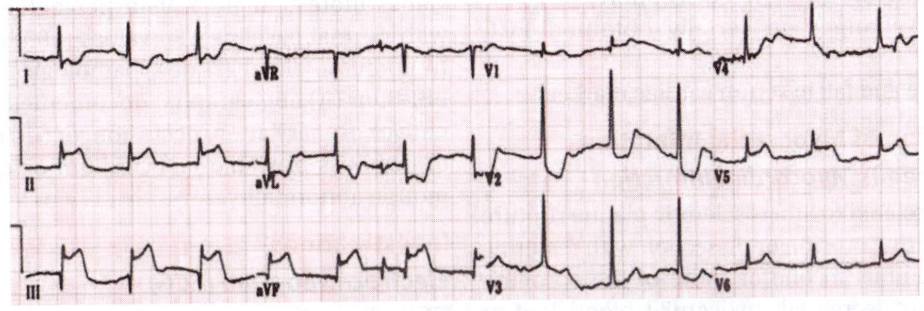

Fig. 127.4: ECG showing inferior and posterior wall MI. ***Note:*** ST-elevation in 2, 3, aVF and ST depression in 1, aVL. Also tall R waves with upright T waves in V1 and V2

generation, and ultimately, thrombus formation. The resultant thrombus that is formed interrupts blood flow and leads to an imbalance between oxygen supply and demand and, if this imbalance is severe and persistent, it results in myocardial necrosis. Plaque erosion is another mechanism, less abrupt than plaque rupture which can lead to acute MI. This is more common in women.

Clinical Features

This is characterized by occurrence of severe retrosternal pain with characteristic radiation. The pain is usually severe and excruciating, but at times it may be mild and rarely pain may be absent. The pain is described as crushing, tearing, bursting, burning, lancinating or vague. The pain generally lasts for more than 30 minutes and generally occurs during rest. Several phenomena are associated with this pain. These are severe anxiety and a feeling of impending death, profuse sweating, dyspnea, shock, cardiac arrhythmias, syncope, nausea, vomiting, and epigastric pain. MI follows the circadian rhythm in that a good number of cases occur in the early hours of the morning. In some patients, especially diabetics and elderly, there may be no chest pain. They may be totally asymptomatic or present with symptoms, like dyspnea, extreme fatigue, syncope, confusion, arrhythmia or peripheral embolism.

Signs

In 20% of cases, the symptoms may be trivial and physical examination may be unrewarding. In the majority, the findings are diagnostic. Coldness of limbs, sweating and sudden onset of pulmonary edema are suggestive of acute LV failure. In cardiogenic shock, the extremities are cold and cyanosed and the BP is low and often unrecordable. Heart rate is variable. In the initial stages, severe bradycardia may occur in some cases as a result of increased vagal tone. Others show tachycardia and arrhythmias, such as frequent ventricular ectopics, atrial fibrillation (AF), ventricular tachycardia (VT) or ventricular fibrillation (VF). BP drops in most cases, but sometimes it may remain normal or even be elevated as a result of intense vasoconstriction. The jugular venous pressure (JVP) may be elevated if there is congestive heart failure (CHF) or RV infarction. About 24–48 hour after the infarct, fever may occur as a response to tissue necrosis.

Physical examination of the heart reveals muffling of sounds, presence of gallop suggesting ventricular failure, arrhythmias and accentuation of the pulmonary second sound (P2), as a result of rise in pulmonary artery pressure. On the 2nd or 3rd day, pericardial friction rub may be heard. If complications develop, these will be clinically evident.

Diagnosis

Strong clinical suspicion is needed for early diagnosis. It should be remembered that in the middle-aged and elderly, one of the common causes for chest pain is MI. Clinical suspicion is strengthened by the presence of characteristic radiation and associated phenomena. Even in the absence of pain, MI should be suspected if a middle-aged person develops any of the complications suddenly.

The World Health Organization (WHO) criteria for diagnosis of acute MI requires at least two of the following three elements to be present:

1. A history of ischemic-type chest discomfort
2. Evolutionary changes on serially obtained ECG tracings
3. The typical rise and fall in serum cardiac markers.

New Classification of Myocardial Infarction

Type 1: Spontaneous Myocardial Infarction

Spontaneous MI related to atherosclerotic plaque rupture or ulceration assuring erosion or dissection with resulting intraluminal thrombus in one or more of the coronary arteries leading to decreased myocardial blood low or distal platelet emboli with ensuing myocyte necrosis. The patient may have underlying severe CAD but on occasion nonobstructive or no CAD.

Type 2: Myocardial Infarction Secondary to an Ischemic Imbalance

In instances of myocardial injury with necrosis where a condition other than CAD contributes to an imbalance between myocardial oxygen supply and/or demand, e.g. coronary endothelial dysfunction, coronary artery spasm, coronary embolism, tachyarrhythmia/bradyarrhythmia, anemia, respiratory failure, hypotension and hypertension with or without left ventricular hypertrophy (LVH).

Type 3: Myocardial Infarction Resulting in Death when Biomarker Values are Unavailable

Cardiac death with symptoms suggestive of myocardial ischemia and presumed new ischemic ECG changes or new left bundle branch block (LBBB), but death occurring before blood samples could be obtained, before cardiac biomarker could rise, or in rare cases cardiac biomarkers were not collected.

Type 4a: Myocardial Infarction Related to Percutaneous Coronary Intervention

MI associated with percutaneous coronary intervention (PCI) is arbitrarily defined by elevation of cardiac troponin (cTn) values more than 5 × 99th percentile URL (upper reference limit) in patients with normal baseline values (< 99th percentile URL) or a rise of cTn values more than 20% if the baselines values are elevated and are stable or falling. In addition, either (i) symptoms suggestive of myocardial ischemia, or (ii) new ischemic ECG changes or new LBBB, or (iii) angiographic loss of patency of a major coronary artery or a side branch or persistent slow- or no-flow or embolization, or (iv) imaging demonstration of new loss of viable myocardium or new regional wall motion abnormality are required.

Type 4b: Myocardial Infarction Related to Stent Thrombosis

MI associated with stent thrombosis is detected by coronary angiography or autopsy in the setting of myocardial ischemia and with a rise and/or fall of cardiac biomarkers values with at least one value above the 99th percentile URL.

Type 5: Myocardial Infarction Related to Coronary Artery Bypass Grafting

MI associated with coronary artery bypass grafting (CABG) is arbitrarily defined by elevation of cardiac biomarker values more than 10 × 99th percentile URL in patients with normal baseline cTn values (<99th percentile URL). In addition, either (i) new pathological Q waves or new LBBB, or (ii) angiographic documented new graft or new native coronary artery occlusion, or (iii) imaging evidence of new loss of viable myocardium or new regional wall motion abnormality.

Investigations

Electrocardiogram (ECG)

ECG taken within a few hours of symptoms shows diagnostic changes in over 80% of cases. More than 95% show positive ECG findings if recorded 12–24 hour after the onset of symptoms. The changes depend upon the type of infarction, site of infarct, presence of arrhythmias and conduction defects. NSTEMI produces depression of the ST-segment or T wave inversion in ECG. Presence of STEMI is recognized by elevation of ST-segment in ECG. Later, majority of them will develop Q waves and inversion of the T waves. The site of infarct can be determined depending on the leads which show abnormalities (Table 127.1).

Note:

- In true posterior infarct, V1 will show upright R and T waves, unlike as in RV hypertrophy in which T is inverted.
- Right ventricular infarction has to be suspected when there are jugular venous changes resembling constrictive pericarditis and shock without hypovolemia. In such

Table 127.1: Location of infarct depending on the ECG leads

Electrocardiogram (ECG) leads showing changes	Location of infarct
V1 to V3	Anteroseptal
V4 to V6, L1 and aVL	Anterolateral
aVF, L2 and L3	Inferior wall
ST depression in V1 and V2	–––––
Presence of tall R-waves and upright T in V1 and V2	True posterior infarct
ST-elevation in right-sided chest	Right ventricular (RV)
Leads and Q waves (V3R, V4R)	Infarct

circumstances, right-sided leads should be taken to demonstrate RV infarction. Presence of RV infarction calls for special management.

It should be remembered that in a small proportion of cases ECG may not show any diagnostic change even in the presence of the typical pain and enzyme changes.

Biochemical Markers of Myocardial Infarction

Several enzymes and other components of cardiac muscle are liberated into circulation from injured and necrotic myocardium. Their presence above diagnostic levels, their peak levels in the plasma and the pattern of their rise and fall, have all been studied in detail and their reliability in the diagnosis of MI has been established. It is a routine practice to estimate these components to establish or exclude the diagnosis of MI (Table 127.2).

Aspartate transaminase

Serum glutamic oxaloacetic transaminase (SGOT), also known as *aspartate transaminase*, is liberated from the myocardium when it undergoes infarction. The levels start rising in 8–12 hours, peak at 18–36 hours and come down in 3–4 days. Their estimation is cheap and freely available in several laboratories.

Creatine kinase

The level rises within 4–8 hours of infarction, reaches its peak in 24 hours and falls to normal levels within 2–3 days. Creatine kinase (CK) shows three isoenzymes: (1) MM, (2) BB and (3) MB which can be identified electrophoretically. MM is more specific to skeletal muscle, BB to brain and kidney, and MB to the heart, though there is some degree of overlap. Thrombolytic therapy, percutaneous revascularization or spontaneous thrombolysis leads to early rise in the enzyme levels. CK is present in several other tissues and therefore non-MI conditions also cause increase in CK levels, e.g. muscle diseases, alcoholic bouts, DM, muscle injury, vigorous exercise, convulsion,

intramuscular (IM) injections, thoracic outlet syndrome and pulmonary embolism. Estimation of the cardiac-specific isoenzyme, creatine kinase-MB CK(MB) is more specific for MI.

Creatine kinase-MB shows two isoforms CK(MB1) and CK(MB2). Elevation of CK(MB2) is more suggestive of cardiac infarction in the absence of other obvious reasons. Levels of CK(MB) isoform more than 1.0 U/L or a ratio of CK(MB2)/CK(MB1) more than 1.5 is diagnostic of acute MI.

Cardiac-specific troponins

The troponin complex usually consists of three subunits that regulate the calcium-mediated contractile process:

1. **Troponin C:** Binds to calcium
2. **Troponin I (TnI):** Binds to actin and inhibits actin-myosin interactions
3. **Troponin T (TnT):** Binds to tropomyosin.

Myocardial injury leads to a rapid rise in cTn in plasma. TnI and TnT are released into the plasma so that reliable diagnostic sensitivity is reached by 12–16 hours and maximal activity is reached by 24–36 hours. The levels return to normal within 10–12 days.

Troponin is the preferred marker for the diagnosis of MI because of the increased specificity and sensitivity compared to CK(MB). However, elevated troponin must be interpreted in the context of clinical history and ECG findings because it can be elevated in several noncardiac conditions. The values of troponins vary depending on the assays used. Values more than 99th percentile of the URL should be considered abnormal. Recently, high-sensitivity cardiac-specific troponin I (hs-cTn-I) is used and diagnosis of MI can be made within 2–3 hours of presentation. The upper limit of normal for hs-cTn-I, according to the European Society of Cardiology (ESC) algorithm is defined as 26.2 ng/L.

In some patients with chest pain, cTn-T may be raised but CK(MB) is in the normal range. The term 'minor myocardial damage' has been used to denote this condition. Such patients have adverse outcome on follow-up including fatal and nonfatal MI.

Lactate dehydrogenase (LDH)

It was done frequently before the availability of specific markers, such as cTn. It is an enzyme found in the heart muscle, along with several other tissues in the body. It consists of five isoenzymes, among which LDH1 is principally seen in the heart. Levels of LDH1 increases following myocardial necrosis. Several other disorders also lead to rise in LDH, e.g. hemolysis, megaloblastic

Table 127.2: Common biochemical markers which diagnose MI

Marker and normal level	Time to show rise (hours after onset)	Peak levels in serum	Time to return to normal	Time for collection of blood
SGOT (5–40 IU/L)	8–12	18–36 hours	3–4 days	Once in 12 hours
LDH (20–220 IU/L)	10	24–48 hours	10–14 days	24 hours
CK(MB)	3–12	24 hours	48–72 hours	Every 12 hours for 3 days
cTn-T	3–12	12 hours to 2 days	5–14 days	Once at least every 12 hours
cTn-I	3–12	24 hours	5–10 days	Once at least every 12 hours

Abbreviations: SGOT = Serum glutamic oxaloacetic transaminase; LDH = Lactate dehydrogenase; CK = Creatine kinase; cTn-T = Cardiac-specific troponin T; cTn-I = Cardiac-specific troponin I

anemia, leukemia, hepatic disorders, renal disease, muscle disorders, pulmonary embolism, shock and others. Estimation of the ratio of LDH1/LDH2 has been accepted as a more reliable test for diagnosing acute MI. Ratios of LDH1/LDH2 more than 1 are diagnostic. However, routine LDH isoenzyme analysis for the diagnosis of acute MI is no longer recommended.

At present the diagnosis of acute MI can be established within 12 hours of onset by estimation of CK(MB), cTn-T or cTn-I at intervals of 8–12 hours. Several other biochemical markers, such as heart fatty acid binding proteins (hFABP), myosin light chains (MLC), myosin heavy chains (MHC) and glycogen phosphorylase isoenzymes are being studied for their promptness and reliability in diagnosis.

Imaging Procedures

Chest X-ray film: Since the patient should not be moved, portable X-ray machine may be required. When present, prominent pulmonary vascular markings on the X-ray reflect elevation of pulmonary venous pressure indicating LV failure. The chest film may also assist in excluding other causes of chest pain, such as pneumothorax, pulmonary infarction with effusion, aortic dissection and skeletal fractures.

Echocardiography: It is particularly valuable in assessing the patient with an equivocal ECG. The presence of a regional wall motion abnormality provides strong supportive evidence of acute coronary ischemia. Echocardiography also provides an assessment of ventricular function. It can provide information on complications, like ruptured chordae tendineae with mitral regurgitation (MR) and ventricular septal defect (VSD). It can help to estimate cardiac hemodynamics by using color Doppler studies.

Nuclear imaging: Radionuclide imaging, angiography, perfusion imaging, infarct avid scintigraphy and positron-emission tomography (PET) are all in use to study the nature of the myocardial lesion, its viability and prognosis.

Computed tomography (CT) scan: It can be used to reveal cavity dimensions, wall thickness, aneurysms and intracardiac thrombi.

Multislice CT angiography: It is useful in getting information on the extent of coronary calcification and coronary artery narrowing.

Magnetic resonance imaging (MRI) scan: It can be made use of to assess the perfusion of infarcted and non-infarcted tissue as well as the state of reperfused myocardium. It can also identify areas of jeopardized but not infarcted myocardium.

Both CT scan and MRI are generally reserved for subsequent evaluation after the acute condition is managed.

Differential Diagnosis

Acute chest pain may occur in pleurisy, pneumonia, pericarditis, pneumothorax, preherpetic neuralgia, dissecting aneurysm of the aorta or lesions on the chest wall. Pericarditis may closely resemble acute MI in respect of the pain and its radiation. Fever, leukocytosis and pericardial rub occur early in pericarditis, whereas these develop only 24 hours after the onset of MI. Dissecting aneurysm of the aorta is uncommon. It causes tearing pain, which is abrupt in onset and severe from the beginning.

Pain may radiate to the back, epigastrium, flank and lower extremities. Ventricular dysfunction is less common to develop.

Sometimes, the pain of MI may be felt mainly under the jaws, shoulder, or epigastrium and these may be mistaken for primary disease at these sites.

Complications

Several complications can occur the following acute MI and can lead to morbidity and mortality.

- ***Arrhythmias:*** Several arrhythmias develop. These include frequent ventricular ectopics, VT, VF, sudden cardiac arrest, AF and varying grades of heart block. The incidence of arrhythmias is higher in those patients seen earlier after the onset of symptoms. The treatment of tachyarrhythmias involves not only the use of antiarrhythmic drugs, but also correction of abnormalities of plasma electrolyte concentrations, acid-base balance disturbances, hypoxemia, anemia and digitalis intoxication.

- ***LV failure:*** LV dysfunction remains the single most important predictor of mortality after acute MI. Clinical manifestations of LV failure become more common as the extent of the injury to the LV increases. In addition to infarct size, other important predictors of the development of symptomatic LV dysfunction include advanced age and diabetes. Apart from myocardial necrosis, another condition which can lead to LV failure is myocardial stunning.

- ***Myocardial stunning:*** The term 'myocardial stunning' defines a prolonged but reversible contractile dysfunction observed after transient myocardial ischemia, i.e. even after blood supply to the myocardium is restored. The recovery of contractile function may take hours or days.

- The term 'hibernating myocardium' is used to denote the condition in which cardiac function is depressed due to persisting ischemia and which recovers fully on restoration of blood supply.

- ***Cardiogenic shock:*** It is a severe form of LV failure. Infarction of 40% or more of the ventricular myocardium leads to cardiogenic shock. Features of cardiogenic shock include systolic BP less than 80 mm Hg, markedly reduced cardiac index (<1.8 L/min/m^2) and an elevated pulmonary capillary wedge pressure (PCWP). Mortality in cardiogenic shock is more than 70%.

- ***Pericarditis:*** It may occur as early as the 1st day and as late as 6 weeks after MI. This develops in 15–20% of patients. It is seen in full-thickness infarcts. The development of pericarditis appears to be correlated with a larger infarct and greater hemodynamic compromise. Treatment of pericarditis pain consists of aspirin. Doses of 650 mg orally every 4–6 hours may be needed.

- ***Phlebothrombosis and pulmonary embolism:*** These develop as a result of prolonged recumbency, venous stasis and tendency for venous thrombosis.

- ***Arterial embolism:*** Mural thrombi develop on the infarcted endocardium and these may embolize into several arterial trunks. This risk starts a day or 2 days after the infarction and persists for a few weeks.

- ***Papillary muscle dysfunction and rupture:*** Ischemia and infarction of the papillary muscles lead to MR. Rupture of the papillary muscles results in the development of acute mitral incompetence which tips the patient into acute pulmonary edema.
- ***Rupture of the IVS:*** This condition leads to acquired VSD. A ruptured IVS is characterized by the appearance of a new harsh, loud holosystolic murmur that is heard best at the lower left sternal border and that is usually accompanied by a thrill. Biventricular failure generally ensues within hours to days.
- ***Cardiac rupture:*** This may develop by the 3rd to the 5th day. The infarcted area gives way giving rise to hemopericardium, cardiac tamponade and death in majority of cases. Rupture of IVS carries a mortality of 24% in the first 24 hours, 46% at 1 week and 67–82% at 2 months. Surgical closure improves the prognosis.
- ***Delayed complications***
  - ***Cardiac aneurysm:*** Weakening of the scar leads to bulging out of the ventricle and the development of ventricular aneurysm. The common sites are the anterior and apical regions. This leads to persistent congestive failure, recurrent embolism and VT. On palpation of the precordium, the aneurysm can be felt as a see-saw pulsation in relation to the apex beat. The condition can be confirmed by X-ray examination, echocardiography and angiocardiography.
  - ***Dressler's syndrome:*** This is probably an immune-mediated reaction in which pericarditis, pleurisy, fever, arthritis and elevation of erythrocyte sedimentation rate (ESR) develop 1–6 weeks after the infarction.
  - ***Shoulder-hand syndrome:*** May develop in a few cases weeks to months after the acute event.

Prognosis

MI is a serious disease with an overall immediate mortality ranging up to 25%, if proper management is not instituted. About 50% of the deaths associated with acute MI occur within 1 hour of the event and are attributable to arrhythmias, most often ventricular fibrillation (VF). For the first 6 months after infarction, the risk of developing sudden death is still high, but this risk falls after this period. Anterior infarction carries a grave prognosis if accompanied by conduction disturbances. All the major complications worsen the prognosis. Age above 70 years, hypertension, diabetes mellitus (DM) and heavy cigarette smoking worsen the outlook further. Women below the age of 75 years have higher mortality rates after acute MI compared to men of similar age.

Several ECG criteria have been employed to predict increased risk of fatal arrhythmias and death in the postinfarct period. These include signal averaged late potentials, heart rate variability and Q-T dispersion.

Patients who had sudden cardiac death and required cardiopulmonary resuscitation during the course of the illness run a higher risk of fatal arrhythmias in the first few years after discharge from hospital.

Management

Prehospital care is an important factor in preventing sudden death and immediate complications and also improving long-term outcome. No time should be lost in seeking hospital admission after the initial symptoms manifest. The time elapsed between the onset of chest pain and reaching the appropriate hospital (pain to hospital time) and the time elapsed between the arrival at hospital and receiving the first dose of medication (door to needle time) are the most important factors which reduce immediate and in-hospital mortality and complications. Several attempts have been made from time-to-time to educate the public on the need to get immediate hospitalization. Provision of special trained teams with coronary care ambulances which can reach the patient's home within minutes and administration of thrombolytics in the ambulance with minimum delay have reduced early mortality in many countries.

Recently total ischemic time, i.e. the time elapsed between the onset of symptoms to the treatment (thrombolysis or primary PCI) has been recognized as the most important prognosticating factor. A total ischemic time of more than 120 minute is associated with bad outcomes.

Emergency Room Management

Aspirin is given straight away in a dose of 325 mg to be chewed. A rapid decision as to the need for thrombolysis should be taken depending on the indication. Clopidogrel [adenosine diphosphate (ADP-receptor antagonist) is given and loading dose of 300 mg followed by 75 mg/day as maintenance dose. A 12-lead ECG forms the cornerstone in decision-making regarding thrombolysis in acute MI. Presence of ST-segment elevation of 1 mm or more in two or more contiguous leads with a history compatible with acute MI are the indications for starting thrombolytic therapy if there are no absolute contraindications. There is no benefit in giving thrombolysis in the absence of ECG showing ST-segment elevation. Before giving thrombolytic agents, blood is collected for biochemical parameters.

If the ECG is suggestive of ischemia without infarction, i.e. ST-depression or T wave inversion, start on anti-ischemic therapy.

If the ECG is not diagnostic, observe the patient repeating the ECG at 2 hour intervals, estimate the serum markers and, if necessary, echocardiography. If there is no evidence of infarction on observation for 24–48 hours, the patient should be subjected to a stress test to provoke ischemia.

Drug Therapy

Aspirin

It is the first-line drug in the initial management of acute MI and all other forms of IHD. Initial dose of aspirin should be 162–325 mg to be chewed to ensure rapid buccal absorption. Subsequent dose of aspirin is 75–162 mg.

Recent studies have shown that addition of clopidogrel to aspirin in acute MI is beneficial. Clopidogrel (ADP-receptor antagonist) is given as loading dose of 300 mg followed by 75 mg/day as maintenance dose. In elderly patients above the age of 75 years, loading dose is avoided.

Control of Cardiac Pain

Pain relief has to be achieved as early as possible. Persistent pain perpetuates sympathetic overactivity, especially so in the early phases of acute MI. Control of pain is achieved by a combination of narcotic analgesics, nitrates and β-blockers. Morphine is the analgesic of choice.

Morphine

Its mode of action includes central narcotic action, depression of vasomotor and respiratory centers, reduction of sympathetic tone, and reduction of histamine release from the periphery. Administration of morphine leads to reduction of pain, anxiety, vasodilation, reduction of the heart rate and effort for breathing, all helping to reduce oxygen demand.

In the intensive cardiac care unit (ICCU), morphine should be given intravenously (IV), initial dose of 4–8 mg and subsequently in doses of 2–8 mg repeated at intervals of 5–15 minutes until the pain is relieved or adverse effects appear. The adverse effects include hypotension, respiratory depression, vomiting, urinary retention and constipation. Maximum dose should not exceed 2–3 mg/kg in 24 hours.

Adverse effects of morphine are managed as follows: Hypotension is counteracted by maintaining the supine position and elevating lower extremities if the systolic BP is less than 100 mm Hg. Administration of atropine 0.5–1.5 mg helps to reduce the vagomimetic effects of morphine. Respiratory depression is treated with naloxone in dose of 0.1–0.2 mg IV, repeated after 15 minutes if needed. Nausea and vomiting can be treated with a promethazine.

Oxygen

It was a routine practice to give oxygen to all patients with anginal pain for 24–48 hours based on the empirical assumption of hypoxia. However, augmentation of the fraction of oxygen in the inspired air does not elevate oxygen delivery significantly in patients who are not hypoxemic. Furthermore, it may increase systemic vascular resistance and arterial pressure and thereby lower cardiac output slightly. In view of these considerations, arterial oxygen saturation may be estimated by pulse oximetry and oxygen therapy may be given if oxygen saturation is less than 90%.

Nitrates

These are used for immediate relief of anginal pain, as well as prevention of its recurrence. For immediate action, nitroglycerine (glyceryl trinitrate) is used IV or sublingually. The vasodilatory effect is immediate and the action is of short duration. For maintenance therapy other preparations are used. Their action is more prolonged.

Actions: Nitrates dilate the epicardial coronary arteries and collaterals, and improve the blood supply. It reduces the preload and also the myocardial oxygen demand. Blood flow of normally perfused areas is redistributed to ischemic areas of the myocardium. Other actions include inhibition of platelet aggregation, limitation of infarct size and improvement in exercise capacity.

Indications: In acute MI with continuing pain, heart failure, or hypertension, nitrates are given for the first 24–48 hours. Maintenance dose is continued in patients with recurrence of angina and persistent pulmonary venous congestion.

Glyceryl trinitrate is available in vials of 5 mg and 25 mg at concentrations of 1 or 5 mg/mL. One vial is diluted in 500 mL normal saline prior to infusion and run at a rate of 5–10 μg/min to start with. It is increased by 5–10 μg/min until clinical effect is manifest. This includes relief of angina, fall of BP by 10% in normotensive, and up to 30% in hypertensive patients.

Sublingual dose: Glyceryl trinitrate is available as tablets containing 0.5 mg, 2.6 mg and 6.4 mg. It is given initially at doses of 0.3–0.6 mg. Additional doses of 0.3 mg may be repeated every 5 minutes to a maximum of 1.2 mg in 15 minutes.

Other preparations are buccal spray containing 400 μg metered doses, 2% skin ointment and transdermal patches containing 2.5 mg, 5.0 mg and 15 mg, released over 24 hours.

Side effects of glyceryl trinitrate: These include headache and flushing, hypotension, hypovolemia and ventilation-perfusion imbalance in the lungs. Methemoglobinemia may develop after large doses.

In general, reduction or withdrawal of the dose helps to relieve the side effects. Hypotension and hypovolemia are managed by elevation of the foot end of the bed and IV fluids.

Tolerance to nitrates develops after all forms of nitrate administration if given continuously even within 12–24 hours, but generally it is delayed. The loss of effect is limited to the capacitance and resistance vessels. Large conductance vessels including epicardial coronary arteries and radial arteries are not affected.

Tolerance to nitrates is prevented by giving the drug at eccentric intervals allowing 10–12 hours of nitrate-free interval in between, e.g. 8 am and 2 pm. Transdermal preparation should not be used continuously for more than 12 hours.

Isosorbide dinitrate: This is available as 5 mg, 10 mg and 20 mg sustained release tablets, or 1.25 mg metered dose buccal spray.

Isosorbide 5-mononitrate tablets of 10 mg and 20 mg tablets and long-acting tablets of 40 mg, 50 mg and 60 mg are available. These are used for maintenance therapy and prevention of angina after the emergency is tided over.

Beta-adrenergic Blockers

Beta blockers relieve pain and reduce the need for analgesia in many patients and reduce infarct size. When used in the early hours of infarction, they limit infarct size; reduce the incidence of ventricular arrhythmias, AF and cardiac arrest. They reduce the incidence of recurrent ischemia and reinfarction within the first 6 weeks of initial MI. Generally, β-blockers are started orally. Metoprolol, bisoprolol or carvedilol are the usual β-blockers used. In presence of severe heart failure, acute pulmonary edema with hemodynamic instability, β-blocker should be avoided.

In the acute phase IV, β-blockers may be considered if there is hypertension and sinus tachycardia. IV metoprolol is the drug of choice. If there are no contraindications, metoprolol is given IV in 3 boluses of 5 mg each at intervals of 2–5 minutes if the heart rate is more than 60 beats/min. If hemodynamic stability continues for 15 minutes after the last IV dose, oral metoprolol 50 mg is given 6 hourly for 2 days and then changed to 100 mg bid.

Contraindications for β-blockers include cardiac failure evidenced by the presence of rales heard over the lower parts of the chest 10 cm above the level of the diaphragm, hypotension (BP < 90 mm Hg), bradycardia (heart rate < 60 beats/min), prolonged PR interval more than 0.24 second or third-degree heart block. Other commonly used β-blockers include atenolol 50–100 mg daily and bisoprolol 5 mg daily, given orally.

Esmolol

The ultra short-acting drug esmolol can be used in an emergency in a dose of 500 μg/kg/min for 4 minutes IV.

Thrombolytic Therapy

Plaque rupture and thrombus formation play a major role in the genesis of acute coronary occlusion leading to acute MI. The introduction of thrombolytic (fibrinolytic) therapy was a major advance in the treatment of acute STEMI, since over 90% of such patients have complete occlusion of the culprit artery. Early reperfusion of the ischemic myocardium has brought down the immediate post-MI mortality from 10–15 to 5–10%. Several randomized trials have upheld its benefit and safety. Whenever possible, thrombolytic drugs should be given by the first attending physician irrespective of the speciality, if the indications are clear.

Classification of Thrombolytic Agents

- ***First-generation drugs:*** Streptokinase (SK) and uro-kinase (UK) act on all sites where fibrin is formed. In addition to dissolution of the clots locally, they also produce generalized hemorrhagic state.
- ***Second-generation drugs:***
  - tPA (tissue plasminogen activator): Single chain-alteplase and double chain-duteplase
  - APSAC (anisoylated plasminogen streptokinase activator complex)
  - SCU-PA (single chain urokinase-type plasminogen activator)
  - TCU-PA (two chain urokinase-type plasminogen activator)
  - These are clot-specific agents acting at the site of fibrin formation with very little or no generalized hemorrhagic tendency.
- ***Third-generation drugs:***
  - Reteplase [recombinant plasminogen activator) (rPA)]: Recombinant tPA
  - Tenecteplase (TNK-tPA).

Though several thrombolytic agents are available, the first-generation drugs are the ones widely used in India on account of their free availability, effectiveness, safety and above all, the lowest cost. A course of SK costs ₹ 3,000, whereas UK costs ₹ 10,000. All the others are more expensive.

Indications

- In those with ST-elevation in the ECG, more than 0.1 mV (1 mm) in two or more contiguous leads within 12 hours of onset of symptoms.
- In those with new onset or presumably new-onset LBBB within 12 hours of onset of symptoms.

Best results are obtained if thrombolysis is done within 6 hours of onset, earlier the better. Benefit may occur even up to 12 hours of onset, though in a smaller proportion.

Dosage and Administration

SK is available as lyophilized powder in vials containing 250,000, 750,000 or 1,500,000 units. It has to be stored at 15–25°C. The initial dose is 1.5 million units diluted in 100 mL normal saline and infused over 1 hour.

Occurrence of thrombolysis and reperfusion of the myocardium is evidenced by the following features:
- Relief of chest pain
- Resolution of the ST-segment elevation of more than 50% by 60–90 minutes
- Evidence of reperfusion phenomena, such as:
  - Arrhythmias: Ventricular premature complexes (VPCs), accelerated idioventricular rhythm (AIVR) or bradycardia
  - Abrupt rise in serum CK activity
  - Recanalization of the coronary artery demonstrable by angiography.

Contraindications

- Absolute contraindications:
  - Previous hemorrhagic stroke at any time
  - Ischemic stroke within 3 months
  - Known intracranial neoplasm, structural cerebrovascular lesion (AV malformation)
  - Suspected aortic dissection
  - Active internal bleeding or bleeding diathesis (other than menstrual bleeding)
  - Significant closed head or facial trauma within 3 months
- Relative contraindications:
  - Hypertension with BP more than 180/110 mm Hg
  - History of prior cerebrovascular accident or known intracerebral pathology
  - Current use of anticoagulants in therapeutic doses and other known bleeding diatheses
  - Recent trauma including head trauma or major surgery within 3 weeks
  - Noncompressible vascular puncture
  - Occurrence of internal bleeding within 2–4 weeks
  - For SK and anistreplase, previous history of use of the same drug within 5 days to 2 years, or history of allergic reaction
  - Pregnancy
  - Active peptic ulcer.

Complications of SK Therapy

- Allergic reactions, such as angioneurotic edema, hypotension, bronchospasm, urticaria, rashes and fever, may develop. Administration of 4 mg betamethasone IV helps to reduce the allergic reactions. Presence of antibodies to SK reduces its therapeutic effects and increases allergic reactions.

- ***Bleeding complications:*** Minor bleeding occurs in 3–4% and major bleeding in 0.4–1%. Intracranial bleed may occur in less than 0.6%.
- ***Hemodynamic effects:*** Transient hypotension and bradycardia.
- ***Reperfusion adverse effects:*** These are the effects of sudden reperfusion into areas of ischemic myocardium. They are caused partially by the effect of free radicals. Adverse effects include arrhythmias, such as VPC, AIVR, VT, VF and bradyarrhythmias. Cardiac rupture may occur due to further damage to infarcted myocardium and hemorrhage into it.
- ***Coronary reocclusion:*** Fifteen percent of recanalized vessels undergo thrombotic occlusion within a few hours to 3 days.

Other Thrombolytic Agents

Urokinase

It is a double chain glycoprotein (GP) which acts as a trypsin-like protease and occurs in two molecular forms. It was first isolated from human urine and hence, its name. It is also obtained by recombinant DNA technology from cultured human renal cells. It is non-antigenic. It is not fibrin-specific and therefore it causes generalized bleeding tendency. Its half-life is 10 minutes. It produces less sustained systemic fibrinolysis. Dose for IV use is 3 million units given over 45–60 minutes. Different dosages of 1.5 million, 2 million and 3 million units have been used in several trials. Patency at the end of 1 hour is 60%. Infusion is similar to that of SK. Anaphylactic reactions are practically nil. It is more expensive than SK and therefore it may be reserved for patients allergic to SK or who have received SK previously.

Tissue plasminogen activator

It is a naturally occurring enzyme that binds to fibrin with greater affinity than SK, without increasing generalized bleeding tendency. It has been in use since 1984. (Recombinant tissue-type plasminogen activator) rt-tPA is produced by recombinant DNA technology. Several dosage schedules are in use. Total dose should not exceed 100 mg. It should be accompanied by IV heparin 5,000 units bolus followed by 1,000 units/hour with the dose adjusted to keep the partial thromboplastin time (PTT) at 1.5–2.0 times the normal. This helps to prevent reocclusion of the coronary arteries.

APSAC and anistreplase

It is a preformed complex of SK and plasminogen, which is spontaneously activated after IV administration. Once activated it behaves identical to SK, except that it has a longer half-life. It has a spectrum of activity and incidence of complications similar to SK. It is easy to administer. Hence, it is used for prehospital thrombolysis in acute MI patients. Dose is 30 Units IV over 2–5 minutes. The half-life is 30–90 minutes and it retains its effect for 4–6 hours.

Tenecteplase

It is a genetically engineered variant of the alteplase molecule. It is the most fibrin-specific thrombolytic agent available. The advantages are:

- Resistance to plasminogen activator inhibitor (PAI)
- Less of bleeding risk

- Greater efficacy compared to SK
- Ease of administration.

Dose is 0.3–0.5 mg/kg administered as single bolus IV. It is however more expensive.

Comparison of Thrombolytic Therapy

Several International Trials, Gruppo Italiano per lo Studio Streptokinase nell'Infarto Miocardico (GISSI-2), International Study of Infarct Survival (ISIS-3), Global Utilization of SK and tPA for Occluded Arteries 1 (GUSTO-1)] TIMI-4 (Thrombolysis in Myocardial Infarction 4) have compared different modes of thrombolytic therapy. Based on their evidence, consensus on this form of therapy has been arrived at.

Choice of Agent

In patients presenting within 4 hours of onset of symptoms, the speed of reperfusion of the occluded vessels is of paramount importance and a high-intensity thrombolytic regimen, such as tPA or APSAC, is the preferred treatment, except in those individuals in whom the risk of death is low.

For those patients presenting between 4 and 12 hours after the onset of chest discomfort, the speed of reperfusion of the occluded vessel is of lesser importance and therefore SK and tPA are equivalent options. Cost is the main factor for choice.

Late Therapy

There is no definite reduction in mortality if thrombolytic drugs are routinely administered to patients presenting after 12 hours of onset. Still we consider it reasonable to give thrombolytic therapy in selected patients with persistent symptoms and ST-elevation in ECG beyond 12 hours.

Since elderly patients are at increased risk of cardiac rupture if thrombolytic drugs are given later than 12 hours after the onset of symptoms, it is better to restrict late thrombolysis to patients younger than 65 years with ongoing ischemia, especially those with large anterior infarctions. Older patients with ongoing ischemic symptoms who come in after 12 hours of onset are probably better managed with percutaneous transluminal coronary angioplasty (PTCA) than with thrombolytic therapy.

Coronary Revascularization

Percutaneous Transluminal Coronary Angioplasty

The cornerstone of treatment of acute ST segment elevation MI is reperfusion therapy. Thrombolysis has been used as the method of reperfusion earlier. With the introduction of angioplasty as a revascularization method, it has been utilized in opening up the occluded infarct-related artery in STEMI. This is known as primary angioplasty where it is done without the use of thrombolytic agents. Several studies, PAMI (Primary Angioplasty in Myocardial Infarction), GUSTO IIb (Global Use of Strategies to Open Occluded Coronary Arteries in Acute Coronary Syndromes) and others have confirmed the advantage of primary angioplasty over thrombolytic therapy.

Advantages include reduction of mortality, preventing re-infarction and a recanalization rate of more than 90%.

Indications

- As an alternative to thrombolytic therapy in patients with ST-segment elevation or new-onset LBBB. PTCA can be done within 12 hours of onset of acute MI or even later if symptoms persist. Success rate of PTCA depends upon the skill of the operator and facilities in the hospital.
- Patients below the age of 75 years who present with shock within 36 hours onset of acute MI should also be considered for PTCA.
- In those presenting with severe CHF and/or pulmonary edema.

PTCA is a radiological intervention procedure undertaken by cardiologists in which the stenotic segment of the arteries are dilated by suitable balloons passed through catheters, percutaneously though the radial or femoral artery, retrograde into the aorta and then into the coronary arteries. By inflating the balloon, the atheroma is crushed and the arterial lumen is restored. The lumen is maintained patent by the use of different types of stents. The number of stents depends on the number of occlusions. Reocclusion by thrombus is prevented by using antiplatelet drugs, like aspirin and clopidogrel. In addition to aspirin and clopidogrel, several newer drugs including GP-IIb to GP-IIIa receptor blocking agents are used. These agents have considerably improved the results of PTCA by maintaining luminal patency in much higher proportion of patients. In well-equipped centers, the success rate exceeds 90%. Even complicated lesions can be treated by angioplasty by skilled operators (Figs 127.5A and B; 127.6A and B).

The original stents introduced in 1987 were simple metallic stents. In them, the reocclusion rate was 30% and above within 1 year. Subsequently drug-eluting stents were introduced. These elute drugs, such as sirolimus, tacrolimus, everolimus, zoterolimus, paclitaxel and others, which serve to inhibit reocclusion. The chance of in-stent restenosis with the newer generation drug-eluting stents is less than 10%. The overall chance of stent thrombosis is approximately 1.0–1.5%. Drug-eluting stents are considerably more expensive than the plain stents. The cost is ₹150,000–300,000 per procedure depending on the number of stents required. Drug-eluting stents have delayed endothelialization, and hence the metallic stent struts remain exposed to the flowing blood for longer periods of time. This is responsible for the slightly higher chance of very-late stent thrombosis (beyond 1 year) with drug-eluting stents compared with bare-metal stents.

In the early days of angioplasty, the PCIs were done as elective procedures in stabilized and chronic patients. With the accumulation of experience and technology, many cases of complex and acute MI have been taken up for emergency angioplasty. PCIs are done as lifesaving and myocardium-saving procedures. The results of such emergency procedures are often dramatic. The complication of restenosis following PCI has been treated by options, such as further balloon angioplasty, intracoronary radiation therapy (brachytherapy) and implantation of further drug-eluting stents.

Pharmacoinvasive treatment: Many patients could be treated with thrombolytic agents and then could be transferred to a center with facilities for primary angioplasty which could be performed within 24 hours of after thrombolysis. This is known as pharmacoinasive treatment and has been shown to be as effective as primary angioplasty.

Coronary Artery Bypass Graft (CABG)

This operation is being done in India for about 40 years and many centers have gained considerable expertise and experience in the procedures. CABG remains the standard care for patients with three-vessel disease and left main CAD. The intra- and perioperative mortality is around 2–3% in good large volume centers. Surgery is indicated for stenosis of left main stem, multivessel disease, especially in presence of LV dysfunction, in which the clinical benefit and coronary disease-related mortality are significantly improved. Several grafts (3–5 or even more) are introduced at the same session, which connect the root of the aorta to the coronary artery distal to the occlusion.

Originally, saphenous vein was used as the conduit. At present in addition to this vein, internal mammary artery and other arteries are also being employed. The results are better with arterial grafts. Several modifications of the original technique have been introduced including keyhole surgery on the beating active heart.

Both bypass surgery and angioplasty may be complicated later by reocclusion. In case of stents, the restenosis is due to smooth muscle proliferation. Several

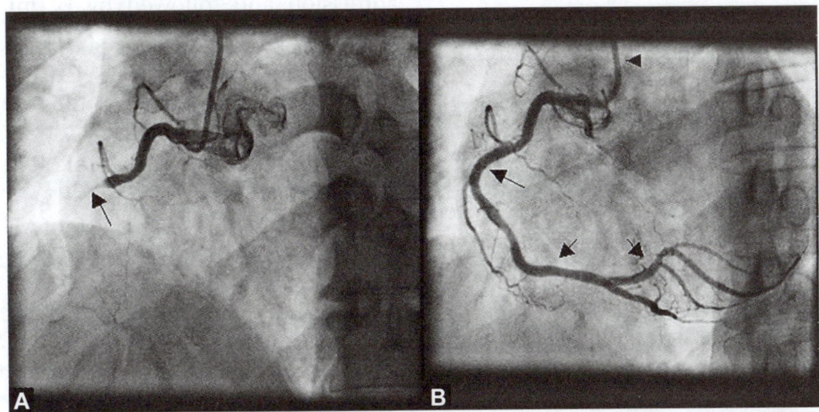

Figs 127.5A and B: Coronary angiogram in a patient with acute inferior wall myocardial infarction showing RCA: **A.** Before primary PTCA, RCA was totally occluded with thrombus (arrow); **B.** After primary PTCA, showing RCA with good flow and the branches (arrows)

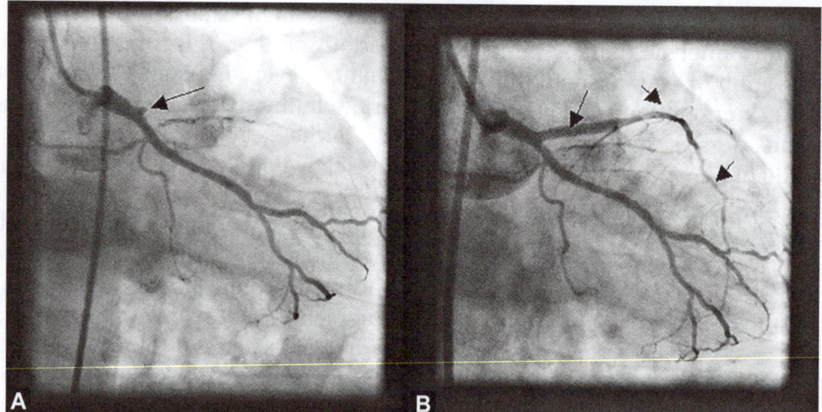

Figs 127.6A and B: Coronary angiogram in a patient with acute anterior wall myocardial infarction showing LAD: **A.** Before primary PTCA, LAD was totally occluded from ostium with thrombus and is not seen (arrow); **B.** After primary PTCA, showing LAD with good flow and the branches (arrows)

newer techniques are being experimented upon to prevent reocclusion of the stent. These include irradiation of the stented artery by γ- or β-radiations and impregnation of the stents with antiproliferative drugs, like sirolimus, actinomycin D and paclitaxel (drug-eluting stents), which prevent smooth muscle cell proliferation. All these innovations are being evaluated for their long-term results.

The procedure followed in most of the centers to pick up cases requiring revascularization is to subject patients who have angina or who have suffered an acute MI (after 2–3 weeks of convalescence) to a stress test on the treadmill. Stress test is taken as positive if it provokes angina or produce ST-segment depression in ECG of 1 mm or more from the baseline, which recovers on rest. Such patients with positive stress test are taken up for coronary angiography. Cases with limited number of stenosis are ideal for coronary angioplasty. Those with multiple-vessel disease and multiple occlusions require bypass graft surgery.

Follow-Up Therapy

ACE-I or Angiotensin-Receptor Blockers

Indications

Indications include:

- Patients seen within 24 hours of acute MI with ST-segment elevation, in the absence of contraindications.
- In those patients with MI and clinical heart failure or LV ejection fraction (LVEF) less than 40% during and after convalescence from acute MI.

Angiotensin-converting enzyme inhibitor (ACE-I) or angiotensin-receptor blocker (ARB) are important group of drugs to be considered in the treatment of acute MI. These drugs have proved to reduce the mortality if started within the first 24 hours of acute MI, especially if the LVEF is less than 40%. It is preferable to start with small and frequent dose and titrates up to the maximum doses which are found to be effective is large trials. Captopril could be started as 6.25 mg 3 times daily and titrate up to 50 mg 3 times daily. Other ACE-I is used are as follows: enalapril, ramipril or lisinopril. Valsartan and losartan are the usually used ARBs in the setting of acute MI.

Lipid-lowering Agents

All patients recovering from acute MI should be considered potential candidates for modification of their lipid profile. The target LDL-cholesterol in patients with IHD is less than 100 mg/dL. More aggressive LDL reduction to a goal of less than 70 mg/dL may be considered in a diabetic with acute coronary syndrome (ACS). Initial therapy should consist of dietary modification (< 7% of total calories as saturated fat and cholesterol < 200 mg/dL). In patients with an LDL-cholesterol level greater than 130 mg/dL on admission, it is better to start lipid-lowering drugs. 3-hydroxy-3-methylglutaryl-coenzymeA (HMG-CoA) reductase inhibitors (statins) are the first-line lipid-lowering drugs.

Magnesium Salts

The available data suggests that routine use of IV magnesium in STEMI has no place in current practice. Magnesium is useful only in known or suspected hypomagnesemic states and especially when these are associated with severe ventricular arrhythmias or QT prolongation.

Anticoagulants

Heparin is used in the acute stage in those undergoing PTCA, those who have received tPA or rPA and those at high risk for systemic emboli (large or anterior MI, AF, LV thrombus). The dose is 5,000 units given as IV bolus admission and followed by IV infusion at the rate of 800–1,000 units/hour.

The indication for routine use of long-term anticoagulation after acute MI is not clear. It may be given for the following conditions:

- Prevention of recurrence of MI in patients who cannot tolerate aspirin
- Post-MI patients in persistent AF
- Presence of LV thrombus (*See* Section 15, Ch 176).

General Measures

To reduce risk of vomiting early after infarction and reduce risk of aspiration, during the first 4–12 hours after admission patients should receive a clear liquid diet. Thereafter diet with 50–55% of calories derived from complex carbohydrates and up to 30% from mono- and unsaturated fats should be given. The diet should contain fruits and vegetables which are rich in potassium and magnesium. The foods should be small in quantity and given at frequent intervals.

Resumption of Physical Activity

Graded and supervised physical activity is encouraged as early as the patient can tolerate. In the absence of complications, such as shock, cardiac failure or serious arrhythmias, mobilization of the patient should be started on the 2nd day itself.

Before allowing the patient to get up and walk, vital signs should be checked and safety of mobilization should be ensured.

Stage 1: First 2 Days

Use bed pan or commode for toilet purposes. The patient is allowed to feed from the food tray with arm and back supported. All joints are given active and passive movements. The ankle joint is exercised actively. The patient may be allowed to sit in a chair for short periods.

Stage 2: Days 3–4

The patient is allowed to walk out of the room under supervision. The upper part of the body can be bathed with the patient sitting in a chair with back supported. Bed to chair transfer for 20–30 minutes may be allowed daily.

Stage 3: Days 5–7

Patient can walk up to 200 m 2 or 3 times a day. Before the patient is discharged, an exercise tolerance test is performed so that the schedule of exercise at home can be advised.

Early ambulation reduces the risk of deep venous thrombosis (DVT), pulmonary embolism and prolonged invalidism, in addition to improving the morale of the patient.

Mineralocorticoid Receptor Antagonists

Drug like spironolactone or selective mineralocorticoid receptor antagonists (MRAs) like *eplerenone* 25 mg daily has been effective in prolonging survival in patients with acute MI and LV dysfunction (LVEF < 40%).

RIGHT VENTRICULAR INFARCTION

The RCA is the major source of blood flow, supplying the RA, RV, inferior wall and posterior wall of LV and posterior part of the IVS. RV is supplied by the RV branches of the RCA. The RV has a more favorable oxygen supply to demand ratio compared to the LV. In addition, the collateral circulation in the RV is also better.

RV infarction may occur in nearly half of all inferior MIs, although only 10–15% of patients show classic hemodynamic abnormalities of clinically significant RV infarction. RV infarction with hemodynamic abnormalities accompanying inferior STEMI is associated with a significantly higher mortality (25–30%) than inferior MI alone.

RV infarction results from occlusion of RCA proximal to the RV branches. Majority of cases of RV infarction occurs in association with inferior wall infarction. Isolated RV infarction accounts for less than 2% of the total.

Physical Findings

The diagnostic triad includes hypotension, clear lung fields and elevation of JVP in the setting of an inferior wall infarction. Although this combination of findings is specific, it occurs only in less than a third of the cases.

ECG recorded with right precordial leads may show the features of RV infarction. Demonstration of 1 mm or more ST-segment elevation in lead V1 and in the right precordial leads V3R and V4R is the single most predictive ECG finding in patients with RV infarction (Fig. 127.7). The finding may be transient; half of patients show resolution of ST-elevation within 10 hours of onset of symptoms. Echocardiography gives diagnostic findings. Right heart catheterization may be helpful in diagnosing RV infarction. Confirmation of the diagnosis can be made by radionuclide ventriculography. Complications include shock, which is uncommon but serious when it occurs, varying degrees of heart block, AF, AV asynchrony, septal rupture and development of right-to-left shunt through a patent foramen ovale.

Management

The principles of therapy include:

- *Maintenance of RV preload:* Maintenance of intra-vascular volume
- *Reduction of RV afterload:* Inotropes and intra-aortic balloon counterpulsation
- Inotropic support to the failing myocardium
- *Early reperfusion:* Primary angioplasty or thrombolysis.

Volume loading with IV normal saline helps to maintain RV preload. Measures usually undertaken to treat LV infarction, such as diuretics, nitrates and injection of morphine sulfate, can reduce the RV preload and aggravate hypotension and shock.

Inotropic support is given by infusion of dopamine or dobutamine in usual doses. If AV asynchrony occurs, it has to be corrected by AV sequential pacing. AF demands prompt cardioversion.

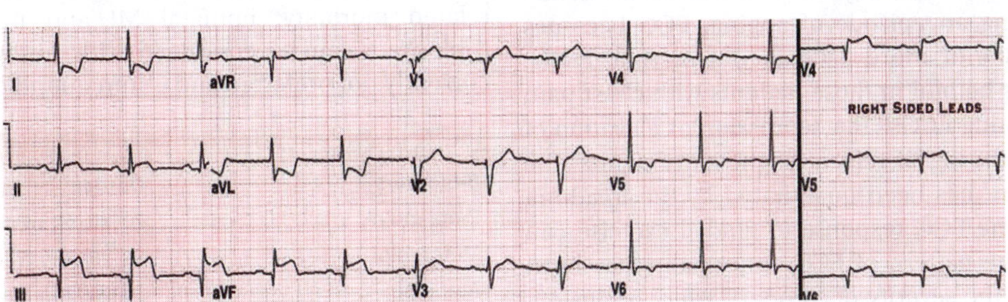

Fig. 127.7: ECG showing inferior MI with right ventricular MI. ***Note:*** ST-elevation in 2, 3, aVF, V1 and right chest leads. ST depression in I, aVL

If there is concomitant LV failure the RV afterload is increased and this further depresses RV function. In such circumstances, measures such as sodium nitroprusside infusion or an intra-aortic balloon counterpulsation which serves to improve LV function should be undertaken. Improvement in LV function automatically leads to fall in afterload as well.

Measures aimed at reperfusing the occluded coronary artery such as fibrinolytic therapy and emergency angioplasty have been found to improve RV function early. Emergency revascularization by angioplasty improves survival.

Prognosis

When inferior MI is complicated by RV infarction, the mortality may go up to 30% compared to 6% in inferior infarction without involvement of the RV. In survivors of RV infarction, generally the RV function recovers on follow up.

STABLE ANGINA PECTORIS (CHRONIC STABLE ANGINA)

The term 'angina pectoris' is used to denote pain or discomfort produced by reversible myocardial ischemia brought on by exertion or emotion and relieved by rest. Coronary atherosclerosis is the most common cause. Other causes include AS, aortic incompetence, syphilitic aortitis, polycythemia vera, rapidly developing anemia and others.

Clinical Features

Ischemic cardiac pain starts and increases with exertion or emotion and forces the patient to stop activity. With rest, the pain completely subsides within a few minutes. The quality of pain, its location and radiation are similar to that described under MI, but it is milder. At times the manifestation may be only undue dyspnea or vague chest discomfort rather than clear cut pain.

Physical Examination

Physical examination in between the attacks is unrewarding in most cases, but during the attacks of pain, elevation of BP, a third or fourth heart sounds, and evidence of mitral incompetence due to papillary muscle dysfunction may be detectable.

Diagnosis

Angina pectoris should be diagnosed by history. Resting ECG may be normal in approximately half of patients with chronic stable angina. The most common ECG changes are nonspecific ST-T wave changes with or without abnormal Q waves. During an episode of angina, ECG becomes abnormal in 50% or more patients with normal ECGs. Exercise ECG is helpful in those patients with chest pain and normal resting ECGs. The depression or elevation of the ST segment during exercise is diagnostic of angina. The whole procedure has been quantitated by the treadmill test, in which the ECG response to graded exercise can be recorded. The pattern of ECG abnormality has been correlated with the severity of coronary artery occlusion. Myocardial perfusion imaging using radioactive isotopes and stress echocardiography are also useful in diagnosis of myocardial ischemia.

Prognosis

Annual mortality in patients managed by medical therapy is about 4%. The mortality is 3%, 7% and 11% with affection of one, two or three coronary arteries respectively. Presence of resting ECG abnormalities and congestive cardiac failure worsen the prognosis.

Management

General measures include control of hypertension and diabetes, treatment of thyrotoxicosis and anemia, weight reduction, and avoidance of smoking and caffeine (coffee and tea in excess of 3 cups a day).

Drugs

Antiplatelet Agents

The use of aspirin is associated with a 33% reduction in the risk of adverse cardiovascular events. In the absence of contraindications, aspirin 75–150 mg daily should be used routinely in all patients with acute and chronic IHD with or without manifest symptoms.

Lipid-lowering Agents

One percent reduction in total cholesterol would reduce coronary events by 2%. Continued treatment is associated with angiographically demonstrable arrest of progression, more stabilization and even regression of the plaque lesions and decreased incidence of clinical events. Both mortality rate and major coronary events are reduced by 30–35%. Lipid-lowering therapy should be recommended even if the elevation of total cholesterol and LDL fraction is moderate. Statins (HMG-CoA reductase inhibitors) are the first choice drugs for the treatment of hyperlipidemia.

Antianginal and Antiischemia Therapy

Drugs in this group include mainly the β-adrenoreceptor blocking agents (β-blockers), calcium antagonists and nitrates. Other classes of drugs include ACE-I and metabolic agents.

β-blockers

Mechanism of action: Inhibition of β-receptors cause decrease in heart rate, decrease in myocardial contractility and lowering of arterial pressure thus decreasing myocardial oxygen demand. Reduction in heart rate also increases diastolic interval thereby improving myocardial perfusion. The β-blockers used commonly are elaborated in Table 127.3.

Other drugs, such as nadolol, acebutolol, nebivolol, are also available. The goal is to reduce the resting heart rate to 50–60 beats/min. β-blockers reduce the rate of cardiac-related mortality, nonfatal MI and unstable angina. β-blockers can be combined with nitrates. Atenolol is currently not preferred and is infrequently used.

Table 127.3: Commonly used β-blockers

β-blockers	Dosage
Propranolol	20–80 mg twice daily
Metoprolol	50–200 mg twice daily
Atenolol	50–200 mg/day
Bisoprolol	5–20 mg/day

Table 127.4: Calcium antagonists

Parameters	Drugs	Release of drugs	Dosage	Side effects
Dihydropyridine group	Amlodipine		2.5–10 mg/day	Headache, edema of the legs and feet
	Felodipine		2.5–10 mg/day	Headache, edema
	Nicardipine		20–40 mg TID	Headache, edema, dizziness, flushing
	Cilnidipine		5–10 mg	Nausea, vomiting, abdominal pain, headache, insomnia
Other groups of drugs	Diltiazem	Immediate	30–90 mg TID	Hypotension, bradycardia release
		Slow	60–180 mg BID	Myocardial depression
	Verapamil	Immediate	80–120 mg TID	Myocardial depression
		Slow	120–480 mg/day	Bradycardia

Advantages: The advantages are:

- Reflex tachycardia seen with nitrates is decreased.
- The increase in LV volume and diastolic pressure and wall tension associated with decreased heart rate caused by β-blockers is counteracted by concomitant use of nitroglycerin.

Side effects: It includes fatigue, inability to perform exercise, lethargy, insomnia, nightmares, worsening of claudication and impotence.

Calcium Antagonists

Mechanism of action

Calcium antagonists (Table 127.4) inhibit calcium ion movement through slow channels in cardiac and smooth muscle membranes by noncompetitive blockade of voltage-sensitive L-type calcium channels. The three major classes of calcium antagonists are (1) the dihydropyridines (nifedipine is the prototype), (2) the phenylalkylamines (verapamil is the prototype) and (3) the modified benzodiazepines (diltiazem is the prototype). All calcium antagonists exert a negative inotropic effect.

The newer second-generation agents, such as amlodipine, felodipine and others, decrease coronary vascular resistance and increase coronary blood flow. They reduce myocardial oxygen demand primarily by reduction of systemic vascular resistance and arterial pressure. The negative inotropic effect of calcium antagonists, like verapamil and diltiazem, also decreases the myocardial oxygen requirement.

Hypotension, depression of cardiac function and worsening heart failure may occur during long-term treatment with all the calcium antagonists. Dependent edema may occur as a troublesome complication. This resolves on withdrawing the drug.

Nitrates

Clinical effects

In patients with chronic stable angina, nitrates improve exercise tolerance, time to onset of angina and ST-segment depression during treadmill exercise test. Combination with β-blockers, or calcium antagonists enhance these beneficial effects (Table 127.5).

Contraindications: Nitroglycerine and nitrates are relatively contraindicated in hypertrophic obstructive cardiomyopathy because in these patients nitrates can increase LV outflow tract obstruction and can precipitate presyncope or syncope. It should also be avoided in cases of critical aortic stenosis.

Other Antianginal Agents

- **Nicorandil** is a potassium channel activator. It has pharmacologic properties similar to those of nitrates and is effective in the treatment of stable angina.
- **Metabolic agents** such as trimetazidine, ranolazine and carnitine, have been observed to produce antianginal effects in some patients. They are still being investigated further.
- **Bradycardiac agents** such as alinidine and zatebradine, have been used for the treatment of stable angina.

Table 127.5: Commonly used nitrates

Nitrates	Mode of action	Dosage
Nitroglycerine	Sublingual tablets	0.3–0.6 mg upto 1.5 mg
	Buccal spray	400 µg as needed
	Transdermal	15 cm × 15 cm patch containing 7.5–40 mg
	Oral slow release (SR)	2.5–13 mg
	Buccal	1–3 mg 3 times daily
	Intravenous (IV)	5–20 µg/min
Isosorbide dinitrate	Sublingual	2.5–15 mg
	Oral	5–80 mg, 2–3 times daily
	Buccal spray	1.25 mg metered doses
	Chewable tablets	5 mg
	Oral SR	40 mg od or bid
	IV	1.25–5.00 mg/hour
	Ointment	100 mg/24 hour
Isosorbide mononitrate	Oral	20 mg twice daily

Other drugs, such as ketanserin and ACE-Is have also been tried successfully.

- ***Xanthine oxidase inhibitors*** can reduce myocardial oxygen consumption for a particular stroke volume. Randomized studies with allopurinol 300 mg BD daily revealed increase in exercise time and reduction of angina. Allopurinol seems to be a promising antianginal agent.

Source: Noman A, Ang DS, Ogston S, et al. Effect of high-dose allopurinol on exercise in patients with chronic stable angina: a randomised, placebo controlled crossover trial. Lancet. 2010;375(9732):2161-7.

- ***Ranolazine:*** It is a new unique antianginal drug approved for use in chronic stable angina. It is a selective inhibitor of the late sodium influx. It attenuates the abnormalities of ventricular repolarization and contractility associated with IHD. ***Dose:*** 500–1,500 mg bd.
- ***Ivabradine*** is a heart rate lowering agent that inhibits the 'if' current in the pacemaker cells of the SA node. It improves exercise duration, reduces angina, but does not prevent death.

Risk Factor Modification

Risk factor modification includes:

- Cessation of cigarette smoking
- Management of hyperlipidemia
- Control of hypertension
- Control of DM
- Treatment of obesity
- Physical exercise-graded regimen
- Relief of anxiety.

Revascularization Procedures

Coronary revascularization procedures, like PCI and CABG, are indicated when angina is refractory to medical management. They improve the quality of life and prolong survival.

Transmyocardial Laser Revascularization

This is an operative treatment for refractory angina pectoris when CABG or PTCA are not feasible. This method has been proved to be beneficial in those with no other treatment options.

UNSTABLE ANGINA PECTORIS

Introduction

CAD presents a spectrum of conditions with acute transmural infarction at one end and nontransmural infarction, unstable angina, chronic stable angina and silent ischemia at the other end. Unstable angina (previously also known as preinfarction angina, crescendo angina, acute coronary insufficiency and intermediate coronary syndrome) is at the center of this spectrum.

Definition

The condition is diagnosed under the following circumstances:

- ***Crescendo angina:*** Angina that is more severe, prolonged or more frequent, superimposed on a preexisting pattern of relatively stable exertion-related angina pectoris

- Angina pectoris of new onset usually within 1 month
- Angina pectoris at rest as well as with minimal exertion.

Classification

Based on the severity, clinical features and response to treatment, Braunwald et al. have classified unstable angina as follows:

Based on Severity

- ***Class I: New-onset severe or accelerated angina:***
  - The duration is less than 2 months. Anginal attacks are more severe, more frequent occurring more than thrice a day and the threshold of exertion to cause angina is less. There is no rest angina.
- ***Class II: Angina at rest—subacute:***
  - Patients with one or more episodes of angina at rest during the preceding month, but not within the preceding 48 hours.
- ***Class III: Angina at rest—acute:***
  - Patients with one or more episodes of angina at rest within the preceding 48 hours.

Based on Clinical Circumstances

- ***Class A: Secondary unstable angina:***
  - This is a clearly distinct condition caused by extrinsic factors which worsen myocardial ischemia, e.g. anemia, infection, fever, hypotension, tachyarrhythmias, thyrotoxicosis and hypoxemia secondary to respiratory failure.
- ***Class B: Primary unstable angina:***
- ***Class C: Postinfarction unstable angina:*** This occurs within 2 weeks of documented MI.

Based on Response to Intensity of Treatment

- Absence of treatment or minimal treatment
- Occurring in the presence of standard therapy with conventional dose of oral β-blockers, nitrates and calcium antagonists for chronic stable angina
- Occurring despite maximally tolerated doses of all three categories of oral therapy and IV nitroglycerine.

This classification can be correlated with the underlying disease, e.g. class III patients are more likely to have intracoronary thrombus and heparin may be of greater value in such patients than in classes I and II. A clinical score based upon this classification is available. It is an important predictor of intracoronary thrombus and complexity of the lesions.

Pathophysiology

The majority of patients with unstable angina have significant obstructive coronary atherosclerosis. Rupture or erosion of an atherosclerotic plaque with superimposed nonocclusive thrombus is by far the most common cause of unstable angina. The type of plaque that ruptures, the so-called vulnerable plaques, are usually lesions with less than 50% stenosis. A patient having a small increase in myocardial oxygen demand, in conjunction with a reduction in coronary blood flow due to the plaque rupture can lead to an episode of ischemia. Other important mechanisms, contributing to aggravation of ischemia, include platelet aggregation, thrombosis and coronary vasoconstriction.

Clinical and Laboratory Findings

Symptoms

The chest discomfort in unstable angina is similar in quality to that of classic effort-induced angina, but it is more intense. There is an abrupt and progressive reduction in the threshold of physical activity required to provoke angina and this should be taken as a warning for the onset of unstable angina. Rest angina or nocturnal angina may occur in many cases. Radiation of pain to an additional site and onset of new associated features, such as sweating, nausea, vomiting, palpitation and dyspnea, should all be taken as suggestive symptoms.

Physical Examination

This may reveal nonspecific findings, such as transient third and fourth heart sounds, dyskinetic apical impulse suggesting LV dysfunction, and transient murmur of mitral regurgitation during or immediately after an ischemic episode. Features of congestive cardiac failure may occur. There may be hypotension during the episodes of pain. These indicate adverse prognosis.

Electrocardiogram

In unstable angina, ST-segment depression (or transient ST-segment elevation) and T wave changes occur in up to 50% of patients. New ST-segment deviation, even of only 0.05 mV, is a specific and important measure of ischemia and prognosis. T wave changes are sensitive but nonspecific of acute ischemia. An unusual finding is the presence of transient inverted 'U' waves. Continuous ECG monitoring can be used for two purposes in unstable angina: (1) to detect arrhythmias in association with the acute episode and (2) to monitor the ST-segment for evidence of recurrent ischemia.

Laboratory Parameters

Laboratory parameters include the following:

- *Cardiac troponins T and I:* The degree of increase of troponins has prognostic implication in unstable angina.
- *C-reactive protein:* This is a sensitive indicator of inflammation and the level of this marker is correlated with adverse prognosis.
- Serum amyloid A protein
- Fibrinogen.

Coronary Angiography

Three-vessel disease is found in approximately 35%, two-vessel disease in 25%, single-vessel disease in about 25% and left main CAD in approximately 5–10%. Critical obstruction may not be demonstrable in any vessel in 15% of patients with unstable angina. Coronary angiogram demonstrating eccentric lesions with scalloped or over-hanging edges are more characteristic of unstable angina.

Adverse Prognostic Factors

Adverse prognostic factors include:

- Older age
- Continuing rest pain despite medical therapy
- Ischemia detected by Holter's monitoring
- Significant ST-T wave changes on ECG at initial presentation
- Troponin-positive cases
- Levels of markers of inflammation, such as CRP, serum amyloid A and fibrinogen
- Multivessel disease, presence of thrombus or complex coronary morphology at coronary angiography.

Management

Comprehensive management of unstable angina or non-Q MI includes the following:

- Antithrombotic therapy including antiplatelet drug and anticoagulants
- Antianginal drugs
- Revascularization procedures
- Risk factor modification and pharmacologic measures to slow or halt progression of atherosclerosis.

Antiplatelet Agents

Aspirin is the drug of choice. It should be started in a dose of 162–325 mg given orally as early as possible. Maintenance dose of aspirin is 75–162 mg/day. Aspirin reduces the risk of MI by 35% at 6 months and 40% at 1 year.

Clopidogrel is a thienopyridine derivative that inhibits platelet aggregation by inhibiting ADP action on platelet receptors. Recent studies have shown that addition of clopidogrel to aspirin in high-risk unstable angina decreases the mortality and further cardiovascular events. Benefit of clopidogrel has been established in both ST and non-ST-elevation in acute coronary syndromes (ACSs). Initial loading dose is 300–600 mg clopidogrel, 2–4 hours prior to PCI and follow-up by 75 mg daily for 12 months or more to prevent stent thrombosis. Clopidogrel genetic testing has been employed to test the efficacy of clopidogrel in individuals since the action of clopidogrel is related to genetic factors. Presence of the gene *CPY2C19*2 allele* in the patient inhibits the action of clopidogrel and therefore the drug is ineffective in them. Prasugrel and ticagrelor are not affected by this gene.

Other newer antiplatelet drugs

- *Prasugrel:* It is more rapid-acting and potent than clopidogrel, is more effective in preventing stent thrombosis in MI patient undergoing coronary revascularization. It is not to be used for patients who do not undergo coronary intervention.
- *Ticagrelor:* Is non-thienopyridine cyclopentyl triazole pyrimidine ADP-receptor antagonist is more potent and rapidly acting than clopidogrel in patients in whom early intervention is planned. Dose of ticagrelor is 180 mg loading dose and 90 mg BD as maintenance.
- *Other antiplatelet drugs:* These are abciximab, eptifibatide and tirofiban which are inhibitors of GP-IIb to GP-IIIa receptors on platelets. Their indication is only under very special circumstances. These are expensive and have significant bleeding potential.

Source: Freedman JE, Hylek EM. Clopidogrel, genetics, and drug responsiveness. New Engl J Med. 2009;360(4):411-3.

Anticoagulants

Heparin given in doses intended to keep the activated PTT at 1.5–2.0 times the normal value reduces the incidences of nonfatal MI from 1.9% to 1.2% and refractory angina from 22.9% to 9.6%. In the acute phase, heparin is more effective than aspirin but a combination is even better. After the acute phase, heparin is withdrawn and aspirin is continued. Low molecular weight heparin is found to be superior and easier to be administered than unfractionated heparin in unstable angina.

Direct thrombin inhibitors: Such as hirudin, hirulog and argatroban dabigatran and rivaroxaban, are effective anticoagulants which could be considered when heparin is contraindicated. These drugs are used only in limited situations at present.

Oral anticoagulants are not routinely used on a long-term basis. Thrombolysis is not indicated for patients with uncomplicated unstable angina. Combined prophylaxis with warfarin and antiplatelet drugs is more effective than using single drugs alone (*See* Section 15, Ch 176).

Antianginal Therapy

Nitrates, calcium-channel blockers and β-adrenergic blockers are used for this purpose.

Nitrates: They form the mainstay of therapy. IV nitroglycerine controls the angina and prevents recurrence. They also improve global and regional LV function. Nitrates may be given sublingually, orally, topically or intravenously (IV). IV nitroglycerine is started in a dose at 5–10 µg/min by continuous infusion and increased by 10 µg/min every 5–10 minutes until relief of symptoms is achieved or limiting side effects appear. Headache, fall of systolic BP below 90 mm Hg or more than 30% below the initial mean arterial pressure are indications for stopping the infusion. Patients controlled with IV nitroglycerine should be switched on to an oral or topical nitrate preparation when they are symptom-free for 24 hours. Tolerance to continuous IV nitroglycerine therapy develops within 24–48 hours.

Beta adrenergic blockers: These drugs are standard therapy for unstable angina. They reduce the risk of developing MI by 13%. For immediate effect IV esmolol or metoprolol can be used. This can be followed by oral drugs, the dose of which can be titrated to keep resting heart rate between 50 and 60 beats/min.

Calcium-channel blockers: These drugs are as effective as β-blockers in relieving symptoms. They do not prevent the development of acute MI or reduce mortality. Even an increased risk of MI has been reported if short-acting nifedipine is used as monotherapy in unstable angina.

Diltiazem has been found to be effective in reducing reinfarction and postinfarction ischemia in non-Q MI. Calcium antagonists should be used as a second-line therapy in patients with continued ischemia despite treatment with nitrates and β-blockers. Particular caution should be taken in adding a calcium antagonist to β-blocker in patients with LV dysfunction.

The antianginal effects of nitrate, β-blockers and calcium-channel blockers are often additives. Triple therapy is recommended in refractory unstable angina. Antithrombotic therapy is generally used concurrently.

Percutaneous Coronary Interventions

Patients with suspected unstable coronary syndromes should be assessed for the risk based on clinical history, physical examination and presenting ECG. Patients considered to be at low risk may be treated with nitrates, aspirin and β-blockers as outpatients. They can undergo stress testing after 48 hours and should undergo coronary angiogram if indicated. Medium- and high-risk patients should be admitted and treated aggressively with heparin, aspirin, clopidogrel, nitrates and β-blockers. Platelet receptor antagonists (GP-IIb to GP-IIIa) should be considered in higher risk groups. Cardiac catheterization and revascularization should be performed early in the high- and medium-risk patients with elevated troponin levels. The sensitivity and specificity of diagnosis can be improved with addition of thallium imaging, single photon emission computed tomography (SPECT) imaging or stress echocardiography.

Role of Ventricular Assist Devices: Intra-aortic Balloon Pump

This increases diastolic flow through the stenotic segment and this may prevent complete occlusion. It also improves ventricular function. Intra-aortic balloon pump (IABP) is extremely effective in controlling.

- Recurrent ischemia
- Complications in very high-risk patients.

Up to 5% of patients may require IABP to control severe recurrent ischemia and to stabilize ventricular function.

Coronary Artery Bypass Grafting

The subsets of patients in whom CABG offers better control of symptoms and survival benefits are those who have:

- Left main stem disease
- Three-vessel disease with LV dysfunction.

Risk Factor Modification and Pharmacological Measures

This includes cessation of smoking, control of hypertension and diabetes, lipid-lowering agents, weight reduction and dietary modifications. Long-term treatment with aspirin, β-blockers and lipid-lowering agents (statins) should be emphasized.

Measures to lower serum lipids should be undertaken in patients with dyslipidemias. Aim should be to keep LDL levels below 100 mg/dL. Drug therapy should be instituted also in marginally abnormal patients if other measures fail to control the lipid levels.

Statins are used more liberally in this group of patients. Statins have the additional benefit of stabilizing the plaques in the vessels.

PRINZMETAL'S ANGINA

Syn: Variant angina

In 1959, Prinzmetal et al. described an unusual syndrome of cardiac pain secondary to myocardial ischemia that occurs almost exclusively at rest, not precipitated by physical exertion or emotional stress and also associated with ST-segment elevation in the ECG. This is known as Prinzmetal's angina or variant angina. It may be associated with AMI, severe cardiac arrhythmias including ventricular tachycardia and fibrillation as well as sudden death.

Pathogenesis

Angina is caused by spasm occurring in normal or diseased coronary arteries. Spasm is usually focal and involves a single site usually adjacent to an atheromatous plaque.

The possible *mechanisms* include:

- Hypercontractility of arterial wall associated with atherosclerotic process itself
- Endothelial injury
- Myocardial sympathetic dyssynergia.

Cigarette smoking, use of cocaine, hyperinsulinemia and insulin resistance are known risk factors. Anginal episodes show a circadian rhythm, peak attacks occurring during early morning hours between midnight and 8 am.

Clinical Features

Patients with variant angina tend to be younger than patients with chronic stable angina or unstable angina and many do not exhibit classic coronary risk factors, except that they are often heavy cigarette smokers. The anginal discomfort which is extremely severe may be accompanied by syncope, the latter presumably due to arrhythmias. Occasionally, the angina is accompanied by other vasospastic disorders, such as migraine and Raynaud's phenomenon.

Electrocardiogram: ECG changes are characteristic. The diagnostic feature is the elevation of ST-segment during pain. A pattern of alternating ST-segment elevation between the precordial and inferior leads is associated with angiographically documented multivessel spasm involving both the left anterior descending and right coronary systems. Conduction disturbances and ventricular arrhythmias may occur during the anginal attacks.

Arteriographic Studies

Spasm of a proximal coronary artery with resultant transmural ischemia and abnormalities in LV function has been convincingly documented arteriographically and is the diagnostic hallmark of Prinzmetal angina. Significant fixed proximal coronary obstruction of at least one major vessel occurs in the majority of patients, and in these patients spasm usually occurs within 1 cm of the obstruction. The remainder has normal coronary arteries in the absence of ischemia. Several provocative tests for coronary spasm have been developed. These tests are not routinely performed as potential for prolonged coronary artery spasm and consequent MI exists.

- *Ergonovine test:* This test has 100% sensitivity.
- *Acetylcholine test:* Sensitivity 99%
- Methacholine test
- *Miscellaneous:* Other provocative agents are exercise, cold pressor test and induction of alkalosis by hyperventilation.

Prognosis

Long-term survival is good. Survival at 5 years is 89–97%. The extent, severity and activity of CAD have adverse influence on prognosis for long-term survival and freedom from MI. Nonfatal MI occurs in up to 20% of patients and death in up to 10% during this period. Patients with variant angina are at a higher risk of sudden cardiac death.

Management

Drugs acting in Prinzmetal's angina bring about relief predominantly by the relief of coronary vasospasm:

- In Prinzmetal's angina nitrates are beneficial, the action being exclusively direct vasodilating effect of spastic coronaries.
- Calcium antagonists are very effective in preventing the coronary artery spasm of variant angina and they should be used in maximally tolerated doses. Calcium antagonists along with long- and short-acting nitrates are the mainstay of therapy. Even after surgical revascularization procedures these drugs should be continued as maintenance therapy.
- *Beta blockers:* Response to β-blockers is variable. They may even cause deterioration in Prinzmetal's angina.
- Prazosin, which is a selective α-adrenoceptor blocker, is beneficial in Prinzmetal's angina.
- Aspirin in dose of 75-mg daily should be given. Larger doses of aspirin inhibit the synthesis of the naturally occurring coronary vasodilator prostacyclin. This may even increase the severity of ischemic episodes.
- Coronary angioplasty and CABG are helpful in variant angina with discrete proximal fixed obstructive lesions. PTCA and CABG are contraindicated in patients with only isolated coronary artery spasm without accompanying fixed obstructive lesions.

Ischemic Cardiomyopathy

Multiple small infarcts and extensive diffuse fibrosis of the myocardium present a picture of cardiomegaly and congestive cardiomyopathy. There may be accompanying mitral incompetence. End-stage ischemic cardiomyopathy is an indication for cardiac transplantation.

ASYMPTOMATIC CORONARY ARTERY DISEASE

This is not uncommon even in apparently normal individuals. Routine stress testing may bring out the abnormality. Such cases may develop acute MI or die suddenly as a result of ventricular fibrillation or cardiac arrest. Significant abnormalities in the treadmill test are indications for coronary arteriography. Occlusion of the left main coronary artery or all the three vessels is an indication for early bypass surgery.

Prevention of Coronary Artery Disease

Primary prevention can be achieved by:

- Proper dietary manipulation to avoid high intake of saturated fats and overnutrition
- Avoidance of smoking
- Regular exercises
- Regular medical check-up.

Diseases of the Myocardium

K Suresh, CG Bahuleyan

Chapter Summary

- Myocarditis
  - Acute Myocarditis
  - Chronic Myocarditis
- Cardiomyopathy
  - Dilated Cardiomyopathy
  - Hypertrophic Cardiomyopathy
  - Obliterative (Restrictive) Cardiomyopathy
  - Endomyocardial Fibrosis

MYOCARDITIS

ACUTE MYOCARDITIS

Myocarditis is defined as inflammation of heart muscle due to any injury. Most commonly it results from an infectious process, the most common being viral infection, notably is coxsackie B, but also including other adenoviruses, parvoviruses and cytomegaloviruses (CMVs). Myocarditis can also be caused by radiation, chemicals, hypersensitivity to drugs or autoimmune reactions. In majority of patients, active myocarditis remains unsuspected because the cardiac dysfunction is subclinical, asymptomatic and self-limited.

Pathophysiology of myocarditis by cardiotropic viruses involves three phases. The first is the viral phase, where the virus reaches the myocardium through hematogenous or lymphatic spread and enters the cells with the help of specific receptors. The second is the immunologic response phase including innate and acquired immunity. Innate immunity is the earliest response, with the help of toll-like receptors (TLRs), resulting in the production of cytokines and interferons (IFNs); whereas acquired immunity results in B- and T-cell activation. Third is the cardiac remodeling phase, which may lead to cell death, hypertrophy or dilated cardiomyopathy, depending on the host-virus response.

Causes

Infectious

- ***Viruses:*** Coxsackievirus, adenovirus, echovirus, influenza virus, herpes simplex virus (HSV), varicella zoster virus (VZV), Epstein-Barr virus, CMV, human immunodeficiency virus (HIV), hepatitis (A and B), poliovirus, mumps, rabies, respiratory syncytial virus (RSV), arbovirus and parvovirus B19 infection.
- ***Bacteria:*** *Corynebacterium diphtheriae, Streptococcal* and *Staphylococcus* species, *Haemophilus influenzae, Bartonella, Brucella, Neisseria gonorrhoeae, Actinomyces, Chlamydia* species, *Treponema pallidum, Leptospira, Borrelia burgdorferi.*

- ***Fungi:*** *Candida* species, *Aspergillus* species, *Histoplasma, Blastomyces, Cryptococcus* and coccidioidomycosis.
- ***Parasites:*** *Trypanosoma cruzi, Toxoplasma, Schistosoma* and *Trichinella.*

Noninfectious

Noninfectious causes include the following:

- Drugs causing hypersensitivity reactions
- ***Antibiotics:*** Sulfonamides, penicillins, chloramphenicol, tetracycline, amphotericin B.
- ***Anti-tuberculous (INH):*** Isoniazid, para-aminosali (PAS) cylic acid
- ***Anti-convulsants:*** Phenytoin, carbamazepine
- ***Anti-inflammatory:*** Indomethacin, phenylbutazone
- ***Diuretics:*** Acetazolamide, chlorthalidone, hydrochloro thiazide, spironolactone
- ***Others:*** Lithium, doxorubicin, emetine, cocaine, numerous catecholamines, acetaminophen, zidovudine
- Wasp, scorpion, spider stings
- Radiation
- Connective tissue disorders such as systemic lupus erythematosus (SLE), rheumatoid arthritis, dermatomyositis, Kawasaki disease, sarcoidosis and giant-cell arteritis (GCA)
- ***Nutritional disorders:*** Deficiency of thiamine—beri-beri.

Clinical Features

Clinical manifestations of myocarditis are variable ranging from asymptomatic electrocardiogram (ECG) changes to symptoms of heart failure or hemodynamic collapse and profound cardiogenic shock. Most patients have a self-limited disease. Most common symptoms include fatigue (82%), dyspnea on exertion, palpitations and chest pain at rest. The viral prodrome like fever, chills, myalgias and other constitutional symptoms occur in 20–80% of the cases, but may be missed by the patient and thus cannot be relied on for diagnosis. Unexplained tachycardia, arrhythmias, hypotension, cardiomegaly, and evidence of cardiac failure occurring in the presence of any of the etiological disorders should suggest the possibility of myocarditis. The disease process affects the impulse producing and conducting tissues and produces arrhythmias and varying grades of conduction defects. Sudden cardiac death can be the initial presentation of myocarditis in some patients, presumably from complete heart block or ventricular tachycardia (VT).

The ECG shows sinus tachycardia, nonspecific changes in ST and T waves, conduction defects, low-voltage complexes and sometimes myocardial infarction (MI) pattern. X-ray may reveal cardiomegaly. Increase in the level of cardiac markers, like creatine kinase-MB (CK-MB) and troponin, are observed in 15–20%; troponin assays are proven to be more sensitive. Echocardiography can reveal left ventricular (LV) systolic dysfunction in patients with a normal-sized LV cavity. Endomyocardial biopsy is the critical test to confirm the diagnosis.

Prognosis

Myocarditis is a serious condition associated with mortality. Death occurs as a result of sudden cardiac failure, heart block or fatal arrhythmias. The prognosis depends upon the extent of cardiac involvement and the underlying cause.

Management

The condition should be anticipated and early treatment instituted. The patient is put to absolute bed rest with cardiac monitoring in an intensive cardiac care facility. Complications such as cardiac failure, heart block and arrhythmias are managed as they arise. Immunosuppressive therapy is not routinely recommended for infective myocarditis. Standard heart failure treatment remains the mainstay of therapy.

CHRONIC MYOCARDITIS

This condition may follow the acute condition or arise de novo. The clinical picture resembles one of cardiomyopathy, but milder. Mainly, it presents with cardiomegaly and congestive heart failure (CHF).

CARDIOMYOPATHY

It is a primary disorder of the heart muscle that causes abnormal myocardial performance and is not the result of disease or dysfunction of other cardiac structures. Thus, the term cardiomyopathy excludes cases of myocardial failure due to MI, systemic arterial hypertension, valvular stenosis or regurgitation and congenital heart disease (CHD).

The currently used clinical classification of cardiomyopathy was developed by the World Health Organization (WHO) and the International Society and Federation of Cardiology.

WHO classification of cardiomyopathy is as following:

- ***Dilated cardiomyopathy:*** This condition is characterized by dilatation and impaired contraction of the left or both ventricles.
- ***Hypertrophic cardiomyopathy (HCM):*** This condition is characterized by left and/or right ventricular hypertrophy (RVH), which is usually asymmetric and involves the interventricular septum (IVS). Typically, the LV volume is normal or reduced. Mutations in sarcomeric contractile protein genes cause disease.
- ***Restrictive cardiomyopathy:*** This entity is characterized by restrictive filling and reduced diastolic volume of either or both ventricles with normal or near normal systolic function and wall thickness.
- ***Arrhythmogenic right ventricular cardiomyopathy (ARVC):*** The disorder is characterized by progressive fibrofatty replacement of RV myocytes.
- ***Unclassified cardiomyopathies:*** This include a few cases which do not fit readily with any group, e.g. fibroelastosis, systolic dysfunction with minimal dilatation, mitochondrial involvement, etc.

SPECIFIC CARDIOMYOPATHIES

Specific cardiomyopathies include the following:

- Ischemic cardiomyopathy
- Valvular cardiomyopathy
- Hypertensive cardiomyopathy
- Inflammatory cardiomyopathy
- Metabolic cardiomyopathy
- General system disease
- Muscular dystrophies
- Neuromuscular disorders
- Sensitivity and toxic reactions
- Peripartum cardiomyopathy.

DILATED CARDIOMYOPATHY

Fifty percent cases are idiopathic and 50% due to secondary causes, like alcoholic (most common), ischemic or hypertensive heart disease. Idiopathic dilated cardiomyopathy (IDC) is diagnosed by excluding the secondary causes. It is noted that many of these IDC result from underlying genetic abnormalities or environmental factors, which are difficult to detect at the time of presentation. It is a relatively common cause of heart failure, with an estimated prevalence rate of 0.04% and incidence rates varying from 0.005% to 0.006%. The incidence increases with age and males are afflicted at a higher rate than females. IDC may be familial in as many as 35–50% of the patients when first-degree relatives are carefully screened. Majority is autosomal dominant due to mutations of the cardiac actin or desmin gene, but in the majority of cases, the disease causing gene is still unknown.

Clinical Features

Main symptoms are shortness of breath, orthopnea, dyspnea upon exertion, fatigue, palpitation and edema. Atrial fibrillation (AF) and ventricular dysrhythmias may be early signs of myocardial disease. Some patients may present with systemic embolism or stroke. On examination, there may be tachycardia, narrow pulse pressure and jugular venous distention (JVD). There may be cardiomegaly, LV third heart sound, and murmurs of mitral and tricuspid regurgitation. ECG demonstrates sinus tachycardia or AF, varying degrees of ST-T wave changes and intraventricular conduction disturbances. Chest X-ray usually demonstrates LV and left atrial enlargement. Echocardiography will show dilatation of left ventricle (LV) and left atrium (LA) and sometimes of right sided chambers and LV systolic dysfunction (Figs 128.1 and 128.2).

Management

In general, treatment consists of use of angiotensin converting enzyme (ACE) inhibitors in asymptomatic or symptomatic patients, the use of diuretics in volume-overloaded subjects and use of digoxin in subjects who remain symptomatic on the former medications. In mild to moderately symptomatic subjects, β-adrenergic

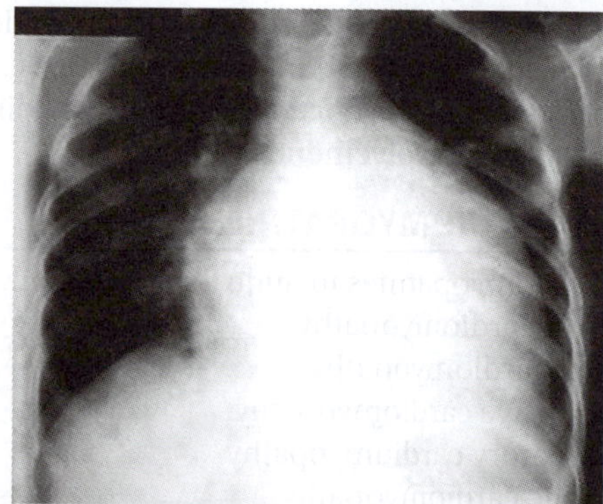

Fig. 128.1: Chest X-ray of a patient with dilated cardiomyopathy showing cardiomegaly, left and right atrial enlargement

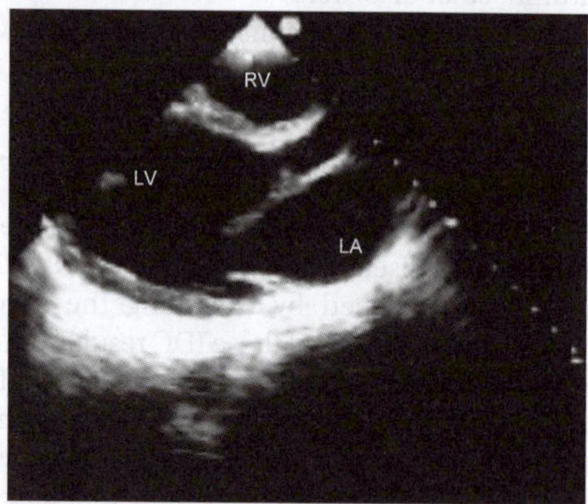

Fig. 128.2: 2D-echo picture of a patient with dilated cardiomyopathy showing dilated LV and LA

Abbreviations: LV = Left ventricle; LA = Left atrium; RV = Right ventricular

blocking agents improve symptoms and reduce mortality. Adjunctive therapy includes anticoagulation in subjects with lower LV ejection fractions to prevent thromboembolic complications, amiodarone to treat symptomatic arrhythmias and maintaining potassium levels in the normal-high (4.3–5.0 mmol/L) range. Those with malignant ventricular arrhythmias may benefit from implantable cardioverter defibrillator (ICD). Those who are resistant to medical therapy are candidates for cardiac transplantation. Newer methods, like stem-cell therapy for cardiac regeneration and gene therapy approaches are emerging.

HYPERTROPHIC CARDIOMYOPATHY

It is known previously as idiopathic hypertrophic subaortic stenosis (IHSS) or hypertrophic obstructive cardiomyopathy (HOCM). HCM has a prevalence of 1/500 in the general population. It is genetically heterogeneous caused by mutations in any 1 of the 11 genes that encode contractile proteins of the cardiac sarcomere, involving thick filaments β-myosin heavy chains (MyHC), first identified and most common, and regulatory myosin light chains (RMyLC), thin filaments cardiac troponin T (cTnT), cardiac troponin I (cTnI), α-tropomyosin (a-TM) and α-actin and cardiac myosin-binding protein C (cMyBP-C). More than 1,000 mutations involving the 11 genes have been reported. HCM has an autosomal dominant pattern of inheritance (Table 128.1).

Table 128.1: Location of common genetic alterations and their relative frequency of occurrence in familial hypertrophic cardiomyopathy (HCM)		
Gene	*Chromosome*	*Frequency (%)*
β-myosin heavy chain	14q1	35–45
Cardiac troponin T	1q31	15
α-tropomyosin	15q2	5
Myosin-binding protein C	11p 13–q 13	10

Asian patients with HCM 70% have mutations in two genes β-MyC7 and myosin-binding protein C3 (MyBPC3). Troponin-T gene (TNNT2) and several other genes account for 5% or less of cases.

Clinical Diagnosis

The clinical diagnosis of HCM is based on the most characteristic morphologic feature of the disease, i.e. thickening of the LV wall associated with a nondilated cavity in the absence of another cardiac or systemic disease capable of producing LV hypertrophy (LVH) (e.g. systemic hypertension or aortic stenosis). The most important features of HCM are the heterogeneous nature of the LVH, which predominantly involves the IVS and the dynamic left ventricular outflow tract (LVOT) obstruction caused by the systolic anterior motion of the anterior mitral leaflet.

LVH is the gross anatomic marker of HCM. The distribution of hypertrophy is almost always asymmetric, with wall thickening dominantly involving the anterior IVS. Dynamic obstruction to LV systolic outflow develops. The main physiologic consequence is caused by the bulge of the asymmetric septal hypertrophy into the LVOT and the systolic anterior motion of the anterior mitral leaflet. In some patients, the pattern of hypertrophy is diffuse, involving both septum and substantial portions of the lateral free wall. In some, concentric LVH can be observed. The generalized form shows hypertrophy without obstructive features (Fig. 128.3).

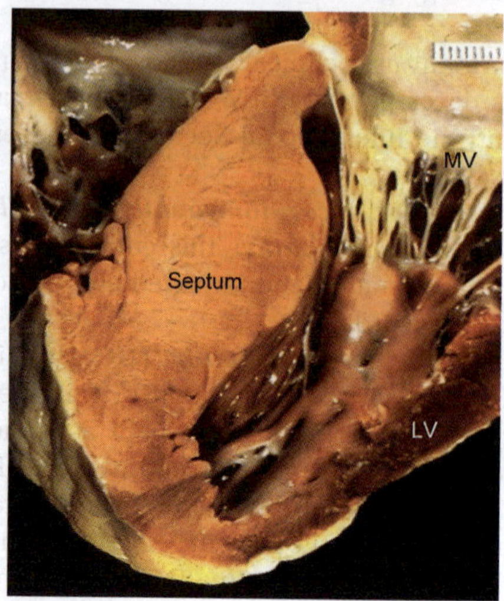

Fig. 128.3: Pathological specimen of hypertrophic cardiomyopathy showing asymmetric septal hypertrophy (ASH) of IVS and normal thickness LV free wall.

Courtesy: JP Veinot: Cardiomyopathy and Pericardial diseases

Abbreviations: IVS = Interventricular septum; LV = Left ventricular free wall, MV = Mitral valve

HCM has to be distinguished from physiological LVH (*athletics heart*) by screening for risk in affected families members.

The pathophysiological abnormalities determine the clinical outcome. These include:

- LV diastolic dysfunction
- Dynamic LVOT obstruction
- Myocardial ischemia
- Arrhythmias particularly AF, VT and sudden cardiac death.

Clinical Features

The onset of symptoms is often between 20 and 40 years of age, although they can become evident at any age. They include exertional dyspnea, orthopnea, paroxysmal nocturnal dyspnea (PND), fatigue, chest pain (which may be atypical of angina pectoris) and palpitation. Impaired consciousness including dizziness, near syncope and syncope or sudden death may occasionally be the first manifestation.

Those with LVOT obstruction may have a brisk carotid pulse, double or triple apical impulse, fourth heart sound and the characteristic diamond-shaped systolic murmur, best heard at the lower left sternal border and apex.

ECG: It shows LVH, ST-segment changes and T wave inversion, LA enlargement, abnormally deep Q waves, and diminution or absence of R waves in the right precordial leads. Chest X-ray may show cardiomegaly and pulmonary venous congestion.

Echocardiogram is the main diagnostic tool in HCM. The asymmetric hypertrophy of the septum (ASH) and the systolic anterior movement (SAM) of the anterior mitral leaflet can be visualized. In addition, the dynamic LVOT obstruction can be quantified. Doppler echocardiography can assess the LVOT pressure gradient and values above 30 mm Hg across the LV outflow are diagnostic.

Assessment of risk: Features which predict higher risk of major cardiovascular events in patients with HCM include the following:

- Family history of sudden death
- Specific mutations in sarcomeric proteins e.g. Troponin-T (TnT) mutation
- History of resuscitation after cardiac arrest, recurrent syncope
- Presence of VT on Holter monitoring
- Extreme LVH (> 3 cm thick)
- Rise in hemodynamic outflow pressure gradient more than 30 mm Hg
- Fall in blood pressure (BP) with exercise
- Limitation of myocardial reserve
- Bridging of the left anterior descending coronary artery in children
- LV apical aneurysm.

Prognosis: Many patients enjoy normal health and life-span with minimal or no disability. In a few, HCM may present with a fatal cardiac event as the first manifestation in an unsuspected case. A frequent cause for unexpected sudden death during competitive sports activities is HCM. In a low-risk patient, the overall annual mortality is less than 1%. It is generally accepted that entrants into vigorous competitive sports should have a preliminary check to exclude conditions like HCM.

Management

Symptomatic patients with HCM may benefit by drugs such as β-blockers, verapamil and disopyramide. Judicious addition of diuretic agents in those with severe symptoms of heart failure despite treatment with beta-blockers or verapamil leads to symptomatic improvement. Beta-adrenergic blocking agents or verapamil are usually efficacious in controlling heart rate in patients with chronic AF. If AF develops, anticoagulant therapy should be started and continued indefinitely. In those patients who are symptomatic despite medical management, septal ablation is one method, which reduces the outflow gradient and symptoms. This is a method to induce infarction of the hypertrophied septum by injecting alcohol into the septal artery. Surgical septal myectomy may be required in some patients (*Morrow's operation*). Infective endocarditis (IE) prophylaxis should be given to those with LVOT obstruction. Prophylactic measures to reduce symptoms include avoidance of dehydration and drug therapy using beta-adrenergic blockers.

Competitive sports and strenuous exertion should be avoided since sudden death may occur during these activities. All first-degree relatives should be screened by echocardiography.

Genetic testing: Rapid automated deoxyribonucleic acid (DNA) sequencing provides opportunities for commercially available genetic tests, but positive results are obtained only in 50% of probands. Genetic tests identify affected family members. Unaffected family members can be reassured to undertake sports activities. General consensus about the schedule for testing:

- At age less than 12 years, optional, but necessary under special circumstances
- Age 12–21 years, screening every 12–18 months
- Age more than 21 years, either at onset of symptoms or routinely at 5 years.

Role of commercial genetic testing for long-term benefit is being evaluated.

Special Variants

Apical HCM

Syn: Takotsubo cardiomyopathy (broken heart syndrome)

Hypertrophy confined to the LV apex (*apical HCM*) has been reported most commonly by Japanese investigators. It is characterized by isolated apical hypertrophy and is common in Japan where it constitutes 25% of all cases of HCM. Outside Japan, it constitutes only 1–2% of cases. Clinical presentation is similar and patients experience chest pain, dyspnea, fatigue and in rare instances, sudden death. The diagnosis is made by the typical ECG, echocardiographic and angiographic features. ECG shows giant negative T waves in precordial leads and LVH. Echocardiogram shows localized hypertrophy in the distal LV, increase in thickness in the apical region of at least 15 mm, or a ratio of maximal apical to posterobasal thickness greater than 1.5 and absence of outflow tract obstruction.

LV angiogram shows spade-like configuration of the LV cavity at the end of diastole, obliteration of apical LV cavity at the end of systole.

Takotsubo Cardiomyopathy

It is an acute stress-related reversible cardiomyopathy characterized by apical ballooning. The contractions of the basal segments are usually preserved. This has been called **Takotsubo cardiomyopathy**. The name comes from the Japanese word for a kind of octopus trap because of the resemblance of the affected LV to that during imaging, either by angiocardiography or echocardiography. It is also called **Broken heart syndrome** because of the relation to psychological stressful event. Coronary angiogram shows normal epicardial vessels or only minor disease. The cardiac markers are normal or only minimally elevated. Treatment consists of β-blockers and calcium-channel blockers. It is generally associated with good prognosis.

OBLITERATIVE (RESTRICTIVE) CARDIOMYOPATHY

The term restrictive cardiomyopathy refers to either an idiopathic or systemic myocardial disorder characterized by impaired diastolic filling of ventricles, normal or reduced LV and RV volumes, and normal or nearly normal systolic (LV and RV) function. The hemodynamic and clinical manifestations may mimic those produced by constrictive pericarditis, which in contrast to restrictive cardiomyopathy, is a surgically curable disorder (Box 128.1).

ENDOMYOCARDIAL FIBROSIS (EMF)

A particularly common form of this disorder, EMF is prevalent in Kerala, certain other states of India, Africa and Brazil. This condition is characterized by fibrosis and obliteration of the ventricular inflow tract and restriction to ventricular filling. Males are affected more, especially children and young adults and more among the poor. The etiological agent is not yet identified for certain, though several factors such as malnutrition, dietary deficiency of trace elements such as selenium, infection, filariasis, eosinophilic infiltration and an imbalance of trace elements (magnesium versus cerium) have been implicated. Pathologically, the disease is characterized by fibrosis affecting the inflow tracts and apices of one or both ventricles; outflow tracts of ventricles are conspicuously unaffected. The disease predominantly affects the endocardium and subjacent myocardium. Combined RV and LV disease occurs in half of the cases, pure LV involvement in 40% and pure RV involvement in 10%.

Clinical features: The onset is slow and symptoms may be present for a few months to several years before presentation. Children and adolescents are affected more.

LVEMF: Patients with LV involvement present very early with varying grades of dyspnea and palpitation–clinically they may resemble mitral incompetence. Physical examination reveals cardiomegaly, loud apical third heart sound and pansystolic murmur in the mitral area. Complications include pulmonary hypertension and left heart failure. ECG may reveal LVH. Myocardial calcification may develop and this may be detected by imaging studies. Echocardiography is diagnostic. The characteristic plastering of the posterior mitral leaflet to endocardium, marked endocardial thickening, obliteration of cavity and sparing of outflow regions are features of endomyocardial disease. Hypercontracting basal segments with obliteration of apex (***Merlon sign***) are typical of EMF. Cardiac catheterization may reveal raised LV end diastolic pressure and pulmonary hypertension.

RVEMF: These cases develop features of RV inflow tract obstruction resulting in back pressure in the right atrium which dilates to aneurysmal levels. Tricuspid incompetence may develop. The patients present with long duration of fatigue and abdominal distension due to hepatomegaly and ascites. Long-standing cases may develop cardiac cirrhosis. Ascitic fluid shows high protein content. Physical examination reveals rise in jugular venous pressure (JVP), loud third heart sound and features of tricuspid regurgitation. AF, thromboembolism, pericardial effusion and cardiac cirrhosis may develop as complications (Fig. 128.4).

Box 128.1: Classification of restrictive cardiomyopathy

Noninfiltrative
- Idiopathic
- Scleroderma
- Diabetic cardiomyopathy
- Pseudoxanthoma elasticum (PXE)

Specific heart muscle disease
- Endomyocardial fibrosis (EMF)
- Eosinophilic endomyocarditis
- Infiltrative
  - Amyloidosis: Common
  - Sarcoidosis: Common
  - Hemochromatosis (dilated left ventricle with restrictive physiology): Rare
  - Glycogen storage disease: Rare
  - Fatty infiltration

Malignancy
- Metastatic endocardial and myocardial infiltration
- Carcinoid heart disease

Iatrogenic
- Following heart transplantation
- Following mediastinal radiation
- Drugs: Anthracyclines and drugs causing fibrous endocarditis (serotonin, methysergide, ergotamine, etc.)

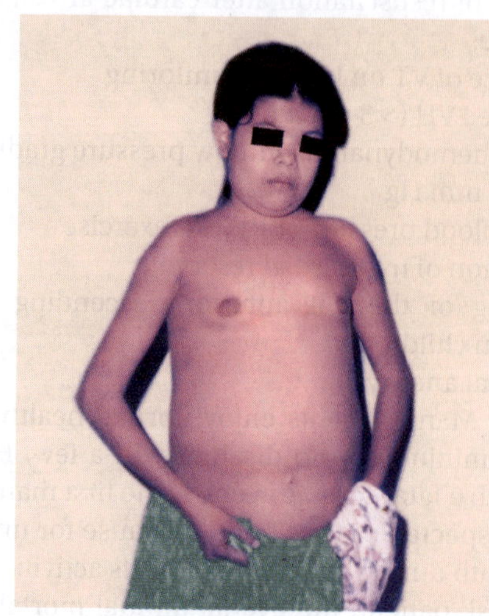

Fig. 128.4: 18-year-old female with endomyocardial fibrosis

ECG may show QR pattern in right precordial leads, indicating right atrial enlargement (RAE). Chest X-ray reveals gross cardiomegaly, mainly due to the aneurysmal RA (Fig. 128.5).

Echocardiography is diagnostic, with the RV cavity obliteration, dimpling of the apex, outflow dilation and huge RAE. RV end diastolic pressure is increased.

Differential diagnosis includes other forms of cardiomyopathy, pericardial diseases, infiltrative lesions of the myocardium and valvular heart disease. Biopsy studies help to exclude infiltrative diseases.

Treatment: Treatment is symptomatic. Measures to control CHF using diuretics and inotropes help to relieve symptoms in early cases. Surgical excision of endocardium, valve replacement, etc. has been tried in selected cases.

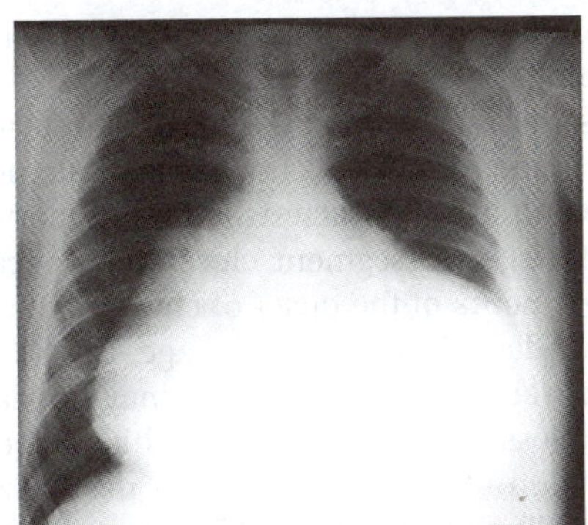

Fig. 128.5: Chest X-ray in right ventricular EMF showing gross cardiomegaly and enlarged right atrium

Abbrevitation: EMF = Endomyocardial fibrosis

CHAPTER
129

Diseases of the Pericardium

CG Bahuleyan, K Suresh

Diseases of the Pericardium

Chapter Summary

- General Considerations
- Acute Pericarditis
- Pericardial Effusion and Tamponade
- Pericardial Aspiration
- Constrictive Pericarditis

GENERAL CONSIDERATIONS

The pericardium is the serous membrane covering heart and root of the great vessels. The visceral layer is closely apposed to the heart and parietal layer encloses the pericardial space which contains a thin film of fluid which lubricates the surfaces. Function of the pericardium is to keep the heart in position and allow smooth and controlled movements within thorax.

ACUTE PERICARDITIS

Acute fibrinous or dry pericarditis is a syndrome, resulting from pericardial inflammation of no more than 1–2 weeks duration and characterized by typical chest pain, a pathognomonic pericardial friction rub and specific electrocardiography (ECG) changes. A variety of conditions are associated with acute pericarditis. However, the majority of cases are idiopathic, i.e. no specific etiology could be identified with routine diagnostic testing. Most such cases are due to viral etiology.

Causes

- ***Idiopathic***
- ***Infections***
  - Viral infections, e.g. Coxsackie B
  - Bacterial infections, e.g. rheumatic fever, tuberculosis, Pneumococci, Staphylococci, Streptococci, Salmonellae, *Actinomyces, Nocardia*
  - Protozoal, e.g. *Entamoeba histolytica, Toxoplasma.* In tropical countries, amebic liver abscess may give rise to pericarditis and effusion.
  - Fungal, e.g. histoplasmosis
- ***Connective tissue disorders***
  - Disseminated lupus erythematosus
  - Rheumatoid disease
  - Scleroderma
  - Polyarteritis nodosa (PAN)
- ***Myocardial infarction (MI)***
- ***Immune-mediated disorders:*** Postmyocardial infarction and postcardiotomy syndromes
- ***Traumatic:*** Blunt injury to chest, penetrating injuries, following paracentesis of pericardium.
- ***Metabolic disorders:*** Uremia, myxedema
- ***Malignancy:*** Leukemias, lymphomas, secondary deposits from the primary tumors
- ***Other causes:*** Rupture of aortic aneurysm, dissecting aneurysm of the aorta, irradiation, cardiomyopathy.

Clinical Features

Acute pericarditis typically produces sharp retrosternal pain that radiates to the trapezius ridge and is aggravated by lying down and relieved by sitting up; its onset frequently is heralded by a prodrome of fever, malaise, and myalgia. The pain of pericarditis is often worse with inspiration and is difficult to distinguish from pleurisy. The hallmark of acute pericarditis is the pericardial friction rub. It has a superficial, creaky, or scratchy character. It is usually heard between the lower left sternal edge and the cardiac apex with patient leaning forward. Pericardial rub usually has three components—during ventricular systole, during ventricular diastolic filling and during atrial systole, resulting in a triphasic rub. Sometimes, it may be monophasic, with only the systolic component or it may be biphasic.

ECG is the most important diagnostic test in acute pericarditis. The ST-T wave changes in acute pericarditis are diffuse and have characteristic evolutionary changes. In the first stage, ST-segment elevations typically occur within a few hours of the onset of chest pain and persist for hours or days. In the second stage, the ST-segments return to baseline and the T waves may appear normal or exhibit a loss of amplitude. In the third stage, tracings show inversion of T waves. The ECG normalizes in the fourth stage. The occurrence of ST-elevation and T wave inversion at the same time is uncommon. The ECG is a very important and reliable tool to distinguish between acute MI and acute pericarditis. In uncomplicated acute pericarditis, the chest radiograph is generally normal. An enlarged cardiac silhouette may occur because of a moderate or large pericardial effusion. Echocardiographic identification of pericardial effusion confirms the clinical diagnosis of acute pericarditis, but a patient with purely fibrinous acute pericarditis often has a normal echocardiogram.

Diagnosis

Acute pericarditis has to be suspected when a patient gets chest pain associated with other signs of infections such as fever and other general symptoms. Fever and signs of infection arise before or along with pericardial findings in pericarditis whereas in MI in which pericarditis can occur as a complication, the pain and features of MI precede the development of pericardial rub and effusion. Serological markers of MI will help to distinguish the two conditions.

Treatment

Acute idiopathic pericarditis is a self-limiting disease in 70–90% of individuals. Symptomatic patients should be treated with nonsteroidal anti-inflammatory drugs (NSAIDs). Aspirin 650 mg q4h or ibuprofen 600–800 mg q6h are the commonly used drugs. Narcotic analgesics may be required for severe pain. Those who do not respond to NSAIDs may require steroid therapy (prednisolone 60–80 mg/day) for a week to control pain, with the dose tapered rapidly thereafter. Colchicine is also found to be effective in severe cases. Patients in whom pericarditis is a manifestation of systemic illness, such as sepsis, uremia, connective tissue disease (CTDs), or neoplasia, in addition to symptomatic treatment, therapy directed towards the primary disorder is required. But in post-MI pericarditis, aspirin is preferred as NSAIDs and steroids may interfere with healing process. If symptoms of pericardial tamponade develop, aspiration will be required.

PERICARDIAL EFFUSION AND TAMPONADE

Accumulation of transudate, exudate, or blood in the pericardial sac is a common complication of pericardial disease and should be sought in all patients with acute pericarditis. Idiopathic pericarditis and any infection, neoplasm, autoimmune diseases and radiation, which can cause acute pericarditis, can cause pericardial effusion. Effusions are common after cardiac surgery.

Hydropericardium can occur in severe cardiac failure. Bleeding into the pericardial sac (hemopericardium) can occur following blunt or penetrating chest trauma and due to cardiac rupture in post-MI patients. Those effusions with high chance of progression to tamponade are caused by bacterial, fungal and human immunodeficiency virus (HIV) associated infections.

Clinical manifestations of pericardial effusion are highly dependent upon the rate of accumulation of fluid in the pericardial sac. Rapid accumulation of pericardial fluid may cause elevated intrapericardial pressures with as little as 80 cc of fluid, while slowly progressing effusions can grow to 2 L without symptoms.

When sufficient amount of pericardial fluid accumulates, it can increase the intrapericardial pressure, cause obstruction to inflow of blood into the ventricles, fall in cardiac output and result in cardiac tamponade. In cases of trauma, rapid accumulation of small quantity of blood can cause tamponade, while in cases of chronic effusions large quantity of fluid accumulates before tamponade develops.

Clinical Features

Many patients with pericardial effusion also have pericardial pain. However, effusions do not by themselves cause symptoms unless tamponade is present. Patients with tamponade may develop dyspnea. They also have chest tightness and dizziness. In the most severe cases, consciousness may be impaired and except for the raised venous pressure, such patients appear to be in hypovolemic shock.

A careful general examination in case of pericardial effusion may give clue to the etiology. In effusions without tamponade, cardiovascular examination is normal, except in very large effusions where the cardiac impulse is difficult to palpate and heart sounds are muffled. If tamponade is present, patient will be uncomfortable with dyspnea, tachypnea, diaphoresis, cold extremities, peripheral cyanosis and depressed sensorium, due to low cardiac output (Fig. 129.1). Tachycardia is the rule. Hypotension is usually present. A paradoxical pulse is present in most cases. Paradoxical pulse is the exaggerated inspiratory fall

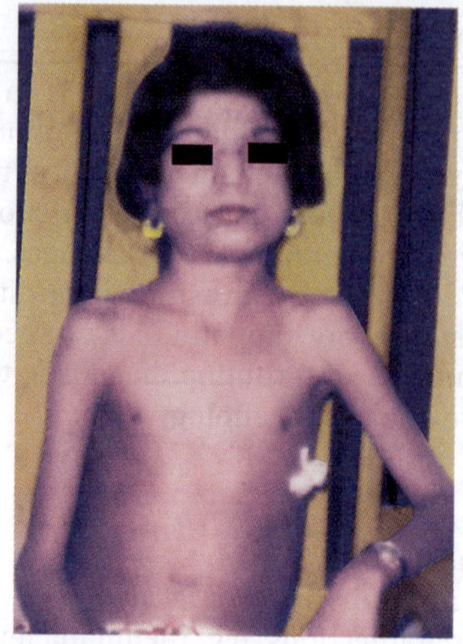

Fig. 129.1: 14-years-old female with chronic pericardial effusion. The cotton seal is over the site of aspiration

in systolic blood pressure (BP), often exceeding 10 mm Hg. Jugular venous pressure (JVP) is markedly elevated and Y descent is absent. Normal decrease in venous pressure on inspiration is maintained. Physical examination reveals reduced force or absence of the apical impulse, enlargement of the area of cardiac dullness, muffled heart sounds and pericardial rub. The elevated JVP, muffled heart sound and hypotension constitute classical **Beck's triad** in acute cardiac tamponade.

Diagnosis

ECG usually shows sinus tachycardia, reduced voltage and sometimes, electrical alternans of the QRS complex. In chest X-ray, cardiac silhouette assumes a flask-like appearance in moderate to large effusions (Fig. 129.2).

Echocardiography is the procedure of choice for diagnosis of pericardial effusion. Pericardial effusion appears as an *echo-free* space between the visceral and parietal pericardium. Early diastolic collapse of right atrium (RA) and right ventricle (RV) seen in echo indicate presence of tamponade (Fig. 129.3). If a definite etiology is not evident by noninvasive testing, pericardiocentesis is required.

Management

In pericardial effusions without tamponade, the aim is to establish the etiology by a careful history including

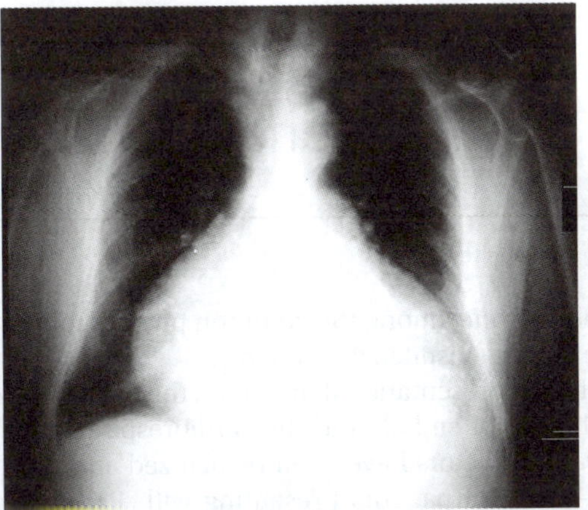

Fig. 129.2: Chest X-ray in pericardial effusion showing flask-shaped enlargement of heart and stenciled appearance of cardiac borders

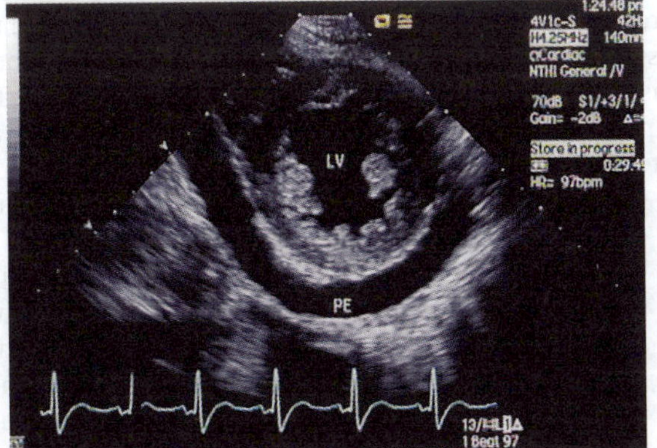

Fig. 129.3: 2D–echocardiographic picture of PE which is seen as echo-free space behind the LV.

Abbreviations: LV = Left ventricle; PE = Pericardial effusion

medication review and radiation therapy, general physical examination and investigations. Depending on the circumstances, the investigations should include, skin testing for tuberculosis, screening for neoplastic and autoimmune diseases, infections and hypothyroidism. Drainage of the pericardial effusion is usually unnecessary unless purulent pericarditis is suspected or cardiac tamponade supervenes.

PERICARDIAL ASPIRATION

Those patients with tamponade should be considered as having a medical emergency. Volume expansion should be done with blood, plasma, dextran, or isotonic sodium chloride solution, as necessary to maintain adequate intravascular (IV) volume. Removal of pericardial fluid is the definitive therapy for tamponade. Removal of small amounts of pericardial fluid (~50 mL) produces considerable symptomatic and hemodynamic improvement. Most commonly employed method for closed pericardiocentesis is the subxiphoid approach. A 16- or 18-gauge needle is inserted at an angle of 30–45° to the skin, near the left xiphocostal angle, aiming towards the left shoulder. Surgical creation of a pericardial window, which involves the surgical opening of a communication between the pericardial space and the intrapleural space, is sometimes required in recurrent effusions.

CONSTRICTIVE PERICARDITIS

It is a condition in which a thickened, scarred and often, calcified pericardium forms a tough cover around the heart limiting diastolic filling of the ventricles. Although acute pericarditis from most causes may eventuate in constrictive pericarditis, the most common causes are idiopathic conditions, cardiac trauma and surgery, tuberculosis and other infectious diseases, neoplasms (particularly lung and breast), radiation therapy, renal failure and CTDs. Rare causes include Dressler's syndrome, sarcoidosis, Whipple's disease, amyloidosis, methysergide therapy and dermatomyositis.

Patients generally complain of fatigue, dyspnea, weight gain, abdominal discomfort, nausea, increased abdominal girth and edema. Physical findings include ascites, hepatosplenomegaly, edema and, in long-standing cases, severe wasting. This general appearance often leads to an erroneous diagnosis of hepatic cirrhosis. Misdiagnosis is avoided through a careful examination of the neck veins. In constrictive pericarditis, the venous pressure is elevated and displays deep Y and often deep X descents. Kussmaul's sign is usually present. Often the heart is normal-sized. Infrequently, a pericardial knock can be detected on auscultation. Since, the myocardium is unaffected, early ventricular filling during the first-third of diastole is unimpeded. Accordingly, the ventricular pressure initially decreases rapidly (producing a steep Y descent on RA pressure waveform tracings) and then increases abruptly to a level that is sustained until systole (the dip-and-plateau waveform or square root sign seen on right or left ventricular pressure waveform tracings).

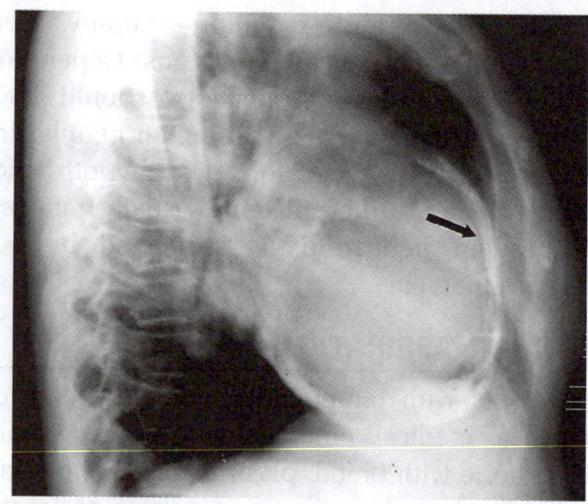

Fig. 129.4: X-ray chest lateral view in constrictive pericarditis showing calcification around the cardiac silhouette (arrow)

ECG will show atrial fibrillation (AF) in approximately one-third of cases. Low QRS voltage, nonspecific T wave changes, and P mitrale are common. Chest X-ray usually shows normal or mildly enlarged cardiac silhouette. Pericardial calcification may be present, best seen in lateral view (Fig. 129.4). Echocardiographic findings of thickened pericardium and abnormal Doppler flow patterns can point to the diagnosis of constriction. Computed tomography (CT) is a highly accurate method of evaluating pericardial thickness and therefore plays an essential role in the diagnosis and management of constrictive disease. Because of the close physiologic similarities of constrictive pericarditis and restrictive cardiomyopathy, increased pericardial thickness detected by CT scan is the most reliable means of distinguishing between the two disorders, as normal pericardial thickness excludes most cases of constrictive pericarditis.

Treatment

Medical therapy in constrictive pericarditis plays only a small role. In some patients, constrictive pericarditis resolves either spontaneously or in response to various combinations of NSAIDs, antituberculous drugs, steroids and antibiotics. Digoxin is useful in patients with AF who are not fit candidates for pericardiectomy. Diuretics can be used but cautiously. In general, beta-blockers and calcium channel blockers are avoided.

Pericardiectomy is the definitive treatment for constrictive pericarditis. Surgery is not indicated in very early stages of constriction or in severe, advanced disease (functional class IV), when the risk of surgery is excessive.

CHAPTER
130

Pulmonary Embolism

A George Koshy, K Suresh

Chapter Summary

- General Considerations
- Risk Factors for Venous Thromboembolism
- Clinical Features
- Investigations
- Management

GENERAL CONSIDERATIONS

(Also Refer to Section 15, Ch 176)

Pulmonary embolism (PE) is obstruction of the main pulmonary arteries or one of its branches by any substance that has traveled from elsewhere in the body through the venous system and the bloodstream. More than three-fourth of cases arise from the embolization of blood clots formed in the deep veins of the legs—iliofemoral and pelvic veins. Deep vein thrombosis (DVT) and PE are considered as a continuum and are collectively described by the term—venous thromboembolism (VTE). Rare causes include fat, air and amniotic fluid embolism and septic embolization from the right-sided valves and other foci in infective endocarditis and tumor embolization. The exact incidence is unknown, but it is a still underdiagnosed entity despite of increased awareness in modern times. At least 5% of in-hospital deaths are contributed by PE. This is probably one among the common preventable cause of death among hospitalized patients.

Clinical presentation depends on the number, size and distribution of emboli and the cardiorespiratory reserve. Several risk factors have been recognized and more than three-fourth of patients presenting with PE will have at least one risk factor.

RISK FACTORS FOR VENOUS THROMBOEMBOLISM

Virchow's triad (stagnation of blood, abnormalities in the vessel wall and factors affecting the properties of the blood) classically describes the three factors that lead to VTE. The important risk factors and predisposing conditions are listed as follows:

- ***Surgery and prolonged immobilization:*** Hip and knee surgery, major abdominal and pelvic surgery
- Procoagulant state associated with pregnancy, puerperium or the use of estrogens and oral contraceptives
- ***Genetic causes of thrombophilia:*** Factor V Leiden abnormality, protein C and protein S deficiency, antithrombin deficiency, hyperhomocysteinemia and others
- ***Acquired thrombophilia:*** Antiphospholipid antibody (APLA) syndrome, paroxysmal nocturnal hemoglobinuria

- Malignant disease
- Congestive heart failure and chronic obstructive pulmonary disease (COPD)
- Stroke and spinal cord surgery
- Increasing age, obesity
- Previous history of VTE
- Hemoconcentration and polycythemias.

CLINICAL FEATURES

Several distinct patterns of clinical presentations have been recognized. These include massive, submassive and small PE and chronic thromboembolic pulmonary hypertension.

Massive PE: At least half of the pulmonary vascular bed is involved and the patient is in hypotension and heart failure. Patients are prone for multisystem organ failure including renal and hepatic dysfunction. It can lead to loss of consciousness and sometimes sudden cardiac death. Acute onset dyspnea is the most striking symptom and patients are tachypneic and cyanosed when seen initially.

Submassive PE: One-third to half of the pulmonary vascular bed is involved and the patient develops right heart failure with elevated jugular venous pressure (JVP). Normal systemic arterial pressure (SAP) is maintained unlike in massive PE. Serum troponins as well as brain natriuretic peptide (BNP) are usually elevated in both massive and submassive PE.

Small to moderate PE: Less than one-third of the pulmonary vascular bed is involved and the patient has preserved right ventricular (RV) function and preserved hemodynamics. The blood pressure (BP) is maintained and the serum biomarkers are negative. RV function is normal.

Symptoms and signs of PE have been shown in Table 130.1.

Chronic thromboembolic pulmonary hypertension: Chronic recurrent small PE causes progressive occlusion of the pulmonary microvasculature leading to pulmonary arterial hypertension and eventually right heart failure. If the embolus lodges in the peripheral pulmonary arterial tree near the pleura, it can lead to pulmonary infarction. This is characterized by pleuritic chest pain and hemoptysis. It can be accompanied by fever, leukocytosis and elevated erythrocyte sedimentation rate (ESR).

Tachypnea is the most common sign in PE. Clinical examination will reveal hypotension and distended neck veins in massive PE. Despite dyspnea, chest will appear clear. Pulmonary component of second heart sound is accentuated indicating pulmonary hypertension.

Table 130.1: Symptoms and signs of pulmonary embolism

Symptoms	Signs
• Dyspnea	• Tachycardia
• Cough	• Tachypnea
• Substernal chest pain	• Crackles
• Sweating	• Wheezes
• Syncope	• Jugular venous pressure (JVP) elevated
• Hemoptysis	• Right ventricular (RV) gallop
• Later pleuritic pain	• Loud pulmonic second sound

INVESTIGATIONS

Chest Radiography

It is useful in ruling out other clinical conditions like pneumothorax, pneumonia and pulmonary edema which can mimic PE. Positive radiological findings in PE include focal oligemia *(Westermark's sign)*, a peripheral wedge-shaped density above the diaphragm *(Hampton's hump)* and an enlarged right descending pulmonary artery *(Palla's sign)*. Chest X-ray may show a wedge-shaped shadow suggestive of pulmonary infarction, but often chest X-ray is unremarkable even in massive PE (Fig. 130.1).

Electrocardiography (ECG)

The usual findings include sinus tachycardia, right axis deviation, right bundle branch block (RBBB), ST-depression and T-inversion in RV leads (V1–V3) indicative of RV strain and appearance of terminal S wave in lead I and Q wave with T-inversion in lead III ($S_1Q_3T_3$) (Fig. 130.2). T is usually upright in lead II. Supraventricular arrhythmias can occur. ECG is helpful in excluding other conditions like acute myocardial infarction (acute MI) and pericarditis simulating PE.

Echocardiography (ECHO)

Bedside ECHO can reveal dilated right atrium, RV and pulmonary arteries in those with massive and submassive

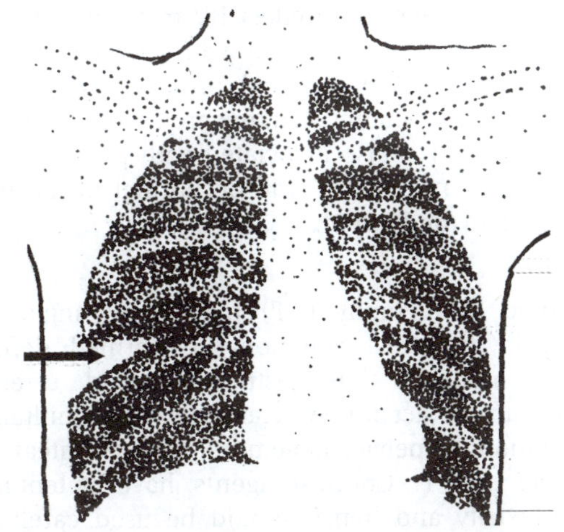

Fig. 130.1: Chest X-ray: Pulmonary infarct. ***Note:*** The triangular opacity with the base towards the pleura (arrow)

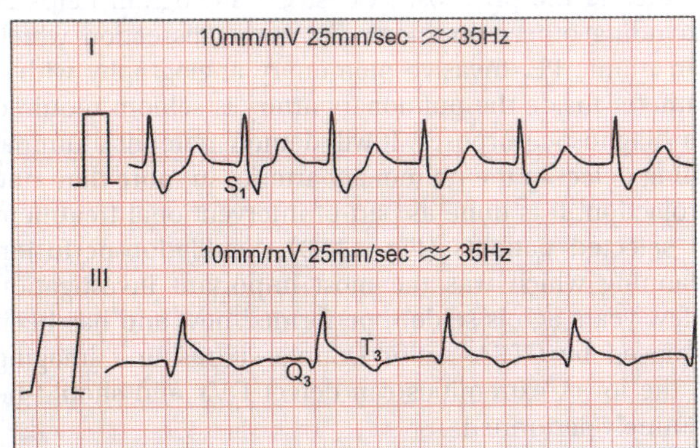

Fig. 130.2: Acute pulmonary embolism: ECG showing sinus tachycardia and the classical $S_1Q_3T_3$ pattern

Courtesy: Professor George Koshy

PE. Tricuspid regurgitation can be detected and quantified by Doppler studies. Hypokinesia of the RV free wall can be identified often with preserved contractility of the apical region (***McConnell's sign***). ECHO is useful in excluding other cardiovascular causes for chest pain and dyspnea like acute MI, LV failure, pericarditis and aortic dissection.

Arterial Blood Gases

Reduced arterial partial pressure of oxygen (PaO_2), normal or reduced arterial partial pressure of carbon dioxide ($PaCO_2$) and an increased alveolar arterial oxygen gradient are the typical findings. Those with acute massive PE and cardiovascular collapse will show metabolic acidosis.

Biomarkers

D-dimer is a specific degradation product released into the circulation when cross-linked fibrin undergoes endogenous fibrinolysis. It is elevated both in DVT as well as in PE. Elevated D-dimer is not specific for VTE as it is elevated in a variety of conditions including MI, sepsis and pneumonia. It can also be elevated in the second and third trimester of pregnancy and also in the postoperative state. However, it is very sensitive in excluding diagnosis of PE. A value below 500 ng/mL measured by enzyme-linked immunosorbent assay (ELISA) practically rules out PE in low-risk individuals. It is not useful in evaluation of high-risk individuals with high probability of PE who anyway require further investigations. Serum troponin T and troponin I elevation reflect RV microinfarction and dysfunction and is associated with adverse outcome. Elevated BNP and N-terminal pro-BNP (NT-proBNP) which are hemodynamic markers are correlated with RV dysfunction and is also associated with poor prognosis. Serum troponin and BNP will be normal in those with acute small to medium PE.

Imaging

Computed tomography (CT) pulmonary angiography (CTPA) is the most commonly performed definitive imaging modality. The distribution and extent of emboli can be accurately characterized. Simultaneous visualization of pelvic, iliofemoral and popliteal veins can detect DVT. Contrast agents have potential for nephrotoxicity and hence should be used carefully in those with renal impairment. Assessment of RV size and function is also possible with CTPA and helps in predicting the prognosis. Chest CT angiogram helps in excluding other conditions like aortic dissection which can mimic PE. Invasive pulmonary angiography with a catheter inside the pulmonary artery is seldom required for diagnostic purposes. It will demonstrate intraluminal filling defect in the pulmonary arteries in more than one projection. It is done as part of interventional treatment in selected patients (Fig. 130.3). Ventilation-perfusion scanning which was the most important investigation a few years ago is seldom performed now and has been replaced by CTPA. Color Doppler ultrasound imaging of the lower extremities can detect DVT and should be routinely performed.

Lung Scan Findings

Isotope lung scan is a useful investigation to demonstrate segmental perfusion defects (Fig. 130.4).

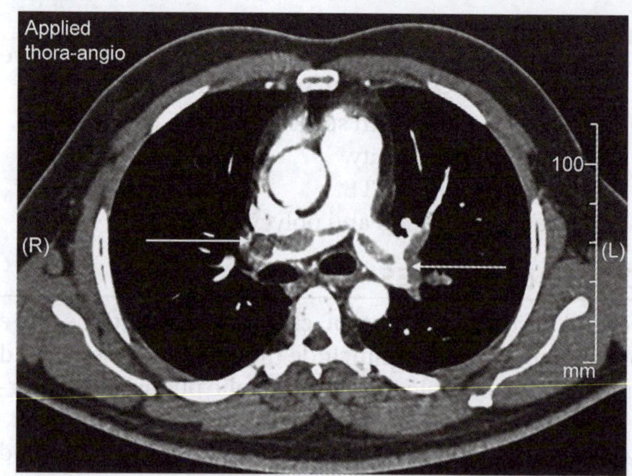

Fig. 130.3: Acute pulmonary embolism—CT. PA showing filling defect in both right and left pulmonary artery branches suggestive of thrombus (arrows)

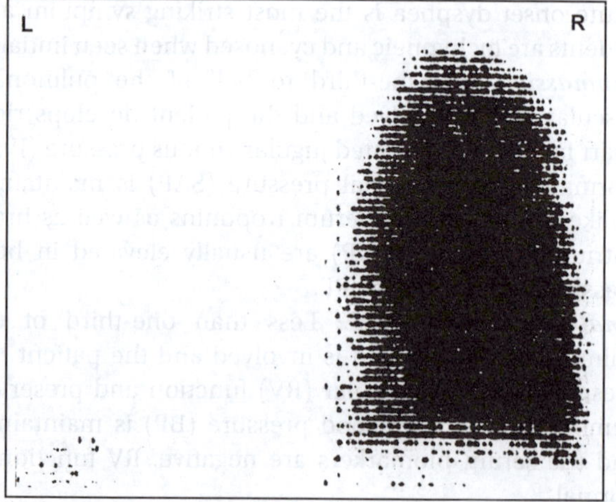

Fig. 130.4: Scintiscan pulmonary embolism. ***Note:*** The isotope does not reach the affected side (left side)

MANAGEMENT

General Measures

Oxygen administration to all hypoxemic patients to maintain arterial oxygen saturation above 90%. Hypotension and shock should be corrected by intravenous (IV) fluids and plasma expanders. Inotropic agents may be required in those who remain in hypotension and shock, but they are seldom useful. Diuretics and vasodilators should generally be avoided.

Thrombolytic Therapy

It is the first-line treatment in patients with high-risk PE presenting with cardiogenic shock and/or persistent arterial hypotension. It rapidly resolves thromboembolic obstruction and exerts beneficial effects on hemodynamic parameters. This is reflected as an increase in cardiac index and a fall in pulmonary artery pressure. The absolute contraindications for thrombolytic therapy include hemorrhagic stroke or stroke of unknown origin at any time, ischemic stroke in preceding 6 months, central nervous system neoplasms, recent major trauma, surgery or head injury (within preceding 3 weeks) and gastrointestinal bleeding within the last month. The relative contraindications include transient ischemic attack in preceding 6 months, oral anticoagulant therapy, pregnancy or within 1-week postpartum, noncompressible punctures, traumatic resuscitation, uncontrolled hypertension (systolic BP above 180 mm Hg), advanced liver disease, infective endocarditis and active peptic ulcer. Routine use of thrombolysis in non high-risk patients is not recommended. Those with cardiogenic shock derive the maximum benefit. Those with ECHO evidence of RV dilatation and hypokinesia of the free wall can also be administered thrombolytic therapy even in the absence of hypotension. Streptokinase can be given as 250,000 IU as a loading dose, followed by 100,000 IU/hour infusion for 12–24 hours. The infusion can be administered for longer periods up to 48 hours. Recently, accelerated regimen of streptokinase of 1.5 million units diluted in 100 mL normal saline administered over a period of 2 hours has been found to be more effective. IV urokinase as well as fibrin-specific agents like tPA and tenecteplase can also be given. Urokinase is administered as 4,400 IU/kg as a loading dose over 10 minutes followed by 4,400 IU/kg/hour infusion. Urokinase can also be given as an accelerated regimen of 3 million units over 2 hours. Recombinant tissue-type plasminogen activator (rtPA) can be given in a dose of 100 mg over 2 hours. Alternatively 0.6 mg/kg over 15 minutes (maximum of 50 mg) can also be given. Tenecteplase is also used in PE. Thrombolytic therapy is associated with approximately 5–8% risk of major bleed and 1–2% risk of intracranial or fatal bleed. More than 90% of patients can be classified as responders to thrombolysis based on clinical and ECHO improvement within the first 36 hours. The greatest benefit is observed when treatment is initiated within 48 hours of symptom onset but thrombolysis can still be useful in patients who have had symptoms for 6–14 days.

Surgical and Catheter-based Techniques

Pulmonary embolectomy is a valuable therapeutic option in patients with high-risk PE in whom thrombolysis is absolutely contraindicated or has failed. Percutaneous catheter embolectomy or fragmentation of proximal pulmonary arterial clots may be considered as an alternative to surgical treatment in high-risk PE patients in experienced centers. This is especially, useful in those who are at high risk for surgery (Fig. 130.5).

Initial Anticoagulation

It is the cornerstone in the treatment of VTE. Rapid anticoagulation can only be achieved with parenteral anticoagulants such as IV unfractionated heparin (UFH), subcutaneous low-molecular-weight heparin (LMWH) or subcutaneous fondaparinux. Considering the high-mortality rate in untreated patients, anticoagulant treatment should be considered in all patients with suspected PE while awaiting definitive diagnostic confirmation. Treatment with parenteral anticoagulants is usually followed by the administration of oral anticoagulants vitamin K antagonists (VKAs). If IV UFH is given, a weight-adjusted regimen of 80 U/kg as a bolus injection (maximum of 5,000 U) followed by infusion at the rate of 18 U/kg/hour should be preferred to fixed

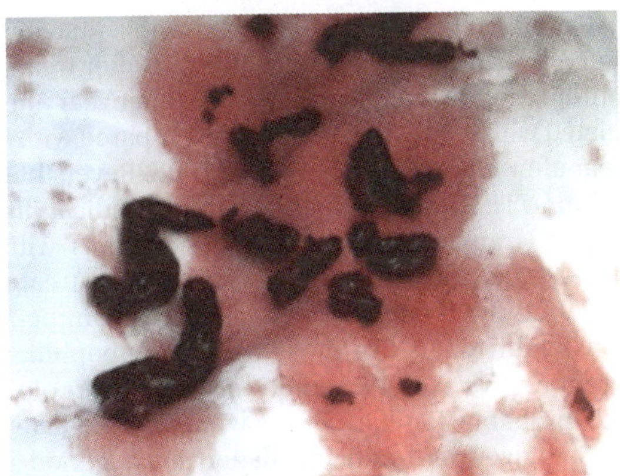

Fig. 130.5: Acute pulmonary embolism: Thrombus obtained from pulmonary arteries after surgical pulmonary embolectomy
Courtesy: Professor George Koshy

dosages of heparin. Subsequent doses of UFH should be adjusted using an activated partial thromboplastin time (aPTT)-based nomogram. The aPTT should be measured 4–6 hours after the bolus injection and then 3 hours after each dose adjustment and should be maintained between 1.5 to 2.5 times control. LMWH and fondaparinux can also be used. LMWH has several advantages over conventional unfractionated heparin. It has better bioavailability, can be administered subcutaneously twice a day and does not generally require monitoring. Enoxaparin is given in a dose of 1 mg/kg (maximum of 60 mg) twice daily. LMWH should be avoided in those with renal impairment. It is better to give LMWH for at least 5 days. Because of the risk of heparin induced thrombocytopenia (HIT), monitoring of the platelet count is necessary during treatment with UFH or LMWH. As fondaparinux does not lead to HIT, routine monitoring of platelet count may not be required. Except for patients at high risk of bleeding and those with severe renal dysfunction, subcutaneous LMWH or fondaparinux rather than IV UFH should be considered for initial treatment. UFH is preferred in high-risk patients who are in shock. Oral anticoagulant usually warfarin is started along with heparin or within the initial 1–3 days. It is discontinued once prothrombin time international normalized ratio (INR) is more than 2. The initial recommended dose of warfarin is 5 mg/day. The INR should be maintained in the therapeutic range of 2–3.

Long-term Anticoagulation for Secondary Prophylaxis

The long-term anticoagulant treatment of patients with PE is aimed at preventing fatal and non-fatal recurrent VTE events. VKAs are used in the vast majority of patients, while LMWH may be an effective and safe alternative to VKAs in cancer patients. VKAs should be given at doses adjusted to maintain a target INR of 2.5 (range 2.0–3.0). The duration of anticoagulation is decided based on the clinical context. Active cancer is a major risk factor for recurrence of VTE, the rate of recurrence being about 20% during the initial year after the index event. Therefore, cancer patients are candidates for indefinite anticoagulant treatment after a first episode of PE. LMWH is probably more effective than oral anticoagulants and hence is preferred at least for the initial 6 months. Follow-up of patients with a first episode of acute PE found that the recurrence rate after treatment discontinuation was approximately 2.5% per year after PE associated with reversible risk factors compared with 4.5% per year after idiopathic (unprovoked) PE. Reversible risk factors for VTE include surgery, trauma, medical illness, estrogen therapy and pregnancy. For patients with PE secondary to a transient reversible risk factor, treatment with a VKA for 3 months is generally recommended. High-risk individuals like those with thrombophilia and recurrent unprovoked PE should receive it for prolonged period, probably for life. Those with intermediate risk should be given oral anticoagulation for a period of at least 6 months. Newer anticoagulants with no need for laboratory monitoring and dose adjustment are currently being evaluated for long-term management of PE. Dabigatran is a selective thrombin inhibitor. Rivaroxaban and apixaban are factor Xa inhibitors.

Venous Filters

Inferior vena cava (IVC) filters may be used when there are absolute contraindications to anticoagulation and a high risk of recurrence of VTE. But routine use of IVC filters in PE is not recommended. Filters are usually placed in the infrarenal portion of the IVC. If thrombus is identified in the IVC below the renal veins, it may have to be placed more superiorly. Permanent and retrievable devices are available. Common complication is thrombosis involving the device.

Prevention

Pulmonary embolism is the most preventable cause of in-hospital mortality. Early ambulation and low fixed dose anticoagulant prophylaxis are certainly helpful in reducing PE. Low dose of heparin, usually LMWH, is used for this purpose. Intermittent pneumatic compression devices reduce the risk of DVT by almost 50%.

CHAPTER
131

Diseases of the Aorta

N Sudhayakumar

> **Chapter Summary**
> - Anatomy
> - Aortic Diseases
> - Aneurysms of Aorta
> - Dissecting Aneurysms of Aorta
> - Aneurysms of Sinuses of Valsalva
> - Cholesterol Crystal Embolism

ANATOMY

The largest and strongest artery of the human body, **aorta**, allows the flow of about 200 million liters of blood in one's lifetime. It extends from its origin at the aortic annulus in the thorax to its bifurcation into the two common iliac arteries in the mid-abdomen. Basically, it is divided into thoracic and abdominal aorta (Fig. 131.1). The thoracic part is subdivided into ascending aorta, aortic arch and descending segments; the ascending aorta (AAo) having two parts: (1) aortic root (from the annulus to the sinotubular junction) and (2) tubular segment (from the sinotubular junction to the arch). Aortic root is the widest part of aorta measuring about 3.5 cm in adults and it contains three pouches called sinuses of Valsalva; two of the sinuses which give origin to the two coronaries are called **coronary sinuses** (left and right) and the third is the **noncoronary sinus**. Structurally, aorta has three layers: (1) Intima, (2) media and (3) adventitia.

AORTIC DISEASES

The common pathology involving aorta is atherosclerosis. Other pathologies include infections and inflammations,

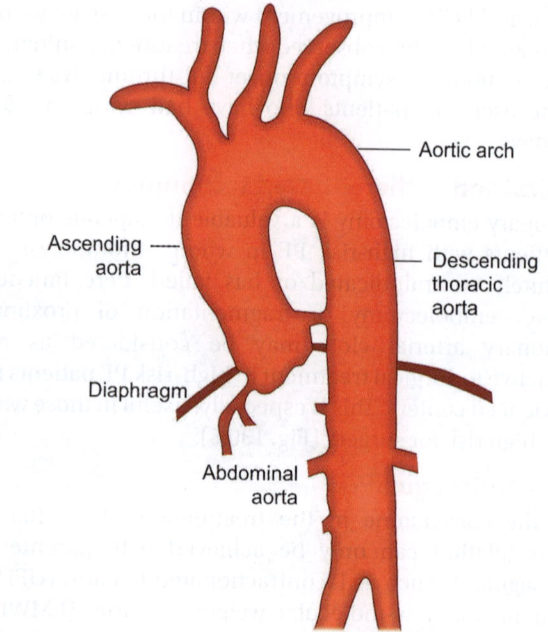

Fig. 131.1: Anatomy of aorta

degenerative changes, trauma, tumors, etc. However, the most dreaded complication is dissection of aorta. An inflammatory process involving the aorta and its major branches may occur as a primary abnormality as in Takayasu arteritis or it may occur in association with conditions such as connective tissue disorders, Hodgkin's disease or infections—bacterial or viral.

Takayasu's Arteritis

Syn: Pulseless disease, young female arteritis, reversed coarctation

(Refer also to Section 12, Ch 110 and Section 16, Ch 187)

This condition is named after Japanese ophthalmologist who first described changes in the central vessels of the retina in 1905. Women are affected eight times more than men. More than half the patients are under 20 years of age. The disease is prevalent in India, Japan, southeast Asia, South and East Africa, South America and Mexico. Aorto arteritis is the common form of large vessel vasculitis. It is also one of the causes for renovascular hypertension (RVHT).

Takayasu's disease is a chronic vasculitis involving mainly the aorta and its large branches such as the brachiocephalic, carotid, subclavian, vertebral and renal arteries as well as the coronary and pulmonary arteries. The etiology is not fully known, though tuberculosis has been strongly considered. Symptoms are caused by stenotic lesions or thrombus formation. More acute progression leads to destruction of the media and consequent aneurysm formation and arterial rupture.

Pathology

The disease courses through three stages: (1) An active inflammatory phase, (2) quiescent phase and (3) fibrotic phase. The histological findings include polyarteritis, fibrous scarring, intimal proliferation, thrombosis and aneurysm resembling syphilitic aortitis (SA), but there is no clinical or serologic evidence to suggest syphilitic etiology even remotely. Current thinking favors an auto-immune process to be operative. In addition to the aorta, arteries of the neck, renal arteries and arteries of the lower limbs are also frequently affected. These may lead to strokes in the young, renal hypertension, limb ischemia and thromboembolic episodes. Based on the distribution of pathology, Takayasu's arteritis is classified as follows:

- *Type I:* It involves proximal aorta, ascending and arch
- *Type II:* It involves descending aorta
- *Type III:* It involves ascending and descending aorta (the most common type)
- *Type IV:* Involvement of pulmonary artery also
- *Type V:* Involvement of coronary arteries also.

Clinical Features

The disease may remain asymptomatic for a long period. The clinical features depend on whether the patients present during the acute inflammatory phase or in the fibrotic phase. The manifestations of the inflammatory phase include fever, myalgia, arthralgia, headache, other constitutional and nonspecific symptoms. Erythrocyte sedimentation rate (ESR) and C-reactive protein (CRP) levels are raised in the early stages. Clinical findings include tenderness of the arteries especially of the head and neck and small tender arterial aneurysms. Rarely, manifestations of myopericarditis may be present.

In the fibrotic phase, the manifestations depend on the arterial system involved. Presenting symptoms may be those of associated hypertension. When the arch and its vessels are involved, symptoms are due to ischemia to the brain and upper extremities such as jaw and upper limb claudication, symptoms of cerebral ischemia and of subclavian steal syndrome. Pulse is absent or feeble in the upper limbs and there is hypertension in the lower extremities (reversed coarctation). Signs of aortic regurgitation (AR) may be present. It is important to look for arterial bruit over major vessels.

Type III aortoarteritis (middle aortic syndrome)

This is the most prevalent type in India, and it involves the ascending and descending aorta. The picture may mimic coarctation of aorta (CoA), but presence of abdominal, subclavian or carotid bruit, asymmetry of blood pressure (BP) in the four limbs, absence of collaterals around the scapula and the lack of rib notching in X-ray suggest the diagnosis of aortoarteritis. Angina pectoris due to coronary arterial involvement, abdominal angina due to mesenteric involvement and pulmonary artery involvement occur uncommonly. Early occurrence of unilateral cataract is often seen in Indian patients. During pregnancy, AR and heart failure may aggravate.

Investigations

During the early inflammatory stage, acute phase reactants like leukocyte count, ESR, CRP, etc. will be elevated. Investigations for tuberculosis as an etiology are also done, but seldom contributory. Diagnosis and typing can be achieved by noninvasive imaging like echocardiography, contrast computed tomography (CT) and magnetic resonance angiography (MRA) (Figs 131.2 and 131.3). Cardiac catheterization and angiography are seldom needed. Positron emission tomography (PET) scan is considered to be highly sensitive to pick up active inflammatory aortitis. The diagnosis and extent of involvement can be confirmed by CT angiography. Echo Doppler studies help in detecting AR and in assessing left ventricular (LV) function. Angiography is required for identifying pulmonary as well as coronary involvement.

Management

Twenty percent remit spontaneously, 75% respond to therapy, short segments of stenosis are treated surgically or by percutaneous intervention.

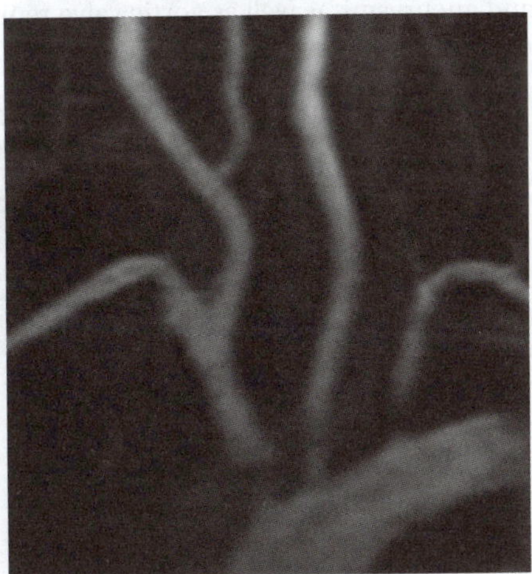

Fig. 131.2: MRA of aortoarteritis showing narrowing of the proximal parts of arch vessels

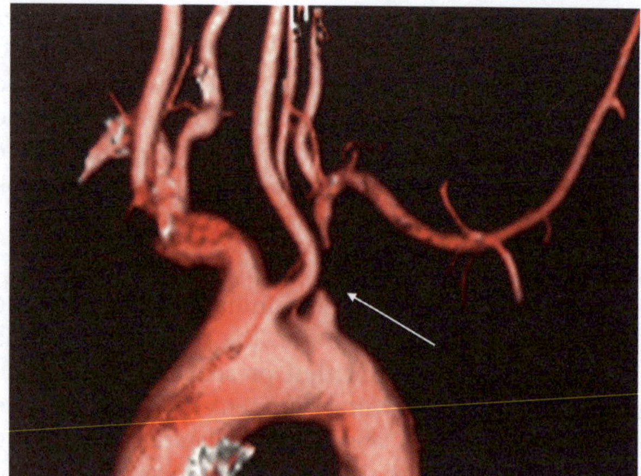

Fig. 131.3: Takayasu's arteritis: Reconstructed CT angiogram showing narrowing and occlusion of the left subclavian artery. This patient presented with left upper limb claudication

Medical therapy

Early institution of steroid therapy and low-dose aspirin have been advocated in the acute inflammatory phase. Most patients with Takayasu's arteritis in the active phase improve with high-dose of steroids, usually prednisolone 1 mg/kg. Long-term maintenance steroid is required and the dose usually, varies between 5 and 20 mg per day. Relapses are common while the steroid dose is tapered. If response is not satisfactory, immunosuppressant drugs like cyclophosphamide and methotrexate are added on to the regimen in selected cases. The results are not uniformly predictable. Monoclonal antibodies like infliximab have been tried in selected cases with partial benefit.

Surgical intervention

In established cases, surgical or percutaneous procedures may have to be considered as palliative measures, especially in localized lesions. Renal artery stenting has been done in cases with severe RVHT, with variable results and high incidence of restenosis. Interventional treatment aimed at relieving the arterial obstruction is useful in several symptomatic patients. Angioplasty and stenting can be done in the subclavian, carotid, renal as well as coronary arteries. Surgical interventions for critical stenosis and aneurysms as well as aortic valve replacement may be required in some patients.

ANEURYSMS OF AORTA

The term aortic aneurysm refers to a pathological dilatation of the aortic lumen involving one or several segments. Aortic aneurysm may be defined as a permanent dilatation of the aorta having a diameter of at least 1.5 times that of the expected normal diameter of that given aortic segment. Morphology of an aortic aneurysm is either fusiform or saccular (Figs 131.4A and B).

Pathogenesis

Elasticity and distensibility of aorta decreases with age resulting in widening of the pulse pressure which leads to progressive dilatation of aorta. Fragmentation of elastin occurs with concomitant increase in collagen; thus, the ratio of collagen to elastin increases with loss of distensibility of aorta.

Seventy-five percent of all aneurysms involve the abdominal aorta and the most common site is below the renal arteries. The vast majority are caused by atherosclerosis. In 60% of cases, there is associated hypertension. Other causes include arteriosclerosis, traumatic false aneurysms, mycotic aneurysms and tertiary syphilis. The most frequent cause of aneurysms of the AAo is cystic medial necrosis secondary to Marfan's syndrome; other causes include atherosclerosis, aortitis, bicuspid aortic valve (BAV), Ehlers-Danlos syndrome and others.

Clinical Features

Majority of aortic aneurysms regardless of their location are asymptomatic. They are discovered accidentally when being evaluated for other diseases. When these aneurysms suddenly enlarge or rupture, they produce dramatic symptoms. Rapidly enlarging aneurysms produce severe pain depending on the location. On examination, a pulsating mass is discovered. Thoracic aortic aneurysms (TAAs) produce pressure symptoms by impingement on other structures. It can produce compression of superior vena cava (SVC) resulting in SVC syndrome (nonpulsatile engorgement of jugular veins with congestion); compression on recurrent laryngeal nerve can produce hoarseness of voice. Traction on trachea produces the characteristic sign, ***tracheal tug***. Ruptured aneurysm should be suspected if the patient presents with severe pain followed by shock. Rupture into esophagus will present as massive

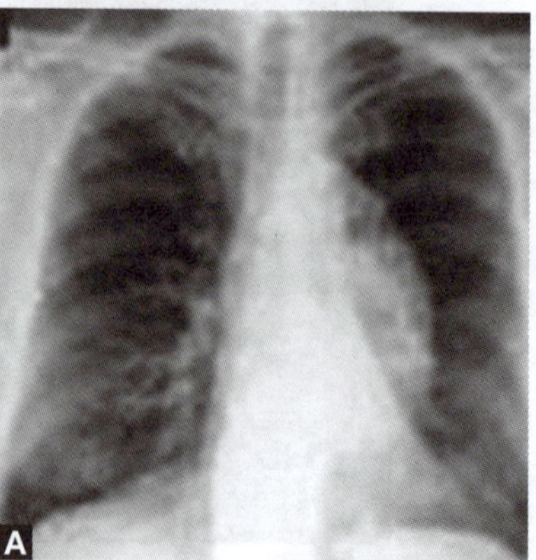

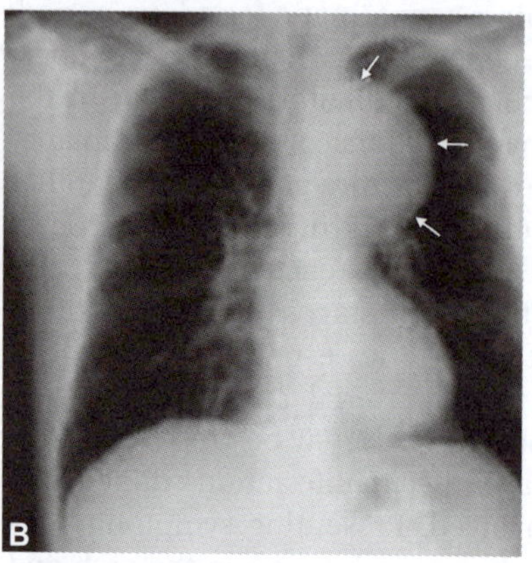

Figs 131.4A and B: Chest X-ray PA view of aortic aneurysms. **A.** Fusiform; **B.** Saccular

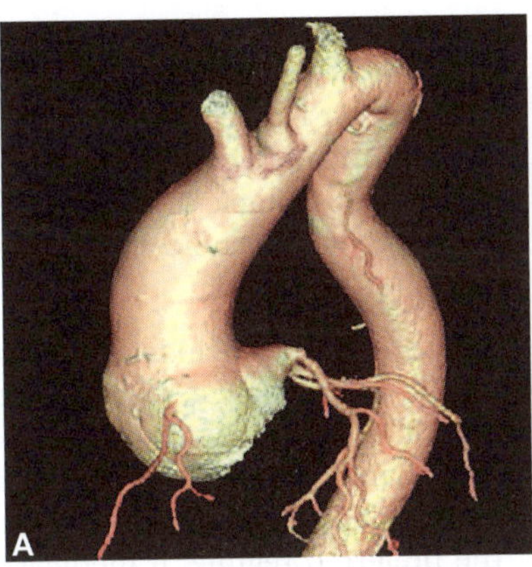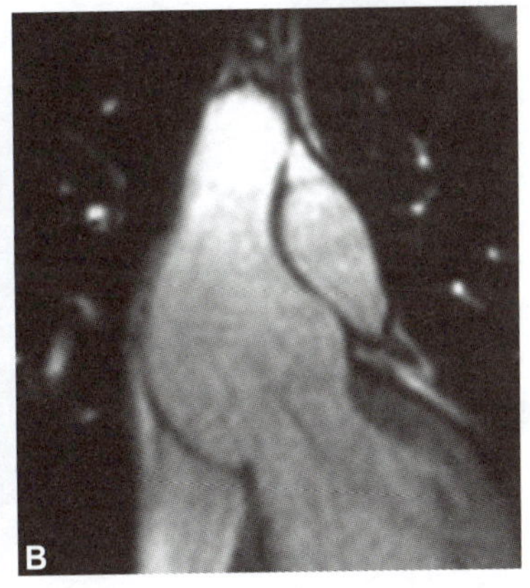

Figs 131.5A and B: A. MRA; **B.** CT image of ascending aortic aneurysm (AAA)

hematemesis, while rupture into pleural or peritoneal space would present as hemothorax or hemoperitoneum.

Investigations

Chest X-ray (CXR) may show aneurysms and calcification along its margins. CT is the investigation of choice and it clearly delineates the extent, size and integrity of the aneurysm. MRA is an alternative for the preoperative evaluation of aortic aneurysms (Figs 131.5A and B). Aortography has several limitations and its use in the evaluation of aortic aneurysms has declined.

Natural History

Rupture is the most frequent cause of death and occurs in 40–70%. Untreated, the 5-year survival rates for thoracic, thoracoabdominal and abdominal aneurysms range from 13 to 39%. Aneurysms of the arch grow faster than those of the ascending and abdominal aorta.

Prognosis

Aneurysms greater than 6 cm in diameter have faster growth rates and higher tendency to rupture. Coexistence of hypertension and cardiac ischemia worsens the prognosis.

Treatment

Treatment depends on the site involved, size of the aneurysm and the propensity for rupture. All TAAs larger than 6 cm and those producing symptoms should be repaired with Dacron graft. If the patient has Marfan's syndrome, then aneurysm should be repaired if it is greater than 5 cm. Abdominal aortic aneurysm (AAAs) should be repaired if it produces symptoms or is greater than 5.5 cm in size.

Repair is done either by endovascular devices (grafts) or by open surgery. Endovascular procedures are associated with lower surgical and postoperative mortality, though total mortality is the same for both methods on follow-up. Endovascular method is associated with greater frequency of long-term complications requiring interventions.

DISSECTING ANEURYSMS OF AORTA

Aortic dissection is a catastrophic illness produced by intimal tear resulting in flow of blood between and along the laminar planes of the media, with formation of a blood-filled channel within the aortic wall. This will lead to creation of a true and false lumen. It may rupture causing massive fatal hemorrhage.

Causes

- **Hypertension:** More than 90% of the patients suffer from chronic hypertension.
- Conditions that cause cystic medial necrosis, e.g. Marfan's syndrome, Ehlers-Danlos syndrome, etc.
- **Other structural disorders of the aorta:** CoA, aortoarteritis, SA and giant-cell arteritis.
- Higher incidence in BAV.
- **Trauma:** Blunt trauma to the chest as in automobile accidents, e.g. steering wheel injury and iatrogenic causes such as catheterization.

Pathogenesis

Aortic dissection is believed to begin with the formation of a tear in the aortic intima that directly exposes an underlying diseased medial layer to the driving force of the intraluminal blood. This blood penetrates the diseased medial layer and cleaves the media longitudinally, there by dissecting the aortic wall.

Clinical Features

The clinical features depend on the site of involvement based on which aortic dissection is classified. There are two major classifications: (1) The DeBakey classification and (2) the Stanford classification (Fig. 131.6).

DeBakey classification divides dissection into three types:
- **Type I:** Dissection starts in the AAo and extends at least to the arch and quite often to the descending aorta
- **Type II:** Dissection involves only the AAo
- **Type III:** Dissection is in the descending aorta and it usually, starts just distal to the left subclavian artery (LSA).
  - **Type IIIa:** Dissection stops above the diaphragm
  - **Type IIIb:** Dissection extends below the diaphragm.

Stanford classification is based on whether AAo is involved or not and is into types A (proximal) and B (distal).
- Type A dissections involve AAo with or without involvement of descending aorta.
- In type B, the dissection is confined to descending aorta.

Men are affected twice as commonly as women. Main symptom is sudden onset of severe pain in the chest,

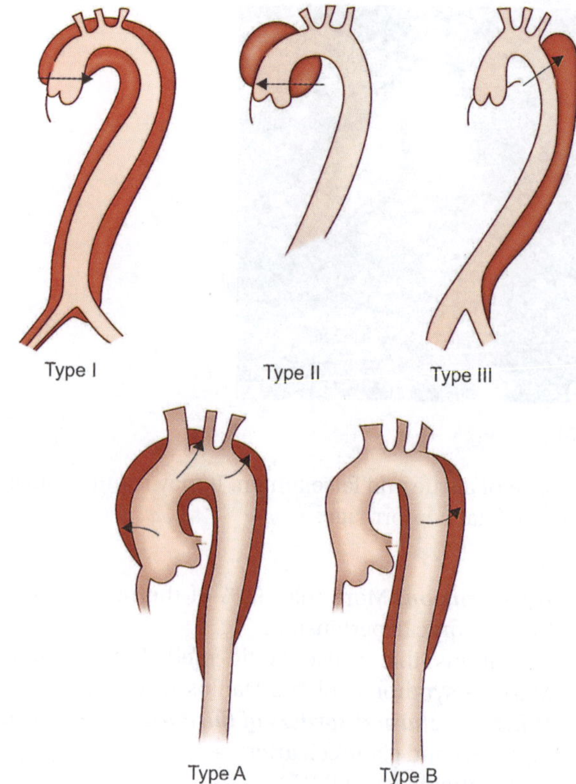

Fig. 131.6: Classification of aortic dissection

interscapular region, neck, mid-back, abdomen, sacral region and lower limbs depending on the site of intimal tear. The pain may be mistaken for myocardial infarction (MI). Unlike the pain of acute MI, the chest pain produced by aortic dissection is usually, abrupt in onset, very severe from the onset itself and unremitting. Dissections involving AAo may involve the right coronary artery (RCA) ostium producing acute inferior wall MI. Dissection can compromise the branches arising from aorta, and hence, can have other manifestations like syncope, stroke, renal failure, lower limb ischemia and mesenteric ischemia. Rupture into the pleural or pericardial spaces will present as acute dyspnea; bleeding can occur into gastrointestinal tract (GIT) and rarely into trachea or bronchus.

Physical Examination

Asymmetry of pulses and difference in BP (anisosphygmia) help to clinch the diagnosis. The jugular vein may be engorged unilaterally. Proximal dissection is one of the causes for acute aortic regurgitation [acute (AR)]. Other features include left-sided hemothorax, cardiac tamponade, silent abdomen due to paresis of intestines, presence of arterial bruits and variable neurological deficits.

Diagnosis

Aortic dissection should be suspected in all cases of intense chest pain associated with signs of shock, especially if the clinical features and electrocardiogram (ECG) do not suggest MI. CXR may show widening of mediastinal shadow; calcium sign is characteristic (intimal tear separates the intimal calcium from the adventitia; hence, the distance from the intimal calcium to the outer border of aorta will be increased to > 1 cm). Transesophageal echocardiography (TEE) is diagnostic in majority of thoracic dissections. Contrast-enhanced CT is the procedure of choice to confirm dissection.

Treatment

Supportive care includes careful monitoring and control of BP, maintenance of fluid intake and output. Pure vasodilators should be avoided as they enhance dissection by enhancing the rate of rise of pressure in the aorta. A combination of sodium nitroprusside and β-blocker is the preferred regime. If medical treatment fails to arrest progression, emergency surgery may be required.

Dissection of the AAo, irrespective of whether it originates there or extends from other sites is most likely to be fatal. Such patients should be taken up for emergency surgery. Distal dissection can be managed medically; if it fails to arrest the progression, surgical management has to be considered. Recently, endovascular procedures have been found to be successful in selected cases.

ANEURYSMS OF SINUSES OF VALSALVA

Congenital abnormality of the media of aortic root can result in progressive dilatation of the sinuses of Valsalva; rarely this could be acquired also. It is seen more often in males in a ratio of 4:1; it is five times more common in Asians. Right coronary sinus is commonly affected followed by noncoronary sinus (Fig. 131.7). It remains unruptured in majority; however, rupture occurs in about 35%, most commonly to right ventricle (RV). Acute rupture results in sudden onset of congestive heart failure (CHF) and the typical auscultatory finding is a superficial loud continuous murmur with diastolic accentuation heard along the left sternal border. The rupture can be corrected surgically or by percutaneous devices.

CHOLESTEROL CRYSTAL EMBOLISM

This occurs when cholesterol crystals derived from atheromatous plaques existing in the major arteries embolize to microvasculature. The precipitating events are intimal

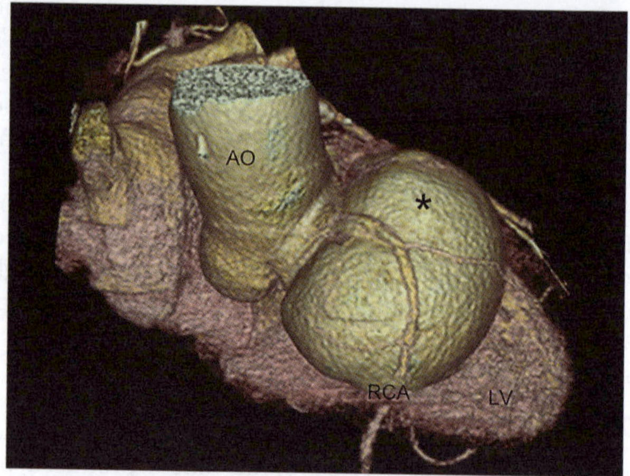

Fig. 131.7: Aneurysm of sinus of Valsalva—from the right coronary sinus

Abbreviations: AO = Aorta; RCA = Right coronary artery; LV = Left ventricle trauma related to aortic surgery and percutaneous aortic procedures or drug induced (anticoagulants, thrombolytics). Typical features include ischemic damage to the kidneys or lower limbs. Ischemia to lower limbs with palpable arterial pulsations and the livedo reticularis pattern of the skin are the classical features (Fig. 131.8). Blood counts show eosinophilia; urine sediment may show cholesterol crystals. Renal failure occurs in 50% and intestinal bleeding in 10%. Reported mortality is 60–80%. Biopsy of skin lesions is diagnostic in cholesterol crystal embolism. Treatment consists of supportive measure, cessation of anticoagulant therapy and institution of corticosteroids in selected cases.

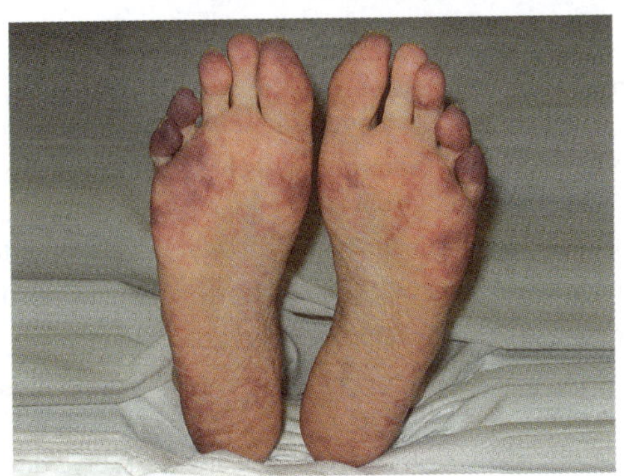

Fig. 131.8: Livedo reticularis (purple toe syndrome)

CHAPTER
132

Cardiac Manifestations of Systemic Diseases

A George Koshy, Sajan S Ahmed

GENERAL CONSIDERATIONS

Systemic disorders can affect the heart and the cardiovascular system (CVS), with diagnostic, therapeutic and prognostic implications (Table 132.1).

NEUROLOGIC DISORDERS

Stroke

Cerebrogenic cardiac arrhythmias and myocardial changes can occur during ischemic strokes producing electrocardiography (ECG) abnormalities like ST-segment elevation or depression and T wave abnormalities. Subarachnoid hemorrhage may be associated with deep T wave inversions, QT prolongation and transient ST-segment elevation, especially in the initial 48 hours. Raised intracranial tension can cause bradycardia and hypertension (Cushing's reflex).

Guillain-Barré Syndrome (GBS)

The dysautonomia in GBS can cause wide fluctuations in blood pressure (BP) hypertension, orthostatic hypotension, resting sinus tachycardia or bradycardia and even life-threatening arrhythmias. The risk of deep vein thrombosis (DVT) and pulmonary embolism (PE) is increased in non-ambulatory patients.

Muscular Dystrophies and Myopathies

- ***Duchenne muscular dystrophy (DMD):*** It is the most common inherited neuromuscular disorder. Up to 90% of patients older than 18 years have a dilated cardiomyopathy (DCM) on ECG, with predominant involvement of the inferobasal and the lateral walls of the left ventricle (LV). Posterior papillary muscle dysfunction can lead to mitral regurgitation (MR). Most patients have an abnormal ECG, the classic pattern being tall R waves in lead V1 and deep narrow

Table 132.1: Systemic disorders and diseases with cardiovascular involvement

Category	Diseases with cardiovascular involvement
Neurologic disease	Stroke, Guillain–Barré syndrome, muscular dystrophies and myopathies
Psychiatric disorders	Depression, mental stress, type A and type D personality, Da Costa syndrome, effects of psychiatric pharmacotherapy
Vasculitis	Takayasu arteritis, giant-cell arteritis, Kawasaki disease, Churg-Strauss syndrome, PAN
Rheumatologic disorders	Rheumatoid arthritis, SLE, HLA-B27 associated spondyloarthropathies, scleroderma, Sarcoidosis Kawasaki's disease

Contd...

Contd...

Endocrine diseases	Diabetes mellitus, hypothyroidism, hyperthyroidism, acromegaly Cushing's syndrome, Carney complex, Conn syndrome, Addison's disease, pheochromocytoma
Infections	Leptospirosis, diphtheria, Lyme disease, Chagas disease, tuberculosis, HIV, syphilis, dengue fever, yellow fever, mumps, rubella
Renal disease	Chronic kidney disease, renal artery stenosis, cardiorenal syndrome
Respiratory disease	COPD, pulmonary hypertension, obstructive sleep apnea
Hepatic disease	Portopulmonary hypertension, hemochromatosis obstructive jaundice
Cancer	Pericardial disease, valvular heart disease, myocardial disease, SVC obstruction, effects of chemotherapy and radiation therapy
Metabolic disorders	Glycogen storage disease, Fabry's disease, amyloidosis
Electrolyte abnormalities	Hypo/hypercalcemia, hypo/hyperkalemia, hypo/hypermagnesemia
Genetic syndromes	Marfan's syndrome, Down syndrome, Noonan's syndrome, Turner's syndrome
Miscellaneous	Hypothermia, fever, Takotsubo syndrome, alcohol exposure

Abbreviations: HLA = Human leukocyte antigen; SLE = Systemic lupus erythematosus; COPD = Chronic obstructive pulmonary disease; HIV = Human immunodeficiency virus; SVC = Superior vena cava; PAN = Polyarteritis nodosa

Q waves in left precordial leads. Sinus tachycardia is very common.

- ***Myotonic dystrophy:*** It is the most common inherited neuromuscular dystrophy in adult patients. The primary cardiac involvement is in the form of arrhythmias, with most patients having ECG abnormalities [first-degree atrioventricular (AV) block in 42%, right bundle branch block (RBBB) in 3%, left bundle branch block (LBBB) in 4%, nonspecific intraventricular conduction delay in 12% and abnormal Q waves]. ECG may show left ventricular dysfunction (LVD) and left ventricular hypertrophy (LVH). The most common electrophysiological abnormality is a prolonged H-V (His–Ventricular) interval and many patients may progress to symptomatic heart block requiring permanent pacemaker implantation. The most common arrhythmias are atrial fibrillation (AF) and atrial flutter (AFL). There is also an increased risk of ventricular tachycardia (VT) (especially bundle branch re-entrant VT) and sudden cardiac death.

- ***Emery-Dreifuss muscular dystrophy (EDMD):*** The classic triad includes early contractures, muscular weakness with atrophy and cardiac disease (most commonly arrhythmias and DCM). ECG abnormalities include first-degree AV block, AF or more typically permanent atrial standstill.

- ***Facioscapulohumeral muscular dystrophy (FSHD):*** Significant clinical cardiac involvement is rare in this muscular dystrophy.

- ***Friedreich's ataxia:*** It is the most common inherited spinocerebellar degenerative disease. It can cause concentric hypertrophic cardiomyopathy (HCM). Asymmetrical septal hypertrophy and myocardial fiber disarray are not commonly seen.

- ***Periodic paralysis:*** Arrhythmias occur mainly in hyperkalemic periodic paralysis (hyperPP) and Andersen-Tawil syndrome (ATS). Bidirectional VT is independent of attacks of muscle weakness and does not correlate with serum potassium levels. ECG abnormalities can be very often picked up in hypoPP.

- ***Mitochondrial myopathy:*** Kearns-Sayre syndrome is characterized by the triad of progressive external ophthalmoplegia, pigmentary retinopathy and AV block.

PSYCHIATRIC DISORDERS

Depression

Depression is associated with increased cardiovascular disease (CVD) risk. Contributing factors include association with other CVD risk factors like smoking, sedentary lifestyle and hypertension, lower adherence to therapy and delay in seeking treatment. Sympathoadrenal (SA) activation with increased release of cortisol and norepinephrine, reduced parasympathetic flow, autonomic dysfunction, enhanced platelet activity, endothelial dysfunction and inflammation are implicated.

Mental Stress

Stressful emotional episodes can trigger acute cardiac ischemia by disrupting a vulnerable atherosclerotic plaque through sympathetic activation, coronary vasoconstriction, inflammation and prothrombotic effects. ***Mental stress ischemia*** is the term used to describe a transient ischemic response to a psychological stress challenge like mental arithmetic or public speeches.

Type A Personality

Anger and hostility as part of a type A personality may be associated with CVD risk, especially among men.

Type D Personality

Type D or ***distressed*** personality combines negative affect and social inhibition and is associated with adverse CVD outcomes.

Da Costa's Syndrome

It is also known as ***neurocirculatory asthenia*** or ***irritable heart syndrome***, it is disorder characterized by breathlessness, chest discomfort, nervousness and palpitations. It was initially described in male soldiers exposed to wartime stress.

Psychiatric Pharmacotherapy

- ***Tricyclic antidepressants (TCAs)*** (e.g. imipramine, amitriptyline) can prolong the PR interval, QRS duration and the QT interval. They should be avoided in patients with pre-existing conduction disease, heart failure or recent myocardial infarction (MI). QT prolongation more than 440 msec may increase risk of malignant ventricular arrhythmias (torsades de pointes). Elderly patients may also be susceptible to orthostatic hypotension.
- ***Monoamine oxidase inhibitors (MAO)*** (e.g. phenelzine, tranylcypromine) can cause a ***wine*** and ***cheese reaction*** with life-threatening hypertension when taken along with foods rich in tyramine like wine, cheese, chocolate and beer.
- ***Selective serotonin reuptake inhibitors*** (**SSRIs**) (e.g. fluoxetine, citalopram, sertraline) are the antidepressant medications of choice in cardiac patients as they do not have significant effects on BP and the heart.
- ***Lithium*** exposure during antenatal period (for treatment of bipolar mood disorder) may increase the risk of Ebstein anomaly in the fetus.

VASCULITIS

Takayasu arteritis: This large vessel vasculitis of young adults (female preponderance) affects the aorta and its major branches. Patients may present with hypertension, upper limb claudication, aortic root aneurysms and aortic regurgitation (AR). Type 5 Takayasu arteritis is associated with involvement of the coronary arteries. Pulmonary arteries can also get involved.

Giant-cell arteritis: It is a granulomatous arteritis of large and medium-sized vessels. Aortitis with involvement of the subclavian arteries and thoracic and abdominal aortic aneurysms (AAA) may occur.

Kawasaki disease: It is an acquired febrile systemic illness of childhood. The most dreaded cardiac complication is the development of coronary artery lesions, with coronary artery aneurysms occurring in 20–25% of untreated cases within 2 weeks. Giant aneurysms (> 8 mm) may get occluded with thrombus and cause MI. Other cardiac features include pericardial effusion, myocarditis, MR, heart failure and arrhythmias.

Churg-Strauss syndrome: It is a vasculitis affecting medium or small-sized vessels associated with atopy, usually asthma. Cardiac involvement can occur in 15–55% of cases. These include pericarditis, myocarditis, coronary arteritis and heart failure.

Polyarteritis nodosa (PAN): It is a nongranulomatous arteritis of medium-sized vessels. Hypertension (30%) and heart disease (infarction, pericarditis) may occur.

SYSTEMIC RHEUMATOLOGIC DISORDERS

Rheumatoid Arthritis (RA)

It is the most common form of chronic inflammatory polyarthritis. Pericarditis and pericardial effusions may occur in 40% of patients. Usually, there is a neutrophil predominance with low glucose levels in the pericardial fluid when compared to the serum glucose levels. RA and aortic valvulitis causing AR is rare. Even though coronary arteritis is rare, patients with RA have an increased incidence of coronary artery disease (CAD), probably related to chronic inflammation, proatherogenic lipid profiles and adverse effects of pharmacotherapy. Pulmonary hypertension (PH) may occur secondary to rheumatoid lung disease.

Systemic Lupus Erythematosus (SLE)

The most common cardiac involvement is pericarditis (30% clinically and 60% by imaging and autopsy). Pericardial fluid usually shows neutrophil predominance, increased protein and low or normal glucose levels, along with low complement levels. Libman-Sacks endocarditis (nonbacterial endocarditis) with valve thickening and regurgitation can occur. The vegetation are usually located on the atrial side of the mitral valve (more common) and the atrial side of the aortic valve.

Coronary involvement may be due to coronary arteritis, thrombosis due to antiphospholipid antibody (APLA), coronary embolism from Libman-Sacks endocarditis or accelerated atherosclerosis related to anti-endothelial cell antibodies (AECAs).

PE can occur, especially in the setting of APLA syndrome. PH may be secondary to chronic thromboembolism, pulmonary arteritis or lung disease.

Infants born to mothers with SLE with positive anti-Ro and anti-La antibodies can develop complete heart block.

HLA-B27 Associated Spondyloarthropathies

Ankylosing spondylitis (AS) patients can develop aortic root disease, dilatation and AR with the murmur of AR being best heard along the right sternal border.

Scleroderma

Cardiac features are fibrinous pericarditis, pericardial effusions and patchy myocardial fibrosis with contraction band necrosis resulting from intermittent ischemia by microvascular occlusion or spasm. PH secondary to lung involvement, (usually interstitial fibrosis) is common.

Sarcoidosis

Granulomatous infiltrative myocarditis can cause arrhythmias VT, conduction system disease (heart block) and rarely DCM with heart failure. The LV, especially the upper septal area is most commonly involved. Cardiac magnetic resonance imaging (MRI) with gadolinium contrast may be useful to demonstrate the mid myocardial and epicardial late gadolinium enhancement (LGE). Pericarditis is usually subclinical. PH may be secondary to lung disease. Sarcoid vasculitis affecting the aorta may mimic Takayasu arteritis.

ENDOCRINE DISORDERS

Diabetes Mellitus (DM)

It is considered as a ***coronary heart disease equivalent***. CVD is the most common cause for mortality in diabetic individuals. It is usually in the form of CAD, but can also be due to stroke, peripheral vascular disease and heart failure. Diabetes accelerates atherosclerosis, causes endothelial dysfunction (hallmark of diabetic vascular disease), and causes vascular damage mediated by advanced glycation end products and free fatty acids. ***'Diabetic dyslipidemia'*** is characterized by high triglycerides (TG) levels, high-density lipoprotein (HDL) levels and increased atherogenic small dense low-density lipoprotein (LDL) particles. The prothrombotic and proinflammatory milieu in diabetes also contributes to increased CVD events.

Hypothyroidism

Cardiac manifestations include sinus bradycardia, diastolic hypertension, pericardial effusion, increased total cholesterol, LDL cholesterol and hypertriglyceridemia. Low-voltage complexes may be seen on ECG. Accelerated atherosclerosis is common.

Hyperthyroidism

The most common cardiovascular manifestation is sinus tachycardia, often associated with palpitations. High cardiac output, bounding pulse and wide pulse pressure may be seen. AF is the most common rhythm disturbance. Long-standing uncontrolled hyperthyroidism can lead to heart failure.

Acromegaly

Cardiac features include hypertension (20–40%), LVH and LVD. ECG abnormalities occur in more than 50% of individuals.

Cushing's Syndrome

Cardiac involvement includes hypertension, dyslipidemia, accelerated atherosclerosis and LVH. On ECG, the PR interval is inversely correlated with adrenal cortisol production.

Carney Syndrome

It combines Cushing syndrome, cardiac myxoma and pigmented dermal lesions.

Conn's Syndrome and Hyperaldosteronism

It causes increased sodium retention, hypertension and decreased vascular compliance. ECG may reveal evidence of hypokalemia.

Addison's Disease

Acute Addisonian crisis is an endocrine emergency and it is characterized by hypovolemia, hypotension, hyperkalemia and loss of vascular tone. Adrenal insufficiency causes a low-diastolic BP and orthostatic hypotension. Cardiac atrophy with reduced LV dimensions is called ***teardrop heart***.

Pheochromocytoma

Hypertension may be episodic or more often constant. Orthostatic hypotension may be seen. Catecholamines are toxic to the heart and can lead to DCM. Hypertensive crisis and direct depressant effect of catecholamines on the myocardium can lead to acute pulmonary edema.

INFECTIONS

Dengue Fever

The most common cardiac manifestation is sinus bradycardia. In addition, premature complexes, transient AV blocks and myocarditis may be seen. Clinically, significant myocarditis is relatively uncommon.

Yellow Fever

Relative bradycardia (bradycardia despite fever) in yellow fever is called ***Faget sign*** or ***sphygmothermic dissociation***.

Leptospirosis

It can produce myocarditis with LVD and troponin elevation, pulmonary edema, AV blocks and ST-T changes on ECG.

Diphtheria

Diphtheritic myocarditis (10–20%) causes ST-segment and T wave abnormalities, AV block or bundle branch block (BBB). Diphtheria toxin is directly cardiotoxic with diphtheritic myocarditis being the most common cause of death in diphtheria (mortality rate of 60–70%).

Lyme Disease

The heart is involved in up to 50% of cases. Ten percent of patients with Lyme carditis develop AV conduction block usually reversible.

Chagas Disease

Acute Chagas myocarditis, chronic Chagas DCM and a form of cardiomyopathy with LV apical aneurysm are seen. ECG abnormalities include RBBB, left anterior fascicular block (LAFB) or AV blocks.

Tuberculosis

The most common cardiac involvement in tuberculosis is pericarditis with pericardial effusion, which may progress to effusive-constrictive pericarditis or constrictive pericarditis. The effusion may be straw-colored or hemorrhagic with fibrinous strands and pericardial thickening. Pericardial involvement may be by retrograde lymphatic spread or by hematogenous spread. The four pathologic stages are fibrinous exudation (predominantly neutrophilic), serosanguinous effusion (predominantly lymphocytic), granulomatous caseation with pericardial thickening and constrictive scarring.

Human Immunodeficiency Virus (HIV)

Patients with HIV infection may have myocarditis, DCM, right-sided valvular endocarditis, marantic endocarditis or PE. HIV infection may also be associated with pulmonary artery hypertension (PAH) (incidence of 1/200 of HIV-infected patients). Highly active antiretroviral therapy (HAART) may increase the risk of CAD, mainly related to the atherogenic effects of protease inhibitor therapy.

Syphilis

Clinical evidence of cardiovascular involvement occurs in approximately 10% of patients with syphilis. It is a manifestation of the tertiary stage of the disease. This is most common in men and can occur at an earlier age compared to women. Though the causative organism, *Treponema pallidum* can involve the *tunica adventitia* of the aortic wall soon after the primary infection, it takes 10–30 years for the disease to progress and manifest clinically. Cardiovascular involvement includes aortitis, AR due to annuloaortic ectasia, AAA, coronary ostial stenosis or atresia (COSA), syphilitic gumma and endarteritis.

Syphilitic aortitis can occur in up to three-fourth of untreated cases. Endarteritis of the vasa vasorum is the underlying mechanism which leads to necrosis of the elastic and connective tissues of the tunica media. This more often involve the ascending aorta (AAo) and the proximal arch. The descending aorta is usually spared. This leads to weakening of the wall and consequent formation of aneurysm which can be quite large. Generalized dilatation can lead to fusiform dilatation and localized dilatation can lead to saccular aneurysm. Symptoms and signs of the aneurysm are related to the pressure effects on the adjacent structures. Surgery is required in such patients to relieve the pressure effects as well as to avoid potentially lethal complication of rupture. AR in syphilis is classically accompanied by loud ringing aortic valve closure sound. Ascending aortic pulsations may be palpable in the second upper right sternal border and the early diastolic murmur of AR tend to be louder along the right sternal border than the left sternal border. The chest X-ray can demonstrate dilated AAo and cardiomegaly. *Egg shell calcification* involving the AAo is a well-described feature. ECG helps in identifying the dilated aortic root and AAo and in detecting and quantifying AR. The left ventricular (LV) function can also be assessed and is very useful for follow-up. Anti-syphilitic treatment initiated early can prevent the progression of the disease. Coronary ostial disease is usually a slowly progressive disease and is almost always associated with significant AR. This can lead to angina and arrhythmias though acute MI is uncommon. Gumma can involve the myocardium, endocardium as well as the conduction system and can lead to heart blocks. Early and prompt treatment of the primary infection can prevent CVD in later life. Because of the better awareness and widespread availability of diagnostic facilities and use of antibiotics, cardiovascular syphilis has become less common in clinical practice.

Mumps

Intrauterine exposure to mumps virus may be associated with endocardial fibroelastosis.

Rubella

Maternal exposure to rubella leads to congenital rubella syndrome, with patent ductus arteriosus (PDA) and branch pulmonary artery stenosis being the most common cardiac defects.

RENAL DISEASE

See also Section 16, Ch 180

Chronic Kidney Disease (CKD)

CVD risk is increased in CKD patients, related to accelerated atherosclerosis, vascular calcification, hypertension, hyperparathyroidism, anemia and prothrombotic state. CKD contributes to heart failure through three major mechanisms: Pressure overload related to hypertension, volume overload due to fluid retention and cardiomyopathy. CKD is linked to mitral annular calcification and aortic valve sclerosis. Uremic pericarditis may also occur. ECG may show the classic triad of LVH with features of hyperkalemia and hypocalcemia. Microalbuminuria and albuminuria are independent risk factors for major cardiovascular events.

Renal Artery Stenosis (RAS)

Atherosclerotic RAS can produce refractory hypertension, renal dysfunction and flash pulmonary edema. Unilateral RAS produces vasoconstrictor mediated hypertension, while bilateral RAS produces hypertension caused by volume overload.

Cardiorenal Syndrome

Acute or chronic dysfunction of the heart or kidneys can induce acute or chronic dysfunction in the other organ. It is classified as follows:

- *Type 1:* Acute cardiorenal syndrome (e.g. acute heart failure causing acute kidney injury)
- *Type 2:* Chronic cardiorenal syndrome (e.g. chronic heart failure producing chronic kidney damage)
- *Type 3:* Acute renocardiac syndrome (e.g. acute glomerulonephritis or ischemia causing cardiac dysfunction)
- *Type 4:* Chronic renocardiac syndrome (e.g. CKD causing coronary disease, heart failure or arrhythmia)
- *Type 5:* Secondary (e.g. systemic diseases like sepsis and diabetes producing cardiac and renal dysfunction).

RESPIRATORY DISEASES

Pulmonary Hypertension (PH)

Hypoxemic lung diseases like chronic obstructive pulmonary disease (COPD), interstitial lung disease (ILD), sleep disordered breathing and chronic exposure to high altitude can cause PH (category 3 in the clinical classification of PH).

Chronic Obstructive Pulmonary Disease (COPD)

ECG may show right atrial abnormality, RV hypertrophy, poor progression of R wave in the precordial leads and low-voltage complexes. Patients may present with multifocal atrial tachycardia (MAT). Chest X-ray may show a tubular heart.

Obstructive Sleep Apnea

It is a sleep related breathing disorder leading to obstruction of the upper airways and consequent hypoxemia. This can lead to sympathetic stimulation and is associated with increased cardiovascular risk. This is usually observed in obese individuals with short neck. Hypertension, insulin resistance, AF, diastolic dysfunction, heart failure and sudden cardiac death are commoner in obstructive sleep apnea syndrome compared to the general population.

HEPATIC DISEASE

Portopulmonary Hypertension

The prevalence of PH in patients with portal hypertension is 2–6%. It is often progressive and irreversible.

Hemochromatosis

The classic features include liver disease, hyper-pigmentation, diabetes, cardiac disease, impotence and arthropathy. Cardiac toxicity is due to free iron moiety. The most common cardiac manifestation is congestive heart failure (CHF) (10%) with a clinical picture simulating DCM.

Obstructive Jaundice

Obstructive jaundice has traditionally been linked to sinus bradycardia, probably due to sinus node suppression by bile salts.

Pericardial Disease

Pericardial effusion in a cancer patient could be due to malignant effusion with pericardial infiltration or metastasis, radiation or drug-induced pericarditis, infectious (tuberculosis, bacterial or fungal) or iatrogenic. Pericardial effusion can progress to cardiac tamponade with hemodynamic compromise, requiring emergency pericardiocentesis. Malignant pericardial effusions (MPEs) are often hemorrhagic, with a high likelihood of rapid reaccumulation. Constrictive pericarditis may occur as a late (7–13 years later) complication of chest irradiation, especially in breast cancer and Hodgkin disease.

Valvular Heart Disease

Cardiac valves may be involved by tumors, infections, or as a late effect of radiation therapy. Nonbacterial thrombotic endocarditis or marantic endocarditis is most commonly seen along with adenocarcinomas of gastrointestinal tract (GIT) and lung. Carcinoid syndrome can produce white fibrous carcinoid plaques most extensive on the right side of the heart, especially on the ventricular surface of the tricuspid valve resulting in tricuspid regurgitation (TR) or the combination of TR and tricuspid stenosis (TS). Carcinoid plaques can involve the right ventricular outflow tract (RVOT) and produce PS or the combination of PS and PR.

Myocardial Disease

Its causes include direct tumor infiltration, myotoxicity secondary to chemotherapy and myocardial fibrosis following radiotherapy. Myocardial dysfunction and arrhythmias may occur.

Superior Vena Cava (SVC) Obstruction

SVC obstruction occurs due to compression of the SVC by tumors or lymph nodes, the most common causes being lung cancer, lymphomas and breast cancer. Endovascular stenting of the SVC may be done for relief of obstructive symptoms.

Adverse Effects of Chemotherapy

Cardiomyopathy: The most cardiotoxic chemotherapeutic agents are the anthracyclines (doxorubicin or adriamycin, daunorubicin) which produce oxidant stress and cellular damage via free radicals. The dose-related toxicity profile includes LVD, heart failure, arrhythmias and pericarditis. Anthracycline cardiomyopathy often occurs within the first year of completing therapy. Risk factors for cardiotoxicity are: Doses more than 450 mg/m^2, pediatric age group, advanced age, history of heart disease and prior mediastinal irradiation. LV diastolic dysfunction may be the first abnormality noted. Endomyocardial biopsy is the most sensitive method to detect anthracycline cardiotoxicity. Epirubicin, a stereoisomer of doxorubicin is less cardiotoxic (toxicity at a dose > 900–1000 mg/m^2). Prophylactic angiotensin converting enzyme (ACE) inhibitor therapy is being tried to prevent progression to heart failure. Cardiotoxicity is also seen with trastuzumab, imatinib, dasatinib and bortezomib.

Ischemic syndromes: 5-fluorouracil (5-FU) and cisplatin can cause acute ischemic syndromes, mainly related to vasospasm. Bevacizumab vascular endothelial growth factor (VEGF receptor antagonist) increases thromboembolic events.

Venous thrombosis: DVT and pulmonary embolism may be seen in patients treated with cisplatin/thalidomide.

Hypertension: Cisplatin and bevacizumab can cause hypertension, which may be severe.

Adverse Effects of Radiation Therapy

Late cardiovascular effects of radiation therapy include valvular heart disease (most commonly affecting the aortic valve), premature CAD, stroke, cardiomyopathy, heart failure, constrictive pericarditis and complete heart block. The pathophysiology involves endothelial dysfunction of the microvasculature, premature atherosclerosis and myocardial fibrosis with diastolic dysfunction and restrictive cardiomyopathy.

METABOLIC DISORDERS

Glycogen Storage Disease

Types 2, 3, 4 and 5 may have cardiac involvement, typically in the form of LVH. Pompe's disease (type 2) is due to deficiency of the enzyme α-glucosidase and classically shows LVH and short PR interval on ECG. The ECG will simulate HCM.

Fabry's Disease

It is an X-linked recessive disorder (deficiency of the enzyme α-galactosidase: A leading to accumulation of glycosphingolipids). Cardiac manifestations include myocardial and valvular (most commonly mitral) deposits and deposition of lipid species in the coronary endothelium.

Amyloidosis

Cardiac amyloidosis is seen in up to one-third of primary amyloidosis due to plasma cell dyscrasias and in one quarter of transthyretin (TTR) induced or familial amyloidosis. Senile systemic amyloidosis (SSA) may cause restrictive cardiomyopathy. Amyloidosis may present with conduction system disease or autonomic dysfunction and orthostatic hypotension. ECG characteristically show low-voltage complexes but echocardiography may show severe degree of LVH. Doppler studies can demonstrate the restrictive filling pattern.

ELECTROLYTE ABNORMALITIES

Hypocalcemia

It prolongs phase 2 of the cardiac action potential and prolongs the QT interval.

Hypercalcemia

It shortens QT interval. Severe hypercalcemia (> 15 mg/dL) can cause decreased T wave amplitude. It can also simulate acute ischemia by producing a high takeoff of the ST-segments in leads V1 and V2.

Hyperkalemia

The earliest change is narrowing and peaking of the T wave (tenting). The QT interval shortens. The QRS widens and P wave amplitude reduces. PR prolongation, followed by AV blocks may occur. Complete loss of P wave can occur due to atrial paralysis (sinoventricular rhythm). Moderate to severe hyperkalemia can produce ST-segment elevation in V1 and V3. Very severe hyperkalemia causes disappearance of the initial R wave in right precordial leads and classical sine wave pattern, followed by asystole. The ECG can mimic acute anterior wall MI and LBBB.

Hypokalemia

Features are ST depression, flat T waves and prominent U waves, especially in the mid precordial leads. True QT prolongation can also occur and can predispose to torsades de pointes polymorphic ventricular tachycardia (PVT). Hypokalemia also predisposes to digitalis induced tachyarrhythmias.

Hypermagnesemia

If severe, it can cause AV conduction delay, complete heart block and cardiac arrest (>15 mEq/L).

Hypomagnesemia

Similar to hypokalemia, it can prolong the QT interval, predispose to torsades and increase the risk of digitalis toxicity.

GENETIC SYNDROMES

Marfan's Syndrome

Cardiovascular abnormalities are the most common cause of morbidity and mortality in these patients. The major features include mitral valve prolapse (MVP) with MR and dilated aortic root with AR, aortic dissection and rupture.

Down Syndrome

Trisomy 21 is the most common defect of human chromosome dosage. Forty to fifty percent of cases have major congenital heart malformations. The prototypic abnormality is atrioventricular canal defects (AVCD). This includes complete atrioventricular canal (CAVC) or partial AVC characterized by primum atrial septal defect (ASD), inlet ventricular septal defect (VSD), cleft anterior mitral leaflet with MR, atrioventricular septal defects (AVSD) and tricuspid valve abnormalities.

DiGeorge Syndrome

Chromosome 22q11 deletion syndrome or velocardio-facial syndrome (VCFS) is characterized by outflow tract defects of the heart, hypocalcemia and thymic hypoplasia.

Noonan's Syndrome

Dysplastic valvular pulmonary stenosis (PS) (40%) is the most common cardiac defect. The other defects are HCM, ASD (30%), VSD and PDA (10% each). Severe valvular PS with interatrial communication (Trilogy of Fallot) is also described.

Turner's Syndrome

Heart defects are seen in 20–50% of patients. The most common is coarctation of aorta (CoA) (50–70%). Bicuspid aortic valve (BAV) and aortic root dilatation are common associations. The affected individuals are prone for aortic dissection.

MISCELLANEOUS

Takotsubo Syndrome

It also known as, **broken heart syndrome** or **apical ballooning syndrome**, is an acute and mostly reversible cardiomyopathy produced by a stressful or emotional situation or an acute systemic illness. It is most commonly seen among middle-aged females and is thought to be mediated by catecholamine release.

Hypothermia

The classic ECG finding is the J wave or Osborn wave (a distinctive convex elevation at the junction or J point of the ST-segment and the QRS complex). Significant hypothermia produces bradycardia, hypotension and even ventricular fibrillation (VF) and asystole.

Fever

The most common finding is sinus tachycardia. Brugada pattern (RBBB pattern and coved ST-segment elevation in leads V1–V3) on ECG may be unmasked by febrile episodes in affected patients, sometimes causing ventricular arrhythmias, syncope or sudden cardiac death.

Alcohol Exposure

Alcoholic cardiomyopathy is a dose-related DCM. Alcohol exposure also increases risk for hypertension, stroke, AF and sudden death. **Holiday heart syndrome** refers to episodes of AF occurring after binge drinking, usually on weekends or holidays.

CHAPTER
133

Pregnancy and Heart Disease

N Sudhayakumar, K Suresh

Chapter Summary
- General Considerations
- Hemodynamics of Pregnancy
- High-risk Pregnancies
- Management
- Cardiovascular Drugs in Pregnancy
- Mitral Stenosis and Pregnancy
- Pregnancy and Prosthetic Valves

GENERAL CONSIDERATIONS

Maternal cardiovascular diseases (CVD) pose an increased risk to mother and fetus in view of the extra hemodynamic burden to the mother. Over the last few decades, change in the pattern of heart disease with complicating pregnancy has occurred with reduction in the frequency of valvular heart diseases, and a dramatic increase in operated heart diseases and in the application of devices. About 2% of pregnancies are complicated by heart disease, majority being relatively well-tolerated. Following are the issues to be addressed by the obstetrician and clinician.

- Is she pregnant or anticipating pregnancy?
- Is the heart normal or diseased?
- Heart disease, if present, is significant or not?
- Hemodynamics of the cardiac lesion, hemodynamics of pregnancy and their interaction
- Problems to mother or fetus; how to prevent the problems?
- Management issues.

HEMODYNAMICS OF PREGNANCY

A clear understanding of the hemodynamic changes during normal pregnancy is of extreme importance to answer the problems raised above. Blood volume starts rising by the sixth week itself and peaks by about 40–45% by midtrimester, after which it plateaus. Increase in plasma volume is more than the rise in red blood cells (RBCs) resulting in hemodilution (physiological anemia of pregnancy). Increase in heart rate (by 10–20%) and stroke volume and reduction in systemic arterial resistance contribute to an increase in cardiac output by more than 30% (Fig. 133.1). All these changes are unfavorable in majority of the heart diseases. Blood pressure (BP) usually, remains unchanged or may fall slightly during normal gestation.

Hemodynamics worsen during labor and in the postpartum period. With each uterine contraction, up to 500 mL of blood is released into the circulation, causing an acute rise in cardiac output and BP. Approximately 400 mL of blood is lost during normal vaginal delivery; it is as high as 800 mL with cesarean section. After delivery, the venous return abruptly increases by two mechanisms— autotransfusion from uterus (which may continue for about 72 hours) and release of inferior vena caval compression by uterus.

HIGH-RISK PREGNANCIES

Many lesions are well-tolerated in pregnancy, especially when they are mild and with normal left ventricle (LV) function. New York Heart Association (NYHA) functional status is a good predictor of outcome; higher the class, worse the outcome. In general, regurgitant lesions are better tolerated than stenotic ones [as the reduction in systemic vascular resistance (SVR) reduces mitral and aortic regurgitation]. Indicators of the clinical situations which predict high-risk pregnancies in those with heart disease.

Indicators of high-risk pregnancy	
Severe PAH	RV systolic pressure > 70 % of LV systolic pressure
LV dysfunction	LV ejection fraction < 40 %
Symptomatic	Obstructive lesions especially of left heart; mitral stenosis, aortic stenosis, coarctation of aorta, Marfan syndrome with aortic root diameter > 40 mm, Cyanotic congenital heart disease (CCHD), Mechanical prosthesis.

Abbreviations: LV = Left ventricle; PAH = Pulmonary artery hypertension; RV = Right ventricle

A Canadian multicentric study in 599 pregnancies proposed a risk scoring for maternal cardiac events in those with heart diseases. Four parameters were considered and one point each was assigned: (1) Prior cardiac event like cardiac failure or stroke before pregnancy; (2) baseline NYHA functional class > II or presence of cyanosis; (3) moderate or severe mitral or aortic stenosis; and (4) left ventricular (LV) systolic dysfunction (ejection fraction < 40 %). The estimated risk for cardiac event in pregnancy was 5% for risk score of 0, 27 % for risk score of 1 and 75 % when the risk score was higher than 1.

MANAGEMENT

A detailed clinical evaluation has to be done with the view to assess the problems that can occur during pregnancy. The common complications during pregnancy are hemodynamic decompensation leading to cardiac failure, arrhythmias, infective endocarditis (IE), drug-related issues, aortic dissection, etc. Normal pregnancy

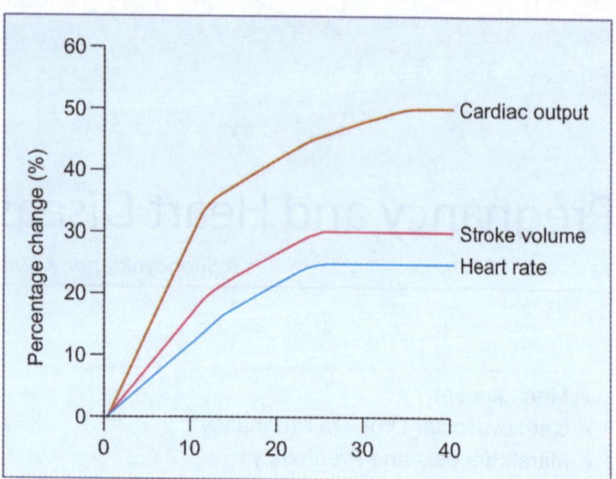

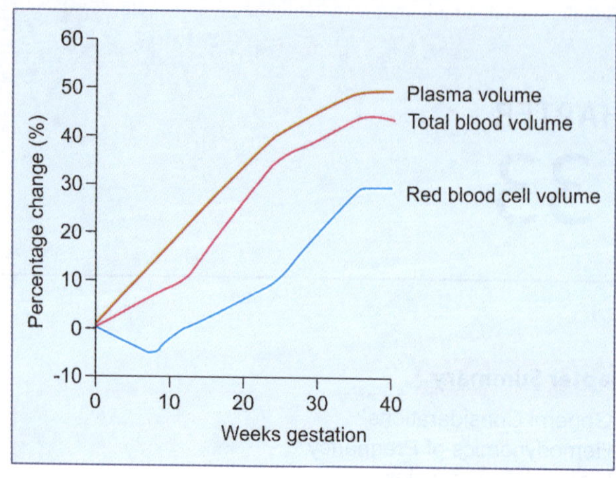

Fig. 133.1: Maternal circulatory changes in pregnancy

can mimic heart disease in many ways. Symptoms like dyspnea, palpitation and edema are common. Pulse is relatively fast and brisk; jugular venous pressure (JVP) can be elevated with sharp descends. Apex beat may be displaced due to increase in heart size and pushing up of the heart by the gravid uterus. Both first and second heart sounds are accentuated; third heart sound and basal midsystolic murmur related to the hyperdynamic circulation are common. Continuous murmur of venous hum or mammary souffle also may be audible. However, fourth heart sound and diastolic murmurs indicate abnormality.

Chest X-ray is avoided, especially during first trimester. Electrocardiogram (ECG) is useful in assessing the underlying cardiac rhythm. Arrhythmias like ectopic beats are common in normal pregnancy. Detailed transthoracic echocardiography (TTE) gives almost all the necessary information needed for diagnosis as well as for risk stratification and planning the management. Fetal ECG is indicated in conditions where there is a high risk for congenital cardiac malformations.

Prepregnant counseling is of extreme importance, especially in patients with high-risk factors. It is better to advise against pregnancy in those with severe pulmonary artery hypertension (PAH) or congestive heart failure (CHF). Patients who are asymptomatic, and at low risk do not require any specific care. Patients in NYHA class II require restriction of the activity; those in class III or IV may require hospitalization for stabilization of cardiac status and safe confinement. Adequate rest and supplementation of iron and vitamins to minimize the anemia of pregnancy are essential. Cardiac failure, if present, has to be meticulously controlled. Role of early termination of pregnancy has to be discussed in high-risk cases.

Vaginal delivery is feasible and preferred in majority of cases; cesarean section being indicated only for obstetric reasons. Second stage should be assisted with forceps or vacuum extraction to avoid long labor. However, elective cesarean section is indicated in the following situations:

- Patients on anticoagulation with vitamin K antagonists like warfarin—fetus is also anticoagulated, hence, the risk to fetus of intracranial hemorrhage (ICH) is high.
- Patients with dilated unstable aorta as in Marfan syndrome, coarctation of aorta (CoA) and bicuspid aortic valve (BAV), in view of risk of aortic dissection
- Patients with severe PAH
- Patients with severe obstructive lesions like aortic stenosis (AS) or mitral stenosis (MS).

Antibiotic prophylaxis is not usually recommended if strict aseptic precautions are taken; however, it may be implemented in cases at high-risk for endocarditis like cyanotic congenital heart diseases (CHD), mechanical prosthetic valves and history of previous endocarditis.

Maternal problems during pregnancy in those with heart disease: The major maternal complications in various heart diseases are summarized (Table 133.1).

Cardiovascular Drugs in Pregnancy

Many drugs used for the management of the heart disease can create problems for both the mother and baby. Aspirin

Table 133.1: Maternal complications during pregnancy in a cardiac patient	
Mitral stenosis	Pulmonary edema, especially during midtrimester, labor and postpartum; AF; thromboembolism
Aortic stenosis	Hypotension or shock; acute LV failure
BAV	Aortic dissection
Coarctation of aorta	Aortic dissection, rupture of Berry aneurysm, hypertension-related complications
Pulmonary hypertension	Hypotension or shock, cardiac arrest, CHF
LV dysfunction	Acute pulmonary edema, CHF, arrhythmias, cardiac arrest
Marfan syndrome	Dissection of aorta
Mechanical valves	Valve thrombosis, embolism
Cyanotic CHF	Worsening of cyanosis, venous or arterial thrombosis, paradoxical embolism

Abbreviations: AF = Atrial fibrillation; LV = Left ventricular; BAV = Bicuspid aortic valve; CHF = Congestive heart failure

crosses the placenta and by its effect on prostaglandin synthesis, it may produce premature closure of ductus arteriosus; however, in small doses, it is safe. β-blockers, especially atenolol, can produce intrauterine growth retardation and neonatal bradycardia and hypoglycemia. However, if definitely indicated, selective β-blockers like metoprolol can be given. Angiotensin converting enzyme (ACE) inhibitors and angiotensin receptor blockers (ARB) are contraindicated in pregnancy as they produce oligohydramnios, intrauterine growth retardation and fetal renal hypoplasia. Risk of intracranial hemorrhage with warfarin has already been mentioned. After discontinuation, reversal of anticoagulant effect is slow in baby due to the immature liver. Hence, it is mandatory to switch over to heparin well before delivery. Drugs like digoxin, calcium channel blockers, nitrates, α-blockers and diuretics are relatively safe in pregnancy; however, high-dose of diuretics should be avoided as it can produce hypovolemia and placental ischemia.

MITRAL STENOSIS AND PREGNANCY

Though the incidence of rheumatic fever is coming down, MS with complicating pregnancy continues to be a major problem in developing countries. The increase in blood volume, cardiac output and heart rate are deleterious in MS; all result in elevation of left atrial (LA) pressure. Tachycardia shortens diastole and hence, LA emptying is reduced leading to LA hypertension. Hence, pregnant women with significant MS are at risk of developing pulmonary edema especially during midtrimester, labor and early postpartum when the hemodynamic burden is high. Onset of atrial fibrillation (AF) also precipitates pulmonary edema by raising the LA pressure due to fast heart rate and loss of atrial contraction. Pregnancy is a hypercoagulable state which adds to the high-risk for thromboembolism.

The cornerstone in the medical therapy of MS is to control the heart rate with β-blockers or nondihydropydrine calcium channel blockers like verapamil or diltiazem. Symptoms of pulmonary congestion can be controlled with judicious use of diuretics. Optimal dose of anticoagulation has to be instituted in patients whose are in AF. If the patient cannot be stabilized on medication, percutaneous mitral balloon commissurotomy (PMBC) can be performed. Rarely, surgery may be needed.

PREGNANCY AND PROSTHETIC VALVES

Pregnancy is a hypercoagulable state, and hence, the risk of prosthetic valve thrombosis (PVT) is high. Valve thrombosis can lead to valve malfunction and embolization; hence, optimal anticoagulation status is mandatory for mechanical prosthetic valves. Aspirin should be continued in those with biological prosthesis. The conventional anticoagulation regime for mechanical

prosthesis during pregnancy is to discontinue warfarin, and switch over to heparin (unfractionated or low molecular weight) in the first trimester. However, from the second trimester onwards, warfarin maybe continued with an optimal international normalized ratio target. About two weeks before anticipated delivery, once again switch over to heparin. After delivery, restart warfarin (combining with heparin for 3–5 days) at the earliest in the postpartum period. However, there are many who believe that the risk of warfarin embryopathy and other fetal complications with continued and uninterrupted oral anticoagulation during pregnancy are minimal and the safest option for the mother with a prosthetic valve is to continue oral anticoagulants without break.

Cardiac Tumors

A George Koshy, Sajan Z Ahmed

Chapter Summary

- General Considerations
- Clinical Presentations
- Benign Tumors
- Malignant Cardiac Tumors
- Cardiac Lymphomas
- Secondary Cardiac Tumors

GENERAL CONSIDERATIONS

Primary cardiac tumors are rare across all age groups. Secondary deposits are 20–40 times commoner and are seen in 1% of postmortem examinations. Most of such individuals have widely disseminated malignancy. Atrial myxomas are the most common (75%) primary cardiac tumor in adults and rhabdomyoma is the most common cardiac tumor in children. A quarter of all cardiac tumors are malignant; the majority of which are angiosarcomas or rhabdomyosarcomas.

The **diagnosis** of primary cardiac tumors is frequently challenging. The symptoms associated with most primary cardiac tumors are very often nonspecific. Many cases are found incidentally during evaluation of an unrelated medical condition. A high index of suspicion is required for a positive diagnosis.

CLINICAL PRESENTATIONS

Primary cardiac tumors can mimic many commonly encountered cardiac and systemic diseases. Depending on the location, size, mobility and friability, cardiac tumors can produce a variety of symptoms and clinical findings. Atrial myxomas, in particular, may cause systemic symptoms mimicking collagen vascular disease, malignancy or infective endocarditis (IE).

The various clinical manifestations of cardiac tumors can be divided into following categories:

Embolic Phenomenon

The tumor itself or adherent thrombi can embolize. Both systemic as well as pulmonary embolism (PE) can occur depending on the site of the tumor. Multiple small emboli can mimic vasculitis or endocarditis. Cardiac myxomas are most frequently associated with embolic findings. The brain is the most common site of involvement for systemic emboli and the involvement of both hemispheres and multiple regions is not uncommon. Histological examination of the retrieved embolic material can give clue regarding the diagnosis and nature of the tumor. Right-sided tumors naturally embolize to the lungs and can result in PE, pulmonary hypertension (PH) and right-sided heart failure.

Cardiac Manifestations

Atrial tumors, once they are large enough, usually lead to obstruction of atrioventricular (AV) flow and behave like AV valve stenosis. Left atrial myxomas very often mimic mitral valve disease. Symptoms can be related to body positions. Gradually progressive exertional dyspnea and posture-related syncope and worsening of breathlessness are characteristic features. Ventricular tumors, though less common, can produce outflow tract obstruction leading to breathlessness, angina or syncope.

Arrhythmias

Conduction abnormalities and arrhythmias can also occur depending on the location of the tumor. Intramyocardial and intracavity tumors may both affect cardiac rhythm, either through direct infiltration of the conduction tissue, or through irritation of the myocardium itself. Sudden cardiac death can occur both due to arrhythmias and conduction abnormalities as well as due to valvular obstruction.

Metastasis

Symptoms secondary to the metastatic disease may represent the initial clinical manifestation of the malignant primary cardiac tumors. Common sites of metastasis include lung, brain and bone.

Before the advent of echocardiography, diagnosis of cardiac tumors was extremely difficult. Now, echocardiography—transthoracic and transesophageal—as well as 3-dimensional imaging modalities have made the diagnosis easy in most of the cases. Cardiac computed tomography (CT) and magnetic resonance imaging (MRI) can provide additional information in certain cases.

BENIGN TUMORS

Myxomas

Atrial myxoma is the most common primary cardiac tumor, comprising 50% of all primary tumors of the heart. Occurring more commonly in women, myxomas are usually diagnosed between the ages of 50 and 70 years. Ninety percent are left atrial in location and 90% are solitary. *Syndrome myxoma* should be suspected in patients younger than 40 years who present with multiple cardiac myxomas. These can include biatrial, ventricular and recurrent myxomas. Multiple acronyms have been proposed for such syndromes. These include LAMB (lentigines, atrial myxomas, mucocutaneous myxomas, and blue nevi) and NAME (nevi, atrial myxomas, myxoid neurofibroma and ephelides). Familial myxomas with a genetic background are collectively described as Carney complex. If diagnosed, all first-degree relatives should be screened for the condition.

The cell of origin of the myxoma is not known. Macroscopically, they appear irregular, shiny and pedunculated. The majority of myxomas are attached to the left side of the interatrial septum around the fossa ovalis.

Clinical Features

Symptoms include breathlessness, fever, weight loss, syncope, hemoptysis and sometimes sudden death. Sometimes patients with transient ischemic attacks or stroke are found to have an isolated myxoma during echocardiographic evaluation. Anemia, raised acute phase reactants and erythrocyte sedimentation rate (ESR) are frequently present. The clinical presentation of left atrial myxoma simulate mitral valve disease with loud first heart sound and mid-diastolic murmur (MDM) with presystolic accentuation. The characteristic **tumor plop** may be audible in diastole in some patients. It is lower pitched compared to opening snap. Pansystolic murmur indicative of mitral regurgitation (MR) may also be audible. The murmur can sometimes show postural changes related to the mobility of the mass.

Diagnosis depends on a high index of suspicion and can almost always be made by echocardiography. Both transthoracic and transesophageal imaging will demonstrate the tumor and its site of attachment to the interatrial septum (Fig. 134.1). MR, if present, can be detected and quantified. Myxoma should be differentiated from left atrial thrombus, vegetations and markedly myxomatous mitral valve tissue itself.

Management

The treatment of choice is early surgical resection on cardiopulmonary bypass (CPB). Surgical outcome is generally good, with a 20-year survival rate of 85%. However, recurrence rate after resection is approximately 5%. Therefore, careful, serial follow-up is required. Because of the risk of embolism, excision should be done at the earliest.

Fibromas

Cardiac fibromas are low-grade connective tissue tumors. They are usually intraventricular in location and mostly occur in children. Pathologically, they appear as firm gray white masses. The size is variable with some tumors reaching almost 10 cm in diameter. They can present

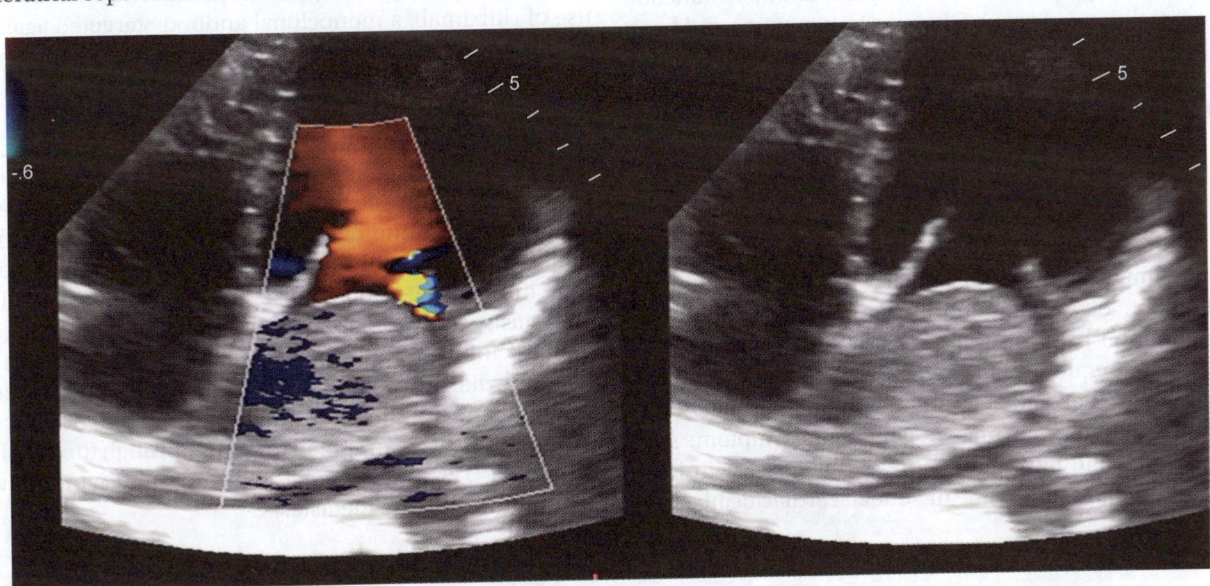

Fig. 134.1: Echocardiogram of left atrial myxoma showing a large mass in the left atrium which is attached to the interatrial septum

Courtesy: Professor George Koshy

with obstructive symptoms, arrhythmias and sometimes sudden cardiac death. Heart failure can also occur. Multiple foci of calcification is common and can be picked up by echocardiography and fluoroscopy. Surgical excision is the recommended treatment but may not be possible in all cases.

Papillary Fibroelastomas

They are the most common valvular tumor but are often asymptomatic during life and are incidentally detected during autopsy. They have a male preponderance with the mean age of detection of 60 years. They rarely cause valvular dysfunction. However, left-sided tumors can embolize to coronary and cerebral arteries leading to acute coronary syndrome (ACS), transient ischemic attacks and stroke. Typically, it has a *sea anemone* appearance, with a short attaching pedicle. Echocardiographically, this may be mistaken for vegetations. *Treatment* is by surgical excision.

Rhabdomyomas

They are the most common primary cardiac neoplasm in children. They are usually multiple and ventricular. They may be seen echocardiographically as a pedunculated mass producing obstruction to ventricular inflow or outflow. Symptoms may result from arrhythmias or mechanical complications due to obstruction of blood flow. Sudden cardiac death is unusual. Spontaneous tumor resolution is common and treatment is therefore usually conservative. Majority of children with cardiac rhabdomyoma have tuberous sclerosis. Surgical resection may be sometimes required in children with severe obstructive symptoms.

Lipomas

Cardiac lipomas can occur, sporadically at all ages with equal frequency in both sexes. They may occur anywhere in the heart. They can occur in the pericardium, sub-endocardium, subepicardium and interatrial septum. They are usually asymptomatic but arrhythmias and conduction abnormalities can occur. Obstructive symptoms and heart failure are less common. Lipomatous hypertrophy of the interatrial septum is a separate, non-neoplastic condition. It is usually found in obese patients, in whom the atrial septum is heavily infiltrated with adiposity.

MALIGNANT CARDIAC TUMORS

Sarcomas

Approximately 25% of primary cardiac tumors are malignant, of which majority are sarcomas. Sarcomas are common between the third and fifth decades of life and most frequently affect the right atrium (RA). They have variable presentations and early diagnosis is often difficult. Patients may present with vague symptoms such as dyspnea and fatigue, or more dramatically with heart failure, cardiac tamponade or sudden cardiac death.

Angiosarcomas

These tumors have male preponderance and are almost exclusively seen in the RA. The tumor can be large and infiltrative, replacing the atrial wall and extending into the chamber. The tumor can sometimes completely fill the RA producing obstruction and right heart failure. They can invade the vena cava, tricuspid valve and pericardium. *Treatment* with chemotherapy or radiation does not relieve symptoms. Even surgical resection is not associated with favorable outcome.

Rhabdomyosarcomas

Cardiac rhabdomyosarcomas are the most common primary sarcoma of the heart in children. The average age at disease presentation is in the second decade of life, but it can also occur in young adults. A slight male predominance exists, especially in the pediatric population. They are rapidly-growing very aggressive tumors which can involve any cardiac chamber. Pericardial involvement is common at the time of initial diagnosis. These tumors have a dismal prognosis and survival is usually less than one year.

Leiomyosarcomas

These are rare tumors found in the left atrium (LA). Their histology demonstrates spindle-shaped cells. Presenting symptoms include arrhythmias, sudden death and hemo-pericardium. They are highly aggressive tumors, which spread systemically and have early local recurrence. Overall prognosis is very poor.

CARDIAC LYMPHOMAS

Primary cardiac lymphomas account for 1–2% of all primary cardiac tumors. Immunocompromised individuals are more commonly involved than immunocompetent individuals. This is particularly known to occur in human immunodeficiency virus (HIV) infections and post-transplant lymphoproliferative disorder (PTLD). Main presentation is as intractable heart failure. Anthracycline-based chemotherapy with or without radiation is the mainstay for treatment of primary cardiac lymphomas. The use of rituximab, a monoclonal antibody targeted against CD20, in combination with conventional chemotherapy, has shown some promise in improving survival.

SECONDARY CARDIAC TUMORS

Secondary involvement of the heart by extracardiac tumors is 20–40 times more common than by primary cardiac tumors. The development of tachycardia, arrhythmias, cardiomegaly or heart failure in a patient with malignancy should raise the suspicion of cardiac metastasis. Carcinoma of the lung or breast can spread by local infiltration to the pericardium, leading usually to pericardial effusion. Carcinoma of the lung can invade the pulmonary veins and grow into the LA. Renal cell carcinoma (RCC) can spread to the RA through the inferior vena cava (IVC). Melanoma, leukemias and lymphomas can produce cardiac metastasis.

An Introduction to Interventional Cardiology

A George Koshy, Sajan Ahmed

Chapter Summary

- Brief History
- Coronary Artery Disease (CAD)
- Valvular Heart Disease
- Cardiomyopathy
- Pacing and Electrophysiology
- Congenital Heart Disease (CHD)
- Miscellaneous
- Interventional Cardiology: Relevant Issues

BRIEF HISTORY

The first cardiac catheterization of a living person was performed by Werner Forssmann on himself in 1929. The percutaneous technique for interventions was developed by Seldinger in 1953. Percutaneous transluminal coronary angioplasty (PTCA) using balloons was introduced by Gruentzig in 1977. The first intracardiac therapeutic catheterization procedure for pediatric congenital heart disease (CHD) was the balloon atrial septostomy by Rashkind and Miller in 1966 (Table 135.1).

CORONARY ARTERY DISEASE (CAD)

Coronary Angiography and Percutaneous Coronary Interventions (PCI)

The most common interventional procedure in the cardiac catheterization laboratory is coronary angiography with or without angioplasty. After an arterial access, a sheath is inserted into the artery, through which special catheters are introduced into the origins of the coronary arteries under fluoroscopic guidance. Contrast agents are injected into the coronary arteries thereby facilitating visualization of intraluminal obstructions produced by atheromatous plaques. Coronary wires are tracked across these stenotic lesions. These lesions are dilated with balloons and then stented with either bare-metal stents (BMSs) or drug-eluting stents (DESs) that provide a stable scaffold and prevent restenosis.

Vascular Access Routes for Coronary Interventions

- **Femoral route:** The target for puncture is the common femoral artery, commonly the right
- **Radial route:** The target for puncture is the radial artery, commonly the right.
- **Contrast media:** Radiographic contrast agents are injected during coronary arteriography to visualize the lumen of the coronary arteries under fluoroscopy. Ionic and nonionic contrast agents may be used, although the preferred agent is the nonionic iso-osmolar iodixanol.

Table 135.1: Interventional cardiology overview

Coronary artery disease (CAD)	Coronary angiogram, angioplasty, stenting, FFR, IVUS, OCT and rotablator
Valvular heart disease	PBMV, Percutaneous mitral valve repair, TAVI, PPVI
Cardiomyopathy	Alcohol septal ablation in HOCM
Pacing and electrophysiology	Pacemaker implantation—PPI, TPI, CRT, ICD, Electrophysiological studies (EPS), Radiofrequency ablation (RFA)
Congenital heart disease (CHD)	Device closure of ASD, VSD, PDA, Balloon dilatation of valvular aortic and pulmonary stenosis, Balloon dilatation and/or stenting of coarctation, Balloon atrial septostomy
Miscellaneous	Renal sympathetic denervation, PFO occlusion, Left atrial (LA) appendage exclusion, IABP, percutaneous LVAD IVC filter, Noncoronary vascular interventions, Pericardiocentesis

Abbreviations: FFR = Fractional flow reserve; IVUS = Intravascular ultrasound; OCT = Optical coherence tomography; HOCM = Hypertrophic obstructive cardiomyopathy; PPI = Permanent pacemaker implantation; TPI = Temporary pacemaker implantation; ASD = Atrial septal defect; VSD = Ventricular septal defect; PDA = Patent ductus arteriosus; PFO = Patent foramen ovale; IABP = Intra-aortic balloon counter-pulsation; LVAD = Left ventricular assist device; IVC = Inferior vena cava; PBMV = Percutaneous balloon mitral valvulopathy; TAVI = Transcatheter aortic valve implantation; PPVI = Percutaneous pulmonary valve impantation; CRT = Cardiac cardioverter defibrillator

Drugs Commonly used During PCI

- **Loading dose of antiplatelet agents:** Aspirin + clopidogrel or prasugrel or ticagrelor
- **Glycoprotein IIb/IIIa inhibitors:** Abciximab, tirofiban, eptifibatide; these are less frequently used now
- **Anticoagulants:** Unfractionated heparin (UFH), low-molecular-weight heparin (LMWH), enoxaparin, direct thrombin inhibitor—bivalirudin
- **Intracoronary agents:** Nitroglycerin, adenosine, sodium nitroprusside and nicorandil.

Coronary Stents

Coronary stents are implanted at sites of coronary obstructions to maintain the long-term patency of the vessel. There are two basic types of stents: (1) BMSs and (2) DESs. BMSs have a higher risk of restenosis. DES consists of a metallic stent that is coated with a polymer which releases an antiproliferative agent capable of preventing restenosis (sirolimus or paclitaxel in first-generation DES and everolimus or zotarolimus in second-generation DES). However, DES is associated with a higher risk of late stent thrombosis, thereby requiring a longer duration of treatment with dual antiplatelets. A newer category of stents is Bioresorbable Vascular Scaffold

(BVS) with a poly-L-lactic acid (PLLA) polymer that elutes everolimus and then resorbs naturally into the body.

Primary Angioplasty

It is the catheter-based reperfusion strategy for the management of ST-elevation myocardial infarction (STEMI). Instead of thrombolysis, the patient undergoes an emergency coronary angiogram in the catheterization laboratory to identify the culprit vessel for the STEMI. The occluded coronary artery is then reopened with the help of thrombus aspiration catheter, balloon angioplasty and stenting.

- *Window period:* 12 hours from the onset of chest pain
- *Target first medical contact (FMC) to device time:* 90 minutes
- *Target FMC to device time if transfer to PCI capable hospital:* 120 minutes
- *Primary PCI beyond the window period is done if:* Ongoing chest pain (12–24 hours), cardiogenic shock, or heart failure.

Adjunctive Technology for PCI

- *Fractional flow reserve (FFR):* It is defined as maximum flow down a vessel in the presence of a stenosis compared to the maximal flow down that vessel in the hypothetical absence of the stenosis. It is estimated using an FFR wire inserted through a catheter into the coronary artery, with maximal hyperemia being induced by the administration of adenosine.
  - *FFR = Pd/Pa,* where Pd = coronary pressure distal to the stenosis and Pa = aortic pressure
  - *FFR values to remember:* 1 (normal), less than 0.75 (significant stenosis and ischemia), more than 0.8 (excludes significant stenosis and ischemia).
- *Intravascular ultrasound (IVUS):* IVUS imaging of the coronary arteries with special IVUS imaging catheters helps in characterizing the obstructions better, especially in left main CAD.
- *Optical coherence tomography (OCT):* OCT catheters utilize light energy sources to provide superior images during PCI, especially regarding the presence of thrombus dissection flaps and the optimal deployment of stents.
- *Rotablator:* It is a device that uses a high-speed rotating diamond coated burr to cut through hard and calcific atherosclerotic plaques (CAP) in coronary arteries.

VALVULAR HEART DISEASE

Balloon Procedures and Surgical Repairs

- *Balloon mitral valvotomy (BMV):* Percutaneous BMV is recommended for moderate to severe symptomatic mitral stenosis (MS) with favorable characteristics [no or mild mitral regurgitation (MR), pliable, non-calcified valve and no left atrial (LA) thrombus]. After gaining access into the LA through a trans-septal puncture, a mitral valve balloon (e.g. Inoue-balloon) is dilated across the stenosed mitral valve with resultant splitting of the fused mitral commissures. The balloon size (in mm) is calculated by the formula: height of the patient in cm/10 + 10.

- *Mitral valve repair:* Percutaneous treatment of MR can target the mitral valve (e.g. MitraClip; improves leaflet coaptation) or the mitral annulus (e.g. percutaneous mitral annuloplasty with Monarc or Carillon device).
- *Balloon aortic valvotomy:* In the adolescent or young adult with severe congenital aortic stenosis (AS), BAV is recommended for all symptomatic patients and asymptomatic patients with a transvalvular gradient higher than 60 mm Hg or electrocardiographic (ECG) ST-segment changes at rest or with exercise. However, in the adult patient with degenerative aortic valve disease, it is associated with high restenosis rates and is therefore not preferred.
- *Balloon pulmonary valvotomy:* It is the standard therapy for valvular pulmonary stenosis with peak gradient more than 50 mm Hg and evidence of right ventricular hypertrophy (RVH). The most commonly used technique is using the Tyshak balloon.
- *Transcatheter aortic valve implantation (TAVI):* It is a new approach to the treatment of aortic valve stenosis in patients who are at a high-operative risk for traditional aortic valve replacement. A percutaneous or transapical route is used to implant a prosthetic aortic valve (e.g., Edward-Sapiens, core valve).
- *Transcatheter pulmonary valve replacement:* The Melody valve *(Bonhoeffer valve)* is a bovine jugular venous valve sutured within a stent and mounted on a balloon. It is primarily used in the treatment of dysfunctional right ventricular outflow tract (RVOT) conduits, in the setting of postoperative CHD patients.

CARDIOMYOPATHY

Alcohol septal ablation: It is an alternative treatment strategy (surgical myectomy being the preferred treatment) for severely symptomatic hypertrophic obstructive cardiomyopathy (HOCM). About 1–3 mL of 95% ethanol is injected into the septal branch of the left anterior descending coronary artery to produce a limited myocardial infarction (MI) and thinning of the proximal interventricular septum (IVS), thereby reducing the left ventricular outflow tract (LVOT) obstruction.

PACING AND ELECTROPHYSIOLOGY

- *Permanent pacemaker implantation (PPI):* It is indicated in symptomatic sick sinus syndrome and advanced atrioventricular (AV) block (Mobitz type 2 and complete heart block) in the setting of symptoms, asystole more than 3 seconds, and/or escape rate less than 40 beats/minute. It can be single chamber or dual chamber pacing. The usual procedure is to insert the ventricular pacing lead via the left subclavian venous approach across the tricuspid valve into the right ventricle (RV). The atrial lead is also inserted through the left subclavian vein and is usually positioned in the right atrial appendage (RAA). The pulse generator of the pacemaker is implanted in a left infraclavicular pocket that is created by blunt dissection. The average lifespan of a standard pacemaker is around 10–12 years.

- ***Cardiac resynchronization therapy (CRT):*** It is a new modality of treatment for patients with heart failure with an LV ejection fraction (LVEF) of 35% or less, sinus rhythm and New York Heart Association (NYHA), functional class III or ambulatory class IV symptoms, despite recommended optimal medical therapy and who have cardiac dyssynchrony, which is currently defined as a QRS interval of 120 milliseconds or longer. Patients with left bundle branch block (LBBB) in the ECG and significant prolongation of the QRS generally respond best. Here, in addition to the RV lead, the LV is also paced via a lead placed in a tributary of the coronary sinus.
- ***Implantable cardioverter defibrillator (ICD):*** It is a device that is implanted within the heart, which detects and terminates life-threatening arrhythmias, like ventricular tachycardia (VT) and ventricular fibrillation (VF) by delivering an intracardiac direct-current (DC) shock, thereby preventing sudden cardiac death. The electrodes for delivering the shock are positioned at the RV apex and at the superior vena cava-right atrial (SVC-RA) junction.
- ***Electrophysiology study (EPS) + radiofrequency ablation (RFA)*** using special catheters can be used to identify substrates for arrhythmias in the heart. These may be subjected to RFA. Supraventricular tachycardias (SVT), like AV nodal re-entrant tachycardias and Wolff-Parkinson-White (WPW) syndromes, and VTs, like RV outflow tachycardias or scar VTs, may be treated in this manner.
- ***Temporary pacemaker implantation (TPI):*** A TPI is sometimes required as an emergency procedure in patients with MI and complete heart block or in odollam poisoning. A pacing lead is inserted via the femoral vein into the RV.

CONGENITAL HEART DISEASE (CHD)

- ***Balloon atrial septostomy:*** It is a lifesaving procedure done in infants younger than 1 month with dextro-transposition (d-TGA of the great arteries—parallel circulation) to allow adequate intercirculatory mixing. Through a femoral venous approach, a balloon septostomy catheter (Rashkind or Miller-Edwards) is advanced through a patent foramen ovale (PFO), dilated in the LA and pulled back to produce a tear and wide opening in the interatrial septum.
- ***Atrial septal defect (ASD) device closure:*** Device closure of hemodynamically significant ostium secundum ASDs can be done percutaneously under fluoroscopic or transesophageal echocardiogram (TEE) guidance, provided the stretched diameter of the defect is less than 41 mm, there are adequate rims around the ASD to secure the device in position and there is normal pulmonary venous drainage (e.g. Amplatzer ASD Occluder device).
- ***Ventricular septal defect (VSD) device closure:*** Muscular, especially mid-muscular VSDs may be amenable to device closure. Device closure of perimembranous VSDs may be associated with a higher risk of complete heart block.

- ***Patent ductus arteriosus (PDA) device closure or coil occlusion:*** Ducts smaller than 8 mm can be treated with device closure [e.g. Amplatzer duct occluder (ADO)]. Single or multiple coils (e.g. Gianturco coils) may also be used. Closure is not warranted in asymptomatic patients with a silent PDA (absent murmur) detected only by Echo Doppler studies.
- ***Coarctation of aorta (CoA):*** Surgery is the preferred treatment for native coarctation in infants and small children. However, balloon dilatation, with or without stenting may be feasible for selected patients, especially for recurrent coarctation after surgery.

MISCELLANEOUS

- ***Renal sympathetic denervation:*** It is a catheter-based technique for the treatment of resistant systemic hypertension. Specially designed catheters (e.g. Simplicity catheter) are used to ablate the sympathetic nerve fibers in the renal arteries.
- ***Patent foramen ovale (PFO) closure:*** Closure of PFO with a device (e.g. Amplatzer PFO Occluder) may be done in case of a documented paradoxical arterial embolism in the setting of venous thrombosis.
- ***LA appendage exclusion:*** LAA exclusion with a device (e.g. Watchman device) may be done to prevent embolic stroke in atrial fibrillation (AF) as most emboli might originate from the LA appendage.
- ***Intra-aortic balloon counter-pulsation (IABP):*** It is a method of temporary mechanical circulatory support, which is useful in cardiogenic shock or ventricular septal rupture complicating MI, or in acute MR. The IABP catheter is inserted via the femoral artery and the tip is positioned below the level of left subclavian artery and above the level of the renal arteries. Timing of balloon inflation is at onset of diastole, and of balloon deflation is at the onset of systole. The IABP helps by improving the coronary perfusion and the hemodynamics. Contraindications are aortic regurgitation and aortic dissection.
- ***Percutaneous left ventricular assist device (LVAD):*** Percutaneous LVADs help in reducing preload and augmenting cardiac output (e.g., TandemHeart and Impella).
- ***Inferior vena cava (IVC) filter:*** IVC filter (e.g. Greenfield filter) is useful to prevent pulmonary embolism (PE) in case of recurrent PE despite optimal anticoagulation or if there is a contraindication for anticoagulation.
- ***Noncoronary vascular interventions:*** Obstructive lesions causing peripheral arterial disease of lower limbs (iliac or femoral arteries), renal artery stenosis, carotid artery disease, mesenteric ischemia (celiac or mesenteric arteries) may be amenable to treatment with angioplasty with or without stenting under fluoroscopic guidance. Uterine artery embolization (UAE) for hemorrhage and hepatic artery embolization (HAE) for treatment of hepatic tumors are also being tried.
- ***Pericardiocentesis:*** Aspiration of fluid from the pericardial cavity is required for the treatment of cardiac tamponade due to any cause and also for diagnostic purposes. A subxiphoid approach is often

used. A pigtail catheter can be retained in the pericardial cavity for a few hours for continuous drainage.

INTERVENTIONAL CARDIOLOGY: RELEVANT ISSUES

- *Patient selection:* Proper selection of the patient, the indication and the procedure, including the cost-benefit ratio is at the heart of every intervention in the catheterization laboratory.
- *Radiation hazards:* The patient and the operators should be adequately protected from the hazards of radiation from the fluoroscopy machine. Lead aprons, neck shields and goggles are often used for this.

- *Contrast-induced nephropathy:* The use of contrast agents may be associated with risk of renal injury in high-risk patients (e.g. diabetes, pre-existing renal disease).
- *Procedural complications:* These may be vascular (hematoma, pseudoaneurysm, AV fistula), coronary (dissection, perforation, tamponade), valvular (acute MR during BMV), device related (embolization), or electrical (complete heart block following RFA). Rarely complications can also lead to mortality.
- *Medical management and follow-up:* Continued optimal medical management and follow-up is essential for success and safety of any interventional procedure.

Cardiac Surgery

A George Koshy, CG Bahuleyan

Chapter Summary

- Surgical Treatment
- Congenital Heart Disease
- Coronary Artery Surgery
- Surgery for Chronic Valvular Diseases
- Cardiac Assist Devices
- Cardiac Transplantation

INTRODUCTION

At present, cardiac surgery has reached to a very high level of technical perfection. This has been made possible by advancements in anesthesia, maintenance of extracorporeal circulation by pumps and oxygenators, hypothermia, methods to control cardiac arrhythmias, better methods of myocardial preservation, availability of newer prosthetic materials and progress in intensive postoperative care including circulatory assist devices.

SURGICAL TREATMENT

Surgical treatment is available for the following conditions:

- Congenital heart diseases (CHDs)
- Acquired valvular diseases
- Ischemic heart disease (IHD)
- Constrictive pericarditis
- Cardiac tumors
- Heart block and serious arrhythmias—pacemaker implantation, implantable cardioverter defibrillator (ICD)
- Correction of abnormal conducting tissues in the heart producing recurrent tachyarrhythmias, e.g. Wolff-Parkinson-White (WPW) syndrome
- Heart failure (HF)—implantation of cardiac resynchronization therapy (CRT) device
- Cardiac tamponade
- Cardiac aneurysms

- Cardiogenic shock not amenable to inotropic drugs—urgent revascularization
- End-stage cardiac failure—transplantation
- Endomyocardial fibrosis
- Hypertrophic cardiomyopathy (HCM)—myotomy and myectomy
- Aortic aneurysms and dissection

In addition to several acute conditions, such as rupture of valves or chordae, obstruction of aorta and pulmonary artery, traumatic lesions and infective endocarditis (IE) resistant to medical therapy, emergency surgical measures may be required.

CONGENITAL HEART DISEASE

Most of the CHD are amenable to surgical correction or palliation now, the present stress being on early detection and correction of congenital cardiac defects. Pediatric cardiac surgery, especially in infants and neonates has so progressed that defects like ventricular septal defects (VSD), tetralogy of Fallot (TOF), aortic stenosis, transposition of great arteries (TGA), tricuspid atresia and total anomalous pulmonary venous drainage are all operable in infancy or early childhood. Most of the cases of persistent ductus arteriosus and secundum atrial septal defects (ASD) are at present managed by nonsurgical means using coils and devices in the cardiac catheterization laboratory. Sinus venosus and primum type of ASD are not suitable for device closure and hence, require surgical intervention. Large secundum ASD and those with defective rims are also not amenable for device closure. Majority of VSD require surgical closure. The surgical closure for septal defects should be done at a young age, before the development of pulmonary obstructive vascular disease. Ideal age of surgical intervention is decided by the clinical status, weight of the child and the experience of the surgeon and the center.

Life-saving palliative surgical procedures may be required in the neonates in the first few days of life in conditions, which threaten life, e.g. transposition of great vessels (TGV), hypoplastic left heart syndromes (HLHS). Those sick infants with TOF and recurrent cyanotic spells with unfavorable pulmonary arteries anatomy may require a palliative systemic to pulmonary artery shunt to increase the pulmonary blood flow. Modified Blalock-Taussig shunt is performed using a side to side anastomosis between one of the subclavian arteries and right or left pulmonary artery. Definitive intracardiac repair can be done at a later date.

In many situations, when two functional ventricular circulations cannot be achieved, bypassing the right ventricle (RV) by anastomosing the vena cava to the pulmonary artery, i.e. total cavopulmonary connection (TCPC) is done. This achieves good functional capacity. Such circulation where in the RV function is bypassed is called *Fontan circulation*.

CORONARY ARTERY BYPASS SURGERY

The technique of coronary artery bypass using saphenous vein grafts was an epoch-making discovery in the management of severe IHD. At present, coronary revascularization procedures include coronary angioplasty and bypass surgery. In the surgical procedure, blood from the aorta is diverted through a conduit to the coronary artery distal to the occlusion. The common materials used are the saphenous vein, the internal mammary arteries (IMA) and the radial arteries. Synthetic prosthetic materials are also being tried upon. Revascularization procedures promptly relieve angina, reduce the extent of infarction and reinfarction, improve the quality of life and also prolong life compared to medical therapy in a selected subset. In good centers, the intra and perioperative mortality is less than 3%.

Long-term results are good. Percutaneous angioplasty techniques are undergoing refinement and perfection. Except in a few situations, angioplasty is able to achieve effective revascularization in the majority of lesions. The major disadvantages of angioplasty include abrupt closure of the vessel and late restenosis, both of which have been brought down to a great extent by routine use of stents, which help us to retain the lumen patent. Use of newer antiplatelet drugs such as prasugrel, ticagrelor, glycoprotein receptor antagonists and newer antithrombotic agents have further reduced the occurrence of acute and delayed thrombotic occlusion of the stents. The restenosis rate following percutaneous coronary interventions (PCI) has been significantly reduced by drug-eluting stents.

At present, the major surgical load in cardiovascular surgery is contributed by coronary revascularization procedures. The long-term patency rate for left IMA as a conduit is excellent. But the venous grafts tend to degenerate and occlude after several years. Almost half of venous grafts get occluded by 10 years. Coronary artery bypass graft (CABG) surgery can be performed without cardiopulmonary bypass (CPB) (Off-pump) and the results are comparable to conventional CABG surgeries performed with the help of CPB. Minimally invasive surgery and robotics-assisted surgery are also available in limited centers.

SURGERY FOR CHRONIC VALVULAR DISEASES

Hemodynamically significant valvular heart disease tends to progress with time in many cases and end up with cardiac failure, if the valvular abnormality is not corrected. All the acquired and congenital valvular diseases are amenable to surgical correction. Stenotic lesions are corrected by valvotomy which can be done either by a closed or open heart procedure. Valve tissue which is not grossly damaged and which will lend itself to dilatation can be corrected by this method. Balloon valvotomy is a standard procedure for the management of pulmonary stenosis and mitral stenosis (MS).

Three types of surgical interventions are available for rheumatic MS. Closed mitral valvotomy is an infrequently performed procedure at present. This is because of the widespread availability and excellent outcome of percutaneous transmitral commissurotomy (PTMC) (balloon mitral valvotomy). Closed procedures are reserved for those with relatively thin and pliable valves with minimal or no calcification and minimal subvalvular pathology. Presence of left atrial (LA) thrombus, moderate to severe mitral regurgitation (MR) and significant involvement of other valves are contraindications to closed procedure. Open mitral valvotomy, where commissurotomy and repair of the subvalvular pathology is performed under direct vision still has a place in the management of rheumatic MS. Heavily calcified mitral valve, those with severe subvalvular pathology and presence of significant MR are indications for mitral valve replacement. Mitral valve repair, where the native mitral valve apparatus is preserved is always preferred over mitral valve replacement. Myxomatous mitral valves with mitral valve prolapse and MR (usually involving the posterior mitral leaflet) are usually amenable to repair whereas, MR due to rheumatic etiology is unsuitable for repair and may require replacement.

Valve replacement has to be undertaken for regurgitant lesions and when the valve tissue is grossly damaged. Prosthetic valves are in use for about 40 years. There are two types of prosthetic valves: (1) Mechanical prosthesis and (2) bioprosthetic valves. The most commonly used mechanical valves are the Starr-Edwards ball-in-cage valve and tilting disc valves (single tilting disk valve, like Chitra valve and bileaflet valve like St. Jude valve). Tissue valves obtained from cadavers or from pig's aorta and valves made from tissues like dura mater, pericardium and fascia lata are also employed at times, depending on the individual circumstances. Stentless prosthesis is also available for the aortic position. Each type of valve has its own advantages and problems. Mechanical prosthetic valves require lifelong anticoagulation with vitamin K antagonists (usually Warfarin) and patients require frequent monitoring of the prothrombin time (PT) to adjust the dose. The International Normalized Ratio (INR) in relation to the PT should be kept around. Inadequate anticoagulation can lead to thromboembolic episodes whereas excessive anticoagulation is associated with bleeding risk. Bioprosthetic valves require oral anticoagulation only for the initial 3–6 months. If the patient remains in sinus rhythm, anticoagulation can be stopped after that. Other problems related to prosthetic valves include IE—both early and late. Bioprosthetic valves can degenerate and may require repeat surgery after 10 or 15 years. In-growth of fibrous tissue (pannus formation) can produce progressive narrowing of the valve orifice in a mechanical valve. Individuals with prosthetic valves require IE prophylaxis prior to procedures, which can lead to bacteremia. In rheumatic mitral valve disease and severe pulmonary arterial hypertension (PAH), the tricuspid annulus may be markedly dilated with severe tricuspid regurgitation and dilated right-sided chambers. Such patients are benefited by tricuspid annuloplasty usually with Carpentier ring. Those patients older than 40 years of age and those with multiple risk factors should undergo coronary angiogram preoperatively to detect any associated CHD. Those with significant epicardial atrial narrowing can undergo CABG surgery along with the valve replacement.

Reports of large series on valve surgery reveal that over 90% of them are well at 5 years and over 70% of them are well at 10 years follow-up. Among those with implanted artificial valves, 38% of deaths are valve problem-related, 20% are due to other cardiac causes, which are not directly attributable to the valve. The remaining patients die of noncardiac causes.

CARDIAC ASSIST DEVICES

Several attempts have been made from time-to-time to assist the failing ventricle to increase its output. From the early part of this decade, artificial hearts have been implanted into individuals suffering from irrecoverable congestive cardiac failure (CCF) and the initial success in keeping such patients alive for weeks to months have encouraged the development of newer and newer devices.

An artificial heart is typically used to bridge the time to cardiac transplantation or to permanently replace the heart in case of transplantation is impossible. Artificial hearts made of inert chemical substances are now available. The first artificial heart to be successfully implanted in a human was the Jarvik-7, designed by a team including Robert Jarvik and implemented in 1982. Maximum clinical experience has also been with Jarvik-7, developed by the cumulative efforts of Willem Kolff, Donald Olson and Robert Jarvik, and the surgical experience of William DeVries and his associates. This device has been used as a permanent cardiac replacement and life has been prolonged for 20 months or more, though complications are frequent.

Leading French heart transplant specialist Alain F Carpentier in association with the biomedical firm, Carmat developed a fully implantable artificial heart and was implanted on December 20, 2013 in a 75-years-old patient in Paris. Though it was successful, the patient died 75 days after the surgery. In Carmat's design, two chambers are each divided by a membrane that holds hydraulic fluid on one side. A motorized pump is used to move the hydraulic fluid in and out of the chambers. This leads to flow of blood through the other side of each membrane. The side of the membrane in contact with the blood is made of tissue obtained from a sac that surrounds a cow's heart, to make the device more biocompatible. The Carmat device also uses valves made from cow heart tissue. It has sensors to detect pressure changes within the device, which is used to adjust flow rate in response to increased demand. It is expected that with further modifications, the Carmat device can be used in cases of terminal HF and not as a bridge to transplantation.

Patients who have some remaining heart function but who can no longer live normally may be the candidates for ventricular assist devices (VADs) which do not replace the human heart but complement it by taking up much of the function.

CARDIAC TRANSPLANTATION

It is performed on patients with end-stage HF or severe CHD not amenable to any revascularization procedure. The functioning heart from a brain-dead organ donor maintained on ventilation and fluid support for oxygenation, circulation and other major organ functions (cadaveric allograft) is implanted into the patient. The patient's own heart is usually removed (orthotopic procedure). Less commonly, it is left in place to support the donor heart (heterotopic procedure). The donor's heart is injected with potassium chloride (KCl) to stop its beating before it is removed from the donor's body and it is then packed in ice. Ice can usually keep the heart viable for around 4 hours. The failing heart is removed by transecting the great vessels and a portion of the LA. A circular portion of the LA containing the pulmonary veins is left in place. The donor heart is trimmed to fit onto the patient's remaining LA and the great vessels are sutured in place. Those who undergo cardiac transplantation require life-long immunosuppressive medications to prevent rejection. Postoperative complications include infection, sepsis, organ rejection as well as the side-effects of the immunosuppressive medications. Cardiac transplantation can be considered as a rational and socially acceptable therapy for patients with incurable cardiac failure, if surgical expertize and donor organ are available. The techniques of cardiac transplantation have improved progressively during the last 3 decades. These advances include better definition of criteria for selection of patients, more effective immunosuppression, improved myocardial preservation and better surgical techniques. The current survival following cardiac transplantation at the end of 3 years is 78% and at the end of 5 years is 72%. Survival overall is slightly better in males compared to females.

The world's first human heart transplant was performed by a South African cardiac surgeon, Christiaan Barnard on December 3, 1967 at the Groote Schuur Hospital in Cape Town, South Africa. Worldwide, about 3,500 heart transplants are performed annually. More than half of these are performed in the United States. Cedars-Sinai Medical Center in Los Angeles, California currently is the largest heart transplant center in the world. The first successful heart transplant in India was done at the All India Institute of Medical Sciences at New Delhi in September 1994. In Kerala, more than 20 transplants have been performed till the end of 2015. The first transplant in the state was done at Lisie hospital, Kochi by a team headed by Jose Chacko Periappuram. The initial experience is encouraging. The same team has also done a cardiac retransplant using heart from a second donor. The prospects for this type of surgery are good in India.

Preventive Cardiology

K Suresh, CG Bahuleyan

Chapter Summary
- General Considerations
- Coronary Heart Disease
- Rheumatic Heart Disease
- Cardiomyopathy
- Congenital Heart Disease

GENERAL CONSIDERATIONS

Many cardiovascular disorders like ischemic heart disease (IHD), hypertension, rheumatic heart disease (RHD), congenital heart disease (CHD) and cardiomyopathy are preventable to a great extent by therapeutic intervention and alteration in the lifestyle. The management of these diseases once established is at best only partly successful and associated with high cost. Therefore, science of preventive cardiology has grown remarkably in the recent past.

CORONARY HEART DISEASE

There are three levels of prevention: (1) Primordial, (2) Primary, and (3) Secondary.

Primordial prevention is the earliest stage of intervention aimed at preventing even the development of atherogenic risk factors in a subject who has no established heart disease or coronary risk factors. *Primary prevention* refers to modification of all the atherogenic risk factors in a subject who has yet no clinical evidence of heart disease but has one or more risk factors that predispose to occurrence of heart disease. *Secondary prevention* includes methods adopted to prevent recurrences or delay progression of the disease in patients with clinically manifest CHD.

Primordial Prevention

This refers to attempts at targeting the young population and inculcating heart-healthy lifestyle practices. Educating the young regarding various atherogenic risk factors, avoidance of exposure to these factors especially tobacco, adoption of healthy eating habits with plenty of fruits, vegetables, nuts and the Mediterranean type of diet, regular aerobic exercise and maintenance of optimal body weight and avoidance of obesity are all encompassed in primordial prevention.

Primary Prevention
Modifiable Risk Factors
Plasma lipids: The relation of plasma cholesterol to the development of atherosclerotic CHD and to coronary mortality is already established. Higher levels of plasma cholesterol cause higher risk. The relationship between dietary and plasma cholesterol is also well-established; the higher the dietary cholesterol content, greater the serum level of cholesterol. Adjustment in the total calorie intake and reduction of saturated fat content in the diet can lower serum level of cholesterol and thereby arrest the progression and also lead to regression of coronary atherosclerosis. It has been found that specific lipid subfractions are involved in the pathogenesis and are considered targets of treatment. Low-density lipoprotein (LDL) is the primary lipoprotein which is associated with atherogenesis. High-density lipoprotein (HDL), which scavenges the cholesterol to liver, is considered *good cholesterol*. Adult treatment panel IV (ATP IV) has revised the guidelines for evaluation and treatment of hypercholesterolemia.

Detailed recommendations of various organizations are available for the various risk categories regarding ideal levels of total cholesterol, LDL cholesterol and HDL cholesterol. These may be referred for further details. In general, total cholesterol less than 200 mg/dL, LDL cholesterol less than 100 mg/dL and HDL cholesterol above 60 mg/dL are desirable.

Regular physical exercise also helps to reduce total serum cholesterol triglycerides and other lipid fractions. Increased consumption of fish and fish oils which contain eicosapentaenoic acid (EPA) and docosahexaenoic acid (DHA) help to lower LDL and elevate HDL in the plasma, thus reducing the atherogenic risk further.

First step in the management of high lipid levels would be to initiate therapeutic lifestyle changes (TLC). These include:
- Cessation of smoking and abstinence or reduction (limited to two pegs of spirits a day) of alcoholic beverages
- *Dietary modification:* Saturated fat less than 7% of the total calories; cholesterol less than 200 mg/day; soluble fiber 10–25 g/day; and inclusion of fruits about 600 g/day
- Reduction of body weight to the ideal or ± 5% of the ideal body mass index (BMI)
- Graded physical activity in the form of exercises such as walking 3 km in 35–40 minutes daily—at least 5 sessions a week. Other desirable exercises include cycling 5–7 km of level ground in 30–40 minutes, swimming, treadmill exercises and sports activities depending upon the cardiovascular status. Additional benefits will be obtained by practicing yoga exercises, which bring in mental and bodily relaxation and also help to avoid mental tension.

In selected cases where the general measures do not achieve reduction of the blood cholesterol to the full target levels, drug prophylaxis should be started. However, the cutoff levels to initiate primary prophylaxis with drugs is different from the cutoff levels for secondary prophylaxis. The drugs used for lipid management in general include the statins, bile acid sequestrants and ezetimibe (to reduce LDL cholesterols). Nicotinic acid and fibric acid derivatives help to reduce triglycerides (*See* Section 10, Ch 94). At present, statins are the most widely sold drugs in the world market, mainly used for lipid-modulating therapy.

Metabolic syndrome: It is a constellation of risk factors which in concert increase the risk for atherogenesis. (For further details refer to Section 10, Ch 94).

Cigarette smoking: Smoking is unquestionably the most important of all preventable cardiovascular risk factors. (Refer to Section 4, Ch 26).

Hypertension: Elevated systolic or diastolic blood pressure (BP) is an independent contributor to coronary risk, especially in people with hypercholesterolemia. It is essential to control hypertension along with modification of other risk factors to minimize progression of coronary atherosclerosis.

Nonpharmacologic measures for control of hypertension include reduction in dietary intake of salt below 4 g/day, foods containing high-content of saturated fats and transfats instituted from childhood. Yoga exercises, transcendental meditation and participation in leisure activities are particularly helpful in reducing BP levels.

Secondary Prevention

These methods are undertaken in patients who have already developed clinical IHD. The measures are aimed at either preventing the recurrences of the disease or at minimizing the complications and progression of the disease. All the preventive measures adopted for primary prevention have a role in secondary prevention also. In addition, included in the scope of secondary prevention are methods to salvage the myocardium by the use of drugs like antiplatelet drugs, β-blockers, renin-angiotensin-aldosterone blockers, or interventional treatment like coronary angioplasty and coronary artery bypass (CAB) surgery. Since the mortality and morbidity from acute myocardial infarction (acute MI) depends mainly on the quantum of myocardial damage, all the methods adopted to reduce the infarct size such as thrombolytic therapy, angioplasty, or myocardial revascularization surgery undertaken in the acute stage also can be included under the broad purview of secondary prevention.

Other recently identified atherosclerotic risk factors include the following:

- High level of C-reactive protein (CRP), especially high-sensitivity-CRP
- Increase in lipoprotein(a)
- Alterations in tissue plasminogen activator and plasminogen activator inhibitor (PAI) levels
- Small, dense LDL and LDL-C particle size and number
- Increase in fibrinogen levels
- Hyperhomocysteinemia
- Higher levels of troponin in the absence of active IHD.

Wherever possible, management of these potential atherogenic influences would contribute to the prevention of heart diseases.

Trials of use of drugs which lower cholesterol and studies on lowering both BP and cholesterol in persons without cardiovascular disease (CVD) have been published.

Findings

Treatment with rosuvastatin at a dose of 10 mg/day resulted in a significantly lower risk of cardiovascular events than placebo in an intermediate risk ethnically diverse population without CVD.

Source: Yusuf S, Bosch J, Dagenais G, et al. Cholesterol Lowering in Intermediate-Risk Persons without Cardiovascular Disease. N Engl J Med. 2016;374(21):2021-31.

Combination of rosuvastatin (10 mg/day), candesartan (16 mg/day) and hydrochlorothiazide (12.5 mg/day) was associated with a significant lower rate of cardiovascular events than dual placebo among persons at immediate risk who did not have CVD.

Source: Lonn EM, Bosch J, López-Jaramillo P, et al. Blood-Pressure Lowering in Intermediate-Risk Persons without Cardiovascular Disease. N Engl J Med. 2016;374(21):2009-20.

Editor's Note: These publications throw light on the present thinking on preventive measures against ischemic heart disease. It is left to the physicians to decide the best method for his/her patients.

RHEUMATIC HEART DISEASES

See also Section 6, Ch 37

Prevention of rheumatic valvular heart diseases may be addressed at three levels—preprimary, primary and secondary levels. ***Preprimary level*** refers to factors that lead to the occurrence of epidemics of streptococcal infections. ***Primary prevention*** refers to prompt treatment of even seemingly harmless sore throats and streptococcal infections particularly in children. ***Secondary prevention*** refers to the use of drug therapy such as long-term oral or intramuscular (IM) penicillin administration for the prevention of recurrences of rheumatic fever. In such patients, secondary prophylaxis with penicillin is recommended, usually for the first 10 years even in the absence of rheumatic carditis. In those with established rheumatic valvular heart disease, it is prudent to continue lifelong prophylaxis.

CARDIOMYOPATHY

The preventive aspect assumes an important role in hypertrophic cardiomyopathy which is transmitted as autosomal dominant. Genetic counseling may help to reduce the birth of affected children.

Deficiency of nutritional factors such as selenium and probably, infection has been implicated in the etiology of endomyocardial fibrosis (EMF). Further studies are in progress.

CONGENITAL HEART DISEASES (CHD)

Refer to Section 13, Ch 122

The etiology of most CHD is multifactorial. Clearly, identifiable genetic factors or environmental factors are responsible only in the minority. Whenever possible, genetic counseling is helpful in high-risk scenarios. Consanguinity is a preventable predisposing factor that can be addressed by proper counseling. Special care to avoid infections like rubella and avoidance of potentially incriminating agents or drugs especially in the antenatal period is important to prevent CHD. Nutritional supplementation with proteins, minerals and vitamins especially folates, and avoidance of potentially harmful hypervitaminoses especially vitamin A and D have been found to reduce the incidence of cardiovascular and neurological defects.

CHAPTER 138

Respiratory System: General Considerations

C Sudheendra Ghosh, CP Murali

Chapter Summary

- General Considerations
- Pulmonary Physiology
- Assessment of Pulmonary Function
- Symptomatology in Respiratory Diseases
- Physical Examination
- Investigations in Respiratory Diseases

GENERAL CONSIDERATIONS

The main function of the respiratory organs is to provide a constant supply of oxygen (O_2) to the tissues and to remove carbon dioxide (CO_2) from them through the lungs. Ultimately, this gas exchange occurs between the alveolar air and mixed venous blood in the capillaries across the alveolocapillary membrane. The alveolocapillary membrane has a total area of 75 m² in an adult. Air is taken in through the air passages comprising the nose, pharynx, larynx, trachea, bronchi and bronchioles. The terminal portions of the air passages—the respiratory bronchioles and alveolar ducts—subserve the function of gas exchange. The part above the vocal cords is termed as upper respiratory tract and the parts below form the lower respiratory tract.

The trachea which is 11 cm long is kept permanently open by the presence of C-shaped cartilages on its wall. Several mucous glands present in the mucous membrane provide mucus which moistens the surface and facilitates ciliary action. The trachea divides into the right and left bronchi.

The bronchi are similar to the trachea in structure. The right main bronchus is 1.0–2.5 cm in length and it is in direct line with the trachea. This fact makes it more vulnerable for obstruction by foreign bodies entering through the trachea. The right main bronchus divides into branches which supply the right upper lobe, middle lobe and lower lobe. The left main bronchus is longer (5 cm) and it forms an angle of 50–100° with the right main bronchus. It divides into two branches which supply the upper and lower lobes. Further division of the lobar bronchi gives rise to segmental bronchi which supply bronchopulmonary segments (Figs 138.1 and 138.2A and B).

Bronchopulmonary Segments

The bronchopulmonary segment is a wedge of lung tissue supplied by each segmental bronchus along with the

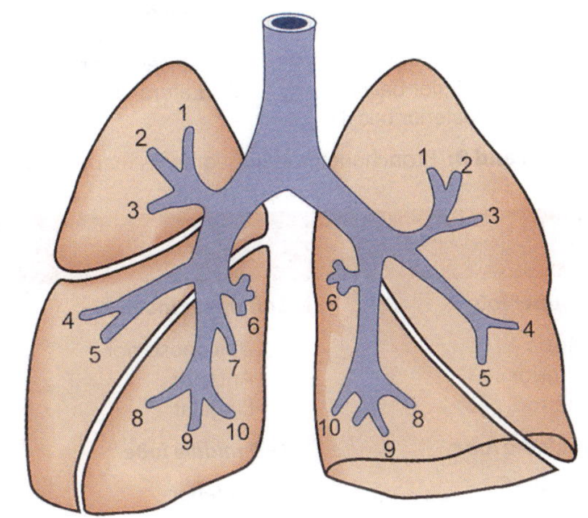

Right upper lobe
1. Apical
2. Posterior
3. Anterior

Right middle lobe
4. Lateral
5. Medial

Right lower lobe
6. Apical lower lobe
7. Medial basal
8. Anterior basal
9. Lateral basal
10. Posterior basal

Left upper lobe
1. Apical
2. Posterior
3. Anterior

Lingular lobe
4. Superior
5. Inferior

Left lower lobe
6. Apical lower lobe

8. Anterior basal
9. Lateral basal
10. Posterior basal

Fig. 138.1: Divisions of bronchi

corresponding branches of the pulmonary artery and vein. They act as independent units and are separated by fibrous septa (Table 138.1).

Divisions of the Bronchial Tree

After 8–13 successive divisions, the segmental bronchi break up into the smallest bronchi. They continue further as bronchioles. The bronchioles have no cartilage and mucous glands on their walls. The bronchioles divide further and the terminal bronchioles are formed after the fourth division. The terminal bronchioles give rise to respiratory bronchioles. Alveoli begin to appear on the walls of the respiratory bronchioles. As the respiratory bronchioles divide further, the number of alveoli, i.e. arising from them it progressively increases. Normal adult lung contains about 300 million alveoli. Rapid division of the respiratory bronchioles results in enormous increase in surface area. The terminal portions of the respiratory

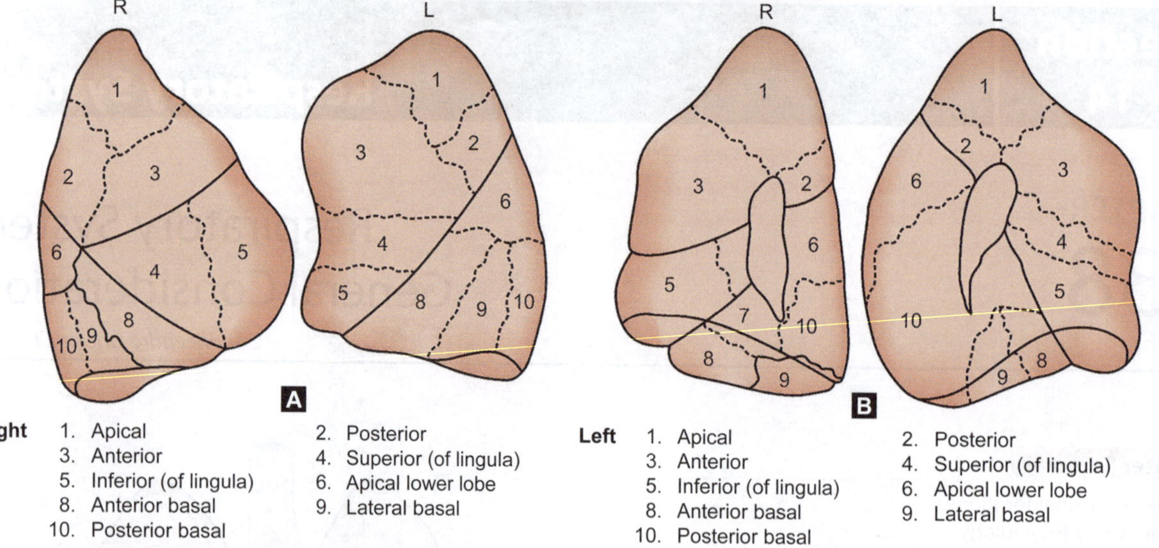

Right	1. Apical	2. Posterior
	3. Anterior	4. Superior (of lingula)
	5. Inferior (of lingula)	6. Apical lower lobe
	8. Anterior basal	9. Lateral basal
	10. Posterior basal	

Left	1. Apical	2. Posterior
	3. Anterior	4. Superior (of lingula)
	5. Inferior (of lingula)	6. Apical lower lobe
	8. Anterior basal	9. Lateral basal
	10. Posterior basal	

Figs 138.2A and B: Bronchopulmonary segments marked on the surfaces of the lungs. **A.** Lateral; **B.** Medial

Table 138.1: Segmental bronchi and the bronchopulmonary segments

Right upper lobe	Left upper lobe
• Apical	• Apicoposterior
• Posterior	• Anterior
• Anterior	• Lingular
Right middle lobe	**Left middle lobe**
• Lateral	• Superior
• Medial	• Inferior
Right lower lobe	**Left lower lobe**
• Apical	• Apical
• Anterior basal	• Anterior basal
• Lateral basal	• Lateral basal
• Posterior basal	• Posterior basal
• Medial basal or cardiac	• Medial basal (absent)

bronchioles divide into alveolar ducts and sacs. Alveoli are 0.1–0.2 mm in diameter. Up to the respiratory bronchioles, the airways only conduct air passively, but beyond this they also take part in gaseous exchange. The part supplied by a single terminal bronchiole is called an *acinus*. An alveolar duct with its distal connections is called a *primary lobule*. A group of primary lobules separated by connective tissue septa form a *secondary lobule*.

Pores of Kohn and Canals of Lambert

- ■ *Pores of Kohn:* They are the openings connecting alveoli, which allow communication between them and sometimes even between adjacent segments.
- ■ *Canals of Lambert:* They are short communications lined by epithelium which exist between distal bronchioles and some of the neighboring alveoli. These may take part in collateral ventilation between different regions of the lung. The lining of the trachea, bronchi and bronchioles consists of ciliated columnar epithelium containing goblet cells. The respiratory bronchioles are lined by non-ciliated cuboidal epithelium. The lining epithelium of the alveoli is flattened and it comprises two types of cells—type I and type II pneumonocytes arranged on a basement membrane. Type I pneumonocytes are numerous and they cover most of the inner surface of the alveoli. Gas exchange occurs mainly across these cells. Type II pneumonocytes are smaller in number. They contain lamellated eosinophilic inclusion bodies which are thought to be of lysosomal nature. Surfactant is produced or stored in them.

Secretions of the Airways and Ciliary Action

Mucus is secreted by the mucous glands and goblet cells. Mucous glands are seen all along from the trachea to the smallest bronchi. They are most numerous in the medium-sized bronchi and are absent from bronchioles. Sixty percent of the submucous glands comprise of mucus cells. Seventeen genes in the human genome encode for the mucins. In the bronchioles, there are only a few goblet cells. Vagus is secretomotor for the mucous glands. The goblet cells respond to direct irritation. The mucus contains acid and neutral polysaccharides mainly, and variable quantities of sodium, potassium, albumin, globulin, specific antibodies, lysozyme and transferrin. Healthy mucus has the consistence of egg-white containing 3% solids. In thick mucus, the solid content may reach 15%. Proteins from homotypic polymers structured as long chains get entangled in a mesh work and by non-covalent calcium-dependent cross-linking of the adjacent polymers lead to formation of the mucus gel. Healthy mucus is a gel with low viscosity and elasticity, abnormal mucus has higher viscosity, abnormal contents of salt and water, increase in mucins, infiltration by inflammatory cells—these occlude air passages and predispose to infection. In addition to its antibacterial action, the mucus provides a milieu for the cilia to function. Ciliary action helps to remove particulate matter. Each cell contains about 200 cilia, each being 6–7 μ long. By successive rhythmic movement, they produce a wave motion passing regularly from cell to cell. An optimum amount of mucus of the correct thickness (5 μ) and optimum viscosity is essential for proper ciliary function.

Drying up of tracheal secretions, increase in thickness and viscosity of the mucus layer, inhalation of irritants, excessive intake of alcohol and drugs like cocaine impair ciliary function and predispose infection of the respiratory tract. Ciliary function is impaired in inherited disorders such as Kartagener's syndrome in which several other defects including loss of motility of the sperms are seen.

Surfactant

This is a substance produced by type II pneumonocytes from the 30th week of intrauterine life. It lines the alveoli and contains an insoluble lipoprotein (dipalmitoyl lecithin) which forms a thin layer at the air-fluid interface and lowers surface tension. Pulmonary surfactant is a mixture of phospholipids and surfactant-specific proteins (SP) which reduce alveolar surface tension during respiration. SP-A, B, C and D contribute to the biophysical properties of surfactant. SP-A and SP-D also have antimicrobial properties. In infant respiratory distress syndrome (IRDS), surfactant is deficient from birth. In adult respiratory distress syndrome (ARDS), surfactant deficiency develops as an acquired defect caused by sepsis, pneumonia, traumatic damage and major surgery. Surfactant has beneficial therapeutic effects only if, it contains the phospholipid as well as the SP. Activated neutrophils clear the surfactant and lead to its dysfunction. Surfactant prevents the alveoli from collapsing by reducing surface tension within the alveoli. Absence of surfactant results in the collapse of small alveoli during expiration and hyperinflation of the larger alveoli during inspiration; in addition to increase in surface tension leads to transudation of fluid from capillaries into the alveoli. Absence of surfactant leads to formation of hyaline membrane disease (HMD) in the newborn. Impairment of pulmonary blood flow and prolonged administration of dry O_2 or air leads to reduction in surfactant.

Pleura

The lung is covered by visceral pleura on its surface and the thoracic cavity is lined by the parietal pleura. The space between them contains 10–20 mL of serous fluid having a protein content of 1.77 g/dL. Pleural cavity is only a potential space. During inspiration, the lung fills the pleural space. The pleural space is under negative pressure so that the lung is kept in apposition with the parietal pleura. At the end of a quiet expiration, the pleural pressure is about 5 cm of water. The pressure inside the pleural cavity is not uniform throughout. The negative pressure is higher at the apices than at the bases. The pleural fluid is formed at the parietal pleura.

Pulmonary Circulation

The main pulmonary artery divides into the right and left pulmonary arteries which divide successively along with the bronchi. The proximal divisions of the artery contain muscular and prominent elastic coats but the branches corresponding to the bronchioles have more prominent muscular coats than elastic layers. The arterioles accompanying the terminal bronchioles and respiratory bronchioles are thin-walled and consist of an endothelial lining with elastic lamina without the muscular layer. These end up as capillaries. The alveolar wall is supplied by a dense capillary network which provides a large perfusing area.

The venous ends of the capillary bed join to form veins which traverse in the interlobar septa. They do not follow the bronchial tree. The veins end up finally as the four main pulmonary veins which drain into the left atrium (LA).

Bronchial Circulation

The bronchi and their branches derive their nutrition from the bronchial arteries which usually arise from the descending aorta, but they may arise from intercostal, subclavian or internal mammary arteries (IMA) as well. The bronchial arteries and their branches supply only up to the level of the respiratory bronchioles. Beyond this, the vascular supply is derived from the pulmonary vessels. Veins arising from the bronchial tree drain into the azygos veins, but some may also enter into the pulmonary veins. Though the bronchial veins drain venous blood into the pulmonary vein, this is not significant in health. In conditions like bronchiectasis and lung abscess, these bronchial capillaries proliferate and larger volumes of venous blood may be added to pulmonary venous circulation.

Lymphatic Drainage

The lungs and pleura are drained by three groups of lymphatics. These are:

1. Lymphatics arising from the visceral pleura and interlobular septa drain the peripheral portions of the lung. These lymphatics follow the pulmonary veins to the hilum.
2. Lymphatics draining the acini form the peribronchial lymphatics and pass to the hilum.
3. Anastomotic channels are formed between the two lymphatic systems.

The lymphatics from the upper part of the left lung drain into thoracic duct while those from the lower part of the left lung and entire right lung drain into the right lymphatic duct.

Protective Mechanisms of the Airways

The innate defense mechanism of the respiratory tree include epithelial barrier, mucociliary clearance, humoral factors such as antimicrobial peptides, complement proteins and surfactant proteins and cellular defenses consisting of macrophages, dendritic cells, natural killer cells (NKC) and mast cells. Apart from ciliary action, the cough, sneeze and gag reflexes serve to protect the air passages.

- *Cough reflex:* All irritating stimuli arising from the respiratory passages below the pharynx evoke cough. Mucus gives rise to cough due to stimulation of vagal afferents and dyspnea due to airways obstruction. Cough reflex is triggered off by stimulation of the subepithelial receptors situated in the trachea and bronchi. Sequences of events during cough are:
  - Closure of the glottis
  - Muscular contraction to increase intrathoracic pressure
  - Sudden release of air by opening of the glottis.
- *Sneeze:* Irritant stimuli from the nose evoke sneeze. The mechanism is same as for cough reflex, but the air is expelled through the nose.

- ***Gag reflex:*** This reflex prevents entry of materials into the trachea and this is associated with closure of the glottis.

Lung Microbiome

In addition to culture of bronchoalveolar lavage (BAL) specimen, high-throughput screening of the 16S rRNA (ribonucleic acid) gene which is a small and highly conserved locus in bacterial deoxyribonucleic acid (DNA) is a reliable method to assess the microbiome quantitatively and qualitatively.

The linear distance from external nares to the alveolar membrane in the adult is 0.5 m in an average adult. The internal surface area of the alveoli is 30 times the skin surface area. Each day this area is exposed to 8,000 L of inhaled air carried to the alveolocapillary interface with 0.1 µm of a tenth of the body's whole blood volume. Lungs have the most intimate and extensive interface with the external environment. The oral and respiratory microbiome share common members due to direct contact and transfer of oropharyngeal organisms by microaspirations and mucosal dispersion. Surfactant has an antimicrobial activity against a few microbes but not all. Chronic respiratory diseases, such as chronic obstructive pulmonary disease (COPD), asthma, cystic fibrosis, noncystic fibrosis—bronchiectasis, idiopathic pulmonary fibrosis (IPF)—all alter the respiratory microbiome, this influences the pattern and outcomes of exacerbations and disease progressions. Viral infections precipitate exacerbations of COPD. ***Chronic azithromycin*** therapy reduces exacerbations in COPD. COPD exacerbations are associated with proliferations of *Haemophilus*, *Pseudomonas* and *Moraxella*.

Exacerbation of asthma is associated with viral infections, especially rhinovirus. *Chlamydia pneumoniae* and *Mycoplasma pneumoniae* infection exacerbate asthma. In noncystic fibrosis bronchiectasis, chronic macrolide (erythromycin) therapy gives relief of the frequency and severity of exacerbation. In IPF, acute exacerbations are a major cause of mortality, though no specific pathogens have been incriminated.

Analogy between exacerbations of chronic respiratory disease and inflammatory bowel disease (IBD): In both, the role of particular pathogens has not been clearly defined. In both, exacerbation can be prevented by long-term macrolide therapy since macrolides have both antimicrobial and immunomodulatory effects.

Source: Dickson RP, Martinez FJ, Huffnagle GB. The role of the microbiome in exacerbations of chronic lung diseases. Lancet. 2014;384(9944):691–702.

PULMONARY PHYSIOLOGY

Gas exchanged between blood and alveoli is brought about by different processes which include ventilation of the alveoli, mixing of inspired air and alveolar air and diffusion of gases across the alveolar membrane. Under resting conditions, 5 L of blood perfuse the pulmonary capillaries, and 6 L of air enter and leave the lungs every minute. 250–300 mL of O_2 is taken by the pulmonary capillary blood to the tissues and 200–350 mL of CO_2 is

released into the alveolar air. With exercise these go up considerably.

Control of Breathing

Nervous Control of Breathing

Respiration is controlled by the respiratory center situated in the medulla and pons. The respiratory center consists of inspiratory center, expiratory center and pneumotaxic center which control the rhythm, depth and rate of respiration. Principle muscles of respiration are diaphragm and intercostal muscles. When there is demand for increasing, ventilation or effort for respiration is higher, the accessory muscles of respiration come into play. These include the muscles attached to the thoracic inlet and abdominal muscles.

Chemical Control of Breathing

Rise in CO_2 tension in the arterial blood is the strongest direct stimulus to the respiratory center to increase ventilation. Next in importance is hypoxia. Hypoxia stimulates the chemoreceptors of the carotid and aortic bodies attached to external carotid artery (ECA) and ascending aorta (AAo), respectively. A fall in pH stimulates breathing directly by its action on the respiratory center (Table 138.2).

Modes of Breathing

- ***Quiet breathing (eupnea):*** This type of breathing occurs at rest due to the diaphragm and external intercostal contraction; it remains under autonomic control and does not require the cognitive thought (Fig. 138.3A).
  - ***A deep breath (diaphragmatic breathing):*** It occurs mainly due to contraction and relaxation of the diaphragm.

Table 138.2: Regulation of ventilation

System component	Function
Medullary respiratory center	Sets the basic rhythm of breathing
VRG	Generates the breathing rhythm and integrates data coming into the medulla
DRG	Integrates input from the stretch receptors and the chemoreceptors in the periphery
PRG	Influences and modifies the medulla-oblongata functions
Aortic body	Monitors blood pCO_2, pO_2 and pH
Carotid body	Monitors blood pCO_2, pO_2 and pH
Hypothalamus	Monitors emotional state and body temperature
Cortical areas of the brain	Control voluntary breathing
Proprioceptors	Send impulses to joint and muscle movements
Pulmonary irritant reflexes	Protect the respiratory zones of the system from foreign materials
Inflation reflex	Protects the lungs from overinflating

Abbreviations: VRG = Ventral respiratory group; DRG = Dorsal respiratory group; PRG = Pontine respiratory group; pCO_2 = Partial pressure of carbon dioxide; pO_2 = Partial pressure of oxygen

- ***A shallow breath (costal breathing):*** This type of breathing occurs due to contraction of the intercostal muscles.
- ***Forced breathing (hyperpnea):*** This type of breathing occurs during exercise and acts like singing. During inspiration and expiration, accessory muscles of respiration come into play.

- ***Cheyne-Stokes breathing:*** In this type of abnormal rhythm of respiration, there is increase in the rate and depth of respiration, which reaches a maximum and then they come down to reach a period of apnea. These cycles repeat. Cheyne-Stokes respiration is indicative of serious functional impairment of the respiratory center. It is seen in cardiac failure, metabolic acidosis, increased intracranial tension, narcotic poisoning and sometimes even during sleep (Fig. 138.3B).
- ***Biot's breathing:*** This is a type of irregular breathing in which 3–4 respirations occur in clusters with apneic pauses. The respiration resembles sighs. This is commonly seen in meningitis and brain damage (Fig. 138.3C).
- ***Kussmaul's breathing:*** In this type, the patients breathe with large tidal volume (Vt) and so rapidly that there is virtually no pause between breaths. This is seen in all forms of metabolic acidosis, particularly diabetic ketoacidosis, renal failure and others (Fig. 138.3D).

Hyperventilation: The rate and depth of ventilation are increased. This occurs commonly in major pulmonary embolism (PE), anxiety, neurocirculatory asthenia, meningitis, encephalitis, therapy with drugs like epinephrine, poisoning with salicylates or aspirin, hyperthyroidism, hypoxia and acidosis. This results in excessive removal of CO_2 and consequent alkalosis. ***Kussmaul's respiration*** occurring in metabolic acidosis is a compensatory mechanism.

Hypoventilation: When ventilation is not in balance with perfusion, O_2 exchange is compromised. Reduction in respiratory drive or neuromuscular competence or substantial increase in respiratory load can diminish minute ventilation, resulting in hypoventilation leading to hypercapnia.

The causes of alveolar hypoventilation are:

- ***Obstruction to the airways:*** Both structural as in foreign body or secretion and functional as in bronchospasm.
- ***Paralysis of respiratory muscles,*** e.g. poliomyelitis, Guillain-Barre syndrome or myasthenia gravis.
- ***Impairment of activity of respiratory center,*** e.g. narcotic poisoning, brainstem hemorrhage, coning of the brainstem.
- ***Alteration in the anatomy of the thoracic cage preventing effective ventilation,*** e.g. severe kyphoscoliosis, diaphragmatic paralysis, pectus excavatum, ankylosing spondylitis, flail chest injuries.
- ***Diseases which affect the lungs and pleura,*** e.g. pneumonia, atelectasis, pulmonary cysts, emphysema, acute pulmonary edema, malignant secondaries, pulmonary fibrosis, pleural effusion, pneumothorax.
- ***Conditions which interfere with movement of the thoracic cage and diaphragm,*** e.g. severe obesity, tense ascites.

Ventilation of Lung and CO$_2$ Elimination

As noted earlier, the respiratory control system that sets the rate of ventilation which responds to chemical signals including (pCO$_2$) dissolved in arterial blood (PaCO$_2$),

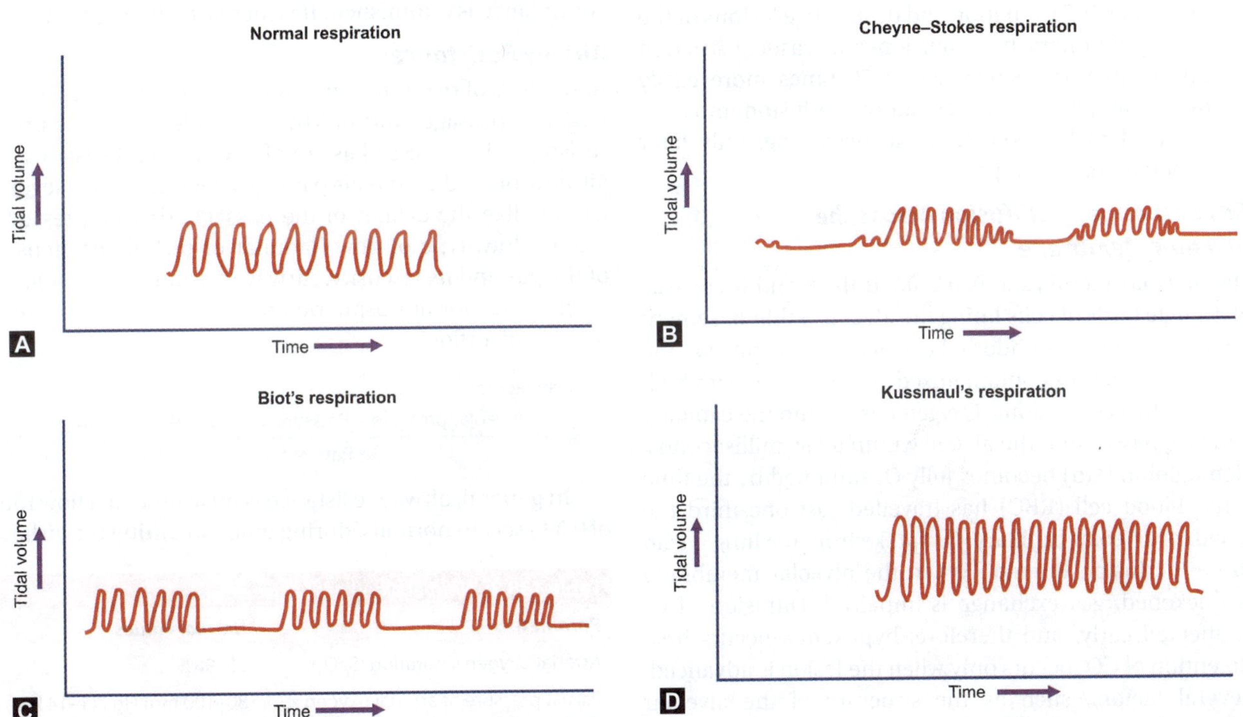

Figs 138.3A to D: **A.** Normal respiration. ***Note:*** The regular pattern, the tidal volume (Vt) remains the same; **B.** Cheyne-Stokes respiration: Apneic spells interpose between episodes of waxing and waning respiratory movements; **C.** Biot's respiration: Apneic spells interpose between episodes of respiratory movements of similar amplitude; **D.** Kussmaul's respiration: Rapid and high-volume respiratory movements occur continuously

partial pressure of oxygen dissolved in arterial blood (PaO_2) and pH.

Gas Exchange in the Alveoli

Air in the conducting airways is functionally inert and its volume is called **anatomical dead space**. Functionally effective ventilation that the alveoli receive is called **alveolar ventilation**. When the alveoli are not perfused with blood, ventilation becomes ineffective. Ventilation occurring in alveoli, which are not properly perfused with blood, is called **physiological dead space**. In normal person, anatomical dead space is equal to physiological dead space. Dead space in typical adult male is equal to 150 mL.

Gas exchange in the alveoli is adversely affected by uneven ventilation, uneven perfusion or defective diffusion.

Ventilation Perfusion Abnormalities

Ventilation of unperfused alveoli leads to increase in dead space. Perfusion of unventilated alveoli results in addition of unoxygenated blood to pulmonary venous blood. Taking effective minute ventilation to be 4 L and pulmonary blood flow to be 5 L, the normal ventilation perfusion ratio is 0.8.

Several Conditions Lead to Imbalance in Ventilation

- **Normal variations:** The upper parts of the lungs receive less blood than the bases, the hydrostatic pressure of the blood being higher at the base. Though the perfusion is unequal in different portions of the lung, ventilation is more or less uniform with only minor differences.
- **Obstruction to pulmonary blood flow:** Pulmonary blood flow is obstructed in PE, vascular changes due to chronic inflammation and destructive lesions of the lung, pulmonary hypertension and vasoconstriction due to hypoxia. Since CO_2 is 20 times more easily diffusible than O_2, the ventilation-perfusion imbalances lead to hypoxia from the beginning, only later hypercapnia develops.

Gas Exchange by Diffusion Across the Alveolar Membrane

The alveolar membrane is 0.2–0.7 μ thick and it consists of a single layer of cells lining the alveoli, a thin basement membrane and the endothelial cells of the capillary. The alveolar capillaries contain mixed venous blood with high CO_2 and low O_2 tensions. Oxygen passes into the capillary and CO_2 passes into the alveoli within a few milliseconds. Hemoglobin (Hb) becomes fully O_2 saturated by the time a red blood cell (RBC) has travelled just one-third the length of alveolar capillary. O_2 uptake from the lung is said to be 'perfusion limited'. When the alveolar membrane is thickened, gas exchange is impaired. Diffusion of O_2 is affected early, and therefore, hypoxemia occurs first. Retention of CO_2 occurs only when the lesion is advanced. Several factors, such as the structure of the alveolar membrane and ventilation perfusion abnormalities, affect the diffusion capacity to a great extent. Hence, the term 'transfer factor' is used instead of diffusion capacity.

Blood Gases

The rate of O_2 uptake is related to the average rate of metabolic CO_2 produced and this ratio is called the 'respiratory quotient'. Both O_2 and CO_2 are carried by blood. Diffusion across the alveolar membrane depends upon the partial pressure of these gases on either side or the diffusing capacity of these gases. Since, CO_2 is much more readily diffusible than O_2, the level of CO_2 in blood closely follows the pCO_2 in alveolar air. The pattern of oxygen dissociation curve of Hb is such that PaO_2 does not fall significantly even when the pO_2 in the alveoli falls from 100 mm Hg to 80 mm Hg. But when the alveolar pO_2 falls below 80 mm Hg, then the arterial pO_2 falls steeply. The arterial pO_2 does not closely follow the alveolar pO_2 due to this phenomenon. Oxygen is carried by blood mainly in combination with Hb (1.34 mL/g) and a small quantity as the dissolved form (0.003 mL/100 mL blood/mm Hg of oxygen tension). The oxygen content in blood can be expressed either as the percentage saturation (SO_2) or PO_2. Arterial CO_2 level is expressed in terms of its partial pressure ($PaCO_2$). Alveolar gas concentrations are expressed in terms of their partial pressures (Table 138.3).

Pulmonary Mechanics: Work of Breathing

The total work involved in moving the thoracic cage, expanding the lungs and moving the gases in and out is known as **work of breathing**.

Pulmonary Compliance

The elastic property of the lung is expressed in terms of pulmonary compliance. It is the distensibility of the lung per unit change in intrapleural pressure. Normal pulmonary compliance is about 0.2 L/cm of water. In conditions like pulmonary fibrosis and pulmonary edema, compliance is diminished. It is increased in emphysema.

Airway Resistance

About 90% of resistance to flow of air is contributed by the larger air passages and 10% by the smaller airways. Airway resistance is expressed as cm of H_2O/L/sec. Resistance to air flow offered by the air passages depends upon several factors, like the caliber of the passage, driving pressure, rate of flow, type of flow (laminar or turbulent), density of the gas and its viscosity. Airway resistance is calculated from values for atmospheric and alveolar pressures and the rate of airflow.

$$\text{Airway resistance} = \frac{\text{Alveolar pressure} - \text{Pressure at the airway opening}}{\text{Rate of flow}}$$

In general, airway resistance is measured at a flow rate of 0.5 L/sec. In normals, during quiet breathing the airflow

Table 138.3: Normal blood gas values

Parameters	Normal values
Arterial oxygen saturation (SaO_2)	95–98%
Partial pressure of arterial oxygen (PaO_2)	80–100 mm Hg (11–14 kPa)
Partial pressure of arterial carbon dioxide ($PaCO_2$)	35–45 mm Hg (4.5–6.0 kPa)

resistance varies between 1.5 and 3 cm of $H_2O/L/sec$. It reaches high values (> 10 cm of $H_2O/L/sec$) in obstructive airway disease.

ASSESSMENT OF PULMONARY FUNCTION

Different aspects of respiratory function can be subjected to investigational study. These include:

- Gas transport down the airways
- Gas mixing within alveoli
- Gas transfer across the alveolocapillary membrane
- Lung perfusion.

Gas Transport down the Airways

Entry of air down the airways and its return can be measured using static and dynamic spirometry. Body plethysmography is employed to measure lung compliance and airways resistance. Several parameters are used to determine the ventilatory capacity of the lung.

Spirometry

It is a measure of airflow and lung volume during a forced expiratory maneuver from full inspiration. It is the simplest test of all respiratory functions. Forced expiratory volume in 1 second (FEV1) and vital capacity (VC), which are the most important parameters to assess the ventilatory capacity, are estimated by spirometry (Fig. 138.4). Other clinical uses of spirometry include the following:

- Additional information to help to establish the *clinical diagnosis* in a patient
- Assess the *prognosis* in a patient
- Assess whether disease is present at *an early stage*, i.e. prior to overt clinical disease
- Assist in quantifying the *severity of airway disease*
- Assess the *effect of therapy*
- Delineating *risk factors*, e.g. the odds of developing future respiratory disease or operative risks
- Monitoring whether there is normal pattern of *lung growth* or *aging*.

Standard abbreviations are used while describing pulmonary function test (PFT) (Tables 138.4 and 138.5).

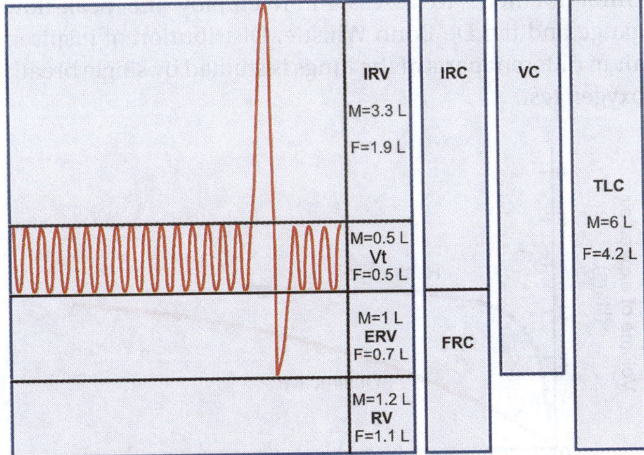

Fig. 138.4: Static lung volumes

Abbreviations: IRV = Inspiratory reserve volume; Vt = Tidal volume; ERV = Expiratory reserve volume; RV = Residual volume; IRC = Inspiratory reserve capacity; FRC = Functional reserve capacity; VC = Vital capacity; TLC = Total lung capacity

Table 138.4: Abbreviations and definitions of pulmonary function test (PFT)

Abbreviations	Definitions
FVC (forced vital capacity)	Volume of air expired with a maximal effort after deep inspiration
FEV1 (forced expiratory volume in 1 second)	Volume of air expired in the first second after deep inspiration
VC (vital capacity)	Maximum amount of air that can be expelled from the lungs after the deepest possible breath; TLC minus RV or maximum volume of air exhaled from maximal inspiratory level (60–70 mL/kg) (3,100–4,800 mL)
PEF (peak expiratory flow)	Volume of forcibly expired air during the first 10 seconds after deep inspiration
TLC (total lung capacity)	Sum of all volume compartments or volume of air in lungs after maximum inspiration (4–6 L)
FRC (functional residual capacity)	Sum of RV and ERV or the volume of air in the lungs at end-expiratory tidal position (30–35 mL/kg) (2,300–3,300 mL). Measured with multiple-breath closed-circuit helium dilution, multiple-breath open-circuit nitrogen washout or body plethysmography. It cannot be measured by spirometry
RV (residual volume)	Volume of air remaining in lungs after maximum exhalation (20–25 mL/kg) (1,700–2,100 mL) Indirectly measured (FRC–ERV) It cannot be measured by spirometry
IRV (inspiratory reserve volume)	Maximum volume of air inhaled from the end-inspiratory tidal position (1,900–3,300 mL)
ERV (expiratory reserve volume)	Maximum volume of air that can be exhaled from resting end-expiratory tidal position (700–1,000 mL)
VT (tidal volume)	Volume of air inhaled or exhaled with each breath during quiet breathing (6–8 mL/kg)
IC (inspiratory capacity)	Sum of IRV and TV or the maximum volume of air that can be inhaled from the end-expiratory tidal position (2,400–3,800 mL)
EC (expiratory capacity)	TV + ERV
DLCO (diffusing capacity of lung for carbon monoxide)	Medical test that determines how much oxygen travels from the alveoli of the lungs to the bloodstream

Table 138.5: Parameters used in pulmonary function tests (PFTs)

PFT tracings have:
- Four lung volumes: Vt, IRV, ERV and RV
- Five capacities: IC, EC, VC, FRC and TLC (Fig. 138.5)
- Flow-volume curves
- Blood gases and pulse oximetry
- Transfer factor (diffusion)
- Exercise tests
- Exhaled nitric oxide

Abbreviations: Vt = Tidal volume; IRV = Inspiratory reserve volume; ERV = Expiratory reserve volume; RV = Residual volume; VC = Vital capacity; EC = Expiratory capacity; FRC = Functional residual capacity; TLC = Total lung capacity

Lung Volumes

- ***Tidal volume:*** It is the volume of gas inspired or expired during each respiratory cycle. Normally, it is 0.5 L in men and women.

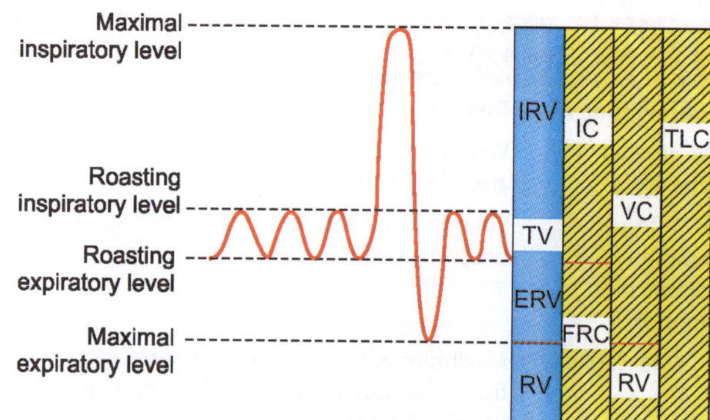

Fig. 138.5: Normal record on induced deep breathing

- ***Inspiratory reserve volume (IRV):*** It is the maximal volume of gas that can be inspired from the end of tidal inspiration. Normal value is 2–3 L in men.
- ***Expiratory reserve volume (ERV):*** It is the maximal volume of gas that can be expired from the end of tidal expiration. Normal value is 1.3 L in men.
- ***Residual volume (RV):*** It is the volume of gas still remaining in the lungs after maximal expiration. Normal value is 1.6 L in men. In women, the values are slightly lower.

Lung Capacities

- ***Total lung capacity (TLC):*** It is the volume of gas contained in the lung at the end of maximal inspiration. Normal value is 5.4 L.
- ***Vital capacity (VC):*** It is the maximal volume of gas that can be expelled from the lung by forceful effort after maximal inspiration. In health, VC is influenced by factors such as age, sex, position, body frame and state of physical conditioning. Average normal value is 3.8 L in men.
- ***Inspiratory capacity (IC):*** It is the maximal volume of gas that can be inspired from the resting expiratory level. Normal value is 2.5 L in men.
- ***Functional residual capacity (FRC):*** It is the volume of gas remaining in the lung at the end of tidal expiration. Normal value is 2.9 L in men.

Forced Expiratory Volume in one Second (Timed VC)

The volume of air expelled in the first 1 second of a forcible expiration following a full inspiration is called FEV1. Normally FEV1 is above 75% of the total VC, FEV2 is above 85%, and FEV3 is above 95%. Airways obstruction is indicated by FEV1 below 70% of normal. Volume-time curve is a very useful spirogram (Fig. 138.6A). FEV1 is the most useful and reproducible measurement. It is the volume of air expelled in the first second of forced expiration after a full inspiration. FEV1 depends on the effort made by the patient, the elastic recoil of the lungs and the positive thoracic pressure applied around them by the expiratory muscles. In patients with obstructive airway disease, successive FEV1 measurements yield reproducible results. FEV1 reflects severity of airway obstruction and correlates approximately with maximal exercise capacity (Fig. 138.6B). Rate of decline is influenced by tobacco smoke (Fig. 138.7).

COPD: It is mainly due to narrowing of the airways, is diagnosed when FEV1 is less than 80% of the predicted value and the FEV1/FVC (forced vital capacity) or FEV1/VC is less than 70%. Improvement or reversibility of airflow obstruction is defined as an improvement in FEV1 by more than 15% and more than 0.3 L after administration of the β-adrenergic agonist, salbutamol, 200 µg by inhalation.

Bronchial challenge studies are very useful in demonstrating airway hyper reactivity which is characteristic of asthma. Patients with asthma characteristically react to small doses of pharmacological bronchoconstrictors, exhibiting transient decreases in FEV1 and increases in airway resistance. The most commonly reported measurements are the dose of methacholine or histamine needed to provoke a 20% reduction of FEV1 (PD_{20}). Healthy non-asthmatic subjects require doses that are, on an average, several orders of magnitude greater.

Forced expiratory time (FET): It is the total time taken for completing a forced expiration. Normally it is 4–6 seconds.

Peak expiratory flow rate (PEFR): It is the maximum rate that can be sustained during the first 10 minutes of a sudden forced expiration after a full inspiration. The PEFR depends upon the height and surface area of the individual. Nomograms are available for reference. It is measured using Wright's peak-flow meter. This is an easy and convenient method to assess airways obstruction. Other methods to assess PEFR employ the peak-flow gauge and the De Bono Whistle. Distribution of inspired air in different parts of the lungs is studied by single breath oxygen test.

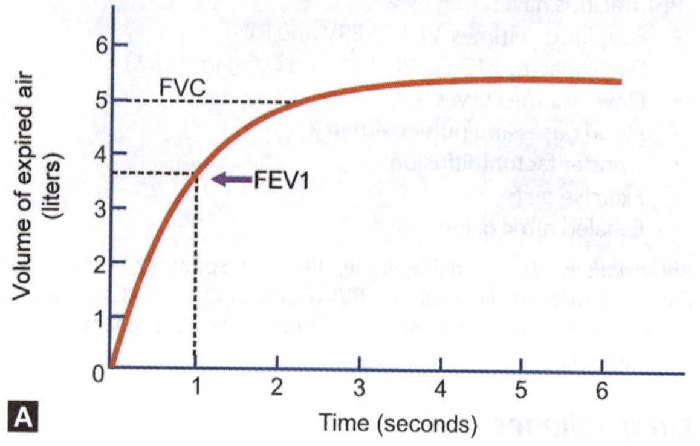

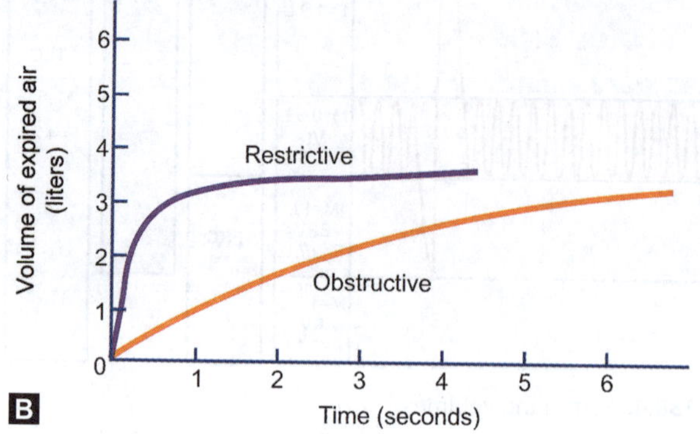

Figs 138.6A and B: Volume-time curves obtained during forced expiration: **A.** Normal; **B.** Restrictive and obstructive lung diseases. It shows the percentage of reduction in the volume of air during the first second

Abbreviations: FVC = Forced vital capacity; FEV1 = Forced expiratory volume in 1 second

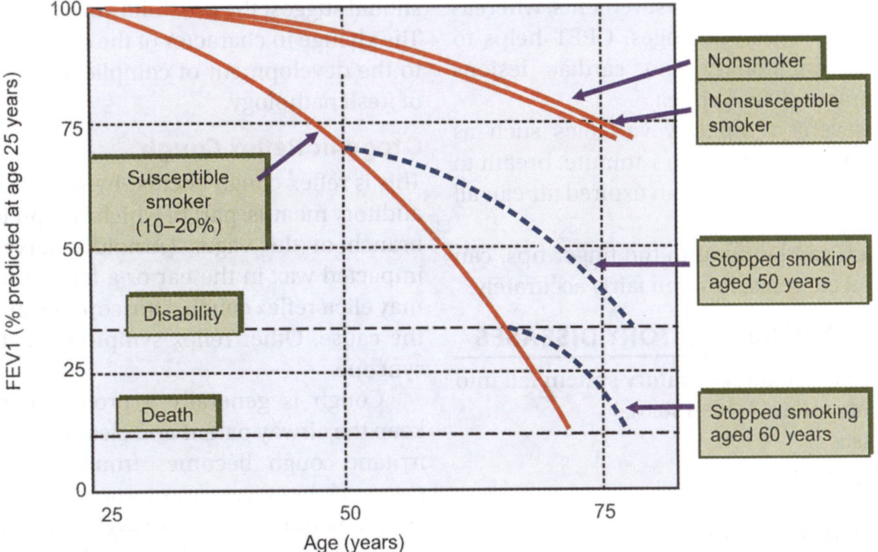

Fig. 138.7: Annual decline in lung function. ***Note:*** The relation between decline in forced expiratory volume in 1 second (FEV1) in the normals (nonsmokers) and smokers. Rate of decline in FEV1 is many times higher in smokers and also improvement in FEV1 on stopping smoking

Forced expiratory flow (FEF 25–75%): It is the velocity of air expressed as liters per second during the middle-third of the total expired volume. In normals the values vary with age and height of the individuals. Average values lie between 1.5 and 5.5 L/sec in men. Determination of FEF 25–75% helps to detect borderline cases of airway obstruction.

Maximal voluntary ventilation (MVV) or maximal breathing capacity: It is the total volume of air breathed by a subject using maximum effort over a period of 1 minutes.

Diffusing capacity: This is the volume of a gas transported across the alveolocapillary membrane in 1 minute for 1 unit of pressure gradient. It is expressed as mL/min/mm Hg difference in partial pressure.

Closing capacity: During inspiration the air enters different portions of the lung in a definite order. The upper portions fill first and then the middle and lower parts in order. During expiration, air escapes in the reverse order, the basal portions emptying first and the apical regions being the last. As a result, the smaller airways at the bases start to close even for a while air from apices is escaping. The volume of air contained in the lungs at the point where the airways first start to close is called closing capacity.

Closing volume (CV): The difference between the closing capacity and the RV is termed as CV. This is often expressed as a percentage of the VC. In normal subjects below 40 years it is less than 20%. The CV increases with age. In many cases increase in CV may be the only detectable abnormality in impending airway obstruction. CV may denote small airway function as well.

Entry of air down the airways and its return can be measured using static and dynamic spirometry. Body plethysmography is employed to measure lung compliance and airways resistance. FEV1 and VC, which are the most important parameters to assess the ventilatory capacity, are estimated by spirometry.

The modern equipment used for estimating the respiratory parameters, such as VC, PEFR, TLC, FEV and

FEF 25–75% which represent different functional aspects of lung function, are computerized and the results are given as graphs or loops (e.g. flow-volume loop), which can be easily interpreted. In normal individuals, the maximal expiratory flow rate decreases steadily throughout forced expiration. Reduction in maximal expiratory flow during the middle of forced expiration is caused by small-airway diseases and can be an early sign of small-airway disease. When tracheobronchial collapse occurs in emphysema or rare disorders of bronchial cartilage, flow rate decreases early in expiration. In obstruction of the airway outside the thorax, flow tends to be constant throughout the first part of expiration rather than decelerating.

Instantaneous flow values are easily read off from such graphs. These can distinguish between obstructions at different levels in the respiratory tree.

Gas Mixing within Alveoli

These measurements demand rapid analysis of expired air. The measurement of alveolar and arterial CO_2 tension is the method employed for this purpose.

Gas Transfer across Alveolar Membrane

Estimation of transfer factor is conducted by using carbon monoxide which has a very high diffusing capacity (DLCO).

Lung Perfusion

It is studied by isotopic methods. This is helpful in assessing function of lung surface area, thickness of alveolar membrane and pulmonary circulation.

Cardiopulmonary Exercise Test

It involves the measurement of oxygen uptake (VO_2), carbon dioxide output (VCO_2), minute ventilation V or VE, and other variables in addition to the monitoring of 12-lead electrocardiogram (ECG), blood pressure (BP) and pulse oximetry during a maximal symptom limited exercise test. When appropriate, measurement of arterial blood gases provides important information about pulmonary gas exchange. During standard cardiac stress testing the focus is primarily on ECG and BP measurements, whereas in CPET the focus is on gas exchanges. CPET helps to distinguish between pulmonary and cardiac lesions responsible for symptoms like dyspnea.

During CPET several ventilatory variables such as VT, respiratory rate and ventilation in 1 minute, breath to breath variation in O_2 and CO_2 levels in expired air can all be estimated.

Oximeters, which can be fitted to the finger tips, can give values of arterial oxygen saturation fairly accurately.

SYMPTOMATOLOGY IN RESPIRATORY DISEASES

The majority of diseases of the respiratory system fall into one of four major categories (Table 138.6):
1. Infectious diseases
2. Obstructive lung diseases
3. Restrictive disorders
4. Abnormalities of the vasculature.

Cough with or without expectoration, chest pain, dyspnea and hemoptysis are the most frequent respiratory symptoms.

Cough With or Without Expectoration

Cough with expectoration is a prominent symptom in inflammatory lesions, such as bronchitis and pneumonia or in irritative and allergic lesions of the respiratory tract. Pharyngitis, laryngitis, tracheitis and early stages of bronchitis give rise to ***cough without expectoration***. In some infections, like *Bordetella pertussis*, *Klebsiella* and some viruses, paroxysms of cough are followed by a long inspiratory whoop caused by laryngeal spasm. Cough elicited by change of posture (postural cough) is characteristic of bronchiectasis, lung abscess and bronchopleural fistula. ***Bovine cough*** or ***gander cough*** is the term used to denote cough devoid of its explosive (tussive) phase. This occurs in bilateral adductor paralysis of the vocal cords. In asthma, cough and dyspnea tend to recur regularly at night. In left-sided heart failure with pulmonary edema, cough occurs in the recumbent posture. Development of a sudden and uncontrollable paroxysm of cough in, an otherwise, healthy person should suggest the possibility of an aspirated foreign body. The change in character of the cough may be an early clue to the development of complications or superimposition of fresh pathology.

Otogenic Reflex Cough

This is reflex cough elicited by stimulation of the external auditory meatus, part of which is supplied by the auricular branch of the vagus (Arnold's nerve). In a rare case, impacted wax in the ear or a foreign body in the meatus may elicit reflex cough. Otoscopic examination may reveal the cause. Other reflex symptoms include vomiting and syncope.

Cough is generally a protective reflex designed to keep the airway patent and clear the exudates. Sometimes irritant cough becomes troublesome, interfering with sleep causing severe annoyance. Other untoward effects of cough include syncope (***cough syncope***), pneumothorax, mediastinal and surgical emphysema and rib fractures ***(cough fracture).*** In children, paroxysmal cough may lead to subconjunctival hemorrhage.

Sputum

The material expectorated from the respiratory tract is called sputum. In healthy individuals, the secretion of the respiratory passages is just adequate to provide a protective lining, and there is no expectoration. Expectoration in excess of 10–25 mL of sputum in 24 hours should raise the possibility of disease. Copious amounts in excess of 300 mL are seen in bronchiectasis and lung abscess. Character of the sputum often suggests the underlying pathology. Sputum is serosanguinous in pulmonary edema, mucoid and sticky in asthma and chronic bronchitis, thick and purulent in bronchiectasis and lung abscess, creamy yellow in pulmonary tuberculosis, blood stained in carcinoma, tuberculosis, bronchiectasis, mitral stenosis and pulmonary infarction, rusty in pneumonia and black in coal worker's pneumoconiosis lung abscess or gangrene of the lung. Copious watery sputum occurs in alveolar cell carcinoma; this is known as bronchorrhea. Sputum is chocolate-colored in hepatopulmonary amebiasis.

Hemoptysis

Presence of blood in the sputum is termed as ***hemoptysis.*** In true hemoptysis, blood is derived from the airways or the lungs. The quantity of blood may be small as in mitral stenosis or massive as in cavitary pulmonary tuberculosis or bronchiectasis. In neoplasms, bleeding is usually brisk. Sometimes blood is derived from the upper respiratory passages or mouth and this is termed as ***spurious hemoptysis***. Hemoptysis before middle age brings to mind tuberculosis, pneumonia, bronchiectasis and mitral stenosis. After 40–45 years of age, bronchogenic carcinoma and tuberculosis top the list. Hemoptysis is a manifestation of serious underlying disease warranting full investigation. Massive hemoptysis may be defined as loss of more than 10% of blood volume or hemoptysis requiring blood transfusion. Though rare, massive hemoptysis demands emergency management. Nonrespiratory causes of hemoptysis include pulmonary hypertension occurring in mitral stenosis, acute pulmonary edema, pulmonary infarction,

Table 138.6: General categories of respiratory disease	
Categories	**Examples**
Infectious disease	Tuberculosis, pneumonia, bronchitis, tracheitis
Obstructive lung disease	Asthma, COPD, bronchiectasis, bronchiolitis
Restrictive pathophysiology—Parenchymal disease	IPF, asbestosis, DIP, sarcoidosis
Restrictive Pathophysiology—neuromuscular weakness	Guillain-Barre syndrome, ALS
Restrictive pathophysiology—Chest wall/pleural disease	Kyphoscoliosis, ankylosing spondylitis, fibrothorax
Malignancy	Bronchogenic carcinoma
Pulmonary vascular diseases	PE, pulmonary arterial hypertension

Abbreviations: COPD = Chronic obstructive pulmonary disease; IPF = Idiopathic pulmonary fibrosis; DIP = Desquamative interstitial pneumonia; ALS = Amyotrophic lateral sclerosis; PE = Pulmonary embolism

trauma and hemorrhagic diseases. Rarely massive and fatal hemoptysis may develop when an aortic aneurysm erodes into the trachea or a bronchus. **Spurious hemoptysis** is commonly resorted to by hysterical individuals to attract medical attention.

Management of Hemoptysis

The patient should be hospitalized as an emergency and a rapid clinical examination is done to determine the cause. It is important to avoid percussion, which may worsen the hemoptysis.

The patient is kept in bed rest and sedated with diazepam 10 mg administered intramuscularly. Respiratory depressants such as morphine should be avoided since they impair expectoration. Blood loss and its effects are assessed by monitoring the volume of blood expectorated and the pulse, respiration and BP. If the blood loss exceeds 200–300 mL in 24 hours and it is persistent, blood transfusion is indicated.

In majority of cases, the underlying cause can be made out by clinical examination and chest radiography. Specific treatment is instituted early (e.g. antituberculosis drugs in tuberculosis, antibiotics in pneumonia and lung abscess) in conditions where such treatment is available. Majority of cases subside with rest, sedation and blood transfusion. In conditions like pulmonary neoplasms, bleeding tends to persist. In such cases, emergency bronchoscopy is done to locate the lesion and decide upon further management. If the site of bleeding is located, bronchial artery embolization is a very effective method to arrest the bleeding promptly, but recurrence can occur.

Digital Clubbing

Syn: Hippocratic Fingers

This is caused by increase in the volume of soft tissue in and around the distal phalanges of the fingers and toes, especially the nailbeds (Table 138.7). This leads to increased curvature of the nails. Severity of clubbing varies and this has been graded for clinical purposes.

- **Grade 1:** Fluctuation of the nail can be elicited on the nailbed.
- **Grade 2:** The normal angle between the nail and nailbed is lost.
- **Grade 3:** The terminal portion of the phalanx and nail appears as a drumstick or a parrot beak.
- **Grade 4:** In addition to digital clubbing, other regions show pulmonary osteoarthropathy.

Being highly subjective, the value of grading is at best minimal in borderline cases. More than the severity of clubbing, the period taken to develop the clubbing may be more important. Occurrence of clubbing within weeks should suggest conditions like lung abscess, bronchogenic carcinoma and infective endocarditis. In these conditions the nails are painful. At times clubbing may be unilateral (Table 138.8).

Common Conditions Associated with Clubbing

- **Respiratory diseases:** Suppurative lesions like bronchiectasis, lung abscess, empyema and infected cysts; advanced tuberculosis with bronchiectatic changes, bronchogenic carcinoma, pneumoconiosis, fibrosing alveolitis and pleural fibroma.
- **Cardiovascular disorders:** Cyanotic CHD and infective endocarditis.
- **Alimentary disorders:** Malabsorption states, ulcerative colitis, cirrhosis of the liver, hepatomas and amebic liver abscess.
- **Miscellaneous groups:** Clubbing may develop in thyrotoxicosis. At times it may occur nonpathologically in several members of a family (familial clubbing). Repeated trauma to the finger tips as occurring in carpenters and blacksmiths leads to occupational clubbing.

In pachydermoperiostosis which is a rare familial disorder, clubbing occurs in association with thickening of the ends of long bones and coarse thickening of the skin over several regions.

Dyspnea

Difficulty in breathing or shortness of breath associated with marked awareness of the effort of respiration is called **dyspnea**. The severity of dyspnea can be graded and this gives clue to the severity of the disease and its progression. The Medical Research Council (MRC) Breathlessness Scale designates five progressively more severe grade of dyspnea based on the answers to questions about common activities of daily life.

Medical Research Council Breathlessness Scale

- **Grade 1:** Are you ever troubled by breathlessness except on strenuous exercise?
- **Grade 2: If yes:** Are you short of breath when hurrying on level ground or walking up a slight hill?
- **Grade 3: If yes:** Do you have to walk slower than most people of your own age on level ground? Do you have to stop after 30 minutes on level ground at your own pace?

Table 138.7: Common causes of clubbing

Causes	Symptoms
Respiratory	• Bronchogenic carcinoma (especially squamous cell carcinoma) • Bronchiectasis • Lung abscess • Empyema • Asbestosis (with mesothelioma) • Sarcoidosis • Cystic fibrosis • Long-standing tuberculosis • Pulmonary atrioventricular (AV) fistula • Interstitial lung diseases
Cardiovascular	• Infective endocarditis • Cyanotic congenial heart diseases
Alimentary	• Inflammatory bowel disease (ulcerative colitis and Crohn's disease) • Biliary cirrhosis • Hepatoma
Miscellaneous	• Hereditary, idiopathic • Thyrotoxicosis • Acromegaly • Unilateral clubbing in Pancoast's tumor, subclavian artery aneurysm and hemiplegia • Unidigital clubbing occurs in repeated trauma

Table 138.8: Some of the common conditions leading to unilateral clubbing

Types of clubbing	Indications	Conditions
Unilateral clubbing	Asymmetrical clubbing usually indicates impaired regional blood flow caused by localized vascular disease or hemiplegia	• Hemiplegia • Aneurysm of subclavian artery, brachiocephalic trunk, aortic arch, axillary artery, palmer arch • Presubclavian coarctation of aorta (left-sided clubbing) • Pancoasts tumor • Unilateral erythromelalgia (a rare neurovascular peripheral pain disorder commonly associated with myeloproliferative disorders in which blood vessels, usually in the lower extremities, are episodically blocked, then become hyperemic and inflamed) • AV fistula used for hemodialysis • Infected arterial graft
	Morphology of clubbing gives information about the diagnosis. The different morphological forms of clubbing are:	• Drumstick type clubbing: Bronchiectasis, congenital cyanotic heart disease (mnemonic: BCD) • Parrot-beak type clubbing: Bronchogenic carcinoma • Painful clubbing: Bronchogenic carcinoma, SBE, lung abscess • Reversible clubbing: Lung abscess, empyema thoracis • Unidigital clubbing: Hereditary, repeated local trauma, median nerve injury, sarcoidosis • Clubbing with cyanosis: Cyanotic heart disease, pulmonary AV shunt, pulmonary disease like lung abscess, bronchiectasis, cystic fibrosis • Acute clubbing (clubbing within 2 weeks after onset of illness): Lung abscess, empyema thoracis • Recurrent clubbing: May occur in pregnancy in otherwise healthy females
Differential clubbing	This type of clubbing is limited to upper or lower limbs alone and is often associated with cyanosis	• Clubbing limited to upper extremity: Chronic obstruction of veins of the upper extremity (IV drug users) • Clubbing limited to lower extremity: Patent ductus arteriosus (PDA) with reversal of shunt (Eisenmenger's PDA), infected abdominal aortic aneurysm
Pseudoclubbing	Several occupations involving heavy activity with hands and minor trauma sustained during such activities give rise to 'clubbed appearance' of the fingers, e.g. masons, blacksmiths and loading workers. Pseudoclubbing is characterized clinically by asymmetrical involvement of fingers and may show radiological abnormalities, such as resorption of the terminal tufts (acro-osteolysis)	

Abbreviations: AV = Atrioventricular; BCD = Binary coded decimal; SBE = Subacute bacterial endocarditis; IV = Intravenous; PDA = Patent ductus arteriosus

- **Grade 4: If yes to either:** Do you have to stop for a breath after walking about 100 yards (or after a few minutes) on the level ground?
- **Grade 5: If yes:** Are you too breathless to leave the house or breathless after undressing?

In left-sided heart failure and in hypoventilatory states, the patient becomes more dyspneic in the recumbent posture and considerable relief is obtained by sitting-up. This is referred to as **orthopnea.** Attacks of severe breathlessness occurring during sleep at night may awaken the patient and assumption of the erect posture gives relief. This is termed **paroxysmal nocturnal dyspnea.** This is also characteristic of left-sided heart failure.

Respiratory disorders that lead to dyspnea may fall into different groups:

- Central causes for dyspnea affect the respiratory center, e.g. encephalitis or cerebrovascular accidents.
- Significant airways obstruction is a common cause for dyspnea. Obstruction to the airway may be mechanical as due to a foreign body or functional as due to spasm. Larger airways may be obstructed by aspirated foreign bodies, diphtheritic membrane, tumors, blood or secretions. Obstruction to the larynx produces inspiratory stridor and indrawing of the chest wall. Dyspnea is felt both during inspiration and expiration. Obstruction to the smaller airways occurs in asthma, emphysema, chronic bronchitis and extensive bronchiectasis. In these conditions, the difficulty is felt more for expiration and the characteristic expiratory wheeze may be heard.
- Disorders that impair the process of gas exchange, e.g. massive pulmonary collapse, PE, respiratory distress syndrome (RDS), fibrosing alveolitis, pulmonary fibrosis (PF) and extensive parenchymal diseases, such as tuberculosis, cystic disease and malignancy.
- Diseases that prevent expansion of the lung, e.g. pneumothorax, pleural effusion, kyphoscoliosis, injury to the chest wall, paralysis of respiratory muscles.
- Dyspnea is commonly the first symptom when the inspired air does not supply adequate amounts of oxygen to the individual. This happens when the oxygen tension is low as in high altitudes or in gas poisoning.
- Hysterical hyperventilation may present as dyspnea. In this, the subject voluntarily hyperventilates. Other traits of the hysterical personality may be evident. Excessive removal of CO_2 due to overventilation leads to respiratory alkalosis and tetany.
- In diseases like pneumonia and pleurisy, painful restriction of respiratory movements leads to hypoventilation and dyspnea.

Cyanosis

Bluish discoloration of the skin and mucous membranes due to the presence of excess of reduced hemoglobin in peripheral blood is called cyanosis. In extensive diseases of the lungs, central cyanosis occurs due to defective oxygenation of arterial blood or the development of functional arteriovenous (AV) shunts. In chronic bronchitis and emphysema, the main defects are those of ventilation and perfusion. In fibrosing alveolitis, the defect is mainly one of diffusion. Differentiation between respiratory and cardiac causes of cyanosis can be made on clinical grounds in many cases. In respiratory diseases, inhalation of oxygen clears the cyanosis, whereas this is not so in cardiac lesions with right to left shunts.

PHYSICAL EXAMINATION

Examination of the respiratory system should be preceded by a careful general examination. Dyspnea, cyanosis, digital clubbing and cervical or axillary lymphadenopathy may suggest a primary respiratory disorder.

For purposes of physical examination, chest is divided into different areas with a view to enable anatomical localization of the lesion (Table 138.9). The anterior part is divided into supraclavicular, infraclavicular, mammary and inframammary regions. The lateral aspect is divided into the axillary and infra-axillary regions and the back is divided into suprascapular, interscapular and infrascapular regions.

Physical examination is carried out sequentially from inspection to palpation, percussion and auscultation. Measurement of the chest for its expansion is a simple and reliable clinical method for assessing the ventilatory capacity. Normal expansion in an adult ranges from 6 to 8 cm.

Percussion

The note raised by percussion and the vibration felt by the pleximeter finger give valuable clues to the state of the underlying lung and pleura. By percussion it is possible to assess the relative proportion of air, solid tissue or fluid underlying the area (Table 138.10).

Special forms of percussion include *tidal percussion* and *elicitation of shifting dullness*. The former is employed to distinguish dullness caused by the upper border of the liver from that caused by pleural fluid or consolidation of the lower portion of the lungs. Shifting dullness occurs when there is fluid which is free to move with changing positions of the patient. This occurs in hydropneumothorax or in a large cavity containing fluid and air.

Auscultatory Findings

Breath sounds, vocal resonance and whispered pectoriloquy are elicited by auscultation. Breath sounds are produced by oscillation set-up in the larger air passages (trachea and larger bronchi) by turbulent flow of air. Over the larger air passages the character of breath sounds is bronchial. In the lower regions of the lungs, the parenchyma acts as a low-pass filter which filters off the higher frequency components (200 Hz and above) and this changes the character of the breath sounds to vesicular. When this filtering effect is lost, the sounds are directly transmitted to the chest wall and the breath sounds become bronchial. This occurs in consolidation of the lungs. This is the acoustic basis of bronchophony and whispered

Table 138.9: Relationship of the clinical areas with the underlying lung

Views	Clinical areas	Indications
Anterior	• Supraclavicular region and infraclavicular region (from the clavicle down to the third rib) • Mammary region (from the third to the sixth rib)	• Corresponding to the apical and anterior segments of the upper lobe respectively • Correspond to the anterior surface of the middle lobe on the right and the lingula on the left
Lateral	• Axilla (from the apex of the axilla down to the sixth rib) • Infra-axillary region (from the sixth rib to the costal margin)	• Major part of the lateral aspect of the upper lobe and part of the lower lobe • Lateral segments of the lower lobe
Posterior	• Suprascapular region (above the spine of the scapula) • Interscapular region (second to seventh dorsal spines) • Infrascapular region (below the seventh dorsal spine)	• Part of the apical segment and contiguous posterior segments of the upper lobe • Apical segment of lower lobe and contiguous posterior portion of the upper lobe • Posterior basal segments of the lower lobes on both sides

Table 138.10: Clinical significance of alteration in percussion note

State of lung	Percussion note
Normal lung	Resonant normally
Hollow viscus, pneumothorax	Tympanitic
Moderate pneumothorax, emphysema, bullae	Hyper-resonant
Consolidation collapse, fibrothorax	Impaired resonance to moderate dullness
Pleural effusion, empyema, thick fibrothorax	Stony dullness

pectoriloquy as well. Adventitious sounds heard during auscultation may be *wheezes* (previously called *rhonchi*) and *crackles* (used to be known as *crepitations*).

Breath Sounds

Normal breath sounds are vesicular and is produced by turbulence of air at carina and major divisions of bronchi. This is characterized by the phase of inspiration, closely followed by a short expiratory phase (one-third of the inspiration) and the quality being rustling. In bronchial breathing, the expiratory and inspiratory phases are equal with a pause in between and the quality is guttural or aspirate. Normally, bronchial breathing is heard over the trachea, when auscultated over the front and back of the neck. Pathological associations of the bronchial breathing include pulmonary consolidation, collapse adjoining a patent bronchus or rarely other conditions. Based on the pitch, bronchial breathing has been described as *tubular* (high pitched), *cavernous* (low pitched) and

amphoric (low-pitched breath sounds with high-pitched overtones). ***Tubular breathing*** is heard over pneumonic consolidation, ***cavernous breathing*** over communicating cavities and large air passages, and ***amphoric breathing*** over open pneumothorax and large communicating cavities. ***Bronchophony*** (increased vocal resonance) occurs over areas of consolidation. ***Whispering pectoriloquy*** (whispered sounds being heard distinctly on auscultating the chest) can be elicited over areas of bronchial breathing. When only high frequency sounds of a spoken voice are transmitted to the chest wall, the vocal resonance attains a nasal quality and this is termed ***egophony***. This may be elicited above the level of a pleural effusion.

Adventitious sounds may be continuous or interrupted. Continuous adventitious sounds include ***stridor*** occurring in laryngeal and bronchial obstruction, and ***wheezes*** arising from narrowed air passages. Wheezes are musical lung sounds. When heard by auscultation, they are termed ***rhonchi***. Interrupted adventitious sounds include crackles (which may be fine, medium or coarse), and pleural rubs. Crackles (crepitations) are produced by explosive equilibration of gas pressure between boluses of air in the air passage and the sequential opening up of airways during respiratory cycles. Coarse crepitations may be due to the presence of exudate in the larger air passages and these disappear with coughing and expectoration.

Pleural friction rub: This is a leather-creaking sound heard superficially in pleural diseases. It may be heard both during inspiration and expiration at the same part of the respiratory cycle. It is not altered by coughing.

Pleuropericardial sounds: These are better heard when the breath is held in full inspiration, as rubbing sounds. They suggest the presence of pleurisy and pericarditis.

Crunching sounds: These are heard when auscultating over areas of surgical emphysema and sometimes over pericarditis.

Knocks: These are sharp adventitious sounds heard in pneumothorax caused by the movement of the collapsed lung over the mediastinum.

INVESTIGATIONS IN RESPIRATORY DISEASES

General investigations of importance which points to diseases of the respiratory organs include peripheral blood picture, total and differential leukocyte counts and determination of erythrocyte sedimentation rate (ESR). Lymphocytosis is suggestive of chronic inflammatory diseases like tuberculosis whereas neutrophil leukocytosis occurs in acute infections like pneumonia. Increase in eosinophils above 10% calls for estimation of the absolute eosinophil count. Mild and moderate increase in eosinophils is very common in Indian subjects. This is caused by factors such as helminthiasis and external allergens. In susceptible subjects, even moderate eosinophilia may present with symptoms of respiratory allergy. Higher eosinophil counts are found in bronchial asthma, hydatid disease and pulmonary eosinophilia. Chronic hypoxemia results in the development of secondary polycythemia. Elevation of ESR is a nonspecific indicator of inflammatory and neoplastic lesions in the lungs. ESR is not specific for diagnosis, but in the follow up of chronic diseases like tuberculosis, ESR is a helpful parameter.

Sputum Examination

- ***Sputum:*** It should be examined macroscopically, microscopically after proper staining and bacteriologically. Total quantity of sputum in 24 hour, color, consistency and other characteristics like odor and presence of blood are of great value in diagnosis. Presence of fungi in mycotic infections, asbestos bodies in asbestosis and motile amoeba in pulmonary amebiasis can be detected by direct microscopy of fresh sputum. ***Gram's stain*** and ***Ziehl-Neelsen*** stain are employed to identify the bacterial and mycobacterial pathogens in the smear. Malignant cells can be detected by cytological examination. Wet preparations stained with methylene blue may suggest the presence of malignant cells. Staining with Leishman's stain helps to identify leukocytes in sputum. Presence of numerous neutrophils suggests infective basis whereas predominance of eosinophils suggests allergic etiology. This distinction is very helpful in the management of asthma. ***Papanicolaou staining*** technique helps to identify the malignant cells further. Giemsa stain reveals *Pneumocystis carinii*.

- ***Bacteriological tests:*** Sputum culture is done to identify the organisms and their sensitivity to various antibiotics. Proper collection of the specimen is essential for getting reliable results. Sputum should be taken directly into sterile receptacles. Contamination by oropharyngeal organisms leads to fallacious results on culture. Uncontaminated specimens of sputum can be obtained by transtracheal aspiration. Bronchial washings collected through a bronchoscope or smears collected by a brush during bronchoscopy are ideal specimens for cytological and microbiological studies, wherever facilities are available.

Radiological Studies

Plain X-ray of chest (posteroanterior view): Radiographs are taken in full inspiration with the film placed in front of the chest and the source of X-ray kept 1.5–2.0 m behind the patient. In addition to posteroanterior (PA) views, lateral views are also taken with the affected side close to the film to locate the bronchopulmonary segment which is the seat of disease. In normal skiagrams, the lungs appear as translucent zones in which bronchovascular markings are clearly detectable and can be traced almost to the periphery.

The trachea, mediastinum, costophrenic and cardiophrenic angles and the level of the diaphragm are taken as landmarks in the interpretation of chest skiagram. On either side, the lung fields are compared zone by zone. For purposes of description, the lung fields are divided into the upper, middle and lower zones. A horizontal line at the level of the lower margin of the anterior end of the second rib separates the upper from middle zone, and a horizontal line passing through the lower margin of the anterior end of the fourth rib separates the middle from the lower zone. Chest radiographs give evidence of morphological lesions. In many instances, radiological appearances help to infer the etiology as well.

Radiological Appearances Caused by Physical Abnormalities in the Lungs

Consolidation: Presence of homogenous opacities with well-defined margins indicate pulmonary consolidation. Radiological consolidation is characterized by presence of air bronchogram that is seen through the consolidated lung. Since there is no change in the volume of the lung, trachea and mediastinum are not shifted.

Collapse: Pulmonary collapse throws a homogenous opacity with clear-cut concave margins. The trachea, mediastinum and interlobar fissures are shifted towards the area of collapse. The dome of the diaphragm on the affected side is elevated. The unaffected portions of the lung show hypertranslucency due to compensatory emphysema.

Fibrosis: Presence of streaky linear or reticular shadows with shift of trachea and mediastinum to the same side and compensatory emphysema of the unaffected regions is suggestive of fibrosis.

Pleural effusion: Presence of small quantities of fluid (< 300 mL) in the pleura causes only obliteration of the costophrenic angle. As the quantity of fluid increases, more extensive homogenous opacity appears with obliteration of the costophrenic and cardiophrenic angles. The upper margin tends to be concave with its higher level towards the axilla and the lower level towards the mediastinum. Midline structures are shifted to the opposite side.

Presence of fluid and air **(hydropneumothorax)** is diagnosed by the presence of a horizontal level of fluid below, with hypertranslucency (due to air) above. The lung markings are not visible since the lung is collapsed towards the hilum.

Pneumothorax: Presence of air in the pleural cavity leads to hyperlucency and absence of lung markings on the affected side. The margin of the collapsed lung is seen towards the hilum. The midline structures are pushed to the opposite side.

Cavities: They are seen as areas of central translucency within areas of consolidation or fibrosis.

Morphology of the cavities varies with different lesions. Tuberculous cavities are thin-walled and empty. Thick-walled cavities containing fluid and air suggest the possibility of lung abscess or neoplasms.

Opacities in the lung: Opacities may be single or multiple. Depending on their size and distribution, multiple opacities are grouped as **miliary mottling** (1–2 mm size), **nodularity** (1 cm or above) and **cannon balls**. Their size, density, distribution and number give clues to their pathological nature. The lungs are hypertranslucent in emphysema and less translucent in conditions, such as interstitial fibrosis or pulmonary edema.

Lesions in the apices of the lungs are brought out better by taking lordotic views or penetrated views. By this method, parts concealed behind ribs are visualized. The exact spatial location of any lesion can be obtained by taking the PA and lateral views. Oblique views may be required for further localization. Radiographs taken in the lateral decubitus are necessary to detect conditions such as infrapulmonary effusions. In cases where X-ray pictures are not conclusive, more informative procedures like high-resolution computed tomography (CT) are done.

Fluoroscopy: This procedure helps in assessing the respiratory movements and the movements of mediastinal structures. Due to the risk of the radiation and want of accuracy in diagnosis, this procedure is seldom used at present.

Contrast radiography: The technique of visualizing the bronchial tree using radiopaque dyes is called **bronchography**. This is the only reliable method to assess the total extent and type of bronchiectasis.

Pulmonary angiography: It is performed to study the pattern and distribution of the pulmonary arteries and their branches. Arteriography is the method of choice to demonstrate PE and AV malformations.

Ultrasonography: Recently ultrasonography has become an important investigational modality in respiratory diseases. Though lung tissue does not echo the ultrasound, the artifacts produced by scattery and reverberations provide specific patterns that can be utilized in identifying pneumothorax, pulmonary parenchymal lesions, mediastinal lesions, pleural fluid and other pleural lesions, cardiac and pericardial lesions. Endobronchial ultrasound provides images of extraluminal pathologies, which can be safely sampled. Ultrasound directed biopsies and aspiration are also more effective than blind procedure.

Radioisotopic investigations: Isotopic techniques have made it possible to obtain visual images as well as precise quantitative information about the regional distribution of ventilation and perfusion. These methods are generally noninvasive. New machines incorporating computer facilities are available.

Perfusion imaging: This is employed to study the state of the pulmonary vasculature. The main clinical uses are in the investigation of PE, atresia or hypoplasia of pulmonary artery, presence of right-to-left intracardiac shunts and pulmonary venous hypertension.

Ventilation imaging: This can be made by using ^{133}Xenon.

Aerosol inhalation studies: Aerosolized radioactive particles can be administered for inhalation. Commonly technetium-99 (^{99m}Tc) labeled phytate, lactose, albumin or sulfur colloids are used. The radioactive particles are distributed in the lungs depending upon the patency of the air passages. The concentration or radioactivity is diminished in areas of poor ventilation. Another use of labeled aerosol particles is to study the efficiency of mucociliary function. When mucociliary function is impaired, the clearance of radioactivity from the lung is delayed.

Using perfusion and ventilation imaging studies, valuable information can be obtained. In PE, ventilation is normal but perfusion is diminished, whereas both ventilation and perfusion are diminished in parenchymal, pleural or obstructive airway disease.

Isotopic localization of pulmonary tumors: Isotopes such as ^{52}Gallium citrate and ^{57}Cobalt-labeled bleomycin which are concentrated by tumors are used to study neoplastic lesions.

CT scan: This is employed to detect abnormalities in the pleura, lungs, major blood vessels and mediastinal structures. CT scan distinguishes between cysts, tumors and vascular lesions. It is very helpful to diagnose bronchiectasis. It is a valuable adjunct when skiagrams are not conclusive. CT has become a regular investigation modality in respiratory medicine. High-resolution CT (HRCT) is more useful to detect pulmonary infiltrative diseases and bronchiectasis early.

Magnetic resonance imaging (MRI): It is also very helpful to bring out structural lesions of intrathoracic organs. The advantages over CT are its capacity to give pictures in the sagittal, coronal and transverse planes with higher resolution. Lesions occurring at the apices of the lungs and thoracoabdominal junctions are picked up better by MRI. It can also distinguish between vascular and nonvascular structures at the hilum even without contrast.

Endoscopic studies: Several endoscopic procedures are available to study respiratory disorders. These include laryngoscopy, bronchoscopy, mediastinoscopy and thoracoscopy. Laryngoscopy visualizes the upper respiratory tract up to the larynx and the trachea.

Bronchoscopy: It is the endoscopic procedure used to visualize the trachea, bronchi and their branches, aspirate secretions for investigations, obtain biopsy material and remove obstructions. Clinical indications for bronchoscopy include bronchial obstruction, pulmonary neoplasms, unresolved pneumonia, lung abscess and recurrent hemoptysis. Bronchoalveolar lavage can be done during bronchoscopy and the specimen can be examined further.

Availability of flexible fiberoptic bronchoscopes with facilities for aspiration and biopsy procedures has increased their importance in diagnosis and therapy in recent years. Flexible bronchoscopes can reach up to the second or third division of the bronchi whereas rigid bronchoscopes reach only up to the first division.

Video bronchoscope gives better clarity of the lesion. Advances in bronchoscopy include transbronchial biopsy to grade peripheral lung cancers, application of transbronchial stents to relieve obstruction and autofluorescence bronchoscopy for early detection of lung cancer. Newer instruments incorporating ultrasound and high magnification equipments give better diagnostic results.

Mediastinoscopes: It is used to inspect the superior mediastinum and perform biopsy procedures under direct vision.

Thoracoscopy: It is inspection of the thoracic contents with a thoracoscope after producing a partial pneumothorax. Video-assisted thoracoscopic surgery (VATS) is useful for conducting procedures like lung biopsy and lung volume reduction surgery.

Investigations using aspirated material: In the diagnosis of pleural diseases, the examination of pleural fluid is most important. So, also examination of bronchial aspirates and material from other sites gives valuable diagnostic clues. Macroscopic appearance, microscopy, cytology, microbiological studies and biochemical investigations are helpful in diagnosis.

Biopsy Studies

Lymph node biopsy: Biopsy of the appropriate scalene lymph node or palpable axillary or cervical lymph nodes helps to diagnose granulomatous and neoplastic lesions.

Lung biopsy: Lung tissue can be obtained by percutaneous biopsy, bronchoscopically or by open biopsy under vision. Percutaneous biopsy using a Vim-Silverman needle or a trephine is performed to diagnose diffuse lesions and peripherally situated localized lesions. When the lesions are small and not accessible superficially, thoracotomy and open biopsy are preferable.

Pleural biopsy: This is resorted to when pleural lesions have to be diagnosed. ***Cope's needle*** or ***Abram's pleural biopsy punch*** is used for obtaining material from the parietal pleura. ***Vim-Silverman needle*** or ***Menghini's needle*** can be used in the absence of the specialized needles. Aspiration and biopsy can be done as ultrasound or CT guided procedures for greater diagnostic yield.

Bronchoalveolar lavage: This procedure is adopted to obtain material from the terminal portions of the respiratory tree and alveoli. The specimen is subjected to microscopy and cytological examination. Organisms such as *Pneumocystis carinii*, cytomegalovirus (CMV), *Legionella*, fungi and mycobacteria can be identified in the washings. Bronchoalveolar lavage has been used therapeutically to remove occluding plugs in cystic fibrosis and severe asthma. In alveolar proteinosis, lavage using heparin and acetylcysteine helps to remove the proteinaceous material.

CHAPTER
139

Respiratory Failure

C Sudheendra Ghosh, CP Murali

Chapter Summary

- General Considerations
- Management of Acute Respiratory Failure
- Chronic Respiratory Failure
- Acute Respiratory Distress Syndrome (ARDS)
- Respiratory Distress Syndrome (RDS) of Newborn

GENERAL CONSIDERATIONS

Respiratory failure is defined as inability of the lungs to maintain normal blood gases and pH. Gas exchange is inadequate during rest as well as exercise. Respiratory failure is one of the most common reasons for admission of patients in the intensive care unit (ICU). In this condition,

Box 139.1: Causes of respiratory failure	
Causes	**Signs and symptoms**
Interference with the mechanics of the chest wall	Severe kyphoscoliosis, obesity, flail chest injury with multiple rib fractures, paralysis of the chest wall muscles and diaphragm, immobility of the chest wall as in progressive systemic sclerosis
Pleural disorders	Large collection of pleural fluid, tension pneumothorax, gross thickening of the pleura and others
Diseases of the airways	Severe asthma, advanced chronic bronchitis and emphysema, laryngeal edema, mechanical obstruction of air passages
Pulmonary diseases	Pulmonary interstitial fibrosis, neonatal and adult respiratory distress syndrome, allergic alveolitis, extensive malignancy, bilateral pneumonia
Diseases of pulmonary vasculature	Primary pulmonary hypertension, polyarteritis nodosa, repeated pulmonary embolism
Metabolic	Metabolic alkalosis
Depression of the respiratory center	Injury to brainstem, raised intracranial tension and narcotic poisoning lead to central respiratory failure

the resting partial pressure of oxygen in the arterial blood (PaO_2) falls below 60 mm Hg (60 torr or 8 kPa) and/or the partial pressure of carbon dioxide in arterial blood ($PaCO_2$) rises above 49 mm Hg (49 torr or 7 kPa), when breathing room air at sea level. Lowered PaO_2 alone is not adequate to make the diagnosis of respiratory failure. In right-to-left shunt lesions, the PaO_2 may be lowered without respiratory failure. Causes of respiratory failure are many (Box 139.1). Interference with any of the major processes—ventilation, perfusion or diffusion—may result in respiratory failure.

The **clinical picture** depends on the speed of onset, cause and severity. Acute respiratory failure produces more dramatic symptoms whereas chronic respiratory failure may even remain asymptomatic. Respiratory failure may or may not be associated with dyspnea. Though in the early stages, CO_2 retention causes dyspnea, with the passage of time the respiratory center becomes adapted and unresponsive to elevated level of CO_2. At this stage, the lowered PaO_2 (60 mm Hg or below) is the effective stimulus for respiration. There is no direct correlation between the blood gas levels and severity of dyspnea.

In majority of cases, patient has a long-standing respiratory problem such as chronic obstructive airway disease and respiratory failure is precipitated by infection. The increased secretions and mucosal edema caused by infection aggravate the airway obstruction and this results in alveolar hypoventilation. As a result, hypoxia and hypercapnia (rise in level of arterial CO_2) develop. As the respiratory failure progresses, the PaO_2 falls from 60 mm Hg (mild) to 20 mm Hg (severe). Respiratory failure can be categorized mechanistically, based on pathophysiologic derangements in respiratory function. Accordingly, four different types of respiratory failure can be described.

Type I Respiratory Failure

This type is characterized by lowered PaO_2 and normal or low $PaCO_2$. This is usually a result of conditions in which ventilation is normal, but there is defective diffusion or ventilation-perfusion imbalance. This occurs when alveolar flooding and subsequent intrapulmonary shunt physiology occur. Conditions like pulmonary edema, respiratory distress syndrome (RDS), hypersensitivity pneumonitis (HP) and interstitial pulmonary fibrosis lead to type I respiratory failure.

Type II Respiratory Failure

In this condition, PaO_2 is reduced and $PaCO_2$ is elevated. **Hypoxia** is the more prominent feature. This results from conditions characterized by defective ventilation occurring along with ventilation-perfusion imbalance. There is alveolar hypoventilation leading to inability to eliminate CO_2 effectively. Alveolar hypoventilation occurs in chronic bronchitis, emphysema, asthma and respiratory paralysis. **Hypercapnia** develops only when the FEV1 goes down below 1.2 L. With higher values of FEV1, hypercapnia is rare. If the respiratory failure is of acute onset, retention of CO_2 leads to acidosis and fall of pH. If the respiratory failure becomes chronic, compensatory mechanisms come into play. Renal conservation of bicarbonate restores the pH to near normal.

Type III Respiratory Failure

This form of respiratory failure occurs as a result of lung atelectasis. Because lung atelectasis occurs so frequently in the perioperative period, this is also called **perioperative respiratory failure**. After general anesthesia, decrease in functional residual capacity leads to collapse of dependent lung. Chest physiotherapy and noninvasive ventilation are used to reverse regional atelectasis.

Type IV Respiratory Failure

This type of respiratory failure results from hypoperfusion of respiratory muscles in patients in shock. Patients in shock often experience respiratory distress due to pulmonary edema, lactic acidosis and anemia. In this setting, up to 40% of cardiac output may be distributed to the respiratory muscles. Intubation and mechanical ventilation can allow redistribution of the cardiac output away from the respiratory muscles and back to vital organs while the shock is treated.

CLINICAL FEATURES

Respiratory failure may be acute or chronic. In the latter, exacerbating factors lead to acute manifestations. The main biochemical factors are hypoxia and hypercapnia, which in turn give rise to various other abnormalities in acid-base balance and electrolyte disturbances. The manifestations of hypoxia and hypercapnia vary from each other.

Manifestations of Hypoxia

Hypoxia is more harmful to tissues than hypercapnia. Vital organs such as the brain, heart, liver and kidney, and the pulmonary vessels are adversely affected. Neurological symptoms include headache, irritability, insomnia, drowsiness, mental confusion and coma. Objective evidence of cerebral dysfunction can be demonstrated by the electroencephalogram (EEG). If hypoxia is severe, fatty change, tissue necrosis and focal hemorrhages develop in the myocardium. Cardiac arrhythmias are precipitated. Constriction of pulmonary arteries leads to pulmonary hypertension (PH) and this may precipitate right-sided heart failure. Liver cells become edematous and necrosed. In chronic hypoxia, the liver shows fatty change and fibrosis. Severe hypoxia may give rise to renal tubular damage. Secondary polycythemia develops in chronic hypoxic states.

Manifestations of Hypercapnia

In the initial stages, hypercapnia stimulates the respiratory center and the resultant hyperventilation helps to lower the $PaCO_2$ to normal levels. In established hypercapnia, the respiratory center becomes insensitive to raised $PaCO_2$. In such cases, the stimulus for the respiratory center is hypoxia. Injudicious administration of oxygen may abolish this hypoxic stimulus and this may give rise to further depression of respiration and CO_2 narcosis. Hypercapnia causes cerebral vasodilatation, headache, and rise in intracranial tension. As a result, papilledema may occur in severe cases. Peripheral vasodilatation develops and this gives rise to warm extremities, flushing, and rapid high volume pulse. When $PaCO_2$ levels exceed 50 mm Hg, drowsiness, confusion, muscle twitching, and flapping tremors develop. The deep tendon reflexes become sluggish. The patient lapses into coma when $PaCO_2$ rises above 80 mm Hg.

MANAGEMENT OF ACUTE RESPIRATORY FAILURE

This should be managed as an emergency in an intensive respiratory care unit, if facilities are available. Proper monitoring includes the record of heart rate, respiratory rate, blood pressure (BP), temperature, serum electrolytes and blood gas levels. In addition to general supportive care, special attention should be paid to the airways and proper oxygenation.

Maintenance of the airway: Irrespective of the cause, in all cases of respiratory failure, the upper air passages should be fully inspected and foreign bodies and secretions should be removed. In the recumbent comatose patient, the chin should be pulled up to prevent the tongue from falling back and obstructing the pharynx. If the patient cannot expectorate freely, secretions should be aspirated. If the patient can cooperate, removal of secretions should be aided by postural coughing, gentle tapping on the chest, steam inhalation and administration of drugs like bromhexine hydrochloride. Bromhexine hydrochloride can be administered orally in a dose of 8 mg thrice daily. Mucolytic agents can be administered as aerosols, e.g. acetylcysteine. Adequate hydration is necessary, since it helps to loosen the secretions for easy expectoration. If bronchospasm is present, it can be relieved by drugs like salbutamol given 2–4 mg orally or 0.5 mg intramuscularly (IM). Parenteral corticosteroids (betamethasone 4 mg) may have to be given if bronchospasm is not relieved by simple measures. Salbutamol and beclomethasone can also be given as metered aerosols. Tracheostomy may be required in some cases where the tidal volume is low.

Antibiotics: Since infection is a very common precipitating factor, antibiotic therapy is indicated. Preliminary assessment of the infecting agent can be made by Gram-staining and culture of the sputum and suitable antibiotic can be started. Antibiotic therapy may have to be reviewed when microbiological results are obtained.

Correction of hypoxia: This is the mainstay in the management of respiratory failure. Oxygen is administered with nasal catheter, or by more effective methods such as masks or tents. If given by nasal catheter, the rate is 2–3 L/min and the catheter tip should be located 15 cm from nostril. The *venturi mask* which delivers oxygen at a preset low concentration is ideal if available. The concentration of oxygen can be adjusted at 24, 28 or 35% by giving oxygen at rates ranging from 4–8 L/min. It is desirable to bring the PaO_2 level above 50 mm Hg and pH above 7.25. In chronic respiratory failure, administration of oxygen should be closely supervised to avoid the development of CO_2 narcosis. Once the emergency has been tided over, the patient is weaned off from oxygen gradually. Long-term oxygen therapy may be required in selected cases of chronic respiratory failure.

Supportive measures: Administration of fluid and electrolytes, preferably with monitoring of central venous pressure (CVP) and maintenance of nutrition are important.

Assistance to ventilation: Mechanical assistance should be considered when the patient's own effort is inadequate to maintain oxygenation. If the PaO_2 remains below 60 mm Hg and $PaCO_2$ remains above 55 mm Hg while receiving oxygen therapy, respiratory assistance is indicated.

The decision to assist ventilation should be individualized depending on several factors. Noninvasive positive pressure ventilation (NIPPV) is delivery of mechanical ventilation to the lungs without an invasive (endotracheal) airway. This can be delivered with the use of either negative pressure ventilators or NIPPV. Intubation is indicated when NIPPV has failed or contraindicated. Contraindications include inability to protect the airway, patient intolerance, and hemodynamic instability or cardiac arrest (Box 139.2).

Different types of ventilators are available. Volume-cycled ventilators are superior since these are more efficient and safe. If the patient's respiratory mechanism is active, it is desirable to assist it (assisted ventilation). On the other hand, in patients in whom spontaneous respiration is abolished, controlled ventilation using a preset volume and rate is employed. Modern respirators are designed to assist respiration when the patient's own respiratory effort goes down and they are reciprocally inhibited when the patient's breathing recovers.

Positive end-expiratory pressure (PEEP): One of the problems encountered in patients with respiratory failure maintained on assisted respiration is premature closure of the terminal airways during expiration, giving rise to air trapping. This is prevented by maintaining a PEEP. In addition, it helps to reopen bronchioles and alveoli which remain closed. The tidal respiration is improved. PEEP also helps to reduce the functional intrapulmonary shunts, thereby increasing the PaO_2. The disadvantage of PEEP is reduction in venous return to the heart due to increased intrathoracic pressure and consequent cardiac

Box 139.2: Indications for mechanical ventilation

- Cardiac or respiratory arrest
- Tachypnea or bradypnea with respiratory fatigue or impending arrest
- Acute respiratory acidosis
- Refractory hypoxemia [when the PaO_2 could not be maintained above 60 mm Hg with inspired O_2 fraction (FIO_2) >1.0]
- Inability to protect the airway associated with depressed levels of consciousness
- Shock associated with excessive respiratory work
- Inability to clear secretions with impaired gas exchange or excessive respiratory work
- Newly diagnosed neuromuscular disease with a vital capacity <10–15 mL/kg
- Short-term adjunct in management of acutely increased intracranial pressure (ICP)

Consider noninvasive ventilation particularly in the following settings:

- Chronic obstructive pulmonary disease (COPD) exacerbation
- Cardiogenic pulmonary edema (CPE)
- Obesity hypoventilation syndrome (OHS)
- Noninvasive ventilation may be tried in selected patients with asthma or noncardiogenic hypoxemic respiratory failure

failure. Assistance to ventilation should be carried out by specially-trained teams. As the patient improves, he is gradually weaned off the ventilator under supervision. Ventilatory support is a highly skilled job, which has to be undertaken by a team trained to establish the airway, activate the machines and monitor the progress of the patient clinically from blood gases and acid-base values. In many centers, this is done under the supervision of the anesthetist, intensivist and pulmonologist.

Ventilatory support is lifesaving in conditions like acute respiratory distress syndrome (ARDS). Special methods have to be employed in ventilation as well as weaning from the ventilator. Long-term study of cases of ARDS (5 years or more) has revealed exercise limitations, physical and physiological sequela, decreased quality of life and increased healthcare costs.

Extracorporeal membrane oxygenators (ECMO) are being employed in the management of severe hypoxemic respiratory failure when conventional methods fail. Solutions containing perfluorocarbon which dissolve oxygen and deliver it to tissues are also being introduced into the management of respiratory failure. As the patient improves, he is encouraged to undertake mild exercises. Respiratory exercises are advised to increase the tidal volume and help expectoration. He is also instructed on methods to avoid the precipitating factors. Incurable cases should be considered for lung transplantation.

CHRONIC RESPIRATORY FAILURE

Some patients with progressive respiratory disease eventually enter a state in which the arterial O_2 and CO_2 are persistently abnormal. Acute respiratory infection tips them into severe respiratory failure. In such cases, prompt treatment of infections, bronchodilators and management of respiratory failure help to tide over the crisis. In irreversible chronic ventilatory failure, provision of continuous oxygen in the house is very beneficial in giving symptomatic relief. Lung transplantation is indicated in many cases. This has to be considered when the chances of functional recovery sufficient to sustain life are improbable with other therapies.

ACUTE RESPIRATORY DISTRESS SYNDROME (ARDS)

Syn: Shock lung, Wet lung

ARDS was first formally described by Ashbaugh and colleagues in 1967.

This is a syndrome characterized by a fairly acute onset of severe respiratory distress in adults who have normal pulmonary functions. Clinically, it resembles RDS of the newborn but in the latter, changes in surfactant are the primary mechanisms for disease. This is not so in adults.

Diagnostic Criteria

- Acute onset of respiratory failure
- ***PaO_2/FIO_2:*** <300 mm Hg = acute lung injury
- ***PaO_2/FIO_2:*** <200 mm Hg = ARDS
- ***Chest radiograph:*** Bilateral alveolar infiltrates consistent with pulmonary edema
- Pulmonary capillary wedge pressure (PCWP) <18 mm Hg or no clinical evidence of increased left atrial (LA) pressure

Etiology

Many factors contribute to the picture of ARDS, which may follow several unrelated pathological conditions. These include prolonged shock, cardiopulmonary bypass (CPB) surgery, severe infections like septicemia, viral, bacterial, fungal or pneumocystis pneumonia (PCP), inhalation of irritant fumes, drugs like nitrofurantoin, methadone and morphine, trauma to chest including major surgery, acute pancreatitis, fat embolism, massive blood transfusions, prolonged administration of oxygen in high concentrations and immunological disorders like Goodpasture's syndrome (Table 139.1).

Pathogenesis

The natural history of ARDS is marked by three phases—exudative, proliferative and fibrotic—each with characteristic clinical and pathologic features. The initiating factor is damage to the pulmonary capillaries leading to extravasation of fluid into the interstitium and alveoli. This results in ventilation-perfusion imbalance. Work required for respiration increases since the edematous lung is less compliant. Disseminated intravascular coagulation (DIC) which may occur in shock favors the development of ARDS. Other pathogenetic mechanisms include microemboli produced from extracorporeal circulation, immune complexes and presence of excess of catecholamines. The lungs are airless, congested, hemorrhagic and edematous. In the acute phase, interstitial and alveolar edema is present. Unlike as in left heart failure where pulmonary capillary pressure is high, it is normal in ARDS. Type I pneumocytes desquamate and are replaced by hyaline membrane. Type II pneumocytes suffer damage resulting in the depletion of surfactant. This results in widespread microatelectasis. Vascular damage leads to interstitial edema. If the condition persists for more than 10 days, the epithelium undergoes cuboidal transformation and

Table 139.1: Clinical disorders commonly associated with ARDS	
Direct lung injury	*Indirect lung injury*
Pneumonia	Sepsis
Aspiration of gastric contents	Severe trauma
Pulmonary contusion	• Multiple bone fractures
Near-drowning	• Flail chest
Toxic inhalation injury	• Head trauma
	Burns
	Multiple transfusions
	Drug overdose
	Pancreatitis
	Post cardiopulmonary bypass

progressive interstitial fibrosis. This may be manifested functionally as alveolocapillary defects.

Clinical Features

ARDS sets in on a background of any of the various clinical conditions mentioned earlier. Early features include tachypnea and dyspnea. Auscultation may reveal diffuse wheezes and crackles. The arterial oxygen saturation falls progressively. Arterial CO_2 is maintained normal for considerable periods by hyperventilation. The chest X-ray shows progressive haziness of lung fields due to increasing quantity of fluid (Fig. 139.1). The fully established picture is one of severe respiratory failure which may be fatal. Prognosis depends upon the underlying condition and the stage at which respiratory support is given. The mortality used to be 50–60%, but with modern treatment, it has come down. Those who recover do so with or without sequela. Rarely emphysema may result.

Management

Prompt treatment of the predisposing factors like shock and infection may help to prevent the development of ARDS and if already established, to prevent deterioration. The general management is the same as for respiratory failure. Fluid therapy should be carefully controlled as the lungs are already edematous. Administration of salt-free albumin along with furosemide has been beneficial. Institution of PEEP ventilation and more efficient cardiovascular support help to reduce mortality. PEEP

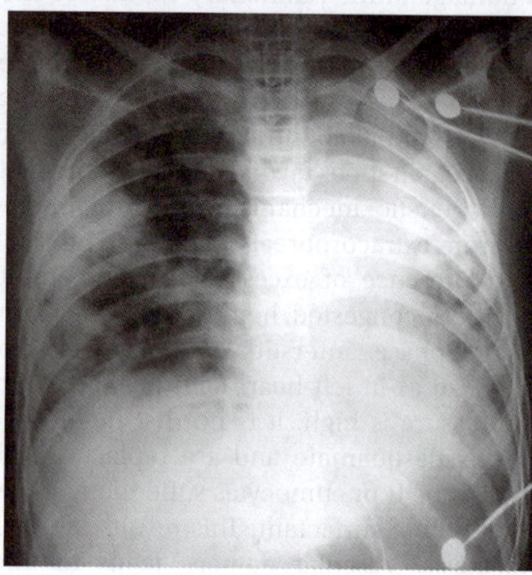

Fig. 139.1: Chest X-ray shows bilateral alveolar infiltrate consistent with pulmonary edema

serves to increase the lung volume, reduce intrapulmonary shunting and collapse of alveoli. ECMO is lifesaving in selected cases.

Inhalation of nitric oxide as a pulmonary vasodilator has been tried. Corticosteroids are indicated in cases where the primary disorder is immune-mediated.

RESPIRATORY DISTRESS SYNDROME (RDS) OF NEWBORN

This is a syndrome characterized by tachypnea, expiratory grunt and cyanosis caused by the lack of surfactant and often with a fatal outcome seen most frequently in premature babies below 38-week gestation. Fetal causes include neonatal asphyxia, acidosis and hypothermia. Antepartum hemorrhage (APH), uncontrolled diabetic state in the mother, hypoxia, gross anemia and cesarean section done for fetal distress are the maternal causes associated with higher incidence of RDS.

Pathogenesis

The level of surfactant in the alveoli is reduced. This results in atelectasis of the alveoli. In addition to the reduction in surfactant, other abnormalities such as alterations in the pulmonary and systemic circulation, coagulopathy, fibrinolysis, interstitial edema, decreased plasma proteins and disordered pulmonary mechanics are important contributory factors leading to the final picture. The effort required to distend the alveoli during inspiration is greater. Reduction in compliance leads to rapid shallow breathing, inspiratory indrawing of intercostal spaces and cyanosis. Histopathologically, there is extensive alveolar atelectasis, dilatation of alveolar ducts, interstitial edema and presence of a hyaline membrane covering the respiratory bronchioles, alveolar ducts and alveoli. The hyaline membrane is formed by desquamated epithelial cell debris and fibrin.

Clinically, the baby has tachypnea, grunting expirations, indrawing of the intercostal, subcostal and suprasternal spaces and cyanosis. Untreated, the mortality is very high. Children who survive RDS are predisposed to various chronic respiratory problems in later life.

Treatment

Neonatal intensive care units (NICUs) have reduced the mortality from RDS. The airway is maintained patent by careful suction of secretion and physiotherapy. Controlled administration of oxygen, PEEP respiration, correction of acidosis and maintenance of normal body temperature (36.5°C skin temperature) are important supportive measures. Antibiotics are indicated in the presence of infection. Corticosteroids have been employed, based on subjective observations.

Surfactant therapy: Instillation of surfactant directly into the airways helps to relieve the condition. Exosurf neonatal (Burroughs Wellcome) is a protein-free synthetic lung surfactant. The contents of a vial is reconstituted with 8 mL preservative-free sterile water. This solution contains 13.5 mg of dipalmitoylphosphatidylcholine (DPPC). Surfactant should be administered only in centers where facilities for assisted ventilation and respiratory monitoring are available. The dose is 5 mL/kg body weight, repeated after 12 hours.

The baby is put on endotracheal ventilation and the surfactant solution is delivered into the infant's trachea through the sideport of the endotracheal tube, taking several minutes for the administration. The first dose should be administered as early as possible on diagnosing RDS.

Prenatal estimation of the lecithin—sphingomyelin (L:S) ratio in amniotic fluid (obtained by amniocentesis) is useful to predict the chances of developing RDS. If L:S ratio is less than 1.5, the risk is high. If L:S ratio is over 2, the risk of RDS is minimal.

Administration of corticosteroids to mothers who go into premature labor helps to reduce the chances of RDS in the newborn.

Diseases of the Upper Respiratory Tract

CHAPTER 140

Diseases of the Upper Respiratory Tract

KE Rajan

Chapter Summary

- Rhinitis
- Epistaxis
- Pharyngitis
- Acute Tonsillitis
- Sinusitis
- Acute Laryngitis
- Chronic Laryngitis
- Laryngeal Paralysis
- Obstruction to the Respiratory Tract
  - Acute Laryngeal Obstruction

RHINITIS

Inflammation of the nasal mucosa is called rhinitis. The most frequent cause is allergy to inhaled substances such as pollen, dust, hair or animal dander. In India, 20–26% people suffer from allergic rhinitis. Symptoms of allergic rhinitis were noted in 75% of children with asthma, while it was 80% among asthmatic adults.

An immediate hypersensitivity reaction occurring on the nasal mucous membrane leads to sneezing, itchy nose, nasal obstruction, and watery nasal or eye discharge. Ingested allergens may also lead to rhinitis. Rhinitis may be a predominant symptom in coryza and other respiratory viral infections. Edema of the mucosa occurring in rhinitis may lead to obstruction and infection of the paranasal sinuses. Other symptoms include frequent sore throat, hoarseness of voice, persistent mouth breathing in children, recurrent otitis media, halitosis and snoring.

Similar symptoms can be produced by physical irritants such as cold air, dry atmosphere or chemicals such as strong perfumes. This condition is called ***vasomotor rhinitis***.

Treatment: Allergic rhinitis responds to antihistamines, chromones and topical steroids. Vasoconstrictor nasal drops (xylometazoline 0.1%) may also be used, but for not more than 3 days at a stretch. Continued use of nasal drops containing sodium cromoglycate may help to desensitize the nasal mucosa (Table 140.1). Eosinophilia, when present, must also be treated.

Table 140.1: Treatment of allergic rhinitis

Drug	Dose	Route	Frequency
Antihistamines			
Loratadine	5 mg	po	Daily
Desloratadine	10 mg	po	Daily
Cetirizine	10 mg	po	Daily
Sodium cromoglycate	2% solution, metered-dose	Nasal spray po	4–6 hourly
Montelukast	10 mg		Daily
Topical steroids			
Beclomethasone	2 doses of 50 µg	Nasal spray	12 hourly
Budesonide	32 µg		
Fluticasone	50 µg		
Mometasone	50 µg		

Abbreviation: po = per os

Prevention: An attempt must be made to avoid known allergens or agents as far as possible.

EPISTAXIS

Epistaxis is bleeding from the nose. It is derived from the Greek word ***epistazo*** which means ***drip from above***. Usually bleeding occurs from the blood vessels over the anterior part of the nasal septum and anterior nares, areas easily examined by a nasal speculum. Epistaxis may result from local or systemic causes (Box 140.1).

Epistaxis is a frightening symptom. In majority of cases, it is self-limiting.

Box 140.1: Causes of epistaxis

Local causes
Rhinitis, foreign bodies, sinusitis, carcinoma, trauma, rhinosporidiosis, insufflation of drugs (cocaine), prolonged use of nasal sprays
Systemic causes
Infections: Influenza, typhoid, pertussis, malaria and rheumatic fever, snake bite
Other systemic diseases: Hypertension, hemorrhagic disorders and cirrhosis liver with hepatic failure

Treatment: It consists of sedation, rest in bed and packing the nose with gauze soaked in adrenaline solution. Local vasoconstriction arrests the bleeding. If bleeding tends to be recurrent, the bleeding spot must be cauterized. In all cases of epistaxis, look for an underlying systemic disorder. Management of the systemic disorder is very important.

PHARYNGITIS

It is the most common cause of simple *sore throat*. In agranulocytosis and acute leukemia, necrotic ulceration of the tonsils and pharynx may be the presenting symptom. Excessive smoking, noxious fumes, corrosives and unaccustomed spicy foods are common irritants, leading to pharyngitis. It may also be caused by allergy to inhaled or ingested allergens (Table 140.2).

Clinical features: Pharyngitis gives rise to sore throat and dysphagia. The posterior and upper cervical lymph nodes may be enlarged and tender. Redness and edema over the pharynx and adjoining areas may be seen. Pharyngitis may form part of the clinical picture of several systemic infections.

Treatment: Appropriate antimicrobial drugs are indicated in pharyngitis due to bacterial infections. Most cases respond to penicillin. Rest, steam inhalation and analgesics give rapid symptomatic improvement. Throat lozenges containing menthol or eucalyptus oil give considerable relief to the pain and discomfort. Gargles with warm saline or 150 mg soluble aspirin are effective for local symptoms.

ACUTE TONSILLITIS

Inflammation of the tonsils is more common during childhood. However, all age groups can be affected.

Table 140.2: Common microbial causes of acute pharyngitis		
Infective agent	*Disease produced*	*Frequency (%)*
Viruses		
Rhinovirus	Common cold	10
Coronavirus	Common cold	10
Adenovirus	Pharyngoconjunctival fever	5
Herpes simplex	Gingivitis, stomatitis, pharyngitis	4
Parainfluenza	Common cold, croup	1
Bacteria		
Streptococcus pyogenes	Pharyngitis, tonsillitis	15–30
Mixed aerobic infection	Gingivitis, stomatitis (Vincent's angina), peritonsillitis, peritonsillar abscess	1
Neisseria gonorrhoeae	Pharyngitis	1
Candida diphtheriae	Diphtheria	1
Mycoplasma pneumoniae	Pneumonia, tracheobronchitis, pharyngitis	1
Fungi		
Corynebacterium albicans	Thrush	5

Box 140.2: Complications of tonsillitis

- ***Extension of infection due to contiguity:*** Pharyngitis, laryngitis, tracheobronchitis, pneumonia, sinusitis, Eustachian catarrh, suppurative otitis media and secondary septic thrombophlebitis
- ***Systemic spread of infection:*** Septicemia, pyemia
- ***Local complications:*** Chronic tonsillitis, peritonsillar, parapharyngeal or retropharyngeal abscess and obstructive sleep apnea in children
- ***Immunological complications:*** Rheumatic fever and glomerulonephritis

Hemolytic *Streptococcus* of Lancefield group A is the most common agent. Other pathogens causing pharyngitis may affect the tonsils as well. Tonsillitis is more common in poorer socioeconomic groups, where chances for cross infection are high.

Clinical features: Symptoms start with sore throat, pain over region of the tonsils, high fever and dysphagia. Examination of the throat with a tongue depressor reveals enlarged, red tonsils covered with yellowish pus in the crypts on one or both sides. The exudate can be easily removed by a swab and the underlying mucosa does not bleed. Tonsillar and adjoining lymph nodes are moderately enlarged and tender. There is moderate neutrophilic leukocytosis.

Even if untreated, the acute symptoms and the tonsillar inflammation may partially may subside in 7–10 days. In many patients, the streptococci persist within the crypts and give rise to recurrence of symptoms over several years. This is referred to as *chronic tonsillitis*.

Complications: Acute tonsillitis may lead to several complications (Box 140.2).

In India and other neighboring countries, acute streptococcal tonsillitis is the most common cause of rheumatic fever.

Diagnosis: Acute tonsillitis is diagnosed from the characteristic appearance of the tonsils, acute febrile onset, and neutrophilic leukocytosis. Confirmation and isolation of the organism must be attempted by culture of the pus taken before antibiotic therapy. Acute tonsillitis has to be differentiated from faucial diphtheria. In neutropenic states, necrotic ulceration of the throat may also develop.

Treatment: Aspirin relieves the pain and fever. Drug of choice is penicillin. Crystalline penicillin G sodium is given in a dose of 1.0 mega unit every 6 hours intravenously (IV). Erythromycin, ampicillin or cotrimoxazole may be given in appropriate doses as alternate therapies. It is important to administer the full course of treatment and repeat bacteriological study at the end of the course to ensure that organisms are eradicated. Indications for tonsillectomy include recurrent exacerbations of tonsillitis (more than four times in one year), or where chronic tonsillitis is complicated by otitis media.

SINUSITIS

It is the acute, subacute or chronic inflammation of the paranasal sinuses. Maxillary sinusitis is the most common type. The ethmoid, frontal and sphenoid sinuses are affected less frequently.

It is caused by a variety of bacteria such as *Streptococci, Staphylococci, Pneumococci, Haemophilus influen-*

zae and anaerobic bacteria. Viruses such as influenza and parainfluenza virus and less commonly fungi such as *Aspergillus* also may produce sinusitis (Table 140.3).

Anatomical abnormalities interfering with the normal draining mechanisms predispose to infection. Often, the disease starts as an acute respiratory infection (ARI). It may follow dental procedures or swimming in contaminated water. Smoking and second-hand smoke are associated with chronic sinusitis.

Infection reaches the sinuses from the nose, mouth, tonsils, nasopharynx and upper canines or molars. The lining mucosa of the nose and sinuses is inflamed. Obstruction of the opening of the sinus leads to accumulation of secretion, which may get infected. Sinuses may become filled with pus.

Clinical features: Malaise, fever, frontal headache and nasal discharge are the presenting symptoms. In maxillary sinusitis, pain may be felt in the maxillary area of the face.

- Frontal sinusitis causes pain around the eyebrows.
- Ethmoid sinusitis causes pain behind the eyes and frontal headache.
- Sphenoid sinusitis causes pain in the occipital region. Tenderness may be elicited over the sinuses. Pus may be seen pouring from the opening of the affected sinus on speculum examination.
- Chronic sinusitis leads to recurrent headache, which shows a diurnal periodicity. The headache starts in the morning and worsens by mid-day, and subsides by evening. Foul-smelling purulent nasal discharge may occur. Once established, the condition persists for months or even years. Box 140.3 gives the complications.

Diagnosis: History of chronic headache and demonstration of purulent discharge from the nose coupled with tenderness over the sinuses should suggest the clinical diagnosis. Worsening of pain on bending the head forwards helps to differentiate sinusitis from pulpitis. Transillumination of the involved sinus produces a dark shadow while the normal one produces a light shadow. X-ray examination of the paranasal sinuses shows haziness or opacities in the region of the infected sinuses. Computed tomography (CT) scan may be required for confirmation in chronic sinusitis, especially in the case of ethmoid or sphenoid sinuses. Fiber-optic nasal endoscopy makes possible the visual examination of the nasal passages and sinuses. The discharge from the sinus on culture isolates the causative organism. Fungal scrapings and smears as well as fungal cultures are done if a fungal etiology is suspected.

Treatment

Conservative: Viruses cause a significant number of acute sinusitis. Symptomatic measures are sufficient for these cases. Drinking adequate fluids, steam inhalation and judicious use of oxymetazoline nasal drops or sprays give relief by reducing the mucosal edema. Drainage of secretions from the involved sinuses gives symptomatic relief.

Medical: Specific therapy is to administer antibiotics depending on bacteriological results. In the acute stage, one of the newer generation cephalosporins is effective. Combine it with conservative management. Aspirin gives symptomatic relief.

Surgical: Surgery is recommended if relief is inadequate from optimal medications. Functional endoscopic sinus surgery reduces tissue disruption and minimizes postoperative complications. In chronic sinusitis, the pus has to be removed by irrigation and drainage, if conservative measures are inadequate. Caldwell-Luc radical antrostomy for chronic maxillary sinusitis helps those patients who have failed medical and the functional endoscopic approaches.

ACUTE LARYNGITIS

Inflammation of the larynx may result from bacterial or viral infection or inhalation of irritant gases. It often results as a complication of acute coryza. Unaccustomed overuse of the voice leads to edema of the vocal cords. Laryngitis is characterized by hoarseness or loss of voice and pain during attempted speech. Irritant nonproductive cough may be present. In children, acute laryngitis manifests as *croup* secondary to partial obstruction of the small larynx.

Treatment consists of rest to the voice, steam inhalations, avoidance of smoking and administration of analgesics (paracetamol 500 mg, 6 hourly). In many cases, the condition is self-limiting with rest and analgesics. Antibiotics are indicated only if bacterial infection is present. Rarely complications do occur, leading to chronic laryngitis, tracheitis, bronchitis or pneumonia.

CHRONIC LARYNGITIS

It is characterized by hoarseness of voice or aphonia in association with throat irritation and dry cough. This may result from repeated attacks of acute laryngitis, excessive use of voice, tobacco smoking or chronic sinusitis. Laryngoscopy is a must to exclude local tumors or vocal

Table 140.3: Causative organisms in acute maxillary sinusitis

Organism	Frequency (%)
Streptococcus pneumoniae	30
Haemophilus influenzae	25
Anaerobic bacteria	6
Staphylococcus aureus	4
Streptococcus pyogenes	2
Branhamella catarrhalis	2
Gram-negative bacteria	9

Box 140.3: Complications of sinusitis

- *Maxillary sinus:* Osteomyelitis
- *Intracranial infection:* Meningitis, thrombophlebitis of the intracranial veins, thrombosis of the cavernous sinus and sagittal sinus, extradural abscesses
- *Infection of the eye socket:* Orbital cellulitis
- *Infection of ethmoid sinus:* Third nerve palsy
- *Frontal sinus:* Osteomyelitis of the frontal bone and edema over the region (*Pott's puffy tumor*)
- *Respiratory tract:* Aspiration of pus into the respiratory tract leading to recurrent bronchitis, aspiration pneumonia, bronchiectasis, and lung abscess

cord palsy. ***Treatment*** consists of absolute voice rest, abstinence from smoking and use of steam inhalations.

LARYNGEAL PARALYSIS

Paralysis of the vocal cords may be organic or functional. The abductors and adductors are supplied by the recurrent laryngeal nerves (RLNs), which are branches of the vagus nerves. In organic paralysis, the abductors, tensors and adductors are affected in the order of sequence. The completely paralyzed vocal cord lies immobile midway between abduction and adduction ***(cadaveric position)***. Abductor paralysis is always organic in nature and it may be unilateral or bilateral. On the other hand, pure adductor paralysis is always bilateral and it is functional in nature. This is frequently seen in hysteria.

Causes of organic laryngeal paralysis: Involvement of the left RLN is common in mediastinal tumors, aortic aneurysm and enlargement of the left atrium occurring in mitral stenosis. One or other of the RLNs may be affected in the neck by enlargement of the cervical lymph nodes, goiter or other surgical causes (Box 140.4).

Paralysis of the vagus may occur in infective polyneuritis, fractures of the base of the skull, space occupying lesions in the posterior fossa, or diphtheria.

Vagal nuclei are affected in brainstem lesions. These include basilar artery insufficiency, bulbar poliomyelitis, motor neuron disease, syringobulbia and tumors.

Clinical features: Usual symptoms are hoarseness of voice, cough, dyspnea and alteration in the quality of the cough. Vocal fatigue, reduced vocal volume, and pain in throat when speaking are other symptoms. Aspiration of liquids with its complications may be seen in some. Organic paralysis is accompanied by cough, whereas hysterical paralysis is not. In bilateral abductor paralysis, the cough loses its explosive phase ***(bovine cough)***. In unilateral vocal cord paralysis, the hoarseness and loss of voice may disappear with time, since the opposite vocal cord crosses the midline and restores the vocal aperture. Laryngeal paralysis is confirmed by laryngoscopy.

Treatment of the cause of laryngeal paralysis must be instituted wherever possible. Otherwise management is symptomatic. Bilateral abductor paralysis results in obstruction of glottis and it is fatal if the airway is not established by tracheostomy or intubation. Surgery to medialize the vocal cords in severe voice weakness is being attempted at some centers. Persons with laryngeal paralysis should avoid swimming as they cannot hold breath and, therefore, they run the risk of drowning.

Box 140.4: Causes of vocal cord paralysis

- ***Vagus nucleus:*** Brainstem lesions, cerebrovascular disease, bulbar poliomyelitis, motoneurone disease, syringobulbia
- ***Vagus nerve:*** Infective polyneuritis, skull-base lesions, posterior fossa lesions
- ***Other neurological diseases:*** Parkinson's disease, multiple sclerosis, myasthenia gravis
- ***Neoplasms:*** Benign/malignant neoplasms around the vocal cords; mediastinal tumors involving recurrent laryngeal nerve
- ***Trauma:*** Larynx, vocal cords, or their nerve supply involved by trauma or surgery/intubation for anesthesia
- ***Inflammation:*** Local inflammation or scarring of larynx/cords

---

OBSTRUCTION TO THE RESPIRATORY TRACT

Acute Laryngeal Obstruction

Acute laryngeal obstruction may present as a life-threatening emergency. Foreign bodies may get impacted in the larynx. This may include dentures or large chunks of meat. Obstruction by bolus of food is more common under alcohol intoxication. This is called ***cafe coronary*** (Box 140.5).

Clinical features: Stridor, aphonia and dyspnea are the hallmarks of laryngeal obstruction. Acute obstruction in children leads to cyanosis and inspiratory indrawing of the trachea. The movement of a foreign body within the larynx may be palpable during respiratory efforts. When obstruction due to large bolus of food occurs at the table, the victim becomes anxious, restless and cyanosed. He tries to cry, but the voice is lost. If the obstruction is not relieved immediately, he falls unconscious and death may occur within minutes.

Diagnosis: Acute laryngeal obstruction should be suspected when an otherwise healthy individual suddenly becomes choked and cyanotic with loss of voice.

Management: First-aid consists of the removal of the foreign body manually or with a pair of tongs. The impacted foreign body can be dislodged by a sudden forcible thud on the chest with the head lowered.

Heimlich maneuver: This effective method is to be learnt by all first-aid teams. The patient is hugged from behind with the rescuer's hands crossing each other over the patient's epigastria and the chest is compressed suddenly. This helps in dislodging the obstruction (Fig. 140.1).

Box 140.5: Causes of laryngeal obstruction

- Foreign body
- Inflammatory or allergic edema (including angioneurotic edema due to food, irritant fumes, corrosives or insect stings)
- Acute laryngitis and epiglottitis (especially in infants)
- Exudates
- Laryngeal muscle spasm
- Inhaled blood clot/vomitus in the unconscious
- Tumors: Chronic progressive obstruction—especially carcinoma
- Bilateral vocal cord paralysis

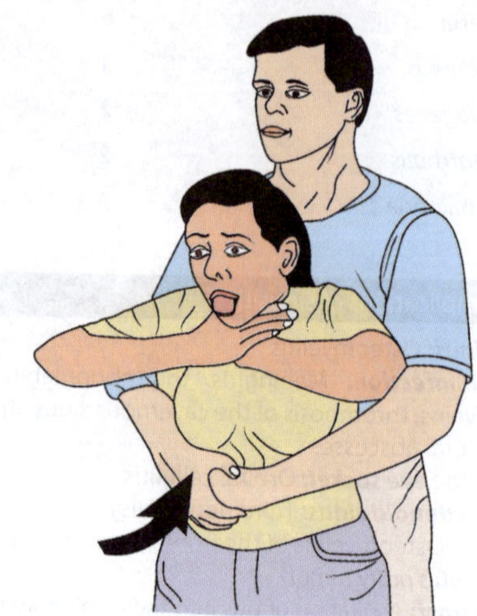

Fig. 140.1: Heimlich maneuver. Application of sudden pressure over the abdominothoracic region may dislodge the laryngeal foreign body

If the above attempt fails, the airway should be made patent by tracheostomy or by inserting a few large-bore hypodermic needles into the trachea. The patient is transported to hospital for further management.

Management of chronic obstruction depends upon the cause.

Tracheal Obstruction

Total tracheal obstruction is rare but may be caused by a foreign body. More often, it is partial and is caused by external pressure due to mediastinal masses, goiter, mediastinitis, mediastinal fibrosis or aortic arch aneurysm. New growths, especially adenomas or polyps arising from the wall cause intermittent obstruction.

Tracheal obstruction leads to stridor, viz. noisy breathing with a harsh crowing sound mainly during inspiration and dyspnea. In the case of pedunculated growths, the obstruction may be postural. Tracheal obstruction has to be distinguished from asthma and other causes of dyspnea.

Treatment is surgical, after confirmation by bronchoscopy and computed tomography scan.

Bronchial Obstruction

It can occur in the larger bronchi or in the bronchioles and may be acute or chronic. The clinical manifestations vary accordingly. *Acute obstruction* is mostly intraluminal. It may be caused by aspiration of vomitus, blood, pus, mucus plugs, foreign bodies, or edema and exudates from the inflamed bronchial wall itself. *Chronic obstruction* is due to extraneous pressure from glands or intraluminal adenoma or bronchogenic carcinoma. Bronchial obstruction leads to collapse of the lung with subsequent infection of the distal parenchyma, bronchiectasis and fibrosis.

Treatment: Put the patient with head low so as to drain any fluid that may be present. Gentle tapping on the chest helps drainage. Aspiration of the tracheobronchial tree is needed, if secretions are copious.

Endoscopic examination with removal of the obstruction should be done without delay. Surgery may be required if the condition does not clear with endoscopic aspiration.

CHAPTER
141

Pneumonias

C Sudheendra Ghosh, CP Murali

Chapter Summary

- General Considerations
- Other Organisms Causing Pneumonia
  - Staphylococcal Pneumonia
- Klebsiella Pneumonia
- Mycoplasma Pneumonia
- Aspiration Pneumonia
- General Guidelines to Start Initial Antibiotic Regimens
- Hypostatic Pneumonia
- Bronchopneumonia
- Prognostic factors in Pneumonia

GENERAL CONSIDERATIONS

Pneumonia is the sixth leading cause of death in the world today. It is also the major cause of death from infectious diseases. The mortality resulting from severe pneumonia varies from 20 to 40%. Mortality is more common among the elderly and patients with comorbidities like diabetes mellitus (DM), chronic obstructive pulmonary diseases (COPD), congestive heart failure (CHF), coronary artery disease (CAD), interstitial lung disease (ILD) and carcinoma. Depending on the severity of the disease, the average cost of treatment varies from small to very large amounts (*See* also Ch 37 Pneumococcal Infection).

Inflammation of the lung is called *pneumonia*. Depending upon the circumstances of onset of the case, several terms have been employed for practical management.

Clinical setting in which the infection occurs (if no pathogen can be isolated).

- Community-acquired acute pneumonia
- Community-acquired atypical pneumonia
- Nosocomial pneumonia or hospital-acquired pneumonia
- Pneumonia in immunocompromised host
- Healthcare-associated pneumonia.

Community-acquired acute pneumonia (CAP): It is defined as an infection that begins outside of the hospital or is diagnosed within 48 hours after admission to the hospital in a patient who has not resided in a long-term facility for 14 days or more before the onset of symptoms. Up to 20% of patients with CAP require hospitalization (Figs 141.1 to 141.3).

Hospital-acquired pneumonia (HAP): It is defined as infection of lung parenchyma occurring more than 48 hours after admission to a hospital. When HAP occurs in a subset of patients receiving mechanical ventilation, it is termed *ventilator-associated pneumonia (VAP)*. VAP usually occurs at 48–72 hours following intubation.

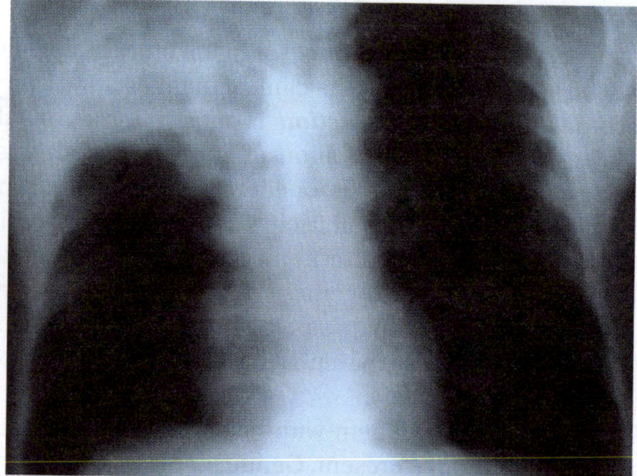

Fig. 141.1: Chest X-ray showing lobar pneumonia. ***Note:*** The consolidation of the upper zone right lung uniform opacity with clear-cut margins, midline structures not shifted

Fig. 141.2: High-resolution CT (HRCT) pneumococcal pneumonia. ***Note:*** The CT= Computed tomography dense consolidation and air spaces in between

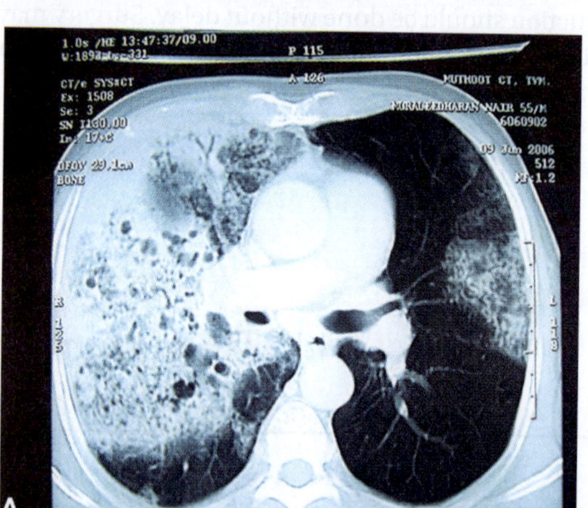

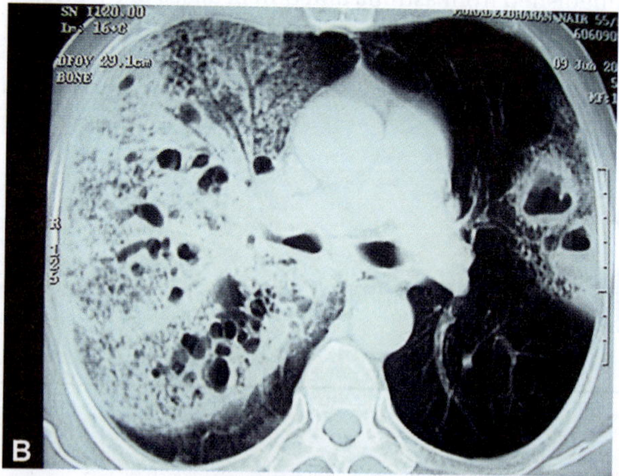

Figs 141.3A and B: Double pneumonia HRCT: **A.** Massive pneumonia right and smaller lesions left; **B.** Cavitation (abscess formation)

Healthcare-associated pneumonia (HCAP): It is defined as pneumonia following admission to an acute care hospital during the previous 90 days or residence in a long-term care facility or recent intravenous (IV) antibiotic therapy.

HAP is a common nosocomial infection with a rate between 5 and 10 cases per 1,000 hospital admissions. The incidence in patients who require mechanical ventilation is 6–20 times higher. It is the leading cause of death from hospital-acquired infections.

Pneumonia may be caused by specific pathogens like *Pneumococcus* or *Klebsiella* or by mixed flora which reach the lungs due to aspiration of infected material from the upper respiratory passages, stomach or exterior (Table 141.1). The latter group is called aspiration pneumonia.

Till a decade ago, invariably the organism causing pneumonia sporadically in the community used to be pneumococcus. There has been a change in the pattern of causative organisms more recently. Due to the increase in number of immunosuppressed individuals in the community and more opportunities for cross infection between hospitalized patients and their home contacts, the microbial pattern has changed even for CAP.

Table 141.1: Causes of community-acquired pneumonia	
Organism	**Frequency (%) (in young adults)**
Pneumococcal	50–80
Aerobic Gram-negative bacilli	3–11
Klebsiella pneumonia	2–6
Staphylococcus aureus	1–10
Mixed anaerobes	2–12
Mycoplasma pneumonia	3–44
Haemophilus influenzae	2.5–15
Viral-influenza A and B, parainfluenza, adenovirus,	1–16
Streptococcus pyogenes	1

Note: Pneumococcal pneumonia is described in Section 6, Ch 37.

OTHER ORGANISMS CAUSING PNEUMONIA

Staphylococcal Pneumonia

This is more frequently seen in debilitated subjects and in hospitalized patients. Respiratory viral infections predispose to staphylococcal pneumonia. This is a dreaded complication in children with cystic fibrosis and in patients receiving immunosuppression therapy. The organisms reach the lung through the bloodstream (pyemia) or along the respiratory passages leading to pulmonary sepsis.

Clinical Features

The onset is with mild symptoms, but soon the condition worsens to produce grave toxemia, purulent and blood stained sputum and cyanosis. The lesions are generally multiple, giving rise to thin-walled abscesses. It may frequently spread to the pleura to produce empyema or pneumothorax. Signs of lobar consolidation may not be evident. Diagnosis should be suspected from the clinical setting and presence of toxemia far out of proportion to the pulmonary signs. Gram staining of sputum and culture reveals the organisms. Mortality varies from 20 to 25%.

Treatment

At present, most strains of hospital-acquired staphylococci produce penicillinase. Hence penicillinase-resistant drugs such as cephalothin, cloxacillin or vancomycin may be necessary.

- Cloxacillin   0.25–0.5g oral, intramuscular (IM) or IV 6 hourly
- Cephalothin   2 g IV 6 hourly
- Vancomycin   0.5 g IV 6 hourly
- Nafcillin   1–1.5 g IV 6 hourly

Early diagnosis and prompt treatment ensures cure.

Klebsiella Pneumonia

Syn: Friedlander's pneumonia

This is a grave illness seen in patients above the age of 40 years. Debilitating diseases, alcoholism and malnutrition predispose this condition. Common site of involvement is the posterior segment of the upper lobe. The right lung is involved more frequently. The condition sets in with sudden chills, rigors, fever, dyspnea and cough with gelatinous thick sputum streaked with blood. The course may be subacute or fulminant and fatal. Abscess formation is a common complication (Fig. 141.4). Mortality is high, ranging around 30%.

Treatment

Once the condition is suspected, urgent treatment with cephalexin 1–4 g per day 6 hour IM should be started. Gentamicin in a dose of 5–8 mg/kg may be added as a second antibiotic. Treatment may have to be continued for 2 weeks or more to ensure cure.

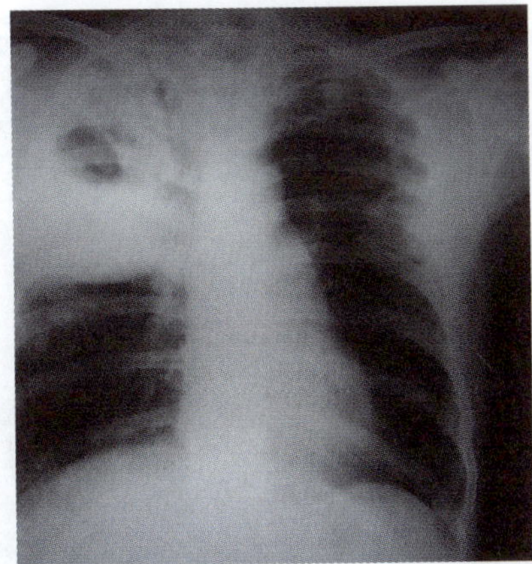

Fig. 141.4: Klebsiella pneumonia chest X-ray showing lobar consolidation with abscess formation right and pneumonitis left. **Note:** The bulging fissure

Mycoplasma Pneumonia

Syn: Primary atypical pneumonia, Eaton agent pneumonia, Cold-agglutinin-positive pneumonia

This is caused by *Mycoplasma pneumoniae* which is a bacterium devoid of cell wall. It spreads in closed communities and in families through the respiratory secretions. Clinically, it maybe present as—tracheobronchitis or pneumonia (in 30%). The disease starts insidiously with lassitude, headache, myalgia and chest pain. Expectoration is scanty. Hemoptysis may occur. Physical examination of the chest may reveal only minimal findings. The skiagram shows extensive lesions, not made out clinically. Over 50% of patients develop cold agglutinins in their serum in a dilution of 1:32 or more by the second week. These nonspecific antibodies agglutinate human O group erythrocytes at 4°C. These antibodies may be present for long periods. Complement fixation tests help to demonstrate specific antibodies. Tetracycline and erythromycin are effective against this organism.

Haemophilus influenzae pneumonia occurs principally in patients with underlying chest diseases such as chronic bronchitis emphysema syndrome, bronchiectasis and others. The organisms show resistance to aminopenicillins. Combination with co-amoxiclav is effective. Pneumonitis is a part of the general picture of infections by *Chlamydia*, rickettsiae, several viruses including acquired immune deficiency syndrome (AIDS) and systemic fungal infections.

Aspiration Pneumonia (Nonspecific Pneumonia)

Infective material may be aspirated into the trachea and bronchi.

Causes

- Conditions which suppress the cough reflex, e.g. coma, alcoholic intoxication, general anesthesia.
- Spill over of pus or gastric contents into the respiratory tract, e.g. sinusitis, tonsillitis, achalasia cardia, pharyngeal paralysis, tracheoesophageal fistula.
- Violent contraction of abdominal muscles forcing gastric contents into the respiratory tract, e.g. epilepsy, tetanus.
- Aspiration from outside, e.g. drowning.

The microbial flora is mixed, depending on the source of infection. The pulmonary lesion may be a localized massive pneumonia or a bronchopneumonia.

Clinical Features

Aspiration of large volumes presents as pulmonary collapse or as pneumonia. In the presence of any of the predisposing factors, aspiration pneumonia should be suspected. Right lower lobe is more often affected because of the disposition of its bronchus. The upper lobe is also not infrequently involved in alcoholics and comatose subjects. If the obstruction is not removed by coughing or by other means, the consolidation tends to persist and proceed to lung abscess so that, it may also tends to recur aspiration pneumonia, if primary cause is not removed.

Treatment

The general principles of treatment of pneumonia are applicable. In addition, prompt attention should be given to clear the respiratory passages of obstructing material. This can be achieved by postural drainage, physiotherapy to the chest to encourage coughing, suction using a mechanical sucker, or by bronchoscopic aspiration.

GENERAL GUIDELINES TO START INITIAL ANTIBIOTIC REGIMENS

Empirical selection of antimicrobial agents for treating patients with community-acquired acute pneumonia (CAP) is recommended as follows:

Outpatients: Generally, preferred antimicrobial drugs are (not in any particular order) doxycycline, macrolides, or fluoroquinolones. Judicious use of fluoroquinolones is to be recommended as indiscriminate use may lead to development of drug-resistance in tuberculosis.

Selection considerations: These agents have activity against the most likely pathogens in this setting, which include *Streptococcus pneumoniae*, *Mycoplasma pneumoniae* and *Chlamydia pneumoniae*. Selection should be influenced by regional antibiotic susceptibility patterns for *S. pneumoniae* and the presence of other risk factors for drug-resistant *S. pneumoniae*. Penicillin-resistant pneumococci may be resistant to macrolides and/or doxycycline.

For older patients or those with underlying disease, a fluoroquinolone may be a preferred choice; some authorities prefer to reserve fluoroquinolones for such patients. For hospitalized patients, an extended spectrum cephalosporin combined with a macrolide or a β-lactam/β-lactamase inhibitor combined with a macrolide or a fluoroquinolone (alone) is generally preferred.

For intensive care unit (ICU), an extended-spectrum cephalosporin or β-lactam/β-lactamase inhibitor plus either fluoroquinolone/macrolide is generally more effective. In patients with structural lung disease, the preferred choice includes antipseudomonal agents (piperacillin, piperacillin-tazobactam, carbapenem, or cefepime) plus a fluoroquinolone (including high-dose ciprofloxacin). In patients allergic to β-lactam, the preferred agents include fluoroquinolone or clindamycin. For suspected aspiration pneumonia, fluoroquinolone with clindamycin or metronidazole are the drugs of choices.

HYPOSTATIC PNEUMONIA

This is seen in elderly debilitated persons who are bedridden. It is a form of aspiration pneumonia. Inadequate cough reflex, excessive respiratory secretions and pulmonary congestion favor the development of hypostatic pneumonia. Microbial flora is derived from the upper respiratory secretions. The lesion is a bronchopneumonia. Hypostatic pneumonia acts as a preterminal event in many elderly debilitated individuals. Avoidance of prolonged recumbency, frequent change of posture (once in 2 hours) in comatose and debilitated subjects and regular breathing exercises help to prevent this condition.

BRONCHOPNEUMONIA

Syn: Acute lobular pneumonia, Diffuse pneumonia

Inflammation of the bronchial wall and pulmonary parenchyma is the essential lesion in bronchopneumonia. This leads to patchy consolidation of the lung. The disease is more common during infancy and old age.

Causes

It may occur as a complication of several diseases such as whooping cough, measles and other viral infections in children. Chronic bronchitis, emphysema and viral infections of the respiratory tract may be complicated by bronchopneumonia. Rarely bronchopneumonia may occur as the primary lesion.

Pathology

The common organisms are *Staphylococci*, *Streptococci*, *Pneumococci* and *H. influenzae*. Rarely rickettsiae, viruses and fungi may cause bronchopneumonia. The inflammatory lesions are widespread and patchy over both lungs, more in the lower lobes. The terminal bronchioles are affected initially and the alveoli are involved secondarily. There is collapse and consolidation in the affected lobule. Confluence of lesions may give rise to larger areas of consolidation. The exudate shows neutrophils and fibrin. Interstitial edema develops. There is compensatory emphysema around the collapsed alveoli.

Clinical Features

The extent of pulmonary involvement and virulence of the infective agent determine the clinical picture. Generally, the onset is insidious. In the majority of cases, bronchopneumonia follows the primary illness after a period of apparent improvement. The temperature goes up and tachypnea, and cough may develop. The child may be cyanosed. Unlike, as in lobar pneumonia, pleural involvement and herpes labialis are rare. Physical examination of the chest reveals widespread rales. Signs of extensive consolidation are rare. X-ray shows bilateral irregular and patchy shadows, more in the lower zones (Fig. 141.5 and Table 141.2). Pneumonia severity scores like pneumonia severity index (PSI), CURB-65 and patient outcomes research team (PORT) are helpful in patient assessment and guiding management.

Rarely bronchopneumonia may lead to bronchiectasis, pulmonary fibrosis, lung abscess or empyema. Mortality is higher in patients with chronic respiratory or cardiovascular disease (CVD).

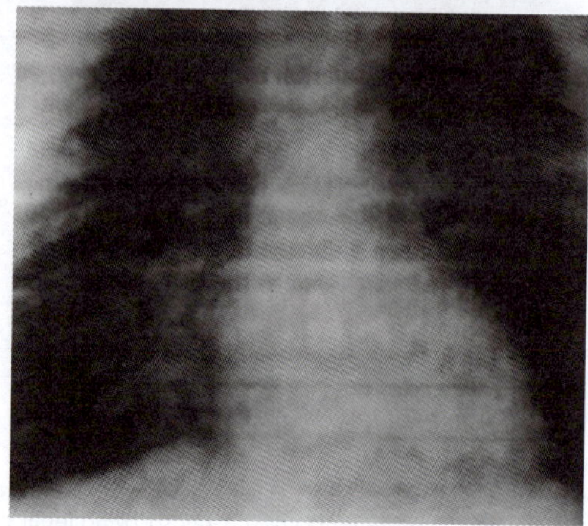

Fig. 141.5: Chest X-ray bronchopneumonia. **Note:** The patchy opacities with indistinct margins

Table 141.2: Relationship between chest X-ray (CXR) patterns and possible pathogens

CXR patterns	Possible pathogens
Lobar	*Streptococcus pneumoniae, Klebsiella pneumoniae, Haemophilus influenzae*, Gram-negative
Patchy	Atypicals, viral, *Legionella*
Interstitial	Viral, *Pneumocystis carinii* pneumonia (PCP), *Legionella*
Cavitatory	Anaerobes, *Klebsiella*, tuberculosis, *Staphylococcus aureus*, fungi
Large effusion	*Staphylococcus*, anaerobes, *Klebsiella*

Box 141.1: CURB-65 rule

- Confusion: New mental confusion
- Urea > 7 mmol/L
- Respiratory rate > 30 breaths per minute
- Blood pressure (BP): Diastolic BP < 60 mm Hg or systolic BP < 90 mm Hg
- Age ≥ 65 years of age

Note: Score 1 point for each feature.
- Group 1: 0 or 1 of the above; mortality low—1.5 %. Likely suitable for treatment at home
- Group 2: 2 of the above; mortality—9.2 %. Hospitalization for treatment
- Group 3: 3 or more of the above; mortality—22 %. Likely requires admission to ICU

Treatment

Prompt use of the appropriate antibiotic brings down the fever and helps in resolution of the lesions. In children suffering from measles and other viral infections, occurrence of bronchopneumonia should be anticipated and early therapy started. In underdeveloped communities, respiratory infections lead to severe setback in the growth and development of children and also predispose to prolonged morbidity and malnutrition.

PROGNOSTIC FACTORS IN PNEUMONIA

Prognostic factors in pneumonia are given by the CURB-65 rule which is given in (Box 141.1).

CHAPTER
142

Lung Abscess and Pleuropulmonary Amebiasis

C Sudheendra Ghosh, Davis Paul

Chapter Summary
- Lung Abscess
- Pleuropulmonary Amebiasis

LUNG ABSCESS

It is suppurative necrosis of lung parenchyma caused by a microbial organism resulting in cavitation with a fluid level. Tuberculosis and cystic cavities, though secondarily infected by pyogenic organisms, are not usually included under this term.

Causes

- ***Aspiration pneumonia:*** Aspiration of gastric contents or materials from the upper respiratory tract occurs during coma, anesthesia or deep sleep
- Other types of pneumonias
- Systemic pyemia
- Secondary infection of pulmonary infarcts
- Postobstructive, e.g. bronchogenic carcinoma, foreign body
- Spread of amebic liver abscess and primary pulmonary amebiasis
- Bronchial obstruction leads to collapse, infection and abscess formation distally.
  Impairment of cough due to painful conditions in the chest or during postoperative period and conditions which impair ciliary function (heavy smoking or bronchitis)

predispose to abscess formation. Right lower lobe is a common site for aspiration and suppuration. In the supine comatose patient, the posterior segment of the right upper lobe and apical segment of the right lower lobe being the most dependent parts suffer more frequently. Next in frequency, corresponding segments are on the left.

Factors Predisposing to Lung Abscess

- ***Aspiration of material occurring in dental sepsis:*** Depressed consciousness, alcoholic bouts, epilepsy, head injury, coma, disturbances of swallowing, esophageal stricture, bulbar palsy, achalasia cardia, and pharyngeal pouch.
- Necrotizing pneumonias
- Hematogenous spread
- ***Pre-existing lung disease:*** Bronchiectasis, cystic disease, bronchial obstruction
- Immunodeficiency.

Pathology

Suppuration and necrosis of lung tissue constitute the basic pathological process. The abscess is lined by granulation tissue which limits the spread of infection. Common organisms are those derived from the upper respiratory tract and mouth. These include ***aerobic*** and ***anaerobic organisms***. Most common anaerobes are *Peptostreptococcus, Bacteroides, Fusobacterium* and *Microaerophilic streptococci*. The aerobic bacteria that frequently cause lung abscess are *Staphylococci, Streptococcus pyogenes, Klebsiella* and *Pseudomonas aeruginosa.* Less commonly *Escherichia coli, Clostridia* and *B. Proteus* may be present. When the abscess ruptures into a bronchus, pus is expectorated. The cavity contains pus and air. The wall is thick and ragged compared to tuberculous cavity or cyst. Chronic abscesses may be multiloculated. When the contents are discharged, healing occurs by fibrosis.

Clinical Features

Early symptoms are those of pneumonia with fever, cough, rigor, malaise and pleuritic chest pain. Initially cough may be unproductive. Hemoptysis is not uncommon. When the abscess ruptures into a bronchus, the cough become postural. The sputum is large in volume (300–500 mL/day), purulent, bloodstained and foul-smelling. Systemic symptoms depend on the virulence of the organisms and general condition of the patient. In a moderately severe case, the patient is febrile, toxic and dyspneic. Painful clubbing of fingers and toes develops in a few weeks.

Physical examination may reveal presence of consolidation due to the surrounding of pneumonic process. Pleural rub may be heard. Once the abscess opens into a bronchus, the auscultatory signs of cavitation are found. The breath sounds are cavernous and coarse. Post-tussive crepitations are heard.

Laboratory Findings

Neutrophil leukocytosis is present in most cases.

Sputum: Once the abscess starts discharging pus, the sputum is large in volume, purulent, foul-smelling and bloodstained. On allowing it to stand in a conical glass, the sputum settles into the three typical layers (froth above, serous portion in the middle and thick nummular particles below). The organisms can be identified by Gram-staining and culture. Blood culture may help in identifying the organism in some patients.

Chest X-ray reveals consolidation with clearance in its center. A partially drained abscess is seen as a cavity containing fluid and air. Both posteroanterior and lateral views are necessary to locate the abscess (Figs 142.1 and 142.2).

High-resolution computed tomography (HRCT) gives better details about the abscess as well as the surrounding pulmonary parenchyma (Fig. 142.3).

Diagnosis

Clinical diagnosis is made from the history, physical signs of consolidation and cavitation and the presence of copious amounts of purulent sputum. Chest X-ray confirms the diagnosis in almost all cases. Location of the abscess can be made by taking the lateral view skiagram as well. Microbial flora can be determined by sputum examination and microbiological tests. In vast majority of cases, these are sufficient to institute treatment and follow-up the case to recovery.

Bronchoscopy is indicated, if there is likelihood of bronchial obstruction and malignancy or doubt about the etiology. Bronchoscopy will help to remove obstruction, drain the pus, collect the secretions for microbiological studies and also for biopsy.

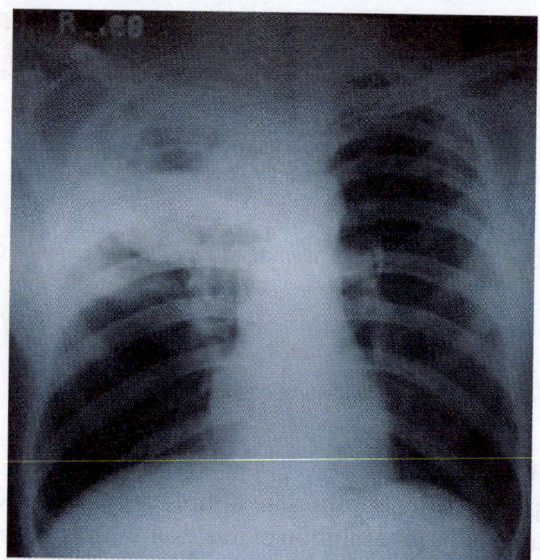

Fig. 142.1: Pyogenic abscess. Chest X-ray lung abscess right upper zone. *Note:* The abscess cavity containing air and fluid

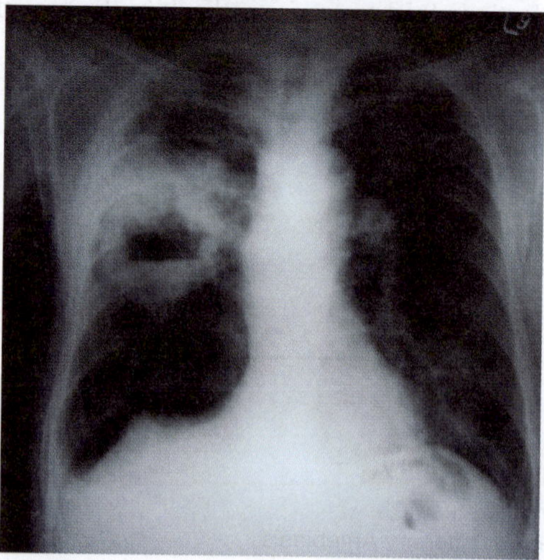

Fig. 142.2: Chest X-ray tuberculosis abscess with secondary infection

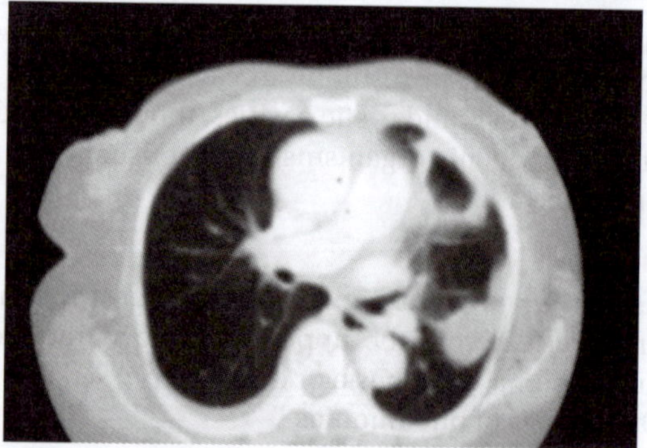

Fig. 142.3: High-resolution computed tomography (HRCT) pulmonary abscess left upper lobe. *Note:* The abscess cavity with the area of consolidation around

Further investigations such as computed tomography (CT) scan or magnetic resonance imaging (MRI) will be required in a few cases which do not run true to type.

Complications

Pulmonary complications: (1) Severe hemoptysis; (2) extension to other parts of the lung and to the other side;

(3) pleurisy, empyema and pneumothorax; and (4) local fibrosis and bronchiectatic changes.

Extrapulmonary complications: Brain abscess may develop due to metastases of septic emboli from the lung which reach the cerebral circulation through the vertebral system of the veins (Batson's system).

Other complications include pulmonary osteoarthropathy, emaciation and cachexia due to loss of large amounts of proteins (in the form of purulent sputum) and infection. If left untreated, lung abscess proves fatal.

Differential Diagnosis

Lung abscess has to be differentiated from bronchiectasis, bronchogenic carcinoma, pulmonary tuberculosis, fungal infection, pulmonary cysts and secondary neoplasms. Bronchiectasis is more chronic and usually bilateral. A cavitating bronchogenic carcinoma may resemble an abscess clinically and radiologically. Carcinoma is more common in smokers. The sputum is seldom profuse or purulent. It is more often bloodstained with necrotic tissue being expectorated at times. Presence of hilar lymphadenopathy is suggestive of carcinoma. In cavitary pulmonary tuberculosis, the sputum is mucoid and often not foul-smelling. Digital clubbing is less common. Tuberculosis affects the upper lobes more often, whereas abscess usually occupies the lower lobes. X-ray reveals thin-walled cavities, without free fluid level.

In endemic areas, lung abscesses should be investigated for fungal pathogens by sputum tests and immunological studies. Cystic disease of the lung is often bilateral and present from early life. Radiologically, the cysts appear thin-walled. Rarely, cysts may be solitary. Digital clubbing is less marked in cystic disease of the lung. Fibrocystic disease of the pancreas may present with severe infection of the cystic spaces mimicking multiple abscess.

Treatment

Principles of therapy include antimicrobial drugs, drainage of the abscess cavity and surgery in intractable cases.

Antibiotics

A properly collected sputum uncontaminated by oropharyngeal microbes should be sent for culture and sensitivity studies and antibacterial drugs should be given in appropriate dosage till radiological clearance is complete. In most of the cases, recovery is full in 4–6 weeks. Treatment of choice in anaerobic infection is clindamycin 600 mg intravenous (IV) 8th hourly initially followed by oral clindamycin 150–300 mg three to four times daily. Injection crystalline penicillin and metronidazole are the other alternate drugs commonly used. Drainage of the abscess is achieved by ***postural drainage*** and gentle tapotement over the chest. Respiratory physiotherapy to stimulate cough and help expectoration is instituted early. If clearance of the abscess is unsatisfactory, bronchoscopic aspiration may help. With proper medical treatment, majority get cure.

Surgery

It is indicated in circumstances such as failure of medical treatment, residual fibrosis with bronchiectatic changes, suspicion of bronchogenic carcinoma, severe hemoptysis and pleural suppuration. If a reasonable course of medical treatment fails to bring about recovery, surgical resection of the abscess should be considered without undue delay. Risks of surgery are greater if the general condition of the patient has deteriorated.

Prevention

Lung abscess is a largely preventable disease by preventing aspiration pneumonia. Other measures include prompt removal of bronchial obstruction, complete treatment of pneumonia and early diagnosis of pulmonary suppuration.

PLEUROPULMONARY AMEBIASIS

(*See* Section 6, Ch 65)

Involvement of pleura and lung used to be common complications of amebic liver abscess. With the reduction of amebiasis in the community, this condition is much less commonly encountered at present, especially in Kerala. Though primary metastatic infection of the lung can occur rarely, in over 90% of cases, the infection is transdiaphragmatic. Direct spread from liver through transdiaphragmatic lymphatics results in pleural and pulmonary amebiasis. The common lesions are mild pleurisy, pleural effusion, empyema, consolidation, abscess formation, bronchopleural fistula and rarely bronchobiliary fistula. The empyema shows a tendency for encystment.

Clinical Features

It is commonly seen in the age group of 20–40 years and is more common in men, invariably in alcoholics. The initial symptomatology is that of liver abscess with fever, chills and pain over the right hypochondrium. The liver is enlarged, acutely tender and there is intercostal tenderness. Bulging and edema of the chest wall are also occasionally seen. Pleural and pulmonary involvement are accompanied by pleuritic pain, dyspnea, chocolate-colored sputum and hemoptysis. When there is a bronchobiliary fistula, the sputum is bile-stained. Examination of the chest reveals signs of pleural effusion or consolidation depending on the lesion.

Diagnosis

The diagnosis should be suspected in right lower lobe lesions and right-sided pleural effusions. Liver enlargement is present in most cases. Trophozoites of *Entamoeba histolytica* can be demonstrated in 20% of cases in the sputum or pleural fluid. X-ray shows elevated right hemidiaphragm with pleural effusion or pulmonary consolidation or abscess formation. Ultrasound examination is most helpful to reveal the abscess in the liver and other lesions in the abdomen. CT scan will reveal the lesion accurately.

Treatment

The condition responds to medical therapy which should be instituted early. Systemic therapy with metronidazole 400 mg three times a day for 10 days orally and chloroquine 500 mg bd for 2 days and thereafter 250 mg bd for 19 days helps to localize the lesion and full resolution in mild or even moderate cases. In severe cases, metronidazole can be given as IV drip 500 mg bd till the acute condition subsides. Presence of secondary infection can be confirmed by examination of the aspirated pus. It has to be treated with appropriate antibiotics.

In many cases, medical treatment suffices to clear the lesions. In moderate and large collections of pus with presence of high fever and toxemia, suggestive of secondary infection, early aspiration of the liver abscess and pleura are indicated.

CHAPTER

143

Allergic Disorders of the Lung

KE Rajan

Chapter Summary

- Bronchial Asthma
  - Pathology
  - Clinical Features
  - Diagnosis
  - Treatment
- Acute Severe Asthma
  - Prevention of Recurrence
- Extrinsic Allergic Alveolitis
- Tropical Pulmonary Eosinophilia
- Allergic Bronchopulmonary Aspergillosis

BRONCHIAL ASTHMA

The term *asthma* in Greek means *breathless* or *breathe with open mouth*. Asthma ranks amongst the most common chronic ailments of the globe. It is estimated that 300 million people worldwide suffer from asthma. Annually, 250,000 deaths are attributed to asthma, and its complications. Indian Council of Medical Research (ICMR) established the prevalence of adult bronchial asthma to be 2.38%. In our country, the disease is under-recognized and undertreated. The World Health Organization (WHO) estimates that asthma contributes to the loss of 15 million disability-adjusted life years (DALY).

Global Initiative for Asthma

Asthma is currently defined by reversible airflow obstruction, airway hyper-reactivity and airway inflammation. It is a common chronic inflammatory condition of the airways. Epidemiological studies suggest that multiple genetic and environmental factors contribute to the causation of asthma, a clinical condition that is viewed as a cluster of related disorders. Many cells and cellular elements play a role in its genesis. It may be defined as 'chronic inflammation of airways, associated with airway hyper-responsiveness that may leads to recurrent episodes of wheezing, breathlessness, chest tightness and coughing. There is a widespread, variable and often reversible airflow limitation'.

There is a strong genetic component as more than 100 genes have been implicated in asthma susceptibility and pathogenesis. Genetic factors which may contribute to the variability with regard to age of onset, sensitivity of environmental causes, and response to treatment. Chromosome 17q21 is considered to be of importance as asthma susceptibility locus. One study has identified a metalloprotein, ADAM-33 that may have a role in inflammatory response to smooth muscle hypertrophy or hypersensitivity.

Airway inflammation is associated with airway hyper-responsiveness, reversible airflow limitation, and respiratory symptoms. Airway inflammation leads to limitation of airflow by acute bronchoconstriction, edema of the airway wall, formation of mucus plugs, and airway remodeling. The characteristics are widely variable and unpredictable.

Interleukin-5 (IL-5) produces eosinophilic inflammation resulting in eosinophilia in sputum. Mepolizumab (an IL-5 antagonist monoclonal antibody) reduces the number of eosinophils in tissues, blood and sputum, and hence used in therapy of such cases.

The tracheobronchial tree shows increased responsiveness to immunological and nonimmunological factors. Several organic dusts, fumes and chemicals precipitate immunological mechanisms. Nonimmunological stimuli include thermal, chemical or psychological factors.

Bronchial asthma used to be classified into the *extrinsic (atopic)* and *intrinsic (cryptogenic)* types (Table 143.1). In extrinsic asthma, allergens such as pet dander or pollens triggering the attack are identifiable. Extrinsic asthma tends to be seasonal, as allergies are also seasonal. The serum of such individuals may show elevated levels of specific antibodies belonging to the immunoglobulin E (IgE) and sometimes IgG classes. Persons developing extrinsic asthma have other atopic manifestations like eczema. The dermatological and respiratory manifestations show a see-saw relationship. In many cases, family history of bronchial asthma may be present. Extrinsic asthma generally sets in by the age of 10–15 years. This type has a better prognosis from the point of response to therapy and mortality.

The age of onset for intrinsic asthma is after 30 years. Precipitating causes or raised antibody levels are not evident but, these patients show a higher frequency of eosinophilia, aspirin sensitivity and nasal polyposis.

Common stimuli which precipitate extrinsic asthma are inhaled allergens, like house dust, pollens, fungi,

Table 143.1: Clinical features between atopic and nonatopic asthma

Features	Early-onset (atopic) asthma	Latest-onset (nonatopic) asthma
Onset	Early age usually begins in childhood	Late age
Individuals	Atopic individuals	Nonatopic individuals
Role of external allergens	Have strong role	No role
Family history	Positive history of asthma or allergic diseases (e.g. eczema, urticaria or hay fever)	Less common or absent
Triggering events	Environmental allergens (e.g. dusts, pollens, animal dander and foods)	Respiratory infections due to viruses (e.g. rhinovirus, parainfluenza virus) Inhaled air pollutants (e.g. smoke, fumes)
Serum level of immunoglobulin E (IgE)	Increased	Normal
Skin hypersensitivity test to common inhalant allergens	Positive	Negative
Response to provocation tests	Positive	Negative

Box 143.1: Common trigger factors for asthma

Allergic triggers
- Dust at home/work place
- Pollens, spores
- Animal/pet dander
- Agriculture-related
- Food additives (sulfites)

Nonallergic triggers
- Some forms of exercise, hyperventilation
- Automobile/industrial fumes, sulfur dioxide
- Foods/drinks
- Viral infections
- Drugs
- Smoke, active/passive, tobacco/nontobacco
- Gastroesophageal reflux disease
- Occupational triggers
- Weather changes
- Psychosocial factors

animal hairs, insect scales and industrial fumes, and foods and drugs which are consumed in day-to-day life (Box 143.1). Once sensitization occurs, these antigens release chemical mediators from the mast cells by interacting with the IgE molecules on their surface. Type I hypersensitivity reaction ensues. Asthma can also be caused by type three (delayed) hypersensitivity mechanism mediated by IgG. In some individuals, both type 1 and type 3 reactions occur, the former leading to an immediate asthmatic paroxysm and the latter leading to a delayed episode.

Exercise-induced bronchoconstriction (also known as exercise-induced asthma) is a problem in children and young adults, in which bronchoconstriction is provoked by various forms of exercise such as running or climbing stairs, but others such as swimming may not do so. Provocation of bronchoconstriction by cold inspired air is a possibility in such cases. In many cases, the attacks are brought on after 4–5 minutes of exercise, peak in 10–15 minutes, and resolve within an hour. In the others, asthma sets in several hours after the exercise. The mechanism is a type I hypersensitivity reaction. A fall in forced expiratory volume in the first second (FEV1) by more than 10% after exercise confirms the diagnosis. Short acting β_2-agonists (SABA) are used to prevent exercise-induced asthma. Inhaled corticosteroids (ICS) are indicated and are useful. Systemic steroids are seldom necessary.

Respiratory infection and psychological stress play important roles in precipitating asthmatic paroxysms in both types. Both viral and bacterial infections may trigger off a paroxysm, and the episodes tend to recur as long as the infections persist. In children, asthma may be the presenting symptom in primary tuberculosis. In adults, asthma may be aggravated by coexistent pulmonary tuberculosis. Cigarette-smoking and air pollution act as aggravating factors. The role of psychological stress is more in perpetuating the asthma than initiating the condition.

Many cases show familial predisposition. The atopic background may be inherited. Members of such families show asthma, eczema, hay fever and similar manifestations. The genetic locus for IgE, which is a mediator of type I anaphylaxis, is situated in the long arm of chromosome 11q. Obesity worsens asthma.

Pathology

Inflammation of the airways is brought on by several factors. Eosinophils, T-lymphocytes (CD4$^+$), macrophages and mast cells infiltrate the bronchial wall. The epithelium is vacuolated, and the ciliated cells desquamate. Several cellular factors play their roles in the inflammatory process. Neuropeptides such as bradykinins, substance P and neurotensin A lead to bronchoconstriction, and excessive secretion of mucus.

Mast cells initiate the response on exposure to allergens, excessive osmotic changes and variations in temperature. Macrophages produce cytokines, which are either bronchoconstrictor or bronchodilator. Presence of eosinophils in the inflammatory exudate is characteristic of asthma. Interleukin-5 action leads to eosinophilic inflammation leading to higher eosinophilic count in sputum. Mepolizumab, an IL-5 antagonist monoclonal antibody, reduces the number of eosinophils in tissues, blood and sputum. Eosinophils are derived from bloodstream. Major basic proteins and cationic proteins of eosinophils lead to destruction of mucosal surface. T-lymphocytes, especially CD4$^+$, produce cytokines IL-3, IL-4, IL-5, and granulocyte-macrophage colony-stimulating factor (GM-CSF) which modify the inflammation. Tumor necrosis factor (TNF) which is an inflammatory cytokine is expressed in greater amounts by mast cells. The bronchoalveolar secretions contain higher levels of TNF. Possibly, platelet-derived humoral factors also modify the inflammation. IL-13 is a pleiotropic cytokine produced by Th2 cells. It is related to many of the key features in asthma. IL-13 induces bronchial epithelial cells to secrete periostin which is a matrix cellular protein. Activated epithelial cells produce large amounts of periostin into the underlying matrix where it has autocrine effects on epithelial cells and paracrine effects on fibroblasts. Periostin is a systemic biomarker of eosinophilic airway inflammation in asthmatics. Serum periostin levels are significantly increased in patients with Th2-high asthma. Lebrikizumab, a monoclonal antibody against IL-13, produces clinical improvement in patients with high level of periostin.

The main chemical transmitters which alter the airways are histamine, prostaglandin and leukotrienes. In the asthmatic patient, the airway wall shows increased smooth muscle mass, mucous gland hypertrophy and vascular congestion. The result is thickening of airway wall and marked reduction of airway calibre. These changes lead to contraction of bronchial muscle, increase in vascular permeability and excessive secretion of abnormal mucus (Fig. 143.1). Healthy mucus has the consistency of egg white containing 3% solids; in thick mucus, the solid content may reach 15%. Proteins from homotypic polymers structured as long chains get entangled in a meshwork and by noncovalent calcium-dependent cross-linking of the adjacent polymers leads to formation of the mucus gel. Healthy mucus is a gel with low viscosity and elasticity, abnormal mucus has higher viscosity, abnormal contents of salt and water, increase in mucins, infiltration by inflammatory cells (these occlude air passages) and predispose to infection. Increased amounts of mucus and inflammatory exudate together block the airway passages. Mucus gives rise to cough due to stimulation of vagal afferents and dyspnea due to airways obstruction. They also increase surface tension favoring airway closure.

Airway inflammation persists for several years. Its severity correlates with the severity of asthma. Hyper-responsiveness of the inflamed airways is aggravated by autonomic and neural mechanisms. The final result is obstruction of the small- and medium-sized airways brought about by mucosal edema, tenacious mucus and bronchoconstriction. In chronic cases, airway may undergo structural remodeling.

Clinical Features

The attacks start with dyspnea (often at rest), expiratory wheeze and cough. The onset is abrupt in most cases.

These attacks may occur seasonally or during all times of the year (perennial asthma). The attacks may last for several hours, if untreated; severity of the paroxysm varies. In a moderately severe case, the patient is orthopneic and cyanosed and the accessory muscles of respiration are active. There may be ineffective cough with only very scanty and tenacious mucoid expectoration. The asthmatic paroxysm in many individuals is ushered in by a bout of coughing and sneezing on exposure to the allergen. The pulse is rapid. Blood pressure (BP) is normal or elevated. In severe cases, pulsus paradoxus may occur. Expansion of the chest is considerably diminished, often to less than 2 cm during the attack. The diagnostic feature of bronchial asthma is the presence of polyphonic expiratory wheeze heard all over the chest.

Once asthma occurs, the tendency is for the condition to persist for varying periods, even life-long, with remissions and exacerbations. About 50–60% of patients get a cure or considerable relief by altering their lifestyle such as change of residence, change of jobs, exercise programs including yoga exercises, changes of diet and others. Appropriate medication may improve the quality of life in the vast majority. Approximately, 20–30% of patients are not free from asthma. However, attacks can be suppressed considerably by drugs. About 10% have severe disability despite active treatment. Allergic bronchopulmonary aspergillosis (ABPA) may develop in some asthmatic individuals.

Laboratory Findings

These are often nonspecific and they help to identify the coexisting disease. Some cases may show moderate eosinophilia (10–15%). Examination of feces may reveal helminths, which may also contribute to the allergic reaction and increase in eosinophils. Sputum may reveal numerous eosinophils, mucus plugs and Curschmann's spirals (casts of smaller airways). Purulent sputum is indicative of respiratory infection. Culture reveals the infecting organisms. A simple method to infer whether infective or allergic causes trigger off paroxysm is to examine a Leishman's stain preparation of the sputum smear. Predominance of neutrophils suggests an infective cause whereas, predominance of eosinophils suggests allergic etiology.

Identification of the allergen: Several tests have been introduced to identify the precipitating allergen. Intradermal tests are performed by using a battery of antigens prepared from the common allergens prevalent in the area. In many instances, the causative agent can be detected by the positive skin tests. These tests are of help in long-term management after tiding over the paroxysm.

Skiagram taken during the acute attack may show hypertranslucency due to emphysema, but there may be no abnormality in between the attacks. It should be remembered that the radiological appearances and clinical severity show wide disparity in bronchial asthma. X-rays often help to identify complications such as pneumothorax and pneumomediastinum. It is a valuable tool in excluding complications such as pneumonia and asthma mimics, especially during exacerbations.

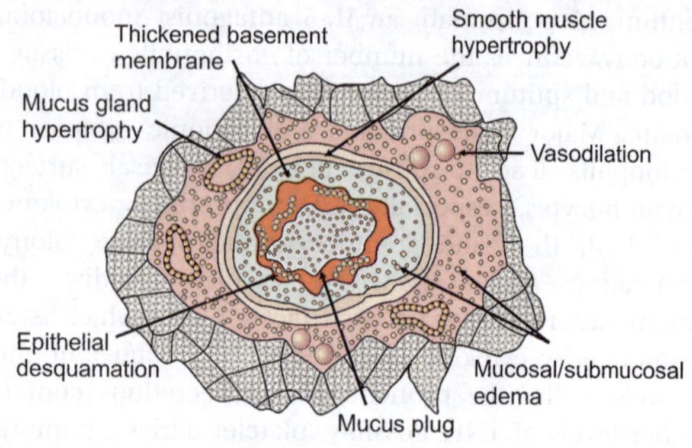

Fig. 143.1: Pathological features of asthma

High-resolution computed tomography (HRCT) findings in bronchial asthma includes bronchial wall thickening, bronchial dilatation, cylindrical and varicose bronchiectasis, reduced airway luminal area, mucoid impaction of the bronchi, centrilobular opacities, linear opacities, air trapping, and/or focal and regional areas of decreased perfusion.

Diagnosis

Diagnosis of bronchial asthma is clinical, supported with spirometry. The history of sudden attack of paroxysmal dyspnea, cough, and the auscultatory hallmark of expiratory wheeze heard all over the chest are diagnostic. Long duration of complaints, history of allergy and positive family history are other helpful clinical points.

The severity of airways obstruction and response to bronchodilator therapy can be objectively assessed with *spirometry*. It also helps to distinguish asthma from chronic obstructive pulmonary disease (COPD). Pulmonary function tests in asthmatics show reduced FEV1, and decrease in FEV1 or forced vital capacity (FVC) ratio with a fall in peak expiratory flow rate (PEFR). In a subject, FEV1/FVC ratio of less than 0.70 is diagnostic of airway obstruction.

Peak expiratory flow rate refers to the maximal rate at which the subject can exhale during a short, maximal expiratory effort, following a full inspiration. PEFR can be assessed using a *bedside peak flow meter.* Using a nebulizer or metered dose inhaler, SABA (e.g. salbutamol or levosalbutamol) is given after basal spirometric assessment. If a repeat spirometry 20 minutes later shows 12% (or 200 mL) improvement in FEV1, it supports the diagnosis of asthma (Fig. 143.2). In asthma patients, the forced expiration time is increased beyond the normal value of 4 seconds. Bedside peak flow meter tests give a quick assessment of airway obstruction. For those who have near-normal spirometry during day time, peak flow meter helps in establishing diurnal variability. It is also useful to monitor severity of asthma at home or work place.

Confirmation of the diagnosis of asthma is usually achieved by serial PEFR monitoring. PEFR in majority of cases shows a diurnal variation of more than 15%

and improvement with therapy. When it is necessary to investigate for provocative factors, bronchial challenge testing or bronchial provocation testing (BPT) may be desirable. Incremental doses of triggering agents are given as inhalation to assess airway hyper-responsiveness. The dose at which FEV1 falls by 20% is known as the provocative dose 20% (PD20). Methacholine, histamine, adenosine or mannitol can act as triggers. Exercise or hyperventilation too can elicit bronchial hyper-reactivity. A methacholine PD20 below 8 mg is consistent with the diagnosis of asthma.

The flow-volume loop gives a graphic representation of airway obstruction (Fig. 143.3).

Other Investigations

Exhaled nitric oxide levels are high in asthma. Viral respiratory infections, sputum eosinophilia, and acute airway inflammation may also raise exhaled nitric oxide levels. High levels of eosinophils in sputum reflect the magnitude of airway inflammation. Assessment of cytokine levels in sputum (induced with inhaling hypertonic saline where necessary) is employed in selected centers.

Clinical features which indicate severe ventilatory impairment are given in Box 143.2 and Table 143.2.

Differential Diagnosis

Chevalier Jackson stated, 'All that wheezes is not asthma'. Bronchial asthma has to be differentiated from other causes of paroxysmal dyspnea. These include chronic bronchitis emphysema syndrome (CBES), acute left-sided heart failure, acute bronchitis, tropical pulmonary eosinophilia (TPE), metabolic acidosis, and tracheal obstruction by

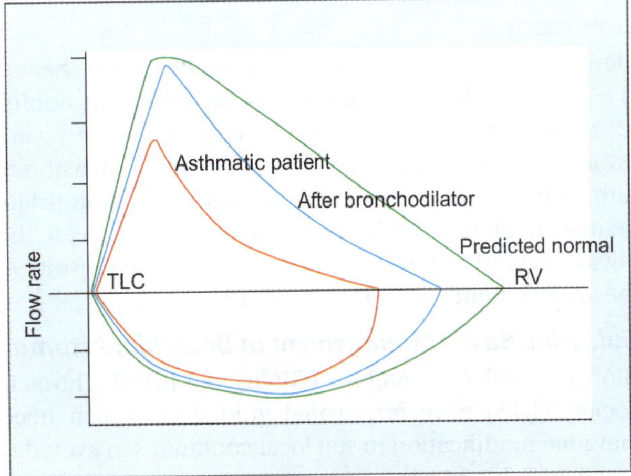

Fig. 143.3: Flow volume curve in normal and asthma

Abbreviations: RV = Residual volume; TLC = Total lung capacity

Box 143.2: Severe ventilatory impairment

- Inability to narrate history continuously or severe distress even on mild exertion
- Cyanosis, flapping tremors
- Mental confusion
- Respiratory rate above 25 breath/minute
- Heart rate persistently above 110 beat/minute
- Inspiratory fall in BP exceeds 16 mm Hg
- PEFR less than 40% of predicted value
- Feeble breath sounds

Abbreviation: PEFR = Peak expiratory flow rate

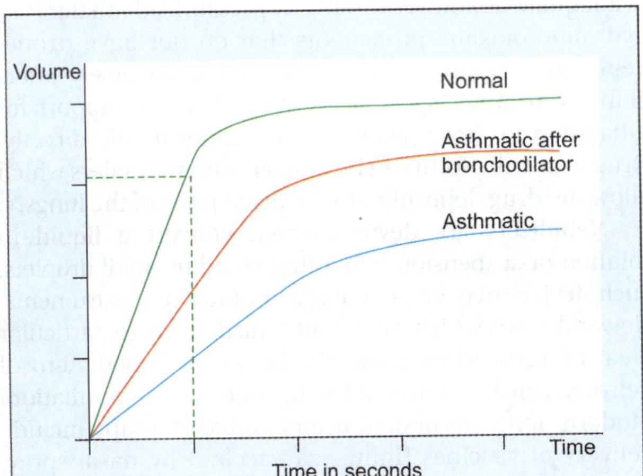

Fig. 143.2: Time-volume curve: bronchial asthma

Table 143.2: The assessment of severity of asthma

Components of severity	Inter-mittent	Persistent		
		Mild	Moderate	Severe
Symptoms	≤ 2 days/week	> 2 days/week but not daily	Daily	Throughout the day
Night time awakenings	≤ 2 × per month	3–4 × per month	> 1 × per week but not nightly	Often 7 × per week
*Using Short-acting β_2-agonists for symptom control	≤ 2 days per week	> 2 days per week but not daily	Daily	Several times per day
Interference with normal activity	None	Minor limitation	Some limitation	Extremely limited

foreign bodies or tumors. Diffuse panbronchiolitis (DPB), prevalent in Japan and the far East, may mimic asthma.

It is important to distinguish left-sided heart failure (cardiac asthma) from bronchial asthma. Left-sided heart failure complicates valvular heart disease, systemic hypertension or ischemic heart disease (IHD). It causes paroxysmal dyspnea in the first half of the night whereas bronchial asthma is more common in the early hours of the morning. In bronchial asthma, there is generalized wheeze all over the chest, whereas in cardiac failure, basal crepitations are more prominent, though generalized bronchospasm may also be evident at times. In heart failure, gallop rhythm may be evident. Careful search for the underlying disease may reveal the etiology.

Treatment

Management may be described under three heads: (1) Guideline based management of asthma in adults, (2) treatment of the acute attack, including acute severe asthma and (3) follow-up and prevention of asthma. Although, there is no cure for asthma, appropriate management that includes a partnership between the physician, and the patient or family most often results in the achievement of control (Box 143.3).

Guideline Based Management of Bronchial Asthma

Global Initiative for Asthma (GINA) and British Thoracic Society (BTS) have formulated guidelines, which need marginal modification to suit local conditions in everyday practice (Table 143.3).

Pharmacological Agents

Asthma medications are classified into controller medications and reliever medications. Box 143.4 for the list of recommended pharmacological agents.

Aerosol Drug Delivery

This aims at delivering the drug in the form of aerosols into the distal parts of the lung and air passages. Four types of devices are available:

1. Pressurized metered dose inhaler (pMDI)
2. Spacers and holding chambers
3. Dry powder inhalers (DPIs)
4. Nebulizers.

Box 143.3: Goals of asthma treatment

- Achieve and maintain control of symptoms
- Maintain normal activity levels including exercise
- Maintain pulmonary function as close to normal levels as possible
- Prevent asthma exacerbations
- Avoid adverse effects from asthma medications
- Control cost of management
- Avoid complications
- Prevent asthma mortality

Table 143.3: Steps in the management of bronchial asthma adapted and simplified

Step 1	Inhaled short-acting β_2-agonists, as required
Step 2	Inhaled corticosteroids (ICS) Low dose: Up to 400 µg/day *or* leukotriene modifier
Step 3	ICS, low dose: Up to 400 µg/day + long-acting β_2-agonists *or* ICS medium/high dose up to 800 µg/day *or* ICS low dose + leukotriene modifiers
Step 4	Step 3 + leukotriene modifiers/theophylline
Step 5	Step 4 + systemic steroids/anti-IgE therapy

Abbreviation: IgE = Immunoglobulin E

Box 143.4: Controller and reliever drugs in asthma

Controller medications
- Inhaled glucocorticosteroids
- Leukotriene modifiers
- Long-acting inhaled β_2-agonists in combination with inhaled glucocorticosteroids
- Systemic glucocorticosteroids
- Theophylline
- Chromones
- Anti-IgE

Reliever medications
- Rapid-acting inhaled β_2-agonists
- Systemic glucocorticosteroids
- Anticholinergics
- Theophylline
- Short-acting oral β_2-agonists

Abbreviation: IgE = Immunoglobulin E

Devices used in the past delivered only 10–37% of the drug to the lungs. If proper technique is employed, the currently available devices can deliver 48–50% of the drug into the deeper airways. In patients with airway narrowing, the drug may not reach the obstructed areas in adequate quantity. Present day pressurized inhalers use hydrofluoroalkane propellants that do not have ozone-depleting properties, and thus do not adversely affect global warming. 'Spacers' provide effective support for inhalation to those patients who cannot inhale directly. Drug in powder form can be inhaled with rotahalers which allow the drug deposition to the distal parts of the lungs.

Nebulizers are devices which convert a liquid in solution or suspension into a thin cloud of small droplets. Such devices may be pneumatic or ultrasonic instruments. Newer devices which can target drug delivery to particular areas of diseased lungs are also being developed. Aerosol delivery can be combined with mechanical ventilation. Modern nonconventional use of aerosol therapy include delivery of vaccines (influenza vaccine) by nasal spray, prostanoids in pulmonary artery hypertension (PAH) and cyclosporine in lung transplant.

Individual Classes of Drugs

Corticosteroids: Glucocorticosteroids are currently the most effective anti-inflammatory medications for the treatment of asthma. They effectively improve lung function, decrease airway hyper-responsiveness, reduce symptoms, reduce frequency and severity of exacerbations, and improve quality of life. ICS form the backbone and foundation of asthma therapy. Patients with asthma of all levels of severity respond to ICS. Patients requiring SABA more than 2–3 times a day should be treated with inhaled steroids. It is recommended, that a starting dose of 400 mg/day for adults, and 200 mg/day for children (beclomethasone equivalent) be employed. The dose must be titrated to the lowest dose, which maintains effective control of asthma. Parenteral, oral or nebulized steroids may be used in acute severe asthma, where they are life-saving.

Table 143.4 gives comparative dosage of commonly used inhaled steroids. Ill-effects of ICS include oropharyngeal candidiasis and dysphonia. Systemic side effects develop, though this is less common than with oral preparations. Cataract may develop in some.

Indications for short-course oral corticosteroid therapy

- Symptoms and PEFR deteriorate day by day (all acute forms of asthma)
- PEFR less than 60% of the patient's best PEFR
- Insomnia due to asthma
- Morning wheeze persists up to mid-day or even beyond
- Other treatments fail.

β_2-agonists

Short acting β_2-agonists (SABA) (called reliever medications) have no significant effect on the inflammatory response. Overdependence on these agents has been established as one of the causes for fatal or near-fatal asthma attacks. Monotherapy with SABA must be limited to step 1 asthma management. Patients need to be educated regarding the side effects, especially tremor, tachycardia and dysrhythmia. Common members of this group are salbutamol, levosalbutamol and terbutaline. Most of these can be given orally, many of them as inhalations (aerosol or powder) and few of them parenterally. The oral dose is effective within 15–20 minutes and the action lasts for 4–6 hours. The oral dose is salbutamol 2–4 mg, levosalbutamol 1–2 mg and terbutaline 2–4 mg. The dosage may be repeated up to thrice daily. They are also available in pMDIs, each puff delivering 50–200 mg per actuation. Good coordination of inhalation and pressure-actuation of canister is necessary for proper drug delivery. The drugs are also available as DPIs of equivalent dosages. Dry powder inhaler devices are delivery systems which provide the dose in powder form (rotahalers, accuhalers, turbohalers, spinhalers and diskhalers). The dosages may be repeated up to 8 inhalations per day. Adverse side effects such as palpitation and tremors may occur up to 50% of patients. Inhalational route for drug delivery may lead to hoarseness of voice in some patients.

Long-acting β_2-agonists (LABA) formoterol/arformoterol, salmeterol, indacaterol and bambuterol. Bambuterol can be given orally in a single dose of 10–20 mg. Most of these drugs can be given as pMDIs and/or DPIs. These have to be used prophylactically and therapeutically at the slightest warning of an impending attack. Their duration of action lasts for 12 hours or more. They may relax as airway smooth muscle, enhance mucociliary clearance, decrease vascular permeability, and it may modulate mediator release from mast cells and basophils. LABA are indicated when initial doses of ICS fail to achieve control of asthma. LABA must be combined with ICS to control airway inflammation. Addition of LABA to ICS improves symptoms, decreases nocturnal asthma, improves lung function, decreases the use of rapid-acting inhaled β_2-agonists, and reduces the number of exacerbations. The inhaled dose being small, adverse side effects are only minimal.

To avoid the chance of inadequate inhalation using aerosol sprays, spacers are utilized. The metered dose can be sprayed into the spacer, from which the patient can inhale it comfortably. Dry powder devices are easier to operate as no coordination is required. Irrespective of the type of delivery system, the patient has to be instructed, demonstrated and reinforced the proper method of usage of the device. In any case, the drug has to reach the lower airways, in order to be optimally effective.

Nebulizers, which can be carried by the patient or operated in the emergency room are available for administration of these drugs. These can deliver larger doses as required. The drug solution is nebulized by passing oxygen or air under pressure through it, either by means of a pump or using ultrasonic vibrations.

Table 143.4: Comparative daily dosage of commonly used inhaled steroids (in mg)

Drugs	Low daily dose		Medium daily dose		High daily dose	
	Adult	**Child**	**Adult**	**Child**	**Adult**	**Child**
Beclomethasone	200–500	100–250	500–1,000	250–500	1,000	500
Budesonide	200–600	100–200	600–1,000	200–600	1,000	600
Ciclesonide	80–160	80–160	160–320	160–320	320–1,280	320
Flunisolide	500–1,000	500–750	1,000–2,000	500–1,250	2,000	1,250
Fluticasone	100–250	100–200	250–500	200–500	500	500
Mometasone	200–400	100–200	400–800	200–400	800–1,200	400
Triamcinolone	400–1,000	400–800	1,000–2,000	800–1,200	2,000	1,200

Long-acting β_2-agonists (LABA) form a major component of asthma control, playing a pivotal role. Their addition to ICS has revolutionized current asthma follow-up and therapy. SMART (Single maintenance and reliever therapy) approach advocates a single inhaler for rescue medication as well as regular use as controller therapy. Formoterol with ICS (budesonide) has found clinical utility in this respect.

Parenteral preparations of SABA are helpful when the paroxysm is severe, and immediate relief is required. They are less often utilized, compared to nebulizations.

Sympathomimetic drugs

Acute asthma readily responds to sympathomimetic drugs. *The time-honored drug, adrenaline 0.5–1 mL of 1:1,000 aqueous solution given subcutaneously (SC) relieves bronchospasm, and terminates the paroxysm in minutes*. Adverse effects include rise in BP, tachycardia, palpitation and precipitation of angina, especially in the elderly. Hurst's method of administration is to deliver adrenaline SC in a dose of 1 drop every minute till the bronchospasm is relieved. With the advent of safer drugs, the use of adrenaline has been reduced but, still in some cases where other drugs fail, adrenaline may give immediate relief. In pediatric practice, nebulized adrenaline has a place for relieving acute bronchospasm.

Ephedrine, widely used in the past, is not commonly used at present even though several antiasthmatic preparations containing ephedrine are still in vogue.

Sympathomimetic drugs should be used with caution in hypertensives, and elderly subjects with coronary artery disease (CAD) or urinary obstruction. Fatal arrhythmias may be precipitated by repeated doses of these drugs.

Leukotriene modifiers

These include several molecules divided into two classes. The first class (cysteinyl leukotriene-receptor antagonists) prevents leukotriene binding to the type 1 receptors. Montelukast (4–10 mg), zafirlukast (10–20 mg) and pranlukast (5–10 mg) are members of this group. The second class of leukotriene modifiers prevents the synthesis of leukotrienes by inhibiting 5-lipoxygenase. Zileuton (600 mg 4 times daily) is an example of this class of drugs. The use of montelukast is particularly effective, where allergic rhinitis coexists with asthma. Montelukast is popular in the management of pediatric asthma, where association with allergic rhinitis is considerable. Usually, it is given as a 10 mg bed-time dose alone or in combination with oral bambuterol for adult asthma. It is indicated in step 2 of asthma treatment onward. It reduces the dose of ICS in moderate to severe asthma. It may also be used to prevent exercise- or drug-induced asthma (e.g. aspirin-sensitive asthma). It is less effective than long-acting inhaled β_2-agonists as add on therapy. Zileuton may cause reversible chemical hepatitis, and is contraindicated in patients with hepatic dysfunction.

Methylxanthines

The common preparations include theophylline and etophylline. They can be given orally or as intravenous (IV) injections, singly or in combination. They are used as add on to ICS + LABA therapy.

Dose: Combination vials of etophylline 169.4 mg and theophylline 50.6 mg are to be given as slow IV injections or as IV drip in 5% dextrose, 2–3 times daily. Tablets containing etophylline 77 mg, and theophylline 23 mg are available for oral use to be taken 3–4 times daily. Sustained release tablets containing etophylline 150 mg, and theophylline 35 mg are available to be taken twice daily.

Their beneficial effects include bronchodilation, synergistic action on the movement of the diaphragm, stimulation of the respiratory center and mild diuresis. When combined with β_2-agonists they act synergistically. Sustained-release preparations are preferred for oral therapy. Long-term treatment with sustained-release theophylline is effective in controlling asthma symptoms and improving lung function. It is also useful in the control of nocturnal symptoms, and as an additional bronchodilator in patients with severe asthma. Theophylline may be used in patients with milder disease, and as an add-on therapy to low or high doses of ICS where further asthma control is needed.

Some patients with severe asthma attacks may benefit from IV aminophylline. For those who were not previously on oral xanthines, 5 mg/kg body weight is administered over 20 minutes, followed by an infusion at the rate of 0.5–0.7 mg/kg/h. Higher incidence of side effects such as palpitation, vomiting and arrhythmias is met within some cases receiving IV aminophylline. Sometimes sudden vasomotor collapse or allergic manifestations may develop.

Anticholinergic agents

Since vagal tone accounts for bronchial muscle tone, anticholinergic drugs have been found to be beneficial in asthma. Inhaled ipratropium bromide and oxitropium bromide are bronchodilators that block the effect of acetylcholine released from cholinergic nerves in the airways. These agents produce bronchodilation by reducing intrinsic vagal cholinergic tone to the airways. They also block reflex bronchoconstriction caused by inhaled irritants. They have no effect on airway inflammation. They are less potent bronchodilators than inhaled β_2-agonists. They have a slower onset of action (30–60 minutes to maximum effect), but the effect is more sustained in duration.

Ipratropium bromide has an additive effect when nebulized together with rapid-acting β_2-agonists for exacerbations of asthma. Usual dose is 0.25–0.5 mg by nebulizer every 4–6 hours or 20–40 mg from a metered dose inhaler. It is useful as an alternative bronchodilator for patients who experience adverse effects of tachycardia, arrhythmia or tremors from rapid-acting β_2-agonists. Inhalation of ipratropium or oxitropium may cause dryness of the mouth and a bitter taste. Unlike atropine, they do not cause mucociliary dysfunction, bladder neck obstruction or rise in intraocular pressure. Tiotropium bromide which is similar to ipratropium is available as rotacaps for inhalation. The dose is 18 µg/inhalation. It is usually, given once daily.

Novel Therapeutic Approaches

Allergen immunotherapy: Specific immunotherapy is administered by the subcutaneous route or sublingual route. Injection of increasing doses of allergen extracts induces immunological and clinical tolerance. Antibodies of IgE class are produced by hyposensitization. These bind the allergen, and eliminate them without causing any allergic symptoms. Sublingual administration of allergen extracts has been successfully tried in the treatment of pollen allergy.

Anti-immunoglobulin E—omalizumab: Binding of specific allergens to receptor-bound IgE on mast cells and basophils signals. These cells may release to preformed mediators (e.g. histamine) and synthesize other proinflammatory molecules (e.g. leukotrienes, cytokines and chemokines). Subcutaneously administered anti-IgE antibody blocks such as a pathway in patients with moderate to severe asthma, and with an allergic component. Omalizumab reduces circulating levels of IgE to values below 10 IU/mL, at which level allergic reactions are reduced. It allows for reduction of oral or ICS and improves asthma control. Omalizumab is a recombinant-DNA (rDNA) and anti-IgE antibody. Dosage depends upon the patient's weight and blood IgE levels. It is given as a slow subcutaneous injection every 2–4 weeks. It is recommended in the treatment of moderate, and severe persistent asthma of the allergic IgE-mediated type. GINA guidelines recommend it as an additional agent in step 5 treatment (Table 143.5). Anti-IgE appears to be safe as add-on therapy, and may reduce features of airway inflammation. Anaphylaxis can occur with omalizumab. It is an expensive modality of treatment, costing \$ 10,000–30,000 per year.

Anti-IL-13: It induces bronchial epithelial cells to secrete periostin, which is a signaling protein. Periostin influences bronchial hyper-responsiveness, bronchial inflammation, and activation as well as proliferation of airway fibroblasts (involved in airway remodeling). Lebrikizumab, a monoclonal antibody against periostin, produces clinical improvement in asthmatics with high level of periostin.

Thromboxane A_2 receptor antagonist: It is a bronchoconstrictor prostanoid. Seratrodast is a thromboxane A_2 receptor antagonist. It is given in 80 mg once daily dose. It causes airway smooth muscle and vascular dilatation. GINA guidelines recommend its use as a controller therapy for long-term management.

New long-acting β_2-agonists—indacaterol: It is ultra long-acting β_2-agonists with high intrinsic efficiency. The dose is 200–800 µg once daily as a dry powder inhalation (DPI). It has the potential to cause paradoxical bronchospasm, and is contraindicated in acute asthma.

Phosphodiesterase-4 inhibitor—roflumilast: Administered orally by once daily dose of 500 µg, roflumilast inhibits phosphodiesterase-4. It produces anti-inflammatory effects in asthma as well as COPD patients.

Bronchial thermoplasty: Radiofrequency ablation of airway smooth muscle mass reduces smooth muscle-mediated bronchoconstriction. Statistically and clinically significant improvement in airway hyper-responsiveness has been demonstrated by this novel technique.

Table 143.5: Stepwise management of asthma

Steps	Management
Step 1: Only for intermittent/less frequent symptoms	Short-acting inhaled β_2-agonist as required (required in all steps)
Step 2: Daily symptoms	Regular inhaled preventer therapy: • Low-dose inhaled corticosteroids (ICSs) up to 800 µg daily or • Leukotriene receptor antagonists (LTRAs), (if patient develops side effects to ICSs)
Step 3: Severe symptoms	ICSs and long-acting inhaled β_2-agonist: • Continue low-dose ICSs plus long-acting β_2-agonist or • Medium or high dose ICSs or • Low-dose ICSs plus LTRAs or • Low-dose ICSs plus sustained-release oral theophylline
Step 4: Severe symptoms uncontrolled with high-dose inhaled corticosteroids	High-dose ICS and regular bronchodilators • Medium or high-dose ICSs (up to 2,000 µg daily) plus long-acting β_2-agonist • May add LTRAs. • May add sustained-release theophylline
Step 5: Severe symptoms deteriorating	Regular oral corticosteroids • Add oral corticosteroids (prednisolone 40 mg daily) • Consider anti-IgE treatment (omalizumab)
Step 6: Severe symptoms deteriorating in spite of prednisolone	Hospital admission

ACUTE SEVERE ASTHMA (PREVIOUSLY KNOWN AS STATUS ASTHMATICUS)

Acute severe asthma is a medical emergency. This lifethreatening emergency places the patient at risk of developing fatal respiratory failure. This condition is generally unresponsive to conventional drugs administered in the usual manner. Clinical assessment of the severity can be made from the intensity of dyspnea, cyanosis and inability of the patient to speak uninterruptedly. They may be often moribund. At this stage, many of them are unresponsive to the ordinary bronchodilators. Dehydration may be evident. Estimation of PEFR gives an objective assessment of the condition (Table 143.6).

Any patient of asthma may develop acute severe asthma as a complication. It may be precipitated by infection, allergic factors or psychological stress (Box 143.5). Even in mild cases such paroxysms may supervene without warning. The attacks usher in either as progressive worsening of an existing paroxysm or sudden onset of severe dyspnea and air-hunger in a mild or moderate asthmatic. The attack may be so severe that the patient may not even be able to cry for help.

Emergency Management

General Measures

Patients should be hospitalized and managed in acute care facility as an emergency.

Table 143.6: Signs to assess severity of asthma

Signs	Mild	Moderate	Severe
Breathless	Walking	Talking	At rest
	Can lie down	Prefer sitting	Hunched forward
Talk in	Sentences	Phrases	Words
Alertness	May be	Usually agitated	Agitated
Central cyanosis	Absent	Absent	Present
Use of accessory muscle	Absent	Moderate	Marked
Sternal retraction	Absent	Moderate	Marked
Wheeze on auscultation	Moderate, often end expiratory	Loud	Loud à silent chest
Pulsus paradoxus	Not palpable	May be palpable	Often palpable
Initial peak expiratory flow (PEF)	More than 80%	60–80%	Less than 60%
Oximetry on presentation	More than 95%	91–95%	Less than 90%

Box 143.5: Common risk factors for acute severe asthma

- Use of more than two canisters per month of inhaled short-acting β_2-agonist
- Two or more hospitalizations for asthma in the previous year
- Past history of sudden severe exacerbations
- Prior admission for asthma to an intensive care unit (ICU)
- Prior intubation and ventilation for asthma
- Current use of/or recent withdrawal from systemic corticosteroids
- Comorbidity such as cardiovascular diseases or COPD
- Serious psychiatric disease or psychosocial problems

- Propped up position in bed
- IV normal saline infusion, for fluid replacement as well as to serve as a port for drug administration
- Electrolyte balance must be considered, while managing the acutely ill asthmatic (steroids and inhaled β_2-agonists can induce hypokalemia).

Oxygen: Hypoxemia must be corrected using high-flow mask or nonrebreathing mask with high concentrations of oxygen. Aim is to maintain oxygen saturation above 92%. Hypercapnia is a poor prognostic sign in asthma.

β_2-agonist bronchodilators: Drugs of choice employed to stop an acute attack are SABA drugs. Salbutamol (2.5–5 mg) or levosalbutamol (0.65–1.25 mg) is given, preferably using an oxygen-driven nebulizer. This dose may be repeated thrice at 15–30 minutes intervals. They act mainly on the bronchial muscle as relaxants without much effect on the cardiovascular system. If no threat to life is perceived, 4–6 metered dose inhaler puffs in a large volume spacer every 10–20 minutes will be useful, till nebulization can be arranged. If inhalational therapy is not reliable, give salbutamol 500 mg IV. IV salbutamol helps to build up the blood level rapidly. For children, IV dose is 15 mg/kg body weight.

Steroids: They are life-saving in acute cases, if administered early. IV hydrocortisone, 200 mg or any equipotent analogue (betamethasone 8 mg, dexamethasone 8 mg or methyl prednisolone 80 mg) is given as an IV push. Nebulized budesonide 0.5 mg every 12 hours may be of help to many patients. Prednisolone 10–15 mg is started simultaneously and repeated 6 hourly. Continue prednisolone 40–50 mg daily for at least 5 days.

Ipratropium bromide: They given either as nebulization (0.5 mg) or as aerosol in a dose of 20–40 mg, repeated at 4–6 hourly intervals. Combination of ipratropium with β_2-agonists in nebulization gives greater bronchodilation than either agent alone.

Magnesium sulfate: 1–2 g of IV magnesium sulfate given as a slow syringe pump infusion (over 30 minute) is a useful adjunct, where response to β_2-agonists, ipratropium and steroids is inadequate.

Aminophylline: IV aminophylline 5 mg/kg loading dose, with infusion of 0.5 mg/kg/h adds to bronchodilation brought about by the previously mentioned drugs. Vomiting, palpitations and arrhythmias pose problems in a significant number of patients.

Routine prescription of antibiotics is not indicated for acute asthma. Sudden death may occur any time within 3–5 days of the acute episode, and therefore, such patients should be under surveillance for this period.

Ventilatory Assistance

If the condition does not respond to treatment or the respiratory embarrassment is increasing, ventilation should be assisted. A significant number of asthma patients admitted to ICU will need mechanical ventilatory support. Ventilation is aimed at minimizing hyperinflation. Small tidal volume, slow respiratory rate and fast inspiratory time help to achieve this. There are some studies to show utility of noninvasive ventilation to reduce hospitalization. It is not recommended as a treatment modality.

If the secretions are tenacious and difficult to be expectorated, throat suction or bronchoscopic aspiration and bronchoalveolar lavage may be required. The indications for ventilatory assistance are summarized in the Box 143.6.

Levels of severity of acute asthma exacerbations: Based on the severity of symptoms and signs, acute asthma exacerbations may be classified into five levels of severity, as detailed in Box 143.7.

Indications for ICU management of patients not responding to initial therapy are summarized in Box 143.8.

Special Considerations

Effect of smoking on asthma: Prevalence of asthma is high among smokers and passive smoke inhalers. Childhood asthma is casually related to in utero exposure to maternal smoking or exposure of mother to second-hand smoke in pregnancy. Smoking has a negative impact on treatment outcomes in asthma. Smokers require more dosage of drugs, develop more severe airway remodeling, and are prone to fixed airway obstruction. Age-related lung function decline is exaggerated in all exposed to tobacco smoke in any form.

Box 143.6: Indications for ventilatory assistance

- Pulsus paradoxus
- Central cyanosis despite O_2 inhalation
- Deterioration of arterial blood gases despite treatment:
  - PaO_2 < 60 mm Hg (8 kPa) and continuing to fall
  - $PaCO_2$ > 40 mm Hg (6 kPa) and continuing to rise
  - pH of 7.3 and falling further
  - Extreme physical exhaustion.
- Clouding of consciousness, confusion and drowsiness
- Coma
- Respiratory arrest

Box 143.7: Levels of severity of acute asthma exacerbation

Brittle asthma
- Wide PEF variability despite intense therapy
- Sudden severe attacks on a background of well-controlled asthma

Moderate exacerbation
- Progressively worsening symptoms
- PEF 50–70% of best for individual or predicted values

Acute severe asthma
- PEFR 33–50% of best for individual or predicted vales
- Respiratory rate > 25 breath/minute
- Heart rate > 110 beat/minute
- Inability to complete a sentence in one breath

Life-threatening asthma
- PEF < 33% of best for individual or predicted vales, PEF not recordable
- Finger pulse oximeter reading < 92%
- PaO_2 < 60 mm Hg, especially on oxygen
- $PaCO_2$ normal, 35–45 mm of Hg
- Low arterial blood pH
- Silent chest, cyanosis and feeble respiratory effort
- Bradycardia, dysrhythmia and hypotension
- Exhaustion, confusion and coma

Near fatal asthma
- Raised $PaCO_2$
- Requiring mechanical ventilation

Abbreviations: PEF = Peak expiratory flow; PEFR = Peak expiratory flow rate; PaO_2 = Partial pressure of arterial oxygen; $PaCO_2$ = Partial pressure of arterial carbon dioxide

Box 143.8: Indications for intensive care unit management of patients not responding to initial therapy

- Worsening PEF
- Persisting hypoxia or worsening PaO_2
- Worsening hypercapnia
- Worsening acidosis
- Deteriorating respiratory effort, exhaustion
- Coma, respiratory arrest

Abbreviations: PaO_2 = Partial pressure of arterial oxygen; PEF = Peak expiratory flow

Steroid-resistant asthma: Among the asthma patients, even after optimal management, 5–10% does not respond adequately. These patients are labeled as having refractory asthma. Type I steroid resistance results from reduced affinity of glucocorticoid receptors to steroids. They may respond to higher doses of steroids. Reduced number of cells with glucocorticoid receptors constitutes the type II steroid resistance. Higher doses of steroids are ineffective. Cytokine-based therapies and bronchial thermoplasty may prove to be useful in such cases in the future.

Brittle asthma: Brittle asthma is a severe clinical type of the disease. Type I brittle asthma shows wide PEF variability, despite maximal doses of ICS. Type II Brittle asthma presents as sudden acute attacks occurring in a well-controlled asthmatic, in less than 3 hours without an obvious trigger. Smooth muscle contraction and edema of the airways in the background of chronic airway inflammation is believed to be the cause. The spectrum of specific symptoms, trigger factors, personal or family history and spirometric PEF monitoring help in the diagnosis. Brittle asthma is managed with high doses of ICS and/or oral steroids, subcutaneous injections of SABA and inhaled LABA. Triggers must be identified and avoided.

The pregnant asthmatic: Asthma is the most common potentially serious medical condition met with in pregnancy. Estimated incidence of asthma is 8% among women in childbearing age-group. Uncontrolled asthma can cause serious maternal complications, viz. systemic hypertension, toxemia, premature delivery and rarely death. For the baby, complications include increased risk of stillbirth, fetal growth retardation, premature birth, low-birth-weight and a low Apgar score at birth. It is imperative to control asthma in pregnancy adequately. Budesonide is the safest ICS for use in pregnancy and lactation. Inhaled cromolyn sodium does not have significant maternal or fetal side effects, but is less effective than ICS. SABA are considered safe during pregnancy. No large scale studies are available to support the use of LABA in pregnancy. However, inhaled LABA may be used during pregnancy for patients not controlled on ICS. Theophylline in pregnancy does not show any significant adverse effects to the mother. New born may have tachycardia, jitters or vomiting, if maternal blood levels of theophylline are high.

Allergic rhinitis and asthma: Association of allergic rhinitis with asthma is well-known to clinicians. Both have overlapping epidemiology, pathophysiology and clinical features. When asthma control remains poor inspite of good compliance, investigate for coexistent allergic rhinitis. Leukotriene modifiers are found to be useful in management of both conditions. Cure of rhinitis may prevent some cases of new-onset asthma. Subcutaneous or sublingual immunotherapy may benefit a subset of patients of allergic rhinitis or asthma with elevated IgE.

Gastroesophageal reflux disease (GERD): Cough, recurrent bronchitis, pneumonia, wheezing and asthma are associated with GERD. GERD is the regurgitation of contents of the stomach into the esophagus. GERD can lead to lung damage, esophageal ulcers and Barrett's esophagus, a premalignant condition. Regurgitated acid may cause injury to the mucosa of the throat, airways and lungs, making inhalation difficult, and often causing a persistent cough. Behavioral and dietary adjustments help those with GERD and asthma.

Cough-variant asthma: It is a type of asthma in which the main symptom is a dry, nonproductive cough. Patients with cough-variant asthma may not have wheezing or shortness of breath. Coughing increases with exercise or when exposed to asthma triggers, including cold air. It is common in young kids with childhood asthma. Some may progress to typical asthma. Treatment is the same as asthma. SABA, ipratropium and/or ICS may be necessary for control of symptoms.

Complications of Asthma

Though mortality is low, severe asthma may result in respiratory failure and death even in the most unexpected situation. Other complications include frequent respiratory infections, pulmonary collapse due to obstruction by viscid secretions, pneumothorax, mediastinal emphysema and cough fractures (fractures of ribs due to violent coughing). Children with asthma may show retardation of growth, especially, if treated with systemic corticosteroids on a long-term basis. Long-standing bronchial asthma, punctuated with frequent respiratory infections may lead on to emphysema and chronic cor pulmonale. Chronic inflammation of the airway, eventually leads to permanent structural changes called 'airway remodeling'. These changes may lead to permanently reduced lung function and a chronic cough. Allergic bronchopulmonary aspergillosis (ABPA) and bronchiectasis are also complications.

Prevention of Recurrence

It is important to avoid known allergens which can be identified. In case of some allergens like house dust and pollen, desensitization can be achieved by repeated challenges (*See* Immunotherapy on page 991 for details).

Inhaled corticosteroids: 200–800 mg per day has been recommended as the treatment of choice for regular preventive therapy of asthma.

Long-acting inhaled β_2-agonists: As explained earlier, LABA act as preventer therapy for asthma attacks.

Chromones: A group of nonsteroidal anti-inflammatory medications. Administered as an inhalation, they prevent IgE-mediated mediator release from the mast cells. Sodium cromoglycate or nedocromil sodium may be used as preventive therapy in mild persistent asthma. Administered as a prophylaxis, these formulations inhibit allergen-induced airflow limitation after exposure to exercise, cold dry air and sulfur dioxide. Therapy has to be continued for 4–6 weeks to determine its efficacy in individual patient. Usual dose of sodium cromoglycate is 20 mg every 6 hours. This drug should not be used during an acute attack since it may cause aggravation of the symptoms.

Anti-IgE treatment—omalizumab: It prevents asthma attacks through cytokine modulation.

Anti-IL-5 treatment—mepolizumab: It is a monoclonal antibody against IL-5. It is effective in reducing the eosinophilic inflammation, thereby reduces the dose of corticosteroids. It is administered as a monthly infusion of 750 mg each for 5 months. Mepolizumab is generally safe, and reduces exacerbation rates in selecting patients with asthma who have the severe, refractory, eosinophilic subtype.

Anti-IL-4 treatment—dupilumab: It is a monoclonal antibody for the treatment of atopic diseases. It binds to the alpha subunit of the IL-4 receptor, and modulates signaling of both the IL-4 and IL-13 pathway. It induces significant reduction in asthma exacerbations in patients with moderate to severe allergic asthma.

Leukotriene modifiers such as montelukast (4–10 mg) are useful as a preventive therapy for asthma.

Ketotifen: Antiallergic H_1-antagonists have mast-cell stabilizing properties. Ketotifen, when given in a dose of 1 mg twice a day as oral tablets on a long-term basis, reduces asthmatic paroxysms due to its inhibitory effects on the allergic response. It also helps to reduce the severity of allergic diseases of the eyes, nose and lungs. Its effects are fully established only when the drug is given regularly for 2 months or more. Sedation and weight gain are the prominent side effects of ketotifen.

Systemic steroid-sparing therapies: They include immunomodulators and macrolides. Examples include rheumatoid arthritis, methotrexate, cyclosporine, and gold. Their potential steroid-sparing effect may not outweigh the risk of serious side effects. IV immunoglobulin has been shown to have some steroid-sparing effect, but this treatment is very expensive and has a high-frequency of adverse effects.

Other modalities of prevention: Respiratory and other systemic infections should receive prompt attention. The appropriate antibiotic should be selected, based on microbiological tests. Tranquilizers, psychotherapy or suggestion under hypnosis may be useful adjuncts in persons with prominent emotional overlay. Yoga and controlled breathing exercises are of considerable benefit in allaying the paroxysms in selected set of patients.

Points to Remember

Bronchial asthma is a very common disease. It may be mistaken for cardiac failure, hysterical hyperventilation or metabolic acidosis. Correct diagnosis and institution of emergency management in acute severe asthma is absolutely essential to save life. The common mistake committed by patients, and doctors is to overlook the seriousness and emergency that can be caused by acute severe asthma.

EXTRINSIC ALLERGIC ALVEOLITIS

This is a group of disorders caused by the inhalation of organic dusts (Table 143.7). These organic substances induce a diffuse immune complex reaction in the walls of alveoli and bronchioles, leading to bronchiolo-alveolitis.

Clinically all these disorders cause dyspnea and systemic disturbances such as headache, muscle pain, fever and malaise within a few hours of exposure to the antigen. Physical examination may reveal wheeze and end-inspiratory crepitations. X-ray of the chest may reveal diffuse small nodular shadows, predominantly involving the upper lobes (Fig. 143.4). HRCT thorax shows bilateral consolidation (Fig. 143.5). Pulmonary function studies

Table 143.7: Some common types of bronchioloalveolitis

Condition	Source
Farmer's lung	Mouldy hay, straw and grain dust
Bagassosis	Sugarcane dust
Byssinosis	Cotton dust
Mushroom worker's lung	Mushroom compost
Malt worker's lung	Mouldy barley, malt dust
Maple bark stripper's lung	Mouldy bark
Bird fancier's lung	Bird's droppings
Cheese worker's lung	Mouldy cheese

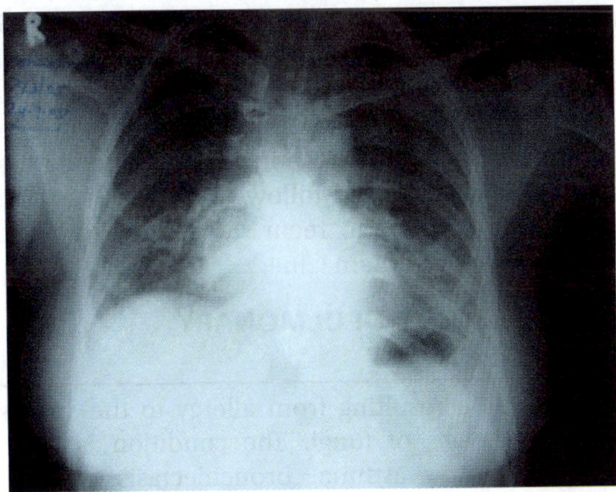

Fig. 143.4: Chest X-ray: Extrinsic allergic alveolitis. **Note:** Bilateral defuse opacities lower zones

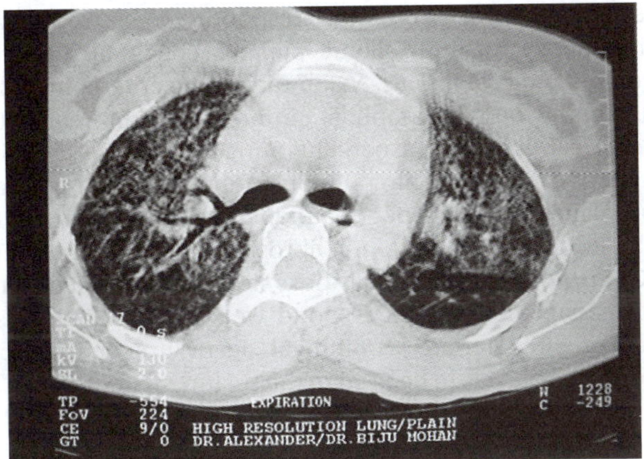

Fig. 143.5: High-resolution computed tomography (HRCT) extrinsic allergic alveolitis. **Note:** The diffuse thickening of the interalveolar septa and honeycombing

show restrictive ventilatory defect with normal FEV1/FVC ratio. Avoidance of the allergen causes relief of symptoms and recovery in the early stages, but in advanced cases the symptoms continue. Diffuse pulmonary interstitial fibrosis develops in those cases, where exposure to the antigen continues. Further, complications include pulmonary hypertension and cor pulmonale.

Treatment consists of avoidance of the allergen and bronchodilators. In acute cases, oral prednisolone 40 mg per day is indicated for 3–4 weeks, along with oxygen supplementation for hypoxemic patients.

Apart from these well-defined conditions, several forms of extrinsic allergic alveolitis occur in different occupational groups, e.g. coir workers, cashew workers, workers in godowns and others.

TROPICAL PULMONARY EOSINOPHILIA

Syn: Weingarten's syndrome, Pulmonary eosinophiliosis

This common disease of the tropics is an immune hyper-response to filarial infection. It is characterized by an absolute eosinophil count of 2,000/mm³ or more in peripheral blood, pulmonary symptoms and radiological changes, fever, dyspnea and loss of weight. The disease is prevalent in India, Sri Lanka, Malaysia, Pakistan, Bangladesh and several other tropical countries.

Etiology

Current evidence suggests that eosinophilia is an allergic reaction to helminthic parasites, particularly filarial worms. It is considered to be an immunologically mediated response to lymphatic filariasis in India. The role of filarial worms in the causation of tropical eosinophilia is suggested by several epidemiological, histopathological and serological studies (*See* also Section 6, Ch 70).

A constant and characteristic feature of TPE is peripheral blood eosinophilia (2,000–50,000 cells/mm³) in the presence of circulating filarial antibodies. A rapid response to diethylcarbamazine or positive serology will be diagnostic. If TPE goes untreated, there may be progression to chronic pulmonary fibrosis.

Pathology

Microscopically, the lesion consists of inflammatory cell infiltration of several tissues. Lymphocytes and histiocytes are the initial invaders, later to be replaced by eosinophils. Lung biopsy shows an eosinophilic bronchitis, and bronchopneumonia, with multiple small granulomas, and areas of necrosis. Foreign body giant cells form tubercle-like nodules, surrounded by mononuclear cells. The extent of lesion is related to the duration of the disorder. While intact microfilaria are not generally seen, there may be fragments in the granulomas. The histological changes are not pathognomonic for tropical eosinophilia, since similar lesions may result from allergy to several other allergens.

Clinical Features

The onset is insidious and the patients may come for treatment with several months history. Males are affected more than females. The severity of symptoms does not correlate with the eosinophil counts. Many patients with high eosinophil counts may remain asymptomatic. In some cases, the onset may be acute resembling influenza, bronchial asthma or gastrointestinal disturbances. Patients may present with severe breathlessness, and nocturnal paroxysmal cough, accompanied by little sputum production. There is often a low-grade fever with occasional hemoptysis. Extrapulmonary manifestations occur in about 15% of patients and include splenomegaly, hepatomegaly and lymphadenopathy. Blood samples show eosinophilia. No microfilaria is seen in peripheral blood. High-IgE levels, seropositivity to filarial antibody and rapid clinical improvement with administration of diethylcarbamazine are the hallmarks of TPE.

The chronic form may present with exertional dyspnea, vague ill-health or asthmatic symptoms. Auscultation over the chest may show rhonchi with crepitations. Some cases present with fever, loss of weight, generalized lymphadenopathy, splenomegaly and bleeding tendencies. The absolute eosinophil count ranges from 2,000 to 10,000/mm³. In some cases the total leukocyte count may go as high as 30–40,000/mm³, and the eosinophils may form 70–90% of the total. All of them are mature eosinophils. The bone marrow shows infiltration by eosinophils, and their precursors. If TPE goes untreated, there may be progression to chronic pulmonary fibrosis. Vast majority of cases are self-limiting and symptoms subside.

Skiagram of the chest reveals diffuse fine mottling with nodules 2–3 mm in size bilaterally in about 50% of cases.

Miliary nodules or nonsegmental, patchy opacities may be seen. Rarely, the radiological features may be unilateral.

Diagnosis

Tropical eosinophilia should be suspected in all cases of respiratory disorders presenting with asthmatic symptoms of short duration. An absolute eosinophil count above 2,000/mm³ is essential for making the diagnosis. Many patients show impaired lung function with reduction of vital capacity, total lung function and residual volume. Some show combination of restrictive and obstructive features.

Tropical eosinophilia has to be distinguished from other parasitic infections, which cause lower degrees of eosinophilia, Löffler's syndrome, aspergillosis, allergic alveolitis, bronchial asthma and pulmonary tuberculosis. In bronchial asthma too, the eosinophils may be increased but the counts seldom reach the levels seen in tropical eosinophilia. Helminthic infections also cause moderate eosinophilia. These may be associated with respiratory symptoms. In these cases, eosinophilia clears up with deworming. Löffler's syndrome is the allergic respiratory features occurring during larval migration.

The course of tropical eosinophilia is benign with remission and exacerbation extending over several months or years. Death is rare, though a few cases have been reported.

Treatment

Drug of choice is diethylcarbamazine in a dose of 4–12 mg/kg/day for 10–14 days. In most of the cases the eosinophil count and symptoms subside promptly. Side effects are mild. These may include headache, joint pains, anorexia, nausea, and vomiting. In a few cases, there may be slight aggravation of respiratory symptoms at the start of treatment. Such cases respond to bronchodilators or corticosteroids. Prolonged follow-up is necessary, since the condition is likely to recur. Relapses also respond promptly to diethylcarbamazine.

ALLERGIC BRONCHOPULMONARY ASPERGILLOSIS

It is a condition resulting from allergy to the spores of *Aspergillus* species of fungi. The condition is seen as a complication in asthma, bronchiectasis and cystic fibrosis. ABPA causes airway inflammation, leading to bronchiectasis. Clinical features are shortness of breath, coughing and wheezing. Chest X-ray shows pulmonary infiltrates, which do not respond to conventional treatment of asthma. Some patients cough up brown-colored plugs of mucus. Major diagnostic criteria include asthma, blood eosinophilia, immediate skin reactivity and/or antibodies to aspergillus antigen, raised serum IgE, history of radiographic pulmonary opacities and central bronchiectasis. If proper treatment is not instituted, ABPA can lead to permanent lung fibrosis. In the management, ICS are not useful. Oral high-dose steroids are the mainstay of management. ABPA respond well to glucocorticoids. Along with steroids, antifungal agent itraconazole or voriconazole has to be used in the treatment of ABPA.

CHAPTER

144

Diseases of the Lower Airways

C Sudheendra Ghosh, Davis Paul

Chapter Summary

- Acute Bronchitis
- Chronic Obstructive Pulmonary Disease
  - Pathogenesis
  - Diagnosis
  - Treatment
  - Acute Exacerbations of COPD
- Bronchiectasis
- Emphysema
- Alpha-1 Antitrypsin Deficiency
- Pulmonary Collapse

ACUTE BRONCHITIS

This is an acute inflammation of the bronchi and its ramifications. This is characterized by cough, discomfort behind the sternum, scanty expectoration to start with, later developing productive cough. In healthy individuals, the infective agents are viral to start with later bacteriae such as *Pneumococcus* or *Haemophilus influenzae* may complicate the picture. At this time, the sputum becomes purulent. In patients with underlying disease such as chronic bronchitis and emphysema, and in heavy smokers bacterial superinfection is the rule. Physical examination of the chest reveals wheeze and at times scattered crepitations.

In otherwise healthy subjects, the disease subsides in 1–2 weeks with simple therapy with analgesics, expectorants and simple antibiotics such as ampicillin and azithromycin. In those with underlying parenchymal diseases, the primary condition is exacerbated and recovery is much slower.

CHRONIC OBSTRUCTIVE PULMONARY DISEASE

Chronic obstructive pulmonary disease (COPD) is defined as a disease state characterized by airflow limitation that is not fully reversible. COPD includes *emphysema*, an anatomically defined condition characterized by destruction and hyperinflation of the lung alveoli,

chronic bronchitis, a clinically defined condition with hypersecretion of mucus sufficient to cause cough and sputum on most days for at least 3 months in a year for 2 or more consecutive years, and ***small airways disease***, a condition in which small bronchioles are narrowed. The airflow limitation is usually both progressive and associated with an abnormal inflammatory response of the lungs to noxious particles or gases. COPD is a disease of increasing frequency and estimates suggest that COPD will rise from the sixth to the third most common cause of death worldwide by 2020. The ***Global Initiative for Chronic Obstructive Lung Disease (GOLD)*** was created to increase awareness of COPD among health professionals, public health authorities, and the general public, and to improve prevention and management through a concerted worldwide effort.

GOLD criteria has defined COPD as a preventable and treatable disease with some significant extrapulmonary effects that may contribute to the severity in patients. Its pulmonary component is characterized by airflow limitation that is not fully reversible.

In the initial stage, the inflammation of the bronchi is intermittent and recurrent, later it becomes established. The larger air passages are affected during the early part of the disease, later obstructive features set in when the smaller airways are also affected. Infection leads to periodic aggravation of the symptoms and the sputum which is mucoid and becomes purulent during these episodes. As the airways obstruction progresses, emphysema sets in. These two processes become established in majority of cases so that the condition is termed ***chronic bronchitis emphysema syndrome*** (CBES). The disease is more common in damp, cold and dusty regions. Atmospheric pollution is accompanied by a higher incidence of COPD.

The most important risk factor for COPD is cigarette smoking. Pipe, cigar and other types of tobacco-smoking popular in many countries are also risk factors for COPD. Passive exposure to cigarette smoke also contributes to respiratory symptoms and COPD.

Other documented causes of COPD include occupational dusts and chemicals (vapors, irritants and fumes) when the exposures are sufficiently intense or prolonged. Indoor air pollution from biomass fuel used for cooking and heating in poorly ventilated dwellings and outdoor air pollution, which adds to the lungs' total burden of inhaled particles, although their specific role in causing COPD is not well understood.

Symptoms of COPD

- Cough
- Sputum production
- Dyspnea on exertion.

Episodes of acute worsening of these symptoms often occur. Chronic cough and sputum production often precede the development of airflow limitation by many years, although not all individuals with cough and sputum production go on to develop COPD.

Pathogenesis

COPD is a descriptive term given to the syndrome seen mostly in the elderly, who have airflow obstruction, not completely relieved by therapy. At least three distinct pathological processes may occur concurrently or separately in different subjects lead to COPD. These are:

- Emphysema which is due to destruction of alveolar walls
- Chronic bronchitis with hypersecretion of mucus
- Asthma with airway remodeling.

COPD disease encompasses chronic obstructive bronchitis with obstruction of small airways and emphysema with enlargement of air spaces, destruction of lung parenchyma, and loss of lung elasticity and closure of small airways.

The inflammatory process in COPD differs from that in asthma in several ways. The type of inflammatory cells, inflammatory mediators, final outcome and response to treatment are different. In COPD, the inflammation affects the peripheral airways, the bronchioles. The cells are macrophages, CD8 lymphocytes and neutrophils. The lung parenchyma is affected. Unlike as in asthma, there is no preponderance of eosinophils.

Oxidative stress also plays a significant role in the pathogenesis. Even though the lungs bear the main brunt of the disease, systemic effects also occur. Muscle weakness and wasting may develop as part of the systemic disorder.

Pathology

The bronchial mucosa shows hypertrophy and increase in the mucous glands and goblet cells with consequent overproduction of viscid mucus. The distal airways show narrowing of lumen caused by increased height of the epithelium, and increased thickness of the muscle and connective tissue. The mucosa becomes ulcerated and when the ulcers heal, fibrosis occurs resulting in distortion of the lumen with stenosis and dilatation.

Distortion of the airways leads to permanent obstruction. Secondary infection occurs in the later stages. The ciliary movement is further impaired by the abnormally viscid mucus. This aggravates infection and a vicious cycle is established.

Infections in COPD

Viral and bacterial infections contribute to exacerbation of COPD. With increasing obstruction to airflow, frequency of infection increases. More than 50% of infections are due to bacteriae, *Haemophilus influenzae, Streptococcus pneumonia* and *Moraxella catarrhalis*. In severe cases, *Pseudomonas aeruginosa* precipitates exacerbation. Viral infection occurs in 10–15% during the stable and 30–60% during the exacerbated phases. Most common viruses are rhinoviruses and influenza virus.

Severe recurrent infections cause development of microabscesses in the bronchial wall, heal with fibrosis. Squamous metaplasia occurs. Distortion and obstruction of the bronchial lumen result in air trapping and emphysema of the alveoli, some show collapse and fibrosis. The main pathological process can be summarized as follows:

- Inflammation of the bronchi with enlargement of mucous glands and smooth muscle hyperplasia, all leading to wall thickening

- Acinar distension due to the destruction of lung parenchyma probably mediated by imbalance of protease-antiprotease (alpha-1 antitrypsin) enzymes causing loss of support of small airways
- Fibrosis and narrowing of the airways leading to increase in airway resistance.

The capillary bed is distorted and truncated and this aggravates progression of pulmonary arterial hypertension (PAH). The pulmonary arteries become distended and atheromatous. Pulmonary hypertension gives rise to right ventricular hypertrophy and dilatation. Chronic cor pulmonale supervenes as time passes. The forced expiratory volume 1 (FEV1) declines at the rate of 33.2 mL/year in patients with COPD. It can be as high as 64 mL/year in severe cases.

Clinical Features

The clinical picture is varied depending on the severity and duration. The most frequent early symptom is cough recurring year after year, especially so in winter months. Later the cough becomes constant. Expectoration is mucoid and the sputum is tenacious, especially on waking up in the morning. Main complaint is feeling of tightness of the chest. *Physical examination* reveals mild wheeze which disappears as the patient clears the bronchi by expectoration. Variable degrees of bilateral rhonchi and coarse crepitations are heard as adventitious sounds. Initially, acute infections give rise to fever and purulent sputum. As the infection becomes established, fever and other general symptoms come down. At this stage, the quantity and character of the sputum are more reliable indicators of infection. The sputum becomes copious in amount when bronchiectatic changes develop.

With the development of emphysema, the chest assumes the inspiratory position and the respiratory excursions are considerably diminished. At this stage, dyspnea is far out of proportion to the physical findings in the chest.

Co-morbidities in COPD

Among the extrapulmonary manifestations, severe skeletal muscle dysfunction is common. This manifests as muscle wasting out of proportion to any neurological cause and extreme weakness. This is taken care of by ensuring adequate nutrition, attention to pulmonary disease and physiotherapy undertaken by a trained team. Exercise programs including, endurance exercises, such as cycling, walking, treadmill and the like produce benefit.

Other than skeletal muscle wasting, comorbidities include cachexia, pulmonary hypertension, ischemic heart disease (IHD), endothelial dysfunction, congestive heart failure (CHF), osteoporosis, normocytic anemia, type 2 diabetes mellitus (DM) and metabolic syndrome. Lung cancer, both small cell and non-small cell types occur more frequently in them.

Key Indicators for Considering the Diagnosis of COPD

Chronic cough: Present intermittently or every day. Often present throughout the day; seldom only nocturnal

Chronic sputum: Any pattern of chronic sputum production may indicate COPD

Acute bronchitis: Repeated episodes

Dyspnea: Progressive (worsens overtime)
- Persistent (present everyday)
- Worse on exercisex
- Worse during respiratory infections.

History of exposure to tobacco smoke (including risk factors–popular local preparations): Occupational dusts and chemicals and smoke from home cooking and heating fuel.

Diagnosis

COPD should be diagnosed from history of recurrent cough extending over several years, mucopurulent sputum and physical findings of bronchial obstruction and emphysema. X-ray is normal in the early stages, but features of emphysema may be evident later. X-ray may be helpful in identifying precipitating conditions like pneumonia, pneumothorax during the time of an exacerbation. High resolution computed tomography (HRCT) is useful in quantifying the severity of emphysematous changes and locating areas with bronchiectatic changes. Lung function tests show reduction in vital capacity, increase in the closing volume and features of airway obstruction.

Assessment of COPD

The goals of COPD assessment are to determine the severity of the disease, its impact on patient's health status and risk of future adverse disease events in order to guide therapy (Fig. 144.1). The following aspects are assessed separately:

- Symptoms—by validated COPD assessment test (CAT) or clinical COPD questionnaire (CCQ)
- Degree of airflow limitation [using spirometry (Table 144.1).
- *Risk of exacerbations:* Best predictor is previous treatment events like hospitalization
- *Co-morbidities:* Cardiovascular disease (CVD), DM, depression, skeletal muscle dysfunction and lung cancer.

Based on the spirometry values, severity of obstruction can be categorized as mild, moderate severe and very severe (Table 144.1).

Combined Assessment of COPD

Symptoms
- Less symptoms (mMRC 0–1 or CAT< 10): Patient is (A or (C)
- More symptoms (mMRC > 2 or CAT > 10): Patient is (B) or (D)

Airflow limitation
- Low risk (GOLD 1 or 2): Patient is (A) or (B)
- High risk (GOLD 3 or 4): Patient is (C) or (D)

Exacerbations
- Low risk: < 1 per year and no hospitalization for exacerbation: Patient is (A) or (B)
- High risk: > 2 per year or > 1 with hospitalization: Patient is (C) or (D)

Note: Combining above assessments will improve COPD management.

Differential diagnosis: Chronic bronchitis has to be distinguished from asthma. Differentiation is easy in the early stages, but there is considerable overlap of symptoms and signs in the advanced stages, and therefore, the clinical assessment is difficult.

Other conditions like pulmonary tuberculosis, bronchiectasis, heart failure and bronchogenic carcinoma,

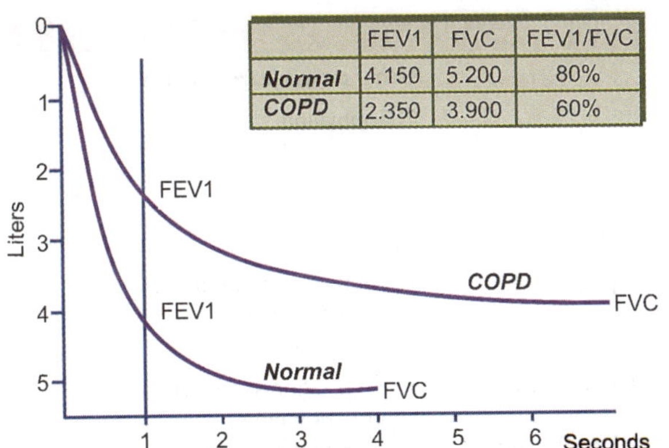

	FEV1	FVC	FEV1/FVC
Normal	4.150	5.200	80%
COPD	2.350	3.900	60%

Fig. 144.1: Example of spirometric tracings and calculation of FEV1. FEV1/FVC ratio in normal and COPD

Table 144.1:	Classification of severity of airflow limitation in (based on postbrochodilator FEV1)	
In patients with FEV1/FVC < 0.70		
GOLD 1	Mild	FEV1 > 80% predicted
GOLD 2	Moderate	50% < FEV1 < 80% predicted
GOLD 3	Severe	30% < FEV1 < 50% predicted
GOLD 4	Very severe	FEV1 < 30% predicted

obliterative bronchiolitis, diffuse panbronchiolitis have to be ruled out in atypical cases.

Course and prognosis: Established chronic bronchitis is incurable. Over several years, the condition progresses to produce complications and death. Each infective exacerbation leads to further deterioration in lung function and precipitates the development of respiratory failure and cor pulmonale. Exacerbation can occur as a result of bacterial infection of the lower respiratory passages, viral infections of the respiratory tract or due to non-infective causes such as environmental allergens and pollutants.

Complications

These include:

- Frequent respiratory infections
- Respiratory failure
- Right-sided heart failure (cor pulmonale)
- ***Mucopurulent relapses:*** It may develop due to secondary bacterial infection by *S. pneumoniae, H. influenzae* or *M. catarrhalis*. Presents with fever and increased production of purulent sputum.
- ***Carbon dioxide narcosis:*** Persistent retention of CO_2 (hypercarbic: high $PaCO_2$) manifests as clouding of consciousness, altered behavior, drowsiness, headache and papilledema.
- ***Respiratory failure***
  - ***Type I respiratory failure (low PaO_2 normal $PaCO_2$):*** Mild to moderate COPD.
  - ***Type II respiratory failure:*** Acute or chronic in severe COPD.
  - ***Features:*** Deep cyanotic, edemas and stupor with respiratory failure.
- ***Secondary polycythemia:*** Due to hypoxemia which stimulating erythropoiesis.
- ***Pulmonary hypertension and right ventricular failure (cor pulmonale):*** Pulmonary hypertension →

chronic afterload on the right ventricle → right ventricular hypertrophy → right ventricular failure and cor pulmonale.

Management

General measures: Most effective single step to prevent deterioration is to stop smoking. This single measure itself affords considerable relief of symptoms. Flu vaccination and pneumococcal vaccinations are useful in preventing infective exacerbations. Environmental allergens and pollutants must be avoided by the patient.

Other general measures include improvement in general health, regular exercise, deep-breathing exercises, adequate sleep, treatment of obesity and eradication of foci of sepsis in the throat, nose and paranasal sinuses. If these measures are started during the early phase of the disease, further progression can be arrested.

Apart from the general measures, no active treatment is indicated in the early stages (Box 144.1).

Treatment of COPD

Only three interventions namely; smoking cessation, oxygen therapy and lung volume reduction surgery (LVRS) in selected patients have been found to influence the natural history of patients with COPD. Current therapies are directed at improving symptoms and decreasing the frequency and severity of exacerbations (Table 144.2).

The institution of these therapies should involve combined assessment as shown above.

Smoking cessation: It has been found to improve the rate of decline in pulmonary function in middle-aged smokers. Conventional smoking cessation therapy can be combined with pharmacotherapy using bupropion, nicotine replacement therapy (NRT) or varenicline (Refer Section 14, Ch 150).

Bronchodilators: Used for symptomatic relief in COPD. The inhaled route is preferred.

β-agonists: The use of short-acting bronchodilators such as salbutamol or long-acting β-agonist like salmeterol are found to be effective when combined with inhaled steroids.

Anticholinergic agents: Ipratropium bromide is an anticholinergic muscarine receptor blocker, which blocks vagal reflexes, responsible for bronchoconstriction. It is indicated when bronchospasm is troublesome. Ipratropium

Box 144.1:	Therapies improving symptoms and decreasing the frequency and severity of exacerbations

- β₂-agonists
  - Short-acting β₂-agonists (SABA)
  - Long-acting β₂-agonists (LABA)
- Anticholinergic/muscarinic antagonists
  - Short-acting muscarinic antagonists (SAMA)
  - Long-acting antagonists antagonists (LAMA)
- Combination of short-acting β₂-agonists + anticholinergic in one inhaler
- Methylxanthines
- Inhaled corticosteroids (ICS)
- Combination of long-acting β₂-agonists + corticosteroids in one inhaler
- Systemic corticosteroids
- Phosphodiesterase-4 inhibitors

Table 144.2: Pharmacologic therapy for stable COPD

Patient group	Recommended first choice	Alternative choice	Other possible treatments
A	SA anticholinergic prn or SA β_2-agonist prn	LA anicholinergic or LA β_2-agonist or SA β_2-agonist and SA anticholinergic	Theophylline
B	LA anicholinergic or LA β_2-agonist	LA anicholinergic and LA β_2-agonist	• SA β_2-agonist and/or SA anticholinergic • Theophylline
C	ICS + LA anicholinergic or LA β_2-agonist	LA anicholinergic and LA β_2-agonist or LA anicholinergic and PDE-4 inhibitor or LA β_2-agonist and PDE-4 inhibitor	• SA β_2-agonist and/or SA anticholinergic • Theophylline
D	ICS + LA anicholinergic and/or LA β_2-agonist	ICS + LA anicholinergic and LA β_2-agonist or ICS + LA β_2-agonist and PDE-4 inhibitor or LA anicholinergic and LA β_2-agonist or LA anicholinergic and PDE-4 inhibitor	• Carbocysteine • SA β_2-agonist and/or SA anticholinergic • Theophylline

Abbreviations: SA = Short-acting; LA = Long-acting; ICS = Inhaled corticosteroid; PDE-4 = Phosphodiesterase-4; prn = when necessary

bromide delivered by a metered dose inhaler (MDI) in a dose of 40–80 µg 6–8 hours helps to relieve bronchospasm without appreciable side effects. In COPD, response of the airways to ipratropium is excellent. Tiotropium is a newer long-acting analogue that can be given once daily by inhaler at a dose of 18 µg. It is superior to ipratropium and is considered as the best bronchodilator in COPD.

Inhaled glucocorticoids: Inhaled corticosteroids have been found to be useful in reducing frequent exacerbation in COPD.

Theophylline: It found to produce modest improvement in lung function and blood gas levels in COPD.

Inhibitors of inflammatory response: Since inflammation plays a major role in the pathogenesis of COPD newer pharmacological agents are under trial. These include mediator antagonists which are capable of counteracting the effects of leukotrienes, lipoxygenases, interleukin B, tumor necrosis factor (TNF) and the like. Other group of drugs includes protease inhibitors which inhibit neutrophil elastases, cathepsin and anti-inflammatory agents such as phosphodiesterase inhibitors. Several newer drugs especially phosphodiesterase-4 (PDE-4) inhibitors are under trial. Roflumilast is a drug of this class given in a dose on 250 or 500 mg orally daily for 24 weeks. Results are encouraging.

Use of N-acetylcysteine, bromhexine hydrochloride, dornase alpha or 7% hyper tonic saline are given as aerosols to liquefy the sputum. N-acetylcysteine and bromhexine hydrochloride given orally thrice daily also help to loosen the sputum and clear the airway. Steam inhalations help to open up the airways and improve vital capacity.

Treatment of infective episodes: A broad spectrum antibiotic should be employed for 7–10 days during an infective episode. Azithromycin or β-lactum agents may be started initially. Depending on the microbiological tests, the antibiotic may have to be changed.

Commonly used formulations of bronchodilator drugs are explained in Table 143.3.

Nonpharmacological measures—management of COPD is according to the individualized assessment of the symptoms and exacerbation as shown in Table 144.4.

Annual influenza vaccination and 1–2 doses of pneumococcal vaccination during the patient's lifetime help to prevent fatal infections.

Oxygen therapy: Long-term oxygen therapy (LTOT) in patients with chronic respiratory failure has shown improved survival with better quality of life. It is indicated if PaO_2 is below 55 mm Hg or oxygen saturation measured by pulse oxymetry (SpO_2) is below 88% during the stable state at rest. Here oxygen has to be used at least 18 hours per day. Oxygen therapy helps to reduce pulmonary hypertension and allay cor pulmonale. Noninvasive positive pressure ventilation (NIPPV) can be tried at home to improve the respiratory failure. Twelve to eight hours of continuous oxygen inhalation, especially during sleep in order to raise the oxygen saturation to 90% or more improves the quality of life. Maintenance of arterial oxygen saturation at 90–93% has been recommended by National Institute of Clinical Excellence (NICE), UK. NIPPV can improve ventilation without endotracheal intubation. It is commonly used in managing respiratory failure associated with acute exacerbation of COPD.

Pulmonary rehabilitation: Structured program of education and exercises is very effective. Blowing into an air pillow repeatedly for 10–15 times twice a day and bending over a pillow held firmly on to the abdomen, in order to push the diaphragm up during expiration are simple maneuvers which can be practiced at home.

Lung volume reduction surgery (LVRS): This has been found to be useful in selected cases. The rationale for this technique is to reduce the volume of overinflated emphysematous lung by 20–30%, in order to improve the

Table 144.3: Commonly used formulations of bronchodilator drugs

Drug	Metered dose inhaler (µg)	Nebulizer (µg)	Oral (µg)	Duration of action (µg) (hours)
β_2-agonists				
Fenoterol	100–200	0.5–2.0	–	4–6
Salbutamol (albuterol)	100–200	2.5–5.0	4	4–6
Terbutaline	250–500	5–10	5	4–6
Formoterol	12–24		–	12+
Salmeterol	50–100		–	12+
Anticholinergics				
Tiotropium	18			
Ipratropium bromide	40–80	0.25–0.5	–	6–8
Oxitropium bromide	200		–	7–9
Methylxanthines				
Aminophyline (SR)	–	–	225–450	Variable, up to 24
Theophylline (SR)	–	–	100–400	Variable, up to 24

Table 144.4: Nonpharmacologic management of chronic obstructive pulmonary disease

Patient group	Essential	Recommended	Depending on local guidelines
A	• Smoking cessation (can include pharmacologic treatment)	Physical activity	• Influenza vaccination • Pneumococcal vaccination
B, C, D	• Smoking cessation (can include pharmacologic treatment) • Pulmonary rehabilitation	Physical activity	• Influenza vaccination • Pneumococcal vaccination

elastic recoil of the lungs, to improve the configuration of the diaphragm, chest wall mechanics and gas exchange.

Lung transplantation: This procedure is in vogue for more than a decade in advanced countries; it is still not available in India. Transplantation of a single lung or both heart and lungs as a whole is possible. Transplantation should be considered if the recipient is below 55 years of age, and is free from underlying conditions such as advanced diabetes, malignancy, hepatic or renal failure and conditions which impair mechanics of the chest wall.

The donor should be air-breathing organ (ABO) and human leukocyte antigen (HLA) compatible with normal lungs, preferably between 12 and 50 years of age and with normal cardiopulmonary anatomy. Usually, cadaver lungs are used for transplantation. Complications may occur as in the case of any other major organ transplantation.

Indications for Lung Transplantation

- ***Incurable respiratory failure:*** Chronic or acute due to pulmonary causes

- Irreversible structural and functional abnormalities in the lung such as fibrosis, extensive bronchiectasis, cystic disease, emphysema and others.

Acute Exacerbations of COPD

Indications for hospital assessment or admission for acute exacerbation of chronic obstructive pulmonary disease (COPD)

- Marked increase in intensity of symptoms, such as sudden development of resting dyspnea
- Severe background COPD
- Onset of new physical signs (e.g. cyanosis, peripheral edema)
- Failure of exacerbation to respond to initial medical management
- Significant comorbidities
- Newly occurring arrhythmias
- Diagnostic uncertainity
- Older age
- Insufficient home support.

Medical Research Council modified dyspnea scale for breathlessness during daily activities

- ***Grade 0:*** No breathlessness
- ***Grade 1:*** Breathless with strenuous exercise
- ***Grade 2:*** Short of breath when hurrying on the level or walking up a slight hill
- ***Grade 3:*** Walks slower than people of the same age on the level or stops for breathe while walking at own pace on the level
- ***Grade 4:*** Stops for breath after walking about 100 yards
- ***Grade 5:*** Too breathless to leave the house or breathless when dressing or undressing.

Hospital discharge criteria for patients with acute exacerbations of COPD

- Inhaled β_2-agonist therapy is required no more frequently than every 4 hours
- Patient, if previously ambulatory, is able to walk across the room
- Patient is able to eat and sleep without frequent awakening by dyspnea
- Patients have been clinically stable for 12–24 hours
- Arterial blood gases have been stable for 12–24 hours
- Patient (or home caregiver) fully understands correct use of medications
- Follow-up and home care arrangements have been complemented (e.g. visiting nurse, oxygen delivery and meal provisions)
- Patients, family and physician are confident patient can manage successfully.

Assessment of Bronchodilator Response

If there is an increase of at least 12% of the baseline FEV1 and 200 mL, it is considered as a sign of reversibility of airway obstruction (British Thoracic Society).

BRONCHIECTASIS

Permanent dilatation and distortion of the bronchi is called bronchiectasis.

Etiology and Pathogenesis

Most of the cases of bronchiectasis result from acquired causes.

- Obstruction to the bronchus due to any cause leads to distal collapse of the pulmonary segment. The pull on the bronchi by the collapsed alveoli leads to dilatation of the bronchi. In the initial stages, this is reversible, and the bronchi regain their normal size when the lung expands. If the obstruction persists, accumulation of mucus occurs distally, infection supervenes and the bronchial wall is destroyed permanently. This results in permanent dilatation. The infective organisms are *Streptococci*, *Pneumococci*, *Klebsiella* and *Anaerobes*.

- Bronchiectasis may follow several viral infections without passing through the obstructive phase.
- Primary ciliary dyskinesia (PCD) can lead to bronchiectasis. The classical example is **Kartagener's syndrome (KS)**, which is characterized by dextrocardia, situs inversus, sinusitis, and defects of ciliary function in the bronchi and non-motile sperms.
- Middle lobe bronchiectasis is a sequel to pulmonary tuberculosis. This is caused by obstruction to the middle lobe bronchus by tuberculosis glands. This is called **middle lobe syndrome** or **Brock's syndrome**.
- Congenital defects in bronchial wall can also lead to bronchiectasis, e.g. William-Campbell syndrome.

Pathophysiology

Bronchiectasis is primarily a disease of bronchi and bronchioles involving a vicious circle of transmural infection and inflammation with mediator release. Bronchial mucosa shows infiltration by neutrophils and T lymphocytes. The expectorated sputum has higher content of elastase and chemoattractants, interleukin-8, TNF-α and prostanoids. The lesions may be localized or diffuse and generalized.

Clinical Features

The clinical picture is very chronic, extending over several years. The common site of lesion is the left lower lobe. Though children may be affected, usually symptoms manifest in early adulthood or middle age. Males are affected more than females. Digital clubbing is a prominent sign, sometimes being associated with hypertrophic pulmonary osteoarthropathy (HPOA).

Postural cough with the production of large quantities of purulent and foul smelling sputum is the presenting complaint in most cases. On standing, the sputum settles into three layers as described under lung abscess. Hemoptysis may occur frequently. This may be mild or severe. Recurrent infections such as pneumonia may develop. Repeated affection of the same lobe or segment should suggest the possibility of underlying bronchiectasis. **Bronchiectasis sicca** is the condition in which the patients present with mild or severe hemoptysis without significant sputum production. This is common in bronchiectasis occurring in upper lobes as in tuberculosis.

Physical examination may reveal impairment of the percussion note and diminution of respiratory sounds over the affected area. The diagnostic finding is the presence of coarse and persistent leathery rales.

Complications

At times bronchiectasis may present with one of its complications. These include massive hemoptysis, recurrent pneumonia, emphysema, septicemia, brain abscess and cor pulmonale. Anemia develops in long-standing cases due to chronic sepsis and recurrent hemoptysis. In untreated cases secondary amyloidosis may develop.

Diagnosis

Bronchiectasis should be diagnosed by the long history, presence of clubbing, postural cough, coarse leathery rales over the affected part and reasonably normal general health. Once established, bronchiectasis is not curable by medical treatment.

Differential Diagnosis

Bronchiectasis should be distinguished from chronic bronchitis and emphysema, lung abscess, tuberculosis, congenital cystic disease of the lung, pulmonary sequestration, interstitial lung disease (ILD) and malignancy.

Lung abscess generally develops acutely. The right lower lobe is affected more often and the signs are localized. Tuberculosis is more common in the upper lobes and clubbing is not prominent in uncomplicated cases. Features like digital clubbing and copious sputum are seen in tuberculosis bronchiectasis. Cystic disease is not uncommon. All age groups are affected. A long history of recurrent respiratory disease is present in the majority of cases. Clubbing is not prominent. The cysts may be localized or generalized. Clinical distinction from bronchiectasis is difficult. Presence of cysts in other organs like the kidneys, liver, etc. suggests the probability of congenital cystic disease of the lung. X-ray reveals the presence of soap bubble-like or ring shadows (Fig. 144.2).

Pulmonary sequestration is a developmental anomaly where a portion of the lung receives aberrant blood supply usually from the abdominal aorta. Patient may present with recurrent hemoptysis and other features of bronchiectasis (Figs 144.3 and 144.4).

Diagnosis can be confirmed by bronchography which helps to determine the extent and type of bronchiectasis. The lesion may be cystic, saccular, cylindrical or varicose. Plain X-ray of the chest is not a reliable investigation to assess the site and extent of bronchiectasis. HRCT has become the investigation of choice to assess the lesions in bronchiectasis. Availability of HRCT has eliminated the need for bronchography.

Management

General measures include high protein diet, treatment of intercurrent infections and removal of focal sepsis from the upper respiratory tract.

Principles of specific therapy include postural drainage, administration of antibiotics, respiratory exercises and in selected cases, surgical excision. Postural drainage helps to clear the bronchi and bring about relief. The patient should be instructed to practice postural drainage regularly. This gives relief of cough and also the foul smell. The fetid odor of the sputum can be controlled by administering clindamycin and steam inhalations. In patients without foul smelling sputum, the choice of antibiotic is determined by microbiological studies. Intermittent antibiotic therapy is required to clear infection, and prevent exacerbation. The site of lesion may have to be excised, if medical treatment fails.

Indications for Surgery

- The disease is localized to one lung or one segment and is not amenable to medical therapy
- Socioeconomic factors such as noncompliance by the patient
- Uncontrollable hemoptysis in which the site of origin of blood may be detected by emergency bronchoscopy and surgical resection has to be planned

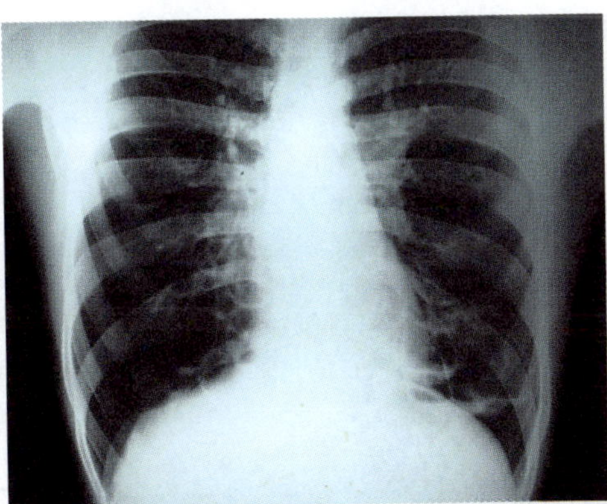

Fig. 144.2: Cystic bronchiectasis. ***Note:*** The cystic areas in both lower zones

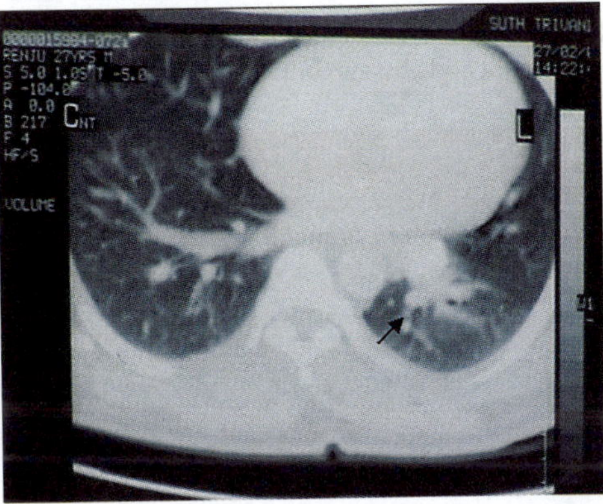

Fig. 144.3: Pulmonary sequestration HRCT. ***Note:*** The vascular anomaly at the site of sequestration (arrow)

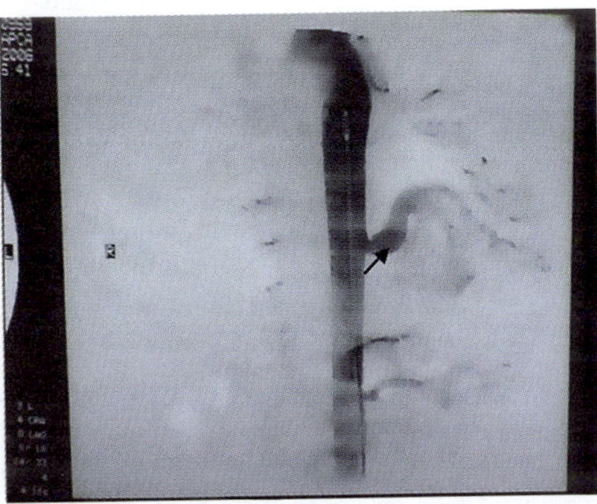

Fig. 144.4: Pulmonary sequestration. Aortogram showing aberrant arterial supply from thoracic aorta (arrow)

- To reduce the area of infection. Even in bilateral disease, sometimes surgical resection may have to be done on the more affected side, with a view to reduce the surface area of infection.
- To remove an obstructive lesion which tends to perpetuate the condition, e.g. bronchial growth or bronchostenosis.

EMPHYSEMA

Emphysema is defined as a pathological increase in the size of airspaces distal to the terminal bronchioles, with destruction of the alveolar walls. The term 'hyperinflation' is used to denote nonpathological overdistension.

Etiology

Diseases of the airways: Chronic bronchitis, prolonged exposure to irritants and dusts (heavy cigarette smoking), and chronic partial bronchial obstruction.

Conditions associated with α-1 antitrypsin deficiency: Persons who have α-1 antitrypsin deficiency develop emphysema by the third or fourth decade of life.

Chronic bronchial asthma leads on to emphysema as a sequel. Persons who have to hold breath for prolonged periods for diving underwater for collecting shells, clay and the like develop emphysema over a period of 15–20 years. *Bidi* or cigarette smoking and repeated respiratory infections accelerate the process.

Several pneumoconioses give rise to emphysema as part of the pathological process or as compensatory mechanism, e.g. coal worker's pneumoconiosis, silicosis.

Occupational causes: Several occupations which require forced expiratory effort as seen in furnace blowers, goldsmiths, and users of wind instruments predispose to the development of emphysema in susceptible subjects. Exposure to cadmium leads to the development of emphysema and pulmonary fibrosis.

Pathology

The lungs are in the inflated position occupying the whole of the pleural cavity. Since the elastic tissue is damaged, the lungs lose their elasticity and they fail to collapse when the chest is opened during autopsy. The diaphragm is depressed and respiratory excursions are diminished. The alveoli are overdistended. The septa rupture and neighboring alveoli coalesce to form air cysts. The pulmonary vascular bed is progressively diminished and PAH results. Reduction of alveolar surface area leads to impairment of gas exchange. Right ventricular hypertrophy and cor pulmonale may develop. Emphysematous bullae may rupture to produce spontaneous pneumothorax.

Clinical Features

The main symptom is exertional dyspnea. As the condition progresses, even ordinary activity like talking, eating or lying flat may cause dyspnea. The chest is distended in the position of full inspiration. Expansion is diminished and the accessory muscles of respiration are active. Expiration becomes an active process due to loss of elasticity of the lung. Infective episodes occur frequently.

Physical Examination

It reveals barrel-shaped chest with diminished expansion, hyper-resonance on percussion, obliteration of cardiac and liver dullness, and diminished breath sounds with prolonged expiration. Due to increased intrathoracic pressure especially during expiration, the neck veins become distended during expiration, and collapse during inspiration. The apex beat is felt feebly because of interposition of the distended lung. Right ventricular hypertrophy produces a heaving impulse in the epigastrium and subxiphoid region. Left parasternal heave may not be evident on account of the inflated lung covering the heart (Fig. 144.5).

Special Forms of Emphysema

Compensatory emphysema: This is a condition in which the normal lung tissue undergoes hyperinflation to com-

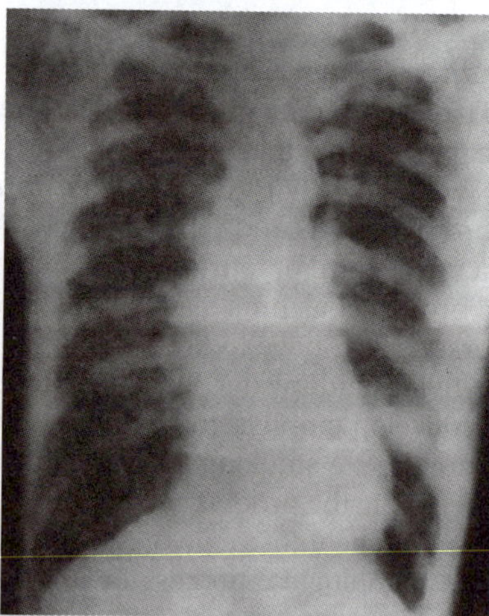

Fig. 144.5: Chest X-ray—emphysema. **Note:** Inflated position of the rib cage, lower level of the diaphragm and hypertranslucent lung fields

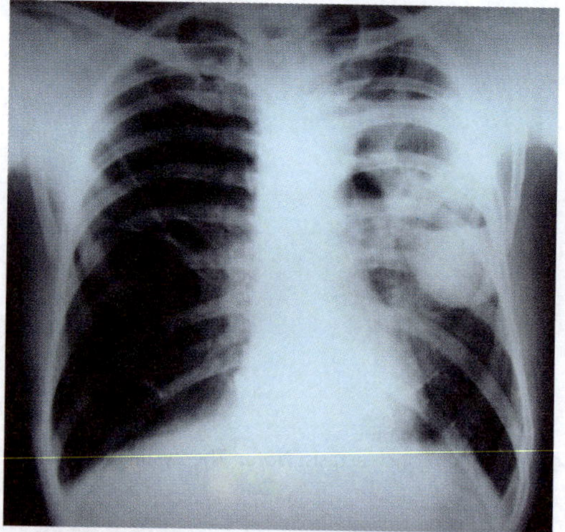

Fig. 144.6: Multiple bullae-infected. **Note:** Large thin walled cystic spaces on the right and abssess containing air and fluid in the left lung

pensate for extensive damage to the other lung or other parts of the same lung. Being a compensatory phenomenon, this is asymptomatic. The respiratory excursion of the normal lung is increased in this case.

Atrophic emphysema: This condition is the result of senile atrophy of interalveolar septa. The total lung volume is not increased.

Bullous emphysema: In this condition, air spaces exceeding 1 cm in diameter develop either congenitally or as a part of acquired generalized emphysema. With passage of time these enlarge bullae and become giant bullous emphysema. They may rupture to produce pneumothorax. At times the bullae may get infected to produce abscesses (Fig. 144.6).

Difference in clinical features between chronic bronchitis and emphysema is given in Table 144.5.

ALPHA-1 ANTITRYPSIN DEFICIENCY

Alpha-1 antitrypsin (α-1AT) is the one among the serine protein inhibitors which occurs in the plasma. It is an inhibitor of neutrophil elastase. It has also got anti-inflammatory properties. α-1AT is a glycoprotein normally secreted by the liver and circulating in blood. It moves with the α-1 band on serum protein electrophoresis. About 90% of the trypsin-inhibitory activity of serum is attributable to α-1AT.

From the plasma, α-1AT diffuses into lung tissues, where it acts as an anti-elastase, the elastase being secreted by neutrophils. Elastase is capable of destroying the connective tissue framework of alveolar walls. Excessive destruction of alveolar walls may lead to emphysema. Cigarette smoking which predisposes to accumulation of neutrophils in the lung aggravates the destructive process. Cigarette smoke also inhibits α-1AT directly. α-1AT deficiency may be congenital or acquired. The gene frequency of the defect occurs in 1 in 2,000 to 1 in 5,000 of the population. In the congenital form it is transmitted as an autosomal recessive. More than 75 alleles of α-1AT gene are known. In the inherited form the hepatic production of α-1AT is less than 15% of normal.

Patients with α-1AT deficiency develop panacinar emphysema by the third or fourth decade of life. The congenital form may also be associated with hepatitis and jaundice in the newborn, and cirrhosis liver in adults. Such patients show accumulation of abnormal α-1AT in hepatocytes.

α-1AT deficiency can be treated by replacing α-1AT by IV infusion weekly or monthly to individuals whose serum α-1AT levels are below 1 mmol/L and who have abnormal lung functions. α-1AT for therapeutic purposes is obtained from pooled plasma. α-1AT can also be administered as an aerosol.

Table 144.5: Difference in clinical features between chronic bronchitis and emphysema

Features	Chronic bronchitis	Emphysema
Cough	Frequent	With exertion
Sputum	Copious	Scant
Hematocrit	Elevated	Normal
PaCO$_2$	Often elevated (> 40)	Usually normal (< 40)
Chest radiograph	Increased lung markings	Hyperinflation
Elastic recoil	Normal	Decreased
Airway resistance	Increased	Normal to slightly increased
Cor pulmonale	Early	Late
Mechanism of airway obstruction	Decreased airway lumen due to mucus and inflammation	Loss of elastic recoil
Dyspnea	Moderate	Severe
FEV1	Decreased	Decreased
PaO$_2$	Marked decreased 'blue bloater'	Modest decrease 'pink puffer'
PaCO$_2$	Increased	Normal to decreased
Diffusing capacity	Normal	Decreased
Hematocrit	Increased	Normal
Cor pulmonale	Marked and early	Mild and late
Prognosis	Poor	variable

Abbreviations: PaCO$_2$ = Partial pressure of carbon dioxide in arterial blood; PaO$_2$ = Partial pressure of oxygen in arterial blood; FEV1 = Forced expiratory volume 1

PULMONARY COLLAPSE

When a portion of the lung becomes airless, it is termed collapse or atelectasis. Collapse may be present from birth, when a portion of the lung fails to expand. Acquired collapse is more common, and this is caused by absorption of air from a previously normal lung.

Causes

Obstruction to the air passages: The air passages may be obstructed by intraluminal or extraluminal causes.

- Foreign bodies which may be inhaled accidentally or aspirated by comatose patient
- Tumors of the bronchus—carcinoma, adenoma, bronchial stenosis
- Copious secretions and thick plugs of mucus
- Extrinsic pressure on the bronchus by lymph nodes, tumors, etc., e.g. middle lobe syndrome in pulmonary tuberculosis
- Pneumothorax and pleural effusion.

    In bronchial obstruction, the air already present in the alveoli is absorbed. The lobe or segment shrinks due to its inherent elastic recoil. Functional impairment depends upon the extent of lung tissue affected.

Clinical Features

Symptoms depend upon the extent of collapse and its onset. Acute lesions are more symptomatic than chronic ones. Small areas of atelectasis may be asymptomatic. Massive collapse gives rise to dyspnea with or without cyanosis. The movement of the affected side is reduced and the chest is flattened. Trachea and cardiac apex are shifted to the same side. Percussion note over the affected side is diminished. Breath sounds are absent or diminished. Adventitious sounds are usually absent.

Investigations

- ***Radiology:*** Skiagrams show the collapsed portion as homogenous opacities with sharp concave borders.

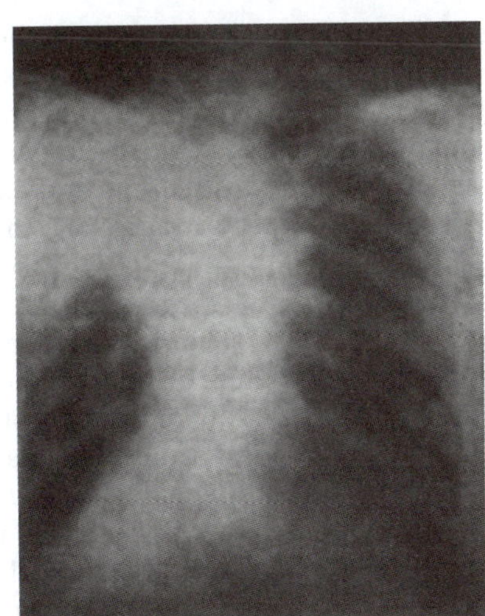

Fig. 144.7: Chest X-ray—pulmonary collapse. ***Note:*** 1. The uniform opacity with clearcut concave margins, 2. Shift of trachea to the affected side

Both the posteroanterior and lateral views are required for proper localization (Fig. 144.7).

- ***Bronchoscopy:*** It is necessary to visualize the affected bronchi.
- ***Bronchography:*** It reveals the actual site and nature of the block.

Complications and sequelae: Pulmonary collapse leads on to infection, abscess formation and fibrosis of the affected segment. Bronchiectasis may develop as a late sequel.

Management: Emergency measures include removal of the obstructive cause and physiotherapy to expand the lung. Antibiotic therapy should be started to prevent aspiration pneumonia. Pleural diseases must be treated promptly to prevent permanent damage to the lungs.

Prevention: Proper physiotherapy and measures to protect the respiratory tract from aspiration of gastric contents go a long way to prevent pulmonary collapse.

CHAPTER 145

Occupational Lung Diseases
Syn: Pneumoconiosis

KE Rajan

Chapter Summary

- General Considerations
- Silicosis
- Coal Worker's Pneumoconiosis
- Asbestosis
- Byssinosis

GENERAL CONSIDERATIONS

Pneumoconioses constitute a group of interstitial lung diseases (ILD), caused by occupational inhalation of dusts. The term ***pneumoconiosis*** was coined by Zenker in 1866 to define a group of diseases caused by inhalation of dusts-organic or inorganic. Inorganic dusts such as silica, asbestos or coal dust and organic dusts such as mouldy hay, cotton dust or sugarcane dust may lead on to pneumoconiosis. At present, several occupations are known to be associated with this risk. More and more entities are likely to be recognized with the expansion of industry. Pneumoconiosis resulted in about 125,000 deaths across the globe during the year 2010. National Institute of Occupational Health (NIOH) investigated cases of nonoccupational pneumoconiosis reported from certain villages of Ladakh. The chest radiographs were indistinguishable from those of miners and industrial workers suffering from pneumoconiosis. The disease amongst the villagers was attributed to dust storms and exposure to soot from domestic fuels used for cooking and heating.

PATHOGENESIS AND PATHOLOGY

Development of the pathological lesions depend upon several factors such as the nature of the substance inhaled, the concentration in the atmosphere, duration of exposure, particle size and responsiveness of the individual. Particles within the range of 1–5 μm penetrate deepest into the lung. Alveolar macrophages carry them to the interstitial space where inflammatory reaction sets in. The process continues over the years and leads to gross functional and structural changes resulting in severe morbidity.

Lesions caused by inorganic dusts range from minimal inflammatory reaction around the dust particle to more marked changes like focal emphysema, interstitial fibrosis and calcification. Some dusts like asbestos are carcinogenic. In some disorders such as silicosis, the host's immune mechanism is altered making them more susceptible to develop tuberculosis.

Several organic dusts are widely distributed in the agricultural belts of India. They exert deleterious effects by local irritation, sensitization to the components of the dust or sensitization to fungal contaminants. They cause damage principally on the alveolar ducts to produce extrinsic allergic alveolitis (Fig. 145.1).

The factors which lead to the final picture depend upon the substances inhaled. In general, they lead to:

- Mechanical blockage
- Chemical irritation of the airways, chlorine and acid fumes
- Direct toxicity to the lung parenchyma, e.g. phosgene, methyl isocyanate (MIC)
- Fibrosis, e.g. silica
- Sensitization, e.g. by animal dander, fungi, cotton dust
- Chronic granulomatous processes, e.g. beryllium toxicity
- Predisposition to secondary infection, e.g. silicosis predisposes to tuberculosis
- Neoplasia, e.g. asbestos.

Genetic factors modify the susceptibility to develop pneumoconiosis. On exposure, susceptible persons show early signs of ill-health, whereas the others are relatively immune. Other factors such as tobacco smoking, nutrition, and infections also may have roles in determining the final outcome in individual subjects. Industrial legislation requires adequate protective steps to be undertaken by establishments to safeguard against the development of pneumoconiosis amongst the workers (Table 145.1).

SILICOSIS

It is the irreversible fibrosis of the lungs caused by inhalation of free silica dust (silicone dioxide). Over 3 million people working in various types of mines, ceramics, potteries, foundries, metal grinding, stone crushing, agate grinding, slate pencil industry, etc. are

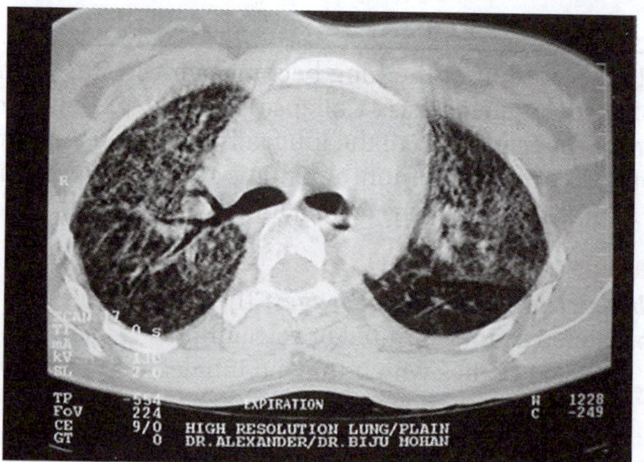

Fig. 145.1: HRCT extrinsic allergic alveolitis. *Note:* The diffused thickening of the interalveolar septa and honeycombing

Abbreviation: HRCT = High-resolution computed tomography

Table 145.1: Common types of pneumoconiosis in India	
Types	**Industry**
Silicosis	Mining, ceramics, potteries, foundries, metal grinding, stone crushing, agate grinding, slate pencil industry, mica
Coal workers' pneumoconiosis	Coal mining (anthracosis, Miner's lung)
Asbestosis	Asbestos cement, asbestos textile, asbestos mining and milling
Byssinosis	Cotton textile industry
Bagassosis	Sugar-cane industry

occupationally exposed to free silica dust and are at potential risk of developing silicosis. Silicosis may occur in combination with anthracosis. This is a major cause of permanent disability and mortality. In India, it was first reported from Kolar gold mines, Karnataka in 1947. Prevalence of silicosis may vary from 12% (stone crushing) to 54.5% (slate pencil industry).

The silica particles are ingested by the phagocytes, which accumulate and block lymphatic channels. The lesions produced by silica dust are similar to those produced by coal dust, but the lesions are larger. In addition, silicosis also gives rise to pleural thickening and adhesions. Sometimes, silicosis produces acute respiratory manifestations with dyspnea and impairment of gas exchange in the alveoli.

Clinical Features

In the acute form, the disease manifests with dyspnea, cyanosis and constitutional disturbances. In the chronic form, the prominent manifestations are cough and hemoptysis. Physical signs may be those of bronchitis, emphysema and pleural thickening. Silicosis predisposes to the development of tuberculosis and two diseases may coexist (silicotuberculosis). The functional impairment is a combination of restrictive and obstructive features. Immunological abnormalities such as the presence of rheumatoid factor may develop in 50% of cases.

Radiology: Diffuse miliary or nodular lesions are found in simple silicosis. Chest radiograph may show snow-storm pattern. Development of progressive massive fibrosis

(PMF) leads to the presence of dense shadows in the upper zones and this is termed as **complicated silicosis**. Hilar lymph nodes may show peripheral calcification. Occasionally, patients with silicosis develop scleroderma.

COAL WORKER'S PNEUMOCONIOSIS

Syn: Anthracosis

Prolonged exposure to coal dust causes anthracosis among miners. These particles give a black color to the lesions. Coal particles reaching the alveoli are ingested by the alveolar macrophages. The phagocytes are activated by the presence of substances like silica. Fibrosis develops at these regions. The affected lobules undergo centrilobular emphysema. On prolonged exposure, PMF develops and this is the characteristic lesion in complicated pneumoconiosis. Radiologically, the lesions of PMF appear as sausage-shaped densities exceeding 1 cm in diameter, in the upper and mid zones of both lung fields (Fig. 145.2). Further complications such as chronic bronchitis, bronchiectasis, and ischemic necrosis, thrombosis of pulmonary veins, pulmonary hypertension, cor pulmonale, or lymphatic obstruction may supervene. Prevalence may vary from 2 to 3% among those who work in coal mines.

Clinical Features

Gradual onset of dyspnea and cough with purulent expectoration mark the onset of the disease. Expectoration is more copious when bronchiectasis is also present. Dyspnea worsens when PMF supervenes. Cavitation of these lesions gives rise to expectoration of huge amounts of black sputum. Large nodular lesions develop in the lungs in subjects with rheumatoid disease who develop pneumoconiosis. These lesions are 1–5 cm in diameter and detectable on X-ray of the chest (Caplan's syndrome, or rheumatoid pneumoconiosis) (Fig. 145.3).

ASBESTOSIS

Inhalation of asbestos dust leads to asbestosis. It is a complex silicate containing silicon, oxygen, hydrogen and metals like calcium, magnesium and iron. The raw material is obtained by mining. Different varieties of asbestos such as chrysotile, crocidolite, amosite and anthrophylite are obtained from different regions. Up to 11% of those engaged in mining and milling asbestos may suffer from this disease.

Asbestos particles are needle-shaped and on account of this shape these preferentially settle in the lower lobes. They may reach the alveoli or may be arrested at the small air passages. They give rise to alveolar epithelial hyperplasia and interstitial fibrosis. Eventually, fibrosis develops around the asbestos particles and this obliterates the alveoli. Fibrosis in asbestosis is due to mechanical irritation. It is peribronchial in distribution and of diffuse character.

Asbestos bodies are seen on histology of the lesions. These consist of asbestos fibers coated by proteinaceous material and ferritin granules derived from macrophages. Asbestos bodies may be demonstrable in sputum. Mere presence of asbestos bodies in sputum is not sufficient to diagnose asbestosis. Asbestos fibers occur in two forms.

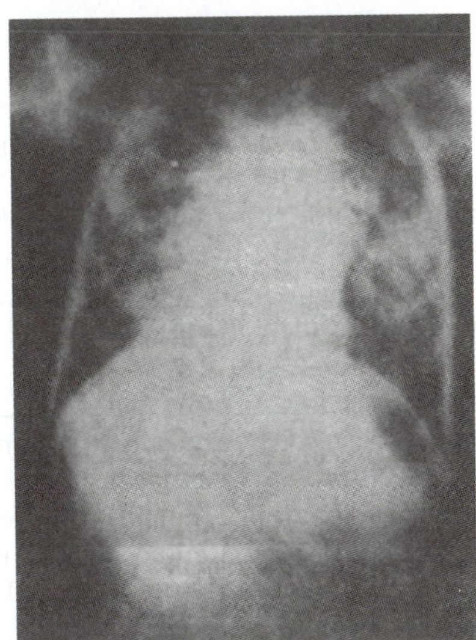

Fig. 145.2: Chest X-ray—progressive massive fibrosis

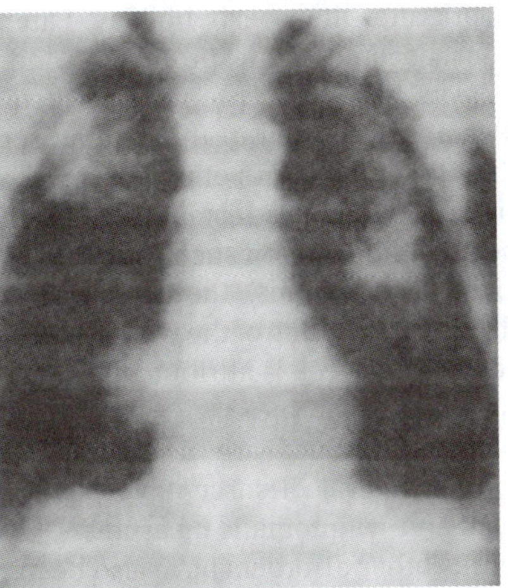

Fig. 145.3: Chest X-ray Caplan's syndrome. **Note:** The large nodular shadows

The long thin fibers are called **amphiboles** (blue asbestos). Other one is the feathery form known as **chrysotile** or **white asbestos**. Both are carcinogenic, the former is more so.

Asbestosis predisposes to bronchogenic carcinoma (especially in smokers) and mesothelioma of the pleura and peritoneum. The pathogenesis of mesothelioma in the pleura involves four steps. These are (1) Irritation of tissue, (2) damage to mitotic spindle, (3) generation of iron-related reactive oxygen molecules and damage to deoxyribonucleic acid (DNA) and (4) phosphorylation of kinases. Pleural mesothelioma is an aggressive tumor of the serosal surface of the pleura. Widespread exposure to asbestos has increased the incidence of pleural and peritoneal mesotheliomas. Asbestosis also predisposes to pulmonary tuberculosis. Malignancies of distant organs such as kidneys and breasts are more common in subjects with asbestosis.

Clinical Features

The symptoms start with increasing dyspnea on exertion, cough, malaise, and weight loss. As the condition proceeds, cyanosis and digital clubbing supervene. The pulmonary function test (PFT) shows restrictive defect and impairment of diffusion. The clinical picture differs from case-to-case, depending on the extent of the lesion and presence of other coexistent conditions such as emphysema, bronchiectasis, tuberculosis, malignancy or pleural disease.

Fine mottling and prominent streaky fibrosis are seen in the middle and lower zones in chest X-ray. Pleural thickening, pleural effusion, pleural plaques and calcification may be evident in some cases.

BYSSINOSIS

Pulmonary disease caused by exposure to cotton dust, flax or hemp is termed **byssinosis**. Among textile mill workers, 30–38% prevalence has been noted. Jute workers too can develop byssinosis. Some authors prefer to include byssinosis as an **occupational lung disease**, but not as pneumoconiosis.

In the early stages, the symptoms are tightness of the chest and wheeze usually felt by the patient when he resumes work after the weekly holiday. Later on, cough and dyspnea becomes more prominent and persistent. Some subjects develop chronic obstructive airways disease. Persons employed in the carding section suffer more than those employed in other areas.

Cotton dust stimulates histamine release from mast cells in the lung. Pure cotton such as surgical cotton does not provoke the symptoms. The occurrence of dyspnea and cough at the beginning of the week and its subsidence during the working week is attributed to depletion of the mast cells of their histamine.

Radiological findings are nonspecific. **Treatment** consists of withdrawal of susceptible persons from the environment and symptomatic measures.

Numerous other disorders have also been recognized as resulting from occupational exposure to different materials. Bauxite fibrosis, siderosis, stannosis and beryl-liosis are other occupational disorders. Wood dust, flour and noxious gases (sulfur dioxide, nitric oxide) could incite occupational disorders. It is beyond the scope of this text to describe all of them. Industrial medicine has assumed the importance of a subspecialty, which includes occupational health hazards, trauma, exposure to toxins, effects of physical agents on health and legal problems arising out of these.

MANAGEMENT

Once established, pneumoconiosis is treated symptomatically since specific therapy is lacking. Bronchodilators, oxygen and management of secondary bacterial or mycobacterial infections are useful in some cases. A retrospective study noted good clinical outcomes after lung transplantation in a small group of patients with coal worker's pneumoconiosis.

PREVENTION

Workers who are employed in industry should be recruited only after proper pre-employment medical examination. Persons with family history of allergic respiratory disorders and those who have features of obstructive airway disease are more likely to develop permanent ill effects. Periodic examination of the workers to facilitate early detection and removal from the harmful environment is required by legislation. Industrial establishments where the risk of pneumoconiosis is present have to follow specifications intended to reduce the concentration of dust in the environment and also for giving protection to the workers. Many of the pneumoconiosis attributable to occupational exposure are eligible for compensation from the employers.

Criteria for diagnosis of occupational lung disease

- There should be an exposure to known, documented, hazardous agent
- The timing of exposure and onset of symptoms should be appropriate
- The clinical syndrome should be consistent with the syndrome related to exposure
- There should be no other more likely explanation for the signs and symptoms.

CHAPTER
146

Sarcoidosis

KV Krishna Das

Chapter Summary

- General Considerations
- Pathology
- Clinical Features
- Diagnosis
- Investigations
- Course and Prognosis
- Treatment

GENERAL CONSIDERATIONS

Sarcoidosis is an immunologically-mediated disease with genetic susceptibility and unknown cause. The pathogenesis is mainly due to exaggerated immune response to unidentified antigens which may have varied genetic factors involving the major histocompatibility complex (MHC-2) genes showing susceptibility phenotype and prognosis of sarcoidosis. Human leukocyte antigen (HLA-

DRB1-14 or HLA DRB1-15) predispose to a chronic course. Other genes may also be involved.

The disease occurs worldwide affecting both sexes, younger ages being affected more. Several suggested etiological agents include viruses, bacteria and exposure to environmental antigen including clay, soil, pine tree pollen, talc and metals such as beryllium, zirconium and aluminum.

PATHOLOGY

The classic feature of sarcoidosis is the formation of non-caseating granulomas made up of collection of macrophages and epithelioid cells surrounded by lymphocytes. Macrophages transform to epithelioid cells which fuse to form multinucleated giant-cells. These granulomas remain chronic (with exacerbation at times) and may resolve spontaneously in 4–5 years or persist longer.

Sarcoidosis lesions affect several organs, especially lungs, lymph nodes, mucous membranes, liver, myocardium, central nervous system (CNS), skin, joints and secretory glands like the parotid and lacrimal. Reticulin fibers are preserved in the granuloma and in chronic cases fibrosis is the end result. In over 80% of cases, the lung is affected. In 16–20% of cases, the lesions either remain active or progress to severe fibrosis.

CLINICAL FEATURES

It may affect any/and all organ systems and, therefore, may be present as a generalized systemic illness or present to various specialties.

Systemic Illness

General symptoms include cough, fever, night sweats, fatigue, weakness, anorexia and weight loss. It is a not-uncommon cause of pyrexia of unknown origin (PUO), fatigue and erythema nodosum.

More Acute Presentations may Occur

These include bilateral mediastinal lymphadenopathy (Löfgren's syndrome) cough with dyspnea, chest pain, wheezing mimicking asthma and mild to severe and crippling disability. Chest X-ray may show prominent bilateral hilar lymphadenopathy and varying stages of diffuse pulmonary fibrosis (PF). At times, the X-ray picture may show advanced lesions but symptoms could be mild. Uncommonly, pleural involvement may occur.

In advanced cases, ventilation and pulmonary gas exchange may be defective. Sarcoidosis may progress and in a few, produce advanced PF.

In a small proportion of cases, diagnosis may be suggested by the presence of prominent bilateral hilar lymphadenopathy in chest X-ray done for routine investigation of other illnesses.

Involvement of other Organ Systems

Skin: Papules, nodules, plaques, scar sarcoidosis, lupus pernio and subcutaneous lesions. The term **lupus pernio** refers to the hyper- and hypo-pigmented erythematous skin lesions usually found over the nose, cheeks and malar regions.

Eyes: Anterior and posterior uveitis, conjunctival nodules, lacrimal adenitis and retinal vascular lesions.

Lymph nodes: All superficial groups may be generally or selectively enlarged moderately and painless usually.

Heart: Cardiomegaly, conduction defects, cardiac failure, pericardial involvement.

Kidney is only rarely involved; lesions include hypercalcemia, nephrocalcinosis, renal stones and increase in serum creatinine.

Parotid gland: Symmetrical bilateral parotid enlargement sometimes associated with uveitis, facial palsy and fever, Heerfordt's syndrome (uveoparotid syndrome).

Nervous system: Polyneuropathy, small-fiber neuropathies, cranial nerve palsies (especially facial nerve), CNS involvement, hypothalamic lesions leading to diabetics insipidus (DI), hypopituitarism and others.

Locomotor system: Myalgia, vague rheumatological manifestations and radiological abnormalities.

DIAGNOSIS

Clinical suspicion of sarcoidosis should be strong when encountering the following clinical problems which elude straight forward diagnosis:

- PUO with or without obvious organ involvement
- **Skin manifestations** such as erythema nodosum, generalized or localized lesions and lupus pernio
- Enlargement of secretory glands such as the parotid and lacrimal and unexplained uveitis
- **Neurological manifestations** involving peripheral nerves and CNS
- **Cardiac manifestations** such as cardiac enlargement, heart failure, conduction defects and pericarditis
- **Respiratory manifestations** such as persistent cough, dyspnea, signs of interstitial lung disease (ILD), pulmonary fibrous and pleural lesions. Respiratory signs may predominate in chronic lesions
- **Vague rheumatological manifestations** like polyarthralgia and arthritis.

INVESTIGATIONS

Chest X-ray shows bilateral intrathoracic and hilar lymphadenopathy or diffuses micronodular pulmonary infiltration. The term **galaxy sign** is given to findings in computed tomograhy (CT) of the chest showing typical nodules with irregular margins and the presence of satellite nodules around. Pulmonary involvement is shown in Figures 146.1 and 146.2.

Endobronchial USG-guided transbronchial needle aspiration in cases of mediastinal lymphadenopathy, transbronchial lung biopsies, ^{18}F-FDG PET (fluorodeoxyglucose positron emission tomography) scan can accurately assess the inflammatory activity. Cardiac lesions can be demonstrated by ^{18}F-FDG PET scan. In cases of localized lesions such as skin lesions, lymph nodes and conjunctival nodules, biopsy samples show noncaseating granuloma. If such superficial lesions are not obvious, flexible bronchoscopy with bronchoalveolar lavage should be undertaken. It shows moderate lymphocytosis (20–50%) in 80% of cases of sarcoidosis. T lymphocyte CD4/CD8 ratio is more than 3.3 in over 50% of cases.

Biopsy of a minor salivary gland (even though not enlarged) may help in some cases.

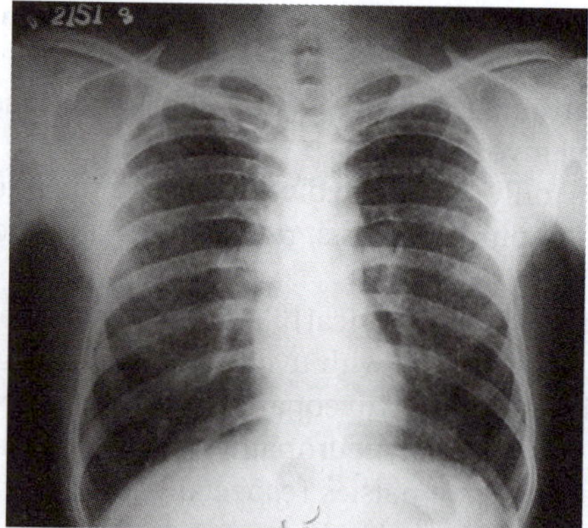

Fig. 146.1: Chest X-ray sacoidosis. **Note:** Bilateral hilaradenopathy with miliary lesions

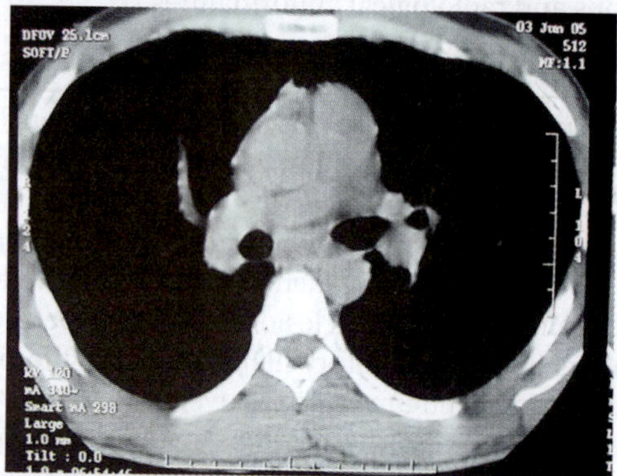

Fig. 146.2: HRCT sarcoidosis. **Note:** Hilar lymph nodes
Abbreviation: HRCT = High-resolution computed tomography

Granulomatous lesions in sarcoidosis have to be differentiated from tuberculosis and pneumoconiosis such as berylliosis. Serum markers such as serum angiotensin converting enzyme (ACE) concentration which used to be done have been discarded due to unreliability. Hypercalcemia may be a useful adjunct to monitor therapy.

COURSE AND PROGNOSIS

In 50% of cases, spontaneous recovery occurs in 2–4 years, even if untreated. In the rest, the disease may progress and give rise to varying degrees of PF (20%). Four percent may develop severe PF and become continuously oxygen-dependent. Development of pulmonary hypertension (PH) portends death.

Fibrosis and dysfunction occur in several other organs, leading to disabling symptoms and considerable morbidity.

Death is due to respiratory and cardiac failure, hepatic causes and massive hemoptysis from pulmonary aspergillosis.

Pregnancy occurring in sarcoidosis patients does not significantly alter the clinical status, but sarcoidosis may flare up after delivery.

Source: Valeyre D, Prasse A, Nunes H, et al. Sarcoidosis. Lancet. 2014;383(9923):1155-67.

Treatment

At present, treatment is palliative, given with a view to retard progress of the disease. Most drugs target tumor necrosis factor (TNF)-α which has a crucial role in perpetuating the granulomatous response.

Drug Therapy Includes

- Glucocorticoids in appropriate dosage given for long duration
- Antimalarials such as chloroquine 200 mg bd to reduce fibrosis
- Methotrexate as a corticosteroid sparing drug and immunosuppressant
- Leflunomide, an antifibrotic agent especially in those intolerant to methotrexate
- Biological anti-TNF α agents such as infliximab, adalimumab or rituximab, as is available and effective.

Personalized choice of drugs and appropriate adjustments of dose and duration are necessary to ensure success.

147

Pulmonary Fibrosis

C Sudheendra Ghosh, Davis Paul

Chapter Summary

- General Considerations
- Replacement Fibrosis
- Focal Fibrosis
- Interstitial Fibrosis
- Newer Modalities of Treatment

GENERAL CONSIDERATIONS

The term describes abnormal formation of fiber-like scar tissue in the lungs. There are over 140 known causes or associations with pulmonary fibrosis (PF). The lung reacts to the insult by inflammation and subsequent fibrosis.

Lung parenchyma has no power of regeneration. Hence, destructive lesions lead on to fibrosis. Fibrosis of the lung parenchyma may take three forms: ***Replacement fibrosis, focal fibrosis*** and ***interstitial fibrosis*** (Table 147.1).

REPLACEMENT FIBROSIS

In this form, fibrous tissue is laid down over areas of lung destruction. The fibrosis is often localized and its extent depends on the extent of parenchymal destruction.

Table 147.1: Causes of pulmonary fibrosis

Type of fibrosis	Causes
Replacement fibrosis	Pulmonary tuberculosis Bronchiectasis Lung abscess Pneumonias Fungal infections Pulmonary infarction Atelectasis Chronic pleural effusion Empyema Lipoid pneumonia Irradiation of lung
Focal fibrosis	Pneumoconiosis
Interstitial fibrosis	Fibrosing alveolitis Allergic alveolitis Connective tissue diseases (CTDs) • Progressive systemic sclerosis • Rheumatoid lung Asbestosis Sarcoidosis Radiation injury Pulmonary hemosiderosis Chronic pulmonary edema of long-standing

The most common cause in India is pulmonary tuberculosis. The upper lobes are affected more frequently.

Clinical Features

The chest is asymmetrical with flattening of the affected side, drooping of the shoulder and diminution of movement. Trachea and mediastinal structures are pulled toward the same side, unless they were already fixed by pre-existing disease. The percussion note is diminished. Vocal fremitus and resonance depend upon the severity of fibrosis. In extensive fibrosis, they are reduced. If a major bronchus lies subjacent to the fibrotic area, the vocal fremitus and resonance are increased and breath sounds become bronchial. In extensive fibrosis, especially fibrothorax, the breath sounds are considerably diminished.

Adventitious sounds may be heard and these are variable. Symptoms and hemodynamic disturbances depend upon the extent of pulmonary lesions and the cause.

Replacement fibrosis has to be distinguished from pulmonary collapse in which there may be ipsilateral shift of midline structures. Pulmonary collapse is usually of shorter duration and the underlying cause may be evident.

FOCAL FIBROSIS

This is seen in pneumoconiosis such as silicosis. The extent of fibrosis may vary from small nodular lesions to extensive areas PMF.

INTERSTITIAL FIBROSIS

Interstitial lung disease (ILD) may result from connective tissue disorders like progressive systemic sclerosis, collagen vascular diseases, hypersensitivity pneumonitis, sarcoidosis, radiation injury, asbestosis, pneumoconiosis, chronic pulmonary edema [as in mitral stenosis (MS)] and idiopathic pulmonary hemosiderosis. Around 50% of ILD occur without any identifiable cause and they are known as IPF. In all these diseases, there is increased fibrous tissue deposition in the interstitium which can affect the diffusion of oxygen across alveolar membrane resulting in hypoxemia and poor exercise tolerance.

Pathogenesis

A common pathogenetic sequence occurs in most of the conditions leading to interstitial fibrosis, regardless of the etiology. An inhalational injury like cigarette smoke, environmental pollutants and other noxious agents can lead to uncontrolled activation of alveolar epithelial cells which leads to migration, proliferation and activation of fibroblast or myofibroblast leading to interstitial fibrosis. Previously, it was thought that fibrosis is the result of an ongoing uncontrolled inflammation (Table 147.2).

Clinical Features

The symptoms are those of ventilatory and diffusion defects, predominantly characterized by dyspnea, cyanosis, frequent respiratory infections and chronic cor pulmonale. Physical examination may reveal gross clubbing, tachypnea, cyanosis and diminished respiratory movements. Since these changes affect both lungs, there is no marked shift of midline structures. Breath sounds are diminished. Diffuse rales (crackles) which persist after coughing are characteristic. The classical end-inspiratory velcro crackles are present in IPF. X-ray of the chest may show generalized loss of translucency and increased reticulation. Pulmonary function test (PFT) will show restrictive pattern, usually decreased vital capacity (VC) (Box 147.1). Earliest change may be reduction in diffusion capacity. High-resolution computed tomography (HRCT) is very useful in assessing the nature of the lesion, extent of disease, and monitoring progress (Fig. 147.1). In advanced cases, traction bronchiectasis and subpleural honeycombing may be seen. Lung biopsy is useful for confirmation.

Cardiac findings include right ventricular (RV) enlargement and hypertrophy and loud pulmonic second sound indicating pulmonary hypertension (PH).

Course and Prognosis

Replacement fibrosis does not usually progress further. The course of the disease and longevity depend on the extent of the lesion, occurrence of secondary infections

Table 147.2: Current clinical terminology and histopathological terminology

Current clinical terminology	Current histopathological terminology
Idiopathic pulmonary fibrosis (IPF)	Usual interstitial pneumonia (UIP)
Acute interstitial pneumonia	Diffuse alveolar damage (DAD)
Nonspecific interstitial pneumonia (NSIP)	NSIP pattern
Desquamative interstitial pneumonia (DIP)	DIP pattern
Lymphoid interstitial pneumonia (LIP)	LIP pattern
Respiratory bronchiolitis interstitial lung disease (ILD)	Respiratory bronchiolitis
Cryptogenic organizing pneumonia	Organizing pneumonia

Box 147.1: ATS/ERS criteria for diagnosis of IPF in absence of surgical lung biopsy

Major Criteria
- Exclusion of other known causes of ILD such as certain drug toxicities, environmental exposures and connective tissue diseases (CTDs)
- Abnormal pulmonary function studies that include evidence of restriction (reduced VC, often with an increased FEV1/FVC ratio) and impaired gas exchange [increased $P(A\text{-}a)O_2$, decreased PaO_2] with rest or exercise or decreased **carbon monoxide diffusing capacity** (DL_{CO})
- Bi-basilar reticular abnormalities with minimal ground glass opacities on HRCT scans
- Transbronchial lung biopsy or BAL showing no features to support an alternative diagnosis.

Minor Criteria
- Age >50 years
- Insidious onset of otherwise unexplained dyspnea on exertion
- Duration of illness >3 months
- Basilar inspiratory crackles (dry or **velcro** type in quality.

Abbreviations: ATS/ERS = American Thoracic Society/European Respiratory Society; IPF = Idiopathic pulmonary fibrosis; ILD = Interstitial lung disease; VC = Vital capacity; FEV1 = Forced expiratory volume in one second; FVC = Forced vital capacity; HRCT = High-resolution computed tomography; BAL = Bronchoalveolar lavage

and the development of cor pulmonale. In general, with reasonable care, localized fibrosis is compatible with prolonged survival. IPF is progressive in most series. 5-year survival is only < ± 20%. Death is due to respiratory or cardiac failure.

Management

General measures include avoidance of smoking, treatment of intercurrent infections, reduction of weight and respiratory exercises. No definite treatment is available at present. Disease has a variable course. Some patients may remain stable for many years without much worsening of the symptoms. Most will progress and die within 5 years. Few have rapid progression and die within months. **Treatment** is primarily symptomatic. Long-term oxygen therapy is beneficial in those with respiratory failure.

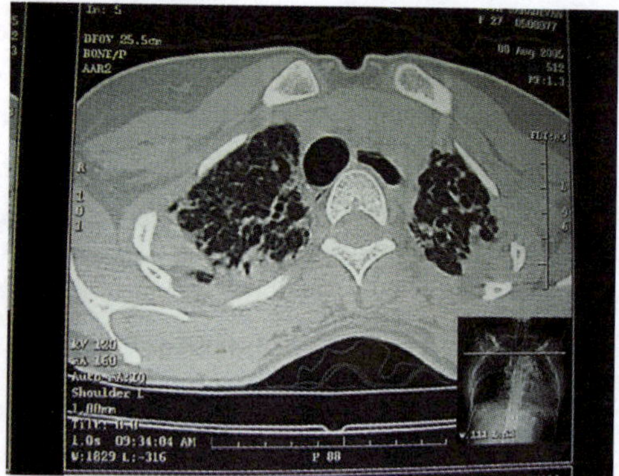

Fig. 147.1: HRCT of pulmonary interstitial fibrosis. **Note:** The thickening of interalveolar septa

Abbreviation: HRCT = High-resolution computed tomography

Treatment of gastroesophageal reflux disease (GERD) is recommended even in patients without reflux symptoms. Corticosteroids, azathioprine and N-acetyl cysteine are other drugs that have been tried with variable response.

Lung transplantation is the only answer in those who do not improve with medical treatment.

NEWER MODALITIES OF TREATMENT

Pirfenidone is a synthetic anti-fibrotic drug but it is not routinely used. [5 methyl 1-phenyl-2-(1H)–pyridone]. It has action on transforming growth factor (TGF) and tumor necrosis factor (TNF). In the ASCEND Trial, conducted in Japan and multinationally, it was shown that pirfenidone acts by inhibition of expression of TGFβ-1. It delays the fibrotic process, improves deterioration of forced expiratory volume in one second and 6 minutes walking distance in PF. Dose of the drug used was 2,403 mg or 1,197 mg given orally daily, the higher dose was more effective. Duration of treatment was for 1 year.

Source: Bouros D. Pirfenidone for idiopathic pulmonary fibrosis. Lancet. 2011;377(9779):1727-9.

148 Circulatory Disturbances in Lungs

C Sudheendra Ghosh, Davis Paul

Chapter Summary
- Pulmonary Edema
  - Acute Pulmonary Edema
  - Chronic Pulmonary Edema
- Pulmonary Thromboembolism
  - Chronic Thromboembolic Pulmonary Hypertension
- Pulmonary Arterial Hypertension (PAH)
  - Primary Pulmonary Hypertension
  - Functional Classification of PH

PULMONARY EDEMA

Acute Pulmonary Edema

It is a common medical emergency which can be brought about by diverse causes. There is accumulation of extravascular fluid within the lung. The mechanisms include rise in the pulmonary wedge pressure (PWP), changes in the dynamics of flow of fluids and protein through the capillary walls and changes in the interstitium. Fluid may accumulate in the interstitium or in the alveoli.

Common Causes

- Left-sided heart failure, e.g. acute myocardial infarction (acute MI), hypertensive cardiac failure or mitral stenosis (MS)
- Aspiration of gastric contents (Mendelson's syndrome)
- Neurogenic disorders such as subarachnoid hemorrhage, meningitis, encephalitis or brainstem injury with resultant depression of respiratory center
- Fluid overload, e.g. over transfusion of fluids, acute nephritic syndrome
- Drug hypersensitivity, e.g. hexamethonium, nitrofurantoin, busulfan
- Change in permeability of capillary wall, e.g. acute glomerulonephritis (GN)
- Narcotic poisoning with depression of respiratory center
- Irritant gases, e.g. phosgene, chlorine, acid fumes
- Other forms of poisoning like paraquat, weedicides, organophosphorus
- Pulmonary embolism (PE) (Fig. 148.1)
- Uremia
- Aspiration of pleural effusion.

Rarer causes: Hanging, near drowning, high-altitude pulmonary edema, hypoproteinemia, disseminated intravascular coagulation (DIC), falciparum malaria and pneumothorax.

Clinical Features

Acute pulmonary edema ushers in with intense dyspnea, anxiety and sweating. At its early phase, the only obvious abnormality may be tachypnea. When fluid collects in the alveoli, the patient expectorates copious amounts of white or pink frothy sputum. Auscultation reveals widespread rales and occasional rhonchi. Initially, the lower lobes are affected. Cyanosis may develop and it becomes deeper. Death occurs due to respiratory failure. Examination of the heart may reveal evidence of left-sided heart failure such as gallop rhythm or the presence of valvular lesions (*See* also Section 13, Ch 120).

Management

Emergency management is indicated to save life. Cardiac causes have to be treated as for acute left-sided heart failure. The main steps in treatment include administration of oxygen, furosemide, digitalis, aminophylline and vasodilator drugs. Continuous positive airway pressure (CPAP) using noninvasive ventilation (NIV) is very useful in relieving symptoms of pulmonary edema. Physiological or open venesection may be required as an emergency, rarely. The underlying cause should be attended to, after instituting the life-saving emergency measures. When pulmonary edema follows inhalation of irritant fumes, massive doses of corticosteroids may be beneficial. In narcotic poisoning, use of antidotes such as naloxone may help in bringing about dramatic improvement. Artificial ventilation is indicated in cases where respiratory failure develops. In addition, all the general principles of management of poisoning have to be adopted.

Chronic Pulmonary Edema

This occurs in chronic heart failure caused by MS or left ventricular (LV) cardiomyopathy. The lungs are edematous, congested and brown on section ***(brown induration).*** Hemosiderosis may occur in long-standing cases. X-ray shows signs of chronic pulmonary venous congestion (Fig. 148.2). Dilated interlobar septal lymphatics (Kerley's B lines) are seen. When pulmonary hemosiderosis develops, miliary shadows are seen in the radiograph. In early cases, treatment of cardiac failure clears the pulmonary edema also.

Hypostatic congestion: This condition may develop in chronically bed-ridden patients due to diminished circulation, local anoxia and infection. Hypostatic congestion can be prevented by early ambulation, respiratory physiotherapy and adequate treatment of infection.

PULMONARY THROMBOEMBOLISM

Chronic Thromboembolic Pulmonary Hypertension (CTEPH)
(*See* also Section 13, Ch 130)

This is a result of multiple and recurrent microemboli obstructing the pulmonary vasculature. Patients who have thrombophilia and those with sources for recurrent emboli are possible candidates. The clinical picture may resemble that of primary pulmonary hypertension (PH) from which this condition has to be differentiated. The pulmonary artery (PA) pressures are elevated. Pulmonary

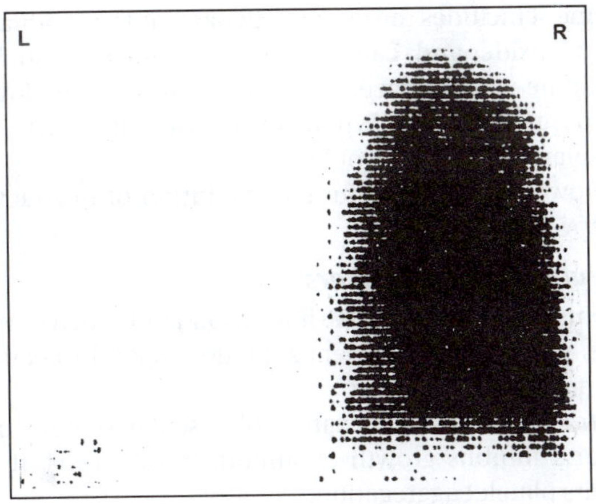

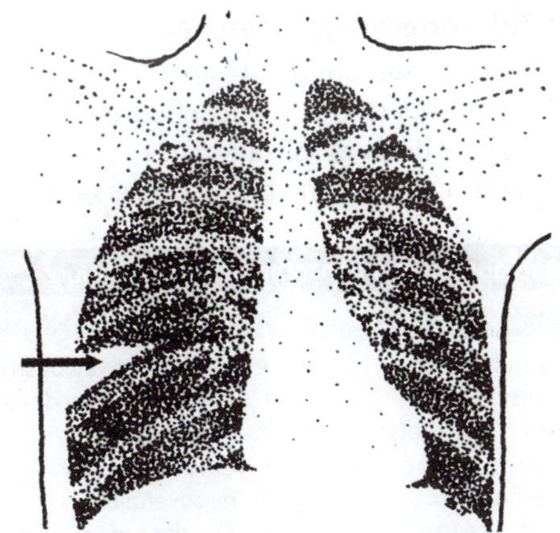

Fig. 148.1: Scintiscan pulmonary embolism. ***Note:*** The isotope does not reach the affected side (left side)

Fig. 148.2: Chest X-ray: Pulmonary infarct. ***Note:*** The triangular opacity with the base towards the pleura

angiography may help to delineate the vascular lesion in some cases, but not in the majority. Isotope scans and right-heart catheterization help to determine the extent and severity of the lesions. Electrocardiography (ECG) helps to demonstrate the degree of enlargement and hypertrophy of the right-sided cardiac chambers. Echocardiography can be used to estimate the PA pressure and for serial follow-up.

Source: Piazza G, Goldhaber SZ. Chronic thromboembolic pulmonary hypertension. N Engl J Med. 2011;364(4):351-60.

PULMONARY ARTERIAL HYPERTENSION (PAH)

It is a disease of the small pulmonary arteries that is characterized by vascular proliferation and remodeling. It leads to progressive rise in pulmonary vascular resistance and ultimately to right ventricular (RV) failure and death. It is of two types: Primary and secondary. The pulmonary vascular bed is a high-flow, low pressure circuit that has the capacity to dilate and recruit unused vasculature in order to accommodate increase in blood flow. In PH, this capacity is lost resulting in elevation of PA pressure at rest and further elevation during exercise.

Criteria for diagnosis for PAH: Mean PA pressure more than 25 mm Hg at rest and more 30 mm Hg at exercise and pulmonary capillary pressure less than 15 mm Hg.

The pathological processes include proliferation of vascular smooth muscle cells and asymmetric neointimal hyperplasia in small pulmonary arteries and arterioles. Resistance to PA blood flow results from mechanical occlusion and vasoconstrictor response of small vessels leading to arteriopathy and obstruction.

Causes

The causes of PAH are listed in Box 148.1.
- Increased pulmonary vascular resistance
- Increased pulmonary venous pressure
  - Mitral valve disease
  - Left ventricular (LV) failure
  - Dilated cardiomyopathy
  - Left atrial (LA) myxoma
- Increased pulmonary blood flow (PBF):
  - Atrial septal defect (ASD)
  - Ventricular septal defect (VSD)
  - Patent ductus arteriosus (PDA)

Primary Pulmonary Hypertension

This is a less common condition seen more frequently in women of child-bearing age and children. The etiology is not clear. Microembolization of the pulmonary arterioles and capillary bed and adverse reaction to drugs, such as appetite suppressants, may very closely mimic primary PH. The normal PA pressure in health is 18–25 mm Hg/6–10 mm Hg. In PAH, the mean pressure is more than 30/20 mm Hg.

Pathological features include medial hypertrophy, fibrinoid necrosis and occlusion of the pulmonary arterial bed. This leads to rise in PA pressure, RV hypertrophy and cardiac failure.

Symptoms are vague until the lesion is advanced. Dyspnea of varying severity and signs of right heart failure develop. Anoxemia develops on exertion and this can be demonstrated by arterial oxygen studies. The six-minute walk test is a clinical test used to assess the progress of the disability and prognosis. Hemodynamic evaluation is done by right-heart catheterization and invasive pulmonary angiopathy.

Functional Classification of PH

Modified after the New York Heart Association (NYHA) Functional Classification according to the World Health Organization (WHO) 1998.
- ***Class I:*** Patients with PH but without resulting limitation of physical activity. Ordinary physical activity does not cause undue dyspnea or fatigue, chest pain or near syncope.
- ***Class II:*** Patients with PH resulting in slight limitation of physical activity. They are comfortable at rest. Ordinary physical activity causes undue dyspnea or fatigue, chest pain or near syncope.
- ***Class III:*** Patients with PH resulting in pronounced limitation of physical activity. They are comfortable at rest. Less than ordinary activity causes undue dyspnea or fatigue, chest pain or near syncope.
- ***Class IV:*** Patients with PH with inability to carry out any physical activity without symptoms. These patients manifest signs of right heart failure. Dyspnea and/or fatigue may even be present at rest. Discomfort is increased by any physical activity.

Prognosis

Prognosis for recovery is poor. Majority die within 2–3 years of onset of symptoms. Death is due to RV failure.

Treatment

General measures include oxygen therapy. Symptomatic treatment includes the use of anticoagulants, vasodilators, nitrous oxide and calcium channel blockers such as nifedipine and diltiazem, sildenafil and its analogues, and oxygen therapy. When facilities permit, early lung transplantation may be of help.

Flowchart 148.1 useful for institution of prostacyclin therapy.

Calcium Channel Blockers

Patients responding to first-line vasodilators such as nitric oxide, prostacyclin or adenosine, do respond to calcium channel blockers.

Prostacyclin causes relaxation of vascular smooth muscles and inhibits growth of smooth muscle cells. It also inhibits platelet aggregation.

Side effects include joint pain, headache, flushing and diarrhea. The drug is expensive.

Box 148.1: Causes of pulmonary arterial hypertension	
Obstructive	***Hypoxic***
• Primary pulmonary hypertension • Collagen vascular diseases • Thromboembolism • Tumor embolism • Sickle cell disease • Drug-induced: Fenfluramine, phenformin	• Chronic airway obstruction • Restrictive lung diseases • High altitude • Chronic alveolar hypoventilation • The dose of IgG in these conditions is very large.

Flowchart 148.1: Management of pulmonary arterial hypertension

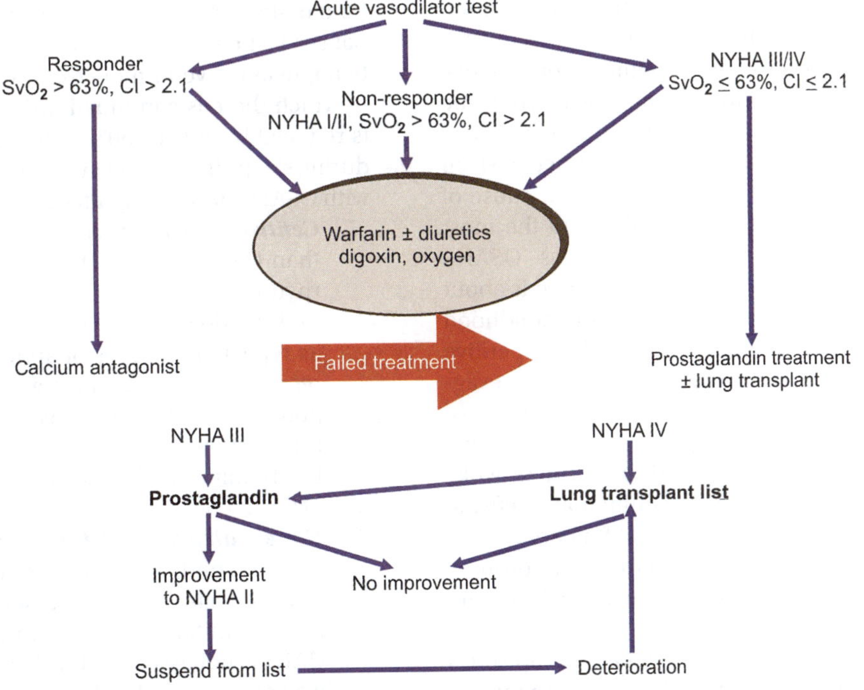

Abbreviations: CI = Cardiac index; SvO2 = Pulmonary arterial oxygen saturation; NYHA = New York Heart Association

Endothelin Receptor Antagonists (ERAs)

Bosentan: It is an orally active dual endothelin receptor blocker. Dose is 62.5 mg bd for 1 month, then 125 mg bd thereafter.

Other ERA drugs in use for moderate-to-severe cases include sitaxsentan and ambrisentan. Inhaled prostacyclin analogue—iloprost and the subcutaneous prostacyclin analogue—treprostinil are also effective.

Sildenafil and its analogues belong to the group of phosphodiesterase type 5 inhibitors. When given orally in doses of 25–50 mg orally repeatedly, it causes pulmonary vasodilatation. These drugs are being used more frequently. Sildenafil 20 mg tds oral, or tadalafil up to 40 mg/day oral. They lead to PA vasodilation and antiproliferative and proapoptotic effects that reverse PA remodeling, both increase 6-minute walking distance. Both drugs are indicated in patients with symptomatic PH. Its adverse effects are hypotension, flushing, heart burn, priapism and others.

A newer drug under trial is ***riociguat***, which is a soluble guanylate cyclase stimulator. Riociguat has dual actions: (1) Stimulating soluble guanylate cyclase independently of nitric oxide; and (2) increasing the sensitivity of soluble guanylate cyclase to nitric oxide. This drug has been tried for both thromboembolic PH and other types of PH de novo and for those who had recurred after PA endarterectomy. Dose of drug is 1–2.5 mg/tds.

Source: Ghofrani HA, Galiè N, Grimminger F, et al. Riociguat for the treatment of pulmonary arterial hypertension. N Engl J Med. 2013;369(4):330-40.

CHAPTER
149

Obstructive Sleep Apnea Syndrome

C Sudheendra Ghosh, CP Murali

Chapter Summary

- General Considerations
- Definitions
- Spectrum of Disease and Risk Factors
- Mechanism of Obstruction
- Clinical Features
- Screening
- Consequences
- Diagnosis
- Treatment

GENERAL CONSIDERATIONS

Sleep-disordered breathing (SDB) is an extremely common medical condition; the clinical significance of which was identified only during the last 50 years. Clinical descriptions of SDB were made by Hunter, Cheyne and Stokes in the 19th century. But, it was in 1965 that Gastaut and associates first recognized obstructive sleep apnea (OSA). The terms sleep apnea syndrome and obstructive sleep apnea syndrome (OSAS) was coined by Guilleminault, et al. in 1976. Obstructive sleep apnea/hypopnea syndrome (OSAHS) is a major cause of morbidity, a significant cause of mortality and the most common medical cause of daytime sleepiness. OSAHS occurs in around 1–4% of middle-aged males and is about 1–2% in females. The syndrome also occurs in childhood as well as elderly. It is characterized by repetitive apneic episodes during sleep leading to hypoxia, exaggerated negative intrathoracic pressure and arousals. These noxious stimuli lead to depression of myocardial contractility, depress parasympathetic activity, provoke oxidative stress and systemic inflammation, activate platelets and impair vascular endothelial function. There are independent associations with hypertension, coronary artery disease (CAD), arrhythmias, heart failure and strokes.

SDB is present when there are repetitive episodes of cessation of respiration (apnea) or decrements in airflow (hypopnea) during sleep, associated with sleep fragmentation, arousals and reduction in oxygen saturation. Apnea can be obstructive (absence of airflow but continued respiratory effort), central (absence of airflow and respiratory effort) or mixed. A mixed apnea starts as a central event and then becomes obstructive event during the latter portion of the same episode. Majority of patients with OSA have both obstructive and mixed apnea.

DEFINITIONS

- **Hypopnea** is defined as a decrement in airflow of 50% or more associated with a 4% fall in oxygen saturation and/or electroencephalographic arousal. Hypopnea has been shown to produce identical clinical consequences as *apneas*.
- A **respiratory effort related arousal (RERA) event** is a sequence of breath characterized by increasing efforts leading to an arousal from sleep that does not fulfil the criteria for apnea or hypopnea. It should last for at least 10 seconds and is terminated by an arousal.
- **Apnea-hypopnea index (AHI)** is the number of apneas plus hypopneas per hour of sleep. It is the standard metric used to quantitate the severity of OSA. An AHI greater than 5–10 events per hour is indicative of OSA. The following criteria are used to define severity of sleep apnea based on AHI events.
  - Mild sleep apnea, AHI: 5–15 events per hour
  - Moderate sleep apnea, AHI: 15–30 events per hour
  - Severe sleep apnea, AHI: Greater than 30 events per hour

  For evaluation of OSAHS, it is also important to assess other indicators like the degree of desaturation, degree of hypoventilation and total number of arousals.
- **OSAHS** is defined as the coexistence of unexplained excessive daytime sleepiness with at least five obstructed breathing events (apnea or hypopnea) per hour of sleep. Apneas are defined in adults as breathing pauses lasting more than or equal to 10 seconds and hypopneas as events more than or equal to 10 seconds, in which there is continued breathing but ventilation is reduced by at least 50% from the previous baseline during sleep. Three other syndromes can either coexist with OSAHS or present independently.

1. **Central sleep apnea (CSA)** is less common than OSAHS and is characterized by a transient rhythmic cessation of breathing. Ventilator muscles do not receive central input. It is defined as repeated episodes of apnea in the absence of respiratory muscle effort and is observed in the polysomnogram (PSG) as an absence of nasal-oral airflow and thoracoabdominal excursion. Heart failure and stroke are important etiologies of CSA.

2. **Upper airway resistance syndrome (UARS):** In this condition, there is increasing negative intrathoracic pressure associated with upper airflow limitation resulting in arousals from sleep. UARS is not associated with apneas or significant oxyhemoglobin desaturation. The arousal results in sleep fragmentation and daytime sleepiness. UARS may represent milder form of OSA spectrum.

3. **Obesity hyperventilation syndrome (OHS) or the Pickwickian syndrome:** It is defined by morbid obesity [Body mass index (BMI) >40 kg/m²] and chronic hypoventilation with hypercapnia ($PaCO_2$ greater than 45 mm Hg) during wakefulness. Other features include awake resting hypoxemia, hypersomnolence, signs of cor pulmonale and nocturnal hypoventilation. The diagnosis of OHS requires a demonstration of at least 10 mm Hg increments in $PaCO_2$ during sleep. This can also coexist with OSAHS.

SPECTRUM OF DISEASE AND RISK FACTORS

OSAHS is part of a spectrum of abnormalities ranging from snoring to obesity hypoventilation syndrome. Several risk factors exist for OSAHS (Box 149.1).

OSA is caused by loss of pharyngeal muscle dilator tone during sleep leading to recurrent pharyngeal collapse and temporary cessation of breathing—at least five or more apneic or hypopneic episodes per hour of sleep. Often, there is habitual snoring. OSA leads to pulmonary vasoconstriction, free-radical production, triggering of inflammatory pathways leading to endothelial dysfunction, vasoconstriction, sympathetic activity and impaired fibrinolytic activity. **Treatment** is done by applying continuous or intermittent positive air pressure by nasopharyngeal mask during sleep. Prevention is by weight reduction.

Epidemiologic studies demonstrate the prevalence of OSAHS to be 2–3 times higher in men than women but postmenopausal women are at a higher risk for OSAHS. The sex difference is related to the body fat distribution. Men exhibit a more central fat distribution, including

Box 149.1: Risk factors for obstructive sleep apnea

- Gender (male/female 2:1)
- Obesity (>120% ideal body weight)
- Neck size (>17 inches in males, >15 inches in females)
- ***Upper airway anatomy***
  - Macroglossia
  - Lateral peritonsillar narrowing
  - Elongation/enlargement of the soft palate
  - Tonsillar hypertrophy
  - Nasal septal deviation
  - Retrognathia, micrognathia
  - Narrowing of the hard palate
  - Class III/IV modified Mallampati airway
- ***Specific genetic diseases:*** Treacher Collins syndrome, Down's syndrome, Apert syndrome, Pierre-Robin Syndrome and Ehlers-Danlos syndrome (EDS)
- Genetic factors
- ***Endocrine disorders:*** Hypothyroidism, acromegaly
- Alcohol, sedative or hypnotic use

neck, thereby increasing the risk for narrowing and closure of the airways. Numerous studies have shown correlation between the prevalence of OSAHS and obesity. Obesity also increases the rate of progression of OSAHS. In nonobese individuals, craniofacial features such as retroposed mandible, micrognathia and narrowing of the hard palate are primary risk factors for apnea. In children, tonsillar and adenoid hypertrophy are important risk factors. Nasal abnormalities like septal deviation and allergic rhinitis also increase apnea risk. Several chromosomal disorders like Treacher Collins syndrome, Down's syndrome, Ehlers-Danlos syndrome (EDS), Apert syndrome and Pierre-Robin syndrome are associated with craniofacial and upper airway soft tissue abnormalities. Hence, they are associated with increased risk for OSAHS. Hypothyroidism is associated with increased frequency of obstructive and central sleep apnea. OSAHS is more common and severe among patients with acromegaly due to the upper airway narrowing by their large tongue. Alcohol reduces the upper airway tone and exacerbates OSAHS. Similarly, sedatives and hypnotics aggravate OSAHS by reducing the arousal mechanism.

MECHANISM OF OBSTRUCTION

OSA is caused by loss of pharyngeal muscle dilator tone during sleep leading to recurrent pharyngeal collapse and temporary cessation of breathing. Apnea and hypopnea are caused by the airway being sucked and closed on inspiration due to relaxation of the dilating muscles during sleep. During sleep, the muscle tone falls and airway narrows. These patients have narrow upper airways and muscle tone is maintained during wakefulness by increased activity that is lost during sleep. Snoring may commence before the airway occludes, and apnea results. Apnea and hypopnea terminate when the subjects arouses from sleep. This arousal is subtle and is associated with cardiac acceleration, blood pressure (BP) elevation, and increased sympathetic tone. Often there is habitual snoring. OSA leads to pulmonary vasoconstriction, free-radical production, triggering of inflammatory pathways leading to endothelial dysfunction, vasoconstriction sympathetic activity and impaired fibrinolytic activity.

CLINICAL FEATURES

OSAHS usually presents with daytime sleepiness, impaired vigilance and cognitive performance, depression of driving ability, disturbed sleep and hypertension. Daytime sleepiness varies in severity and may be indistinguishable from narcolepsy. The sleepiness may cause inability to work effectively, damage interpersonal relationships and prevent socializing. The somnolence is dangerous, with a 3–6-fold risk of road accidents. Other symptoms include difficulty in concentrating, unrefreshing nocturnal sleep, nocturnal choking and decreased libido. Partners report nightly loud snoring in all postures, which may be punctuated by the silence of the apneas. Nocturia is fairly common and is related to atrial natriuretic peptide (ANP) release. Excessive daytime sleepiness is a chief clinical consequence among patients with OSAHS.

Clinical presentation of obstructive sleep apnea

- Habitual loud snoring
- Excessive daytime sleepiness
- Witnessed apneas
- Nocturnal awakening
- Gasping or choking episodes during sleep
- Nocturia
- Irritability, memory loss, personality change
- Decreased libido
- Impotence
- Unrefreshing sleep, morning headaches
- Automobile or work-related accidents

Severity of OSAHS can be assessed by using the ***Epworth sleepiness scale*** (Box 149.2), which is a standard instrument for measuring the degree of self-rated sleepiness. The score ranges from 0 to 24. A value above 10 is considered abnormal. Physical exam in OSAHS focusses on neck circumference, obesity (BMI >28 kg/m^2), upper respiratory tract to visualize crowding and soft tissue dimensions, craniofacial structures and BP. Neck circumference greater than 40 cm predicts OSAHS with a sensitivity of 61% and specificity of 93%.

SCREENING

Standardized questionnaire such as multivariable apnea prediction (MAP) has been found to be an excellent tool in predicting OSA. By computing the total score of MAP with age, sex and BMI, the pretest likelihood of apnea can be calculated. Conditions where sleep apnea should be considered for evaluation.

- Systemic hypertension
- Obesity
- Myocardial infarction (MI)
- Cerebrovascular accident
- Pulmonary hypertension
- Type II diabetes mellitus (DM)
- Nocturnal cardiac arrhythmias
- Driver involved in a sleep-related automobile crash
- Preoperative anesthesia evaluation

CONSEQUENCES

Neurocognitive Function

Excessive daytime sleepiness and sleep fragmentation associated with sleep apnea lead to diminished cognitive

Box 149.2: Epworth sleepiness scale to assess disability

How often are you likely to doze off or fall asleep in the following situations, in contrast to feeling just tired?
This refers to your recent way of life in recent times; even if you have not done some of these things recently, try to work out how they would have affected you. Use the following scale to choose the most appropriate number for each situation.
0 = Would never doze
1 = Slight chance of dozing
2 = Moderate chance of dozing
3 = High chance of dozing

Situation	*Chance of dozing*
Sitting and reading	_________________
Watching TV	_________________
Sitting inactive in a meeting	_________________
As a passenger in car for 1 hr without a break	_________________
Lying down to rest in the afternoon when circumstances permit	_________________
Sitting and talking to someone	_________________
Sitting quietly after lunch without alcohol	_________________
In a car while stopped for a few minutes in traffic	_________________
TOTAL	

function. As a consequence, there is increased risk of motor vehicle accidents among these patients.

Hypertension

OSAHS increases BP. Increase in BP is related to nocturnal hypoxemia. This increase in BP would increase the risk of MI and stroke.

Diabetes Mellitus (DM)

Recent data suggest that increased apnea and hypopnea during sleep are associated with insulin resistance. Trials show that OSAHS can aggravate diabetes and that treatment of OSAHS decreases the insulin requirements in diabetic patients.

Hepatic Function

Patients with apnea and hypopnea show features of elevated liver enzymes and hepatic fibrosis.

Anesthetic Risk

Patients with OSAHS are at increased risk perioperatively. During recovery period or as a consequence of sedation, upper airway obstruction can occur.

DIAGNOSIS

Diagnosis is by taking a good sleep history from patient and partner, completion of sleep questionnaire including Epworth sleepiness score (score >11 indicates sleepiness). Physical examination must include assessment of obesity, jaw structure, the upper airway, BP and possible predisposing causes including hypothyroidism and acromegaly. Diagnosis of OSAHS is established by PSG. Four types of PSG based on supervision and diagnostic equipment can be employed. In full PSG, there is recording of multiple respiratory and neurophysiological signals during sleep. In *limited sleep studies*, there is overnight recording of respiratory and oxygenation patterns done without neurophysiological recording.

Differential Diagnosis

Depression is a major cause of sleepiness in India. Sedative and stimulant drugs can induce sleepiness. Narcolepsy is less common but seen from childhood and is associated with cataplexy. Idiopathic hypersomnolence and phase alteration syndromes can also present with long duration of sleepiness.

TREATMENT

First-line therapy for sleep apnea syndrome remains medical. The medical treatment options are listed in Box 149.3.

General measures include good sleep hygiene, avoidance of alcohol, hypnotics and sedatives. Weight loss is recommended in all overweight patients. It has been shown that 1% change in weight is associated with a 3% change in AHI. For patients with position-dependent sleep apnea, symptoms can be alleviated by promoting sleep in the lateral decubitus position. Specific measures to increase upper airway caliber include position therapy and positive airway pressure (PAP) therapy. Main treatment modality is by continuous positive airway pressure (CPAP) therapy. CPAP works by blowing the airway open during sleep, usually with pressures of 5–20 mm Hg. Clinical trials have shown that CPAP therapy offers better quality of life by controlling most of the associated symptoms. CPAP therapy can be applied by different types of machines applied to mask over the mouth and nose during sleep. These work on different principles. Each case has to be prescribed the appropriate instrument for full benefit and patient compliance.

Box 149.3: Medical treatment of obstructive sleep apnea/hypopnea syndrome

- General measures
  - Avoidance of alcohol, sedatives and hypnotics
  - Weight loss
- Specific measures to increase upper airway caliber
  - Position therapy
  - Positive airway pressure
    - Continuous Positive Airway Pressure (CPAP)
    - Bi-level systems
    - Auto-CPAP
- Oral appliances

Various surgical procedures are tried for those cases not responding to above therapy and in persons with specific anatomic defects. Mandibular repositioning splint (MRS) is an oral device found to be useful in some cases.

For patients with problems in the management of CPAP therapy, management is done with stimulation of the hypoglossal nerve by surgically implanted upper airway stimulation device. In this uncontrolled study, upper airway stimulation resulted in significant improvements in objective and subjective measurements of the severity of OSA.

Source: Malhotra A. Hypoglossal-nerve stimulation for obstructive sleep apnea. N Engl J Med. 2014;370(2):170-1.

CHAPTER
150

Neoplasms of the Lung

C Sudheendra Ghosh, Murali CP

Chapter Summary

- Benign Tumors
  - Bronchial Adenoma
- Malignant Tumors
- Bronchogenic Carcinoma
- Small Cell Lung Cancer

Pulmonary tumors may be benign or malignant, the latter may be primary or secondary. Malignant tumors far outnumber the benign ones.

BENIGN TUMORS

The benign lesions include hamartoma, chondroma arising from the bronchi, bronchial adenoma, fibroma, neurofibroma, myxoma and lipoma. Sclerosing angiomas, lymph cysts, histiocytomas and endometriosis may be seen rarely. Hamartomas are tumors in which normal components of the lungs are combined in a disorganized manner.

Bronchial Adenoma

These constitute 1–6% of all pulmonary neoplasms. Females are affected more than males and age group is lower than that of bronchogenic carcinoma. There is an association between bronchial adenomas and multiple endocrine neoplasia (MEN). Histologically, the tumors may be carcinoids, cylindromata, mucoepidermoid tumors or mixed tumors which resemble mixed parotid tumors.

Adenomas occur in the larger bronchi. They may be silent, or they produce symptoms such as cough, hemoptysis, bronchial obstruction and recurrent pneumonia. Hemoptysis may be massive and intractable.

The *diagnosis* should be suspected in any healthy young individual presenting with recurrent and massive hemoptysis and confirmed by bronchoscopy. *Treatment* is surgical excision.

MALIGNANT TUMORS

Primary carcinomas are fairly common all over the world. The main types are carcinoma of the bronchus and alveolar cell carcinoma (*bronchiolar carcinoma, pulmonary adenomatosis*).

The lungs are commonly the seat of secondary deposits from malignant tumors arising from many organs. Carcinomas of the breast, kidney, liver, gastrointestinal tract (GIT), testes, prostate, female genital tract and thyroid, and sarcomas from bone and soft tissues may all produce extensive metastases in the lungs.

BRONCHOGENIC CARCINOMA

This tumor originates from the basal cell layer of the bronchial wall. Bronchogenic carcinoma is the most common cause of cancer-related to mortality in the world.

Epidemiology

The disease is more common in the western world and the highest prevalence has been reported from Scotland. In India, also the number of cases reported is steadily increasing and bronchogenic carcinoma accounts for 0.14–0.15% of all medical admissions in the major general hospitals. Incidence in males is 10–15 times more than that in females. The disease is most frequent in fifth and sixth decades.

The role of external factors such as carcinogens derived from cigarette smoke and from atmospheric pollution in the pathogenesis has been established by several epidemiological studies. In addition to cigarette smoke, exposure to several substances such as 3, 4-benzopyrene from automobile smokes, asbestos, nickel chromate, arsenic, vinyl chloride, uranium and radioactive materials increase the risk of developing pulmonary cancer (Flowchart 150.1 and Table 150.1). Among these, the most widely investigated factor is cigarette smoking. Fifteen percent of male smokers develop lung cancer. Following cessation of smoking, risk of developing cancer decreases by 10–20 years, but the risk is still 2.5 times that of nonsmokers.

Cigarettes and beedies, considerably increase the risk of developing bronchogenic carcinoma, especially the squamous and small cell types. Adenocarcinoma and large cell carcinomas do not show this direct relationship. Smoking more than 20 cigarettes daily for 20 years or more, increases the risk of developing bronchogenic

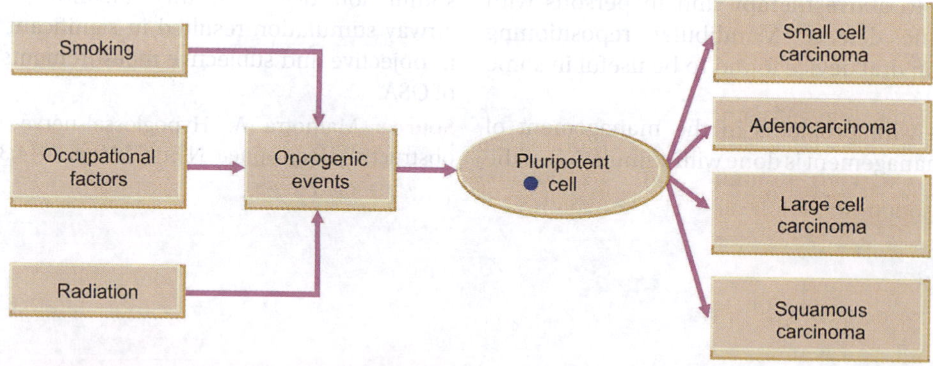

Table 150.1: Risk associated with occupational carcinogens

Occupational carcinogens	Risks
Asbestos	Insulation and shipyard workers, increase in risk of lung cancer after 10 years of exposure, with concurrent smoking increases risk 90-fold
Arsenic	Smelters and vineyard workers, Upper lobe predominance
Nickel	SCC–MC
Radiation	Uranium mining, oat cell carcinoma–MC
Hematite mining	Due to radon exposure
Hard rock mining	Chromium exposure, squamous cell–MC
Chloromethyl	Oat cell–MC
Ethers and mustard gas	Squamous and undifferentiated–MC
Soots, tars	Coke oven workers
Oils and cokes	Gas house workers, roofers

carcinoma 8–20 times above that of nonsmokers. Cigar and pipe-smoking is less harmful. Many substances present in tobacco and the components of the paper have been found to increase the risk cumulatively. Both direct smoking and passive smoking, i.e. inhalation of smoke exhaled by others in a closed environment, are found to be harmful (*See* Ch 26).

Histological Classification

Histologically, the tumors are classified into small cell type otherwise known as oat cell carcinoma and non-small type which includes squamous cell carcinoma (SCC), adenocarcinoma and large cell carcinoma (Flowchart 150.2). Oat cell carcinomas are invariably disseminated

at the time of presentation. In contrast, large cell carcinomas which are detected early may be localized and hence, amenable to surgical resection. One variety of adenocarcinoma is bronchioloalveolar cell carcinoma. In some tumors, both epidermoid and adenocarcinomatous patterns are seen. Around 50% of tumors are situated centrally proximal to a segmental bronchus and the rest are peripheral. Site of predilection is the right upper lobe. In some cases, adenocarcinoma may supervene on areas of infarction or scars of tuberculosis. Lung tumors have been staged, taking into account the size, location, local effects, local lymphadenopathy and distant metastases.

The incidence of SCC is coming down and that of adenocarcinoma is going up (Table 150.2).

Over 90% of the total number is constituted by SCC, adenocarcinoma, small cell carcinoma and anaplastic large cell type. Histological diagnosis is important since the different types have different biological behavior.

Squamous cell or epidermoid carcinoma: Arises from the central bronchi in over 80% of cases. Among superior sulcus tumors, it forms 30% or more. These tumors undergo cavitation readily. Metastasis occurs later in the disease.

Adenocarcinomas: They are more commonly associated with previous scars in the lungs. They form acinar and glandular patterns. They are situated more peripherally. Metastasis occurs early. Bronchioloalveolar carcinoma (BAC) is a variant of adenocarcinoma, forming about 5% of the total primary malignant tumors. It may arise from the mucin-secreting bronchial epithelial cell, nonciliated secretory bronchiolar cells or type 2 alveolar epithelial cells. It is more common in women. Local spread throughout the airspaces occurs early. In many cases, the origin may be multicentric.

Flowchart 150.2: Classification of lung cancer

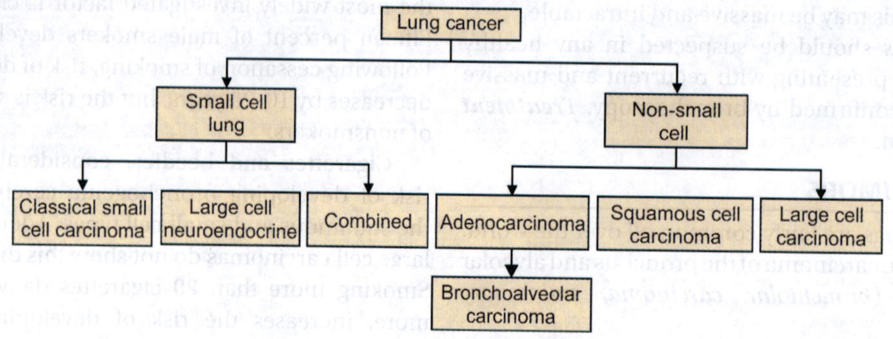

Table 150.2: Frequency and features of non-small cell lung cancer subtypes

Features	Squamous Cell Carcinoma	Adenocarcinoma	Large Cell Carcinoma	Bronchoalveolar variant of adenocarcinoma
Prevalence number of people suffering from the disease in a year	Accounts for about 25% of NSCLC cases	Accounts for about 40% of NSCLC cases	Accounts for about 10% of NSCLC cases	Occurs in about 3% of all lung cancer patients
Incidence number of new cases developing in a year	Decreasing	Increasing		Increasing (corresponds to increase in adenocarcinoma)
Location	Usually central	Usually more peripheral but can be multifocal	Central or peripheral location	
Risk Factors	Highly correlated with smoking (~90% of those with SCC are smokers)	Most common type seen in non-smokers Precursor is atypical alveolar hyperplasia		Typically affects younger, female and non-smoking patients
Histologic Features	Cancer of squamous epithelial cells	Cancer of bronchial mucosal (glandular) tissue or the alveolar surface epithelium. Cancer may produce glandular patterns	Diagnosis of exclusion (i.e. doesn't have features of adenocarcinoma or SCC)	Cancer of type 2 pneumocytes grows along alveolar septa. ('lepidic' or scale-like growth)
Prognosis	Slow-growing tumor may be poorly or well-differentiated	Faster doubling time than squamous cell. Often early metastasis. Usually worse prognosis than squamous cell	Can cavitate Metastasize early (often to GIT). Prognosis is similar to that for adenocarcinoma	Often radio and chemoresistant. Less frequently metastasizes to lymph nodes compared to other NSCLC variants. Better prognosis than non-BAC adenocarcinoma

Abbreviations: NSCLC = Non-small cell lung cancer; SCC = Squamous cell carcinoma; BAC = Bronchoalveolar carcinoma; GIT = Gastrointestinal tract

Large cell carcinoma: These consist of anaplastic large cells without squamous or glandular differentiation. They also occur more peripherally. Local spread and metastasis occurs early. These tumors tend to cavitate. Though distinct histological patterns can be identified in most cases, some may show overlap in cell types, e.g., adenosquamous carcinoma.

Small cell lung carcinoma (SCLC): They are also known as oat cell carcinoma are made up of cells containing large nuclei in relation to their cytoplasm. These are also seen more centrally in the lungs. Compared to SCC, the evolution of the disease is more rapid and metastasis occur earlier (Table 150.3).

Several cytogenetic abnormalities are being elucidated. Oncogenes play a role in malignant transformation. Several tumors produce autocrine secretions which enable them to proliferate autonomously. World Health Organization (WHO) has introduced classification of lung tumors. In 2004, the classification also took into account genetic details. Much effort is under way to detect genetic susceptibility to lung cancer, especially on chromosome 15A–24, 25.

Clinical Features

In many cases, a long latent period may elapse before the tumor produces symptoms. Sometimes the radiological abnormality may be the finding that draws attention. In some cases, metastases are the first to produce symptoms (Fig. 150.1). Clinical features may be described as:

- Intrathoracic manifestations
- Symptoms due to metastases
- Paraneoplastic syndromes.

General symptomatology includes nonspecific manifestations such as tiredness, anorexia, weight loss, clubbing of fingers and toes, fever, and pulmonary osteoarthropathy (Table 150.4).

Table 150.3: Comparison of small cell and non-small cell lung cancer

SCLC	NSCLC
• 10–15% of lung cancers	• 85–90% of lung cancers
• Classically, three subtypes	• Many subtypes
• Usually centrally located	• Centrally or peripherally located
• More aggressive	• Fast or slow growing
• Staged as limited or extensive disease	• Staged using TNM staging
• Treatment usually chemotherapy with or without radiation	• Treatment is surgical, medical or radiation

Abbreviations: SCLC = Small cell lung cancer; NSCLC = Non-small cell lung cancer; TNM = Tumor-node-metastasis

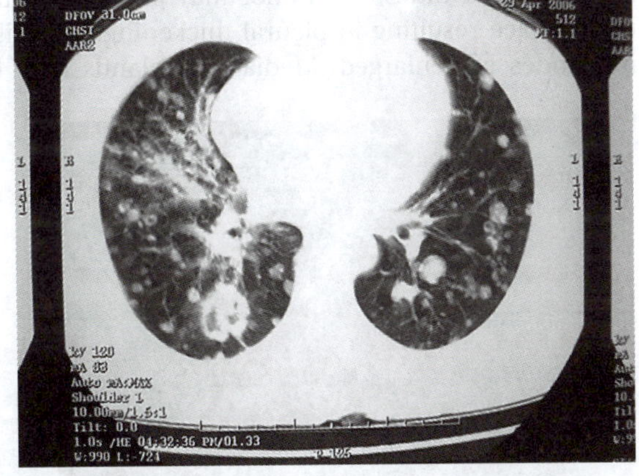

Fig. 150.1: HRCT—Metastases

Abbreviation: HRCT = High-resolution computed tomography

Pulmonary Manifestations

Cough due to irritation of the bronchus may be troublesome, interfering with sleep. In the chronic smoker, this is likely to be mistaken for cough due to

Table 150.4: Common presenting signs and symptoms of lung cancer

Symptoms	Signs
• Cough	• Clubbing
• Weight loss	• SVC obstruction
• Dyspnea	• Dysphagia
• Chest pain	• Wheezing and stridor
• Fever	• Features of paraneoplastic syndromes
• Hemoptysis	• Features of mass lesion
• Bone pain	• Features of collapse
• Weakness	• Features of obstructive pneumonia

Abbreviation: SVC = Superior vena cava

excessive smoking. Hemoptysis occurs in many cases. Bleeding may be from the tumor or from other pulmonary complications. The tumor may block the bronchus and lead to obstructive symptoms like unilateral or localized wheezing, atelectasis, recurrent pneumonia or lung abscess. Further complications like pleurisy or empyema may be evident. At times, obstruction to the bronchus becomes valvular and affected segment undergoes localized emphysema.

In some cases, a peripheral tumor undergoes central liquefaction and abscess formation.

Tumors of the apical region of the lung may invade the pleura, the brachial plexus and cervical sympathetic chain. In most cases, the tumor is a SCC and this is called ***Pancoast's tumor*** or ***superior sulcus tumor (Fig. 150.2)***. Involvement of the brachial plexus leads to intense neuralgic pain along the arm. Paralysis of the sympathetic chain gives rise to ipsilateral Horner's syndrome.

Pancoast's syndrome: It is a constellation of characteristic symptoms and signs that include pain over the shoulder and arm along the distribution of the C8, T1 and T2 nerve roots, Horner's syndrome, weakness and atrophy of muscles of the hand, most commonly caused by extension of an apical lung tumor at the thoracic inlet.

Malignant pleural effusion: It may develop due to spread to the pleura. At times, the tumor may grow along the pleural surface resulting in pleural thickening. The hilar lymph nodes are enlarged. Mediastinal glands may be affected and enlargement of these structures gives rise to mediastinal syndrome. Compression of the phrenic nerve gives rise to diaphragmatic paralysis. Malignant pericardial effusion may develop. Direct spread to the ribs may lead to their destruction.

- Manifestation due to the location of the primary tumor/growth (Table 150.5)
- Manifestation due to the regional spread of tumor in the thorax
  - The regional spread of tumor in the thorax may occur by direct extension or by metastasis to regional lymph nodes. The clinical effects of such spread are listed in Table 150.6. Hematogenous, lymphatic or direct spread to pleura results in malignant pleural effusion.

Physical Examination

Physical examination of the chest may reveal signs of consolidation, cavitation, atelectasis or pleural effusion.

Table 150.5: Manifestation due to the location of the primary tumor

Due to a central or endobronchial growth	Due to a peripheral growth
• Cough • Hemoptysis • Wheeze and stridor • Breathlessness/dyspnea • Post-obstructive pneumonitis presenting with fever and productive cough	• Chest pain from pleural or chest wall involvement • Dyspnea on a restrictive basis • Symptoms of lung abscess due to cavitation of tumor

Table 150.6: Manifestations of lung cancer due to regional spread of tumor in the thorax

Pathological basis	Local effects
Obstruction of airway by tumor	Pneumonia, abscess, atelectasis, focal emphysema
Tracheal obstruction	Stridor (a harsh inspiratory noise) and dyspnea
Local spread into pleura	Pleuritis and malignant effusion
Local spread to pericardium	Pericarditis, effusion, tamponade
Compression of SVC by tumor	SVC syndrome
Invasion of structures	**Effects**
RLN	Hoarseness of voice and 'bovine' cough
Phrenic nerve	Diaphragm paralysis and dyspnea
Sympathetic ganglia	Horner syndrome ((ipsilateral partial ptosis, enophthalmos, miosis and hypohidrosis of the face)
Esophagus	Dysphagia
Chest wall (direct extension)	Destruction of rib producing rib pain, pathological fractures and intercostal neuralgia
Superior sulcus tumor (destruction of the T1 and C8 roots in the lower part of the brachial plexus by an apical lung tumor)	Pancoast's syndrome (pain in the inner aspect of the arm, sometimes with small muscle wasting in the hand)
Pericardial and cardiac	Cardiac tamponade, arrhythmias or cardiac failure

Abbreviations: SVC = Superior vena cava; RLN = Recurrent laryngeal nerve

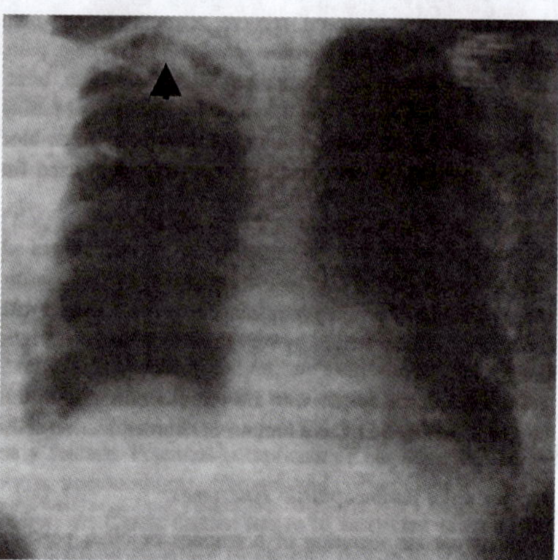

Fig. 150.2: Pancoast's tumor. ***Note:*** The rounded opacity in the right upper region—arrowhead

Enlargement of pretracheal and scalene lymph nodes and recent onset of finger clubbing should suggest the possibility of malignancy.

Extrathoracic Manifestations

Widespread secondaries may occur in the liver, bone, adrenal glands, brain, kidney, spleen, peritoneum, skin and other organs. Manifestations caused by metastases may be the presenting features in many. For example, late onset seizures or a pathological fracture may be the first evidence of a bronchogenic neoplasm.

Nonmetastatic metabolic or neuromuscular manifestation of lung cancer is known as paraneoplastic manifestation.

Diagnosis

Bronchogenic carcinoma should be considered in the diagnosis of all respiratory disorders. Malignancy can mimic virtually all common pulmonary diseases such as tuberculosis, pneumonia, lung abscess, atelectasis, localized emphysema and pleural effusion.

The term **lymphangitis carcinomatosa** is given to the condition where the cancer has spread extensively through the lymphatics into the adjacent part of the lung giving rise to a picture of pneumonia or bronchopneumonia. X-ray shows characteristic streaky shadowing possibly representing the lymphatic spread (Fig. 150.3).

When a solitary pulmonary nodule (**coin shadow**) is detected and diagnosis is not evident, the patient should be followed up to see the progress of the lesion. In general, malignant lesions have a doubling time of 20–400 days. More rapid growth is suggestive of inflammatory lesions. Calcification is in favor of nonmalignant lesions.

Investigations

Radiological Findings

Radiological findings may be varied. The presence of a circular or irregular shadow in an asymptomatic patient may be the only finding. The classic circular shadow is called **coin lesion**. In more advanced cases, the lesion may be more extensive. Hilar glands are enlarged. The growth may undergo central cavitation and the resulting abscess shows thick and ragged walls. The presence of hilar adenopathy should suggest the malignant nature of the lesion. Presence of diaphragmatic paralysis along with a hilar mass should strongly suggest the possibility of bronchogenic carcinoma. Other features like collapse, consolidation, localized emphysema and pleural and pericardial effusion may also be present.

Golden 'S' Sign

This is a radiological sign seen in central bronchogenic carcinoma obstructing the upper lobe bronchus. This produces collapse. The margin of the collapse segment produces the inward curve of 'S' and mass will produce the outward curve of the 'S' in the lower part. Radiologically, this is a characteristic of upper lobe carcinoma (Fig. 150.4).

High-resolution computed tomography scans (HRCT) and magnetic resonance imaging (MRI) give good delineation of the tumor and its extensions in the thoracic cavity and thoracic cage (Fig. 105.5). Positron emission

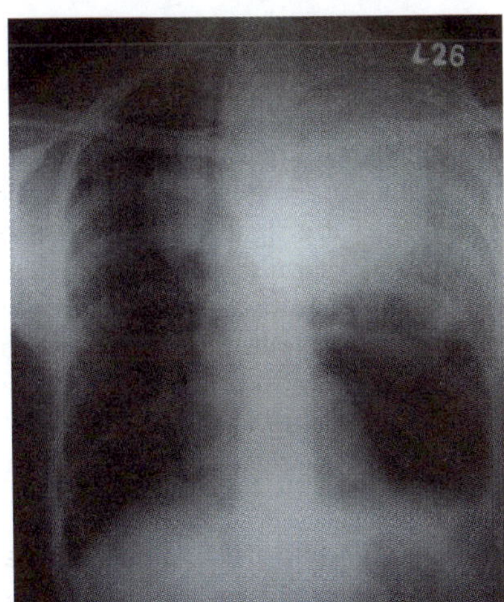

Fig. 150.3: Chest X-ray—Bronchogenic carcinoma. **Note:** Tumor with bilateral massive lymph node metastases

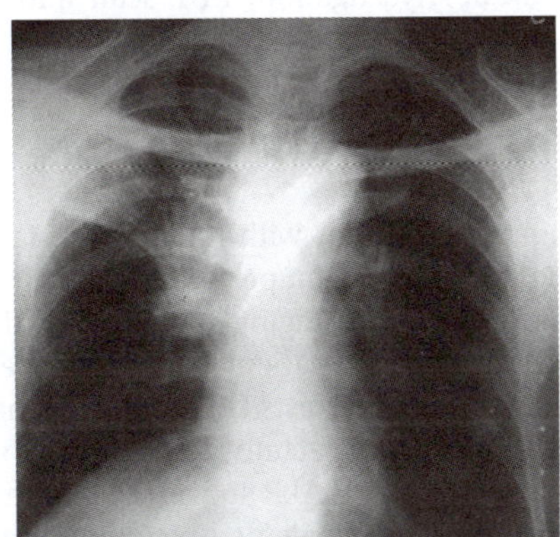

Fig. 150.4: Golden 'S' sign

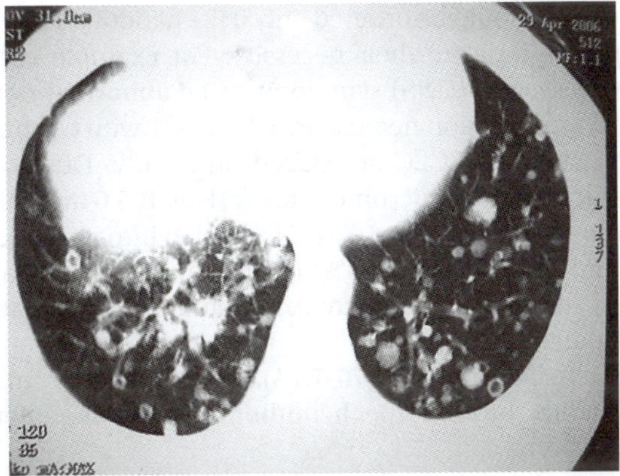

Fig. 150.5: HRCT cavitating metastasis

tomography (PET) scans improve the rate of detection of local and distant metastases, especially in patients with non-small cell lung cancer (NSCLC). PET scan using 18F-fluorodeoxy glucose, a new investigative modality to detect mediastinal and distant metastases in NSCLC.

Sputum Examination

Hemoptysis is present in many cases and the sputum is typically described as **currant jelly**. Malignant cells may be detected in the sputum by examining a wet preparation with methylene blue staining and this can be confirmed by **Papanicolaou's method**.

Other Diagnostic Procedures

Other diagnostic procedures include bronchoscopy, needle biopsy of peripherally placed tumors, biopsy of palpable lymph nodes in the neck and axilla and *scalene fat pad biopsy*. The right scalene node should be biopsied in cases of lesions of the right lung and left lower lobe. The left scalene node should be biopsied for left upper lobe neoplasms. Mediastinoscopy and biopsy of nodes is a more rewarding procedure. Fluorescent bronchoscopy is a specialized form of bronchoscopy in which the malignant tissue emits fluorescence. This enables more easy detection of the lesions and helps to make more accurate biopsy.

Modern Ultrathin Fiber-optic Bronchoscopes

Those that can reach beyond the eighth generation bronchi are available. These help to diagnose peripheral lesions. When the nature of the lesion cannot be confirmed by the common investigation, PET scan allows precise diagnosis and risk stratification. Measurement of tumor markers will also help in the diagnosis of carcinoma lung.

Special Tests to Stage the Diseases

Staging

Correct staging of patients with lung cancer is crucial in determining the proper therapeutic approach. One of the most important parts of staging is thorough history and physical examination. All patients need serum electrolyte estimation, liver function tests (LFTs) [including alkaline phosphatase (ALP) and lactate dehydrogenase (LDH)], and chest X-ray. Elevated ALP suggests bone metastases. In the past, patients routinely had head computed tomography (CTs) and radionuclide bone scans as part of the diagnostic workup, but large studies have shown that these tests should be ordered only if the patient's signs and symptoms indicate their necessity. For example central nervous system (CNS) symptoms or an abnormal neurological examination necessitate a brain CT with contrast.

NSCLC and SCLC are staged differently. Due to the high incidence of micrometastases (Figs 105.6 and 105.7) early in the disease state, SCLC is divided into two stages:

1. Limited disease (25–30%), in which the tumor is limited to ipsilateral hemithorax (including contralateral mediastinal nodes)
2. Extensive disease (70–75%), in which the tumor extends beyond the hemithorax (including pleural effusions).

SCLC is treated with chemotherapy and radiation therapy. NSCLC is staged using the TNM staging system (T is tumor size, N is nodal involvement, and M is presence or absence of metastases). TNM descriptors and staging for lung cancer are given in Tables 150.7 and 150.8.

Prognosis

Since most of the cases are diagnosed late in the disease, overall prognosis in bronchogenic carcinoma is poor. Asymptomatic subjects detected by investigations have the best prognosis. Next in line are subjects with symptoms referable to the primary tumor with duration of less than six months. Metastases in CNS and liver confer a poor outcome. Small cell carcinomas have a poor

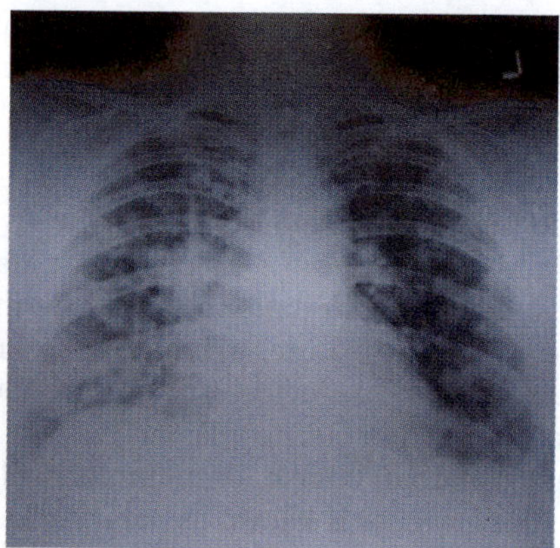

Fig. 150.6: Non-small cell lung carcinoma

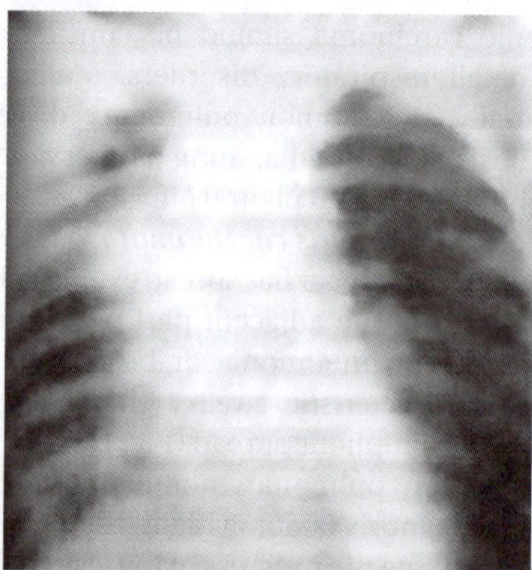

Fig. 150.7: Chest X-ray—carcinoma lung. **Note:** The mass with hazy margins extending outwards from the right border of the mediastinum

Table 150.7: TNM descriptors	
T (primary tumor)	
T_0	No evidence of primary tumor
T_x	Tumor proven by presence of malignant cells in bronchopulmonary secretions
T_{is}	Carcinoma *in situ*
T_1	Tumor <3 cm (not in main stem bronchus)
T_2	Tumor >3 cm or present in main stem bronchus but not within 2 cm of carina, invasion of visceral pleura, associated atelectasis or pneumonitis extending to hilar region
T_3	Tumor of any size that invades the chest wall, diaphragm, mediastinal pleura and parietal pericardium. Tumor <2 cm from carina is associated with atelectasis or pneumonitis of entire lung
T_4	Tumor of any size with invasion of mediastinum, heart, great vessels, trachea, esophagus, vertebral body or carina; malignant pleural or pericardial effusion; satellite tumor nodules in the same lobe
N (nodal Status)	
N_0	No nodal involvement
N_1	Metastases to ipsilateral peribronchial or ipsilateral hilar region (including direct extension)
N_2	Metastases to ipsilateral mediastinal and/or subcarinal lymph nodes
N_3	Metastases to supraclavicular or contralateral mediastinal, hilar, or scalene nodes
M (distant metastases)	
M_0	No distant metastasis
M_1	Distant metastasis

Table 150.8: Staging of bronchogenic carcinoma

Stage	TNM Descriptor
Occult carcinoma	$T_x N_0 M_0$
0	T_{is} (carcinoma *in situ*)
IA	$T_1 N_0 M_0$
IB	$T_2 N_0 M_0$
IIA	$T_1 N_1 M_0$
IIB	$T_2 N_1 M_0$ or $T_1 N_0 M_0$
IIIA	$T_1 N_1 M_0$ or $T_{1-3} N_2 M_0$ (N_2 disease)
IIIB	Any $TN_3 M_0$ or T_4 any NM_0
IV	Any T any N M_1

prognosis since metastases develop early. In the majority of patients, only palliative therapy is possible. Five-year survival figures for SCC vary from 40 to 50% for stage 1 to less than 10% for stages III and above. Five-year survival rate in resected NSCLC ranges from 35 to 73%. Adjuvant chemotherapy improved survival further.

Treatment

Management depends on the stage of the tumor on diagnosis, histological type and presence of complications. *Treatment* may consist of surgery, irradiation and chemotherapy.

Surgery

When the primary is small and is detected before clinical manifestations develop and there are no metastases, surgical treatment is ideal. Contraindications for surgery include infiltration of the trachea, carina, superior vena cava (SVC), recurrent laryngeal nerve (RLN) paralysis and pleural effusion. Involvement of the mediastinal nodes precludes the chance of resection in non-small carcinoma. Staging of the tumor by the presence of mediastinal lymph node involvement is absolutely essential for deciding on surgery. Stage I with N_0 (i.e.) no lymph node involvement and stage II with N_1 (i.e.) only ipsilateral mediastinal or bronchopulmonary node is present, are amenable to surgical resection which is the treatment of first choice. Surgical results are less satisfactory in those cases which have developed symptoms and those with small cell carcinoma.

Radiotherapy

Radical radiotherapy is preferred in selected cases. In practice, in the majority of cases radiotherapy is given as a palliative measure in inoperable cases with local spread or distant metastases. Several recent advances in radiotherapy techniques such as split dose radiotherapy, use of radiosensitizers and the availability of radiation equipment like linear accelerator, betatron, neutron beams and meson beams have made radiotherapy more effective with less of hazard. In some centers, radiotherapy is also used prophylactically to the brain to prevent the development of metastases.

Chemotherapy

It is indicated in 90% of patients with bronchogenic carcinoma. The choice of drugs is based on the tumor histology, facilities for supportive therapy and tolerance by the patient. Chemotherapy may be used as the sole modality of treatment in advanced cases or as an adjuvant to surgery and radiotherapy. Commonly used chemotherapeutic agents are methotrexate, cyclophosphamide, vincristine, CCNU, adriamycin, etoposide and cisplatin. Small cell cancer responds well whereas the others do not.

Other modalities of treatment are laser therapy which is employed in order to reduce the tumor mass and relieve obstructive symptoms. Incurable cases should receive terminal care which includes the provision of comfort, analgesics to relieve pain, management of symptoms, maintenance of nutrition, treatment of infection and proper attention by friends and family members. Preoperative radiotherapy followed by in enbloc surgical resection is the most common treatment used for Pancoast's tumor.

Newer Developments

Monoclonal antibodies (mAbs) has been used with benefit. Bivacizumab, is an antibody against vascular endothelial growth factor (VEGF). Cetuximab is a mAb against epidermal growth factor-receptor (EGFR).

SMALL CELL LUNG CANCER

It forms 20% of all primary lung cancers. It is associated with smoking. It is characterized by very rapid local and metastatic spread.

Paraneoplastic Syndromes

They are more common with this subtype. Possibly SCLC is a tumor of neuroendocrine cells.

Mechanism of Paraneoplastic Syndromes

- Inappropriate secretion of hormones or other peptides such as growth factors, cytokines and prostaglandins by the tumor
- Immunological cross-reaction of antitumor antibodies with normal tissues.

In SCLC, the genes encoding these hormones and humoral agents are not mutated, but they are deregulated, so that secretion goes on without feedback inhibition. Moreover, biologically inactive forms of hormones may result from aberrant processing of the ribonucleic acid (RNA) peptide.

Hormonal Abnormalities

Syndrome of inappropriate antidiuretic hormone (SIADH) occurs in 10% cases.

Peptide Hormones Produced by SCLC

Atrial natriuretic peptide (ANP), corticotropin, beta-endorphin, beta-human chorionic gonadotropin (β-hCG), calcitonin, granulocyte-colony stimulating factor (G-CSF), erythropoietin, gastrin releasing peptide, glucagon, growth hormone, interleukin-10 (IL-10), melanocyte stimulating hormone (MSH), neuron-specific enolase (NSE), neuro-physin, neurotensin, parathyroid hormone, physalemin, somatostatin, vasoactive intestinal peptide (VIP), vaso-pressin and others.

Immunologically-Mediated Paraneoplastic Neurological Syndromes

These result from the cross-reaction of antitumor antibodies with antigens present in neural tissue, neuromuscular junction or muscle, e.g. Lambert-Eaton myasthenic syndrome (LEMS) occurs in 6% of SCLC cases and myasthenia gravis (MG) may also occur rarely.

Myasthenia results from autoantibody-mediated functional blockade of the calcium channels involved in the release of acetylcholine at nerve terminals.

Peripheral Nervous System

- Autonomic neuropathy
- Intestinal pseudo-obstruction

Sensorimotor Peripheral Neuropathy

- Subacute motor neuropathy
- Subacute sensory neuropathy

Central Nervous System

Angioendotheliosis, dementia, encephalomyelitis—(brainstem encephalitis, limbic encephalitis), myoclonus-opsoclonus, optic neuritis, cancer-associated retinopathy (CAR), subacute cerebellar degeneration (SCD), subacute necrotizing myelopathy occur in CNS-related syndromes.

Cachexia

The most common paraneoplastic phenomenon is cachexia which is a complex metabolic syndrome probably resulting from a host response to tumor.

Treatment

Chemotherapy is the first-line of treatment. The common regimens are:

> A – Adriamycin (doxorubicin)
> C – Cyclophosphamide
> E – Etoposide and
> A – Adriamycin
> C – Cyclophosphamide
> V – Vincristine

About 70–90% get effective symptom relief. SCLC is highly radiosensitive but relapse occurs frequently and rapidly. Combination of chemotherapy and radiotherapy is more useful. SCLC is common to produce brain metastasis and, therefore, prophylactic cranial irradiation (PCI) may help to prevent intracranial metastases. Still, life is not prolonged since metastases at other sites prove fatal. At the time of diagnoses, brain metastases are seen in 10%, liver metastases in 25% and bone metastases in 20%.

Two-year survival rate is about 30% in the cases with limited spread whereas it is below 10% in more advanced cases. SCLC—the median survival without treatment is 6–8 weeks for limited disease. At presentation, less than 30% have limited disease.

Tyrosine kinase group of drugs are tried for the treatment of bronchogenic carcinoma. Gefitinib is an oral tyrosine kinase inhibitor which shows promise has been employed with success. Crizotinib which is another oral tyrosine kinase inhibitor is more effective.

Prophylaxis

Bronchogenic carcinoma is at least partially preventable by avoidance of smoking. The risk of cancer comes down quantitatively with the reduction in the number of cigarettes smoked and in those who give up smoking completely the increased risk of cancer comes down after a period of a few years.

Occupational exposure to asbestos, environmental pollutants and radioactive materials should be reduced to the minimum and persons engaged in these industries should receive protection.

CHAPTER
151

Pulmonary Cysts

C Sudheendra Ghosh

Chapter Summary

- Congenital Cysts
- Acquired Cysts

CONGENITAL CYSTS

These cysts are of three varieties:

1. **Bronchogenic** may be solitary or multiple.
2. **Alveolar cell types** may also be solitary or multiple.
3. **Mixed types** having elements of both bronchogenic and alveolar cysts.

These may vary in size and may be unilateral or bilateral. They may be located anywhere in the lung. They are filled with fluid at birth, but air enters the cavity later when bronchial communications develop. The cysts may be thick- or thin-walled.

Cystic disease of the lung: This may occur in association with fibrocystic disease of the pancreas. This is common in Western countries, but is rare in India.

ACQUIRED CYSTS

These may present as bullous emphysema, subpleural cysts or parasitic cysts, which include hydatid disease and paragonimiasis.

Clinical Features

The severity of symptoms is determined by the extent, size, time of diagnosis and presence of complications. When the lung parenchyma is grossly reduced, respiratory embarrassment and respiratory failure may develop. Superadded infection is common and this is characterized by fever, cough, purulent sputum and even hemoptysis.

Though pulmonary osteoarthropathy may occur, it is a late feature. This is in contrast to bronchiectasis, in which clubbing is an early feature. Potential complications are infection, hemoptysis, pneumothorax, fibrosis and cor pulmonale.

Diagnosis

Cystic disease has to be suspected when a child presents with recurrent respiratory infections. Presence of other congenital abnormalities should strengthen this suspicion. X-ray shows thin-walled cysts, which may be single or multiple. High-resolution computed tomography (HRCT) is very useful in locating the lesion and confirming the diagnosis. Tuberculosis, bronchiectasis and lung abscess have to be differentiated.

In congenital cystic lung, bronchography delineates the lesions. In the case of single noncommunicating cysts, the dye does not enter the cavity.

Treatment

A large single cyst producing respiratory embarrassment from infancy has to be excised. Video-assisted thoracoscopy is used at present for the surgical excision of cysts. When the cysts are too numerous, surgery is contraindicated. Medical management is on the same lines as for bronchiectasis.

CHAPTER

152 Pulmonary Involvement in Systemic Diseases

C Sudheendra Ghosh, Davis Paul

> **Chapter Summary**
> - Collagen Diseases
> - Ankylosing Spondylitis
> - Wegener's Granulomatosis
> - Pulmonary Involvement in Goodpasture's Syndrome

COLLAGEN DISEASES

Systemic lupus erythematosus (SLE), dermatomyositis, progressive systemic sclerosis, rheumatoid arthritis (RA), polyarteritis nodosa (PAN) and Sjögren's syndrome involve the lung in varying degrees. Out of these RA is most common.

RA: Pleurisy, nodular intrapulmonary lesions, diffuse interstitial fibrosis, rheumatoid pneumoconiosis (Caplan's syndrome) and pulmonary hypertension (PH) are the common manifestations. Diagnosis depends on the total clinical picture and laboratory tests.

SLE: Pleurisy with or without effusion which may be unilateral or bilateral, lupus pneumonia, diffuse interstitial fibrosis, pulmonary hemorrhage and PH are the usual manifestations. Diagnosis is based on other clinical features and demonstration of antinuclear antibodies (ANAs).

PAN: In this, there is a necrotizing vasculitis affecting the systemic arteries. In addition, it may affect the pulmonary arteries as well, producing PH. This condition has to be distinguished from Goodpasture's syndrome. X-ray shows patchy infiltrates or nodular type of lesions and pleural effusions. Steroids are the mainstay in the management.

Progressive systemic sclerosis: Pulmonary fibrosis (PF) starts in the lower lobes and is seen as a honeycomb pattern of the lungs in the skiagram. Spontaneous pneumothorax is a common complication. Alveolar cell carcinoma may develop in some.

Dermatomyositis: Lung involvement is rare. The early lesions are in the form of a lymphocytic interstitial pneumonia (LIP) of the lower lobes which gradually leads on to interstitial fibrosis.

Sjögren's syndrome: Pulmonary lesions are in the nature of LIP leading on to interstitial fibrosis. Secondary bacterial pneumonias and later bronchiectasis occur. Infections are more common due to drying up of the secretions.

ANKYLOSING SPONDYLITIS

Here, the upper lobes are involved. The initial lesion is consolidation which progresses to cavitation and fibrosis. The lesions are considered to be part of the disease process itself.

WEGENER'S GRANULOMATOSIS

Syn: Granulomatous polyangiitis

Clinical Features

It may manifest at any age, the mean age of onset is 40 years and males are more affected. Initial symptoms are headache, sinusitis, rhinorrhea and vague general ill-health. Cough and hemoptysis may occur. Pulmonary manifestations are pneumonitis, hemoptysis, pleurisy, pneumothorax or cavitation. Acute glomerulonephritis syndrome may occur.

Treatment

Corticosteroids and immunosuppressant drugs like cyclophosphamide and azathioprine are effective. Fifty percent get full remission, 30% get partial remission and 10–20% may die of the disease. Therapy with cotrimoxazole (160 mg trimethoprim and 800 mg of sulfamethoxazole) bd for 24 months has been found useful to reduce the frequency of relapses.

PULMONARY INVOLVEMENT IN GOODPASTURE'S SYNDROME

Syn: Lung purpura, Antiglomerular basement membrane disease

The disease is common between ages 18 and 30 years and again between 50 and 60 years. It is more common among men. The disease initially begins with mild cough and breathlessness. Patient seeks medical help when hemoptysis develops. There can be associated renal symptoms like hematuria. **Diagnosis** is made when they develop fairly advanced disease with renal failure. Iron deficiency anemia (IDA) occurs due to blood loss. Occasionally, clubbing of fingers, enlargement of liver, spleen and lymph nodes may occur. Confirmation of the disease is by renal biopsy and antiglomerular basement membrane (anti-GBM) antibody estimation. Renal lesion is progressive and death occurs due to renal failure (*See* Section 16, Ch 181).

Treatment is with moderate to high doses of corticosteroids. Immunosuppressants and plasmapheresis can be tried. Overall prognosis is poor.

CHAPTER

153

Diseases of Pleura

C Sudheendra Ghosh, Davis Paul

Chapter Summary

- General Considerations
- Pleurisy
- Pleural Effusion
  - Tuberculous Pleural Effusion
  - Empyema
  - Tumors of the Pleura
- Pneumothorax
- Chemical Pleurodesis

GENERAL CONSIDERATIONS

Both visceral and parietal pleura have a single layer of mesothelial cells. Mesothelial cells contain abundant microvilli that are present diffusely over the entire pleural surfaces. They are 0.1 μm in diameter and about 1.5 μm length. They produce collagen, elastin, fibronectin and laminin. The visceral pleura can be considered to consist of three layers. The *endopleura*, which is the continuous mesothelial layer; then *external elastic lamina*; and the third layer *vascular layer* consisting of connective tissue containing lymphatics and blood vessels. This lies over the internal elastic lamina. In health, the surfaces of the pleural cavity are coated with a thin layer of pleural fluid that allows frictionless apposition of visceral and parietal pleura during each respiratory cycle. Pleural fluid is formed as ultrafiltrate of plasma just enough to wet the pleural surfaces. The rate of production of pleural fluid is 0.01 mL/kg/hr and it maintains a balance between production by the systemic vessels of the parietal pleura and removal by the parietal pleural lymphatics. Pleural fluid does not enter the visceral pleural lymphatics. The pressures vary during the entire respiratory cycle from -5 cm H_2O at mid chest at full expiration to -30 cm H_2O at mid chest at full inspiration.

PLEURISY

Inflammation of the pleura is called **pleurisy**. In dry pleurisy, the pleural surfaces are inflamed without fluid in between them. In many cases, pleurisy is associated with effusion. Both dry pleurisy and pleural effusion may develop at different stages of the same disease process. **Dry or fibrinous pleurisy:** In this condition, the lesion in the underlying lung spreads to the pleura. Trauma to the chest may also lead to pleurisy. The suggestive symptom is the catching pain felt acutely over the affected area by inspiratory movements brought about by deep breathing, coughing or sneezing.

Etiology of Pleurisy

- Pulmonary tuberculosis
- Pneumonia, lung abscess, bronchiectasis
- Bronchogenic carcinoma with secondaries
- Pulmonary infarction
- Connective tissue disorders such as systemic lupus erythematosus (SLE), polyarteritis nodosa (PAN), and rheumatoid disease
- Rheumatic fever
- Viral infections, especially Coxsackie (Bornholm disease)
- Hepatopulmonary amebiasis
- Uremia
- Pleural malignancy-mesothelioma
- Secondaries from other malignancies
- Lymphomas
- Lymphatic obstruction, especially filariasis
- Trauma to chest wall
- Complication of surgery in the abdomen or thorax
- Pleural effusion in association with tense ascites
- Pancreatitis.

PLEURAL EFFUSION

In this condition, fluid accumulates between the two layers of the pleura. Normally, pleural cavity contains only a small amount of fluid. Movements of the lung favor the movement of the fluid in and out of the pleural space. Normal composition of pleural fluid is:

- Volume—0.1–0.2 mL/kg
- Cells per mm^3—1,000–5,000
  - Mesothelial cells—3–70%
  - Monocytes—30–70%
  - Lymphocytes—2–30%
  - Granulocytes—10%
- Protein—1–2 g%
  Albumin—50–70
- Lactate dehydrogenase (LDH)—<50% of plasma LDH
  pH—7.6.

In most of the disease states, absorption of the fluid is reduced. The fluid may be contained in the general pleural space or it may be loculated in the interlobar fissure, infrapulmonary space or may remain adjacent to the mediastinum. The fluid progressively compresses the adjacent lung which undergoes collapse.

Clinical Features

The development of symptoms depends upon the speed of accumulation of fluid and its quantity. Common symptoms include dyspnea, pleuritic pain, or symptoms of the underlying disorder. High fever may occur in acute pyogenic infections. Tuberculosis may be associated with low grade fever.

Physical Examination

Physical examination reveals diminution of movement on the affected side and the presence of pleural friction rub on auscultation. Pleural rub has a superficial grating quality. The rub is heard better by gentle pressure of the chest piece of the stethoscope on the chest wall. Unlike rales, it is not altered by coughing. With the development of pleural effusion, the rub may disappear in many cases. Pleural rub has to be distinguished from crepitations and sounds arising from movements of the chest wall. Other painful conditions like myalgias, myocardial infarction (MI), and herpes zoster have to be differentiated from pleurisy.

Pleural fluid is clinically detectable only when it is about 500 mL in volume, but radiologically it may be detected even when the volume is 300 mL. A fully developed moderate or massive effusion reveals fullness of the intercostal spaces and restriction of respiratory movements on the same side. Midline structures are shifted to the opposite side. Percussion elicits stony dullness with the highest level in the axilla and lower levels in front and back *(S-shaped curve of Ellis)*. This is the most constant physical sign. The Traube's space which is the area overlying the gas bubble of the stomach, is obliterated in left-sided effusions. Breath sounds, vocal fremitus and vocal resonance are diminished or absent. Egophony may be present above the level of effusion. At times, bronchial breathing may be heard over a pleural effusion.

Complications

These include: (1) Respiratory embarrassment, (2) massive bilateral effusions which may be fatal due to respiratory failure, (3) secondary infection of the pleural fluid which converts it into empyema, (4) organization of fibrin from the fluid on the surface of the collapsed lung *(cortication)* that *(prevents re-expansion),* and

(5) fibrosis of the pleura and obliteration of the pleural space *(fibrothorax)* which develop as a sequel to long-standing pleural effusions.

Characteristics of uncomplicated and complicated effusion are shown in Table 153.1.

Radiographic appearances: If the fluid volume is small, only the costophrenic angles are obliterated. As the fluid accumulates further, it throws a triangular lateral opacity obscuring the hemidiaphragm. Large pleural effusions shift the midline structures to the opposite side (Fig. 153.1). An interlobar effusion in the oblique fissure produces an elongated cigar-shaped shadow seen well in the lateral view. Fluid in the horizontal fissure throws a rounded shadow seen in the posterior-anterior view. The term ***vanishing pulmonary tumor*** has been used for interlobar effusions since they clear up with treatment.

- Character of the fluid may be transudate or exudate
- The light criteria help to identify exudates.

Light criteria
- Pleural fluid/serum protein ratio >0.5
- Pleural fluid LDH >200 U/L
- Pleural fluid/serum LDH >0.6

Abbreviation: LDH = lactate dehydrogenase

Causes of transudate and exudate pleural effusions are shown in Table 153.2 and differentiation of transudative effusion from exudative effusion is shown in Table 153.3.

Tuberculous effusion is straw-colored. The fluid is hemorrhagic in malignancy and infarction and it is chylous (milky) in lymphatic obstruction due to filariasis and lymphomas. Collection of purulent fluid in the pleura is called ***empyema***.

Microscopy: In acute bacterial infections, neutrophils predominate, while lymphocytes predominate in tuberculo-

Table 153.1: Characteristics of uncomplicated and complicated effusion

Features	Uncomplicated	Complicated
Appearance	Clear fluid	Cloudy/turbid
pH	>7.30	7.1–7.29
Glucose (mmol/L)	>2.2	<2.2
LDH (IU/L)	<1,000	>1,000
Organism	negative	negative/positive

Abbreviation: LDH = lactate dehydrogenase

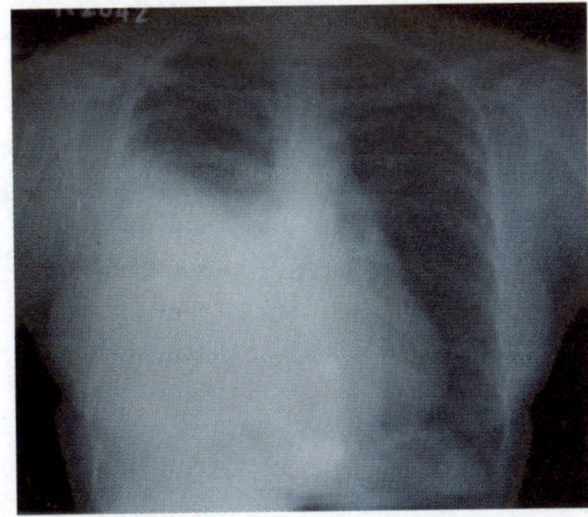

Fig. 153.1: X-ray pleural effusion (right side). **Note:** The homogenous opacity on the right hemithorax with highest level in the axilla. Costophrenic and cardiophrenic angles are obliterated

Table 153.2: Causes of transudate and exudate pleural effusions

Causes of transudate pleural effusion	Causes of exudate pleural effusion
• LVF	• Tuberculosis
• Cirrhosis	• Parapneumonic
• Nephrotic syndrome	• Malignancy (primary and metastatic)
• Hypoalbuminemia	• Collagen vascular diseases
• Hypothyroidism	• RHD disease, SLE
• PE	• PMIS
• Meig's syndrome	• Pulmonary infarction
• Peritoneal dialysis	• Pancreatitis
	• Pseudopancreatic cyst
	• Esophageal rupture
	• Drugs
	• Chylothorax, pseudochylothorax

Abbreviations: LVF = Left ventricular failure; RHD = Rheumatic heart disease; SLE = Systemic lupus erythematosus; PE = Pulmonary embolism; PMIS = Postmyocardial infarction syndrome

sis. Eosinophils may predominate in dyscollagenoses and pulmonary infarction.

Examination of a wet preparation stained by methylene blue reveals malignant cells in over 90% of cases of malignant effusions. Identification of the nature of the malignant cells is done by Papanicolaou's technique.

The nature of chylous fluid is confirmed by demonstrating the presence of fat.

Elevated amylase levels are suggestive of acute pancreatitis (500 units/mL or higher). High elevation of pleural fluid amylase may occur in pancreatitis, esophageal rupture or adenocarcinomas metastating in the pleura. Pancreatic and salivary amylase (in esophageal rupture) can be distinguished by isoenzyme estimation. If these are excluded, markedly elevated pleural fluid amylase > 1,000/L should suggest malignancy and less commonly

other conditions. Levels of LDH are raised in exudates. The chemical nature and cellular content of the fluid may give clues about the cause of the effusion in many cases. Examples are given below.

- Low glucose concentration in the pleural fluid (15–60 mg/dL) may suggest empyema, malignancy or tuberculosis or rheumatoid effusions.

- Excess of eosinophils in pleural fluid (>10% of the total cells) should suggest resolving infections, pneumothorax, hydropneumothorax, hemothorax and pleural effusion occurring in mesothelioma, paragonimiasis, Churg-Strauss syndrome or as side effects of drugs like dantrolene, bromocriptine, nitrofurantoin.

Gram-staining, Ziehl-Neelsen staining and culture help to identify the causative microbes.

When the diagnosis is not arrived at by these investigations, pleural biopsy may be attempted. Biopsy is done with a **Cope's needle** or **Abram's needle**. Pleural biopsy can also be done under direct vision using a thoracoscope. This will help to visualize the pleura and biopsy can be taken from the lesions that are present in the pleural cavity. Thus the yield of diagnosis is improved. Though a positive biopsy is diagnostic, a negative biopsy does not exclude pleural malignancy.

Management

Pleural effusion may rarely present as an emergency with respiratory embarrassment. In such cases, emergency measures are required to give relief especially, if the effusion is massive or bilateral.

Emergency Aspiration

Aspiration is done to get a specimen of fluid for diagnostic tests and to relieve distress.

Table 153.3: Differentiation of transudative effusion from exudative effusion

Characteristics	Transudative effusion	Exudative effusion
Appearance	Clear, serous	Cloudy/purulent/hemorrhagic/chylous
Color	Straw yellow	Yellow to red
Specific gravity	< 1.018	>1.018
Protein		
• Absolute value	Low, < 2 g/dL, mainly albumin	High, >2 g/dL
• Pleural fluid: serum ratio	< 0.5	>0.5
Clot	Absent	Clots spontaneously because of high fibrinogen
Leukocytes		
• Total leukocytes	<1,000/mm³	>1,000/mm³
• Type of cells: Differential leukocytes	> 50% lymphocytes or mononuclear cells and mesothelial cells	>50% lymphocytes (tuberculosis, malignancy) >50% polymorphs (acute inflammation)
• Erythrocytes	<500/mm³	Variable
Bacteria	Absent	Usually present
Lactate dehydrogenase (LDH)		
• Absolute value	<200 IU/L	200 IU/L
• Pleural fluid: serum ratio	<0.6	>0.6
Glucose	>60 mg/dL (usually same as in blood)	<60 mg/dL (variable)
Examples	Seen in CCF	Pus
Character of edema	Pitting type	No pitting

Abbreviation: CCF = Congestive cardiac failure

The fluid is aspirated by thoracentesis done in the eighth or ninth intercostal space in the posterior axillary line after anesthetizing the part. Sufficient fluid is removed to relieve the distress. Whenever pleural fluid is aspirated, it is also subjected to diagnostic investigations.

Elective Aspiration

Medical therapy is instituted depending on clinical features and pleural fluid analysis. It is ideal to aspirate the fluid after instituting specific drug therapy for 3–4 days.

Indications for Aspiration

Indications include (1) to make the diagnosis, (2) to relieve distress and (3) to remove the exudate so as to hasten full recovery of the pleura and avoid complications. It is generally advisable to restrict the volume of fluid removed at one sitting to 1 liter or less in order to avoid pulmonary edema. Aspiration has to be repeated at times. Two or three aspirations will be adequate in most of the cases of tuberculous effusion. In malignant pleural effusion and pulmonary infarction, the pleural fluid tends to reaccumulate even after repeated aspirations. Sometimes aspiration of the pleural cavity may give rise to complications. These include pleural shock, anaphylactic shock due to anesthetic, bleeding into the pleural cavity, pulmonary edema, infection and accidental introduction of air into the pleura.

- **Pleural Shock:** The patient develops vasomotor collapse on puncturing the pleura. Inadequate local anesthesia may be a predisposing factor. Urgent resuscitatory measures include the injection of adrenaline, parenteral steroids and intravenous (IV) fluids. Pleural shock may be fatal, if not recognized in time.
- **Bleeding into the pleural cavity** is from vessels on the pleural surface. Bleeding should be suspected when the aspirated fluid becomes progressively blood-stained. In severe cases, hypovolemic shock may ensue. When bleeding is evident, it is advisable to stop the procedure.
- **Entry of air inadvertently during aspiration** converts a simple pleural effusion into hydropneumothorax. Rarely subcutaneous emphysema or air embolism may develop.
- **Pulmonary edema** occurs in some cases of chronic effusion when the lung expands on removal of the fluid. Slow aspiration and limiting the volume of fluid aspirated at one sitting to 1 liter helps to reduce these complications. Onset of pulmonary edema is heralded by troublesome cough with frothy expectoration. Auscultation reveals the presence of rales. Onset of pulmonary edema is an indication for stopping aspiration.

Pleural effusion which is a part of generalized edema clears up when the underlying condition is treated. Unless there is respiratory embarrassment, thoracocentesis is required only for diagnostic purposes.

Tuberculous Pleural Effusion

Tuberculosis is perhaps the most common cause of pleurisy occurring in younger adults in India (below the age of 60 years). The pleura may be directly involved by the tuberculous process. In most cases, it spreads from an underlying pulmonary focus and the effusion is almost always on the side of the pulmonary lesion. Sometimes a caseous subpleural focus may rupture into the pleural cavity or the pleura may be the seat of miliary lesions. In the majority of cases, the classic adolescent pleural effusion is a postprimary tuberculous phenomenon though rarely it may occur in primary tuberculosis. The effusion may develop rapidly or insidiously. Strongly positive tuberculin test favors tuberculous etiology. The fluid is an exudate. The cells are mainly lymphocytes. Tubercle bacilli are difficult to demonstrate in serous effusion by conventional methods. Culture and animal inoculation may be positive. In tuberculous empyema, the organisms are more easily demonstrable. Needle biopsy is helpful, but this is not required in the ordinary case.

Management

Standard antituberculosis treatment is started. Pleural aspiration is done electively. Repeated aspiration may be required to make the pleural cavity dry. Respiratory physiotherapy is essential to restore function promptly.

Empyema

Collection of pus in the pleural cavity is called **empyema**. Pus may be free in the pleural space or loculated.

Pathogenesis

Empyema may result from the extension of infection from the underlying lung, or it may complicate chest injuries, thoracentesis, or generalized pyemia. Pneumonia, lung abscess, bronchiectasis, tuberculous cavities, hepatopulmonary amebiasis, bronchogenic carcinoma, osteomyelitis of the ribs, fungal infections and actinomycosis are all common causes. Thoracic and upper abdominal surgery may lead to empyema (Flowchart 153.1). Common bacterial flora includes *Streptococcus, Staphylococcus, Pneumococcus, Pseudomonas, Klebsiella, Haemophilus influenzae* anaerobes, *Mycobacterium tuberculosis* and *Actinomycetes.*

Clinical Features

All ages may be affected, but children suffer more. Onset is marked by high fever, pleuritic or dull chest pain and dry cough. Physical signs of pleural effusion may be evident. Unlike as in simple pleural effusion, the chest wall becomes edematous. Digital clubbing is common. Sometimes the empyema communicates with the bronchus **(bronchopleural fistula)**. In this case, postural cough is a troublesome symptom and the findings are those of pyopneumothorax. The pus may work its way outside and point on the chest wall. This is called **empyema necessitans**. Left-sided empyema may pulsate due to transmitted pulsation from the heart—**pulsating empyema**.

Radiologically: The findings closely resemble those of pleural effusion (*See* Fig. 153.1). Demonstration of pus in the pleural cavity by aspiration confirms the diagnosis. The causative organism can be identified by examination of the pus.

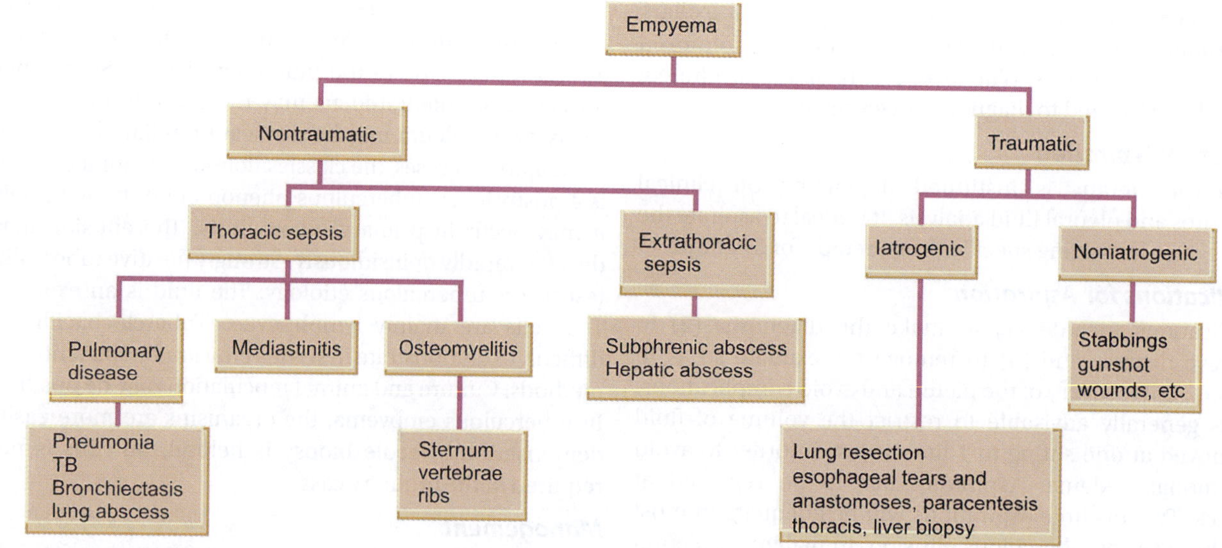

Abbreviation: TB = tuberculosis

Clinically, a large lung abscess may resemble an empyema or encysted pyopneumothorax and these two conditions have to be differentiated. Fever, toxemia and digital clubbing occur in both. Shift of the mediastinum to the opposite side and stony dullness on percussion are in favor of empyema. Radiological techniques like computed tomography (CT) of the thorax may be necessary to differentiate them. In a loculated pyopneumothorax, the air-fluid interphase may transgress anatomical boundaries of lobes, whereas a lung abscess is limited by the interlobar fissures (Fig. 153.2).

Complications of empyema include severe toxemia, cachexia, anemia, pulmonary fibrosis, pleural fibrosis, metastatic brain abscesses and in longstanding cases, secondary amyloidosis. The overall mortality is 10–11%.

Treatment

After determining the infecting organism, antimicrobial treatment is instituted. The fluid has to be removed at the earliest by aspiration. This will not only relieve the fever and toxemia but also prevent the encystment of empyema fluid which may later lead to difficulties in further aspiration. When the pus is too thick to be aspirated, or if it re-accumulates rapidly; underwater tube drainage has to be established. Clearance of the pleural space and full re-expansion of the lung may take several weeks to

complete. Thick pus which is difficult to be aspirated can be liquefied by instillation of proteolytic enzymes like streptokinase and streptodornase. In patients not responding to this treatment, thoracoscopic evacuation pus from pleural cavity and release of pleural adhesion may help in the re-expansion of lung. Rarely, few may need surgical intervention with decortications of pleura.

Tumors of the Pleura

Primary tumor (mesothelioma) is rare, whereas secondary tumors are common. Mesothelioma may be benign or more commonly malignant. Pleural malignancy is more common in persons chronically exposed to asbestos. Secondary tumors arise from carcinomas of the bronchus, stomach, liver and other structures. Malignant lesions in the pleura give rise to hemorrhagic pleural effusion.

PNEUMOTHORAX

Presence of air in the pleural cavity is known as ***pneumothorax***. Pneumothorax may be spontaneous, traumatic, and iatrogenic ***(artificial).*** Another classification is to divide them into ***open, closed*** and ***valvular pneumothorax (tension pneumothorax).*** In open pneumothorax, there is a free rent on the surface of the lung through which air gets in and out of the pleural cavity during inspiration and expiration. In closed pneumothorax, the pleura does not communicate with the exterior. In tension pneumothorax, there is a valvular slit on the surface of the lung through which air enters the pleural cavity, but does not escape. As a result, tension pneumothorax develops leading to respiratory and cardiac embarrassment.

Spontaneous Pneumothorax

This results from rupture of pulmonary lesion leading to escape of air into the pleura. Pneumothorax may be primary where there is no obvious underlying lesion or secondary to pulmonary lesions such as cavitation, emphysema, bullae and others.

Subpleural blebs or bullae, pulmonary tuberculosis, congenital cystic disease of the lungs, chronic bronchitis

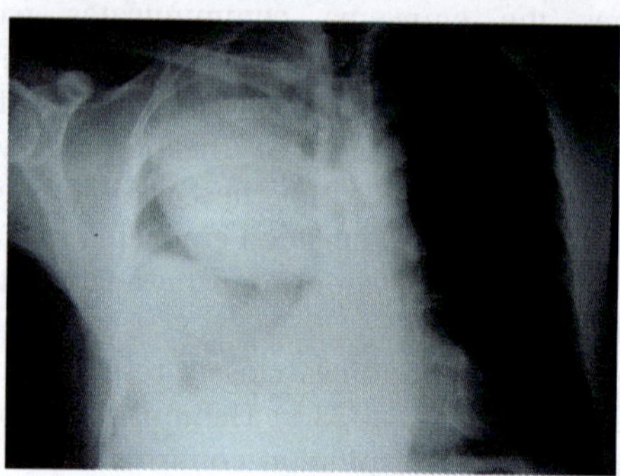

Fig. 153.2: Chest X-ray multiple encysted empyema right.
Note: Multiple well-defined rounded shadows

with emphysema, bronchial asthma, pneumoconiosis and *Staphylococcal pneumonia* are the common medical causes. Fracture of a rib, thoracotomy, puncture of the lung at needle biopsy and rupture of a bronchus are the common surgical causes. Sometimes pneumothorax is produced artificially for diagnostic radiology of the lungs or as a therapy to arrest massive hemoptysis. The lung collapses toward the hilum, when air enters the pleura and abolishes the negative pressure.

Clinical Features

Onset is with unilateral pleuritic pain and dyspnea. A feeling of something having given way is complained of by many. Shortness of breath and unproductive cough develop soon. In tension pneumothorax, respiratory embarrassment and cyanosis may be evident.

The affected side is prominent and it does not move with respiration. Midline structures are shifted to the opposite side. Percussion note is hyper-resonant. Breath sounds are absent in many cases. If air enters the pleural cavity as in brochopleural fistula, amphoric breath sounds may be heard. A special percussion phenomenon is the coin sound. A coin kept firmly over the front of the chest wall is struck with another coin. Auscultation at the back of the chest reveals a metallic note. Adventitious sounds like clicking sounds synchronous with the heart beat may be heard in a left sided pneumothorax.

Differential Diagnosis

Differential diagnosis of pneumothorax includes other painful conditions associated with dyspnea such as MI and pulmonary infarction. Severe emphysema, large bullae and diaphragmatic hernia may cause problems in diagnosis.

Radiological Features

The radiological features are diagnostic in a well-developed case. The affected side is hypertranslucent due to the collection of free air in the pleural cavity and absence of normal lung markings. The outer margin of the collapsed lung is seen as a sharp margin against the background of air. There is shift of the trachea and mediastinum to the opposite side (Fig. 153.3). Skiagram should be taken in the erect posture so that even small collections of air will not be missed. High-resolution computed tomography (HRCT) gives the state of the lung parenchyma as well (Fig. 153.4).

Complications

Though in majority of cases, spontaneous pneumothorax is uncomplicated, serious complications may develop in some cases. These are: (1) severe cardiorespiratory embarrassment due to compression of the normal lung by the displaced mediastinum in cases of tension pneumothorax; (2) air embolism; (3) surgical emphysema; (4) infection of the pleural cavity resulting in the formation of hydro- or pyopneumothorax; (5) pneumothorax on the opposite side from pre-existing disease of the lung and (6) failure of expansion of the collapsed lung.

Hydropneumothorax

When both air and fluid are present in the pleural cavity, it is known as hydropneumothorax. This is usually a result of rupture of a pulmonary lesion letting in air and exudates into the pleural cavity. In many cases, it is caused by tuberculosis. Other causes include lung abscess, bronchiectasis, bronchogenic carcinoma and trauma to the chest. Some cases of pneumothorax get converted into hydropneumothorax when effusion develops as a result of infection (Fig. 153.5).

In hydropneumothorax, a horizontal upper level of dullness caused by the fluid can be demonstrated which shifts when the patient is made to adopt different positions *(shifting dullness)*. On shaking the patient gently while auscultating on the air-fluid interphase, a *succussion splash* is heard. Chest radiograph reveals a horizontal upper level of fluid with the findings of pneumothorax above it (Fig. 153.6)

Management of Pneumothorax

Small closed pneumothorax which is not severely symptomatic can be left alone with bed rest and analgesics, since the air will be absorbed within a few days. Simple aspiration may hasten recovery.

Tension pneumothorax may present as a life-threatening emergency. Unless the tension is relieved by letting out the air, the patient may die of cardiorespiratory failure.

Emergency Management

The air is let out by inserting a wide bore hypodermic needle into the second intercostal space 2–3 cm outside the lateral border of the sternum. The needle is connected

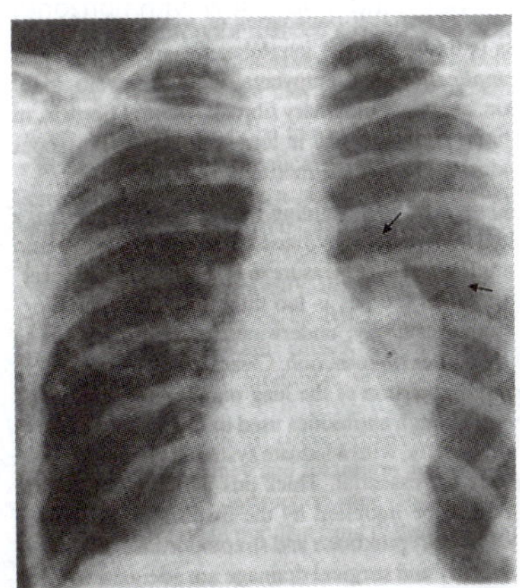

Fig. 153.3: Chest X-ray—Pneumothorax (left). *Note:* (1) The airfilled thoracic cavity; (2) collapsed lung (arrows)

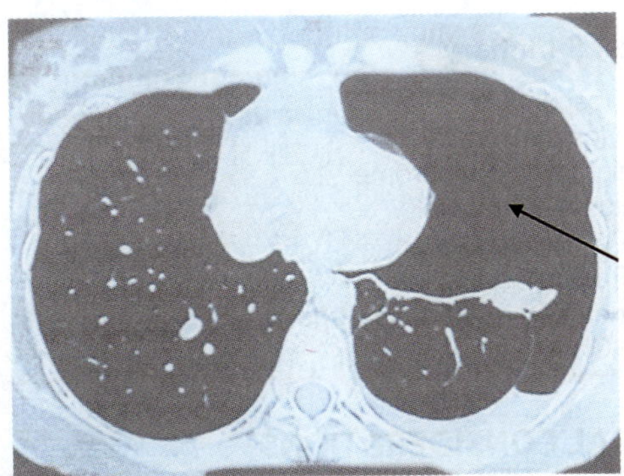

Fig. 153.4: HRCT showing open pneumothorax left pleura (arrow). *Note:* The absence of lung markings in the area of pneutmothorax

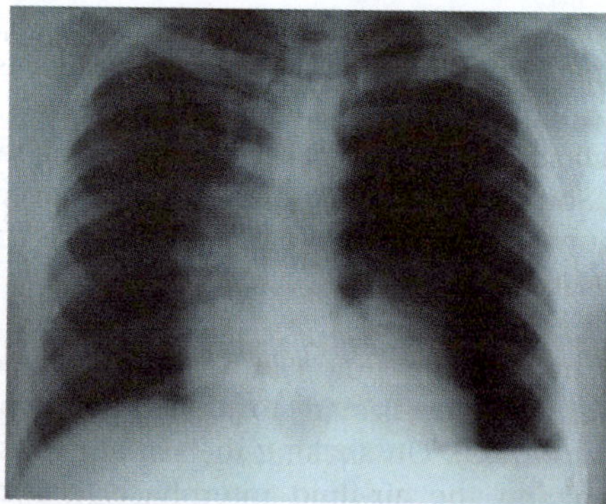

Fig. 153.5: Chest X-ray pneumothorax (left). ***Note:*** (1) Hypertranslucency left hemithorax, (2) collapsed lung adjacent to the left cardiac border, (3) shift of mediastinum to the right and (4) horizontal level of fluid in the left pleural cavity (the pneumothorax is complicated by the development of effusion)

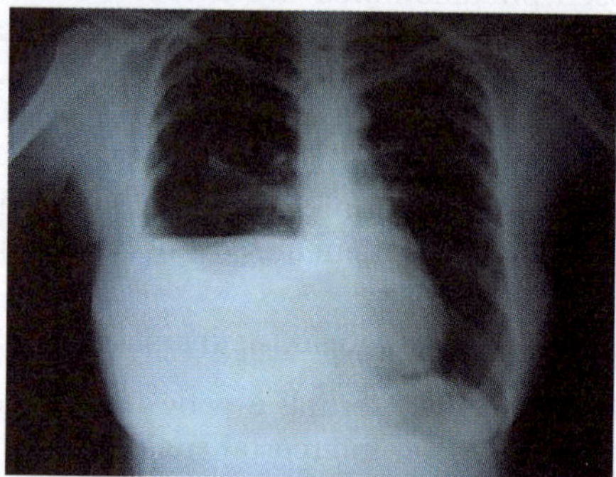

Fig. 153.6: Hydropneumothorax with collapsed lung. ***Note:*** On the right side, (1) air above and fluid below with horizontal level of fluid, (2) shift of mediastinum to the left and (3) collapsed lung on the right hilum

to a rubber tube which is led under water, to prevent re-entry of air (underwater seal). This procedure may have to be instituted even outside the hospital at times. Though this procedure may save life in an emergency, sooner or later the needle gets blocked and air reaccumulates with recurrence of symptoms. It is ideal to hospitalize the patient for further management.

In the hospital, the ideal procedure is to establish drainage of the pleura by a rubber tubing connected to an underwater seal. The tube may have to be kept in place for a few days or weeks. Antibiotics are given to prevent secondary infection of the pleura. Any obvious underlying condition is treated with specific drugs. Recovery of pulmonary function is facilitated by starting physiotherapy at an early stage.

If the lungs fail to expand spontaneously, suction of the pleural cavity may help. Surgical repair of the pleural surface may be required in intractable cases.

In recurrent pneumothorax, pleurodesis with sclerosing agents are useful.

CHEMICAL PLEURODESIS

Production in pleural inflammation and adhesion between parietal and pulmonary pleura by sclerosing agents helps to prevent recurrence of pneumothorax.

- ■ *Indications:*
  - Persist air leak and repeated pneumothorax
  - Bilateral pneumothorax
  - Pneumothorax complicated with bullae
  - Occupations where pneumothorax should not occur—drivers, pilots
- ■ Commonly used sclerosing agents include tetracycline, minocycline, doxycycline, erythromycin and talc. *Corynebacterium parvum* induces biological pleurodesis.

Physical pleurodesis is achieved by creating mechanical abrasions on the pleural surfaces.

CHAPTER 154

Diseases of the Chest Wall

KE Rajan

Chapter Summary

- Kyphoscoliosis
- Ankylosing Spondylitis
- Straight Back Syndrome
- Pectus Deformities
  - ▪ Pectus Excavatum
  - ▪ Pectus Carinatum
- Injuries to the Thoracic Cage
- Flail Chest

GENERAL CONSIDERATIONS

The integrity of the chest wall and muscular action of the intercostals muscles and diaphragm are necessary to ensure proper ventilation. Though minor deformities may not be functionally significant, gross bony deformities and muscular paralysis impair ventilation and give rise to respiratory embarrassment.

KYPHOSCOLIOSIS

Kyphosis is the abnormal curvature of the thoracic spine with convexity directed posteriorly. Scoliosis denotes gradual lateral curvature of the thoracic spine, with rotation of the vertebrae in their longitudinal axis. In kyphoscoliosis, there is progressive deformity of spine consisting of lateral and posterior curvatures. Spine is curved in both coronal and sagittal planes.

Kyphoscoliosis may be congenital or acquired. In majority of patients, it is idiopathic in origin. Congenital kyphoscoliosis results from developmental anomalies. Acquired kyphoscoliosis results from poliomyelitis, myopathies, muscular dystrophies and diseases of the vertebrae such as osteoporosis. Primary respiratory diseases like pulmonary fibrosis (PF) or atelectasis may be associated with this deformity. Causes of acquired kyphosis include ankylosing spondylitis, infections like tuberculosis, connective tissue disorders, disk degeneration, Paget's disease and tumors.

Clinical Picture

The deformity may remain asymptomatic for variable periods of time. It may result in shortening of height. A relative may observe the deformity and bring the patient to medical attention. Mobility of chest wall is impaired. The lung on the narrowed side is compressed. The opposite lung shows compensatory emphysema. Position and relationship of mediastinal structures are altered. Physical examination may demonstrate displaced apical impulse, pulsations at unusual locations, altered tactile/vocal fremitus and variations in intensity of breath sounds.

Chest X-ray shows distortion of spine. Spirometry shows reduction of vital capacity (VC) and total lung capacity (TLC) with preservation of forced expiratory volume in 1 second (FEV1). Breathing is shallow and rapid with low tidal volumes. The ventilation-perfusion ratio is grossly reduced and this results in hypoxemia. These subjects are prone to develop repeated respiratory infections. In severe cases, respiratory failure may develop. Cardiorespiratory embarrassment develops in severe kyphosis where the angle of curvature exceeds 20° and in severe scoliosis with the angle less than 100°. Advanced kyphoscoliosis may lead to chronic cor pulmonale.

Management

Milwaukee brace controls moderate deformities. Surgical correction is attempted in selected cases to fix the spine and arrest progression of the deformity. Respiratory physiotherapy improves ventilation. Domiciliary oxygen on a long-term basis may be necessary in patients with significant hypoxemia. Special attention must be paid to prevent respiratory infection.

ANKYLOSING SPONDYLITIS

Refer Section 12, Ch 113

In this condition, there is marked flexion and rigidity of the thoracic spine. Ventilation is carried out mainly by diaphragmatic movement. Though the vital capacity is reduced, signs of frank respiratory embarrassment are few.

STRAIGHT BACK SYNDROME (SBS)

It is a benign abnormality of the spine in which the normal upper dorsal kyphosis is abolished, giving rise to diminution of anteroposterior diameter of the chest. The heart is shifted to the left and forwards giving rise to prominent parasternal impulses on the second to fourth intercostal spaces and grade 1–3 pulmonary systolic ejection murmur (SEM). Pulmonary second sound may be split so as to mimic atrial septal defect (ASD).

Diagnosis can be made from X-ray of the chest. There is greater incidence of SBS in association with mitral valve prolapse (MVP). It is important to recognize this condition so as to avoid unnecessary invasive investigations.

PECTUS DEFORMITIES

These deformities usually result from a genetic disorder, which causes an abnormal growth of four or more pairs of costal cartilages.

Pectus Excavatum

It is also known as funnel chest. In this, the sternum is pushed inward. The thoracic cage may be flattened anteroposteriorly. A furrow develops in front of the chest, which is deepest just above the xiphoid process. In many cases, it is a familial deformity. Though present at birth, the deformity may aggravate during adolescence. Their severity usually remains the same after the age of 18 years (Fig. 154.1).

Symptoms include cosmetic problems, shortness of breath, discomfort/pain in the lower anterior chest and decreased exercise endurance. The heart is rotated and displaced to the left to varying degrees. This may give rise to systolic murmurs along the left sternal border. Compression of the heart will reduce the stroke volume and cardiac output in moderate to severe deformities leading to early fatigue. There is compensatory tachycardia during exercise. The sternal depression decreases the intrathoracic volume. Respiratory movements are shallow and rapid.

Pectus Carinatum (Pigeon Chest)

In this, the sternum gets pushed forwards with the ribs sloping steeply on either side. This deformity used to be a sequel to childhood rickets. There is increased incidence of respiratory infections. Pectus carinatum prevents complete expiration of air from the lungs and significant air trapping. These patients often experience wheezing and occasionally mild to moderate asthma. On exercise, carinatum patients develop tachypnea.

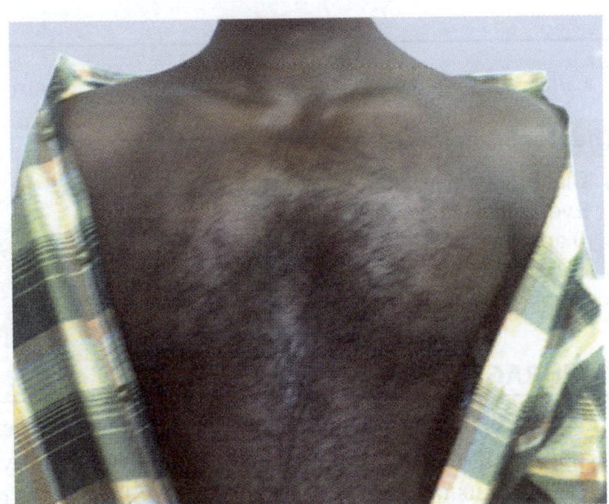

Fig. 154.1: Pectus excavatum. **Note:** The abnormal hollow in the midline below the sternal angle

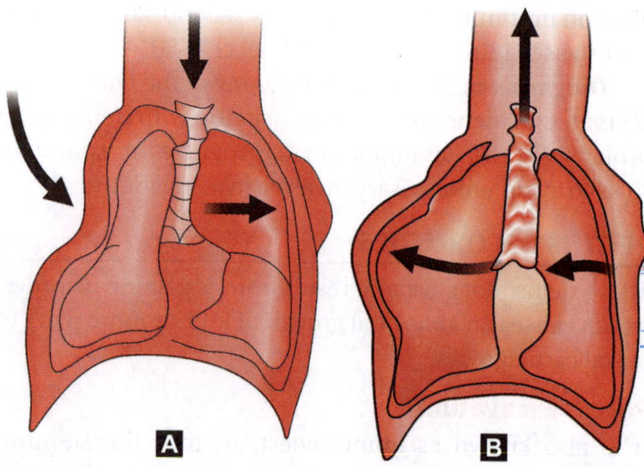

Figs 154.2A and B: Flail chest. *Note:* Paradoxical movements of lung

Management

Surgical correction is needed in symptomatic patients. It consists of removal of a small segment of the deformed cartilages medially and laterally on each side of the sternum and bringing the sternum to the desired position with a metal bar support.

INJURIES TO THE THORACIC CAGE

The thoracic cage is often injured in accidents. Fractures of individual ribs, contusion of the chest wall/lungs, open wounds (which lead to pneumothorax or hemothorax) and surgical emphysema may be seen. In comatose subjects, injury to the chest wall or viscera may be missed, resulting in fatalities. The need for careful examination to exclude thoracic and abdominal injuries in cases of accidental injuries cannot be overemphasized since at the first examination they may be missed.

FLAIL CHEST

It results when ribs are fractured in two places. The fractured segment of the thoracic wall floats independently of the rest of the chest wall and moves paradoxically. The negative intrathoracic pressure during inspiration causes the fractured ribs to be sucked in, thereby preventing expansion of the lung. During expiration, this segment moves outwards. When the injury is unilateral, air from the lung of the affected side passes into the opposite healthy lung during inspiration and air is sucked into it from the normal lung, during expiration. This type of paradoxical respiration is called ***pendulum breathing*** (Figs 154.2A and B). This results in serious respiratary insufficiency and respiratory failure.

Management

As first-aid, the chest wall should be stabilized to avoid suffocation. Immediate requirement is to prevent the flail segment from moving out paradoxically during expiration. A firm chest wrap is used to support the flail segment. Making the patient lie down with the flail segment against the cot or trolley surface may help. Applying towel clips to the area of paradoxical movement and exerting traction during inspiration is another method. Oxygen supplementation is advisable in all symptomatic patients.

The patient is transported to hospital at the earliest. Stabilization of the flail segment has to be maintained by weight traction. Definitive treatment of flail chest depends upon the degree of respiratory distress. Local anesthetic block is useful to relieve pain. In severe cases where the flail segment is impairing gas exchange or contributing to hypoxemia, internal fixation is done surgically.

CHAPTER
155

Diseases of the Diaphragm

KE Rajan

Chapter Summary

- Diaphragmatic Paralysis
- Eventration of Diaphragm
- Diaphragmatic Hernia
- Hiccough
- Diaphragmatic Flutter

DIAPHRAGMATIC PARALYSIS

The diaphragm is supplied by the phrenic nerve, which has a long intrathoracic course. Involvement of this nerve anywhere in its course is a common cause of paralysis of the diaphragm. The paralyzed dome is pushed up by the intra-abdominal pressure. It moves paradoxically with respiration, i.e. during inspiration it is drawn up and vice versa.

Diaphragmatic paralysis may be unilateral or bilateral. Table 155.1 gives causes of diaphragmatic paralysis.

Rarely rheumatic fever, typhoid, pneumonia, mediastinitis, pericarditis and encephalitis lethargica may lead to diaphragmatic paralysis. Apart from full diaphragmatic paralysis several neural disorders give rise to varying degrees of diaphragmatic dysfunction (Table 155.2). It is important to look for any degree of diaphragmatic paralysis with respiratory involvement in all conditions involving neuromuscular system, generally or selectively.

Table 155.1: Causes of diaphragmatic paralysis

Unilateral	Birth injuries
	Viral infections (e.g. *Herpes zoster*)
	Carcinomatous infiltration
	Trauma
Bilateral	Guillain-Barré syndrome (GBS)
	Cervical cord lesions
	Motor neuron disease
	Poliomyelitis
	Myasthenia gravis (MG)
	Muscular dystrophies

Table 155.2: Causes of diaphragmatic dysfunction in neurological disorders

Level of impairment	*Part of nervous system affected*
Multiple sclerosis Stroke Arnold-Chiari malformation	Brain
Quadriplegia Amyotrophic lateral sclerosis Poliomyelitis Spinal muscular atrophy Syringomyelia	Cervical cord
Guillain- Barré syndrome Tumor compression Neuralgic neuropathy Critical illness polyneuropathy Chronic inflammatory demyelinating polyneuropathy Charcot-Marie-Tooth diseases	Spinal cord
Hyperinflation (chronic obstructive pulmonary disease and asthma)	Primary disease of the lung
Myasthenia gravis Lambert-Eaton syndrome	Neuromuscular junctions
Botulism Organophosphorus poisoning Drugs	Autonomic nerves
Muscular dystrophy Myositis (infection, inflammatory, metabolic dyscollagenosis) Acid maltase deficiency Glucocorticoids Disuse atrophy	Muscle

Abbreviations: ALS = Amyotrophic lateral sclerosis; SMA = Spinal muscular atrophy; CIP = Critical illness polyneuropathy; CIDP = Chronic inflammatory demyelinating polyneuropathy; COPD = Chronic obstructive pulmonary disease; MG = Myasthenia gravis; AMD = Acid maltase deficiency; GBS = Guillain- Barré syndrome

Clinical Features

Unilateral diaphragmatic paralysis may reduce ventilatory capacity by 20%. Otherwise healthy subjects may remain asymptomatic and may be detected during physical examination or by radiology. Sometimes left sided paralysis may produce gaseous dyspepsia. In bilateral diaphragmatic paralysis, dyspnea may occur because of ventilatory insufficiency. During inspiration, the lower part of the chest moves horizontally, the subcostal angle widens, and the epigastrium and hypochondria recede. Absence of the normal peeling movements of the diaphragm visible on the thoracic cage is known as ***Litten's sign***. Abdomen is drawn in during inspiration.

Radiologically, the dome of the diaphragm on the paralyzed side is seen to be elevated. Unilateral diaphragmatic paralysis has to be differentiated from other causes of elevated hemidiaphragm. Pulmonary fibrosis (PF), atelectasis, eventration of the diaphragm, pulmonary infarct, subphrenic abscess and large space occupying lesions of the liver may cause elevation of the dome. Screening or ultrasound study may confirm the diagnosis by asking the patient to perform sniffing during the procedure. In diaphragmatic paralysis, the movement is paradoxical, whereas in PF and atelectasis the movement of the elevated diaphragm is considerably restricted.

Treatment

Respiratory embarrassment caused by acute diaphragmatic paralysis may have to be treated by intensive respiratory care and ventilatory support.

EVENTRATION OF DIAPHRAGM

Eventration is the abnormal elevation of the diaphragm at a site of weakness. It is seen more often on the left side. This may be a congenital or acquired condition. Congenital diaphragmatic eventration results from defective development of septum transversum. Affected areas include the vertebrocostal triangle and the central tendon. Acquired eventration is more common, resulting from atrophy of muscle fibers secondary to phrenic nerve injury. In eventration, the diaphragmatic movement is paradoxical. The absence of any underlying cause and, persistence over several years should suggest the possibility of eventration (Fig. 155.1). Infants with extensive muscular defect of the diaphragm may present with acute respiratory distress. Many patients remain asymptomatic till accidentally found out by skiagram in adult life. Eventration has to be differentiated from a Morgagni's hernia.

DIAPHRAGMATIC HERNIA

The diaphragm acts as a musculotendinous partition between the thoracic and abdominal cavities. The peritoneum and pleura on either side strengthen it further. Inferior vena cava (IVC), esophagus and aorta pass through the diaphragm. The apertures through which they pass are

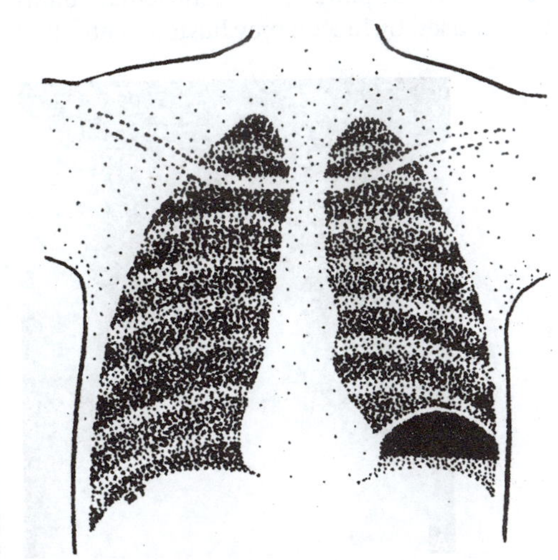

Fig. 155.1: Chest X-ray. Eventration of diaphragm

Textbook of Medicine

covered and sealed by the serous membranes. When the apertures become lax or other defects develop, abdominal contents herniate into the thoracic cavity.

Herniation may be spontaneous without any known cause or it may be traumatic. Traumatic hernia is more common on the left side. Though any part may be ruptured, the common site is between the central tendon and ninth rib laterally.

Nontraumatic hernias may occur congenitally or may be acquired. Maldevelopment of the diaphragm or laxity of the apertures occurs in congenital hernias.

Common sites of hernia occurrence

- Esophageal hiatus
- Foramen of Morgagni (between the sternal and costal slips of origin of the diaphragm)
- Foramen of Bochdalek (pleuroperitoneal hiatus)
- Areas of partial absence of the diaphragm

Among these, in more than 75% cases, herniation occurs through the esophageal hiatus (Figs 155.2 and 155.3).

Herniation of abdominal viscera into the thorax produces clinical features of decreased intensity of breath sounds on the affected side. Bowel sounds may be heard in the thorax. Congenital hernias may be associated with other anomalies such as dextrocardia. The diagnosis is confirmed by a barium meal follow through examination, which will show the presence of stomach and/or intestines above the diaphragm.

HICCOUGH

Syn: Hiccup

This is a common reflex phenomenon resulting from sudden spasmodic involuntary contraction of the diaphragm with the glottis remaining closed. The afferent limb of the reflex arc is the vagus and the sensory fibers of the phrenic nerve. The efferent limb is the motor part of the phrenic nerve. The reflex center is in the upper cervical cord. The increased intrathoracic pressure forces air through the glottis. This produces the characteristic sound of hiccough. In most cases, the onset and termination of hiccup may be spontaneous and abrupt. Hasty ingestion of food and fluids may trigger off an attack.

In a gravely ill-patient, the muscular effort and discomfort caused by hiccup may hasten death. In hiccup

due to central causes both sides of the diaphragm contract. In conditions caused by local irritation, the contraction may be unilateral.

Causes of Hiccough

- Local
  - Irritation of diaphragm
    - Gaseous distension of stomach and intestines
    - Diaphragmatic pleurisy
    - Pneumonia
    - Subphrenic abscess
    - Peritonitis
    - Acute myocardial infarction (MI)
    - Pregnancy
  - Irritation of phrenic nerve
    - Pericarditis
    - Mediastinitis
    - Compression by tumors
    - Surgery of thorax or upper abdomen
- Metabolic
  - Renal failure
  - Hepatic failure
  - Diabetic ketoacidosis
  - Respiratory failure
  - Electrolyte disturbances
- Others
  - Cerebrovascular accidents
  - Encephalitis
  - Brain tumors
  - Psychogenic.

Persistent hiccough is one which lasts for more than 2 days. It has to be distinguished from diaphragmatic flutter.

Management

Though many cases stop spontaneously, in resistant cases treatment is unsatisfactory. Simple physical measures such as drinking cold water, pressure over the eyeball, Valsalva maneuver, pull on the tongue, stimulation of the phrenic nerve by pressure in the neck or rebreathing into a paper bag may stop the hiccup in many cases. If there is associated gastroesophageal reflux disease (GERD), proton pump inhibitors (PPI) are useful. Inhalation of 5–10% carbon dioxide is effective. Unilateral hiccup can be arrested by local infiltration of the phrenic nerve with procaine. In cases with abdominal distension, aspiration

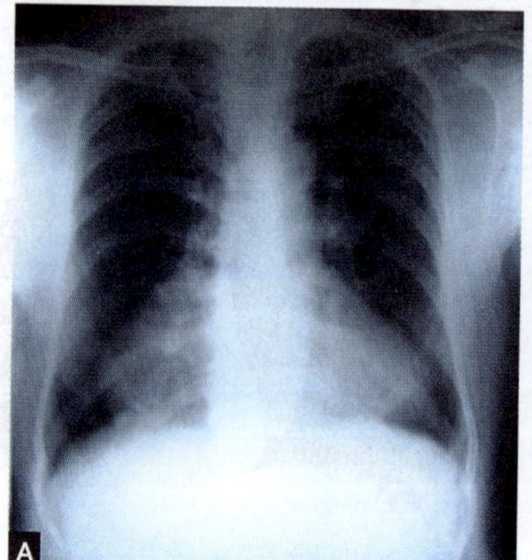
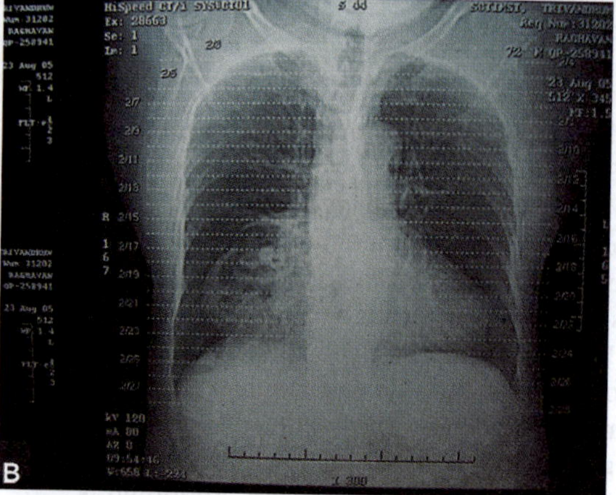

Figs 155.2A and B: A. Chest X-ray showing diaphragmatic hernia right side; **B.** High-resolution CT (HRCT) scan

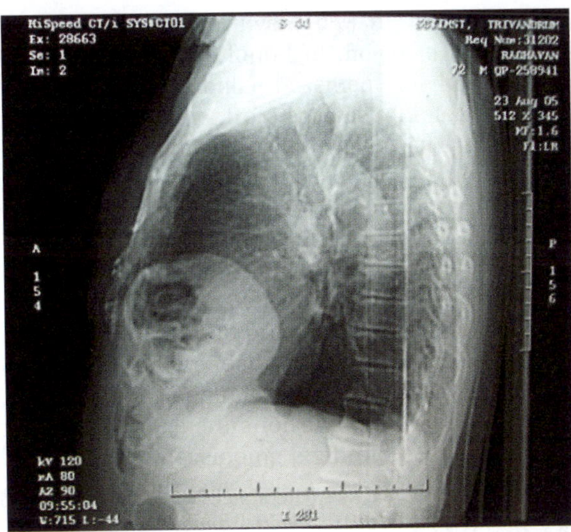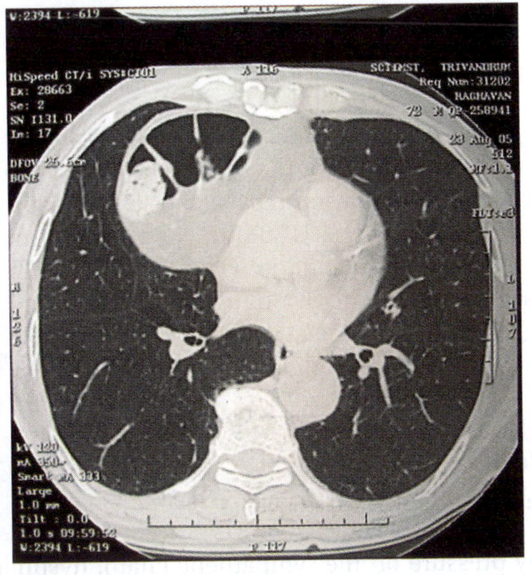

Figs 155.3A and B: X-ray lateral view of diaphragmatic hernia (left) and HRCT scan of the same. **Note:** The presence of abdominal viscera above the diaphragm

of gastric contents through a nasogastric tube may provide prompt relief. Some cases are distressing when the attacks cannot be terminated by simple measures. Chlorpromazine given intramuscularly (IM) in a dose of 25–50 mg brings about sedation and relief of the hiccough. Other drugs, which may be tried, are metoclopramide in a dose of 10 mg or domperidone in a dose of 10 mg. Some cases recover when sedated for 8–12 hours.

DIAPHRAGMATIC FLUTTER

Sometimes, the diaphragm manifests paroxysmal wave-like rhythmic movements at rates going up to 100/min or more. The exact mechanism or cause is not clear. When the condition persists, ventilation may be jeopardized. The term *diaphragmatic tic* is given to flutter occurring at a slower rate. Diaphragmatic flutter is seen more frequently in patients recovering from cerebrovascular accidents or encephalitis.

Treatment

The condition responds to anticonvulsant drugs such as dilantin sodium or carbamazepine. In intractable cases, temporary phrenic paralysis may have to be induced by crushing the nerve.

CHAPTER
156

Diseases of the Mediastinum

C Sudheendra Ghosh, Davis Paul

Chapter Summary

- Mediastinal Tumors
- Cysts
- Pneumomediastinum

MEDIASTINAL TUMORS

An imaginary plane at the lower border of the manubrium sterni divides the mediastinum into superior mediastinum above and anterior, middle and posterior mediastinum below (Fig. 156.1). Space-occupying lesions in the mediastinum are not uncommon. Due to their location, they produce characteristic clinical picture, totally referred to as the mediastinal syndrome. Diseases of the mediastinum may affect any or all structures within the chest. It is broadly classified as (a) non-neoplastic disorders, (b) neo-plastic disorders, (c) congenital cysts and developmental anomalies.

Common non-neoplastic diseases of the mediastinum are acute mediastinitis, due to mediastinal perforation, post-ternotomy mediastinitis and fibrosing mediastinitis. Pneumomediastinum can be spontaneous or associated with mechanical ventilation.

Tumors: The most common mediastinal tumors are metastases from bronchogenic carcinoma and lympho-mas. Neurofibromas, ganglioneuromas, schwannomas, neuroblastomas, teratomas, dermoids, thymomas and cysts are seen less commonly. The majority of cases are asymptomatic. Symptoms are caused by obstruction and infiltration. These are lymphatic and superior vena caval (SVS) obstruction, hoarseness of voice due to recurrent laryngeal nerve (RLN) paralysis, Horner's syndrome

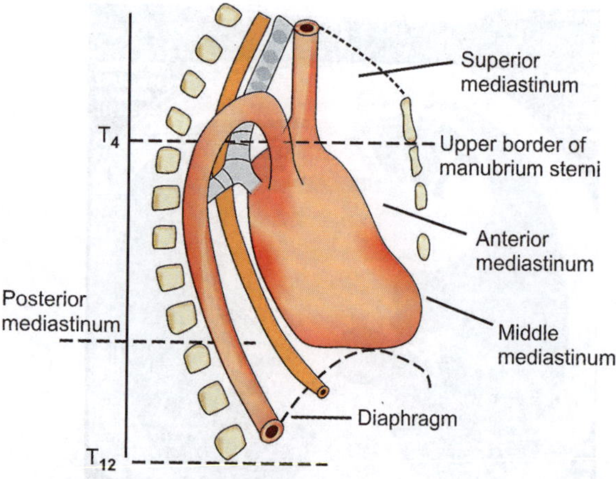

Fig. 156.1: Subdivisions of mediastinum

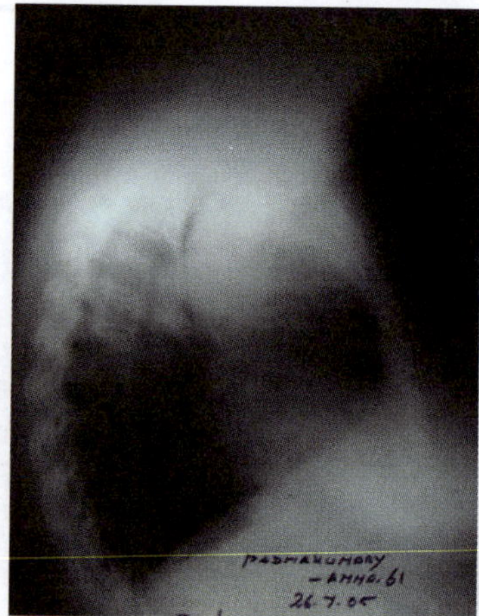

Fig. 156.3: Chest X-ray lateral view. **Note:** The opacity of the superior mediastinum due to retrosternal tumor

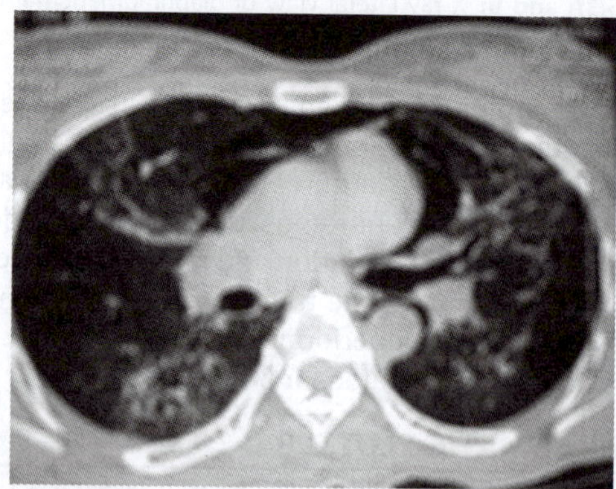

Fig. 156.4: Pneumomediastinum; high-resolution computed tomography (HRCT)

caused by pressure on the sympathetic chain, dysphagia due to pressure on the esophagus and cough and dyspnea due to pressure on the trachea. Neural tumors may elaborate hormones, e.g. pheochromocytoma.

Investigations

Both invasive and noninvasive procedures are needed for detailed evaluation. Noninvasive are skiagrams in different views (Figs 156.2 and 156.3), computed tomography (CT), magnetic resonance imaging (MRI), ultrasonography (USG), radionuclide scanning and biochemical tumor markers. Invasive procedures include bronchoscopy, mediastinoscopy and biopsy of nodes by thoracotomy. Vast majority of the mediastinal lesions can be detected clearly by MRI and CT.

CYSTS

The anterior and middle mediastinum may be the seat of benign cysts, the majority of which are asymptomatic. ***Bronchogenic cysts*** are seen by the side of the trachea or the carina most frequently. These cysts do not communicate with the air passages.
Enteric cysts develop in relation to the esophagus. Their lining may resemble the gastric or intestinal mucosa.
Pericardial cysts develop by the side of the pericardium without communicating with its cavity.

PNEUMOMEDIASTINUM

Syn: Mediastinal emphysema

Presence of air within the planes of the mediastinum is called ***pneumomediastinum***. This may occur spontaneously or results from trauma to the chest or perforation of the trachea and esophagus. Surgical emphysema occurring in the fascial planes of the neck or retroperitoneal region may spread to the mediastinum. In emphysema and conditions associated with violent cough, alveolar air may enter the interstitium and reach the mediastinum through the hilum. Other rare causes include Caisson disease and perforation of the esophagus during instrumentation.

Clinical Features

The condition may be asymptomatic in many cases. Others complain of retrosternal pain, dyspnea, cough and dysphagia. Crepitus may be felt over the upper part of the chest. Crunching adventitious sounds may be heard on auscultating the heart (Hamman's sign). In severe cases, cardiac failure may develop. Skiagrams reveal the air in tissues (Fig. 156.4).

Treatment

Measures to abolish pain and prevent infection are sufficient in spontaneous cases. In traumatic cases, the surgical defects have to be repaired.

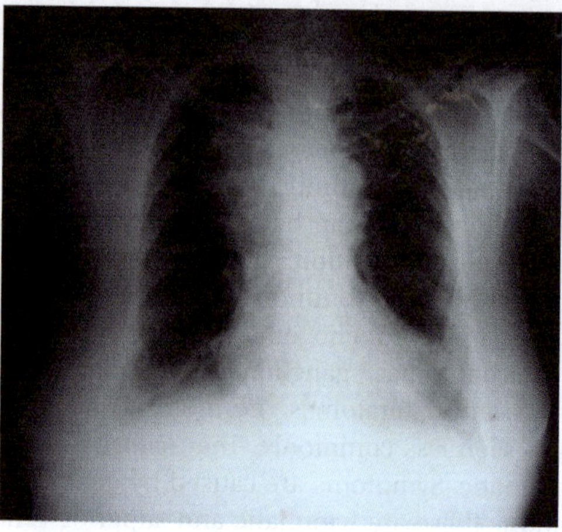

Fig. 156.2: Chest X-ray: Mediastinal tumor widening of the mediastinum

Pulmonary Rehabilitation and Respiratory Physiotherapy

KE Rajan

Chapter Summary

- General Considerations
- Education
- Airway Clearance
- Relaxation Techniques
- Respiratory Re-Education
- Muscle Training
- Nutrition/Occupation
- Pulmonary Rehabilitation and diseases
  - Chronic Obstructive Pulmonary Disease
  - Asthma
  - Bronchiectasis

GENERAL CONSIDERATIONS

The American Thoracic Society and the European Respiratory Society (ATS/ERS) define pulmonary rehabilitation as an evidence-based, multidisciplinary and comprehensive intervention for patients with chronic respiratory diseases who are symptomatic and often have decreased daily life activities. Pulmonary rehabilitation is designed to reduce respiratory symptoms, optimize functional status, increase participation and reduce healthcare costs through stabilizing or reversing systemic manifestations of the disease. Respiratory physiotherapy, exercises and rehabilitation have become integral parts of many disciplines in medicine, especially, major abdominal and thoracic surgeries, trauma surgery, organ transplantations and several others.

Key Components of Pulmonary Rehabilitation

- *Education:* Respiratory physiotherapy
- *Muscle training:* Lower limb/upper limb/muscles of respiration
- *Psychosocial:* Nutritional support, occupational therapy.

Pulmonary rehabilitation involves assessment of the patient, exercise training, education, nutritional intervention and psychosocial support. Pulmonary rehabilitation improves exercise tolerance and quality of life as well as reduces dyspnea in patients with respiratory diseases. Respiratory physiotherapy forms an integral component of education in a pulmonary rehabilitation program. Respiratory physiotherapy includes techniques to improve regional ventilation, gas exchange and respiratory muscle function.

EDUCATION

Physiotherapists play a key role in the delivery of pulmonary rehabilitation including noninvasive ventilation (NIV) service, delivery of oxygen and utilization of nebulized medications. Physiotherapy should be offered to all patients with chronic respiratory conditions. The aim of pulmonary rehabilitation is management of breathlessness and symptom control, mobility and function improvement or maintenance, and airway clearance and cough enhancement or support. Physiotherapy may be helpful for postural and/or musculoskeletal dysfunction and pain. It provides help in improving continence, especially during coughing and forced expiratory maneuvers.

Respiratory physiotherapy consists of three groups of techniques: (1) To improve airway clearance, (2) to relax the patient and (3) to provide breathing training in the form of respiratory re-education. Together, these measures aim to improve mucociliary clearance. In addition, they optimize respiratory function by enhancing respiratory muscle efficiency and improving chest wall compliance.

AIRWAY CLEARANCE

Several methods can be adopted to enhance clearance of airways. These include positioning of the patient, shock waves to chest wall, compression techniques and use of positive pressure.

Examples of airway clearance:
- ***Positioning of patient:*** Postural drainage, postural coughing
- ***Shock waves to thorax:*** Chest percussion and vibration
- ***Compression:*** Manual chest compression, forced expiration (huffing)
- ***Use of positive pressure:*** Continuous positive airway pressure (CPAP) and bi-level CPAP.

RELAXATION TECHNIQUES

The patient is advised how to relax the body and avoid getting into panic situations. Yoga and meditation have been observed to be of use in this direction.

RESPIRATORY RE-EDUCATION

Patient is taught to breathe more effectively, with incurring less energy expenditure. Controlled, slow, rhythmic breathing can be more energy efficient. Pursed lip breathing is aimed to improve intra-airway pressures. The patient needs to understand how to control breathing during daily activities to the optimum level.

MUSCLE TRAINING

Muscle training improves dyspnea, exercise tolerance and quality of life in patients with chronic obstructive pulmonary disease (COPD) or other respiratory diseases. Lower limb and upper limb exercise training give maximum benefit in improving dyspnea and bettering the quality of life. Recent randomized controlled trials

(RCTs) indicate that training can improve strength and respiratory muscle resistance. There is significant cost reduction in healthcare delivery for these patients who are willing to carryout muscle training. It is still controversial whether a survival benefit is always obtained with muscle training. ATS/ERS statement recommends emphasizing self-management skills in the educational component of rehabilitation, particularly in managing exacerbations in terms of both detection and treatment. Guidelines advocate that specific respiratory muscle training should be included as part of general training for patients presenting with weak respiratory muscles.

NUTRITION/OCCUPATION

Nutritional support and occupational therapy are the two key components that need to be included in any pulmonary rehabilitation program. Excess weight and malnutrition are both problems for the patient with chronic respiratory ailment, especially in COPD.

The success of pulmonary rehabilitation program depends upon the transformation of physiological improvements into benefits that are important to patients; a transformation facilitated by occupational therapy. Reduction of the dyspnea caused by activities of daily living is mandatory. The occupational therapist teaches the patient how to simplify routine activities to ensure greater efficiency and lower calorie expenditure. Recent recommendations are there to include energy conservation and work simplification techniques in patient education programs.

PULMONARY REHABILITATION AND DISEASES

Chronic Obstructive Pulmonary Disease (COPD)

The patient with COPD will benefit from breathlessness management advice. Maneuvers include positioning to fix the shoulder girdle passively and forward lean postures to lengthen the diaphragm and improve its length-tension ratio. A wheeled walking aid will reduce the ventilatory requirements of walking.

A variety of breathing techniques can be used to reduce dyspnea and panic at rest or during exertion. Energy conservation strategies can aid activities of daily living. Endurance and strength training exercises of both upper and lower limbs are very rewarding. Inspiratory muscle training may help some patients. Airway clearance techniques can be used, especially during an infective exacerbation. NIV should be considered in hypercapnic respiratory failure, with proper training and support for the effective delivery of NIV. Intermittent positive pressure breathing (IPPB) may be considered in acute exacerbations of COPD where patients present with retained secretions but are too weak or tired to generate an effective cough.

In patients with COPD, malnutrition worsens pulmonary impairment and diminishes physical capacity. Malnutrition affects one-third of patients with moderate to severe COPD. Obesity and malnutrition have adverse effects on COPD. A reduction in the body mass index (BMI) of COPD patients is an independent mortality risk factor.

Asthma

Some form of breathing retraining (breathing exercises and relaxation) should be considered as an appropriate treatment for patients with asthma to reduce symptoms and improve quality of life, along with their prescribed medication. There is insufficient evidence for inspiratory muscle training, or the use of airway clearance techniques in asthma. Many asthmatics report benefit of relaxation therapy though evidence is inconclusive. Yoga, Tai Chi, acupuncture or acupressure all may be useful in some subset of patients who prefer them.

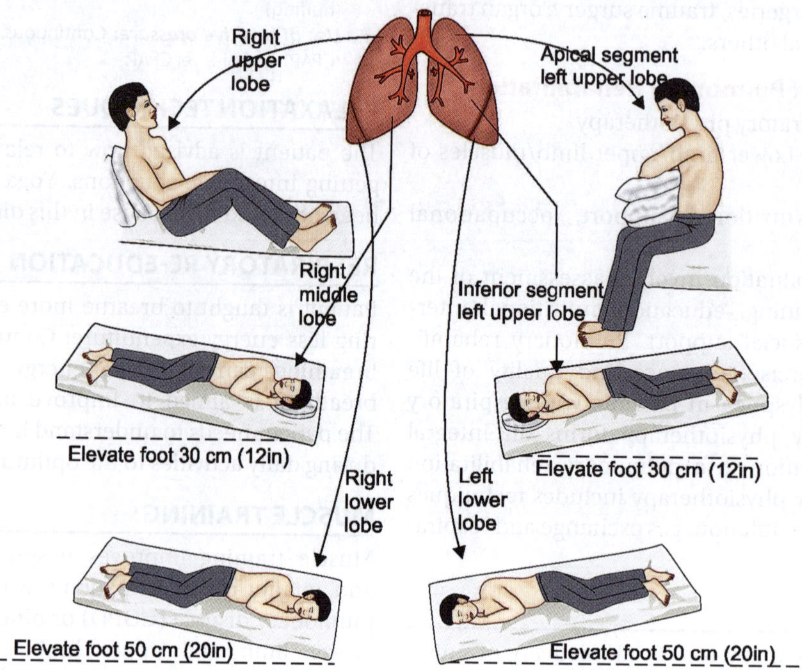

Fig. 157.1: Postural drainage of different areas of the lungs

Bronchiectasis

Physiotherapy has a key role in the management of the person with bronchiectasis. Pulmonary rehabilitation is to be offered to all patients of bronchiectasis with breathlessness affecting activities of daily living. Inspiratory muscle training is recommended. Airway clearance techniques may be offered and taught for use as necessary. Accurate and appropriate postural drainage must be explained. Nebulized therapies enhance airway clearance. Use of NIV and IPPB should be considered if needed (Fig. 157.1).

In addition to pure physiotherapy, special forms of drug therapy act synergistically to clear the respiratory passages. These are listed below—treatment modalities for mucus hypersecretion:

- Glucocorticoids in respiratory allergy and asthma
- Botulinum toxins may be used to inhibit mucin secretion
- *Physical measures:* Aerosol, hypertonic saline 7% as aerosol and mannitol
- Inhaled bronchodilators mucolytics such as dornase α which can be inhaled, N-acetyl cysteine which breaks the disulfide bond in mucin and helps in expectoration. When applied intrabronchially through a scope.
- Antibiotics to clear airway infection through all routes—oral, IV or inhalation.

In addition, pulmonary rehabilitation may play a part in the management of several disorders such as cystic fibrosis (CF), ventilated pneumonia patient, kyphoscoliosis and restrictive lung defects. Patients with vocal cord dysfunction, neuromuscular disorders and spinal cord disease or injury may also benefit from chest physiotherapy.

Source: British Thoracic Society. Concise BTS/ACPRC guidelines physiotherapy management of the adult, medical, spontaneously breathing patient. [online] Available from www.brit-thoracic.org.uk [Accessed Sept 2016].

CHAPTER

158

Hematology: General Considerations

KV Krishna Das

> **Chapter Summary**
> - Blood Formation
> - Erythrocyte
> - Hematopoietic Growth Factors
> - Leukocytes
> - Platelets
> - Clinical Aspects of Hematological Disorders
> - Laboratory Investigations

BLOOD FORMATION

As early as the 3rd week of gestation, blood cells are formed in the yolk sac outside the embryo. Hematopoiesis is taken up by the liver and spleen after a few weeks. The bone marrow progressively takes over this function after the 20th week.

Red Cell Production

In early embryonic life, a cohort of red blood cell (RBC) precursors appear in the blood islands of the yolk sac. Definitive stem cells which lead to hematopoiesis [hematopoietic stem cells (HSCs)], which persists throughout fetal and adult life emerge from the ventral wall of the dorsal aorta. By about 60 days of gestation, they migrate to the fetal liver and first fetal red cells are released into the circulation to replace embryonic red cells. During fetal life, the HSCs migrate to the bone marrow which is the seat of hematopoiesis, later on senescent RBCs are replaced by younger forms continuously. About 2–3 million RBCs have to be produced every second in order to maintain normal RBC count in adult.

After birth, hepatic and splenic hematopoiesis ceases and bone marrow is the only site for blood formation. Normally, in adults only the marrow in the axial skeleton, skull and ends of long bones is active, the rest remains in a dormant stage, but it can become active in times of need. In the adult, 30% of hematopoiesis takes place in the pelvic bones.

The bone marrow is a highly organized tissue supported by reticular cells and anchored on a spoke-like vascular structure. Functionally there are two components:

1. ***Microenvironment*** consists of the stromal cells, accessory cells and extracellular matrix formed by them. The stromal cells include fibroblasts, macrophages, endothelial cells and adipocytes. The macrophages elaborate a wide range of cytokines which influence growth of marrow cells—either stimulatory or inhibitory. Function of stroma is to provide a structural framework for the blood-forming cells and to produce cytokines.

2. ***HSCs in various stages of proliferation and maturation:*** A rich network of blood vessels empties blood into sinuses. The hematopoietic cells lie in cords or islands between the vascular sinuses in a meshwork of reticular cells. Erythrocytes, myeloid cells and megakaryocytes (MKCs) develop outside the vascular compartment. The marrow contains a rich supply of nerve cells which are sensitive to changes in intramedullary pressure. They are packed into fronds consisting of a network of reticular fibroblastoid cells surrounded by endothelial cells. As the blood cells mature, they extricate themselves from this network, pass through the gaps between the endothelial cells and are liberated into the sinusoidal blood. From the sluggish circulation in the sinusoids, ultimately they reach the mainstream of circulation. Each day an adult produces 200 billion erythrocytes, 100 billion leukocytes and 100 billion platelets. These rates can be increased by 10-fold in times of need.

The pluripotent stem cell differentiates first into the myeloid cell progenitor or CFU-S (colony-forming unit spleen). From this cell, the progenitors of erythroid burst-forming unit (BFU-E), myeloid and monocytic cells (CFU-GM) and MKCs (CFU-MK) arise. CFU-GM further differentiates into the precursors of macrophages (CFU-M) and granulocytes (CFU-G) (Figs 158.1 and 158.2).

The stem cells and their progeny show distinct surface-antigen expression as they proliferate and differentiate (Table 158.1).

Several growth factors and differentiating factors are produced by different cells which help in proliferation of the hematopoietic cell precursors.

Lymphoid cells arise in the bone marrow from the lymphocyte precursors.

ERYTHROCYTE

The most primitive committed erythropoietic precursor cells are called BFU-E since they give rise to multiple subcolonies when they are grown *in vitro*. The burst-promoting activity is brought about by the secretions of specific types of T-cells and monocytes occurring in close proximity to each other. As the primitive progenitor cells replicate and mature, they become increasingly sensitive

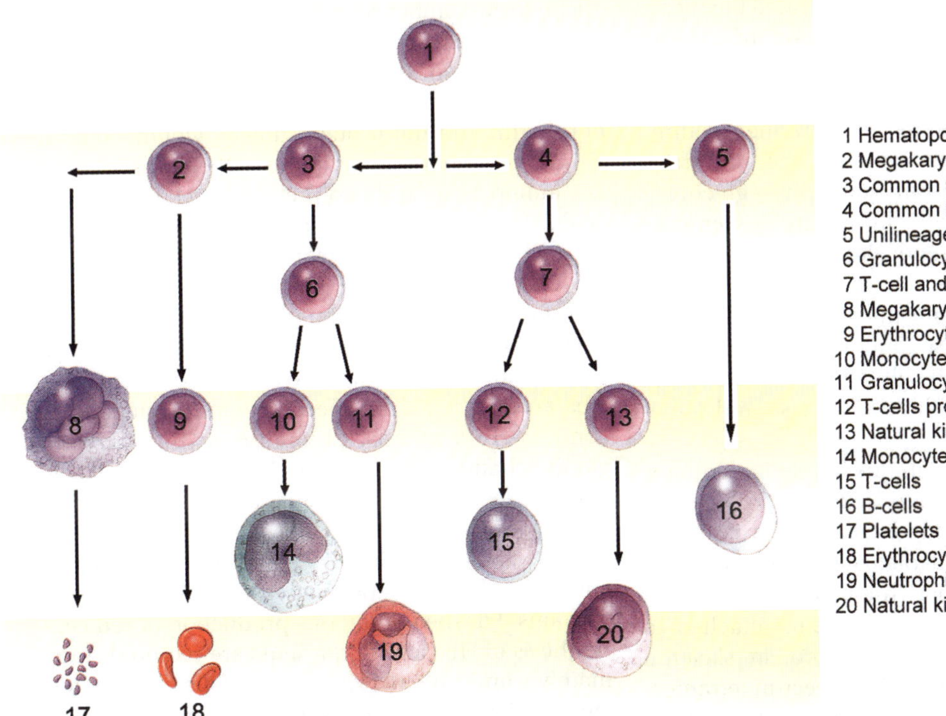

Fig. 158.1: Scheme of hematopoiesis: Diagrammatic representation of hematopoieses from a precursor stem cell

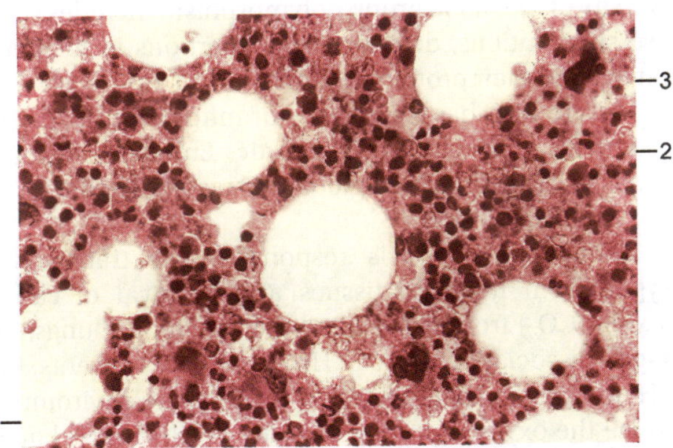

Fig. 158.2: Normal bone marrow × 400. **Note:** 1. Erythroid cell, 2. Granulocyte and 3. Megakaryocyte (MKC)

Table 158.1: Surface antigen expression of different types of cell	
Type of cell	**Surface antigen expression**
Pluripotent stem cell	CD34–, CD90+, CD123+, CD117+, CD135+
HSCs	CD34+, CD33–, CD38–, CD45RO+, CD45RA–
Myeloid progenitor cell (CFU-GM)	CD64+
CFU-M	CD34+, CD33+, CD13+
CFU-G	CD45RA+, MPO+
Lymphoid progenitor	
β-cell progenitor	CD34+, CD10+, CD19+
Common lymphoid progenitor and T-cell progenitor	CD34+, CD45RA+, CD33–, CD7+
Progenitor for NK-cell and dendritic cell	CD34+, CD33–, CD44, CD5±

Abbreviations: HSCs = Hematopoietic stem cells; CFU = Colony-forming unit; GM = Granulocyte-monocyte; CD = Clusters of differentiation; NK = Natural killer; MPO = Myeloperoxidase

to erythropoietin (EPO) and form erythroid colonies more rapidly [erythrocyte CFU (CFU-E)]. These develop into **erythroblasts** and **erythrocytes**. EPO is the main hormone which controls the proliferation and maturation of erythroid precursors.

Stages in the Development of the Erythrocyte

Different stages are recognizable in the process of maturation of the erythrocyte. These are the proerythroblast, basophilic, polychromatophilic, eosinophilic normoblasts, reticulocytes and mature erythrocytes. The nucleus of the normoblast degenerates and it is extruded to give rise to the reticulocyte. In this cell, ribosomes, mitochondria and Golgi apparatus persist for a short time. These cytoplasmic organelles reveal a granular or strand-like pattern when stained with vital stains like brilliant cresyl blue or aqueous methylene blue. These are called reticulocytes. The remnants of the degenerating nucleus, which are in the process of extrusion, are demonstrable as **Howell-Jolly bodies** and **Cabot's rings**.

In the normal adult, 2×10^{11} erythrocytes die every day. In replacing this number, the marrow synthesizes 4×10^{14} molecules of hemoglobin (Hb) every second. Hb consists of heme and globin. Heme is synthesized by inserting an atom of iron into an intensely colored ring of protoporphyrin IX by the developing erythroblast. Simultaneously, the developing red cell produces α- and β-globin chains which are joined to the heme molecule. This process proceeds in a precisely programed manner. Heme is formed in the mitochondria from where it has to move out into the cytoplasm where globin chains are formed. Disruption of these processes leads to disorders such as thalassemias where globin chain synthesis is defective and sideroblastic anemias where incorporation of iron into heme is defective.

The ***mature erythrocyte*** is a non-nucleated biconcave disk most suited to perform the function of gaseous exchange. It is a highly specialized, metabolically active cell which obtains energy by utilizing glucose by anaerobic pathways. It is provided with enzymes required for metabolism of glucose. Some of the important enzymes, which take part in anaerobic glycolysis are hexokinase, glucose-6-phosphate isomerase (GPI), phosphofructokinase and aldolase. Those taking part in oxidative glycolysis are glucose-6-phosphate dehydrogenase (G6PD), 6-phosphogluconate dehydrogenase (6PGD), transketolase and transaldolase. This pathway is connected with glutathione metabolism through the enzymes glutathione reductase and glutathione peroxidase.

The ***red cell membrane*** is unique in that it maintains the biconcave shape of the red cell; it is capable of accommodating increase and decrease of volume of the contents, and it is deformable so as to pass through blood vessels of smaller caliber. The membrane consists of a bilayer of lipids and interval proteins attached to an underlying protein skeleton. The protein skeleton consists of a two-dimensional mesh of spectrin tetramers and oligomers, cross-linked by protein 4.1 and ankyrin. Spectrin is a cytoskeletal protein that lines the intracellular side of the plasma membrane in eukaryotic cells. It forms a scaffolding and plays an important role in maintaining plasma membrane integrity and cytoskeletal structure. Ankyrins are a family of adaptor proteins that mediate the attachment of integral membrane proteins to the spectrin-actin cytoskeleton. They comprise at least 12 families of integral membrane proteins with binding sites for the β-subunit of spectrin. The protein skeleton is attached to the membrane by the binding of spectrin to ankyrin, and of ankyrin to another protein called band-3 which is an anion exchanger. Other membrane proteins include palladin. Abnormalities of these membrane proteins lead to early destruction of the erythrocytes.

The protein skeleton helps to maintain the shape of the red cell. The deformability is grossly affected in defects of membrane of the erythrocyte as occurs in spherocytosis and elliptocytosis and also when abnormal Hbs, such as Hbs-induced polymerization under anoxic environment. Normal erythrocyte does not freely adhere to endothelium while in circulation. Under abnormal conditions the adhesive properties of the membrane also changes, rendering them more adherent to endothelium.

The erythrocyte membrane has a major role in ion transport which is mediated by several membrane channels or pumps that can maintain the osmotic gradient within the cell. These functions which require energy can be modified by hormones, cyclic nucleotides, calcium and calmodulin.

Anaerobic metabolism supplies 90% of the energy requirement and only 10% is supplied by the aerobic or pentose-phosphate cycle. The mature red cell is incapable of protein synthesis. The full complement of Hb and enzymes present in erythrocytes is handed down by the erythroblast. Life of the red cells is 120 days. They are destroyed in the reticuloendothelial system subsequently.

The red cell number remains nearly constant in the range of 5–6 millions/mm³ ($5–6 \times 10^{12}$/L) throughout life.

Hemoglobin is a complex molecule consisting of the heme moiety (the red pigment) comprising iron and porphyrin, and the protein moiety, globin. In adult Hb (HbA), the globin consists of two α-chains, each containing 141 amino acids and two β-chains each with 146 amino acids. The fetal Hb (HbF) consists of two α-chains and two γ-chains. After birth, within 5–6 months the synthesis of γ-chains stops and β-chains are formed in the required amounts. By the age of 6 months 98–99% of Hb is made up of HbA. The rate and amount of production of the α, β and γ-chains and their synthesis to form normal and abnormal Hbs are controlled by specific genes. Multigene cluster controls Hb synthesis. Chromosome 16 controls α-like globin chains, chromosome 11 controls β-like globin chains. Several other genetic loci promote or inhibit the expression of the different globin chains. In normal persons, the production of γ-chains fall rapidly after birth and give place to rapid increase in the production of β-chains. For the continuous production of red cells and synthesis of Hb, several nutrients are required. These are mainly iron, proteins, vitamin B_{12}, folic acid, pyridoxine, vitamin C, nicotinic acid, copper and cobalt.

The blood group antigens are attached to the red cell membrane. The molecular basis for the remarkable diversity of the blood group polymorphism includes single base substitutions, deletions and insertions in the genes that encode their protein products.

Mature RBC has no nucleus or mitochondria. Energy is derived through the glycolytic Embden Meyerhof Parnas pathway in which glucose is metabolized with the production of lactate.

Hemoglobin (Hb) is responsible for transport of oxygen from lungs to tissues and removal of carbon dioxide (CO_2) from tissues and delivery to the lungs. The oxygen dissociation curve of Hb depicts these events. Rise in H^+ ion concentration and CO_2 levels in the environment reduce the oxygen-binding capacity of Hb. This is known as the Bohr's effect. Increase in oxygenation of Hb reduces its affinity to CO_2. This is known as the Haldane effect.

Androgens also stimulate the production of EPO and also directly activate the stem cells. Estrogens suppress EPO production and hence depress erythropoiesis. Thyroxine probably stimulates erythropoiesis by producing tissue anoxia. Hypothyroidism leads to a mild degree of anemia, which can be corrected by thyroxine.

HEMATOPOIETIC GROWTH FACTORS

The expansion of the stem cell pool, maturation and expansion of precursor cells and their liberation into circulation are all under control of well-defined humoral influences. These include EPO, granulocyte colony-stimulating factor (G-CSF), macrophage colony-stimulating factor (M-CSF), granulocyte-macrophage colony-stimulating factor (GM-CSF) and interleukin-3 (IL-3) (also known as multicolony-stimulating factor).

Erythropoietin

During fetal life, it is produced in the liver. In postnatal life, by far the main source is kidneys (90%), a small amount is also produced in the liver (10%). In the kidneys the EPO-producing cells are found in the renal cortex, lying outside the renal tubular basement membrane. These cells are derived either from a subset of interstitial cells or capillary endothelial cells which can sense oxygen levels by a complicated mechanism. Action of EPO on the erythroid precursor cells is receptor mediated.

It is a glycoprotein with a molecular weight of 30,000 Daltons. Its principal actions are on the developing erythroid precursor cells after they have become sensitive to EPO. The erythroid precursors are stimulated to proliferate and differentiate and thus accelerate erythropoiesis. Normal apoptotic mechanisms play a role in regulating erythrocyte maturation and disposal.

The viability of the developing erythroid cells is also maintained by this hormone. It is a survival factor for them. EPO production is tightly controlled to prevent inappropriate rise in red cell mass. Main stimulus for EPO production is anoxia. Rise in red cell mass and viscosity of blood depress EPO production independent of the tissue oxygenation status. Small rise in EPO levels do occur with slight fall in Hb, up to 10 g/dL, but not beyond the normal ranges. The normal range of plasma EPO is 5–25 U/L. In response to anemia or arterial hypoxemia, the serum level of EPO may go above 25 U/L.

There is only one form of circulating EPO. Production is controlled at the gene level. There are no stores and the production and clearance are independent of the plasma levels. EPO gene transcription is inhibited by inflammatory cytokines, such as IL-1 and tumor necrosis factor (TNF).

Actions of EPO

Actions of EPO include the following:

- EPO leads to proliferation of erythroid precursors which differentiate into normoblasts, which leave the bone marrow after extrusion of the nucleus. Reticulocyte counts start rising within 1–2 weeks of EPO administration.
- EPO crosses blood-brain barrier and it plays a protective role in ischemic neurons. It also has tissue-protecting activity in the myocardium and the kidney.

Various conditions, such as renal parenchymal diseases, hyperviscosity, cancer, infection, inflammation, chronic liver diseases, surgery, pregnancy and prematurity, suppress EPO production without regard to tissue oxygenation. EPO is metabolized by erythroid progenitor cells. In hypoplastic anemia, due to defective utilization of EPO, the serum levels are relatively high. EPOs, their analogues and mimetics are produced by recombinant technology. These include recombinant EPO, darbepoetin-α which has longer duration of action compared to EPO, continuous EPO-receptor activator (CERA), synthetic EPO protein, EPO fusion protein and EPO-mimetic peptides. All these are under different stages of drug development and are introduced for therapeutic use.

Hematopoietic growth factors other than EPO are produced by fibroblasts, endothelial cells, monocytes and lymphocytes which are widely distributed. In experimental studies, stimulation with bacterial endotoxin, monokines and lectins increase the production of these growth-promoting factors. They act on progenitor cells to produce precursor cells and simultaneously expand the progenitor pool.

Clinical Uses

EPO is very successful in correcting anemia and improving the general well-being in chronic renal failure (CRF) when given in a dose of 75–150 IU/kg bw thrice a week (total dose required annually for an adult being 2–12 mg). It is also used to stimulate red cell production preparatory to autologous transfusion at a later date.

EPO is given by subcutaneous injection. Indications for EPO include:

- ***Anemia of CRF***
- ***Anemia of cancer:*** Patients with Hb less than 10 g/dL benefit by EPO which also prolongs life.
- ***In patients recovering from myelosuppressive chemotherapy***, induces apoptosis both in cancer cells and erythroid precursors. EPO blocks the apoptosis of erythroid precursor cells.

Repeated use over long periods may lead to the development of anti-EPO antibody which neutralizes endogenous and exogenous EPO. The patient becomes unresponsive to the use of EPO and may develop pure red-cell aplasia (PRCA). This condition responds to immunosuppressive therapy. Another adverse side effect is the development of hypertension with rise in erythrocyte counts.

A long-acting analogue of EPO which is also used in therapy is darbepoetin-α.

Granulocyte-macrophage Colony-stimulating Factor

It acts on the precursors of granulocytes, monocytes, macrophages, erythrocytes and also MKCs.

GM-CSF is produced by several cell types. It stimulates the proliferation of several myeloid cell lines and MKCs. The result is increased production of neutrophils and other granulocytes and monocytes and improvement in neutrophil survival. GM-CSF stimulates the production of neutrophils, eosinophils, basophils, monocytes and dendritic cells in culture and activates most of these cells into action.

Clinical Uses

GM-CSF is employed in doses of 10 µg/kg bw, in order to stimulate neutrophils, monocytes and circulating stem cells, and thereby reducing the duration of dangerous neutropenia following intensive chemotherapy and bone marrow transplantation. For harvesting, circulating stem cells preliminary to stem cell transplantation which is an alternative to bone marrow transplantation, GM-CSF is employed. It is also used in some cases of cyclical neutropenia and agranulocytosis where other therapeutic measures are not fully effective.

Granulocyte Colony-stimulating Factor

G-CSF is produced by endothelial cells, fibroblasts and macrophages in virtually all organs. It stimulates growth of neutrophil colonies *in vitro* and stimulates neutrophils into activity, such as phagocytosis and bacterial killing. It leads to release of young neutrophils into the circulation leading to shift to the left of neutrophil distribution. It also causes presence of toxic granules in the neutrophils in peripheral blood, which is a morphological correlate of their heightened functional state. In inflammation, cytokines such as TNF-α, IL-1 and IL-6, derived from activated monocytes stimulate G-CSF production. Recombinant G-CSF is available for therapy as injection containing 30 MU (300 μg)/mL. After injection, peripheral blood neutrophil count rises within 48 hours. Monocytes and eosinophils may show slight rise. The dose is 0.5 MU (5 μg)/kg bw (twice a day) given SC or as intravenous (IV) infusion.

G-CSF mobilizes stem cells from the bone marrow to peripheral blood and therefore increases the yield of stem cells from peripheral blood. G-CSF therapy helps to prevent chemotherapy-induced neutropenia.

Hemopoietic growth factors are administrated for four groups of conditions:

1. Correction of cytopenias
2. For harvesting stem cells and progenitor cells
3. Augmentation of hematopoiesis to compensate for accelerated cell destruction
4. Activation of mature hemopoietic cells.

Clinical Uses

G-CSF is also used extensively in leukopenic states and chemotherapy-induced neutropenia, both prophylactically and therapeutically.

LEUKOCYTES

White blood cells (WBCs) originate from pluripotent-hemopoietic stem cells. Under the influence of various external stimuli including cytokines, matrix proteins and accessory cells, the stem cells differentiate into hemopoietic progenitor cells (Table 158.2) (Refer also Section 1, Ch 3). Broadly they may be divided into phagocytes and lymphocytes. The former includes the neutrophils, eosinophils, basophils (granulocytes) and monocytes (Table 158.3).

The granulocytes are formed from the stem cell through the stages of myeloblasts, promyelocytes, myelocytes and metamyelocytes. As the neutrophil ages, the number of lobes in the nucleus increases and age of the cell can be assessed this way. The cytoplasmic granules are lysosomal in origin and are of two types—the *primary granules* which appear at the promyelocytic stage and *secondary granules* which appear at the myelocytic stage. Primary granules contain myeloperoxidases, acid

Table 158.2: Cytokines involved in the production of different leukocytes

Cell type	Cytokine involved
Neutrophil	G-CSF, GM-CSF, IL-3 and M-CSF
Monocytes	GM-CSF and M-CSF
Eosinophils	GM-CSF, IL-3 and IL-5
T-lymphocytes	A complex process, IL-2 and IL-3
B-lymphocytes	IL-7

Abbreviations: G-CSF = Granulocyte colony-stimulating factor; GM-CSF = Granulocyte-macrophage colony-stimulating factor; IL = Interleukin; M-CSF = Macrophage colony-stimulating factor

Table 158.3: The normal distribution of leukocytes in peripheral blood

Parameters	Range (× 10⁹/L)	Percentage of total (%)
Total leukocytes (adults)	5–10	–
Neutrophils	3.5–7.0	60–70
Eosinophils	0.1–0.6	2–6
Basophils	0.01–0.10	0–1
Monocytes	0.2–0.5	2–5
Lymphocytes	1.5–3.0	25–35

Note: 1×10^9/L = 1,000 cells/mm³. Children have slightly higher leukocyte counts

phosphatases and other acid hydrolases. Secondary granules contain alkaline phosphatase and lysozyme. The latter predominates in the mature neutrophil. Myeloblasts are the earliest recognizable precursors seen in the bone marrow. The nucleus contains 2–5 nucleoli and the cytoplasm is clear, nongranular and basophilic. In normal marrow, the myeloblasts do not exceed 4%. Promyelocytes are formed by division of myeloblasts. The nucleoli disappear and the cytoplasm acquires primary granules. The promyelocytes give rise to myelocytes which show specific secondary granules in the cytoplasm. The nucleus is more condensed and nucleoli are absent. Neutrophils, eosinophils and basophils arise from corresponding myelocytes. Myelocytes divide to form metamyelocytes which do not divide further. Metamyelocytes have indented or horse shoe-shaped nucleus and cytoplasm filled with primary and secondary granules. These cells develop into *band forms* or *juvenile neutrophils* in which the nucleus starts to show lobulation, but the distinct filamentous constriction between the lobes is absent.

Myeloblasts, promyelocytes and myelocytes are together known as the proliferative or *mitotic pool*, and the metamyelocytes, band forms and segmented neutrophils are known as the *postmitotic maturation pool*. The store of granulocytes present in the marrow is 10–15 times the circulating pool. Majority of the marrow granulocytic cells are myelocytes and neutrophils. After release from the bone marrow, granulocytes circulate in the peripheral blood for about 10 hours and then enter tissue for phagocytosis. In the peripheral blood, half of the neutrophils circulate freely (*circulating pool* included in the blood count) and the other half forms the *marginating pool* which adheres to vessel wall (not included in the blood count). In the tissues, the granulocytes remain for 4–5 days before they perish during defensive action or due to aging.

The various compartments in the peripheral blood, tissues and bone marrow are regulated by a feedback mechanism. Leukopoietins, analogous to EPO, have been described.

Neutrophils

Functions of Neutrophils

These include chemotaxis, phagocytosis, intracytoplasmic killing, and destruction of foreign particles and microbes. Neutrophils are phagocytic and this activity is of prime importance in microbial killing. In many inflammatory diseases, further processes mediated by the cytokines liberated by neutrophils tend to perpetuate the inflammatory and tissue destructive processes. Functional defects of neutrophils may occur at times. In this condition, there will be defects of any or all the functions.

Neutrophils adhere to cells and surfaces by receptor-mediated activity and the cell surface glycoproteins are important for this function. Neutrophils activated by phagocytic stimuli or chemoattractants produce large amounts of microbicidal oxidants. The neutrophils contain cytoplasmic granules of different sizes. The azurophil granules are lysozyme-like, and contain various enzymes and other proteins possessing antibacterial and antifungal properties. The lysosomal granules contain myeloperoxidase. Neutrophil-specific (secondary) granules are rich in glycoproteins. Deficiency of the contents of granules makes the neutrophils functionally defective (Refer also, Section 1, Ch 3).

Functional Defects of Neutrophils

This may be acquired or congenital.

Defect in chemotaxis (lazy leukocyte syndrome): It occurs in alcoholism, hyperosmolar states, myelogenous leukemia, abnormalities of complement, and rarely as a congenital condition. Drugs, like aspirin and corticosteroids impair chemotaxis further.

Defective phagocytosis: It occurs in hypogammaglobulinemia, hypocomplementemia, postsplenectomy states and sickle cell anemia.

The killing function: It is reduced in granulomatous disease, myeloperoxidase deficiency, Chédiak-Higashi syndrome, acute and chronic granulocytic leukemias, preleukemia and myelodysplastic states.

Alteration in Neutrophil Counts

Neutrophil leukocytosis (count > 7.5 × 10⁹/L): This condition occurs in many bacterial infections, inflammations, tissue necrosis, metabolic disorders such as renal failure, gout, acidosis, toxemias of pregnancy, malignant neoplasms, acute hemorrhage, acute hemolysis and corticosteroid therapy. Myeloproliferative disorders are characterized by very high granulocyte counts. A rapid increase in the production of neutrophils is generally associated with the appearance of many young forms (shift to the left) and presence of myelocytes in peripheral blood.

Neutropenia (counts < 1 × 10⁹/L) develops as a toxic reaction to several drugs or as a part of pancytopenias. Milder grades of transient neutropenia occur in many viral infections and bacterial infections like typhoid, hypersensitivity, anaphylaxis, autoimmune disorders like disseminated lupus erythematosus, and in hypersplenism. When neutropenia is caused by reduction in the formation of cells, most of the neutrophils in peripheral blood are the older forms. They show four or more lobes in the nucleus (shift to the right), the younger forms being particularly absent.

Reduction of neutrophil counts to below 500 cells/mm³ is associated with increased risk of several opportunistic infections. Neutropenia associated with fever is a dreaded complication in chemotherapy of malignancy, organ transplantation and others. This calls for special therapeutic intervention.

Cyclical neutropenia is a rare disorder showing periodic reduction in neutrophils at 3–4 week intervals. It is characterized by a regular 21-day cyclic fall and rise in the numbers of circulating neutrophils, monocytes, eosinophils, lymphocytes, platelets and reticulocytes. This is caused by a defect of the stem cells. During the leukopenic phase, the bone marrow shows paucity of myeloid elements. Neutropenia by itself does not cause symptoms, but it predisposes to infection when the neutrophil count falls below 500 cells/mm³ and persists so for above 10–14 days.

During these episodes, infections may develop leading to oral ulceration, gingivitis, pharyngitis, lymphadenopathy and skin infections. Human G-CSF given in a dose of 3 µg/kg daily SC has been found to be effective in correcting the neutropenic state.

Sometimes neutrophils migrate from the circulating pool to the marginating pool and the neutrophil count in peripheral blood falls. There is no increased tendency for infections in this condition. This is referred to as ***idiopathic benign neutropenia***.

Eosinophils

Eosinophils are derived from CD34– progenitor cells in the bone marrow. They differentiate in response to T-cells derived cytokines including IL-5, IL-3 and GM-CSF. The mature eosinophils can persist for up to 24 hours in the circulation before they migrate into extravascular sites where they can survive up to a few days.

Eosinophils are generally similar in morphology to neutrophils, with eosinophilic granules in the cytoplasm. The nucleus contains only two or rarely three lobes. Eosinophils develop through the same stages as the neutrophils. Distinguishing features develop at the stage of myelocyte.

Four processes are distinguishable in the development of eosinophils:

1. Differentiation of progenitor cell and proliferation in the bone marrow
2. Interaction between eosinophils and endothelial cells that include rolling, migration and adhesion of eosinophils
3. Chemoalteration which directs eosinophils to specific locations
4. Activation and destruction.

Three cytokines—IL-3, IL-5 and GM-CSF are particularly involved in the development of eosinophils. Among these three, IL-5 is the most important. It is also called eosinophil differentiation factor.

Eosinophils in tissues survive for varying periods, up to 12–24 days.

Several enzymes, such as arylsulfatase, phospholipidase, acid phosphatase, β-glucuronidase, peroxidase and cathepsins are present in the cytoplasmic granules. The function of eosinophils has been extensively studied and their importance recognized. They phagocytose a variety of substances such as immune complexes, mast cell granules, mycoplasma, ferritin and others. But this activity is considerably less than that of neutrophils. Eosinophils suppress allergic inflammatory processes. They play an important role in defense against parasites and in the removal of fibrin formed during inflammation.

Larval forms of parasites, like filaria and schistosomes, are killed by eosinophils. They kill parasites by releasing cationic proteins and reactive-oxygen metabolites into the extracellular fluid. They also secrete leukotrienes, prostaglandins and various other cytokines. Their life in peripheral blood is longer than that of neutrophils. In many conditions like hypersensitivity reactions, parasitic diseases, drug sensitivity and polyarteritis nodosa, eosinophil counts are moderately increased (0.4–2.0 $\times 10^9$/L). Marked increase (over 3×10^9/L) occurs in tropical eosinophilia which is common in India. Asthma, polyarteritis nodosa, Churg-Strauss syndrome and helminthiasis are associated with eosinophilia. Primary hypereosinophilic syndrome and eosinophilic leukemia cause high eosinophilia, but these are rare.

Definitions

Eosinophilia: Absolute eosinophil count more than 500 cells/mm³.
Hypereosinophilia: Absolute eosinophil count more than 1,500 cells/mm³.

Causes of Eosinophilia

- ***Infections:*** Parasites, lymphatic filariasis (tropical eosinophilia), dirofilaria, strongyloides, echinococcus, schistosoma, trichinella, toxocara, human immuno-deficiency virus (HIV) and human T-cell lympho-trophic virus.
- ***Allergic conditions:*** Atopic dermatitis, allergic asthma, drug allergy.
- ***Rheumatological:*** Churg-Strauss syndrome, idiopathic eosinophilic synovitis.
- ***Adrenal insufficiency:*** Sarcoidosis, ulcerative colitis.
- ***Malignant conditions:*** Solid tumors.
- ***Nonmyeloid hematological cancers:*** T-cell lymphoma, Hodgkin's disease, acute lymphocytic leukemia (ALL).
- ***Myeloid cancers,*** such as chronic myelogenous leukemia (CML), systemic mastocytosis, myeloid and lymphoid neoplasms producing platelet-derived growth factor (PDGF) receptor α or β and fibroblast growth factor receptor.

Idiopathic Hypereosinophilic Syndrome

Hypereosinophilic syndrome occurs as a result of growth factors elaborated by a clone of immunophenotypically aberrant T-cells. In many cases underlying cause may not be evident (idiopathic). Morphological abnormalities, such as hypogranulation and hyperlobation may occur in reactive eosinophils. They do not always suggest clonal abnormality.

This is a pathological condition characterized by eosinophilia associated with affection of multiple organ systems. Lesions involve the skin, and cardiac, neuro-logical and hematological systems. This represents a heterogeneous group of disorders. The cardinal features are long continued eosinophilia and multiorgan dys-function.

Clinical Features

Clinical features vary. It presents with fatigue, cough, dyspnea, angioedema, rash, fever and rhinitis. Absolute eosinophilic count may vary from 1,500 to 400,000 cells/mm³. Systemic complications may occur in hypereosinophilic syndrome.

Gastrointestinal system: Eosinophilic gastroenteritis characterized by abdominal pain, diarrhea, gastrointestinal (GI) bleeding and colitis.

Cardiac complications: Eosinophilic myocarditis, micro-vascular compromise, subendocardial fibrosis, arrhythmias, hypersensitivity myocarditis, fulminant heart failure, pericarditis and effusion. Chronic cardiac lesions include endomyocardial damage due to thrombo-embolism, valvular dysfunction and restrictive cardiomyo-pathy leading to endomyocardial fibrosis (Davies' disease).

Survival varies from 9 months to 3 years. Common causes of death are due to cardiac complications.

Bad prognostic features include male sex, total leukocyte count (TLC) more than 100,000 cells/mm³, circulating blasts in peripheral blood, refractoriness to glucocorticoids and presence of cardiac lesions.

Management of Hypereosinophilic Syndrome

- Glucocorticoids
- If response to glucocorticoids is poor, drugs like hydroxyurea, vincristine, imatinib or dasatinib may be tried
- Interferon-α has been used with glucocorticoids or hydroxyurea
- Anti-IL-5 monoclonal antibody mepolizumab has been tried
- Hematological stem cell transplantation have to be done in desperate cases.

Source: Fathi AT, Dec GW, Richter JM, et al. Case 7-2014: A 27-year-old man with diarrhea, fatigue, and eosinophilia. N Engl J Med. 2014;370(9):861-72.

Basophils

Basophils form up to 1% of the total leukocytes. They are identified by the presence of coarse basophilic granules which often overlie the nucleus which is bilobed. The granules are rich in histamine, serotonin and leukotrienes. Mast cells are related to, but distinct from basophils. They are long-lived cells which reside in tissues rather than in peripheral circulation, and they can divide further. Both basophils and mast cells participate in immediate allergic reactions, such as urticaria, anaphylaxis, asthma and allergic rhinitis. Increase in basophil leukocytes (counts > 0.1×10^9/L) is uncommon, but this is seen in myeloproliferative disorders, such as chronic myeloid leukemia and polycythemia vera. Disorders, like myxedema, smallpox, chickenpox and ulcerative colitis, also may be associated with basophil leukocytosis.

Monocytes

Syn: Mononuclear phagocytes

Mononuclear phagocyte system is made up of peripheral blood monocytes, their precursors in the bone marrow and tissue macrophages. Though their nomenclature indicates that they are predominantly phagocytic, they also mediate several other functions including induction of acute phase responses, regulation of hematopoiesis, activation of immune and coagulation systems, killing of micro-organisms and tumor cells, and tissue repair.

The precursor of the monocyte is the monoblast which resembles the myeloblast but can be distinguished histochemically and immunologically. From their sites of origin in the bone marrow, the monocytes circulate in the peripheral blood for about 3 days and enter the tissues where they are known as macrophages. The numbers of tissue macrophages are several 100 times that of the circulating monocytes and their lifespan is around a few months. The macrophages are seen in all tissues, but they are particularly prominent in the spleen, lymph nodes, pulmonary alveoli, liver **(Kupffer's cells)**, peritoneum and skin **(Langerhan's cells)**. Once the monocyte enters the tissues, it does not return to the circulation.

Mononuclear macrophages secrete several substances (numbering about a hundred) and these take part in several functions ranging from induction of cell growth to cell death. The major functions mediated by monocyte macrophages are listed below:

- *Inflammation:* The acute phase response which is a systemic inflammatory reaction resulting from infection or injury consists of fever, tachycardia, shock and changes in the concentrations of circulating proteins, such as C-reactive protein, fibrinogen, IL-1, TNF and IL-6. These are secreted by the monocytes and they form important mediators of this response.
- *Regulation of hemopoiesis:* Monocyte products, such as G-CSF and M-CSF directly stimulate cell production. IL-1 and TNF activate T-lymphocytes to produce GM-CSF and IL-3 which also stimulates hemopoiesis.
- *Hemostasis:* Monocytes and macrophages can activate the blood coagulation process in response to several stimuli including bacterial endotoxin, immune complexes and complement components. Mononuclear phagocytes synthesize tissue thromboplastin which can activate the extrinsic coagulation pathway.
- *Lymphocyte activation:* Some B- and T-lymphocytes cannot recognize free antigens themselves. Mononuclear phagocytes are capable of taking up such antigens and converting them into immunogenic fragments which are presented to B- and T-lymphocytes which are activated in turn.
- *Microbial killing:* Mononuclear phagocytes are attracted towards an infective focus by several substances including bacterial components and endotoxins, complement components, immune complexes and collagen fragments. Once they reach the site, they remain there under the influence of a migration inhibitory factor secreted by T-lymphocytes and phagocytose the microbes. After ingestion the organisms are killed.
- *Destruction of tumor cells:* Mononuclear phagocytes infiltrate tumors and lead to lysis of tumor cells. This forms a major defensive mechanism against tumors. TNF produced by the mononuclear phagocytes has been synthesized by recombinant DNA technology and it is used therapeutically.

- *Tissue repair and remodeling:* The collagenase and elastase secreted by mononuclear phagocytes help to debride wounds. They also release substances which stimulate the proliferation of fibroblasts and new vessels.

Macrophages in tissues are quiescent under normal conditions, but in times of need they are activated by several stimuli including endotoxin, immune complexes, complement components and products of T-cells. Interferon-γ secreted by lymphocytes is an important activator of macrophages. Macrophage function is essential to life. It is impaired in immunosuppressed states, diabetes mellitus, chronic granulomatous disease and several others.

Bacterial infections such as tuberculosis, brucellosis, bacterial endocarditis and typhoid, and protozoal infections like amebiasis may lead to moderate monocytosis ($> 0.8 \times 10^9$/L). Other causes of monocytosis are neutropenia, Hodgkin's disease and monocytic leukemia.

Lymphocytes

Lymphocytes and plasma cells are together known as immunocytes. Their role is to assist the phagocytes in defense mechanism and add specificity to the attack (Refer also to Section 1, Ch 3).

Lymphocytes are formed in the bone marrow and thymus during postnatal life. In the fetus, the yolk sac and liver produce lymphocytes. In the lymphopoietic tissues, the stem cells undergo spontaneous division without depending on antigenic stimulation. Other lymphoid tissues include lymph nodes, spleen, organized lymphoid tissues of the alimentary and respiratory tracts and the lymphocytes seen in blood and tissue spaces. They constitute secondary lymphoid tissues. In the bone marrow, the precursor of the lymphocyte is the lymphoblast. Maturation to the lymphocyte stage occurs without any distinct stages in between.

B-lymphocytes are derived from bone marrow stem cells. When activated by antigens, the B-cells proliferate and mature into plasma cells which secrete specific immunoglobulins (Igs), the antibodies.

The *primordial T-cells* are produced in the bone marrow and the cortex of the thymus, where they are conditioned to recognize the body's antigenic make-up. T-cell precursors migrate from the bone marrow to the corticomedullary regions of the thymus where they begin to differentiate, rearrange their variable region genes and proliferate. This process is completed in the medulla of the thymus from which the mature T-cells exit, 98% of the cells undergo apoptosis during their maturation in the thymus and only 2% emerge as functionally competent T-cells.

They are the main cells responsible for cell-mediated immunity. *Helper T-cells* (CD4+) are specific lymphocytes which instruct B-cells about specific antigens. The T-cell population also contains *suppressor cells* (CD8+) which reduce B-cell responses. The *killer cells* (K cells) cause damage to cells recognized as 'foreign'. Lymphocytes migrate to the lymph nodes and spleen through postcapillary venules. The T-cells are seen in the perifollicular areas of the cortex of lymph nodes (paracortical areas) and in the periarteriolar sheaths surrounding the central arterioles of the spleen. The majority of lymphocytes in the thoracic duct and peripheral blood are T-cells. B-cells selectively accumulate in the subcapsular periphery of the cortex and medullary cords of lymph nodes, and germinal follicles of lymph nodes and spleen. Majority of B-cells remain for long periods in these sites.

Most of the lymphocytes in peripheral blood are small with scanty nongranular cytoplasm and a central nucleus with coarse chromatin. Larger lymphocytes, which may also occur in peripheral blood, are probably stimulated by antigenic challenge from viruses or foreign proteins.

T- and B-lymphocytes are not distinguishable morphologically in the smear. The large lymphocytes, which form about 10%, characterized by abundant cytoplasm and reddish granules are the natural killer (NK) cells. They can destroy virus-infected cells and human leukocyte antigen (HLA) incompatible target cells. They can be distinguished by surface molecular configuration (CD+ characteristics).

Cytokines

In addition to specific antibodies produced by specifically stimulated cells, the cytokines constitute another type of mediators. They act as messengers both within the immune system and between the immune system and other systems of the body forming an integrated network that is highly involved in the regulation of immune responses.

B-lymphocytes

Bone marrow stem cells migrate to the gut lymphoid tissue associated with the alimentary and respiratory tracts and develop into B-lymphocytes. These are concerned mainly with the production of antibodies. B-cells differentiate into plasma cells which produce the antibodies. Antibodies consist of two identical heavy chains and two identical light chains that are held together by disulfide bonds. The amino acid sequence of the constant region of the heavy chain specifically determines the class of immunoglobulins IgG, IgA, IgM, IgD and IgE, and the subclasses of IgG and the IgA. Each type of antibody can be produced as a circulating molecule or a stationary molecule. The latter, which is anchored to the B-lymphocyte cell membrane, acts as the B-cell receptor. It has been estimated that both B-cells and T-cell can produce about 10^{15} different antibody variable regions and T-cell receptor regions, respectively. Unlike antibodies, T-cell receptors are produced only as transmembrane molecules. Peptides held by the major histocompatibility complex (MHC) molecule are recognized by specific receptors on T-cells.

The extreme diversity of antibody production is achieved by less than 400 genes which are located on three chromosomes 14, 2 and 22. The sequence of receptors on T-cells remains unaltered during cell division whereas the B-cells can undergo further rearrangement in the genes, their receptors and their antibody-producing capacity, in the germinal centers of the secondary lymphoid organs. This process is referred to as ***receptor editing***.

When B-lymphocytes meet an antigen presented by the MHC class I molecule, they proliferate to produce a few thousands of cells. Each B-cell is capable of producing only the same type of antibody. The term pre-B-cell denotes the immature B-lymphocyte in which Igs have not appeared on the surface. On exposure to an antigen the clone of specific B-cells proliferates rapidly and produces antibodies promptly. Primary immune response occurs on first encounter with the antigen. During this phase all the three types of cells: (1) Cytotoxic and helper T-cells, (2) B-cells (antibody-secreting plasma cells) and (3) memory T- and B-cells proliferate.

The memory T- and B-cells enable a quantitatively superior immune response on subsequent exposure to the same antigen. The germinal centers of lymph nodes and spleen are discrete areas where B-cell responses occur. Ig class switching of B-cells, production of memory cells and plasma cell precursors occur within the germinal centers. The final stage of differentiation of B-cell into antibody-producing plasma cells occurs outside the germinal centers.

When B-cells undergo terminal differentiation into plasma cells they acquire the ability to produce and secrete large amounts of antibodies. The antibody can be directly protective if it can inhibit the binding of the micro-organisms or its toxin to the target tissue. In most instances, in addition to this effect, the antibodies also recruit other arms of the immune system for defense.

Activation of the complement cascade helps to enhance phagocytic activity of neutrophils. NK-cells, monocytes, macrophages and neutrophils can all function in IgG-mediated antibody-dependent cellular cytotoxicity. Macrophages, eosinophils and platelets are involved in IgE-mediated antibody-dependent cellular cytotoxicity. If the target cell is too large for phagocytosis, the mechanisms employed include perforins (which perforate the cell wall), granzymes which destroy the cell components and reactive oxygen intermediates.

In normal adults, 3–4 g of secretory IgA is produced every day, by plasma cells located under mucosal surfaces. This is transported to mucosal surface. It offers protection against adhesion by microbes on the luminal surface.

In general, plasma cells are short-lived with a half-life of only a few days, but some of them, located within the bone marrow survive for weeks.

T-lymphocytes

Formation of T-cells in the thymus occurs throughout life even when the thymus has involuted. MHC class I molecules are expressed on all nucleated cells in the body. This allows infected cells to signal their plight to cytotoxic CD8 T-cells and establish intimate intercellular contact by presenting the complex of foreign peptides and MHC molecules to the T-cell receptors.

T-cell function and migration

T-cells respond to pathogens when they get contact with pathogen-derived antigens. This is achieved by the T-cell receptors, recognizing the peptide or lipid antigen bound to a MHC or CD1 respectively on the surface of another cell. The dendritic cells, which are derived from monocytes present in skin, epithelial surfaces and subepithelial tissues are the antigen-presenting cells. These cells engulf antigens, break them down to peptides and display them on their surface with the help of MHC complexes, also known as HLA molecules. The site of engagement of the antigen-presenting cell and the T-lymphocyte is called the immunological synapse. The MHC molecules help to transport intracellular antigenic material to the surface of the cell.

The T-cells are capable of detecting antigens occurring in any part of the body promptly. The dendritic cells present in various tissues and secondary lymphoid organs trap antigens produced in their territories. Naive (unstimulated) T-cells reach these lymphoid organs preferentially, being attracted by inflammatory cytokines. This is called homing. Maturing dendritic cells also home to the T-cell areas of lymph nodes. They ready their apparatus for antigen presentation and also secrete cytokines which make them attractive to T-cells which have arrived in the lymph nodes. On meeting the antigen, the T-cells proliferate to produce 1,000 times the number of original activated T-cells. Eventually these activated T-cells 'home' to sites of inflammation. They interact with antigen-bearing tissues, parenchymal cells and leukocytes. For allergic reactions, eosinophils and basophils are recruited. For inflammatory response, neutrophils and macrophages are involved. Most of the effector cells die after the antigen is cleared, but a few antigen experienced T-lymphocytes persists for long-term protection as memory cells.

Clusters of differentiation 4 (CD4) T-cells are mainly cytokine-producing helper cells. CD8 T-cells are mainly cytotoxic killer cells. CD4 T-cells (helper) can be subdivided into two major types based on their cytokines:

1. Type 1 T helper (Th1) T-cell secrete IL-2 and interferon, but not IL-4, IL-5 or IL-6.
2. Type 2 (Th2) T-cells secrete IL-4, IL-5, IL-6 and IL-10, but not IL-2 or interferon-γ.

Type 1 helper T-cells (Th1 cells) facilitates cell-mediated immunity including activation of macrophages and T-cell-mediated cytotoxicity. On the other hand, Th2 cells help B-cells to produce antibodies.

The null cells, which do not possess either T or B markers, are also members of the immune system.

Interaction between T- and B-cells

There is close interaction between T- and B-lymphocytes at several stages of the immune response. Some of the T-cells influence B-cells for humoral responses. Leukocytes engage several sequential-adhesion pathways to leave the circulation and enter tissues. Adhesion is affected with the help of selectins and integrins which are adhesion proteins. Chemokines are produced by activated endothelial cells, epithelial cells, leukocytes and several other types of cells. They direct the migration of leukocytes to the sites of antigens.

Some of the T-cells proceed to eliminate pathogens, whereas others find pathogen-specific B-cells which need the help of T-cells for efficient antibody response.

The killer T-cells CD8 (T-cells) kill virus-infected cells. The viruses are deprived of the cellular enzymes needed for their replication and they are also deprived of their sanctuary within the host cell. Any virus that is released is destroyed by the antibodies.

In addition to direct killing of infected cells, the CD8 T-cells also produce cytokines such as TNF (TNF-α), lymphotoxin (also known as TNF-α), interferon-γ and others. The interferon-γ renders neighboring cells resistant to viral infection. To a minor extent, CD4 cells (both Th1 and Th 2) can become cytotoxic on recognizing peptides presented by MHC class II molecules.

A successful immune response eliminates the inciting antigen, and once rid of the stimulus, the concerned cells go back to their prestimulatory state.

Plasma cell series: Plasma cells form about 2–3% of cells in the bone marrow. Though they are not usually seen in the peripheral blood, they may appear occasionally. Plasma cells accumulate in chronically inflamed tissues. Such plasma cells contain eosinophilic (acidophilic) smooth-hyaline spherical-cytoplasmic bodies called ***Russell bodies***. These bodies are composed mainly of gammaglobulin. Plasma cells constitute the main source of antibodies. They are formed from stem cells in the bone marrow though B-lymphocytes and then migrate to other tissues. Plasma cells synthesizing IgA migrate to GI tissues while cells producing IgG and IgD go to tonsillar tissue.

PLATELETS

Platelets are formed from MKCs. About 10 billion platelets/L of blood are produced everyday in an adult. This can be increased 10-fold in times of need (Figs 158.3 to 158.8).

Myeloid stem cells give rise to megakaryoblast which resemble myeloblast morphologically.

Pro-MKCs develop from them by endoreduplication. This is the process in which nucleus divides without cell division. As the MKCs mature, the capacity for endoreduplication increases. This leads to the formation of large cells resembling multinucleated giant cells containing basophilic cytoplasm and a few basophilic granules.

Mature MKCs are large cells 30–80 μm in diameter and containing 4–16 lobes in the nucleus. The cytoplasm is protruded into the sinusoids of the bone marrow and the platelets are detached and liberated into the circulation. Platelets themselves are nonmotile, but they possess intrinsic contractile activity.

The final product of thrombopoiesis is a platelet which is nonnucleated and is 1–4 μm in diameter. The central

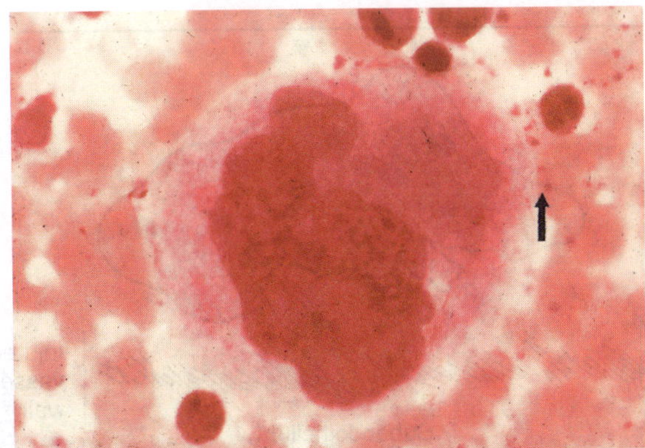

Fig. 158.3: Normal bone marrow × 1,000. **Note:** Platelets escaping from the margins of the megakaryocyte (MKC) (arrow)

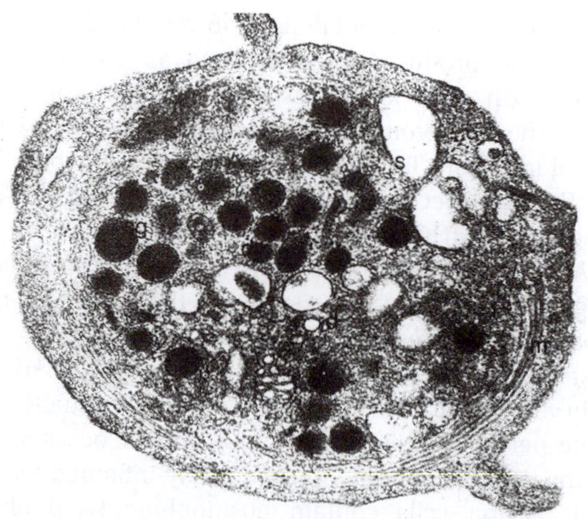

Fig. 158.4: Ultrastructure of the platelet electron microscopy

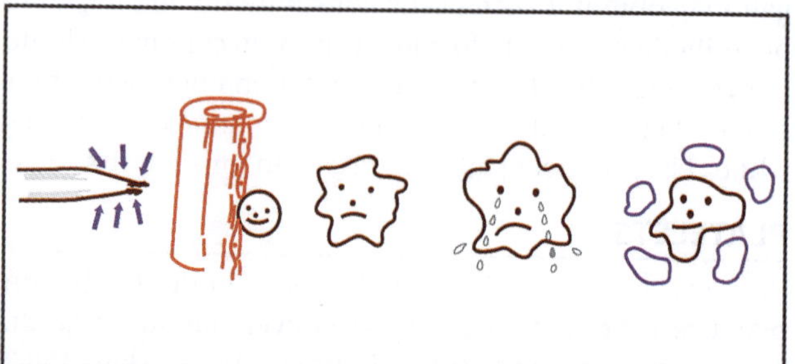

Fig. 158.5: Morphological changes in platelet on vessel injury

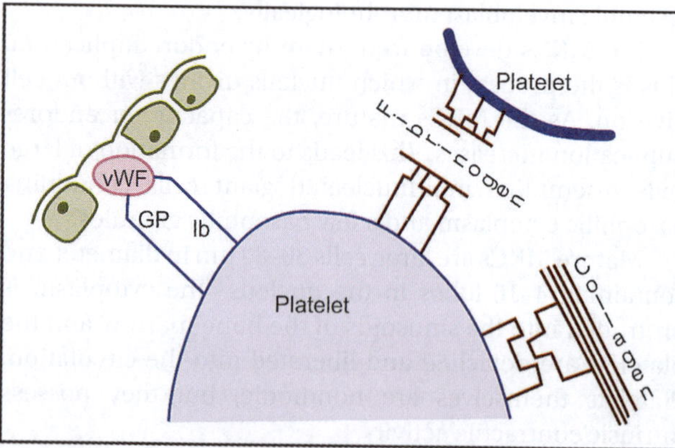

Fig. 158.6: Platelet surface receptors
Abbreviations: vWF = von Willebrand factor, GP = Glycoprotein

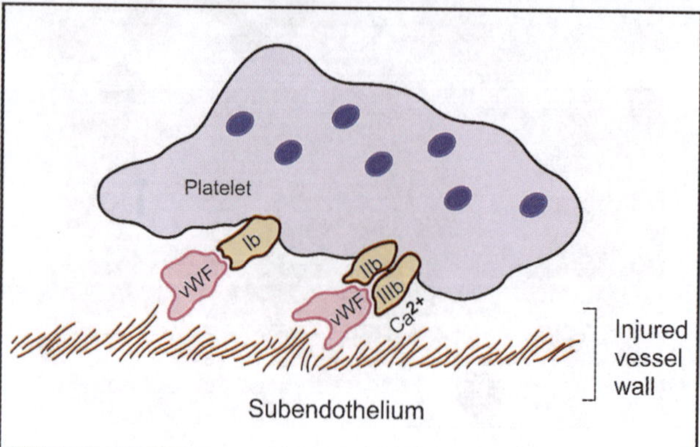

Fig. 158.7: Mechanism of adhesion to vessel wall

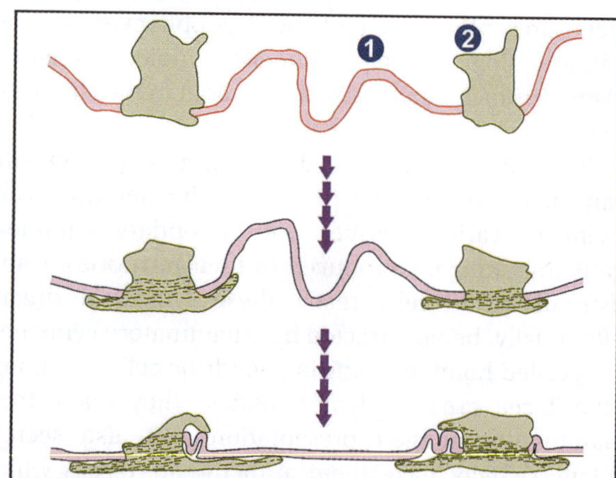

Fig. 158.8: Platelet physiology—action on fibrin to stabilize it; (1) Fibrin threads and (2) Activated platelets

part contains red purple granules and the cytoplasm is light blue. Normal platelet count ranges from 150 to 300,000 cells/mm³ of blood.

Thrombopoiesis occurs under the influence of thrombopoietin (TPO) which controls the proliferation and development of MKCs precursors. TPO is a polypeptide growth factor containing 353 amino acids. Plasma levels of TPO vary inversely with the platelet mass in circulation. It acts as a M-CSF including the proliferation of the committed precursors. It also promotes platelet production and release.

Freshly formed platelets are nonnucleated; they contain ribonucleic acid (RNA) and are able to synthesize small amounts of proteins. Platelet with elevated nucleic acid content can be detected by flow cytometry. These are called reticulated platelets (RPs). The RNA content can be identified by using the fluorescent dye thiazole orange, and platelet surface markers, such as CD41 and CD61. Estimation of the proportion of RPs gives an idea of the rate of platelet production. Normal RP is 7.7%. In conditions such as immune thrombocytopenia, the RP may go up as high as more than 20%.

About 30% of platelets are in the splenic pool. The rest are in circulation. Under normal conditions, in the absence of overt or occult bleeding, the lifespan of platelets is 8–14 days. They are used up in the hemostatic process. Old and effete platelets are destroyed, especially in the spleen.

Thrombopoietin (TPO) is produced mainly from the hepatocytes (50%) and sinusoidal endothelial cells of the liver. Small amounts are produced by the kidneys, brain, testes and skeletal muscles. It is a polypeptide growth factor containing 353 amino acids. TPO is the primary regulator of platelet production. It supports the survival and proliferation of MKC progenitors. *In vitro*, TPO induces the differentiation of progenitor cells into large MKCs each of which produces thousands of platelets. TPO is a potent stimulator of platelet production and it also enhances the aggregating activity of the platelets. Fall in platelet counts leads to rise in TPO levels by 50% or more within 8 hours and reach a peak by 24 hours. Platelets have receptors for TPO and they take up TPO from the circulation. TPO levels are low in immune thrombocytopenic purpura and they are high in aplastic anemia. TPO acts synergistically with EPO to stimulate erythrocyte production.

Thrombopoietin also enhances the survival and expansion of HSCs. It is used to stimulate stem cell production in the bone marrow and peripheral blood.

Hepatic TPO production is enhanced by inflammatory cytokines such as IL-6 and therefore platelet levels increase in infections, inflammations, chronic diseases like rheumatoid arthritis and others.

Thrombopoietin has a half-life of 30 hours in circulation. Pegylation increases the half-life 10-fold. Platelet counts start rising in 3–5 days after administration of TPO and reach a peak in 10 days. TPO is available commercially for therapeutic use as recombinant TPO. Prolonged use of TPO leads to production of antibodies which suppress endogenous TPO, thereby leading to thrombocytopenia. This can be reversed by the use of immunosuppressants.

Therapeutically TPO is indicated in thrombocytopenic states, chemotherapy for malignancy, and to improve the yield of platelets and stem cells for therapy.

Thrombopoietin Stimulating Protein

This is a protein moiety (AMG 531) which has been developed to stimulate thrombopoiesis. It is quite different from TPO. It has been employed to stimulate thrombopoiesis in immune thrombocytopenic purpura. Initial results are encouraging. At present, drugs which stimulate platelet production can be used in thrombopenic states are available, e.g. eltrombopag and romiplostim.

CLINICAL ASPECTS OF HEMATOLOGICAL DISORDERS

Pallor

Pallor of the mucous membranes and skin occurs when the Hb level is below 10 g/dL. Skin color also depends on other factors such as state of peripheral circulation and pigmentation. Mucous membrane over the soft palate is the most suitable area to assess pallor since this is least likely to be influenced by other factors. Though there is general agreement between pallor and the severity of anemia, these show wide disparity in many cases. Some clinician assess pallor from the color of the palms.

Jaundice

Jaundice is an important finding in hemolytic anemia. The severity of jaundice depends on the level of bilirubin in the blood and this corresponds to the severity of hemolysis. In the majority, jaundice is only mild-to-moderate, but deep jaundice may occur in hemolytic crises. In hemolytic jaundice, the serum contains unconjugated bilirubin and the urine is loaded with urobilinogen, but bile pigments are absent. In severe cases, methemalbumin may be present in the serum and urine may contain Hb. In fulminant cases, renal failure may occur.

Hepatosplenomegaly

Many hematological disorders are associated with hepatosplenomegaly. Mild or moderate hepatosplenomegaly occurs in 10–20% of cases of nutritional anemias, 60–80% of acute leukemias, 90% of hemolytic anemias, 80% of infectious mononucleosis and practically never in idiopathic thrombocytopenic purpura. Gross splenomegaly exceeding 15 cm is seen in thalassemias, hemoglobinopathies, chronic granulocytic leukemia, lymphomas and myelofibrosis. The liver also shows variable degrees of enlargement in these cases.

Moderate enlargement of lymph nodes occurs in acute leukemias and infectious mononucleosis. Lymphomas, chronic lymphatic leukemia and blastic transformation of chronic granulocytic leukemia are characterized by gross lymphadenopathy.

Fever

Fever is a common nonspecific accompaniment of many hematological disorders. In anemia, when the Hb level goes below 7 g/dL, fever is common. The temperature reverts to normal on correcting the anemia. Hectic rise of temperature may accompany hemolytic crises. In all forms of leukemia, fever may occur. Often this is due to infection, less commonly it may be due to the malignant process itself. Presence of fever in lymphomas is of diagnostic and prognostic importance.

Bleeding Tendency

Hemorrhagic manifestations may be the primary symptom in disorders like immune thrombocytopenic purpura and hemophilia. In acute leukemia and aplastic anemia, secondary thrombocytopenia may occur resulting in bleeding. Purpuric hemorrhage into the skin, mucous membranes or tissues is commonly seen if the abnormality affects the platelets or blood vessels. In disorders of coagulation, spontaneous bleeding occurs into deep tissues and joints. Bleeding from cuts and wounds tends to be prolonged markedly.

LABORATORY INVESTIGATIONS

- ***Hemoglobin estimation:*** It is now accepted that this procedure should be done with internationally accepted standards by the cyanmethemoglobin method using a photoelectric colorimeter. Other visual methods are only approximate at best.
- ***Cell counts:*** Automated instruments, which give several parameters, are available commercially. Their advantage is reliability of the result and reproducibility, provided the operator is skilled and the machine is kept in good condition and the laboratory is under quality control organizations. As far as possible, manual testing should be avoided.
- ***Reticulocyte count:*** The reticulum in the erythrocyte is the remnant RNA present in the developing erythroblast continuing into the erythrocyte. Increase in reticulocyte above 1.5–2.5% of the total erythrocyte count indicates activated erythropoiesis and release of early erythrocytes into the peripheral circulation. Reticulocyte count is done directly in the wet preparation after staining with brilliant cresyl blue which is a vital stain or by the dry method.
  - ***Corrected reticulocyte count:*** This is also known as absolute reticulocytes percentage. This is a formula which is used to correct the variations of

Table 158.4: Maturation time in relation to hematocrit (HCT) values

HCT values	Maturation time (in days)
40%	1
30–40	1.5
20–30	2
< 20	2.5

reticulocyte count in relation to total erythrocyte count or packed cell volume (PCV).

$$\text{Corrected reticulocyte count} = \frac{\text{Observed reticulocyte count (\%)} \times \text{Patient's PCV}}{\text{Normal PCV for that age and sex}}$$

$$\text{i.e. } \frac{\text{\% of reticulocytes} \times \text{(Patient's PCV)}}{45 \text{ (Normal PCV)}}$$

- **Reticulocyte proliferation index (RPI)** is a measure of erythrocyte regeneration. RPI is obtained by the following formula:

$$\text{Reticulocyte proliferation index (RPI)} = \text{Corrected reticulocyte count} \times \text{Maturation time in peripheral blood (in days)}$$

The maturation time for reticulocytes varies in relation to the hematocrit (HCT) values which are given in Table 158.4.

$$\text{Reticulocyte proliferation index (RPI)} = \frac{\text{Corrected reticulocyte count}}{\text{Shift factor}}$$

Where the shift factor is a constant depending upon the PCV.

- **Absolute reticulocyte count:** It is obtained by using the formula:

$$\text{\% of reticulocyte count} \times \text{RBC (count/mm}^3\text{)}$$

Normal value is 50,000–75,000 cells/mm^3.

- **Estimation of PCV:** Venous hematocrit.
- **The red cell indices:** These are calculated from PCV, Hb and red cell count. They are mean corpuscular hemoglobin concentration (MCHC), mean corpuscular hemoglobin (MCH) and mean corpuscular volume (MCV).

  - **MCHC:** This represents concentration of Hb in the red cell. It is calculated as follows:

$$\text{MCHC (g/dL)} = \frac{\text{Hb (in g/dL)} \times 100}{\text{PCV}}$$

Normal range is 32–36 g/dL.

  - **MCH:** It represents the average weight of Hb in each cell and is calculated as follows:

$$\text{MCH (pg)} = \frac{\text{Hb (in g/dL)} \times 100}{\text{RBC count (in million/mm}^3\text{)}}$$

Normal range is from 27 to 32 pg (picogram).

  - **MCV:** It gives the average volume of red cells and is calculated as follows:

$$\text{MCV (fL)} = \frac{\text{PCV} \times 10}{\text{RBC count (in million/mm}^3\text{)}}$$

Normal value varies from 76 to 94 fL (femtoliters).

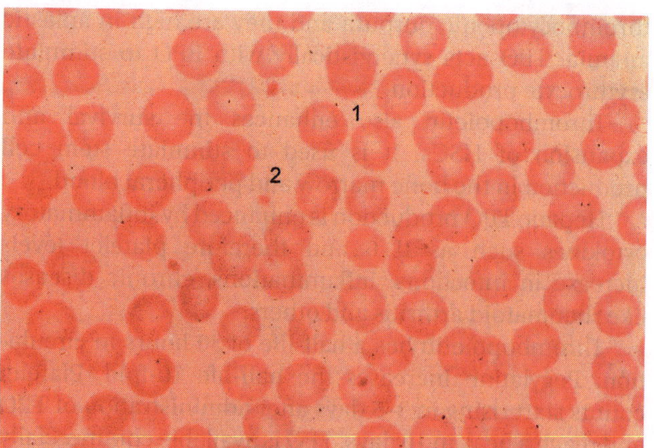

Fig. 158.9: Normal blood film: 1. Red blood cells (RBCs) and 2. Platelets

- **Osmotic fragility of erythrocytes:** It is determined by estimating the hemolysis when a standard volume of erythrocytes is added to increasing dilutions of sodium chloride. Osmotic fragility is increased in spherocytosis and decreased in thalassemia, generally related to the volume of the erythrocyte.
- **Peripheral blood smear:** This is the most useful single investigation which will help in diagnosis (Fig. 158.9). All the cellular elements are examined systematically. Erythrocytes may be small (microcytes), large (macrocytes) or normal in size (normocytes). Variation of size is called anisocytosis. **Poikilocytosis** refers to difference in shape. The cells may be pear-shaped, elliptical or sickle-shaped. **Schistocytes** are fragmented red cells. **Acanthocytes** (spur cells) show numerous spiny projections. Both are seen in hemolytic anemias. Burr cells show short projections on their surface. These are seen in renal failure.
- **Bone marrow examination:** It is an important and integral part of hematological examination. Bone marrow examination is absolutely necessary to establish the diagnosis of leukemias, myeloma, myelofibrosis, hypersplenism, lymphomas, aplastic anemia, megaloblastic anemia and other dyshemopoietic states. It is helpful in the diagnosis of kala-azar, histiocytosis, amyloidosis, secondary carcinomatosis and several other conditions.

Commonly used site for bone marrow aspiration and biopsy is the posterior superior iliac spine or other regions on the iliac crest. With proper techniques, in almost all cases, successful aspiration can be done from this region.

The posterior superior iliac spine overlies actively cellular marrow tissue. The needle used for aspiration is the Cox needle. For trephine biopsy, the Jameshidi needle or Islam's needle is used. Suitable sizes for adult and children are available. It is better that trephine biopsy is done for the proper morphological diagnosis of the marrow which is confirmatory in lymphomas, granulomas, metastases, tumors, myelofibrosis and hypoplastic anemia. A core of marrow tissue 1.5 cm long is taken and processed as tissue for histopathological studies. Imprints, touch smears and smears from blood obtained from the biopsy needle are helpful in the diagnosis of general hematological disorders,

Anemias: General Considerations

Table 158.5: Normal hematological values

Parameters	Category	Normal values
Hemoglobin (Hb)	Infants	16–18 g/dL
	Men	13–16 g/dL
	Women	11–14.5 g/dL
Red cells	Infants	5–6×10^{12}/L
	Men	4–6.6×10^{12}/L
	Women	3.5–4.5×10^{12}/L
PCV	Men	40–54%
	Women	35–47%
MCV		76–94 fL
MCH		27–32 picogram (pg)
MCHC		32–36 g/dL
Reticulocytes		0.2–2.5%
ESR	Males	0–10 mm 1st hour (Westergren)
	Females	0–20 mm 1st hour (Westergren)
White cells	Infants	15–16×10^{9}/L
	Adults	5–10×10^{9}/L
Differential leukocyte count (adults):	Neutrophils	40–75%
	Lymphocytes	20–45%
	Monocytes	2–9%
	Eosinophils	1–5%
	Basophils	0.0–1%
Platelets		150,000–400,000/mm³ (1.5–4×10^{11}/L)
Bleeding time		(Ivy's method) up to 10 min
Coagulation time		(Lee and White method at 37°C) 5–11 min
Prothrombin time		12–14 sec
Plasma fibrinogen		150–400 mg/dL
Serum iron		60–160 µg/dL
TIBC (transferrin)		280–400 µg/dL

Contd...

Contd...

Serum ferritin	Males	40–340 µg/dL
	Females	14–148 µg/dL
Serum folate		6–20 ng/mL
RBC folate		160–640 ng/mL
Serum vitamin B_{12}		100–1,000 pg/mL

Abbreviations: PCV = Packed cell volume; MCV = Mean corpuscular volume; MCH = Mean corpuscular hemoglobin; MCHC = Mean corpuscular hemoglobin concentration; ESR = Erythrocyte sedimentation rate; TIBC = Total iron-binding capacity; RBC = Red blood cell

such as leukemia, anemia and myeloma. Conditions, such as myelofibrosis, myelodysplastic syndromes, hairy cell leukemia, lymphomas, secondaries and marrow necrosis, can be diagnosed only with marrow biopsy. The biopsy material can be used for electron microscopy and immunophenotyping studies. In nonhematological conditions such as typhoid fever and miliary tuberculosis, the success rate of culturing the organisms is higher with bone marrow than blood.

In extreme obesity, the iliac crest may not be easily accessible. Other sites for aspiration are the manubrium sterni and body of the sternum, ribs, vertebral spines and tibial shaft in children. These alternate sites are seldom used now due to higher risks involved and more chances for procedural failure. Failure to get marrow tissue by aspiration is called 'dry tap'. This may be due to:

- Faulty techniques
- Aplasia of marrow or solid marrow as occurs in fibrosis, osteopetrosis or
- Extreme cellular hyperplasia where the marrow assumes the consistency of solid tissue.

Contraindications to bone marrow aspiration include defects of coagulation and sepsis at the site of aspiration. Complications of bone marrow puncture include prolonged bleeding, formation of hematoma and periostitis. Sternal puncture may be complicated by injury to mediastinal structures and mediastinitis. Aortic aneurysm is a contraindication for sternal puncture. Table 158.5 lists the various hematological values.

CHAPTER
159

Anemias: General Considerations

KV Krishna Das

Chapter Summary

- Classification
- Clinical Aspects
- Investigations
- Course and Prognosis
- Management of Anemia

INTRODUCTION

Anemia is defined as a reduction of hemoglobin (Hb) levels below the normal values for the different age and sex groups. The normal values of Hb for different age groups accepted by the World Health Organization (WHO) are as follows:

Children	6 months–6 years	11 g/dL and above
	6–14 years	12 g/dL and above
Adult males		13 g/dL and above
Adult female	(nonpregnant)	12 g/dL and above
Adult female	(pregnant)	11 g/dL and above

In full health, there is no racial variation in Hb. In India, any Hb level below 12 g/dL in adult males and 11.5 g/dL in adult females should be diagnosed as anemia and investigated. In general, reduction of Hb is associated with a fall in erythrocyte count and packed cell volume (PCV). In anemic subjects, hemoconcentration, as occurring in dehydration, tends to mask the severity of anemia, so also when there is increase in plasma volume as in pregnancy there is an apparent fall in Hb level even though the total Hb mass remains normal.

CLASSIFICATION

Based on erythrocyte morphology as seen in the stained blood film, anemias may be classified into microcytic hypochromic, normocytic normochromic, macrocytic normochromic and macrocytic hypochromic (Table 159.1).

CLINICAL ASPECTS

General Features

Irrespective of the etiology or type, anemic subjects develop a group of symptoms on account of reduction in Hb. The severity of symptoms depends on the rapidity of fall of Hb. When anemias develop slowly, the subject adapts to the lower levels of Hb by reducing his physical activity and the symptoms are less pronounced. With falling levels of Hb, the oxygen carrying capacity of blood diminishes. This is partly compensated by increasing the blood flow to organs by vasodilatation. The cardiac output is increased. Most of the general symptoms are attributable to the diminished oxygen carrying capacity of blood and hyperdynamic circulation. These symptoms include fatigue, disinclination to work, mental apathy, pallor, exertional dyspnea, effort angina and cardiac failure in severe cases. Symptoms are referable to all systems. Alimentary symptoms include loss of appetite, constipation and abdominal distension. The liver is enlarged and tender due to fatty change. Cardiovascular changes include tachycardia, cardiomegaly, high volume pulse, prominent third heart sound, ejection systolic murmurs heard over the pulmonary and aortic areas and in advanced cases, signs of cardiac failure. Cardiac murmurs are produced as a result of decreased viscosity of blood and increased cardiac output. Pallor is most marked

Table 159.1: Classification of anemia based on erythrocyte morphology	
Microcytic hypochromic anemia	Iron deficiency, thalassemias, hemoglobinopathies, hemolytic anemia
Normocytic normochromic anemia	Aplastic anemia, anemia of chronic diseases
Macrocytic normochromic anemia	Folate deficiency, vitamin B_{12} deficiency, hypothyroidism
Macrocytic hypochromic anemia (dimorphic)	This picture is due to combined deficiency of iron and folate or B_{12}

Table 159.2: Classification of anemia based on etiopathogenesis	
Dyshemopoietic (disorders of erythrocyte formation)	• Nutritional anemias due to deficiency of essential nutrients such as folate, vitamin B_{12}, proteins, vitamin C • Hypothyroidism • Sideroblastic anemia due to metabolic blocks in the synthesis of hemoglobin
Hemorrhagic	• Acute hemorrhage, e.g. APH and PPH bleeding esophageal varices, bleeding peptic ulcer, hematemesis and melena, traumatic or surgical bleeding • Chronic blood loss, e.g. due to intestinal parasites such as hookworms, whipworms and histolytica hemorrhoids, excessive menstrual blood loss and repeated pregnancies, chronic peptic ulcer, erosions (drug-induced), cancers in the GIT
Hemolytic	Anemias developing because of increased destruction of erythrocytes— various causes
Hypoplastic	Anemias developing because of decreased formation of erythrocytes— various causes
Myelophthisic	Anemias developing as a result of replacement of normal erythropoietic tissue by abnormal tissue, e.g. acute leukemias, lymphomas, multiple myeloma, malignant secondaries in bone marrow, myelofibrosis and storage diseases

Abbreviations: APH = Antepartum hemorrage; PPH = Postpartum hemorrage; GIT = Gastrointestinal tract

over the mucous membranes, skin and nails. There may be graying of hair and premature baldness. Neurological manifestations include apathy, loss of mental alertness, paresthesia over the extremities and brisk tendon reflexes. When severe anemia develops rapidly, signs resembling raised intracranial tension may be rarely encountered. These include headache, papilledema and retinal hemorrhages. All these regress with improvement in the Hb levels.

Several other criteria have also been employed for classification. Etiological classification is given in Table 159.2.

Splenomegaly occurs in many cases and the frequency and extent depends on the type of anemia. Whereas in iron deficiency anemia (IDA), 10% may show mild splenomegaly, in hemolytic anemias it is over 90%.

Diagnosis

Any patient with anemia should be approached with the aim of determining the type, severity and cause of the disorder. Anemia may be the only apparent general feature of several underlying disorders and attempts should be made to detect the etiology. Symptomatic treatment of anemia without identifying the cause should be avoided since in many instances, a serious underlying disorder like gastrointestinal (GI) malignancy or renal failure may be missed at an early stage when effective treatment is possible.

Detailed history should include the onset, course and duration of anemia. Periodic fluctuation in intensity is common in nutritional and hemolytic anemias. In general, they are of longer duration than aplastic and myelophthisic anemias. Nutritional anemias affect several members of the same family or household. Hemolytic anemias such

Table 159.3: Signs suggesting etiology of anemia

Sign	Probable etiology
Angular stomatitis cheilitis, koilonychia	Iron deficiency anemia (IDA)
Glossitis	Iron, vitamin B_{12} and folate deficiency anemia
Neurological changes (neuropathy, dementia, ataxia), Knuckle pigmentation	Vitamin B_{12} deficiency
Jaundice	Hemolytic anemia, megaloblastic anemia—it may be caused by nonhematological conditions (e.g. hepatitis)
Splenomegaly	Malaria, chronic hemolytic anemia, acute infection, leukemia, lymphoma, portal hypertension, megaloblastic anemia, IDA (rare)
Frontal bossing, dental malocclusion, skin ulcers	Chronic hemolytic anemia

as spherocytosis, hemoglobinopathies and red cell enzymopathies reveal characteristic genetic patterns.

Common bleeding foci such as hemorrhoids, menorrhagia, peptic ulcer and esophageal varices should be excluded by interrogation and full physical examination. Rectal and pelvic examinations should be undertaken in all cases. Signs suggesting etiology of anemia have been listed in Table 159.3.

INVESTIGATIONS

Preliminary Investigations

The following investigations are carried out to detect the severity and type of anemia.

Hemoglobinometry and Blood Counts

The standard procedure is the cyanmethemoglobin method using a reliable standard for comparison. When the Hb level is below 12 g/dL, full investigations should be undertaken. Absolute counts of erythrocytes, leukocytes and platelets and calculation of the erythrocyte indices should be done by automatic machines which are accurate.

Packed Cell Volume (PCV)

It (hematocrit) is a reliable parameter which should be done in all cases. The mean corpuscular hemoglobin concentration (MCHC) is calculated by:

$$MCHC = \frac{(Hb \text{ in g/dL} \times 100)}{PCV}$$

It helps to determine the type of anemia in a borderline case and also in the follow-up of the case. Values below 27 g/dL suggest microcytic hypochromic types.

Examination of Blood Smear

This is the easiest and reliable method to determine the morphology of erythrocytes. Microcytic hypochromic erythrocytes are smaller than normal [normal mean corpuscular diameter (MCD) is 7.5 ± 0.3 μm] and the center is empty with only a ring of Hb taking up the stain. Considerable anisocytosis and poikilocytosis are seen. Macrocytic erythrocytes are larger with the center also showing uniform staining. Normocytic normochromic erythrocytes are normal in size and staining. Reticulo-cytes appear as polychromatophilic macrocytes in Romanowsky's stained films, but when stained in the fresh state with brilliant cresyl blue, the cytoplasmic reticulum is visualized. Normal value for reticulocytes in Indian subjects is 0.5–2.5%. Anisocytosis, poikilocytosis, polychromasia and reticulocytosis indicate active regeneration of erythrocytes. When erythropoiesis is very much accelerated, normoblasts may appear in peripheral blood. In myelophthisic anemias, normoblast may be released from the bone marrow even without active regeneration of erythrocytes. The leukocyte picture is often helpful. Neutropenia and relative lymphocytosis may suggest aplastic anemia. Presence of eosinophilia suggests helminthic infestation.

Examination of the platelets will give additional clues regarding the type of anemia and its cause. Normally functioning platelets occur in small- or medium-sized clumps. Absence or considerable reduction in the platelets shows up as scanty platelets in the smear and absence of clumps.

In microcytic hypochromic anemia, presence of excess platelets generally suggests blood loss. Thrombocytopenia indicates the possibility of hypoplastic anemia. In the tropics, special attention should be given to detect malarial parasites in all cases, specially *Plasmodium falciparum*.

Red blood cell distribution width (RDW): With the availability of automated counting machines and recording instruments in hematology, red blood cell (RBC) distribution curves are provided along with the counts. A routine measurement obtained from these curves is the RDW. Depending upon the technology employed in the machine, RDW can be expressed as RDW-SD or RDW-CV. The different technologies employed to count and size the RBCs determine the shape of the RDW distribution curves. These denote the homogeneity or heterogeneity of erythrocyte size, i.e. anisocytosis. Manual determination of anisocytosis by light microscopy is at best only approximate.

The values obtained by RDW-SD and RDW-CV differ. The RDW is a reliable parameter to distinguish between IDA and other microcytic anemias. Values of RDW-CV greater than 17 are suggestive of iron deficiency. In thalassemias and anemia of chronic disease, the RDW-CV is below 17. Increase in RDW is one of the early findings in IDA. In aplastic anemia, leukemia and megaloblastic anemia, the leukocytes also show morphological changes which are diagnostic.

Examination of the Bone Marrow

Examination of bone marrow will reveal the type of erythropoiesis and the underlying cause in secondary anemias. Normoblastic hyperplasia suggests iron deficiency. Megaloblastic hyperplasia should suggest primary or secondary deficiency of folate or vitamin B_{12}. Normoblastic, but hypoplastic erythropoiesis occurs in aplastic anemia, anemia of chronic disease and others. Leukemia, myeloma, disseminated lymphomas, parasitic infections such as visceral leishmaniasis and several other conditions can be diagnosed by marrow examination.

Investigations to Detect Etiology

- Microscopic examination of feces for parasites and chemical examination for occult blood to identify GI blood loss, rectal examination, proctoscopy. Repeated examination of feces may have to be undertaken to detect occult blood since bleeding from the alimentary tract may be intermittent at times. Negative results may exclude bleeding foci in most of the cases, though not in all.

- Skiagram of the chest to detect tuberculosis.
- *Investigations for gastric lesions*—barium meal, endoscopy and biopsy.
- Studies for detecting malabsorption states.
- *Investigation of the large intestine*—barium enema, endoscopy and biopsy.
- *Blood chemistry*—blood urea, serum proteins, serum creatinine, levels of nutrients in blood.
- *Skeletal survey*—multiple myeloma, secondary deposits, thalassemias and myelosclerosis produce characteristic skeletal changes. Skiagram of the skull, vertebrae, long bones and hands are taken for this purpose.
- *Isotope studies*
  - Schilling's test for determining the absorption of vitamin B_{12}.
  - Determination of life span of red cells using ^{51}Cr labeled erythrocytes.
  - Determination of ferrokinetics (absorption, utilization and disposal of iron) using ^{59}Fe.
  - Whole body scanning for bone marrow activity and presence of secondaries or tumors.
- *Other imaging procedures*—ultrasonography (USG), computed tomography (CT) scanning and magnetic resonance imaging (MRI) may be needed in cases where organomegaly, lymph node enlargement, collection of fluid in natural cavities or neoplasms are suspected.

COURSE AND PROGNOSIS

This largely depends upon the type of anemia. Nutritional anemias are generally very insidious in onset and course. Periodic exacerbation results from intercurrent infection or physiological stresses like puberty, growth, or pregnancy. The disease progresses over several years and death is due to intercurrent illnesses or rarely severe anemia per se.

Hemolytic anemias exhibit wide variability in their course, ranging from fulminant hemolysis ending fatally within weeks to very slow chronic course with periodic exacerbations, extending over several years. Aplastic anemias have an intermediate course. The onset is within months and course extends over months to a few years with either recovery or death within a few months in the majority of cases if left untreated. In myelophthisic anemia, the course and outcome depend entirely on the primary disorders.

MANAGEMENT OF ANEMIA

The specific management depends on the etiology.

General principles: Hospitalization is advisable when the Hb drops below 7 g/dL. With Hb levels below 3 g/dL, severe disability occurs and cardiac failure at this stage may be fatal. In such a case, emergency transfusion with packed erythrocytes to raise the Hb above 5 g/dL is life-saving. When cardiac failure is present, intramuscular

(IM) administration of furosemide 40 mg prior to the transfusion serves to prevent fluid overloading. Specific treatment depends upon the cause and the severity. The duration of treatment also varies depending upon the type. Details are given in the respective Chapters.

Peripheral Blood Slides (Figs 159.1 to 159.14)

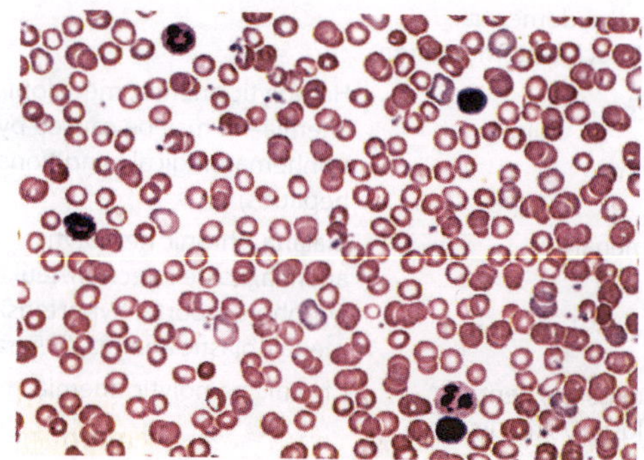

Fig. 159.1: Peripheral blood iron deficiency anemia

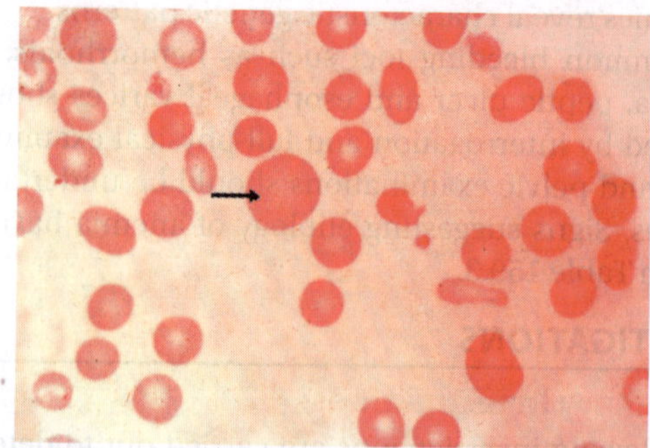

Fig. 159.2: Peripheral blood megaloblastic anemia. *Note:* Macrocyte (arrow)

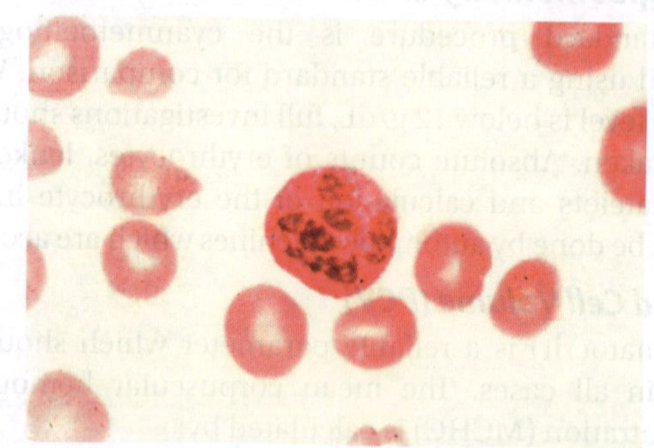

Fig. 159.3: Peripheral blood megaloblastic anemia with hypersegmented neutrophil

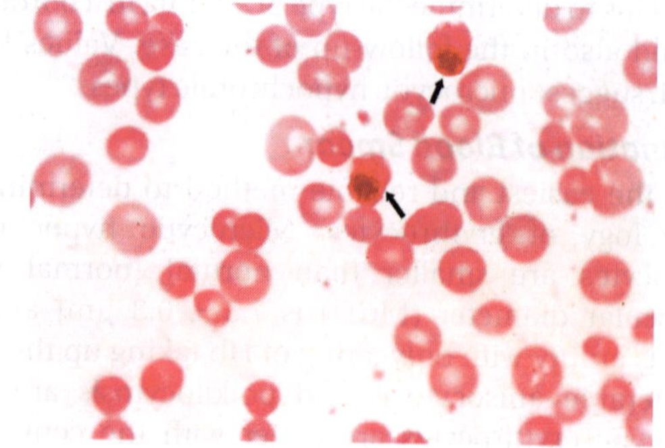

Fig. 159.4: Peripheral blood hemolytic anemia with hemolytic crisis. *Note:* Normoblasts (arrows)

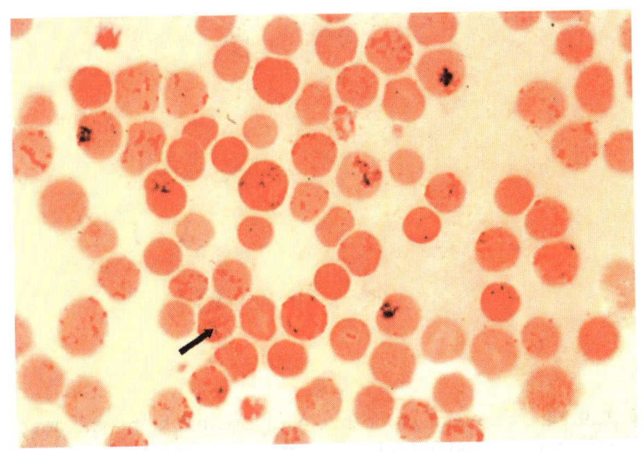

Fig. 159.5: Peripheral blood reticulocytes in hemolytic anemia (arrow)

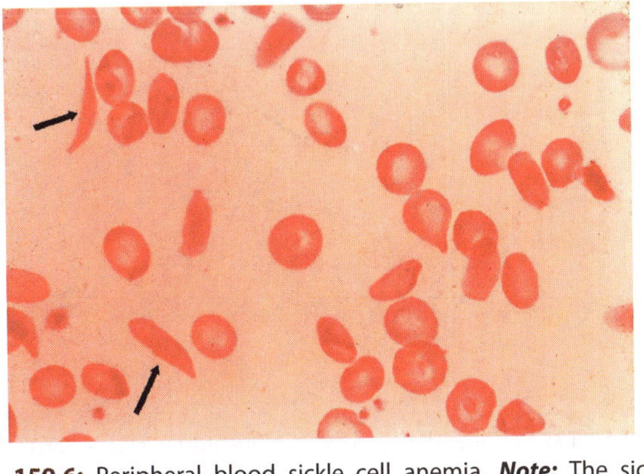

Fig. 159.6: Peripheral blood sickle cell anemia. ***Note:*** The sickle-shaped erythrocytes (arrows)

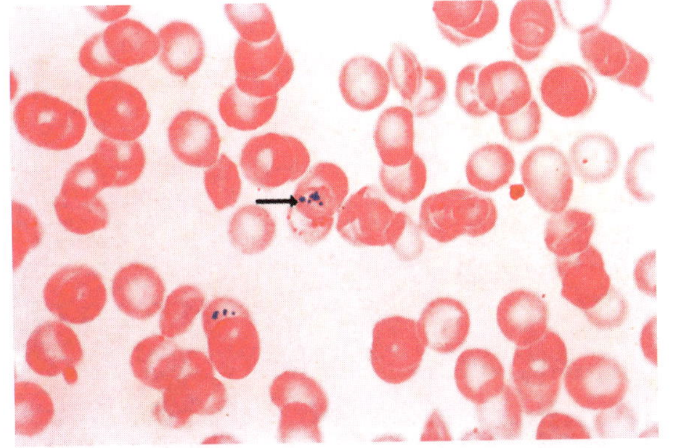

Fig. 159.7: Peripheral blood sideroblastic anemia. ***Note:*** Sideroblast (arrow)

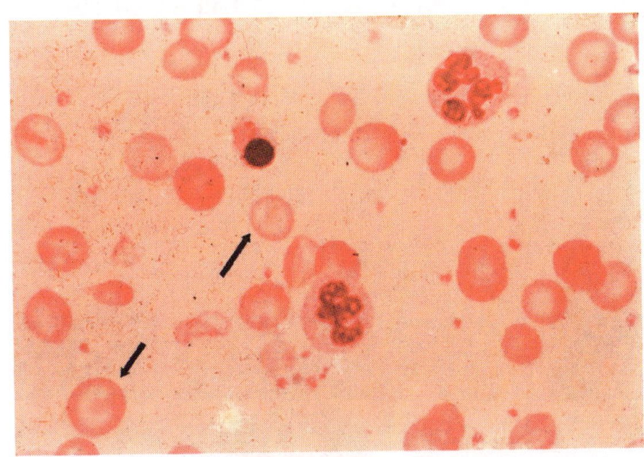

Fig. 159.8: Peripheral blood thalassemia major. ***Note:*** Microcytosis-anisopoikilocytosis, target cells (arrows)

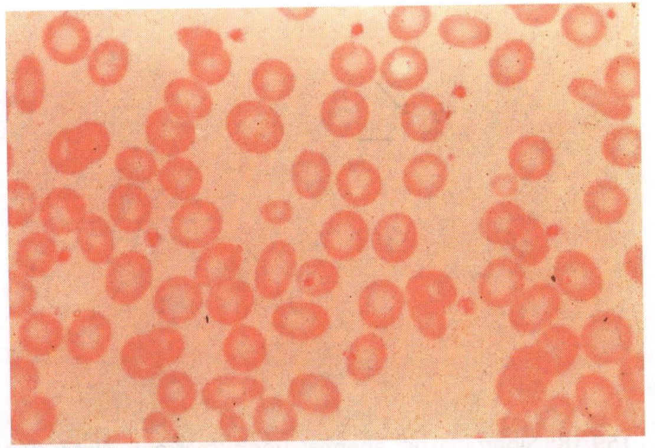

Fig. 159.9: Peripheral blood thalassemia minor. ***Note:*** Mild hypochromia

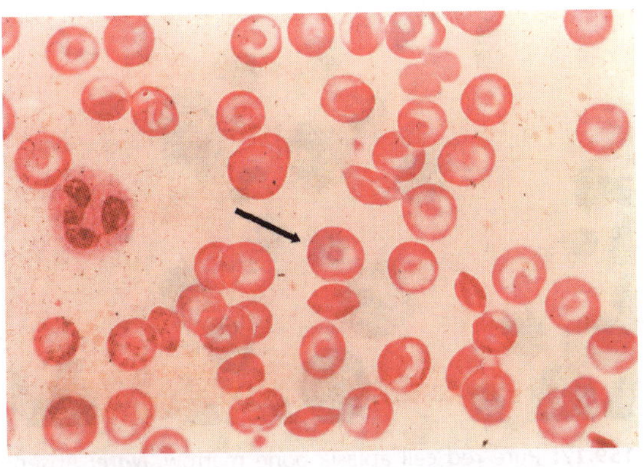

Fig. 159.10: Peripheral blood target cells in thalassemia (arrow)

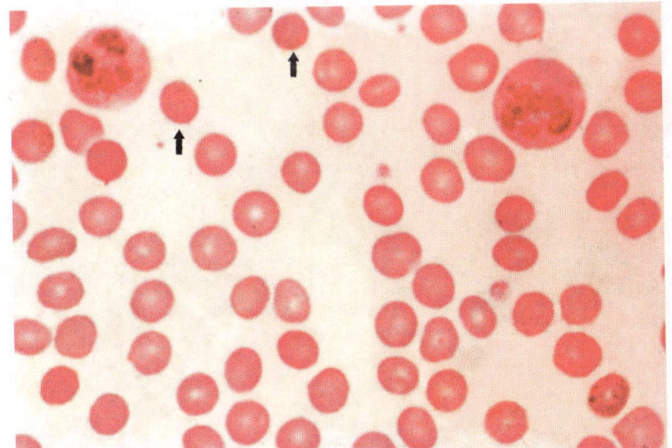

Fig. 159.11: Peripheral blood spherocytes in hereditary spherocytosis—spherocyte is a smaller dark erythrocyte biconvex (arrows)

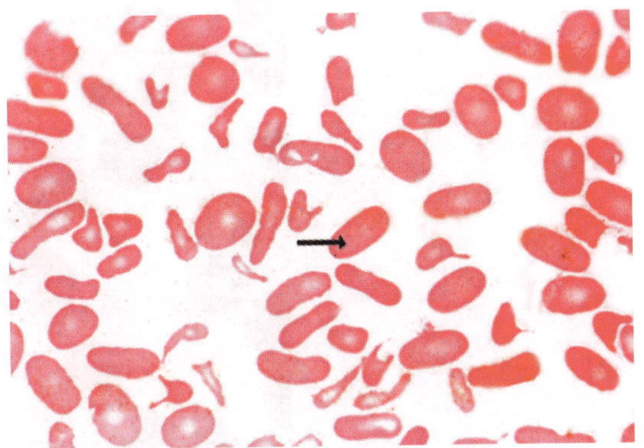

Fig. 159.12: Peripheral blood ovalocytes. ***Note:*** The elongated oval erythrocytes (arrow)

Anemias: General Considerations

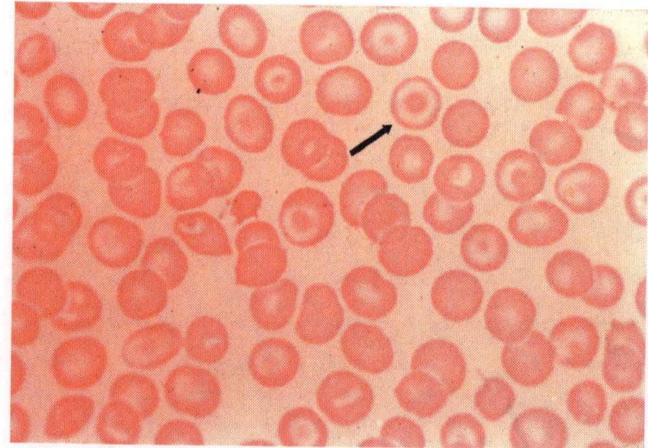

Fig. 159.13: Peripheral blood postsplenectomy states target cell (arrow)

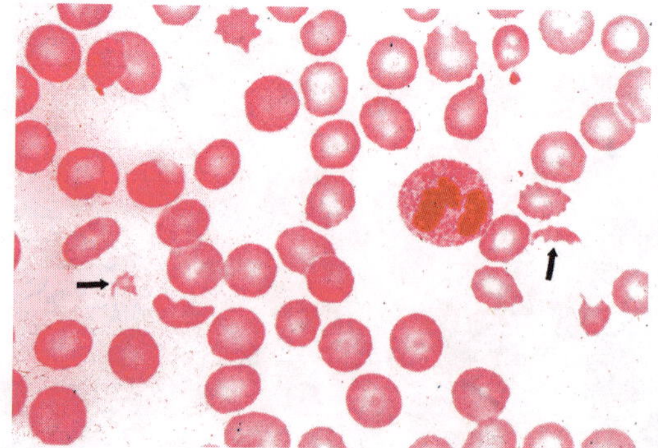

Fig. 159.14: Peripheral blood microangiopathic hemolytic anemia. **Note:** The fragmented red cell—schistocyte (arrows)

Bone Marrow (BM) Slides (Figs 159.15 to 159.19)

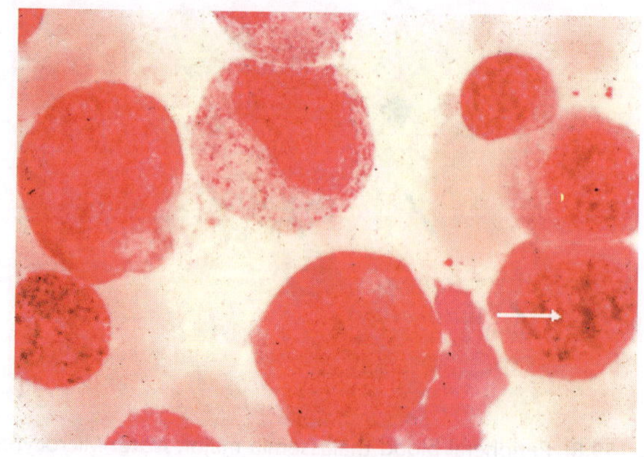

Fig. 159.15: Megaloblastic bone marrow—megaloblast (arrow)

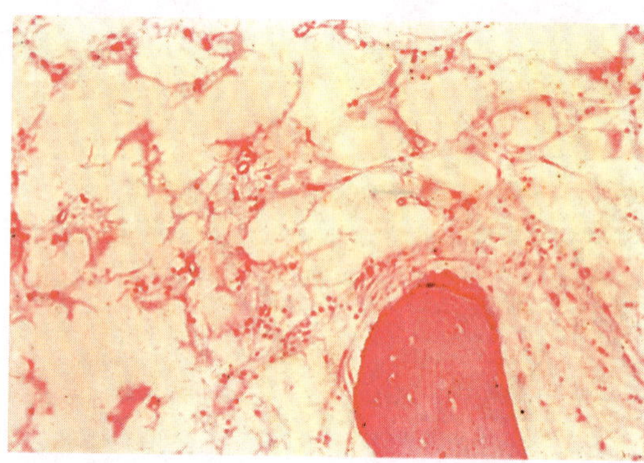

Fig. 159.16: Aplastic anemia bone marrow. **Note:** The reduction in cellularity of the marrow

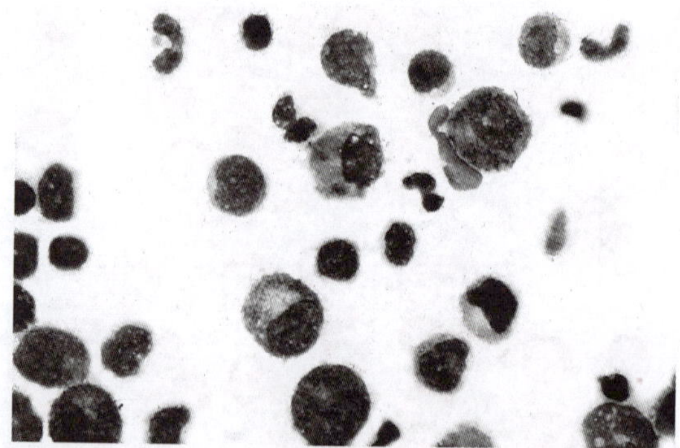

Fig. 159.17: Pure red cell aplasia bone marrow. **Note:** Absence of erythroid precursors, other elements being present

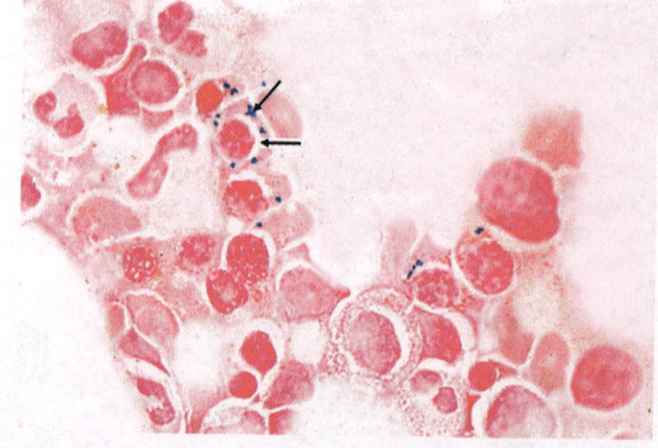

Fig. 159.18: Sideroblastic anemia bone marrow. **Note:** Ringed sideroblast stained by Prussian blue method (arrows)

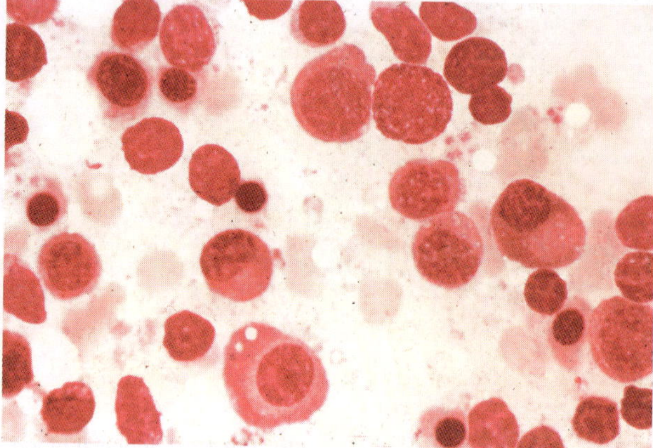

Fig. 159.19: Agranulocytosis bone marrow. **Note:** The reduction in granulocyte precursor

CHAPTER 160

Nutritional and Other Anemias

KV Krishna Das

Chapter Summary

- Iron Deficiency Anemia (IDA)
- Symptomatic Iron Deficiency Anemia
- Macrocytic Anemias
- Addisonian Pernicious Anemia
- Congenital Megaloblastic Anemias
- Rarer Causes of Nutritional Anemia
- Anemia in Systemic Diseases
- Anemia of Chronic Diseases

IRON DEFICIENCY ANEMIA (IDA)

Microcytic hypochromic anemia occurring in India is mostly due to iron deficiency. Less commonly, thalassemias and other hemoglobinopathies also produce similar morphology. In India and other developing countries, IDA far outnumbers all the other types of anemias put together, as it constitutes 90–95% of the total. IDA is one of the most widespread diseases all over the world.

Epidemiology

In India, 5–6% of general population suffers from this disease. It is prevalent in 3% among men and 10–14% among women. About 10% of attendance in the general hospitals is accounted by anemias. In specific groups like slum dwellers, plantation laborers and pregnant women, the prevalence rate is 30–50% or even more. Iron deficiency is prevalent in 30–50% of the adolescent and young adult women due to their unsatisfactory food habits and moderate or heavy blood loss during menstruation. Even though iron deficiency is mainly caused by inadequate iron intake in food, IDA is not exclusively a disease of the poor. Food faddism and other diseases which cause blood loss account for the majority of anemia cases occurring in the rich.

Data from 107 countries reveal that global mean hemoglobin (Hb) improved slightly between 1995 and 2011 as follows 125–126 g/L in nonpregnant women, 112–114 g/L in pregnant women and from 109 to 111 g/L in children. Anemia prevalence varied from 23–29% in nonpregnant women, from 43–38% in pregnant women and from 47–43% in children. The mean Hb levels were lowest and prevalence figures were highest in South Asia and Central and West Africa.

Source: Stevens GA, Finucane MM, Luz Maria De-Regil, et al. Global, regional, and national trends in haemoglobin concentration and prevalence of total and severe anaemia in children and pregnant and non-pregnant women for 1995–2011: a systematic analysis of population-representative data. The Lancet. Global Health. 2003;1(1). Available from http://www.thelancet.com/journals/langlo/article/PIIS2214-109X(13)70001-9/fulltext.

Causes (*See* also Section 5, Ch 32)

- ***Nutritional inadequacy:*** It is present in more than 80% of cases, specially in the poorer groups. Meat, poultry and fish form good dietary sources of heme iron. Milk is low in its iron content. Among vegetable sources, grapes, dates, prunes, amla (gooseberry), green leafy vegetables, onions, jaggery and betel leaf are moderate sources of iron. Due to the cereal-based dietary habits, the optimum intake of dietary iron recommended by Indian Council of Medical Research (ICMR) is 20 mg for adults. Many diets do not contain the optimum amount of bioavailable iron. Cooking in cast iron vessels and iron from water sources supplement iron intake to some extent. Replacement of cast iron kitchen vessels from many households has probably deprived this source of iron, though it may be small. There is a direct correlation between the quality of food ingested and the available iron in it (6 mg/1,000 cal). Amount of dietary iron required for replacing normal loss from the body amounts to ±10 mg in men and ±15 mg in women with normal menstrual periods. Absorption of iron in the normal state is up to 20% from dietary heme iron (of animal source) and only up to 10% dietary nonheme iron in foods from vegetable sources. During pregnancy, daily iron requirement rises to 5–6 mg in the second and third trimesters. If this supply is not met, the women is bound to get her iron stores depleted. This deficiency persists into later life unless precautions are taken to replace this increased loss.

- ***Blood losses:*** Sources of chronic blood loss are ancylostomiasis, hemorrhoids, menstrual losses, repeated pregnancies in women and ulcerating lesions in the gastrointestinal tract (GIT). Normal menstrual blood loss is about 60 mL per period. Periods which are heavy and which occur more frequently than once a month predispose to iron deficiency. About 750 mg of iron is utilized from the mother for each pregnancy and lactation. Successive pregnancies occurring at short intervals without supplementation of iron during pregnancy and lactation are bound to deplete the iron stores of the mother.

Hookworms and other soil-transmitted helminths lead to chronic blood loss from the upper intestinal region. Though most of this iron is absorbed, a small part is lost in feces. Hence, heavy infestations are bound to cause anemia. *Ancylostoma duodenale* is more pathogenic than *Necator Americanus.* If nutritional status is good, anemia may not occur even with moderate worm loads, but in majority of cases, hookworms act as the most common aggravating factor in the presence of undernutrition. In many states of India, hookworm infestation rates have come down considerably due to general improvement in sanitation, provision of sanitary latrines and safe drinking water. In some areas, *Trichuris trichiura* (whipworm) which has established as a common intestinal nematode, causes blood loss and even malabsorption states. Bleeding caused by whipworms is considerably less than that due to hookworms (*See* Ch 67). In most parts of Kerala, the prevalence of soil-transmitted helminths—roundworm, hookworms, whipworms and strongyloides—has come down considerably, but it may still be prevalent in tribal areas and among nomadic tribes.

Loss of iron from surface epithelium increases with excessive sweating. This is a significant source of iron loss in the tropics, specially in the working classes.

Iron absorption is controlled at the level of the intestinal mucosal epithelium. Excess of dietary or medicinal iron is not absorbed normally, but in the presence of iron deficiency, higher amounts of iron are absorbed till the deficiency is corrected. When loss of iron from the body exceeds absorption, the tissue stores gradually become depleted. This phase is asymptomatic and when anemia develops, there is considerable depletion of iron stores. So also when iron is supplied, the anemia recovers first but it requires prolonged supplementation to replenish the tissue stores, usually up to 1 year and often, continuously. Bone marrow shows normoblast hyperplasia (Fig. 160.1).

In IDA, the transferrin saturation is lowered and is often below 15%. Iron is present in plasma also as ferritin. The serum levels of ferritin reflect the iron stores of the individual more reliably than either serum iron or transferrin saturation.

Normal levels of serum ferritin	
Adult male	40–340 µg/L
Adult female	14–148 µg/L
Children	7–142 µg/L

In iron deficiency states, it is below 12 µg/L. Very high levels are reached in siderosis. Normally, there is stainable iron in the marrow. When there is iron deficiency, this form of storage iron disappears. Absence of stainable iron in the bone marrow is a reliable evidence of iron deficiency state which helps to distinguish IDA from hemolytic and hypoplastic anemias in which there is increase in stainable iron. Gross iron deficiency leads to depletion of the iron containing enzymes in tissues and

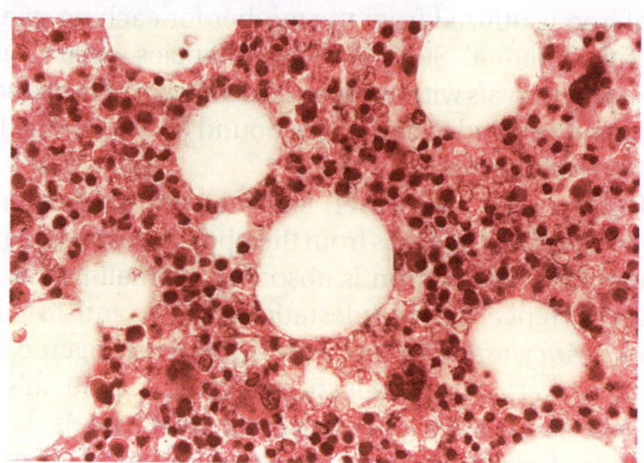

Fig. 160.1: Normoblastic bone marrow. *Note:* All elements are present

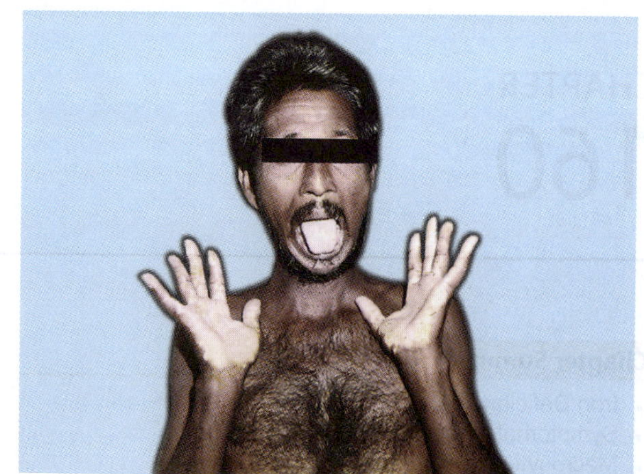

Fig. 160.2: Male iron deficiency anemia. *Note pallor:* Small pale tongue

this probably accounts for the generalized tissue effects. These are promptly restored by iron therapy even before the Hb level improves. As the Hb levels fall below 3 g/dL, compensatory mechanisms fail and death is usually due to cardiac failure or infection of the respiratory or GIT.

Clinical Features

In addition to the general features of anemia described earlier, special features particular to IDA are described below.

- Onset is gradual over months or years. Special features include loss of appetite; pica, especially for eating sand, raw cereal or lime ($CaCO_3$), glossitis, sideropenic dysphagia and koilonychia. About 10% of cases may show mild splenomegaly. Extreme pica may itself lead to further nutritional deficiency (Fig. 160.2).
- The tongue is pale and small. Dysphagia takes the form of a feeling of obstruction and food sticking at the upper end of the esophagus specially on swallowing liquids. It is called ***Plummer-Vinson syndrome (PVS)*** or ***Paterson-Kelly syndrome***. Probably dysphagia is produced by loss of afferent impulses for the swallowing reflex due to degeneration of the lining epithelial cells. Sometimes constriction, spasm, or even bands may be detected, but in general, local examination is unrewarding. In one-third cases, barium swallow may reveal the narrowed area. Clinical features and the radiological abnormalities clear up easily within months of iron therapy, but in a few neurotic individuals vague symptoms may persist. There is increased incidence of postcricoid and oropharyngeal carcinoma in these subjects, specially in women.
- ***Nail changes*** are characteristic of IDA of long-standing and in many cases these are diagnostic. The initial changes are thinning, cracking and brittleness of the toe and finger nails, later becoming typically spoon-shaped ***(koilonychia)***. With correction of iron deficiency, normal nail grows and replaces the affected nail.
- ***Alimentary system:*** Gastric acid is reduced, but histamine fast achlorhydria is rare. Motility of the alimentary tract is reduced and this results in constipation. Gastric secretion and GI motility recover with treatment.

Diagnosis

Clinical Diagnosis

Clinical diagnosis of IDA is simple. In areas where thalassemia and other hemoglobinopathies occur, these have to be differentiated. Though iron deficiency is by far the most important etiological factor, latent deficiency of folate (20–40%) and/or vitamin B_{12} (5–10%) may occur simultaneously. These become manifest as megaloblastosis, when the iron deficiency is corrected by treatment. In such cases, iron therapy produces initial rise in Hb, but full correction can be achieved only with supplementation of folate and/or vitamin B_{12}.

Laboratory Diagnosis

The erythrocytes are microcytic hypochromic (Table 160.1). Presence of eosinophilia usually points to a helminthic etiology and thrombocytosis to chronic or acute blood loss. IDA itself can lead to mild thrombocytosis but more severe levels are generally due to blood loss. Reticulocytes are mildly increased (2–3%) even before specific treatment is started, but when therapy is started, their count rises to 15–30% within days and remains elevated at lower levels till anemia is corrected. In severe iron deficiency, erythropoiesis may be suppressed and reticulocytes may be scanty. The mean corpuscular hemoglobin concentration (MCHC) is below 27 g/dL. Red cell distribution width (RDW) is above 17. Bone marrow shows normoblastic hyperplasia with absence of stainable iron. It is not feasible, nor is it necessary to do bone marrow examination in all cases of IDA. The serum iron is usually below 80 µg/dL (normal 60–160 µg/dL). Transferrin levels are normal (280–400 µg/dL) or increased. Transferrin saturation is about 14–15% or less. Estimation of serum ferritin is helpful to assess the iron stores in the body and therefore, wherever facilities permit, this should be done. Values below 15 µg/L suggest depletion of stores. Based on the several metabolic steps undergone by dietary and transport iron, specific sophisticated tests are available. These help to distinguish anemia due to iron deficiency from anemia of chronic disease, thalassemias and others. These tests may be required only in exceptional circumstances.

Free erythrocyte protoporphyrin (FEP): Elevation of FEP, mainly the erythrocyte zinc protoporphyrin (EZP) is a very sensitive index of iron deficiency. In uncomplicated IDA, EZP levels reach 100–1,000 µg/dL.

Soluble transferrin receptor (STfR): Serum levels of STfR are elevated in iron deficiency. The assay is done by enzyme linked immunosorbent assay (ELISA)—normal serum levels of STfR range from 2.8 to 8.5 mg/L.

For all practical purposes, the beneficial response of oral iron in correcting microcytic hypochromic anemia may be taken as a suggestive evidence of iron deficiency, retrospectively. Search for the cause of iron deficiency should be continued and this should be corrected to prevent relapse.

Complications

- Infections are more common in IDA, specially those of the respiratory, GI or urinary tracts. These are associated with higher mortality. Tuberculosis is more common in them. Cell-mediated immunity is reduced in these subjects.
- Chronic anemia reduces the efficiency in work and study and therefore, widespread nature of this disease in the community impairs efficiency for work and productivity. Deficiency of tissue iron and presence of anemia have been shown to lead to impairment of cognitive function of the brain and retardation of learning ability and motor skills in children. This may persist for long periods even after correction of the anemia. Reversible diminution of functional reserve of heart, muscles and other organs has been demonstrated.

Symptomatic Iron Deficiency Anemia

Even though IDA is caused by nutritional inadequacy and GI blood loss due to intestinal parasitism in the vast majority of patients, in a small proportion it may be the warning symptom of carcinomas, specially of the GIT—stomach, colon and other sites. Slowly proceeding blood loss as occurring in menorrhagia, hereditary hemorrhagic telangiectasia, angiodysplasia of the GIT, hemoptysis due to bleeding into the respiratory tract as in Goodpasture's syndrome and chronic purpura should be looked for, if an obvious nutritional cause is not forthcoming.

Treatment of IDA

This can be considered under two heads: (1) Correction of anemic state and replenishment of iron stores and (2) elimination of the cause.

Table 160.1: Various differentiating features of hypochromic microcytic anemias

Features	Iron deficiency anemia	Thalassemia trait	Anemia of chronic disease	Sideroblastic anemia
MCV	Reduced	Very low for degree of anemia	Low normal or normal	Low in inherited type but often raised in acquired type
Serum iron (normal 60–170 µg/dL)	Reduced (<30 µg/dL)	Normal to high	Reduced (<50 µg/dL)	Raised
Serum TIBC (normal 300–350 µg/dL)	Raised (>350 µg/dL)	Normal	Reduced (<300 µg/dL)	Normal
Serum ferritin (normal 15–300 µg/dL)	Reduced (<15 µg/dL)	Normal (50–300 µg/dL)	Normal or raised (30–200 µg/L)	Raised
Serum soluble transferrin receptors	Increased	Normal or raised	Normal	Normal or raised
Iron in marrow	Absent	Present	Present	Present
Iron in erythroblasts	Absent	Present	Absent or reduced	Ring forms
Hemoglobin A_2 (normal <3%)	Reduced	Increased	Normal	Reduced

Abbreviations: MCV = Mean corpuscular volume; TIBC = Total iron binding capacity

Correction of Anemia

Overall correction of nutrition with articles rich in iron is most important. For the poorer sections of society, proper dietary advice, including indigenously available sources of food, is most important. Meat, liver, green vegetables, onions, grapes and jaggery are good sources of iron.

Iron deficiency is corrected by administration of *medicinal iron*. Ferrous sulfate given as 300 mg tablets thrice daily after food is ideal and least expensive. The response is evident within a week as improved well-being and activity, return of appetite and increase in reticulocytes and Hb. On an average, the Hb rises at a rate of 1% every day. Ferrous sulfate is well-tolerated in most cases but 10% of cases may show side effects such as nausea, vomiting, abdominal pain, metallic taste in the mouth, staining of the tongue (Fig. 160.3), diarrhea and constipation. Side effects are reduced if the drug is administered after food, but absorption is better if given on empty stomach. Rarely oral iron may not be tolerated.

Other preparations are available for administration to those who show intolerance to ferrous sulfate (Table 160.2).

The gastric delivery system (GDS) technology consists of controlled release of drug which is incorporated into a matrix with inert materials which form the outer capsule. In contact with gastric juice, the outer capsule becomes semipermeable. It releases the drug slowly. The capsule floats over the gastric contents and remains for several hours in the stomach. GDS ensures good absorption of the drug with less side effects. These pharmaceutical manipulations may be marginally more beneficial in practice.

Chelated iron is available as iron choline citrate. None of the iron preparations is totally free from side effects. Iron salts have to be continued for at least 6 months after

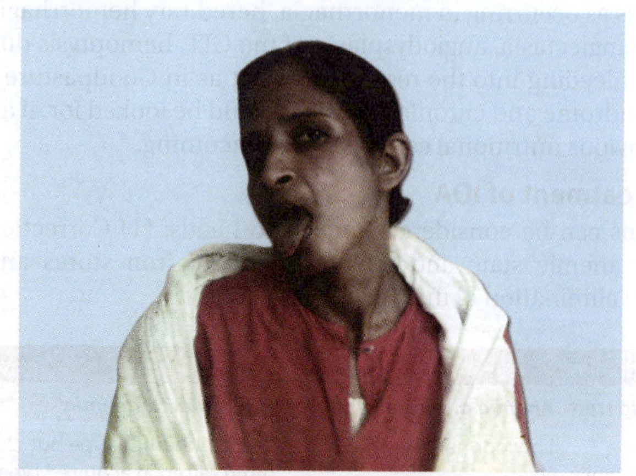

Fig. 160.3: Female staining of tongue by oral iron therapy

the Hb level reaches normal with a view to replete the iron stores. In multiple deficiency, the other nutrients also have to be supplemented.

Parenteral iron is indicated when oral medication becomes impossible because of side effects or when the anemia has to be corrected within a shorter period. Parenteral iron raises Hb by 2% everyday. The preparations are iron dextran complex, iron sorbitol complex, ferric gluconate and iron-sucrose complex. All preparations are effective, but iron dextran complex is more popular. The total dose required for correcting the iron deficiency is calculated using a specific formula and this total dose is given intravenously (IV) slowly or given by repeated intramuscular (IM) injections over a few weeks.

> **Formula for calculating total iron requirement:**
>
> Total dose of iron required in mg =
> (weight of patient in kg) × (deficiency in Hb%) × (0.66)

IM injection: Iron dextran complex is given in doses of 100 mg of elemental iron given in areas usually covered by clothing, once in 3 days till the total dose is reached. Thereafter only nutritional therapy is continued along with oral supplementation. Hb reaches normal levels in course of time when the administered iron is used up.

When a large dose is decided to be administered within a shorter period to save the pressure on hospital beds and avoid frequent injections, IV route is adopted. The *total dose infusion (TDI)* is given as a slow drip in which 500–1,000 mg of iron dextran complex is diluted in 5% glucose after testing for hypersensitivity with the pilot ampoule supplied by the manufacturers. The whole requirement can be administered in 2 or 3 sessions. In general, only mild side effects occur, but rarely, they may be catastrophic.

Side effects of parenteral iron include fatal anaphylactic reactions, iron encephalopathy, local thrombophlebitis, tissue necrosis, pyrexia, arthralgia, arthritis, serum sickness like reactions and pigmentation over injection sites. Anaphylaxis is more frequent with TDIs and more so if oral iron is concurrently administered. It is advisable therefore, to stop oral iron therapy for a week before parenteral iron is administered. Administration of excessive doses of parenteral iron leads to hemosiderosis.

Iron sorbitol citrate (Jectofer): Each mL contains 50 mg of elemental iron. Thirty percent of the injected drug is excreted in urine within 24 hours. This loss has also to be taken into consideration while calculating the total dose. The total dose of Jectofer is given as 10–20 deep IM injections.

Ferric gluconate (Globac, Efficient): It is safer than iron dextran complex and iron sorbitol complex. Two strengths are available 62.5 mg/mL and 125 mg/mL. It is given in split doses as IV infusions, the total dose being determined beforehand.

Iron sucrose (Encifer): This is a complex of polynuclear iron (111) hydroxide in sucrose. It is available as 5 mL vials, each mL containing 20 mg of elemental iron.

It can be given as slow IV injection over 5 minutes or as an infusion mixed with 100 mL normal saline and given over 15 minutes. TDI should not be undertaken.

Table 160.2: Iron preparations

Iron preparations	Weight per tablet (mg)	Elemental iron (mg)	% of elemental iron
Ferrous sulfate	300	80	20
Ferrous gluconate	300	40	12
Ferrous fumarate	200	60	33
Ferrous succinate	150	35	23

Compared to iron dextran complex injections, the newer preparations are safer and the utilization time may also be shorter.

Ferric carboxymaltose 500 mg in 10 mL solution (Orofer FCM injection): 10–20 mL can be given diluted in normal saline, given over 15–30 minutes IV.

Rarely, a case of anemia with Hb level below 3 g/dL may require packed cell transfusion and management for cardiac failure.

Prophylaxis

Iron has to be given prophylactically to vulnerable groups which are likely to develop iron deficiency. These include:

- Premature infants and infants fed solely on unfortified milk formulas
- Pregnant and lactating women
- Patients who had surgical operations on the stomach.

Measures to Eradicate IDA in the Community

Several attempts have been made in India to eradicate IDA from large sections of the population. Improvement in nutrition, elimination of helminthic parasites, provision of protected water and sanitary latrines and prompt treatment of respiratory and GI infections should all be taken up as a comprehensive program to eliminate anemia at the community level. Several studies have shown that isolated programs of deworming or nutritional supplementation are of only marginal and temporary benefit. Attempts have been made to fortify cooking salt with iron.

The problem is to incorporate a stable, at the same time absorbable form of iron in the salt without altering its cooking properties. Iron pyrophosphate has been identified as a suitable salt for this purpose. Wheat flour with iron salt and folic acid is available in more than 70 countries. Field trials have being undertaken by the ICMR and the findings are encouraging.

In many centers in India, tablets containing iron and folic acid are distributed among vulnerable groups specially pregnant women and adolescents and this measure has also proved successful in improving Hb levels.

MACROCYTIC ANEMIAS

These constitute about 5% of nutritional anemias seen in India. In these, the red cells are larger in size. The mean corpuscular volume (MCV) reaches above 110 fL or more. These cells are usually fully hemoglobinized and MCHC is normal. Mean corpuscular Hb is increased. In some cases, the macrocytes may also be hypochromic due to concomitant deficiency of iron (dimorphic). Megaloblastosis results when deoxyribonucleic acid (DNA) synthesis is impaired in the presence of normal ribonucleic acid (RNA) and protein synthesis. Synthesis of protein, RNA and Hb continues in the cytoplasm. When DNA synthesis is impaired, cell division is retarded but the cell grows more in between mitotic cycles, and this accounts for the larger size of the megaloblasts and macrocytes. As the deficiency becomes more pronounced, many early forms of erythroblasts are destroyed in the marrow and ultimately erythropoiesis becomes almost totally ineffective.

Macrocytic anemias may be associated with megaloblastic erythropoiesis or normoblastic erythropoiesis. Macrocytic anemia with normoblastic marrow is seen when there are numerous reticulocytes in peripheral blood. Other less common causes include hypothyroidism, liver disease, renal failure and chronic infections. The vast majority of macrocytic and dimorphic anemias in India are due to nutritional deficiencies of folates and/or vitamin B_{12}. Addisonian pernicious anemia, which is more common in the Caucasian races is less common, though there are several reports of proved cases in the Indian subcontinent.

Megaloblasts

The defect of DNA synthesis is most pronounced in marrow cells, but it is also present in varying degrees in all rapidly proliferating cells. The nucleus of the megaloblast has a finer reticular pattern which distinguishes it from normoblast. Megaloblastic anemia is common in nutritional deficiency of folate or vitamin B_{12} or when the metabolic pathways of these nutrients are blocked.

Causes of megaloblastic anemia due to folic acid deficiency

- Nutritional deficiency
- Increased demand such as pregnancy, infancy and infection
- Protein-calorie malnutrition
- Malabsorption states
- Drugs with antifolate action, e.g. phenytoin, methotrexate, trimethoprim and pyrimethamine.

Nutritional Megaloblastic Anemia (NMA)

In India, this is the most common form of megaloblastic anemia and is caused by deficiency of folic acid, vitamin B_{12} or both. Folate deficiency is more frequent than vitamin B_{12} deficiency in all parts of the country. In many cases, there is also iron deficiency and so the blood picture is dimorphic.

Folic acid is obtained from dietary sources such as green vegetables, sprouted cereals or pulses, liver, meat, yeast and others. The daily requirement of folic acid is 200 µg. Excessive demand occurs during growth spurts, pregnancy and convalescence from illnesses. Folic acid is absorbed from the small intestine. Malabsorption states such as celiac disease, sprue and others lead to folate deficiency. In communities in which nutritional status is marginal, diarrheal diseases precipitate folate malnutrition. Several drugs such as phenytoin sodium, methotrexate and sulfonamides exert their therapeutic effects by interfering with the metabolic pathways in the utilization of folate. Such drugs are liable to lead to folate deficiency on prolonged administration.

Since folate is rapidly used up by the system and body stores are relatively less compared to vitamin B_{12}, folate deficiency manifests within weeks to months of onset of dietary deficiency.

Requirement of vitamin B_{12} (cyanocobalamin) is 1 µg/day. It is obtained mainly from animal foods such as liver and meat. Smaller amounts are obtained from milk and fermented milk products such as buttermilk and yoghurt or curds, which form an important component of Indian diets. Dietary deficiency occurs in those who are vegans, i.e. those who consume only diets of plant origin excluding even dairy products. In general, the serum vitamin B_{12} levels of vegetarians are lower than those of persons consuming adequate amounts of meat products.

Uptake of vitamin B_{12} (cobalamins) in the GIT depends upon (A) supply, (B) intrinsic factor, synthesized by gastric parietal cells and (C) cubam receptor in the distal ileum.

Normal absorption of vitamin B_{12} in the GIT

Cobalamin (CBL) present in food is released by peptic action→binds to haptocorrin (HC) in the stomach and travels in the duodenum where pancreatic protease digests the HC releasing CBL which binds to intrinsic factor. The **B_{12} + intrinsic factor** complex binds to a specific receptor (cubam receptor) in the ileum and is internalized and eventually released from lysosomes and transported in the blood in combination with HC (80%) and transcobalamins (20%). The latter is the form in which B_{12} is delivered to the target cells.

Pathophysiological effects of vitamin B_{12} deficiency

Vitamin B_{12} is cofactor for only two enzymes—methionine synthase and 1-methylmalonyl-coenzyme A mutase. Interaction between folate and vitamin B_{12} is responsible for the development of megaloblastic anemia seen in both vitamin deficiencies. Dyssynchrony between the maturation of the cytoplasm and the nucleus leads to macrocytosis, immature nuclei and macropolycytes in peripheral blood. Criteria for macropolycyte are the presence of 1% of total neutrophils with 6 lobes or 5% with 5 lobes. Ineffective erythropoiesis leads to intramedullary hemolysis and rise in lactate dehydrogenase (LDH). Vitamin B_{12} is necessary for the initial myelination of central nervous system (CNS) and for maintenance of its function. Demyelination may involve cervical and thoracic dorsal columns of spinal cord, occasional demyelination of cranial and peripheral nerves and white matter in the brain. The pyramidal tract and posterior column are affected and their dysfunction leads to neurological deficit depending on which tract is affected more (combined degeneration). Pathologically, the loss and swelling of myelin sheaths appear as spongy degeneration. MRI can pick up the lesions. For unknown reasons, the severity of megaloblastic anemias is inversely related to the severity of neurological lesion.

In normal subjects, there is adequate store of vitamin B_{12} which may last for several years and therefore dietary deficiency of the vitamin manifests clinically only after several months or even years.

Folate and cyanocobalamin are required for normal metabolic activities of almost all growing cells in the body, and therefore, widespread dysfunction of several organs systems occurs in deficiency states. Maximal effects are seen in bone marrow, epithelial cells and others.

Clinical Features

The onset is insidious. Pregnant women and children are more affected. In addition to the general features of anemia certain, distinguishing features seen are: (1) Large beefy tongue, (2) dark pigmentation over the palms, soles, face and tongue, (3) hepatosplenomegaly and (4) mental changes and neurological involvement in vitamin B_{12} deficiency. Neurological abnormalities include peripheral neuropathy and degeneration of the posterior columns and pyramidal tracts—subacute combined degeneration. Psychiatric disturbances and optic neuritis may occur in a few. The neurological manifestations can develop in nutritional deficiency of vitamin B_{12} also, if the condition persists for long periods, but compared to pernicious anemia this complication is less frequent and milder. Nutritional deficiencies of folate and/or vitamin B_{12} may lead to hyperhomocysteinemia which, in turn, induces thrombophilia and pathological thrombosis in arteries and veins. Stroke occurring in young persons in developing countries is caused by hyperhomocysteinemia in a small proportion of cases. This risk is abolished by nutritional supplementation.

Infantile B_{12} deficiency: In breastfed children of mothers with B_{12} deficiency, failure of brain development, developmental regression, hypotonia, lethargy, tremors, hyperirritability, feeding difficulties and coma may develop. MRI may reveal the lesion in the CNS. Early replacement therapy rapidly corrects the picture, delay leads to residual defects.

Investigations

Hb level may vary from 5 to 8 g/dL or less, MCHC is within the normal range (28–32%) while MCV is increased and may be as high as 120 fL. Macrocytosis and anisopoikilocytosis are easily recognizable. Some red cells may show punctate basophilia due to the presence of remnants of RNA. Nuclear material may be present in erythrocytes. These are seen as **Howell-Jolly bodies** and **Cabot's rings**. Leukocytes may be normal or decreased in number. Granulocytes are larger than normal, showing increased lobulation with the average lobe count higher than 5 **(macropolycytes)**. This change in leukocytes is very helpful in diagnosis when the morphology of erythrocytes is equivocal. Platelet count may be decreased at times. Platelet function may also become defective.

Bone marrow is hyperplastic due to erythroid hyperplasia. All stages of megaloblasts are present. Normoblastic erythropoiesis may also be present simultaneously. In the absence of iron deficiency, hemosiderin content of marrow is increased. Life span of red cells is moderately decreased. Megaloblasts defer qualitatively from normoblasts (the erythroid precursor formed in normal health with the availability of all nutrients) in their nuclear pattern. The nucleus of the megaloblasts consists of thin reticulate chromatin whereas nucleus of the normoblasts is composed of condensed chromatin (Figs 160.1 and 160.4).

Levels of serum folate and red cell folate are diminished. The normal level of folate in serum is 6–20 ng/mL and that in red cells is 160–640 ng/mL. Serum levels below 3 ng/mL and red cell levels below 100 ng/mL indicate deficiency of folate. Serum vitamin B_{12} values below 100 pg/mL are indicative of deficiency.

In pure megaloblastic anemia due to B_{12} or folate deficiency, serum iron values and ferritin levels are normal. Concomitant iron deficiency presents as transferrin saturation less than 100% and ferritin level 30 ng/mL. If transferrin saturation is less than 15% and ferritin levels are more than 200 ng/mL, it suggest inflammatory block in iron utilization.

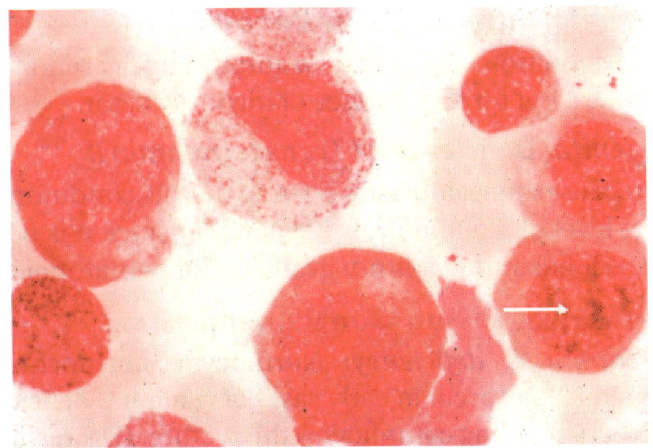

Fig. 160.4: Megaloblastic bone marrow. *Note:* Megaloblast—nuclear chromatin is loose (arrow)

Treatment

Overall dietary correction should be undertaken. Oral administration of 1 mg or more of folic acid daily is adequate to correct folate deficiency. Supplementation of folic acid will improve the anemia due to deficiency of vitamin B_{12} also, but not the neurological complications. In the later stages of therapy, deficiency of iron may develop and iron may have to be given.

Vitamin B_{12} deficiency can be rapidly corrected by IM injection of 1,000 µg of hydroxocobalamin. Oral doses of 2–3 µg are curative in most cases if continued over a few months.

Prevention

Oral supplementation of folates to 0.1 mg/day to growing children and subjects receiving antiepileptic drugs, helps to prevent folate deficiency. In pregnancy, a daily dose of 0.5 mg of folic acid should be given prophylactically from the first trimester. When megaloblastic anemia has developed, 5 mg should be given orally daily throughout the pregnancy and puerperium. Infants require 1 mg of folic acid orally daily as supplement. Therapeutic administration of folates (400 µg/day) to pregnant women, irrespective of their nutritional status reduces the risk of development of neural tube defects in the baby. If absorption is defective, folic acid has to be given by IM injection in a dose of 5 mg daily for a few days.

Prophylactic oral supplementation of vitamin B_{12} is given as 1–2 µg either singly or along with the other deficient factors during pregnancy and in those with marginal nutritional states. When absorption is defective, IM injection of 1,000 µg is given once a week for 3–4 weeks.

Addisonian Pernicious Anemia

Syn: Pernicious anemia, Biermer's anemia

Etiology

It is more common among the Caucasian population, but is rare in Indian subjects, though there are definite cases reported from several parts of India. Study of anti-intrinsic factor blocking antibody was positive in 19 out of 50 patients and antiparietal cell antibody was positive in 28 out of some 50 patients studied by Pradeep G Divate and Rashida Patanwala from Pune. It is found more often in the older age groups and only rarely before 30 years of age. It may be familial and affects both sexes. Antibodies directed against the gastric parietal cells are present in the serum in 85–90% of cases and antibodies against intrinsic factor are demonstrable in the serum as well as in the gastric juice in a smaller proportion of cases. This is an autoimmune disease. Other disorders like myxedema, type 1 diabetes mellitus (DM), Addison's disease, thyrotoxicosis, Hashimoto's disease and vitiligo which all have an autoimmune basis may occur along with pernicious anemia. Antibodies to parietal cells develop and destroy them leading to fall in gastric hydrochloric acid (HCl) and intrinsic factor. The gastric mucosa undergoes atrophy resulting in the absence of intrinsic factor and gastric acid—*Achylia gastrica*. Dietary vitamin B_{12} is not absorbed. This leads to megaloblastic erythropoiesis. Several other tissues are also affected, particularly the nervous system. Demyelination of the pyramidal tracts and posterior columns develop (*See* also Section 17, Ch 198). Carcinoma of the stomach develops in 4% of cases on follow-up.

Source: Divate PG, Patanwala R. Neurological manifestations of B_{12} deficiency with emphasis on its aetiology. J Assoc Physicians India. 2014;62(5):400-5.

Clinical Features

The onset is insidious. In addition to symptoms of anemia, special features include soreness of the tongue, paresthesia of hands and feet, diarrhea and yellowish tinge of skin and mucous membranes. The tongue is atrophic. Spleen is palpable in 25% of cases. Spinal cord involvement results in subacute combined degeneration manifesting as varying combination of dysfunctions of the pyramidal tracts and posterior columns. In adults, most common neurological symptoms is symmetrical paresthesia and gait problems.

Psychiatric symptoms are common. These include melancholia, depression and behavior disorders which may be mistaken for primary psychiatric disorders.

If left untreated, the disease follows a prolonged course, ending fatally due to severe anemia or its complications. The megaloblastic change and anemia are rapidly correctable by the parenteral administration of vitamin B_{12} or oral administration of folate. The neurological changes tend to remain permanent once they have developed. Only vitamin B_{12} is capable of preventing their occurrence and arresting their further progress, once they have set in. Folate does not prevent this neuropathy; in some it may even aggravate the lesion.

Laboratory Findings

Erythrocytes are macrocytic with marked anisopoikilocytosis. The bone marrow is megaloblastic. Bone marrow biopsy may be even misleading—since pancytopenia, hypercellularity, increased erythroblasts and even cytogenetic abnormalities may occur. In a florid case, Hb is usually below 7 g/dL. Leukopenia and thrombocytopenia are common. Gastric juice analysis shows histamine fast achlorhydria and absence of intrinsic factor (*Achylia gastrica*). Serum vitamin B_{12} is below 80 pg/mL. In the laboratory estimation of vitamin B_{12}, the antibody to intrinsic factor (if present) may vitiate the test and give a spurious high value of B_{12} even in the presence of B_{12} deficiency. Vitamin B_{12} assays in the lab are subject to vagaries and the lab values may not correspond to the clinical situation. Normal or even high values of B_{12} may be seen in pernicious anemia patients. Recent assays estimating holotranscobalamins (saturation by B_{12} or transcolabamines) are being developed, but not yet commercially available. Since vitamin B_{12} assays may be altered by methodological problems, measurement of methylmalonic acid (MMA) and homocysteine may help in diagnosis. Normal level of MMA is less than 400 mmol/L and homocysteine is less than 14 mmol/L. Serum and red cell folate are normal. Serum iron levels are elevated.

Measurement of MMA and total homocysteine

These are elevated in untreated B_{12} deficient patients in more than 98% of cases. Levels of MMA often reach more than 500–1,000 mmol/L. Levels of homocysteine are also elevated; these are nonspecific since this occurs in folate deficiency, classic homocystinuria and renal failure. With treatment, the levels fall. Sometimes false low values may be obtained.

Defect of absorption of vitamin B_{12}, and its correction by addition of intrinsic factor present in normal gastric juice can be demonstrated by Schilling's test using radioactive vitamin B_{12}. Parietal cell antibodies which are detectable in the serum are helpful in diagnosis. Gastroscopy and biopsy confirm the diagnosis.

Serum iron and total iron binding capacity (TIBC) levels: Serum iron levels and ferritin levels can be low in concurrent iron deficiency but occasionally the value of ferritin may be high even in the presence of iron deficiency. The ferritin levels in this case do not reflect the true iron status in pernicious anemia.

MRI studies

Though MRI imaging of spinal cord is not needed in an ordinary case, characteristic hyperintensity on T2-weighted imaging described as inverted V-shaped pattern of the cervical or thoracic spinal cord may be evident.

Therapy

In severe cases where Hb is below 5 g/dL, transfusion of packed erythrocytes may be required to improve the oxygen carrying capacity of blood. Specific therapy is to give hydroxocobalamin 1,000 µg IM every week till Hb level becomes normal. Reticulocyte response is noticed within 2–3 days of the first injection. Folic acid is contraindicated since it is known to precipitate the neurological complications, if administered alone.

Maintenance

Subjects with pernicious anemia should receive life-long supplementation of parenteral vitamin B_{12}, 1,000 µg every month. In pernicious anemia, if B_{12} therapy is stopped, neurological features return within 6–12 months, whereas megaloblastosis takes longer time to return. Oral supplementation of 100 µg vitamin B_{12} may be tried with benefit in patients who wish to avoid injections. Some may respond adequately.

Congenital Megaloblastic Anemias

Though in vast majority of cases of pernicious anemia, the defect in intrinsic factor is an acquired one, it can be congenital in some rare cases.

Congenital Intrinsic Factor Deficiency

In this condition, the gastric histology and secretions are normal except for the absence of intrinsic factor.

Congenital Deficiency of Transcobalamin II

It also causes megaloblastic anemia. In this condition, the serum level of vitamin B_{12} is normal, but since it is bound to transcobalamin I; it is not available for hematopoiesis.

Rarer Causes of Nutritional Anemia

- ***Vitamin C deficiency:*** Normocytic normochromic anemia may occur in early cases of vitamin C deficiency. When bleeding complicates the picture, IDA results.
- ***Protein deficiency:*** It can lead to anemia due to diminished production of erythrocytes and possibly reduced lifespan of these cells. The anemia is mild, and Hb levels range from 8 to 10 g/dL.
- ***Copper deficiency:*** This leads to hypochromic microcytic anemia in experimental animals. Copper deficiency may occur in infants fed solely on milk or due to severe malnutrition. In adults, this is not a significant clinical problem.

ANEMIA IN SYSTEMIC DISEASES

- ***Thyroxine (T4) deficiency:*** This produces a mild to moderate type of anemia in 20–60% of cases. T4 deficiency per se causes a normocytic normochromic anemia or slightly macrocytic anemia. There is mild hypoplasia of erythroid precursors.
- ***Anemia in rheumatoid arthritis (RA):*** There is mild to moderate anemia with Hb levels ranging from 9 to 10 g/dL. Blood picture is usually normocytic hypochromic. Anemia may be partly due to GI bleeding resulting from excessive ingestion of antirheumatic drugs. In addition to concomitant nutritional deficiencies, RA per se produces a resistant type of normocytic hypochromic anemia, which is relatively resistant to oral iron. Parenteral iron therapy results in significant improvement.
- ***In acute renal failure (ARF):*** Normocytic normochromic anemia develops with reticulocytopenia and depression of erythroblasts in bone marrow. Erythropoietin (EPO) levels are low.
- ***In chronic renal failure (CRF):*** Severity of anemia correlates well with the glomerular filtration rate (GFR) and to a lesser degree with blood urea nitrogen (BUN). Anemia is mainly due to reduction in EPO levels and diminution in erythropoiesis. Blood loss and nutritional deficiency contribute in varying proportions. Hemodialysis aggravates the blood loss. When the blood urea exceeds 280 mg/dL hemolysis may develop. The anemia is generally resistant to treatment, but EPO produces marked improvement in Hb level and several other parameters as well (*See* also Section 16, Ch 184).
- ***In chronic liver disease:*** There is mild anemia which may be multifactorial in origin. The factors are GI bleeding, ineffective erythropoiesis and hemolysis. The anemia may be hypochromic or macrocytic normochromic. Usual hematinics are not very effective. Improvement may take place with improvement of liver function.

- ***Malignant neoplasms:*** These cause anemia at some stage or the other during their course. Different types of anemia are encountered since multiple factors operate. These are:
  - ***IDA*** due to GI hemorrhage or malabsorption.
  - ***Folic acid deficiency anemia*** due to increased requirement of the vitamin caused by extensive tumor growths or due to chemotherapy or radiation therapy. Folinic acid therapy together with vitamin B_{12} is helpful.
  - ***Hemolytic anemia*** may occur in lymphomas or ovarian neoplasms due to development of antibodies.
  - ***Hypoplastic anemia*** may result from bone marrow suppression caused by immune mechanisms, e.g. thymoma and lymphoma.
  - ***Myelophthisic anemia*** caused by invasion of the marrow by tumor tissue, e.g. malignant secondaries, lymphoma and myelofibrosis.

ANEMIA OF CHRONIC DISEASES

Syn: Anemia of Inflammation

Anemia may complicate several chronic, and at times, acute inflammatory disorders. These are not uncommon. These may masquerade as other types of anemia. Activation of the immune system by chronic and acute inflammatory disorders leads to anemia of chronic diseases (ACD).

Causes

Chronic and acute infections—bacterial, parasitic, fungal and viral including human immunodeficiency virus (HIV) and acquired immunodeficiency syndrome (AIDS).

- ***Neoplasms:*** Hematological malignancies and tumors of solid organs
- Autoimmune diseases, specially rheumatoid disease, systemic lupus erythematosus (SLE), vasculitis, sarcoidosis, inflammatory bowel disease, transplant rejection after solid organ transplantation
- Chronic renal diseases
- Other forms of chronic inflammation
- Anemia developing after trauma, blast injury, DM, sepsis, myocardial infarction (MI), heart failure and others.

Mechanism

Immune-mediated cytokines and immunocytes are activated which adversely affect iron metabolism, erythroid progenitor development, production of EPO and red blood cell (RBC) lifespan. All these factors contribute to the development of anemia. Bleeding, conditioned deficiencies of hemopoietic factors and autoimmune hemolysis aggravate the anemia. The proliferation and differentiation of the proerythroblast, erythroid burst-forming unit and colony-forming unit are impaired. Interferon-γ is one of the potent inhibitors. Stimulation by EPO is inadequate to compensate for the inhibition. The response of the erythroid progenitor cells to EPO is inhibited in proportion to the severity of the underlying chronic disease and inhibitor cytokines. Erythrophagocytosis (phagocytosis of RBC by macrophages) develops and this worsens the anemia by reducing RBC life span in some cases of ACD.

Hepcidin-induced alteration in the iron metabolism is now considered as the main mechanism of reduced RBC production. Increased hepcidin produced in many conditions of ACD decreases iron absorption from the intestine and traps the iron in the macrophages. The serum iron is decreased (hypoferremia) and iron becomes unavailable for hemoglobin synthesis.

There is also an inability to increase erythropoiesis in response to anemia though there is some increase in the erythropoietin produced by the renal cells.

Table 160.3: Clinical parameters to distinguish between IDA and ACD

Parameter	ACD	IDA	Combined ACD + IDA
Iron	Reduced	Reduced	Reduced
Transferrin	Reduced	Increased	Reduced
Transferrin saturation	Reduced	Reduced	Reduced
Ferritin	Normal	Reduced	Reduced or normal
STR	Normal	Increased	Normal or increased
STR/log ferritin	<1	>2 high	>2
Cytokine levels	Increased	Normal	Increased

Abbreviations: IDA = Iron deficiency anemia; ACD = Anemia of chronic diseases; STR = Soluble transmembrane receptor

Laboratory Findings

The anemia is mild (Hb 6–9.5 g), normocytic, normochromic or microcytic. Where iron absorption is impaired, the anemia resembles IDA. In IDA, serum ferritin levels are generally less than 30 ng/mL. Ferritin levels are higher in ACD due to the increase in storage iron in reticuloendothelial (RE) cells and also the acute inflammatory reaction raising ferritin levels (Table 160.3).

A specific distinguishing test to differentiate between IDA and ACD is the level of soluble transmembrane receptor (STR) in serum. STR is a truncated fragment of the membrane receptor that is increased in iron deficiency when the availability of iron for erythropoiesis is diminished. In ACD, the STR levels are normal. Another measurement is the determination of the ratio of the STR to the log of ferritin. Ratios above 2 suggest IDA whereas ratios below 1 suggest ACD. STR can be estimated easily using commercially available test kits.

Hemoglobin levels below 8 g/dL double the chances of death in CRF.

Treatment

- To raise Hb up to 12 g/dL
- Attention to the underlying disorder.

Management consists of supplementation of iron in those with iron deficiency. Iron should not be administered to those without evidence of iron deficiency, since this may lead to the production of highly active toxic hydroxyl radicles which can worsen tissue damage. EPO is indicated in those in whom attention to the primary disease is not fully successful. The dose of EPO should be adjusted to keep Hb levels around 12 g/dL. Overuse of EPO is contraindicated since erythrocytosis can lead to thrombotic complications specially in the CNS.

Anemia of infections: Infections suppress EPO production nonspecifically. Inflammatory cytokines also depress the production of EPO. In addition, iron availability is blocked by inflammatory mediators and acute iron deficiency results.

CHAPTER
161

Hemolytic Anemias

KV Krishna Das

Chapter Summary

- General Considerations
- Acquired Hemolytic Anemias
  - Autoimmune Hemolytic Anemia
- Secondary Hemolytic Anemias
  - Hemolytic Disease of Newborn
- Inherited Disorders of the Erythrocytes
  - Red Cell Membrane Disorders
    - Hereditary Spherocytosis
  - Other Red Cell Membrane Disorders
    - Hereditiary Elliptocytosis
- Red Cell Enzymopathies
- Hemoglobinopathies (Thalassemias and Thalassemia Syndromes)
  - Sickle Cell Disease
  - Acute Chest Syndrome
  - Hemoglobin E Disease
- Thalassemias
- Thalassemia Syndromes

GENERAL CONSIDERATIONS

Normal lifespan of red cells is 120 days. Old erythrocytes are removed from the circulation. Mildly deformed cells are phagocytozed in the spleen, severely injured cells are removed by the liver macrophages, and grossly damaged cells are destroyed in the circulation itself. When destruction of erythrocytes exceeds the normal rate, their lifespan diminishes and compensatory hyperplasia of erythroid precursors develops. For considerable periods this compensates and hemoglobin (Hb) level is kept up. Since the marrow can compensate by enhanced erythropoiesis up to seven times the normal rate, anemia need not follow in all cases. When hemolysis is severe and the lifespan of the erythrocyte falls below 18 days, anemia is bound to develop. Rarely marrow erythropoietic activity may fail, aggravating the anemia. The term hemolytic anemia is reserved for those disorders where the anemia is caused predominantly by excessive destruction of erythrocytes.

Hemolysis occurs due to several pathogenetic mechanisms (Box 161.1).

- A decrease in the surface area/volume ratio, e.g. hereditary spherocytosis, autoimmune hemolytic anemia (AIHA) and drug-induced hemolysis.
- Defect in structure of the erythrocyte membrane, e.g. paroxysmal nocturnal hemoglobinuria (PNH) and drug-induced hemolytic disorders.
- Increased internal viscosity inside the red cell, e.g. sickle cell anemia and Heinz-body hemolytic anemia.
- Hypersplenism.

Box 161.1: Classification of hemolytic disorders

- Inherited hemolytic disorders
  - Red cell membrane defects, e.g. hereditary spherocytosis, hereditary elliptocytosis, hereditary acanthocytosis, hereditary stomatocytosis
  - Red cell enzyme deficiencies, e.g. deficiencies of pyruvate kinase, hexokinase, glucose-6-phosphate dehydrogenase (G6PD) and glutathione reductase
  - Defects in amino acid configuration of globin chains, e.g. sickle cell anemia and other hemoglobinopathies including unstable Hb
  - Failure to switch over of beta or alpha globin chains in post-natal life, e.g. thalassemias
- Acquired hemolytic anemia
  - Immunologically-mediated hemolytic anemia, e.g. incompatible blood transfusion, hemolytic disease of the newborn (HDN), AIHA (warm antibody and cold antibody types)
  - Microangiopathic hemolytic anemia, e.g. disseminated intravascular coagulation, hemolytic uremic syndrome, thrombotic thrombocytopenic purpura, mechanical causes like implantation of cardiac prosthesis and march hemoglobinuria
  - Caused by infections, e.g. malaria, *Clostridium welchii* infections and bartonellosis
  - Caused by drugs, chemicals, and toxins, e.g. nitrofurantoin, sulfonamides, viper venom and formic acid poisoning
  - Paroxysmal nocturnal hemoglobinuria

Hemolytic anemia contributes 4% of the total anemias seen in South India. Hemolysis may occur intra- or extravascularly. Intravascular hemolysis takes place in many cases of acquired hemolytic anemias whereas in the inherited form, hemolysis is generally extravascular.

In intravascular hemolysis, it is usually a complement mediated antigen-antibody reaction. It is seen in conditions such as black water fever in *P. falciparum* malaria, and favism-induced hemolysis. This may lead to presence of Hb in the plasma, methemalbuminemia and hemoglobinuria in addition to hyperbilirubinemia. Acute massive intravascular hemolysis leads to hemoglobinuria and renal failure.

Extravascular hemolysis is generally caused by destruction of the erythrocytes in reticuloendothelial organs, particularly in the spleen. In these, hyperbilirubinemia and jaundice are more prominent.

Clinical Features

In addition to the general symptomatology of anemia, hemolysis leads to distinctive features which differ from each other in the acute and chronic forms. Chronic hemolysis leads to jaundice, hemolytic facies, chronic leg ulcers, splenomegaly, cholelithiasis, cutaneous pigmentation, and iron overload states. On the other hand, acute hemolytic episodes are characterized by sharp rise in temperature and marked prostration. They may be accompanied by hemoglobinuria, acute renal failure (ARF), disseminated intravascular coagulation and shock. In many cases, the hemolysis is secondary to other underlying conditions such as lymphomas, leukemia, malignancy or dyscollagenosis.

- *Jaundice:* Hemolytic jaundice is generally mild, but at times this can be very severe, e.g. Rh incompatibility. The degree of jaundice and the extent of hemolysis may not always correlate.
- *Facies:* It is characteristic in chronic hemolytic anemias specially thalassemia. There is enlargement of the skull with frontal and parietal bossing. The malar bones are prominent with flattening of the bridge of the nose, widely set eyes and malocclusion of the teeth. The appearance may be mongoloid. All these changes are caused by enlargement of the marrow tissue.
- *Chronic leg ulcers:* Chronic non-healing ulcers develop over the malleoli in severe hemolytic states such as sickle cell anemia and hereditary spherocytosis. These heal when the anemia improves.
- *Splenomegaly:* It is invariably seen in all cases of hemolytic anemia though the size of the spleen may be variable. Massive splenomegaly occurs in thalassemia and this may lead to hypersplenism.
- *Cholelithiasis:* Pigment stones in the biliary tree are occasional complications seen in chronic hemolysis, caused by the excessive presence of bilirubin in bile.
- *Hemolytic crisis:* The course of chronic hemolytic anemias may be punctuated by acute episodes called crisis (Fig. 161.1). These may be aplastic, megaloblastic, hemolytic, sickling and sequestration crisis. Aplastic crisis is due to sudden marrow failure precipitated generally by viral infection specially parvoviruses. Megaloblastic crisis is produced by folate deficiency resulting from excessive demand brought about by accelerated erythropoiesis. Hemolytic crisis is rare, which may develop spontaneously or may be an adverse reaction to drugs or viral infections. Sickling crisis occurs in sickle cell anemia when exposed to hypoxic environment. This leads to vascular occlusion of many organs such as lungs, spleen, kidney and brain. In sequestration crisis, sudden splenomegaly develops because of pooling of blood within the organ and severe anemia ensues rapidly.

- *Darkening of skin and other iron overload syndromes:* Chronic hemolytic anemia leads to iron overload due to liberation of excessive iron which is taken up by the macrophages or deposited in the parenchymal cells of several organs. The absorption of iron from the GIT is also increased in thalassemia. Repeated blood transfusion adds to iron overload. These result in hemosiderosis characterized by grayish complexion of the skin, cirrhosis of liver, diabetes mellitus and cardiomyopathy.

Investigations

Proper laboratory investigations are necessary to establish the diagnosis of hemolytic anemia.

- *Tests to detect the presence of hemolysis:* The direct method is to measure the red cell lifespan and the rate of erythrocyte destruction. The presence of hemolysis can be inferred by demonstrating: (1) Reticulocytosis (Fig. 161.2), (2) rise in serum bilirubin, (3) reduction of serum haptoglobin and (4) increase in serum lactic dehydrogenase. Normal haptoglobin levels in serum range from 100 to 300 mg/dL.
  - Hemolytic anemia must be suspected wherever the reticulocyte count is above 2.5% and this is not accountable by other causes like recent blood loss or hematinic therapy. Rarely, reticulocytosis may be absent even in hemolytic states when there are antibodies against red cell precursors or bone marrow aplasia.
  - *Bilirubin:* Presence of unconjugated hyperbilirubinemia (above 1 mg/dL) in the absence of primary hepatobiliary disease strongly suggests hemolysis. The metabolic products of bilirubin like urobilinogen in the urine and stercobilinogen in feces are also increased. Presence of excess pigment in feces makes it darker—polycholia.
  - *Serum haptoglobins:* These are alpha-2 glycoproteins which are normally present in serum at a concentration of 60–160 mg/dL. They combine with Hb liberated from red cells to form complexes which are rapidly destroyed. Consequently, haptoglobin level in serum is lowered in active hemolysis.
  - *Serum lactic dehydrogenase level:* This is invariably elevated above the normal range (70–240 IU/mL)

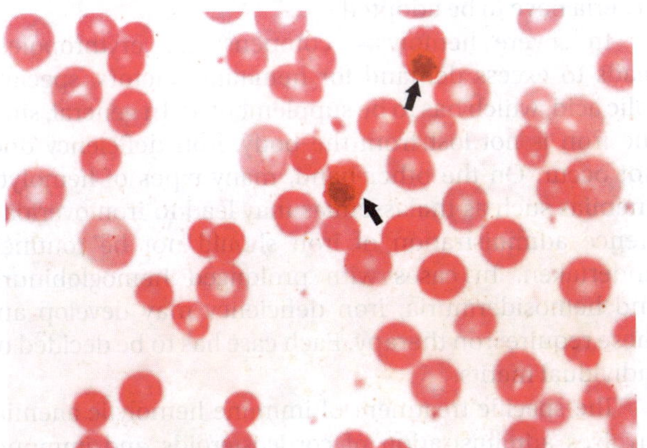

Fig. 161.1: Hemolytic crisis: peripheral blood. *Note:* Anisopoikilocytosis and presence of normoblasts (arrows)

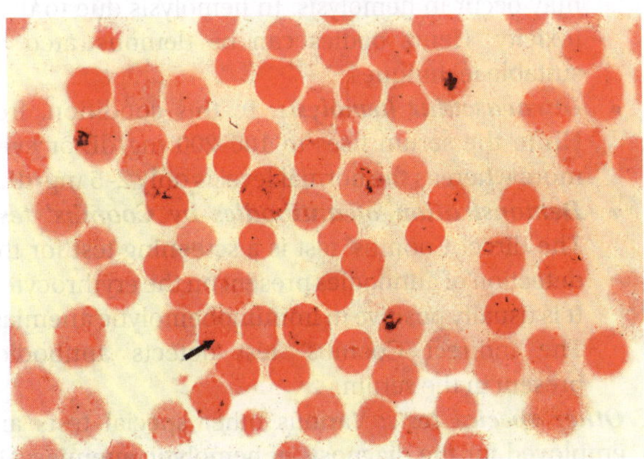

Fig. 161.2: Hemolytic anemia pheripheral blood × 1000 reticulocytes increased. *Note:* Reticulum within erythrocytes (arrow)

in hemolytic anemia. This is more marked in intravascular hemolysis.

- ***Bone marrow:*** The bone marrow shows erythroid hyperplasia in vast majority of cases. Megaloblastosis occurs when there is associated folate deficiency. Chronic overactivity of erythroid tissue leads to expansion of marrow volume and deformity of several bones such as the skull, facial bones, metacarpals, phalanges and others.
- ***Isotopic methods:*** Red cell survival and the sites of hemolysis can be studied isotopically using ^{51}Cr. The severity of hemolysis can also be established by this method. The rate and pattern of hemolysis can be demonstrated by isotopic studies which can reveal the rate of destruction of the erythrocytes and also the sites where this occurs. These investigations are not needed for routine purposes but are of value in special situations.

■ ***Tests to detect the cause:*** History and physical examination help to reveal the cause in most of the cases. Examination of the peripheral blood film, tests for intravascular hemolysis and demonstration of antibodies serve to identify the underlying factors.

- ***Examination of a peripheral blood film*** gives the most valuable clues to the etiology in most of the cases. Large number of spherocytes is suggestive of hereditary spherocytosis or immune hemolytic anemias. Gross alteration of red cell morphology and the presence of basophilic stippling, hypochromia and target cells favor the diagnosis of thalassemia and hemoglobinopathies. Schistocytes, which are fragmented erythrocytes, are seen characteristically in microangiopathy and mechanical causes for hemolysis. Stomatocytosis is seen in hereditary stomatocytosis and hepatic disorders. Acanthocytes are seen in abetalipoproteinemia and in chronic liver diseases. In elliptocytosis, the erythrocytes are oval—hence called ovalocytes. In India, no examination of blood film is complete without careful search for malarial parasites which may be the cause of hemolysis in many cases in endemic areas.
- Anisopoikilocytosis, polychromasia, punctate basophilia and Cabot's rings are suggestive of active erythropoiesis and also dyserythropoiesis which may occur in hemolysis. In hemolysis due to drug toxicity, Heinz bodies can be demonstrated by suitable techniques.
- ***Intravascular hemolysis:*** In this condition, free Hb in the serum rises to 100–200 mg/dL or even more whereas the normal level is only 2–5 mg/dL.
- ***Demonstration of antibodies by Coombs' test:*** The direct Coombs' test is a screening test for the detection of antibodies present on the erythrocytes. It is usually positive in immunohemolytic anemias. The indirect Coombs' test detects antibodies present in the serum.

■ ***Other special tests:*** Various other special tests are employed for the diagnosis of hemolytic anemias: (1) Osmotic fragility is increased and autohemolysis is present in spherocytosis, (2) sucrose-hemolysis test

and Ham's acid serum test are positive in paroxysmal nocturnal hemoglobinuria, (3) detection of abnormal Hb, assays for erythrocyte enzymes, demonstration of Heinz bodies and immunological studies are all employed in specific cases.

Box 161.2 shows the features of increased red blood cell (RBC) destruction.

Course and Prognosis

Prognosis in hemolytic anemias is very variable. Mild cases may extend over several years with aggravation of hemolysis during periods of stress. On the other hand, acute fulminant hemolysis can be fatal. Death is due to severe anemia and shock or ARF. The course of secondary hemolytic anemias depends on the primary cause.

Management

General measures: When the drop in Hb is severe, it has to be restored by transfusion of packed erythrocytes. In acute intravascular hemolysis, emergency transfusion is needed to avoid cardiorespiratory failure. Packed cell transfusion obviates the risk of volume overloading and also the risk of sensitization by plasma proteins. When the hemolysis is aggravated by complement, as in paroxysmal nocturnal hemoglobinuria, washed erythrocytes should be given. The modern trend is to limit the packed cell transfusion to the levels at which the patient is comfortable and not dyspneic (around 10 g/dL), but in case of thalassemias and sickle cell disease, different criteria have to be adopted.

In severe hemolysis, compensatory erythropoiesis leads to excess demand for hematinic factors, specially folic acid, which has to be supplemented. In general, since the iron is not lost from the body, iron deficiency does not occur. On the other hand, many types of hemolytic anemias such as thalassemias may lead to iron overload. Hence administration of iron should not be routinely undertaken. In cases with prolonged hemoglobinuria and hemosiderinuria, iron deficiency may develop and these require iron therapy. Each case has to be decided on individual merits.

The specific treatment of immune hemolytic anemias involves administration of corticosteroids and immunosuppressants. Splenectomy is the treatment of choice in hereditary spherocytosis, immune hemolytic anemia

---

Box 161.2: Features of increased red blood cell destruction

Extravascular hemolysis

- Anemia
- Unconjugated hyperbilirubinemia (jaundice)
- Increased urobilinogen in urine leading to high colored urine
- Shortened red cell lifespan (demonstrated by ^{51}Cr-labelled red blood cells)
- Decreased plasma haptoglobin and hemopexin
- Splenomegaly

Intravascular hemolysis

Increased plasma LDH, hemoglobinemia, hemoglobinuria, hemosiderinuria (demonstrated by Prussian blue reaction) and methemoglobinemia (in some)

Note: Normal serum hepatoglobin level is 60–160 mg/dL. Normal hemopexin level in serum is 500–1000 mL both are heme binding plasma glycoproteins. Their levels fall when hemolysis occurs

refractory to medical treatment, and in the presence of hypersplenism. In enzyme deficiencies and hemoglobinopathies, splenectomy is not generally indicated.

Intravenous (IV) immunoglobulin given in a dose of 0.4 g/kg bw daily for 3–4 days is effective in acute hemolytic episodes. This should be reserved for intractable cases since its cost is high and the results are also only temporary.

ACQUIRED HEMOLYTIC ANEMIAS

Autoimmune Hemolytic Anemia

Autoantibodies develop against the erythrocytes. The antibody may agglutinate the red cells at 37°C (warm antibody) or at lower temperatures 0–4°C (cold antibody). Warm antibodies generally belong to IgG class whereas cold antibodies are immunoglobulin M (IgM).

In the warm antibody type, hemolysis takes place extravascularly in the spleen, while in the cold antibody type, hemolysis occurs intravascularly or in the liver. Warm antibody type may vary in its course from mild chronic anemia to explosive and life-threatening hemolytic crisis. Sometimes there may be both warm and cold antibodies (mixed antibody type).

Etiology

Table 161.1 lists the causes of warm antibody type autoimmune hemolytic anemias.

Pathogenesis

The antibody is usually of IgG class which is an agglutinin reacting with the erythrocyte Rh antigen complex. Complement activation may or may not occur. The antibody coated cells may be removed by the splenic macrophages. Partially damaged erythrocytes may escape destruction, these repair themselves and appear as spherocytes, which is a finding in many types of hemolytic anemias.

Clinical Features

The majority of cases present symptoms like anemia, jaundice and splenomegaly. In secondary AIHA, features of the underlying disorder may be evident. Acute massive hemolysis with shock and renal failure may develop in some cases.

Cold Antibody Type of Hemolytic Anemia

Hemolytic anemia of the cold antibody type may give rise to two clinical syndromes on exposure to cold environment: (1) Cold agglutinin syndrome and

Table 161.1: Causes of autoimmune hemolytic anemias (warm antibody type)

- Idiopathic (primary)
- Drugs, e.g. penicillin and methyldopa
- Systemic lupus erythematosus and other collagen disorders, AIDS
- Antiphospholipid syndrome, organ transplantation, allogeneic red cell transfusion
- Lymphomas and chronic lymphatic leukemia
- Immune deficiency states
- **Venom:** Arthropods and snakes
- **Infections:** Direct damage, malaria, *Bartenellosis*, *Leishmaniasis*, *Trypanosomiasis*, *Babesiosis*
- **Toxic damage:** *E. coli*, Anerobic sepsis, sepsis syndrome

Table 161.2: Causes of cold agglutinins diseases

Cold agglutinins diseases	Infections
Waldenstrom's macroglobulinemia	HIV
Viral infections	Influenza viruses
Infections Mycoplasma	*Mycoplasma pneumoniae*
Multiple myeloma	
Kaposi's sarcoma	Cytomegalovirus
• Autoimmune diseases • Rheumatological disorders • Bacterial infections • Protozoal diseases	Rubella, varicella, mumps *E. coli*, syphilis infective endocarditis, malaria and probably others

(2) Paroxysmal cold hemoglobinuria. Cold agglutinins are generally IgM antibodies directed against red cell antigens and may develop in adults. Cold agglutinins may be primary as occurring in elderly patients (above 70 years) and the antibody is of monoclonal kappa IgM type. Secondary cold agglutinin disease may be caused by a variety of conditions. Cold agglutinin syndrome occurs in older patients and presents with acrocyanosis, Raynaud's phenomenon, gangrene of fingertips and a mild chronic hemolytic anemia. In paroxysmal cold hemoglobinuria, sudden hemolysis develops leading to hemoglobinuria. Paroxysmal cold hemoglobinuria is the first identified autoimmune disease described by Karl Landsteiner, a pathologist from Vienna. The antibody reacts with erythrocytes in the cold.

Causes of cold agglutinins diseases are given in Table 161.2.

The peripheral blood film shows marked anisopoikilocytosis, polychromasia, spherocytosis, and increase in reticulocytes. ***Neutrophil leukocytosis*** is common. Rarely platelets may be reduced due to the development of antibodies against them (Evan's syndrome). The antibodies present on erythrocytes can be demonstrated by ***direct Coombs' test*** and free antibodies in the serum can be identified by the ***indirect Coombs' test***. The thermal characteristics are demonstrable by suitable tests.

Treatment: In secondary hemolytic anemia, treatment is directed towards the underlying cause. If blood transfusion is necessary, properly cross-matched erythrocytes should be given.

Majority of cases of primary AIHA responds to prednisolone in a daily dose of 1–2 mg/kg bw. Once the acute episodes are controlled, the dose should be tapered off but the maintenance dose may have to be continued for prolonged periods. Methylprednisolone in doses of 1–2 g/day given IV as infusion may prove to be superior to other steroids in some cases. In cases where steroids fail or the maintenance dose is high, splenectomy has to be considered. If erythrocyte destruction can be demonstrated in the spleen by isotopic methods, such cases benefit promptly by splenectomy. In the others, although the response is unpredictable, 33–50% still derives benefit.

Immunosuppressive drugs like azathioprine (2–3 mg/kg bw), cyclophosphamide (1–2 mg/kg bw) or cyclosporine may be required, if steroids given alone are not fully effective. Rituximab, a human monoclonal anti-CD20 antibody which acts against B-cells (mature and precursor lymphocytes) is employed in cases resistant to the first line immunosuppressants. It may be beneficial in 30–50% of resistant cases. Doses given should be 40–500 mg IV infusion per hour in graded doses.

In paroxysmal cold hemoglobinuria, the antibody binds to the erythrocytes in the cooler parts of the circulation and also fixes complement. When the sensitized erythrocytes reach the warmer parts of the circulation, they undergo complement-mediated lysis. The syndrome manifests as a dramatic illness characterized by fever, myalgia of the back and legs, followed by varying severities of hemoglobinuria. The episodes are self-limiting.

In cold antibody type, if the hemolysis is mild, only general measures such as avoidance of cold may be necessary. If transfusions are necessary, the blood should be warmed to body temperature before infusion. Steroids and splenectomy are less effective in this type, compared to warm antibody type of AIHA. Severe hemoglobinuria may lead to formation of Hb casts in the renal tubule and consequent renal failure. Adequate hydration and monitoring of renal function should be implemented.

SECONDARY HEMOLYTIC ANEMIAS

Syn: Symptomatic hemolytic anemia

These include several infections, adverse effects of drugs and physical causes which lead to erythrocyte destruction.

Hemolysis may develop in the course of infections such as malaria, viral hepatitis, infectious mononucleosis, and mycoplasma infection. Collagen disorders, leukemia, lymphomas, and other malignancies may be associated with immune hemolysis. Several drugs like penicillin and methyldopa are associated with the production of antibodies and hemolytic anemias. Drugs act in several ways: (1) Drugs like penicillin may act as haptens and make the erythrocyte antigenic, (2) drugs like stibophen, quinine, quinidine, para-aminosalicylate (PAS), isoniazid (INH) and sulfonamides lead to the development of immune complexes which get attached to the erythrocytes and lead to complement-mediated hemolysis (innocent bystander type) and (3) drugs like methyldopa lead to production of antibodies directed against specific antigen sites in the erythrocyte and lead to hemolysis.

Rarely hemolysis may be due to physical factors. Prosthetic cardiac valves lead to mechanical injury and damage of red cells. Long marches and severe physical exertion lead to hemolysis by the same mechanism—march hemoglobinuria. Severe burns lead to extensive hemolysis.

Hemolytic Disease of Newborn

The newborn may suffer from Rh incompatibility or ABO incompatibility if there is Rh or ABO incompatibility between the parents. If the father is Rh positive, the fetus may also sometimes be Rh positive and entry of fetal erythrocytes into the Rh negative mother leads to production of anti-negative-Rh antibodies which reach the fetus and destroy its erythrocytes. A similar phenomenon may occur in ABO incompatibility as well.

Rh Incompatibility

This accounts for the vast majority of isoimmune hemolytic anemias of the newborn and manifests as jaundice on the first day of life. Among the Rh antigens, 'D' is most antigenic. Fetuses with this phenotype cause more severe immunization of the mother and greater degrees of hemolysis in the fetus. In India, 8% of population is Rh negative, unlike in the West where the frequency is 15%. About 17% of Rh negative women get immunized during pregnancy if the fetus is Rh positive.

Pathogenesis

The Rh isoimmunization occurs when an Rh negative individual receives Rh positive blood by transfusion or by other sources. When an Rh negative mother carries an Rh positive fetus, there is transplacental exchange of small quantities of fetal blood into the maternal circulation during the later weeks of pregnancy and during labor. Therapeutic obstetric procedures increase this risk. The fetal cells immunize the mother and antibodies of IgG class are produced depending upon the amount of fetomaternal transfer. Usually the first born child escapes unless the mother is previously sensitized due to Rh incompatible blood transfusions during childhood or due to previous abortions. With successive pregnancies and abortion, the antibody titer in the mother progressively rises. Spontaneous or induced abortions, ectopic pregnancy, amniocentesis and other similar procedures increase the risk. The maternal antibodies pass back into the fetus and lead to hemolysis of fetal erythrocytes, resulting in hemolytic disease of the newborn. Severity of hemolysis depends upon the amount of maternal antibody and the period of gestation at which the fetus is affected.

Hemolysis leads to the development of marrow hyperplasia and extramedullary hematopoiesis. Hepatosplenomegaly occurs. Hepatic function suffers and therefore hypoalbuminemia, ascites and hydrops fetalis develop. In the severe form, there is congestive heart failure, impairment of placental circulation, intrauterine growth retardation and stillbirth. The excess of bilirubin resulting from excessive hemolysis is handled both by the liver and placenta during fetal life, but after birth, this bilirubin load has to be handled by the liver alone. Unconjugated bilirubin crosses the blood-brain barrier (BBB) when the serum levels are high. It gets deposited in neural cells when the serum level exceeds the binding capacity of serum albumin. It interferes with mitochondrial function and leads to cell death and permanent-neurological defects. Neurones in the brainstem, basal ganglia and other regions are affected most. Neurotoxicity of bilirubin may also lead to nerve deafness, seizures, athetoid movements, spasticity and death (kernicterus).

D-phenotypes cause maximum sensitization and lead to most severe disease. Factors determining the extent and severity of the disease are the timing, number and extent of fetomaternal exchanges of blood. Fetal cells which are both ABO and Rh incompatible are more rapidly destroyed in the maternal circulation than purely Rh-incompatible cells. Hence the latter type is more immunogenic and it leads to clinically more serious type of disease. The unconjugated bilirubin formed by hemolysis is bound to albumin, but when the bilirubin level exceeds 20 mg/dL, the binding capacity of albumin is exceeded and the unbound bilirubin passes to the central nervous system (CNS) and causes damage, which is most pronounced in the basal ganglia. The unbound bilirubin is the fraction that is toxic to neural structures. Bilirubin binds avidly to myelin-rich membranes making neurons the primary targets for bilirubin toxicity. Bilirubin-induced oxidative stress and mitochondrial injury may be the nexus of neuronal injury. The toxic effects of bilirubin on the neurons depend on the concentration of unconjugated bilirubin, especially more than 140 nm/L. Non-neuron cell types of the CNS such as astrocytes, microglia, oligodendrocytes, brain microvascular endothelial cells of the BBB and the choroid plexus epithelial cells which form the blood-CSF barrier, all play a role in bilirubin neurotoxicity. They produce inflammatory cytokines of various types which contribute to neuronal damage. The exact final picture of the production of neural damage is not still fully known. The globus pallidus, subthalamic nucleus, brainstem nuclei, hippocampal carbonic anhydrase 2 (CA2) neurons and cerebellar Purkinje cells show lesions.

Bilirubin neurotoxicity is clinically characterized by:

- Extrapyramidal movement disorders—dystonia, choreoathetosis or both
- Hearing loss due to auditory neuropathy spectrum disorders
- Oculomotor paresis.

Other comorbid conditions in the neonates which aggravate hemolysis increase the risk of bilirubin neurotoxicity, e.g. G6PD deficiency, Rh isoimmunization and sepsis.

Clinical Presentation

The mild form manifests as moderate hemolytic anemia in the first days of life. Hepatosplenomegaly may be just detectable. The moderately severe form presents as *icterus gravis neonatorum*. This leads to jaundice within 24 hours of birth and this feature distinguishes it from physiological jaundice. Anemia may progress and lead to cardiac failure. Hepatosplenomegaly may be more evident. Neurological abnormalities develop in severe cases. This is known as *kernicterus* which is characterized by a high-pitched cry, opisthotonus and convulsions. Sequelae include choreoathetosis, deafness, cerebral palsy and mental deficiency which become evident as the child grows.

The severe form manifests as *hydrops fetalis*. Usually the affected baby is born dead or it dies soon after birth. Gross edema, hepatosplenomegaly, anemia and effusions into serous cavities are the common stigmata.

Investigation in a suspected case of Rh isoimmunization: The mother's blood shows the presence of antibodies by the indirect Coombs' test. Titers above 1/64 or rising titers are indicative of risk to the fetus. Further adjuncts to diagnosis are amniocentesis and analysis of bile pigments in amniotic fluid. Unlike normal amniotic fluid which is colorless, in Rh hemolytic disease, the amniotic fluid is bright yellow and this can be quantitated spectroscopically.

Postnatal diagnosis: The baby's blood shows positive direct Coombs' test, elevated serum bilirubin, reticulocytosis, anemia and presence of large number of erythroblasts (over 10% of nucleated cells).

Management

Rh immunization is a preventable disease by proper Rh typing during the prenatal check up.

Prenatal Management

- When the mother is not immunized or the Rh antibody titer is low and static, the pregnancy is allowed to continue.
  - The Rh-D antibody titers are estimated at the first month itself in at-risk pregnancy and repeated. If the titer exceeds 1/16 at 20 weeks or the titers double from the original value, amniocentesis is done to estimate the bilirubin level in amniotic fluid. Polymerase chain reaction (PCR) has been employed to determine the fetal genotype using amniotic cells or fetal blood or maternal plasma collected early in the second trimester.
  - Other investigations to be undertaken include ultrasonography and two-dimensional Doppler studies to detect fetal ascites and hydrops. If the risk of hydrops fetalis or stillbirth before 34 weeks is high, blood transfusions have to be given to the fetus to ameliorate anemia, reduce ascites and hydrops and suppress erythropoiesis. With modern techniques, direct intravascular transfusion is possible in up to 80% of cases. The alternative is to give intraperitoneal infusion of blood.
- If the risk of hydrops fetalis or stillbirth is high, induction of labor between 34 and 38 weeks is indicated.

  Test for pulmonary maturity is carried out by estimating the lecithin sphingomyelin (L/S) ratio of the amniotic fluid. If the L/S ratio is above 2, the pulmonary surfactant will be normal and so there is no risk of acute respiratory distress syndrome in the newborn.

Postnatal Management

The principles of management include correction of anemia, acidosis, hypoglycemia and hyperbilirubinemia. When the serum level of unconjugated bilirubin is above 20 mg/dL in term babies or 15 mg/dL in preterm babies, exchange transfusion with Rh negative group O blood is indicated. By this procedure, antibody coated erythrocytes and excess bilirubin are removed and anemia is corrected. Hb level below 14 g/dL and serum bilirubin above 3 mg/dL in cord blood are also indications for immediate exchange transfusion. Usually, 150 mL/kg bw of compatible blood is used for each exchange.

Other forms of therapy: Mild or even moderate cases can be controlled by ***phototherapy*** and ***phenobarbitone***. Natural sunlight and fluorescent light oxidize bilirubin to biliverdin and then to nontoxic water-soluble products. Phototherapy reduces indirect bilirubin level and helps to reduce the need for exchange transfusion. Phenobarbitone induces liver enzymes to conjugate bilirubin and favor its excretion. Tin mesoporphyrin is effective in reducing total bilirubin levels and use of this drug is under trial. Minocycline (a second generation tetracycline) is effective in neuroprotective effect over several neuron groups and is useful to reduce the damage, but being a tetracycline, it has harmful effect in developing bones and teeth. Double volume exchange transfusion intravenous immunoglobulin (IVIG) is also tried.

Prevention: Rh negative mothers who are at risk are protected from getting immunized by the administration of 300 µg of anti-D gammaglobulin (Rhogam) within 72 hours of delivery or abortion, amniocentesis or rupture of ectopic gestation. Rh immunoglobulin is prepared from plasma obtained from persons with Rh D antibodies. It agglutinates and destroys the circulating fetal cells.

ABO Hemolytic Disease

In 15–20% of pregnancies, ABO incompatibility occurs between the mother and fetus. IgG antibodies against fetal red cells are produced in the mother. Group O mothers produce antibodies more readily than A or B group mothers. The ABO hemolytic disease of the newborn is mild compared to Rh hemolytic disease. Further differences are: (1) The first pregnancy may be affected as frequently as subsequent pregnancies and (2) even if one pregnancy is affected, the subsequent one may escape.

The clinical features are milder compared to Rh hemolytic disease and they may subside spontaneously. Phototherapy and exchange transfusion may be required at times.

Non-Rh Hemolytic Anemias

Other alloantibodies are increasingly being recognized as causes of non-Rh hemolytic anemia. These include antibodies of the Kell system (K and K), Duffy (Fy), Kidd (JKa and Jk[6]) and MNSs systems (M, N, S and S). Some women get immunized to more than one system of antigens. Next to anti-D, anti-Kell is the most common. Six to eight weeks after the recovery from the hemolytic process with treatment, hyporegenerative anemia may develop in the infant. This may require transfusion.

Findings suggestive of autoimmune hemolytic anemia include positive direct antiglobulin test, warm reacting and cold reacting antibodies, presence of spherocytes (but no schizocytes) in peripheral blood and normal coagulation results.

Autoimmune hemolytic anemia may be associated with connective tissue diseases, especially SLE, viral infections (HCV), drug use (cephalosporin, piperacillin), malignant disease (CLL), immunodeficiency (common variable immune deficiency), previous blood transfusions and organ transplantation.

Evan's Syndrome

Thrombocytopenia with autoimmune hemolytic anemia constitute Evan's syndrome. If intravascular hemolysis is incomplete, spherocytes are formed. Evan's syndrome may be primary (idiopathic) or associated with SLE, immune disorders, immunodeficiencies or lymphoproliferative disorders. SLE is the most common cause (50% or more). Antibodies can be present in SLE for as long as 10 years before the onset of symptoms and continue to develop even after onset of symptoms. Warm reacting antibodies act at 37°C and cold reacting antibodies are active between 0 and 4°C. Cold reacting antibodies may have a wider thermal range.

Management

- If the Hb is low to produce symptoms, packed red cell transfusion is required.
- **Glucocorticoids:** 1–2 mg/kg/bw daily till packed cell volume (PCV) is 30% and Hb is more than 10 g/dL and then tapered to a maintenance dose of 20 mg/day.

If the is less than 10 g and PCV < 30%, second line treatment should be started.

Second line treatment

- IVIG in usual doses
- Therapeutic antibodies—rituximab which is a monoclonal antibody to the B cell antigen CD20 dose of rituximab is 375 mg/m² body surface area weekly for 4 weeks
- Splenectomy—remission rate 20–40%
- Danazol
- Immunosuppressants—mycophenolate mofetil, cyclosporine
- Chemotherapy—vincristine, cyclophosphamide or azathioprine
- Bone marrow transplantation.

In practice, Evan's syndrome is a difficult condition to treat and fatalities are common.

INHERITED DISORDERS OF ERYTHROCYTES

Red Cell Membrane Disorders

Hereditary Spherocytosis

Hereditary spherocytosis is the most common inherited disorder of erythrocyte membrane. It is an autosomal dominant disorder presenting as a chronic hemolytic anemia with the presence of spherocytes in peripheral blood, intermittent jaundice and splenomegaly. In 80% cases, family history indicates hereditary involvement.

Pathogenesis: Though the exact molecular lesion in spherocytosis is yet unknown, several alterations in structure and function of the cell membrane have been noticed. These include: (1) Reduction in membrane lipid, (2) increased permeability to sodium and (3) defective phosphorylation of the membrane protein—**spectrin**. Abnormalities in membrane proteins such as spectrin, ankyrin, paladin (protein 4.2) and band 3 have been identified. The spherocytes are erythrocytes which assume a spherical shape due to inability to maintain the normal biconcave shape.

Hereditary spherocytosis is a heterogeneous disorder showing variations in the nature of the protein defect and in the pattern of inheritance. Table 161.3 shows the specific protein defect and the inheritance pattern.

Loss of deformability of the erythrocyte in the circulation and action of an intact spleen together accounts for the hemolysis. Membrane loss in hereditary spherocytosis is associated with the defects in several membrane proteins. The biochemical phenotype of combined spectrin and ankyrin accounts for 40–65%.

Spleen destroys defective erythrocytes. Bone marrow shows erythroid hyperplasia. In long-standing cases, gallstones are common.

Table 161.3: Red blood cell membrane protein abnormalities leading to hereditary spherocytosis

Protein defect	Frequency	Autosomal inheritance	Clinical severity of hemolysis
Spectrin beta chain	± 20%	Dominant	Mild to moderate
Ankyrin defect	Common > 60%	Dominant	Mild to severe
Band 3 defect	Common ± 20%	Dominant	Mild to moderate
Spectrin alpha chain	Rare	Recessive	Severe

Note: Defect of protein 4.1 occurs as a mild autosomal dominant hemolytic disorder in North Africa. Defect of protein 4.2 occurs as a moderate to severe autosomal recessive hemolytic disorder in Japan

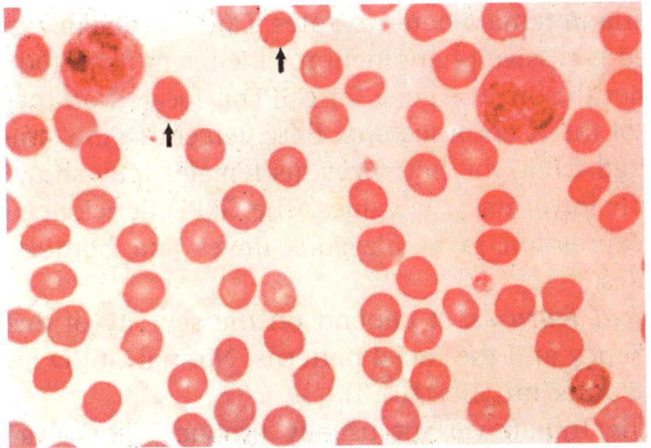

Fig. 161.3: Spherocytosis: peripheral blood. **Note:** The small densely stained RBCs (spherocytes)—(arrows)

Clinical Manifestations

In vast majority, the condition presents in the second and third decades with mild hemolytic anemia and recurrent jaundice. Occasionally, it may manifest as persistent anemia and failure to thrive in infants. Many cases remain asymptomatic throughout life. Hemolytic and aplastic crises may occur from time-to-time. Aplastic crisis are caused by parvovirus B_{19}. Megaloblastic crisis may occur at times. Extreme cases may present as neonatal hyperbilirubinemia requiring exchange transfusion.

Laboratory Findings

Hb level is usually 8–10 g/dL. Reticulocyte count ranges from 5 to 20%. Over 30% of erythrocytes in the peripheral blood are spherocytes (Fig. 161.3). They are smaller in diameter, thicker and appear uniformly stained with loss of the central pallor. Mean corpuscular volume is increased.

The osmotic fragility is increased. Normal osmotic fragility in hypotonic saline starts at 0.4–0.35% and is complete at 0.35%. In a classic case of spherocytosis, osmotic fragility starts at about 0.6% and is complete by 0.5%. In 25% of cases, osmotic fragility may be normal. When the red cells are incubated at 37°C for 24 hours, the osmotic fragility increases. This is a reliable test for hereditary spherocytosis. When there is concomitant presence of iron deficiency, recovery from aplastic anemia and obstructive jaundice, osmotic fragility is not increased Autohemolysis occurs in stored blood and this is corrected by the addition of glucose or adenosine triphosphate (ATP). Coombs' test is negative.

Diagnosis

Recurrent anemia, jaundice, splenomegaly, and spherocytosis should suggest this diagnosis, though spherocytosis may occur in other types of hemolytic anemias also as an acquired defect. Occurrence of spherocytosis and hemolysis in siblings or parents strengthens the diagnosis. In addition, demonstration of autohemolysis and its correction by glucose or ATP are diagnostic, since these tests are specific for hereditary spherocytosis.

Flow cytometry has been found to be a good tool to detect hereditary spherocytosis.

Hereditary spherocytosis may be associated with other genetic disorders which complicate the clinical picture. It may coexist with thalassemia and Gilbert's disease in which cases thalassemia is more severe. Aplastic crisis or megaloblastic crisis may occur. Stomatocytosis may be present in addition to spherocytosis. Differential diagnosis includes AIHA, congenital dyserythropoiesis type 2 and hereditary stomatocytosis.

Treatment

Hereditary spherocytosis is functionally curable by splenectomy in almost all cases. Poor response to splenectomy or relapse suggests a wrong diagnosis or development of accessory splenic tissue. Children have a higher tendency to develop pneumococcal and other types of septicemia after splenectomy and therefore, splenectomy should be avoided in children below 10 years of age. In some intractable cases, splenectomy may have to be done but this should be preceded by pneumococcal vaccination and prophylactic penicillin therapy when infections are likely to occur. Target cells appear in peripheral blood after splenectomy (Fig. 161.4).

Other Red Cell Membrane Disorders

Hereditary Elliptocytosis

This is a specific autosomal dominant disorder where mild or moderately severe hemolysis occurs, but may remain unnoticed in about 90% cases. The clinical presentation may resemble that of hereditary spherocytosis. Almost all the red cells are elliptical in shape (elliptocytes) (Fig. 161.5). This confirms the diagnosis. Diminished spectrin interactions, deficiencies or dysfunction of protein 4.1 and glycophorin deficiency have been identified. Treatment is symptomatic. Results of splenectomy are unpredictable. The term hereditary pyropoikilocytosis is given to a condition of double heterozygous inheritance

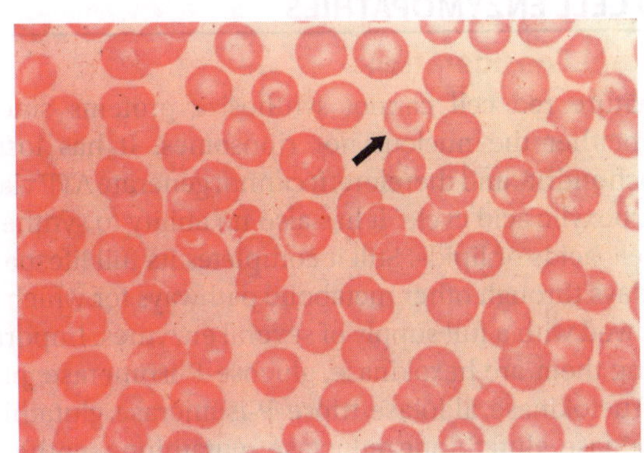

Fig. 161.4: Peripheral blood-post postsplenectomy. **Note:** Target cells (arrow)

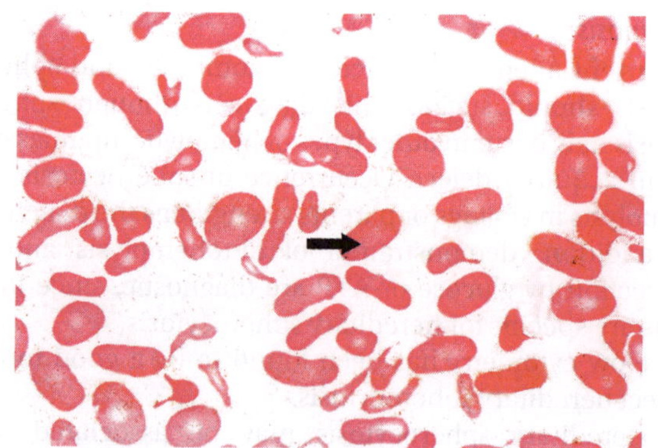

Fig. 161.5: Ovalocytosis peripheral blood × 1000 (elliptocytosis). **Note:** The oval erythrocytes (arrow)

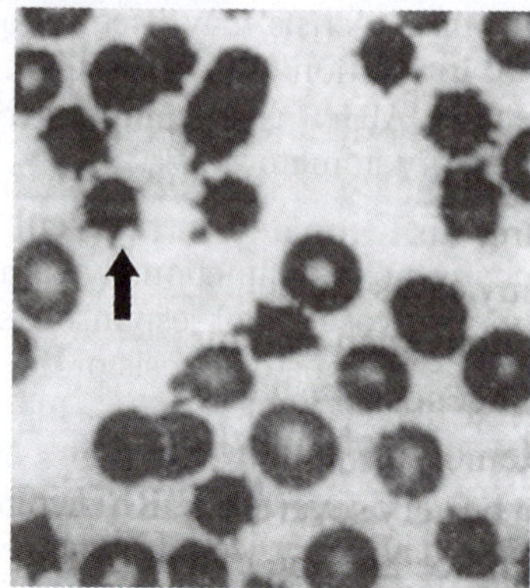

Fig. 161.6: Acanthocytes (arrow)

of elliptocytosis which may manifest as a most severe hemolytic anemia.

Acanthocytosis: They are abnormal erythrocytes showing projections of variable width and length on their surface. They are seen in abetalipoproteinemia and severe liver disorders (Fig. 161.6). Both hereditary and acquired conditions may present with acanthocytes.

Conditions Producing Stomatocytosis

Recessive hereditary stomatocytosis due to homozygous mutation in protein 4:2 gene is common in Japan but not in other countries. These show ovalocytes and stomatocytes in addition to spherocytes.

Rh deficiency syndrome: In the absence or deficiency of Rh antigen expression. Peripheral blood shows stomatocytes and occurrence of hemolysis.

RED CELL ENZYMOPATHIES

General Considerations

A mature red cell cannot synthesize proteins since it has neither the nucleus nor ribosomes. It has lost its mitochondria, and therefore, it cannot generate ATP via the tricarboxylic acid cycle. It has also no ability to synthesize nucleic acids or lipids. Still it completes its full lifespan of 120 days through other metabolic pathways for which it is endowed with a full supply of several enzymes. Important among them are hexokinase, glucose-P-isomerase, phosphofructokinase, aldolase, triose-P-isomerase, glutathione peroxidase, glutathione reductase, glutathione synthetase, glucose-6-phosphate dehydrogenase (G6PD) and many others. Most enzymopathies are inherited in an autosomal

recessive manner but some are sex-linked or autosomal dominant. Hemolytic anemias caused by enzymopathies are also known as ***hereditary nonspherocytic hemolytic anemias***.

Glucose-6-Phosphate Dehydrogenase Deficiency

Prevalence: G6PD deficiency is prevalent in different parts of the world, commonly in the Mediterranean population. In India, the incidence varies from 1 to 2% in different ethnic groups, the highest incidence being in Naga Tribals, Parsees and others. Three common variants of G6PD have been identified. These are G6PD Kerala, G6PD West Bengal and G6PD Jammu. At present, over 400 isoenzymes of G6PD have been recognized. G6PD deficiency gives partial protection against falciparum malaria in female heterozygotes. G6PD deficiency is sex-linked recessive phenomenon which is transmitted from mother to son. The gene for G6PD is located on the long arm of the X chromosome. Fifty percent of the sons are affected while the heterozygous females may show only slightly lower enzyme values. The G6PD deficiency finds full expression in hemizygous males and homozygous females.

Clinical features: It depend on the severity of enzyme deficiency and the racial patterns. Normal G6PD level is 12–18 units/mL (Box 161.3).

The Indian variant usually produces hemolysis on exposure to several drugs and infections. Drug-induced hemolysis may present as a life-threatening disorder in such subjects. Rarely neonatal jaundice may occur—icterus neonatorum.

Common Drugs Causing Hemolysis in G6PD Deficiency

Antimalarials	Quinine, primaquine, chloroquine, mepacrine and the newer anit-hypnozoite drugs for malaria
Sulfa group	Sulfanilamide, sulfapyridine, acetylsulfanilamide, sulfacetamide, sulfafurazole, thiazosulfone, salazosulfapyridine, aldesulfone sodium, sulfamethoxypyridazine, cotrimoxazole
Analgesics	Acetanilide, acetylsalicylic acid, phenacetin, phenazone, aminophenazone
Other drugs	Furozolidone, nitrofurantoin, chloramphenicol, para-aminosalicylic acid, naphthalene, vitamin K, probenecid, quinidine, trinitrotoluene, methylene blue, dimercaprol, phenylhydrazine

In addition, several articles of food may precipitate hemolysis, e.g. fava beans.

Box 161.3:	Clinical severity of glucose-6-phosphate dehydrogenase (G6PD) deficiency disorders
Class I	Enzyme activity is below 10% and these results in chronic hemolysis
Class II	Enzyme activity is below 10% but there is no chronic hemolysis, e.g. G6PD B
Class III	Functional activity 10–60%. Here hemolysis occurs only after exposure to drugs or infections, e.g. G6PD A
Class IV	Normal functional activity
Class V	Increased activity

Classes IV and V are of no clinical significance.

Clinical Features

The subjects carrying the enzyme defect do not show any evidence of disease but exposure to oxidant drugs and/or infection may lead to hemolysis. Drug-induced hemolysis starts 24–72 hours after administration of the drug. Urine is dark and jaundice may be present. Hemolysis stops when the drug is withdrawn and the Hb level improves. Sometimes spontaneous arrest of hemolysis occurs even when the drug is continued. Babies with G6PD deficiency may develop severe icterus neonatorum.

Laboratory findings

Severe anemia may result. Red cells may show **Heinz bodies** before the onset of hemolysis. These are refractile inclusions which are seen in the erythrocyte in the wet unstained preparation. They are indistinguishable by the Romanowsky stains, since they stain uniformly with the surrounding Hb. Hemoglobinuria may develop and this may result in renal failure. Reticulocytes are increased. Red cell morphology is generally normal. Estimation of the enzyme helps to establish the diagnosis. Since reticulocytes are generally rich in G6PD, the enzyme activity may be normal in the presence of active reticulocytosis. In such cases the enzyme assay should be repeated after the reticulocytosis has subsided.

Course

In the majority of G6PD deficiency patients, it is a self-limiting phenomenon and it tends to subside when G6PD levels increase with the onset of reticulocytosis.

Therapy

Mild cases are self-limiting and demand only withdrawal of the offending drugs. In severe cases, blood transfusion may be required. Renal failure should be managed on its own merits. Subjects who are G6PD deficient should be informed of the condition to prevent further recurrence.

Other important inherited enzymopathies include the following:

Pyruvate kinase deficiency: This is an autosomal recessive disorder with several different mutations of the gene. It also manifests as hemolytic anemia. Splenectomy may benefit some cases.

Triose-phosphate deficiency: This leads to hemolytic anemia as well as neurological defects, cardiomyopathy and susceptibility to infections. Many cases die in childhood.

Red cell enzymopathies should be suspected in children with hemolytic anemia which is not associated with abnormalities of Hb and morphological abnormalities of erythrocytes and absence of antibodies against erythrocytes.

HEMOGLOBINOPATHIES (THALASSEMIAS AND THALASSEMIA SYNDROMES)

General Considerations

Pauling and colleagues identified electrophoretic abnormalities in HbS and coined the term molecular disease in 1949. WHO estimated that 1.5% of world's population might be carriers of β^0/β^+ thalassemia. Sixty thousands severely affected infants are born annually. Considerable amount of studies on various aspects of these diseases is taking place all over the world with frequent interaction among them. The studies on Hb genetics are proceeding in several centers globally at rapid paces and since 1978, leading research groups meet at the 'Hemoglobin Switching Conference' to report and discuss developments once in 2 years.

Hemoglobinopathies are among the most widespread genetic disorders seen in humans. The Hb in normal individuals is made up of three components. These are HbA_1 (94–97%), HbA_2 (1–3.5%) and HbF (0–2%). During fetal life, HbF is the main Hb and it is replaced by HbA within the first six months of life. This transformation is under genetic control. Failure of formation of adult Hb to replace the fetal Hb results in thalassemias.

The Hb molecule is made up of heme and globin. Chemical changes in the heme lead to the production of methemoglobin, sulfhemoglobin (SulfHb) and carboxyhemoglobin. The globin contains four polypeptide chains. The polypeptide chains are alpha, beta, gamma and delta. HbA_1 has 2 alpha and 2 beta, HbF has 2 alpha and 2 gamma and HbA_2 has 2 alpha and 2 delta chains. The genes for beta, gamma and delta chains are located in a closely linked cluster on the short arm of chromosome 11. Alpha and beta chains are produced on separate ribosomes in nearly equal amounts. Each polypeptide chain has a specific amino acid constitution. When the sequential order of amino acids is altered or the chain is altered by deletion or addition, abnormal Hb are formed. For example, substitution of valine for glutamic acid at sixth residue of beta chain results in the formation of HbS and lysine for glutamic acid results in formation of HbC. Such alterations result in the change of electrical charge of the molecule and consequently the electrophoretic mobility alters. This property enables these abnormal Hb to be separated by electrophoresis. Abnormal Hb and thalassemias are inherited as autosomal dominant trait, but their expressivity and penetrance vary considerably. This factor accounts for the very heterogeneous mode of transmission. Many authors consider that inheritance of abnormal Hb may clinically resemble that of autosomal recessives. Variants of HbA have been identified.

Hemoglobinopathy in India

Several Hb variants are encountered in India. These are Hbs D, E, F, H, I, J, K, L, M, S, Q, Norfolk and Lepore. Of these, prevalence of Hb S, E, D, J, K, and Q have been studied in detail in population groups. HbS is found mostly in the tribals. HbE is seen in Bengal and Assam; Hbs D, J, and K are seen in *Punjabis* and *Gujaratis* and HbQ is seen in *Sindhis*. Among these only HbS and HbE are widely prevalent. The sickle cell gene is widespread in India. In some tribal populations, the frequency is up to 45%. HbC is not reported from India.

The cumulative gene frequency for HbS, E and D in India is 5.45. For HbS it is 4.5, for HbD it is 0.86, and for HbE in the northern states it is 10.9. In Wynad district of Kerala, *Kurumas, Paniyas, Adiyas* and *Wynad Chettys* have HbS disease. Hbs has been detected to be prevalent among the tribals in Attapadi tribal belt of Kerala. The disease is mild in 52.2% of cases. Crisis occurs in 43% of cases. Splenomegaly and leg ulcers occur with a frequency of 4.3% in these tribes.

Source: Balgir RS. Genetic epidemiology of the three predominant abnormal hemoglobins in India. J Assocn Phys India. 1996;44(1):25–8.

Sickle cell β⁺ thalassemia has HbA levels of 20-30% whereas sickle cell β⁰ thalassemia has only much lower levels of HbA and therefore the former is less severe. Sickle cell β⁺ thalassemia and sickle cell HbC disease tend to be milder than sickle cell anemia.

Inheritance Pattern

If both parents carry one each HbS gene, 25% of children develop SS disease and the others will be heterozygous for S. All pregnancies carry the same risk. If one parent is SS and the other is heterozygous (AS), the risk of having SS for the offspring is doubled. The study of the structure of DNA flanking the beta-globin locus has helped to classify population groups who possess the HbS gene. The genetic constitution of HbS patients in India belongs to the Asian haplotype. This is the same seen in eastern Saudi Arabia too.

Hemoglobinopathies lead to physical and chemical alterations in the function of the Hb molecule depending on the site and nature of the amino acid substitution. Many lead to hemolytic anemia, e.g. HbS. Substitution of certain nonpolar amino acids within the Hb molecule makes it unstable so that even in the heterozygous state it leads to hemolytic anemia. Certain substitutions lead to congenital methemoglobinemia.

Some substitutions lead to increased affinity of the Hb to oxygen and this prevents the release of oxygen to the tissues. Tissue anoxia leads to polycythemia. Abnormal Hbs can be separated by electrophoresis in suitable buffers. In comparison with the mobility of HbA, they can be classified as slow moving, fast moving and very fast moving types as given below.

Electrophoretic mobility at pH 8.6		
Very fast	H group	H, I, Barts
Fast	J group	J, K, No, Norfolk
Normal	A group	A, M, F
	G group	G, L, P, Q
Slow	S group	S, D, Stanville-2, Lepore
	C group	C, E, A₂, O, F, Alexandra

Sickle Cell Disease

It is one of the most common monogenic disorders in the world and is the most widespread hemoglobinopathy. Sickle cell anemia has been recognized as a global public health problem by the UN and WHO in 2010. In India, more than 25,000 neonates are born with SSHb disease. Weatherall, Herald and colleagues estimated that about 2,16,000 babies were born in Africa with sickle cell anemia and between 60,000 and 100,000 outside Africa.

Sickle-shaped red cells were first described by Harrick in 1902. Sickle cell disease is the most widespread hemoglobinopathy in India. Though nationwide epidemiological data is not available for India, it is known to be widely prevalent in many areas, particular communities being affected. Many tribal populations of Tamil Nadu, Assam, Andhra Pradesh, Orissa, Madhya Pradesh, Kerala (particularly *Paniyas*), Maharashtra and all other states do suffer from the disease. Occurrence among high caste population in Kerala has also been reported. HbS may constitute more than 50% of the contents of the red cell.

Sickle Cell Anemia

Homozygous sickle cell disease: It leads to sickle cell anemia. In sickle cell trait the condition is heterozygous and the levels of HbS are much lower. HbS offers partial protection against falciparum malaria **(balanced polymorphism)** accounting for the persistence and relative increase in HbS hemoglobinopathy in regions has high prevalence of falciparum malaria.

The genetic variants are:

Sickle cell anemia	Homozygous SS
Sickle cell trait	Heterozygous AS
HbS-thalassemia	Heterozygosity between HbS and thalassemia Thalassemias may be B⁰ or B⁺ HbS + B⁰ has severe manifestations whereas HbS + B⁺ give rise to milder manifestations
HbS-C disease	Heterozygosity between S and C
HbS-D disease	Heterozygosity between S and D
HbS with hereditary	The clinical manifestations are milder persistence of fetal hemoglobin

Pathology

HbS is formed by the substitution of valine in place of glutamic acid in the sixth residue of the beta chain of adult Hb and it is slow-moving Hb. Oxygenated HbS is normally soluble and the erythrocyte carrying it behaves normally. On deoxygenation, the abnormal hydrophobic valine becomes exposed. On encountering another deoxygenated HbS molecule, polymerization occurs at an explosive rate. Higher concentration of HbS and low pH favor polymerization. This leads to change of shape of the erythrocyte—sickling. The erythrocyte loses its deformability due to stiffening.

On reoxygenation, the polymerized HbS promptly fall apart instantaneously.

The polymerization of HbS is central to the pathogenesis of the disease. Polymerization which occurs in anoxic environment stiffens the sickled erythrocytes, changing it from a flexible and deformable biconcave disk to an unyielding obstacle that blocks the circulation leading to the anoxic and nutritional damage to distal tissues. The polymerized HbS forms liquid crystals (tactoids) which distort the erythrocytes and make them assume the sickle shape (Figs 161.7A and B).

Only deoxygenated HbS polymerizes. On reoxygenation the processes are promptly reversed. Organs with relatively sluggish circulation, high level of oxygen extraction and low pH such as the spleen and bone marrow are the most vulnerable to polymerization and anoxic damage. Vaso-occlusion and tissue ischemia are caused by other factors as well, which are triggered by sickling and adhesion of erythrocytes. These include interaction between erythrocytes, endothelium, platelets, leukocytes

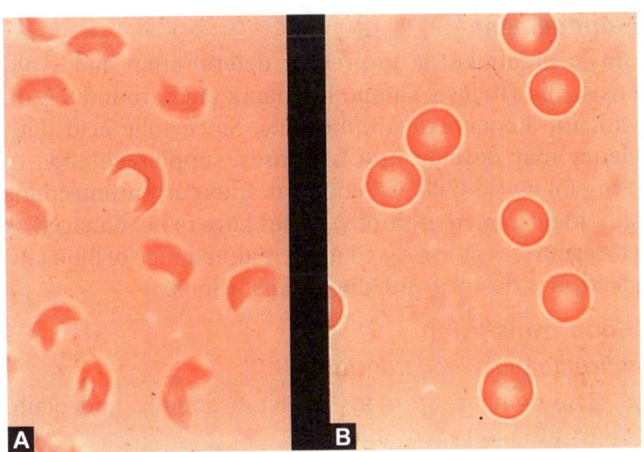

Figs 161.7A and B: Sickle cell anemia (HbS). **A.** Sickling (arrow); **B.** Oxygenated blood

and plasma factors. Endothelial dysfunction also plays a major role in the final outcome of vaso-occlusion. High molecular weight von Willebrand's factor favors adhesion of red cells and platelets to endothelium. Reticulocytes release free oxygen radicals which lead to endothelial damage and further changes. These pathological changes are most marked in SS disease. They are milder in HbS-β⁺ thalassemias and HbS⁺ persistence of HbF.

The painful episodes in the spleen and bones are caused by anoxic infarction. As a result of repeated infarcts the spleen may shrink and become functionless (autosplenectomy). In the bone marrow periodic infarction leads to fat necrosis and fat embolism and embolization in the lungs is one of the precipitating factors for acute chest syndrome.

Normally the lung is the depolymerizing organ which protects the arterial side of the circulation from blockage by sickled erythrocytes.

Vaso-occlusion by sickle cells is a two step process that begins with adhesion of red cells to endothelium, probably in the postcapillary venules. This is followed by a propagation phase caused by accumulation of poorly deformable red cells behind the site of adhesion.

In addition to the abnormalities in sickled red cells, several other factors also favor their adhesion to the endothelium. These include endothelial injury caused by release of cytokines liberated by granulocytes, thrombospondin released by activated platelets leading to adhesion, and the influence of young reticulocytes called 'stress reticulocytes'. These cells express adhesive ligands that facilitate interaction between sickle cells and endothelial cells. Expression of adhesion receptors on endothelial cells is accelerated by hypoxia, thrombin, tissue necrosis factor, platelet activating factor and interleukin-1 (IL-1). Among the various hemolytic anemias, the vaso-occlusive component in sickle cell anemia is unique.

Lifespan of the erythrocyte is reduced to 10–12% of normal. A new equilibrium with Hb around 6–9 g/dL and reticulocytes forming 10–15% gets established.

Sickled cells are easily destroyed and this leads to hemolytic anemia. Factors which precipitate sickling are hypoxia, acidosis, dehydration, fever and infections. Occlusion of the microcirculation resulting from sickling aggravates acidosis further, thereby establishing a vicious circle. Maximal lesions are seen in the heart, lungs, spleen, bone marrow, brain and placenta. Pulmonary hypertension (PH) demonstrable by Doppler studies is common in adults with sickle cell disease. Hemolysis seems to be the causative factor, stimulating procoagulant activity leading on to microvasculopathy and thrombosis. Primary pulmonary hypertension (PPH) is also not uncommon. Presence of PH confers higher mortality.

Obstruction of the microcirculation of the bone marrow leads to ischemic necrosis, marrow embolism and fibrosis. Priapism occurs due to occlusion of the corpora of the penis. This may be persistent, painful and troublesome. Retinitis proliferans may develop in children.

In HbS-thalassemia, presence of large amounts of HbF protects against sickling.

Clinical Features

Most of the clinical features can be explained on the basis of anemia, hemolysis, obstruction to microcirculation and siderosis of parenchymal organs. Sickle cell disease may present in different ways, with a wide spectrum ranging from subclinical cases to mild, moderate and severe manifestations. The child may appear normal at birth. The disease becomes evident after six months of age, by which time; normally adult Hb takes over completely from HbF. The defects in the synthesis of the chains are manifest by this period. Severe cases of HbS disease have higher neonatal and perinatal mortality due to pneumococcal infections. Untreated, severe cases die within 10 years. When the disease is severe, growth is retarded with delay in skeletal maturation giving rise to the characteristic picture of stunted growth, long limbs, narrow hips and exaggerated lordosis. Anemia, mild or moderate splenomegaly, swelling of fingers and a characteristic appearance develop.

Sickling crises supervene frequently involving several organs, and untreated cases are fatal before the third decade. This extreme form is more common in Negros and many tribals. In mild cases there may be only mild anemia, growth and development being normal. This variety is more common in the Middle East. In India, the cases show an intermediate severity.

Splenic sequestration syndrome is characterized by sudden painful splenomegaly associated with rapid fall in Hb and hypotension. This is seen more frequently in children. The condition may be fatal if left untreated. As a result of repeated infarction, the spleen may shrink and be converted into a fibrous streak. This is referred to as ***autosplenectomy***. The infarcts may become calcified. The spleen becomes impalpable in sickle cell anemia by the age of 10–12 years. In other sickle cell syndromes such as S-thalassemia, S-C and S-D, the spleen remains palpable throughout life.

Acute Chest Syndrome

Three major causes of the acute chest syndrome include pulmonary infection, embolization of bone marrow fat and intravascular sequestration of sickled erythrocytes in pulmonary capillaries. Necrosis of bone marrow leads to embolization of its contents—fat, cells and even bony spicules leading to acute PH, severe lung inflammation and hypoxemia. Pulmonary infarction occurs. Free Hb leads to resistance to nitrous oxide and triggers vasculopathy.

Pulmonary Hypertension

Both acute and chronic develops in sickle cell anemia leading to further cardiac complications and increasing mortality. The PH may resemble PPH as well as thrombo-embolic PH due to bone marrow embolism, platelet activation and tissue factor activation.

Source: Gladwin MT, Vichinsky E. Pulmonary complications of sickle cell disease. New Eng J Med. 2008;359(21):2254-65.

Renal involvement manifests as hematuria, hyposthenuria, acute nephritis or occasionally nephrotic syndrome. *Priapism* may occur due to obstruction to corpora cavernosa. *Skeletal symptoms* are common. These include bone pain, arthralgia, backache, dactylitis, salmonella osteomyelitis and multiple bone infarcts. *Dactylitis* is seen in young children. The femoral and humeral heads may undergo avascular necrosis. Neurovascular accidents develop due to occlusion of intracranial vessels.

Stroke is a very disabling complication occurring in 10% of patients annually. This occurs around the age of 10–20 years and this confines them to a life of morbidity up to the age of 30. *Blindness* may develop due to repeated vitreous hemorrhages, and retinal tears and detachment. *Aplastic crisis* occur rarely and it is characterized by rapid development of severe anemia due to marrow hypoplasia and accelerated hemolysis is usually the result of parvovirus B19 infection. It is self-limiting if the crisis is tided over.

Complications

Include anemia with Hb levels below 6 g/dL, cholelithiasis, aplastic crisis, sickling crisis, acute chest syndrome, stroke, infections by *Str. pneumoniae, E. coli* and gram-positive cocci, Salmonella osteomyelitis and adverse effects of repeated blood transfusion.

Diagnosis: In endemic areas, the clinical diagnosis can be easily confirmed by demonstrating the sickling phenomenon. One drop of blood is mixed with an equal volume of 2% sodium metabisulfite solution. A cover slip is applied and the edges are sealed with vaseline. After incubation at 37° for 30 minutes, sickle cells are demonstrable. Sickling may occur with other Hbs also in some cases, e.g. HbC group and Hb Barts. Electrophoresis of Hb at pH 8.6 shows HbS as a slow-moving band.

Course and prognosis: Majority of severe cases die in childhood before reaching five years of age. Only one-fourth live up to 30 years or more. Acute splenic sequestration, chest syndrome, septicemia, meningitis, stroke and gastroenteritis account for most of the morbidity and deaths. Pregnancy carries increased risk to mother and fetus. By proper transfusions and chelation therapy, the risk of stroke can be reduced to 1% annually. Proper transfusion therapy even helps to reduce the narrowing of the cerebral blood vessels. Those with lower levels of HbS develop painful crises and chest syndrome and they may live up to 40–45 years.

Cases with thalassemia with higher levels of HbF live up to 40 years or more and may have only minor episodes of crisis. Their transfusion requirements are also low.

Management

Aim of treatment is to prevent deterioration and avoid crisis. The Hb level should be maintained around 8 g/dL with the hematocrit around 25%. Since folic acid deficiency may develop in a few cases, supplementation of 1 mg folic acid daily is beneficial. Intercurrent infections should be treated promptly. Crises have to be managed as emergencies with rest, sedation, maintenance of fluid and electrolyte balance and blood transfusions.

Blood Transfusion

Indications for blood transfusion

- Symptomatic episodes of acute anemia and acute sequestration syndromes
- Prevention of recurrent strokes in children
- Surgery, eye complications.

The aim of transfusion is to raise the general level of Hb and also reduce the relative proportion of HbS to below 30%. Partial exchange transfusion may be needed during hemolytic or sickling crises if other methods fail.

In severe cases, exchange transfusions and simple transfusions in milder cases are life-saving. In case of stroke, exchange transfusion should be adequate to lower HbS level below 30%. Follow up transfusions to prevent rise of HbS above 30% are required. Packed cell transfusions are preferable. The transfused packed cells should be sickle cell negative and preferably leukocyte depleted.

Priapism can be managed by packed cell transfusion and alpha adrenergic agonists like terbutaline. Surgery may be required in resistant cases. Iron overload occurs and this has to be treated with iron chelating agents. This is detailed on p 51.

Hydroxyurea (hydroxycarbamide) given in a dose of 500 mg bd orally improves the production of HbF and this helps to reduce the frequency and severity of sickling crisis. Reduction in level of neutrophils and platelets reduces the adhesion of sickled cells to vascular endothelium. The drug also reduces the frequency and severity of painful episodes, hospitalization, chest syndrome and need for transfusions. Increasing the level of HbF is the most widely studied method to prevent sickling. In addition to hydroxyurea, 5-azacytidine, decitabine, erythropoietin, short chain fatty acid like valproic acid and others are also active in this respect.

Sickling is precipitated by cellular dehydration caused by injury to cell membrane. Substances which modulate the ion transport systems of RBC membrane have been tried. Such drugs include **clotrimazole** and **magnesium pidolate**. Nitric oxide (NO) has shown antisickling activity. A drug which improves blood flow in the microcirculation is **polaxamer**, which a copolymer surfactant copolymer.

Bone marrow transplantation (BMT) is curative in over 70% of cases and this is the only modality which is curative. It is ideal if suitable donors are available. Transplantation of cord blood stem cells is an alternative.

Gene therapy has been tried with success; but the progress has been slow. These forms of treatment are available in a few centers in India.

Prophylactic measures: These include: (1) Screening of babies born to carriers of HbS, with a view to make an early diagnosis and prevent crises, (2) detection of an affected fetus by amniocentesis and termination of the pregnancy and (3) genetic counseling to avoid marriage between heterozygotes.

Since pneumococcal infection leads to septicemia, meningitis and pneumonia in children with sickle cell disease, long-term penicillin prophylaxis has been tried. Oral penicillin (penicillin V potassium) given in a dose of 125 mg bd introduced before four months of age prevents infection and reduces morbidity and mortality. *Pneumococcal infection* is common to produce crisis in sickle cell anemia and therefore antipneumococcal vaccination should be given.

Hemoglobin E Disease

This is the common hemoglobinopathy in the eastern parts of India, specially Bengal and Assam. HbE results from the substitution of an amino acid β 26GU→Lys in Hb. The disease may exist in the homozygous and heterozygous states and also as HbE-thalassemia. HbE disease causes mild anemia even in the homozygous state, but the HbE β-thalassemia gives rise to severe anemia, splenomegaly and jaundice.

THALASSEMIAS

In normal intrauterine life, fetal Hb made up of alpha and gamma polypeptide chains constitutes more than 95% of the total. After birth, there is a switch over to beta globin chains which are produced in progressively increasing amounts, substituting gamma chains, thereby giving rise to the transition from HbF to HbA by the age of six months. Fetal Hb is not as efficient as adult Hb for oxygen transport in postnatal life, though it is ideally suited for the intrauterine environment.

Thalassemias are genetic disorders in which the synthesis of normal polypeptide chains forming adult Hb is suppressed. Though the adult Hb level does not come up, the production of gamma chains subsides, and therefore, the absolute level of HbF falls even though its level may be proportionately higher.

Selective deficiency of one or more polypeptide chains has two consequences.

- Reduction in Hb leading to anemia and exaggerated erythropoiesis.
- Imbalance between alpha and non-alpha chains, which is even more dangerous. In the absence of the complementary globin chains, the normally produced chains form aggregates precipitate within the cytoplasm, damage cell membranes and leads to premature destruction of cells. In β-thalassemias where β-chains are not formed normally, α-chains are in excess, and they precipitate in the erythroid precursors to form structures similar to Heinz bodies. True Heinz bodies contain denatured Hb (α 2-β 2) whereas the precipitates in beta thalassemia contain only α-chains with some amount of attached heme. In an ordinary case of β-thalassemia, only 15–30% of cells escape destruction in the marrow. The condition manifests with varying degrees of severity. In decreasing order of severity, they may be classified as *thalassemia major, thalassemia intermedia, thalassemia minor* and *thalassemia minima*.

β-thalassemia major	In this there are major clinical abnormalities with profound anemia
β-thalassemia intermedia	Anemia is not so severe as to necessitate regular blood transfusion
β-thalassemia minor	This is seen in parents of children with thalassemia major who have genetic abnormalities and morphological abnormalities in erythrocytes but no anemia
β-thalassemia minima	This is the condition in which the person who is an obligate carrier of the abnormal gene manifests neither anemia nor abnormal erythrocyte morphology

Another scheme of nomenclature takes into account the polypeptide chain involved. The condition is designated α or β-thalassemia if the synthesis of α chain or β-chain is depressed respectively. In some cases of β-thalassemia, the adjacent δ chain gene is also affected and this gives rise to δ-β-thalassemia.

Several genetic mechanisms have been shown to be responsible for thalassemia. These are gene deletion, gene loss due to unequal crossover, defective transcription of messenger ribonucleic acid (mRNA), unstable mRNA and nucleotide mutation leading to premature termination of polypeptide chain synthesis. More than 100 different mutations have been identified giving rise to thalassemia, and therefore, genetically and clinically the disease has a highly varied presentation. The single nucleotide mutation produces defects in transcription, RNA splicing and modification and abnormalities of translation, in β-thalassemia either no β-chains are produced (β°) or β-chain production is only impaired (β–). In α-thalassemia there are two main abnormal forms. In α+ thalassemia there is deletion of only one α-chain gene, and therefore, some amount of alpha chains are produced. In α° thalassemia both α-chain genes are deleted and therefore there is no α-chain formation. In the homozygous state only γ-chains are produced. The γ-chains combine with each other to form Hb Barts ($\gamma 4$). In the heterozygous form some α-chains are produced. Excessive production of β-chains without corresponding production of α-chains leads to formation of tetramers of β-chainsHb-H ($\beta 4$). Interaction of the genes for abnormal Hbs and thalassemia gives rise to heterozygous states showing the characteristics of both. Homozygous thalassemia presents as a severe hemolytic anemia, whereas in the heterozygous state β-thalassemia is asymptomatic or only mildly symptomatic. It is β-thalassemia which is most commonly seen in India.

Pathophysiology of Thalassemia

Defects in synthesis of one globin chain leads to excess of the unpaired other globin chain leading to unpaired chain precipitation and membrane damage (Flowchart 161.1).

Molecular Genetics of Hemoglobinopathies

Genetic loci on chromosome 16 controls α-like globins and genetic loci on chromosome 11 control β–like globins. These are acted on by other genes which promote, inhibit, or alter the expression of the various globin chains. Mutations which abolish expression of β globin chains lead to β° thalassemia. Those in which β globin chains are only diminished, result in β⁻ thalassemia. Structural variations in β globin expression (β^e) can also lead to

Flowchart 161.1: Pathophysiology of thalassemia

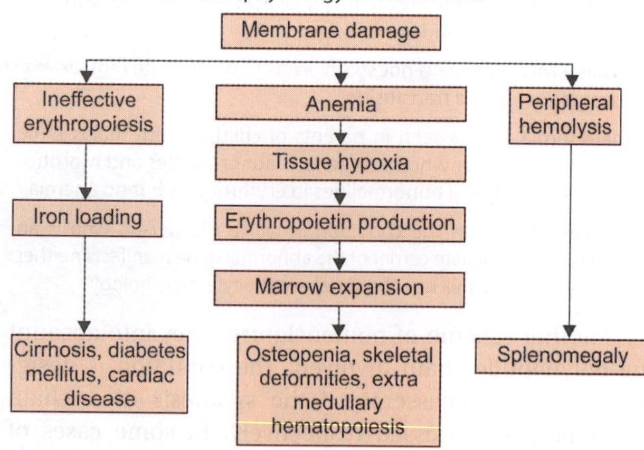

thalassemic effects since their interaction with β° and β⁻ thalassemias can result in many forms of severe β thalassemias (β^E β^1).

Mutations which promote γ-globin expression lead to increased production of HbF as occurring in hereditary persistence of fetal HB (HPFH). Several genome wide association studies (GWAS) have revealed that several factors can regulate the pattern of globin–gene expression. More than 200 β-thalassemia alleles have been described in the database of human Hb variants and thalassemias. In severe cases of thalassemias erythropoiesis is ineffective since many of the precursors fail to reach maturity.

Beta Thalassemia Major

Syn: Cooley's anemia

Also known as homozygous β-thalassemia, this is the most severe form of thalassemia, and is reported from all parts of India. In homozygous β° thalassemia, there is no synthesis of β-chains, while in homozygous β⁺ thalassemia, β-chains are present, but only in small amounts. In most cases the formation of γ-chains is also reduced.

Pathogenesis: Due to the absence of β-chain synthesis, the α-chains which are in excess are precipitated to form inclusions within the erythroid precursors. These α-globin inclusions lead to impairment of erythroid cell replication, membrane function, migration from bone marrow and red cell survival. Such cells are selectively destroyed in the bone marrow. Erythropoiesis becomes ineffective and this, in turn, stimulates further erythropoiesis.

The relative excess of α-chains determines the clinical severity. In those cases in which production of gamma chains continues, some of the alpha chains combine with them to form fetal Hb and such cases are clinically less severe.

Hyperplasia of erythroid marrow leads to skeletal changes, thalassemic facies, increased cardiac output, hyperdynamic heart failure, arthralgia and recurrent fractures. Because of diversion of a major part of the cardiac output to the marrow and consequent hypoperfusion of other parts, muscular development is poor.

There is considerable increase in absorption of iron from the intestines and together with iron introduced by blood transfusion, iron-overload results. On an average, 19–21 mg of iron accumulate everyday from both sources. The body stores of iron may reach 40–60 g or above. This leads to deposition of iron in several organs such as liver, pancreas, spleen, gonads, heart, muscles and others. These organs develop hemosiderosis and dysfunction. Secondary diabetes, hypogonadism and skin pigmentation may develop. Cardiac dysfunction and intractable cardiac failure set in later and this is a major cause of death in those cases which live up to adolescence or more. Serum ferritin is raised to very high levels and this indicates the tissue iron load.

By transfusion of 250 mL erythrocytes, 250 mg of elemental iron is introduced into the recipient. The end organ manifestations of iron overload include hepatic cirrhosis, cardiac failure, diabetes mellitus, hypo-pituitarism and hepatocellular carcinoma. These shorten life-expectancy in the same manner as hereditary hemo-chromatosis. Cirrhosis occurs in β-thalassemia when the hepatic iron concentration rises above 15 mg/g (0.268 μmol/g) dry weight.

Clinical Features

The child is quite normal at birth and for the first few weeks or months of life, but anemia appears and gradually increases from the 6 to 24th week. Gross hepatosplenomegaly causes protuberance of the abdomen (Fig. 161.8). The limbs are thin. Overgrowth of malar bones, depression of the nasal bridge, protrusion of the upper row of teeth and bossing of the frontoparietal regions contribute to the ***classic thalassemia (chipmunk) facies***. There is increased susceptibility to infection. Intercurrent infection may be the presenting complaint, anemia being detected incidentally. Anemia and hepatosplenomegaly increase with time. The Hb level is generally 3–4 g/dL on presentation. Erythrocytes are hypochromic and microcytic with the presence of anisopoikilocytosis, schistocytes, target cells, basophilic stippling and normoblasts (*See* Fig. 159.10). Presence of target cells in large numbers is suggestive of the diagnosis. Other features indicating hemolysis are the presence of Howell-Jolly bodies, Cabot's rings and reticulocytosis. Leukocyte count is generally normal but in some cases leukemoid blood picture may occur. Osmotic fragility of red cells is decreased. Marrow is hypercellular with marked erythroid hyperplasia. 'Hair-on-end' appearance on skull X-ray

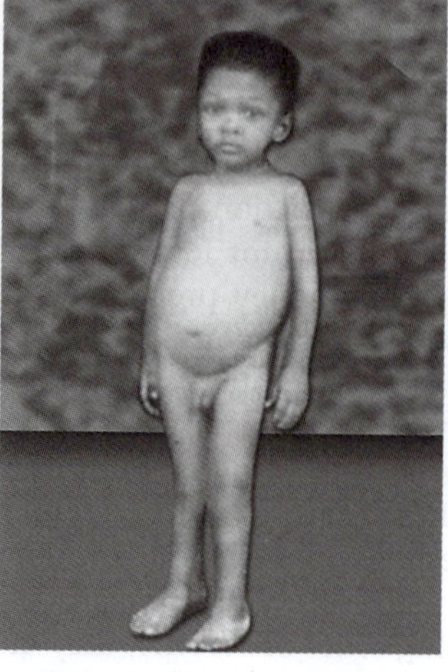

Fig. 161.8: 4-year-old boy (thalassemia major). **Note:** The gross splenomegaly

and thinning and widening of metacarpal shafts indicate enlargement of marrow tissue. Primary pulmonary arterial hypertension develops in majority of cases. Main endocrine disturbances include retardation of growth, hypogonadism, osteopenia and osteoporosis. These lead to bone pains and fractures.

Diagnosis

Thalassemia should be looked for in all children showing persistent or progressive anemia, hepatosplenomegaly and the characteristic facies. Positive family history strengthens the diagnosis. Microcytic hypochromic anemia unresponsive to iron therapy and the presence of numerous target cells and other evidences of hemolysis are strongly suggestive of thalassemia.

The diagnosis is established by estimating the fetal Hb level which forms even up to 80% of the total. Fetal Hb is easily estimated by alkali denaturation test. HbA is considerably diminished. HbA_2 may be increased in most of the cases though it can be normal at times. Normal level of HbA_2 in adults ranges from 1.8 to 3.2%. The abnormal Hb are identified by electrophoresis in paper, cellulose acetate or starch block, using appropriate buffer solutions. Further identification is done by studying the polypeptide chains. Genetic characterization is facilitated by gene mapping and DNA splicing techniques or chain synthesis studies using reticulocytes. In iron deficiency anemia which is the most common cause for hypochromic microcytic anemia in India, HbA_2 levels are subnormal. The red cell distribution width (RDW) is small unlike as in iron deficiency anemia in which the RDW is above 17.

Course and prognosis: Children do not survive without adequate blood transfusions. With passage of time hemosiderosis eventually develops. Damage to several organ systems manifests as delayed puberty and maturation, diabetes, cirrhosis of liver and heart failure. Cardiac failure is the result of accumulation of iron in the myocardium and the increased demands caused by anemia. The majority of patients succumb before the age of 20 years. Ferritin levels below 2000 ng/mL indicate better prognosis. Rise in levels of tissue iron in the liver and the heart is associated with poorer prognosis. ***Magnetic susceptimetry*** is a noninvasive method to measure the iron content of the liver. This investigation is not available in India at present.

In addition to the damage done by tissue iron, non-transferrin bound serum iron is highly toxic since it catalyzes the formation of reactive oxygen and leads to tissue damage.

Management

Blood transfusion

Blood transfusion is the mainstay of therapy. If Hb level is maintained above 10.0 g/dL all the time by regular transfusions, erythroid hyperplasia is suppressed. If the treatment is started early, skeletal deformities are prevented and growth and development continue normally. ***Hypertransfusion*** is the use of packed red cell transfusion in doses adequate to keep the Hb above 10 g/dL. This method helps to ensure near-normal growth, physical and mental development and sexual maturity. Splenomegaly, cardiac failure, infective episodes, bone

marrow hyperplasia and hypogonadism can be prevented. The average requirement of packed cells is 200 mL/kg/year. If hypertransfusion is started around 3 years of age, bony deformities can be prevented and near-normal growth ensured. If the program is started after 4 years, the catch-up growth may not be complete. Even in ideally transfused subjects the growth lags behind the ideal due to the ill-effects of iron overload.

Super transfusion programs aim at keeping the Hb level above 14 g/dL. This allows the bone marrow volume to shrink further. Growth pattern also becomes normal. When the Hb rises, intestinal absorption of iron is reduced.

Refinements in transfusion techniques include the following:

- Proper compatibility testing of ABO and RhD and matching for other components of Rh system and Kell system
- Use of packed cells within 7 days of collection: This ensures longer survival
- Phenotypically matched donor
- Use of leukocyte depleted packed red cells, this reduces the incidence of nonhemolytic transfusion reactions
- Use of washed packed red cells, this reduces allergic reactions caused by plasma proteins
- Transfusion of neocytes, which are young red cells selectively harvested and transfused. They have longer *in vivo* survival and therefore the number of transfusions and total annual quantity of packed cells are reduced.

Iron chelation therapy should be started when the serum ferritin levels reach more than 2000 ng/mL.

Transfusional hemosiderosis

One unit of packed erythrocytes (250–300 mL) contains 250–300 mg iron (1mL $\equiv$ mg). Patients who have received >100 units of packed RBCs would have invariably developed iron overload. The ferritin and hemosiderin levels increase, organ dysfunction develops—early glucose intolerance, delay in puberty, cirrhosis, cardiomyopathy pericarditis, pump failure and arrhythmias develop. If untreated, cardiac failure portends death usually within one year. Hence long-term repeated transfusion therapy should be accompanied by institution of iron chelating therapy.

Iron chelating agents

These are employed to mobilize tissue iron from iron stores and eliminate it in urine. The original drug desferrioxamine is in use for over 5 decades. It has to be given parenterally, preferably as continuous subcutaneous infusion lasting for 8–12 hours at night over the abdominal wall or other regions. Infusion pumps are available. The dose is 1.5–2 g (up to 12 g) daily.

Infusions are given 5–6 times a week. Prior administration of 100 mg vitamin C increases the mobilization of iron and its excretion. The drug is available as Desferal in vials and the daily injection costs ' 200–500.

Though generally safe, the adverse effects include local pain and visual and auditory impairment. Posterior capsular cataract may develop in some and it is essential to monitor vision to avoid toxic damage.

Patients with β-thalassemia have fewer cardiac related complications, iron overload and better survival when the serum ferritin is kept below 2500 µg/L or hepatic iron concentration is kept below 15 mg/g dry weight.

Oral iron chelating agent: 1-2-dimethyl-3-hydroxy-pyridin-4-one (deferiprone) is a good chelator of iron. It is available as 0.5 g tablets and it is given an hour before food. The total dose is up to 100 mg/kg bw, the average being 2–3 g/day. In short-term studies, the drug is safe. Concurrent administration of vitamin C enhances iron excretion. This drug chelates iron selectively without leading to loss of calcium, zinc and magnesium. Toxic side effects include agranulocytosis, arthralgia, arthritis and drug-induced lupus erythematosus. Daily elimination of iron in urine may reach up to 36 + 19 mg, if the drug is given daily in a dose of 100 mg/kg bw. The commercial preparation is Deferiprone. The drug is available as Kelfer, 250 and 500 mg tablets.

Long-term observations on this drug show that even though it eliminates iron, accumulation of hepatic iron is not prevented to the same extent as desferrioxamine. Deferiprone removes myocardial iron effectively. When regular therapy with desferrioxamine is not possible due to economic reasons and lack of facilities, deferiprone is the next best alternative. This drug is also expensive, a day's treatment costing more than ₹60.

A newer iron chelating agent is a tridentate orally active iron chelator (ICL670) which is still under trial. When given in a dose of 20 mg/kg bw it is effective and well-tolerated.

Splenectomy is indicated if transfusion requirements exceed 250 mL/kg of packed cells annually.

BMT: Allogeneic BMT done early in the disease before iron accumulation develops, is effective in curing the disease in over 80% of cases when followed up for 3 years or more. If the procedure is done after siderosis of the liver has started, the cure rates are lower. Facilities for BMT are available on a limited scale in India. The cost is around ₹6–10 lacs or more.

Stem cell transplantation

If HLA-matched stem cell transplantation is done before complications and iron overload occurs, success rate is 80–90%. If done in adults after complications have started, success rate falls to less than 70%.

Cord blood transplantation in thalassemia is approaching that of BMT and disease-free survival of up to 90% is achievable. Stem cell transplantation has converted thalassemias a chronic survivable disease with life-expectancy > 50 years.

Gene therapy

Using viral vectors this has been developed and it shows promise in future.

Induced pluripotent stem cells (IPSC)

In 2007, skin fibroblasts were induced and reprogramed to form multipotent cells resembling embryonic stem cells. Research in programing them as hemopoietic stem cells are in progress.

Source: Higgs DR, Engel JD, Stamatoyannopoulos G. Thalassemia. Lancet. 2012;379(9813):373-83.

Considerable interest has developed in recent years to increase contents of fetal Hb so that the severity of the disease may get allayed both in hemoglobinopathies and thalassemias. The aim of drug therapy has been also to increase β globin chain production and suppress α globin chains.

Drugs therapy

- Hydroxy carbamide (hydroxyurea)
- DNA dimethylating agents, azacitidine and decitabine
- Deacetylase inhibitors, sodium butyrate—results are variable.

Work in India and abroad have indicated at least partial reduction in severity of the disease and complications. Studies are progressing.

Attempts have been made to increase the production of gamma chains, with a view to increase the content of fetal Hb. Drugs such as 5-azacytidine, cytarabine and hydroxyurea have been shown to increase the production. At present these methods have not gained universal acceptance, though individual cases they may show benefit.

THALASSEMIA SYNDROMES

In a population where genes for abnormal Hbs and thalassemia are present, random mating gives rise to offspring carrying both the abnormal genes. Such double heterozygocity may lead to HbE thalassemia, HbS thalassemia, and so on. The term thalassemia syndrome is used to include these double heterozygote conditions as well as the classic homozygous thalassemia. The double heterozygote states present with milder manifestations compared to thalassemia major. In such subjects the presence of abnormal Hb as well as the elevation of fetal Hb can be demonstrated by suitable tests.

Lepore Hemoglobins

Lepore Hbs are formed when normal alpha chains combine with chains consisting of the N-terminal residues of Δ chain and G terminal residues of β-chains. Three variants of Hb Lepore have been identified. In the homozygous state, clinical picture is that of Cooley's anemia, the Hb consisting of 75% HbF and 25% Hb Lepore.

Hereditary Persistence of Fetal Hemoglobin

In this condition the gene for HbF persists beyond the neonatal period, resulting in the production of large amounts of HbF throughout life. The hematological picture varies. In homozygous subjects, HbF constitutes 100% and in heterozygotes it forms about 25%. Except for slight morphological abnormalities of erythrocytes, the clinical picture is almost normal. It is important to distinguish them from thalassemia syndromes which have different courses and prognosis.

Prevention: Considerable progress has been achieved in the treatment and prevention of thalassemia. Chorionic biopsy and amniocentesis done during pregnancy help to make accurate prenatal diagnosis in the fetus at risk. Such pregnancies can be terminated. This is done on a wide scale in many countries where thalassemias are rampant.

Other hemoglobinopathies: Several other hemoglobinopathies have been described from time to time in India. Except HbE these are less common and hence not described in this book. The student should refer to larger monographs for further details.

Anemias Characterized by Defective Erythrocyte Production

CHAPTER 162

Anemias Characterized by Defective Erythrocyte Production

Mathew Thomas, KV Krishna Das

Chapter Summary

- Aplastic Anemia
- Special Forms of Aplastic Anemia
  - Fanconi's Anemia
  - Pure Red Cell Aplasia (PRCA)
  - Sideroblastic Anemia
- Paroxysmal Nocturnal Hemoglobinuria (PNH)
  - Venous Thrombosis

APLASTIC ANEMIA

Anemia resulting from failure to produce the formed elements of blood by the bone marrow is called aplastic anemia. Morphologically, in vast majority of cases, the bone marrow is hypocellular or even totally acellular (Fig. 162.1). Generally, all the formed elements are affected; though at times, the affection may be selective. Aplastic anemia can result from either inherited or acquired causes. The incidence of aplastic anemia is, therefore, triphasic with one peak in childhood at 2–5 years (due to inherited causes), and two peaks in adulthood, 20–25 years and majority of patients presenting beyond 55–60 years of age (typically due to acquired causes).

Major Causes of Pancytopenia Secondary to Bone Marrow Failure

Congenital Aplastic Anemia

- Fanconi's anemia (FA)
- Dyskeratosis congenita
- Shwachman-Diamond syndrome
- Amegakaryocytic thrombocytopenia
- Reticular dysgenesis
- Others.

Acquired Aplastic Anemia

- Drugs or chemicals
- Radiation
- Viral infections
- Immune disorders
- Idiopathic
- Paroxysmal nocturnal hemoglobinuria (PNH)
- Hypoplastic myelodysplastic syndromes
- Large granular lymphocytic leukemia.

Classification Based on Pathogenesis

The classification based on pathogenesis is given in Box 162.1.

Aplastic anemia can be defined as absent or diminished hematopoietic precursors in the bone marrow due to an injury to the pluripotent stem cells. Maturing precursor cells and mature cells are easily recognizable under a microscope. But more primitive progenitors and

---

Box 162.1: Classification based on pathogenesis

Congenital
- Fanconi's anemia (FA)
- Diamond-Blackfan anemia
- Telomerase defects

Acquired

Idiopathic
- Acquired defects in stem cell
- Immune-mediated

Secondary
- Chemical agents:
  - Dose-related
    - Cytotoxic drugs (alkylating agents, antimetabolites)
    - Benzene
    - Inorganic arsenicals
    - Chloramphenicol
  - Idiosyncratic
    - Chloramphenicol
    - Phenylbutazone
    - Penicillamine
    - Carbamazepine
    - Gold salts
    - Organic arsenicals
    - Methyl-phenyl-ethyl-hydantoin
- Physical agents: Whole-body irradiation
- Viral infections:
  - Hepatitis (unknown type)
  - EBV infections
  - CMV infections
  - Herpes zoster (varicella zoster)
  - HIV

Abbreviations: EBV = Epstein-Barr virus; CMV = Cytomegalovirus; HIV = Human immunodeficiency virus

Note: Chloramphenicol can produce bone marrow—aplastic anemia by different mechanisms: (1) Idiosyncrasy and (2) direct toxic effect of the precursors.

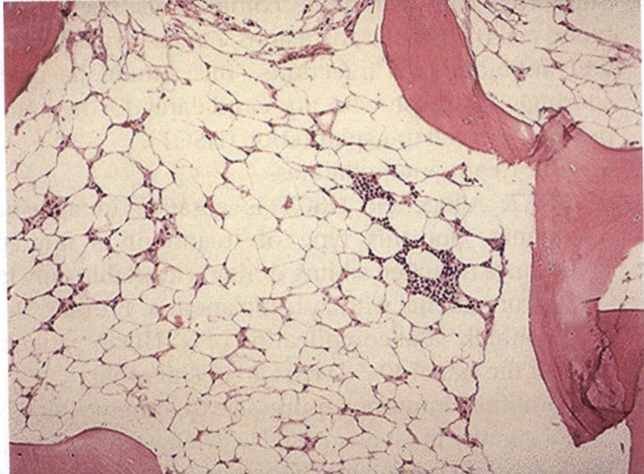

Fig. 162.1: Aplastic anemia with marked hypocellularity of the bone marrow

hematopoietic stem cells (HSCs) are morphologically indistinguishable. They require functional assays in which progenitor cells form colonies of maturing cells of different lineage, if they are grown in a medium containing methyl cellulose or agar. They can also be identified by surface antigenic characteristics. The most frequently used markers are CD34 antigen expressed on HSC and progenitors, and CD38 expressed on subset of mature progenitors. Hematopoietic pluripotent stem cells can self-renew (forming new pluripotent stem cells) and differentiate (into lineage-specific progenitors)—self-renewal and differentiation. When the pluripotent stem cell mass falls below a critical mass, the balance of these two processes cannot be maintained and leads to stem cell or bone marrow failure and the clinical condition is called aplastic anemia. In 2000 AD, skin fibroblasts were induced and reprogramed to form multipotent cells resembling embryonic stem cells [induced pluripotent stem (iPS) cells]. Research in programing them as HSC is still in progress.

Causes

Bone marrow failure is a broader term that describes pancytopenia due to different causes, e.g. replacement by tumor and myelodysplasia. Aplastic anemia is a more specific condition reflecting deficiency of HSCs resulting in peripheral pancytopenia and bone marrow aplasia.

Major causes include idiopathic, cytotoxic drugs and chemicals (cancer treatment), drug reaction (carbamazepine, hydantoins, chloramphenicol, phenylbutazone, indomethacin, propylthiouracil, gold, arsenicals).

Toxic Chemicals: Benzene

Viral infections: Epstein-Barr virus (EBV), human immuno-deficiency virus (HIV), herpes, hepatitis, cytomegalovirus (CMV) infections.

Immune disorders: Systemic lupus erythematosus (SLE), graft-versus-host disease (GVHD), eosinophilic fasciitis (EF).

Miscellaneous: PNH, thymoma and pregnancy.

Most of the causes of aplastic anemia that we see in clinical practice are idiopathic. Several observations are consistent with the destruction or suppression of the stem cells by an autoimmune mechanism.

Observations suggestive of autoimmune mechanism are as follows:

- Many patients respond to immunosuppressive therapy.
- Aplastic anemia is associated with other autoimmune diseases and conditions such as EF and GVHD.
- Blood lymphocytes from aplastic anemia patients inhibit hematopoiesis when cultured with patient's or normal marrow.
- Expansion of CD8+ T cells have been found in patients with idiopathic aplastic anemia.

Interferon gamma (IFN-γ), tumor necrosis factor alpha (TNF-α) and many other cytokines are found to be increased in patients with aplastic anemia. Damage induced by chemicals, drugs, viruses or antigens lead to lymphocytic activation in patients with aplastic anemia.

There is a close association of aplastic anemia with other clonal multilineage hematopoietic disorders like PNH and myelodysplastic syndrome (MDS) (refractory anemia).

Flow cytometry has shown a population of cells in aplastic anemia to be PNH type cells (CD59).

Mutations in telomerase RNA component (TERC) and variations in telomere length were detected in some patients with aplastic anemia. FA is a type of congenital aplastic anemia (described later in this chapter).

Clinical Features

The disease is insidious in onset. The peak age groups are 10–25 years and above 60 years. Symptoms are slow in onset, taking 1–2 months for manifestation. Sometimes, bleeding and infection may set in early. Symptoms are due to the consequences of pancytopenia. Varying grades of anemia develop and often it is severe. Hemorrhagic manifestations occur due to thrombocytopenia. Common presentations are purpura, ecchymosis, epistaxis, bleeding from the gums, gastrointestinal (GI) bleeding and vaginal bleeding. Bacterial infections occur due to neutropenia. These present with fever or other localized infections.

Diagnosis

Bone marrow biopsy is done in all suspected cases in addition to other hematological investigations. Diagnostic criteria for moderate and severe aplastic anemia are as follows:

Moderate aplastic anemia: Bone marrow cellularity <30%. Absence of severe pancytopenia. Depression of at least two or three blood elements below normal.

Severe aplastic anemia (SAA): Bone marrow biopsy showing <25% or <50% of normal cellularity in which fewer than 30% of the cells are hematopoietic and at least two of the following are present, reticulocyte count (<1%) or absolute reticulocyte count <40,000/µL, absolute neutrophil count (ANC) <500/µL or platelet count <20,000/µL.

Very severe aplastic anemia (vSAA): SAA + ANC <200/µL.

Treatment

If no treatment is offered for patients with SAA and vSAA, 70% die within one year.

Treatment consists of:

- Withdrawal or stopping of any offending chemicals or drugs.
- Supportive care with blood components, packed red blood cells (PRBCs) transfusions, platelet transfusions and antibiotics for infections. This should be used sparingly for those who are candidates for hematopoietic stem cell transplantation (HSCT).
- Specific treatment modalities—
  - ***HSCT:*** Allogeneic HSCT is curative in aplastic anemia. But this type of treatment is limited because matched sibling donor is available only in 30% of patients with aplastic anemia. Further, the potentially fatal complication of GVHD in patients over the age of 40–50 years is considerable.
  - Combined immunosuppressive treatment which is not curative but is associated with long-term survival.

The recommended immunosuppressive treatment consists of ATG (antithymocyte globulin—horse ATG is now found to be superior to rabbit ATG). The dose of ATG is 40 mg/kg as intravenous (IV) infusion (in 500 mL saline) over 4–6 hours daily for 4 days.

Cyclosporine, the second immunosuppressive drug, is given in a starting dose of 10–12 mg/kg/day as two equally divided doses, reducing the dose by about 5–7 mg/kg/day to have a trough level between 200 and 400 mg/day. Cyclosporine is usually continued for a duration of 6 months.

Prednisolone or methylprednisolone 1 mg/kg/day is also given from the beginning which is tapered and stopped over one month.

Age below 20 and 20–50 years: In patients with SAA and vSAA with human leukocyte antigen (HLA) matched sibling, allogeneic HSCT is the treatment of choice. If this is not available, unrelated donor HSCT is undertaken.

Above the age of 50 years, both for SAA and vSAA, the use of immunosuppressive treatment is recommended over HSCT because of the very high-risk of GVHD in patients above 45 years.

Prognosis

Prognosis depends on two main factors—disease severity and patient's age.

Disease severity depends on how severe the formed elements of blood are reduced, especially the ANC. Age is inversely related to the prognosis. Response rate of immunosuppressive treatment is about 62% at 12 months. At 5-year, survival rate depends on age; survival being 72% below 49 years and 50% above 60 years. With HSCT, the 5-year survival rate below 49 years has increased over the years. It was 56% in the period of 1974–79 and 89% in the period of 1990–97.

Approximately, 15–40% of aplastic anemia patients with immunosuppressive treatment develop PNH which may be mild, transient or progress to full-blown disease.

Relapse rate for patients treated with immunosuppressive treatment is about 35% at 14 years. Immunosuppressive treatment may be given again and 50% of patients will show a good response.

Newer Directions in the Treatment of Aplastic Anemia

Alemtuzumab plus cyclosporine is found to produce good response.

Another interesting treatment regime in refractory or resistant cases of aplastic anemia was the use of a thrombopoietin mimetics eltrombopag. The drug was given on a dose of 50 mg/day (up to 150 mg) to patients with aplastic anemia who did not respond to immunosuppressive treatment. Out of total, 40% showed good response both bi- and tri-lineage. This may be a good choice for Indian patients who cannot afford HSCT and immunosuppressive treatment.

SPECIAL FORMS OF APLASTIC ANEMIA

The term constitutional aplastic anemia is used to denote congenital, genetic or familial aplastic anemias.

Fanconi's Anemia

Syn: Congenital pancytopenia

It is the most common type of inherited aplastic anemia. In this syndrome, congenital abnormality like hyperpigmentation, absence or hypoplasia of the thumbs and radii,

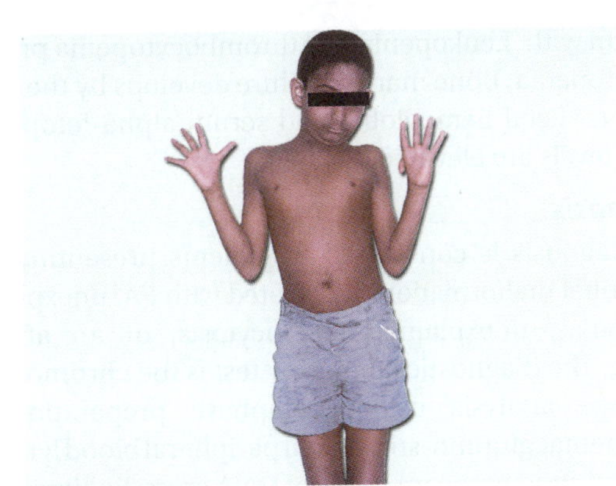

Fig. 162.2: Fanconi's anemia, 12-year-old boy. ***Note:*** Hypoplastic thumb left hand

strabismus, mental retardation, deafness and dwarfism are seen (Fig. 162.2). Pancytopenia and bone marrow hypoplasia develop by the age of 5–10 years. Untreated, the mortality is high.

FA is an autosomal recessive disorder characterized by developmental abnormalities, bone marrow failure and cancer predisposition, specially squamous cell carcinoma (SCC) and acute myeloid leukemia (AML).

It is usually lethal by the age of 20 years. The underlying defect in FA is not fully known. Multiple genes are responsible for aplastic anemia. Many of them are tumor suppressor genes responsible for gene repair. Cultured fibroblasts from these patients show increased generation time and increased cell death. More than eight groups of FA have been distinguished genetically (termed FA—A to H), each carrying a distinct genetic lesion. FA-A gene which is found in 60% of patients with aplastic anemia is located on chromosome 16q23.3. Germ-line mutations in six different genes have been identified. Cell lines established from FA patients show two unique characteristics:

1. Accumulation of broken and misshaped chromosomes that originate from deoxyribonucleic acid (DNA) replication.
2. Increased sensitivity to the action of DNA cross-linking agents like mitomycin-C which trigger chromosomal abnormalities.

Clinical Features

Patients with FA are diagnosed between 6 and 9 years of age. Out of total, 60–70% of them will have:

- Short stature
- Hypopigmented spots
- Abnormality in thumbs
- Microcephaly or hydrocephaly
- Hypogonadism
- Developmental delay.

Rest of them may not have congenital abnormalities. Patients with FA are at a high risk of developing malignancies like MDS, AML and SCC of the head or vulva. Malignancy can be first manifestation of FA. Some of them may have clonal the chromosomal changes in the bone marrow.

Laboratory Findings

The hematological abnormalities may take years to evolve. They may have only a mild anemia or thrombocytopenia to begin with. Leukopenia and thrombocytopenia precede pancytopenia. Bone marrow failure develops by the age of 10 years. Fetal hemoglobin and serum alpha-fetoprotein (AFP) levels are elevated.

Diagnosis

The diagnosis is considered in patients presenting with congenital malformations associated with FA, unexplained cytopenias, unexplained macrocytosis, or an affected sibling. The diagnostic laboratory test is the chromosomal breakage analysis using metaphase preparations of phytohemagglutinin-stimulated peripheral blood lymphocytes cultured in the presence of DNA cross-linking agents such as mitomycin. Spontaneous chromosome breakages are demonstrable in up to 70% of lymphocytes and 25–50% fibroblasts. Such an abnormality is not present in Diamond-Blackfan syndrome, another cause of anemia in children. Prenatal diagnosis is possible by chromosome breakage studies done by chorionic villus sampling (CVS) at 9–12 weeks gestation, amniocentesis at 16 weeks or by fetal blood sampling done later.

Treatment

Anabolic steroids

Mild cases may benefit by administration of anabolic agents such as oxymetholone 2–3 mg/kg bw given orally for 2–3 months. Adverse side effects such as virilization and fluid retention may develop. Dose may be tapered to the minimum effective dose. The drug should be stopped if there is no response within 3 months. Hematopoietic growth factors (HGFs)—granulocyte colony-stimulating factor (G-CSF) and granulocyte-macrophage colony-stimulating factor (GM-CSF) may increase the neutrophil counts in neutropenic patients. Blood component therapy may be required for symptom relief. Bone marrow transplantation from HLA matched normal donors is the only curative treatment for the bone marrow failure. This is better than using mismatched donors. Umbilical cord blood is a good source of stem cells for transplantation.

Pure Red Cell Aplasia (PRCA)

It is a rare form of aplasia selectively affecting the erythroid precursors, reticulocytes and red cells; the other formed elements and their precursors being normal. The causes may be inherited or acquired.

Acquired PRCA in Adults

This is a rare chronic condition of profound anemia, reticulocytopenia and absence of erythroid precursors in the bone marrow. Usually, the onset is insidious. If red cell aplasia supervenes on hemolytic states where the life span of the red cell is considerably shortened, the onset is much more rapid and the condition is more serious. This is what happens in sickle-cell anemia and other acquired or inherited hemolytic anemias when aplastic crisis develops as a result of parvovirus B19 infection.

Patients with acquired PRCA present with severe anemia without any bleeding tendencies or infective episodes. Reticulocytes are very low, often absent. Bone marrow shows pure aplasia of the erythrocyte progenitors. Fifteen percent of the patients have spontaneous recovery (drugs, pregnancy). Others recover with treatment. Some others follow a prolonged course and end fatally.

Etiology

Majority of cases are immune-mediated and various autoimmune mechanisms have been postulated. Antibodies against erythroblasts and erythropoietin (EPO) may develop and selectively suppress and destroy them. T-cells may produce selective cytokines inhibiting erythroid precursors or leading to their lysis. Another mechanism is loss of major histocompatibility complex (MHC) class 1 expression on the erythroid progenitor cells which become increasingly susceptible to destruction by natural killer-T lymphocytes. Autoimmune PRCA may be primary (idiopathic) or secondary. Secondary causes for acquired PRCA may be due to:

- **Infections:** Parvovirus B19, acquired immunodeficiency syndrome (AIDS), viral hepatitis
- Autoimmune diseases like rheumatoid disease and SLE
- Neoplasms such as thymoma, lymphoma, chronic lymphocytic leukemia (CLL), chronic myeloid leukemia (CML) or carcinoma
- A preleukemic or premyelodysplastic manifestation
- Drug induction or during pregnancy.

Prolonged use of EPO in chronic renal failure (CRF) may lead to development of neutralizing antibody against EPO by about 1 year after the start of therapy. This happened specially with one brand of EPO called Eprex due to the stabilizing agent, methods of storage and administration. These cases present as PRCA. Treatment with corticosteroids, other immunosuppressants and IV immunoglobulins (Igs) is successful. With changes made in the preparation of EPO, the incidence of this condition has considerably declined.

Occasionally, ABO incompatibility between donor and recipient of bone marrow transplantation or stem cell transplant can lead to antibody-mediated PRCA.

PRCA has to be differentiated from aplastic anemia, in which all the blood cell precursors are affected. Early stages of MDS may produce diagnostic difficulty. In MDS, dysplasia is evident in all cell lines. The anemia in PRCA is normocytic and normochromic. There is no ineffective erythropoiesis or hemolysis. Underlying causes should be investigated. Bone marrow is characteristic with normal cellularity and complete absence of red cell precursors.

Management

Transient cases are self-limiting. In other cases with prolonged anemia and with evidence of parvovirus infection, idiopathic causes and with underlying immunological processes; steroids, immunosuppressants such as glucocorticoids, cyclosporine or mycophenolate mofetil are beneficial. In intractable cases, IV immunoglobulin in a dose of 0.4 g/kg bw for 6–8 days is effective. In those with thymoma, thymectomy may be beneficial. In those with other underlying disorders, treatment of the primary disease relieves the PRCA as well.

Red Cell Aplasia in Children

Syn: Diamond-Blackfan anemia (DBA), Congenital hypoplastic anemia, Chronic congenital aregenerative anemia, Erythrogenesis imperfecta

This is a form of congenital PRCA developing in infancy or in early childhood. The children during their infancy or early childhood develop normochromic and more commonly macrocytic anemia caused by selective aplasia of erythroid precursors beyond the stage of proerythroblasts, and reticulocytopenia. Leukocyte and platelet counts and their precursors are generally normal. Seventy five percent of cases are sporadic, 25% show inheritance patterns. Both dominant and recessive inheritance has been identified. DBA is considered as a ribosomopathy caused by genetic mutations affecting ribosome synthesis. As a result, there is stabilization and activation of the TP53 (tumor protein p53) tumor suppressor pathway. This is the cause of all clinical manifestations including impaired erythropoiesis. Chromosomal abnormalities, mainly involving chromosomes 19 and 13 (translocation or deletions), have been reported. Congenital abnormalities occur in about 50%. These include short stature, atrial or ventricular septal defects (ASDs or VSDs), urogenital abnormalities, craniofacial abnormalities, ophthalmological abnormalities, thumb abnormalities, pre- and postnatal growth failure and others. Fetal hemoglobin and erythrocyte adenosine deaminase (eADA) levels may be increased. eADA is an enzyme involved in purine metabolism and it is elevated in the erythrocytes of DBA. Elevated eADA levels have a sensitivity of 84% and specificity of 95% for diagnosis. eADA levels have positive and negative predictive values for the diagnosis of DBA. DBA patients have tendency to develop malignancies such as MDS, AML, solid tumors like colon cancer, female genital cancers and osteogenic sarcoma.

Diagnostic criteria include age less than 1 year, macrocytic anemia, reticulocytopenia, normal marrow cellularity with paucity of erythroid precursors. Major supporting criteria include presence of a gene mutation associated with DBA and a positive family history. Minor supporting criteria include increase in eADA activity, congenital abnormalities and elevated fetal hemoglobin. Elevated ADA activity is seen in 80–85% of cases with DBA. The levels are more than three standard deviations higher than normal. This parameter is not a strong independent predictor for the presence of the disease because it can be seen in other conditions of immune deficiencies, hemolytic anemia, chronic myeloproliferative neoplasia, dyskeratosis and megaloblastic anemia.

Differential diagnosis include transient erythroblastopenia of childhood (TEC), FA and dyskeratosis.

Management

Spontaneous remission occurs in 25% of cases. Corticosteroids and red cell transfusion form the mainstay of the treatment. Response to corticosteroids is found in 50–75% of cases but this drug is avoided until 6 months to 1 year. Patients containing the mutations have the least response to steroids. Many studies suggest that HLA-identical sibling donor HSCT is effective in the treatment of DBA that is unresponsive to immunosuppressive therapy. However, it is unclear whether alternate donor HSCT is a reasonable option in the treatment of DBA unresponsive to immunosuppressive therapy.

Transient Erythroblastopenia of Childhood (TEC)

This is an acquired form of PRCA in previously healthy children. TEC is a transient or temporary red cell aplasia occurring in children older in age than DBA even though the majority is below 1 year of age. Etiology is not very clear but possible causes include viral infections, inhibitors to progenitor cells, cell-mediated suppression of erythropoiesis or other autoimmune mechanisms as in adults. Mild neutropenia is found in 50% of cases. There is a temporary cessation of red blood cell (RBC) production. Serum titers for parvovirus IgM and IgG and viral antigen by polymerase chain reaction (PCR) may be undertaken. The condition is generally benign with spontaneous recovery within 4–8 weeks. Management is symptomatic with red cell transfusion, and immunosuppression in severe cases.

Sideroblastic Anemia

It is characterized by congenital or acquired defects affecting the biosynthesis of heme, iron-sulfur (Fe-S) cluster generation or mitochondrial protein synthesis, within red cell precursors. In a large number of patients, the underlying mechanism remains undefined. Eighty-five percent of body heme is generated by the erythron. Defective heme synthesis in the red cells leads to decreased hemoglobin production with the formation of hypochromic and microcytic red cells. The term sideroblast denotes an erythroblast containing one or two stainable iron granules in the cytoplasm. When such stainable non-hemoglobin iron granules are present in the erythrocyte, it is called ***siderocyte***. Even under normal conditions, a few of these iron granules may be seen lying free in the cytoplasm without relation to any particular organelle within the cell. But under pathological conditions, iron granules accumulate in the mitochondria and they appear in the form of a perinuclear ring in the late erythroblasts and such cells are called ***ringed sideroblasts (Figs 162.3 and 162.4)***. Sometimes pathological nonring sideroblasts occur, with excess of free iron granules in the cytoplasm.

Ineffective erythropoiesis is found in this type of anemia. Iron delivery to the developing erythroid cells is not down regulated even though heme synthesis is impaired, leading to accumulation of mitochondrial iron

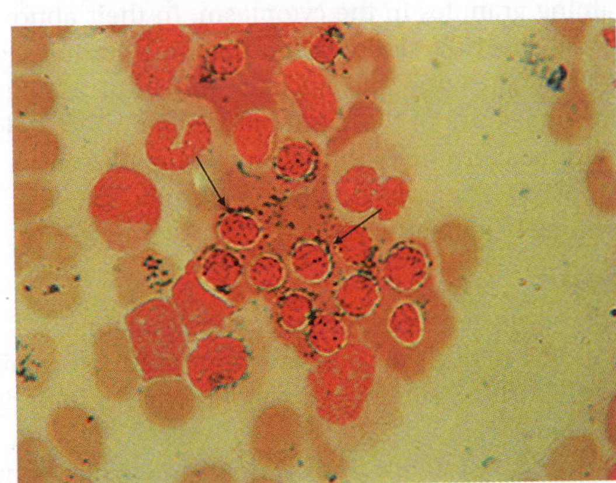

Fig. 162.3: Prussian blue stain of the bone marrow in a patient with refractory anemia and ring sideroblasts. Blue stained ferritin iron deposits form an apparent ring around the nucleus (arrows)

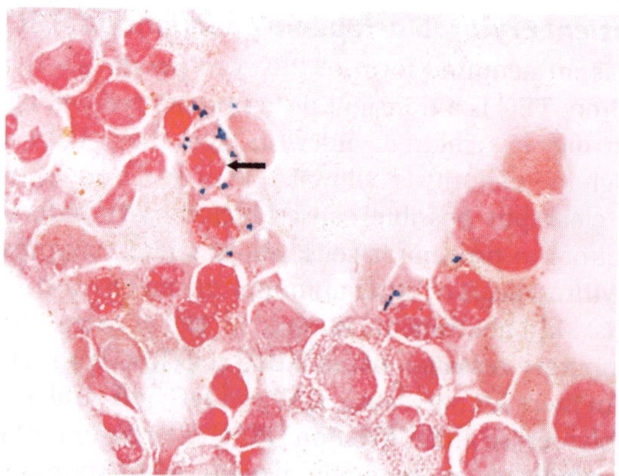

Fig. 162.4: Sideroblastic anemia—bone marrow × 1000. **Note:** Ringed sideroblasts (arrow)

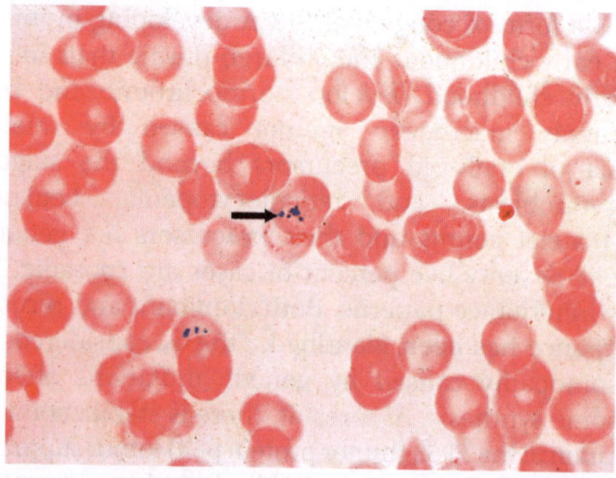

Fig. 162.5: Sideroblastic anemia peripheral blood × 1000. **Note:** Siderocytes (RBC containing iron pigment) Prussian blue stain (arrow)

and formation of ring sideroblasts. Iron overload is due to suppressed production of hepcidin by ineffective erythropoiesis and related to the degree of marrow erythroid hyperplasia, patient's age and duration of abnormality.

Causes

Congenital

- **Nonsyndromic:** X-linked defect in ALAS (5-aminolevulinate synthase)
- **Syndromic:** X-linked with ataxia
- **Syndromic or nonsyndromic:** Autosomal of unknown cause.
- Sporadic congenital

Acquired—clonal or neoplastic

- Refractory anemia with ring sideroblasts and thrombocytosis (RARS-T)
- Refractory cytopenia with multilineage dysplasia and ring sideroblasts (RCMD-RS)
- Metabolic or reversible
- Drugs (e.g. isoniazid, chloramphenicol, linezolid)
- Copper deficiency (zinc toxicity)
- Hypothermia.

The metabolic or reversible conditions are fully reversible when the offending factors are removed.

Sideroblasts are found in small numbers in the bone marrow of normal iron-sufficient subjects as nucleated RBC precursors (erythroblasts) with one or more iron-containing granules in the cytoplasm. In their abnormal form, i.e. the ring sideroblasts, the iron granules may completely surround the nucleus and form a singular diagnostic feature of the sideroblastic anemia. It reflects the various aberrations in the processing of iron by the erythroblasts. Patients develop a chronic anemia not responding to hematinics.

Diagnosis

- Microcytic, normocytic or macrocytic anemia.
- Presence of ring sideroblast on bone marrow examination. At times, siderocytes may be present in peripheral blood (Fig. 162.5).
- Presence of systemic iron overload unless there is iron deficiency.

The most frequent form of microcytic or hypochromic sideroblastic anemia is X-linked sideroblastic anemia (XLSA), caused by mutations in the erythroid-specific ALAS2 gene found in males. This gene is located at chromosome Xp11.21. The most common normocytic or macrocytic sideroblastic anemia is the acquired clonal type refractory anemia with ringed sideroblasts (RARS). Molecular studies can be done for the diagnosis.

Management

In nonsyndromic forms of congenital sideroblastic anemia, close to normal survival can be achieved in patients by controlling the symptoms of anemia and early institution of treatment programs to prevent organ damage associated with iron overload.

The acquired clonal sideroblastic anemia predisposes to leukemic evolution but the congenital and acquired reversible forms do not. Definite curative treatment is not available. Allogeneic HSCT has been successful in seven patients. Gene therapy is difficult due to problems involving transducing HSCs.

XLSA may respond to pyridoxine supplement in about two-thirds of cases. Vitamin B_6 (pyridoxine) in oral doses of 50–100 mg/day over and above the adult daily requirement of 1.2–2 mg/day will produce the maximal response. Maintenance treatment is necessary to prevent relapse.

Iron overload associated with sideroblastic anemia requires treatment to prevent organ damage due to iron excess.

Treatment should be started when serum ferritin is more than 500 µg/L. Therapeutic phlebotomy (in patients who have responded to pyridoxine supplements) if hemoglobin is greater than 9 g or iron chelation for anemic patients should be undertaken to minimize organ damage.

Sideroblastic anemia occurs in one-third of cases of heavy alcoholism and this will disappear on stopping alcohol. The drug-induced sideroblastic anemia which occurs with treatment with drugs like isoniazid, chloramphenicol, linezolid and melphalan clears up on withdrawal of the drug.

Copper deficiency occurring in prolonged parenteral nutrition, intestinal malabsorption, use of copper chelating agents and nephrotic syndrome (due to urinary loss of ceruloplasmin) and after prolonged zinc administration can be corrected by copper supplementation. Copper deficiency produces neurological manifestation like central nervous system (CNS) demyelination, peripheral and optic neuropathy or myeloneuropathy.

Thiamine-responsive megaloblastic anemia (TRMA) syndrome is an autosomal recessive inherited disorder that is characterized by megaloblastic anemia, sensorineural hearing loss and diabetes mellitus (DM). Onset of megaloblastic anemia is between infancy and adolescence.

PAROXYSMAL NOCTURNAL HEMOGLOBINURIA (PNH)

This is an acquired hemolytic disease with an intracorpuscular abnormality. It is a clonal disorder with various clinical manifestations. The name is derived from the fact that intravascular hemolysis is observed at night and hemoglobinuria occurs more frequently in the morning, intermittently.

Pathogenesis

The fundamental pathogenic defect in PNH is an inability of hematopoietic cells to produce the glycosylphosphatidylinositol (GPI) anchor due to a defect in PIGA gene. There are many important (about 20) proteins which are tethered or attached to GPI anchor tail of the hematopoietic cells (mainly the RBCs, granulocytes, lymphocytes, monocytes and platelets). CD59 [membrane inhibitor of reactive lysis (MIRL)] is one of the proteins which is completely missing in PNH. Another protein missing is CD55 (decay accelerating factor). According to the status of GPI-linked proteins, different populations of red cells have been defined in PNH.

- PNH type 1 cells normal
- PNH type 2 cells partial absence of GPI-linked proteins
- PNH type 3 cells complete absence of GPI-linked proteins.

The deficiency of GPI-linked proteins increases the sensitivity of the red cells in PNH to the hemolytic action of complement. The clinical manifestations of PNH are related to the abnormalities in hematopoietic function including hemolytic anemia, a hypercoagulable state, bone marrow hypoplasia or aplasia and progression to MDS or acute leukemia.

Hemolytic Anemia

In PNH, CD55 and CD59 are deficient on RBC surface. Normally, these inhibit complement activation. Normal alternate pathway starts with the activation of complement C3 and C5 which lead to the formation of the final product. Membrane attack complex (MAC) causes lysis of RBC. Normally, CD55 and CD59 inhibit this process. In their absence, complement activation and RBC lysis occurs. Hemolysis occurs due to the destruction of complement-sensitive RBCs. In type 3 PNH, the GPI-linked proteins are absent in majority of the cells and so the hemolysis is marked. Hemolysis also depends on the degree to which complement is activated. Intravascular hemolysis produces hemoglobinuria or iron deposition in the kidneys.

Clinical Features

Clinical features of hemolysis like high-colored urine, jaundice and hepatosplenomegaly may be seen. Many patients with PNH have a distressing degree of fatigue that is not related to the hemoglobin level.

The free hemoglobin released causes sequestration of nitric oxide (NO) necessary for smooth muscle relaxation. Decrease in NO leads to erectile dysfunction in males, esophageal spasm and dysphagia and tightness of the chest. Mild arterial spasm also leads to the reduction in renal function and an element of pulmonary hypertension (PH).

Venous Thrombosis

PNH is associated with a marked increase in venous thrombosis in the hepatic, other intra-abdominal and peripheral veins. The risk of thrombosis depends on the size of the PNH clone of cells (PNH granulocytes). Venous thrombosis is less in Asians since this clone is less in them. There is a low grade in vivo activation of clotting but the exact mechanism is not clear. High expression of tissue factor, absence of GPI-linked protein tissue factor pathway inhibitor and delayed fibrinolysis is all postulated for this hypercoagulable state. It is postulated that leukocyte-derived microparticles initiate thrombosis. The microparticles are derived from complement injured CD55- and CD59-deficient monocytes and macrophages expressing tissue factor.

Diminished Hematopoiesis

PNH can lead to granulocytopenia or thrombocytopenia. *Clinical features* may be infection and bleeding tendency. In extreme cases, it can manifest as aplastic anemia. On the other hand, patients with aplastic anemia can develop PNH. The GPI-deficient cells can be detected in aplastic anemia up to 70% of patients. Patients with aplastic anemia treated with ATG or cyclosporine can develop PNH.

Patients with PNH may develop MDS (5–9%) or AML (<5%).

Diagnosis

Diagnosis should be suspected if the patients are having any one of the following findings: Acquired hemolytic anemia, hemoglobinuria, negative direct Coombs test, granulocytopenia, thrombocytopenia, venous thrombosis, aplastic anemia, MDS, episodes of dysphagia or abdominal pain.

In the past, PNH was screened and diagnosed by sucrose lysis test and Ham acid hemolysis test, respectively.

But now, PNH is diagnosed by finding out the deficiency of GPI-linked proteins by using monoclonal antibodies (mAbs) to the GPI-anchored proteins CD55 and CD59 followed by flow cytometry. A bacterial toxin, aerolysin which binds specifically to the GPI anchor may be used with fluorescent label called fluorescein-labeled proaerolysin (FLAER) to detect the deficiency of the GPI anchor by high-sensitivity flow cytometry. FLAER is available only in a few centers and can detect even a very small clone of PNH cells.

Treatment

The only curative treatment for PNH is allogeneic HSCT. All other treatments are supportive in order to alleviate the various manifestations of the disease.

Asymptomatic patient with a PNH clone of less than 10% need not to be treated but the clone should be checked once in 6 months to 1 year period to see if the clone is progressively increasing. Supportive treatment includes iron, folic acid, blood components, erythropoiesis-stimulating agents, corticosteroids and treatment of venous thrombosis by anticoagulation.

Prophylaxis of thrombosis in PNH is not well-established. Those patients with severe disabling symptoms or recurrent venous thrombosis should be treated with eculizumab, a humanized mAb against C5 component of the complement, which inhibits terminal complement activation and formation of the MAC. Intravascular hemolytic episodes and transfusion requirements are reduced. Thromboembolic events are also reduced. It improves the hemoglobin concentration and the quality of life. Eculizumab 600 mg is given by infusion every week for 4 weeks followed by 900 mg every two weeks for 26 weeks. The treatment can be given long term also but it is very expensive (400,000 dollars per year).

Follow-up of patients unresponsive to eculizumab:

PNH patients were studied in Japan who received eculizumab. Eleven of them had a poor response. These had a single missense C5 heterogeneous mutations C26545→A, which predicts the polymorphism of p.Arg885HIS. This mutation occurs in 3.2% of patients with PNH. Both nonmutant and mutant C5 cause hemolysis but only nonmutant C5 is bound and inactivated with eculizumab. Both mutant and nonmutant C5 were completely blocked with the use of a new mAb (N19-8) which binds to a site different from that of eculizumab on C5.

Cyclosporine and ATG are also used in some patients, specially those resembling aplastic anemia.

Source: Nishimura J1, Yamamoto M, Hayashi S, et al. Genetic variants in C5 and poor response to eculizumab. N Engl J Med. 2014;370(7):632-9.

Prognosis

Overall survival of patients who have undergone treatment with HCT is 70–86%. Now, it is concluded that HSCT is not suitable for PNH patients with thrombosis. They should be preferably treated with eculizumab.

Future Direction

The defective PIGA gene in PNH has been cloned. It is possible now theoretically to correct the defect in the abnormal stem cells by using gene therapy.

CHAPTER

163

Blood Transfusion

KV Krishna Das, Mathew Thomas, Jaisy Mathai

Chapter Summary

- General Considerations
- Blood Group Antigens
- Blood Group Antibodies
- Blood Group Systems
- Blood Bank Procedures
- Indications for Transfusion
- Erythrocyte Preparations
- Platelet Transfusions
- Fresh Frozen Plasma (FFP)
- Hazards of Transfusion Therapy
- Transfusion Transmitted Infections
- Cord Blood Transfusion
- Blood Substitutes
- Stem Cell Transplantation
- Important Points in Blood Banking Procedures

GENERAL CONSIDERATIONS

Transfusion medicine has become a major specialty encompassing several subspecialties such as immuno-hematology, blood banking, component preparation, genetic studies and so on. Many of the present day state-of-the-art technologies such as complicated cardiac surgery, other major surgical procedure, traumatology, organ transplantation, cancer chemotherapy, management of hematological and immunological disorders, prenatal and neonatal interventions and several others owe their existence and development to sound transfusion medicine practices. The present day problems of transfusion transmitted infections including acquired immunodeficiency syndrome (AIDS) has given further impetus to the growth of this specialty. The general approach to the quantitative and qualitative aspects of transfusion products in different clinical situations have also changed based on randomized controlled trials (RCTs).

BLOOD GROUP ANTIGENS

The outstanding landmark in the history of blood transfusion is the discovery of human ***ABO blood group system*** in 1900 by Landsteiner. He differentiated human blood into four distinct groups on the basis of two antigens A and B.

Following the discovery of the ABO system in 1900, Landsteiner and his coworkers described further blood group systems. The human MN and P antigens were described, but those systems seemed to have only little clinical importance. In 1937, Landsteiner and Wiener discovered the Rhesus (Rh) factor by a new method.

Subsequent workers have identified several other antigens present on the red cell surface and these form the basis of blood grouping.

On the basis of different antigens, about 15 different red cell blood group systems are known with wide distribution in different radical groups. These are ABO, MNSs, P, Rh, Lutheran, Kell, Lewis, Duffy, Kidd, Diego, Yt, Xg, Ii, Dombrock and Cotton system. Except Xg system, which is determined by genes on the X chromosome all the others are determined by genes located on autosomes.

Among all the different blood group antigens, ABO and Rh system are the most important in clinical transfusion practice. The others which are less prevalent assume importance when dealing with hemolytic states developing in multiple transfused individuals and while cross-matching blood for patients who may require life-long transfusion therapy.

BLOOD GROUP ANTIBODIES

Two types of antibodies against red cell antigens occur. These include:

1. *Naturally occurring antibodies* which develop even without external antigenic stimulus, e.g. anti-A and anti-B. These antibodies which are present in the serum are directed against antigens which are not present on the red cells of the same individual.
2. *Immune or acquired antibodies:* These develop as a result of immunization by a red cell antigen which is foreign to the same individual. These develop as a result of mismatched transfusion or pregnancy, e.g. Rh antibodies, ABO antibodies. All red blood cell (RBC) antigens are capable of stimulating antibody production, but some, such as Rh antigen are more powerful than others. Even among the Rh antigen, group D is more antigenic.

In addition to red cell antigens, other immunizing antigens such as tetanus toxoid, typhoid-paratyphoid A and B (TAB) vaccine, pneumococcal vaccine and others which contain substances closely mimicking A and B antigen stimulate the production of immune anti-A and anti-B antibodies. These assume clinical importance in persons who have been repeatedly immunized against infections and those who receive transfusions repeatedly.

Naturally occurring red cell antibodies belong to immunoglobulin M (IgM) class and they react best at temperature below 37°C. In contrast, immune antibodies are mainly immunoglobulin G (IgG) or IgM and their optimal temperature for reaction is 37°C. Immune antibodies produced early during the process of immunization are IgM class, whereas the antibodies produced long-term are IgG. IgM does not cross the placenta whereas IgG readily crosses it.

Antibodies are detected in the laboratory by four types of tests:

1. Saline agglutination
2. Agglutination in colloid solutions-albumin
3. Tests using enzyme treated cells
4. Indirect antiglobulin test (Coombs test).

Complete antibodies are detectable by saline agglutination. Incomplete antibodies are detectable by the other three methods. The various immune antibodies behave differently in the various tests. Their detection and cross-matching in their presence involve very delicate and highly developed laboratory techniques.

Blood group systems form the cornerstone of transfusion medicine. The study of blood groups helps to:

Table 163.1: Distribution of ABO blood groups in the Caucasian population and Indians

Blood group	Caucasian	Indian
O	47%	40%
A	42%	22%
B	8%	33%
AB	3%	5%

- Perform blood banking
- Anthropological studies
- Performance of medicolegal investigations in paternity disputes [at present molecular studies involving deoxyribonucleic acid (DNA) are more popular]
- Correlate with prediction of diseases. Several diseases show associations with particular blood groups (Table 163.1).

BLOOD GROUP SYSTEMS

ABO System

This comprises of four main blood groups A, B, AB and O designated according to the presence or absence of A or B antigens on the red cell surface. In the O group, there is neither A nor B antigen. In addition to the presence of the antigen on the red cell surface, in the natural state itself the plasma contains antibodies against the A or B antigen that is not naturally present in the same individual (Table 163.2).

The formation of A and B antigen is controlled by three allelic genes A, B and D located on the long arm of chromosome 9. The A and B genes are codominant. O gene is an amorph, i.e. it has no effect on antigenic structure. Another gene, the H gene controls the formation of a precursor H-substance which is present in the serum. Action of A and B genes leads to the formation of A and B antigen and in the process, the H-substance is consumed. The O gene does not act on the H-substance therefore O group individuals have higher levels of H-substance in the serum. Conversely, AB group individuals have the lowest levels of H-substance. Very rarely some of the O group subjects not possessing the H-substance in the serum develop antibodies against H-substance as well. There are several subgroups of A, among which A_1 and A_2 are important. Eighty percent of A group subjects possess A_1 and 20% possess A_2. Correspondingly, AB subjects also fall into the subgroups A_1B and A_2B. Compared to A_1, A_2 cells react only weakly with the antiserum. It is therefore necessary to use strong antisera which will agglutinate both A_1 and A_2 cells in order to detect A_2 subtypes. Rarely, A_2 subgroup persons may produce anti-A_1 antibody which can destroy transfused A_1 cells.

Table 163.2: Antigens and antibodies present in each of the four main groups of the ABO system

Blood group	Antigen in red cell	Antibodies in plasma
O	Nil	Anti-A, anti-B
A	A	Anti-B
B	B	Anti-A
AB	A and B	Nil

Table 163.3: Specific ABH substances present in the saliva of secretors

ABO group of red cells	Soluble antigen in saliva
O	H
A	A and H
B	B and H
AB	A, B and H

The Bombay Blood Group

O group individuals normally possess serum antibodies against A and B antigens only. O group individuals who have antibodies against H-substance are designated as the Bombay blood group, being described first by HM Bhatia and his colleagues from the Blood Group Reference Centre, Bombay.

Secretors are individuals who secrete these blood group substances or antigens in the body secretions (80%) whereas nonsecretors are those who do not secrete blood group antigens in body secretions (20%). For purposes of testing, saliva is examined (Table 163.3).

Rhesus System (Rh System)

Next in importance to the ABO system are the Rh antigens. The Rh antigens (C, c, D, d, E and e) are inherited through three closely linked allelic genes C or c, D or d and E or e, located on chromosome 1. One set of three genes is inherited from each parent giving rise to various combinations of genotypes, e.g. CDE/CDE or CDe/CDe. The antigens produced by the genes are given similar notations. All the genes except *d* express their corresponding antigens, while *d* being an amorph, there is no *d* antigen.

Among these antigens, the presence or absence of D antigen is most important and Rh positive and negative are decided by the presence or absence of D antigen.

Among Caucasians, 85% are Rh positive and 15% are Rh negative. Among Indians, 4–10% (average 7) are Rh negative. A study from Bangalore in 2001 gave the prevalence of Rh positive as 94.25% and Rh negative as 5.75%.

Unlike the ABO blood groups, antibodies to the missing Rh-antigens do not occur naturally, but Rh negative persons can be alloimmunized to produce anti-Rh antibodies on challenge with the foreign Rh antigen obtained either through transfusion or during pregnancy (*See* Rh hemolytic disease, page 1078).

Leukocyte Groups

Human leukocyte antigens (HLAs) are present on the surface of granulocytes and lymphocytes. ABO antigens may be present on lymphocytes and possibly, granulocytes, in very small quantities.

Platelet Groups

ABO, HLA-A, HLA-B, and HLA-C are present on platelet surface in addition to several other platelet specific antigens. Platelet antibodies may be detectable in multitransfused persons and these shorten the lifespan of transfused platelets.

Lewis System

These antigens are glycosphingolipids which are produced in the plasma and are absorbed to the red cell surface.

There are two subtypes Lewis a (Le-a) and Lewis b (Le-b). Though they are independent systems, often they interact with other systems. This system does not lead to hemolytic diseases of the newborn.

Ii Blood Group System

This system consists of two antigens I and i. At birth, the neonatal red cells are rich in i antigen and are low in I. There is a gradual change over from i to I antigen up to the age of 2 years. In some persons, this change over may not take place and i antigen predominates. In hemoglobinopathies and dyshemopoietic states also, the red cells may contain more of i antigen.

MNS System

This system is made for anthropological and genetic studies, and also for medicolegal purposes. This group is not generally responsible for hemolytic anemia.

BLOOD BANK PROCEDURES

These include:

- Collection of blood
- Preservation of blood
- Separation of components
- Cross-matching
- Monitoring the adverse reactions.

At present, blood is collected in citrate phosphate dextrose with adenine solution. In this medium, the blood can be stored for 35 days.

Coomb's Test

ABO and Rh groupings may be done by slide method, tube method, or tile method using specific known antisera and red cells. Detection of incomplete antibodies in the serum and red cells is done by the indirect Coombs test and direct Coombs test respectively.

Indirect Coombs Test

This is used for detecting the presence of incomplete antibodies in the serum, e.g. Rh antibodies or antibodies in autoimmune hemolytic anemia. The test serum is incubated with saline washed O group Rh positive cells for 1 hour at 37°C, washed, and 2% suspension of the sensitized washed red cells is made. One drop of washed cell is mixed with one drop of Coombs serum and examined for agglutination by microscopy. A positive test indicates the presence of antibody in the test serum.

Direct Coombs Test

It is done to find out whether the cells are already sensitized by an incomplete antibody *in vivo*. The washed red cells are suspended in saline and one drop of Coombs serum is added to one drop of red cell suspension. Agglutination indicates that the cells are already sensitized by the antibodies *in vivo*.

INDICATIONS FOR TRANSFUSION (TABLE 163.4)

- Replacement of whole blood—sudden loss of 30% of the blood volume (1.5 L) demands urgent replacement.

    Whole blood provides all the components of normal blood. It serves to replace volume loss (as in blood loss) and oxygen carrying capacity which is

Table 163.4: Blood components: use and abuse

Component	Indications	Abuse
Red cells	To increase oxygen carrying capacity in anemic patients	• As a volume expander • To improve general well-being
Platelets	To control or prevent bleeding associated with deficiencies in platelet number or function	• Routine treatment of immune thrombo-cytopenic purpura • Prophylactically in other conditions
Fresh frozen plasma	As a replacement of clotting factors when specific deficiency is demonstrated	As a simple volume expander

Examples

- Anemia
- Thrombocytopenia
- Fibrinogenopenia
- Hypogammaglobulinemia
- Hypoalbuminemia
- Deficiency of clotting factors

- Packed erythrocytes
- Platelets
- Fibrinogen
- Gammaglobulin
- Albumin
- Coagulation factor concentrates

Table 163.5: Storage requirements and shelf-life of blood products

Blood product	Storage specification	Shelf-life
Red cells	2–6°C	35 days
Frozen red cells (reconstituted)	2–6°C	24 hours
Washed red cells	2–6°C	6 hours
Granulocyte concentrates	Room temperature	24 hours
Platelet concentrates	Room temperature with agitation	5 days
Fresh frozen plasma	−20–40°C	12 months
Cryoprecipitate	−20–40°C	12 months

diminished when the hemoglobin (Hb) falls below 10 g/dL. Oxygenation sufficient to support life during rest (without exertion or metabolic stress) can be maintained even with Hb level as low as 7g/dL. Even though up to a decade ago blood losses such as traumatic or surgical conditions were replaced to the full normal level, it is now realized that in many cases correction of Hb up to 10 g/dL is sufficient to keep the oxygen supply from being critically low. Therefore, it is the general policy to refrain from full replenishment of the Hb level, but to top up the level to 10 g/dL or nearabouts. Several studies have also shown that it is not necessary to reach the normal levels and that patients do better if the replenishment is kept around 10 g/dL.

- Specific components are indicated under special circumstances when there is selective deficiency of these components.

Many of the coagulation factors are produced by recombinant DNA technology at present.

Present policy is to separate blood into its components such as erythrocytes, plasma, coagulation factor concentrates, platelets and fibrinogen and give them selectively when indicated. These components are useful for specific indications. Whole blood is given mainly for replacement of extravasated blood. Plasma fractions are coagulation factor concentrates, immunoglobulins and albumin. In many situations, specific component therapy is more effective and safer than whole blood. Component therapy serves to raise the missing coagulation factor rapidly and predictably with a small volume of the concentrated material. In many cases, the exact dose to be transfused can be calculated so that the coagulation factor level can be raised to the desired level and maintained for long periods depending on the specific requirement.

Collected whole blood retains all the stable coagulation factors for 7 days. The labile factors disappear rapidly and only 30% of factors V and VIII will be present in stored blood. RBC maintains their oxygen carrying capacity for 7–10 days, after which the oxygen dissociation curve shifts to the left due to reduction in the levels of diphosphoglycerate. Platelets lose their viability rapidly, unless stored under special conditions. Granulocytes undergo degeneration and become nonfunctional after 24 hours (Table 163.5).

The term *massive transfusion* refers to the transfusion equal to the patient's blood volume within 24 hours.

At present, donor blood is collected in polythene bags. By using appropriate bags, a single unit of blood can be fractionated into packed red cells, platelet concentrates and plasma. From the plasma, further preparations such as cryoprecipitate, fibrinogen and coagulation factors are produced. Erythrocyte fraction is also processed further.

ERYTHROCYTE PREPARATIONS

- Packed cells with or without the buffy coat
- Partially packed red cells
- Washed red cells
- Frozen red cells
- Leukocyte-poor and platelet-poor red cells.

PLATELET TRANSFUSIONS

These are frequently used to tide over periods of thrombocytopenia occurring during anticancer chemotherapy, naturally occurring disease such as thrombocytopenia and thrombocytopathy and to prevent excessive bleeding during and after surgery on thrombocytopenic individuals. Many infections such as dengue hemorrhagic shock, toxic shock syndromes (TSS) and septic shock demand platelet replacement from time-to-time.

The original method was to concentrate platelets by centrifugation of freshly collected blood. This preparation has the disadvantage of lower yield of platelets and presence of excessive amounts of leukocytes and plasma. Moreover several donors have to be recruited for optimal therapy.

Present method is to separate platelets by apheresis in a cell separator from a single donor. On an average, 5×10^{11} platelets are removed in each sitting. Platelets lose their ability to aggregate if stored at refrigerator temperature. They can be stored at +22°C for up to 5 days with constant shaking in order to facilitate gas exchange. Infused platelets may remain viable in the system for short periods. Presence of antibodies directed against class I HLA antigens on platelet surface, or specific antiplatelet alloantibodies developing as a result of repeated transfusions result in rapid destruction of transfused platelets.

Table 163.6: Indications for prophylactic use of platelets in common conditions

Condition	Threshold platelet count
Chronic thrombocytopenic states, e.g. ITP aplastic anemia	5,000/mm³
Stable acute leukemia with bleeding tendency	10,000/mm³
Infection, sepsis, toxemia	20,000/mm³
Preparing the patients for invasive procedures, minor or moderately severe surgery	50,000/mm³
Brain surgery, eye surgery, major and prolonged surgeries	100,000/mm³ or even higher, depending on the clinical condition

Abbreviation: ITP = Idiopathic thrombocytopenic purpura

This can be avoided to some extent by making the platelet concentrate as pure as possible without admixture of leukocytes. Another method is to expose the platelet concentrate to ultraviolet (UV) light, which inhibits lymphocyte function while sparing platelet function.

Indications for Platelet Transfusion

- Prophylactic in bleeding thrombocytopenic patients when the platelet count is < 50,000/mm³.
- In head injury when platelet count is < 100,000/mm³.
- Idiopathic thrombocytopenic purpura (ITP) when other measures do not help to bring up the platelet count and arrest bleeding.
- ITP with pregnancy when the maternal and fetal platelet counts are low.
- In cancer chemotherapy when iatrogenic thrombocytopenia is likely.
- In leukemia patients when platelets count is less than 20,000/mm³.

Platelets can be administered as platelet concentrates obtained by apheresis using a cell separator from single donor or as platelet rich plasma (PRP). One unit of PRP raises the platelet count by 5,000–10,000/mm³. One unit of platelet concentrate obtained by apheresis is equivalent to 6-8 units of PRP.

Several indications for prophylactic use of platelets in common conditions are given in Table 163.6.

One unit of random donor platelet concentrate raises the platelet count by 5,000–10,000/mm³. One apheresis unit of platelet raises the count by 30,000–60,000/mm³.

FRESH FROZEN PLASMA (FFP)

This is prepared form fresh blood by separating and freezing the plasma within 6 hours. It can be stored at –20°C or below for up to 1 year. The volume of one unit of FFP is 200–250 mL. It contains mainly factors V and VIII, but other factors as well. FFP is given usually in conditions such as disseminated intravascular coagulation (DIC), liver disease with bleeding tendency, emergency treatment of coagulation defects when the specific component therapy is not available and reversal of bleeding tendency in warfarin overdose. The usual dose is 10–15 mL/kg bw. One unit of FFP raises the missing coagulation factor by 8–10% for varying periods. FFP should be thawed immediately prior to use and once thawed, it should be used within 6 hours.

Table 163.7: Various coagulation factors and their amount in one unit of cryoprecipitate

Coagulation factor	Quantity/unit
Fibrinogen	150–250 mg
Factor VIII	80–150 units
von Willebrand factor	100–150 units
Factor XIII	50–75 units

Cryoprecipitate

This is prepared from single donor plasma by controlled precipitation from fresh plasma, at 4°C. It is rich in factors VIII, von Willebrand factor (VWF), factor XIII, fibrinogen and fibronectin. Before transfusion, it is thawed at 30°C. One mL of cryoprecipitate contains 10 units of factor VIII compared to 1 unit/mL in FFP. The dose of cryoprecipitate is 1 unit for every 10 kg bw. Once it is thawed to room temperature it should be used within 6 hours (Table 163.7).

Plasmapheresis

In this process, only plasma is removed from the donor. Plasmapheresis can be used as a therapeutic measure to treat circulatory overload, hyperviscosity syndromes, or for removal of circulating immunoglobulins and immune complexes and macroglobulins. Plasmapheresis and plasma exchange are accepted methods of treatment for myasthenic reactions, Guillain-Barré syndrome (GBS), hemolytic uremic syndrome (HUS), thrombotic thrombocytopenic purpura (TTP) and others. This method is also employed to obtain high titer immunoglobulins from suitable subjects.

Leukapheresis

Therapeutically, leukapheresis, i.e. removal of leukocytes, can be done to reduce leukocytes load in extreme leukocytosis.

Plateletpheresis

In addition to prepare platelet concentrates from selected donors for massive platelet transfusion, this method can be used as temporary measure to reduce extremely high platelet counts which may precipitate thrombotic complications.

HAZARDS OF TRANSFUSION THERAPY

Febrile Reactions

These are caused by pyrogenic substances present in the material or in the infusion set. Sometimes these indicate bacterial contamination.

Allergic Manifestations

Allergic reactions like urticaria and edema may occur due to antigen-antibody reactions.

Bacterial Contamination

If the blood is heavily infected, severe reactions set in even with the introduction of a small quantity of blood. Shock may ensue which may be followed by DIC.

Mechanical Complications

Circulatory overloading, air embolism, thrombophlebitis and pulmonary embolism (PE) may develop if the infusion is not carefully supervised.

Metabolic Complications

These develop due to citrate toxicity, potassium toxicity, toxic substances eluted from synthetic containers and vasoactive substances, specially after massive transfusion.

Hemolytic Reactions

These reactions usually develop due to the presence of incompatible antibody in the recipient's plasma which causes destruction of donor red cells. Less commonly, potent antibodies such as anti-A or anti-B present in donor plasma may react with the homologous antigens present in the recipient's red cells and provoke hemolysis.

Hemorrhagic Reaction

This complication may be encountered after massive transfusions using stored blood. Post-transfusion purpura follows massive transfusion of stored blood poor in platelets or after 7–10 days of collection. The latter is due to immune destruction of allogenic and autologous platelets caused by antiplatelet HPA antibodies.

Immune Reactions

Various types of immunological reactions may develop varying in severity from fatal to mild symptoms. Among this, hemolytic reactions due to transfusion of incompatible blood or hemolyzed blood are the most common. This manifests with pain in the back, dyspnea and circulatory collapse. At times, persistent hypotension may be the only finding. In severe cases jaundice, hemoglobinuria and anuria develop within 24 hours. Renal failure may be fatal. Rarely DIC may follow ABO incompatibility.

Nonhemolytic Reactions

These may vary from simple allergic reactions to fatal anaphylaxis. Antibodies to drugs such as penicillin may be present in the donor's blood causing allergic reactions in the recipient.

It is a rule that all transfusion should be supervised by trained competent personnel and all adverse effects occurring during the procedure and for a week subsequently should be recorded and attended to.

Immune-mediated Problems

These include transfusion associated graft-versus-host disease (GVHD) and transfusion-related immune modulation (TRIM).

The former is due to recognition of the recipient's antigen as foreign, by the donor T-lymphocytes. This leads to pancytopenia and dermatological, gastrointestinal (GI), and hepatic symptoms. The exact pathogenesis of TRIM is not clear. It leads to increase in cytokine stimulation of donor leukocytes and improved survival of renal allografts. Adverse effects include the precipitation of infections and recurrence of tumors.

TRANSFUSION TRANSMITTED INFECTIONS

- ***Viral infections:*** Human immunodeficiency virus (HIV) I and HIV II. Data from Delhi gave seroprevalence for HIV rate as 0.71–0.77% for blood donors. In Trivandrum, the seroprevalence of HIV is 0.2%. In Punjab, it was 0.26%.

- ***Hepatitis viruses:***
  - All the hepatitis viruses—hepatitis B virus (HBV), hepatitis C virus (HCV), delta virus, hepatitis A virus (HAV), hepatitis G virus (HGV) and hepatitis E virus (HEV) can be transmitted. HBV and HCV are clinically the most important in this group. The approximate risk for transfusion associated hepatitis (TAH) in India for HBV is 0.07% and for HCV is 0.04%.
  - Transfusion-associated hepatitis should be diagnosed if there is elevation of serum glutamic-pyruvic transaminase (SGPT) levels in the recipient to 1.5 times the normal value or more, on two occasions at 5 days interval when estimated at 14–180 days after the transfusion.

- ***Other viruses:*** Human T-cell lymphotropic virus (HTLV) I and II, cytomegalovirus (CMV).
- ***Parasitic infections:*** Malaria, trypanosomiasis, toxoplasmosis, babesiosis.
- ***Bacterial infections:*** *Yersinia enterocolitica*, *Staphylococcus epidermidis*, *Bacillus cereus*, syphilis and others. *Treponema pallidum* can remain viable in refrigerated blood for up to 5 days.

The risk of infection from needle stick injuries to medical personnel handling infective blood is given below:

HIV	3/1,000
HBV	30%
HCV	1.2–10%

- The rates are much higher if infected blood is transfused.
- Apart from extreme care in selecting donors, proper methods to sterilize the equipment are absolutely essential to avoid microbial contamination of the blood and blood products and infection of the medical and laboratory personnel. Common norms to be followed include:
  - Proper handwashing before and after handling every patient
  - Use of protective gloves
  - Use of mask and eye-protectors when blood or body fluids are likely to splash
  - Handling all infective fluids and tissues with the same precautions as for blood, e.g. semen, vaginal and cervical secretions, amniotic fluid, cerebrospinal fluid (CSF), other aspirated fluids, saliva, tissues and organs including the cornea.

Disinfection

Most of the disinfectants available in India are capable of destroying almost all microbes including HIV, if used properly. Since blood and tissue fluids will protect the microbes embedded within them, they have to be properly cleaned before applying the chemical disinfectant. The following disinfectants are amply effective in the recommended dosage:

- Chlorine releasing compounds
- Iodine compounds—povidone iodine 1% strength
- Ethyl alcohol 70% (denatured spirit)
- Cetrimide (Savlon) 1/1,000 solution
- Dichloroxylenol (Dettol) 1.5% solution.

Gamma Irradiation of Blood

Transfusion-associated GVHD is a rare immunological complication caused by the presence of immuno-competent T-lymphocytes in the donor blood. Gamma irradiation of blood and blood products prevents this complication.

Hemosiderosis: In subjects receiving repeated transfusions, iron overload may occur leading to deposition of iron in reticuloendothelial and parenchymal tissue. Usually this complication is seen in persons who have received 100 units or more of blood.

Each unit of 250 mL of erythrocytes introduces 250 mg of elemental iron into the recipient. The end organ manifestations of iron overload include cirrhosis, hepatocellular carcinoma, cardiac failure, diabetes mellitus (DM) and hypothyroidism.

Autotransfusion: This is the use of blood collected from the patient for use at a subsequent occasion such as selective surgery. Several units of blood can be collected from the patient at regular intervals preceding the surgical procedure, to be used at the time of need. Stimulation of erythropoiesis by erythropoietin (EPO) and nutritional supplements helps to increase the yield of blood. Autotransfusion is safe and it is free from several of the drawbacks of external blood.

Any reaction occurring in the patient within 48 hours of transfusion should be reported to the blood bank. Whenever there are good grounds for suspecting any untoward reaction, transfusion should be discontinued, and the patient should be monitored. The blood sample should be taken for tests.

CORD BLOOD TRANSFUSION

Use of blood collected from the umbilical cord after delivery as a source of stem cells has become an established procedure within the past 3 decades. Cord blood contains large number of granulocyte-macrophage progenitor stem cells, sufficient enough to repopulate marrows of irradiated subjects. This has paved way for organized cord blood banking. There are several blood banks undertaking storage and delivery of cord blood, all over the developed countries. In India, there are a few privately-owned cord blood banks. Cord blood can be cryopreserved in the viable state for many years. The services provided include:

- Use of cord blood as a source of stem cells
- Preservation of the cord blood indefinitely for long periods, for use in the same individual if a need for stem cells arises. The donor is charged for this service.

Uses of Cord Blood

- Allogenic transplant
- Autologous transplant
- As a source of pluripotent stem cells for reconstitution and repair of damaged tissues such as the heart after myocardial infarction (MI).

The immunological properties of cord blood stem cells differ from those of adult marrow or peripheral blood.

Cord blood contains a higher proportion of T-cells expressing (CD45 RA$^+$/CD45 RAO$^-$) and CD62L$^+$. These cells are immunologically naive and therefore GVHD is less common. The chemokine receptor CCR5 expressed by Th1 T-lymphocytes is less abundant in cord blood T-cells compared to adult T-cells.

Cord Blood Banking

Pregnant women are recruited as donors after obtaining informed consent and excluding common communicable diseases. Blood is collected from the placental side of the severed umbilical cord either *in utero* before the delivery of the placenta or *ex utero* after its delivery. Long-term storage is done under temperatures below −180°C and released for use on demand after proper cross-matching.

Indications for Cord Blood Transfusions

- Stem cell replenishment in hematological malignancies—acute leukemias, chronic myeloid leukemia (CML) and myelodysplastic syndrome (MDS).
- Nonmalignant conditions—aplastic anemia, thalassemias, hemoglobinopathies, immunodefficiency states.

Advantages of cord blood are its availability, lower incidence of GVHD and good success rate even if mismatched for two antigens. The waiting period for transplantation is also shorter. ***Disadvantages*** are higher infection rates with cord blood stem cells compared to preparations from bone marrow or peripheral blood from adult donors. Future strategies for improving the service include:

- Wider recognition and acceptance of this method and establishment of more cord blood transfusion units in major hospitals.
- Cord blood expansion using cytokines which stimulate stem cell proliferation.
- Combining cord blood and haploidentical bone marrow transplants.
- Nonmyeloablative or reduced intensity conditioning regimen.

BLOOD SUBSTITUTES

Several attempts have been made from time-to-time to find out substitutes for blood, i.e. fluid media which can transport oxygen from the lungs to the tissues and remove carbon dioxide. Perfluorocarbon compounds have the property to transport oxygen and carbon dioxide and these have been studied in detail. Hemoglobin solutions have also been studied for this purpose.

STEM CELL TRANSPLANTATION

Stem cells are capable of pluripotent differentiation when exposed to appropriate chemical or biological influences, both *in vivo* and *in vitro*. Such cells are present in several tissues in the body such as the bone marrow, peripheral blood, skin, periodontal ligament of teeth sockets and others. When transplanted, these cells can reconstitute the cell population of several organs such as the hemopoietic tissue of bone marrow, myocardium, neural tissue, immunocytes, periodontal ligament and others. Stem cells have the unique property of self-perpetuation, i.e. a proportion of the stem cell pool remains in the pluripotent phase without differentiation, and these proliferate and help to perpetuate these primordial capabilities, without decline. Stem cells are immunophenotypically classified as CD34$^+$.

Sources of stem cells include bone marrow, peripheral blood, umbilical cord blood, fetal organs and artificially produced human embryos *in vitro*. Active research is going on in several countries on the potential use and production of stem cells.

Mainly stem cells are used for hematological disorders such as aplastic anemia, leukemia, myeloma, thalassemias, hemoglobinopathies, congenital immunodeficiency syndromes, inherited disorders of metabolism and for repopulating the marrow after intensive chemotherapy for malignancies.

Stem cells have been used for the treatment of nonhematological diseases as well. There include:

- Intracoronary infusion of stem cells for restoration of function of ischemic myocardium
- Restoration of periodontal tissues
- Reconstitution of immunocytes
- Generation of neural precursors using stem cells derived from adult human skin
- Amyotrophic lateral sclerosis
- DM and several others.

Creation of human embryos for purposes of organ donation and stem cell production are matters involving ethical issues and therefore this matter is under discussion and debate.

IMPORTANT POINTS IN BLOOD BANKING PROCEDURES

All containers and equipment have to be pyrogen-free. Blood containers are made of polyvinyl chloride (PVC) and they should allow exchange of oxygen and carbon dioxide.

While collecting blood, the time for a collection is limited to 15–20 minutes and the volume collected is 350–450 mL of blood. The donor should be advised to drink adequate fluids and refrain from smoking tobacco for at least 1 hour. Adverse donor reactions include vasovagal attacks, fainting and even convulsions.

Platelets for Transfusion

For transfusion of platelets in large quantities, apheresis platelet collection from patient's family members is preferable, if possible, from HLA compatible persons. The donor should have platelet count above 150,000/mm^3. Platelet units collected by apheresis should contain at least 3×10^{11} platelets in 90% of the units. If donors for platelet collection are repeatedly summoned and if the platelet sample contains red cells, care should to be taken to limit the RBC loss to less than 200 mL in 8 weeks. If the apheresis procedure leads to a red cell loss of 200–300 mL/session, the donor should be deferred from next donation for 8 and 16 weeks respectively.

Granulocyte Concentrates

Each unit should contain 1×10^{10} cells. Testing for ABO and Rh compatibility should be done by looking for antibodies. Presence of infection should be meticulously prevented. Granulocytes should be stored at 20–24°C only for 24 hours.

Screening for Infections

Risks of acquiring HIV, HBV, HCV, HTLV, CMV and human herpesvirus (HHV) 8 are high in those receiving repeated transfusions. Low transmission rates occur in parvovirus B19. West Nile virus infection has attracted the attention of blood transfusion officers.

Bacterial contamination of blood and blood components are generally derived from donor skin or donor blood and infection during the process. Infection of the blood and blood component leads to production of bacterial toxins. Platelets are more likely to develop bacterial contamination since they are stored at near room temperature. Gram-positive skin saprophytes are the common organisms contaminating platelet units.

Adverse Reactions

All transfusions should be supervised by trained personnel and adverse effects occurring during the transfusion and later should be recorded and attended to.

CHAPTER 164

Leukemias: General Considerations

Salim Shafeek, Kasim Salim, KV Krishna Das, Mathew Thomas

Chapter Summary

- General Considerations
- Classification of Leukemias
- Etiology and Pathogenesis
- Pathophysiology
- General Symptomatology
- Diagnosis of Leukemias
  - Peripheral Blood Film Examination
- Bone Marrow Transplantation (BMT)
  - Peripheral Stem Cell Transplantation

GENERAL CONSIDERATIONS

Leukemias are a group of neoplastic disorders affecting mainly the leukopoietic tissues in the body and characterized generally by the presence of leukocytosis, immature leukocytes in the peripheral blood and proliferation of these immature cells in the bone marrow resulting in the suppression of normal tissues. The abnormal cells infiltrate several organs in the body. Genetic abnormalities transform precursor stem cells into

Table 164.1: Frequency of leukemias in adults seen in India

Leukemias	Percent (%)
Chronic myeloid leukemia	25–30
Acute myeloid leukemia	20–25
Acute lymphatic leukemia	20–25
Chronic lymphatic leukemia	1–2
Other types (megakaryocytic and erythro)	1

potential leukemia cells. The disease process starts in the bone marrow or lymphatic tissue depending on the cell type and peripheral blood is flooded with abnormal cells several years after the formation of the malignant clone. Less commonly, erythroid precursors, megakaryocytes and plasma cells may be involved.

Leukemias may be broadly grouped into two—acute and chronic. ***Acute leukemias*** affect younger age groups more frequently. They run a rapid course and the peripheral blood and bone marrow show presence of large number of blast cells. If left untreated, these are fatal within weeks or months. ***Chronic leukemias*** generally affect the older age groups, they run a more protracted course, and terminate life within 2–3 years of onset. Leukemias account for 0.15–0.6% of the total medical admissions in many general hospitals in India.

It is to be noted that chronic lymphocytic leukemia (CLL) is less common in India and neighboring countries when compared to West (Table 164.1).

CLASSIFICATION OF LEUKEMIAS

Leukemias being heterogeneous diseases, several parameters have been employed for classification. These include morphology, histochemistry, cell surface and cytoplasmic immunological markers and cytogenetic, and immunogenetic studies.

It is important to classify the disease precisely since the clinical behavior, course, prognosis and response to treatment differ in the different types.

In over 80% of cases of acute lymphatic leukemia (ALL) and acute myeloid leukemia (AML), nonrandom chromosomal abnormalities are usually present. At present, the ***French-American-British (FAB) classification*** is one of the accepted systems for acute leukemia (Table 164.2). This has been modified repeatedly including immunological and molecular parameters from time-to-time. AML is classified on the degree of maturation and differentiation of the abnormal cell. ALL is classified on the basis of cell size, nuclear chromatin pattern, nuclear shape, nucleoli, amount and basophilia of cytoplasm, and extent of cytoplasmic vacuolization.

ETIOLOGY AND PATHOGENESIS

Leukemias are multicentric in origin. An abnormal stem cell undergoes mutation and proliferates in a disorderly and unrestrained manner so as to fill the marrow, spill into the peripheral blood, and infiltrate almost all organs in the body. The clone of malignant cells proliferates by division but fails to differentiate and hence, immature forms persist in the marrow and peripheral blood. Though the exact

Table 164.2: Classification of neoplasia involving leukocytes

Chronic leukemias
- Chronic myeloid leukemia (CML)
- Chronic lymphatic leukemia (CLL)
- Hairy cell leukemia (variant of CLL)
- Prolymphocytic leukemia (variant of CLL)
- Plasma cell leukemia
- Chronic myelomonocytic leukemia
- Sézary syndrome—leukemic phase of mycosis fungoides

Acute leukemias: Acute myeloid leukemia French-American-British (FAB) Classification. Differentiation of the immature cells forms the main criteria.

Subclass	Type of cell
M0	Undifferentiated by light microscopy
M1	Poorly differentiated
M2	More differentiated
M3 [acute promyelocytic leukemia (PML)]	Dysplastic promyelocytes M3h-hyper granular PML M3v-inapparent or fine granules M3a-less hypergranular blasts
M4	Both granulocytic and monocytic
M4	Eo-myelodysplastic eosinophils
M5	Monocytic differentiation M5a-predominantly blasts M5b-differentiation into promonocytes and monocytes
M6	Myeloblasts with dysplastic erythroid precursors
M7	Megakaryoblastic

Acute lymphatic leukemia (FAB): When stained with Wright's stain three types, L1, L2 and L3 can be distinguished morphologically.

L1: The blast cells are small and there is no appreciable variation in size and shape. The nuclear chromatin is smooth and the nucleoli are indistinct.

L2: The blast cells vary in size with prominent nucleoli and a variable amount of cytoplasm.

L3: The cells are deeply basophilic with vacuolated cytoplasm. Immunological markers and other cytochemical markers help to identify the cell precisely.

Different hematological cancers can be distinct at the molecular level even though they may appear similar morphologically. This is true for acute and chronic leukemias and lymphomas. ALLs can be broadly grouped into three:
1. Precursor B lymphoblastic leukemia
2. Precursor T lymphoblastic leukemia
3. Burkitt lymphoma or leukemia

In addition, there are acute leukemias of ambiguous lineage. These are:
- Biphenotypic acute leukemias
- Undifferentiated acute leukemias.

The availability of immunological probes like monoclonal antibodies (mAb), techniques like flow cytometry and deoxyribonucleic acid (DNA) microarray analysis have enabled the subtyping of acute leukemias and lymphomas based on immunological markers such as CD positivity (cluster group of differentiation). This has helped to devise specifically effective therapy with less of side effects.

stimulus for the mutation is not clear in an individual case, several factors are known to induce leukemia in experimental animals and humans.
- Genetic factors are important as evidenced by the increased incidence of leukemia in mongolism and Fanconi's anemia.

- Ribonucleic acid (RNA) viruses such as the retrovirus and deoxyribonucleic acid (DNA) viruses such as Epstein-Barr virus (EBV) may induce leukemogenic changes in cells.
- Exposure to ionizing radiation (accidental and therapeutic) and long-term use of drugs and chemicals which depress bone marrow (benzol, chloramphenicol and cytotoxic drugs such as alkylating agents and cyclophosphamide) have been incriminated to be leukemogenic by clinical, experimental and epidemiological observations.
- Occurrence of cases in close relatives or in successive generations and in clusters in closed communities has strengthened the role of environmental factors in leukemogenesis.
- Diseases like multiple myeloma and lymphomas transform into acute myelogenous leukemia in some cases. It is likely that the development of leukemia is the total effect of the environmental factors on the genetically predisposed individual. The clone of leukemic cell multiplies in exponential rates. The cell cycle time is generally longer for leukemias than for many other tumors [AML 80–84 h, chronic myeloid leukemia (CML) 120 h].

The role of oncogenes in the causation of malignancies has been established (*See* Ch 6). Several leukemias show chromosomal abnormalities which point to their basic role in leukemogenesis. The formation of proto-oncogenes, their activation to form oncogenes by translocation, and the production of malignant clone has all been studied. Diagnostic and prognostic information is obtained by chromosomal studies of almost all hematological malignancies, specially, in CML and myelodysplastic syndromes (MDS).

PATHOPHYSIOLOGY

The underlying defect in acute leukemia is the unregulated proliferation of primitive cells without undergoing differentiation. The transformation into a leukemic cell may occur at any point in the maturation and differentiation of the pluripotent stem cell. Both ALL and AML are unicellular in origin and this abnormal cell proliferates to form a clone of malignant cells which populate the marrow and other tissues. AML may develop at any stage of development of the myeloid stem cells colony-forming unit–spleen (CFU-S). If the malignant transformation takes place at the early stage, both erythroid and granulocytic series are involved (M6). Similarly, CML originating from a very primitive precursor which has the capability of differentiating into lymphoid or myeloid cell lines can develop lymphoid blast crisis during transformation. If it occurs at a later stage of development after formation of the committed granulocyte macrophage progenitor (CFU-GM), only the myeloid and monocyte series are involved (M1-M6). In ALL, the committed myeloid progenitor cells (CFU-C) are normal. In acute leukemia, the bone marrow contains both abnormal and normal cells, the latter being considerately suppressed, so that with eradication of the malignant cells, the remaining normal cells can repopulate the marrow. In contrast, in CML almost all the cells in the bone marrow are abnormal.

GENERAL SYMPTOMATOLOGY

Symptoms differ between acute and chronic leukemias. These are summarized in Table 164.3.

Table 164.3: Differences between acute and chronic leukemias

Features	Acute leukemia	Chronic leukemia
Age group	More in the 1st and 2nd decades but can occur in all age groups	Mostly in the 4th, 5th and 6th decades but even young children may be affected rarely
Sex ratio	M:F is 2:1	M:F is 1:1
Duration of symptoms	Weeks to months	Several months to 1 year
Presenting complaints	Anemia, fever, infections, hemorrhagic tendencies or complications, specially neurological	Vague symptoms, loss of weight, mass in the abdomen or lymph nodular masses
Organomegaly	Liver, spleen and lymph nodes are moderately enlarged in 70–80% of cases	Moderate to gross splenomegaly is the rule in CML Moderate to gross lymphadenopathy occurs in CLL
Blood picture	Total leukocyte count is moderately elevated ($15-30 \times 10^9$/L = 15–30,000/mm^3), Blast cells form 10–90% of the total; Platelets are often reduced	Total leukocyte count is grossly elevated, $15-25 \times 10^{10}$/L (150–250,000/mm^3)
Bone marrow	Shows depression of erythroid cells, myeloid cells and megakaryocytes, and infiltration by the abnormal cells. Blast cells form more than 20% and may be even up to 90%	CML shows increase in myeloid cells, specially myelocytes, metamyelocytes, and nertrophils, infiltration by small lymphocytes is seen in CLL, Erythroid and megakaryocytic precursors show variable cellularity
Chromosomal studies	Different patterns in different subtypes	Ph chromosome is demonstrable in over 95% cases of CML
Course and prognosis	Untreated, fatal within weeks to six months due to infections, hemorrhage, anemia or other complications	Untreated, CML has a median survival of 18–24 months, CLL has a generally more prolonged course of several years
Response to treatment	Spontaneous remissions have rarely been reported. With modern treatment, over 90% of cases go into remission and 60–70% get complete cure. ALL in children gives the best results	With modern chemotherapy about 20–30% of CML is cured; With bone marrow transplantation at the ideal-time cure rates exceed 50% CLL follows a variable course with chemotherapy

Abbreviations: M = Male; F = Female; CML = Chronic myeloid leukemia; CLL = Chronic lymphocytic leukemia; ALL = Acute lymphatic leukemia

DIAGNOSIS OF LEUKEMIAS

Acute leukemia should be suspected in all cases of rapidly developing anemia, prolonged fevers, hepatospleno-megaly, lymph node enlargement, hemorrhagic tendency, local tumor formation, neurological manifestations and other bizarre clinical presentations. ALL may be mistaken for rheumatic or rheumatoid arthritis (RA) in children. Early diagnosis is possible only if the clinical suspicion is strong.

It is not uncommon for AML to present with atypical features initially. Local tumor formation (also known as granulocyte sarcomas) without or with blood and bone marrow abnormalities is a rare presentation. Granulocytic sarcomas may develop in AML and less commonly in CML or other myeloproliferative disorders. They can be typed histologically into mature, immature (intermediate) or blastic types according to the cell composition. They may involve any tissues.

As the disease evolves, characteristic bone marrow and blood picture become evident. Aleukemic leukemia cutis (ALC) is such a condition in which the skin lesion appears as an induration, nodule or tumor caused by leukemic cell infiltration, blood and bone marrow remaining normal. ALL is more common to produce local lesions in the bone.

Serum uric acid is elevated during the active phase of leukemias. Uric acid levels are elevated further during treatment with cytotoxic drugs due to rapid cell destruction.

Since early institution of treatment is more effective in curing the disease, specific investigations should not be delayed. Rarely leukemias may be brought out by routine investigations in asymptomatic individuals. This is more so for CML.

Clinical diagnosis has to be followed up with hematological confirmation.

Peripheral Blood Film Examination

The diagnosis of acute leukemia is suggested by the presence of blast cells, which are the precursors of leukocytes. Blast cells are characterized by deep blue nongranular cytoplasm and a rounded or oval nucleus showing pale stained inclusions, the nucleoli, which vary in number from 2 to 5. Though some idea about the nature of the blast can be obtained by morphology, further identification is done by cytochemical and immunological methods (Figs 164.1 to 164.3).

Peroxidase and *Sudan black* are stains which detect the presence of lysosomes containing the primary granules of the neutrophilic and monocytic series. Terminal deoxynucleotidyl transferase is seen most commonly in ALL, occasionally in the blastic phase of CML and rarely in AML (Table 164.4).

Cytological differentiation and immunophenotyping are important since the treatment, complications and prognosis differs in the various subtypes.

Bone marrow examination is mandatory in all cases. Presence of blasts in excess of 30% of the total cells in the marrow confirms the diagnosis of acute leukemia. Elevation above 5% should be taken into account and the

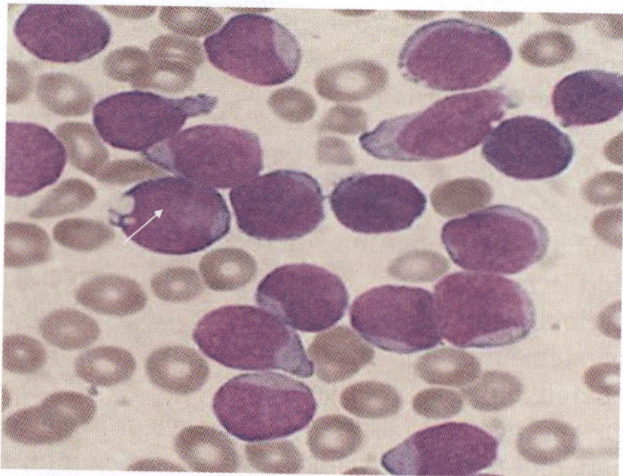

Fig. 164.1: Acute lymphatic leukemia peripheral blood × 1,000. **Note:** The blast cell with nucleolus (arrow)

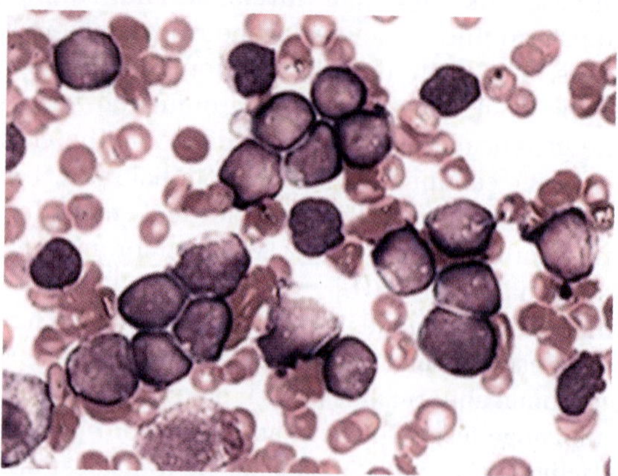

Fig. 164.3: Acute lymphatic leukemia bone marrow × 400. **Note:** Replacement by lymphoblasts

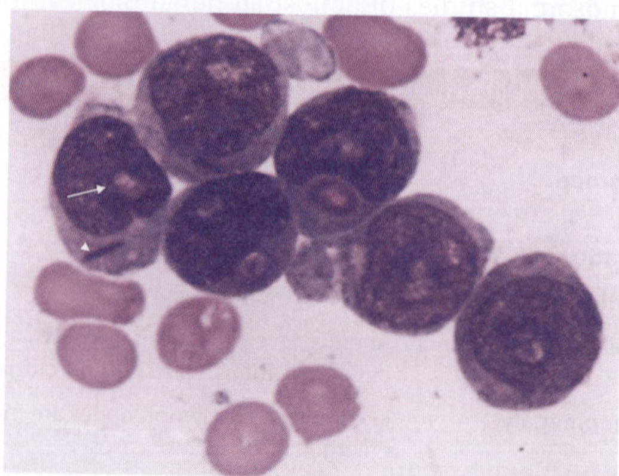

Fig. 164.2: Acute myeloid leukemia peripheral blood × 1,000 myeloblast with Auer's rods (arrow head), nucleolus (arrow)

patient should be followed up with periodic repetition of laboratory tests to detect the onset of florid leukemia at the earliest.

In chronic leukemias, diagnosis is easy by examining the blood film, since the cells show typical differentiating features. In CML, neutrophils and myelocytes predominate in the peripheral blood. In CLL, mature lymphocytes predominate.

Though vast majority of leukemias show leukocytosis, in 10–20%, the count may be normal or low even though immature cells are present. These are termed as *subleukemic leukemias*. When there are no abnormal

Table 164.4: Differences between lymphoblasts and myeloblasts

Features	Lymphoblasts	Myeloblasts
Number of nucleoli	1–2	2–5
Accompanying cells	Lymphocytes and nongranular cells	Promyelocytes, myelocytes and neutrophils
Peroxidase staining	Negative	Promyelocytes, myelocytes and neutrophils are positive; early blasts are negative
Sudan black staining	Negative	Positive
PAS (periodic acid Schiff staining)	Coarsely positive	Finely positive
TdT (terminal-deoxytransferase)	Generally positive	Generally negative

Note: Many more histochemical and immunological markers are available for precise diagnosis

cells in the peripheral blood, the term ***aleukemic leukemia*** is used. Bone marrow is hypercellular in most cases and shows infiltration by abnormal cells irrespective of the leukocyte count in peripheral blood.

Leukemias have to be differentiated from leukemoid reactions which are less common.

Immunophenotyping is mandatory for confirmation of the diagnosis and for accurate differentiation between subtypes in both acute and chronic leukemias. This is the final word in conjunction with morphology, worldwide. This can give a more accurate diagnostic tool separating B-cell from T-cell origin. Specific monoclonal primary antibodies (Abs) for the same antigens are used for assigning cluster of differentiation numbers approved at the International Leukocyte Typing Workshop.

Flow cytometry plot clearly showing the clear cut differentiation acute promyelocytic leukemia (APL) (M3) leukemia on the left and chronic lymphocytic lymphoma on the right (Figs 164.4A and B, see the color tagging).

Curve on the left: Showing the clear cut differentiation of green cell population of hypergranular blasts in APL. Size and granularity pushes the cells to left and upper quadrant.

Compared to the right picture showing the green plot of lymphoid cells in CLL with no granules at all, hence the green uptake is toward right lower quadrant. This is an extremely useful technique used to differentiate the type of leukemia.

Fluorescence *in situ* Hybridization (FISH) used to Detect BCR-ABL (Philadelphia Chromosome)

Karyotype and chromosomal aberrations:

- Tricolor dual fusion translocation probe showing the classical t9:22 BCR/ABL.
- Multicolor banding probe showing clearly the microdissection specific at chromosome 9.
- ***FISH:*** Confirming the complex t9:22 and additional chromosome t10:17 (rare but seen in relapsing CML).
- The deletion of TP53 and deletion 17p, rare but associated with poor prognosis CML, relapsed and resistance to tyrosine kinase inhibitors (TKIs).

Cytogenetics and FISH

Conventional cytogenetics requires dividing cells and can be time-consuming. FISH is more and more commonly used for diagnostics, as it gives results faster (Fig. 164.5).

In situ hybridization, polymerase chain reaction (PCR) and gene expression profiling

- ***In situ hybridization*** uses labeled probes (complimentary DNA or RNA strands) to localize specific DNA or RNA sequences in samples and tissue.
- ***PCR*** enables detection of rearrangements in the immunoglobulin gene in B- and T-cells receptors and determine clonality specifically.
- ***Gene expression profiling*** is the newest technology which has been tried in different diagnostic tools and which has been found to give prognostic information in different leukemias and lymphomas. DNA microarrays and other high throughput technologies improve the diagnostic specificity of leukemias and lymphomas.

This will be the future diagnostic tool for easy and rapid screening. This method is currently used as a part

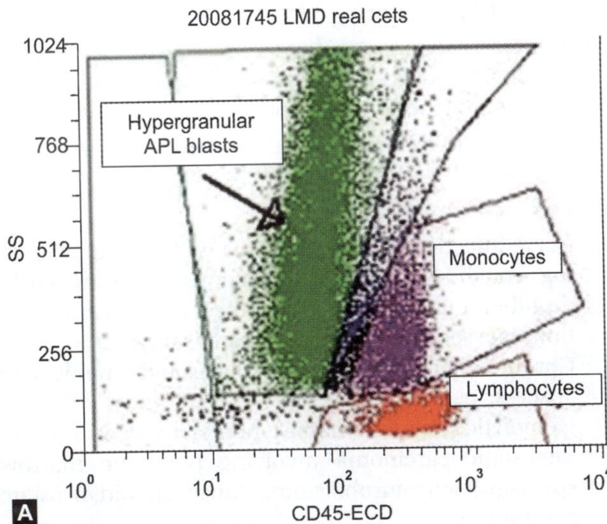

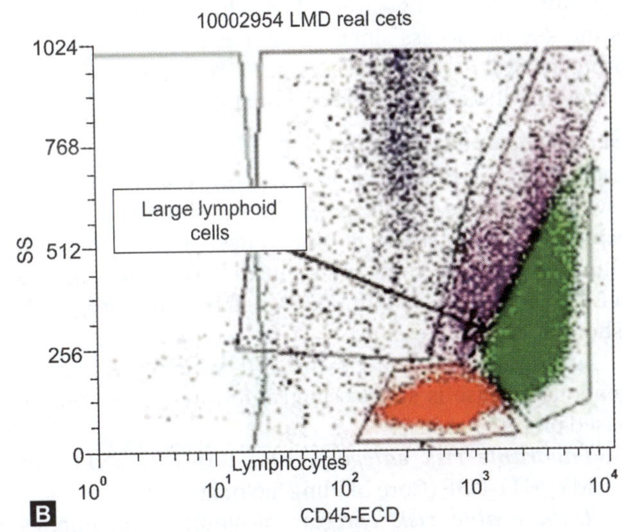

Figs 164.4A and B: Flow cytometry plot

Abbreviation: APL = Acute promyelocytic leukemia

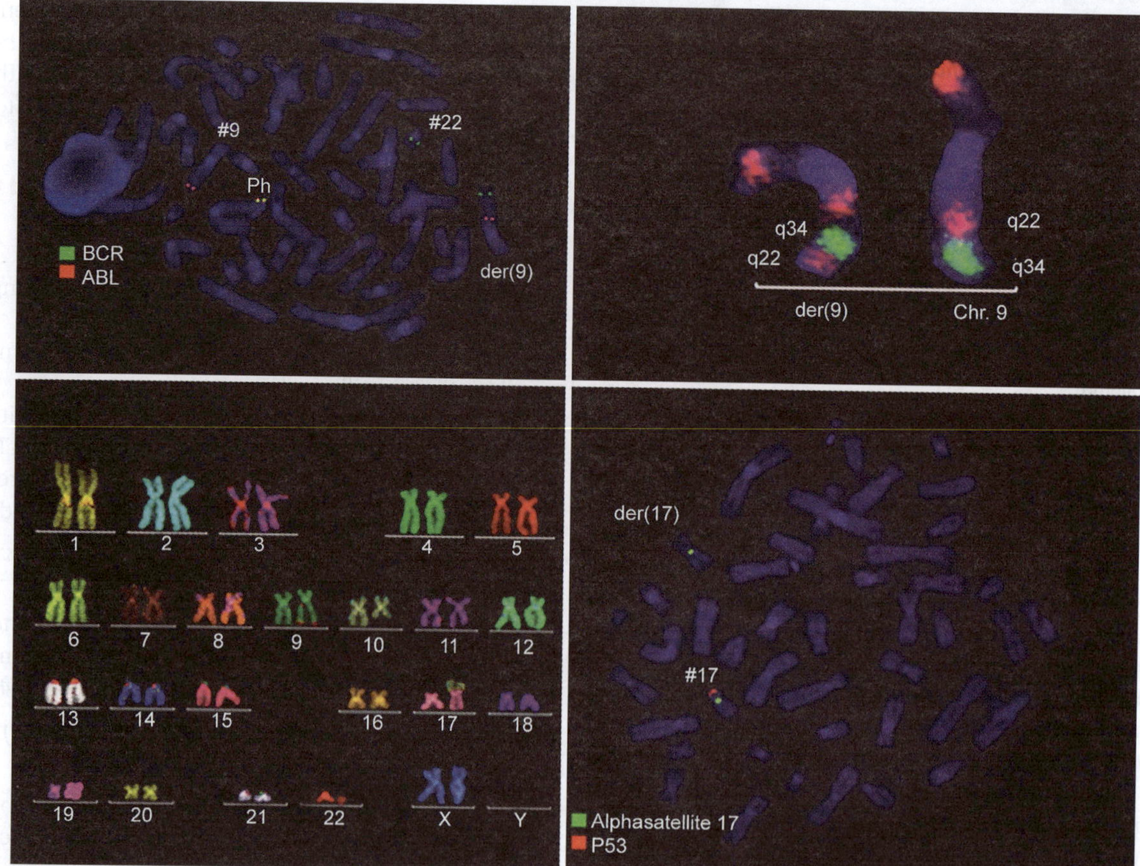

Fig. 164.5: FISH used to detect BCR-ABL (Philadelphia chromosome) in chronic myeloid leukemia

of all European leukemia trials like AML 17 and 18 done through Medical Research Council (MRC), UK.

Colors representing gene activity (red is high, blue is low) show that mixed lineage leukemia (MLL) has a distinct pattern from both ALL and AML. Each vertical column of squares represents a tumor sample. Each horizontal row of squares represents the activity of one gene. MLL has a totally different prognosis from childhood ALL and AML, and it is extremely difficult to differentiate from childhood ALL and AML by morphology and immunophenotyping alone. Risk stratification of MLL is the key to success since treating as per pediatric ALL protocol will not be successful. Tyrosine-kinase gene targeting will be the treatment modality for future.

Gene Expression Profiling (Fig. 164.6)

Each column represents a bone marrow sample and each row corresponds to a gene. Red color shade is elevated expression while shade in blue is decreased expression. This is useful to demonstrate, Fms like tyrosine kinase 3 (FLT3) gene expression in MLL which has poor prognosis (showing over expression).

Epigenetic and genetics in AML which is a heterogeneous disease is subclassified into three risk category based on cytogenetics:

1. ***Favorable risk category:*** PML-RARA/RUNX1T1 or MYTH11-CBF (Core binding factor group)
2. ***Unfavorable risk category:*** Complex cytogenetics (e.g. monosomy karyotype)
3. ***Intermediate risk category:*** Normal karyotype.

AML whole genome profiling showed nine different categories playing role in pathogenesis. Tumor suppressor gene, transcription factor fusion, activated signaling gene and epigenetic modifiers. This gives the AML risk stratification a new front of subdivision even in the group which was classified as intermediate risk due to previous normal karyotype. Further work in this direction are progressing and it is likely that further minute classifications may be detected which will lead to improvement in treatment strategy and survival.

Leukemoid Reaction

Leukemoid reaction is a non-neoplastic reactive leukocytosis characterized by the presence of immature cells of all stages in peripheral blood. This may involve the myeloid, lymphatic or other cell types. Children are affected more frequently than adults.

Causes

- Acute infections like pneumonia, septicemia, whooping cough, chickenpox, infectious mononucleosis, diphtheria and meningitis. In the case of acute infections like sepsis, it indicates greater severity.
- Chronic infections like tuberculosis and amebic liver abscess.
- Hemolytic crisis and massive hemorrhages.
- Metastatic carcinoma involving the bone marrow specially from neuroblastoma, lungs, thyroid, prostate and others.
- Other hematological malignancies, e.g. multiple myeloma, myelofibrosis and Hodgkin's disease.

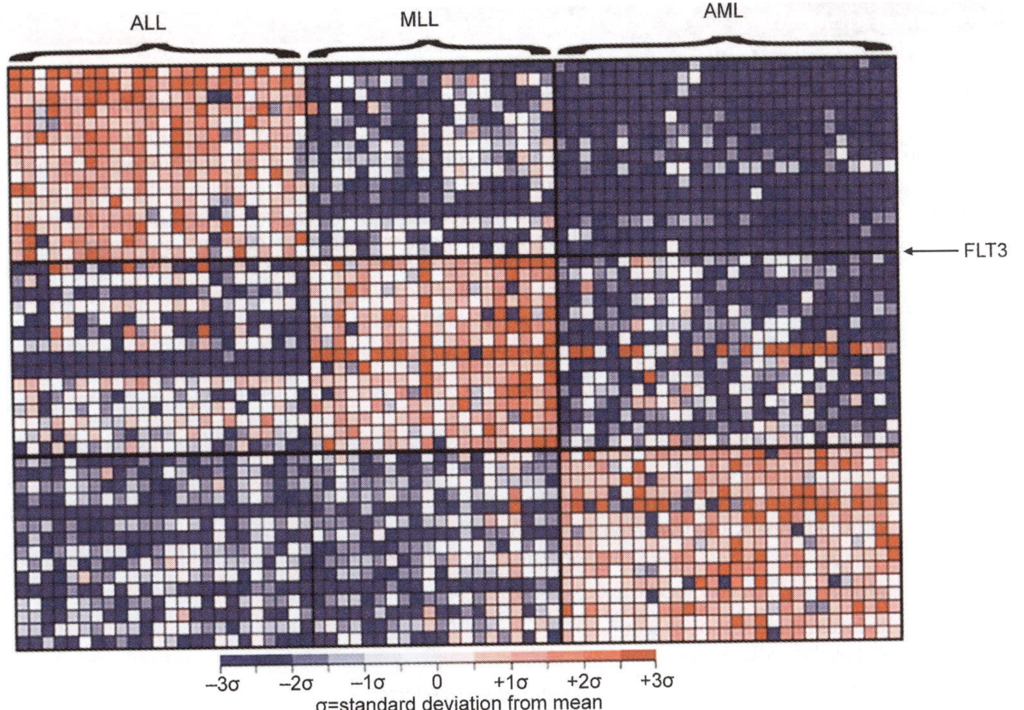

Fig. 164.6: Gene expression profiling includes DNA microarrays. The figure shows the presence of FLT3 internal tandem duplications ITD mutation which predicts less favorable outcome in AML

Abbreviations: DNA = Deoxyribonucleic acid; FLT3 = Fms like tyrosine kinase 3; ITD = internal tandem duplication; AML = Acute myeloid leukemia; MLL = Mixed lineage leukemia; ALL = Acute lymphatic leukemia

- Toxic states like eclampsia, burns and mercury poisoning.

The blood picture is myeloid with mostly neutrophils and their precursors such as myelocytes in pneumonia, meningitis, diphtheria, tuberculosis, amebic liver abscess, metastatic malignancies, multiple myeloma, posthemorrhagic states and hemolysis.

Lymphoid picture occurs in whooping cough, chickenpox, infectious mononucleosis and tuberculosis.

Monocytic reaction rarely occurs in disseminated tuberculosis.

Eosinophilic picture occurs in amebiasis, melanomatosis, and invasive stages of helminthiasis. The bone marrow is normal with accelerated leukopoiesis in leukemoid reaction unlike as in leukemia. Total leukocyte counts may vary widely and overlap with those of leukemia. Liver and spleen are not usually enlarged. Leukocyte alkaline phosphatase (LAP) is increased in leukemoid reaction whereas it is low in CML.

Treatment of the underlying disorder corrects the blood picture also.

Congenital Leukemia

This is leukemia presenting within the first month of life. Almost always it is acute nonlymphatic leukemia. Chromosomal disorders such as Down's syndrome, Turner's syndrome, trisomy 13, monosomy 7, mosaic trisomy 9 and abnormalities of chromosome 11 have a higher incidence of congenital leukemia.

Drugs used in the treatment of Leukemias

Several drugs which have got different modes of action at different phases of the cell cycle have been experimented upon by large multinational leukemia groups and by international random controlled studies and close monitoring over long periods, evidence-based protocols which give best results with acceptable adverse effects have been formulated. Though there are several of them, selection of a particular protocol depends upon various characteristics of the disease such as cell type, age of patient, immunophenotypic and molecular genetic markers and the expertize of the treating group. Conformation to the protocol is absolutely essential to get optimum results. Treatment of acute and chronic leukemias have become highly specialized and technology dependent so that the best results are to be expected only if treatment is undertaken by such teams. There are several centers in India where such specialized treatment is available. Nonconformation of the protocols, however, minor it may appear, leads to suboptimal results. Hence, it is advisable that the physician after making the diagnosis, refers the case to an appropriate specialist center for further management, as is the case with solid tumors.

All the cytotoxic drugs, irrespective of their type, are capable of producing marrow aplasia and this effect is cumulative. This is probably the most serious toxic effect which limits the total dose (Table 164.5). Till the advent of stem cell transfusion therapy intended to repopulate the marrow with normal cells, intense cytotoxic chemotherapy could not be given in eradicative doses due to toxicity on the host. With the support of stem cell transfusion and judicious use of cytokine growth factors it is possible to give more intensive chemotherapy and achieve higher cure rates at present. Specific monoclonal Ab are also being introduced is selected cases.

Table 164.5: Mechanism of action and toxic side effects of antileukemic drugs

Drugs	Mechanism of action	Toxic side effect
Vincristine (oncovin)	Mitotic inhibitor	Alopecia, leukopenia, peripheral neuropathy and myelopathy
Daunorubicin Doxorubicin (adriamycin) Rubidazone Hydroxydoxorubicin	Binds DNA and inhibits mitosis	Alopecia, leukopenia, cardiomyopathy as a sequel. Doxorubicin cardiomyopathy is dose dependent and is more frequent when the total dose-exceeds 550 mg/m^2. It leads to oxidative stress and cellular injury which can be demonstrated by myocardial biopsy studies. Often it occurs after long latent periods, even up to 20–40 years. Echocardiographic studies show reduction in ejection fraction. Slow administration of the drug as IV infusion over a period of 48–96 hours reduces cardiotoxicity. Antioxidants such as probucol have been used as protective drugs
L-asparaginase	Deprives the cells of asparagine	Hypersensitivity, hepatic dysfunction, pancreatitis
6-Mercaptopurine 6-Thioguanine Cytosine arabinoside Methotrexate	Inhibit purine or pyrimidine synthesis or inhibit incorporation into DNA	Ulceration of mouth and GI tract, leukopenia
Cyclophosphamide	Alkylating agent, cross-links DNA and impairs RNA formation	Alopecia, leukopenia, marrow aplasia, pigmentation, hemorrhagic cystitis, pulmonary fibrosis Second neoplasms on follow-up
Corticosteroids	Mechanism of action not clear	Several toxic effect (*See* Ch 5)
All transretinoic acid	Induces differentiation in acute promyelocytic leukemia	
Interferons	Immunomodulation	Several adverse effects

Abbreviations: RNA = Ribonucleic acid; DNA = Deoxyribonucleic acid; GI = Gastrointestinal; IV = Intravenous

Drugs are usually given in combination cyclically or as continuous dosage. The selection, dose and sequence of administration of these drugs depend on the type of leukemia. The dosage is usually calculated in terms of body surface area (which can be read off from nomograms using the height and weight), and this is more reliable than determining the dose on the basis of body weight. Combination of different drugs and intermittent administration has served to reduce the dosage and toxicity of each drug and improve the effectiveness by optimal action at the appropriate phases of the cell cycle several collaborative studies have been conducted and evidence-based protocols have been formulated for different subtypes of leukemia. It is important to follow the protocols strictly. Breaking the protocol or use of individual drugs at random results in suboptimal outcome. Studies on the management of leukemias are continuing. These include:

- The provision of an isolated sterilized environment
- Reverse barrier nursing to avoid infection from the attendants
- Provision of sterilized articles for food and drink
- Special care of intravenous (IV) lines and injection sites
- Prophylactic use of antimicrobial drugs like cotrimoxazole and nystatin with a view to sterilize the gut flora.

Prophylactic antimicrobial drugs are started prior to the induction of remission and are continued during the phase of leukopenia. Systemic infection should be anticipated when there are early symptoms like fever and rigor or any local lesions such as furuncles, cellulitis or ulcers. A combination of powerful bactericidal antibiotics should be instituted early, after taking blood and bacteriological specimens from the nose, throat, mouth, anus and genitalia for culture and sensitivity studies. Fungal infections such as candida and aspergillus are common. Amphotericin used to be the popular antifungal agent. At present, AmBisome 3 mg/kg has replaced the use of amphotericin. Echinocandins like caspofungin, micafungin and anidulafungin are better choices for candida species. They are not that effective treating aspergillus infections and drug of choice for these infections would be amBisome, amphotericin and voriconazole.

BONE MARROW TRANSPLANTATION (BMT)

It has been employed as a therapeutic modality in several diseases for over five decades, to reconstitute stem cells in conditions where there is deficiency (e.g. aplastic anemia and immunodeficiency states) or abnormality of the patient's own stem cells (e.g. leukemias and thalassemia). The success of this procedure and availability of BMT in several centers in many parts of the world have established its place in treatment of a wide variety of apparently unrelated conditions. The pioneer in initiating BMT was ED Thomas who reported success of this procedure in 1959. Later, he was awarded Nobel Prize for his work (Fig. 164.7). Stem cells are obtained from several sources— bone marrow, peripheral blood and cord blood. They have the potential to repopulate the marrow and differentiate into appropriate mature cells.

The indications and ideal time to perform BMT have also been defined. Unlike as in other solid organ transplants, there is no need for a major surgical procedure since the stem cells collected from the donor reach their location in the bone marrow when injected IV. Within a few weeks of marrow donation, the donor's marrow fully regenerates so that there is no organ-loss for the donor. The marrow to be transfused may be homologous or allogenic (derived from another person with nonidentical genetic status), isologous or syngenic (derived from identical

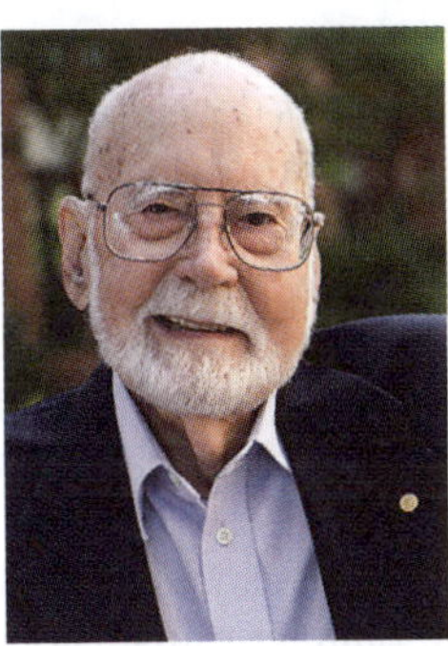

Fig. 164.7: Edward Donnall Thomas: Nobel prize winner and pioneer of bone-marrow transplantation. Born on March 15, 1920, in Mart, TX, USA; he died in Seatle, WA, USA on Oct 20, 2012, aged 92 years

Courtesy: The Lancet 2012, 380, issue 8th December 2012.

twins with the same genetic status) or autologous (marrow recovered from the patient on an earlier occasion and transplanted later). Selection of the donor depends upon the compatibility of the human leukocyte antigen (HLA) complex. Theoretically, a single stem cell can repopulate the entire marrow. The genes for the HLA complex are closely linked on chromosome 6 and they are inherited as haplotypes. Thus, two siblings have a one-in-four chance of being HLA identical. Transplantation between HLA identical persons does not evoke a graft-vs- host disease (GVHD). In selecting donors, siblings are the most suited, next only to identical twins.

Principles in BMT

Conditioning Regimen

Ablation of the recipient's marrow cells: This is done by administration of cyclophosphamide 50 mg/kg bw daily for 4 days along with total body irradiation (TBI) of 14.4 grays (8 fractions over 4 days). At present, depending on the type of marrow or stem cell transplant, different types of ablating regimens are in vogue. This regimen destroys all or most of the hematopoietic cell lines in the patient, including most of the leukemic cells. The present trend is to use less aggressive regimen to ablate the recipient's marrow since such regimen are associated with better success rates and survival. Other regimes include the use of busulfan/fludarabine with cyclophosphamide-TBI and antithymocytic globulin.

Infusion of donor marrow: About 750 mL of marrow withdrawn from the HLA matched donor by multiple punctures over the iliac crest, vertebrae or the long bones under anesthesia. It is processed for infusion and administered IV at a dose of $2–6 \times 10^6$ donor marrow cells per kg bw.

In the vast majority, the recipient's marrow increases in cellularity within 2–4 weeks. Thereafter, all the hematopoietic cells, plasma cells, tissue macrophages and immunological cells are derived from the transplanted marrow.

Though in principle BMT appears to be simple, elaborate equipment, facilities to control infection of the recipient during the pretransplant preparation and during the leukopenic phase before the donor marrow proliferates, need for powerful antibiotics and hyperalimentation during the critical period, make BMT a highly specialized and very expensive procedure which can be undertaken only in advanced institutions where trained teams are available. Several institutions undertake BMT in India. The approximate cost is ₹ 10–12 lacs ($ 22,000).

Complications

An immunological complication that develops in all successful transplants is GVHD, if the donor happens to be other than an identical twin. The immunocompetent T-lymphocytes in the donor marrow derived from the stem cells proliferate and attack recipient's tissues and give rise to the clinical picture of GVHD. GVHD may be acute or chronic. Acute GVHD occurs within 1–2 months of BMT. The incidence ranges from 10–80% depending upon the initial disease and technique of preparation of bone marrow. Main targets of attack of GVHD are the immune system, skin, gastrointestinal tract (GIT), liver and brain. Profound immunosuppression occurs as a result of GVHD, leading to fatal infections. Selective epithelial damage occurs in the target tissues.

Chronic GVHD occurs after about 3 months or persists for more than 100 days. Two stages may be recognized in the pathogenesis. ***First step*** is activation of donor T-lymphocytes by recipient tissues. ***Second step*** is the production of cytokines by the activated T-cells, recruitment of more cells and mounting the immune response in the host's tissues.

Administration of immunosuppressants, particularly methotrexate and cyclosporine helps to suppress GVHD by inhibiting donor T-cell activation. Corticosteroids and cyclosporin inhibit the synthesis of interleukin (IL). Methotrexate blocks cell proliferation. After varying periods, these drugs can be discontinued. Newer immunosuppressants such as tacrolimus and mycophenolate mofetil are also used whenever they are indicated.

The occurrence of GVHD is associated with more complete eradication of the leukemia clone and therefore, better long-term results. Cases that survive successful management of GVHD have longer leukemia-free survival.

Other fatal complications include graft rejection, severe infections, pulmonary complications including acute respiratory distress syndrome (ARDS) and interstitial pneumonia and iatrogenic problems. Availability of growth promoting factors such as granulocyte-macrophage colony-stimulating factor (GM-CSF) has enabled earlier reconstitution of recipient's neutrophils and macrophages, thus reducing infections and mortality. The mortality in the post-transplant period used to be 30–40% at the initial periods and the main causes are infection, marrow failure or GVHD. Refinements in techniques have given better results, lower failure rates and better survival.

A major offshoot of this procedure is the employment of ***autologous marrow transplant***. This is the procedure in which bone marrow of the patient is harvested prior to administration of aggressive chemotherapeutic regimen. The harvested marrow is treated with monoclonal antileukemia Ab which help to remove the intrinsic malignant cells contained in it. This procedure is called purging the marrow. This treated marrow is infused back after chemotherapy is administered. This helps to repopulate the marrow after ablating cancer tissue. Use of autologous marrow obviates both the problems of donors and GVHD.

Peripheral Stem Cell Transplantation

Another modality that is more popular is stem cell transplantation. Peripheral blood normally contains stem cells which can be used to repopulate marrow after chemotherapy. The stem cell pool is allowed to proliferate under stimulation by appropriate colony stimulating factors (GM-CSF or G-CSF) and the harvested stem cells are infused into the patient instead of bone marrow.

Cord blood is a rich source of pluripotent stem cells. They are less likely to mount immunological reactions. Cord blood stem cell infusion has become more popular and cord blood banking is practiced in several institutions.

Prophylactic use of fluconazole and ganciclovir ensure prophylaxis against fungal and cytomegalovirus (CMV) infections respectively.

Indications

- Acute and chronic leukemias, MDS
- Multiple myeloma
- Lymphomas which have relapsed after initial chemo-therapy
- Aplastic anemia, radiation injury, paroxysmal nocturnal hemoglobinuria (PNH)
- Hemoglobinopathies, thalassemias
- Immunodeficiency states—severe combined immuno-deficiency, Wiskott-Aldrich syndrome, Chédiak-Higashi syndrome, chronic granulomatous disease
- Other genetic disorders such as malignant osteo-petrosis, Gaucher's disease, infantile metachromatic leukodystrophy and X-linked adrenoleukodystrophy.

Table 164.6 gives the present indications for BMT and survival rates.

Blood Component Therapy

Chemotherapy-induced thrombocytopenia and anemia are promptly reversed by transfusion of platelets and

Table 164.6: Indications for bone marrow transplantation (BMT) and survival rates

Disease	Time for BMT	Survival rate
ALL	Second relapse	70%
AML	First relapse	70%
CML	Within 1 year of diagnosis, while in CML phase	70%
CLL	Variable	50%
Multiple myeloma	Stage I	66%
	Stage II	33%
Poor prognosis lymphomas	Failure of initial or second course of treatment	Over 50%
Hemoglobinopathy, Thalassemia	As early as possible	Over 80%
Severe aplastic anemia	As early as possible	Over 60%

Note: There are several other conditions in which BMT is an accepted treatment modality at present. A complete list is not attempted in this table. Supportive stem cell transplantation given along with intensive cancer chemotherapy has improved the curability of several malignant diseases.

Abbreviations: ALL = Acute lymphatic leukemia; AML = Acute myeloid leukemia; CML = Chronic myeloid leukemia; CLL = Chronic lymphatic leukemia

packed red cells. Coagulant factors may be needed as and when bleeding tendencies develop.

Use of colony-stimulating factors such as G-CSF and GM-CSF help to reconstitute the neutrophil and mac-rophage population early, shorten the period of danger-ous neutropenia and risk of severe infections. Adverse side effects of colony-stimulating factors include-worsening of autoimmune disorders, inflammation of ocular structures and allergy.

Other supportive measures include red cell trans-fusions for anemia, platelet transfusions for hemorrhage, and whole blood to correct blood loss.

Hyperuricemia may lead to secondary gout and renal failure during treatment. Prompt use of allopurinol 100 mg thrice daily orally during the initial phases of treatment helps to keep the uric acid levels normal. Febuxostat is a newer xanthine oxidase inhibitor effective in daily dose of 80–120 mg given orally in divided doses. Adequate hydration and maintenance of urine output of at least two liters daily help to minimize the risk of nephropathy.

Prognosis

Leukemia is invariably fatal if untreated. Modern treatment has helped to prolong useful life in the vast majority of cases of acute leukemias and in about 50–60% of cases to bring about cure. Best results are obtained in ALL in children. Those who are not curable by chemotherapy are subjected to BMT which is curative in more than two-thirds of the cases. Stem cell transplantation is a more readily available alternative to repopulate the marrow which is the preferred treatment in many centers at present.

Favorable Prognostic Factors

- Initial leukocyte count below 20,000/mm³
- Platelet count above 100,000/mm³
- Absence of organomegaly, i.e. lymph nodes, spleen, and liver are impalpable
- Null cell (common ALL) leukemia, promyelocytic leukemia
- Absence of complications
- Absence of mediastinal lymphadenopathy in ALL
- Younger age groups
- Institution of proper therapy from the beginning
- Availability of trained teams for management and BMT.

Unfavorable Prognostic Factors

- Older age groups
- Initial leukocyte count above 20,000/mm³
- Thrombocyte count below 100,000/mm³
- Organomegaly
- Presence of complications
- T-cell ALL
- Presence of mediastinal lymph nodes in lymphatic leukemia.

Cases which fall in the poor-prognosis group are given more intensive induction regimen using a larger number of drugs and early bone marrow transplant.

Diagnostic Work-up and Disease Classification

Based on revised World Health Organization (WHO) pub-lication—WHO Classification of tumors of hematopoietic and lymphoid tissues, a total of seven entities are defined within the subgroup.

- ***Acute myeloid leukemia with recurrent genetic abnormalities***
  - AML with t(8;21)(q22;q22); RUNX1-RUNX1T1
  - AML with inv(16)(p13.1q22) or t(16;16)(p13.1q22); CBFB-MYH11
  - APL with t(15;17)(q22;q12); PML-RARA
  - AML with t(9;11)(p22q23); MLLT3-MLL
  - AML with t(6;9)(p23;q34); DEK-NUP214
  - AML with inv(3)(q21q26.2) or t(3;3)(q21q26.2); RPN1-EVI1
  - AML (megakaryoblastic) with t(1;22)(p13;q13); RBM15-MKL1
  - AML with mutated NPM1*
  - AML with mutated CEBPA*
- ***AML with myelodysplasia-related changes***
- ***Therapy-relayed myeloid neoplasms***
- ***AML, not otherwise specified***
  - AML with minimal differentiation
  - AML without maturation
  - AML with maturation
  - Acute myelomonocytic leukemia
  - Acute monoblastic/monocytic leukemia
  - Acute erythroid leukemia
    - Pure erythroid leukemia
    - Erythroleukemia, erythroid/myeloid
- Acute megakaryoblastic leukemia
- Acute basophilic leukemia
- Acute panmyelosis with myelofibrosis (also known as acute myelofibrosis or acute myelosclerosis).

Myeloid sarcoma (also known as extramedullary myeloid tumor, granulocytic sarcoma or chloroma).

- ***Myeloid proliferations related to Down syndrome***

Transient abnormal myelopoiesis (also known as transient myelo-proliferative disorder).

Myeloid leukemia associated with Down syndrome.

- ***Blastic plasmacytoid dendritic cell neoplasm***
- ***Acute leukemias of ambiguous lineage***
- ***Acute undifferentiated leukemia:***
  - Mixed phenotype acute leukemia with t(v;11q23); MLL rearranged
  - Mixed phenotype acute leukemia, B/myeloid, NOS
  - Mixed phenotype acute leukemia, T/myeloid, NOS
  - Provisional entity natural killer cell lymphoblastic leukemia/lymphoma.

Acute Leukemias

Salim Shafeek, Kasim Salim, KV Krishna Das, Mathew Thomas

Chapter Summary

- Acute Lymphatic Leukemia (ALL)
  - Neuroleukemia
  - Testicular Leukemia
- Acute Myeloid Leukemia (AML)
  - Acute Promyelocytic Leukemia
  - Acute Myelomonocytic Leukemia
  - Erythroleukemia (Di Guglielmo's Syndrome)
  - Acute Megakaryoblastic Leukemia

ACUTE LYMPHATIC LEUKEMIA (ALL)

Syn: Acute lymphoblastic leukemia

This type of leukemia, which is more common in children, arises from lymphoid tissue. About 75% cases are null-cell type, 20–25% T-cell type and a few are B-cell type. Maximum incidence is in the first two decades. There is also a peak in the fourth and fifth decades. Male to female ratio is 2:1.

Clinical Features

The presenting features are fever, pallor, lymphadenopathy and bleeding tendencies. Some cases present with neurological involvement. These take the form of meningitis, cranial nerve palsies, focal neurological deficits, convulsions or coma. About 20% present with arthralgias and arthritis resembling rheumatic or rheumatoid arthritis (RA). Moderate lymphadenopathy, especially the posterior cervical and mediastinal groups,

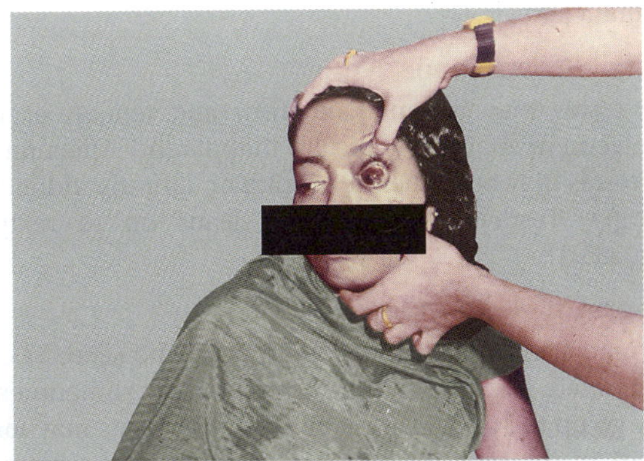

Fig. 165.1: Acute leukemia; subconjunctival hemorrhage

mild hepatosplenomegaly (spleen 2–5 cm) and pallor are detectable on physical examination. Bone involvement is more common.

Ophthalmoscopic examination reveals pallor of the optic disk, venous engorgement, hemorrhages and exudates. Vitreous hemorrhage and subconjunctival hemorrhage may occur in severe cases (Fig. 165.1).

T-cell leukemia is more serious since it is less responsive to therapy. It is characterized by higher total leukocyte count (TLC) and enlargement of mediastinal lymph nodes. There are reports that the frequency of T-cell lymphatic leukemia is higher in India. A subgroup of acute lymphoblastic leukemia, also known as acute lymphocytic leukemia or acute lymphoid leukemia (ALL), specially in adults shows the Philadelphia chromosome (Ph1) positivity on karyotyping. Probably these arise from a very early totipotent stem cell which has the capacity to develop toward the myeloid cell line as in chronic myeloid leukemia (CML). Ph1-positive ALL has a poorer prognosis compared to Ph1-negative ALL.

Neuroleukemia

Neuroleukemia occurs in 50% of ALL and 10–12% of acute myeloid leukemia (AML) cases, if neuroprophylaxis is not given along with initial therapy.

Pathological lesions include infiltration by leukemic cells, hemorrhage and demyelination. In addition, drug toxicity and occlusion of cerebral microcirculation due to leukostasis add to the total neurological picture. When the leptomeninges are infiltrated, cerebrospinal fluid (CSF) shows the presence of a large number of blast cells, rise in protein and increased pressure and this may be mistaken for meningitis. Neuroleukemia may manifest during remission or this may even be the presenting symptom in some.

Clinical features may be those of meningitis, raised intracranial tension with papilledema, stupor, coma, focal neurological symptoms like convulsions or paralysis, cranial nerve palsies (Fig. 165.2), spinal cord or spinal root compression, or intracranial hemorrhage. Sometimes hyperviscosity syndrome develops because of very high leukocyte counts above 200×10^9/L (200,000/mm³). Symptoms of cellular hyperviscosity include auditory and visual disturbances, ataxia, headache, profound lethargy and coma. Leukapheresis relieves these symptoms dramatically.

Testicular Leukemia

The testes may be enlarged, firm and tender, or the involvement may be clinically inapparent. Affection of the testes may occur before, during or after the induction therapy. Testicular involvement leads on to relapse (Fig. 165.3).

Laboratory Findings

Normocytic normochromic anemia may be seen. TLC is moderately elevated (20–30,000/mm³) but sometimes it may go up to 100–200,000/mm³. Lymphoblasts may form 5–95% of the total. Platelets are reduced. Bone marrow shows infiltration by lymphoblasts.

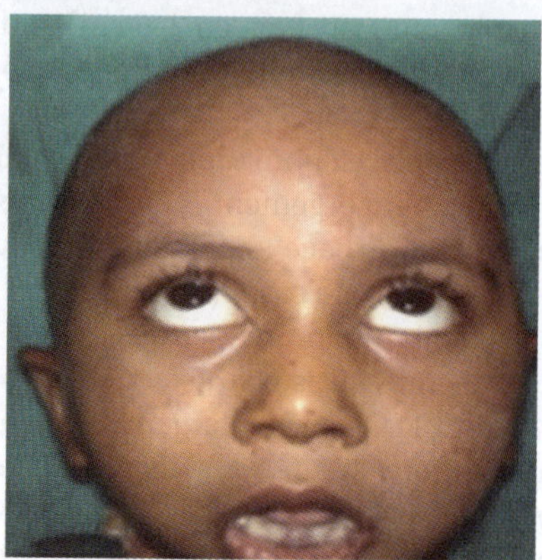

Fig. 165.2: Bilateral facial palsy

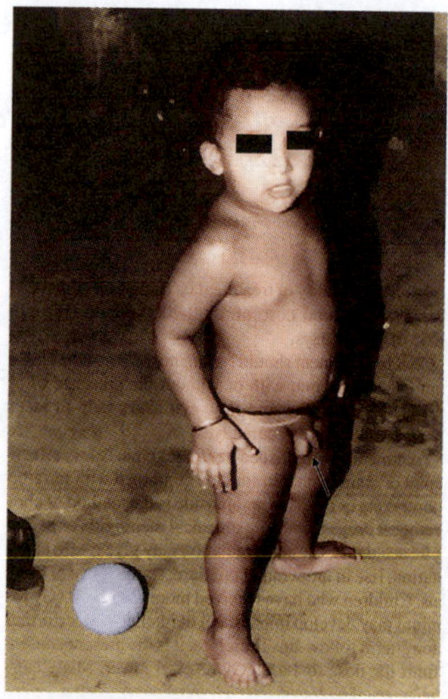

Fig. 165.3: Testicular leukemia. Boy aged 2 years with acute lymphatic leukemia. *Note:* The enlarged testes (arrow)

Table 165.1: ALL immunophenotypic classification			
	Frequency		
Lineage	**Children**	**Adults**	**Markers**
Precursor B cell			CD19+, cCD22+, TdT+, plus
• Pro-B ALL			CD10–, clg–
• Common ALL	65–70%	50–60%	CD10+, clg–
• Pre-B ALL	15–20%	15–25%	clg+
Mature B-cell	<5%	<5%	slg+, IgM+(usually), TdT–
T-cell ALL	10–15%	20–25%	cCD3+, CD7, plus others depending on maturity

Abbreviations: TdT = Terminal deoxynucleotidyl transferase; CD = Cluster of Differentiation; slg = Surface immunoglobulin; clg = Cytoplasmic immunoglobulin; IgM = Immunoglobulin M

Immunophenotyping is a key diagnostic tool in ALL (Table 165.1).

Treatment

Principles of Treatment of Acute Leukemias

Management of leukemia requires the coordinated efforts of a physician, oncologist, radiotherapist, clinical psychologist and blood bank officer. The services of a well-equipped laboratory are absolutely essential for proper workup of the case and follow-up. The prime requirements expected of the general physician are to detect leukemias early and arrange treatment for them under the specialist team. In the following description, only principles of diagnosis and management are given, omitting practical details. Monographs on the subject should be consulted for more practical information.

When the disease is clinically evident, the tumor load is heavy and malignant tissue proliferates rapidly. At this stage, it is essential to reduce the tumor load within a short time by the use of intensive chemotherapy. This phase is called *induction of remission*. The patient is deemed to have achieved remission when the clinical and hematological abnormalities (both blood and bone marrow) have disappeared. Even at this stage, although tumor cells are not demonstrable by the usual laboratory techniques, 10^5–10^6 tumor cells persist in the body which are capable of proliferating and repopulating the bone marrow and blood. This is the common cause for relapse.

Many tissues in the body such as the brain, meninges, CSF cisterns and testes act as sanctuaries for the leukemic cells since the systemically administered drugs do not freely reach them. The residual leukemic tissue in the brain and CSF is destroyed by drugs like methotrexate or cytosine arabinoside (Ara-C) introduced intrathecally or intravenously (IV) in high doses. This constitutes neuroprophylaxis.

Testicular involvement occurs in 10–15% of ALL cases before the onset of therapy. This usually clears up with chemotherapy. Next to the central nervous system (CNS), testis is the most frequent sanctuary site where leukemic cells proliferate. Though overt testicular leukemia is treated by local irradiation, at present there is no consensus regarding testicular prophylaxis.

Consolidation: After the induction and cranial prophylaxis, another course of chemotherapy, meant to decrease the leukemic burden and to avoid the development of resistance is given, employing a different combination of drugs.

The present schedules of chemotherapy do not eradicate the leukemic cells completely. Hence, ***maintenance therapy*** is given after the achievement of remission to prevent the surviving cells from proliferating and leading to relapse. Maintenance therapy is generally given for varying periods after which it could be withdrawn. During maintenance, regular short intensive regimens as given for induction are included in many treatment protocols. These pseudoinduction regimens are given to ensure that the leukemic cells do not reach significant numbers. It is possible that if the leukemic cell population is kept low, immunological defenses of the host will eliminate them.

Maintenance therapy is more commonly employed for ALL. For AML, the success depends more on the effectiveness of induction therapy.

A modern approach to the problem of eradicating the residual leukemic cells is the use of monoclonal immunoglobulins (Ig) which selectively destroy the malignant cells. Monoclonal antibodies (mAbs) have been employed therapeutically and diagnostically in clinical situations rarely. Their greater use is for the removal of leukemic cells from harvested marrow before transplantation.

The total duration of treatment is generally limited to 5 years since the majority of patients attain freedom from the leukemic process by this period. Many of those who remain in the first remission without relapse achieve long-term survival (above 10 years) and cure, though a few may relapse even after this interval. In those in whom relapse occurs, survival is considerably shortened. Relapses are treated on the same lines as initial induction. If relapse occurs, the therapeutic modality of choice is marrow transplantation. If this is not available, the next best is chemotherapy. Box 165.1 and Table 165.2 give the details of drugs used to treat acute leukemias.

Supportive treatment: Infections are very common in the active phase of acute leukemia, specially during the induction phase, because of impairment of cellular and humoral defense mechanisms. They account for 80% of deaths during induction and remission. The common

Box 165.1: Drugs used for the treatment of acute leukemias

- ***Antimetabolites***
    - Methotrexate
    - Cytosine arabinoside
    - 6-mercaptopurine
    - 6-thioguanine
- ***Antimitotic drugs:*** Vinca alkaloids (vincristine)
- ***Antibiotics***
    - Daunorubicin (daunomycin)
    - Doxorubicin (adriamycin)
    - Rubidazone
    - Bleomycin, mitomycin
- ***Enzymes:*** L-asparaginase
- ***Alkylating agent:*** Clophosphamide
- ***Corticosteroids:*** Prednisolone

Table 165.2: Dose and their route of administration

Dose	Route	Interval	Total number of courses
Vincristine	1–1.5 mg/m² intravenous	7-day intervals	4–8
Prednisolone	40 mg/m² oral		Daily
L-asparaginase	10,000 units/m² intravenous		Daily × 5 days

Flowchart for the management of ALL

	Consolidation		
Induction of remission	Neuroprophylaxis	Intrathecal drugs	Maintenance Consideration of bone marrow transplant (BMT)

infective agents include the pyogenic cocci, Gram-negative bacilli, *Pseudomonas aeruginosa,* anaerobes, *Candida* species, *Aspergillus* and herpes viruses. Relatively avirulent organisms such as *Mycoplasma pneumoniae, Pneumocystis carinii* and *Cryptococcus neoformans* become invasive and account for many deaths. The risk of tuberculosis flaring up during treatment with corticosteroids is also high. Fulminant infections are seen most frequently during the stage of induction. Bacterial infections are common when the neutrophil count is below 1000/mm³. Reduction of absolute neutrophil counts below 500/mm³ is dangerous, unless prompt antimicrobial therapy is instituted. Infection may be nosocomial or endogenous from the flora inhabiting the alimentary tract. Several methods have been employed to prevent such infections.

Medications commonly used to treat childhood ALL include methotrexate, thiopurines, glucocorticoids, vincristine, L-asparaginase, anthracyclines, antibiotics, alkylating agents and others. Treatment approach in ALL has been shown in Flowchart 165.1.

Antiviral drugs such as vidarabine 5 mg/kg/day or acyclovir 5 mg/kg/day IV every 8 hourly may be given for treating herpes and other viral infections. *P. carinii* infection responds to co-trimoxazole in a daily dose of 9–12 g given in divided doses.

Delay in starting antimicrobial therapy results in heavy mortality and hence, it is necessary to start treatment on clinical grounds, even before bacteriological evidence is obtained. The advent of newer antimicrobial agents has been a great help in treating these patients.

Flowchart 165.1: Treatment approach in ALL

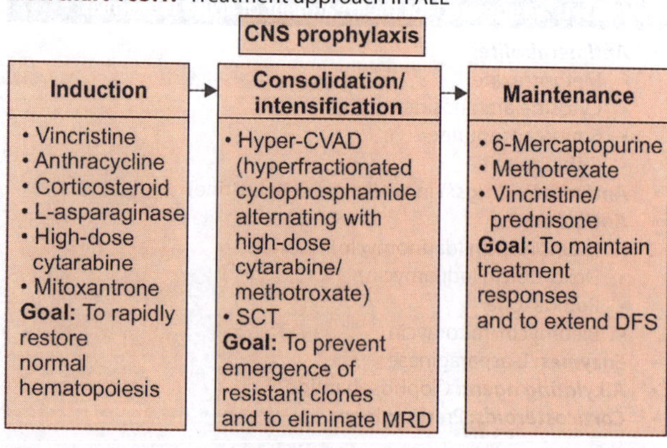

Abbreviations: DFS = Disease-free survival; SCT = Stem cell transplantation; MRD = Minimal residual disease; CNS = Central nervous system

Remission is induced by a combination of vincristine, prednisolone and L-asparaginase. Several other drugs such as doxorubicin (adriamycin), etoposide and cytosine arabinoside are also used for induction in high-risk cases. Newer modalities and treatment protocols are still being developed.

About 95% of children and 90% of adults respond to this regimen and achieve complete remission. Poor prognostic factors include the following:

- Age less than 1 and greater than 10 years
- Male sex
- Presence of mediastinal mass in X-ray
- Presence of organomegaly involving the spleen, liver, lymph nodes and other organs
- Laboratory features:
  - TLC exceeds 50,000/mm^3
  - Blasts are of T-cell phenotype, which do not express CD34 or CD10 with a hypodiploid, diploid or near diploid karyotype
  - Presence of Ph1 chromosome.

Remission is consolidated by giving one or two doses of the drugs used in the induction regimen.

Maintenance: Methotrexate in a dose of 15 mg/m^2 as a single weekly dose and 6-mercaptopurine in a total dose of 600 mg/m^2/week divided into daily doses are given orally. Vincristine 1.5 mg/m^2 is given IV every month. Maintenance therapy has to be continued for 2 years.

Allogenic (Allogeneic) Transplantation for Acute Leukemia

Allogenic transplantation constitutes curative treatment for acute leukemia and high-risk myelodysplasia. Its therapeutic effects are to a large extent mediated by graft-vs-leukemia (GVL) effects, but partially offset by treatment-related mortality and loss of quality of life caused by acute and chronic graft-vs-host disease (GVHD). Although severe acute and chronic GVHD are associated with a reduction in relapse risk, they are not associated with improved survival. Recent efforts to modulate the GVL-GVH balance include novel methods of *in vitro* or *in vivo* T-cell depletion that are associated with a minimal impact on rates of disease recurrence and a dramatically decreased risk for GVHD.

Donor selection algorithms may also have a significant impact on transplantation outcomes. Low expression HLA alleles, particularly HLA-DP, should be incorporated in selection of adult unrelated donors. High-resolution HLA typing and the importance of fetal-maternal interactions in umbilical cord transplantation play a major role.

Nonmyeloablative Transplants/Reduced Intensity Conditioning Allografts

This method is more popular at present due to the reduction in the risk and complications during the recipient's bone marrow ablation phase. By this method, it is possible to extend the age limit for marrow transplantation. Common conditioning regimen is fludarabine/melphalan/Campath (Flu-Mel-Campath). Campath is alemtuzumab developed in the United States of America (USA). It is a humanized mAb that selectively binds to CD52, a protein found on the surface of normal and malignant B- and T-cells of the immune system. By binding the CD52 protein on the malignant B-cells, the antibody removes them from the circulation. Reduced intensity conditioning (RIC) regimens have increased the availability of alternate donors and have transformed the management of AML, myelodysplastic syndrome (MDS) and ALL.

UKALL XII/ECOG (Fig. 165.4) showed data on the overall survival (OS) l for non-Philadelphia ALL depending on the availability of stem cell donor versus no stem cell donor. There was no clear benefit in poor risk cytogenetics ALL.

Risk-Stratified Approach in ALL Treatment

Cytogenetics provide reliable risk stratification for treatment. The genetics of ALL are becoming well-understood. The incidence of individual chromosomal abnormalities varies considerably with age. High hyperdiploidy and ETV6-RUNX1 are good risk subjects, whereas BCR-ABL1, mixed-lineage leukemia (MLL) rearrangements and hypodiploidy are poor risk. Lab procedures such as single nucleotide polymorphism arrays and next generation sequencing have revolutionized the risk stratification of ALL. Several new abnormalities are identified including intrachromosomal amplification of chromosome 21 (iAMP21) which carry poor prognosis with standard treatment (Fig. 165.5).

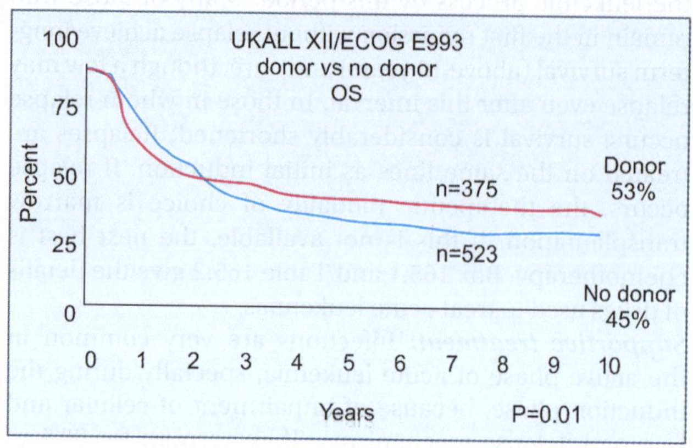

Fig. 165.4: Survival rates after bone marrow transplantation

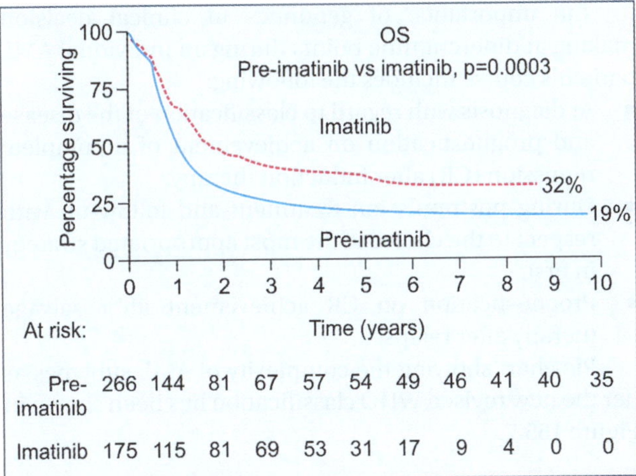

Fig. 165.5: The response of BCR-ABL1-positive ALL with and without imatinib in the treatment regimen

Use of Tyrosine Kinase Inhibitors (TKIs) in Ph1-Positive ALL

With the successful use of TKIs in the treatment of BCR-ABL1-positive ALL, patients with alternative ABL1 trans-locations and rearrangements involving PDGFRB show benefit from treatment with TKIs.

Neuroprophylaxis: It is started along with induction regimen and is a must in ALL. Intrathecal methotrexate in a dose of 10–12 mg/m^2 should be given twice a week for a total of six doses. A single dose should not exceed 15 mg. An alternative is Ara-C 50 mg intrathecally given twice a week for six doses.

CNS involvement should be diagnosed when the CSF cell count exceeds 5/mm^3 with or without the presence of blast cells. Cytospin studies and flow cytometry help to identify abnormal cells more accurately.

Treatment of established neuroleukemia is less effective. Cranial or craniospinal irradiation combined with intrathecal methotrexate or Ara-C used to be the method of choice. Intrathecal drugs may cause chemical meningitis or neuroparalytic accidents. Many centers have stopped cranial irradiation due to serious sequelae. Drugs such as methotrexate when given IV in high doses reach the CSF in therapeutic concentrations.

At present, results in the management of the primary disease are very good. However, neuroleukemia once it occurs, worsens the prognosis for long-term survival. Therefore, prevention of this complication has an important place in overall management.

Treatment of Testicular Leukemia

Treatment of testicular lesion is by irradiation with 1,000–2,000 rads over a period of 2–10 days. This leads to sterility, still this remains the treatment of choice since drug treatment is not effective due to nonpenetration of the drugs at the site of disease. Presence of testicular leukemia at the initial stage of diagnosis demands concurrent radiotherapy along with systemic drug treatment. Development of testicular leukemia in the maintenance phase is treated with local radiotherapy and institution of reinduction. There is no consensus regarding testicular prophylaxis.

Treatment of Relapse

Reinduction can be achieved by the same regimen as for the initial presentation. After achieving remission a second time, the possibility of bone marrow transplantation (BMT) should be explored since the chances of long-term survival with medical therapy are less in such cases. With the improvement in the results of bone marrow and stem cell transplantation (SCT), these modalities are considered even earlier.

Genomic variation in ALL: Genomic variation that is somatically acquired in ALL blasts that is inherited in the germline can affect interindividual variability in response, whereas adverse effects are affected by inherited variations. All phenotypes can be affected by several nongenetic features, so controlling and adjusting for these nongenetic features in genome-wide association studies (GWAS) of ALL is critical.

New Immune Strategies for Treatment of ALL

Antibody-Based Therapies

Prognosis of adult ALL remains poor and hence novel therapies are needed with antibody-based therapy approach. There are four major classes of antibody therapy.

1. ***Naked antibodies:*** For example, rituximab CD20, epratuzumab CD22, alemtuzumab CD52.
2. ***Bispecific T-cell engager (BiTE) antibodies:*** BiTE single-chain antibodies are a class of artificial mAbs used in anticancer treatment. They direct T cell's cytotoxic activity against malignant cells, e.g. blinatu-momab CD19.
3. ***Immunotoxins/immunoconjugates:*** BL22 and CAT-8015-CD22, Combotox (CD19 and CD22), SAR3419 anti-CD19, inotuzumab ozogamicin-CD22.
4. ***Chimeric antigen receptors:*** CAR-T-ALL more than B-ALL.

At present, several protocols are being tried for treatment in ALL and almost all hematological malignancies with a view to make the drug combination more effective, safer and less expensive. A few protocols that are being developed and still being studied are indicated.

Minimal residual disease monitoring in ALL is a key part of monitoring in adult and pediatric ALL treatment (Fig. 165.6). Various techniques using flow cytometry and polymerase chain reaction (PCR) are being employed.

ACUTE MYELOID LEUKEMIA (AML)

Syn: Acute nonlymphocytic leukemia

It also known as acute myelogenous leukemia or acute nonlymphocytic leukemia (ANLL), arises from a common precursor stem cell and it is subdivided into seven types—M1 to M7. Risk factors include exposure to ionizing radiations, benzene and cytotoxic chemotherapy, specially alkylating agents. Cigarete smoke is a common cause of benzene exposure. AML blast cells develop from normal blasts which have undergone genetic damage. Marrow blasts are protected by the marrow stroma from apoptosis induced by chemotherapy.

AML shows various cytogenetic abnormalities. The World Health Organization (WHO) has proposed the WHO

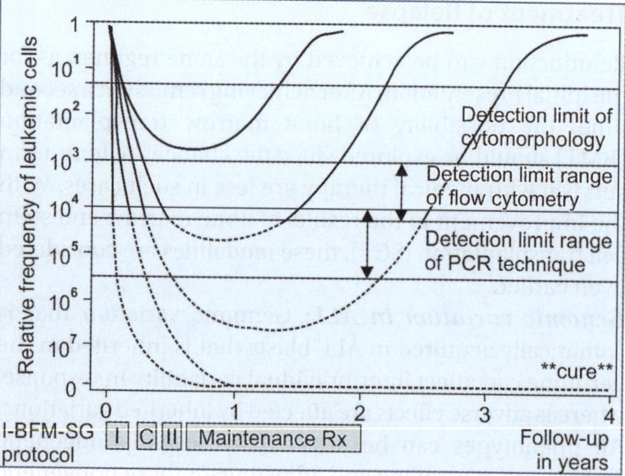

Fig. 165.6: Detection levels of minimal residual disease by various techniques

Abbreviation: PCR = Polymerase chain reaction

Table 165.3: Prognostication of response to induction therapy in AML

	Complete remission (CR) rate		
	Age < 60 years; intensive induction	Age ≥ 60 years; intensive induction	Age ≥ 60 years; nonintensive treatment
Favorable marker			
RUNX1-RUNX1T1'	80–90%	70–80%	N/A
CBFB-MYH11'	80–90%	70–80%	N/A
NPM1-mut	80–90%	80–90%	50%
CEBPAdm	80–90%	N/A	N/A
Unfavorable marker			
Monosomal karyotype	30–35%	30–35%	N/A
TP53 alteration	25–30%	25–30%	N/A
Inv(3) or t(3;3)	31%	N/A	N/A

classification of AML, based on genetic abnormalities. This helps to select the best therapeutic approach and to assess the prognosis. Cytogenetic markers help to categorize the therapeutic response in AML as favorable, intermediate or adverse. The myeloid blast cells have surface markers CD33 or CD13 (Table 165.3).

All age groups are affected, though the second and third decades show a higher incidence. Both sexes are equally affected.

AML is heterogeneous disorder and characterized by accumulation of somatically acquired genetic changes in hematopoietic progenitor cells that alter normal mechanism of self-renewal, proliferation and differentiation. According to recommendations from an international expert panel, on behalf of the European LeukemiaNet (ELN), AML can be grouped into four risk groups as shown here.

1. Acute promyelocytic leukemia (APL) (M3)
2. Acute myelomonocytic leukemia (M4)
3. Erythroleukemia (Di Guglielmo's syndrome) (M6)
4. Acute megakaryoblastic leukemia (M7).

The importance of genomics in clinical decision making at different time points during an individual AML patient's course includes the following:

- At diagnosis with regard to classification of the disease and prognostication on achievement of a complete remission (CR) after induction therapy.
- During postremission treatment and follow-up with respect to the choice of the most appropriated strategy in first.
- Prognostication on CR achievement after salvage therapy after relapse.

Pie chart showing the complexity of AML subtypes as per the new revised WHO classification has been shown in Figure 165.7.

Clinical Features

The disease presents with progressive anemia, fever and focal or general infections or hemorrhages (Fig. 165.8).

Usual sites of infection are gums, mouth, throat, skin, perianal regions, genitalia and respiratory tract. In many cases, lymphadenopathy and hepatosplenomegaly may be absent. Atypically, the disease may present with affection of unusual sites. Sites of extramedullary involvement include:

- Bilateral or unilateral retro-orbital masses producing exophthalmos (Figs 165.9 and 165.10).
- Breasts—uniform or localized enlargement occurs in one or both sides (Figs 165.11 and 165.12).
- Skin—nodular or diffuse lesions. Chloromas are cutaneous manifestations of myeloid leukemia. They appear as reddish blue thickening of the skin. On pressing out the blood from the area, a greenish hue is noticeable for a few seconds due to the presence of myeloperoxidase.
- Bones—diffuse osteoporosis or localized tumors affecting the long bones.

Acute Promyelocytic Leukemia (M3)

About 15–20% of AML fall under this group. The predominant cells are promyelocytes with coarse granules in the cytoplasm. In addition to the general features of acute leukemia, APL is characterized in most cases by major bleeding tendency, caused by disseminated intravascular coagulation (DIC).

In APL, there is translocation between chromosomes 15 and t(15:17). The genes for retinoic acid receptor (RAR)-alpha on chromosomes 15 fuses with the promyelocytic leukemia gene (PML) on chromosome 17, resulting in the formation of PML-RAR fusion product. All-trans retinoic acid (ATRA) acts at this fusion product and normalizes it.

Acute Myelomonocytic Leukemia (M4)

It shows a high proportion of monoblasts and monocytes. Hypertrophy and infection of gums are prominent features. Neuroleukemia is more common in this group.

Erythroleukemia (Di Guglielmo's Syndrome) (M6)

In this variety, abnormal erythroid precursors proliferate. Erythroleukemia forms 5–7% of all (ANLL). It presents as progressive anemia, hepatosplenomegaly and presence of numerous erythroblasts in peripheral blood. Marrow

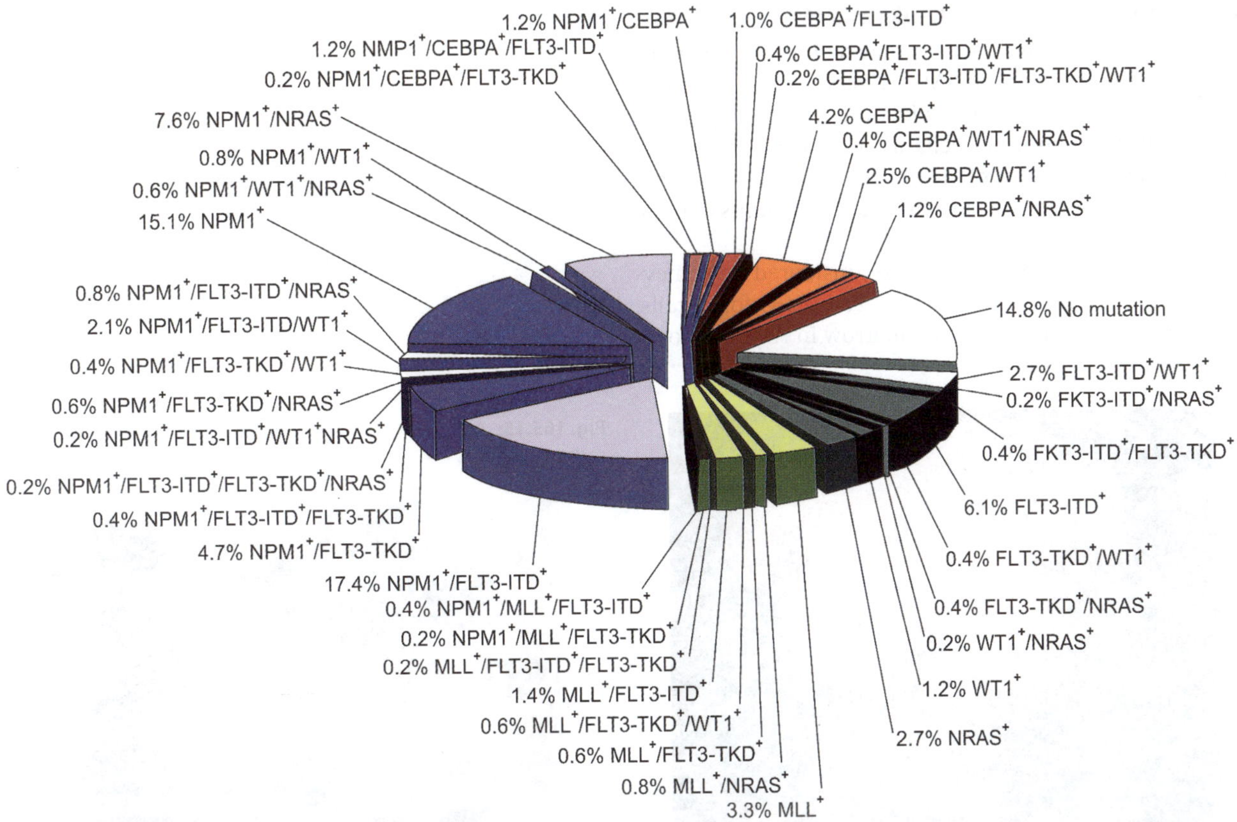

Fig. 165.7: Complexity of AML subtypes as per the new revised WHO classification

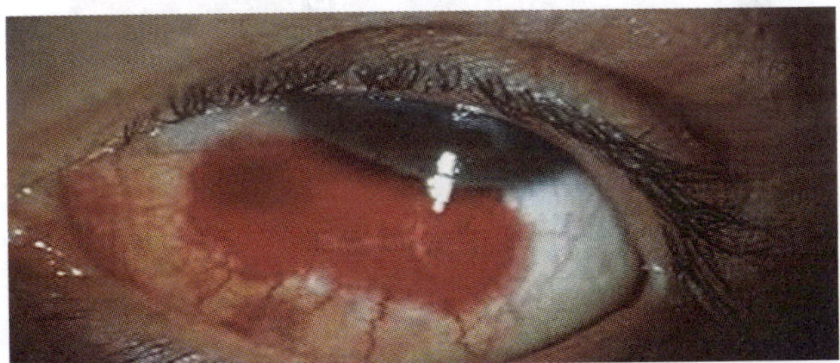

Fig. 165.8: AML subconjunctival hemorrhage. **Note:** The more extensive nature of the bleeding

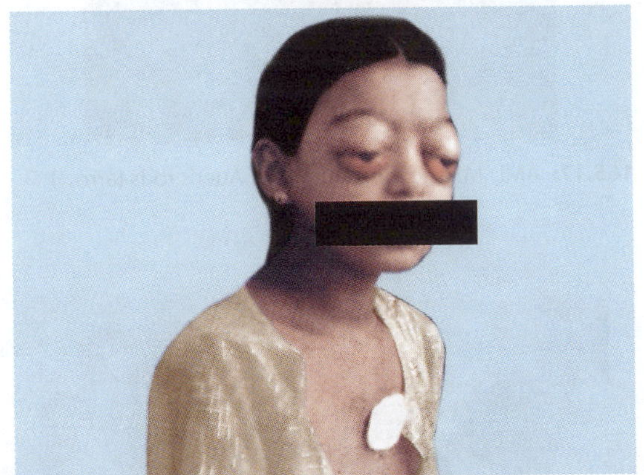

Fig. 165.9: AML female retro-orbital tumors

shows gross hyperplasia of erythroblasts, many of which have a superficial resemblance to megaloblasts (hence, termed as megaloblastoid). As the condition progresses, numerous myeloblasts also appear in peripheral blood.

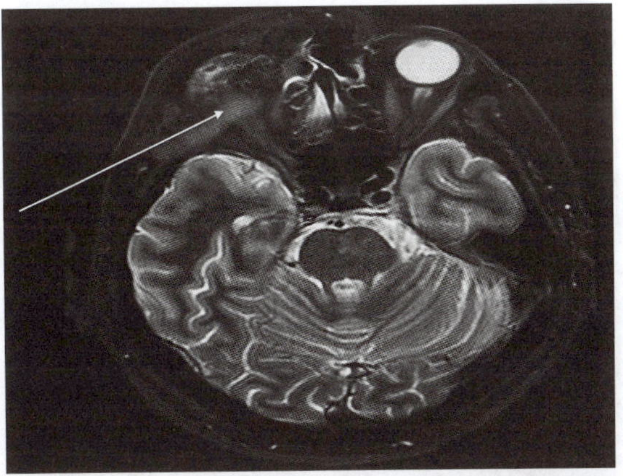

Fig. 165.10: MRI scan AML retro-orbital tumors producing proptosis (arrow)

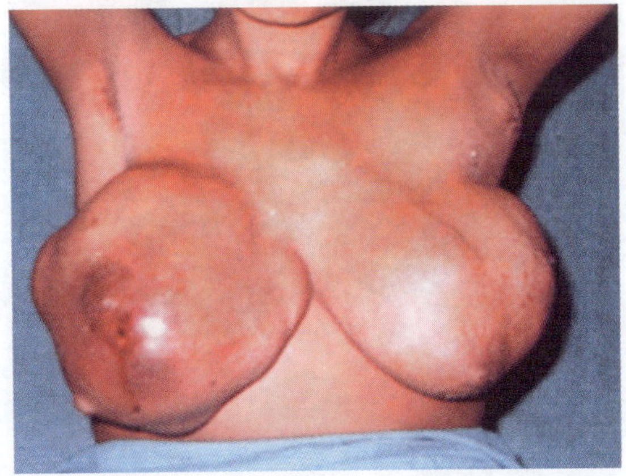

Fig. 165.11: AML female multipara tumor breasts

Acute Megakaryoblastic Leukemia (M7)

This may occur rarely. The cells may be indistinguishable from the other types of AML. Histochemical staining for platelet peroxidase and electron microscopy helps to identify the abnormal cells as megakaryoblasts. The histological appearance of the marrow is similar to that of myelofibrosis with presence of increased amounts of bone marrow reticulin.

Bone marrow or SCT should be considered on achieving first remission. For Diagnosis, *See* Ch 164 for details. Peripheral blood film and bone marrow in AML is shown in Figures 165.13 to 165.19.

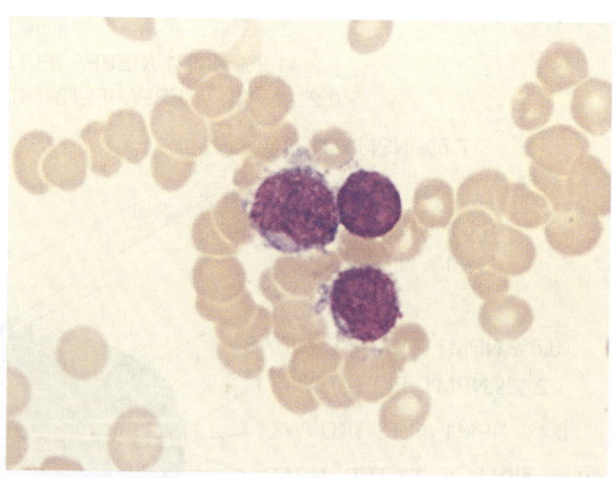

Fig. 165.15: AML- M7-Classical cytoplasmic projections on with Auer's rods myeloblasts

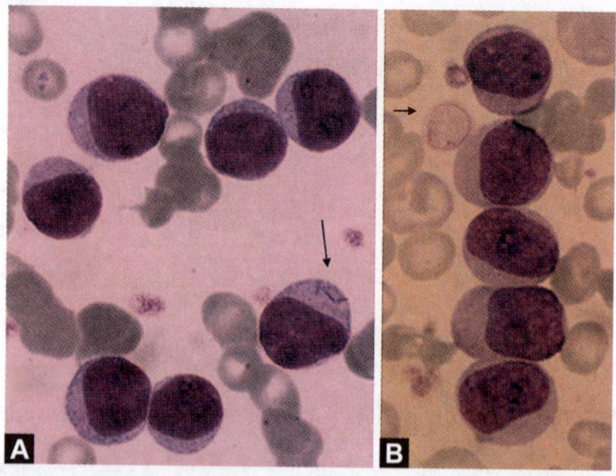

Figs 165.16A and B: Acute myeloid leukemia (AML) peripheral blood × 500: **A.** M1; **B.** M0

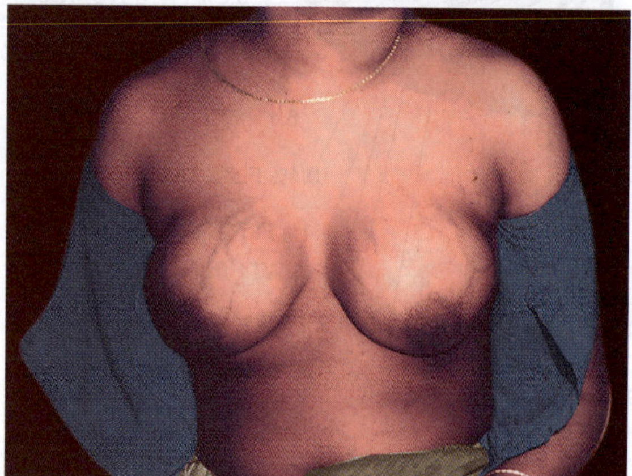

Fig. 165.12: AML adolescent girl tumor breasts

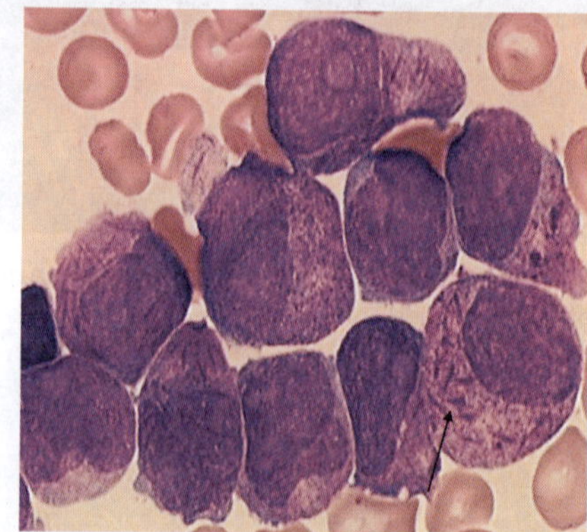

Fig. 165.17: AML: M3 showing clumps of Auer's rods (arrow)

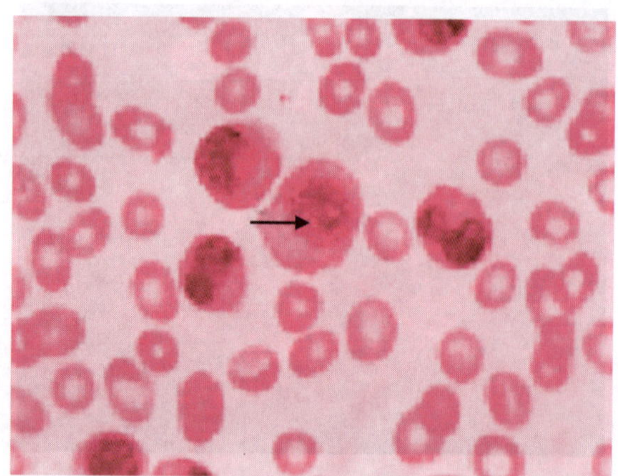

Fig. 165.13: AML peripheral blood × 500. ***Note:*** Myeloblast (arrow)

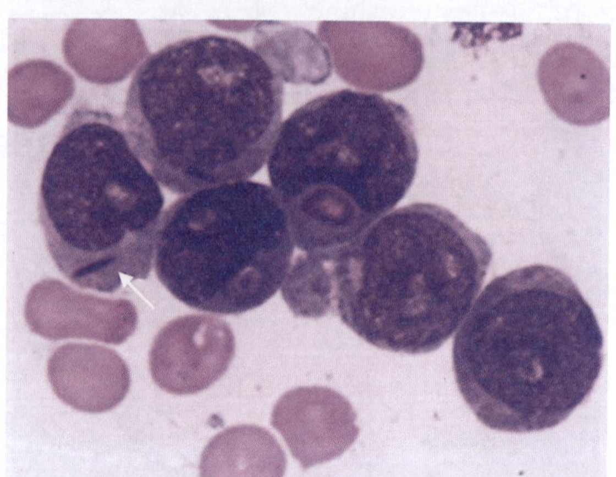

Fig. 165.14: AML peripheral blood × 1000. ***Note:*** Myeloblast (arrow)

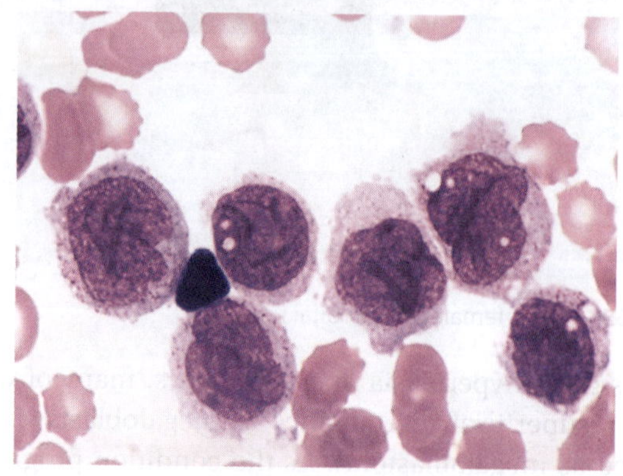

Fig. 165.18: Acute monoblastic leukemia peripheral blood. AML-M5b

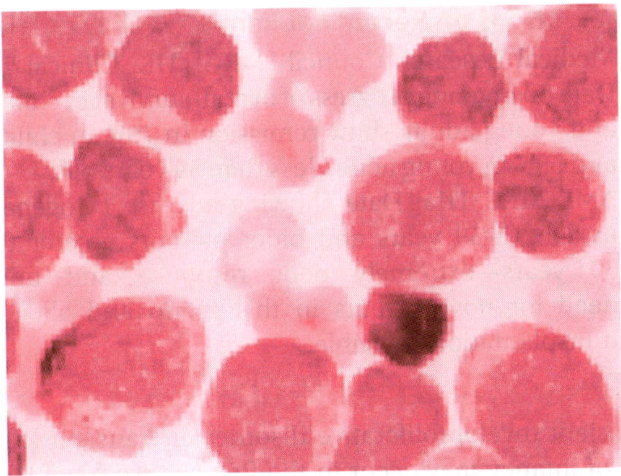

Fig. 165.19: AML: Bone marrow—normal marrow cells are replaced by myeloblasts

Table 165.4: Induction treatment schedule for acute myeloid leukemia (3+7 regimen)

	Dose	Route	Frequency
Daunorubicin	45–60 mg/m²	Intravenous	Daily for 3 days
Cytosine arabinoside (ara-c)	For 7 days	100 mg/m²	Continuous IV infusion or push doses 8 hourly
6-thioguanine or	100 mg/m²	Oral	Given 8 hourly
6-mercaptopurine	100 mg/m²	Oral	Daily

Treatment

Except for APL, the induction regimen consists of daunorubicin and Ara-C (Table 165.4).

Induction therapy: The most popular regimen is the 3+7 combination of daunorubicin 45 mg/m² or 60 mg/m²/IV for 3 days and standard dose cytarabine 100 mg/m² by continuous infusion for 7 days. This combination produces severe neutropenia and when the neutrophil count falls below 0.5×10^9 cells/L fatal infections may occur. Therefore, in order to achieve good results, proper germ-free environment and prophylactic antimicrobial therapy are essential. Judicious use of colony-stimulating factors such as GM-CSF and G-CSF helps to reduce the duration and severity of drug-induced leukopenia. Availability of these cytokines has helped to plan more aggressive and curative chemotherapeutic regimens. Other induction regimens employ idarubicin or mitoxantrone instead of daunorubicin. Therapy-related AML is more resistant to treatment.

The induction of remission and its maintenance depends mainly on the effectiveness of initial inducing regimen. The value of maintenance regimen is not as clear-cut as in the case of ALL. Therefore, many centers do not follow a continuous maintenance regimen.

Neuroprophylaxis may be indicated for acute myelomonocytic leukemia even though the incidence of neuroleukemia is much less compared to ALL. BMT has to be considered earlier than in the case of ALL.

Special Points in the Treatment of APL

ATRA induces differentiation of the immature cells into mature granulocytes. APL responds very satisfactorily to initial treatment with ATRA which is the treatment of choice

Table 165.5: Genetic findings in relation to prognosis

Genetic group	Subset
Favorable	T(8;21)(q22;q22); RUNX1-RUNX1T1' inv(16)(p13.1q22) or t(16;16)(p13.1;q22) CBFB-MYH11' Mutated NPM1 without FLT3-ITD (CN-AML) Mutated CEBPA (CN-AML)
Intermediate-I'	Mutated NPM1 and FLT3-ITD (CN-AML) Wild-type NPM1 and FLT3-ITD (CN-AML) Wild-type NPM1 without FLT3-ITD (CN-AML)
Intermediate-II	t(9;11)(p22;q23); MLLT3-MLL Cytogenetic abnormalities not classified as favorable or adverse†
Adverse	inv(3)(q21q26.2) or t(3;3)(q21;q26.2); RPN1-EVI1 t(6;9)(p23;q34); DEK-NUP214 t(v;11)(v;q23); MLL-rearranged -5 or del(5q); -7; abnl(17p); complex karyotype††

Notes:

t(8;21) and inv(16)/t(16;16) are frequently denoted as core binding factor-acute myeloid leukemia (CBF-AML)

'Includes all AMLs with normal karyotype except for those included in the favorable subgroup.

†For most abnormalities, adequate numbers have not been studied to draw firm conclusions regarding their prognostic significance.

††Three or more chromosome abnormalities on the absence of one of the WHO-designated recurring translocations or inversions: t(15;17), t(8;21), inv(6) or t(16;16), t(19,11), t(v;11)(v;q23),t(6;9), inv(3) or t(3;3).

Abbreviations: CN-AML = Cytogenetically normal acute myeloid leukemia; NPM1 = Nucleophosmin1; CEBPA = CCAAT/enhancer-binding protein alpha; FLT3 = fms-like tyrosine kinase 3 gene; ITD = Internal tandem duplication; MLL = Mixed lineage-leukemia gene

at present. The dose is 45 mg/m² body surface per day for 15 days, once in 3 months as maintenance therapy. This may lead to rise in mature granulocytes which may lead to pulmonary infiltration, so-called retinoic acid syndrome. This is treated by glucocorticoids. The remission induced by ATRA tends to be short lived and therefore, it has to be followed up by chemotherapy.

Arsenic (arsenious oxide) can also induce differentiation of PML cells. Combination of ATRA and arsenic effects better differentiation of APL cells. Prognostic group based on genetics (Table 165.5)

High-risk AML Treatment

High-risk AML constitutes a biologically distinct subset of disease and comprises a sizeable percentage of adult AML. A distinct profile of cytogenetics and molecular features can be used to assign risk. High-risk disease features cluster among clinical phenotypes, such as among patients over age 60, those with antecedent hematological disorders, and those who have received prior treatment with cytotoxic chemotherapy, high-risk karyotype or the expression of mutated flt3, kit and other molecular markers which explain both the poor response to induction chemotherapy and the high relapse rate previously attributed to clinical variables alone (Table 165.6).

New therapeutic regimens and drugs for high-risk AML:
- Cytotoxic agents
  - Clofarabine
  - Elacytarabine
  - CPX-351

Table 165.6: Cytogenetics and mutational findings characteristic of newly diagnosed high-risk AML

Cytogenetic classification	Mutation
Favorable risk t(8;21); inv(16) or t(16;16)	kit
Intermediate risk Normal; +8	FL3-ITD-positive; Mutant TET2, MLL-PTD, DNMT3A, ASXL1, PHF6
Unfavorable risk -5/-7; 11q23, 20q-, 3 or more	

Abbreviations: FLT3 = fms-like tyrosine kinase 3 gene; ITD = Internal tandem duplication; TET2 = Tet methylcytosine dioxygenase 2; MLL-PTD = Mixed lineage-leukemia-partial tandem duplication; DNMT3A = DNA methyl transferase 3A; ASXL1 = additional sex comb-like 1; PHF6 = PHD finger protein 6

- *Immunoconjugate:* Gemtuzumab ozogamicin
- Alternative targeted agents
  - Farnesyl transferase inhibitors
  - Histone deacetylase inhibitors
  - FLT3 antagonists
  - Others
- *Chemosensitizing agents:* CXCR4 antagonist.

Observations on Recent Leukemia Treatment Trials

- Medical Research Council (MRC), UK, Clinical Trial Data on ongoing progress of overall survival in children and young adults show remission in 79% in children and 59% in young adults less than 59 years old.
- AML MRC Trial Data showing adverse cytogenetics in age 15–59 years and older patients greater than 60 years—extremely poor response and unmet need for novel agents in this group and allogenic transplantation if eligible.

Transient Myeloid Disorder of Infancy

Transient myeloproliferative disorder or transient leukemia of infancy may occur in the first few weeks of life. It is always associated with Down's syndrome or trisomy 21. Infants with these disorders have leukocytosis, often with blast cells in peripheral blood, exceeding that in the bone marrow. Most often the blast cells are of megakaryocytic or erythroid lineage and are clonal. Hepatosplenomegaly, pericardial and pleural effusion and liver involvement are common. Majority show spontaneous remission. In 30%, MDS or AML may develop.

CHAPTER
166

Chronic Leukemia

Salim Shafeek, Kasim Salim, KV Krishna Das

Chapter Summary

- Chronic Myeloid Leukemia (CML)
- Chronic Lymphatic Leukemia (CLL)
- Hairy Cell Leukemia
- Prolymphocytic Leukemia (PLL)

CHRONIC MYELOID LEUKEMIA (CML)

It is also known as *chronic granulocytic leukemia*, is the most common type of chronic leukemia affecting adults in India. It forms 30% of the total leukemias. It is clinically characterized by gross overproduction of granulocytes. The disease is rare (less than 5% of total) below the age of 5 years. Maximum incidence is in the age group 40–60 years, men are affected more often than women (3:2). Neutrophilic leukemia forms more than 95% of the total, though rarely eosinophils and basophils may be the affected cells.

Etiology

CML is a neoplastic disorder arising from the malignant transformation of a single hematopoietic stem cell (HSC). Over 95% of CML shows a constant chromosomal abnormality in the myeloid, erythroid and megakaryocytic cells. This abnormal chromosome known as the *Philadelphia chromosome* (Ph) is formed by the reciprocal translocation of the long arms of chromosome 22 and 9. CML arises from a single pluripotent HSC which acquires Ph1 chromosome carrying the BCR-ABL fusion gene which confers a proliferative advantage over normal cells and thus allow the Ph1 carrying cells to proliferate at the expense of other hematopoietic cells. CML cells also live longer since they resist apoptosis.

Ph1 Chromosome

This chromosomal abnormality was identified in 1960 but only in 1973, it was attributed to 9:22 translocation which involves a reciprocal translocation of genetic material (containing proto-oncogene c-abl, from chromosome 9–22, at the break point of the BCR locus) resulting in the fusion gene BCR-ABL which encodes for an abnormal tyrosine kinase with abnormally increased activity. There is clonal expansion of the stem cells with BCR-ABL probably due to reduced adhesion of progenitor cells to stromal elements, as a result of which the stem cells escape the physiological inhibition. Even though the specific cellular disturbances involved are not fully known, it is certain that BCR-ABL is directly involved in the pathogenesis as evidenced from animal experiments. Ph are demonstrable in the dividing cells from the marrow as well as in the circulating cells. Myeloid, erythroid and megakaryocytic cell lines show Ph1 chromosome.

What causes the mutation in human beings with CML is not known; viruses, radiation and toxic chemicals are all implicated.

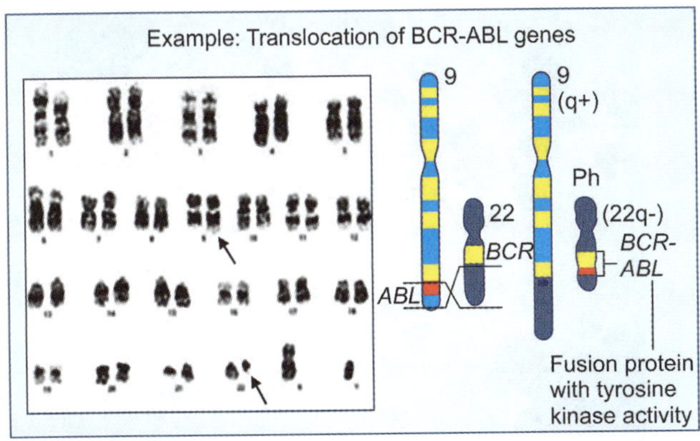

Fig. 166.1: CML karyotype showing Ph t9:22 translocation (arrows)

Molecular Pathogenesis

Molecular consequence of t(9;22) (q34;q11) translocation is the creation of the fusion gene BCR-ABL which encodes for an abnormal tyrosine kinase that mediates an unregulated signal transduction. Depending on the site of breakpoint in the BCR gene, the fusion proteins may vary in size from 185–230 kd. Nearly, all patients with CML express 210 kd BCR-ABL fusion protein. Fusion proteins of different sizes can be related to different outcomes. 190 kd BCR-ABL protein has greater tyrosine kinase activity and is a more potent oncogene than 210 kd protein. Abelson (Abl) kinase can be inhibited by imatinib which is used in therapy. BCR gene is located on the long arm of chromosome 22 and Abl resides in chromosome 9. BCR-ABL fusion protein activates Abl kinase (Fig. 166.1).

The Ph results in the expression of a constitutively active protein tyrosine kinase BCR-ABL that is essential for the hematopoietic cell transformation. As a consequence of increased tyrosine kinase activity, the BCR-ABL protein can phosphorylate several substances, thereby activating multiple signal transduction cascades affecting growth and differentiation of cells. Since the BCR-ABL signal is constitutive, these cells escape the normal constraints of growth and become leukemic. On the basis of these findings, remission in CML can be defined as hematologic, cytogenetic (disappearance or reduction of Ph1 chromosome) and molecular (disappearance of BCR-ABL gene). Modern polymerase chain reaction (PCR) assays enable quantitative monitoring of BCR-ABL messenger ribonucleic acid (RNA) transcripts periodically. This is used for assessing prognosis and predicting cure.

Pathology

There is gross increase in granulocytes and their precursors in the blood and marrow. The bone marrow is filled with granulocytes, myelocytes, metamyelocytes and promyelocytes. Blasts are less than 5% in the chronic phase but can increase in the accelerated and blast phase. Erythroblasts are usually decreased. Megakaryocytes are normal in number or may be increased. The spleen is grossly enlarged and the liver is moderately enlarged. All organs show infiltration by myelocytes and a smaller number of promyelocytes. When blastic transformation occurs, the percentage of blast cells increases in the marrow and peripheral blood. The diagnostic finding in the peripheral blood is gross leukocytosis with total leukocyte count (TLC) often exceeding 50,000–100,000/mm^3 or more and the differential count showing 40–50% neutrophils, 20–30% myelocytes, 10–30% metamyelocytes, 5–10% promyelocytes, an occasional blast and the rest constituted by basophils, lymphocytes and monocytes. Basophil count is increased in CML during the chronic phase and remains elevated even when the patient responds to treatment. Platelet count is increased or normal. Mild anemia may occur. In an occasional case, the peripheral smear may show only leukocytosis with mature neutrophils. This is called ***chronic neutrophilic leukemia (CNL)*** or ***Emil-Weil's CML***.

Serum proteins are elevated with increase in gamma globulin. Leukocyte counts exceeding 300,000 mm^3 may give rise to cellular hyperviscosity syndrome. The serum uric acid is high due to more rapid cell turnover. Basal metabolic rate is increased. ***Leukocyte alkaline phosphatase score (LAP score)*** is low or absent in more than 90% in the chronic phase. Serum vitamin B_{12} and B_{12} binding capacity are elevated due to increase in transcobalamin I and II.

Clinical Features

The disease is insidious in onset and it is almost impossible to assess the duration of illness when the patient comes up for examination. Some asymptomatic cases are picked up by routine blood tests. Majority of patients present with the feeling of a mass and dull ache in the abdomen caused by splenomegaly. The spleen is grossly enlarged in over 95% of cases (Figs 166.2 and 166.3). Splenic size correlates reasonably well with the TLC. Gross splenomegaly is associated with episodes of splenic infarction which present as painful episodes. Some cases reveal bone tenderness. Pallor, exertional dyspnea and tachycardia may occur due to moderate or severe anemia. Hypermetabolism leads to loss of weight, lassitude and night sweats. With progress of the disease, the abdomen becomes distended due to huge splenomegaly and moderate hepatomegaly. Nutritional deficiencies, cachexia and intercurrent infections complicate the picture. When the leukocyte count is high, the ocular fundus shows hyperemia of the disk, venous engorgement and occasionally hemorrhages.

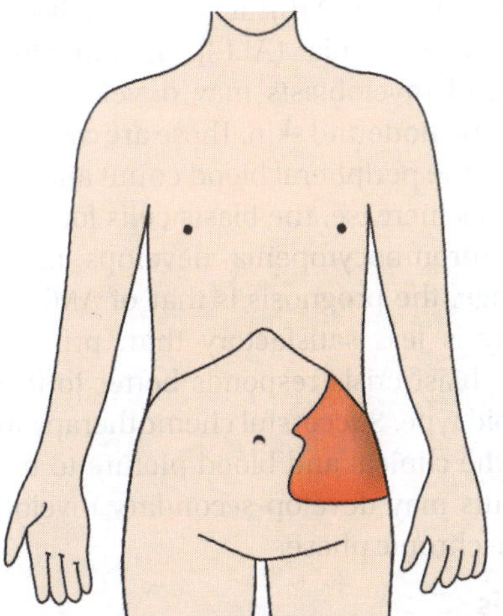

Fig. 166.2: CML—gross splenomegaly in 34-year-old male, without gross impairment of general health

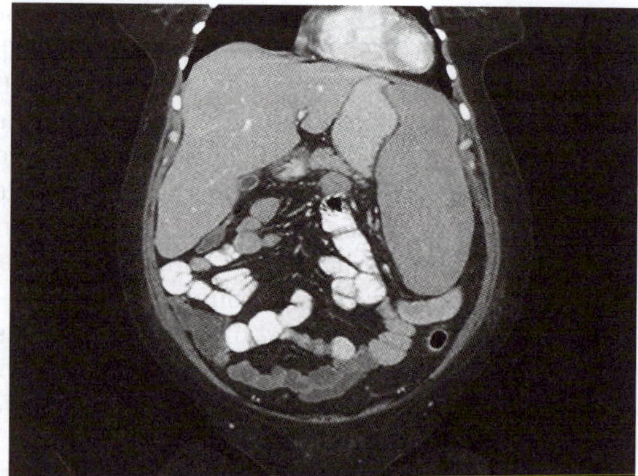

Fig. 166.3: CML—gross splenomegaly shown in CT scan

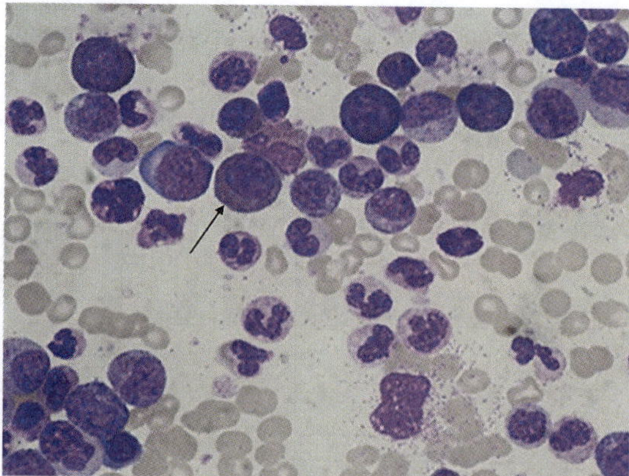

Fig. 166.4: CML—peripheral blood × 1000. ***Note:*** Neutrophil myelocyte, left shifted neutrophils and basophils (arrow)

Complications

Several complications may occur from time-to-time. These are infections, malnutrition, anemia, trauma, infarction of the spleen and secondary gout. Thrombotic tendencies due to high leukocyte counts, consequent leukostasis and associated thrombocytosis develop resulting in venous thrombosis and priapism. Hemorrhagic complications may also occur because of the defective platelet function despite a normal or high platelet count.

Blastic Transformation

Most of the CML patients present in the chronic phase with very few blasts in the peripheral blood and marrow and after a variable period of months to years enter the more serious and inescapable complication of ***blastic transformation*** (blast crisis). A range of additional nonrandom chromosomal changes occur including duplication of Ph chromosome and trisomy 8. Multiplication or deletion of tumor suppressor genes such as p16 and p53 occur with variable frequency. Probably these contribute to the blastic transformation. Blastic transformation is heralded by unresponsiveness to conventional treatment and development of severe anemia, fever, infections, lymphadenopathy, bleeding tendencies and rapid deterioration of general health. In 75% of cases, blast transformation is into myeloid [acute myeloid leukemia (AML)] and in 25% lymphatic [acute lymphocytic leukemia (ALL)]. Extramedullary tumors consisting of myeloblasts may develop specially in the bones, lymph node and skin. These are called ***granulocytic sarcomas***. The peripheral blood count and the proportion of blast cells increase, the blasts cells forming more than 20–30%. Thrombocytopenia develops as well. In the blastic stage, the prognosis is that of AML, but response to therapy is less satisfactory than primary AML. The lymphatic blast crisis responds better to treatment than the myeloid type. Successful chemotherapy in blast phase converts the clinical and blood picture to that of CML. A few patients may develop secondary myelofibrosis even during the chronic phase.

Diagnosis

CML should be considered in the diagnosis when there is moderate to massive splenomegaly in the presence of

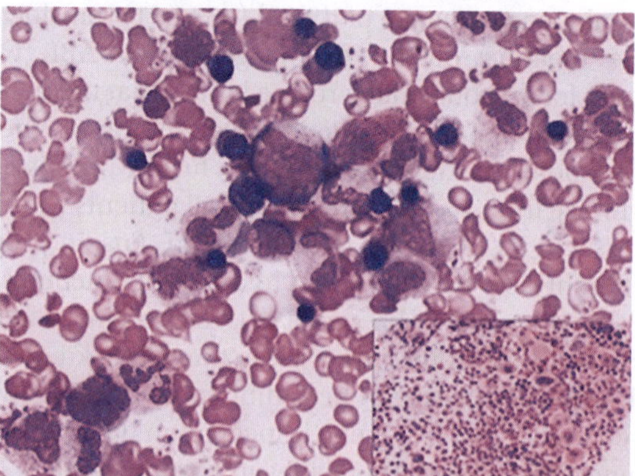

Fig. 166.5: CML—bone marrow × 400. ***Note:*** Myeloid hyperplasia. All the elements are present

reasonably good general health. A very high TLC and blood smear examination confirm the diagnosis (Fig. 166.4). Presence of thrombocytosis and basophilia are supporting evidences. Low or absent LAP score almost confirms the diagnosis. When the diagnosis is in doubt, demonstration of the Ph1 chromosome by karyotyping or fluorescent *in situ* hybridization (FISH) is diagnostic of CML. In addition, highly sensitive and specific molecular probes are now available to detect the presence of BCR-ABL in peripheral blood or bone marrow leukocytes. This helps to diagnose and monitor therapy. PCR testing of peripheral blood, RNA is so sensitive as to detect one Ph positive cell in 106 cells. For clinical purposes, bone marrow examination and genetic studies are not mandatory (Fig. 166.5).

Differential Diagnosis

Other causes of splenomegaly such as myelofibrosis, portal hypertension, chronic malaria, leishmaniasis, and hemolytic anemia should be considered in the differential diagnosis. Leukemoid reactions should be excluded. LAP score is low in CML, whereas in leukemoid reactions it is high. Idiopathic myelofibrosis may pose some difficulty to be distinguished from CML. Myelofibrosis is characterized by gross splenomegaly, only modest elevation of the TLC (15,000–30,000 cells/mm³) and is characterized by a leukoerythroblastic blood picture. Teardrop-shaped erythrocytes are characteristic. Bone marrow is scanty and trephine biopsy reveals fibrosis.

Course and Prognosis

CML runs a relentless course to end fatally in all cases. Unlike as in acute leukemia, medical therapy does not bring about predictable cure. Untreated, the average period of survival used to be 2–3 years in the early 1990s. Treatment given early in the disease brings about clinical relief and clears the blood picture, but the disease is not eradicated, and therefore, relapse is the rule. About 20% patients survive up to 10 years. Death is due to blastic transformation, infection, hemorrhage or rarely drug toxicity. Presence of Ph1 chromosome confers a better prognosis. Ph1 positive cases do better and live longer with an average period of survival of 4 years whereas Ph1 negative cases invariably run a downhill course and die within one year. Ph1 chromosome negative cases have been termed as *atypical CML*, and most of these occur in children.

Bone marrow transplantation (BMT) brings about cure in the vast majority who survive the procedure. With the introduction of the specific tyrosine-kinase inhibitor (TKI), imatinib the disease undergoes clinical, hematological and even molecular remission. Symptoms are completely abolished and quality of life improves.

Treatment

Eradication of residual disease (CML stem cell) in CML that is presumed to arise from malignant Ph1 positive stem cells which should result in permanent cure and long-term leukemia-free survival is the ideal to be achieved. Clinical trials in CML are addressing this issue of depth of molecular remission while on TKIs. Since conventional medical therapy does not eradicate the disease, the aim is to relieve symptoms and bring about clinical and hematological normalcy. The high leukocyte count and organomegaly subside completely with treatment and the patient becomes asymptomatic though a few abnormal cells and Ph1 chromosomes persist.

Drugs

Imatinib (Gleevec)

The inhibition of tyrosine kinase activity is the most effective therapy for CML, if BMT is not available. The signal transduction inhibitor (STI 571), imatinib selectively inhibits the fusion protein tyrosine kinase of the BCR-ABL gene. It has been approved for use in CML patients as first-line therapy. It is given in doses of 400 mg orally as single dose for adults continuously for an indefinite period. At times, up to 800 mg can be given daily. It is still not clear how long the treatment has to be continued. Within weeks of starting therapy, the leukocyte counts, the abnormal cells and splenomegaly come down and full clinical normalcy is restored. The median survival has also improved. Complete cytogenetic response at 12 months was 69% and at 60 months was 87%. Blast crisis develops in 7% even while on treatment. Overall median survival at 60 months in those who were put on imatinib from the start was 89%.

Cessation of therapy promptly brings back the leuko-cytosis and abnormal blood picture. Sixty to eighty percent show full clinical response with 68% showing cytogenetic clearance in the chronic phase. Real time PCR measures the ratio of BCR-ABL transcripts to BCR transcripts. This helps to monitor recovery at the molecular level.

Imatinib may produce response in accelerated and blastic phase as well, even though the results are poorer. In such cases, the duration of response is also shorter. Adverse side effects include peripheral and periorbital edema, muscle cramps, joint pains, neutropenia, elevated liver enzymes and rarely, congestive heart failure (CHF). Resistance to imatinib has been recorded. Administration of hydroxyurea in doses of 1–2 g orally daily in combination with imatinib restores the clinical effects of the latter. Combination therapy with two TKIs is also under evaluation.

Imatinib mesylate is finding its use in several other neoplasms where the tyrosine kinase receptor is expressed prominently. The present cost of imatinib therapy is ₹ 300/day.

Dasatinib (Bristol-Myers Squibb)

It is an ABL kinase inhibitor that differs from imatinib in that it combines to both the active and inactive conformations of the ABL kinase domain. In imatinib resistant cases and in those who are intolerant to imatinib, dasatinib given orally in doses ranging from 15 to 240 mg/day leads to hematological and cytogenetic response. Major adverse effects include reversible myelosuppression and nonmalignant pleural effusion.

Nilotinib (Novartis)

This is a new orally active aminopyrimidine-derivative TKI which is more potent than imatinib *in vitro* against CML. In doses starting from 50 mg oral daily and worked up to 1200 mg od or 400–600 mg bd, this drug is effective during the chronic phase, accelerated phase and blastic phase in diminishing effectiveness. Adverse effects include myelosuppression, transient direct hyperbilirubinemia and rashes. Nilotinib is the standard of care following the randomized trial between imatinib and nilotinib.

Third generation TKI are *bosutinib* (dose 200 mg daily) and *ponatinib* (dose 15–45 mg daily oral). Ponatinib is specific to overcome T315I mutation (Tables 166.1 and 166.2).

Table 166.1: Response of drugs

Response	Definition
CHR	Leukocyte count of < 10 × 10⁹/L; platelet count < 450 × 10⁹/L; normal differential with no early forms; no splenomegaly
MCyR	0–35% Ph + metaphases (BM)
PCyR	1–35% Ph + metaphases (BM)
CCyR	0% Ph + metaphases (BM)
MMR	BCR-ABL1 IS ≤ 0.1%
MR	Undetectable BCR-ABL1 (assay sensitivity ≥ 4.5 or 5.0 logs) BCR-ABL1 IS ≤ 0.0032 (MR 4.5) BCR-ABL1 IS ≤ 0.001 (MR 5.0)

Note: CHR indicates complete hematological response; BCR-ABL1 IS, percent BCR-ABL1 control gene standardized to the IS. Common control genes are ABL1 and BCR.

Abbreviations: MCyR = Major cytogenetic response; PCyR = Partial cytogenetic response; CCyR = Complete cytogenetic response; MMR = Major molecular response; MR = Molecular response; BM = Bone marrow

Table 166.2: Recommendations for disease monitoring

Metaphase bone marrow cytogenetics	BCR-ABL1 transcript levels (IS) peripheral blood	ABL kinase domain point mutation analysis
At diagnosis	At diagnosis to establish baseline	If no partial cytogenetic response at 3 months or BCR-ABL1/ABL is > 10% at 3 months
At 3 months, if QPCR not available	Every 3 months until CCyR	If no CCyR at 12 or 18 months
At 12 months in no CCyR or MMR	Every 3 months after CCyR for 2 years, then every 3–6 months	5–10 fold increase in BCR-ABL1 transcript levels
At 18 months, if no CCyR at 12 months or no MMR	Every 3–6 months after MMR	Disease progression to AP or BC
If increasing BCR-ABL1 transcript levels (5–10 fold) in the absence of MMR	When BCR-ABL1 transcript levels increase by 5–10 fold with MMR, repeat in 1–3 months	Loss of hematologic or cytogenetic response

Abbreviations: CCyR = Complete cytogenetic response; MMR = Major molecular response; AP = Accelerated phase; BC = Blast crisis

Table 166.3: Criteria for accelerated phase (AP) of CML given by different centers

AP criteria	Blasts	Basophils	Persistent thrombocytopenia (unrelated to therapy)	Additional clonal cytogenetic aberrations
WHO	10–19%	≥20%	<100 x 10^9/L	Present
ELN	15–29%	≥20%	<100 x 10^9/L	Present
MD Anderson	15–29%	≥20%	<100 x 10^9/L	Present

Abbreviations: WHO = World Health Organization; ELN = European Leukemia Net

Hydroxyurea (Hydroxycarbamide)

This used to be the drug of choice for over 5 decades for the treatment of CML before the advent of interferon alpha (IFN-α) and imatinib.

The dose varies from 0.5 to 2 g daily orally in divided doses. It brings about a steady fall in TLC with reduction in the immature cells within 1–2 months. The mechanism of action is inactivation of the enzyme ribonucleotide reductase (RNR) with consequent inhibition of cellular DNA synthesis leading to cell death in the S-phase. Adverse side effects include gastrointestinal (GI) upsets, marrow suppression, skin pigmentation, alopecia and ulceration in the feet. These regress on stopping the drug. The cost of treatment is ₹ 70/day.

Busulfan (Myleran)

This alkylating agent belonging to the group of sulfur mustards used to be given orally in the dose of 2–8 mg/day in the 5th–9th decades of the previous century as a main anti-CML drug. The drug has to be continued till the TLC falls below 10,000/mm³, at which stage the splenomegaly also disappears. When the leukocyte count falls below 10,000/mm³, busulfan is withdrawn to avoid marrow suppression. Further treatment is indicated when TLC goes above 50,000/mm³. Busulfan is effective in over 75% of cases to produce symptomatic relief. Relapses also respond to busulfan. Finally, the disease becomes resistant and the blastic crisis sets in which is the terminal stage.

Adverse side effects include bone marrow aplasia, allergic manifestations and pigmentation resembling Addison's disease, but without the endocrine abnormalities. Rarely, busulfan produces extrinsic alveolitis and interstitial pulmonary fibrosis (busulfan lung). This is an absolute contraindication for further busulfan therapy. At present in view of the availability of more effective and safe drugs, busulfan is not used as a primary anti-CML drug.

Interferon Alpha (IFN α)

Interferon was the first-line of therapy for all patients with CML before the advent of imatinib. Sustained disappearance of Ph occurs only in 5–10%. It is not used routinely for CML at present (Table 166.3).

Management of Hyperviscosity State

Leukapheresis

Leukapheresis using a cell separator may be temporarily beneficial in hyperviscosity state and may be required when the TLC exceeds 300–400,000/mm³. The procedure may also bring about temporary hematological remission. For BMT/stem cell transplantation 9 refer to Ch 164.

Since this is the only predictable curative modality of treatment at present, it should be considered as early as possible after diagnosis. BMT done in the chronic phase of the disease and in younger subjects, gives the best results with cure rates well above 70%. The procedure related mortality is a major deterrent in opting for this form of therapy. At present, the cost of BMT in India is ₹ 10–15 lacs. BMT done during the accelerated or blastic phase is less successful and more risky.

Indication in CML for allogenic stem cell transplantation has significantly reduced after the successful use of TKIs. This is currently experimental and used for patients who are young and could not tolerate other TKIs due to side effects or resistance like T315I mutation status. The other indication is blast crisis in CML which has extremely poor prognosis.

Variants of CML

Eosinophilic Leukemia

In this disorder, patients present with marked eosinophilia, often above 100,000/mm³ with the clinical picture of CML. The blood shows eosinophils, eosinophil myelocytes and occasional neutrophil myelocytes. In a few cases, Ph may be found.

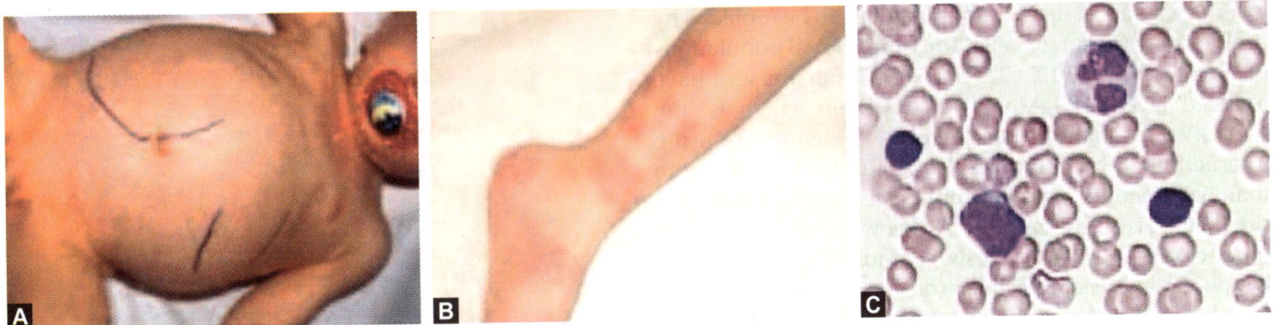

Figs 166.6A to C: Juvenile myelomonocytic leukemia. **A.** Gross hepatosplenomegaly; **B.** Skin lesions; **C.** Blood picture showing neutrophil and monocyte

Chronic Basophilic Leukemia

This clinically resembles CML, but there is gross increase in basophils. A few neutrophils may be present. Ph chromosome may or may not be present.

Chronic Monocytic Leukemia

This term is used to denote the condition in which the monocytes are also considerably increased in addition to the blood picture of CML.

Chronic Myelomonocytic Leukemia

This entity which is considered as one of the myelodysplastic syndromes (MDS) is seen in patients over the age of 50 years and the clinical picture resembles that of refractory anemia with excess of blasts (RAEB). Blood shows absolute elevation of monocytes (2×10^9L or more), many of them being atypical. The spleen enlarges progressively. The main difference from AML (M2, M4 and M5) is that the total count of promyelocyte and blasts in the marrow are less than 30%. Over one-third of the cases develop AML on follow-up (Figs 166.6A to C).

CML in Infants and Children

In children, only less than 5% of leukemia is formed by CML. There are two types:

1. *Ph1 positive CML,* which has the same biological behavior and response to therapy as adult CML.
2. *Ph1 negative CML* which is more frequent. These may occur at any age, between 2 months and 9 years, though the peak incidence is between 1 and 2 years. This is termed juvenile CML.

Juvenile CML

It is characterized by proliferation of myelocytes in bone marrow, peripheral blood and tissues. Both sexes are equally affected. They show marked enlargement of spleen and liver. The peripheral blood shows increase in myelocytes and monocytes, but the TLC may be lower than that in adults. Platelets are often reduced. There is increase in fetal hemoglobin which may form up to 85% of the total. The disease runs a more rapid course and ends fatally within one year of diagnosis (Fig. 166.7).

A diagnostic feature is the finding that, on *in vitro* cultivation of peripheral blood stem cells stimulated by granulocyte-macrophage colony-stimulating factor (GM-CSF), only colonies of monocytes are produced whereas in Ph1 positive CML, both myelocytes and monocytes are

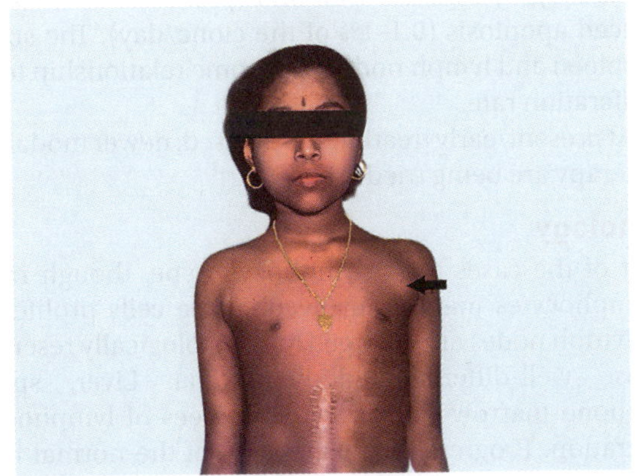

Fig. 166.7: Juvenile CML in blastic crisis. **Note:** The gross lymphadenopathy (arrow)

produced. There is suggestion that juvenile CML may be more akin to acute myelomonocytic leukemia.

Treatment: The response to conventional drugs is less satisfactory. Newer generation TKIs are more effective in treating this condition.

Cytosine arabinoside (Ara-C) and 6-mercaptopurine are found to be partially effective. Isotretinoin given orally in a dose of 100 mg/m² daily is reported to produce durable improvement in clinical and laboratory parameters. The newer drugs and BMT have to be employed when indicated.

CHRONIC LYMPHATIC LEUKEMIA (CLL)

This is the most common type of leukemia occurring in adults in the West, but in India, this is much less common. In the Mongoloid and Chinese races, the incidence is very low. CLL is a neoplasm arising usually from a clone of B-lymphocytes, occurring usually above the age of 45 years, characterized by the presence of excessive number of mature looking lymphocytes in the bone marrow and peripheral blood, and organomegaly due to infiltration by lymphocytes. In around 2% of cases, the neoplastic cells are of T-cell origin and this is termed T-cell prolymphocytic leukemia (PLL). The modern trend is to include CLL and its variants such as hairy cell leukemia and PLL along with primary lymphatic malignancies. This is so, because there is considerable overlap in the cell characteristics and clinical manifestations.

CLL is now considered to be two related entities, both originating from antigen stimulated mature B-lymphocytes which either avoid death through the intercession of external signals or die by apoptosis, only to be replaced by proliferating precursor cells. The monoclonal populations of B-cells show CD19, CD5 and CD23 markers and have reduced levels of IgM, IgD and CD79b which is, the phenotype of mature B-cells. Latest guidelines from the international workshop on CLL criteria require more than 5,000 monoclonal B-lymphocytes/mm³ of blood for the diagnosis. If the number is below 5,000, diagnosis is monoclonal B-lymphocytosis. Pathological features of lymph nodes resemble those of small cell lymphocytic lymphoma. Antigenic stimulation and presence of pro-CLL activating factors have been identified. These cytokines help the CLL cell to proliferate and avoid apoptosis. CLL cells are highly dynamic with brisk proliferation rates and reduced apoptosis (0.1–1% of the clone/day). The size of the spleen and lymph nodes bear some relationship to the proliferation rate.

At present, early treatment is advised; newer modalities of therapy are being tried.

Pathology

Most of the cases are B-lymphocyte type, though rarely T-lymphocytes may be involved. These cells proliferate. The lymph nodes are enlarged and histologically resemble diffuse well-differentiated lymphoma. Liver, spleen and bone marrow show varying degrees of lymphocytic infiltration. Progressive replacement of the normal bone marrow leads to compensatory hyperplasia of the yellow marrow, but finally, the bone marrow fails. Lymphocytes may infiltrate other organs and the skin. At times, monoclonal paraproteins of the kappa or lambda type are produced by the tumor cells even without antigenic stimulation. Normal immune mechanisms of the host are impaired since the abnormal immunocytes are functionally incompetent. Immunity against infection is reduced but autoimmunity is increased. Other autoimmune disorders like hemolytic anemia, autoimmune thrombocytopenia, rheumatoid disease and Guillain-Barré syndrome (GBS) may occur in association with CLL.

Clinical Features

Males are affected twice as frequently as females. Most of the patients are above 50 years. The disease is rare in younger individuals. The onset is insidious with fatigue, tiredness and vague ill health, and on many occasions, the disease is revealed by routine physical examination and/or blood examination in asymptomatic subjects. Clinically, two forms of the disease can be identified—**benign** and **aggressive forms**. In about 80% of cases, the disease presents with painless lymphadenopathy. The nodes are moderate to large in size, rubbery in consistency, discrete, and are most prominent in the neck and axillae. Tonsils may be enlarged considerably. Enlargement of the lacrimal and salivary glands is known as Mikulicz syndrome, but this presentation is more common with lymphoma. Anemia develops due to marrow infiltration by lymphocytes replacing the erythroid series, autoimmune hemolysis, hypersplenism, vitamin B$_{12}$ or folic acid deficiency or even iron deficiency and blood loss.

Spleen is moderately enlarged (5–10 cm) in 75% of cases and in 10% splenomegaly may be the only sign in the absence of lymphadenopathy. Splenic enlargement

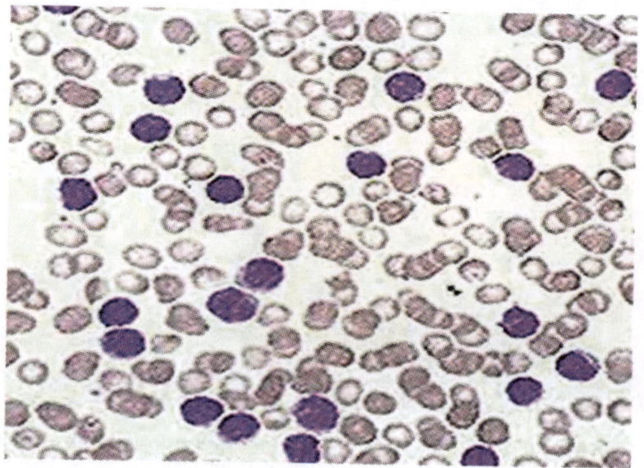

Fig. 166.8: Peripheral blood film of chronic lymphatic leukemia. ***Note:*** Mature looking lymphocytes

can lead onto hypersplenism and associated clinical problems. Cutaneous involvement presents as nodules, or diffuse infiltration producing a picture of erythroderma **(homme rouge)**. Some have an exaggerated cutaneous response to mosquito bites. Immunodeficiency due to poor T-cell function and hypogammaglobulinemia contribute to recurrent infections of the respiratory and urinary tracts. Intractable pruritus is a distressing feature.

Diagnosis

The disease should be suspected from the clinical findings. Diagnostic finding in peripheral blood is the marked leukocytosis (50–200 × 10⁹/L or 50,000–200,000/mm³) consisting almost totally of small mature lymphocytes. The cells are uniform in type and blasts are usually not seen except in the later stages (Fig. 166.8). The TLC does not bear a direct relationship to the tumor load. Many lymphocytes are ruptured and these are termed **smudge cells** or **basket cells**. The bone marrow is replaced by lymphocytes which form 90–95% of the total cells (Fig. 166.9). Pseudohyperkalemia can occur due to severe leukocytosis.

Differential diagnosis includes other causes of lymphocytosis like viral infections—the lymphocytosis in such infections is not persistent, the patients are younger, the clinical setting is different and cells are not monoclonal. Low-grade small lymphocytic B-cell lymphoma comes in the differential diagnosis, since the lymph node histology is similar; the distinction is basically made by clinical evaluation. CLL is associated with blood lymphocytosis and marrow lymphocytosis with or without lymphadenopathy. Whereas lymphoma is primarily

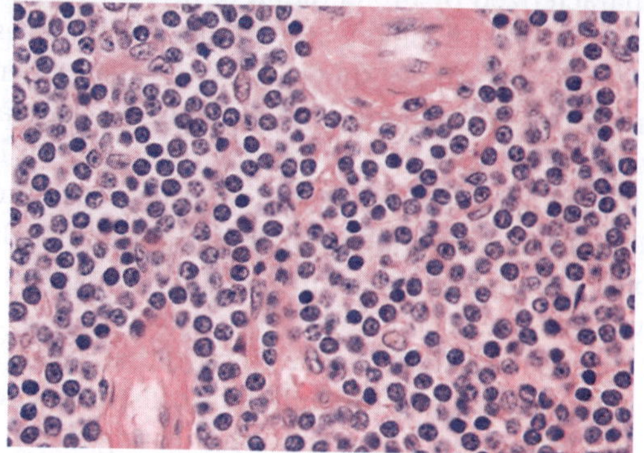

Fig.166.9: Bone marrow trephine biopsy—chronic lymphatic leukemia. ***Note:*** Infiltration by lymphocytes

associated with lymphadenopathy but marrow and blood lymphocytosis are uncommon except in late stages when these organs are involved. Prolymphocytic lymphoma closely mimics CLL but the cells here are larger. Hairy cell leukemia can be differentiated by the larger size of the lymphocytes and electron microscopic hairy projections on the cells. Waldenstörm's macroglobulinemia is another condition to be differentiated from CLL.

A system of *clinical staging* has been accepted since it correlates with the response to treatment and survival.

Course and Prognosis

In the Caucasian races, the disease follows a slow and progressive course, remaining asymptomatic for several years and ultimately ending fatally because of infection, bone marrow failure, cachexia or iatrogenic complications. In general, patients with stages I, II and III disease survive for 150, 101 and 71 months respectively. Stage III and IV do not show any significant difference in survival. Though acute lymphoblastic or even acute myeloid leukemia (AML) may occur terminally in a few cases, unlike CML, terminal blast crisis is much less common. CLL can transform to an aggressive large B-cell high-grade lymphoma at any point in the course of the disease and this is called *Richter's syndrome*.

In 1981, Binet suggested an alternate three stage classification considering total lymphoid mass. *Stage A* having less than three areas of lymphoid enlargement, *stage B* having three or more areas of lymphoid enlargement. The advanced form of *stage C* includes all patients having anemia and thrombocytopenia (Table 166.4).

The aggressive form is more common in Indians. This type follows a more rapidly progressive course, punctuated by episodes of infection. Death occurs within 2–3 years in the advanced stages in majority of cases. Since the TLC does not bear a direct relation to the tumor load, this is not useful in prognosis. High leukocyte count by itself is not an indication for starting therapy. In general, the following are the indications for starting treatment:

- Anemia
- Thrombocytopenia
- Disease-related symptoms
- Markedly enlarged spleen
- Disfiguring or symptomatic lymph node enlargement
- Blood lymphocyte doubling time less than 6 months
- Prolymphocyte transformation
- ***Richter transformation:*** Treatment helps to allay symptoms and relieve suffering and hence, treatment is indicated in all symptomatic cases though it is not clear whether it prolongs life.

A subgroup of CLL is present in which the leukemic cells show deletion of chromosome 13q14 and also contain mutated immunoglobulin heavy chain variable (IgVH) region genes. This subgroup has a better prognosis. It is seen in 50% of cases of CLL. Other conditions where the gene situated at 13q14 is deleted include non-Hodgkin's lymphoma (NHL) and multiple myeloma. Trisomy 12 confers a poor prognosis to CLL.

Treatment

Although it is customary in the West to withhold treatment till the disease reaches stages III or IV, in Indian subjects, treatment may have to be started earlier, depending on the progress and extent of the disease. Prior to the introduction of modern combined chemotherapy tailored to different types of lymphocyte disorders, specific treatment used to be with *chlorambucil (Leukeran Burrough Wellcome)* started usually with 2–4 mg per day continuously till TLC becomes normal and morphological lesions disappear. An alternate dosage schedule is 0.4 mg/kg/bw of total dose divided into 4 equal doses and given on days 1 through 4. This cycle can be repeated every 2–4 weeks. Cyclophosphamide 50–100 mg/day can be used instead of chlorambucil. Corticosteroids, given in cycles, enhance the effect of alkylating agents. Clinical improvement occurs in 1–2 years, though the neoplasm is not eradicated. With the advent of modern investigations and individualized chemotherapeutic regimens, this therapy is no longer practiced.

Fludarabine which is a nucleoside analogue given in a dose of 25 mg/m² body surface area IV daily for 5 days every 28 days is effective in bringing about higher response rates and longer remissions specially in chlorambucil resistant cases. The drug is expensive. Another nucleoside analogue, *Cladribine* also is equally effective. *Pentostatin* which is a purine analogue and *Alemtuzumab* which is a monoclonal antibody (mAb) are occasionally used in patients refractory to common drugs.

System	Stage	Definition	Median survival
Table 166.4: Rai and Binet staging systems for classification of CLL			
Rai staging system			
	0 (low risk)	Lymphocytosis only	11.5 years
	I (intermediate risk)	Lymphocytosis and lymphadenopathy	11.0 years
	II (intermadiate risk)	Lymphocytosis in blood and marrow with splenomegaly and/or hepatomegaly (with or without lymphadenopathy)	7.8 years
	III (high risk)	Lymphocytosis and anemia (hemoglobin <11g/dL or hematocrit < 33%)	5.3 years
	IV (high risk)	Lymphocytosis and thrombocytopenia (platelet count < 100,000/mm³)	7.0 years
Binet staging			
	A	Enlargement of < 3 lymphoid area (cervical, axillary, inguinal, spleen, liver); no anemia or thrombocytopenia	11.5 years
	B	Enlargement of ≥ 3 lymphoid areas	8.6 years
	C	Anemia (hemoglobin < 10 g/dL or thrombocytopenia plateler count <100,000/mm³) or both	7.0 years

Infective episodes demand prompt treatment with antibiotics. Immunoglobulin can be given prophylactically in doses of 50–100 mg/kg/bw periodically to reduce the frequency and severity of bacterial infections.

Leukapheresis has been found to be beneficial in removing the leukemic cells and thereby reducing the tumor load in intractable cases and also to reduce leukostasis.

The role of bone marrow or stem cell transplantation has not been definitely established. Results and evidence-based guidelines have not yet become clear.

Monoclonal antibodies (mAbs) specially campath-1H has been tried in relapsed and refractory CLL. The response rate is around 40%.

Combination Therapy

- Fludarabine 25 mg/m^2/day plus cyclophosphamide 250 mg/m^2/day given IV for 3 days.
- Fludarabine 24 mg/m^2/day plus cyclophosphamide 150 mg/m^2 given orally for 5 days repeated at 4 week intervals for six course has given better remission rates and quality of life, compared to others drug schedules.

Oral fludarabine is widely used now because of the good bioavailability and convenience.

FCR: Fludarabine + Cyclophosphamide + Rituximab (anti-CD20)

Monoclonal antibodies like rituximab (anti-CD20) have been combined with old treatments like chlorambucil. Treatment paradigm in CLL is changing day by day. Following the landmark German CLL8 study, FCR (Fludarabine Cyclophosphamide Rituximab) is the standard of care in younger and older fit patients. All new clinical trials are basing this as the standard of care comparing with new novel combinations including Bruton's tyrosine kinase (BTK) inhibitors like ibrutinib and CAL 101.

Ofatumumab is a fully humanized antibody targeting a unique epitope on CD20 molecule expressed on human B-cells, with increased binding affinity, prolonged dissociation rate and increased cell kill due to greater complement dependent cytotoxicity and antibody–dependent cellular cytotoxicity. It is more effective than rituximab, specially in cells expressing low levels of CD20. It is effective in fludarabine and alentuzumab refractory group with overall response rate (ORR) of 58%. Currently, several trials have been published on the effectiveness of combination with bendamustine and chlorambucil specially in older people with CLL.

Targeting B-cell receptor signaling as a therapeutic strategy in CLL is coming up in a big way as a more definitive treatment of NHL and CLL. Drugs like ibrutinib in CLL and NHL and idelalisib in CLL and NHL are likely to change the treatment in lymphoproliferative disorders into a chemotherapy-free treatment option.

Source: Catovsky D, Richards S, Matutes E, et al. Assessment of fludarabine plus cyclophosphamide for patients with chronic lymphocytic leukaemia (The LRF CLL 4 trial): a randomised controlled trial. Lancet. 2007;370(9583):230-9.

Potential Future Strategies to Achieve Long-term Control of CLL

Treatment algorithm for CLL patients in frontline (A) and second line (B) indications (Flowchart 166.1).

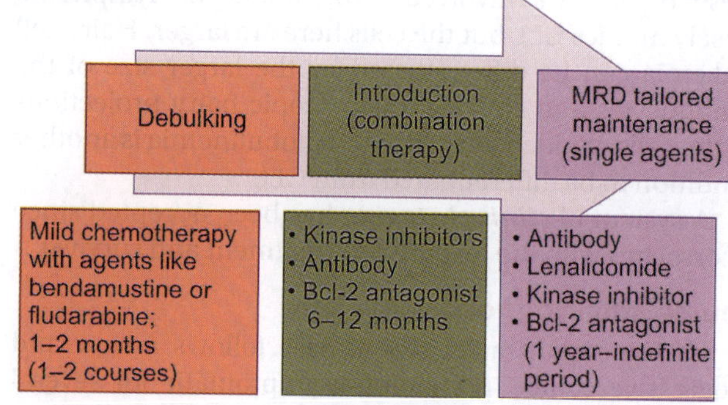

Flowchart 166.1: Potential future strategies to achieve long-term control of CLL

- ***Therapeutic modalities employed:*** AL-Alentuzumab (anti CD52), R-Rituximab, O-Ofatumumab, F-Fludarabine, C-Cyclophosphamide, mAb-monoclonal antibody, Dex-deaxamethasone, Allo-SCT- Allogenic stem cell transplantation.
- ***Agents targeting BCR signaling:*** Idelalisib (CAL-101): Class I P13K selective inhibitor—oral agent or combinations, ibrutinib (formerly called PCI-32765): BTK inhibitor and oral agent. Bcl-2 inhibitors—ABT-263 and ABT-199: Extremely effective as single agent in refractory CLL.

HAIRY CELL LEUKEMIA

Syn: Leukemic reticuloendotheliosis

This is a variant of CLL and is rare. It is seen in the age group 40–80 years and males are affected four times more common than females. Presents with massive splenomegaly, anemia, relative lymphocytosis, more often with a low TLC, often pancytopenia is present. The B-lymphocytes are larger than that in CLL and show the characteristic fine hairy projections which can be detected in peripheral smear and bone marrow, but best brought out by electron microscopy. The cytoplasm shows a number of villi which gives the hairy appearance. The diagnostic histochemical test for hairy cells is acid phosphatase staining reaction resistant to the action of tartrate. Bone marrow is infiltrated heavily and it is difficult to aspirate and often a dry tap is obtained. Marrow biopsy and imprint smears show the hairy cells (Figs 166.10 and 166.11A and B).

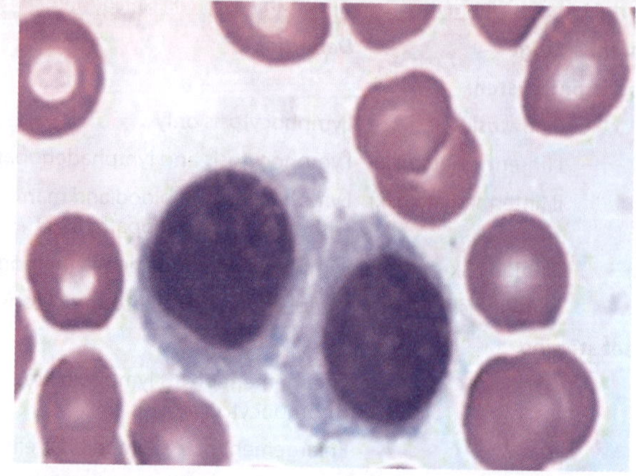

Fig. 166.10: Hairy cell leukemia blood film showing hairy projections

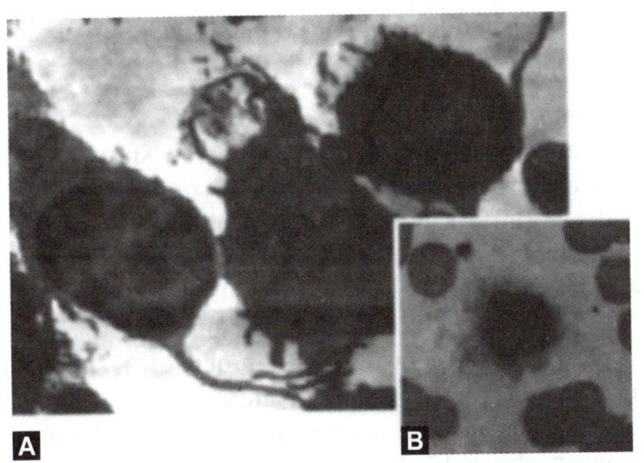

Fig. 166.11: Hairy cell leukemia. **A.** Electron microscopy; **B.** Blood film

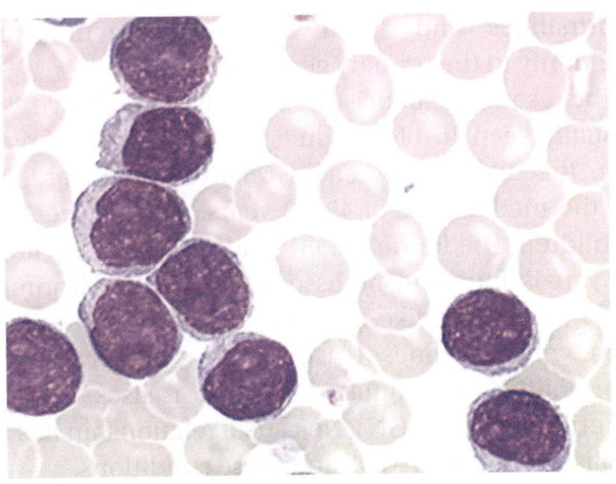

Fig. 166.12: Prolymphocytic leukemia—prominent vacuolation

Treatment

In the early stages, corticosteroids are useful. The disease responds best to splenectomy. Other drugs include pentostatin (deoxycoformycin, Nipent Parke-Davis), a purine analogue and cladribine (2-chlorodeoxyadenosine-Leustatin-Ortho Biotech) which produce lasting remissions.

Dose

Pentostatin: Given 4 mg/m^2/week for three weeks, then once in 2 weeks for 6 weeks followed by once a month for 6 months, given IV.

Cladribine: Given in doses of 0.1 mg/kg/bw by continuous IV infusion for 5 days every month.

Subcutaneous cladribine is convenient and effective and is currently the standard of care.

IFN-α given in doses of two million units/m^2 thrice a week used to be the treatment of choice. It is most probably only palliative.

PROLYMPHOCYTIC LEUKEMIA (PLL)

This is a rare variant of CLL, seen in males above the age of 60 years and showing gross splenomegaly and a very high white cell count, often above 400×10^9/L. Lymphadenopathy is rare. The characteristic cell is the large lymphocyte showing a prominent nucleolus. The course is rapidly downhill and prognosis is poor (Fig. 166.12).

There are T- and B-cell subtypes, both are refractory. Current treatment options are cladribine, subcutaneous, similar dose as hairy cell leukemia.

CHAPTER
167

Myelodysplastic Syndrome

Mathew Thomas, KV Krishna Das

Chapter Summary

- General Considerations
- Pathogenesis
- Clinical Presentation
- Diagnosis
- World Health Organization (WHO) Classification
- Prognosis
- Treatment
- Leukoerythroblastic Blood Picture

GENERAL CONSIDERATIONS

Myelodysplastic syndromes (MDS) comprise a group of potentially malignant hematopoietic stem cell (HSC) or clonal disorders and are characterized by dysplasia and ineffective blood cell production. The risk of acute leukemic transformation is variable. MDS may be primary (de novo) or secondary. Secondary MDS occur years after a potentially mutagenic therapy, e.g. radiation therapy or chemotherapy. Most of the patients will have varying degrees of cytopenias (involving the red cells, neutrophils, or the platelets) due to dysplasia and ineffective blood cell production.

PATHOGENESIS

The pathogenesis of this disorder is not clearly understood. However, it is thought that the dysplasia and ineffective hematopoiesis result from transformation of a single HSC due to multiple acquired mutations. The transformed stem cell multiplies and forms a clone which perpetuates the disease. In about 60–80% of the major subtypes of MDS, somatic mutations occur in the SF3B1 gene, which encodes the components of the ribonucleic acid (RNA) splicing machinery. Haploinsufficiency of the ribosomal proteins and global deoxyribonucleic acid (DNA) hypomethylation with concomitant hypermethylation of gene promoter regions are the other genetic changes observed. Stromal abnormalities and T-cell dysregulations may occur secondarily to the primary genetic lesions.

The exact incidence of MDS is not known. MDS is usually seen in older adults after 65 years of age. In India, the disease is seen in relatively younger people with the median age of 45–50 years. MDS is seen rarely in children (pediatric MDS) and in families (familial MDS). It is found to be associated with environmental factors (chemicals like benzene, radiation and tobacco), genetic abnormalities (trisomy 21), connective tissue abnormalities, inflammatory bowel diseases (IBD) and glomerulonephritis (GN). No causal relationship has been established between MDS and these conditions.

CLINICAL PRESENTATION

Patients have vague symptoms. Many of the patients are asymptomatic at the time of diagnosis because very often they seek medical advice due to an abnormal complete blood count (CBC). Symptoms result from the different cytopenias—anemia, bleeding and infections.

Physical findings are also nonspecific. Organomegaly and lymphadenopathy are uncommon. Infection is due to neutrophil dysfunction, which in turn is due to decreased myeloperoxidase (MPO) and alkaline phosphatase (ALP) activities.

Autoimmune abnormalities like chronic rheumatic heart disease (RHD), rheumatoid arthritis (RA), pernicious anemia, pericarditis, pleural effusion, iritis, myositis, peripheral neuropathy and skin ulcerations may complicate the clinical course of MDS. Acquired hemoglobin H (HbH) disease (acquired alpha thalassemia) is observed in a small percentage of MDS patients.

Two cutaneous syndromes found in MDS are **Sweet syndrome** (acute febrile neutrophilic dermatosis) and myeloid sarcoma (*granulocyte sarcoma or chloroma*). The former may herald transformation to acute leukemia. Excess interleukin-6 (IL-6) and granulocyte-colony stimulating factor (G-CSF) are incriminated for the pathogenesis of Sweet syndrome.

DIAGNOSIS

Diagnosis is made by the findings in the peripheral blood and bone marrow, which should be interpreted in the clinical context. The three main features of diagnosis should be:

1. Changes in one or more of the blood and bone marrow elements (red cells, granulocytes and platelets) which is unexplained by any other disorder. Values for defining the cytopenias are Hb (<10 g/dL), absolute neutrophil count (<1,800 μL) and platelet count (<100,000 μL).
2. Dysplastic changes of blood cells by morphology of the peripheral blood and bone marrow, which should be more than 10% of erythroid precursors, granulocytes or megakaryocytes. Genetic abnormalities in the absence of dysplastic changes could be diagnostic.
3. A blast cell count of less than 20% of the cells of the peripheral blood and bone marrow aspirate. If the blast count is more than 20% the diagnosis is AML. In the presence of certain genetic abnormalities, a diagnosis

of AML is made even with the blast cell percentage of less than 20%.

Hematology

Both peripheral blood and bone marrow show morphological abnormalities.

The important findings are dysplasia (abnormal cell morphology) and quantitative changes in one or more of the blood and bone marrow elements (red cells, granulocytes and platelets). Pancytopenia is found in 50% of MDS.

Anemia (normocytic or macrocytic) is the most common abnormality. It is associated with low reticulocyte response. The red cell distribution width (RDW) may be increased above 15. Peripheral blood smear shows the typical dysplastic changes described later.

Red blood cells (RBCs): Ovalo-macrocytes, elliptocytes, acanthocytes, stomatocytes, teardrop cells, nucleated erythrocytes, basophilic stippling and Howell-Jolly bodies.
Leukopenia: Found in 50% with absolute neutropenia. Peripheral blood may show an occasional blast cell.
Leukocytes: Neutrophils may show pseudo-Pelger-Huët anomaly, Auer rods, hypogranulation, nuclear sticks, hypersegmentation and ring-shaped nuclei.
Thrombocytopenia: It may occur in 25% of cases. Thrombocytosis may occur uncommonly, but when it occurs it is associated with the 5q– syndrome. Platelet abnormalities include giant platelets and hypogranular or agranular platelets.

Bone Marrow Aspirate and Biopsy

Bone marrow is hypercellular with single or multilineage dysplasia. In the bone marrow, the blast cell count may be increased, but unlike acute leukemia blast cell count is below 20% of the total leukocyte precursors. While doing bone marrow cell count, 500 cells should be counted to determine the blast percentage. The paradox of peripheral cytopenia despite hypercellular bone marrow is due to premature cell loss or apoptosis (cell death). Mild to moderate degrees of myelofibrosis may occur in 50% of cases.

Impairment of myeloid maturation and arrest at the myelocyte stage is seen. Specific abnormalities may be seen in all the cell lines. Erythroid changes include megaloblastoid cells, ring sideroblasts (RAS), internuclear bridging and multinucleation. Changes in myeloid series include nuclear budding, cytoplasmic vacuolization increase in blast cells and morphological changes in the early forms.

Abnormalities of megakaryocytes include micro-megakaryocytes, megakaryocytes with multiple nuclei, failure to produce platelet and hypogranularity. Micro-megakaryocyte is smaller platelet precursor cell with agranular cytoplasm, hyalinoplasmic zones (pseudopods), a rounded, dense nucleus and 1–3 small nucleoli (Figs 167.1A to C).

Cytochemistry and Immunocytochemistry

These studies may show loss of myeloid maturation antigens, decreased MPO and ALP, RAS, peroxidase and Sudan black for blast cells. Immunocytochemistry is done for identifying myeloblasts and exclusion of lymphoid blasts and immature megakaryocytes.

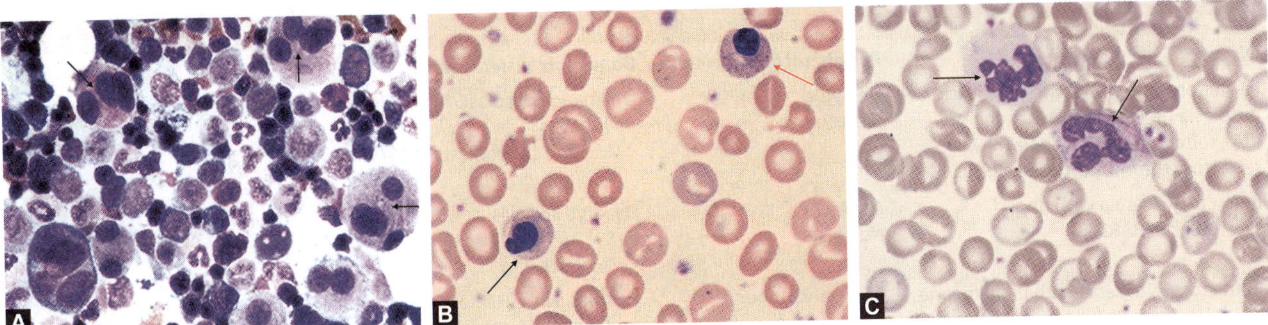

Fig. 167.1A to C: A. Myelodysplastic syndromes (MDS)—dysplasia of megakaryocytes: Multiple small lobes (arrows); **B.** Dysplasia of the red blood cells (RBCs). Abnormal nuclear shape, basophilic stippling (arrows); **C.** Dysplasia of the neutrophils: Agranular cells, abnormal segmentation (arrows)

Flow Cytometry

The observation of dysplastic changes, which is the cornerstone of diagnosis of MDS can be highly subjective. Flow cytometric systems for scoring dyspoiesis in MDS have been developed to overcome this difficulty.

Genetic Studies

Abnormalities like t(8:21), inv(16) and t(15:17) when detected can distinguish acute myeloid leukemia (AML) from MDS even if the blast count is less than 20%. Some other features, like 5q–del, 7del, del(13q) del(11q) point toward MDS even if dysplastic features are not present.

Differential Diagnosis

MDS should be differentiated from other conditions producing cytopenias and/or dysplasia. They are idiopathic cytopenia of undetermined significance, AML, myeloproliferative neoplasms including myelofibrosis, chronic myelomonocytic leukemia (CMML), aplastic anemia, idiopathic thrombocytopenic purpura (ITP), human immunodeficiency virus (HIV) infection and medications.

WORLD HEALTH ORGANIZATION (WHO) CLASSIFICATION (2008)

This is based on morphology, immunophenotype, genetics and clinical features (Tables 167.1 and 167.2).

- Refractory cytopenia with unilineage dysplasia (RCUD): Less than 5%.
- Refractory anemia (RA) with ring sideroblasts (RARS): Less than 5%.
- Refractory cytopenia with multilineage dysplasia (RCMD): 70%.
- Refractory anemia with excess blasts (RAEB): 25%.
- Myelodysplastic syndromes (MDS) with isolated (Del) 5q: 5%.
- Myelodysplastic syndromes (MDS) unclassified: Less than 5%.

PROGNOSIS

Revised international prognostic scoring system (IPSS-R). The prognostic variables in this system are:

- Cytogenetics
- Bone marrow blasts
- Hb
- Platelets
- Absolute neutrophil count.

Each variable has score of 0–4 points. Risk categories are:

- ***Very low risk:*** Less than 1.5 points
- ***Low:*** More than 1.5–3 points
- ***Intermediate:*** More than 3–4.5 points
- ***High:*** More than 4.5–6 points
- ***Very high:*** More than 6 points.

Complete remission requires blast cells less than 5% in the bone marrow with normal maturation of the cell lines, dysplastic changes less than 10%, Hb more than 11 g/dL, platelets more than 100,000, absolute neutrophils more than 1,000 and no circulating blast cells.

There can be partial remission, marrow complete remission, stable disease, disease progression and cytogenetic response.

Median overall survival for patients with a very low IPSS-R score (<1.5) is about 8.8 years and for those with a high score (>6) is 0.8 years.

TREATMENT

Transfusion of packed red cells and platelets and use of erythropoiesis-stimulating agents remained the treatment modalities for many years. But now many drugs have been developed, which are directed against the underlying abnormalities of MDS. Still supportive treatment remains the cornerstone of treatment because of the advanced age of the patients, chronicity of the disease and associated comorbidities.

Asymptomatic patients should not be treated. They should be followed up at regular intervals with blood counts to know the tempo of the disease. Prophylactic antibiotics, platelet or red cell transfusions are not recommended.

For symptomatic patients, there is no consensus regarding a standard treatment protocol.

One of the following treatment strategies can be adopted:

- For low-risk patients, supportive care will be the mainstay. This includes antibiotics for infection, red cell transfusion for symptomatic anemia and platelet transfusion for patients with thrombocytopenia and bleeding symptoms. Supportive care can be given to all patients with MDS as an adjunct.
- Growth factors [erythropoietin (EPO), granulocyte-colony stimulating factor (G-CSF), granulocyte-macrophage colony stimulating factor (GM-CSF)], azacytidine and decitabine (they are referred to as

Table 167.1: World Health Organization (WHO) classification (2008) of myelodysplastic syndromes (MDS)

Disease	Peripheral blood picture	Bone marrow features
Refractory cytopenia with unilineage dysplasia (RCUD): Refractory anemia (RA), refractory neutropenia (RN), refractory thrombocytopenia (RT)	Unicytopenia or bicytopenia[1]	Unilineage dysplasia in > 10% of the cells in one myeloid lineage <5% blasts <15% ring sideroblasts (RAS)
Refractory anemia with ringed sideroblasts (RARS)	Anemia No blasts	Dyserythropoiesis ≥15% RAS <5% blasts
Refractory cytopenia with multilineage dysplasia (RCMD)	Bi or pancytopenia rare blast No Auer rods < 1 × 10⁹/L monocytes	Dysplasia in ≥ 10% of cells in 2 myeloid lineages (neutrophil and/or erythroid and/or megakaryocytes) < 5% blasts No Auer rods +/− 15% RAS
RA with excess blasts-1 (RAEB-1)	< 5% blasts[2] Bi or pancytopenia No Auer rods < 1 × 10⁹/L monocytes	5–9% blasts Unilineage or multilineage dysplasia No Auer rods
RA with excess blasts-2 (RAEB-2)	5–19% blasts cytopenia Auer rods +/−[3] < 1 × 10⁹/L monocytes	10–19% blasts unilineage or multilineage dysplasia Auer rods +/−
MDS-unclassified (MDS-U)	< 1% blasts Cytopenia only	< 5% blasts Unequivocal dysplasia in less than 10% of cells in one or more myeloid cell lines when accompanied by cytogenetic abnormalities considered as presumptive evidence for diagnosis of MDS
MDS with isolated del (5q)	No or rare blasts Anemia Platelets increased or normal	< 5% blasts Increased to normal megakaryocytes with hypolobated nuclei Isolated 5q deletion No Auer rods

1. Bicytopenia may occasionally be observed. Cases with pancytopenia should be classified as MDS-U.
2. If the marrow myeloblast percentage is <5% but there are 2-4% myeloblasts in the blood, the diagnostic classification is RAEB-1. If the marrow myeloblast percentage is <5% and there are 1% myeloblasts in the blood, the case should be classified as MDS-U.
3. Cases with Auer rods and <5% myeloblasts in the blood and <10% in the marrow should be classified as RAEB-2

$$ $$

Table 167.2: Clinical, hematological and molecular features of various types of myelodysblastic syndromes

FAB subgroup	Bone marrow (BM) blasts (%)	Ringed sideroblasts (RAS) (%)	Peripheral blood (PB) monocytes (× 10⁹/L)	Chromosomal abnormalities (%)	Frequently associated karyotype	Rate of leukemic progression (%)	Median survival (mo)
Refractory anemia	<5	<15	<1	30	5q, −7, +8, 20q−	12	32
RA + ringed sideroblasts (RARS)	<5	≥15	<1	20	+8,5q−,20q−	8	42
RAEB	5–20	Variable	<1	45	−7, 7q−, −5, 5q−, +8	44	12
RAEB-t	21–30	Variable	Variable	60	−7, 7q−, −5, 5q−, +8	66	5
CML	1–20	Variable	≥1	30	−7, +8, t(5;12), 7q−,12q−	14	20

Abbreviations: FAB = French-American-British; RAEB = Refractory anemia with excess of blasts; CMML = Chronic myelomonocytic leukemia

DNA hypomethylating agents), immunosuppressive therapy and lenalidomide are low intensity therapies which can be administrated on an outpatient basis. Treatment-related morbidity and mortality are less. They are not curative but can improve the symptoms and quality of life. Lenalidomide is very effective in 5q– syndrome. Azacitidine and decitabine result in a hematologic response in about 50% of MDS patients.

- The high intensity treatment includes intensive combination chemotherapy and allogeneic hematopoietic cell transplantation (HCT). There is high treatment-related mortality and patients have to be hospitalized. These modalities may improve the blood counts more quickly than less intensive treatments, reduce the risk of death from MDS and may alter the disease course.

Patients with a very low (<1.5 points) or low risk (>1.5–3 points) are mainly treated by supportive care or low intensive therapies. Patients with high risk (>4.5–6 points) or very high risk (>6 points) with a good performance status are treated by combination chemotherapy or allogeneic HCT. Patients with intermediate risk (>3–4.5 points) are treated by either of the above mentioned approaches.

LEUKOERYTHROBLASTIC BLOOD PICTURE

This is the simultaneous presence of precursors of both myeloid and erythroid series of cells in peripheral blood (Fig. 167.2).

It is also characterized by abnormal RBC, white blood cell (WBC) and platelet morphology. RBCs appear pear-

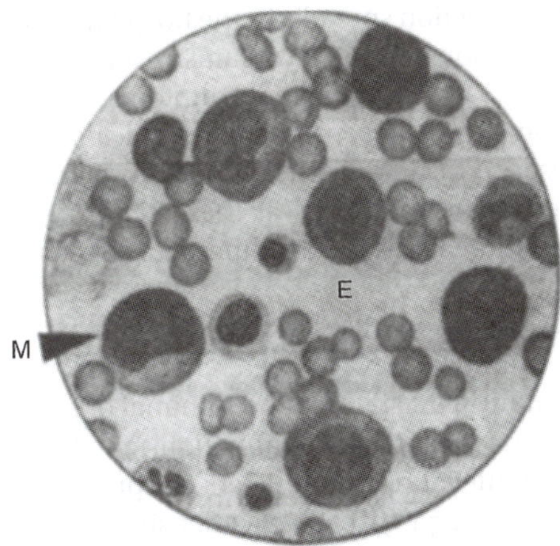

Fig. 167.2: Leukoerythroblastic picture
Abbreviations: M = Myeloid cell; E = Erythroblast

shaped or distorted. Nucleated red cell precursors occur. WBC count is elevated, with immature cells like myelocytes, promyelocytes and even myeloblasts suggesting a leukemoid reaction. Platelets are generally normal, but they may be reduced or increased or may be larger size. All these are the result of hematopoiesis occurring outside the marrow (extramedullary hematopoiesis) in foci such as the spleen, liver and even lymph nodes, consequent to marrow fibrosis, or infiltration by inflammatory or neoplastic tissue. The condition should not be mistaken for leukemia.

The developing cells proliferating in the extramedullary sites enter the bloodstream prematurely without passing through the normal tissues which prevent immature precursors and defective cells from entering the circulation. Normally the spleen destroys and removes deformed erythrocytes from circulation. In the absence of normal splenic function, leukoerythroblastic blood picture may result. The causes of leukoerythroblastic blood picture include:

- Primary idiopathic myelofibrosis
- Secondary myelofibrosis
- Infections like tuberculosis, HIV, fungal infections
- Radiation
- Associated with polycythemia, chronic myeloid leukemia (CML), lymphoma, myeloma, hairy cell leukemia
- Marrow infiltration
  - Carcinoma breast
  - Carcinoma lung
  - Carcinoma prostate
  - Neuroblastoma
  - Sarcoidosis.

All the conditions other than primary idiopathic myelofibrosis can be called ***myelophthisic***. In all these conditions, there are three processes occurring in varying grades:

1. Proliferation of fibroblasts in the marrow space
2. Extramedullary hematopoiesis (myeloid metaplasia)
3. Ineffective erythropoiesis.

Similar blood picture can sometimes occur when a normally functioning marrow is under stress due to acute hemorrhage, hemolysis or disseminated intravascular coagulation (DIC). When megaloblastic anemia is treated with large doses of vitamin B_{12} and folate, there is severe erythroid hyperplasia and the immature cells may come out of the normal marrow in large numbers.

Agranulocytosis (Severe Neutropenia)

CHAPTER
168

Agranulocytosis (Severe Neutropenia)

PK Sasidharan, KV Krishna Das

Chapter Summary
- General Considerations
- Drug-induced Agranulocytosis
- Clinical Features
- Diagnosis of Neutropenia
- Differential Diagnosis
- Treatment

GENERAL CONSIDERATIONS

Agranulocytosis (severe granulocytopenia) refers to decrease in absolute neutrophil count below 500/mm³. Though the term indicates total absence of granulocytes (specially neutrophils), for practical purposes, neutrophil counts below 500/mm³ should be taken as agranulocytosis and remedial measures have to be instituted urgently. Severe neutropenia of this level will predispose to life-threatening infections. It can occur due to various causes such as chemotherapy with anticancer drugs, hypersensitivity to other drugs in common use, infections, bone marrow failure, irradiation by ionizing radiations and at times, without an obvious underlying cause. Though there are several causes of neutropenia as given in Box 168.1 and severe neutropenia (agranulocytosis) is often drug-induced (Box 168.2).

It should be remembered that almost all drugs can cause severe neutropenia, and hence this risk should be anticipated when introducing any new drug. Some drugs have a predilection to cause agranulocytosis.

DRUG-INDUCED AGRANULOCYTOSIS

Pathogenesis: It may be due to direct effect on bone marrow as in the case of several anticancer drugs including

Box 168.1: Major causes of neutropenia

- Drug-induced
- Infections—viral hepatitis, dengue fever, enteric fever, tuberculosis, human immunodeficiency virus (HIV), other viral infections
- Septicemias
- Acute leukemias
- Myelodysplasias
- Aplastic anemia
- Bone marrow infiltration/metastasis
- Autoimmune destruction
- B_{12} or folate deficiency
- Hypersplenism
- Radiation—therapeutic or accidental

Note: Though several conditions lead to neutropenia, many of them do not lead to severe neutropenia or agranulocytosis.

Box 168.2: Common drugs causing severe neutropenia

- Cytotoxic and anticancer drugs
- Immunosuppressants
- Antithyroid drugs—propylthiouracil, methimazole, carbimazole
- Anticonvulsants—phenytoin, carbamazepine
- Antihypertensives—methyldopa, captopril
- Nonsteroidal anti-inflammatory drugs (NSAIDs)—indomethacin, ibuprofen, gold salts
- Antibiotics—chloramphenicol, sulfonamides, rifampicin
- Diuretics—acetazolamide, hydrochlorothiazide
- Others—dapsone, quinine, interferons, allopurinol

Note: It is better to consider that all drugs have a potential to cause hematological toxic effects and monitor this effect during therapy.

methotrexate and 6-mercaptopurine (6-MP) and immunosuppressive drugs like azathioprine (AZA). The unexpected neutropenia is often caused by immunological mechanisms, where the antibody-coated granulocytes are preferentially removed by the reticuloendothelial system. Two clinical patterns are usually seen. Sometimes, it can occur even with administration of the first dose or on intermittent administration and the agranulocytosis occurs abruptly. In the second pattern as exemplified by drugs like phenothiazines, prolonged administration leads to a gradual reduction of neutrophils. Often this neutropenia recovers when the drug is withdrawn or sometimes the neutrophil count can get stabilized at a lower level even when the drug is continued. It is to be noted that no drug is completely free from this form of toxic reaction. All antineoplastic drugs are capable of producing severe neutropenia if administered in sufficient dosage and this is due to direct impairment of cell production. History of drug ingestion may not be forthcoming in 20% of cases.

CLINICAL FEATURES

Irrespective of the cause, the risk of infections is maximum when the absolute neutrophil counts fall below 500/mm³. The neutropenia is often asymptomatic when the counts are above 1000/mm³ and also when it is acute in onset or of brief duration. When neutropenia is chronic, monocytosis may occur and might compensate for the risk of infections. The sources of infection in such patients are usually gums, throat, tonsils, lips, tongue, genitalia, perianal regions, genitourinary tract, gut, skin and lungs and the organisms are the usually suspected ones from these respective sites

from which infection spreads. In the hospital settings, they can have infection by unusual organisms and even by drug-resistant ones. Usual signs and symptoms which suggest an infection may be absent in neutropenic patients owing to the absence of inflammatory mediators and hence, a careful search for infections at these sites is mandatory and it should be continued till the patient recovers from neutropenia.

In severe neutropenia, serious pneumonia can present with only minimal or even absent chest signs, no sputum or only nonpurulent sputum and minimal or no infiltrates on chest X-ray. Signs of inflammation may be absent at sites of skin infections and if ulcers are present they may be covered with grayish-black offensive exudates. The surrounding skin may be red and necrotic without any tendency to localize the lesion. Since these infections are not contained locally, they get disseminated very fast and hence, empirical broad-spectrum antibiotic treatment is warranted without delay. Clinical features are basically those of the primary disorder causing neutropenia and those due to neutropenia which predisposes to severe bacterial and fungal infections. The patient may present with high fever, chills and rigor, sore throat or only extreme prostration without fever. In severe neutropenia, patient can develop septicemia and even acute respiratory distress syndrome (ARDS) without any fever. Therefore, any subtle changes on general examination like extreme fatigue, tachypnea, drowsiness or any change from the previous observation should be taken seriously.

DIAGNOSIS OF NEUTROPENIA

Total neutrophil counts below 1,000/mm³ should alert the physician. Counts below 500/mm³ indicate serious neutropenia. Whenever any unusual symptom develops in a patient who can potentially have neutropenia, or when very low neutrophil counts are documented, bacteriological samples should be collected from the appropriate sites for culture and sensitivity and broad-spectrum antibiotics started without waiting for the culture reports. Culture report might help to modify the regime in a given patient or at least help to plan empirical treatment in a future patient.

DIFFERENTIAL DIAGNOSIS

Agranulocytosis has to be differentiated from acute aleukemic leukemia, aplastic anemia, infectious mononucleosis, Vincent's angina and thrush. Bone marrow study is mandatory only when the cause is not obvious; it is specially needed when it is a bicytopenia or pancytopenia. But it should not be attempted, for fear of introducing an infection, in a severely neutropenic patient where the cause is almost certainly due to a drug.

Examination of peripheral blood reveals leukopenia or absence of neutrophils or presence of only a few old neutrophils with multilobed nuclei. Young forms with less than three lobes in the nuclei are rare or absent. This should suggest suppression of leukopoiesis. Bone marrow examination will show suppression of neutrophil precursors (Fig. 168.1).

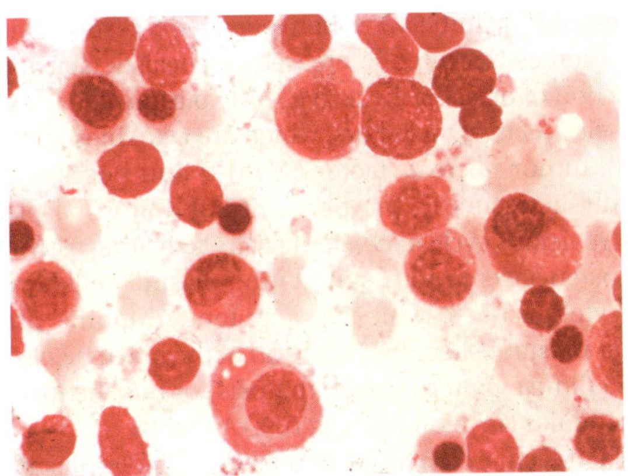

Fig. 168.1: Agranulocytosis bone marrow. ***Note:*** The absence of myelocytes, promyelocytes and neutrophils

TREATMENT

At the earliest clinical suspicion, all potentially offending drugs should be withdrawn. Meticulous oral and dental hygiene, perianal hygiene, hand hygiene, respiratory hygiene and using face mask, proper nutrition and vitamin supplements are essential for preventing infections and for recovery of neutropenia. Otherwise treatment depends on the cause of neutropenia and treatment of infection by powerful bactericidal antibiotic combinations. Empirical broad-spectrum antibiotic therapy should be started without delay whenever infection is suspected. One useful combination is gentamicin, ciprofloxacin and metronidazole, all given intravenously (IV). Other drugs that may be considered for use are piperacillin plus tazobactam and amikacin. Vancomycin or linezolid may be used when infection with methicillin-resistant *Staphylococcus aureus* (MRSA) is suspected. Severe neutropenia in selected situations are benefited by recombinant granulocyte colony-stimulating factor (G-CSF) or granulocyte-macrophage colony-stimulating factor (GM-CSF) but the routine use of these drugs specially to prevent infections is not recommended, except in the setting of potentially toxic anticancer chemotherapy. Antifungal drugs may have to be added if the patient develops neutropenic sepsis or when fungal infection is clinically suspected. Prognosis depends on the cause, prompt diagnosis and timely intervention. Drug-induced agranulocytosis is a preventable disease if it is remembered that all drugs, including even apparently safe drugs are capable of producing this complication.

CHAPTER 169

Plasma Cell Dyscrasias

Salim Shafeek, Kasim Salim, Mathew Thomas, KV Krishna Das

Chapter Summary

- Classification of Plasma Cell Proliferative Disorders
- Multiple Myeloma (Myelomatosis)
- Monoclonal Gammopathy of Undetermined Significance (MGUS)
- Amyloidosis

INTRODUCTION

The term ***plasma cell dyscrasias*** include a group of disorders mainly characterized by: (1) Uncontrolled proliferation of antibody-producing cells and (2) secretion of a structurally homogenous gammaglobulin or its polypeptide chains—the ***M*** component.

CLASSIFICATION OF PLASMA CELL PROLIFERATIVE DISORDERS (BOX 169.1)

Traditionally, multiple myeloma (MM), Waldenström's macroglobulinemia, heavy chain diseases (HCDs), benign monoclonal hypergammaglobulinemia and amyloidosis are included in this group, though Waldenström's macroglobulinemia and HCDs are actually lymphoid dyscrasias.

Characteristic protein abnormalities form the hallmark of these disorders.

Box 169.1: Classification of plasma cell proliferative disorders

Monoclonal gammopathies of undetermined significance (MGUS)
- Benign (IgG, IgA, IgD, IgM and, rarely free light chains)
- Associated neoplasms or other diseases not known to produce monoclonal proteins
- Biclonal gammopathies
- Idiopathic Bence-Jones proteinuria

Malignant monoclonal gammopathies
- Multiple myeloma (IgG, IgA, IgD, IgE and free light chains)
  - Overt multiple myeloma
  - Smoldering multiple myeloma
  - Plasma cell leukemia
  - Nonsecretory myeloma
  - IgD myeloma
  - Osteosclerotic myeloma (POEMS syndrome)
  - Solitary plasmacytoma of bone
  - Extramedullary plasmacytoma
- Waldenström's macroglobulinemia
  - Other lymphoproliferative diseases

Heavy chain diseases (HCDs)
- γ-HCD
- α-HCD
- μ-HCD

Cryoglobulinemia

Primary amyloidosis (AL)

Abbreviations: Ig = Immunoglobulin; POEMS = Polyneuropathy, organomegaly, endocrinopathy, monoclonal protein, skin changes

MULTIPLE MYELOMA (MYELOMATOSIS)

This is the most common disorder among the group of plasma cell dyscrasias. Myeloma is a malignant tumor arising from the plasma cells. The tumor may arise unicentrically or multicentrically from the bone marrow or as localized tumors in other sites.

Genetics of Myeloma

Many cases show a 14q32 translocation (1gH translocation). The immunophenotype in myeloma is characterized by CD38++, CD138+, CD56+, CD20– and FMC7.

Myeloma is a clonal disorder arising from one abnormal clone of plasma cells, secreting only the same type of immunoglobulin (Ig)-monoclonal myeloma. Rarely, myeloma proteins may be biclonal. Any of the Igs—IgG and its subclasses, IgA, IgM, IgE and IgD, or their light chains-kappa or lambda—may be produced in large amounts. The abnormal Igs are produced without antigenic stimulation and the normal Igs are reduced. Hence, infections are common. Rarely abnormal Igs may not be secreted outside the cells—***nonsecretory myeloma***.

Evolution of Myeloma

First step is the emergence of a limited number of clonal plasma cells. This is the stage of monoclonal gammopathy of undetermined significance (MGUS). This is not detected clinically. Annually, 1% of these develop MM or other related malignant diseases. With the progression of MGUS into myeloma, complex-genetic events occur in the abnormal plasma cells and bone marrow microenvironment. These include angiogenesis, suppression of cell-mediated immunity and development of paracrine signaling loops involving cytokines, such as interleukin (IL)-6 and vascular endothelial growth factor (VEGF). The resultant interactions of myeloma cells, bone marrow stromal cells and microvessels contribute to the persistence of the tumor and its resistance to drugs. Asymptomatic cases may become symptomatic in 2–3 years.

Pathology

There is gross hyperplasia of the plasma cells and these almost fill the bone marrow, eroding into bone and leading to pathological fractures. Myelomatous bone disease represents an imbalance between bone resorption and formation as a result of increased osteoclastic activity and reduction of osteoblastic activity. The plasma cells produce osteoclast-activating factors, which are cytokines including IL-1β, tumor necrosis factor (TNF)-α and possibly, IL-6. Osteolysis occurs in the proximity of abnormal plasma cells. A vicious cycle of myeloma cells activating osteoclasts and osteoclasts in turn stimulating plasma cells through the cytokine IL-6, which is a potent myeloma growth factor, is established. Proliferation of the plasma cells may take a diffuse pattern (myelomatosis) or may be localized and nodular (myeloma) (Figs 169.1A and B).

The plasma cells show abundance of cytoplasm with foamy vacuoles and many of them may be multinucleated (myeloma cells). Signs of nuclear immaturity may be evident. Due to increased cell turnover, serum uric acid level is elevated. Primary type of amyloidosis occurs in 10% cases. In over 60% of cases, the light chains appear in urine in demonstrable amounts. These are called Bence-Jones proteins (BJPs). The Bence-Jones proteinuria, amyloidosis and hyperuricemia lead to renal damage resulting in renal failure. The light chains are toxic to renal tubules. Mobilization of calcium from bones causes hypercalcemia, hypercalciuria and nephrocalcinosis. (Refer to Section 16, Ch 187).

Hyperviscosity syndrome (HVS) may develop due to the presence of abnormal Igs. The signs of hyperviscosity include weakness, anorexia, impairment of cerebral circulation leading to neurological deficits and retinal abnormalities. This is more pronounced in IgA myeloma.

Invasion of the bone marrow by plasma cells may cause anemia, leukopenia and thrombocytopenia. In majority of cases, plasma cells occur in small numbers in peripheral blood and can be demonstrated in the buffy coat. In a few, large number of plasma cells and plasmablasts (showing nucleoli) appear in the peripheral blood when the condition may be termed ***plasma cell leukemia.*** At autopsy several organs show infiltration by myeloma cells, but clinical abnormality may not be detectable in many. Chromosomal changes do occur in myeloma. Primary chromosomal translocations occur at the Ig switch region on chromosome 14(Q32.33), which

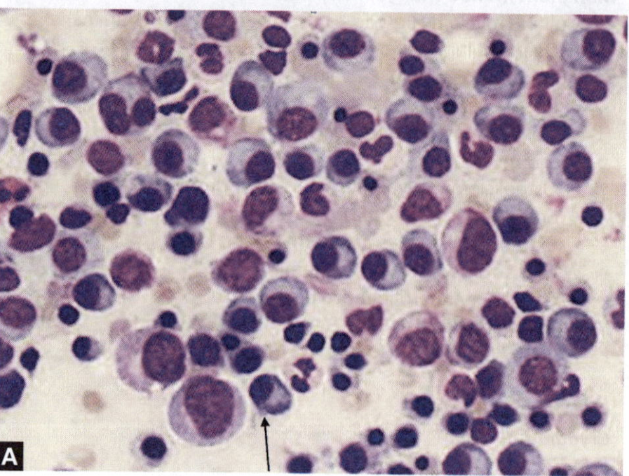

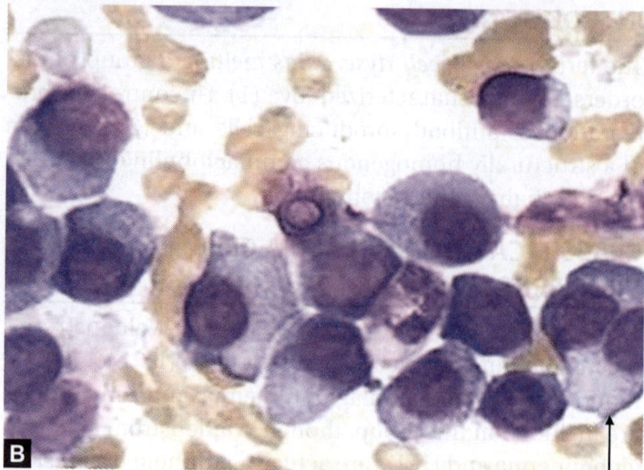

Figs 169.1A and B: A. Normal plasma cells (arrow); **B.** Malignant plasma cells in bone marrow (arrow). ***Note:*** In Figure 169.1A, eccentric, blue cytoplasm without vacuoles and in Figure 169.1B, different shape, blue cytoplasm dividing nucleus vacuoles in cytoplasm

is most commonly juxtaposed to c-musculoaponeurotic fibrosarcoma (c-MAF) [t(14;16(q 32.33;23)] and multiple myeloma set domain (MMSET) on chromosome 4p 16.3. Secondary translocations and gene mutations develop. Gene expression profiling allows classification of MM into different subgroups.

Several cytokines and growth factors are secreted by cells in the bone marrow microenvironment including myeloma cells and regulated by autocrine and paracrine loops.

Clinical Features (Table 169.1)

This disease is more frequent in the middle and older age groups, majority of cases being between 50 and 70 years. It is more common in males. The onset is insidious with symptoms of vague ill-health, back pain, aches and pains, arthralgia and progressive anemia. In majority of cases, diagnosis is made on routine investigation for anemia, raised erythrocyte sedimentation rate (ESR), bone pains or pathological fractures, localized tumors or recurrent bacterial and viral infections. In the more advanced cases, all evidences of myelophthisic anemia may be present. Twenty percent of cases are asymptomatic and detected by routine laboratory workup during health checks.

Bone Changes

Vertebrae, sternum, ribs, skull and clavicles show characteristic osteolytic changes. Localized bony or soft tissue swellings may be detectable over these sites. In some, the disease presents abruptly with the onset of pathological fractures in an otherwise healthy subject. In about 3% of cases, the osseous lesion is confined to a single bone without evidence of generalized marrow involvement. Vertebral compression may result in reduction in height of the individual and compressive myelopathy.

Other Neurological Manifestations

These develop due to demyelination, amyloid peripheral neuropathy, paraproteinemia neuropathy, carpal tunnel syndrome and rarely, cranial nerve palsies.

Splenomegaly occurs in 20%, hepatomegaly in 40%, lymphadenopathy and involvement of organs like thyroid, adrenal, ovaries, testes, lung, pleura, pericardium, skin and others in a smaller proportion of cases. Infections like pneumonia and herpes zoster are more common due to immunodeficiency state.

Renal Failure

It may present as insidious onset of azotemia, which is made out on investigation, or it may occur acutely with renal shut down due to tubular obstruction. Contrast radiography [Intravenous pyelogram (IVP)] may precipitate renal failure due to dehydration. Aggressive chemotherapy is also associated with the development of uric acid nephropathy.

Hematology

Normocytic normochromic anemia may be present and neutropenia and thrombocytopenia may develop later. In addition to thrombocytopenia, qualitative platelet defects occur. These include abnormalities of adhesion, aggregation and platelet factor three release. Inhibitors of coagulation factors may develop. Hyperviscosity develops as a result of increase in paraproteins. This manifests as bruising and bleeding tendency. In 5% of cases, cryoglobulins occur as part of the paraproteins. Such patients may manifest Raynaud's phenomenon. The peripheral blood smear shows marked rouleaux formation, which reflects the high ESR. Plasma cells may be seen in small numbers. Presence of numerous plasma cells suggests plasma cell leukemia. In some cases, plasma cell precursors (plasmablasts) are seen in peripheral blood and bone marrow.

Diagnosis

Myeloma should be suspected in any elderly person presenting with vague rheumatic symptoms, pains and deformity over the spine. Neurological symptoms, pathological fractures, unexplained anemia and recurrent infections should alert the physician to the possibility of myeloma. Investigations are absolutely essential

Table 169.1: Involved organs in multiple myeloma and its clinical feature

Involved organ/system	Features
Bone	• Localized bony swellings over vertebrae, skull, sternum, ribs and clavicle • Bone pain due to pathological fractures • Neurological symptoms of sensory and/or motor loss due to lesion in the vertebrae compressing the spinal cord nerve root
Bone marrow	Anemia, leukopenia and thrombocytopenia
Immune system	Humoral immune deficiency leading to increased susceptibility to infections, particularly of the respiratory system and urinary tract
Renal damage is multifactorial due to Bence-Jones proteinuria, hypercalcemia, humoral immune deficiency	Nephrocalcinosis, amyloidosis, renal insufficiency, infections or nephrotic syndrome
Bleeding tendency	Purpura, epistaxis, gastrointestinal bleeding
Cryoglobulinemia and hyperviscosity (uncommon) syndrome	**Hyperviscosity may affect:** • CNS (leading to confusion headache, vertigo, nystagmus, postural hypotension and dizziness) • Retina (producing blurred vision, retinal venous congestion, papilledema • CVS (congestive cardiac failure)
Neurological manifestations	Amyloid peripheral neuropathy, carpal tunnel syndrome and compressive myelopathy

Abbreviations: CNS = Central nervous system; CVS = Cardiovascular system

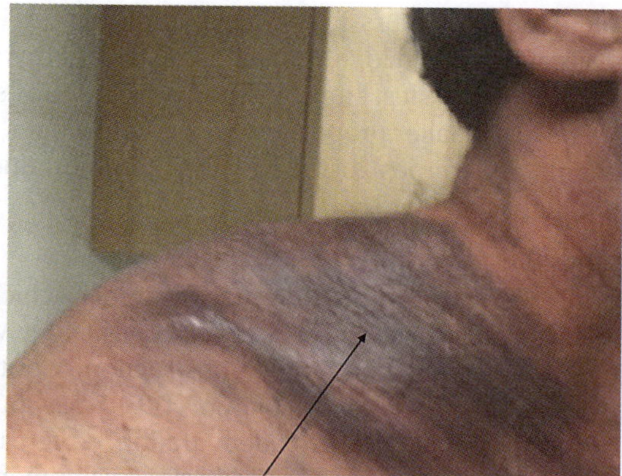

Fig. 169.4: Extramedullary plasmacytoma

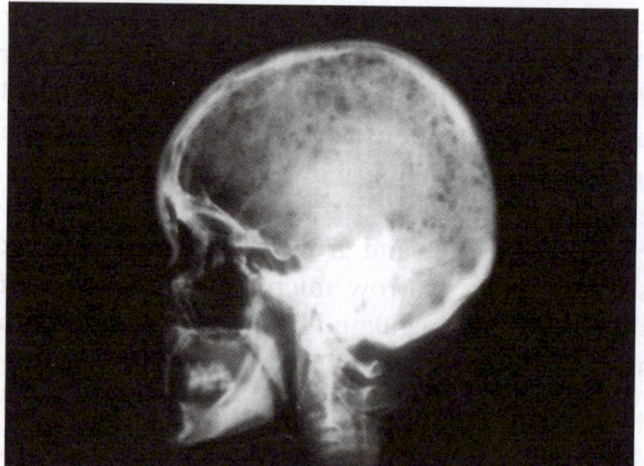

Fig. 169.5: X-ray skull showing punched out areas

to diagnose the condition and assess the extent of the disease. Presence of a very high ESR (often above 100 mm in 1 hour) should suggest the possibility of myeloma, if other more common causes can be excluded.

Plasmacytoma

Localized myeloma could be associated with localized disease or part of systemic myeloma, including relapsing disease (Fig. 169.4).

Urine Examination

Over 50% of cases show Bence-Jones proteinuria. BJPs are made up of light chains, which cross the glomerular filter. On heating acidified urine above 80°C, the protein precipitates, and on continuing heating it redissolves above 90°C. Another method for detection is to add an equal volume of 5% sulfosalicylic acid, which precipitates the proteins.

Immunoelectrophoresis of urine reveals the type of protein. Though BJPs are very suggestive of myeloma, other conditions such as combined light chain nephropathy, lymphomas, leukemias and congenital renal tubular defects may also be associated with this abnormality.

Serum-free Light Chain Estimation

Estimation of free light chains (FLCs), kappa and lambda help to estimate the extent of disease and the prognosis. The proportion of FLCs also gives us diagnostic and prognostic values. New guidelines recommend that screening FLC assays can be used in the initial evaluation of MM. Freelite is a simple blood test to quantitate Kappa-like

and free lambda Ig-like chains. This has revolutionized the field of myeloma and amyloidosis. This will be replacing the traditional urinary BJP estimation. It is extremely useful in diagnosing and monitoring light chain myeloma and oligosecretory myeloma. Previously classed nonsecretory myelomas also have changed since this test arrived. It is also been used toward stringent complete remission (sCR) after autologous transplantation.

Heavy Chain Estimation

This is latest modality of diagnosis and monitoring in myeloma with wider spectrum of globulin molecule.

Radiology

X-rays of the skull, long bones, pelvis, ribs and vertebrae reveal characteristic punched out lesions (Fig. 169.5). One or several vertebrae may be affected. The bone lesions are usually localized. Despite the bone lesions plasma alkaline phosphatase (ALP) is normal (Figs 169.6A and B).

Bone Marrow Examination is Diagnostic

Material aspirated from any site is usually diagnostic, but in case of doubt, aspiration must be done from an area of radiological abnormality. Normally, the proportion of plasma cells ranges from 2 to 10%. Rarely, it may rise even up to 20%. In myeloma, the number of plasma cells is considerably increased (>10%) and the plasma cells show morphological abnormalities (Fig. 169.7).

Some plasma cells show multinucleation and cytoplasmic vacuoles. These are called myeloma cells. Plasmablasts possess nucleoli. Increase in plasma cells

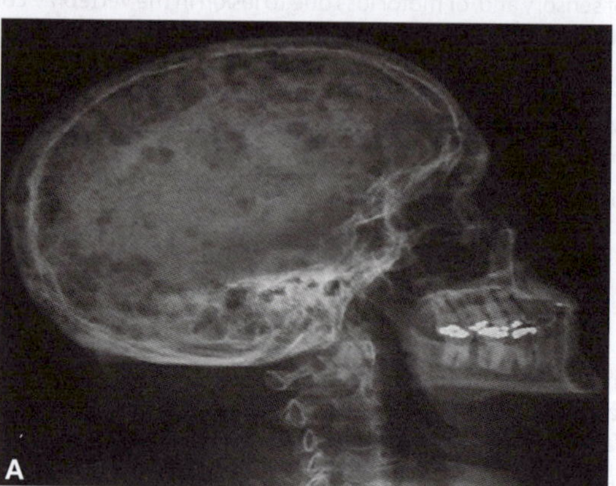

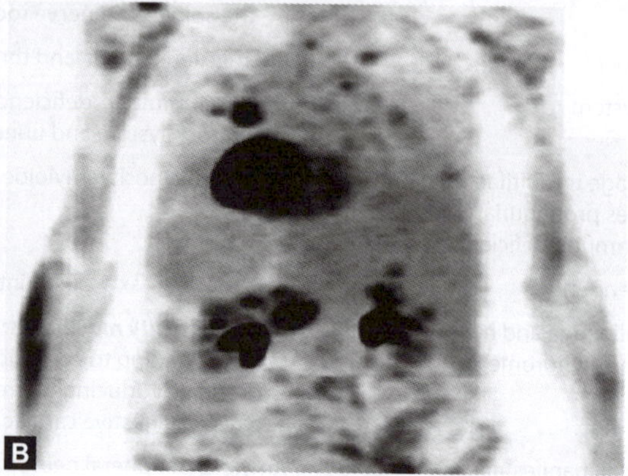

Figs 169.6A and B: **A.** Skull changes in myeloma; **B.** Positron emission tomography-computed tomography scan showing multiple myeloma lesions

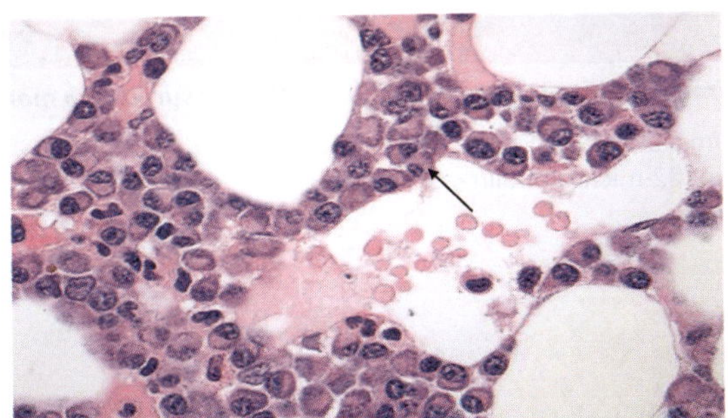

Fig. 169.7: Bone marrow trephine showing plasma cell infiltration (arrow)

Table 169.2: Staging of myeloma

Criteria	Stage I	Stage III
Hemoglobin	Above 10 g/dL	Below 8.5 g/dL
Serum calcium	Below 12 mg/dL	Above 12 mg/dL
X-ray of bones	Normal or sparse lesions	Advanced lytic lesions
M-components IgG IgA	 Below 5 g/dL Below 3 g/dL	 Above 7 g/dL Above 5 g/dL
Urinary M-component	Below 4 g/24 h	Above 12 g/24h

Note: Stage II is between I and III

Abbreviation: Ig = Immunoglobulin

due to myeloma has to be distinguished from reactive plasmacytosis in which plasma cells are increased. Several conditions give rise to reactive plasmacytosis. These include chronic infections like tuberculosis, amyloidosis and secondary neoplasms. In this condition, the plasma cells do not generally exceed 10% of the total. Morphological abnormalities are not produced. The secondary plasmacytosis resolves on removing the cause.

Diagnostic Criteria for Myeloma

- Plasma cells in the marrow more than 10%
- Presence of monoclonal proteins in the serum or urine
- CRAB criteria:
  - **C**alcium level—hypercalcemia more than 11.5 mg/dL
  - **R**enal insufficiency—creatinine more than 2 mg/dL
  - **A**nemia—hemoglobin less than 10 g/dL
  - **B**one lesions—osteopenia, osteoporosis and fractures.

Electrophoretic Studies

Demonstration of paraprotein by electrophoresis and determination of the Ig type by immunoelectrophoresis or diffusion techniques help to confirm the diagnosis and type the myeloma.

Serial measurement of the paraprotein level helps to assess progress since its level reflects the tumor load. Seventy five percent show IgG, 25% IgA and 1% IgD. In younger patients, the proportion of IgD myeloma is slightly more. IgD myeloma is more often associated with hypercalcemia and renal failure. Bence-Jones myeloma is also more common in the younger age group. Assessment of renal function by blood urea, creatinine, uric acid and glomerular filtration rate (GFR) are essential to indicate prognosis and plan therapy. Table 169.2 gives the clinical staging for assessing the prognosis and which is of help to plan therapy.

Differential Diagnosis

Diagnosis of MM includes multiple bony secondaries from carcinoma of the prostate, adrenals, breast, thyroid and other organs. In this condition, protein abnormalities are absent or only minimal. Biopsy from these sites may be required to confirm the diagnosis. Eosinophilic granuloma of bone or other lipidoses like Hand-Schüller-Christian disease and Niemann-Pick disease may produce multiple lytic lesions in the skull.

Genetic analysis helps to differentiate Waldenström's macroglobulinemia from MM.

Box 169.2: High-risk factors at diagnosis and international scoring system

High-risk factors at diagnosis
Cytogenetics: del(13), t(4;14), t(16;16), del(17p), del(1p) and +1q
Renal failure, elevated LDH, plasma cell leukemia, GEP 70, EMC-92
Comorbidities-limiting therapy
International scoring system stage II or III
Cytogenetics: del(13) is high-risk by metaphase karyotyping,
Recommend that FISH be performed after CD138 selection of BM cells to increase plasma cell yield;
GEP 70 is validate;
EMC-92 has early validation and is ongoing;
New molecular genetic tests await validation in multiple datasets.

Abbreviations: LDH = Lactate dehydrogenase; EMC = Erasmus Medical Center; GEP = Gene expression profile; FISH = Fluorescence *in situ* hybridization; BM = Bone marrow

Benign monoclonal gammopathy is a rare disorder in which paraproteins are increased to high levels, but often lower than that in myeloma. Normal immune mechanisms are not suppressed. The stage of the disease can be assessed by the laboratory values.

Stage II is intermediate between stage I and III. Subclass A indicates normal and B indicates impaired renal function based on serum creatinine levels. In A, it is less than 2 mg/dL and in B it is more than 2 mg/dL.

High-risk factors at Diagnosis and International Scoring System stage II or III (Box 169.2).

International Scoring System for staging myeloma and defining prognosis by further genetic analysis is available.

Course and Prognosis

The disease runs a chronic course extending over a few years, but relentlessly progresses to death. Blood urea level above 80 mg/dL (13 mmol/L), hemoglobin below 7 g/dL and hypoalbuminemia are bad prognostic factors. Cases with blood urea above 80 mg/dL rarely survive a few months. Complications include painful pathological fractures, anemia, hypercalcemia, recurrent bacterial infections and renal failure.

Prognosis

It varies with the different types of myeloma and treatment administered. At present, chemotherapy and radiotherapy are only palliative. Bone marrow transplantation (BMT) is curative in a smaller proportion when compared to leukemias. Younger patients do better. Median duration of remission with palliative treatment is 2 years. Less than 10% of cases may survive 10 years. Even this small group ultimately succumbs to the disease (Table 169.3).

Table 169.3: Staging system and survival in multiple myeloma

Stage	Durie-Salmon staging system	International staging system (ISS)	Median survival in months
I	All of: Hemoglobin > 10g/dL Normal serum calcium Low concentration of M-protein (IgG < 50g/L, IgA < 30g/L, Bence-Jones protein < 4g/24 hours) No bony lesions	Serum albumin > 35g/L Serum β2-microglobulin < 3.5 mg/L	62
II	Neither stage I nor stage III		45
III	Any of: Hemoglobin < 8.5 g/dL Serum calcium > 3 mmol/L High concentrations of M-protein (IgG>70g/L, IgA > 50g/L or Bence-Jones protein > 12g/24 hours)	Serum β2-microglobulin > 5.5 mg/L	29
Other prognostic markers	Cytogenetic (by conventional karyotyping and by FISH): Good/Average: Hyperdiploidy, t(11; 14) Bad/Poor: Hypodiploidy, deletion 13q on conventional cytogenetics, t(4; 14), t(14; 16), chromosome 1 abnormalities, 17p deletion Others: Advanced age, poor performance status, high LDH, high CRP, low platelets, M-protein (e.g. IgD having more renal failure and amyloidosis), circulating plasma cell, BM plasma cells > 50%, plasmablastic morphology, high BM plasma cell labeling index (PCLI > 3%), and serum FLC ratio (< 0.03 or > 32 having a significantly shorter survival).		

Abbreviations: LDH = Lactate dehydrogenase; CRP = C-reactive protein; BM = Bone marrow; FLC = Free light chain; Ig = Immunoglobulin; FISH = Fluorescence *in situ* hybridization

Treatment

Drugs

Melphalan: The drug freely available at low cost is melphalan, which is an alkylating agent (phenylalanine mustard). This is the most time-honored specific drug. Several dosage schedules have been used. One of the standard regimens is to give melphalan 8 mg/m² and prednisolone 60 mg/m² orally after breakfast for four consecutive days repeated once in 4 weeks. If the response is not satisfactory, the dosage of both the drugs should be increased by 20%.

Forty percent of cases get clinical remission with reduction of myeloma protein by 75%, Bence-Jones proteinuria by 95% and reduction of bone marrow plasma cells below 5%. Maintenance therapy has to be given by repeating the course. Though this regimen was used for palliation in the prechemotherapy era, this regimen is not used as routine at present.

Vincristine (Oncovin®) Adriamycin® (doxorubicin) and Decadron® (dexamethasone) (VAD) regimen: A combination of vincristine, doxorubicin and dexamethasone may be successful. This is getting outdated currently due to evolving new drugs.

Dose: Vincristine 0.4 mg/day and doxorubicin 9 mg/day are given as continuous intravenous (IV) infusion through a central venous catheter for 4 days along with oral administration of 40 mg dexamethasone on days 1, 9 and 17 of each 28-day cycle. About 30–40% of resistant cases do respond. High-dose dexamethasone and methyl prednisolone (2 g given IV once a week) are very potent drugs, which suppress myeloma in combination with other drugs.

Immunomodulatory Drugs

Thalidomide or alpha-(N phthalimido) glutarimide which is a derivative of glutamic acid has produced very good results in myeloma. When given orally, it is readily absorbed. Its main actions are anti-TNF-alpha activity, antiangiogenesis activity and immunomodulation. It inhibits IL-6, IL-12 and IFN-gamma. It reduces expression of intracellular adhesion molecules. Different doses have been tried. Thalidomide doses have been varying between 50 and 200 mg daily with pulsed dexamethasone 10–40 mg days 1–4 and 15–18. Response rates are 65–70% of newly diagnosed cases and 50% in relapsed cases. Adverse effects include teratogenicity, somnolence, peripheral neuropathy, constipation and others. Thalidomide is also effective in advanced myeloma.

Lenalidomide and pomalidomide: A newer analog of thalidomide, lenalidomide and pomalidomide is an amino substitute variant, which is more potent with less side effects. Combined with steroids is a popular combination specially low-dose dexamethasone rather than high-dose dexamethasone.

Other drugs which can be combined with thalidomide include cyclophosphamide and melphalan. Studies are going on to identify the best regimen.

Proteasome inhibitors: Proteasomes are protein complexes inside all eukaryotes and in some bacteria. The ***proteasome*** is a multisubunit enzyme complex that plays a central role in the regulation of proteins that control cell-cycle progression and apoptosis. The main function of the proteasome is to degrade unneeded or damaged proteins by proteolysis, a chemical reaction that breaks peptide bonds. Proteasomes have been the targets for cancer chemotherapy during the past decade. Proteasome inhibitors are drugs that block the action of proteasomes that have been approved for relapsed and refractory MM.

- ***Bortezomib*** (Velcade), which is a proteasome inhibitor, which inhibits nuclear factors and also induce apoptosis. It is given in a dose 1.3 mg/m² IV over 3–5 minutes on days 1, 4, 8 and 11. Cyclically, every 21 days. Same drug is licensed to be given subcutaneous with less side effects and weekly once schedule called Velcade lite is very popular for older frail patients.

- ***Carfilzomib*** is newer-generation proteasome inhibitors with more potent antimyeloma effect and has been tried in relapse refractory myeloma and recently in combination as front-line treatment. Combinations in front-line are chronic respiratory disease (carfilzomib, lenalidomide and dexamethasone) or complicated chronic respiratory disease with cyclophosphamide combination.

Bone Marrow Transplantation

Allogenic or autologous BMT is an accepted and very useful therapeutic modality employed, when the myeloma is not amenable to chemotherapy. With the present state of technical advancement, persons up to 65–70 years can be considered for successful engraftment. At present, less aggressive bone marrow-ablative regimen to the recipient is being tried in several centers (mini transplant). The post-BMT complications are less severe. With the use of modern immunosuppressive, drugs results are quite encouraging.

Stem Cell Transplantation

Autologous stem cell transplantation: It is preceded by high-dose chemotherapy and is beneficial. This is standard of care in younger patients with myeloma up to the age of 70 years. Major phase III randomized trials like French IFM, Spanish Myeloma trials and Medical Research Council (MRC) Myeloma UK trials have confirmed this role.

Tandem transplantation in myeloma: In this procedure, a second autologous stem cell transplant is given after the patient has recovered from the first. They have much better progression-free survival compared to single autografts. This is not standard of care but only part of clinical trials.

Allogeneic stem cell transplantation in myeloma: It is only used as a part of clinical trials specially in inpatients with extremely bad cytogenetics. The results are not very encouraging.

Relapse of Refractory Cases

This is the most challenging part of myeloma treatment. Combination treatments combining alkylating and nonalkylating agents are the way forward.

DT-PACE/V (Velcade)-DT-PACE regimen: These include combination chemotherapy; extremely strong salvage chemotherapy from little rock group consisting of dexamethasone, thalidomide, cisplatin, adriamycin, cyclophosphamide and etoposide.

Supportive Measures

Bone Resorption-inhibiting Agents

The ***bisphosphonates-pyrophosphate analogs***—suppress osteoclastic activity and indirectly myeloma cells as well. The different members of this group of drugs vary in their therapeutic potential and possibly mode of action as well. Etidronate is the least effective, but the later analogs are definitely beneficial by reducing vertebral and other fractures, bone pains, plasma levels of paraproteins and also serum calcium. Several preparations are available. These include etidronate, clodronate, pamidronate, ibandronate, zoledronate and alendronate in the ascending order of therapeutic potency. They have to be given under supervision. Alendronate is highly effective, the drug is expensive.

It is now clear that patients who have bone lesions, with or without hypercalcemia benefit by the addition of bisphosphonate. Bisphosphonates may lead to osteonecrosis of the jaw. ***Treatment*** consists of withdrawal of bisphosphonates and antibiotics to treat infection. ***Infections*** have to be treated promptly with antibiotic combinations.

Hyperuricemia

It has to be prevented by the oral administration of allopurinol 100 mg tid.

Renal Complications

Renal complications of hyperuricemia can be avoided by hydrating the patient, alkalinizing the urine by the administration of sodium bicarbonate and ensuring a daily urine output of at least 2 liters by the use of furosemide in small doses. Hemodialysis may be required to tide over acute renal failure. Dangerous hypercalcemia may occur. Management of hypercalcemia is given in Section 11, Ch 100.

Hyperviscosity Syndrome

It is treated by plasmapheresis using a blood cell separator. Administration of thiols inhibits the synthesis of myeloma proteins. Bleeding and fractures demand symptomatic treatment in addition. Spinal cord compression demands immediate laminectomy and irradiation to the spine.

Treatment of Localized Myeloma

Local irradiation in a dose up to 4,000 cGy gives rapid pain relief and helps to clear the lesions. This has to be accompanied by chemotherapy.

Extramedullary plasmacytomas may occur, most commonly in the upper respiratory tract, gastrointestinal tract (GIT) and other regions.

Localized plasmacytomas in soft tissues have to be removed surgically and the patients have to be followed-up for several years to watch for the development of MM.

Vertebroplasty and Balloon kyphoplasty: Newer nonsurgical techniques to treat vertebral collapse mainly for pain control. This is done by musculoskeletal invasive radiologist. Balloon kyphoplasty has revolutionized the way we used to treat collapse vertebral bodies.

Variant Forms of Myeloma

Smouldering Multiple Myeloma

This condition presents with the following features:

- Abnormal monoclonal protein in excess of 3 g/dL in serum.
- Presence of abnormal plasma cells in excess of 10% in bone marrow.

BJPs may be present in urine. Levels of normal Igs may be decreased. Many of them follow a prolonged benign course, which may resemble benign ***monoclonal gammopathy***. Risk of developing florid myeloma is 51%, 66% and 73% at 5 years, 10 years and 15 years, respectively. Management consists of close follow-up every 4–6 months.

Plasma Cell Leukemia

In this condition, peripheral blood plasma cells form more than 20% of nucleated cells or absolute count of plasma cells exceed 2,000 mm³. If the presentation of the plasma-cell disorder is with the leukemic phase, it is called primary plasma cell leukemia, and if this phase develops during the course of MM, it is termed as secondary.

Nonsecretory Myeloma

One percent of MMs fall under this category. In this condition, plasma cells may produce abnormal protein, but do not secrete it into the plasma. The presence of monoclonal protein within the plasma cells can be confirmed by immunoperoxidase staining or immuno-fluorescence studies.

Oligosecretory Myeloma

In this subgroup of myeloma, serum and urinary levels of M-proteins are below measurable thresholds. Measurable disease is typically defined as those with serum M-proteins at least 1 g/dL and urinary M-protein of at least 200 mg/day, or both. In these patients, routine serum standard electrophoresis assays are not precise to detect changes with treatment. In many of these patients, the serum-free light chains (SFLC) can be done to monitor treatment progress. FLC levels of at least 10 mg/dL are now defined as having measurable diseases.

Osteosclerotic Myeloma (POEMS Syndrome)

This produces osteosclerotic shadows in skiagrams and accounts for 3–5% of all the myelomas. The lesion may be single or multiple. This is a rare condition in which the number of plasma cells in bone marrow is below 5%, but bone biopsy may show localized plasmacytomas. The components of this syndrome include:

- **P**olyneuropathy, mostly demyelination, motor disability
- **O**rganomegaly—liver, spleen and lymph nodes
- **E**ndocrinopathy—gynecomastia, atrophic testes
- **M**onoclonal protein abnormality
- **S**kin changes—pigmentation and hypertrichosis.

The major disability is due to a chronic inflammatory polyneuropathy. Bone marrow shows only less than 5% of plasma cells. Diagnostic finding is the presence of plasmacytoma on histology of the bone lesion. **Treatment** consists of local radiation of the bony lesion.

MONOCLONAL GAMMOPATHY OF UNDETERMINED SIGNIFICANCE (MGUS)

This is the condition, which is not uncommonly observed, in which there is elevation of serum monoclonal protein (M-protein <3g/dL) with less than 10% plasma cells in BM in the absence of hypercalcemia, renal impairment, anemia and skeletal lytic lesions. Frequency is 3.2% in people more than 50 years and 7.5% in people more than 85 years. MGUS may evolve into MM.

Bence-Jones proteinuria may be a more advanced form of MGUS. With highly sensitive FLC assay, more cases of light chains MGUS and MM are being diagnosed. About one-fifth of patients with MM (20%) produce only light chains. Light chains MGUS may evolve into light chain MM and heavy chain MGUS may evolve into heavy chain MM. Risk of progression to MM in persons with light chain MGUS is 0.3% annually.

Source:

1. Dispenzieri A, Katzmann JA, Kyle RA, et al. Prevalence and risk of progression of light-chain monoclonal gammopathy of undetermined significance: a retrospective population-based cohort study. Lancet. 2010;375(9727):1721-8.
2. Van Rhee F. Light Chain MGUS–Implications in clinical practice. New Eng J Med. 2010;2670-7.

MGUS progresses to myeloma or a related malignancy at a rate of 1% per year. Light chain smouldering MM—previously known as idiopathic monoclonal light chain (Bence-Jones) proteinuria, develops from idiopathic light chain MGUS, proceeding to myeloma. Patients having smoldering myeloma did better on being treated with lenalidomide and dexamethasone.

AMYLOIDOSIS

Virchow coined the term amyloid in the mid of 19th century. Amyloidosis consist of a large group of diseases in which misfolding of the extracellular proteins has a major role. This dynamic process, which occurs in parallel with or as an alternative to physiological folding, generates insoluble toxic protein aggregates that are deposited in tissues as bundles of β-short fibrillar protein. These consist of strands of polypeptides arranged in zigzag manner. The unique feature of amyloidosis is the capacity of these proteins to acquire more than one conformation. Amyloidosis is characterized by the extracellular deposition of amyloid, which appears as a homogenous eosinophilic material in several tissues (Figs 169.8A to C). Amyloidosis may be primary or secondary.

The amyloid fibrils in primary amyloidosis are fragments of Ig light chains. Lambda light chains predominate over kappa light chain in the ratio of 2:1. Different proteins make up the amyloid fibrils in reactive (secondary) and familial amyloidosis.

Clinical Classification (Table 169.4 and Box 169.3)

Familial Amyloidosis

This consists of a group of autosomal-dominant diseases in which a mutant protein forms amyloid fibrils beginning in mid-life. The most common form is caused by mutant transthyretin (TTR). Other genetic and environmental factors may play a role in the phenotypic expression of this disease.

Secondary Amyloidosis

These are due to amyloid formed from serum amyloid A (SAA), which is an acute phase protein produced in response to inflammation. There are several SAA proteins, out of which at least four different molecular forms take part in the formation of amyloid.

Clinical Features

Systemic Amyloidosis

Clinical features depend on the tissues involved. Since the kidneys are affected most frequently in secondary amyloidosis, 60% cases present with nephrotic syndrome. Proteinuria results from damage to the glomeruli and also toxicity of SAA oligomers or profibrils. The rest may be asymptomatic. The common cause of death is chronic renal failure (Refer to Section 16, Ch 187).

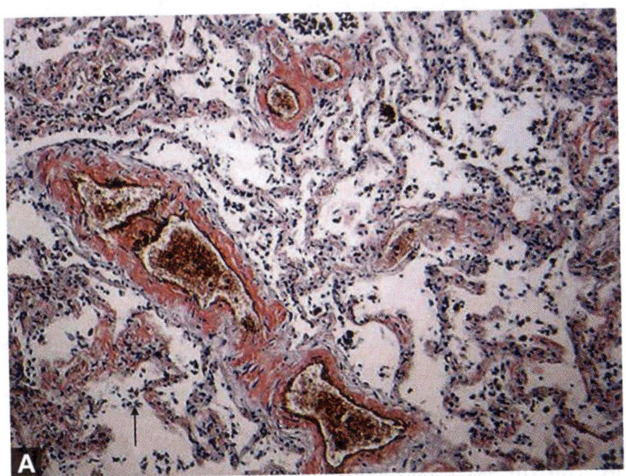

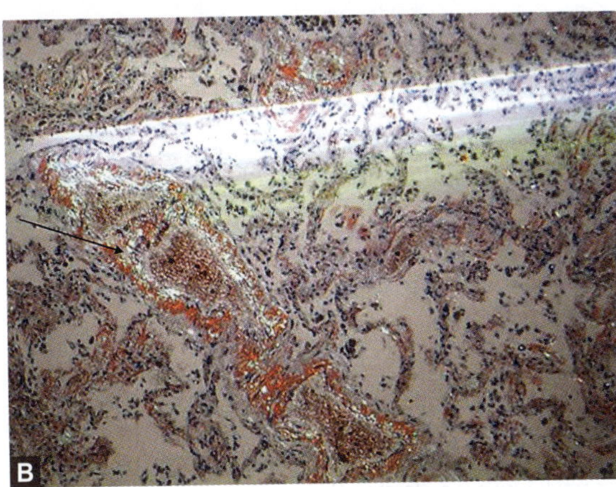

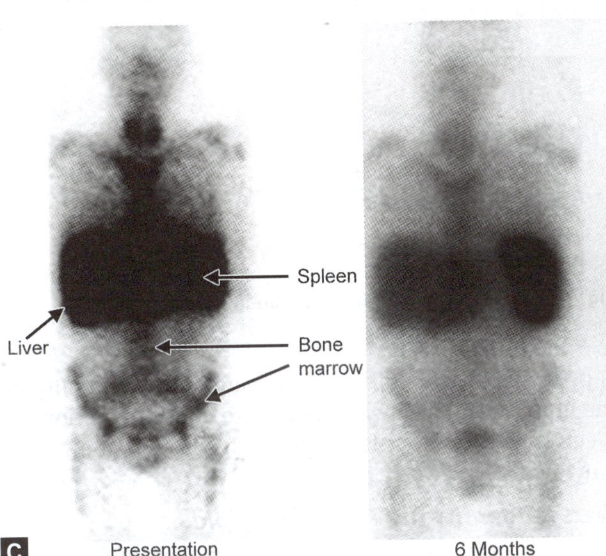

Figs 169.8A to C: A. Bone marrow trephine showing amyloid deposit. **B.** Amyloid deposit showing birefringence. **C.** Serum-amyloid P component scan showing infiltrates in spleen, liver and bone marrow

The heart is affected in 80–90% of cases of primary amyloidosis and this results in restrictive and congestive cardiomyopathy, cardiac failure and arrhythmias (Table 169.5). Amyloid deposition in the heart may lead to biatrial dilatation and thickening of interatrial and interventricular septum (IVS) (Fig. 169.9). Sudden death may occur.

Gastrointestinal Involvement

Macroglossia may interfere with deglutition and respiration. The enlarged tongue may show indentation by the teeth (Fig. 169.10). Involvement of the intestines produces diarrhea, malabsorption, intestinal obstruction and gastrointestinal bleeding.

Liver

It is commonly involved in both types of amyloidosis. The organ is enlarged and firm but functional derangement is not marked.

Spleen

It is commonly enlarged and firm in secondary amyloidosis.

Adrenal Gland

It is affected in secondary amyloidosis and this leads to hypofunction of the gland.

Respiratory Tract

Amyloid deposition may occur in the respiratory passages or in the lung parenchyma.

Nervous Involvement

Common presentations are peripheral neuropathy and carpal tunnel syndrome. Primary cerebrovascular amyloidosis may occur in which amyloid deposits occur in the arteries and arterioles as well as adventitia of the veins and venules. This weakens the vessel wall and accounts for some cases of hemorrhagic stroke. Autonomic neuropathy affecting several organs is common.

Localized Amyloidosis

Nodular masses of amyloid may occur in and around joints, and tendons, particularly around the glenohumeral joints. Large deposits may occur giving rise to the ***shoulder pad sign.***

Arthralgia and arthritis resembling rheumatoid arthritis (RA) may occur. Affection of the skin manifests as lichenoid plaques, nodules or purpura around the orbits.

In 80–90% of persons above the age of 80 years amyloidosis of the heart may occur (senile cardiac amyloidosis).

Table 169.4: Characteristics of systemic amyloidosis			
Type	**Fibril composition**	**Precursor protein**	**Clinical spectrum**
Primary AL	Monoclonal immuno-cardiomyopathy, hepatomegaly, globulin light chains		Lambda or kappa light chain proteinuria, macroglossia autonomic dysfunction, orthostasis, ecchymosis, shoulder pad sign, carpal tunnel syndrome (CNS not affected, peripheral and autonomic nervous system are affected)
Familial ATTR	Transthyretin	Abnormal transthyretin	Mid-life onset of peripheral and autonomic neuropathy, myopathy, vitreous opacities
Secondary AA	Amyloid A protein	Amyloid A protein	Underlying inflammatory disease, hepatosplenomegaly renal failure

Abbreviations: ATTR = Transthyretin-related amyloidosis; AA = Amyloid A; CNS = Central nervous system; AL = Amyloidosis light chain

Box 169.3: Clinical classification of amyloidosis

- ***Primary:*** Without any detectable underlying cause or associated with myeloma
- ***Secondary:***
  - Chronic infections—tuberculosis, bronchiectasis
  - Rheumatoid disease
  - Lymphoma and other neoplasms
- ***Heredofamilial mediterranean fever***
- ***Local amyloidosis***—skin, joints, tendons, nerves and other structures
- ***Senile amyloidosis***

Modern biochemical classification is based on the nature of precursor plasma proteins that form the fibril deposits:
- ***AL amyloidosis:*** Ig light chain-related (AL)
- ***Familial amyloidosis:*** Transthyretin-associated (ATTR)
- ***Secondary amyloidosis:*** Amyloid A protein (AA)

Primary amyloidosis is a plasma cell dyscrasia related to MM. Clonal plasma cells in the BM produce Igs that are amyloidogenic

Abbreviations: MM = Multiple myeloma; BM = Bone marrow

Table 169.5: Common sites of involvement in amyloidosis

Primary amyloidosis	*Secondary amyloidosis*
• Heart	• Kidney
• Tongue	• Spleen
• Gastrointestinal tract (GIT)	• Liver
• Skeletal and visceral muscles	• Adrenal cortex
• Nerves	• Lungs
• Joints, tendons	• Other organs
• Liver	
• Skin	
• Lungs	

Note: Considerable overlap may occur between the two forms

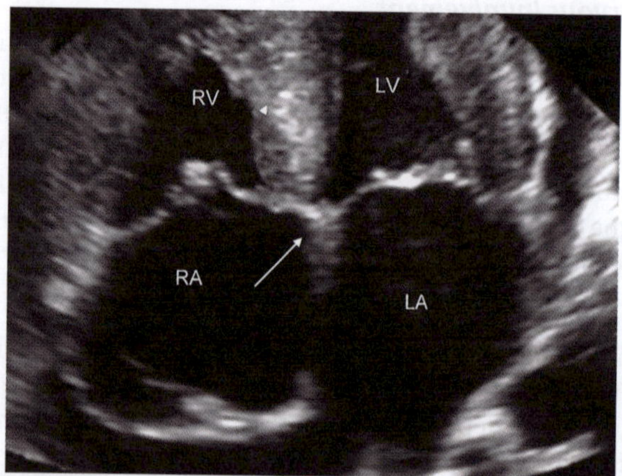

Fig. 169.9: Amyloid heart. **Note:** Biatrial dilation (RA and LA) and thickening of interventricular (arrowhead) and interatrial septum (arrow). Ventricles (RV and LV) not dilated
Abbreviations: RA = Right atrial; LA = Left atrial; RV = Right ventricle; LV = Left ventricle

Amyloid purpura occurs rarely over the chest above the nipple line, neck and eyelids (Fig. 169.11). Amyloid fibrils bind to factor X and lead to factor X deficiency and purpura. Here, Box 169.4 showing typical findings in amyloidosis.

Diagnosis

Amyloidosis is confirmed by biopsy of appropriate tissues. The rectal mucosa is commonly involved in primary amyloidosis and therefore, rectal biopsy is a rewarding procedure. Renal biopsy is usually positive when there

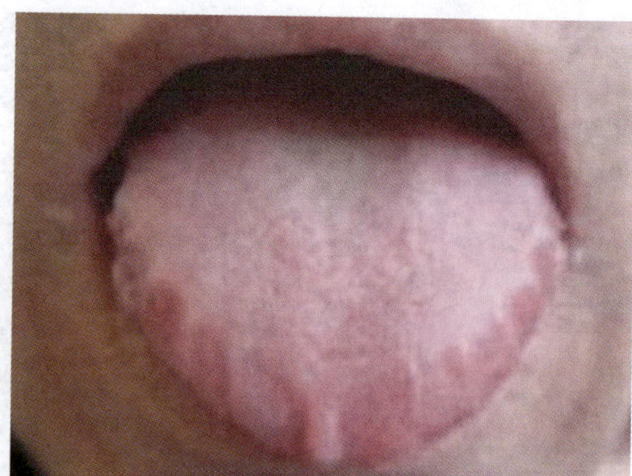

Fig. 169.10: Macroglossia showing teeth indentation in light chain amyloidosis

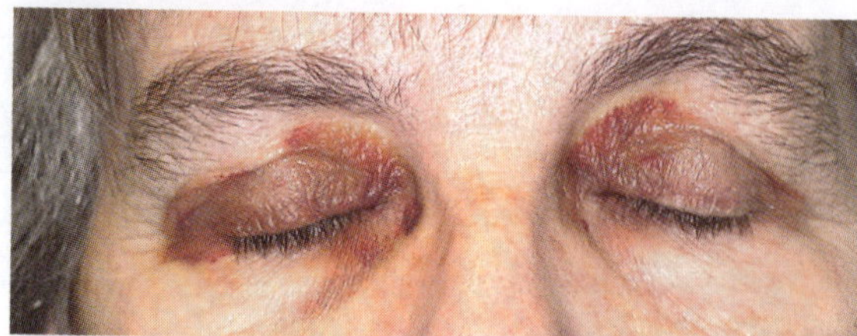

Fig. 169.11: Amyloidosis showing skin involvement purpura above the eyelids

is proteinuria. Amyloid deposits can be demonstrated in the gingival mucosa when gums are clinically abnormal. Electron microscopy of urine and synovial fluid may reveal amyloid fibrils.

Tests to Identify the Type of Amyloid

Light chain amyloid: Immunofixation electrophoresis of urine and serum, bone marrow biopsy with immune histo-chemical staining for lambda and kappa light chains help to diagnose the condition. FLC measurement can also predict the outcome in light chain amyloidosis better than standard paraprotein criteria. Amyloid deposits are identi-fied on the basis of their apple green birefringence under polarized light microscope after staining with Congo red. Under the electron microscope, amyloid fibers appear as rigid nonbranching fibrils 7.5–10 nm in diameter.

Familial ATTR: Serum isoelectric focusing for abnormal TTR or deoxyribonucleic acid (DNA)-based test for mutant TTR gene.

Secondary amyloid A: Elevated concentration of SAA protein, immunohistochemical staining of tissue for AA protein. Normal level of SAA fragments in blood is less than 4 mg/dL. Severity of amyloidosis and prognosis correlate with blood levels of SAA.

Prognosis

Systemic amyloidosis is always fatal, if untreated. Death is due to renal or cardiac failure within 1–2 years of diagnosis. Progress of amyloidosis can be arrested and lesions may even regress with treatment of the underlying condition. AL amyloidosis (primary) has the worst progress with a median survival of 1–2 years. Patients with ATTR amyloidosis may survive up to 15 years and the prognosis for secondary amyloidosis depends upon the underlying condition.

Malignant Disorders of Lymphoid Cells

Box 169.4: Signs and symptoms of amyloidosis

Primarily nonspecific symptoms
- Arrhythmia
- Changes in skin, including purpura (e.g. around the eyes)
- Diarrhea
- Edema in ankles and legs
- Enlarged tongue (macroglossia)
- Fatigue; can be severe
- Numbness and/or tingling hands or feet
- Shortness of breath
- Swallowing difficulties
- Weakness
- Weight loss

More specific symptoms seen with:

Kidney involvement: Nephritic syndrome—initial slight proteinuria, them a symptom complex of anasarca, hypoproteinemia and massive proteinuria

Hepatic involvement: Painless hepatomegaly—occasional portal hypertension (with esophageal varices and ascites); jaundice is rare.

Cardiac involvement: Restrictive cardiomyopathy resulting in heart failure; cardiomegaly; various degress of heart block and arrhythmia

GI involvement: Macroglossia (common in AL); motility abnormalities of the esophagus and small and large intestines, malabsorption, bleeding pseudo-obstruction

Thyroid involvement: Goiter (firm, symmetric, nontender)

Lung involvement: Focal pulmonary nodules, tracheobronchial lesions, diffuse alveolar deposits (AL)

AL and ATTR: Peripheral neuropathy (with paresthesias of fingers and toes) occurs; autonomic neuropathy may cause orthostatic hypotension, erectile dysfunction, sweating abnormalities and GI motility disturbances

Several hereditary amyloidosis: Amyloid vitreous opacities and scalloped papillary margins (bilateral)

A beta-microglobulin amyloidosis: Carpal tunnel syndrome and chronic pain in the fingers, wrist and shoulder; fractures of the humerus and femur

Abbreviations: AL = Primary amyloidosis light chain; ATTR = Transthyretin-related amyloidosis; GI = Gastrointestinal

Treatment

Treatment of the underlying cause is instituted, wherever a cause can be detected. Cytotoxic drugs like melphalan, cyclophosphamide, bortezomib, thalidomide, lenalidomide and pomalidomide are sometimes beneficial in primary amyloidosis, but not in all cases. For all forms, specific therapy directed to the organs affected is essential. For primary amyloidosis, chemotherapy is needed. Largest series in this field comes from Royal Free National Amyloid Centre in London. These plasma cell/light chain dyscrasias are treated similar to myeloma. Velcade (bortezomib)-based combinations are the current frontline treatment. Cardiac monitoring is very essential and multidisciplinary approach is critical, specially nephrology and cardiology. New prognostic criteria based on Mayo criteria are followed in treatment decisions. Autologous and allogeneic transplantation is associated with extremely high transplant-related mortality, hence, not standard of care. Transplants should only be done as a part of clinical trials. New monoclonal antibodies have been developed targeting serum-amyloid P component (SAP) and have been tried in clinical trials.

Diflunisal is effective in familial amyloidosis. Eprosidate inhibits amyloid deposition in tissues. It delays renal damage. The dose is 800–2,400 mg oral daily. Liver transplantation helps in cases with familial amyloidosis. BMT has been tried with varying success.

Newer Antiamyloid Treatment Studies

In systemic amyloidosis, the amyloid deposits always contain the nonfibrilar normal plasma proteins—SAP. The drug R-1-16-[R]-2 carboxy-pyrrolidine-1-[Y]-6-0 x 0 hexyl-pyrrolydine-2-carboxylic acid (CP4PC) efficiently depletes SAP from plasma, but leaves same SAP in amyloid deposits that can be specially targeted by therapeutic IgG and SAP antibodies. A pilot trial using CPHPC followed by an anti-SAP antibody safely triggered clearance of amyloid deposits from the liver and other tissues. This is a novel method, which requires further study.

Source: Richards DB, Cookson LM, Berges AC, et al. Therapeutic clearance of amyloid by antibodies to serum amyloid P component. N Eng J Med. 2015;373(12):1106-14.

CHAPTER 170

Malignant Disorders of Lymphoid Cells

Salim Shafeek, Kasim Salim, KV Krishna Das, Mathew Thomas

Chapter Summary

- Lymphomas
- Hodgkin's Disease
- Non-Hodgkin's Lymphoma (NHL)
- Autologous Peripheral Stem Cell Transplantation (APSCT) in Lymphoma
- Other Rare Forms of Lymphocyte Tumors
  - Angioimmunoblastic Lymphadenopathy (AILD)
  - Hydantoin-Linked Lymphoma
  - Mycosis Fungoides

LYMPHOMAS

GENERAL CONSIDERATIONS

These are malignant tumors arising from lymphoid tissue. In general, lymphomas remain confined to lymph nodes and other lymphoid structures in their early stages. Lymphomatous cells in varying numbers are seen later in the bone marrow and peripheral blood. On the other hand, lymphatic leukemias which are also primary malignancies of the lymphatic cells start in the marrow or in the lymph nodes and become disseminated from the beginning, even though lymph nodes and other lymphoid organs do show lesions simultaneously.

Lymphomas may start unicentrically or multicentrically. They have been classified broadly into Hodgkin's lymphoma (HL) and non-Hodgkin's lymphoma (NHL). HL is characterized by the presence of **Reed-Sternberg cells** which are absent in the latter. The course, prognosis and response to treatment are different in the two types.

Source: Hiddemann W, Longo DL, Coiffier B, et al. Lymphoma classification–the gap between biology and clinical management is closing. Blood. 1996;88(11):4085-9.

In many instances, lymphomas arises de-novo at sites not conventionally included under the lymphoreticular system, such as brain and several other solid organs. These may remain so for long periods without manifesting any tendency for generalized spread and behaving like local tumors.

Etiology

As in the case of leukemias, several possibilities have been postulated. These include genetic predisposition, viral infections, immunological factors, long-term toxicity to drugs like cyclophosphamide and exposure to irradiation and chemicals. There are many reports of lymphomas occurring in clusters in closed ethnic groups and showing a seasonal prevalence. These phenomena suggest a common environmental factor.

Epidemiology

Lymphomas form 1.9% of all cancers in many general hospitals in India. Among the lymphomas, 35–43% are HL and rest are NHL. Lymphatic malignancies formed 4.3% of all cancer cases seen in Tata Memorial Hospital, Mumbai.

Source: Biswas G, Parikh PM, Nair R, et al. Rituximab (Anti-CD20 monoclonal antibody) in lymphoproliferative malignancies: Tata Memorial experience. J Assoc Physicians India. 2006;54:29-33.

Data from the Regional Cancer Centre, Thiruvananthapuram (given in their website in 2010) shows the following data (Table 170.1).

Lymphomas have been the object of intensive studies by oncologists and hematologists and based on the various parameters such as cell morphology, cytology, cytochemistry, immune markers, chromosomal characteristics, gene variation and biological behavior, classification, specific diagnosis, management protocols and follow-up have all assumed great importance just as in the case of leukemias (Flowchart 170.1).

Management of lymphomas is an equally complex exercise requiring sophisticated facilities for diagnosis and treatment. Newer observations lead to changes in classification and management strategies. Only basic principles are given in this chapter.

HODGKIN'S DISEASE

Syn: Hodgkin's lymphoma

Pathology

Hodgkin's disease (HD) generally arises unicentrically and spreads to other lymphatic tissues by contiguity and later to nonlymphatic organs as well.

The pathological hallmark is the presence of **Reed-Sternberg's cells (RS cells)** which are large multinucleated cells with the nuclei being arranged in mirror image fashion in histological slides (Figs 170.1A to C). A causal association between Epstein-Barr virus (EBV) infection and EBV positive subgroup of HD has been identified.

They are clones of neoplastic B-lymphocytes which originate from the germinal centers of lymphoid organs. They appear as modified germinal center B-lymphocytes that have escaped apoptosis. They show rearrangement of immunoglobulin (Ig) variable region (V) genes. RS cells produce cytokines which promote their own growth and are also responsible for the systemic manifestations of the disease. In general, RS cells form only 1% of the cell population even though they constitute the malignant tissue. The rest of the tissue is made up of lymphocytes, macrophage and granulocytes, especially eosinophils.

The lymph node architecture is destroyed and replaced by abnormal tissue. Four histological patterns have been recognized.

Rye (1965) Classification

This classification arrived at by consensus, held its pride of place until recently. Now newer and more elaborated classifications have been introduced. The Rye classification is based on general morphology of the tissue and cell types.

Lymphocyte Predominant (10%)

There is predominance of lymphocytes with a few RS cells. Nodular and diffuse patterns are recognizable. This has the best prognosis. Nodular variety of lymphocyte predominant HD is of B-cell origin.

Nodular Sclerosis (30–40%)

In this form, the tumor is arranged as nodules which are encircled by collagenous bands extending from the capsule. A variant of the RS cell, the lacunar cell, may be present. Mediastinal lymph node enlargement is more common.

Mixed Cellularity (20–30%)

There are numerous RS cells and moderate number of lymphocytes.

Lymphocyte Depleted (10–20%)

The pattern may be reticulate or diffuse fibrosis. In the former, there is dominance of RS cells and depletion of lymphocytes. In the latter, the lymph node is replaced by disorderly connective tissue containing a few lymphocytes and a few RS cells.

Table 170.1: Number and relative proportion of lymphomas in cancer statistics at RCC, Thiruvananthapuram in 2010

Gender	Lymphoma	Number	Percentage (%) among cancer cases
Adult male	do	386	6.7
Adult females	do	206	3.5
Children	do	38	5.5

Flowchart 170.1: B- and T-cell origin from the common lymphoid stem cell

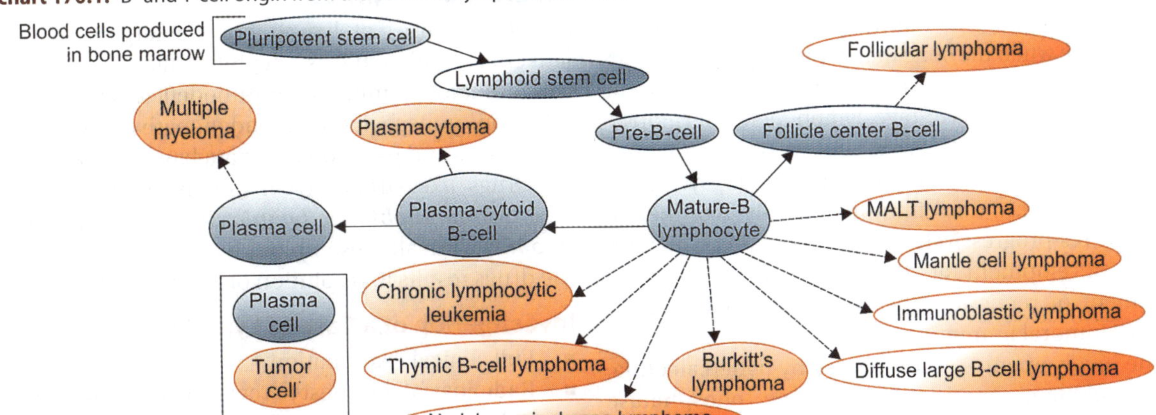

Abbreviation: MALT = Mucosa-associated lymphoid tissue

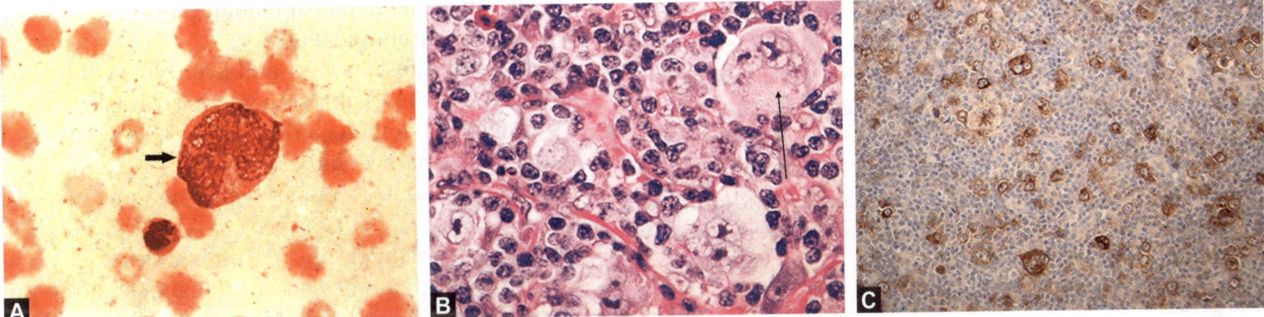

Figs 170.1A to C: A. Bone marrow Hodgkin's disease. **B.** Lymph node showing Hodgkin's disease. **C.** Lymph node showing CD30 positive Reed-Sternberg's cells. *Note:* The Reed-Sternberg's cell (arrow);

The nodular sclerosis type maintains its distinct histology throughout whereas the other types may progress to one or the other or show overlap when followed up. In India, mixed cellularity type is more frequent than nodular sclerosis. The prognosis becomes progressively worse as one moves from the lymphocyte predominant type to the lymphocyte depleted types.

Newer Classifications

Different newer classifications have come in. HD has been broadly classified as two distinct entities: (a) Nodular lymphocyte predominant and (b) the classic HD which is further divided into four subtypes 1–4 shown in below box:

> ***World Health Organization (WHO) classification of lymphoid tumors***
>
> - Nodular lymphocyte predominant Hodgkin lymphoma
> - Classical Hodgkin lymphoma
>   1. Nodular sclerosis classical Hodgkin lymphoma
>   2. Lymphocyte-rich classical Hodgkin lymphoma
>   3. Mixed cellularity classical Hodgkin lymphoma
>   4. Lymphocyte-depleted classical Hodgkin lymphoma.

Clinical Features

Hodgkin's disease may be encountered at any age, but it is more common in the 2nd decade. Males are affected twice as frequently as females. The majority of patients come in an advanced stage, the disease having been present for more than 6 months.

The most frequent symptom is painless asymmetrical circumscribed enlargement of the lymph nodes, which are rubbery in consistency. In over 75% cases, cervical groups are affected. Axillary, mediastinal and inguinal groups are involved less frequently. Involvement of the retroperitoneal lymph nodes is not uncommon. The lymph nodes reach moderate to large sizes. They do not soften, breakdown or ulcerate.

Moderate splenomegaly occurs in over 50% of cases and hepatomegaly in a smaller number. These organs are firm and nontender. Hepatocellular or obstructive jaundice may occur.

Constitutional symptoms occur in the majority of cases in the later stages. Pel-Ebstein fever consists of a few days of high swinging pyrexia followed by an afebrile period. Though Pel-Ebstein type of fever has come to stay as a classic feature of HD, in vast majority, the typical form is not seen. Fever is commonly due to concomitant infection, but less commonly it is due to the malignant process itself. The patient rapidly loses weight and develops toxemia. Sweating, intractable pruritus and anemia develop in many cases.

Alcohol-induced tenderness over the lymph nodes and bone is described as a diagnostic feature, but in Indian subjects it is rare. Horner's syndrome may occur due to pressure on the cervical sympathetic chain. Spinal root and cord compression and development of lymphoma in the central nervous system (CNS) are neurological complications. Opportunistic infections such as herpes zoster, *Mycobacterium tuberculosis,* Cytomegalovirus (CMV), *Cryptococci* and *Candida* species are common.

Investigations

There may be normocytic normochromic anemia. In the advanced stage when the bone marrow is infiltrated, myelophthisic anemia develops. Mild eosinophilia may occur frequently. In the advanced stage, lymphopenia develops.

Bone marrow involvement is seen in 10–20% of cases and this is best demonstrated by trephine biopsy. As the disease progresses, the immunologically competent T-lymphocytes progressively diminish and this coincides with the development of anergy to tuberculin. With achievement of remission, the cell-mediated immunity recovers. Humoral immunity may be normal.

Bone involvement is accompanied by hypercalcemia, hyperphosphatemia and raised alkaline phosphatase (ALP) levels. Hyperuricemia may develop. Hepatic ALP is raised. Serum copper is elevated during the active stages and it falls during remission. Serum lactate dehydrogenase (LDH) is elevated and it is an indicator of the tumor burden.

Several other advanced investigations such as cytochemistry, immunological tests, molecular procedures and imaging modalities such computerized tomography (CT) scan, magnetic resonance imaging (MRI) and positron emission tomography (PET) studies are undertaken for full evaluation of the extent, type of tumor and prognostic information.

Diagnosis

All cases presenting with chronic local or general lymphadenopathy in which a distinct cause cannot be established should be subjected to lymph node biopsy without delay. When several groups of nodes are affected, an entire node which is moderately enlarged should be selected for biopsy.

Differential Diagnosis

All other causes of lymph node enlargement such as leukemias, tuberculosis, syphilis, filariasis, secondary carcinomatosis, human immunodeficiency virus (HIV) infection, nonspecific lymphadenopathy, toxoplasmosis, sarcoidosis and pseudolymphoma have to be excluded.

Drugs like streptomycin and phenytoin produce a type of *immunoblastic lymphadenopathy (pseudolymphoma)* clinically resembling lymphoma. Withdrawal of the drugs results in resolution of the node.

Investigation of a Case of Lymphoma

- Full clinical examination
- Radiology of the chest to reveal mediastinal nodes and pulmonary involvement
- Complete hematological investigations
- Ultrasonography (USG) to detect masses of glands in the abdomen and hepatosplenomegaly
- Bone marrow trephine biopsy
- Liver function tests (LFTs) and liver biopsy if liver is enlarged and shows ultrasonographic changes
- CT scan of abdomen and chest to detect enlarged masses and wherever indicated MRI
- Isotopic liver scan to detect lymphomatous involvement
- Radioisotopic scintigraphy of lymph nodes
- CT-PET scan has replaced all modalities and is the investigation of choice in all lymphomas specially in HL (Figs 170.2A to H).

Staging laparotomy which was a regular procedure in early stage HD has now been abandoned since the necessary information can be obtained by imaging procedures. In addition, systemic chemotherapy is more commonly employed in all stages.

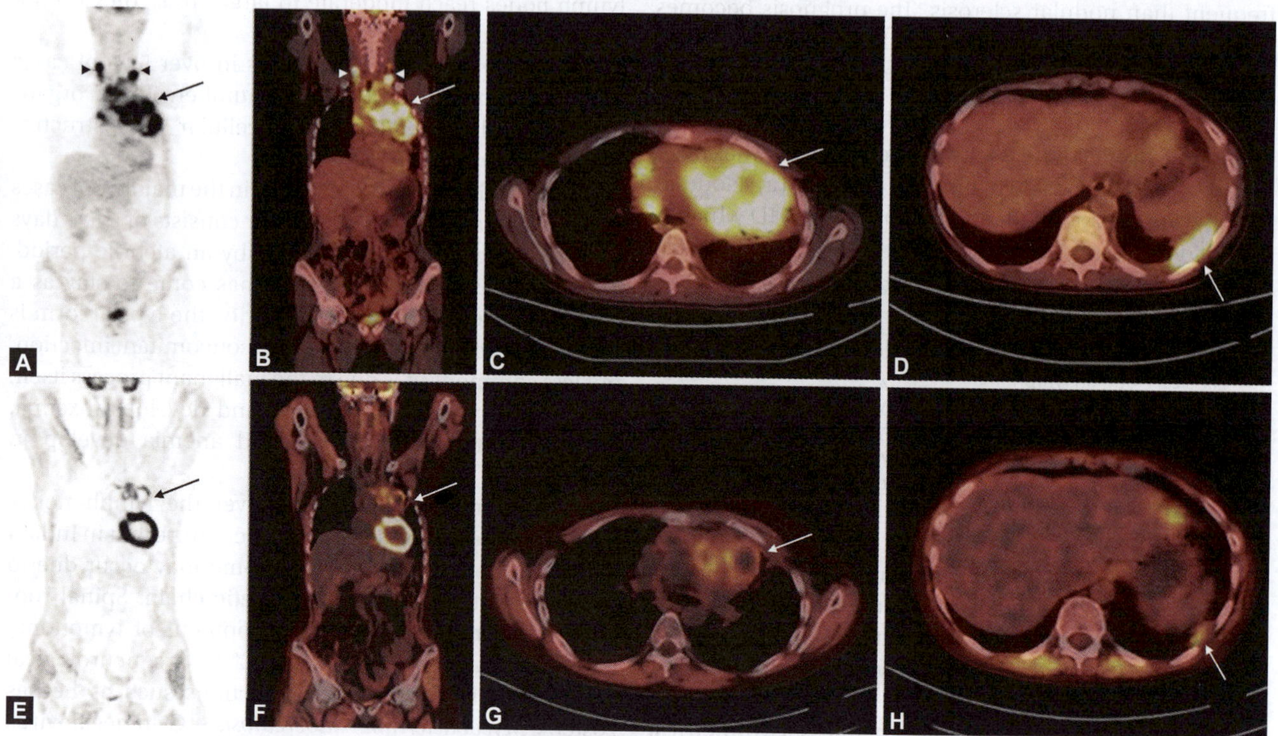

Figs 170.2A to H: CT-PET scan showing mediastinal lymphoma (B, C, G), pleural-based lesions (D and H) showing post-treatment effect (arrows)

Table 170.2: Five-point scale for intrim fluorodeoxyglucose-positron emission tomography (FDG-PET) scan results for standardization used in clinical trials

Score	PET/CT result
1	No uptake above background
2	Uptake ≤ mediastinum
3	Uptake > mediastinum but ≤ liver
4	Uptake moderately increased compared to liver at any site
5	Uptake markedly increased compared to liver at any site
X	New areas of uptake unlikely to be related to lymphoma

Table 170.3: Clinical staging of Hodgkin lymphomas (Cotswold revision of Ann Arbor staging classification)

Stage	Definition
I	Involvement of a single lymph node region or lymphoid structure (e.g. spleen, Waldeyer ring, thymus) or involvement of a single extra-lymphatic site
II	Involvement of two or more lymph node regions on the same side of the diaphragm (the mediastinum is a single site; hilar nodes, when involved on both sides, constitute stage II disease); localized contiguous involvement of only one extranodal organ or site and lymphnode region(s) on the same side of the diaphragm (IIE). The number of anatomic sites should be indicated by suffix (e.g. II_3)
III	Involvement of lymph node regions or structures on both sides of the diaphragm, which may also be accompanied by involvement of the spleen (IIIS) or by localized involvement of only one extranodal organ site (IIIE) or both (IIISE) III_1 with or without splenic, hilar, celiac or portal nodes III_2 with para-aortic, iliac or mesenteric nodes
IV	Diffuse or disseminated involvement of one or more extranodal organs or tissues, with or without associated lymphnode involvement.

Note: E, involvement of a single extranodal site, or contiguous or proximal to known nodal site of disease.

A: No **B** symptoms

B: Place the patient in the **B** category when at least one of the following is observed:

1. Unexplained weight loss >10% of body weight during 6 month before staging
2. Recurrent unexplained fever >38°C during the previous month
3. Recurrent heavy night sweats during the previous month.

The PET/CT scan results can be used for scoring the clinical state of myeloma and initiating treatment (Table 170.2).

Staging of Lymphomas

Staging procedures: Since the choice of initial therapy depends on the stage, full investigation should be undertaken in all cases before deciding the therapeutic schedule. It has been established beyond doubt that proper staging and institution of appropriate therapy from the beginning are most important in bringing about a favorable outcome.

Clinical staging is currently according to the Cotswolds modification of the Ann Arbor classification (Table 170.3).

Lymphatic Structures

It includes lymph nodes, spleen, thymus, Waldeyer's rings, appendix and Peyer's patches; liver and bone marrow are excluded.

Each stage is further divided into A or B based on the absence or presence of systemic symptoms (B symptoms), respectively.

Treatment

Stages I and II: Early stage HL still treated with radiotherapy but inverted Y and mantle radiotherapy is no longer in clinical practice due to long-term side effects, both from the radiation fields and second malignancies. The treatment of choice is to give radiotherapy up to a total dose of 4,000–4,500 cGy in 4 weeks. This is curative in 90% of cases. Newer modalities of radiotherapy are being developed.

Popular regimens used in the treatment of early and intermediate stages of HD are given in Table 170.4.

The 14-days treatment is followed by 14 days rest and the cycle is repeated. Usually six courses are given. There are many other effective regimens which use different drug combinations (Table 170.5).

ABVD (adriamycin, bleomycin, vinblastine and dacarbazine) regimen: A more popular chemotherapeutic regimen consists of doxorubicin, bleomycin, vinblastine and dacarbazine. ABVD is the most common regime. This has been used as standard of care in all randomized trials in HL comparing with German schedule BEACOPP [bleomycin,

Table 170.4: Popular regimens used in the treatment HD

Drugs	Dose	Days
Mustine hydrochloride	6 mg/m² IV	1 and 8
Oncovin (Vincristine)	1.5 mg/m² IV	1 and 8
Procarbazine (Natulan-Roche)	100 mg/m² oral	1–14
Prednisolone	40 mg/m² oral	1–14

Abbreviation: IV = Intravenous

Table 170.5: Other popular regimens for treatment in different stages and clinical situations in Hodgkin's lymphoma

Initial diagnosis of Hodgkin's lymphoma	
• Early stage (I-II) (favorable)	• ABVD 2–4 cycles + involved-field radiation
• Intermediate stage (unfavorable)	• ABVD 4–6 cycles + involved-field radiation
• Advanced disease:	
▪ Nonbulky	• ABVD or Stanford V or BEACOPP + involved-field radiation
▪ Bulky	• ABVD or Stanford V or BEACOPP ± involved-field radiation
Relapsed Hodgkin's lymphoma	
• Late relapse (>12 mo)	• Same treatment initially used
• Early relapse (<12 mo)	• Salvage therapies: ICE, DHAP, ESHAP, ASHAP, Dexa-BEAM, mini-BEAM, high-dose chemotherapy followed by stem cell transplantation, single-agent gemcitabine
Localized site of relapse	• Radiation to site not previously irradiated

Abbreviations: ABVD = Adriamycin, bleomycin, vinblastine and dacarbazine; BEACOPP = Bleomycin, etoposide, doxorubicin, cyclophosphamide, vincristine, procarbazine, and prednisone; ICE = Ifosfamide, carboplatin, etoposide; DHAP = Dexamethasone, high-dose cytarabine and procarbazine, ESHAP = Etoposide, methylprednisolone, cisplatin and cytarabine; ASHAP = Doxorubicin, methylprednisolone, cisplatin and cytarabine; BEAM = Bis-chloroethyl nitrosourea (BCNU), Etoposide, cytarabine and melphalan

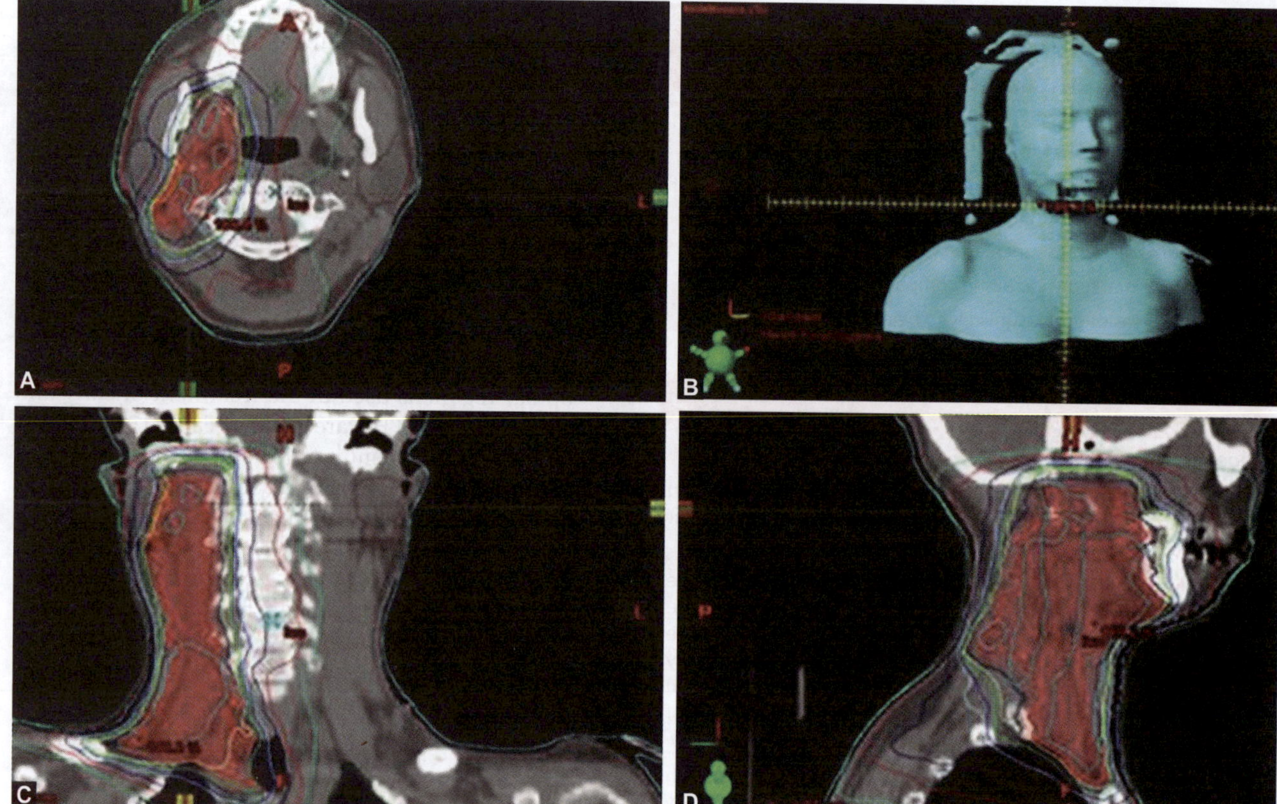

Figs 170.3A to D: Image-guided radiotherapy (IGRT) has more capability in limiting the damage to the involved lymph nodes

etoposide, adriamycin (doxorubicin), cyclophosphamide, oncovin, procarbazine and prednisone].

Stages III and IV: These patients are treated with cyclical chemotherapy.

Newer Modalities of Radiotherapy

Involved Field Radiotherapy (IFRT) and Involved Node Radiotherapy (INRT)

This is standard of care to avoid excess radiation and limiting the field. Limiting the dose to 20–40 Grays over 2–4 weeks. Most likely the radiotherapy is used in conjunction with chemotherapy like ABVD 3–4 cycles and followed by IFRT. More and more are done with the assistance of CT-PET scan. This is standard baseline investigation in HL (Figs 170.3A to D).

Intensity Modulated Radiation Therapy (IMRT)

This is going to be standard of care for some types of lymphoma especially head and neck localized HL and NHL.

Proton therapy is among the latest interventional forms of radiotherapy used for other tumors limiting the toxicities and delivering maximal dose to the tumor sites like lymph nodes.

Stereotactic body radiation therapy is a highly selective form used to deliver radiation to areas like brain stem, upper cervical and brain lymphomas.

Prognosis

The 5-year survival rates differ between the different age groups and stage of the lymphoma at the onset of treatment. Present aggressive modalities of treatment of resistant cases and relapses have helped to improve survival. On an average, the 5-year survival rates reported from several centers is given in Table 170.6.

Histologically, lymphocyte predominant types show the best prognosis. Circumscribed lesions have a better prognosis than diffuse lesions.

Other adverse prognostic factors include:

- Age above 45 years
- Presence of B symptoms
- Mediastinal width exceeding 45% of thoracic width in the skiagram
- Presence of extranodal disease
- Involvement of bone marrow
- Packed cell volume (PCV) below 25% and erythrocyte sedimentation rate (ESR) above 50 mm/hour.

Relapses are managed by same or alternate schedules of chemotherapy. In resistant cases, two regimens can be combined. At present, more aggressive drug combinations are being used in poor-prognosis cases and relapsed cases. This has been made possible due to the availability of supportive services during the phase of neutropenia. Autologous bone marrow transplantation and stem cell transplantation have helped to institute almost curative chemoradiotherapy.

Table 170.6: 5-year survival rates of Hodgkin's lymphoma with treatment

Stages	Below 20 years (%)	21–40 years (%)	Above 40 years (%)
IA and IIA	94	93	78
IB and IIB	93	83	45
III and IV–A and B	80	61	22

Long-term Risks

One percent of patients treated for HD may develop acute myeloid leukemia (AML) which is resistant to therapy. The risk of second malignancies is higher in treated HD patients than in the general population. Several types of second malignancies have been reported. Other complications include reversible azoospermia caused by chemotherapy, serious infective complications in splenectomized patients, amenorrhea and cumulative cardiotoxicity caused by daunomycin and related drugs. The cardiotoxicity may manifest as cardiac dysfunction even several years after recovery from the malignancy.

Advances in investigations and therapeutic modalities introduced during the past decade have made the results of therapy and prognosis much better in India as well, but results in Indian series are not so encouraging since in India, only about 25% of cases are in stages I or II when initially diagnosed and rest come in more advanced stages.

Institution of therapy in special institutions has helped to improve the results. Wherever possible, treatment of lymphoma should be undertaken in tertiary care centers specializing in lymphoma treatment.

Novel therapies in HL include (1) Brentuximab (Anti-CD30) and histone deacetylase (HDAC) inhibitors Panobinostat and Vorinostat; and (2) Brentuximab Vedotin (Anti-CD30) in clinical trials on front-line use in elderly HL cases.

NON-HODGKIN'S LYMPHOMA

Majority of these are B-cell neoplasms, though T-cell NHL also occurs. Unlike HL, the clinical picture is more variable. Extranodal involvement is more common, so also involvement of the blood and bone marrow. The disease often starts multicentrically.

Classification

Classification of NHL has undergone considerable modification from time-to-time. Rappaport (1966) gave the histological classification as mainly nodular and diffuse types. Luke and Collins based their classification on morphology and immunological characteristics.

Newer classifications have come in such as Kiel, International Working Formulation (IWF), Revised European and American lymphoma (REAL) group and WHO. Modern classification takes into account the clinical schema classifying the disease into:

- Indolent lymphoma/leukemias (with survival times measured in years, if untreated)
- Aggressive lymphomas (survival measured in months)
- Highly aggressive lymphomas and leukemias (survival measured in weeks).

Each type is further subdivided into B- and T-cell types and also the histological pattern (Fig. 170.4).

The Kiel classification, which is also in vogue, makes a distinct subdivision into low-grade and high-grade

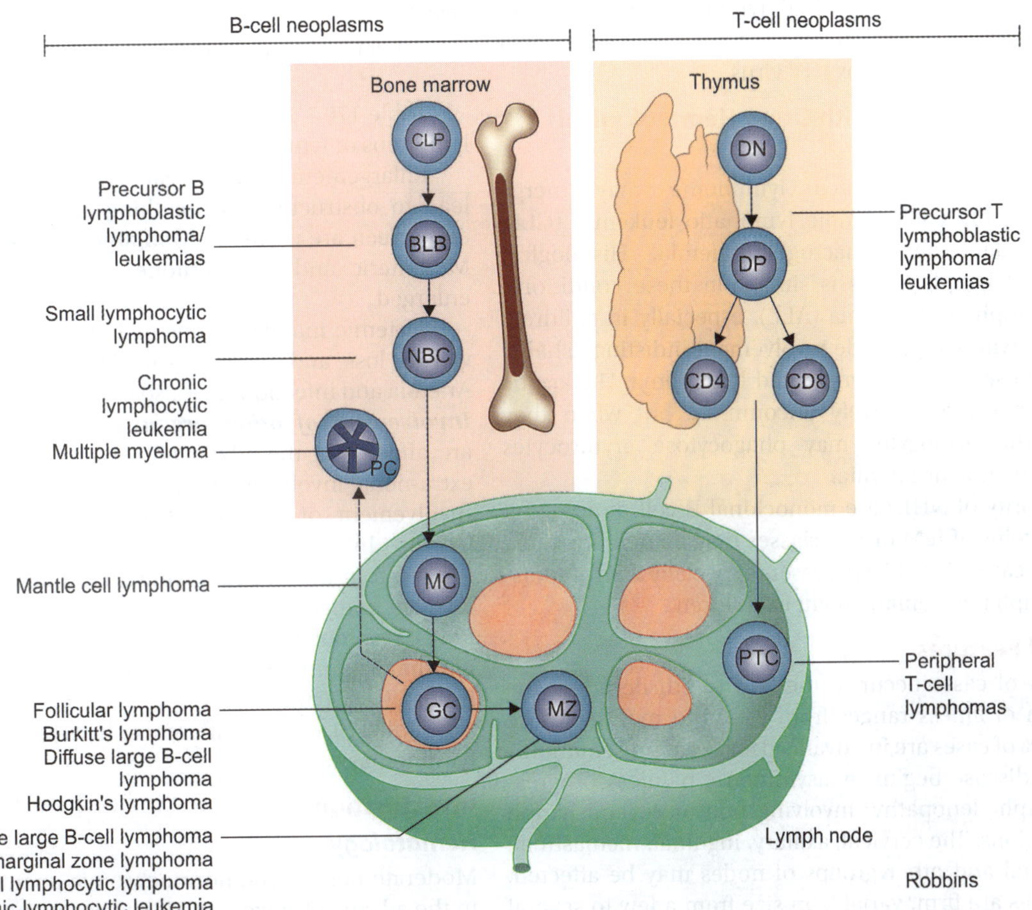

Fig. 170.4: Histological origin for different subtypes of non-Hodgkin's lymphoma according to the lymph node architecture

Abbreviations: CLP = Common lymphoid progenitors; BLB = Pre-B lymphoblast; NBC = Naive B cell; PC = Plasma cells; DN = CD4/CD8 double negative pre-T cell; DP = CD4/CD8 double positive pre-T cell; MZ = Marginal zone B cell; GC = Germinal center B cell; MC = Mantle B cell; PTC = Peripheral T cell

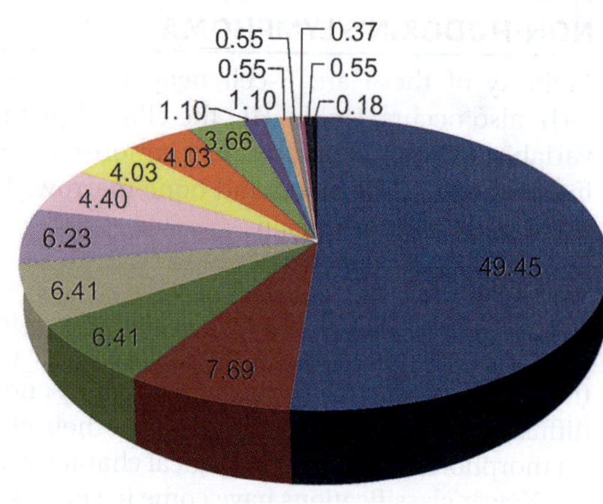

Fig. 170.5: Prevalence of non-Hodgkin's lymphomas subtypes

Abbreviations: DLBCL = Diffuse large B-cell lymphoma; HL = Hodgkin's lymphoma

Textbook of Medicine

lymphomas, the former being composed of relatively small cells, whereas the latter is composed of larger and more rapidly proliferating cells. Different institutions follow a combination of histologic, immunologic (B-cell, T-cell, etc.) and behavioral factors (Kiel) to group the lymphomas for statistical and therapeutic purposes (Fig. 170.5).

NHL occur in all regions. Certain types show geographic differences, e.g. Burkitt's lymphoma (BL) is seen in Africa mainly. Kaposi's sarcoma is a cutaneous lymphoma in some cases triggered by HIV virus.

Coexistence of NHL with Other Hematological Disorders

Diffuse well-differentiated lymphoma may merge imperceptibly with chronic lymphatic leukemia (CLL) and Waldenström's macroglobulinemia. Histological picture of lymph nodes is similar in these conditions. Acute lymphatic leukemia (ALL), especially in children, presents with lymph node involvement indistinguishable from diffuse poorly differentiated lymphoma. Histiocytic lymphomas are relatively uncommon, but when they occur, the histiocytes may phagocytose erythrocytes causing hemolytic anemia.

Majority of NHLs are monoclonal B-cell tumors and paraproteins of IgM or IgG classes may be demonstrable in many cases. T-cell NHL presents specially with mediastinal lymph node enlargement in children.

Clinical Features

Majority of cases occur in the 2nd to 5th decades. The duration of illness ranges from weeks to months. More than 70% of cases are in advanced stages at presentation.

The disease begins as asymmetric painless progressive lymphadenopathy, involving one or several lymph node regions. The cervical, axillary, inguinal, mediastinal, abdominal and other groups of nodes may be affected. The nodes are firm, variable in size from a few to several centimeters and are matted in the later stages. Pressure on neighboring structures may lead to mediastinal syndrome, Horner's syndrome and lymphedema.

Table 170.7: Comparison between HL and NHL lymphomas		
Clinical findings	**HL (%)**	**NHL (%)**
Lymphadenopathy	93	89
Fever	69	29
Abdominal masses	–	16
Cough and dyspnea	20	25
Skin lesions	3	15
Pruritus	14	3
Pleural effusion (*Based on 120 cases*)	6	17

Table 170.7 shows comparison between HL and NHL lymphous or lymphomas.

Enlargement of the tonsils and Waldeyer's ring may lead to obstruction to breathing and swallowing. Liver and spleen are moderately enlarged in majority of cases. Mesenteric and retroperitoneal lymph nodes may be enlarged.

Systemic manifestations include early onset of fever, weight loss and night sweats in about 30% of cases. Anemia and infections are also more common.

Involvement of other organs: Though several organs are affected in the advanced stages of NHL, sometimes extra-nodal involvement may be the presenting symptom. Involvement of the skin leads to nodular or diffuse lesions. Intense pruritus is an early and intractable symptom in a few. Brain, spinal cord and meninges are affected in many cases. Gastrointestinal tract (GIT), liver, lungs, respiratory tract, pleura and bone may be the seat of primary lymphoma. Hemorrhagic pleural effusion may occur (Fig. 170.6).

Table 170.8 shows differences between HL and NHL or lymphomas.

Investigations

Hematology

Moderate normocytic normochromic anemia may occur in the advanced stages. The leukocyte picture is generally unremarkable but in a few cases lymphosarcoma cells are detectable in the circulation. These cells resemble large lymphocytes with lobed or folded nuclei and may

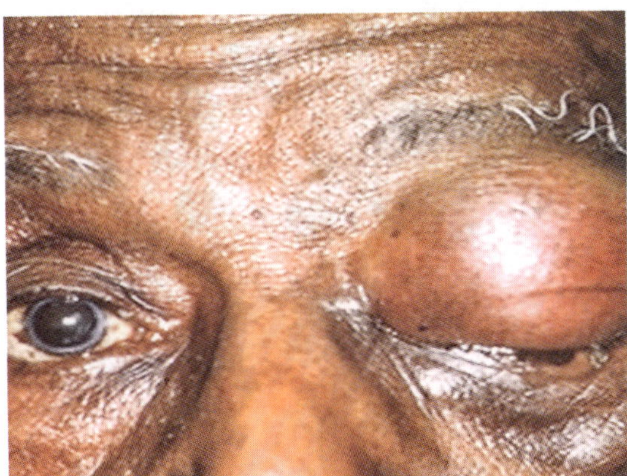

Fig. 170.6: Female with orbital lymphoma

show nucleoli. The condition is termed ***lymphosarcoma leukemia.***

Autoimmune hemolytic anemia develops in a few cases. Infiltration of the marrow results in myelophthisic anemia. Bone marrow involvement is common in stage IV NHL.

Biochemistry

Paraproteins of IgM or IgG class may be detectable in a few cases. Serum uric acid is moderately elevated in the advanced stages. Hepatic involvement is characterized by rise in ALP and transaminases. Obstructive jaundice results from pressure of lymph nodes at the porta hepatis.

Other Investigations Include the Following

Full blood count, LFTs, urea and electrolytes, LDH, immuno-globulin (paraprotein), beta-2 microglobulin, Hepatitis B and C serology, HIV I and II serology.

Staging CT scan/CT-PET, bone marrow aspirate and trephine biopsy (Figs 170.7A to C).

Lymph node biopsy: Histology review of lymphoma by a pathologist (Fig. 170.8).

Histological characterization of the cell type is important in classification, prognostication and decision of treatment modality (Figs 170.9A to C). Gene expression studies help to further characterize the lymphomas and predict their behavior with treatment (Fig. 170.10 and Table 170.9).

Staging Non-Hodgkin's Lymphoma

Ann Arbor staging system	
Stages	**Definitions**
I	Lymphoma in 1 lymph node region or a single localized extranodal site, i.e. thyroid
II	Lymphoma in 2 or more lymph node regions situated either above or below the diaphragm
III	Lymphoma in lymph node regions situated both above or below the diaphragm
IV	Lymphoma in 1 or more extralymphatic organs with or without associated lymph node involvement (diffuse or disseminated)

International Prognostic Index for Follicular NHL and High Grade NHL (DLBCL) (Table 170.10). FLIPI2 Revised Scoring System for Follicular NHL (Table 170.11).

Follicular Lymphoma International Prognostic Index (FLIPI2) risk factors:
- Age >60 years
- Hemoglobin level <12 g/dL
- Serum beta-2-microglobulin (β2M) > upper limits of normal (ULN)
- LoDLIN >6 cm (The longest diameter of the largest involved node)
- Bone marrow involvement

Treatment

Combination Therapy and Radiotherapy

Stages I and II respond to radiotherapy as for HD. In the other stages, chemotherapy is advocated. At present, chemotherapy is given even in the earlier stages.

Combination therapy with cyclophosphamide, vincristine and prednisolone (COP), as in the case of stages II and IV NHL, has been tried with remission rates up to 55–60%. A remission rate of 60% is obtained with mustargen, oncovin, procarbizaine, prednisone (MOPP) regimen. In more advanced cases, adriamycin and

Table 170.8: Differences between Hodgkin's and non-Hodgkin's lymphomas		
Characteristics	**Hodgkin's lymphoma**	**Non-Hodgkin's lymphoma**
Age	Bimodal peak incidence, 15–35 years and 45–70 years	Peak incidence around 60 years
B symptoms	More common	Less common
Alcohol-induced discomfort in lymph nodal region	Common	Not observe
Disease at the time of diagnosis	Usually well-localized	Usually widespread
Site of involvement	Unifocal origin and arises in a single node or chain of nodes (cervical, mediastinal, para-aortic)	Mostly involves multiple peripheral nodes (multicentric origin)
Pattern of spread	Orderly spread by contiguity in a predictable fashion	Noncontiguous spread in an unpredictable fashion
Epitrochlear node involvement	Rare	Common
Mediastinal involvement	Common	Uncommon
Mesenteric nodes and Waldeyer-ring	Rarely involved	Commonly involved
Bone marrow involvement	Late	Early
Extranodal involvement	Uncommon	Common
Characteristic of neoplastic cells	***Neoplastic cells:*** Hodgkin's or Reed-Sternberg's (RS) cells form minor tumor cell mass 1–5%	Neoplastic cells form the major tumor cell mass
Number of neoplastic cells	Few neoplastic cells (RS cells)	Majority of the cells are neoplastic

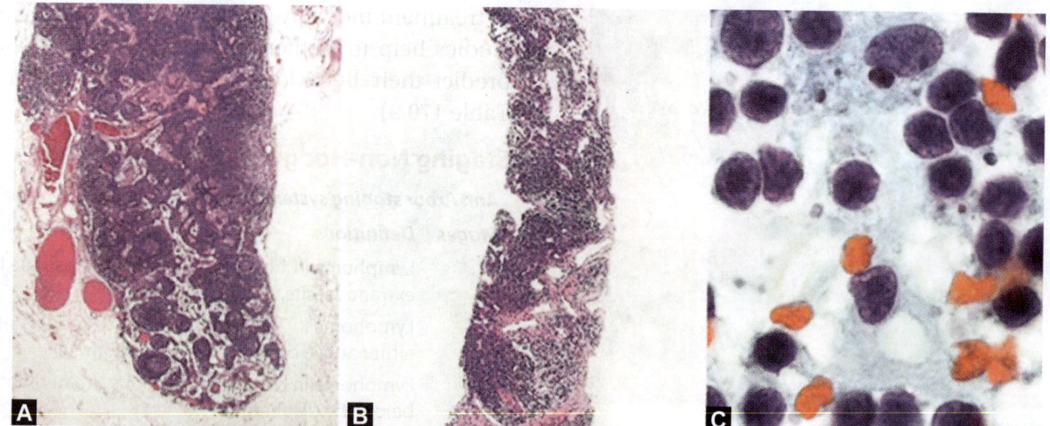

Figs 170.7A to C: Lymph node. **A.** Excisional biopsy; **B.** Needle core biopsy; **C.** Smear for cytology. ***Note:*** In Fig C; cytology is the last resort if there is no other way to obtain appropriate tissue

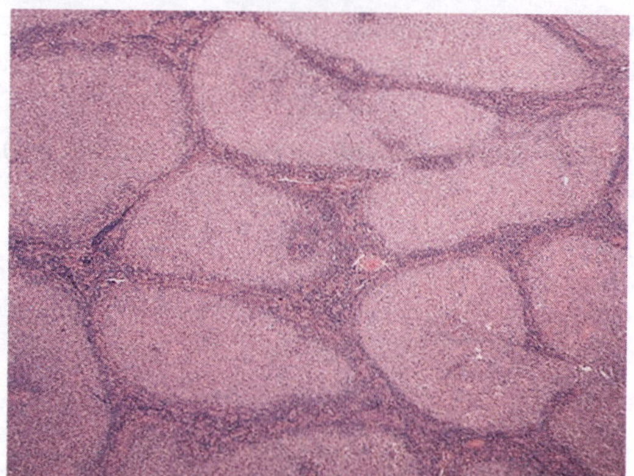

Fig. 170.8: Follicular non-Hodgkin's lymphoma–lymph node histology low power view. ***Note:*** The distinct follicular pattern

bleomycin have been included (BACOP regimen) with remission rates up to 80%.

Local irradiation with 4,000–5,000 cGy to control massive local disease and systemic chemotherapy give better remission rates in diffuse poorly differentiated lymphoma.

Stage I: Follicular NHL and low-grade NHL are treated by IFRT only.

Stage II: Follicular NHL: Asymptomatic cases are treated by watch and wait only.

Symptomatic follicular advanced stage: Rituximab + CHOP/CVP (cyclophosphamide, hydroxydaunorubicin, oncovin, predrisone) is the standard of care, followed by rituximab maintenance for 2 years follow-up every 2 months.

StiL NHL Study has shown beneficial advantage of rituximab in combination with bendamustine (BR) over R-CHOP.

Diffuse Large B Cell Lymphoma (DLBCL)

Stage IA and B: Treated with combination of R-CHOP 3–4 cycles followed by IFRT.

DLBCL stage II–IV A and B

Combination chemotherapy consisting of cyclophosphamide, doxorubicin, vincristine and prednisolone is used most frequently in the aggressive types of NHL due to its better efficacy and predictable results.

Monoclonal antibodies developed against specific CD 20 cells-rituximab (Mabthera) is used to target specific CD 20+B-cells which occur in several forms of NHL. The dose is 375–500 mg/m^2 on day-1 of the cycle. The results are considerably better.

R-CHOP 21 is the standard of care following the landmark trial from GELA group in France. Even though

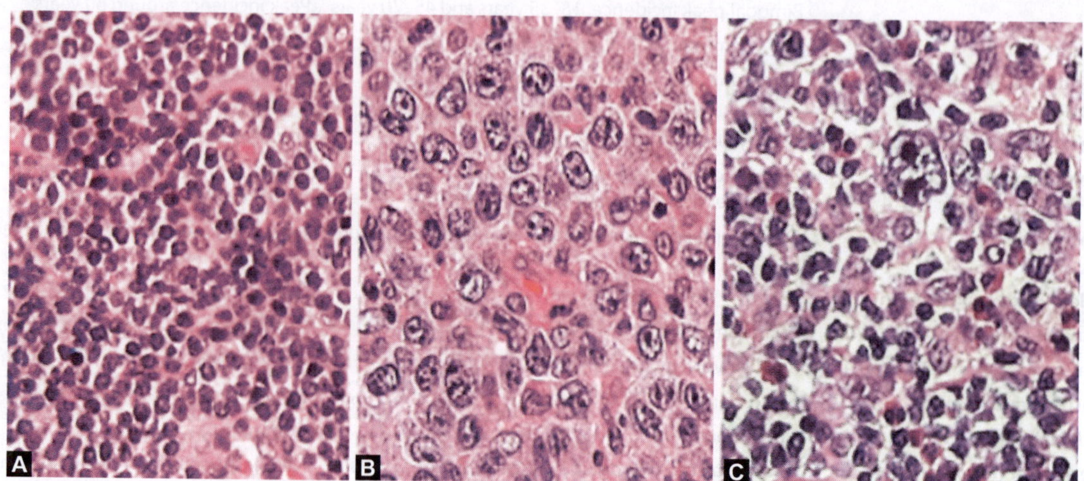

Figs 170.9A to C: Histological characterization of cell type in NHL. **A.** Small cells in small lymphocytic lymphoma; **B.** Large cells in diffuse large B-cell lymphoma; **C.** Hodgkin's cell with inflammatory background

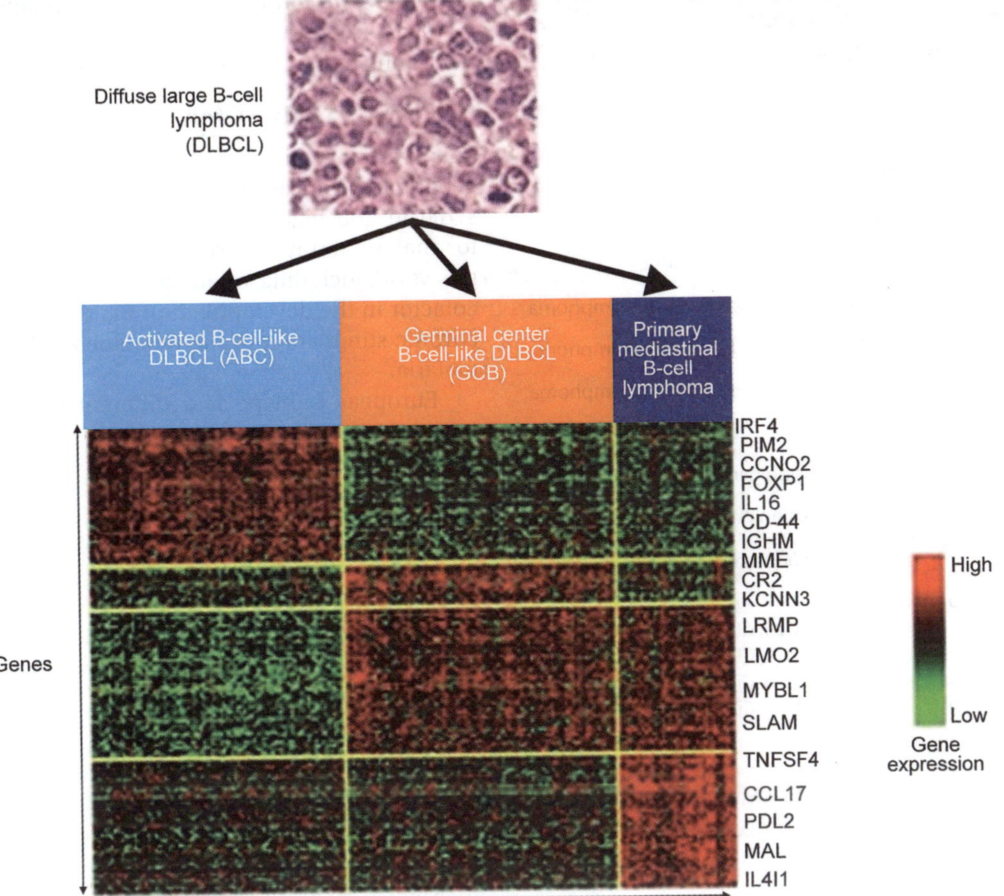

Fig. 170.10: Lymph node: Diffuse large B-cell lymphoma (DLBCL) with the genetic pattern exposed

initial trials like RICOVER-60 showed advantage for R-CHOP 14, latter MRC-BNLI trials has disproved this.

DBCL Subtypes: Activated B-Cell Type (ABC) and Germinal centre type (GCB). Both behave different to standard R-CHOP type of treatment.

New trials and agents are used to target the poor prognostic type which is ABC-DLBCL, some are treating with dose adjusted (DA)-EPOCH in combination with bortezomib.

UK NCRN trial ReMODEL-B trial is looking at randomized data between R-CHOP and R-BCHOP (combined with bortezomib).

Newer agents like ibrutinib (BTK inhibitor) and lenalidomide (IMiD) has been used in clinical trials.

Mantle Cell Lymphoma

This is a rarer type of NHL with broad spectrum of grades varying from low risk indolent forms on one side to aggressive blastoid form on the other end.

Standard R-CHOP may not be the best option for this group. Young fit patients are treated with Nordic protocol alternating R-Maxi CHOP and high dose cytarabine, followed by autologous stem cell transplantation. R-Hyper CVAD (cyclophosphamide, vincristine, adriamycin and dexamethasone) is another popular option.

Relapsed disease is treated with bortezomib (Velcade) and recently by BTK inhibitor ibrutinib.

Marginal Zone Lymphoma

Treated similar to follicular NHL with R-CVP like regime. Role of maintenance rituximab is under clinical trials.

MALT Lymphoma

Treated like indolent lymphoma, but association with *Helicobacter pylori* makes eradication of *H. pylori* essential.

AUTOLOGOUS PERIPHERAL STEM CELL TRANSPLANTATION (APSCT) IN LYMPHOMA

Indications: Age below 70 years; state of the disease.

- In relapsed follicular HL/DLBCL with age below 70 years, APSCT is the standard of care following salvage regimes like IVE, ESHAP or ICE (ifosfamide carboplatin, etoposide). Standard conditioning regime is BEAM chemotherapy.
- ***Mantle cell lymphoma:*** Front-line treatment after nordic type of approach with R-Mega CHOP/high dose Ara-C.
- ***Angioimmunoblastic lymphoma (AILD):*** Front-line treatment after aggressive induction regime like IVE or alternating intermediate dose methotrexate.
- Anaplastic large cell lymphoma (ALK negative).

Allogenic Stem Cell Transplantation (Age <55 years)

- Second relapse after autologous stem cell transplant in HL
- High-grade transformation in follicular NHL

Table 170.9: Genetic and molecular characteristics of lymphomas

Genetic abnormality	Oncogene	Lymphoma
t(8;14)(q24;q32)	MYC	BL, DLBCL
t(8;22)(q24;q11)	MYC	BL, DLBCL
t(8;2)(q24;q12)	MYC	BL, DLBCL
t(14;18)(q32;q21)	BCL2	FL, DLBCL
t(11;14)(q13;q32)	CCND1	MCL
t(11;18)(q21;q21)	API2-MALT Fusion gene	MALT lymphoma
t(14;18)(q32;q21)	MALT1	MALT lymphoma
t(3;14)(p14.1;q32)	FOXP1	MALT lymphoma
t(1;14)(p22.1;q32)	BCL10	MALT lymphoma
t(2;5)(p23;q35)	NPM-ALK fusion gene	ALCL ALK+
t(1;2)(q25;p23)	TPM3-ALK fusion gene	ALCL ALK+

Lymphoma	Characteristic antigen
Mature B-cell lymphomas	
CLL/SLL	CD20, CD79a, CD5, CD23
MCL	CD20, CD79a, CD5, CyclinD1
Follicular lymphoma	CD20, CD79a, BCl2, CD10, BCl6
Burkitt's lymphoma	CD20, CD79a, CD10, BCl6
Mature T- and NK-cell lymphomas	
Peripheral T-cell lymphoma	CD2, CD3, CD4>CD8
ALCL	CD2, CD30, ALK, CD4>CD8, EMA
Angioimmunoblastic T-cell lymphoma	CD2, CD3, CD5, CD4>CD8
Extranodal NK-/T-cell lymphoma, nasal type	CD2, CD56
Hodgkin's lymphomas (HL)	
Classical HL	CD15, CD30
Nodular lymphocytic predominant HL	CD20 (weak), CD79a (weak), CD45

Abbreviations: BCL2 = B-cell lymphoma 2; CCND1 = Cyclin D1; MALT = Mucosa-associated lymphoid tissue; FOXP1 = Forkhead Box P1; NPM-ALK = Nucleophosmin-anaplastic lymphoma kinase; TPM3-ALK = Tropomyosin alpha-3- anaplastic lymphoma kinase; BL = Burkitt lymphoma; DLBCL = Diffuse large B-cell lymphoma; FL = Follicular lymphoma; MCL = Mantle cell lymphoma; ALCL = Anaplastic large cell lymphoma; CLL = Chronic lymphocytic leukemia; SLL = Small lymphocytic lymphoma; NK-cell = Natural killer cells

- ***Young fit follicular NHL:*** First relapse with short event free survival
- Young fit mantle cell lymphoma with sibling donor.

BURKITT'S LYMPHOMA

This lymphoma is more prevalent in Africa showing a geographical localization to areas with altitude below 1,700 m and high rainfall, which are also holoendemic for malaria. Stray reports are available from all parts of the world, including several from India. EBV infection is a cofactor in the development of BL, the other factor being chronic stimulation of the reticuloendothelial system by malaria.

European subtype is a different disease entity and more prevalent in West.

Histology

Histology of the lesion is diagnostic and the tumor is made up of uniform type of lymphoblast-like cells, 10–25/μm in size with rounded nuclei and nucleoli. Phagocytic macrophages with large pale cytoplasm are uniformly distributed among the dark staining cells giving the appearance referred to as the ***starry sky appearance***. Chromosomal abnormalities have been observed, the most frequent being a translocation between 8 and 14 [t,(8,14) (q24,q32)].

Clinical Features

The African cases are seen predominantly in children, mostly in the age group of 3–5 years. Multicentric tumors arise which grow rapidly affecting the jaw, salivary glands, neck, abdominal viscera, long bones and CNS. Spread to bone marrow and lymph nodes and the leukemic phase are uncommon.

Burkitt's lymphoma, as reported from other parts of the world affects older age groups. Lymph node and marrow involvement is more common. Antibodies to EBV are less pronounced.

Course and Prognosis

The disease is rapidly fatal if untreated. The African cases respond dramatically to cyclophosphamide in large doses or combination chemotherapy. Response is less dramatic in cases described from other parts of the globe.

Table 170.10: Differences between International Prognostic Index for FLIPI and IPI

FLIPI (follicular lymphoma)		IPI (large cell lymphoma)	
Age >60 year Ann Arbor stage (III or IV) Hemoglobin level <12 g/dL (120 g/L) Number of nodal* areas >4 Serum LDH level above normal		Age >60 year Stage I or II Performance status 0 or 1 Extranodal involvement >1 site Serum LDH level >1 × normal	
Risk categories (factors)	**5–10-year overall survival (%)**	**Risk categories (factors)**	**5-year overall survival**
Low (0–1)	90/70	Low (0–1)	73
Intermediate (2)	77/50	Low intermediate (2)	51
High (>3)	52/35	High intermediate (3)	43
		High (4–5)	26

Abbreviations: FLIPI = Follicular lymphoma International prognostic Index; IPI = International prognostic index; LDH = Lactate dehydrogenase
*The nodal categories are cervical, mediastinal, axillary, mesenteric, para-aortic, inguinal, epitrochlear and poplit

Table 170.11: FLIPI2 prognostic index by risk group				
Risk group	**Number of risk factors**	**Percentage of patients (%)**	**3-year PFS rate (%)**	**5-year PFS rate (%)**
Low	0	20	91	80
Intermediate	1–2	53	69	51
High	3–5	27	51	19

Abbreviation: PFS = Progression-free survival

European Burkitt's Lymphoma

It is treated aggressively depending on age. Common treatment available is rituximab in combination with intensive regime cyclophosphamide, vincristine, doxorubicin, high dose methotrexate (CODOX-M) and ifosamide, etoposide and high dose cytarabine (IVAC) alternating regime. These are inpatient-based chemotherapy schedule including cyclophosphamide, doxorubicin, steroids, methotrexate, ifosamide, cytarabine in combination with intrathecal chemotherapy using cytarabine (Fig. 170.11).

OTHER RARE FORMS OF LYMPHOCYTE TUMORS

Angioimmunoblastic Lymphadenopathy (AILD)

This is the result of an immunological disorder seen in patients taking drugs for various conditions. The pathological process suggests a borderline between a reactive condition and a neoplasm.

Histology

The lymph node shows loss of normal architecture, pleomorphic cellular infiltrate consisting of immunoblasts, plasma cells, neutrophils and histiocytes and proliferation of small blood vessels.

Clinical Features

The disease starts as an acute or subacute illness characterized by fever, sweating, weight loss, generalized lymph node enlargement and hepatosplenomegaly. Unlike malignant lymphomas, these patients show rise in polyclonal Igs, specially IgM. If left untreated, many cases end fatally due to infective complications or supervening malignancy. The prognosis in individual cases is unpredictable.

Treatment is effective in one-third of the cases. Corticosteroids, alkylating agents and combination chemotherapy have all been employed with variable results.

Hydantoin-Linked Lymphoma

Syn: Pseudolymphoma

Diphenylhydantoin may produce an allergic response characterized by fever, rash, generalized lymphadenopathy and even splenomegaly resembling AILD. The condition remits fully within months of drug withdrawal (Fig. 170.12).

Mycosis Fungoides

This term has been loosely used by different workers. The consensus is to limit the term to the group showing a classical histological picture. Mycosis fungoides and Sézary's syndrome are T-cell NHLs. These are all rare diseases.

Clinical Features

The onset of the disease may be as a lesion resembling pruritic erythroderma, psoriasis, seborrheic dermatitis, eczema, nonspecific exfoliative dermatitis, lichenoid dermatitis, or neurodermatitis. After several years, plaque formation or tumor formation starts. In some cases, the lesions directly start as tumors which may ulcerate. The skin is red and diffusely thickened. Later, the nails may be affected and they may be lost.

The course of the disease is variable. Tumor-like lesions do worse than lichenoid lesions. Advancing age

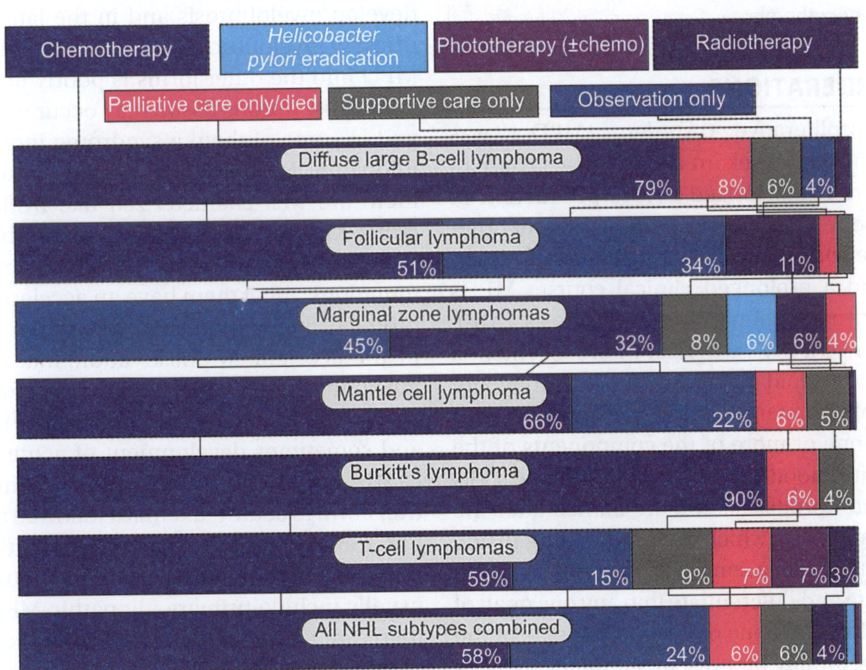

Fig. 170.11: Present treatment modalities given for different types of lymphomas

Abbreviation: NHL = Non-Hodgkin's Lymphoma

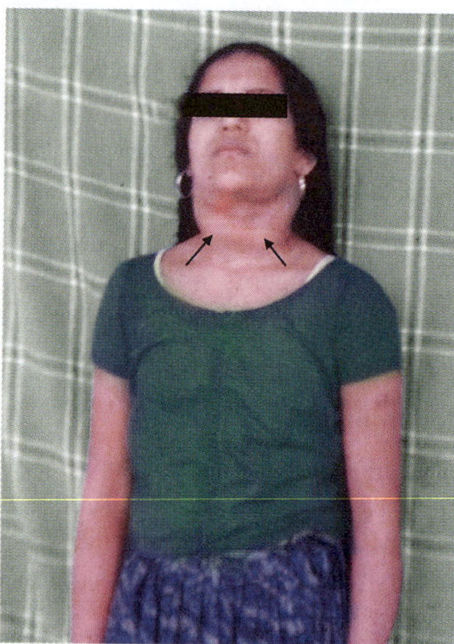

Fig. 170.12: Hydantoin-linked lymphoma. **Note:** The gross lymphadenopathy (arrows), complete resolution with withdrawal of drug

worsens the prognosis. Median survival period is 5 years from diagnosis.

Sézary Syndrome

This is the leukemic phase of mycosis fungoides. It is rare and is characterized by intense pruritus, erythroderma, and later on, enlargement of the liver, spleen and lymph nodes. Skin shows diffuse infiltration by typical *Sézary's cells*. These cells are seen in good numbers in the peripheral blood.

Treatment

The condition responds to alkylating agents like chlorambucil or cyclophosphamide singly. Combination therapy as for NHL has been found beneficial in advanced lesions. Superficial irradiation with rays of low penetrance and surface application of mustine hydrochloride (HN_2) 10 mg dissolved in 60 mL water brings about remission in a good number of cases. Intensive electron beam therapy or photochemotherapy with psoralens and long-wave ultraviolet (UV) light are other modalities employed.

Myeloproliferative Disorders

PK Sasidharan, KV Krishna Das

Chapter Summary

- General Considerations
- Primary Myelofibrosis (PMF)
- Polycythemia Rubra Vera (PV)
- Essential Thrombocythemia

GENERAL CONSIDERATIONS

The term myeloproliferative disorders (MPDs) was coined by William Dameshek in 1951 for a group of neoplastic disorders characterized by overproduction of fibroblasts in the bone marrow or overproduction of other components of the marrow resulting in mature functional blood cells and a prolonged clinical course. MPDs usually include primary idiopathic myelofibrosis (MF), polycythemia rubra vera (PV), essential thrombocythemia (ET) and chronic myeloid leukemia (CML). They are clonal disorders of the stem cells in the marrow with overproduction of one or more of the components of the bone marrow [white blood cells (WBC), red blood cells (RBC), platelets and fibroblasts] and are named after the component or components which are proliferating inside the marrow. They arise from a common precursor stem cell which can proliferate and differentiate into any one or all of these types. Sometimes any one of the components of the marrow or all of them may be present simultaneously as in PV and the component which predominates will decide the clinical presentation too. All of them run an indolent

course and some may show a tendency to transform into one or other type when followed up. All these disorders have some phenotypic similarity. Several patients with ET later on transform to PV; around 30% of cases of PV develop myelofibrosis and in the late stages behave like primary myelofibrosis. What leads to the evolution of one MPD into the other forms is poorly understood. Increase in marrow fibrous tissue may occur with time in PV or ET and in some of them a syndrome indistinguishable from idiopathic MF develops. Genetic mutations in some of them are well-characterized like BCR-ABL in CML and Janus Kinase2 (JAK2) V617F in PV, but in some others there are no definitive well-characterized documented mutations. All of them have an accelerated phase which is probably due to acquisition of additional genetic changes. In the accelerated phase, additional changes occur like myelofibrosis in PV or ET, and a rising total leukocyte count (TLC) with blasts and neutropenia or thrombocytopenia, and sometimes development of acute myeloid leukemia (AML). All these disorders show a higher tendency to transform to acute leukemia if followed up for long periods. But transformation to acute lymphatic leukemia (ALL) is extremely rare in any of these. Though the term MPDs usually include primary idiopathic MF, PV, ET and CML, there are some less common conditions which are also considered as MPDs like systemic mastocytosis, chronic eosinophilic leukemia (CEL), chronic myelomonocytic leukemia (CMML), and chronic neutrophilic leukemia

(CNL). The cardinal features of the main MPDs are an increased WBC count in CML, increased red cell mass in PV, a high platelet count in ET and bone marrow fibrosis in IMF. Since CML is described in Ch 155 this discussion is focusing on the remaining disorders.

After identification of BCR-ABL gene and the role of tyrosine kinase in CML, the Janus kinase 2 (JAK2) mutation is now identified as the genetic marker that is directly associated with the pathogenesis of the MPDs and is emerging as an important tool for analysis of the molecular basis of these disorders. JAK2 is a cytoplasmic tyrosine-kinase and is critical for instigating intracellular signaling by the receptors for erythropoietin (EPO), thrombopoietin (TPO), interleukin-3 (IL-3), granulocyte-colony stimulating factor (G-CSF) and granulocyte-macrophage colony stimulating factor (GM-CSF). JAK2 binds to EPO receptors in the endoplasmic reticulum and aids in their expression on the surface. The JAK2 mutation in MPDs is acquired and it appears to be common to all the MPDs. Experimental evidences have shown that erythroid progenitors from the bone marrow of patients with PV were capable of growing *in vitro* in the absence of EPO.

JAK2 mutation occurs in more than 95% of cases of PV, and in 50–60% of cases of ET and idiopathic MF. The JAK2 mutation is the first detected genetic marker associated with the pathogenesis of MPDs and it has acquired importance in both diagnosis and follow-up and now in therapy as well. The V617F mutation in the JAK gene results in the substitution of phenylalanine for valine at position 617 (hence, called as JAK2 V617F mutation). The causative role of this mutation in the pathogenesis of MPDs is now established. The JAK2 mutation explains many of the cardinal features of MPDs and it can be compared to the role played by BCR-ABL in CML. Mutant JAK2 protein activates multiple downstream signaling pathways with effects on gene transcription, apoptosis, the cell cycle and differentiation. Testing for JAK2 V617F mutation is now widely available and it promises to simplify the diagnostic work up. JAK2 V617F can be identified by allele specific polymerase chain reaction (PCR) assay, pyrosequencing, restriction enzyme digestion and real time PCR. Mouse models of JAK2 V617F mutation have been made by infecting (transfecting) them with a retroviral vector carrying the mutant gene. It has shown all the features of PV. The animals with the mutation have erythrocytosis and leukocytosis and there is evolution to postpolycythemic myelofibrosis. Thrombocytosis is not a reproducible feature in these animal models, perhaps because the high levels of mutant JAK2 generated by the retroviral vector might be inhibiting the differentiation of megakaryocytes. The JAK2 mutation is also assuming importance in classification of MPDs as JAK2 V617F positive and negative MPDs, and determining in targeted therapy. The first JAK2 inhibitor ruxolitinib was launched in 2011. The second JAK2 inhibitor SAR302503 which appears to be more selective is available now and a number of drugs are undergoing trials.

Source: Campbell PJ, Green AR. The myeloproliferative disorders. N Engl J Med. 2006;355(23):2452-66.

PRIMARY MYELOFIBROSIS (MF)

Syn: Chronic idiopathic MF, agnogenic myeloid metaplasia, or myelofibrosis with myeloid metaplasia

It is a neoplastic disorder resulting from clonal expansion of neoplastic multipotent stem cell, characterized by anemia, splenomegaly, mild neutrophilia and thrombocytosis. Peripheral blood shows immature myeloid and erythroid precursors and teardrop-shaped RBCs and bone marrow shows increased reticulin fibers, later developing collagen fibrosis. The characteristic marrow fibrosis is the result of cytokines released locally from abnormally increased number of megakaryocytes derived from the neoplastic clone. But the stromal cells and fibroblasts responsible for increased fibrosis, angiogenesis and new bone formation (osteosclerosis) are not derived from the myeloproliferative clone. The changes in the marrow represent a reaction to cytokines including transforming growth factor-β (TGF-β), basic fibroblast growth factor (bFGF) and vascular endothelial growth factor (VEGF) produced from megakaryocytes and monocytes derived from the neoplastic myeloproliferative clone. There is overproduction of TGF-β and thrombopoietin. As a consequence of proliferation of fibroblasts which replace the marrow with fibrous tissue, there is extramedullary hematopoiesis predominantly in the spleen and liver resulting in moderate to massive splenomegaly and the characteristic leukoerythroblastic blood picture. The etiology of this disorder is not known and there are no specific cytogenetic abnormalities except the JAK2 mutation in 50–60% of cases. Abnormalities like 20q-, 13q- and trisomy-1q are often encountered. Those who are positive for the JAK2 mutations are likely to respond to targeted therapy. The marrow is initially hypercellular with an excess of megakaryocytes and as the disease progresses, the marrow becomes fibrosed and is difficult to aspirate. Before diagnosing idiopathic MF, all the secondary causes of marrow fibrosis have to be excluded. Idiopathic MF is clinically similar to the PV transforming into myelofibrosis (happens in late phases of PV—called as spent phase or accelerated phase of PV) and the diagnostic criteria are similar. For that reason at least some patients who receive the diagnosis of idiopathic MF are having the accelerated phase of previously unrecognized polycythemia or ET.

Causes

- Secondary MF
    - Infections [tuberculosis, human immunodeficiency syndrome (HIV), fungal infections]
    - Lymphomas [Non-Hodgkin's lymphoma (NHL)]
    - Hodgkin's disease
    - Acute leukemia—AML-M7
    - CML
    - PV
    - Systemic mastocytosis
    - Systemic lupus erythematosus (SLE)
    - Hypoparathyroidism
    - Vitamin D deficiency
- Primary myelofibrosis (idiopathic).

In some of the secondary myelofibrosis, clinical features may be present to indicate another disorder, but may not be obvious in hypoparathyroidism and vitamin D deficiency and may look like idiopathic MF only. The so-called idiopathic MF represents the group where the etiology is not obvious or we are in the dark about the true etiology. SLE, chronic infections and other malignancies may be searched for when there are features clinically or when suggested by preliminary evaluation. High index of suspicion and a determined search for secondary causes is essential before labelling a given case of myelofibrosis as primary or idiopathic. In most patients with myelofibrosis irrespective of the etiology, the clinical features are dominated by the cell type causing the marrow fibrosis and the consequent splenomegaly and extramedullary hematopoiesis. Therefore, the clinical features of primary and secondary myelofibrosis may be almost the same in many patients.

Clinical Features of Primary Myelofibrosis

Most patients are over the age of 50 years and they usually come to medical attention for anemia and symptoms due to splenomegaly which is often moderate or massive even at presentation. A dragging sensation in the left upper abdomen or early satiety due to enlarged spleen is a common presentation of the disorder. Symptoms due to anemia may be bringing some patients to clinical attention. Other associated symptoms like fatigue, tiredness, weight loss, night sweats and sometimes low-grade fever due to the hypercatabolic state may also be the presenting symptoms. Many patients are apparently asymptomatic and come to attention due to incidentally detected splenomegaly or abnormal blood counts during a routine examination. Severe left upper quadrant or left shoulder pain due to splenic infarction and persplenitis can occur and sometimes this is what brings the patient to clinical attention. Symptoms of hyperuricemia may develop. The anemia is caused by replacement of the hematopoietic tissue, ineffective erythropoiesis and hypersplenism. Sometimes portal hypertension may develop due to the excessive blood flow through the portal veins from an enlarged spleen. Mild hepatomegaly is also common due to extramedullary hematopoiesis. Other rare sites for extramedullary hematopoiesis include lymph nodes, pleura (resulting in pleural effusion) or peritoneum (leading to ascites) or in paraspinal or epidural spaces with resultant spinal cord or nerve root compression.

Diagnosis

The erythrocytes show marked anisocytosis and poikilocytosis with polychromasia and characteristic **tear drop** cells. Most patients have elevated WBC count at presentation with a leukoerythroblastic blood picture with shift to left suggesting extramedullary hematopoiesis (Fig. 171.1). WBC count can sometimes be normal or even decreased due to hypersplenism. Thrombocytosis can occur in some, suggesting ET or polycythemia with myelofibrosis but others may have normal or even decreased platelet counts. Megakaryocytic fragments may be seen in peripheral blood.

Bone marrow examination is essential to establish the diagnosis. Bone marrow aspiration often results in dry tap. Trephine biopsy of the bone marrow reveals

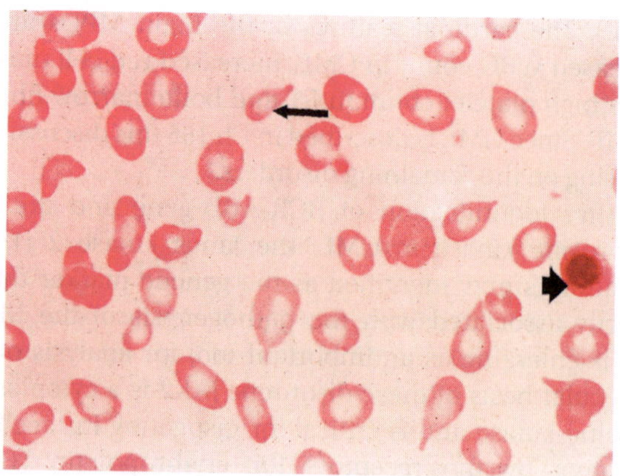

Fig. 171.1: Peripheral smear in myelofibrosis. **Note:** The tear drop cell (arrow). Normoblast (arrowhead)

cellular marrow with granulocytic and megakaryocytic hyperplasia, dysplastic changes in the megakaryocytes and osteosclerosis. When the fibrosis is intense, the cellularity may be decreased but megakaryocytes are prominently present. Foci of extramedullary hematopoiesis can be demonstrated in the spleen, liver and rarely lymph nodes. Radiographs of bones show osteosclerosis with obliteration of marrow cavity. Changes are most markedly seen in the vertebrae, shafts of long bones of the extremities, ribs, clavicles and pelvis. Hyperuricemia and secondary gout can occur due to the hypermetabolic state. Leukocyte alkaline phosphatase (LAP) is high.

Differential Diagnosis

Myelofibrosis should be considered when there is leukoerythroblastic blood picture and massive spleno-megaly. But in myelofibrosis, the WBC counts are only moderately elevated and the counts are usually less than 30,000/mm^3; in CML, the WBC count is usually greater than 50,000/mm^3; but in the early stages of CML, the counts can be lower but at this stage, the spleen may be absent or only just palpable. The hallmark of myelofibrosis at any stage is splenomegaly. When the WBC count is more than 50,000/mm^3 usually it is unlikely to be primary myelofibrosis. In addition, in CML, the spleen size has linear correlation to WBC count. When the spleen is massive, a WBC count of 30,000/mm^3 or less in an untreated case is almost unlikely to be CML. Besides CML all the other conditions with a leukoerythroblastic blood picture need to be excluded by clinical and appropriate laboratory evaluation. When hypersplenism dominates they may present with pancytopenia and if so all the causes of pancytopenia with splenomegaly come in the differential diagnosis; one must remember here that the common causes of pancytopenia does not have splenomegaly. Therefore, this situation has to be differentiated only from the conditions with splenomegaly and pancytopenia-including severe portal hypertension with hypersplenism, hairy cell leukemia, splenic lymphomas and even kala-azar. The overall clinical picture and bone marrow help to differentiate primary MF from all these disorders. With pancytopenia, splenomegaly and myelofibrosis in the marrow, all the secondary causes of myelofibrosis have to be ruled out. Primary autoimmune myelofibrosis is to be considered if it is a young patient, especially young female. Even if it is a definite case of myelofibrosis after evaluation and looks like idiopathic, all the secondary causes of myelofibrosis are to be carefully looked for and excluded before considering it as idiopathic MF. It is important to have good clinical evaluation and clinical judgment to arrive at the correct diagnosis rather than depending blindly on laboratory features alone. In the Medical College Hospital, Kozhikode, by careful clinical examination and appropriate laboratory work up we could pick up cases of vitamin D deficiency, hypoparathyroidism, SLE, polyarteritis nodosa (PAN), kala-azar, tuberculosis and lymphoma presenting as myelofibrosis.

Prognosis

Prognosis is good in most cases and they can be managed with supportive measures for more than 10 years but the survival is shorter than that for PV and ET. With advanced age, anemia and WBC counts more than 30000/mm^3 and blasts in peripheral blood, the survival may be much less (1–2 years). Survival is not related to the degree of splenomegaly. The common disease-related cause of death is leukemic transformation which usually occurs after 10 years, or death could be due to the secondary effects of the cytopenias.

Treatment

About 30% of patients remain asymptomatic for years without any form of treatment. Symptomatic anemia, symptomatic thrombocytopenia and huge splenomegaly need treatment. EPO may help sometimes, but the anemia is usually due to ineffective erythropoiesis and hypersplenism and this may not respond to EPO. Androgens have also been used to correct anemia. Hydroxyurea given in doses of 500 mg daily or up to three times a day is used to control leukocytosis, thrombocytosis and organomegaly. Packed red cell transfusions may be given to correct severe anemia. Splenectomy may be required when the splenomegaly causes disabling symptoms or when there is severe hypersplenism. Splenectomy will be followed by rebound thrombocytosis and progressive hepatomegaly and sometimes extra-medullary hematopoiesis at unusual sites including lymph nodes. Allopurinol has to be used in doses of 100 mg tid to control hyperuricemia. Glucocorticoids are useful when there are coexisting autoimmune phenomena, such as hemolysis, thrombocytopenia, Sweet's syndrome or if autoimmunity is suspected as the primary cause of myelofibrosis. Treatment is thus mainly supportive or palliative, with supplementation of folic acid and at times, pyridoxine. Thalidomide given in doses of 100 mg daily produces benefit in anemia and thrombocytopenia. Bone marrow transplantation (BMT) may be beneficial in 50–60% of young patients.

With the discovery of JAK2 mutation and the availability of specific inhibitors of JAK-STAT pathways, there is some promise in the treatment. Ruxolitinib (also known as INC424 or INCB18424) is an orally administered potent and selective inhibitor of JAK1 and JAK2 that is approved for the treatment of intermediate and high-risk myelo-fibrosis. Ruxolitinib selectively inhibits the proliferation of JAK2 V617F-driven Ba/F3 cells and these effects are correlated with decreased levels of phosphorylated JAK2 and of signal transducer and activator of transcription 5 (STAT5). Ruxolitinib used at a median dose of 30 mg/day orally has shown promising results as compared with patients receiving the best available therapy (hydroxyurea and glucocorticoids). Continuous ruxolitinib therapy has shown marked and durable reduction in splenomegaly and disease-related symptoms, improvements in quality of life with modest toxic effects. But it has failed to show an influence on overall survival. Various causes of secondary myelofibrosis are given in Table 171.1.

Table 171.1: Causes of secondary myelofibrosis

Malignant conditions	Nonmalignant conditions

• Hematological
  ▪ Leukemia
    – Acute leukemia (lymphoid/myeloid)
    – Chronic myeloid leukemia
    – Hairy cell leukemia
  ▪ Multiple myeloma
  ▪ Polycythemia vera
  ▪ Hodgkin's lymphoma
  ▪ Essential thrombocytosis
• Nonhematological
  ▪ Metastasis to marrow
    – Carcinoma breast, lung or prostate
    – Neuroblastoma
	• Infections
	  ▪ HIV infection
	  ▪ Tuberculosis
	• Exposure to thorium dioxide
	• Systemic lupus erythematosus
	• Renal osteodystrophy
	• Hyperparathyroidism
	• Radiation therapy or treatment with radiomimetic drugs
	• Gaucher disease

Abbreviation: HIV = Human immunodeficiency syndrome

Source:

1. Verstovsek S, Mesa RA, Gotlib J, et al. A double-blind, placebo-controlled trial of ruxolitinib for myelofibrosis. N Engl J Med. 2012;366(9):799-807.
2. Verstovsek S, Kantarjian H, Mesa RA, et al. Safety and efficacy of INCB018424, a JAK1 and JAK2 inhibitor, in myelofibrosis. N Engl J Med. 2010;363:(12):1117-27.

POLYCYTHEMIA RUBRA VERA (PV)

Syn: Erythremia, Vaquez's disease, Osler's disease, cryptogenic polycythemia

The word *polycythemia* indicates presence of excess of all three cellular components of blood namely RBCs, WBCs and platelets. In adult men, hemoglobin level more than 17 g/dL or packed cell volume (PCV) more than 50% can be taken as abnormal. In females, the corresponding values are hemoglobin level more than 16 g/dL and PCV more than 45%. Polycythemia may be true or apparent. In true polycythemia, there is increase in red cell mass. Apparent polycythemia occurs when there is an acute reduction in plasma volume following severe dehydration, as happens in diarrhea, vomiting, use of diuretics, capillary leak syndromes and in severe burns.

Polycythemia may be primary or secondary. The latter is more common. When polycythemia occurs in the absence of any physiological stimulus or without a pathological increase in EPO, it is called as primary polycythemia and the most common form of primary polycythemia is PV. This is one of the MPDs.

Secondary polycythemia (erythrocytosis) occurs mainly due to increased amounts of EPO secreted as a physiological response to hypoxic stimulus, or abnormal secretion of EPO from the kidneys or from ectopic foci. Rarely, the erythroid progenitors in the bone marrow may respond in an exaggerated manner to normal levels of EPO. All these constitute secondary erythrocytosis (referred by some authors as secondary polycythemia).

Causes of Secondary Polycythemia (Erythrocytosis)

EPO-Mediated Hypoxia Driven

- Chronic lung diseases leading to hypoxemia
- Chronic carbon monoxide exposure (including cigarette smoking)
- Right to left cardiac shunts
- High altitudes above 2,500 meters
- Hypoventilation syndromes including extreme obesity
- Sleep apnea
- Dysfunction of the respiratory center
- Renal artery stenosis
- High affinity hemoglobin (autosomal dominant) with defective oxygen unloading in the tissues
- Defective oxygen delivery by erythrocytes having deficiency of 2,3-diphosphoglycerate (DPG).

Pathologic EPO Production

- Malignant tumors producing excessive EPO
  - Hepatocellular carcinoma
  - Renal cell cancer
  - Cerebellar hemangioblastoma
- Nonmalignant conditions
  - Uterine leiomyoma
  - Renal cysts
  - Hydronephrosis
  - Adrenal tumors
  - Atrial myxoma
  - Postrenal transplantation.

Miscellaneous Causes

- Androgen over use (specially in hypogonad states), EPO abuse
- Familial polycythemia (autosomal dominant).

Pathogenesis of PRV

The EPO-independent proliferation of multipotent stem cells occurs possibly due to an aberrant signal transduction pathway resulting from mutation in JAK gene (JAK2). The root cause behind the causative mutation is not clear but it certainly lies in lifestyle, diet and environment, issues which we fail to identify. Because of the mutation, there is clonal expansion of multipotent hematopoietic stem cells (HSCs) resulting in overproduction of phenotypically normal RBCs, WBCs and platelets without any physiologic stimulus. The V617F mutation which causes the substitution of phenylalanine for valine at position 617 of the JAK gene is present in 95% of patients with PV. It is also seen in 50–60% of ET and IMF. Upregulation of the JAK2 pathway by natural mutation is a major cause of PV and ET. ***Though PV can be diagnosed with accuracy almost always using clinical skills, JAK2 mutation now defines this distinctive myeloproliferative syndrome.*** JAK2 gene is a signal transduction molecule which influences several cytokine receptors including receptors for EPO. This gene encodes a cytoplasmic tyrosine kinase and the mutation (JAK2 gene V617F mutation), increases JAK2 kinase activity and causes cytokine-independent growth of cell lines and cultured bone marrow cells, allowing the erythroid precursors to grow even in the absence of EPO. Mutant JAK2 transfected into murine (mouse) bone marrow cells produces erythrocytosis and subsequent myelofibrosis in recipient animals, suggesting a causal role for the mutation. PCR can be used to detect the V617F mutation in peripheral blood nucleated cells. By an unknown mechanism, there is suppression of proliferation of the normal stem cells and hence, the formed elements in the patients represent the progeny of the transformed clone. The bone marrow is apparently normal, but there is increase in number of all cellular elements. Two phases of the disease can be seen. The initial one is of cellular proliferation. The latter is one of cytopenias with ineffective hematopoiesis, marrow fibrosis and hypersplenism resembling idiopathic MF (spent phase).

Clinical Features

Usually PV occurs in people above 40 years. The symptoms are vague and are produced by problems related to high blood volume and viscosity of blood and consequent sluggish blood flow to various organs. These include lassitude, loss of concentration, dizziness, vertigo, tinnitus, heaviness of head or headaches and visual disturbances. Sometimes they may present with complications like vaso-occlusive events. These include digital ischemia in upper or lower limbs, cerebral vein thrombosis transient ischemic attack (TIA) or stroke occurring in any territory, myocardial infarction (MI), deep vein thrombosis (DVT) with or without pulmonary embolism (PE), Budd-Chiari syndrome and portal vein thrombosis. Any one of the above problems may bring the patient with high hemoglobin of any etiology to clinical attention and proper clinical examination can pick up the features of high hemoglobin as well as the causes almost always. Easy bruising, epistaxis and gastrointestinal (GI) hemorrhage due to peptic ulceration may be the presenting symptoms in PV. Hypermetabolic state can give rise to weight loss, fatigue, night sweats or hyperuricemia with features of secondary gout or even renal calculi. A symptom that is more specific for PV is pruritus exacerbated by water contact (aquagenic pruritus).

On examination, there is congestion of conjunctiva and palms which are striking even in dark subjects but ruddy complexion may be more obvious only in fair skinned individuals. Systemic hypertension may be present, if present it should lead to search for renal causes of polycythemia (e.g. renal artery stenosis, adult polycystic kidney disease, nephrocalcinosis, hydronephrosis and others) before accepting it as due to PV. Splenomegaly if present helps to differentiate from secondary causes. But splenomegaly may rarely be due to portal hypertension in a patient with other causes of polycythemia. While evaluating a patient with polycythemia or suspected polycythemia, look for features of the known secondary causes for high hemoglobin before considering PV. Absence of features of secondary polycythemia should arouse suspicion of PV. Proper clinical examination and appropriate investigations done in time help to make the diagnosis early in most cases.

Diagnosis

Features that Support the Diagnosis of PV

- Abnormal increase in hemoglobin (above 17 g/dL) and erythrocyte count (> 6.5 million/mm^3) and increase red cell mass (hematocrit > 55%)
- Polycythemia without any known secondary cause
- Splenomegaly
- Elevated WBC count > 12×10^9/L
- Increased basophil count
- Thrombocytosis > 400×10^9/L
- Elevated serum uric acid levels
- Elevated LAP levels (no practical use)
- Elevated serum vitamin B_{12} and vitamin B_{12}-binding protein levels are often seen (no practical use).

Clinical differentiation between PV and secondary polycythemia is shown in Table 171.2.

Note: Very rarely PV can coexist with iron deficiency anemia (IDA) and then, the hemoglobin will not be as high as expected; with massive splenomegaly also hemoglobin may not be high.

Clinically, polycythemia is suspected based on symptoms and signs. Estimation of hemoglobin, PCV and red cell count confirms erythrocytosis/polycythemia. In those with massive splenomegaly, at times the hematocrit values may be normal due to pooling of blood in the spleen. Normal hemoglobin levels in the presence of moderate or massive splenomegaly is an indirect evidence of increased red cell mass. Presence of elevated platelet count and neutrophil count or both without any obvious cause support the diagnosis of PV. Elevated uric acid levels can serve as indirect marker in an appropriate clinical setting. Presence of JAK2 V617F is highly suggestive of PV since it is positive in about 95% of cases. Only less than 5% of cases of PV are negative for this mutation.

Bone marrow study is not required unless myelofibrosis or leukemic transformation is to be excluded. In uncomplicated PV, bone marrow is hypercellular with less of fat spaces and showing marked increase in all the three elements—erythroid, myeloid and megakaryocytic cells. Unlike as in leukemia, the cells are morphologically and immunologically normal. LAP is increased in many. Serum vitamin B_{12} levels and vitamin B_{12} binding protein are elevated but their diagnostic significance is not specific. In the presence of massive splenomegaly, estimation of red cell mass may be needed to differentiate PV from primary myelofibrosis. In the absence of secondary causes for erythrocytosis, presence of the JAK2 mutation is sufficient for a firm diagnosis. For practical purposes until we have an effective targeted therapy against JAK2 kinase, even PCR for JAK2 mutation need not be done routinely for managing these cases since the molecular tests are expensive.

Course and Prognosis

Prognosis is good and majority lives more than 10 years after diagnosis; many live up to 20 years or more. Thrombotic complications occurring in vital tissues may contribute to morbidity and mortality. Death may occur due to fatal thrombosis or hemorrhage and due to leukemic transformation into acute myeloid leukemia or sometimes due to unrelated causes. Secondary myelofibrosis may develop in some on follow-up, with the patient developing cytopenias, massive splenomegaly and intense marrow fibrosis (burned out phase or spent phase of PV).

Treatment

Aims of management include reduction of the red cell mass and thrombocytosis to near normal levels, avoidance of thrombotic complications and reassuring the patient and relatives about the benign nature of the disease; helping the patient and family to learn to live with the disease and to have a near normal life. Counseling and education of the patient and relatives should be part of the management as in any other chronic conditions. Thrombotic complications are prevented by maintaining the hemoglobin at around 15 g/dL (PCV 45%) in males and around 14 g/dL (PCV 42%) in females. This is achieved by repeated venesections (300–400 mL) weekly in the initial stages, sufficient to induce a state of iron deficiency and thereafter, done less frequently (once in 3 months or so). After venesection, the blood volume has to be made up by equal volume of suitable intravenous (IV) fluid (5% dextrose or normal saline depending on the patient characteristics). Anticoagulants and aspirin are relatively contraindicated in these patients for control of thrombotic tendency but may be given if the situation warrants. The importance of adequate hydration (an intake of around 2 L of water per day) is important to prevent thrombotic complications and complications due to hyperuricemia. Allopurinol is also given in doses of 100 mg tid to control hyperuricemia.

Hydroxyurea can be used to reduce or avoid venesections and to control the splenomegaly and extreme thrombocytosis (keeping platelets at around 400,000/mm^3 and the TLC above 3500/mm^3). If the patient is accepting venesections, it is better than treatment with hydroxyurea. Sometimes both venesection and hydroxuurea may be

Feature	Polycythemia vera	Secondary Polycythemia
Oxygen saturation	Normal	Low
EPO (erythropoietin) levels	Decreased	Increased
Blood counts		
Total white cell count	Increased	Normal
Absolute basophil count	Increased	Normal
Platelet count	Increased	Normal
Leukocyte alkaline phosphatase (LAP)	Raised	Normal
Vitamin B_{12} levels	Increased	Normal
Bone marrow	Trilineage (panhyperplasia)	Erythroid hyperplasia
Splenomegaly	Present	Absent

Table 171.2: Clinical differentiation between polycythemia vera and secondary polycythemia

Textbook of Medicine

combined. If there is severe thrombocytosis (levels above 600,000/mm³), hydroxyurea 500 mg one to three times a day may have to be used along with antiplatelet, drugs like aspirin 75 mg/day. Anagrelide can also be used to lower platelet levels at a dose of 0.5 mg daily, but the drug is not superior to hydroxyurea, it is expensive and not freely available in India. Besides the above measures, modifying diet and lifestyle is very important. Ensure adequate water intake and a well-balanced diet in moderation including fruits and vegetables. If the diagnosis of PV was not firmly established or was doubtful, at each follow-up visit it is essential to look for secondary causes including neoplasms which can lead to secondary polycythemia.

Source: Marchioli R, Finazzi G, Specchia G, et al. Cardiovascular events and the intensity of treatment in Polycythemia Vera. N Engl J Med. 2013;368(1):22-33.

Ruxolitinib

It has been found to be useful in treating PV when other treatment do not achieve full remission. It controls the blood counts and all other clinical and laboratory characteristics. The dose is 20 mg twice daily if platelet count is > 200,000/mm³; 15 mg twice daily if the platelet count is between 100,000/mm³ and 200,000/mm³ and 5 mg daily if the count is between 50,000/mm³ and 100,000/mm³.

CHUVASH polycythemia is rare congenital polycythemia caused by homozygous.

R 200W (C598C → T) germline mutation in the von Hippel Lindaw gene (VHL). Symptoms resemble polycythemia vera, with similar complications and early death JAK1 and JAK2 inhibitor. Ruxolitinib given in doses of 5 mg bd orally measured up to 20 mg bd gives relief. Short-term follow up shows continued benefit.

ESSENTIAL THROMBOCYTHEMIA

Syn: Primary idiopathic thrombocytosis, hemorrhagic thrombocythemia, megakaryocytic myelosis

It is a clonal disorder of unknown etiology with cytogenetic abnormalities. There is primary proliferation of megakaryocytes in the marrow, producing apparently normal platelets but having some functional abnormalities which can predispose to either thrombosis or hemorrhage. Increased thrombotic risk in the MPDs is not exclusively due to thrombocytosis or erythrocytosis alone; it is also due to interactions among white cells, platelets, endothelium and other proteins in blood and the status of hydration. It is important to look for all the causes of secondary thrombocytosis before considering ET. Physiological thrombocytosis, mediated by thrombopoietin usually occurs as a response to infections, chronic inflammatory disorders, connective tissue disorders (CTDs), posthemorrhagic states and iron deficiency anemia (IDA) in association with some malignancies or after splenectomy. Thrombocytosis occurring in the absence of any such physiologic stimulus by thrombopoietin is called essential thrombocytosis or ET. This is a myeloproliferative disorder. Apparently, normal looking platelets are seen on the peripheral smear, no specific platelet function defects have been

documented in spite of the bleeding tendency which they may develop at times. Bone marrow biopsy is not required for diagnosis but it usually shows megakaryocyte hyperplasia and sometimes myelofibrosis. Clonal abnormalities of the JAK2 gene (JAK2 V617F) are demonstrable in 50–60% of cases. In the absence of secondary causes, in patients with thrombocytosis, the presence of JAK2 mutation is strongly diagnostic of ET.

Causes of Thrombocytosis

Reactive Thrombocytosis

- Transient
  - Acute blood loss
  - Recovery (***rebound***) from thrombocytopenia
  - Acute infection or inflammation
  - Response to exercise
- Persistent
  - Iron deficiency
  - Hemolytic anemia
  - Asplenia (e.g. after splenectomy)
  - Malignancies, e.g. lymphoma
  - Chronic infections like tuberculosis
  - Vasculitic disorders/CTDs
  - Inflammatory bowel disease
  - Chronic pneumonitis
  - Drug reactions
  - Vincristine
  - All trans-retinoic acid
  - Cytokines ⎤ IL-1, IL-6 C-reactive protein (CRP), granulocyte-colony stimulating factor (G-CSF), granulocyte-macrophage colony-stimulating factor (GM-CSF), all can lead to thrombocytosis
  - Growth factors ⎦

Neoplastic Thrombocytosis

- CML
- PV
- Myelofibrosis
- ET

Clinical Features

It is an uncommon disease seen in adults and older individuals. Patient may present with arterial or venous thrombosis at different sites. These include cerebrovascular accidents, ischemic heart disease (IHD), cerebral cortical vein thrombosis or digital ischemia and gangrene (Fig. 171.2) often mistaken for vasculitis. Hemorrhagic manifestations like mucocutaneous bleeding, easy bruising, epistaxis or GI hemorrhage may occur. Thrombotic complications are more common in patients above 60 years of age and those with previous episodes of vascular complications. Hemorrhage is more common in those with extreme thrombocythemia. Sometimes the disorder is identified when very high platelet count (> 600,000/mm³) is reported on routine investigations for other conditions. Physical findings are usually unremarkable, but sometimes mild splenomegaly may be seen. These are often those patients who are

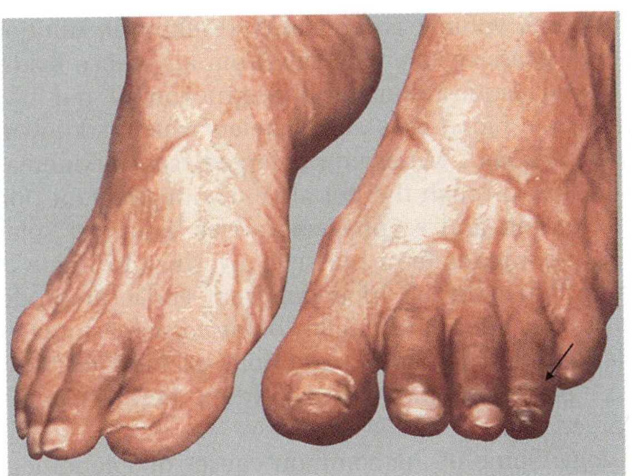

Fig. 171.2: Digital gangrene on the foot due to arterial thrombosis in essential thrombocythemia (arrow)

evolving into PV or have coexisting myelofibrosis. Diagnosis is established by the presence of sustained elevation of platelet counts, usually above 600,000/mm³ without any underlying cause on evaluation and a period of follow-up. In patients with unexplained thrombocytosis presence of JAK2 suggests diagnosis of ET or another MPDs. Patients with ET who are positive for JAK2 V617F mutation are more sensitive to hydroxyurea (but not to anagrelide) than patients who are JAK2, V617F negative.

The course of the disorder is generally benign but occasionally they can have serious complications caused by thrombosis or hemorrhage. The prognosis for survival is good and rarely the disease may transform into PV, idiopathic MF or megakaryocytic leukemia.

Treatment

Asymptomatic patients below 45 years of age with platelet counts below 500,000/mm³ have very low risk of thrombotic episodes. Such patients can be kept under observation without active treatment. Treatment is indicated only when the platelet count goes very high or if clinical features are attributable to the elevated platelet count. Hydroxyurea is effective in reducing the platelet count when given in doses of 1–2 g/day orally. Alpha interferon (α-IFN), given subcutaneously in doses of 25 million units/week in divided doses and tapered off to 8.5 million units/week, is effective in bringing down the platelet count. Anagrelide given in a dose of 0.5 mg daily is an alternative. Both these drugs are more expensive. Low dose aspirin (50–75 mg oral daily) may have to be used to prevent thrombotic tendencies. All the other contributory factors for thrombotic risk need to be addressed and treatment has to be individualized. With the success story of imatinib therapy in CML, now the trend is to develop JAK2 inhibitors which are known to reduce the growth of JAK2 V617F-positive cell lines. Since there are no satisfactory treatments at the moment, they are particularly useful in those patients in accelerated phase, including those with myelofibrosis. In future, JAK 2 inhibitors may prove useful in reducing the risk of vascular events and progression of the disease.

Spleen and its Disorders

CHAPTER
172

Spleen and its Disorders

KV Krishna Das, PK Sasidharan

Chapter Summary
- Functions of the Spleen
- Splenomegaly
  - Hypersplenism
- Tropical Splenomegaly Syndrome
- Hyposplenism

FUNCTIONS OF THE SPLEEN

The spleen is located in the left upper quadrant of the abdomen between the fundus of the stomach and diaphragm and is covered by peritoneum (splenic capsule) all around except at the hilum where the blood vessels enter and leave. Around 10% of people have one or more accessory spleens of around 1 cm size, resembling lymph nodes, located usually near the splenic hilum or near tail of pancreas. Splenic artery and vein are located at the hilum; after the splenic artery pierces the splenic capsule at the hilum, it divides into progressively smaller branches and each branch is called a central artery which is situated at the center of the white pulp; surrounding the central artery is the periarterial lymphoid sheath and around this is the marginal zone which together constitute the white pulp, and surrounding the marginal zone is the red pulp. Spleen is made up of collections of lymphocytes in the white pulp which is composed more of white cells and perform the functions of humoral and cellular immunity, and the red pulp contains more of red blood cells and reticuloendothelial cells (macrophages) performing phagocytic function. A major function of spleen is to remove worn out, damaged or potentially dangerous cells from the bloodstream. It has to be enlarged two to three times the normal size to become distinctly palpable.

White Pulp

This contains lymphocytes and plasma cells that surround the central artery branching off from the splenic artery, each central artery is surrounded by a cuff of lymphocytes (periarterial lymphoid sheath) which are mostly CD4+

T-cells and some memory B-cells. The marginal zone is the area surrounding the periarterial lymphoid sheath; the marginal zone surrounds the white pulp and contains predominantly B-cells, marginal zone is part of the white pulp and it merges imperceptibly into the red pulp which is surrounding the white pulp.

Red Pulp

It is composed of a reticular meshwork of sinuses which surrounds the white pulp and it contains predominantly erythrocytes, but has in addition large number of macrophages and dendritic cells. Spleen serves the following immunological function:

- Spleen is the major site of immune response to blood-borne antigens, whereas lymph nodes are involved mostly in dealing with antigens present in the lymph. The splenic lymphoid tissue gives an environment in which the cells of the immune system (B-cells, T-cells and the macrophages) can interact with one another and with circulating antigens to develop an immune response. T-cell, B-cell interaction is facilitated by the special anatomical configuration. It produces antibodies to circulating antigens from the germinal centers of the white pulp. Milieu of the germinal center provides specific conditions for initiating and halting the production of highly specific clinically protective antibodies by B-lymphocytes.
- *Phagocytic function:* The cells of the red pulp remove aged red cells, abnormally-shaped or damaged or rigid or antibody coated or parasitized red cell, this is called culling. The anatomy of the spleen allows marginal zone and red pulp to cull defective erythrocytes. The phagocytes situated here remove the intraerythrocytic inclusion or nuclear remnants such as Howell-Jolly bodies, and Heinz bodies by a process called pitting. Presence of numerous erythrocytes containing Howell-Jolly bodies would indicate the absence of splenic function. In the splenectomized subject, macrophages of the liver, lymph nodes and bone marrow take over most of these functions.
- The spleen acts as a reservoir for the formed elements of blood and these are released into the general circulation in times of stress. About one-third of the total platelet pool is stored in the spleen. Normal lifespan of platelets is only 9 days and out of this one-third is spent in the spleen. Splenectomy leads to thrombocytosis which may persist for several weeks, sometimes even up to years.
- Hematopoiesis occurs in the spleen normally in fetal life. When there is impairment of normal marrow activity, the spleen takes over hematopoiesis (extramedullary hematopoiesis) but this cannot replace normal hematopoiesis.

SPLENOMEGALY

Various conditions lead to splenomegaly in the tropics. Size of the enlarged spleen is variable and when it is gross, the spleen may even fill almost the whole abdomen. An enlarged spleen can sequester up to 2–30% of the total red cell mass. In splenomegaly, proportionately more red cells are sequestered as compared to plasma and hence the plasma volume is increased, resulting in dilutional anemia. Massive splenomegaly from any cause leads to increased sequestration and destruction of red blood cells, white blood cells and platelets which is known as *hypersplenism*. Massively enlarged spleen increases blood flow through the portal vein with resultant portal hypertension and esophageal varices. Enlarged spleen, when it is moderate or massive, gives rise to vague dull aching pain in the left upper quadrant, and it can produce early satiety due to the inability of the adjacent stomach to distend on taking food. In addition, splenic infarcts with severe pain are commonly seen when there is massively enlarged spleen.

Etiology: Some of the common causes of splenomegaly are listed below:

- *Chronic infections:* Malaria, visceral leishmaniasis, trypanosomiasis, disseminated tuberculosis, brucellosis and systemic mycotic infections. In some of these conditions, the spleen is considerably enlarged and generally firm in consistency. In chronic malaria and visceral leishmaniasis, the spleen may be massively enlarged.
- *Acute infections:* Septicemia, enteric fever, infectious mononucleosis, subacute endocarditis, relapsing fevers, typhus and viral hepatitis, the spleen shows only mild enlargement and is often soft.
- *Venous congestion:* Portal hypertension, splenic vein thrombosis, chronic right-sided heart failure as in chronic constrictive pericarditis and endomyocardial fibrosis. In portal hypertension due to extrahepatic portal vein obstruction, spleen enlarges considerably. Portal hypertension due to cirrhosis of liver usually causes only mild or moderate splenomegaly.
- *Hematological neoplasia:* Chronic leukemias, specially chronic myelogenous leukemia (CML), myelofibrosis, acute leukemias (specially acute lymphoblastic leukemia), lymphomas and polycythemia vera. Massive splenomegaly occurs in CML, myelofibrosis, hairy cell leukemia and primary splenic lymphomas.
- *Reactive splenomegaly with reticuloendothelial hyperplasia:* Hemolytic anemias, ineffective erythropoiesis (vitamin B_{12} deficiency, congenital dyserythropoiesis), thalassemia and hereditary spherocytosis, sickle cell disease and other hemoglobinopathies, bone marrow infiltrating disorders (myelophthisic conditions), tropical splenomegaly and acquired hypogammaglobulinemia.
- *Granulomatous disorders:* Felty's syndrome, SLE, sarcoidosis and berylliosis.
- *Infiltrative disorders:* Lipid storage disease, amyloidosis, histiocytosis and gargoylism.

Note: Several other conditions are also present which produce varying grades of splenomegaly.

Hypersplenism

The spleen is involved in removing aged and abnormal cells from blood and removing intraerythrocytic inclusion bodies (culling and pitting). It sequesters approximately one-third of normal platelet pool. Exaggeration of this normal function can occur in any condition with splenomegaly. Hypersplenism is characterized by the occurrence of anemia, leukopenia and thrombocytopenia (pancytopenia) in a patient with moderate or massive splenomegaly of any etiology. The bone marrow is active and hypercellular. When the splenic size is increased there is increased pooling of blood in an environment with relatively decreased availability of nutrients, but is full of phagocytes, leading to exaggerated sequestration and destruction of cells. In other words, hypersplenism is an exaggeration of its normal filtration and phagocytic function. In addition there may be humoral factors depressing cell maturation as well. The cytopenia recovers promptly on splenectomy. But the thrombocytopenia of chronic liver disease, even in the presence of portal hypertension results primarily from failure of thrombopoeitin synthesis and secretion, and folic acid deficiency. At times, it may be due to immune mechanisms. Splenectomy may be of little benefit in this setting.

Causes of Hypersplenism

All causes of moderate to massive splenomegaly of long duration like portal hypertension, splenic lymphomas, tropical splenomegaly syndrome, myelofibrosis, hemolytic anemias, chronic infection and hairy cell leukemia may lead to this situation.

Treatment

If the pancytopenia is severe or when there is increased need for repeated blood transfusions splenectomy is indicated, irrespective of the cause; the prognosis is decided by the original cause of splenomegaly.

TROPICAL SPLENOMEGALY SYNDROME

The condition is characterized by persistent splenomegaly without any other cause in some residents of malaria endemic areas of tropical Africa and Asia. Probably it is due to an abnormal immunological response to repeated malarial infections. Malarial parasites are not seen in blood, liver or spleen but there is lymphocytic infiltration of splenic sinusoids and they show high titers of immunoglobulin M (IgM) malarial antibody. Anemia and sometimes pancytopenia may occur due to hypersplenism as in any other cause of splenomegaly.

Treatment

Those in endemic areas should receive chemoprophylaxis with proguanil and those who migrate to nonendemic areas should receive antimalarial treatment.

HYPOSPLENISM

This term denotes the condition that develops after splenectomy or after splenic atrophy. As a consequence, alterations of cellular and humoral immunity may develop.

Causes of Hyposplenism

- **Asplenia:** Congenital—may be associated with fatal cardio-vascular anomalies.
- Splenectomy splenic atrophy/or loss of spleen
  - Infarction as in severe sickle cell disease
  - Injury
  - Irradiation

Splenic atrophy is common in sickle cell disease due to repeated splenic infarctions. Rarely ulcerative colitis, Crohn's disease and adult celiac disease may be associated with splenic atrophy.

Diagnosis

The hematologic features include presence of large number of target cells and Howell-Jolly bodies which are normally removed by the phagocytes in the spleen. Moderate leukocytosis and thrombocytosis are present. Diagnosis is based on clinical suspicion and hematological features.

Complications

Splenectomy or asplenia predisposes to infection by capsulated organisms like *Streptococcus pneumoniae*, *Haemophilus influenzae* and meningococci. Children are more susceptible. Protozoal infections such as malaria, babesiosis and toxoplasmosis are also more common.

Management

Asplenic patients should receive bactericidal antibiotics active against pneumococci and *Haemophilus influenzae*, at least at the first sign of infection. Prophylactic vaccination against pneumococcus and *Haemophilus influenzae* is mandatory.

CHAPTER
173

Hemostasis: General Considerations

Mathew Thomas, KV Krishna Das

Chapter Summary

- Normal Hemostasis
- Platelets
  - Ultrastructure of Platelets
- Coagulation
- Fibrinolytic System
  - General Clinical Considerations
  - Laboratory Investigations in Hemorrhagic Disorders

NORMAL HEMOSTASIS

Clotting of blood is one of the host defense mechanisms, which when accompanied by inflammation and repair responses, helps to protect vascular integrity and preserve life. Hemostasis is blood clot formation at the site of a blood vessel injury. The hemostatic response should be quick, localized and very carefully regulated. This is a very delicately balanced mechanism in our body. Abnormal bleeding or a propensity to nonphysiologic thrombosis (thrombosis not required for hemostatic regulation) may occur when delicate elements of this hemostatic process are missing or dysfunctional.

Phases of Hemostatic Process

Though the clotting process is now considered as a dynamic process, for practical purposes it can be divided into four phases:

1. Initiation and formation of the platelet plug. This is considered as primary hemostasis.
2. Propagation of the clotting process resulting in formation of the fibrin clot. This is secondary hemostasis.
3. Termination of the clotting process by antithrombotic control mechanisms. Examples are antithrombin (AT), protein C, etc.
4. Removal of clot by fibrinolysis.

PLATELETS

Ultrastructure of Platelets

The surface of platelets is made of three layers—(1) glycoprotein (GP) layer, (2) phospholipid layer and (3) inner layer. The GP layer contains receptors for the binding of von Willebrand's factor (vWF) and fibrinogen. Defects in the GP layer lead to abnormalities of adhesion and aggregation. The matrix of the platelet is made up of the sol-gel zone and the organelle zone. In the sol-gel zone, the cytoplasm shows fiber systems in various stages of polymerization. These fiber systems help to maintain the shape and also account for the contractile apparatus of platelets. The organelle zone shows various bodies— alpha granules, dense granules and lysosomes. The alpha granules contain several secreted proteins, vWF, fibrinogen, fibronectin, thrombospondin, coagulation factor V, high molecular weight kininogen (HMWK), platelet factor 4, β-thromboglobulin, platelet-derived growth factor (PGDF), albumin and histidine-rich GPs. The dense granules contain calcium, pyrophosphate, serotonin and adenine nucleotides. All these substances are released into plasma when the platelets are activated. Deficiency of α-granules and dense granules lead to platelet dysfunction (*See* Fig. 158.4).

Platelet function requires presence of specific receptors on the platelet surface, which interact with proteins in the plasma including those secreted by the platelets (*See* Fig. 158.7).

Platelets can produce many of the factors taking part in the coagulation cascade, in addition to concentrating them on their surface.

These processes collectively known as contact interactions consist of several processes. Platelet adherence is mediated by the interaction of platelet GP Ib/1x with endothelial vWF under high-shear conditions, and by platelet GP Ia/IIb binding to collagen under low-shear rates. Upon stimulation, adherent platelets recruit more platelets into the growing thrombus by three distinct mechanisms:

1. Platelets concentrate clotting factors on their surface and favor thrombin generation. Thrombin activates further platelets and other clotting factors.
2. The activated platelets liberate adenosine diphosphate (ADP) from their granules and activate further platelets.
3. Activated platelets generate thromboxane A2, which also activates further platelets.

Activation of platelets by an agonist also activates the GP IIb/IIIa receptor conformationally. This receptor also known as integrin binds to fibrinogen.

Fibrinogen is essential for platelet aggregation. Normal inactive platelets do not bind fibrinogen. Once activated by ADP, epinephrine or thrombin then fibrinogen receptors manifest on the surface and bind to fibrinogen. The contractile proteins of the platelets consist of actin and myosin. These help in changing shape, locomotion and extrusion of the contents to the surface.

Apart from mediating primary hemostasis (which includes the retraction and contraction of the injured vessel, and plugging of the injured vessel by platelet plug), the platelets take part in coagulation as well—this is referred to as procoagulant activity. Platelet procoagulant activity is mediated by the following mechanisms:

- Protection of the coagulation factors on the platelet surface from the action of plasma inhibitors and secretion of several coagulation factors
- Activation of factors X, XII and XI
- Platelet factor 4 antagonizes heparin and other inhibitors of coagulation.

Antigenicity of Platelets

The glycocalyx layers on the external membrane of the platelets contain a series of complex GPs numbered I to X. These express several polymorphic antigenic determinants on their surfaces. These are termed as platelet-specific antigens (HPP, PIA-I or HPA-I). These antigens lead to antibody formation resulting in post-transfusion purpura and neonatal autoimmune thrombocytopenia purpura.

Initiation and Formation of the Platelet Plug

The platelet functions are also dynamic and consist of initiation, extension and consolidation.

Initiation

When the endothelium is intact, the platelets cannot adhere due to the action of nitric oxide and prostacyclin. Intimal injury disrupts these processes and platelets become exposed to the subendothelial elements like collagen and leads to adhesion, activation, secretion and aggregation. During the initiation phase after the blood vessel injury, vWF binds to collagen and in turn to platelet membrane receptor GP I complex (Ib-IX-V complex). The platelets adhere to the vessel wall (adhesion). After this more stable monolayers are formed on the collagen mediated by GP VI and integrin alpha-2beta-1.

Extension

In the *extension phase*, prothrombin is converted to thrombin on the platelet surface, initiating platelet activation. The platelets contain alpha and dense granules, which secrete many substances like ADP and serotonin. It also contains other substances like thromboxane A2, fibronectin and thrombospondin. Platelet activation releases contents of the alpha and the dense granules—

both containing prothrombotic components. Proteins are packed in the alpha-granules, whereas ADP and calcium are packed in the dense granules. When ADP and serotonin are secreted (platelet secretion), these act along with substances like thromboxane A2 promoting further platelet activation and secretion.

Consolidation

In the **consolidation phase**, platelet aggregation occurs. There is platelet-to-platelet adhesion. Fibrinogen and/or vWF get bound to platelet integrin alpha-2bbeta-3 (formerly called GP IIb-IIIa). Fibrinogen acts at low-shear rates and vWF at high-shear rates. This is a very important step in the whole process of platelet plug formation. The aggregated platelets form the platelet plug (*See* Figs 158.3 to 158.8).

COAGULATION

Clotting Cascade and Propagation of the Clot

Nomenclature of the coagulation proteins has been accepted internationally.

- Factor I—fibrinogen
- Factor II—prothrombin
- Factor III—tissue thromboplastin
- Factor IV—calcium ions
- Factor V—proaccelerin (labile factor)
- Factor VII—proconvertin (stable factor)
- Factor VIII—antihemophilic globulin or antihemophilic factor
- Factor IX—Christmas factor (plasma thromboplastin component)
- Factor X—Stuart-Prower factor
- Factor XI—plasma thromboplastin antecedent
- Factor XII—Hageman's factor
- Factor XIII—fibrin-stabilizing factor

The numerical order does not represent the sequence of activation. In addition to the above, several other factors, such as prekallikrein (PK) and HMWK and several cytokines, are involved in the activation of coagulation factors at several steps in the intrinsic pathway. The activated factors are represented with suffix 'a'.

The main feature of this process is a sequential activation of a series of proenzymes or inactive precursor proteins to active enzymes resulting in significant stepwise response amplification.

All the procoagulants are synthesized in the liver except vWF, which is synthesized in megakaryocytes and endothelial cells.

Traditionally, the clotting cascade is taught and known as consisting of intrinsic and extrinsic pathways (Fig. 173.1). This view of coagulation is useful for interpreting *in vitro* tests of coagulation [prothrombin time (PT), activated partial thromboplastin time (aPTT)]. It may not be physiologically accurate. Now it is known that coagulation is normally initiated solely through tissue factor (TF), which is expressed by subendothelial cells of the vessel wall like the smooth muscle cells and the fibroblasts. TF is a membrane protein present in cells in different locations and has several actions, initiating coagulation, signaling of intercellular events leading to angiogenesis, tumor progression, metastasis and yolk sac vasculature. The endothelium was thought to be separating the tissue from circulating factor VIIa. However, the TF is

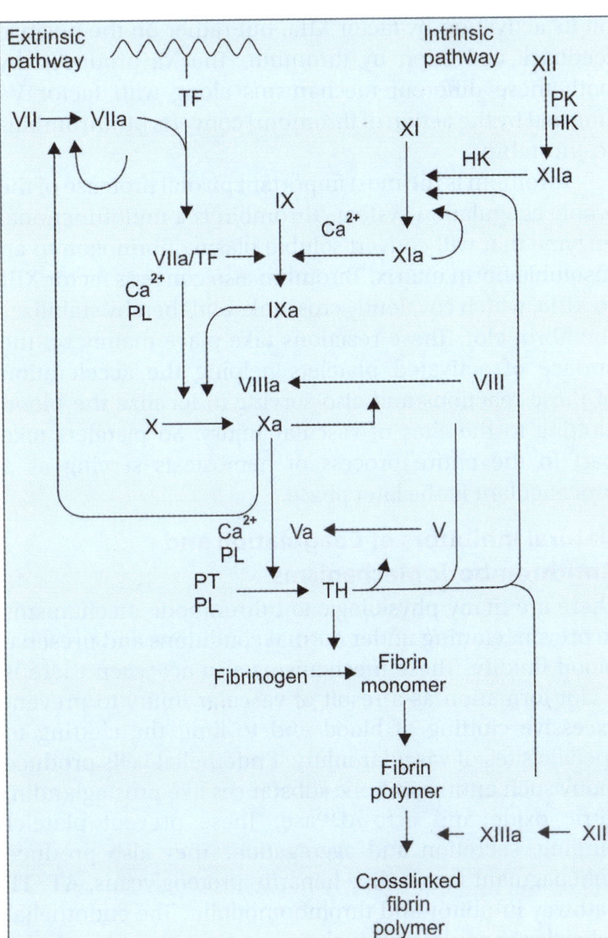

Fig. 173.1: Normal coagulation cascade
Abbreviations: TF = Tissue factor; PT = Prothrombin time; PL = Phospholipids; TH = Thrombin

present in the inactive form in circulating blood as well as associated with protein microparticles less than 1,000 nm in diameter. The TF is captured by the propagating thrombus to facilitate fibrin production. Possibly, activation of TF in circulation occurs as a result of chemicals released by endothelial cells and platelets.

Tissue factor acts through the classic extrinsic pathway, but also gets very important and critical augmentation by the intrinsic pathway. These reactions take place on the phospholipid surfaces like the activated platelets.

The endothelium contains three thromboregulators: (1) nitric oxide, (2) prostacyclin and (3) the ectonucleosidase—all these together protecting against thrombosis. When the vessel wall is injured, exposed collagen favors platelet aggregation, whereas the exposed TF initiates the formation of thrombin, which converts fibrinogen to fibrin and also activates the platelets.

The TF, which is expressed by the subendothelial cells combines with the serine protease factor VIIa (which is formed by the action of thrombin). This TF-VIIa complex activates factor X to Xa. Alternatively, this complex can activate factor X indirectly by activating factor IX to factor IXa. Factor IXa with VIIIa (formed by the action of thrombin) can also activate factor X to Xa. Thrombin converts XI to XIa, which can also convert factor IX to IXa. Participation of factor XI in hemostasis is not dependent on its activation by factor XIIa, but rather on the positive feedback activation by thrombin. The Xa produced by both these different mechanisms along with factor Va (formed by the action of thrombin) converts prothrombin-to-thrombin.

Thrombin is the most important pivotal protease of the whole coagulation system. Thrombin is a multifunctional enzyme that will convert soluble plasma fibrinogen to an insoluble fibrin matrix. Thrombin also converts factor XIII to XIIIa, which covalently crosslinks and thereby stabilizes the fibrin clot. These reactions take place mainly on the surface of activated platelets helping the acceleration of these reactions and also serving to localize the blood clotting to the sites of vascular injury. So platelets take part in the entire process of hemostasis serving as a procoagulant in the later phase.

Natural Inhibitors of Coagulation and Antithrombotic Mechanisms

There are many physiologic antithrombotic mechanisms to prevent clotting under normal conditions and preserve blood fluidity. These mechanisms also act when there is a clot formation as a result of vascular injury to prevent excessive clotting of blood and to limit the clotting to specific sites of vascular injury. Endothelial cells produce many such antithrombotic substances like prostaglandin, nitric oxide and ecto-ADPase. These prevent platelet binding, secretion and aggregation. They also produce anticoagulant factors like heparin, proteoglycans, AT, TF pathway inhibitor and thrombomodulin. The endothelial cells also modulate fibrinolytic mechanisms through the production of plasminogen activator inhibitor (PAI) and annexin-2.

Antithrombin

Antithrombin (previously called AT III) is the most important plasma protease inhibitor of thrombin and many other clotting factors in coagulation. This is present in normal plasma and endothelial cell surfaces. It neutralizes thrombin and the other clotting factors by forming inactivating complexes with the active sites of the clotting factors and thrombin. The formation of these inactivating complexes is enhanced several times by the presence of heparin. Hence, AT used to be known as heparin cofactor. AT has got other activities as well. These include inhibition of the procoagulant factors such as IXa, Xa, XIa, XIIa, VIIa, TF, plasma kallikrein, HMWK and plasmin. Deficiency of AT may lead to thrombotic tendencies. AT has also antiplasmin activity.

Protein C

It is a plasma GP that becomes activated by thrombin. It is a vitamin K-dependent protein synthesized in the liver and is a key component in a physiologically important anticoagulant system. The activation of protein C occurs on thrombomodulin. The thrombin-thrombomodulin complex activates protein C. Activated protein C (APC) cleaves and inactivates factor V and VIII. By inactivating these factors, it controls the conversion of factor X to Xa and that of prothrombin to thrombin, thereby inhibiting the coagulation cascade. Inherited abnormalities of factor V, also known as factor V, Leiden has a glutamine instead of arginine in position 506. Factor V Leiden is resistant to the action of APC. In the white population, the frequency of this genetic defect is 2–15%. In India, this abnormality is not a common cause of thrombophilia. APC, AT and tissue factor pathway inhibitor (TFPI) dampen coagulation, enhance fibrinolysis and remove microthrombi. APC proteolytically inactivates factors Va and VIIIa and decreases the synthesis of PAI-1.

Protein S

The action of protein C is accelerated by a cofactor protein S. This is also a vitamin K-dependent plasma protein synthesized by the liver, which acts as a cofactor for APC and this complex takes part in inhibiting coagulation cascade. Protein S exists in two forms: (1) Plasma-free and (2) combined forms. The former is the functionally active one. Action of protein S is not fully understood. Inherited protein S deficiency leads to thromboembolic complications. Individuals who develop thromboembolic complications due to abnormalities of protein C or protein S, probably require lifelong anticoagulant therapy.

Tissue Factor Pathway Inhibitor

It is a plasma protease inhibitor that regulates the TF-induced extrinsic pathway of coagulation. TFPI inhibits TF-VIIa complex basically by turning off the TF-VIIa initiation of clotting process. This leaves only the weak amplification loop via factors VIII and XI activation of thrombin. Heparin acts by releasing the bound TFPI from the subendothelial cells and platelets.

FIBRINOLYTIC SYSTEM

The fibrin that is formed after a blood vessel injury has to be disposed. Also, any thrombin that escapes the inhibitory action of the normal anticoagulant system may convert further fibrinogen to fibrin. Under these circumstances, the fibrinolytic system gets activated to dispose the intravascular fibrin and to maintain or re-establish the patency of circulation. Plasmin, a protease enzyme is the key player in the fibrinolytic system and it digests fibrin-to-fibrin degradation products. The plasminogen activators, tissue-type plasminogen activator (tPA) and the urokinase-type plasminogen activator (uPA) cleave the bond of plasminogen to generate the active enzyme plasmin. In physiologic fibrinolysis, plasmin is fibrin specific because it binds to very specific sites. Plasmin cleaves fibrin at distinct sites of fibrin molecule leading to the generation of specific fragments during the process of fibrinolysis. The sites of plasmin cleavage of fibrin are the same as those on fibrinogen. But when plasmin cleaves the covalently crosslinked fibrin, characteristic D-dimers are released. So D-dimers can be measured in the plasma and used as a relatively specific test of fibrin (rather than fibrinogen) degradation. D-dimers are sensitive markers of blood clot formation that is clinically used with a negative-predictive value for deep vein thrombosis (DVT) and pulmonary embolism.

Physiologic regulation of fibrinolysis occurs primarily at three different levels:

1. Plasminogen activator inhibitor specifically PAI-1 and PAI-2. They inhibit the physiologic plasminogen activators tPA and uPA

2. The thrombin-activatable fibrinolysis inhibitor limits fibrinolysis

3. Alpha-2 antiplasmin inhibitors, which inhibit plasmin.

General Clinical Considerations

In general, primary hemorrhagic disorders are rare. In majority of cases, abnormal bleeding is due to secondary causes, either localized [surgical conditions or obstetric conditions, like postpartum hemorrhage (PPH)] or generalized, e.g. hepatic failure, renal failure and anti-coagulant overdose. In any patient who gives a history of easy bruising or excessive bleeding from childhood, a congenital hemostatic defect is likely. The acquired form starts at a later age. Even in congenital defects, which are mild, clinical onset may be delayed.

Congenital hemorrhagic disorders are characterized by:

- Purpura, ecchymosis, hematoma or spontaneous bleeding from multiple sites or following minor trauma
- Excessive bleeding after trauma or minor surgery
- Bleeding into joints, gums and mucous membranes of the gastrointestinal and the genitourinary tracts
- Positive family history in many cases
- History of previous episodes of hospitalization and blood transfusions to control the hemorrhage
- Abnormality involving one or only a few coagulant factors.

On the other hand, acquired hemorrhagic tendencies, set in at a later age may be temporary and may reveal deficiencies of multiple coagulation factors.

Broadly the hemorrhagic disorders can be divided into two groups:

1. *Purpuric disorders:* These affect the process of primary hemostasis, i.e. platelet and/or vascular functions are abnormal. These are characterized by bruising, ecchymosis and bleeding from mucous membranes, specially of the gastrointestinal and genitourinary tracts. Bleeding starts soon after injury and it is brisk initially. It is relieved by local pressure. The capillary resistance test (Hess' test) is positive.

    Bleeding time is prolonged. Unless there is severe thrombocytopenia (less than 20,000/μL), coagulation time is not prolonged.

2. *Coagulation defects:* These may be congenital or acquired. In majority of cases, the primary coagulation disorders are congenital. They are characterized by deep tissue bleeding, bleeding into joints, progressive deformity of joints, prolonged coagulation time and normal bleeding time and a negative Hess's test. If the platelets and capillaries are normal, post-traumatic bleeding stops temporarily to be followed by prolonged and gradually increasing bleeding, this may even threaten life.

Laboratory Investigations in Hemorrhagic Disorders

Screening Tests

- Platelet count and morphology
- Prothrombin time—to test the extrinsic coagulation pathway
- Partial thromboplastin time (PTT)—to test the intrinsic coagulation pathway

- Thrombin time—to test the common coagulation pathway.

A stained blood film should show clumped and single platelets at the rate of 1 for 20–25 erythrocytes. Absence of clumping may suggest thrombasthenia.

Further Tests for Platelet Function

- *Bleeding time (Ivy):* Prolongation beyond 12 minutes is definitely abnormal. In dysfunction of platelets and capillaries, the bleeding time is prolonged. Common causes of prolongation of the bleeding time are thrombocytopenia (platelet count below 100,000/μL), functional platelet disorders, von Willebrand's diseases and scurvy. This test is now not used in many centers due to lack of standardization and reproducibility.

- *Hess tourniquet test:* Appearance of more than 30 spots (when examined with a hand lens) within a circle of 2.5 cm diameter is considered a positive test. Hess's test is positive in thrombocytopenia, functional platelet disorders and diseases of the capillaries. This test is less reliable than the bleeding time and, hence, abandoned in many centers.

- *Platelet aggregometry:* This is an *in vitro* test to determine the ability of the platelets to aggregate in platelet-rich plasma. This phenomenon can be studied spectrophotometrically or using an aggregometer. Platelet aggregation in response to ADP, epinephrine, collagen or thrombin is absent in thrombasthenia. Abnormalities of platelet aggregation in certain diseases are given in Table 173.1.

- Tests for platelet adhesion.

- The diagnosis of platelet functional disorders has become easy with the newly introduced platelet functional analyzer-100. The sensitivity and the specificity of this are comparable to the conventional platelet aggregometry.

Tests for Coagulation

Clotting Time

Clotting time (coagulation time-Lee and White)—1 mL blood is drawn into each of three clean dry test tubes and clotting time for each test tube at room temperature is noted and the values are averaged. This test is not done now because it is not sensitive or specific.

Clot Retraction

When kept at room temperature, the clot retracts and the serum separates within 2 hours. When the platelet number is grossly deficient or platelet function is defective, clot retraction is impaired. Normally the serum expressed measures 55–65% of the total quantity of blood.

Table 173.1: Abnormalities of platelet aggregation in certain diseases

Platelet aggregation	Disease process
Normal	Thrombocytopenias and von Willebrand's disease
Absent	Thrombasthenias, especially Glanzmann disease
Diminished	Disorders of platelet release reaction and afibrinogenemia

Prothrombin Time

Prothrombin time (Quick's): This test evaluates the production of thrombin and fibrin polymers by the extrinsic coagulation pathway. PT is prolonged, whenever factors VII, X or V, prothrombin or fibrinogen are reduced to levels below 30% of normal. Normal PT is 10–12 seconds. In order to standardize the test results and avoid interlaboratory variations, internationally standardized thromboplastin is used and the results are expressed as International Normalized Ratio (INR). Normal INR is 1.0.

Partial Thromboplastin Time

Partial thromboplastin time—aPTT measures the time required for the formation of thrombin and fibrin polymers by the intrinsic pathway. Normal aPTT is 35 seconds. Value of aPTT rises whenever the levels of one or more of the coagulation factors other than factor VII is reduced below 30% of the normal. When the common pathway is impaired, both PTT and aPTT are prolonged.

Substitution Tests and Factor Assays

Identification of deficiencies of coagulation factors is done by estimating aPTT in the patient's plasma, and repeating the test with added plasma with known defects till aPTT is corrected. Assays of factors XII, XI, IX and VIII-C, PK and HMWK are done by modified aPTT test.

Thrombin Time

This helps to identify abnormalities in the quantity and quality of fibrinogen. It is prolonged in hypofibrinogenemia and dysfibrinogenemia. Normal level of fibrinogen in plasma is 150–400 mg/dL.

Estimation of Fibrin Degradation Products

Increase in fibrin degradation products (FDPs) in serum and urine indicate increased fibrinolysis.

Euglobulin Lysis Time

This indicates the amount of fibrinolytic activity in the serum, and therefore, it is an indirect indication of plasmin activity. In disseminated intravascular coagulation (DIC) and primary hyperfibrinolytic states, euglobulin lysis time is shortened and serum levels of FDPs are increased.

D-dimer

Elevated levels of D-dimer in plasma are more specific indicators of thromboembolic episodes followed by fibrinolysis. D-dimer is the fibrin fragment in plasma, which is a marker of fibrin formation and reactive fibrinolysis. Normal levels of D-dimer in plasma are less than 500 ng/mL.

Rusven (Russell's Viper Venom)-Clotting Time

It is employed to assay factor X and also for the detection of lupus anticoagulant.

At present test kits are available from many sources, and therefore, these tests can be done even in moderately equipped laboratories.

Detection of Circulating Anticoagulants

In conditions where the abnormality of coagulation is due to deficiency of one or more of the clotting factors, addition of 10–30% by volume of normal plasma corrects the abnormal laboratory tests.

In conditions where circulating anticoagulants or antibodies to coagulation factors are present, substitution with normal plasma fails to correct the abnormality until very large quantities are added. Such antibodies are found in antiphospholipid syndrome and acquired antibodies to the clotting factors.

Automated testing machines are available for performing coagulation tests and platelet function tests. If properly serviced and calibrated using standard specimens, they are reliable and more accurate than manual methods.

CHAPTER 174

Platelet and Vascular Disorders

Mathew Thomas, KV Krishna Das

Chapter Summary

- General Considerations
- Immune Thrombocytopenic Purpura (ITP)
- Neonatal Thrombocytopenia
  - Autoimmune Neonatal Thrombocytopenia
  - Neonatal Alloimmune Thrombocytopenia (NAIT)
- Chronic ITP
- Secondary Thrombocytopenia
- Congenital and Acquired Disorders of Platelet Function (Thrombocytopathies)
  - Acquired Disorders of Platelet Function
- Vascular Purpuras
- Hereditary Hemorrhagic Telangiectasia (HHT)
- Antiplatelet Drug Therapy

GENERAL CONSIDERATIONS

The term purpuric disorder is applied to a hemorrhagic state characterized by bleeding into the skin in the form of dot-like purpura, ecchymosis, or deep hemorrhages, and often associated with bleeding from the mucous membranes of the mouth, nose, gastrointestinal tract (GIT), uterus and urinary tract. Purpuras are caused by primary disorders of blood vessels or thrombocytopenia or functional platelet disorders. Purpura has to be distinguished from macular rashes and telangiectasia. The former does not blanch on pressure whereas the latter does. Palpable purpura occurs in vasculitis, e.g. Henoch-Schönlein syndrome (Table 174.1).

Table 174.1: Distinction between platelet vascular diagnosis and coagulation defects

Characteristics	Platelet/vascular disorders	Coagulation disorders
Onset	Spontaneous and develops immediately after trauma/surgery	Delayed bleeding after trauma/surgery
Type of lesion	Petechiae, ecchymoses	Hematomas
Sites	Skin, mucous membrane	Deep tissues
• Mucous membrane	Common from nose, mouth, gastrointestinal and genitourinary tracts	Uncommon except from gastrointestinal or genitourinary tract
• Into the joint	Absent	Common in severe factor deficiencies
• Into the muscle	Following trauma	Spontaneous
• Local pressure	Effective	Ineffective

When the platelet count falls below 100,000/μL, it is designated as thrombocytopenia. Even at this level mild bleeding tendency may start, but bleeding becomes pronounced when the platelet count falls below 50,000/μL. Severe bleeding occurs when the platelets fall below 20,000/μL. The severity of bleeding does not always correlate with the degree of thrombocytopenia. Bleeding may be spontaneous or may follow minor trauma. Purpuric bleeding usually stops within 24 hours either spontaneously or on local compression.

Causes of thrombocytopenia: Thrombocytopenia may result from either diminished production or increased destruction of platelets (Box 174.1). In some, both may operate. It may also occur in disseminated intravascular coagulation (DIC) and massive transfusion of stored blood.

In ***pseudothrombocytopenia,*** the platelet count is normal but recorded as low in the electronic blood counter. The patient will not have any apparent causes or symptoms of thrombocytopenia. This can be due to an *in vitro* artefact resulting from platelet agglutination via antibody (usually IgG) when the calcium content is decreased by blood collection in ethylenediaminetetra-acetic acid (EDTA) anticoagulant. Pseudothrombocytopenia can also occur when giant platelets when present are counted as red blood cells (RBCs) or when there is platelet satellitism in which platelets rosette around the neutrophils due to antibody coating. The agglutinated platelets are not counted. These errors are avoided by collecting the blood in citrate anticoagulant.

IMMUNE THROMBOCYTOPENIC PURPURA (ITP)

Syn: Idiopathic thrombocytopenic purpura

This is one of the common hemorrhagic disorders seen in clinical practice in India. In vast majority of cases, antibodies develop which coat the platelets and lead to their destruction in the reticuloendothelial system in the spleen, liver, bone marrow and other sites. These antibodies are demonstrable by direct or indirect methods. Though the exact antigenic stimulus for production of the antibodies is not clear, it is seen that they are directed against many of the components of the platelets. Most of the autoantibodies are directed against epitopes on glycoproteins on the platelet surface. The antibody-coated platelets are sequestrated in the spleen, liver, bone marrow and other reticuloendothelial organs and selectively destroyed by macrophages. The antibodies are presumed to be produced in the spleen and bone marrow. They are IgG in 70%, IgM in 5% and IgG and IgM in 20% of cases. In the circulation, they are attached to the platelets. Most of the autoantibodies are directed against epitopes on glycoproteins on the platelets surface. Lifespan of the platelets is reduced and the reduction is inversely related to the amount of platelet-associated IgG.

There is compensatory increase in platelet production brought about by increase in the number of megakaryocytes to 3–5 times the normal, but platelet destruction exceeds the regeneration and ultimately the platelet count falls. The antibody has also action in inhibiting the production and release of platelets from megakaryocytes and in some cases platelet production may be suppressed. In the bone marrow, many megakaryocytes are seen to possess hyaline cytoplasm and entire margins, indicating absence of platelet production. So, the pathogenesis of ITP includes increased platelet destruction and decreased platelet production. In small doses, the antibodies lead to platelet dysfunction. In larger doses, they lead to platelet destruction. Many of the platelets formed under stress are larger than normal. These megathrombocytes have the

---

Box 174.1: Causes of thrombocytopenia

- ***Diminished production of platelets***
  - Aplastic anemia
  - Selective hypoplasia of megakaryocytes or inhibition of platelet production by antibodies
  - Dyshemopoietic states, e.g. megaloblastic anemia
  - Myelophthisic conditions, e.g. acute and chronic leukemia, lymphoma, myelofibrosis, disseminated carcinoma and multiple myeloma
  - Heavy alcoholism (ethanol leads to inhibition of megakaryo-cytes)
- ***Increased destruction***
  - ITP
  - Chronic or acute secondary immune thrombocytopenia following viral infections, SLE, lymphomas and chronic lymphatic leukemia (CLL), acquired hemolytic anemia, AIDS and others
  - Drugs like sedormid, quinine, quinidine, para-aminosalicylic acid, sulfonamides, rifampicin, stibophen, digoxin, strepto-mycin, alpha methyldopa, heroin, carbimazole, chloramphen-icol, tetracycline, mesantoin, troxidone and phenylbutazone
  - Sequestration of platelets, e.g. splenomegaly, giant hemangioma, arteriovenous fistulae, disseminated intravascular coagulation (DIC)
- ***Dilutional thrombocytopenia,*** e.g. transfusion of massive quantities of stored blood poor in platelets

Abbreviations: ITP = Idiopathic (immune) thrombocytopenic purpura; SLE = Systemic lupus erythematosus; AIDS = Acquired immunodeficiency syndrome

same diameter as red cells. They have reduced lifespan which is inversely proportional to their diameter. Presence of antibodies may also contribute to their morphological abnormality.

The incidence of ITP is on the increase. This is because many people with mild thrombocytopenia and without any bleeding manifestations are being diagnosed as ITP due to the regular testing of complete blood count (CBC) by automated blood cell counters which are used widely in laboratories.

Clinical Features

ITP may occur at any age, but younger subjects are affected more. The disease may present as the acute and chronic varieties. In chronic ITP, duration of the disease exceeds 12 months. Acute ITP is more common in children whereas the chronic variety is more common in young women (Table 174.2). Both sexes are equally affected below the age of 12 years, but after that age, females are affected about four times more frequently than males. It is also now found that there is another peak incidence of ITP in older people in their 5th and 6th decades. So it is no longer considered as a disease of children and young females. Currently, ITP is classified as:

- Newly diagnosed ITP (up to 3 months of diagnosis)
- Persistent ITP (3–12 months of diagnosis)
- Chronic ITP (lasting for more than 12 months).

In many cases of ITP in children, purpura may be preceded by an upper respiratory infection or other specific diseases like measles or mumps. Viral infections trigger the formation of antiplatelet antibodies. The acute form is characterized by rapid onset of bleeding from the gums, purpura, ecchymosis and bleeding into deeper tissues. Majority of these patients seek medical help within 1–2 weeks of onset. In the chronic form, the onset is insidious and course is prolonged over several weeks or months, sometimes even years, before they seek medical help. Periods of exacerbations and remissions occur. In women, one of the common presentations is menorrhagia and intermenstrual bleeding (IMB). The menorrhagia tends to be severe and in some cases blood loss may be considerable so as to necessitate blood transfusion. Due to this complication, ITP tends to be more severe in women than in men. Subdural hematoma may occur in chronic ITP.

Physical Examination

It reveals the typical purpuric spots and ecchymosis, particularly over the limbs, chest and sometimes over the neck. Areas of pressure by clothing or minor trauma of rubbing as in the axillae and thighs show more purpuric spots (Fig. 174.1). Spontaneous bleeding is seen from the mouth, nose, urinary tract and genital tract in women. In severe cases, hemorrhagic bullae develop in the mucous membrane of the mouth (*wet purpura*) (Fig. 174.2). The extravasated blood undergoes clotting. Hematemesis and melena may occur. Usually, the bleeding stops within a few days either spontaneously or with treatment. Retinal bleeding occurs in severe cases. Bleeding into the central nervous system (CNS) may present as spontaneous subarachnoid hemorrhage or cerebral hemorrhage. CNS bleeds are likely when the platelet counts fall below $20,000/mm^3$. As a rule, there is no palpable splenomegaly. Presence of moderate or marked splenomegaly should suggest the possibility of leukemia, systemic lupus or other disorders. There is no direct correlation between the platelet count and the clinical bleeding even though patients with lower counts have more marked bleeding tendency and the benefit of therapy is related to the increase in platelet count.

In ITP as a result of accelerated platelet destruction, there is an increased platelet production in most patients. These platelets are young and have greater hemostatic effectiveness. This is not the situation in thrombocytopenia which occurs in bone marrow aplasia. As a result, bleeding manifestations in ITP are less severe than in patients with aplasia having equivalent platelet counts. From observations regarding different etiologies including ITP, there is suggestive evidence that the threshold for serious bleeding manifestations in ITP is $10,000/mm^3$. But since

Table 174.2: Clinical features of idiopathic thrombocytopenic purpura in children and adults

Features	Children	Adults
Occurrence		
Peak age (years)	2–4	15–40
Sex (F:M)	Equal	1.2–1.7
Presentation		
Onset	Acute (most with symptoms <1 week)	Insidious (most with symptoms >2 months)
Symptoms	Purpura (<10% with severe bleeding) less than	Purpura (typically bleeding not severe) more
Platelet count	20,000/L	than 20,000/L
Antecedent infection	Usually follows an antecedent upper respiratory viral infection	Usually no preceding history of viral infection
Course		
Spontaneous remission	83%	2%
Chronic disease	24%	43%
Response to splenectomy	71%	66%
Eventual complete recovery	89%	64%
Morbidity and mortality		
Cerebral hemorrhage	<1%	3%
Hemorrhagic death	<1%	4%
Mortality of chronic refractory disease	2%	5%

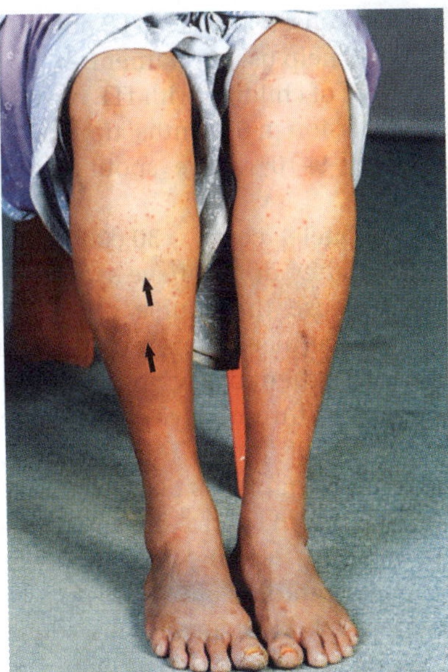

Fig. 174.1: Female purpura over legs (arrows)

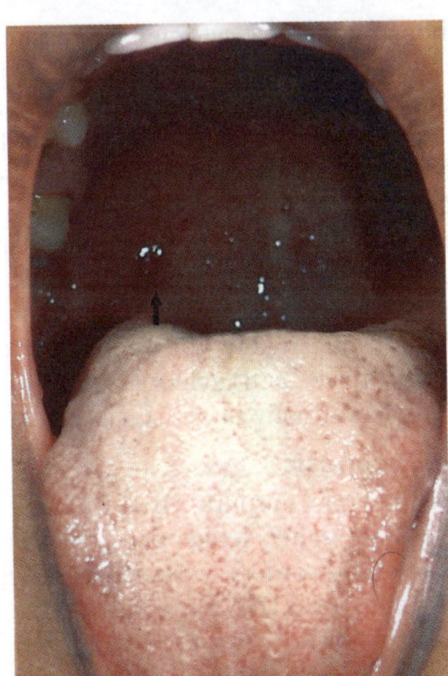

Fig. 174.2: Purpura over the palate (arrow)

the course of ITP and risks for bleeding cannot be predicted at the time of initial diagnosis, treatment in ITP is usually initiated when the platelet count is below 30,000/mm³ and not 10,000/mm³.

Diagnosis

Diagnosis of ITP is mainly clinical. In the majority, it presents as a subacute or chronic disorder, but at times it may present as an acute emergency.

- Isolated thrombocytopenia should be present. The rest of the CBC including examination of the peripheral blood smear is entirely normal [unless other coincidental abnormalities like iron deficiency anemia (IDA) or hemolysis as in Evan's syndrome is present].
- Other causes of thrombocytopenias such as systemic lupus erythematosus (SLE), antiphosphoslipid syndrome (APS), leukemias, myelodysplasias and aplastic anemia are not present. Patients with these associated conditions are described as having a secondary immune thrombocytopenia.
- Drugs including herbal medicines which are very common in India may produce thrombocytopenia and this should be excluded by clinical examination.

Primary or idiopathic ITP is diagnosed when the platelet count is less than 100,000/mm³ and in the absence of any other causes or disorders that may be associated with thrombocytopenia.

It should be remembered that several viral infections present with mild or even moderate thrombocytopenia lasting for days to weeks should not be mistaken for ITP.

Laboratory Investigations

Platelet count is reduced in all cases. It may be below 20,000/μL in severe cases. Under light microscopy, the platelets appear normal, except for the presence of a few large forms—**megathrombocytes** or **giant platelets** (Fig. 174.3). The presence of megathrombocytes indicates disordered thrombopoiesis and possibly the effect of antibodies. Though there is no gross impairment of platelet function, the antibody leads to impairment of

platelet release reaction which can be demonstrated *in vitro*. The hemorrhagic manifestation is mainly due to thrombocytopenia, it is aggravated by platelet dysfunction as well. Bleeding time is prolonged whereas the whole blood clotting time is normal. Clot retraction is deficient if the platelet count is below 50,000/mm³. Hess's test is positive. Examination of the bone marrow is basically normal but it may show increased number of megakaryocytes. Many of them have hyaline cytoplasm, entire margins and are devoid of budding activity. The degree of anemia is proportional to the blood loss which may be superficial or deep.

In over 75% of cases, antiplatelet antibodies can be demonstrated by direct or indirect tests. Different methods used to be employed to detect platelet-associated antibodies. The early tests depended on function defects such as alpha-granule release inhibition, aggregation and agglutination.

Present method for demonstration of platelet specific autoantibodies is by monoclonal antibody immobilization of platelet antigen (MAIPA), antigen captures enzyme-linked immunosorbent assay (ELISA) and its modifications.

Flow cytometry can demonstrate platelet auto-antibodies. Platelet-associated IgG (PAIgG), IgM and IgA

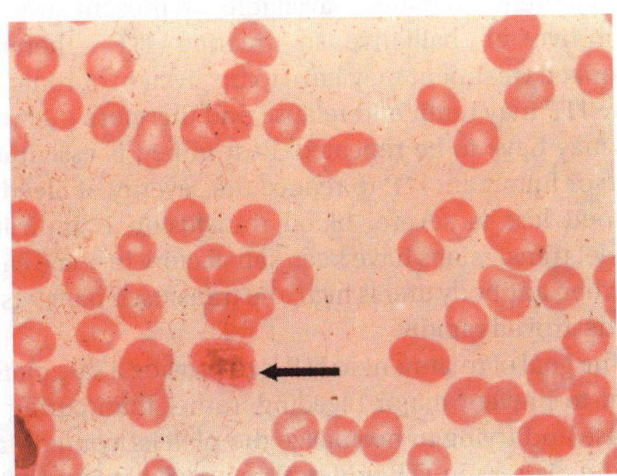

Fig. 174.3: Peripheral blood—ITP megathrombocytes (arrow)

can be demonstrated. Flow cytometry compares well with MAIPA. Acute ITP is associated with higher prevalence of antibodies compared to chronic ITP. The antibodies may be against glycoproteins (GP1a, GP1b, GP2a, GP3a, GP2a3b and so on). Their demonstration is helpful in a doubtful case.

Antiplatelet antibody testing is necessary for the diagnosis or management decisions in ITP. Almost 3–15% of patients with apparent isolated ITP may go on to develop SLE on long follow-up. About 40% of patients with ITP may have antinuclear antibody (ANA) or antiphospholipid antibody as well.

Differential Diagnosis

This includes allergic purpura, drug-induced thrombocytopenia, SLE, acute leukemia, aplastic anemia, functional platelet disorders, vascular disorders, human immunodeficiency virus (HIV) infection and septicemia.

Presence of mild or moderate splenomegaly should suggest the possibility of acute leukemia, lupus erythematosus, or hemolytic anemia. Sometimes ITP may be associated with other autoimmune disorders such as hemolytic anemia (Evan's syndrome). Rarely, ITP may coexist with autoimmune thyroid diseases.

Course and Prognosis

Acute ITP runs a short course and may remit spontaneously in a few of the cases. It may result in serious bleeding with rapid development of anemia. Fulminant cases may be fatal if untreated. Death is due to severe blood loss or bleeding into vital organs such as the brain. Platelet counts below 10,000/mm³, hematuria, retinal hemorrhages and signs of meningeal irritation are grave prognostic signs. Mortality is about 2–3% in large series.

Among the acute ITP cases, 7–28% goes into the chronic form. In the chronic form, periods of remissions and exacerbations alternate and patient suffers only minor disability. Infections, menstruation, or drugs like aspirin may precipitate bleeding episodes. Menstrual and intermenstrual blood loss in women may be severe and even life-threatening and they seek medical help early due to this factor. During pregnancy, the bleeding episodes may aggravate in many cases, though in some cases the condition may remit. Risk of intrauterine death (IUD) of fetus and perinatal fetal loss are high.

Treatment of Acute ITP

All treatment modalities available at present are only supportive or palliative in treating ITP. Therefore, prolonged treatment may have to be given in chronic ITP. Acute ITP may remit and relapse and therefore treatment also may have to be repeated. Rest in bed is essential in acute or fulminant ITP to reduce the severity of bleeding. If blood loss is severe, blood transfusion is indicated. Platelet transfusions have been satisfactory in some cases, but when antibody titer is high, the transfused platelets are also destroyed rapidly.

The goal of treatment in ITP is to provide a safe platelet count to prevent major bleeding, rather than curing the disease and trying to normalize the platelet count. Major bleeding is rare in ITP and occurs usually below 10,000/mm³.

There are many observations in ITP patients in the past decades which will help us in treatment:

- A large number of children with ITP have spontaneous complete remission in 6 months' time.
- In adults only 9–10% have spontaneous complete remission.
- Adults with platelet count <30,000/mm³ should be treated even if they do not have symptoms or minor symptoms because the course of the disease and the risk for future bleeding is not predictable. Avoid unnecessary treatment of asymptomatic patients with mild to moderate thrombocytopenia (platelet counts about 30,000–50,000/mm³). They can be followed up with close monitoring of their platelet count and general advice to avoid trauma and to abstain from drugs such as aspirin and non-steroidal anti-inflammatory drugs (NSAIDs) which inhibit platelet function and also lead to gastrointestinal (GI) bleeding. Presence of serious bleeding requires aggressive treatment.
- Treatment should be tailored to the age, lifestyle, risk for trauma, occupation, comorbid conditions (peptic ulcer disease, cerebrovascular disease and systemic hypertension), disorders requiring treatment with antiplatelet drug or anticoagulant [coronary artery disease (CAD)] or need for surgery and procedures.
- Side effects of treatment are found to cause more morbidity and mortality in ITP, if care is not taken to avoid them.
- All the observations including many follow-up studies suggest that ITP is a more benign disease than originally believed.
- There are only a few prospective controlled trials concerning different therapies for ITP on long-term outcomes.

If a patient is diagnosed to have mild thrombocytopenia on routine blood count, e.g. 70,000/mm³ or 80,000/mm³, the patient should not have any treatment (mild asymptomatic ITP with no symptoms or minor symptoms). If the count is between 30,000/mm³ and 50,000/mm³, follow-up and monitoring of the platelet count is all that is required.

If the patient has severe bleeding and platelet count is less than 10,000/mm³, aggressive measures of treatment may be tried. The options are:

- Intravenous immunoglobulin (IVIg) 1g/kg one or two days
- IV methylprednisolone 1g daily × 3 doses (slow infusion)
- High dose dexamethasone 0.6 mg/kg/bw (40 mg) daily × 5 days—more than one course may be necessary
- Prednisolone 1mg/kg oral as a single dose for 6 weeks
- Rh Ig anti-D (Rhogam), 50–75 µg/kg given once daily is effective in moderately severe cases and it is more easily available and cheaper.

A combination of these different treatments can also be given if the platelet count does not improve and the patient has severe symptoms.

If the platelet count is < 30,000/mm³ with only mode-rate bleeding, oral prednisolone 1mg/kg is the drug of choice. When platelet count improves, the dose should be tapered and if possible the drug stopped in 8–12 weeks' time. About 40% show a good response and go into remission. For others who continue to have severe symptoms and low platelet count after these first-line drugs, second-line of treatment should be initiated. A newer glucocorticoid drug, derivative of prednisone—deflazacort can be used. This drug seems to have lesser side effect profile specially when used for a longer period of time. The dose is 1–2 mg/kg with a maximum oral dose of 120 mg per day for adults.

Second-line Management after Failure of Initial Therapy

Second-line treatment is given for patients who are very symptomatic with low platelet count specially after a trial of glucocorticoid drugs. The choice of treatment should be from the following:

- Splenectomy
- Rituximab
- Thrombopoiesis-stimulating drugs like eltrombopag or romiplostim.

Splenectomy

This treatment works by removing the major site where antibody coated platelets are trapped and destroyed and spleen contains 25% of lymphoid mass of the body and is believed to produce the platelet antibodies.

> **Points to Remember**
> - Long periods of remission occurs after splenectomy in about two-thirds of cases.
> - Splenectomy is preferably done only after 6 months of ITP allowing sufficient time for a definite and confirmed diagnosis and after knowing the response of other drugs.
> - Morbidity and mortality of splenectomy have come down with laparoscopic techniques.
> - Patients should be immunized at least two weeks prior to splenectomy for *Streptococcus pneumoniae*, *Haemophilus influenzae* and *Neisseria meningitidis*.
> - Young patients, prior response to IVIg and splenic sequestration of radiolabelled platelets (only an investigational procedure) are indicators of good response with splenectomy.

Rituximab

This anti-CD20 antibody has been used in a number of situations in ITP specially as a second-line drug and in those who are not good candidates for splenectomy. The dose is 375 mg/m^2/week × 4 weeks. A lower dose of 100 mg/m^2/week × 4 weeks appeared to have similar efficacy in inducing remissions. No trial has directly compared rituximab with splenectomy in patients who are unresponsive to the first-line of drugs specially glucocorticoids. With this drug, complete and overall response rate of 40% and 60% respectively is obtained. Relapse-free survival at 12 and 24 months are 61% and 45% respectively. Side effects are fewer than surgical complications of splenectomy. The serious side effect is multifocal leukoencephalopathy which is rare. Response rate is less than splenectomy and it is a very costly treatment in India. Rituximab has been used in other combinations also and even after splenectomy.

Thrombopoiesis-stimulating agents

Thrombopoietin (TPO) mimetics (thrombopoietic receptor agonists) are approved by US Food and Drug Administration (FDA) for use in adult ITP in patients with insufficient response to corticosteroids, IVIg or splenectomy. These agents are the only treatment for ITP with efficacy and supported by randomized clinical trials. These drugs act through the TPO receptor cMPL and JAK-STAT (Janus kinase and signal transducer and activator of transcription of stem cells). They act on early and late megakaryocytes which produce platelets. These drugs are effective in raising the platelet levels in thrombocytopenia associated with low levels of thrombopoietin.

These agents are best used when all other treatments to achieve a durable remission have failed. These drugs are very expensive and used only in patients who are very symptomatic and having a very low platelet count. Another indication would be patients who cannot undergo splenectomy.

The limitations of these agents apart from the cost are that the increment in platelet count is durable only during the period of drug administration.

Romiplostim: The recommended dose is 1 µg/kg once weekly as subcutaneous injection. The dose is subsequently adjusted to achieve platelet count above 50,000/mm^3 as necessary to reduce the risk of bleeding and not to normalize the platelet count.

Eltrombopag (revolade): The recommended dose is 50 mg tablet once daily and the dose is later adjusted to achieve platelet count above 50,000/mm^3. Apprehension regarding increased reticulin in the bone marrow after using these agents has not been substantiated. This drug is available in India and has proved to be useful when judiciously given to patients with severe symptoms and low platelet count to raise the platelet count to safe levels.

Life-threatening bleeding and surgery: After conventional critical care measures are done, the important modalities that may be employed in such an emergency or preparing a thrombocytopenic patient for surgery include the following:

- Platelet transfusions
- IVIg 1g/kg repeated on the following day if platelet count is less than 50,000/mm^3
- Pulse methylprednisolone 1 g IV repeated daily for 3 days
- Recombinant factor VIIa in life-threatening bleeding.

ITP during Pregnancy and Delivery and Neonatal Thrombocytopenia

About 50% of women develop mild asymptomatic gestational thrombocytopenia during term which needs no treatment. If the platelet counts go below 70,000/mm^3 in early gestation, ITP is the probable diagnosis. Women with ITP should be counseled regarding the risks before they opt to become pregnant. There is higher risk for both the mother and the fetus. Aggravation of bleeding tendency in the mother and risk of fetal loss has to be anticipated. These patients should be monitored every month. Corticosteroids can produce adverse side effects. Early in pregnancy, the management of ITP is the same as if the patient were not pregnant using prednisolone as initial therapy to treat patient with a platelet count less than 30,000/mm^3 with severe symptoms of bleeding.

Patient with ITP with platelet count between 30,000/mm³ and 50,000/mm³ should not be treated. Splenectomy should be deferred in pregnancy and it is recommended to avoid rituximab. IVIg is a good option to increase the platelet count at the time of delivery especially if the patient requires cesarean section. A platelet count of more than 50,000/mm³ is considered safe for delivery (vaginal or C-section). Antiplatelet drugs (aspirin, NSAIDs) should be avoided postpartum in women with thrombocytopenia. In many reports and in our own experience, even women with platelet counts less than 50,000/mm³ or 20,000/mm³ did not have serious bleeding during delivery.

Pre-eclampsia (PE) is associated with thrombocytopenia in 15% of cases. In addition, some women with PE develop microangiopathic hemolysis and liver dysfunction known by the acronym HELLP (hemolysis, elevated liver enzymes and low platelet counts). If severe, plasma exchange may be needed. In the ordinary cases, the platelet abnormality clears after delivery.

NEONATAL THROMBOCYTOPENIA

The neonatal thrombocytopenia could be autoimmune or alloimmune.

Autoimmune Neonatal Thrombocytopenia

It occurs when IgG antibodies from women suffering from ITP, cross the placenta to reach the fetus. The neonate may develop thrombocytopenia and bleeding. Common manifestations include bleeding from the umbilical stump and ecchymosis. The majority of infants recover spontaneously. Very rarely during delivery or soon after, the fetus may die from intracranial bleeding. Maternal platelet count below 100,000/mm³ and/or fetal platelet count below 50,000/mm³ are associated with possible risk of intracranial bleed during delivery. In severe cases, IV hydrocortisone 2–3 mg/kg bw and platelet transfusions are necessary to tide over the crisis. Judicious use of Ig will help to tide over a crisis if other measures fail. Neonatal thrombocytopenia may develop even when the mother is in remission. The newborn infant will have approximately 5 and 10% risk of thrombocytopenia with a platelet count of less than 50,000/mm³ and less than 20,000/mm³ respectively. The only predictors of neonatal thrombocytopenia are:

- Mother has had a splenectomy
- Mother's platelet count has been <50,000/mm³ at sometime during pregnancy
- An older sibling has had neonatal thrombocytopenia.

The mother's platelet count has no effect on neonatal thrombocytopenia. Severe thrombocytopenia can develop in the infant several days after delivery due to the late splenic function in the infant. The incidence of neonatal intracerebral hemorrhage is less than 1%.

Neonatal Alloimmune Thrombocytopenia (NAIT)

It occurs when fetal platelets contain an antigen inherited from the father that the mother lacks. The mother forms IgG class antiplatelet antibodies against the *foreign* antigen; these cross the placenta and destroy fetal platelets, resulting in fetal and neonatal thrombocytopenia. In contrast to Rh sensitization, NAIT often develops in the first pregnancy of an at-risk couple. It is a rare fetomaternal incompatibility in which maternal IgG antibodies directed against fetal platelets reach the fetus transplacentally. The mother is clinically normal and does not have thrombocytopenia. In most children, the platelet count is low at birth, it declines further during the first 48 hours of birth, to reach a nadir below 10,000/mm³ in almost 50%. Hemorrhagic manifestations develop in 90% of cases. NAIT follows a benign course in 90% of cases and spontaneous recovery is the rule. Recurrence rate in subsequent pregnancies is 50%. CNS bleeding may occur in 15% of cases, it may be intracerebral or rarely subarachnoid.

Treatment

Corticosteroids, transfusion of maternal platelets and Igs have been tried with good results. Treatment of choice is transfusion of maternal platelets, washed free from antibody containing plasma and suspended in AB blood group plasma. IVIG therapy should be tried in cases resistant or not fully responding to corticosteroids. Anti-D immunoglobulin is a less effective alternative. It is given in doses of 25 µg/kg IV on two consecutive days.

CHRONIC ITP

Among adults, majority of cases falls under this category. Usually these patients have mild bleeding tendency from mucous membranes of the mouth, genitalia, urinary tract and skin. Any stress, comorbidities, ingestion of antiplatelet drugs and infections may tip them into active bleeding. During these episodes, they may require short courses of glucocorticoids and treatment of the underlying condition. On a long-term basis, they require only advice to avoid precipitation of bleeding. Low dose of corticosteroid can be continued if they are symptomatic. On the whole, the majority can maintain normal hemostasis by these minor measures. In any case if the platelet count goes down below 20,000/mm³, risk of intracranial bleeding (both spontaneous and traumatic) increases and they have to be watched and active treatment instituted.

Chronic Refractory ITP

- ITP persistent for more than 3 months
- Failure to respond to splenectomy and rituximab
- Platelet count less than 50,000/mm³.

About 10% of ITP patient will fall under this category. A low platelet count alone is not a sufficient reason for treatment but they should have clinically significant bleeding symptoms. Management options of these patients are:

- Observation only specially if there is no symptoms
- Thrombopoiesis-stimulating drugs
- Observations with supportive care (short courses of steroids or IVIG for bleeding symptoms) or use of immunosuppressive and other agents, (cyclophosphamide, vincristine, azathioprine, danazol, mycophenolate mofetil, cyclosporine, etc.) may be tried. These drugs are also used in combination.

Autologous hematopoietic stem cell transplantation (HSCT) (lymphocytes depleted) after high dose chemotherapy has been tried in resistant ITP with variable success. Additional experience is needed with this approach.

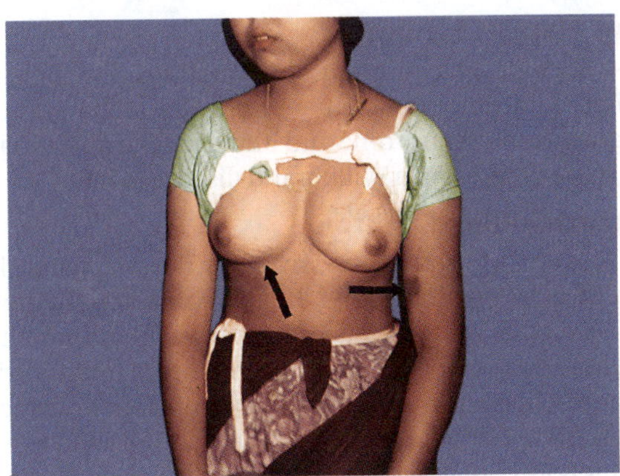

Fig. 174.4: ITP—female long-term steroid therapy striae (arrows)

Treatment of Associated Conditions/Complications

As a result of long use of a number of drugs in the treatment of ITP, patient may develop many complications like diabetes mellitus (DM), systemic hypertension, peptic ulcer, osteoporosis, cataract, various opportunistic infections, neutropenia, bone marrow depression and hepatic toxicity. These complications have to be treated appropriately.

Long-term Outcome and Mortality

Now studies are available where ITP patients have been followed up for 1–2 decades. In many of these studies, it is found that 70–80% of the patients have platelet count above 50,000/mm^3 after many years. Twenty percent had no response to treatment or required continued treatment. Four percent (4 patients in one series) died due to infectious complications of treatment and 25% due to bleeding.

In some follow-up studies even patients with chronic refractory ITP did well even though their platelet count was low. Mortality in published case series ranges from 0.3 to 0.5%. Reports with high mortality are probably not relevant to current clinical practice since:

- These reports are relatively small series of patients
- Many of these series are reported prior to availability of modern treatment and supportive care
- Identification of many asymptomatic patients by routine CBC has shifted the overall clinical spectrum of ITP towards that of decreased severity (Fig. 174.4).

SECONDARY THROMBOCYTOPENIA

Thrombocytopenia may develop as part of the clinical picture in acute leukemia, aplastic anemia, myelodysplastic syndrome (MDS), SLE, acquired immunodeficiency syndrome (AIDS), viral hemorrhagic fevers and several virus infections. In these, major clinical manifestations are those of the primary condition.

Drug-induced thrombocytopenia may be a result of toxic damage to the bone marrow. In this case, thrombocytopenia is a manifestation of marrow hypoplasia. Drugs may lead to immune-mediated thrombocytopenia. Heparin, sedormid, quinine, vancomycin and others may lead to immunologically-mediated platelet destruction. The antibodies can be demonstrated by flow cytometry or ELISA.

In drug-induced thrombocytopenia, very often other signs of drug toxicity may be evident but thrombocytopenia may be the sole manifestation at times. The drug or its metabolites act as haptens which bind noncovalently with albumin or other serum proteins in the plasma to form complete antigens. Antibodies are produced which combine specifically with the protein-bound haptenic drug or its metabolites to form antigen-antibody complexes. These are absorbed on to the platelet glycoproteins such as IIb/IIIa, fibrinogen receptor or glycoprotein 1b/1x (vWF receptor or both).

In some cases, e.g. quinine, the thrombocytopenia may be accompanied by other phenomena such as immune neutropenia and disseminated intravascular hemolysis. They activate complement and this leads to complement-mediated lysis of platelets in the circulation. If the amount of antibody coating the platelets is small, such platelets are destroyed by the macrophages of the spleen and liver. Drug-induced thrombocytopenia is generally severe. Since presence of the drug or its metabolites is essential to perpetuate the immune mechanism, withdrawal of the drug relieves the thrombocytopenia promptly. In severe cases, platelet transfusions are required. Corticosteroids help to arrest platelet destruction by inhibiting macrophage function in the spleen and liver.

Thrombocytopenia occurring as an isolated abnormality in otherwise healthy persons: Thrombocytopenia detected on routine platelet count may remain asymptomatic in many cases. Sometimes congenital thrombocytopenia may occur. Asymptomatic thrombocytopenia may precede myelodysplastic states or immune-mediated diseases like SLE for considerably long periods.

Congenital thrombocytopenia is rare. Commonly, it is associated with morphological abnormalities such as giant platelets.

CONGENITAL AND ACQUIRED DISORDERS OF PLATELET FUNCTION (THROMBOCYTOPATHIES)

These are conditions associated with functional defects of platelets. Platelet counts are normal or even increased in many. The defects may be either congenital or acquired. A classification of these various disorders is given in the Table 174.3.

Functional disorders of platelets are common, though many may be asymptomatic. The acquired disorders are much more common than the inherited conditions because of the very common use of drugs specially antiplatelet drugs and increased incidence of various systemic diseases which are associated with platelet dysfunction. The diagnosis of platelet functional disorders has become easy with the newly introduced platelet functional analyzer-PFA 100. The sensitivity and specificity of this are comparable with the conventional platelet aggregometry.

Storage Pool Disease

This disease is inherited as an autosomal dominant. In this condition, there is no store of adenosine diphosphate (ADP) in the granules of the platelets and so ADP is not released for further aggregation and platelet functions.

Bleeding disorder associated with ***albinism*** and ***Wiskott-Aldrich syndrome*** is also due to deficiency of

Table 174.3: Classification of platelet functional disorders	
Conditions	**Disorders**
Hereditary	• Storage pool disease • Wiskott-Aldrich syndrome • Albinism • Hermansky-Pudlak syndrome • Hereditary thrombasthenia (Glanzmann disease) • May-Hegglin anomaly, gray platelet syndrome • Bernard-Soulier syndrome
Acquired	• Drug effects—anti-inflammatory drugs, e.g. aspirin, phenylbutazone, indomethacin, other NSAIDs, dextran, clofibrate, dipyridamole, beta-lactam antibiotics and antihistamines, clopidogrel, GPIIb/IIIa receptor antagonists • Uremia, hepatic failure, scurvy, cardiopulmonary bypass surgery, trauma • Paraproteinemias—myelomatosis, Waldenström's macroglobulinemia, myeloproliferative disorders • Articles of food such as excess of ginger, garlic and onion

Abbreviations: NSAIDs = Nonsteroidal anti-inflammatory drugs; GP = Glycoprotein

nucleotides in the platelets. **Wiskott-Aldrich syndrome** which is inherited as a sex-linked recessive is usually associated with bleeding from various sites, thrombocytopenia, microthrombocytes, overwhelming infection due to immunodeficiency, eczematous dermatitis and a tendency to develop lymphomas.

In **Hermansky-Pudlak syndrome,** there is lack of storage of adenine nucleotides and a deficiency of serotonin. The associated hemorrhagic disorder is clinically mild.

Hereditary Thrombasthenia

It is a rare autosomal recessive disorder occurring in both sexes. The platelet membrane glycoprotein platelet integrin alpha(IIb) beta(3) (formerly called GPIIb/IIIa) is deficient or defective. The platelets do not bind fibrinogen and cannot aggregate. Bleeding manifestations are purpura, epistaxis, bleeding from wounds and cuts, menorrhagia and excessive bleeding during delivery. The characteristic laboratory finding is the failure of platelets to aggregate in presence of ADP, adrenaline, noradrenaline, thrombin or 5-hydroxytryptamine. Platelet adhesion and clot retraction are also poor. There is deficiency of fibrinogen on the platelet and it does not bind to the platelet surface membrane. Therefore, aggregation is not initiated. Bleeding may be mild or sometimes severe. Platelet transfusion may be required to arrest bleeding.

Diagnosis

Mucocutaneous bleeding, normal platelet count with single isolated platelets without any platelet clumping (in a noncoagulated peripheral blood smear) should raise the possibility of this disorder. In thrombasthenia, the platelets are seen singly in large numbers, without any tendency to form clumps.

Morphological abnormalities of platelets such as larger size may suggest immunological and functional abnormalities. Diagnosis is confirmed by studying platelet aggregation. Positive family history may be obtained in the majority of cases.

Giant Platelet Syndromes

These include glycoprotein abnormalities, e.g. Bernard-Soulier syndrome, deficiency of platelet alpha granules, e.g. gray platelet syndrome and May-Hegglin abnormality, and some types of von Willebrand disease (vWF).

Bernard-Soulier Syndrome

This is a rare autosomal recessive disorder which may lead to mild or severe bleeding. This is characterized by the presence of larger platelets in peripheral blood which fail to adhere to vessel wall. The abnormality is in the surface glycoprotein coat. The platelets have deficient or defective glycoprotein GPIb/Ix complex. They cannot bind to vWF and therefore, platelet adhesion to vascular endothelium is defective.

May-Hegglin Anomaly

In this anomaly, a mild bleeding disorder is associated with basophilic and pyroninophilic inclusion bodies in the leukocytes and an abnormality of the megakaryocytes. Thrombocytopenia may develop. Megathrombocytes may be seen in peripheral blood.

Acquired Disorders of Platelet Function

Drugs such as aspirin, clopidogrel and sulfinpyrazone inhibit platelet activities and they are used as antiplatelet drugs. Several drugs and articles of food produce platelet dysfunction, sometimes leading to mild or even moderate bleeding tendency. These are used as antiplatelet drugs.

Other drugs such as NSAIDs, beta-lactam antibiotics and antihistamines and articles of food such as ginger, onion, garlic and fish oils may give rise to purpura.

Except thrombocytopenia, drug-induced thrombopathies rarely give rise to serious generalized bleeding tendency in normal subjects. In persons who have congenital or acquired defects of hemostasis, more serious bleeding manifestations develop. Withdrawal of the drug for a week may be essential if surgery or similar procedures are to be undertaken. The platelet defect can be compensated by platelet transfusions. Recently, DDAVP (1-desamino-8-d-arginine vasopressin) given in doses of 3 µg/kg/bw (maximum 20 µg IV/SC 12 hourly) is useful in relieving the bleeding tendency. This can be used for short-term use.

Platelet adhesiveness is diminished in scurvy and this factor also contributes to the hemorrhagic tendency.

Paraproteinemias

Platelet dysfunction may develop in Waldenström's macroglobulinemia and myeloma. The abnormal protein in circulation may coat the platelets and lead to dysfunction resulting in disorders of adhesion, aggregation and release reaction.

Metabolic Disorders

The bleeding diathesis in uremia is partly attributable to defects of platelet function. Several abnormalities may be seen. These defects are reversible when the metabolic abnormalities are corrected. In liver failure, variable platelet defects may be encountered.

Treatment of Platelet Functional Disorders

The treatment of the inherited abnormalities is very limited. The offending drugs responsible for platelet dysfunction and bleeding should be stopped. Treatment for the basic disease is undertaken, e.g. hemodialysis for uremia. The other modalities include desmopressin for vWD, oral estrogen 50 mg/kg/day or transdermal estradiol 50–100 mcg/24 hours applied twice daily and erythropoietin (EPO) for uremia. Platelet transfusion may be given if the bleeding is severe but there is always a complication of developing platelet antibodies and later on refractoriness to platelet transfusions. Recombinant factor VIIa has been tried if there is a severe bleeding not amenable to any other treatment.

VASCULAR PURPURAS

These are a group of heterogeneous disorders characterized by bruising and spontaneous bleeding from small vessels. In these, the bleeding is due to abnormality in the capillaries. Except for a prolongation of bleeding time, other tests may be normal.

The number and function of platelets are usually normal, though occasionally platelet dysfunction may coexist. The defects may be hereditary as in Ehlers-Danlos syndrome or acquired as in scurvy.

Henoch-Schönlein Syndrome (IgA vasculitis-IgAV)
(**See** also Sections 12, 16 and 17)

This is an immune complex disease caused by type III hypersensitivity reaction similar to that of rheumatic fever and acute glomerulonephritis (AGN). This is an acute small vessel leukocytoclastic vasculitis. This is not a primary hematological disorder. It belongs to a group of vasculitic disorders, described in Section 12. The current name of this entity is IgA vasculitis (IgAV) and shares many characteristic features of IgA nephropathy. This particular entity is described here because it may be mistaken for thrombocytopenic purpura clinically. Although the cause is unknown, IgA has a pivotal role in the pathogenesis of Henoch-Schönlein purpura (HSP). Among the two subclasses of IgA (IgA_1 and IgA_2), only IgA_1 is involved in HSP. IgA_1 is deposited in the organs affected, e.g. vessel walls and renal mesangium. The IgA_1 molecules are altered so that they aggregate into macromolecular complexes which activate the alternate pathway of complement and then deposit in the renal mesangium.

Histology shows vasculitis involving the small blood vessels. This syndrome is more common in children but occasionally it may be seen in young adults. It is the most common form of systemic vasculitis in children. Eighty to ninety percent occurs in the pediatric age group. Unlike other forms of vasculitis IgAV is self-limited in a great majority of cases. Males predominate. In a small proportion of cases, there is history of preceding B-hemolytic streptococcal infection 10–20 days prior to the onset of purpura. Other precipitating causes are allergic reactions to drugs and food materials. In many, there may be no evidence of a precipitating cause.

Clinical Features
The clinical tetrad of manifestations is:
- Palpable purpura (Fig. 174.5)
- Arthritis/arthralgia
- Abdominal pain
- Renal disease.

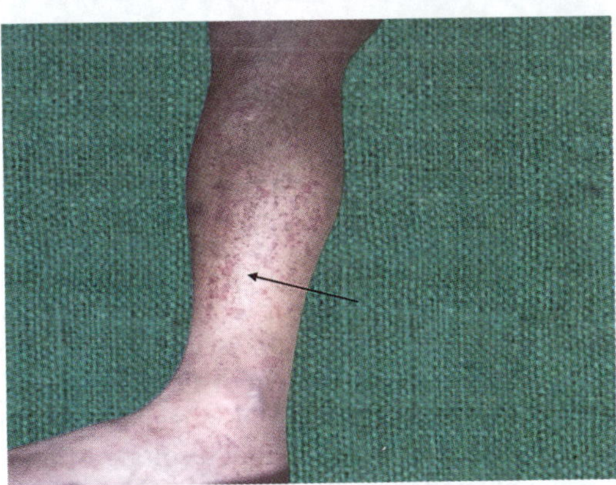

Fig. 174.5: Henoch-Schönlein purpura uncomplicated. *Note:* Purpura most distally (arrow)

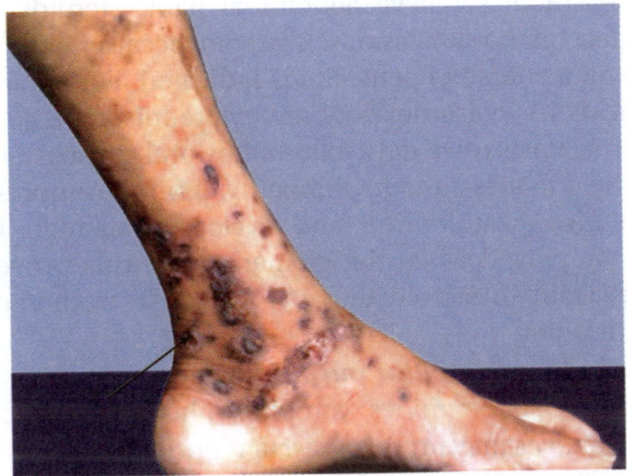

Fig. 174.6: Henoch-Schönlein purpura with skin necrosis and ulceration (arrow)

A purpuric rash which is characteristically palpable develops acutely over the skin of the extensor surface of the forearms, elbows, buttocks and legs distally. The lesions may be urticarial, blotchy and pruritic. Only rarely lesions develop over the trunk and face. Cutaneous purpura in the distal parts of the body is the essential feature (Fig. 174.6). Joint lesions occur in 75%, GI involvement occurs in 50–75% and renal involvement occurs in 40–50%. They share many of the features of IgA nephropathy.

Abdominal symptoms such as colicky pain and vomiting are usual. Hematemesis and melena may develop in severe cases. Children may develop intussusception.

Involvement of joints is common and many large joints are affected. Polyarthralgia, polyarthritis and periarthritis may occur. Hematuria, albuminuria, edema, and hypertension are indicative of renal involvement which may develop in 10–30% of cases. The renal lesions may manifest as AGN. Some of the cases may develop acute renal failure. A small proportion develops persistent and progressive renal lesions. Diagnosis is clinical. There are no pathognomonic laboratory tests. Serum IgA levels are raised in 50% of cases. Skin biopsy is not mandatory but it will show involvement of small blood vessels (postcapillary venules) within the papillary dermis. The predominant cell infiltrates are neutrophils and monocytes. Those having a marked renal involvement, e.g. nephrotic range proteinuria or elevated serum creatinine should undergo a renal biopsy to know the extent of renal involvement. Blood shows neutrophil leukocytosis. Mild eosinophilia may occur at times. Tests of platelet and capillary function are usually normal. HSP is a self-limiting disease. In a third, recurrence may occur. Majority of patients recover completely but recurrence may occur on exposure to the allergen.

Treatment

Symptomatic treatment is adequate in most of the cases since the condition is self-limiting in the majority. Supportive care (rest, hydration, symptomatic relief of pain) and symptomatic treatment of abdominal and joint pain with paracetamol and NSAIDs are given. The role of corticosteroids is controversial. Prednisolone 1 mg/kg per day may benefit patients with abdominal symptoms and it may reduce the risk of recurrence and renal involvement. Steroids should be withdrawn after a short course. Antispasmodics relieve abdominal pain. Steroids have no effect on the skin lesions. If streptococcal sore throat is evident, a course of penicillin is indicated. For persistent nephritis, IV pulse doses of methylprednisolone 30 mg/kg for 3 consecutive days followed by oral corticosteroids may help to arrest the nephropathy. Immunosuppressive drugs like azathioprine and cyclophosphamide have been employed when the glomerulonephritis proves to be resistant to steroid therapy. Response to therapy is unsatisfactory.

Drug-induced vascular purpura: Exposure to drugs like penicillin, sulfonamides, atropine, phenacetin, aspirin, and sedatives may produce vascular purpura.

Senile Purpura

This condition occurs as a chronic disorder of thin elderly people above the age of seventy years. Purpuric and ecchymotic spots occur on the extensor surfaces of the forearms which arise spontaneously or after unnoticed trauma. The purpura is due to traction injury to the small capillaries of the dermis due to loss of dermal collagen and subcutaneous fat. No therapy is effective in this condition. It is important to distinguish this benign disorder from other diseases which may require therapy.

HEREDITARY HEMORRHAGIC TELANGIECTASIA (HHT)

Syn: Rendu-Osler-Weber syndrome

Etiology and Clinical Features

This hereditary bleeding disorder is transmitted as an autosomal dominant trait and affects both sexes. Endoglin is a transferring growth factor-β (TGF-β) receptor which is normally present abundantly on endothelial cells. TGF-β is member of a family of dimeric polypeptide growth factors. TGF regulates the proliferation and differentiation of cells, embryonic development, wound healing and angiogenesis. Endoglin is mutated in patients with HHT. It is believed that most if not all cases of HHT results from endoglin or ALK-1 haploinsufficiency (i.e. lack of sufficient protein for normal function). Multiple telangiectasia are found in the tongue, nasal mucosa, face, lips, conjunctiva, mucous membrane of GIT, kidneys, solid organs and over other parts of the skin (Fig. 174.7). Any of these sites may bleed recurrently since the vessels are fragile. Smaller lesions on exposed parts may lead

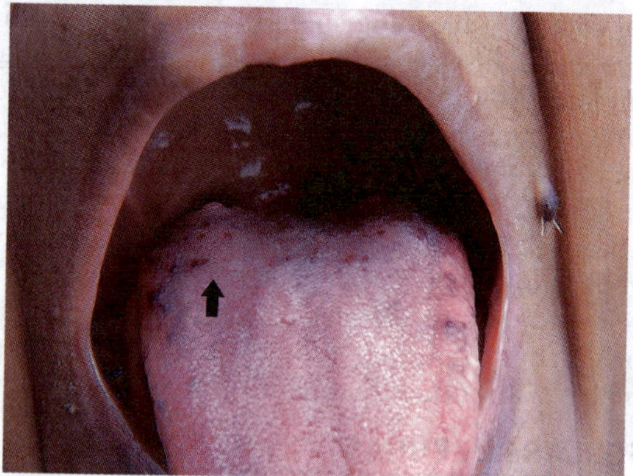

Fig. 174.7: Woman with telangiectasis oral cavity and tongue. **Note:** The telangiectasias (arrow)

to cosmetic problems and bleeding. Larger ones lead to bleeding, embolic manifestations and high output cardiac failure. At the sites of bleeding, there is increased fibrinolytic activity.

Ocular complications include bleeding from the conjunctiva, retinal hemorrhage and retinal detachment. Neurological hepatic and pulmonary complications may develop. These include cerebral or subarachnoid hemorrhage, development of mycotic aneurysms, hepatic cirrhosis, portal hypertension, biliary disease and pulmonary arteriovenous (AV) fistulae. Primary pulmonary hypertension occurs in 15%.

High output cardiac failure, embolization and digital clubbing may follow. As age advances, the number of lesions increases and bleeding becomes more marked.

Diagnosis

Diagnosis is made from the typical telangiectasia, bleeding episodes and family history.

Treatment

Local pressure and application of thrombin help to arrest bleeding. Cauterization and surgical treatment of AV fistula are of limited value but may be required at times. Hematinic therapy is indicated to prevent anemia. Antifibrinolytic drugs have been tried with benefit. Pulmonary AV malformation is treated by embolization. Cerebral AV shunts are surgically excised. Hormones, antifibrinolytic drugs, estrogen, antiestrogens (tamoxifen) angiogenesis inhibitors like bevacizumab are used to treat HHT and its manifestations. Bevacizumab in a dose of 5 mg/kg bw once every 2 weeks gives amelioration of the AV lesions and bleeding episodes.

SYMPTOMATIC PURPURA

Several infections cause purpuric manifestation:

- ***Bacterial infections:*** Meningococcal septicemia, bacterial endocarditis, leptospirosis and Gram-negative septicemias.
- ***Viral infections:*** Dengue fever, measles, influenza, hemorrhagic fevers and smallpox.
- ***Rickettsial infections:*** Typhus and spotted fevers.
- ***Protozoal infections:*** Falciparum malaria.

Bleeding is caused by the direct injury to the vascular endothelium by the infecting agent, bacterial embolism, or due to vasculitis as in bacterial endocarditis. The toxins of infective agents inhibit thrombopoiesis and also accelerate platelet destruction. Other factors like thrombocytopenia and diffuse intravascular coagulation may also be contributory.

ANTIPLATELET DRUG THERAPY

Antiplatelet drugs to prevent thrombosis of the coronary, cerebral and peripheral arteries are widely employed. Antiplatelet drugs acting at different levels of platelet activation are available at present. On many occasions, they are used singly. Often they are combined in order to improve the efficacy. All of them lead to some degree (often minor) of hemorrhagic tendency. The three groups of antiplatelet drugs and their mechanisms of actions are given below.

- Aspirin blocks the enzyme cyclo-oxygenase (prostaglandin H synthase), the enzyme that mediates the first step in the biosynthesis of prostaglandins and thromboxanes (including TxA2) from arachidonic acid. This will inhibit the platelet aggregation.
- The P2Y12 receptor blockers, clopidogrel, ticlopidine, prasugrel, ticagrelor and cangrelor block the binding of ADP to a platelet receptor P2Y12, thereby inhibiting activation of the GPIIb/IIIa complex and platelet aggregation.
- Anti-GPIIb/IIIa antibodies and receptor antagonists inhibit the final common pathway of platelet aggregation (the crossbridging of platelets by fibrinogen binding to the GPIIb/IIIa receptor) and may also prevent adhesion to the vessel wall.

Aspirin blocks synthesis of thromboxane A2 by inhibiting the enzyme cyclooxygenase.

Aspirin in doses of 75 mg/day has been recommended for general use by cardiologists particularly with or without statins and mild antihypertensive drugs as protection against atherosclerotic vascular disease.

Ticlopidine and clopidogrel inhibits GPIIb/IIIa and thus blocks aggregation in response to ADP and other aggregrating agents. Different types of GPIIb/IIIa receptor antagonists are available. These include:

- ***Abciximab:*** It is a monoclonal antibody against IIb/IIIa receptor, it blocks receptor action and also blocks the binding of vitronectin to its receptors on endothelial cells. It inhibits platelet aggregation and the template bleeding time.
- Synthetic inhibitors:
  - ***Eptifibatide:*** This is a heptapeptide
  - ***Tirofiban:*** These are nonpeptides
  - ***Lamifiban***.
  All inhibit IIb/IIIa receptors.

Combination of different antiplatelet drugs produce enhanced activity than using a single drug. This type of different combinations of antiplatelet drugs improves the success rate of stenting in coronary and other arteries and prevents postangioplasty thrombosis.

Temporary Stoppage of Antiplatelet Therapy

This may be required at times when patients receiving long-term antiplatelet have to undergo surgical or dental procedures, due to risk of increased bleeding. The antiplatelet drug has to be stopped for 7–10 days before the surgical procedure and restarted after the surgery. There is a small risk of precipitating the illness for which long-term antiplatelet treatment is instituted, this has to be managed with the help of the cardiologists and/or neurologist.

CHAPTER
175

Defects of Coagulation

Mathew Thomas, KV Krishna Das

> **Chapter Summary**
>
> - Inherited Disorders
>   - Hemophilia A (Factor VIII Deficiency)
>   - Christmas Disease
>   - von Willebrand's Disease
> - Vitamin K Deficiency
> - Circulating Anticoagulants
> - Pathological Fibrinolysis

INHERITED DISORDERS

HEMOPHILIA A (FACTOR VIII DEFICIENCY)

Hemophilia comprises of two clinically indistinguishable coagulation defects—hemophilia A due to deficiency of factor VIII, and hemophilia B due to deficiency of factor IX. Both of these conditions are inherited through the X-chromosome. The pathogenesis and basic defects in the two conditions are different; therefore, treatment schedules are also different. Hemophilia is one of the most common inherited coagulation defects. The disease is worldwide in distribution. In India, it forms two-thirds of all the inherited coagulation defects. About 25–33% of cases may not give any family history and it is presumed that in them the disease arises due to spontaneous mutation either in the patient or his mother. The clinical picture varies widely in affected subjects.

Prevalence of hemophilia in the developed world is around 6/10,000 population. India should have about 50,000 patients with severe hemophilia. In addition, about 1,300 new patients will be added each year.

Hemophilia is transmitted as a sex-linked recessive disorder and the genetic defect is located in the X-chromosome. The gene locus for factor VIII is located at the tip of the long arms of X-chromosome at Xq28. It is divided into 26 exons that spans 186,000 base pairs and has a molecular weight of 267,000. It is one of the largest known genes. It constitutes 0.1% of the bulk of the X-chromosome. Factor VIII gene is very susceptible to undergo abnormalities such as deletion, missense mutation and nonsense mutation. Due to the variability of genetic abnormalities, hemophilia is a heterogeneous disorder varying in severity and clinical behavior. In about 50% of hemophiliacs, factor VIII C is below 5% of normal. In the others, the level ranges from 5 to 20%. It is transmitted by females who act as carriers, but it manifests almost exclusively in males. Half of the daughters of female carriers possess the trait and half of the sons suffer from the disease. Male hemophiliacs pass the trait to all their daughters but their sons are not affected. Carries of hemophilia (A and B) have only 50% of the normal levels of factor VIII and factor IX respectively (Tables 175.1 and 175.2). Clinically, they have no bleeding, but they have decreased coagulability. This may even protect them against fatal ischemic heart disease (IHD). They may show higher bleeding tendencies when exposed to antiplatelet drugs. Females may be rarely affected when an affected male marries a carrier female, when there is an X-chromosome inactivation in the female at an unusually early stage of embryogenesis resulting in low levels of factor VIII or a female with an abnormal karyotype as with loss of part or all of an X-chromosome as in Turner's syndrome.

The basic defect is deficiency, defective function or absence of factor VIII. Levels of factor VIII as low as 0.2 units/mL of plasma is enough for adequate coagulation activity. The bleeding tendency depends to a great deal on the levels of factor VIII in the plasma.

Table 175.1: Classifications of hemophilia based on the severity

Classification	Hemophilia A factor VIII level	Clinical features
Severe	≤1% of normal (≤0.01 u/mL)	• Spontaneous hemorrhage from early infancy • Frequent spontaneous hemarthroses and other hemorrhages, requiring clotting factor replacement
Moderate	1–5% of normal (0.01–0.05 u/mL)	• Hemorrhage secondary to trauma or surgery • Occasional spontaneous hemarthroses
Mild	6–30% of normal (0.06–0.30 u/mL)	• Hemorrhage secondary to trauma or surgery • Rare spontaneous hemorrhage

Table 175.2: Relationship between the levels of factor IX and clinical severity

Classifications	Factor IX levels	Hemophilia B factor IX dose
Mild	5–40% of normal	0.05–0.4 u/mL
Moderate	1–5%	0.01–0.05 u/mL
Severe	<1%	<0.01 u/mL

When the level of factor VIII falls below 30% of normal, bleeding tendencies start. Spontaneous bleeding occurs only when the level falls below 5%. In a severe case, there may be no detectable factor VIIIC during episodes of bleeding.

Factor VIII molecule: This is a protein of large molecular size, $1.5–2 \times 10^6$ daltons. Factor VIII is synthesized primarily by the hepatocytes, but kidneys, sinusoidal endothelial cells and lymphatic tissue can also synthesize small amounts. Its half-life in circulation is 12 hours in adults. It circulates in plasma as a covalent complex with von Willebrand's factor (vWF) which is synthesized by endothelial cells. vWF forms the major bulk of the circulating factor VIII complex. It used to be known as factor VIII-related antigen (VIII RAG) since it could be precipitated by heterologous antisera developed in animals. Combination of vWF with factor VIII helps to increase the synthesis, protect factor VIII from proteolysis and concentrate factor VIII coagulant activity at the required site. Factor VIII has to be released from vWF to enable it to take part in the process of coagulation and form the complex consisting of factor VIIIa, IXa and phospholipid. Factor VIIIa accelerates the rate of cleavage of factor X through IXa. Activated factor VIII is short-lived.

Clinical Features

The clinical severity usually correlates with the assayed factor levels. Approximately 80% of the patients have hemophilia A. Two-thirds of the patients have severe disease. The bleeding tendency is noticed early in life, within the first 2 years of life in severe cases. Few of them do not bleed till they are 4 years. Sometimes, the umbilical stump may bleed. Though bleeding can occur from any site, the common presentations are hematomas, deep tissue bleeding, hemarthrosis or hematuria. Bleeding may be spontaneous, may follow trivial trauma or undue physical exertion. Following cuts or wounds, bleeding is arrested initially, but may soon restart and continue unchecked, leading to fatal blood loss. The extravasated blood does not clot for long periods. Recurrent painful swelling of the knees when the child starts to walk should suggest the possibility of hemophilia.

Bleeding into joints occurs frequently in moderate and severe cases. The knees, ankles, elbows, shoulders, and hips are commonly affected. Bleeding may be spontaneous or follow unaccustomed exertion. The joints show features of acute inflammation. Repeated hemorrhage into joints and deep tissues lead to crippling ankylosis and contractures (Fig. 175.1). Chronic synovitis is seen in 10% of hemophiliacs in India. Among 64% of such patients showed the presence of human leukocyte antigen (HLA) B27 and this is statistically significant. Bleeding can occur in the central nervous system in severe cases.

The disease shows remissions and exacerbations. Physical exertion, infections, trauma or psychological stress lead to exacerbations. With the passage of time, the severity and frequency of bleeding diminishes. Death may result from uncontrolled blood loss or bleeding into vital organs. Patients and carriers of hemophilia appear to have a reduced risk of coronary artery disease (CAD).

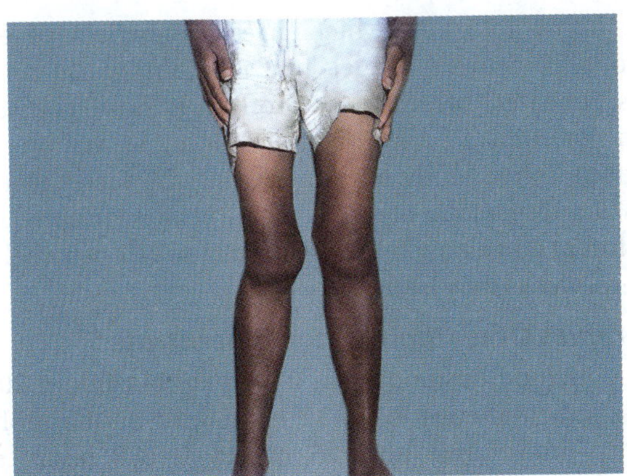

Fig. 175.1: Male—hemophilic arthritis knees. ***Note:*** Swelling and deformity

Diagnosis

Hemophilia should be suspected from the history, evidence of hereditary and from the prolonged coagulation time or activated partial thromboplastin time (aPTT). Clinical hallmarks are joint and muscle hemorrhages, easy bruising and prolonged potentially fatal hemorrhage following trauma or surgery, but no excessive bleeding after abrasions or minor cuts. Normal platelet count, normal bleeding time, normal prothrombin time (PT) and a prolonged aPTT are characteristics of hemophilias.

Differential Diagnosis

Hemophilia has to be differentiated from Christmas disease, von Willebrand's disease (vWD) and acquired coagulopathies. vWD is distinguished form hemophilia by the pattern of bleeding, which is mucocutaneous in the former. The most sensitive laboratory test for the diagnosis of vWD is ristocetin cofactor assay which is difficult to perform. Carrier detection is not necessary if she is an obligatory carrier, e.g. mother of more than one hemophilic sons. But, if necessary, deoxyribonucleic acid (DNA)-based techniques are the preferred method. Bleeding can occur in carriers, since their factor levels can have a wide range. Factor level should be determined in carriers before a major surgery to know their risk of bleeding. Genetic analysis of factor VIII and IX genes can provide accurate prenatal diagnosis but invasive methods like amniocentesis carries risk. Forceps and vacuum should be avoided in pregnant women.

Normal PT and a prolonged aPTT are also found in heparin therapy, acquired inhibitors of factor VIII or IX, deficiency of factors XII, prekallikrein and high-molecular-weight kininogen (HMWK) and in patients with antiphospholipid syndrome (APS). Patients with factor XII, prekallikrein and HMWK deficiencies do not clinically bleed. In APS, the antiphospholipid antibodies interfere with the *in vitro* test prolonging it. Inhibitors and acquired antibodies are differentiated by mixing study in which normal plasma corrects the factor deficiency and the prolonged aPTT while the others do not. Specific factor deficiencies are then detected by assessing the aPTT after mixing the test plasma with commercially available plasmas, deficient in known factors. After determining the factor deficiency as VIII or IX, specific factor assays are done by either one stage or two stage methods. Assay of factors helps to establish the diagnosis and assess the severity. Factor VIII assay also helps to monitor replacement therapy.

Treatment

Modern optimal management of hemophilia is complex and consists of provision of preventive care, use of replacement treatment with coagulation factors during acute bleeding as well as for prophylaxis, treatment of complications of the disease and the complications of antihemophilic therapy. Patients with hemophilia should receive an integrated comprehensive care.

Circumcision: About 50% of undiagnosed hemophilic children bleed during circumcision for the first time. Male children with family history should be diagnosed soon after birth by factor determination by cord blood or a superficial venous blood sample. Fibrin glue is safe and effective during the circumcision and is less costly than factor treatment.

Vaccinations: The routine childhood vaccinations should not be given intramuscularly (IM). Instead, they should be given as subcutaneous injections using the smallest gauge needle. Pressure and ice should be applied to the site for 3–5 minutes after the injection.

Counseling, education, dental care and exercise and athletic participation are to be given to the growing hemophilic children. Comprehensive, multidisciplinary hemophilia centers help the patients with hemophilia in all aspects of their care.

Replacement therapy with clotting factor concentrates forms the cornerstone of treatment. They are given to prevent bleeding and to limit or resolve hemorrhage. Factor VIII and IX products are of two types:

1. ***Plasma derived factor VIII:*** Derived from processed human plasma. These are of intermediate, high and ultra-high purity. Intensity of viral inactivation and the amount of factor content are the markers of purity.
2. ***Recombinant factors VIII and IX:*** Produced from cell lines engineered to express large amounts of the factors. First, second and third generation recombinant factors are now available. The third generation will not have any added human or animal proteins in the manufacturing process or final preparation. Recombinant preparations are more costly.

Strategies are being studied to produce clotting factors with longer half-life by combining it with an immunoglobulin fragment crystallizable domain and reconstitution with pegylated liposomes.

Dosing and Desired Factor Levels

One international unit of clotting factor is the amount present in 1 mL of pooled normal plasma. On an average, a normal person with a plasma volume of 3,000 mL will have 3,000 international units of each clotting factor (100%). So, according to this fact, about 3,000 units of factor VIII would be required to increase the patient's factor level from 1% (severe hemophilia) to 100%.

Practically, the number of units required for a patient with hemophilia depends on his weight, volume of distribution and the desired factor level. Volume of distribution of factor VIII is 0.5 (half of normal plasma

Table 175.3: Dosage of factor VIII

Condition	Initial dose U/kg	Repeat doses U/kg	Total duration of therapy
• Life/limb-threatening bleed • Intracranial bleed • Major tissue bleeds Major surgery	50	25–30 every 8–12 h or 3–4 U/kg/bw as IV infusion	14–21 days
Hemarthrosis	20–30	20 every 12 h	1–2 days
Hematomas—not life-threatening	20–30	20 every 12 h	1–2 days
Dental extraction, minor surgery	20	20 every 12 h	1–2 days

volume) (Table 175.3). The formula for calculating the dose of factor is:

> Dose of the factor (international units) = Weight (kg) × desired percentage increase × 0.5.

For example, in a patient with severe hemophilia (factor level <1%), if the factor level has to be increased to 30% and his weight is 60 kg, the dose required is 60 × 30 × 0.5 = 900 international units. As the half-life of factor is about 12 hours, the factor has to be administered every 12 hours to maintain the desired level. The factor is usually given as an intravenous (IV) bolus infusion. A maintenance continuous infusion can be given at a dose of 2–4 units/kg/hour after the initial bolus dose. Factor IX has a longer half-life and need to be given once in 18–24 hours. The diagnosis of the type of hemophilia should be certain because there is no clinical effect if the factor is administered wrongly.

Primary prophylaxis is regular administration of factor VIII from very early age to maintain factor level above 1% to prevent spontaneous bleeding. The factor is given three times a week up to about 15–20 years of age. Many studies on primary prophylaxis showed excellent results with very few joint and other bleeds and arthropathies. The disadvantages are high cost and inhibitor development.

Desired factor level for various bleeding episodes:
- Early joint and muscle bleeds: 30%.
- Severe joint and muscle bleeds and dental surgery: 50%.
- Intracranial, face, neck and hip bleeds: 80–100%.
- Orthopedic surgery: 80–100% followed by 30% (prophylaxis) after surgery.
- Major surgeries: 60–100% followed by prophylactic 30–60% after surgery.

Therapy in Acute Bleeding Episodes

Rest in bed is essential during a bleeding episode. The inflamed joint should be splinted and cooled with ice packs. Sedatives like diazepam or phenobarbitone or analgesics like dextropropoxyphene may be used to relieve insomnia and pain. Local measures to stop the bleeding include pressure, adrenaline packs and local dressing with fibrin foam or thrombin. Bleeding sites from gums, tooth sockets or nose should be plugged with adrenaline packs.

At the first indication of a joint bleed, factor infusion should be started at home (caregivers are trained to give home infusion) which gives the benefit of early factor replacement. Target joint is a joint which undergoes repeated bleeding. A short high dose course of corticosteroids (5 days) is useful. Joint aspiration may be done infrequently after increasing the factor level to 50%. For target joint bleeding, a short course prophylactic treatment consisting of 3 doses of factor VIII per week for several weeks may be useful.

Therapies Other than Factor Concentrate

These include desmopressin 0.3 μg/kg, maximum 20 μg IV or subcutaneous every 12 hours and antifibrinolytic agents—tranexamic acid 25 mg/kg at 6–8 hours and epsilon-aminocaproic acid (EACA) 75–100 mg/kg per dose every 6 hours. Desmopressin can be also used as an intranasal spray 300 μg and it acts by increasing the circulating factor VIII level 2–4 times above the baseline by releasing the factor from endothelial storage sites. Antifibrinolytic drugs act by inhibiting plasminogen activation in the fibrin clot.

In India where factor concentrates are costly and not easily available, fresh frozen plasma (FFP) and cryoprecipitate are used which contains much less amount of factor VIII and IX. Large volumes will have to be given to increase the factor level at least by a few percentages. At present, many states in India including Kerala provide factor VIII to hemophiliacs free of cost in selected hospitals.

Aspirin and nonsteroidal anti-inflammatory drugs (NSAIDs) are generally contraindicated. Pain management should be with paracetamol, propoxyphene or codeine.

Factor VIII Inhibitors

About 25–30% of hemophilia A patients and 3–5% of hemophilia B patients develop factor inhibitors during treatment. These inhibitors occur more frequently in severe cases and are not usually responsible for frequent bleeding. Inhibitor activity is measured by Bethesda units. High responders have more than 5 units and low responders less than 5 Bethesda units. The high responders are treated by bypassing the deficient clotting factor. The drugs used are activated prothrombin complex concentrates (aPCC)—FEIBA or recombinant factor VIIa. The low responders may be treated by high purity factor concentrates or porcine factor VIII concentrates. Inhibitor eradication [Immune tolerance induction (ITI)] is done by administration of the deficient factor to reset or tolerize the patient's immune system.

Newer Information on Neutralizing Antibodies

Development of neutralizing antifactor VIII alloantibodies (inhibitors) in patients with hemophilia may depend on the concentrate used for replacement therapy. Both groups of patients develop antibodies irrespective of the type of replacement used (natural vs recombinant). The authors found that the plasma-derived natural product was less immunogenic than the recombinant preparations.

Source: Peyvandi F, Mannucci PM, Garagiola I, et al. A randomized trial of factor VIII and naturalizing antibodies in hemophilia A. N Engl J Med. 2016;374(21):2054-64.

Factor VIII Mimetics

Substances other than factor VIII which perform or supersede the functions of factor VIII (factor VIII mimetic) are being developed. Emicizumab (ACE910) functions as a conformational replica of factor VIII, binding to factor IX and X in a thrombin-generating complex. The use of emicizumab as subcutaneous injections would permit a weekly prophylactic therapy avoiding IV infusions. Newer drugs which perform the function of factor VIII without being chemically related to factor VIII C (factor VIII-mimetic function) produced by humanized bispecific antibodies are being introduced. These avoid the present cumbersome management of hemophilia with therapeutic and prophylactic doses of natural or recombinant factor VIII which demand regular injections and both being associated with the risk of producing antibodies which neutralize the administered antihuman globulin. Emicizumab 6 (ACE916) is a humanized bispecific antibody mimicking the cofactor functions of factor VIII developed by Japanese workers. Administration of emicizumab in doses of 0.3, 1.0 or 3.0 mg/kg bw subcutaneously weekly reduced the frequency and severity of bleeding episodes in hemophilias in both patients with and without antibodies. Antibodies have not been detected against emicizumab so far. Serious side effects did not occur in 18 patients studied for 12 weeks. Further studies are indicated.

Source: Shima M, Hanabusa H, Taki M, et al. Factor VIII-mimetic function of humanized bispecific antibody in hemophilia A. N Engl J Med. 2016;374(21):2044-53.

Long-term Complications of Hemophilia

The long-term complications like arthropathies are treated by synovectomy (open or radioactive synovectomy) or total joint replacement arthroplasty. Modern donor screening methods, virucidal techniques, insistence on safety testing and recombinant products have led to factor products with extremely low-risk of transmission of infectious agents. But hepatitis C virus and parvovirus transmission occur very rarely. Till three decades ago prior to the discovery of acquired immunodeficiency syndrome (AIDS), use of infected blood has transmitted AIDS to hemophiliac patients inadvertently. The modern factor VIII preparations are free from human immunodeficiency virus (HIV) contamination. Patients who develop end stage liver disease can undergo liver transplantation which cures the hemophilia in many patients.

Gene Therapy

Currently gene therapy is studied in many clinical trials as a treatment for hemophilia.

- Cells from the patient are taken out, genetically modified to secrete the deficient factor, and reimplanted back to the patient—ex vivo gene therapy.
- Factor VIII or IX encoding vectors are injected into the hemophilic patients.
- Universal cell lines are enclosed in immune-protective devices and implanted into the recipient in a non-autologous therapy.

Prognosis

With the modern knowledge and care, patients with hemophilia are likely to live longer without many disabilities, specially patients who have undergone prophylactic therapy.

Acquired Hemophilia

These are acquired bleeding disorders in which inhibitors are acquired against clotting factors. The most common condition is development of inhibitors against factor VIII. These antibodies suppress factor VIII in nonhemophilic patients and results in bleeding manifestations. Such factor VIII antibodies are detected in postpartum women, rheumatic diseases like rheumatoid arthritis and systemic lupus erythematosus (SLE), in solid tumors and also drug induced. *Clinical features* consist of bleeding manifestations specially after surgical procedures. Many patients have ecchymosis, bleeding gums and hematomas. Spontaneous hematomas which are common in hemophilia are unusual in this disorder. The condition is suspected when there is a prolonged aPTT and a normal PT in a patient with recent onset of bleeding. Mixing studies with normal plasma does not correct the aPTT confirming the presence of inhibitors which can be quantified by Bethesda assay.

Treatment consists of stopping the bleeding by desmopressin, factor VIII concentrates, aPCC and recombinant factor VIIa. The antibody elimination is done by giving drugs like rituximab, cyclophosphamide or prednisone.

CHRISTMAS DISEASE

Syn: Hemophilia B

This is also an X-linked recessive disease, caused by deficiency or abnormality of factor IX. Transmission is similar to that of hemophilia. Factor IX is a 415 amino acid serine protein, synthesized in the liver. It is the largest among the vitamin K-dependent proteins. Plasma concentration of factor IX is 50 times that of factor VIII and its half-life is 24 hours. Factor IX gene is located in the long arm of chromosome X at Xq27.1–q27.2. The gene for factor IX is smaller and less complex than that of factor VIII. More than 2,100 mutations of the gene have been identified.

Preliminary coagulation tests are similar to those of hemophilia. Frequency is one-fourth of that of hemophilia A. The diagnosis can be confirmed by demonstration of reduced levels of factor IX. Fifty percent of daughters of carrier females are carriers. Carriers of hemophilia B have lower levels of factor IX activity compared to normal. Normal level of factor IX activity is 1 u/mL levels less than 0.1 u/mL indicates severe disease. The clinical spectrum resembles that of hemophilia, and it varies depending on the levels of factor IX. Inhibitors to factor IX develop only in 1.5–3% of cases.

Treatment: Factor IX can be administered as the concentrate, prothrombin complex concentrates, recombinant factor IX or FFP. Since the distribution volume of factor IX in the tissues is twice the plasma volume, the dose of factor IX for therapy should be twice that of factor VIII. This has to be administered as IV bolus twice a day.

VON WILLEBRAND'S DISEASE

Syn: Pseudohemophilia

This is the most common inherited bleeding disorder, the next being hemophilia. vWD affects approximately 1% of the population. The disease is due to mutations in vWF which leads to either decreased level or abnormal constitution of the factor. Most cases are transmitted as autosomal dominant. Males and females are affected equally. vWF is encoded by a gene spanning 178 kb of genomic DNA of chromosome 12. More than 250 mutations of the vWF gene have been identified. Normal vWF contains multimers of varying molecular sizes ranging from 850,000 to 12 million daltons. vWF is normally secreted from endothelial cells and megakaryocytes as extra-large polymers of a peptide bound by disulfide bonds. In the plasma, the peptide bonds are cleaved by a metalloproteinase enzyme called ADAMTS13 (a disintegrin and metalloproteinase with a thrombospondin type 1 motif, member 13). This results in the formation of dimers of 176 kD and 140 kD fragments. This protease enzyme is inactive in circulation unless it is unfolded by high shear force or other factors. Inhibition of this enzyme and abnormal configuration of this enzyme leads to abnormalities of function of vWF.

Functions

- Von Willebrand's factor is very important in the initial phase of hemostasis when it binds to both platelets and endothelial components enhancing platelet adhesion and aggregation. Thus it acts as an adhesion protein and helps in the formation of the platelet plug.
- It also helps the fibrin clot formation by acting as a carrier protein for factor VIII. It forms a noncovalent complex with factor VIII in plasma, thereby protecting it from inactivation and clearance.

The basic defect in vWD is reduction of the amount of subendothelial factor VIII: vWF polymers or the presence of abnormal or inadequately polymerized subendothelial factor VIII: vWF. The defective vWF leads to impairment of platelet adhesion to sites of vascular injury. vWF is required for maintaining the integrity of factor VIII in circulation and preventing its rapid destruction. Abnormalities of vWF also lead to impairment in function of factor VIII leading to defects of coagulation, despite normal levels of factor VIII.

Inherited vWD is classified into types 1, 2 and 3.

Type 1 is autosomal dominant and accounts for about 75% of cases. In type 1 disease, there is quantitative vWF deficiencies.

Type 2 is also autosomal dominant and accounts for about 25–30% of cases and divided into 2A, 2B, 2M and 2N. There is qualitative vWF abnormality.

Type 3 is autosomal recessive and leads to severe disease with marked decrease in vWF.

Genetic Transmission of Von Willebrand's Disease (Table 175.4)

Clinical Features

These are similar to that of immune thrombocytopenic purpura, i.e., excessive post-traumatic bleeding, menorr-

Table 175.4: Genetic transmission of von Willebrand's disease

Phenotype mechanism		Transmission
1 (1)	Partial quantitative deficiency of vWF and factor VIII	Autosomal dominant (AD)
2 (A)	Defect in platelet-dependent vWF and lack of large multimers	AD
2 (B)	Heightened platelet-dependent vWF functions associated with lack of large multimers	AD
2M	vWF functions and multimers reduced	AD
2N	Defective vWF binding to factor VIII	AD
3	Severe or complete deficiency of vWF and moderately severe factor VIII deficiency	Autosomal recessive

Note: Rarely vWD can arise as an acquired disease.

hagia, and mucosal bleeding, specially from the nose, gums, GIT, and genitourinary tract. Bleeding time is prolonged. Platelet counts are normal in types I and IIA, but may be moderately decreased in II B. In those with factor VIII C levels below 1% of normal, manifestations of a coagulation defect may also be prominent. Bleeding manifestations are most marked in homozygous type II A which is rare.

Diagnosis

Initial laboratory tests for vWD show prolonged bleeding time and prolonged aPTT. After this, the following tests are useful: Plasma vWF antigen, plasma vWF activity (ristocetin cofactor activity) and factor VIII activity. If any one of them is positive, specialized assays are done for vWF multimers distribution using gel electrophoresis and ristocetin-induced platelet aggregation (RIPA). These tests differentiate the different types of vWD.

Ristocetin cofactor activity is an *in vitro* test to determine the capacity of plasma to aggregate platelets in the presence of the antibiotic—ristocetin. Ristocetin partially neutralizes negative charges on factor VIII:vWF polymers to induce platelet aggregation. This phenomenon is called ristocetin cofactor activity. This is diminished in types I and II A disease.

In patients with type I or II A vWD, the diminution of ristocetin cofactor activity correlates with the defective platelet adhesion to subendothelium *in vitro*. But in type II B disease, this is not so. In type II B, the factor VIII:vWF polymers are abnormally formed and these are incapable of inducing platelets to adhere to vascular endothelium. But even in the presence of small amounts of ristocetin, these abnormal polymers present in platelet poor plasma attach to platelets and induce aggregation *in vitro*.

In homozygous type II A vWD patients with severe bleeding tendency, endothelial polymerization of factor VIII:vWF monomers is defective and only small factor VIII:vWF polymers are present in plasma. In these patients, bleeding time is prolonged and plasma levels of factor VIII:vWF antigen, ristocetin cofactor activity, and factor VIII:C are extremely low. Being heterozygous, the majority of cases of vWD have only mild bleeding tendency.

Factor VIII:C is also reduced in the plasma of majority of patients with vWD. Unlike hemophilia in which the synthesis of factor VIII:C is diminished, in vWD, though factor VIII:C is synthesized, it is not transported effectively in the systemic circulation without adequate levels of polymerized factor VIII:vWF. Further, factor VIII:C molecules which enter the circulation unbound to VIII:vWF polymers are rapidly removed.

Treatment

The five categories of medications used in the treatment are: 1) Desmopressin, 2) replacement with vWF, 3) antifibrinolytic drugs, 4) topical therapy with thrombin or fibrin sealant and 5) estrogen therapy. In severe cases, factor VIII concentrates and recombinant factor VIIa are used.

Cryoprecipitate infusions arrest bleeding promptly and these are employed to arrest bleeding episodes and to prepare the patient for surgery. The largest factor VIII:vWF polymers in the cryoprecipitate get deposited on the injured subendothelial surface and this favors platelet adhesion and hemostasis. The therapeutic effect lasts only for 4 hours and hence cryoprecipitate has to be repeated. Lyophilized factor VIII preparations are not as effective as cryoprecipitate as they do not contain the largest plasma factor VIII:vWF polymer forms.

In type I vWD where synthesis of factor VIII:vWF within the endothelial cells is normal, infusion of 1-deamino-8-D-arginine vasopressin (DDAVP) causes release of VIII:vWF polymers from endothelial cells. DDAVP attaches itself to vasopressin receptors on the endothelial cells and helps in releasing factor VIII:vWF polymers. Both factors VIII and vWF can be temporarily raised. Optimal dose is 0.3 µg/kg bw IV. If given intranasally, the dose is 300 µg in adults and 150 µg in children. The concentration of factor VIII and vWF are doubled or quadrupled within 10–30 minutes of IV use and 60–90 minutes of intranasal use. Side effects include facial flushing, headache and arterial thrombosis. In heterozygous type II A and II B and homozygous type II A vWD, DDAVP is not very effective.

Acquired von Willebrand Disease

In this acquired disorder, antibodies are produced against vWF resulting in its impaired function or increased clearing. The disorders associated with it are:

- Malignant diseases, e.g. monoclonal gammopathy of undetermined significance, multiple myeloma, non-Hodgkin's lymphoma (NHL), chronic lymphocytic leukemia (CLL), chronic myelogenous leukemia (CML), other carcinomas.
- Immunologic disorders, e.g. SLE.
- States of high vascular flow ventricular septal defect (VSD), aortic stenosis, mitral valve prolapse and ventricular assist device.
- Other disorders—hypothyroidism, uremia and hemoglobinopathies.
- Drugs and other agents like valproic acid, ciprofloxacin and griseofulvin.

Plasma antibodies to vWF may not be usually demonstrable, but they are demonstrated by mixing studies of the suspect patient plasma and normal plasma and by showing an inhibition of vWF in a functional assay. It is postulated that vWF may be adsorbed on to the cells (e.g. multiple myeloma) leading to an increased clearance.

Proteolysis of vWD and high intravascular shear forces has been described as the pathogenic factors.

Treatment of acquired vWD depends on the pathogenic mechanism. Desmopressin, vWF replacement therapy or intravenous immunoglobulin (IVIg) and treatment form the basis of management depending on the individual case.

Acquired vWD can also be produced when vWF is excessively cleaved by increase in concentration of the metalloproteinase ADAMTS13. This happens in valvular heart diseases such as aortic stenosis, VSD and patent ductus arteriosus. Reduction or absence of large multimers of vWF causes bleeding from mucous membranes and skin.

Correction of the cardiac defect abolishes the bleeding as well. Acquired vWF does not respond to DDAVP or replacement of coagulation factors.

RARE COAGULATION DISORDERS

Hemophilia A and B, and vWD constitute about 95–97% of inherited coagulation disorders. The remaining defects of coagulation are very rare. They are mainly found in Jewish community (factor XI deficiency), Middle East countries and South India where consanguineous marriages are relatively common. Congenital deficiencies of fibrinogen, prothrombin, and factors V, VII, X, XI and XIII [recessively inherited coagulation disorders (RICDs)] are found rarely. Most of these disorders are characterized by a reduction in both functional and quantitative assays of the affected factor. Quantitative abnormality (type 1 deficiencies) is more common than qualitative abnormalities (type 2 deficiencies).

Clinical Features

The rare bleeding disorders have been classified and bleeding severity of RICDs has been assessed.

> *Asymptomatic:* No documented bleeding episodes.
> *Grade I bleeding:* Bleeding after trauma, antiplatelet or anticoagulant therapy.
> *Grade II bleeding:* Spontaneous minor bleeding.
> *Grade III bleeding:* Spontaneous minor bleeding.

Diagnosis

Prothrombin time and aPTT testing is usually sufficient to identify RICDs of clinical severity. For example:

- A normal aPTT and prolonged PT is typical of factor VII deficiency.
- Prolonged aPTT with normal PT is indicative of factor XI deficiency, provided factor VIII and IX deficiency and vWD can be ruled out by appropriate studies.
- Prothrombin time and aPTT and thrombin time are normal in factor XIII deficiency but the clot will be abnormal and it can be lysed *in vitro* in 5 molar urea, 2% acetic acid or 1% monochloroacetic acid. Specific assays are available to detect minimal deficiencies.
- Both PT and aPTT are prolonged in factor V and X and prothrombin or fibrinogen single deficiency or due to combined factor deficiencies.

Treatment

Plasma concentrates of single coagulation factors are available for replacement therapy in a few European countries. Recombinant factors are also available for factor VII and XIII. If these are not available, prothrombin complex concentrates (containing mainly factor IX, but also factors II, VII and X) or FFP may be used. Adjuvant treatments include antifibrinolytic drugs like EACA and tranexamic acid.

Hemostasis with Newer Agents Activated Factor VII

Under normal conditions, excessive spontaneous bleeding occurring in coagulation disorders can be controlled by the administration of the deficient factors, e.g. bleeding in hemophilia. Sometimes, problems arise when a patient with hemophilia develops excess of factor VIII antibodies and becomes resistant to even large doses of factor VIII. Such patients can be treated with prothrombin complex concentrate (PCC), which contains partially purified and variably activated mixtures of the vitamin K-dependent clotting factors prepared from plasma. Newer products with increased levels of proteases—aPCC are available for clinical use at present. These bypass the activity of the normal clotting factors. There is the risk of unwanted thrombosis for aPCC. Further work showed that the hemostatic efficacy was due to the presence of activated factor VII. Hence, this has been developed into a universal hemostatic agent. Recombinant activated human factor VII is produced by transfection of human factor VII gene into cultured hamster cells. Activated factor VII is commercially available (NovoSeven).

Mechanism of Action

When supraphysiological dose of recombinant factor VIIa is administered, it binds to the surface of the activated platelets (binding to glycoprotein Ib/IX/V complex) independent of tissue factor (TF). It then promotes factor X (FX) activation and thrombin generation on the activated platelet surface. In hemophiliacs, this will restore the platelet surface FX activation which is deficient because of the absence of factor VIIIa/IXa complexes. In nonhemophiliac conditions, platelet bound recombinant factor VIIa increases activation of both factors IX and X and thrombin generation above normal levels. The increased thrombin generation then promotes increased activation and local accumulation of platelets including dysfunctional platelets potentially improving hemostasis in a wide range of bleeding conditions.

Approved indications: The standard dosing is 90–120 μg/kg every 2–3 hours till bleeding stops.

- For treatment or prevention of bleeding in patients with hemophilia A and B who have inhibitors to factors VII or IX respectively.
- Treatment or prevention of bleeding episodes in patients with acquired hemophilia (who has developed acquired antibodies to factor VIII in mostly non-hemophiliacs).
- Treatment and prevention of bleeding episodes in patients with congenital factor VII deficiency.
- Treatment and prevention of bleeding episodes in patients with Glanzmann's thrombasthenia.

Recombinant factor VIIa is also used in several other conditions as off-label uses to enhance hemostasis in patients with bleeding who may or may not have an underlying coagulation defect. But the optimal dose and schedule are not known with certainty.

The conditions for off-label uses are—factor XI deficiency, vWD, inherited disorders of platelet function, excessive warfarin associated bleeding, acute intracerebral bleeding, reduction of perioperative blood loss, post-traumatic hemorrhage, bleeding during treatment with glycoprotein IIb/IIIa antagonists, and coagulopathy of liver dysfunction. In the absence of high quality data favoring off-label use of recombinant factor VIIa, absence of a laboratory test able to predict response to this agent and considering the high cost; these off-label uses of the agent should be considered only when hemorrhage has not responded to transfusion or other conventional therapy. Appropriate uses would include patients who are currently experiencing or are likely to experience life-threatening bleeding and meet one or more of the following additional criteria: 1) No response or inability to tolerate conventional treatment, 2) appropriate blood products (compatible red cells) are unavailable or are refused by the patient, 3) presence of coagulopathic bleeding and 4) bleeding conditions for which no other therapy is available.

Circulating Antibodies to Clotting Factors

Acquired inhibitors of coagulation are antibodies that either inhibit the activity or increase the clearance of a clotting factor. Certain clinical disorders like SLE are associated with antibodies to a variety of clotting factors. In SLE, the antiphospholipid antibodies and antibodies directed against factors II, V, VIII, IX, X, XI, XII, XIII and thrombin may be produced not infrequently. The most common among these is antibodies against factor VIII (acquired hemophilia) which is described in detailed under hemophilia. These conditions with antibodies against the clotting factors produce clinical bleeding varying in severity. Prothrombin antibodies are most often detected in patients with antiphospholipid antibodies. The antibodies bind to nonactive portion of prothrombin resulting in accelerated clearance of prothrombin. Possible presence of these antibodies should be suspected as patients with APS who develop bleeding tendencies instead of thrombosis. Measurement of prothrombin levels suggest the diagnosis. Treatment consists of administration of FFP.

Inhibitors specific for human thrombin are detected only rarely, but inhibitors of thrombin and factor V may develop in patients exposed to topical bovine thrombin or fibrin glue used in surgical procedures. These do not cause clinical bleeding. Thrombin and factor V antibodies can also develop in patients spontaneously without exposure to exogenous thrombin. Such patients may develop severe and even life-threatening bleeding. Treatment consists of platelet transfusion, plasma exchange and immunosuppressive treatment using prednisolone, cyclophosphamide or rituximab.

VITAMIN K DEFICIENCY

(*See* also Section 5, Ch 30)

Clinically, it manifests as ecchymoses, bleeding from injection sites, bruises, gum bleeding, hematemesis, melena or hematuria. Both the PT and aPTT are prolonged. Administration of vitamin K in a dose of 5–10 mg stops the bleeding promptly within 1–2 days. Either the oral water-soluble preparation or parenteral forms may be used. Natural preparations are preferable, being more effective. If blood loss is severe or response to vitamin K is inadequate, fresh blood transfusion or FFP is also indicated. Vitamin K deficiency in the newborn give rise to hemorrhagic disease correctable by vitamin K injections (*See* also Section 5, Ch 30).

CIRCULATING ANTICOAGULANTS

Sometimes, hemorrhagic manifestations develop on account of the presence of anticoagulants in the circulation. Many of these anticoagulants are antibodies to fibrinogen and the other specific clotting substances like factors VIII, IX, V, X, XI and XIII. Antibodies may develop due to repeated transfusions, or as part of an immunological disorder like SLE, rheumatoid disease or generalized penicillin allergy.

Clinical features are similar to those of the primary coagulation disorders with the exception that replacement therapy may be ineffective as long as the antibody persists in the circulation. This can be overcome by giving large doses of the missing factor and removal of the circulating antibodies by plasmapheresis or by immunosuppressant therapy.

Other rare coagulation disorders: Several other inherited deficiencies of coagulation factors exist, though they are rare. These include deficiencies of fibrinogen and defects in the composition of fibrinogen, deficiency of prothrombin, and factors XII, X, XI and XIII. These crop up infrequently and may be mistaken for the more common acquired hemorrhagic disorders. Diagnosis is by specific laboratory tests. Therapy consists of the administration of the specific factors, FFP or PCC.

PATHOLOGICAL FIBRINOLYSIS

Healthy individuals may show minor variations in fibrinolytic activity without any deleterious effects, but gross increase in fibrinolytic activity causes hemorrhage. Excessive fibrinolysis may be a primary phenomenon or develop as a consequence of disseminated intravascular coagulation (DIC) or extensive thrombosis.

Causes of Excessive Fibrinolysis

- *Obstetric causes:* Abruptio placentae and amniotic fluid embolism.
- *Surgical causes:* Gastrectomy, lung resection, nephrectomy, prostatectomy, cardiopulmonary bypass, splenectomy and pancreatectomy.
- *Medical causes:*
  - Liver diseases such as cirrhosis of liver.
  - Leukemias, specially in acute leukemia and chronic granulocytic leukemia.
  - Anaphylactic shock.
  - Autoimmune diseases such as SLE.

Pathogenesis

Fibrinolytic activity may be enhanced as a result of excessive release of plasminogen activator or reduction in the inhibitor. The sequence of events is given in Flowchart 175.1.

Clinical Features

The clinical features depend on the predominant mechanism. If thrombocytopenia is also pronounced, capillary bleeding predominates. If coagulation mechanism is defective, the bleeding is more serious. The severity and clinical presentation may vary from case-to-case.

Diagnosis

Normal bleeding time, slightly prolonged clotting time, and poor quality of the clot should suggest the possibility of excessive fibrinolysis. Primary fibrinolysis has to be distinguished from DIC. In primary fibrinolysis, platelet count is normal and this distinguishes it from DIC in which platelet count is reduced. It is important to distinguish these two conditions since treatment is different (Table 175.5).

Laboratory tests: The tests for fibrinolysis are:
- Euglobulin lysis time for detecting the presence of increased levels of circulating plasminogen activator is shortened.
- The detection of excess of fibrin degradation products (FDP) by immunological methods.
- D-dimer levels in plasma are elevated. D-dimer is the fibrin fragment in plasma which is a marker of fibrin formation and active fibrinolysis.
- Circulating levels of plasminogen which will be low in fibrinolysis.

Treatment

Primary fibrinolysis can be readily controlled by the use of antifibrinolytic agents.

Commonly used antifibrinolytic agents are EACA and tranexamic acid which are synthetic amino acids, and

Flowchart 175.1: Sequence of events in accelerated fibrinolysis

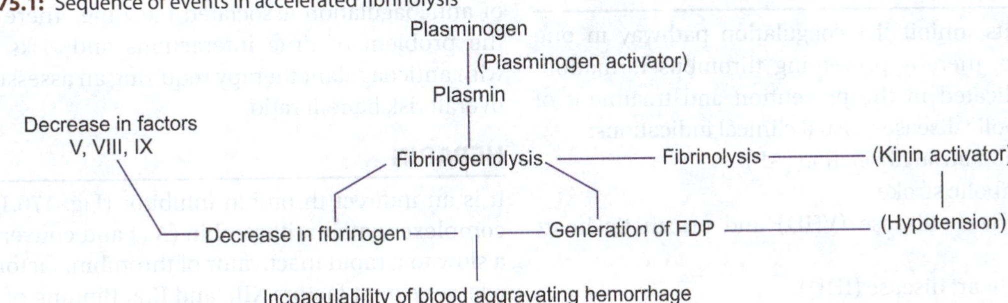

Abbreviation: FDP = Fibrin degradation product

Table 175.5: Differentiation between disseminated intravascular coagulation (DIC) and primary fibrinolysis

Tests	Acute DIC	Primary fibrinolysis
Platelet count	Decreased	Normal
Bleeding time	Prolonged	Normal
Clot retraction	Defective	Clot is dissolved
Red cell fragmentation	Present	Absent
Clotting time	Prolonged	Slightly prolonged
Prothrombin time activated partial	Prolonged	Prolonged
Thromboplastin time	Prolonged	Slightly prolonged
Euglobulin lysis time	Shortened	Shortened
Fibrin split products estimation	High titer	High titer
D-dimer levels	Raised	Raised
Thrombin time	Prolonged	Prolonged

aprotinin (Trasylol) which is a polypeptide. Both EACA and tranexamic acid bind reversibly to plasminogen and thereby block its binding to fibrin and fibrinolysis. Aprotinin inhibits the action of trypsin, chymotrypsin, plasmin and tissue kallikrein. By inhibiting kallikrein, it indirectly blocks the activation of factor XII and thereby prevents the initiation of both coagulation and fibrinolysis. Activity of aprotinin is expressed as kallikrein inactivation units (KIU).

When given orally, EACA is rapidly absorbed and a single oral dose is effective for 4 hours. It is contraindicated in advanced renal disease. For immediate effect, 5–10 g is given IV in the first hour followed by 2 g hourly for the next 2–3 hours. This is then followed by oral therapy with 4 g every 4 hours. The total dose in 24 hours should not exceed 30 g. Since the drug is excreted by the kidneys, its concentration in urine is higher than in plasma. In the presence of active hematuria, this will lead to formation of clot in the bladder and urinary obstruction.

Dose of tranexamic acid is 20–25 mg/kg bw orally bd or tds. The parenteral dose is 0.5 to 1 g IV tds or also as an infusion.

Aprotinin (Trasylol) is used for reducing intraoperative blood loss in cardiac surgery. At times, it may lead to serious nonfatal cardiovascular events and also renal toxicity. The dose is 0.5–1 million units given over 10 minutes, repeated in doses of 0.2 million units till the bleeding is arrested.

Since aprotinin inhibits pancreatic trypsin and chymotrypsin, it is also useful in acute pancreatitis.

In DIC, fibrinolysis occurs as a defense mechanism helping to remove the clots formed, and inhibition of fibrinolysis is harmful since it may lead to widespread thrombosis. Administration of EACA should not be undertaken without concurrent heparin therapy if the distinction between primary fibrinolysis and DIC is not clear. Thrombotic complications, particularly renal cortical necrosis may develop when EACA is used alone in patients with DIC.

CHAPTER
176

Therapeutics of Anticoagulants

Mathew Thomas, KV Krishna Das

Chapter Summary

- Indications of Anticoagulants
- Heparin
  - Heparin-induced Thrombocytopenia
- Warfarin and Other Vitamin K Antagonists
- Anticoagulation with Direct Thrombin Inhibitors and Factor Xa Inhibitors

INDICATIONS OF ANTICOAGULANTS

Anticoagulants inhibit the coagulation pathway in one or other step, thereby preventing thrombus formation. They are indicated in the prevention and treatment of thromboembolic diseases. Usual clinical indications:

- Nonvalvular atrial fibrillation (AF)
- Cardioembolic stroke
- Valvular heart disease (VHD) and prosthetic heart valves
- Ischemic heart disease (IHD)
- Left ventricular dysfunction (LVD)
- **Venous thromboembolic disease:** Thrombophilia including pulmonary embolism and deep vein thrombosis (DVT)
- Peripheral artery disease (PAD).

Many of these conditions are found in older adults who have many comorbid conditions. They also use many drugs especially antiplatelet drugs. All these factors raise questions regarding the appropriate use and safety of anticoagulants as they are at a greater risk of anticoagulation associated bleeding. There also exists the problem of drug interactions and risks associated with anticoagulant therapy requiring an assessment of the overall risk benefit ratio.

HEPARIN

It is an indirect thrombin inhibitor (Fig. 176.1). Heparin complexes with antithrombin (AT) and converts AT from a slow to a rapid inactivator of thrombin, factor Xa and to a lesser extent factors XIIa and IXa. Binding of heparin to the heparin binding site of AT produces a conformational

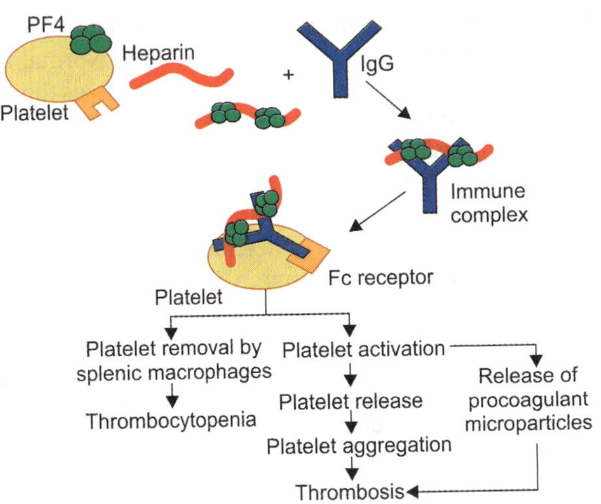

Fig. 176.1: Heparin: Mode of action

Abbreviations: PF4 = Platelet factor 4; IgG = Immunoglobulin G

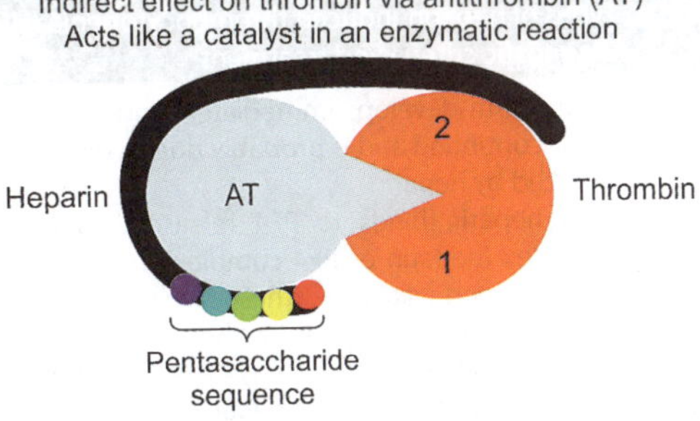

Fig. 176.2: Mechanism of heparin-induced thrombocytopenia

change in AT. This will accelerate the inactivating function of AT 1,000–4,000 folds. This is the indirect action of heparin on thrombin. If heparin is to inactivate thrombin directly, then heparin should be able to bind with both AT and to a binding site of thrombin forming a ternary complex. This can happen only when the pentasaccharide containing chains are at least 18 saccharide units long. Such long chains are present in the most chains of unfractionated heparin (UFH) and are less commonly present in low-molecular-weight heparin (LMWH) and are not present in fondaparinux.

So LMWH and fondaparinux have less AT activity than does UFH. Lesser important actions of heparin include direct platelet binding at high concentration and binding to heparin cofactor II (AT is heparin cofactor I). Heparin does not cross the placenta and is safe in pregnancy.

The dose of UFH in DVT is an initial bolus intravenous (IV) dose of 5,000 U. This is followed by a continuous IV infusion of heparin in a dose of 20–30,000 U in 24 hours. There is also a weight-based nomograms for calculating the dose of UFH.

Heparin has a number of limitations for its clinical use. These include a narrow therapeutic window of adequate anticoagulation without bleeding and a highly variable dose response relation requiring laboratory monitoring. The variable response is due in part to differences in bioavailability of subcutaneous (SC) heparin and to competitive occupation of the binding sites by plasma proteins other than AT, by proteins secreted by platelets [platelet factor 4 (PF4)] and by endothelial cells. It was found that even with very close adherence to the recommended heparin dosing only 34% of the initial activated partial thromboplastin times (aPTTs) were therapeutic (1.5–2 times control), 13% markedly low (<1.25 times control) and 16% were markedly high (>2.75 times control). Heparin has reduced ability to inactivate thrombin bound to fibrin as well as factor Xa bound to activate platelets within a thrombus.

Heparin-induced Thrombocytopenia (Fig. 176.2)

Another potential fatal complication of heparin treatment is heparin-induced thrombocytopenia (HIT)

and heparin-induced thrombocytopenia with thrombosis (HITT). This occurs in 5% of the patients who are exposed to heparin regardless of the dose and route of administration. In a few patients who are given heparin, the heparin forms a complex with PF4 (heparin PF4 complexes). These individuals produce immunoglobulin G (IgG) autoantibodies directed against heparin complex with PF4. Platelet Fc receptors bind the antibody–heparin–PF4 immune complex. This leads to platelet activation and microparticle release that contributes to thrombosis. Thrombocytopenia is due to removal of platelets bound to IgG by splenic macrophages and platelet consumption by thrombus formation. Heparin should be stopped and alternate anticoagulants like, bivalirudin, argatroban or fondaparinux should be used.

The *diagnosis of HIT* is by measurement of the antibodies against the PF4 heparin complexes. The C14 serotonin release assay (SRA) is considered as the gold standard for laboratory diagnosis because of its high sensitivity and specificity. There is also an enzyme-linked immunosorbent assay (ELISA) test for the detection of the antibodies, which is a rapid and sensitive test. Platelets should be monitored from 4th to 14th days after the initial administration, every other day, when therapeutic dose is used and once in 3 days if prophylactically used. Weight-based and other nomograms are available for heparin administration by IV and SC routes for various indications. Protamine sulfate in a dose of 1 mg per 100 units of heparin is used as an antidote for bleeding produced by heparin. The other complications of heparin are skin necrosis, allergic and nonallergic skin lesions, systemic allergic reactions, hypersensitivity, heparin contamination and osteoporosis when used for more than 6 months (Box 176.1).

Low-molecular-weight Heparin (LMWH) and Fondaparinux

There are a number of advantages of LMWH over UFH. Bioavailability of LMWH is much greater when given as SC injection. Duration of action is greater because of the reduced binding to macrophages and endothelial cells. Anticoagulant effect is directly proportionate to the body weight (bw) permitting a fixed dose. Laboratory monitoring is not necessary in nonpregnant patients as it does not prolong aPTT and has lesser effects on thrombin. It is less likely to produce immune thrombocytopenia. LMWH can be safely administered in the outpatient setting. The long half-life of LMWH can be sometimes disadvantageous as rapid discontinuation is not possible (bleeding during

Box 176.1: Types of heparin-induced thrombocytopenia (HIT): Diagnostic criteria and treatment

HIT type I: Benign form develops immediately and often resolves after heparin is discontinued and is probably due to direct platelet-aggregation induced by heparin

HIT type II: The heparin binds to PF4 released from platelets and forms a complex (heparin or PF4 complex) in the circulation. The antibodies formed against these complexes activate platelets, promoting thrombosis even in the presence of marked thrombocytopenia. It develops 5–10 days after starting heparin therapy and can occur with all types of heparin.

- **Diagnostic criteria for HIT type II** includes at least one of the following:
  - Thrombocytopenia
  - Thrombosis (e.g. DVT, pulmonary embolism, adrenal hemorrhage, etc.)
  - Necrotizing skin lesions at heparin injection sites
  - Acute anaphylactoid reaction (usually occurs 5–30 minutes after intravenous heparin or rarely after subcutaneous heparin).
- **Treatment of HIT type II**
  - Immediately stop all heparin administration
  - Start nonheparin anticoagulants—e.g. Lepirudin, a recombinant hirudin, argatroban, danaparoid, fondaparinux and bivalirudin
  - Do not administer warfarin as it can produce gangrene of limb or necrosis of skin. Vitamin K is administered if HIT diagnosed after warfarin has already been started.

Do not administer platelet transfusion even though there is severe thrombocytopenia.

pregnancy around the time of delivery, renal impairment). There are many commercially available LMWHs. They differ according to the different processes of manufacture, chemical structure, pharmacokinetic activity and molecular weight. The different molecules available are enoxaparin, dalteparin, tinzaparin, nadroparin, bemiparin and certoparin.

Fondaparinux is a synthetic highly sulfated penta-saccharide. It is not classified under LMWH but acts in a similar way. It binds to AT with a higher affinity than any heparins and causes a conformational change in AT that significantly increases the ability of AT to inactivate factor Xa. It does not bind to PF4 and does not produce immune thrombocytopenia. Fondaparinux is 100% bioavailable after SC injection. There is no antidote.

LMWH and fondaparinux can be used in all indications as UFH (e.g. treatment of DVT and its prophylaxis, pulmonary embolism and other indications of anticoagulations. Dose of commonly used LMWH and fondaparinux is as follows:

- **Enoxaparin:** 1 mg/kg, twice daily for DVT and once daily for prophylaxis
- **Dalteparin:** 5,000 IU once daily
- **Fondaparinux:** 2.5 mg SC once daily for DVT prophylaxis and 5 mg daily for treating DVT (<50 kg).

Monitoring of LMWH and fondaparinux can be done by antifactor Xa assays if needed. Protamine sulfate though less effective may be used as an antidote for LMWH to reduce the complication of bleeding.

WARFARIN AND OTHER VITAMIN K ANTAGONISTS

These drugs are used in a variety of clinical conditions. Their therapeutic range is narrow and their metabolism is affected by diet, absorption, drug interactions and genetic factors. Time spent with an International Normalized Ratio (INR) above the therapeutic range increases the risk of bleeding and time spent below the range increases the risk of thrombosis.

Common drugs used are warfarin (WARF–for Wisconsin Alumni Research Foundation, where the drug was originally developed), acenocoumarol (acitrom), phenprocoumon and fluindione.

Warfarin

It is a racemic mixture of S and R stereoisomers. The S form is metabolized by CYP269 hepatic microsomal enzyme system, which is inducible by many drugs. It has many genetic variants. So this enzyme system greatly alters the *in vivo* action of warfarin. It is protein bound and only the nonprotein bound form is biologically active. Agents binding to albumin displace warfarin increasing its *in vivo* activity. It is water-soluble and completely absorbed from proximal small bowel. Biological half-life of warfarin is 36–42 hours whereas it is shorter for acenocoumarol (8–11 hours).

Tecarfarin is a new and novel vitamin K antagonist currently used in clinical trials. It has no drug interaction and genetic variation as it is metabolized by esterase and not by cytochrome P450 system.

Mechanism of Action

Warfarin acts by inhibiting of vitamin K-dependent gamma-carboxylation of factors II, VII, IX and X. It also inhibits gamma-carboxylation of proteins C and S producing a biochemical paradox, i.e. inhibition of both procoagulant and anticoagulant factors. Period taken to inhibit vitamin K-dependent clotting factors is not the same. The least to be inhibited is prothrombin and it takes 3 days. So, the ultimate anticoagulant affect is attained only after 3 days. For this reason and that it also inhibits the anticoagulant proteins C and S, parenteral anticoagulants like heparin should overlap by 4–5 days when warfarin is initiated. The equilibrium of inhibited clotting factors is 10–35% of normal at the therapeutic range. Polymorphisms in the genes of the two enzymes hepatic cytochrome P-4502C9 (CYP2C9) and vitamin K epoxide reductase complex 1 (VKORC1) has been associated with altered sensitivity to warfarin. A number of drugs produce increased warfarin effects and others decreased effects.

Drugs which increase warfarin effects: Commonly used drugs are acetaminophen (paracetamol), allopurinol, aspirin, amiodarone, cephalosporins, ciprofloxacin, clofi-brate, clopidogrel, diclofenac, fluconazole, fluorouracil (5-FU), selective serotonin reuptake inhibitors (SSRIs) (fluoxetine), influenza virus vaccine, metronidazole, mac-rolides, omeprazole, cotrimoxazole, tamoxifen and thyroid hormones.

Drugs which reduce warfarin effects: Azathioprine, antithyroid drugs, carbamazepine, haloperidol, oral contraceptives, phenobarbital, rifampin and vitamin K produce decreased warfarin effects. The list is only a partial list. Some drugs can have multiple opposing effects both increasing and decreasing effects depending on which aspect is dominant in that patient.

Warfarin Administration

A baseline INR and an aPTT are to be done. This is important for comparison as the patient is on therapy and for diagnosing pre-existing conditions [e.g. antiphospholipid syndrome (APS) with prolonged aPTT]. Initial dose may be decided by the following suggestions and should be individualized. According to available studies, initial dose of warfarin more than 5 mg is generally not employed (uptodate.com). Initial dose for first 2 days can vary from 2–10 mg.

Dose of 2-5 mg is given to patients with hepatic impairment, debilitation, congestive cardiac failure (CCF), elderly, severe chronic kidney disease and those with high-risk of bleeding.

Doses of 5-10 mg are given in highly selected patients who are stable, reliable patients with a low risk of bleeding and in whom there is a history of prior high maintenance dose. But this high dose has resulted in over anticoagulation in three randomized trials.

Pharmacogenetic testing is currently not recommended before initiating warfarin. Monitoring warfarin treatment is best done by prothrombin time (PT) INR in a standard reliable laboratory. Clinical effect is monitored through a standard PT termed INR. It has to be done frequently when warfarin treatment is initiated and less often when the dose and INR are stabilized. When stabilized, it is done once in 4 weeks. No protocols for adjusting the dose of warfarin have been uniformly accepted. Serial monitoring will detect patients who are under or over coagulated and the dose can be adjusted. But monitoring is not a fool-proof method to prevent warfarin overdose completely.

Maintenance therapy and the target INR depends on the primary condition, which demands anticoagulation. Some patients may require a low dose and others a very high dose over 10 mg. This depends on several factors, like genetic constitution, nutritional status, vitamin K intake, rate of intestinal absorption, hepatic function, medication compliance and drug interactions. Patients on warfarin are usually prescribed a diet with low vitamin K content.

Bleeding: Warfarin is one of the common drugs producing a large number of serious adverse events. The risk of major bleeding episodes in warfarin treated patients is related to their degree of anticoagulation and the presence of pre-existing risk factors present in the patient. These include increased age, female sex, diabetes mellitus (DM), malignancy, hypertension, alcoholism, severe kidney disease, anemia, poor drug compliance, prior hemorrhagic stroke, bleeding lesions like peptic ulcer, bleeding disorders like thrombocytopenia and use of aspirin. INR above 3 and INR above 1.2 at initiation and prior history of hemorrhage during warfarin therapy increase the risk. Sometimes an outpatient bleeding risk index (OBRI) is used.

- Age above 65
- History of stroke
- History of gastrointestinal (GI) bleed
- One of the following–recent myocardial infarction (MI), hematocrit <30%, S creatinine more than 1.5, DM. Patients were divided into low risk (no factors) intermediate (1–2 factors) and high (3 or more).

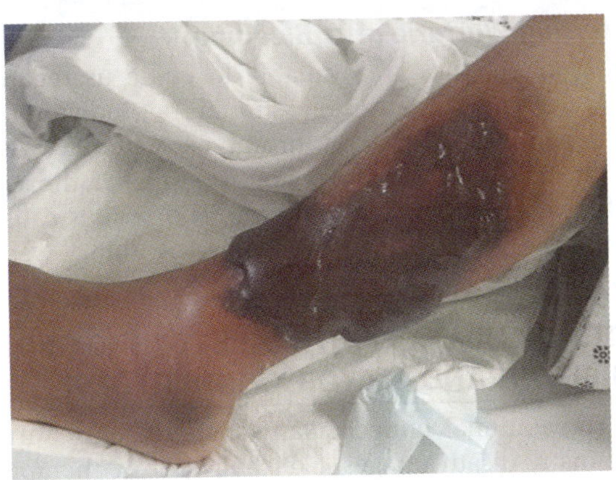

Fig. 176.3: Warfarin skin necrosis: A rare complication of warfarin

Incidence of bleeding was found to be 3%, 12% and 53% in the three groups respectively. Increased blood levels of thrombomodulin are sometimes used to predict major bleeding. Complications other than bleeding include warfarin skin necrosis (Fig. 176.3), teratogenicity during pregnancy, cholesterol embolization, vascular calcification and warfarin-related nephropathy.

Correction of excess coagulation after warfarin: Excess coagulation is mainly due to altered metabolism of warfarin due to various factors already mentioned. INR can be falsely elevated if the drawn blood has any heparin content (e.g. blood drawn from indwelling, central venous catheter).

Treatment

- INR less than 5 without bleeding—next dose of warfarin should be omitted and/or the maintenance dose reduced. There is no need to reduce the dose if the prolongation is only minimal.
- INR 5-9 without bleeding—risk of bleeding in the next 30 days is 1%. Two options are stopping warfarin temporarily or stopping warfarin temporarily for 1–2 days and adding a small dose of oral vitamin K (1–2.5 mg vitamin K). Lower maintenance dose should be reinstituted when INR falls into normal therapeutic range.
- INR less than 9 without bleeding—warfarin should be stopped and 2.5–5 mg of oral vitamin K administered. Monitor INR and review after 48 hours. Additional dose of vitamin K is to be given if needed. Lower maintenance dose should be reinstituted.
- INR less than 9 with minimal bleeding—there is only little guidance regarding this situation. They can be treated like a previous group or those who have significant bleeding according to the clinical judgment.
- Significant bleeding—warfarin is stopped and vitamin K 10 mg given as slow IV infusion over 20–60 minutes. For urgent situations stop warfarin, start vitamin K infusion 10 mg. Fresh-frozen plasma (FFP) or prothrombin complex concentrates (PCCs) should be administered if bleeding continues. Vitamin K can be repeated every 12 hours for persistently elevated INR.

Imaging of brain [noncontrast computed tomography (CT) scan] is advocated for all patients who are seen in emergency room with head trauma.

Restarting Warfarin after Bleeding

Only a few studies are available to guide us regarding this decision. The decision should be individualized and depends on the risk of thrombosis without warfarin and the cause of bleeding. For example, if the cause of bleeding is only trivial and there is a serious cause of thrombosis, warfarin may be restarted within a week of stopping of the bleeding.

ANTICOAGULATION WITH DIRECT THROMBIN INHIBITORS AND FACTOR Xa INHIBITORS

The conventional anticoagulants heparin and warfarin have many disadvantages, like their narrow therapeutic window of adequate anticoagulation without bleeding and a highly variable does response relations among individuals that require laboratory monitoring. Newer anticoagulants are being developed and researched to overcome these difficulties.

Direct Thrombin Inhibitors (DTIs)

Recombinant hirudin, argatroban and bivalirudin are examples of parentally administered DTIs, which are now available in the market. Dabigatran is an orally active DTI. These can inactive clot bound thrombin, which is an important thrombogenic stimulus as in coronary thrombosis, especially following clot disruption by thrombolytic agents. DTIs are AT independent and do not bind to PF4. And hence, some of them like argatroban and bivalirudin are used in HIT. DTIs are also studied in a number of clinical settings including treatment and prophylaxis of DVT, prevention of stroke in AF and acute management of patients with unstable angina or MI (Table 176.1).

Argatroban is parental DTI with a half-life of 24 minutes. Its effect is monitored by aPTT. In subjects with normal liver function, standard starting doses is 2 μg/kg/min by continuous IV injection adjusted to maintain the aPTT 1.5–3 times baseline not to exceed 100 seconds. Transition to warfarin is made as for heparin. The main indication is HIT.

Bivalirudin is similarly used for HIT in a dose of 0.15 mg/kg/h. To achieve an aPTT 1.5–2.4 times baseline. Warfarin should be started only after the patient has been stably anticoagulated and platelet count has increased to at least 150,000/mm³.

Dabigatran is an orally active DTI used to prevent and treat venous and arterial thromboembolic disorders in various settings (prevention of VT in hip surgery, treatment of acute venous thromboembolism (VTE), prevention of stroke in AF. Dabigatran should not be used in pregnancy. Important side effect of dabigatran is nonbleeding GI events (dyspepsia, dysmotility, GI reflux). Dabigatran etexilate the prodrug is converted in the liver to the active drug dabigatran. The half-life of dabigatran is approximately 12–14 hours in adults with normal renal functions. Its absorption is unaffected by food and has to be given twice daily. Renal excretion of unchanged drug is the main elimination pathway. Drug clearance is less in older people and in renal dysfunction. Drug stability is maintained only if the drug is stored in the original bottle or blister package so the capsule cannot be opened or given through nasogastric (NG) tube. It is a substrate for the efflux transporter P-glycoprotein. So it is contraindicated with drugs, which induce P-glycoprotein and drugs which alter its bioavailability (rifampin, quinidine, ketoconazole, verapamil, amiodarone and clarithromycin).

Dose for Treating DVT

DVT is initially treated by LMWH for 7 days and then dabigatran 150 mg twice daily is given for the desired period. No laboratory monitoring is necessary. An antidote for dabigatran is now not available but is in its development. The antidote in development consists of humanized dabigatran specific (Fab) antibody fragments analogous to those used to treat digoxin toxicity.

Factor Xa Inhibitors

Now, there are a number of different factor Xa inhibitors that are developed. They are mainly synthetic analogs of the heparin pentasaccharide required for binding to AT. There are also a number of orally active direct factor Xa inhibitors under clinical development. These new anticoagulants have a rapid onset of action with peak anticoagulant effect achieved within 2–4 hours thus potentially avoiding the need for a parenteral anticoagulant. They also have stable pharmacodynamic profiles so that routine monitoring is not required making them superior to warfarin for long-term use. The direct oral Xa inhibitors should not be used during pregnancy.

Idraparinux is a longer acting analogue of fondaparinux, which need be given only once per week. Idrabiotaparinux is a biotinylated version of idraparinux.

Ultra LMWH—semuloparin with a molecular weight as low as 2,000–3,000 g/mol has nearly pure antifactor Xa activity.

Rivaroxaban is an orally available direct factor Xa inhibitor with a bioavailability of 80%, with a peak plasma concentration occurring 2.5–4 hours after oral

Table 176.1: Properties of available direct thrombin inhibitors (DTIs)

Parameter	r-hirudin	Bivalirudin (Hirulog)	Argatroban (Novastan)	Ximelagatran and melagatran (Exanta)	Dabigatran
Route of administration	IV, SC	IV	IV	Ximelagatran po; melagatran oral IV and SC	Oral
Plasma half-life	60 min (IV) 120 min (SC)	25 min	45 min	Oral 3–5 hours IV and SC, 2–3 hours	12 hours 50–225 mg
Dose	15 mg/day for 8–12 days	—	—	Ximelagatran 24 mg bd × 7–12 days oral melagatran 3 mg/day SC	50–225 mg bd for 6–10 days
Main site of clearance	Kidney	Kidney, liver, other sites	Liver	Kidney	Kidney

Abbreviations: IV = Intravenous; SC = Subcutaneous

administration. For treatment of DVT, it is used in a dose of 20–40 mg/day and for prophylaxis 10 mg/day. There is no platelet activation and does not interact with PF4. So it may be used in HIT. Rivaroxaban is contraindicated if creatinine clearance is less than 30%, in pregnancy and children less than 18 years of age. For VTE prophylaxis after hip surgery, it is given in a dose of 10 mg/day. For the treatment of VTE, the dose is 15 mg twice daily for 21 days and then 20 mg/day if creatinine clearance is more than 30 mL/min. In AF, it is used in a dose of 20 mg/day if creatinine clearance is more than 50 mL. Rivaroxaban interacts with drugs that are potent inhibitors of both CYP3A4 and P-glycoprotein efflux transporter (e.g. systemic ketoconazole, itraconazole, voriconazole or ritonavir, rifamycins and carbamazepine).

Till recently there were no specific antidotes for factor Xa and direct thrombus inhibitors.

At present a drug ANDEXANET alfa which is a recombinant modified human factor Xa decoy protein that has been found to reverse the inhibition of factor Xa in patients with gastrointestinal and intracranial bleed, when the drug was given intravenously in doses ranging from 480–960 mg. Following the administration of Andexanet the bleeding stops in one hour. Andexanet restores the factor Xa levels on follow up for 30 days thrombotic events may occur.

Note: Decoy protein is a protein with similar structure to the substrate of the enzymes in order to make the enzyme bind to the pseudosubstrate instead of the real substrate. Such proteins are in effect, enzyme inhibitors.

Source: Stuart J Cannolly, et al. NEJM. 2016; 375:12;1311–1411.

Apixaban is a similar oral direct factor Xa inhibitor, which does not require monitoring. In acute DVT, the dose is 10 mg twice daily for 7 days followed by 5 mg twice daily for 3–6 months.

Edoxaban is yet another oral direct factor Xa inhibitor, which does not require regular monitoring. Dose for DVT is 60 mg daily for 3–6 months after initial LMWH. A lower dose of 30 mg/day is used for patients with a creatinine clearance of 30–50 mL/min.

Antifactor Xa antidote is in its development. It is catalytically inactive truncated form of factor Xa and binds to factor Xa inhibitor at subnanomolar affinity. This agent seems to be also effective as an antidote for LMWH. A small molecule antidote (PER977) is being developed for heparins, DTIs and factor Xa inhibitors.

The anticoagulants in development are recombinant form of tissue factor pathway inhibitor (TFPI), factor VIII inhibitor (human IgG4 monoclonal antibody with a prolonged antithrombotic effect after a single dose up to 10–14 days) and factors IXa, XI and XIIa inhibitors.

Some suggestions and recommendations regarding the use of new anticoagulants:

- Patients already taking warfarin with excellent INR control and minimal bleeding side effects, may have little to gain by switching to the new drugs.
- Warfarin with once daily dosing is convenient to many patients whereas most of the new drugs have to be taken twice daily.
- Warfarin monitoring with frequent INR checks is less convenient for some patients who can be changed to the new drugs.
- Warfarin is preferred over dabigatran and rivaroxaban in those with reduced renal function.
- Patients with GI disease and bleeding may prefer to avoid new drugs, since they do not have any antidote.
- Patients with unexplained, poor INR control with significant period of time in subtherapeutic INR range, newer drugs may be used.
- Patients with poor level of INR control because of unavoidable drug interactions may do better with the new drugs.
- Older patients with nonvalvular AF (above 80 years) who may not receive warfarin due to concerns about bleeding, the newer drugs may be used.
- Oral DTIs and factor Xa inhibitors should not be used in pregnancy.

Overview of traditional and newer antithrombotic drugs tabular column and antiplatelet drug tabular columns have not been entered.

CHAPTER
177

Fragmentation Hemolysis

Mathew Thomas, KV Krishna Das

Chapter Summary

- Fragmentation Hemolysis
  - Disseminated Intravascular Coagulation
    - Diagnostic Scoring System for DIC
  - Thrombotic Thrombocytopenic Purpura (Hemolytic Uremic Syndrome)
    - Clinical and Laboratory Findings
    - Treatment (TTP-HUS Syndrome)

FRAGMENTATION HEMOLYSIS

Syn: Microangiopathic hemolytic anemia (MAHA), disseminated intravascular coagulation (DIC), thrombotic thrombocytopenic purpura and hemolytic uremic syndrome (TTP-HUS)

New definition of DIC: It is an acquired syndrome characterized by intravascular activation of coagulation with loss of localization arising from several factors.

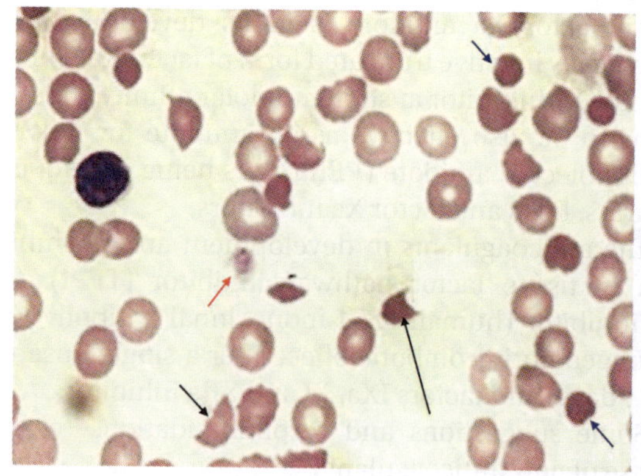

Fig. 177.1: Microangiopathy hemolytic anemia (MAHA)—helmet cell (long arrow), schistocytes (small black arrow), spherocytes (blue arrows), normoblasts (red arrow)

Hemolytic anemia or microangiopathic hemolytic anemia (MAHA) is characterized by reduction in the red cell survival to less than 100 days due to increased rate of destruction of the red blood cells (RBCs). They are broadly classified into intracorpuscular defects (which are usually inherited, e.g. hemoglobinopathies, red cell membrane abnormalities, various enzymopathies) or extracorpuscular defects [which are usually acquired, e.g. autoimmune hemolytic anemia (AIHA), nonimmune hemolytic anemia, systemic diseases, mechanical destruction in fragmentation hemolysis, hypersplenism, action of drugs and toxins].

The **characteristic features** of this type of hemolytic anemia are varying degrees of anemia with evidence of red-cell fragmentation. The fragmented red cells may be schistocytes or helmet cells in the peripheral blood smear. This group of hemolytic anemias is also called MAHA (Fig. 177.1) or thrombotic microangiopathy (TMA) as microvascular abnormalities are frequently involved and sometimes they are associated with thrombotic changes. The following conditions are included under fragmentation hemolysis:

- Disseminated intravascular coagulation (DIC)
- Thrombotic thrombocytopenic purpura (TTP) and hemolytic uremic syndrome (HUS)
- Hemolysis, elevated liver enzymes, low platelet count syndrome (HELLP)
- Malignancy
- Malignant hypertension
- Scleroderma renal crisis
- Malfunctioning cardiac valves and cardiac assist devices
- Kasabach-Merritt syndrome
- Inclusion of foreign bodies, such as cardiac valves, filters, stents and others in the circulation
- Drugs
- Other diseases [eclampsia, PNH (paroxysmal nocturnal hemoglobinuria), scleroderma, vasculitis, catastrophic APS (antiphospholipid syndrome)].

Disseminated Intravascular Coagulation

This is also known as consumption coagulopathy and defibrination syndrome. This is a clinicopathological syndrome characterized by a hematological paradox of both thrombosis and hemorrhage.

The definition by the International Society of Thrombosis and Hemostasis (ISTH) is that DIC is an acquired syndrome characterized by intravascular activation of coagulation with loss of localization arising from different causes. This condition typically originates in the microvasculature. DIC usually presents as hemorrhage, with only 5–10% of cases presenting with microthrombi (e.g. digital gangrene) alone. The condition is initiated by a number of well-defined disorders and the following components are usually observed:

- Exposure of the components of the blood to procoagulants like tissue factor (TF) and cancer procoagulants. Several cytokines also act as procoagulant mediators. Prominent among them is interleukin-6 (IL-6)
- Generation of excess of thrombin and fibrin in the circulation
- Excess of fibrinolysis
- Depletion of coagulation factors and platelets
- End-organ damage due to fibrin deposition in the microvasculature.

There are two forms of DIC—acute (DIC-1) and chronic (DIC-2). This depends on the cause and rapidity with which the initiating event or disorder is propagated. If the activation is slow, the excess of procoagulants which are produced will result in thrombosis. But at the same time if the liver and bone marrow are normal, they produce sufficient clotting factors and platelets as a compensatory mechanism. So the bleeding symptoms are not clinically apparent. This is the picture of chronic DIC. The clinical presentation consists of primarily thrombotic manifestations which can be both venous and arterial, e.g. Trousseau's syndrome, a hypercoagulable state associated with malignancy.

Normally, activation of hemostasis begins with exposure of the blood to procoagulants initially mediated by TF and activated factor VII (TF-factor VIIa complex). This results in localized thrombin generation inducing platelet aggregation and deposition of cross-linked fibrin to form the hemostatic plug. The thrombin generation is tightly balanced by anticoagulant factors like antithrombin (AT) and TF pathway inhibitor. When these mechanisms are overwhelmed by massive activation of hemostatic mechanism, excess thrombin is formed. The excess thrombin circulates leading to acute DIC. There is widespread fibrin deposition in the small vessels (microcirculation) which leads to damage of various organs. The increased amount of FDP (fibrin degradation product) may enhance bleeding by various mechanisms. The causes of DIC are described in Table 177.1.

- **Sepsis:** Both bacterial and nonbacterial infections can produce DIC. Thirty to fifty percent of patients with Gram-positive and Gram-negative sepsis develop DIC (e.g. meningococcemia).
- **Trauma and extensive surgery:** There is a release of tissue enzymes and/or phospholipids from the damaged tissue into systemic circulation triggering activation of cytokines and hemostatic system.
- **Malignancy:** Twenty five percent of patients with malignancy develop DIC, e.g. acute promyelocytic leukemia (APML).

Table 177.1: Causes of disseminated intravascular coagulation (DIC)

Parameters	Causes
Infections	• Gram-negative bacterial sepsis • Meningococcemia and other bacteria • Fungi, viruses, Rocky Mountain spotted fever, malaria
Obstetric complications	• Retained dead fetus • Septic abortion • Abruptio placentae • Amniotic fluid embolism • Toxemia and pre-eclampsia
Neoplasms	• Carcinomas of pancreas, prostate, lung and stomach • Acute promyelocytic leukemia (APML)
Massive tissue injury	• Traumatic • Burns • Fat embolism • Surgery
Vascular disorders	Aortic aneurysm, giant hemangioma
Miscellaneous	Snakebite, liver disease, acute intravascular hemolysis, shock, heat stroke, hypersensitivity, vasculitis

- ***Obstetric conditions:*** Amniotic fluid embolism and abruptio placentae account for 50% of obstetric causes of DIC. Leakage of TF like materials into the circulation occurs which leads to DIC. Twenty percent of HELLP syndrome develops DIC. Other conditions causing DIC include fatty liver of pregnancy, septic abortion and dead fetus syndrome.
- ***Miscellaneous causes*** include giant hemangioma (Kasabach-Merritt syndrome), insertion of peritoneovenous shunts, acute hemolytic transfusion reactions, PNH, hemotoxic snakebite (viperine), fulminant hepatic failure, cirrhosis of the liver, heat stroke, rhabdomyolysis, acute respiratory distress syndrome (ARDS), purpura fulminans and catastrophic APS.

Acute inflammation, infection, sepsis and endotoxemia can all induce a hypercoagulable state. When the coagulation mechanisms are overwhelmed, DIC occurs which leads to consumption coagulopathy and bleeding. In chronic DIC, thrombotic phenomena predominate over hemorrhage. Thrombosis and inflammation are related since the same mediators contribute to both and reinforce each other. The inflammatory markers include endotoxin, tumor necrosis factor (TNF), clusters of differentiation 40 (CD40) ligand, TF exposed monocytes, activated endothelium and the circulating TF-bearing microparticles. A primary cause of thrombosis in DIC is the disruption of endogenous anticoagulant pathways. TF present in microparticles is in an inactive form. It is activated when the microparticles are recruited to the site of injury.

Clinical Features

It includes bleeding and thrombotic manifestation which may overlap. Two types of DIC are recognized: (1) Acute DIC (Table 177.2) and (2) chronic DIC.

Bleeding is in the form of petechiae and ecchymosis. Oozing can occur from wound sites, intravenous lines, catheters and mucosa. Sometimes there can be life-

Table 177.2: Clinical features of acute disseminated intravascular coagulation (DIC)

Parameters	Values (%)
Bleeding	64
Renal dysfunction	25
Hepatic dysfunction	20
Respiratory dysfunction	15
Shock	14
Thromboembolism	7
Central nervous system (CNS) manifestation	2

threatening bleeding from gastrointestinal tract (GIT) or central nervous system (CNS).

Acute renal failure (ARF) is either due to microthrombosis of afferent arterioles leading to cortical ischemia/necrosis or acute tubular necrosis due to hypotension and/or sepsis. Jaundice is common and may be due to both liver disease and hemolysis. Pulmonary hemorrhage with hemoptysis and dyspnea are due to damage of pulmonary vascular endothelium.

Patients with chronic DIC are asymptomatic with increased levels of FDP or have manifestations of venous and arterial thrombosis. They may also have minor skin and mucosal bleeding. Solid tumors are the most common cause of chronic DIC. Most of them are asymptomatic with only laboratory abnormalities. When symptomatic, they present with venous thrombosis—deep vein thrombosis (DVT) or superficial migratory thrombophlebitis (Trousseu's syndrome). Arterial thrombosis leads to digital gangrene, renal infarction or stroke usually due to embolization from nonbacterial thrombotic (marantic) endocarditis of mitral valve. Age above 60 years, male sex, breast cancer, tumor necrosis and advancing stage are the risk factors for chronic DIC.

Diagnosis

After a possible clinical diagnosis, following investigations are helpful in diagnosis and confirmation of DIC. Investigations done are complete blood count (CBC), C-reactive protein (CRP), erythrocyte sedimentation rate (ESR), peripheral blood smear, prothrombin time (PT), activated partial thromboplastin time (aPTT), FDP, D-dimer, fibrinogen, thrombin time and reptilase time, AT, protein C and protein S levels, factor V and VIII levels. Characteristic diagnostic findings are:

- Presence of schistocytes in peripheral blood smear
- Thrombocytopenia
- Prolonged PT, aPTT, thrombin time
- Increase in FDP and D-dimer
- Decreased fibrinogen, factor V and VIII
- Decreased AT, proteins C and S.

D-dimer is the degradation product of fibrin when acted by plasmin. The test is performed on finger prick blood. The test is very sensitive but not specific for DVT but may be specific for DIC when compared to FDP. Raised levels of CRP as a result of inflammation or tissue damage vitiate the D-dimer levels and hence, its value comes down. In suspected DVT, negative D-dimer test excludes

Table 177.3: Diagnostic scoring system for disseminated intravascular coagulation (DIC)

Criteria	Number of points
Platelet count 50,000–100,000/mm³	1
Platelet count < 50,000/mm³	2
No increase in fibrin markers (D-dimer, FDP)	0
Moderate increase in fibrin markers (D-dimer, FDP)	2
Strong increase in fibrin markers (D-dimer, FDP)	3
Prolonged PT increase < 3 seconds	0
Prolonged PT increase > 3–6 seconds	1
Prolonged PT increase > 6 seconds	2
Fibrinogen level > 1 g/L	0
Fibrinogen level < 1 g/L	1

Note: Total score more than 5 points is compatible with overt DIC; less than 5 points suggestive of nonovert DIC. Scoring is repeated daily or on alternate day depending upon the clinical condition.

Abbreviations: PT = Prothrombin time; FDP = Fibrin degradation product

the diagnosis. Normal level of D-dimer in plasma is 80–500 ng/mL. Normal fibrinogen in plasma is 150–400 mg/dL.

Secondary involvement of vital organs, like the liver, heart and kidney, should be looked for frequently and their dysfunction managed appropriately.

Diagnostic Scoring System for DIC

Diagnostic scoring system for DIC is described in Table 177.3.

Treatment

DIC has a high mortality of 40–80%, specially when it is associated with severe sepsis, trauma or burns. The important risk factors are increasing age, severity of the organ dysfunction and hemostatic abnormalities. The most important factor in the treatment of DIC is the detection and treatment of the underlying condition. Use of blood components and heparin may be of value. Antifibrinolytic agents are contraindicated as it can increase the risk of thrombosis. Platelet transfusions and fresh frozen plasma (FFP) are given only if there is bleeding symptoms and not on a prophylactic basis. Heparin used to be given in chronic compensated DIC, especially in malignancy associated with thrombotic manifestations. But currently, there is only insufficient clinical evidence to make a firm recommendation on this issue. Restoration of the natural anticoagulants, like AT and protein C, may be helpful. If bleeding manifestations are not controlled by the above measures recombinant factor VIIa can be used as a last resort.

Thrombotic Thrombocytopenic Purpura (Hemolytic Uremic Syndrome)

Currently, TTP and HUS are considered together. Although these diseases have multiple etiologies, different demographics, different response to different treatments and different prognosis, the presenting features are same in many patients. Most of them have thrombocytopenia and MAHA without another apparent cause and many have neurological and/or renal abnormalities. Patients with dominant neurological abnormalities with minimal

Table 177.4: Causes observed in a large TTP-HUS registry

Parameters	Values (%)
Idiopathic	40
Autoimmune disease, infection, cancer	27
Drug associated	12
Bloody diarrhea	8
Pregnancy/postpartum	7
Hemopoietic stem cell transplantation	6

or absent ARF are considered to represent classical or idiopathic TTP. They are associated with severely deficient ADAMTS13 (a disintegrin and metalloproteinase with a thrombo spondin type 1 motif member 13). In some other patients, ARF is dominant and neurological abnormalities are minimal or absent. These are considered to represent HUS. Some patients will have both severe ARF and neurological manifestations. Some patients may have thrombocytopenia and MAHA without much renal or neurological manifestation. So, all these presentations are now considered as the broad spectrum of TTP-HUS syndrome.

Causes

The incidence of TTP-HUS syndrome is approximately 11 cases/million population per year for suspected cases and 4.5 cases for idiopathic TTP. The causes observed in a large TTP-HUS registry (Oklahoma, 1969–2011) are given in Table 177.4.

Pathogenesis

Reduced ADAMTS13 activity as the underlying cause and the mechanism for platelet consumption is found in some patients with TTP-HUS. They are at a risk of developing recurrent symptoms. von Willebrand's factor (vWF) is synthesized in endothelial cell and is assembled in the normal plasma. These unusually large vWF multimers (ULvWF) are rapidly degraded in the circulation into the normal size range of vWF multimers by a specific vWF cleaving protease called ADAMTS13. The locus of this enzyme is on chromosome 9q34 and up to 12 mutations have been identified which can lead to reduction of activity of ADAMTS13. As a result, there is an accumulation of ULVWF multimers, which lead to platelet aggregation and platelet thrombi which are characteristic of the disease. The enzyme can be absent or there can be severe deficiency in the activity of the enzyme. An inhibitory IgG antibody to ADAMTS13 metalloproteinase has been found in some patients with TTP-HUS syndrome. The presence of these inhibitory antibodies suggests the potential benefit of corticosteroids and rituximab in the treatment of this condition.

Although many cases of TTP-HUS are idiopathic, the following underlying causes have been now identified. Congenital ADAMTS13 mutation leading to congenital or hereditary TTP, congenital hereditary complement mutations (responsible for familial HUS), various types of infections [Shiga toxin producing *Escherichia coli*, human immunodeficiency virus (HIV), *Pneumococcal* infection, flu-like infection, gastroenteritis, ear nose and throat infections, urinary tract infection (UTI), bronchitis, pneumonitis and lung abscess] drugs like quinine, chemotherapy agents [mitomycin, gemcitabine and cisplatin, bevacizumab, bis-chloroethylnitrosourea (BCNU)], immunosuppressive drugs (cyclosporine, tacrolimus), antiplatelet drugs (ticlopidine, clopidogrel), vancyclovir, malignancy, pregnancy, cardiovascular surgery, kidney transplant, allogeneic hematopoietic stem cell transplantation (HSCT). Genetic factors play a role in atypical HUS. Abnormal thrombomodulin have been identified in 5% of cases. Normally, it is ubiquitous endothelial glycoprotein which activates protein C, thereby suppressing clot formation. Protein C has also anti-inflammatory and cytoprotective actions. TMB (tetramethylbenzidine) through its lecithin-like domain interferes with inflammation by suppressing leukocyte trafficking and dampening complement activation.

Clinical and Laboratory Findings

Patients with TTP-HUS may have one or many of the following features:

- MAHA
- Thrombocytopenia
- Renal function may be normal, but ARF may be present
- Fluctuating neurological findings, but some may have no findings
- Fever is rare. If high fever with chills is present, diagnosis of sepsis should be made.

When there was no effective and curative treatment like plasma exchange, full clinical course of the disease was observed. For the diagnosis, a pentad was necessary with pathological evidence of fibrin deposition. The mortality was as high as 90%. Now only thrombocytopenia and MAHA (dyad) without another clinically apparent etiology (DIC, malignant hypertension, severe pre-eclampsia, sepsis, systemic malignancy) are required to suspect the diagnosis of TTP-HUS and to initiate plasma exchange. All the clinical pentad is now rare to be seen in a patient.

MAHA is the hallmark of TTP-HUS and along with thrombocytopenia is the major diagnostic criterion. It is defined as nonimmune hemolytic anemia [direct Coombs test (DCT) negative] with prominent RBC fragmentation (schistocytes and helmet cells). Schistocytosis for the diagnosis of MAHA is now defined as schistocytes more than 1% or more than 2 in an oil immersion field (Fig. 177.2). They have all the other features of hemolysis, such as jaundice, splenomegaly and increase in indirect serum bilirubin, reticulocyte count, lactate dehydrogenase (LDH) and reduced haptoglobin.

Thrombocytopenia is the other major diagnostic criterion. Platelet count before treatment is around 20,000/mm^3.

Renal disease is due to thrombotic microangiopathy (TMA) and urinalysis is near normal with only mild proteinuria (1–2 g/day). In one half (50% of cases), complement activation (hypocomplementemia) and features of glomerular involvement (red cells + RBC casts) and vasculitis may be seen.

Neurological findings are seen in many patients and consist of confusion, headache, focal neurological deficits [transient ischemic attack (TIA), stroke, aphasia] seizures

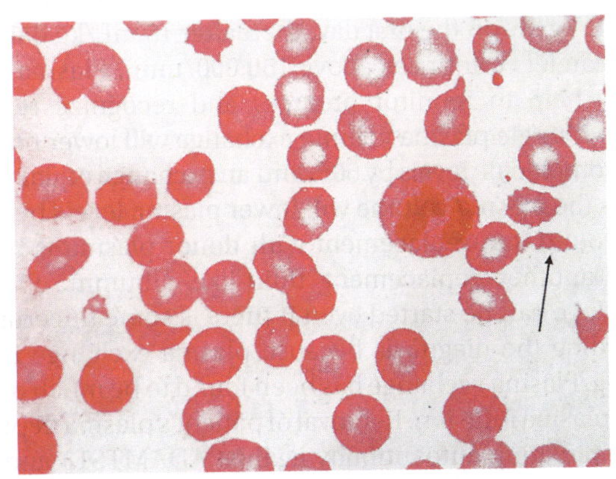

Fig. 177.2: Blood smear—schistocytes in microangiopathic hemolytic anemia (arrow)

or coma. Imaging may be normal or show PRES (posterior reversible leukoencephalopathy syndrome).

Fever is less common in more recent case series. Cardiac involvement, like arrhythmias, sudden cardiac death, myocardial infarction (MI) and cardiac failure, can occur due to hemorrhage and patches of necrosis in cardiac tissue.

Congenital TTP is caused by ADAMTS13 mutation leading to absent or very low levels of its activity. Patients with congenital TTP may present in the neonatal period, childhood or not until adulthood. It may be misdiagnosed as hemolytic disease of newborn or alloimmune thrombocytopenia.

Diagnosis

It is now stressed that the diagnosis of TTP-HUS should be clinical and requires only the presence of thrombocytopenia and MAHA. ADAMTS13 activity is not required for starting the treatment but is better that blood is drawn for this investigation before starting the treatment as the enzyme activity can be increased by treatment. The normal activity of ADAMTS13 is above 50%. If low activity is detected, testing for inhibitors also should be done. Additional investigations to assess the various organ function (renal, hepatic, CNS, cardiac) should be done. If it is less than 10%, it indicates severe deficiency. Most of the cases of TTP-HUS are idiopathic. Associated conditions, like bloody diarrhea, pregnancy and drugs, should be looked into. Systemic diseases mentioned earlier should be differentiated from TTP-HUS. A useful differentiating point from DIC is that in TTP-HUS the coagulation parameters [International Normalized Ratio (INR), aPTT, and factor V and VIII levels] are usually normal.

Treatment (TTP-HUS Syndrome)

If untreated, patients with TTP-HUS will progressively worsen and die. The mortality before the plasma exchange treatment was 90% and now the mortality is reduced to about 25%. It is a medical emergency and if left untreated it is associated with a rate of death of 90% usually from MI due to platelet thrombi in the coronary arteries. The treatment of choice is plasma exchange in which the patient's plasma is removed by apheresis and replaced by donor plasma. Plasma exchange is done using 1.0–1.5 times of the patient's predicted plasma volume. FFP is used, starting with

30 mL/kg bw on the first day, thereafter 15 mL/kg daily till the platelet count rises above 150,000/mm^3. Plasma LDH levels help to monitor progress and recognize relapse early. A single plasma volume exchange will lower plasma macromolecule levels by 60% and an exchange equal to 1.4 times the plasma volume will lower plasma levels by 75%. It is found that replacement with donor plasma is better than another replacement fluid-like albumin. Plasma exchange can be started even if there is some uncertainty regarding the diagnosis because plasma exchange is life saving. Plasma exchange has been found to be much better than plasma infusion. Removal of patient's plasma depletes the circulating autoantibody against ADAMTS13 and the circulating very high-molecular-weight vWF multimers. Donor plasma supplies the deficient ADAMTS13 and its activity. Adult diarrheal HUS also responds well to plasma exchange. Plasma exchange is not usually done for postdiarrheal HUS in children, patients undergoing cancer chemotherapy and HCT and in pneumococcal infections. On an average, 7–16 daily exchanges are required for a remission.

Immunosuppression

Glucocorticoids may be a useful addition to plasma exchange to suppress autoantibodies against ADAMTS13.

Prednisolone 1 mg/kg or methylprednisolone 125 mg intravenous (IV) twice daily is used. It may also help the patients with persistent thrombocytopenia. Rituximab is used in a dose of 375 mg/m^2 weekly for 4 weeks with or without cyclophosphamide for more severe cases and cases who do not respond to plasma exchange (10–20%). The drug should be administered after the plasma exchange so that it is not removed by the exchange. There is no known effective maintenance therapy for this condition. For congenital TTP who have low or absent levels of ADAMTS13 due to genetic mutations, plasma infusion alone is enough for treatment. Plasma exchange is not necessary. Recombinant ADAMTS13 has been developed and is found to normalize vWF-cleaving activity *in vitro* in plasma of patients with acquired TTP. It is not yet used in man, but is likely to be effective in congenital TTP.

Relapse

A number of studies indicate that severe ADAMTS13 deficiency and/or the presence of inhibitors may have prognostic value in predicting the relapse. Such patients are found to have about 40% relapse over the following 7.5 years.

CHAPTER

178

Thrombophilia

Mathew Thomas, KV Krishna Das

Chapter Summary

- Definition
- Causes
- Clinical Presentation
- Diagnosis
- Treatment

DEFINITION

The term 'thrombophilia' denotes an abnormally increased tendency of the blood to undergo thrombosis *in vivo* either spontaneously or due to trivial reasons. Venous system is affected more often than the arterial system. This is a pathological state caused by several inherited and acquired abnormalities.

The most common manifestations of thrombophilia are venous thromboembolism (VTE). The reasons include:

- Alterations in the blood flow
- Vascular endothelial injury
- Alterations in the constituents of blood leading to inherited and acquired hypercoagulable states.

CAUSES

The causes of thrombophilia may be hereditary or acquired.

Hereditary Thrombophilia

The usual inherited hypercoagulable states are:

- Factor V Leiden mutation
- Prothrombin mutation
- Protein S deficiency
- Protein C deficiency
- Antithrombin (AT) deficiency
- Dysfibrinogenemia.

There are many other alleged inherited factors, like heparin cofactor II deficiency, plasminogen deficiency and factor XII deficiency, but it is not clear if these factors have a significant role in the pathogenesis of thrombophilia. Low levels of activated protein C (APC) are associated with greater severity of atherosclerosis. In addition to its anticoagulant properties, protein C pathway exerts protective effects on gene expression profiles involving antiapoptotic and anti-inflammatory responses and stabilizing effect on the endothelial barrier. The role of APC in the pathogenesis of atheroma is being studied.

Acquired Thrombophilia

The acquired risk factors are prior thrombotic event, recent major surgery, presence of a central venous catheter, trauma, immobilization, malignancy, pregnancy, use of oral contraceptives, heparin, tamoxifen, postmenopausal hormone replacement therapy (HRT) with estrogens, myeloproliferative disorders, antiphospholipid syndrome (APS), long air travel, hyperhomocysteinemia, a number of major medical illnesses [congestive cardiac failure, nephrotic syndrome, inflammatory bowel disease (IBD), paroxysmal nocturnal hemoglobinuria (PNH), liver disease, cancer], elevated levels of normal clotting factors [factors VIII, IX, von Willebrand's factor (vWF) and fibrinogen] and other plasma components [reduction of tissue factor (TF) inhibitor, plasma fibrinolytic activity and thrombomodulin], anatomic risk factors, such as [congenital venous malformation of the inferior vena cava (IVC), May-Thurner syndrome-compression of left common iliac vein by the overlying right common iliac artery and the underlying vertebral body, etc.]. Microparticles containing activated TF initiate thrombosis in cancer. Mutation of thrombomodulin or reduction in its amount leads to deficient function of protein C and also leads to thrombophilia.

Causes in India

About 66% of patients seen in India in a center handling 300 thrombophilia patients annually were found to have an identifiable cause. The most common cause detected was isolated elevation of factor VIIIC above 220% in 70% of patients. Isolated lupus anticoagulant (LA) positivity was seen in 10%, decreased protein S in 3% and decreased protein C and AT in 1% each (personal communication). In the western countries, the most common cause of thrombophilia detected is factor V Leiden mutation.

CLINICAL PRESENTATION

The two most common presentations of thrombophilia, both inherited and acquired, are deep venous thrombosis (DVT) of the lower limbs and pulmonary embolism (PE). The venous thrombosis may also occur at uncommon sites as the upper limbs, cerebral veins, portal vein and its branches, hepatic vein, jugular veins and others. Generally arterial thrombosis is uncommon in thrombophilia but occurs in conditions such as APS and hyperhomocysteinemia. Most of the incidents of venous thrombosis are due to acquired hypercoagulable states and less commonly due to inherited causes. In India, in a good number of cases, an underlying hypercoagulable state is not evident. Sometimes in a patient with inherited hypercoagulable state venous thrombosis may be precipitated by an acquired risk factor such as major surgery.

Quantitative risk of DVT in thrombophilic conditions was compared to normals (Table 178.1).

DIAGNOSIS

A strong clinical suspicion is necessary to make a diagnosis of venous thrombosis. Venous thrombosis should be confirmed by definitive investigations, e.g. compression ultrasonography in DVT of lower and upper limbs, pulmonary computed tomography (CT) angiography to diagnose PE and magnetic resonance venography in cerebral venous thrombosis. Cut-off values for D-dimer

Table 178.1: Deficiency of factors causing thrombophilia

Factors	*Occurrence*
Factor V Leiden	7-fold in heterozygotes; 80-fold in homozygotes
Factor II G 20210A	2.8-fold
Antithrombin (AT) III deficiency	8-fold
Protein C deficiency	7-fold
Protein S deficiency	8-fold
High-clotting factor levels:	
• Factor VIII > 150 IU/dL	4.8-fold
• Factor IX > 129 IU/dL	2.8-fold
• Factor XI > 121 IU/dL	2.2-fold
Mild hyperhomocysteinemia	2.7-fold
Pregnancy and puerperium	2–14-fold

Source: Kyrle PA, Eichinger S. Deep vein thrombosis. Lancet. 2005;365(9465):1163-74.

of 500 ng/L have a sensitivity of 100% for DVT, but specificity of only 14%. In suspected cases of DVT, negative D-dimer test almost excludes the diagnosis. The *other investigations* that may be done at this stage are complete blood count (CBC), C-reactive protein (CRP), prothrombin time (PT), International Normalized Ratio (INR), activated partial thromboplastin time (aPTT), anticardiolipin antibody (aCLA), immunoglobulin M (IgM) and IgG, LA, β-2 glycoprotein-1, IgM and IgG, and antinuclear antibody (ANA) screening. Complete thrombophilia screening is not justified for patients with arterial thrombosis since hereditary thrombophilia is principally a risk factor for venous thrombosis. Screening for thrombophilia is also not recommended for patients with recent surgery, active malignancy, systemic lupus erythematosus (SLE), IBD, myeloproliferative disease, retinal vein thrombosis, upper limb and VTE. It is also stressed that most of the screening tests for thrombophilia are not done during the acute phase of the venous thrombosis because there will be some reduction of protein C, S and AT. Screening at a later stage (after 3–4 months) is preferably done for patients less than 50 years of age without any identifiable risk factors, those with a strong family history of venous thrombosis, those with recurrent VTE, thrombosis occurring at unusual sites and prior history of warfarin skin necrosis in whom protein C deficiency is likely. The screening is usually done after stopping the maintenance warfarin for 15 days in a good center where all the screening tests can be done.

TREATMENT

Treatment for any thromboembolic event including DVT should be initiated with heparin [unfractionated or low-molecular-weight heparin (LMWH)] or fondaparinux or one of the newer anticoagulants. This treatment is used to prevent clot extension, prevention of fatal PE, for reducing the risk of recurrent thrombosis and for limiting the late complications, like postphlebitis syndrome. The most common agent used for initiating the treatment is LMWH, e.g. enoxaparin given subcutaneously twice a day. In most cases, the treatment can be done on an outpatient basis. The indications for admission are massive DVT (e.g. iliofemoral DVT), presence of symptomatic PE, high risk of bleeding with anticoagulant treatment, cerebral venous thrombosis and presence of comorbid conditions.

A baseline INR should be done and an oral anti-coagulant, e.g. warfarin, should be started along with or after 1–2 days of heparin treatment. The dose of warfarin should be adjusted according to the INR. The target INR for warfarin maintenance treatment in DVT is 2–3. When the target INR is reached, heparin can be stopped and warfarin is continued with monitoring the INR at frequent intervals (weekly or twice a week). Inferior vena cava (IVC) filters are indicated if there is any contraindication to (recent surgery, hemorrhagic stroke, active bleeding) or failure of anticoagulant therapy at a high risk of VTE and PE. Recurrent thromboembolism despite of adequate anticoagulation is another indication. If there is a contraindication for warfarin, LMWH can be continued for maintenance treatment also.

The newer anticoagulant drugs can also be used in the treatment of venous thrombosis (*See* Ch 176). Rivaroxaban, a factor Xa inhibitor, is used in a dose of 15 mg twice daily for 3 weeks followed by 20 mg daily for 3–6 months. Apixaban 10 mg twice daily for 7 days followed by 5 mg twice daily for 6 months or edoxaban 60 mg daily as maintenance dose after LMWH are other factor Xa inhibitors used. Dabigatran, a direct thrombin inhibitor, is used in a dose of 150 mg twice daily after 7 days of LMWH. When considering these agents, the physician should weigh the apparent benefits of these new agents (no need for monitoring and easy oral administration) as primary or secondary therapies for the treatment of VTE against the risks of uncontrolled bleeding and the cost of therapy. For uncontrolled bleeding caused by factor Xa inhibitors the antidots andexanet is available (*See* Ch 176).

Early ambulation is now strongly advocated after a VTE. Use of elastic graduated compression stockings (GCSs) that provide 30–40 mm Hg of ankle pressure started 2 weeks after anticoagulation prevents post-thrombotic or postphlebitis syndrome.

Duration of Treatment in Thrombophilia after an Episode of Venous Thrombosis

For duration of treatment in thrombophilia after an episode of venous thrombosis, patients are divided into:

- First VTE provoked by surgery
- First VTE provoked by nonsurgical factor (e.g. pregnancy)
- First unprovoked VTE
- Second unprovoked VTE.

Present evidence suggests that the duration of anticoagulant therapy for thrombophilic states does not relate directly to the presence or absence of inherited coagulation abnormalities. For the first VTE provoked by surgery or nonsurgical factors, anticoagulation for 3–6 months is recommended. After this, if the bleeding risks are low the anticoagulation may be continued to prevent recurrence. For second unprovoked VTE (whether any inherited risk factors for thrombophilia are present or absent), anticoagulation should be continued indefinitely unless the bleeding risk is very high. Recurrent thromboembolism in APS after an initial event is approximately 11% per year regardless of warfarin treatment. In untreated patients, the recurrence rate may go up to 19–29% per year. These evidences are strong arguments for lifelong anticoagulation in most patients with APS who had a thromboembolic event.

Role of prophylactic treatment in antiphospholipids syndrome (APS) in the absence of any clinical event is debated. This question was looked into in many clinical trials by using low-dose aspirin. The conclusions were that asymptomatic patients who have persistently positive antibodies have low-annual incidence of thrombosis and that they do not benefit from low-dose aspirin. But strict control of cardiovascular risk factors should be instituted in all patients with high-risk profile of APS. They should also be given thromboprophylaxis with LMWH during high-risk situations, like surgery, prolonged immobilization and puerperium. In patients with SLE and medium-to-high titers of acute promyelocytic leukemia (APML) antibodies, low-dose aspirin and hydroxychloroquine (HCQ) were found to be useful for primary thromboprophylaxis. LAs can sometimes interfere with the phospholipids used in the thromboplastin used for doing the PT. This may cause false elevation of INR. In such situations, thromboplastin containing excess of phospholipids should be used. Alternatively chromogenic factor X levels, factor II levels and prothrombin proconverting time may be done and these tests are not affected by LAs. After the first unprovoked VTE event a patient with other thrombophilic conditions has 5–15% risk of VTE recurrence within the 1st year following discontinuation of the anticoagulation and 30–60% risk of VTE recurrence within the following 5–10 years. For treatment failures in APS (VTE occurring with full anticoagulation) the INR target for warfarin can be increased to 2.5–3.5. Better options are addition of aspirin, HCQ or continuation with LMWH instead of warfarin.

CHAPTER 179

Structure and Function of the Kidneys and Urinary Tract

R Kasi Visweswaran, Susan Uthup

> **Chapter Summary**
> - Development of the Kidneys and Urinary System
> - Structure of Kidney
> - Functions of Kidney

DEVELOPMENT OF THE KIDNEYS AND URINARY SYSTEM

Nephrogenesis starts from the 4th week of intrauterine life. Three sets of excretory organs are formed in mammalian embryos from the intermediate mesoderm. They are the pronephros, mesonephros and metanephros. The pronephros and mesonephros are tubular structures that involute before birth. Only the caudal portion of the mesonephric duct, which opens into the cloaca persists. Metanephros is the direct precursor of the adult kidneys. Nephrons, the excretory units of the kidneys, develop from metanephros. Collecting system of the kidneys develop from the ureteric bud, which starts as an outgrowth of the mesonephric duct close to its entrance to the cloaca (Figs 179.1A and 179.2B).

The ureteric bud penetrates the metanephric tissue (blastema) and blastema appears as a cap molded over its blunt end of the outpouching, which is the ureteric bud. The bud dilates and splits into branches. The trigone of

bladder, ureters, renal pelvis, major and minor calyces and collecting ducts which may develop from the ureteric bud. The glomeruli, proximal convoluted tubule (PCT), loop of Henle and distal convoluted tubule (DCT) and renal interstitium develop from the metanephric blastema. Nephrogenesis is complete at 36 weeks of intrauterine life. The number of nephrons does not increase once the development is complete. At birth, the kidneys have a lobulated appearance (Fig. 179.2). During infancy, the lobulation disappears as a result, of further growth and maturation of the nephrons.

The development of urinary bladder and urethra starts with the formation of a membrane called the urorectal septum. This membrane divides the cloaca into two compartments—dorsal rectal compartment and ventral urogenital compartment. The urogenital compartment communicates with the allantois. The caudal portion of the mesonephros forms the urogenital sinus. The urinary bladder develops from the urogenital sinus and allantois. The trigone of the bladder develops from the ureteric bud.

STRUCTURE OF KIDNEY

The kidneys are paired bean-shaped organs situated in the retroperitoneum on either side of the vertebral column against the psoas major muscle. Each kidney

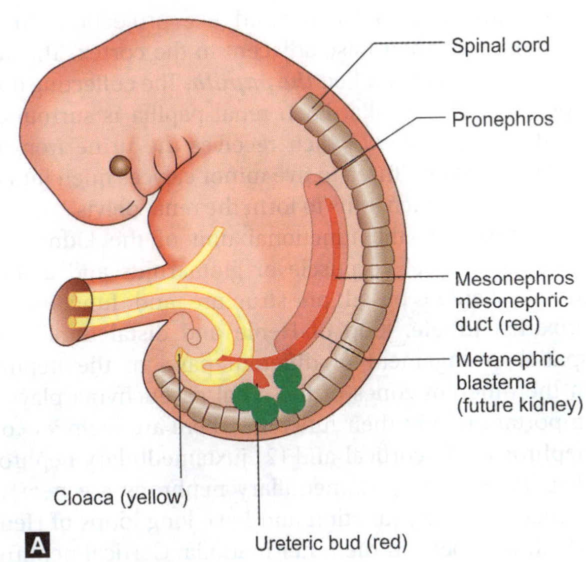

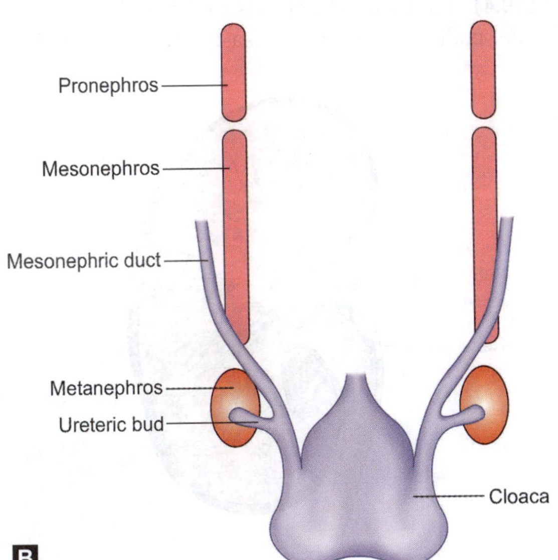

Figs 179.1A and B: Relationship of cloaca, ureteric bud, pronephros, mesonephros and metanephros. **A.** In the embryo during renal development; **B.** In the embryo

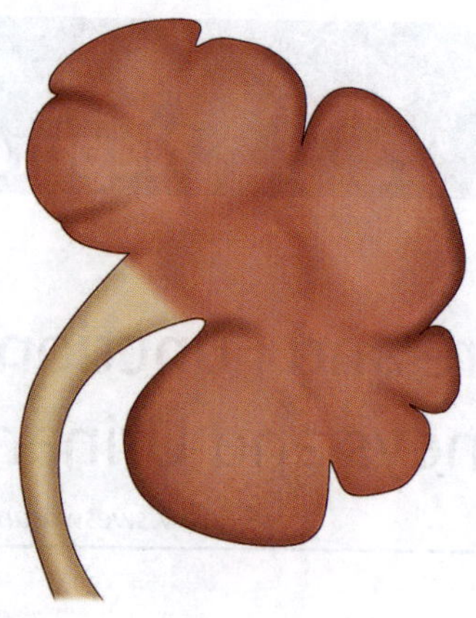

Fig. 179.2: Lobulated appearance of kidney

weighs about 120–170 g and is about 12 cm in length, 6 cm in breadth and 3 cm in thickness. At the concave medial border of each kidney, there is a slit-like aperture—the hilum. The renal artery, renal vein, nerves, lymphatic and the expanded funnel-shaped renal pelvis pass through the hilum. Surrounding each kidney is the tough fibrous capsule, the perinephric fat and perirenal fascia (Gerota's fascia). The Gerota's fascia is fused on all the sides, except inferiorly. Therefore, the perirenal abscesses spread only inferiorly towards the pelvis, psoas muscle or even to the contralateral and retroperitoneal regions. It cannot spread upward or laterally outside the fascia. The kidneys play the major role in maintaining the internal environment (*milieu interior*).

The cut section of the kidney reveals an outer dark zone—the cortex and inner pale zone, the medulla (Fig. 179.3). Corticomedullary distinction can be clearly made out. The cortex is 2–3 cm thick. It is divided into an outer cortex and juxtamedullary cortex. The cortex contains the glomeruli, proximal and distal tubules, blood vessels and interstitium. The medulla is divided into outer and inner parts. The outer medulla adjacent to the cortex is divided into an outer stripe and inner stripe (Fig. 179.4). The medulla consists of the limbs of the loop of Henle, collecting tubules, vasa-recta and interstitium.

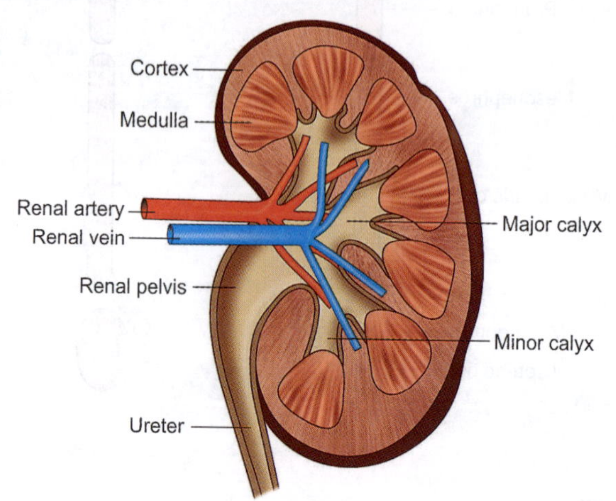

Fig. 179.3: Cut section of adult kidney showing cortex, medulla, renal pelvis and upper part of ureter

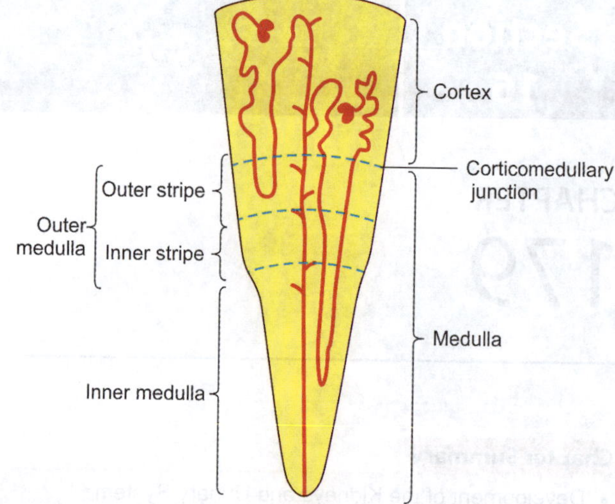

Fig. 179.4: Subdivisions of renal parenchyma

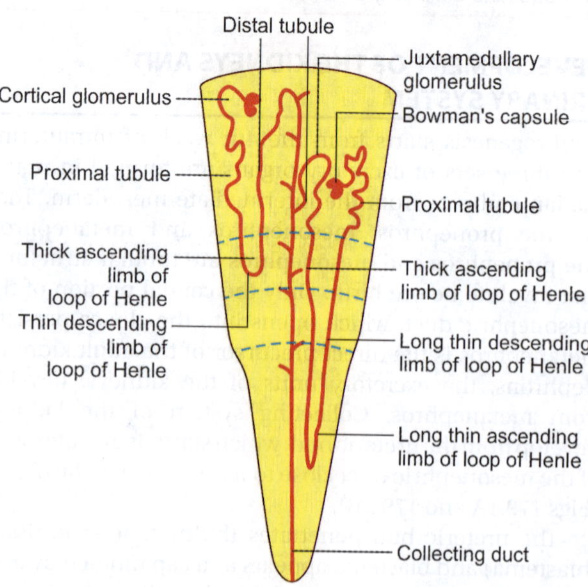

Fig. 179.5: Arrangement of cortical and juxtamedullary nephrons

There are about 8–18 pyramid like projections in the medulla with their base adjacent to the cortex. The apex of each pyramid is called *the papilla*. The collecting ducts open into the papilla. Each renal papilla is surrounded by the minor calyx, which receives the urine from the collecting ducts. Three to five minor calyces open into the major calyx, which joins to form the renal pelvis.

Nephron is the functional unit of the kidney and consists of renal corpuscle or glomerulus and a single tubule divided based on structure and function into proximal tubule, loop of Henle and distal tubule. The spatial arrangement of different parts of the nephron in the different zones of the renal parenchyma plays an important role in their function. There are mainly two of nephrons—(1) cortical and (2) juxtamedullary nephrons (Fig. 179.5). The juxtamedullary nephrons are near the corticomedullary junction and have long loops of Henle, which turn back in the inner medulla. Cortical nephrons have short loops of Henle, which may turn back in the outer medulla.

The glomerulus consists of the central mesangial framework surrounded by a specialized capillary network. This globular structure is encircled by the Bowman's capsule all around, except at the vascular pole. The afferent arteriole enters the glomerulus at the vascular pole and divides into the capillary network. The network of capillaries reunites and forms the efferent arteriole, which leaves the glomerulus. The blood is filtered and the ultrafiltrate moves through the basement membrane into the Bowman's capsular space. The mesangium is the central skeletal framework of the glomerulus. The mesangium consists of the mesangial cells and the matrix. The mesangial cells contain contractile elements, like actin and myosin which enable them to regulate the ultrafiltration. The macrophage derived cells in mesangium exhibit reticuloendothelial function and remove the trapped macromolecules. The wall of the capillary loop is lined by endothelial cells. The endothelial cell cytoplasm is stretched into thin sheets completely encircling the lumen. On electron microscopy, fenestrations are seen in this thin sheet of endothelial cell cytoplasm. Outside the endothelium is the glomerular capillary basement membrane and a layer of specialized visceral epithelial cells called podocytes. The basement membrane consists of a central dense layer called lamina densa with two less dense layers on either side, lamina rara interna on the endothelial side and lamina rara externa on the epithelial side. It is made-up of collagen and negatively charged sialoglycoproteins (Fig. 179.6).

Podocytes are specialized visceral epithelial cells. They resemble an octopus with a central nucleus and numerous cytoplasmic prolongations. The divisions and subdivisions of these cytoplasmic prolongations which interdigitate with the neighboring podocytes. The term podocyte is derived on account of the presence of the foot processes, which are in contact with the basement membrane. The space between two foot processes has a slit pore membrane. The slit in this membrane is the ultimate ultrafiltration barrier, which permits only

substances with less than 60 daltons to pass through. The whole glomerular capillary network is surrounded by the Bowman's capsule. The parietal epithelial cells line the outer surface of the Bowman's capsule. The space between the visceral and parietal cell layers is the urinary space. The urinary space communicates with the lumen of the proximal tubule (Fig. 179.7).

The renal tubules consist of a long tubular system with three main segments, which may differ in their structure and functions. They are the proximal tubule, loop of Henle and distal tubule. The proximal tubule consists of a convoluted and a straight portion. The glomerular basement membrane (GBM) continues as the basement membrane of the proximal tubule. The proximal tubule is lined by a single layer of columnar cells with prominent brush border on the luminal side. These cells contain several mitochondria and are metabolically very active and highly oxygen dependent. Thus, this region is very vulnerable to ischemic injury. The capillary network arising from the efferent arteriole surrounds the proximal tubule. Loop of Henle, is a hairpin, like segment of the tubule which connects the proximal and distal tubules. It consists of the descending limb, bend and ascending limb. The descending limb and 'U' bend of the loop of Henle is lined by a single layer of flat cells with clear cytoplasm. Cortical nephrons have short loops of Henle with short thin descending limbs. The 'U' bends stop short at the outer stripe of the medulla. The juxtamedullary nephrons have long thin descending and ascending limbs with the 'U' bend reaching deep into the inner medulla. A portion of the ascending limb is thick and it is called thick ascending limb. The thick ascending limb is lined by columnar cells and it has specialized function. At the junction of the ascending limb and distal tubule, the glomerulus, afferent and efferent arterioles and the distal tubule are close together to form the juxtaglomerular apparatus (JGA).

The JGA consists of macula densa at the initial part of the distal tubule, the afferent and efferent arterioles of the parent glomerulus and glomerular mesangium at the vascular pole (Fig. 179.8).

The modified smooth muscle cells of the afferent arteriole contain renin stored as granules. The macula densa consists of specialized cells in the tubular wall at the junction between thick ascending limb of loop of Henle and distal tubule. These long and narrow cells have densely packed large nuclei (macula densa). The structural organization of JGA suggests a regulatory function. The macula densa senses the composition of the tubular fluid reaching it. This information is used to regulate the release of renin from the modified smooth muscle cells of the afferent arteriole.

The distal tubule is the continuation of the thick ascending limb of loop of Henle. The lining cells of the distal tubule are cuboidal with microvilli on the luminal side. Unlike proximal tubular cells, they do not have brush border. The collecting ducts are formed by the union of several distal tubules. They pass through part of the cortex and whole length of the medulla to open into the calyxes through slit like openings into the renal papillae. The lining cells of the collecting ducts are of two types—

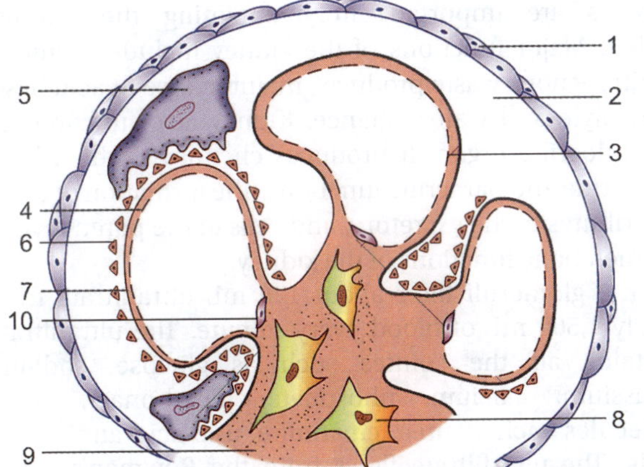

Fig. 179.6: Electron microscopy of the glomerulus

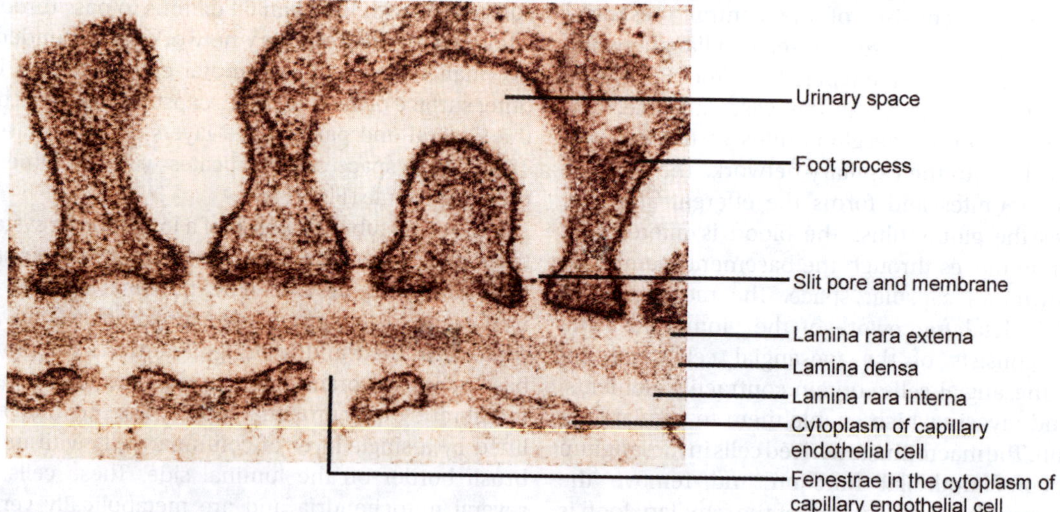

Fig. 179.7: Glomerular capillary filtration barrier

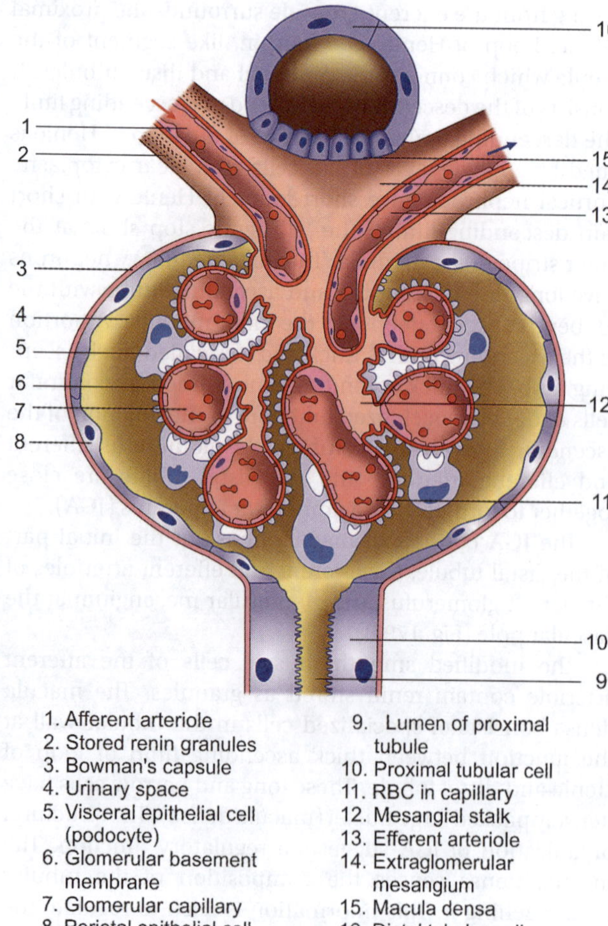

1. Afferent arteriole
2. Stored renin granules
3. Bowman's capsule
4. Urinary space
5. Visceral epithelial cell (podocyte)
6. Glomerular basement membrane
7. Glomerular capillary
8. Perietal epithelial cell
9. Lumen of proximal tubule
10. Proximal tubular cell
11. RBC in capillary
12. Mesangial stalk
13. Efferent arteriole
14. Extraglomerular mesangium
15. Macula densa
16. Distal tubular cell

Fig. 179.8: Juxtaglomerular apparatus

(1) the principal cells and (2) intercalated cells. The principal cells are simple polygonal cells. The intercalated cells are of two types—(1) alpha (type A) and (2) beta (type B) cells. Alpha-cells secrete acid and beta-cells secrete bicarbonate.

The renal interstitium increases in volume progressively from cortex to medulla. The interstitium contains fibroblasts with many lipid droplets especially in the medulla. These are called lipid-laden interstitial cells. They produce prostaglandin and vasodilatory hormones called **medullipin**. The peritubular fibroblasts secrete **erythropoietin (EPO)**. The interstitium also contains dendritic cells, which are of macrophage origin.

The kidney receives about 20% of the cardiac output and each gram of renal tissue receives 3.5–4 mL of blood every minute. Near the renal sinus, the renal artery divides into 6–8 interlobar arteries. At the junction between cortex and medulla, they divide into numerous arcuate arteries, which run along the corticomedullary junction. Interlobular arteries arise perpendicularly from the arcuate artery and traverse the renal cortex. The afferent arterioles arise from the interlobular arteries. The afferent arterioles divide to form the glomerular capillary network and reform as the efferent arterioles. They break up to form the peritubular capillary plexus or vasa recta and ultimately form the interlobular veins, arcuate veins, interlobar veins and renal veins.

FUNCTIONS OF KIDNEY

Kidneys are important in maintaining the internal milieu. Major functions of the kidney include excretion of nitrogenous waste products, maintenance of acid base, electrolyte and water balance. Kidney also functions as an endocrine organ. It produces chemicals which have endocrine and paracrine functions. The formation of urine contributes to the excretory, and cells in the parenchyma, the metabolic functions of the kidney.

The glomeruli filter about 120 mL ultrafiltrate from nearly 1,500 mL of blood every minute. The ultrafiltrate contains all the solutes such as glucose, sodium, potassium, calcium, phosphate, bicarbonate, small molecules such as urea, creatinine, uric acid and amino acids. The ultrafiltrate flows from the Bowman's space through the urinary pole into the PCT. About 60–70% of water and solutes are reabsorbed from PCT. Glucose, bicarbonate, amino acids and phosphate are completely reabsorbed. The proximal tubule is capable of reabsorbing large amounts of fluid. As the fluid reabsorption is iso-osmotic, the concentration of the fluid and osmolality do not change. The proximal tubular cell is also involved in the metabolism and elimination of metabolites like ammonium, drugs and toxic chemicals. The proximal tubule is particularly vulnerable to injury by toxins which reach the tubule in high concentrations either through the tubular fluid or peritubular blood. The tubule cell has to reabsorb or metabolize many substances including drugs and toxins, and is highly vulnerable to chemical injury.

The thin portion of the descending and ascending parts of the loop of Henle are freely permeable to water and urea. Since the medullary interstitium is maintained hyperosmotic (1,100–1,200 mOsm/kg water), there is reabsorption of water and urea from the tubular fluid. Consequently, the osmolality of the tubular fluid progressively increases as the fluid moves down the thin portion, reaching a maximum of approximately 1,200 at the 'U' bend of the loop. The thick ascending limb of loop of Henle is impermeable to water. There is an active chloride pump which helps to remove chloride, and sodium from the tubular fluid into the interstitium. Approximately, 20–25% of the sodium filtered by the glomerulus is reabsorbed in this segment without reabsorption of water. Thus, the tubular fluid leaving this segment is always hypotonic with osmolarity of 50–100 mOsm/kg. So, this segment is also called the ***diluting segment***.

In the distal tubule, reabsorption of sodium in exchange for potassium occurs and is regulated by aldosterone. In the distal tubule, ammonia (NH_3) is converted to ammonium NH_4 by H+ in secreted into the tubule. This segment is permeable to water and the permeability is regulated by the antidiuretic hormone (ADH). ADH completely controls the water reabsorption in the collecting duct. In the presence of ADH, water transport channels called ***aquaporin (two channels)*** are inserted into the tubular cell membrane. Thus, the cell becomes freely permeable to water and reabsorption occurs resulting in formation of smaller volumes of concentrated urine. In the absence of ADH, the aquaporin channels are stored inside the cell and the cell wall becomes impermeable to water. Thus, larger volumes of dilute urine are formed.

The kidney functions as an endocrine organ. It produces hormones with local and systemic effects. The main hormones are:

- Renin-angiotensin
- Metabolites of vitamin D
- EPO (erythropoietin)
- Prostaglandins
- Kallikrein-kinin system.

Angiotensinogen is an alpha-globulin produced by the liver and circulates in the plasma. This is converted by the renin which is released by the modified smooth muscle cells of the afferent arterioles into ***angiotensin I***. This in turn is converted by the angiotensin converting enzyme (ACE) to ***angiotensin II*** which is a powerful vasoconstrictor. It is a trophic hormone for the zona glomerulosa of the adrenal cortex stimulating the release of aldosterone. By selective action of angiotensin II on the smooth muscle cells of the afferent and efferent arterioles, the glomerular filtration can also be regulated by the JGA. This interaction between the tubule and glomerulus is called the ***tubuloglomerular feedback***. The renin-angiotensin system controls the blood pressure and electrolyte balance through the co-ordinated effects on the heart, blood vessels and kidney.

Vitamin D obtained from different sources is converted to 25-hydroxy (25-OH) vitamin D in the liver. This is further converted to 1,25 dihydroxy [1,25 $(OH)_2$] vitamin D in the proximal tubular cells of the kidney. This conversion is under the influence of parathormone which is the rate limiting factor. The most active biological product which acts as a hormone is 1,25 dihydroxy-vitamin D. Renal osteodystrophy may occur in chronic renal disease due to inadequate formation of active vitamin D. Administration of conventional or even high doses of vitamin D may be ineffective in such patients. Administration of 1,25 dihydroxy-vitamin D is therapeutically effective.

EPO is a glycoprotein with a molecular weight of 36,000 produced mainly by the interstitial cells of the kidney and to a lesser extent by the liver. It is secreted in response to hypoxia. It stimulates the proliferation of committed stem cell precursors in the bone marrow and induces differentiation as erythroblasts. Deficiency of EPO causes are generative anemia in chronic renal failure (CRF). Recombinant human EPO is now used for the management of anemia in CRF.

Vasodilator prostaglandins produced in the renal medulla play an important role in autoregulation of renal blood flow. Even in times of hypotension and early shock, they help to maintain glomerular blood flow and filtration. Nonsteroidal anti-inflammatory drugs (NSAIDs) which suppress prostaglandins render the kidney susceptible to hypoperfusion and damage even with mild or transient hypotension. These drugs should be avoided especially in those with compromised renal blood flow and when other nephrotoxic drugs are concurrently used.

The renal kallikrein-kinin system also produces renal vasodilatation and plays important roles in renal hemodynamics and excretory function. They are important in the pathogenesis of essential hypertension. In addition to the primary renal hormones already listed, kidney is also acted upon by other hormones, like parathormone, prolactin, estrogen, progesterone, aldosterone, ADH, growth hormone and several others. Kidney also plays a key role in the metabolism of hormones like insulin.

CHAPTER
180

Clinical Approach: Evaluation and Investigations
Jacob George

Chapter Summary

- Symptomatology in Renal Disease
- Clinical Syndromes in Nephrology
- Investigations in Renal Disease

SYMPTOMATOLOGY IN RENAL DISEASE

An underlying renal disease may be suspected if a patient presents with any of the following symptoms:

- **Oliguria:** The urine output is less than 400 mL/ 24 hours. This is usually seen with renal failure, though some cases of renal failure may be nonoliguric.
- **Anuria:** The urine output is less than 50 mL/ 24 hours and may be seen with severe renal failure, total urinary obstruction, bilateral renal artery occlusion, acute cortical necrosis, rapidly progressive glomerulonephritis (RPGN) and others.
- **Edema** can occur with acute nephritis, nephrotic syndrome or in renal failure. Periorbital edema (Fig. 180.1) is more often seen in renal edema rather than cardiac edema as patients with cardiac failure have orthopnea and hence have more of dependent or pedal edema.
- **Hematuria** can signify a pathology occurring anywhere in the genitourinary tract and may also be due to a urological problem. Cola-colored urine is however more often seen with glomerular diseases. Presence of red blood cell (RBC) casts and dysmorphic RBCs also favor glomerular disease.
- **Anorexia, nausea** and **vomiting** may signify underlying renal failure.
- **Dysuria, frequency** and **urgency** should raise the possibility of a lower urinary tract infection (UTI) irritation by stone.

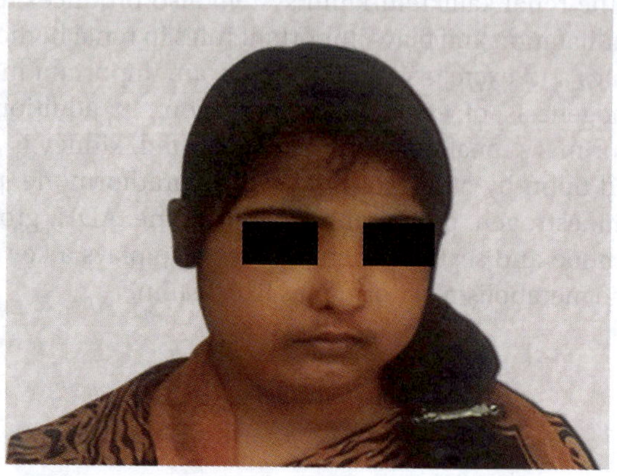

Fig. 180.1: Acute glomerulonephritis—30-year-old woman **Note:** Puffiness of face

- **Nocturia:** Normally, the urine output is more at daytime. In chronic renal failure (CRF), this is altered with patients having to get up more than two times in the night to pass usually large amounts of urine.
- **Polyuria:** This can occur in nephrogenic diabetes mellitus (DM) due to resistance to antidiuretic hormone. This is mainly seen with chronic tubulointerstitial diseases.
- **Frothing of urine:** This may be a sign of proteinuria which reduces the surface tension of urine.
- **Colic:** Stones in the ureter typically produce severe intermittent pain radiating from loin to groin, often associated with nausea and vomiting and this is characteristic of a ureteric colic. A renal calculus usually produces a constant dull ache in the loins and is hence not a typical colic though it is termed as renal colic.

CLINICAL SYNDROMES IN NEPHROLOGY

A constellation of symptoms, signs and abnormal investigation results can constitute a renal syndrome.

The following are some of the syndromes often seen in nephrology practice:

- **Acute nephritic syndrome (acute glomerulonephritis):** This is characterized by varying combinations of edema, hypertension, hematuria and oliguria. Acute postinfectious glomerulonephritis, immunoglobulin A (IgA) nephropathy, lupus nephritis and membranoproliferative nephritis can present with this syndrome.
- **Nephrotic syndrome:** It is associated with massive proteinuria exceeding 3.5 g/1.73 m² surface area, edema, hypoalbuminemia, hypercholesterolemia and lipiduria. Minimal change disease, focal segmental glomerulosclerosis, membranous nephropathy, diabetic nephropathy, amyloidosis and other systemic diseases can present with this syndrome (Fig. 180.2).
- **Rapidly progressive glomerulonephritis:** There is a doubling of serum creatinine within a period of weeks to months with associated glomerular hematuria or RBC casts in urine. Postinfectious glomerulonephritis, Goodpasture syndrome, lupus nephritis and vasculitis can present with this syndrome.
- **Acute kidney injury (formerly termed acute renal failure):** It is characterized by a rapid fall in glomerular filtration rate (GFR) with accumulation of nitrogenous waste products and can be seen in prerenal, renal and obstructive causes.
- **Chronic renal failure (CRF):** It is associated with a gradual but often progressive decline in GFR of

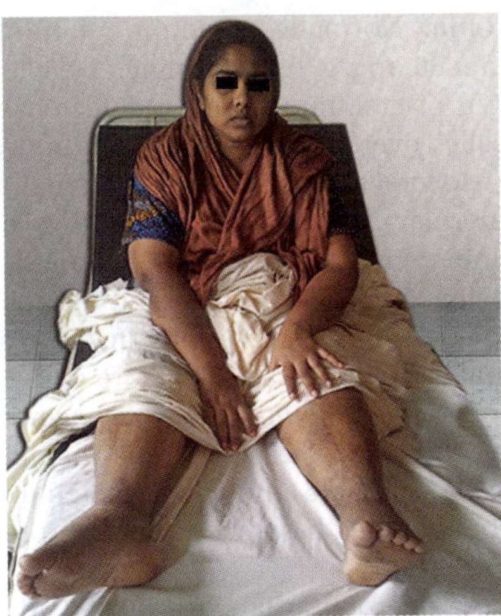

Fig. 180.2: Lady with nephrotic syndrome

more than 3 months. There can be various signs and symptoms in this disorder which are however individually nonspecific, so that several of these patients can present to various other specialties of medicine. The term chronic kidney disease (CKD) is used to represent chronic involvement of kidney with structural or functional abnormalities of clinical significance lasting for over 3 months. Though the term CKD is presently more used than CRF, they are not synonymous and CKD is not a syndromic diagnosis as not all patients with CKD are symptomatic with a low GFR.

- Other syndromes include *UTI, urinary tract obstruction, nephrolithiasis, hypertension,* renal tubular disorders, etc. which are covered in detail in the subsequent chapters.

INVESTIGATIONS IN RENAL DISEASES

They are intended to diagnose the type of renal involvement, quantify the severity, identify the underlying etiology, plan management strategies as well as predict the outcome. Investigations start with routine urinalysis and more sophisticated tests are done if needed.

Urine Examination

This is the most rewarding investigation in renal disease. It is essential, therefore, that the clinician familiarizes himself with all the tests and their critical interpretation. Fresh urine collected directly in a clean container is examined macroscopically and is subjected to biochemical and other tests. The centrifuged deposit is examined under the microscope. Gram-staining of the deposit, cytology and urine culture is undertaken depending on the indication.

The first voided sample in the morning is usually preferred for routine test. For estimating urinary loss of proteins, electrolytes and for calculating creatinine clearance, 24-hour urine is collected in appropriate containers with preservative. If collection and transport of the 24-hour urine sample is difficult, timed samples for 4, 6 or 12 hours is collected. In females, labia are separated and in males, prepuce is retracted to ensure a clean catch specimen. For microbiological culture, a midstream specimen of urine is collected directly into the culture bottle after cleaning the genitalia with water. Since this procedure may not always be practical in children, suprapubic aspiration of bladder may be necessary to get an uncontaminated sample.

Urine sample for culture should not be taken from an indwelling catheter since false results will be obtained due to micro-organisms in the biofilm in the catheter.

A detailed urinalysis includes numerous tests from which the appropriate ones are chosen.

- *Volume:* This is determined by accurate 24-hour urine collection.
- *Color:* Normal urine is amber colored. The color can vary widely in normal persons depending on the concentration or dilution of urine. Presence of substances like bilirubin, blood, drugs, dyes or other coloring agents impart different colors. Common causes for altered colors of urine are listed in Table 180.1.
- *Odor:* Normally, freshly passed urine is odorless. On standing, a pungent ammoniacal odor develops due to splitting of urea to ammonia. In UTIs, even freshly passed urine may be foul smelling. Excretion of substances such as metabolites or other malodorous substances may impart characteristic smells to the urine, e.g. fruity odor of acetone.
- *Turbidity:* Turbid urine may occur in pyuria, chyluria or hematuria. Amorphous phosphate may precipitate on standing and lead to turbidity, which disappears on adding acetic acid. Chyluria has a milky appearance due to fat droplets which clears on addition of ether or chloroform. In pyuria, centrifugation of the urine leaves the supernatant clear.
- *Reaction/pH:* The pH of urine ranges from 4.5 to 8.0. Strongly alkaline urine may denote infection with urea splitting organisms such as *Proteus* or renal tubular acidosis. Estimation of the pH of urine is important in the diagnosis and management of UTIs, renal calculi and others.

Table 180.1: Common causes for altered colors of urine	
Straw yellow	Normal
Deep yellow	Concentrated urine
	Jaundice
Red urine	Hematuria
	Hemoglobinuria
	Myoglobinuria
	Porphyria
	Beet root ingestion
	Drugs—rifampicin, pyridium
Cloudy	Infection
Milky	Chyluria
	Pyuria
	Phosphaturia
Dark on standing	Porphyria
	Alkaptonuria

- ***Specific gravity and osmolality:*** These are indirect indicators of the solute content of urine. Normal specific gravity of urine may vary from 1,002 to 1,030. Specific gravity increases during water deprivation, presence of excessive solutes, excessive fluid losses, and in some cases of acute glomerulonephritis. Increase in specific gravity may occur due to presence of glucose, proteins or radiographic contrast dyes in urine. Specific gravity is low in the diuretic phase of acute tubular necrosis, diabetes insipidus (DI), during clearance of edema and in normal subjects after large volume fluid intake. In chronic glomerulonephritis, where the tubules lose their capacity to concentrate and dilute the urine, the specific gravity becomes fixed around 1,010 (isosthenuria). This is approximately the specific gravity of protein free plasma. Osmolality indicates the amount of osmotically active particles and it is expressed as mOsm/kg. Normal urine osmolality can vary from 50 to 1,200 mOsm/kg.

- ***Water deprivation test:*** This assesses the concentrating capacity of the kidney and is employed in polyuric states. On withholding fluids for a period of 6–8 hours normally the hourly urine output falls and the kidneys produce concentrated urine with a specific gravity of 1,022 or more. In DI, the concentrating power of the kidney is lost and therefore large volumes of dilute urine with specific gravity less than 1,004 are passed. If the DI is due to reduced production of vasopressin (central DI), injection of vasopressin will correct the urine volume and concentration. In nephrogenic DI, where the renal tubules are unresponsive to vasopressin, this does not happen.

- ***Water loading test:*** This tests has diluting ability and is rarely done in clinical practice. The patient is given 1 L of water to drink within 20 minutes. A normal person excretes 80% of this water within 4 hours and the specific gravity of at least one sample should be around 1,002. A normal test suggests that the ability of the kidney to dilute the urine is preserved. Apart from primary renal disorders which impair the excretory capacity of the kidney, deficiency of glucocorticoids (Addison's disease) leads to impairment of diluting function.

- ***Proteinuria and albuminuria:*** They are not synonymous terms. Normally, urine may contain up to 150 mg proteins in 24 hours. In health, two-thirds of the urinary proteins are constituted by protein of tubular origin, particularly the Tamm-Horsfall mucoprotein. This protein is secreted into the tubular lumen by the distal tubular cells and it forms the basic ingredient of urinary casts. Proteins derived from plasma namely albumin, immunoglobulins (Igs), light chains and beta-2 microglobulin constitute the remaining third. Albumin may constitute only up to 10 mg in 24 hours. Such small amounts of albumin are not detectable by the usual side room tests. Specific dipstick tests or radioimmunoassays (RIA) are needed for detecting albumin in such small quantities. Calculation of albumin creatinine ratio is a cheaper and more readily done method to get an idea about the elimination of albumin. Normally, albumin/creatinine ratio is less than 30 mg/g of creatinine. Levels exceeding 300 mg/g of creatinine can be detected by dipstick and is called overt albuminuria. Levels between 30 and 300 mg/g of creatinine are termed microalbuminuria.

In glomerular diseases, the proportion of albumin lost in urine increases. In addition, small quantities of lipoproteins may also be present. Proteinuria may result from renal disorders, lesions in the urinary tract or extra renal causes like cardiac failure and fever. Gross proteinuria associated with the presence of casts is invariably due to renal disease. Presence of blood in urine gives rise to considerable amounts of protein in urine and this has to be excluded before attributing proteinuria to a primary renal lesion.

Selectivity of proteinuria can be used to assess the extent of glomerular damage and predict response to drugs such as corticosteroids in diseases like nephrotic syndrome. The ratio of immunoglobulin G (IgG) excretion to albumin forms the basis for identifying selectivity. In highly selective proteinuria, more of albumin and less of IgG are excreted, suggesting milder glomerular damage and good response to steroids. If the proportion of IgG is high, it suggests greater damage and poorer therapeutic response. A globulin albumin ratio of less than 0.1% suggests highly selective proteinuria. Gross proteinuria, above 3.5 g in 24 hours or 2 g/m^2 body surface occurs in nephrotic syndrome. Serial quantitative estimation of urinary proteins helps to monitor the progress of nephrotic syndrome and other renal diseases. Proteinuria can be assessed from a spot urine sample by estimating the protein-creatinine ratio. A value of 3.5:1 indicates a 24-hour urinary protein of 3.5 g. Estimation of this ratio is useful in children and in situations where an accurate 24-hour urine collection is difficult. In about 50% patients with multiple myeloma, light chains of immunoglobulins called Bence-Jones protein are detected in urine. These may also be seen in other conditions like macroglobulinemia, amyloidosis, lymphoma, leukemia, and other malignancies. The dipstix test does not detect Bence-Jones protein. Immunoelectrophoresis of urine is the ideal method to detect and quantify Bence-Jones protein.

Several terms are used to denote specific types of proteinuria.

- ***Fixed proteinuria:*** Greater than 1 g/24 hours mostly of glomerular origin and mainly albumin.
- ***Tubular proteinuria:*** Less than 1 g/24 hours mostly proteins other than albumin.
- ***Overflow proteinuria:*** Light chains of myeloma.
- ***Orthostatic proteinuria:*** This occurs only when the patient assumes erect posture.
- ***Physiological proteinuria (transient proteinuria):*** This may occur transiently even in normal persons after heavy exertion.

  Among the pathological proteinurias, approximately two-thirds is of glomerular origin and one-third is of tubular origin.

- ***Reducing substances:*** Presence of glucose in urine often suggests a diagnosis of DM. Rarely, glucose may appear in urine in the presence of normal blood sugar and this occurs in renal glycosuria. Glucose oxidase test is specific for glucose and can be used in test stripes for rapid detection of glucose.

- ***Other biochemical tests:*** Specific tests are available for detection of ketone bodies, bile pigments, bile salts, urobilinogen and others. Other tests which are occasionally employed include urinary electrolytes, urea, creatinine, uric acid, calcium, amino acids, phosphates, oxalate, metabolites of hormones, drugs or toxic substances.
- ***Microscopic examination:*** This is done to study the formed elements consisting of various cells, casts, crystals, lipid droplets, microorganisms and parasites. The cells are derived from blood or may be acquired from any part of the urinary tract (Figs 180.3 to 180.6).
  - ***Erythrocytes:*** Presence of more than two erythrocytes in every high power field should suggest microscopic hematuria. Gross hematuria occurs in acute glomerulonephritis, infections, tumors, renal infarction, ulceration in the urinary tract, bleeding disorders and others.
  - ***Leukocytes:*** Neutrophils constitute the majority. They are numerous in UTIs, urologic disorders and in patients with interstitial nephritis. Lymphocytes may appear in urine in smaller numbers. Eosinophils also may occur particularly in acute interstitial nephritis or atheroembolic renal diseases.
  - ***Renal tubular cells:*** These can be differentiated from leukocytes only by transmission electron microscopy.
  - ***Urothelial cells:*** These may be present in small numbers. The cells are derived from the urinary tract. Excessive number of vaginal squamous cells should suggest contamination during collection of urine.
  - Cancer cells from malignancy of the urinary tract or renal carcinoma can be identified by special stains
  - ***Casts:*** Casts are elongated and cylindrical-shaped molds formed in the lumen of the distal tubules where aggregation and gel formation of Tamm-Horsfall glycoprotein occurs. The casts may be hyaline, granular or cellular. ***Hyaline casts*** contain mainly Tamm-Horsfall protein and they may be seen even in normal urine. They have low refractive index and hence they are visible under dim lighting. ***Granular casts*** contain either fine

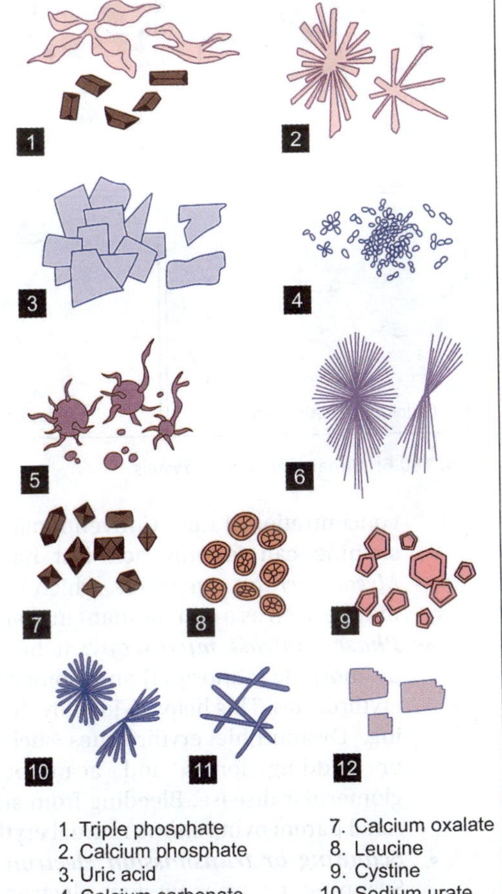

1. Triple phosphate
2. Calcium phosphate
3. Uric acid
4. Calcium carbonate
5. Ammonium urate
6. Tyrosine
7. Calcium oxalate
8. Leucine
9. Cystine
10. Sodium urate
11. Hippuric acid
12. Cholesterol

1. Hyaline cast with white cell inclusion
2. Epithelial cell cast
3. 4. 5. Urinary tract epithelial cells
6. Mucus threads
7. Cylindroids
8. Bacterial cast
9. Granular cast
10. Hyaline cast
11. Waxy cast
12. RBC cast
13. Spermatozoa

Fig. 180.3: Urinary sediments

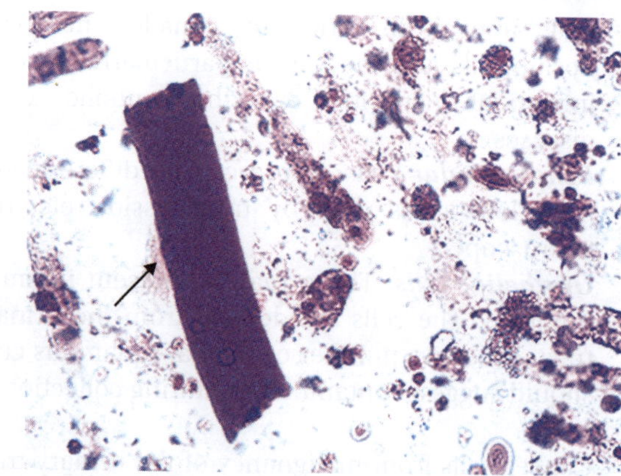

Fig. 180.4: Waxy cast

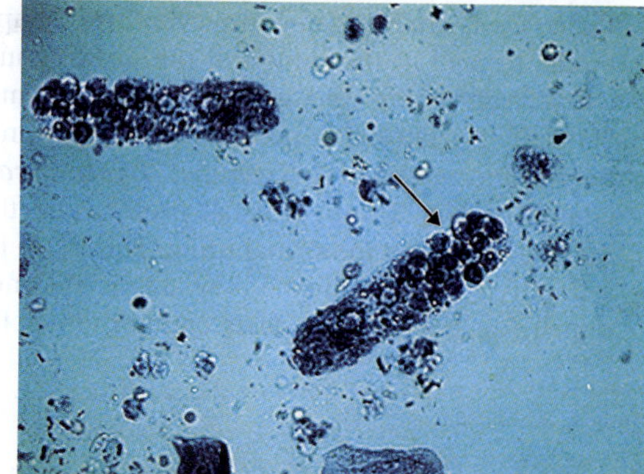

Fig. 180.5: White blood cell cast

Table 180.2:	Clinical significance of urinary casts
Cast	**Clinical significance**
Hyaline	Nonspecific. Present in normal urine
Waxy	Advanced renal failure
RBC	Proliferative glomerulonephritis (GMN)
WBC	Proliferative GMN Interstitial nephritis
Granular	Nephritis with tubular injury
Fatty	Nephrotic syndrome Fabry's disease Other nephritides
Mixed (telescoped)	Proliferative GMN (systemic lupus erythematosus, polyarteritis nodosa)
Bacterial	Bacterial pyelonephritis
Epithelial cell	Acute tubular injury Glomerulonephritis Interstitial nephritis Transplant rejection
Broad	Progressive renal failure with compensatory hypertrophy of nephrons

Abbreviations: RBC = Red blood cell; WBC = White blood cell

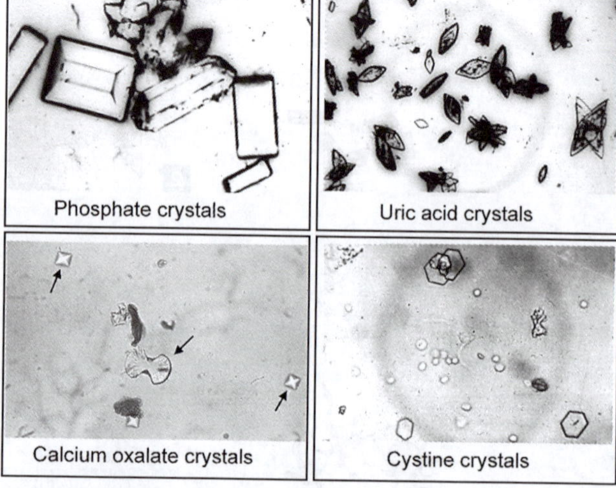

Fig. 180.6: Urinary sediments crystals

or coarse granule like substances. These granules may represent ultrafiltered protein or degenerating cells. Normal urine may show only a few fine granular casts. **Waxy casts** are large and refractile with clean-cut edges (Fig. 180.4). **Broad casts** are formed in the dilated tubules of the surviving hypertrophied nephrons in CKD. **Fatty casts** contain lipids and are characteristic of nephrotic syndrome. **Pigment casts** may contain hemoglobin, myoglobin, bilirubin or other pigments. **Cellular casts** may contain erythrocytes, leukocytes, and renal epithelium in varying numbers.

The significance of urinary casts is shown in Table 180.2.

- **Crystals:** Various types of crystals are seen in the urine and can be identified by their characteristic morphology (Fig. 180.6). Normal urine may contain several crystals depending on the concentration and pH. Under abnormal conditions such as gout, oxaluria and urolithiasis, specific crystals may be present in large numbers and may even suggest the diagnosis. Presence of cystine, leucine, isoleucine and other amino acid crystals occurs in metabolic diseases and in hepatic failure. These are always pathological.

- **Gram-staining and acid-fast staining:** Gram-staining and acid-fast staining are done with centrifuged deposit of fresh urine. If there is likely to be delay in transport to the laboratory, the urine should be preserved with boric acid to give a final concentration of 1.8%. Conventional Ziehl-Neelsen staining can identify acid-fast bacilli in urine. *Mycobacterium smegmatis*, which is also acid-fast may be seen as a contaminant in males.

- **Phase contrast microscopy:** It helps to identify dysmorphic (abnormal) and isomorphic (normal) erythrocytes. This helps to identify the site of bleeding. Dysmorphic erythrocytes such as crenated or budding forms and acanthocytes suggest glomerular disease. Bleeding from sites below the renal parenchyma shows normal erythrocytes.

- **Scanning or transmission electron microscopy:** Scanning or transmission electron microscopy can be used to distinguish between leukocytes and tubular epithelial cells in the urine sediment.

- **Culture:** A clean catch midstream specimen of urine is generally satisfactory for microbiological examination. Urinary catheterization should not be routinely performed for this purpose due to risk of introducing infection. Urine collected from a long standing indwelling catheter for culture is not reliable since the organisms that are present in the biofilm from such a catheter may be grown as contaminants. If the patient has an indwelling catheter for a long time, the catheter may be changed and sample for culture is taken immediately from the new catheter. In addition to routine culture, quantitative determination of the colony count helps to decide whether the organisms exist as contaminant or as active invaders. Bacterial count below 10^4 colony forming units (CFU) per mL of urine is suggestive of contaminants whereas those above 10^5/CFU/mL suggest active infection. For doing colony counts and to facilitate culture, dipsticks coated with the culture media are available commercially. These can be directly inoculated by immersion to the urine and incubated straight away.

- *Hematological tests:* Hemoglobin and packed cell volumes (PCVs) are often low in patients with chronic renal disease. Patients with nephrotic syndrome who develop contraction of plasma volume may have high hemoglobin and PCV. Polymorphonuclear leukocytosis occurs when there is acute infection. High erythrocyte sedimentation rate (ESR) often above 100 mm should suggest the possibility of lupus erythematosus, other forms of collagen disorders, renal tuberculosis or myeloma. In CRF, the erythrocytes are normocytic and normochromic. This is due to deficiency of erythropoietin. In addition to this mechanism, several other factors may also contribute to the development of anemia.

Biochemical Tests

Investigations of the blood and urine are necessary to assess the renal function. These tests also help to assess the functions of the different parts of the nephron.

- *Blood urea or blood urea nitrogen:* Urea is the principal end product of nitrogen metabolism. It is excreted by the kidney and it accounts for 50% of total urinary solutes. Amount of urinary urea is primarily determined by dietary protein intake and it depends upon the amount of urinary flow. Urea is filtered, reabsorbed and secreted by the tubule. Normal blood urea is 20–40 mg/dL and blood urea nitrogen (BUN) is 10–20 mg/dL. BUN is approximately 50% the value of blood urea. Blood urea or BUN gives an approximate estimate of the GFR. In addition to changes in GFR, several other factors like the state of hydration, urine flow rate and protein intake alter the serum levels of blood urea or BUN. Hence, blood urea level or BUN is a less reliable parameter for assessment of GFR compared to creatinine.
- *Serum creatinine and creatinine clearance:* Creatinine is the end product of muscle breakdown and is normally excreted by the kidney. The normal level of serum creatinine is 0.8–1.3 mg/dL (70–113 μmol/L). Creatinine is filtered by the glomerulus and is not reabsorbed from or secreted into tubular lumen in large amounts. Therefore, for all practical purposes, the clearance of creatinine closely reflects the GFR.

The normal creatinine clearance is 115 ± 15 mL/min. The clearance of a substance is the amount of plasma that is completely cleared of the substance in unit time and can be calculated from the formula:

$$C = \frac{UV}{P} \ mL/min$$

where,

C = Clearance of the substance in mL/min,
U = Concentration of the substance in the urine (mg/mL)
V = Volume of urine formed (mL/min)
P = Concentration of the substance in plasma at that time (mg/mL)

Given the 24-hour urinary creatinine in mg/day and serum creatinine in mg/dL, the clearance can be calculated at the bedside as follows:

$$\text{Creatinine clearance} = \frac{\text{24-hour urinary creatinine (mg/day)}}{\text{Serum creatinine (mg\%)}} \times \frac{5}{72}$$

(This is derived from the formula: Clearance = UV/P)

Example: If 24-hour urinary creatinine is 1,200 mg and serum creatinine is 1.0 mg/dL, then

$$\text{Creatinine clearance} = \frac{1200}{1} \times \frac{5}{72} = 83.33 \ mL/min$$

The creatinine clearance reduces with age even though the serum creatinine levels remain within normal range. This is due to the reduction in muscle mass which occurs with age. It is possible to calculate the creatinine clearance from serum creatinine, age and body weight using the following formula *(Cockcroft-Gault formula)*:

$$\text{Cockcroft-Gault formula} = \frac{[140 - \text{age (in years)}] \times \text{body weight (kg)}}{\text{Serum creatinine (mg\%)}} \ \text{(males)}$$

Note: For females, multiply the value obtained for male by 0.85.

This formula helps to calculate the approximate creatinine clearance at the bed side, particularly for adjusting drug dosages. There is a fixed relationship between serum creatinine and creatinine clearance in the same person. When the creatinine clearance falls to 50%, the serum creatinine doubles. Therefore, serial estimations of serum creatinine can give an approximate idea about creatinine clearance. For example, if the creatinine clearance is 120 mL/minute and the serum creatinine is 1.2 mg/dL, when the creatinine clearance comes down respectively to 60 mL/min, 30 mL/min and 15 mL/min the corresponding values of serum creatinine would be 2.4, 4.8 and 9.6 mg/dL in the same patient. Therefore, if the relationship between serum creatinine levels and the corresponding creatinine clearance is known, it will be possible to estimate the creatinine clearance by serial monitoring of serum creatinine alone.

- *Cystatin C:* This is an endogenous substance produced at a constant rate by all nucleated cells and is removed only by glomerular filtration. It is possible to estimate the GFR by measuring cystatin C blood level. This test eliminates the need for 24-hour urine collection.
- *Serum electrolytes:* Estimation of serum sodium, potassium, bicarbonate and pH helps to assess acid-base status and renal function.

- **Serum cholesterol** and lipids are elevated in some types of nephrotic syndrome and in CRF.
- **Uric acid:** Hyperuricemia may be the cause or result of renal failure. High serum uric acid level can itself produce renal damage. In renal failure caused by hyperuricemia, the excretion of uric acid (spot sample) exceeds that of creatinine.
- **Serum calcium:** Serum calcium levels are low in CRF. Secondary hyperparathyroidism may cause bone changes. In advanced cases, tertiary hyperparathyroidism may develop, resulting in elevation of serum calcium and metastatic calcification. Serum phosphorus levels are increased in acute and CRF.

Radiological Investigations

- **Plain X-ray of the abdomen** to include kidney, ureter, bladder and urethra taken after suitable bowel preparation gives a good picture of the kidney and urinary tract. For getting a good skiagram, it is better to ensure proper bowel movement, if necessary by giving antiflatulents like activated carbon and laxative for the previous 2 days and asking the patient to be ambulant so as to avoid excess of gas in the intestines.

  Abnormalities of size, presence of calculi and calcification can be seen (Fig. 180.7). The bipolar length of the normal kidney is about the width of 3½ lumbar vertebrae. The left is about 1 cm longer and is situated higher than the right. In health, the two kidneys do not differ in length by more than 2 cm. An atrophic kidney may be smaller than its normal counterpart. Tumors may lead to enlargement. In addition, bone changes occurring in the spine and pelvis can be seen. Tumors of the kidney may give rise to larger renal shadows. Hydronephrosis and polycystic kidney, though palpable as abdominal masses, may not be seen in the plain X-ray picture. Larger tumors, polycystic kidneys and hydronephrosis may give indirect evidences of their presence such as the displacement of gas-filled bowel.

- **Ultrasonography (USG):** This has become the most popular and easily available imaging procedure for the preliminary assessment of the excretory organs. This is an investigation of choice for assessing renal size and the presence of obstruction, tumor, cysts, and calculi.

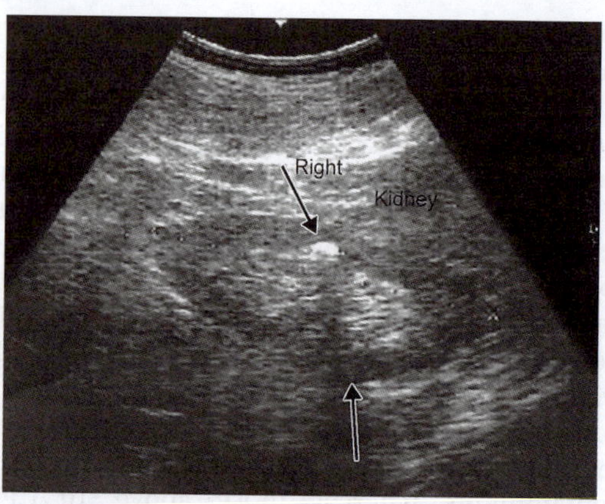

Fig. 180.8: Ultrasonogram showing stone in renal pelvis (arrow). **Note:** The acoustic shadow due to the stone (arrowhead)

Moreover, ultrasonography being noninvasive is used more and more extensively. Ultrasonography is not useful for assessing renal function (Fig. 180.8).

- **Intravenous urography (IVU):** It helps to assess the renal structure, anatomy of the collecting system and function by using radiocontrast agents, which contain iodine. These agents are selectively concentrated and excreted by the kidneys. Originally, hyperosmolar agents like meglumine and iothalamate were used. At present safer and nonionic low osmolar agents like, iohexol, iopamidol and ioxaglate are used. They produce adverse side effects only infrequently. Hypersensitivity to iodine is an absolute contraindication for IVU. Risk of renal failure is high in impaired renal function, multiple myeloma with proteinuria, diabetic nephropathy and concurrent use of other nephrotoxic agents. The risk of contrast nephrotoxicity can be reduced by good hydration with intravenous saline and agents like N-acetyl cysteine (Fig. 180.9).

A plain X-ray of the abdomen is taken for comparison. Then films are taken at 5, 10, 20 and 30 minutes after administration of the contrast agent intravenously (IV) and a final picture after complete micturition.

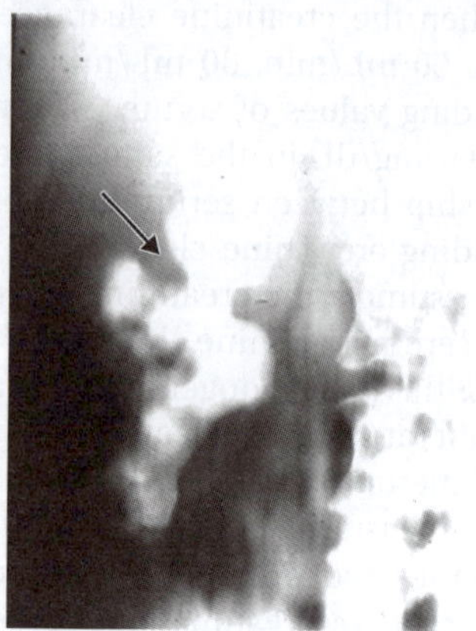

Fig. 180.7: Plain X-ray abdomen—right renal area showing branched radio-opaque staghorn calculus (arrow)

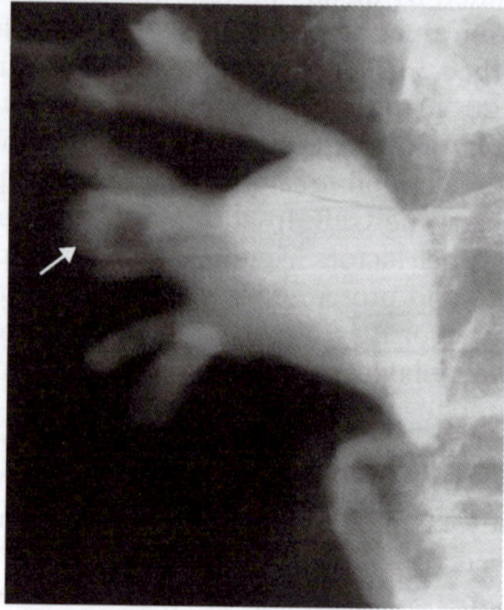

Fig. 180.9: Intravenous urogram showing right renal area with sloughed papilla appearing as a rounded shadow in the middle calyx—arrow (from a case of analgesic nephropathy)

Points to be noted on the IVU are summarized below:

- **Time of initial visualization of the renal outlines.** This depends upon renal circulation and glomerular filtration.
- **Time for maximum opacification of kidneys and visualization of pelvicalyceal system.** This depends upon the excretory function of the kidneys.
- **Size, shape and presence of negative contrast** (stones, tumors, clots) in the pelvicalyceal system.
- **Flow of the dye along the ureters,** their size and presence of obstruction.
- **Time taken for the renal and pelvicalyceal shadow to disappear.** This is usually complete within 20–30 minutes and this gives an idea about the efficacy of the drainage system, as well as vascularity of the kidneys.
- **Size and shape of the bladder,** presence of filling defects caused by calculi, tumors or enlarged prostate and completeness of bladder emptying, as is seen in the postmicturition film.

Several modifications of the IVU have been devised. These include the following:

- **Minute sequence pictures:** When pictures are taken every minute for the first 5 minutes, delay in appearance of nephrogram on one side, decrease the size of the kidney, higher concentration of the contrast in the collecting system and delayed drainage on the same side are all suggestive of unilateral renal artery stenosis.
- **Diuretic urogram:** Diuretic urogram is performed by administration of a diuretic in cases with upper ureteric ballooning or obstruction to confirm or rule out obstruction. A functional obstruction of the pelviureteric junction is relieved by the use of diuretic whereas the ballooning persists if there is a mechanical block.
- **Infusion urogram:** Infusion urogram is undertaken in the presence of renal failure and delayed pictures are taken at intervals of 6 hours up to even 96 hours to delineate the urinary tract in some cases of obstructive uropathy.
- **Retrograde pyelography:** Retrograde pyelography is the procedure by which the ureter is catheterized and the pelvicalyceal system is visualized by direct instillation of radiographic agent.
- **Cystourethrography:** Cystourethrography helps in studying the bladder, urethra, and vesicoureteric junction.
- **Micturating cystogram:** X-ray is taken while the patient passes urine after introducing radiopaque contrast into the bladder. This helps to visualize the urethra, identify lesions such as posterior urethral valve or other obstructions and to establish the presence of vesicoureteric reflux (Figs 180.10A and B).
- **Aortography:** Aortography performed by injecting dye into the aorta delineates clearly the aorta, renal arteries and the renal vascular pattern. Selective angiography can be done after catheterizing the renal arteries. Renal venograms can be obtained by injecting the dye into the renal veins (Fig. 180.11).
- **Isotope renography:** Isotope renography helps to assess renal perfusion and excretory function. It is

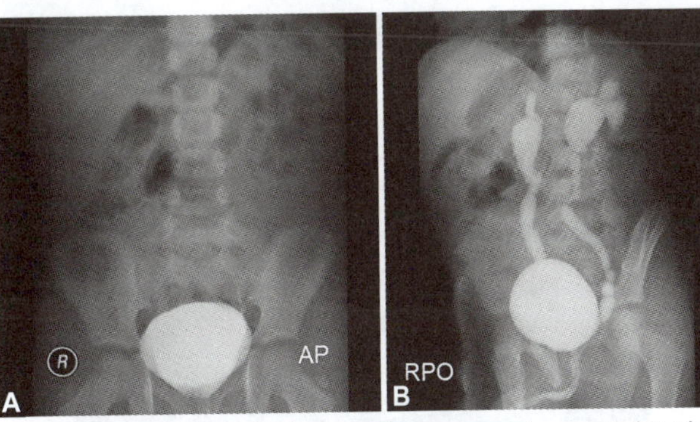

Figs 180.10A and B: A. Cystourethrogram—anteroposterior view showing bladder filled with dye before patient tries to pass urine. Note that there is no filling of the ureters; **B.** Oblique view of the same case when the patient (child) is passing urine. **Note:** Flow of urine through the urethra and simultaneous filling of both ureters and the dilated renal pelvis and calyces (grade V vesicoureteric reflux)

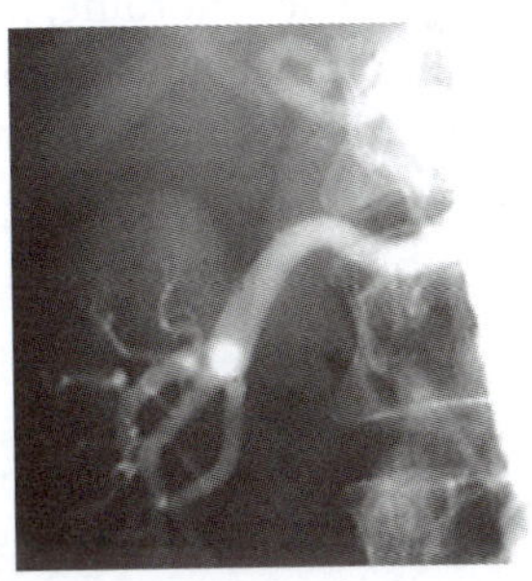
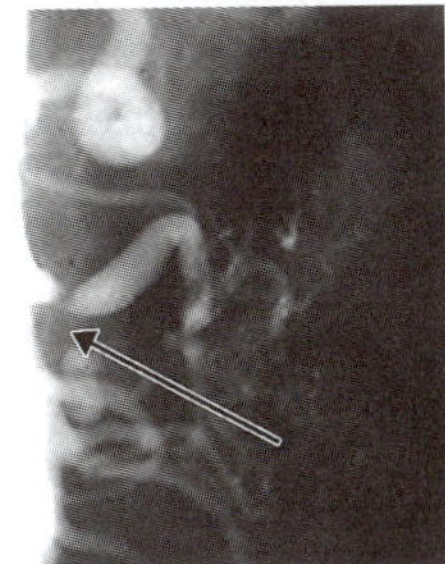

Fig. 180.11: Abdominal aortogram showing aorta and both renal arteries. Note the narrowing of proximal left renal artery (arrow) and poststenotic dilatation

particularly useful to diagnose renovascular hypertension, assess individual kidney function, renal scarring and to confirm pelviureteric junction obstruction. The radiopharmaceutical agents include technetium labeled diethylene triamine pentaacetic acid. Diuretic renogram is performed after administering frusemide helps to differentiate between organic and functional ureteric obstruction. The functional obstruction clears after diuretic. Captopril renogram is performed after administration of 12.5 mg captopril orally and it helps to identify renal artery stenosis. The radiopharmaceutical dimercaptosuccinic acid is concentrated in the renal parenchyma and it is used to identify scars in the parenchyma.

- **Computed tomography scan:** Computed tomography (CT) scan helps to delineate the structural and morphological abnormalities in the kidney, details of tumor, and the relationship to other organs. In the vast majority of cases, CT scan will give adequate information (Fig. 180.12).
- **Magnetic resonance imaging (MRI):** It is employed at times. The advantages are a clear delineation of the corticomedullary junction and better visualization of the renal artery, vein and inferior vena cava.

Renal Biopsy

Renal tissue can be obtained by closed needle biopsy. The tissue is processed for histology, microbiological studies, electron microscopy and for immunofluorescence microscopy. Histological diagnosis is necessary for determining

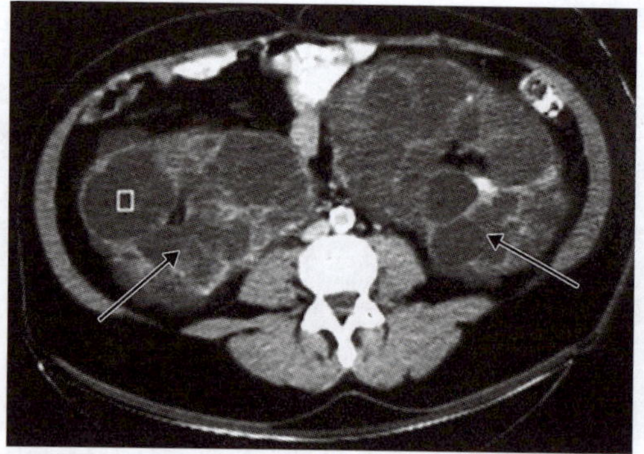

Fig. 180.12: Computed tomography (CT) scan showing bilateral enlarged kidneys due to numerous cysts of varying sizes in both kidneys (arrows) (autosomal dominant polycystic kidney disease)

the management and prognosis of several renal disorders like acute glomerulonephritis, nephrotic syndrome, lupus erythematosus, amyloidosis, and transplant rejection. Since clinical pattern of several different pathological entities may be similar, the ultimate diagnosis in many diseases has to rest on renal biopsy.

Serological Tests

These have to be done in selected cases depending on the clinical picture to confirm the diagnosis. These include antinuclear antibody, antibody to double stranded DNA, antistreptolysin O titer, complement (C3 and C4) levels, antineutrophil cytoplasmic antibodies [perinuclear anti-neutrophil cytoplasmic antibodies (pANCA) and cyto-plasmic antineutrophil cytoplasmic antibodies (cANCA)], antiglomerular basement membrane antibodies, screening for hepatitis viruses especially hepatitis C, hepatitis B (HCV and HBV) and human immunodeficiency virus (HIV).

Urologic Investigations

Urological investigations such as cystourethroscopy help to visualize the urinary tract and enable endoscopic procedures.

Glomerulonephritis
Acute Nephritic Syndrome and Nephrotic Syndrome

Jacob George, Noble Gracious

Chapter Summary

- Introduction to Glomerular Diseases
- Poststreptococcal Glomerulonephritis
- Immunoglobulin A Nephropathy
- Rapidly Progressive Glomerulonephritis
- Lupus Nephritis (LN)
- Pauci-immune Crescentic GN
- Minimal Change Disease (MCD)
- Focal Segmental Glomerulosclerosis (FSGS)
- Membranous Nephropathy
- Membranoproliferative Glomerulonephritis

INTRODUCTION TO GLOMERULAR DISEASES

Glomerular diseases have clinical presentations that may vary from asymptomatic to fulminant illness with acute kidney injury (AKI). The common ways in which glomerular diseases present are shown in Table 181.1.

Asymptomatic Microscopic Hematuria

Microscopic hematuria is defined as the presence of more than two red blood cells (RBCs) per high-power field

Table 181.1: Clinical presentations of glomerular diseases

- Asymptomatic
- Macroscopic hematuria
- Nephrotic syndrome
- Nephritic syndrome
- Rapidly progressive glomerulonephritis (RPGN)
- Chronic glomerulonephritis

(HPF) in a spun urine sediment (3,000 rpm for 5 minutes) or more than 10×10^6 RBCs/L. It is seen in many glomerular diseases, especially immunoglobulin A (IgA) nephropathy and thin basement membrane nephropathy. A glomerular origin should be considered, if more than 5% of the red cells are acanthocytes or if the hematuria is accompanied by red cell casts or proteinuria (Fig. 181.1).

Asymptomatic Non-nephrotic Proteinuria

Urinary protein excretion is less than 150 mg/24 hours in normal persons. Increased urine protein excretion may result from alterations in glomerular permeability or tubulointerstitial disease. Proteinuria can be detected and quantified by dipstick testing or by assay in timed urine collection.

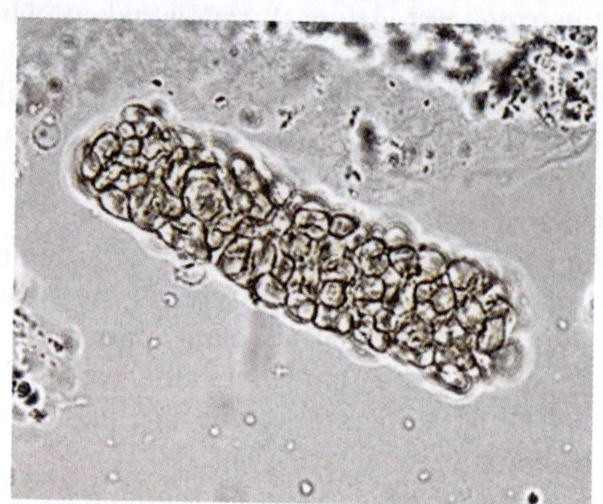

Fig. 181.1: RBC cast seen on urine microscopy

Microalbuminuria

It is defined as the excretion of 30–300 mg of albumin/day, equivalent to urine albumin to creatinine ratio expressed in g/day of 0.03–0.3. It is detected by quantitative immunoassay or by special urine dipsticks. Any protein excretion of more than 300 mg/day is called *significant proteinuria*. If it is between 300 and 3500 mg in 24 hours, it is called non-nephrotic range of proteinuria. Tubulointerstitial diseases may be associated with proteinuria, usually non-nephrotic (<2 g/day). Urine protein excretion exceeds 3.5 g/24 hours only in glomerular diseases and this is called nephrotic range of proteinuria.

Overflow Proteinuria

In this, the blood level of the concerned protein is very high resulting in increased filtration through normal glomeruli. This may occur commonly in paraproteinemias (e.g. multiple myeloma) where there is increased excretion of urinary light-chains.

Tubular Proteinuria

In tubular diseases, low molecular weight proteins [e.g. beta-2-microglobulin (B2M)] are excreted in the urine due to decreased reabsorption resulting in protein loss of less than 2 g/day.

Glomerular Proteinuria

The type of protein lost in urine in glomerular proteinuria is mainly albumin.

Functional Proteinuria

It refers to the transient non-nephrotic proteinuria that can occur with fever exercise, heart failure and hyperadrenergic or hyper-reninemic states.

Orthostatic Proteinuria

In children and young adults, low-grade glomerular proteinuria may be orthostatic, it means that proteinuria is absent when urine is generated in the recumbent position. Total urine protein in orthostatic proteinuria is usually less than 1 g/24 hours.

Fixed Non-nephrotic Proteinuria

It is usually caused by glomerular disease. Renal biopsy is usually done in patients with suspected glomerular disease, if proteinuria exceeds 1 g/day. Renal biopsy is indicated even if urine protein is only 0.5 to 1 g/24 hours, if there is also persistent microscopic hematuria with casts.

Macroscopic Hematuria

It is associated with glomerular disease, is often episodic, painless, brown or smoky rather than red urine and not associated with clots. It must be distinguished from other causes of red or brown urine including hemoglobinuria, myoglobinuria, porphyrias, consumption of food dyes (beetroot) and intake of drugs (in particular rifampin). Macroscopic hematuria caused by glomerular disease is observed primarily in children and young adults. Most cases are caused by IgA nephropathy or infection-related glomerulonephritis (GN). Occasionally, hematuria may occur with other glomerular and nonglomerular renal diseases, including acute interstitial nephritis and in several nonrenal causes like trauma, malignancy, tuberculosis, etc. If macroscopic hematuria occurs in association with pain and/or passage of blood clots, a urological cause such as urinary stones or infection should be looked for.

Nephrotic Syndrome

This is characterized by relatively gradual onset of edema, often severe enough to produce anasarca and associated with massive proteinuria (≥ 3.5 g/day), hypoalbuminemia, hypercholesterolemia and sometimes lipiduria. The common causes of primary nephrotic syndrome are listed below.

Causes of primary glomerular diseases presenting as nephrotic syndrome

- Minimal change disease (MCD)
- Focal segmental glomerulosclerosis (FSGS)
- Membranous nephropathy (MN)
- Membranoproliferative glomerulonephritis (MPGN)
- Amyloidosis
- Diabetic nephropathy

Several terms which have been used to describe and define response to treatment in nephrotic syndrome are shown in Table 181.2. Protein loss in urine leads to severe consequences (Table 181.3).

Nephritic Syndrome

This is characterized by a relative abrupt onset of varying combinations of edema, hematuria, proteinuria, hypertension and renal failure. Clinical points which help to

Table 181.2: Treatment-related definitions in nephrotic syndrome

Term	Adult	Pediatric
Relapse	Proteinuria ≥ 3.5 g/day occurring after complete remission has been obtained for >1 month	Albustix >1+ or proteinuria >40 mg/hour/m^2 occurring on 3 days within 1 week
Frequently relapsing	Two or more relapses within 6 months	Two or more relapses within 6 months of initial episode or > 3 episodes in any 12 months period
Complete remission	Reduction of proteinuria to ≤ 0.3 g/day	< 4 mg/hour/m^2 or < 1+ on dipstick at least 3 occasions within 7 days and serum albumin >3.5 g/dL
Partial remission	Reduction of proteinuria to between 0.21 and 3.4 g/day $\pm$ decrease in proteinuria of $\geq 50\%$ from baseline	Disappearance of edema. Increase in serum albumin >3.5 g/dL and persisting proteinuria >4 mg/m^2 or >100 mg/m^2/day
Steroid-resistant	Persistence of proteinuria despite prednisone therapy 1 mg/kg/day $\times$ 4 months	Persistence of proteinuria despite prednisone therapy 60 mg/m^2 $\times$ 8 weeks
Steroid-dependent	Two consecutive relapses occurring during tapering therapy or within 14 days of completing steroid therapy	Two consecutive relapses of proteinuria within 14 days after stopping or during alternate day steroid therapy

Table 181.3: Consequences of protein loss in urine

Nature of protein loss in nephrotic syndrome	Consequences
Hypoalbuminemia	Edema and may also produce pleural effusion and ascites. Subungual edema may manifest as parallel white lines in the fingernail beds. Increased susceptibility to infections
Urinary losses of plasma proteins like thyroxine-binding globulin	Abnormalities in thyroid function tests Abnormalities in thyroid function tests
Deficiency of antithrombin III (due to urine loss)	Hypercoagulable state and renal vein thrombosis. Consequences of hypercoagulable state include pulmonary embolism, myocardial infarction (MI) and stroke
Loss of globulins in urine	Severe IgG deficiency leading to spontaneous bacterial peritonitis
Loss of cholecalciferol binding protein	Vitamin D deficiency state
Loss of transferrin	Microcytic hypochromic anemia
Loss of metal-binding proteins	Metal deficiency—e.g. zinc, copper
Loss of drug-binding proteins	Altered drug pharmacokinetics

Table 181.4: Differentiation between nephrotic and nephritic syndrome

Typical features	Nephrotic	Nephritic
Edema	++++	++
Blood pressure	Normal or low	Usually raised
Jugular venous pressure	Normal/low	Raised
Proteinuria	Nephrotic range	Often non-nephrotic
Hematuria	Usually absent	Present
Red cell cast	Absent	Present
Serum albumin	Low	Normal or slightly reduced

differentiate nephrotic from nephritic syndrome are shown in Table 181.4.

Common glomerular diseases which present as acute nephritic syndrome are shown below.

- Poststreptococcal glomerulonephritis
- IgA nephropathy
- Other postinfectious diseases
- Infective endocarditis
- Visceral abscess
- Shunt nephritis
- Systemic lupus erythematosus (SLE)

Rapidly Progressive Glomerulonephritis

The term rapidly progressive glomerulonephritis (RPGN) is used to describe acute deterioration in renal function characterized histologically by the presence of crescentic GN. Crescentic GN represents the proliferation of parietal epithelial cells in the Bowman's capsule that appear in the form of a crescent (Figs 181.2A and B) when seen in the renal biopsy section. Common causes of RPGN are shown in Table 181.5.

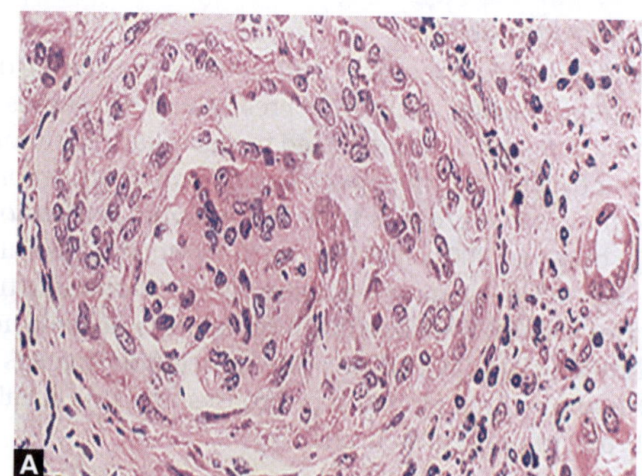

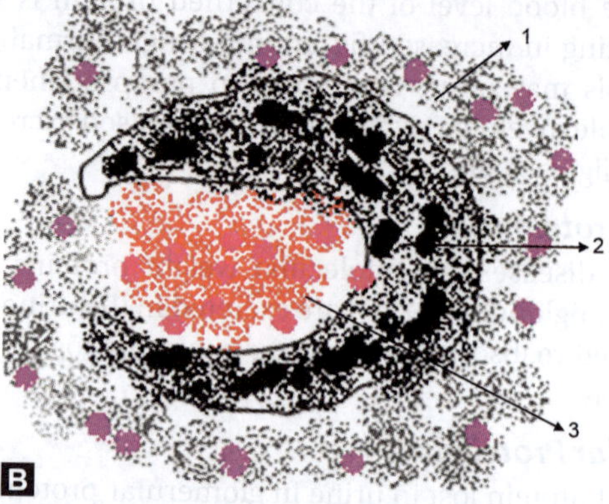

Figs 181.2A and B: A. Renal biopsy under light microscopy H&E stain showing cellular crescent almost surrounding a glomerulus; **B.** Line diagram showing crescent (black), glomerular capillaries (pink) and tubular cells (gray). **Note:** 1. Tubulointerstitial; 2. Crescent; 3. Glomerular capillary tuft

Abbreviation: H&E = Hematoxylin and Eosin

Table 181.5: Immunofluorescence pattern in common types of rapidly progressive glomerulonephritis (RPGN)

Type of RPGN	Immunofluorescence
Type I antiglomerular basement membrane (GBM) antibody	
• Goodpasture syndrome • Idiopathic anti-GBM antibody mediated RPGN (only kidney involvement)	Linear deposits of IgG and C3 in the GBM
Type II (immune complex)	

• Idiopathic immune complex-mediated RPGN
  ▪ IgA nephropathy
  ▪ Membranous glomerulopathy
  ▪ Mesangiocapillary GN
• Associated with secondary GN
  ▪ Postinfectious glomerulonephritis (poststreptococcal GN)
  ▪ Lupus nephritis
  ▪ Henoch-Schonlein purpura
  ▪ Mixed cryoglobulinemia
	Granular fluorescence characteristic of immune complex nephritis

Type III (pauci-immune)	
• Idiopathic • Granulomatous polyangiitis • Antineutrophil cytoplasmic antibody (ANCA)-associated • Microscopic polyangiitis • Renal-limited necrotizing crescentic GN • Eosinophilic granulomatosis with polyangiitis	Neither show anti-GBM antibodies nor immune complexes by immunofluorescence and electron microscopy

Chronic Glomerulonephritis

This is characterized by a slowly progressive renal impairment with urinary abnormalities and hypertension which is present for over 3 months. In very long-standing GN, the kidneys shrink (but remain smooth and symmetric). Renal biopsy at this stage is more hazardous and less likely to provide diagnostic material. For this reason, chronic GN has often been a presumptive diagnosis in patients presenting late with shrunken kidneys, proteinuria and renal impairment. Some of the common glomerular diseases are discussed in this chapter.

POSTSTREPTOCOCCAL GLOMERULONEPHRITIS (PSGN)

It is an acute onset of nephritic syndrome following infection with nephritogenic strains of group A Streptococci. It was described in 1836 by Richard Bright who is considered as 'Father of Nephrology'.

Epidemiology

It is the most common cause of acute nephritic syndrome in children. Peak age of incidence is 2–6 years and occurs predominantly in males. It occurs sporadically or in epidemic form. Subclinical nephritis is 4–10 times more common than overt nephritis. Acute nephritis may follow infection with nephritogenic strains of group A beta-hemolytic Streptococci belonging to M types 1, 2, 3, 4, 5, 12, 18, 25, 49, 55, 57, 59, 60, 61. In the temperate zones, PSGN occurs more in winter months, following pharyngeal infection, whereas in the tropics, it occurs during summer, following skin infections. In India, infected scabies was the most common initiating event during the last century. Development of acute glomerulonephritis (AGN) depends on host factors also. Only less than 10% patients develop overt acute nephritis following infection with nephritogenic strains of streptococci.

Pathogenesis

Two main mechanisms are implicated in the pathogenesis of PSGN:

1. ***Glomerular inflammation secondary to deposition of immune complex containing streptococcal antigen:*** Following streptococcal infection, the bacterial antigens evoke antibody response. The antigens and antibodies form immune complexes (ICs) which circulate in the blood. The ICs produced during the early stages of infection have excess antigen. Such ICs are small and can be cleared from the body easily. The ICs produced later have excess antibody and are large in size. Such antibodies are also cleared by the reticuloendothelial system. The ICs produced at the time of mild antigen excess (which occurs about 2–3 weeks after the infection) are intermediate sized and are trapped in the glomerular capillary filter on the ***epithelial side*** of the basement membrane. Here, they activate the compliment system, recruit polymorphs and initiate the immunologically-mediated acute inflammation of the glomerulus.

2. Molecular mimicry is the mechanism by which host develops an immune response to a foreign antigen that cross reacts with host antigen. The most common streptococcal antigens implicated in PSGN are:
   - NAPLr—Nephritis-associated plasmin like receptor
   - SPEB—Streptococcal pyrogenic endotoxin B.

Pathology

The characteristic light microscopic finding in PSGN is diffuse (>50%) involvement of glomeruli. The glomeruli appear enlarged and the cellularity of the glomerular tuft is increased with neutrophilic infiltration (exudation). The lumen of the capillary loops may not be visible. The pathological picture is described as ***diffuse proliferative glomerulonephritis (DPGN)*** (Figs 181.3A and B). Immunofluorescence shows granular deposition of C3 often with IgG and occasionally IgM. If the immunoglobulin deposits are along the capillary wall, it gives a garland pattern under fluorescent microscope. The immune deposits in the mesangium give diffuse 'starry sky' pattern. Garland pattern is often associated with more proteinuria and worse prognosis. The classic electron microscopic finding is the presence of large dome-shaped subepithelial electron dense deposits (humps) along with small subendothelial and mesangial immune deposits.

Clinical Features

Patients, usually present with acute nephritic syndrome characterized by abrupt onset of puffiness of face, pedal edema, reduced urine output, cola-colored urine (hematuria), volume-dependent hypertension and even renal failure. Rarely, they may present with cardiac failure, hyper-

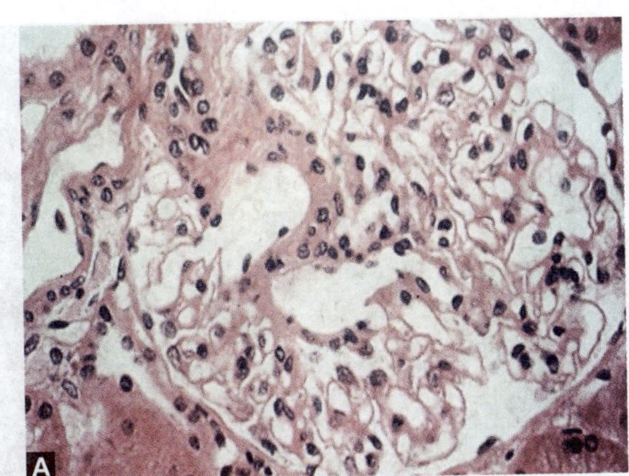
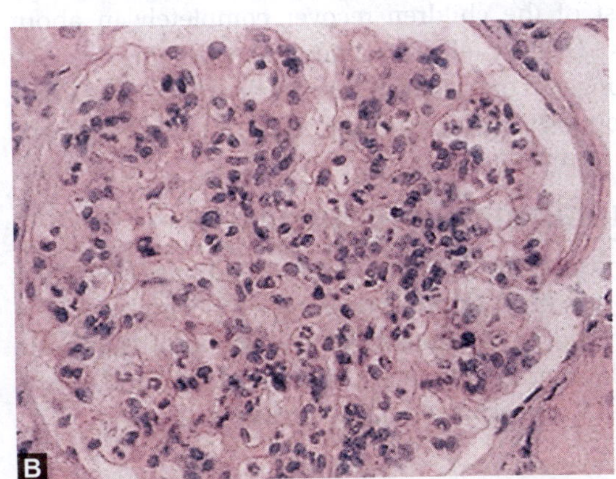

Figs 181.3A and B: Diffuse proliferative glomerulonephritis (DPGN) with neutrophil exudation on the right in comparison with a normal glomerulus on the left

tensive encephalopathy and/or dialysis requiring renal failure (<5%). The latent period between streptococcal infections, following pharyngitis is usually 1–3 weeks, whereas after skin infection it is, usually 3–6 weeks.

Investigations and Diagnosis

Urinalysis shows proteinuria and hematuria. Examination of urinary sediments shows dysmorphic RBCs and RBC casts. Presence of RBC cast indicates active GN. Blood examination may show polymorphonuclear leukocytosis (PMNL) and elevated antistreptococcal antibodies. Anti-streptolysin O (ASO) titer is the frequently employed serological test. Streptozyme test, which detects antibodies to four streptococcal antigens namely, ASO, AntiDNAse-B, antihyaluronidase and anti-nicotylamide-adenine dinucleotidase antibody, is more sensitive in identifying the presence of antecedent streptococcal infection. The cultures are usually negative at the time of presentation. Compliment factors C3 and CH50 levels are low in majority of patients (alternate compliment pathway activation) whereas C4 levels are normal. Renal biopsy is not indicated routinely, but may be diagnostic in atypical presentations or when the patient does not show the expected recovery. Other diseases presenting as acute nephritic syndrome are shown below.

Differential diagnosis of poststreptococcal glomerulonephritis (PSGN)

- IgA nephropathy
- Lupus nephritis
- Infective endocarditis
- Anti-glomerular basement membrane (GBM) disease
- Pauci-immune crescentic glomerulonephritis
- Membranoproliferative glomerulonephritis (MPGN)
- Shunt nephritis

Treatment

Most patients are managed conservatively with control of blood pressure (BP), diuretics for volume overload and salt restriction. Antibiotics are usually not indicated, if the underlying infection has resolved. Pulse steroids are occasionally used in treatment of severe cases and in the presence of crescents in renal biopsy.

Prognosis

Children with PSGN have a favorable prognosis particularly and most of the children recover completely in about 6 weeks. Urinary abnormalities or hypertension may persist longer. If they persist for more than 1 year, the long-term prognosis may be unfavorable and these patients progress to renal failure.

IMMUNOGLOBULIN A NEPHROPATHY

IgA nephropathy is the most common primary GN in the world. It was first described by Berger and Hinglais and is characterized predominantly by deposition of IgA in the glomerular mesangium. It occurs more in men and affects all ages with a peak onset in 2nd decade of life.

Pathogenesis

IgA nephropathy is an immune complex-mediated GN characterized by the presence of IgA deposits diffusely in the mesangium. These are polymeric and of IgA1 subclass. Abnormalities in the glycosylation of IgA may result in decreased clearance of IgA from the circulation and is postulated as the key pathogenetic factor. There is also overproduction of IgA in plasma cells and a defective mucosal immune system. Due to increased levels of circulating IgA, it gets trapped and is deposited in the mesangium leading to IgA nephropathy.

Clinical Features

Patients present with recurrent episodes of macroscopic hematuria, usually in association with an upper respiratory infection (synpharyngitic hematuria) unlike in PSGN where hematuria occurs 2–3 weeks after the episode of infection. Other common presentations are episodes of microscopic hematuria with or without proteinuria. Few cases of IgA nephropathy present with nephrotic-range proteinuria. They can present as AKI because of either crescentic GN or acute tubular necrosis (ATN) caused by gross hematuria. IgA nephropathy is also a common cause of end-stage renal disease (ESRD) requiring long-term renal replacement therapy (RRT).

Diagnosis

Urinalysis reveals microscopic hematuria, usually with dysmorphic RBC and/or RBC casts. Subnephrotic proteinuria without hematuria can also occur. ***Renal biopsy with immunofluorescence study is the gold standard in diagnosis of IgA nephropathy***. Light microscopy shows expansion of mesangial area with proliferation of mesangial cells and increased extracellular matrix. Immunofluorescence shows granular deposits of IgA in the mesangium along with C3 (Fig. 181.4).

Treatment

There is no disease specific therapy for IgA nephropathy. Optimum dose of angiotensin-converting enzyme inhibitor (ACEI)/angiotensin receptor blocker (ARB) with a view to control BP and reduce proteinuria is the mainstay in the treatment. When IgA nephropathy presents as nephrotic syndrome, it may be treated with 6 months course of corticosteroids similar to minimal change disease. If IgA nephropathy presents as RPGN with biopsy showing more than 50% crescents, treatment with cyclophosphamide and steroids similar to treatment of vasculitis may be tried.

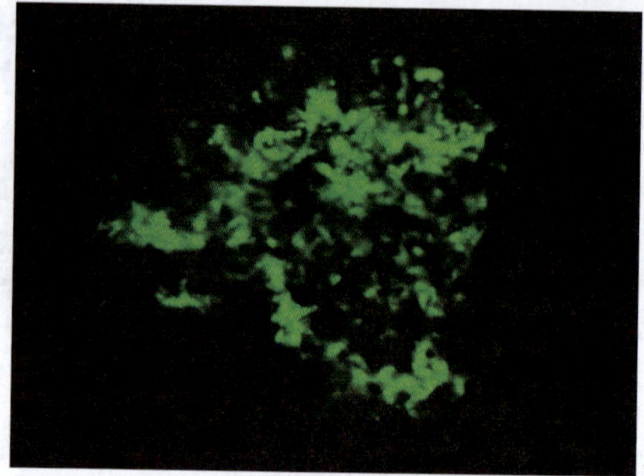

Fig. 181.4: Immunofluorescence microscopy showing mesangial IgA deposits

Supportive therapy with statins is also advocated. Large doses (3 g/day) of fish oil containing omega-3 fatty acids is also used to treat slowly progressive IgA nephropathy or persistent proteinuria and microscopic hematuria, but their effectiveness is not convincing.

RAPIDLY PROGRESSIVE GLOMERULONEPHRITIS (RPGN)

It is a clinical syndrome characterized by rapid loss of renal function accompanied by features of acute nephritic syndrome often with oliguria or anuria. The pathognomonic histological feature of RPGN is crescentic GN, i.e. the presence of crescents in more than 50% glomeruli. Crescent is the proliferation of parietal epithelial cells of the Bowman's capsule which may encroach or/and destroy the capillary tuft.

Classification of RPGN

It is classified into three major types based on immune complex deposits in immunofluorescence (IF) microscopy.

Anti-GBM Disease/Goodpasture Syndrome

Anti-glomerular basement membrane (GBM) disease occurs as a renal limited disease (anti-GBM glomerulonephritis) or as a pulmonary renal syndrome (Goodpasture syndrome). This disease is characterized by circulating antibodies to GBM and deposition of antibodies (usually IgG) along GBM. The antibodies are directed against noncollagenous domain (NCI) of alpha 3 chain of type 4 collagen.

Anti-GBM disease has a bimodal incidence. First peak is in 2nd or 3rd decade of life with male preponderance often associated with lung hemorrhage. Second peak is in 6th to 7th decade of life and is more in women and often have renal limited disease. The typical clinical presentation is with acute nephritic syndrome and oligoanuric renal failure. Unlike with PSGN, hypertension is characteristically absent. Pathological examination show crescentic GN with linear immune complex deposits along GBM in IF. Serological examination reveals high titers of anti-GBM antibody, the levels of which often correlate with severity of illness.

The standard treatment for anti-GBM disease is intensive plasmapheresis combined with corticosteroids and cyclophosphamide. The major prognostic marker for progression to ESRD is serum creatinine level at the time of initial presentation. Aggressive immunosuppression is not advised in patients with renal limited disease whose biopsy shows widespread glomerular and interstitial scarring and those who have a serum creatinine of more than 7 mg/dL at presentation in view of poor treatment response.

Once remission of anti-GBM disease is achieved with immunosuppressive therapy, recurrent disease occurs only rarely, hence, only short-term immune suppression is required. Similarly, the recurrence of anti-GBM after renal transplantation is rare if done 6 months after disappearance of anti-GBM antibody from circulation.

LUPUS NEPHRITIS (LN)

This is seen in around 40% of patients with systemic lupus erythematosus (SLE) and contributes to the high morbidity and mortality of these patients. It is characterized by presence of proteinuria of more than 0.5 g/day, and or presence of RBCs, WBCs or cellular casts in urine. Hence, all patients with SLE should be subjected to screening for renal involvement by urinalysis during follow-up. The popular classification of lupus nephritis proposed by the WHO in 1975 is shown in Table 181.6.

A modified classification by International Society of Nephrology and Renal Pathology Society (ISN-RPS) was suggested in 2002 where further subclassification into active, chronic, segmental and global lesions were included.

Table 181.6: Morphologic classification of lupus nephritis (WHO)	
Class I	Normal—no pathological finding, no glomerular immune complex
Class II	Mesangial lupus nephritis—normal or hypercellular mesangium—mesangial immune complex
Class III	Focal lupus nephritis—less than 50% of glomeruli involved
Class IV	Diffuse lupus nephritis—more than 50% of glomeruli involved
Class V	Membranous lupus nephritis
Class VI	Advanced sclerosing glomerulonephritis

Management

All cases of LN irrespective of class require treatment with hydroxychloroquine and steroids along with renoprotective measures like dietary sodium and protein restriction with RAAS (renin-angiotensin-aldosterone system) blockade therapy (ACEI/ARB). Class I and II seldom need additional cytotoxic drugs. In class III and IV, LN patients are given additional immunosuppressives as induction and maintenance regimen. Induction therapy consists of pulse methylprednisolone followed by oral steroids along with intravenous (IV) cyclophosphamide therapy or oral mycophenolate mofetil (MMF). After attaining remission, maintenance therapy is given, either with MMF or with azathioprine. It is currently unclear how long to continue any regimen of cytotoxic drugs in treatment of lupus nephritis. Some protocols recommend continuing treatment for one year of remission and no longer than 4 years of total treatment duration. Class V LN can be treated with steroids, along with MMF or calcineurin inhibitor.

Prognosis

After successful initial treatment of LN, patients require regular follow-up as they are prone for relapses. Some patients who fail to respond to usual therapy (resistant lupus) can be treated with newer drugs like rituximab, bortezomib, belimumab or plasmapheresis. ESRD occurring as a result of LN requires long-term dialysis or renal transplantation. Recurrence of SLE after renal transplantation is unusual as the disease usually burns out by then.

PAUCI-IMMUNE CRESCENTIC GN

It is characterized by focal necrotizing and crescentic GN with little or no immune complex staining in glomerulus by immunofluorescence. This usually occurs as a part

Table 181.7: Classification of systemic Vasculitis	
Large vessel	• Giant cell arteritis • Takayasu arteritis
Medium vessel	• Kawasaki disease—mucocutaneous lymph node syndrome • Polyarteritis nodosa (PAN)
Small vessel vasculitis	• Granulomatosis with polyangiitis (GPA)—formerly Wegeners granulomatosis • Eosinophilic granulomatosis (EG)—formerly Churg-Strauss syndrome • Microscopic polyangiitis (MPA)

of small vessel vasculitis (affects capillaries, venules, arterioles and small arteries).

The nomenclature of systemic vasculitis approved at a Consensus Conference held at Chappel–Hill in the US is shown in Table 181.7.

Anti-neutrophil cytoplasmic antibody (ANCA) has an important pivotal role in pathogenesis of small vessel vasculitis and testing for ANCA in serum is a useful diagnostic procedure for pauci-immune small vessel vasculitis. There are mainly two types of ANCA based on immunofluorescence staining pattern—cytoplasmic (cANCA) and perinuclear (pANCA). cANCAs are formed against the enzyme proteinase 3 and pANCAs are directed against myeloperoxidase enzyme. cANCA positivity in seen is 70–90% of patients with granulomatosis with polyangiitis (GPA) (earlier known as Wegener's granulomatosis) and in 50% of patients with microscopic polyangiitis. In eosinophilic granulomatosis, 60% show pANCA positivity. These antibodies against neutrophils promote degranulation of neutrophils, macrophages, eosinophils and increase endothelial adherence, thereby damaging the vascular endothelium triggering a vascular inflammatory process.

Treatment

Treatment of pauci-immune GN involves three phases—induction of remission, maintenance of remission and treatment of relapse. Induction therapy involves IV methylprednisolone 7 mg/kg/day (approximately 500 mg in an adult) for 3 days followed by oral prednisolone 1 mg/kg/day tapering to an alternate day regimen and discontinuing within 3–4 months. Corticosteroid treatment is combined with 2 mg/kg/day oral cyclophosphamide at 0.5 g/m²/month. Plasma exchange can also be used for induction therapy in those with life-threatening pulmonary hemorrhage or with dialysis-dependent renal failure at presentation. Cyclophosphamide may be substituted by azathioprine 2 mg/kg/day after 3–6 months to reduce toxic side effects. Other immunosuppressive agents that have been used for maintenance therapy include methotrexate, anti-tumor necrosis factor antibody (antiTNF-Ab, e.g. infliximab, etanercept), anti-CD 20 Ab (Rituximab) and MMF. In case of relapse, reinstitution of treatment similar to induction regimen is most often used.

Transplantation

Risk of recurrence following renal transplantation is approximately 20%. However, ANCA titers at the time of transplantation generally do not correlate with risk of recurrence.

MINIMAL CHANGE DISEASE (MCD)

It is usually a steroid sensitive nephrotic syndrome in the absence of histologic glomerular abnormalities, other than electron microscopic evidence of epithelial cell foot process fusion. It is the cause of nephrotic syndrome in about 90% of children less than 10 years and about 10–15% of adults.

Epidemiology

MCD can appear as early as in the first year of life, but peak incidence is at 3 years of age. In childhood, it occurs twice more commonly in males than in girls, but has an equal sex incidence in adults. Up to two-thirds of initial presentations and relapses follow an infection, most commonly of the upper respiratory tract.

Etiology and Pathogenesis

Most cases of MCD are idiopathic, though occasionally it can be secondary to certain conditions like Hodgkin's disease, use of drugs like interferon-alpha (IFN-α) and nonsteroidal anti-inflammatory drugs (NSAIDs), etc.

The primary abnormality in MCD is a defect in the selective glomerular filtration barrier to albumin. In normal glomeruli, albumin filtration is prevented by both size and charge barriers. In MCD, there is defect in permeability due to alterations in the GBM, particularly a loss of negative charge.

Clinical Features

Patients typically present with edema that develops over days to weeks with fluid retention that often exceeds more than 3% of the body weight. Facial edema is usually the initial symptom. Hypovolemia, pleural effusions and ascites are common in children. Pericardial effusions and pulmonary edema may occur rarely. Gross edema may predispose to ulceration and infection of dependent skin. Clinical examination may also show white nails, sometimes with band called as Muehrcke's lines. Peritonitis due to *Streptococcus pneumoniae, Haemophilus influenzae* and other encapsulated bacteria is another common complication. The risk of thromboembolism is also increased. Renal function is generally preserved, but slight rise in creatinine concentration may be seen in adults.

Diagnosis

Nephrotic syndrome is diagnosed in the presence of edema with nephrotic-range proteinuria [>3.5 g/24 hours in adults or >3 g/m²/24 hours (= 40 mg/m²/hour) in children] or a protein to creatinine ratio of more than 0.25 g/mmol (>2 mg protein/mg creatinine) on a spot urine sample along with hypoalbuminemia (<2.5 g/dL) and hyperlipidemia. Urine analysis reveals hyaline casts and sometimes lipid casts. Minimal change disease is characterized by highly selective proteinuria. Selectivity index is usually derived from the ratio of IgG clearance to albumin clearance. If the selectivity index is less than 0.1, the proteinuria is highly selective and if it is more than 0.2, it is nonselective. In children, renal biopsy is usually not indicated in nephrotic syndrome as more than 90% are steroid responsive and are due to MCD. In adults, a renal biopsy is necessary as only a few are steroid responsive and are often due to causes other than MCD.

Treatment

Oral prednisone is administered as a single daily dose starting at 60 mg/m²/day or 2 mg/kg/day to a maximum 60 mg/day be given for 4–6 weeks followed by alternate day medication as a single daily dose starting at 40 mg/m² or 1.5 mg/kg (maximum 40 mg on alternate days) and continued for 2–5 months with tapering of the dose. Steroid responsive patients who relapse are treated with daily steroids till they attain remission for three consecutive days and then shifted to alternate day steroids for 4 weeks and the dose is then tapered. Treatment of frequently relapsing and steroid-dependent nephrotic syndrome may benefit with addition of either alkylating agents (cyclophosphamide or chlorambucil) or calcineurin inhibitors (cyclosporine, tacrolimus). Levamisole has been tried frequently in children with relapsing nephrotic syndrome.

Natural History

The clinical course of MCD in children is often one with remissions and relapses. Those presenting younger are more likely to have relapses and a longer disease course. Relapses may occur in more than two-thirds of affected children after stopping or reducing dose of corticosteroids. Long-term remission can be expected in 75% of initial responders who do not relapse within 6 months. Less than 5% of children with MCD relapse after entering adulthood. In general, increasing time since last relapse reduces the risk of further relapse. MCD generally does not progress to renal failure. Some patients who present as MCD may have underlying focal segmental glomerulosclerosis (FSGS) which may be revealed in subsequent biopsies. Such cases may develop progressive renal failure. Whether the focal nature of the disease caused a misdiagnosis on initial biopsy or whether MCD progressed subsequently to FSGS is not clear.

FOCAL SEGMENTAL GLOMERULOSCLEROSIS (FSGS)

It is characterized by segmental scarring in the glomerular capillary tuft identifiable in the light microscopy of renal biopsy (Fig. 181.5) and often clinically present with significant proteinuria.

Epidemiology

FSGS is the cause of nephrotic syndrome in less than 10% of children and in around 20% of adults.

Etiology

- Primary (idiopathic) FSGS
- Secondary FSGS (Table 181.8).

Pathogenesis

A circulating permeability factor termed soluble urokinase receptor (suPAR) has been recently implicated as the cause of this disease. It is elevated in two-thirds of subjects with primary FSGS, but not in people with other glomerular diseases. The investigators further found that a higher

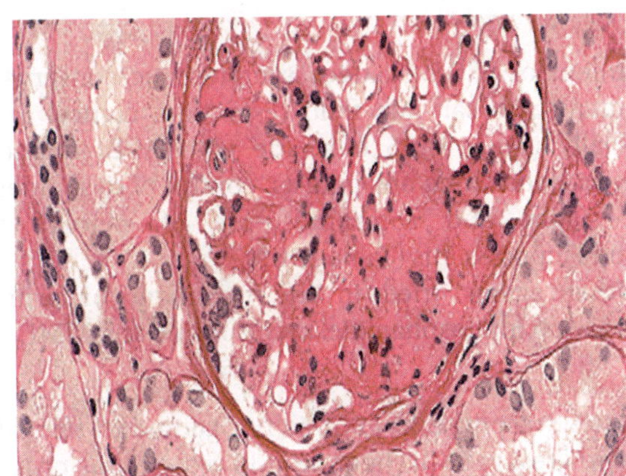

Fig. 181.5: Light microscopy showing focal segmental sclerosis

Table 181.8: Causes of secondary FSGS	
Familial/genetic	Mutation in nephrin, podocin, alpha-actinin 4, TRPC6, etc.
Virus associated	HIV, Parvo virus, CMV
Drugs	Heroin, interferon, lithium, pamidronate
Postadaptive	Unilateral renal agenesis, reflux nephropathy, renal dysplasia

Abbreviations: TRPC6 = Transient receptor potential cation channel 6; HIV = Human immunodeficiency virus; CMV = Cytomegalovirus

concentration of suPAR before transplantation carries an increased risk for recurrence of FSGS after transplantation, thereby leading them to conclude that serum suPAR may be the circulating factor that causes FSGS.

Pathology

Light microscopy: FSGS classically involves less than 50% of glomeruli (focal). The involved glomeruli show scarring only in a segment which is less than 50% of the area of the glomerular tuft (segmental). The capillary of affected segments are obliterated by accumulation of acellular matrix and hyaline deposits. There may be adhesion of the glomerular tuft to the Bowman's capsule. Juxtamedullary glomeruli are typically the first to be affected. The sclerotic segments are often positive for IgM and C3 in immunofluorescence. Electron microscopy shows wide spread podocyte foot process effacement.

FSGS is classified according to the Columbia Classification of into five histological categories as shown below.

Histological types of focal segmental glomerulosclerosis (FSGS)

- FSGS-NOS (not otherwise specified)—most common type
- Perihilar—usually seen in postadaptive FSGS
- Tip lesion—best prognostic variety
- Cellular variant
- Collapsing—worst prognostic of all (reach ESRD in short period and associated with massive proteinuria)

Clinical Presentation

The clinical presentation of patients with FSGS is highly variable. Nephrotic-range proteinuria is seen in approximately 90% of children, but only in 10% of adults. Common associated clinical features include microscopic hematuria (55% in adults and 45% in children) and some amount of renal insufficiency at presentation (20% in children and 30% in adults).

Treatment

Treatment of FSGS includes symptomatic/conservative treatment with salt and fluid restriction, control of BP, especially using RAAS blockade with ACE inhibitors, ARBs or aldosterone antagonists, control of dyslipidemia with statins and sometimes use of steroids and immunosuppressants (Table 181.9).

Other agents tried in the treatment of primary FSGS are cyclophosphamide, cyclosporine and MMF.

Prognosis

Treatment response in FSGS is not good and several of them progress to ESRD by around 10 years. Some progress to ESRD in less than 3 years and are labeled as malignant FSGS. The latter variant has a higher chance of recurrence in the grafted kidney.

MEMBRANOUS NEPHROPATHY

This is the most common cause of nephrotic syndrome in elderly and it in rare is childhood. The peak incidence is between the ages of 30 and 50 years. Idiopathic or primary membranous nephropathy (MN) is characterized by the presence of subepithelial deposition of IgG and C3 with massive proteinuria. It is a glomerular-specific autoimmune disease.

Pathogenesis

Idiopathic MN is a noninflammatory glomerular lesion which results from an autoimmune mechanism. In 70% of the primary MN, there is a circulating autoantibody to the M-type phospholipase A2 receptor (PLA2R). PLA2R is a member of mannose receptor family of transmembrane glycoproteins expressed by the human podocyte. The presence of such antibodies is closely associated with clinical disease activity. Anti-PLA2R antibody tends to disappear with remission of disease and reappear with relapse. Causes of MN are shown below:

- Primary/idiopathic
- Secondary membranous
  - Infections—hepatitis B and C, malaria, leprosy, filariasis, schistosomiasis, syphilis.
  - Cancer—breast, colon, lung, kidney, esophagus, neuroblastoma
  - Drugs—gold, mercury, penicillamine, NSAIDs, probenecid
- Autoimmune diseases—SLE, rheumatoid arthritis (RA), primary biliary cirrhosis, dermatitis herpetiformis, bullous pemphigoid, myasthenia gravis
- Systemic illness—diabetes mellitus (DM), sarcoidosis.

Pathology

The name MN is derived from the histologic appearance of the glomeruli in light microscopy showing diffuse uniform thickening of GBM associated with absence of inflammatory cells. Silver methenamine (Jone's stain) reveals 'spikes' of GBM caused by the non-silver stained immune deposits. This finding is pathognomonic of MN. The finding of granular deposits of IgG with C3 in capillary loop pattern on immunofluorescence is characteristic of the primary and secondary MN. The hallmark of MN in electron microscopy is the presence of subepithelial electron dense deposits. In advanced cases, the glomerular capillary basement membrane will be thickened and shows a ***moth eaten*** appearance under the electron microscope.

Clinical Features

Majority of patients present with insidious onset of edema, proteinuria and other signs of nephrotic syndrome which develop over the course of months. Proteinuria is nonselective as there is increased in immunoglobulins as well as albumin excretion. Microscopic hematuria and hypertension occur in around 30% of patients. Some patients present with thromboembolic complications such as deep vein thrombosis (DVT), pulmonary embolism (PE) or renal vein thrombosis (RVT).

Therapy

Treatment goals in patients with MN include preventing or treating complications of nephrotic syndrome. Preventing deterioration in renal function and limiting the adverse effects of therapy. The treatment can be broadly classified as supportive therapy and disease-specific therapy. The main supportive treatment includes ACEIs or ARBs to maintain BP less than 130/80 mm Hg or less than 125/75 mm Hg, if proteinuria more than 1 g/day, dietary salt restriction and statins. Diuretics are given, if edema is present and anticoagulation may be used, if serum albumin is less than 2.5 g/dL to decrease the risk of vascular thrombosis.

In those with life-threatening symptoms of nephrotic syndrome, proteinuria is more than 8 g/day or with progressive worsening of renal function, immunosuppressive therapy is given if kidney size is normal. Modified ***Ponticelli regime*** for a duration of 6 months is given initially. This treatment regimen consists of IV methylprednisolone 1 g daily for 3 consecutive days followed by oral prednisolone 0.5 mg/kg/day for next 27 days. The above schedule is repeated during third and fifth months. During the second, fourth and sixth months, oral cyclophosphamide in doses of 2 mg/kg/day is given (In the original regimen proposed by Ponticelli, chlorambucil was used but was substituted by cyclophosphamide because of the higher toxicity of the former). Alternative immunosuppressive therapy

Table 181.9: Some factors influencing treatment in focal segmental glomerulosclerosis (FSGS)	
Primary FSGS with subnephrotic proteinuria	RAAS blockade, sodium restriction, statins
Primary FSGS with nephrotic syndrome	Corticosteroids (1 mg/kg/day) to a maximum of 16 weeks or until remission. Calcineurin inhibitors in steroid nonresponsive or those intolerant to steroids
Adaptive FSGS	RAAS blockade and sodium restriction
Secondary FSGS	Treatment of underlying disease
Recurrent FSGS after renal transplant	Plasmapheresis, rituximab

Abbreviation: RAAS = Renin-angiotensin-aldosterone system

includes calcineurin inhibitors (cyclosporine, tacrolimus) and newer monoclonal antibodies like rituximab (anti-CD 20 antibody).

Prognosis

It is generally agreed that patients who have MN with non-nephrotic proteinuria have a good prognosis. In one study, 65% of patients who were followed up for more than 5 years developed spontaneous remission of proteinuria and the estimated 5-year renal survival rate was 88%. Permanent remission and renal survival among untreated patients who had nephrotic syndrome and were followed up for more than 10 years were 33% and 60%, respectively. Deterioration in renal function as indicated by increase in serum creatinine level is invariably associated with progression to ESRD.

MEMBRANOPROLIFERATIVE GLOMERULONEPHRITIS (MPGN)

It is characterized by diffuse mesangial proliferation and thickening, and double contouring of capillary wall under light microscopy. MPGN may be primary (idiopathic) or secondary (associated with specific diseases).

Classification

It is classified into three types based on location of immune deposits on electron microscopy.

1. *Type 1:* Deposit in subendothelium (most common form)
2. *Type 2 (dense deposit disease):* Deposit in basement membrane and mesangium
3. *Type 3:* Deposits in subendothelium and subepithelium.

Etiology

Box 181.1 lists some of the common causes of secondary MPGN.

Pathogenesis

Type 1 MPGN

Type 1 or primary MPGN is primarily an adaptive immune response to chronic antigenic stimulus leading to subendothelial and mesangial deposition of circulating ICs. Once localized, these ICs activate complement via the classical pathway leading to generation of chemotactic factors, opsonins (C3b), membrane attack complex (C5b-9), cytokines and growth factors which lead to mesangial proliferation. This proliferative phase is followed by a reparative phase which results in double contouring of capillary loops.

Type 2 MPGN

It is due to continuous activation of alternate complement pathway due to the absence of inhibitors of complement activation like Factor H or due to the presence of autoantibodies like C3 nephritic factor which prevent the regulation of complement pathway.

Type 3 MPGN

Pathogenesis of type 3 MPGN appears to be similar to type 1 MPGN except that certain characteristics of ICs which is responsible for localizing it to subepithelial space is unknown.

Box 181.1: Common causes of secondary membranoproliferative glomerulonephritis (MPGN)

Infections
- Hepatitis C
- Hepatitis B
- Human immunodeficiency virus (HIV)
- Shunt nephritis
- Visceral abscess

Autoimmune
- SLE
- Scleroderma
- Sjogren's syndrome
- Vasculitis

Monoclonal gammopathy
- Monoclonal gammopathy of unknown significance (MGUS)
- Multiple myeloma
- Chronic lymphocytic leukemia (CLL)
- Waldenstrom's macroglobulinemia

Miscellaneous
- Sarcoidosis
- Sickle cell disease
- Drugs—heroin
- Alpha interferon (α-IFN)
- Transplant glomerulopathy

Pathology

Light Microscopy

Light microscopy of MPGN is characterized by hypersegmentation and lobulation of capillary loops. Diffuse global capillary wall thickening, increased mesangial matrix, endocapillary hypercellularity and double contouring (tram-track) appearance of GBM in silver and PAS stain. Based on immunofluorescence staining of deposits, MPGN is subdivided into two types (Table 181.10).

Electron Microscopy

This is characterized by massive electron dense deposits in subendothelium, mesangium, intramembranous or subepithelial depending on the type of MPGN (Figs 181.6A to C).

Clinical Presentation

MPGN usually presents as nephritic and nephrotic syndrome (hematuria with nephrotic-range proteinuria). There may be associated systemic hypertension. If renal dysfunction is present, it indicates worse prognosis. On evaluation, hypocomplementemia is present in around 80% of patients. Ophthalmic examination reveals deposits

Table 181.10: Classification of membranoproliferative glomerulonephritis (MPGN)

Immune complex-mediated MPGN	Complement-mediated MPGN (C3 glomerulopathy)
- Activation of classical complement pathway - C3 and C4 low - Immunofluorescence-positive for C3 and Immunoglobulins	- Activation of alternate complement pathway - C3 normal, C4 low - Only C3 and absent immunoglobulins
Causes	**Two types**
- Chronic infection - Autoimmune diseases - Monoclonal gammopathies	1. C3 glomerulopathy 2. Dense deposit disease

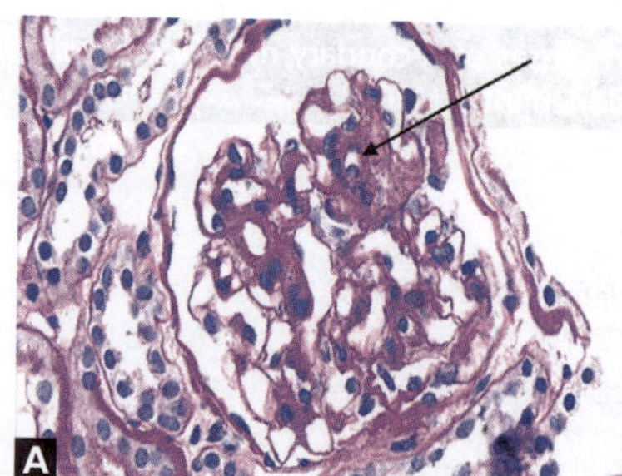
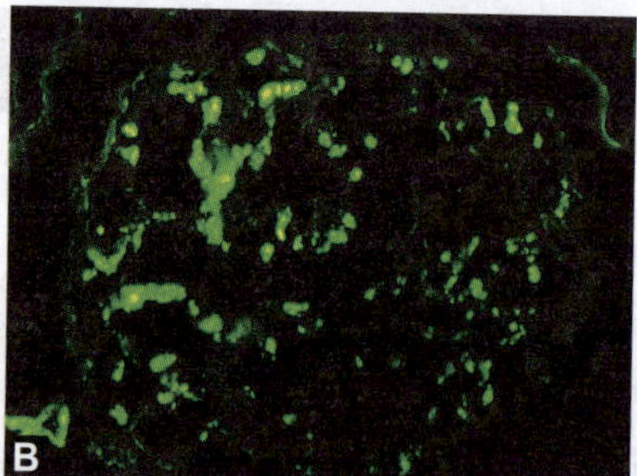
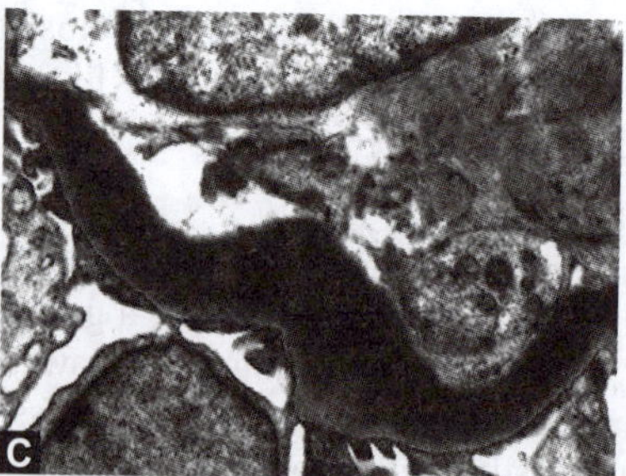

Figs 181.6A to C: A. Membranoproliferative glomerulonephritis (MPGN) light microscopy showing thickened capillary loops (arrow); **B.** Immunofluorescence showing bright C3 staining; **C.** Electron microscopy showing dense intramembranous deposits

along Bruch's membrane in macula called ***Drusen bodies***. Partial lipodystrophy is often seen in association with type 2 MPGN.

Treatment

There is at present no definite recommended primary treatment. In secondary MPGN, treatment is primarily of underlying cause. In idiopathic MPGN, those presenting with normal renal function and subnephrotic proteinuria require only periodic follow-up with dietary modifications, use of RAAS blockers and statins. In presence of nephrotic syndrome or impaired renal function, steroid therapy may be indicated, especially in children. In adults, with nephrotic syndrome or impaired renal function, aspirin 330 mg daily and dipyridamole 75 mg thrice daily have been tried. Significant benefit may not occur in all cases. If renal function continues to deteriorate, steroids may be added. No specific treatment is recommended in the presence of chronic renal failure (CRF) and these patients often need dialysis or renal transplantation.

Prognosis

In childhood, 40–50% develop ESRD by 10 years from diagnosis whereas in adults, 50% reach ESRD by 5 years. Type 2 MPGN has a poor prognosis. Unfortunately, the chance of recurrence of the original disease in the transplanted kidney is high, especially in type 2 MPGN.

C3 Glomerulopathy

It is a term used to describe a range of disorders characterized by isolated deposition of C3 without the presence of immunoglobulin in the glomeruli. This represents uncontrolled activation of the alternate pathway of complement system. There are two main entities of C3 glomerulopathy.

1. ***Dense deposit disease (DDD):*** This is characterized by the demonstration of electron dense deposits in the GBM (intramembranous deposits).
2. ***C3 GN:*** This is defined by presence of glomerular C3 deposition in the absence of immunoglobulin, predominantly in a subendothelial and mesangial distribution but also including subepithelial hump-like deposits. There are many features similar to DDD but the characteristic intramembranous dense deposits are not seen. Clinical courses are highly variable with approximately 50% maintaining normal renal function, while 15% progress to ESRD. Uncontrolled activation of the alternate pathway of complement occurs due to autoantibodies (C3 nephritic factor) and mutations in genes controlling the complement regulatory proteins (factor H, factor I, membrane co-factor protein). Therapy for this condition is mostly supportive. Identification of specific complement abnormalities may result in focused treatments such as plasmapheresis, rituximab or eculizumab (monoclonal antibody against C5a).

CHAPTER
182

Acute Kidney Injury

Jigy Joseph, Vimala A

Chapter Summary

- Incidence and Mortality
- Criteria for Diagnosis of AKI
- Causes
- Pathophysiology
- Clinical Features
- Evaluation
- Newer Markers for AKI
- Management
- Renal Replacement Therapy in AKI

DEFINITION

Acute kidney injury (AKI) is characterized by onset within hours to days of impairment of kidney function which results in retention of nitrogenous waste products that are normally excreted by the kidneys. The earlier term of acute renal failure (ARF) was renamed as AKI by Acute Kidney Injury Network (AKIN) of International Society of Nephrology in 2007. The new definition enables very-early detection of kidney dysfunction and emphasizes the reversible nature of most acute insults. AKI is currently defined by a rise of serum creatinine by at least 0.3 mg/dL or 50% higher than baseline within 24–48 hours or a reduction in urine output (UO) to less than 0.5 mL/kg bw/hour for longer than 6 hours.

INCIDENCE AND MORTALITY

Different values of serum creatinine levels and different definitions were used for diagnosing AKI. There was difficulty in assessing the incidence and mortality of AKI in various studies. By and large, if the AKI is due to community acquired causes, with failure of only the kidneys, as in acute gastroenteritis, snake bite, milder cases of leptospirosis or single nephrotoxic drug/toxin use, the outcome is very favorable. In hospital-acquired AKI, sepsis, nephrotoxic drugs, fluid and electrolyte disorders, acid-base imbalance, cardiovascular instability and multiorgan involvement/failure, the mortality is high. AKI occurs very frequently in the critical care setting and the incidence ranges from 5 to 20%.

CRITERIA FOR DIAGNOSIS OF AKI

The standardized criteria for AKI are necessary because they are useful for risk stratification, interpreting epidemiologic data and in analyzing clinical studies. Early interventions are possible if changes in kidney function can be detected earlier. In order to enable early diagnosis, the 'Acute Dialysis Quality Initiative' has proposed the RIFLE (Risk, Injury, Failure, Loss and End-stage renal disease) criteria for the grading of AKI. The RIFLE criteria provide for a graded definition of the severity of AKI. The acronym 'RIFLE' consists of three-graded level of severity for injury and two outcomes (Table 182.1).

RIFLE criteria have been validated to assess the risk and predict patient's outcome. The inpatient mortality rates are observed as 8.8%, 11.4% and 26.3% for risk, injury and failure, respectively.

AKI Network Criteria

The change in serum creatinine concentrations does not accurately correlate with the percentage decrease

Table 182.1: The RIFLE criteria for diagnosis of AKI

Category	Creatinine/GFR	UO
Risk	Increase in creatinine by 1.5 times or decrease in GFR by ≥ 25%	≤ 0.5 mL/kg/hour for 6 hours
Injury	Increase in creatinine by 2 times or decrease in GFR by ≥ 50%	≤ 0.5 mL/kg/hour for 12 hours
Failure	Increase in creatinine by 3 times or creatinine > 4 mg% or decrease in GFR by ≥ 75%	≤ 0.3 mL/kg/hour for 24 hours or anuria for 12 hours
Loss (outcome)	Persistent ARF = Complete loss of renal function > 4 weeks (but ≤ 3 months)	
ESRD (outcome)	Complete loss of renal function > 3 months	

Abbreviations: RIFLE = Risk, Injury, Failure, Loss and End-stage renal disease; AKI = Acute kidney injury; GFR = Glomerular filtration rate; ARF = Acute renal failure; UO = Urine output; ESRD = End-stage renal disease

Table 182.2: AKIN ereteria for AKI

Stages	Creatinine	UO
1	Increase in creatinine by 1.5 times or ≥ 0.3 mg/dL	≤ 0.5 mL/kg/hour for 6 hours
2	Increase in creatinine by 2 times	≤ 0.5 mL/kg/hour for 12 hours
3	Increase in creatinine by 3 times or creatinine value ≥ 4 mg/dL (with acute rise at least 0.5 mg/dL) patients on RRT	≤ 0.3 mL/kg/hour for 24 hours or anuria for 12 hours

Abbreviations: AKIN = Acute kidney injury network; AKI = Acute kidney injury; UO = Urine output; RRT = Renal replacement therapy

in glomerular filtration rate (GFR) and is a fallacy of the RIFLE classification. In the setting of AKI, even minor increment in creatinine may be associated with fallacies in calculating GFR. The proposed new diagnostic criteria are abrupt (within 48 hours) absolute increase in the serum creatinine concentration of more than or equal to 0.3 mg/dL from baseline, a percentage increase in the serum creatinine concentration of more than or equal to 50%, or oliguria of less than 0.5 mL/kg/hour for more than 6 hours (Table 182.2).

Kidney Disease Improving Global Outcomes Criteria for AKI

Kidney Disease Improving Global Outcome (KDIGO) Clinical Practice Guidelines revised the definition of AKI. In the revised KDIGO definition, the timeframe for an absolute increase in serum creatinine of 0.3 mg/dL is retained as such at 48 hours but the timeframe for a 50% increase in serum creatinine is revised to 7 days. For staging, KDIGO criteria make use of changes in serum creatinine and UO only. Change in GFR, instead of rise in creatinine is made use of only if, the patient is below the age of 18 years. AKI is now staged as follows using the KDIGO criteria:

- **Stage 1:** Increase in the serum creatinine by 1.5–1.9 times baseline or more than or equal to 0.3 mg/dL (≥ 26.5 µmol/L), or UO less than 0.5 mL/kg/hour for 6–12 hours.
- **Stage 2:** Increase in the serum creatinine by 2.0–2.9 times baseline or UO less than 0.5 mL/kg/hour for more than or equal to 12 hours.
- **Stage 3:** Increase in the serum creatinine by 3.0 times baseline or level more than or equal to 4.0 mg/dL (≥ 353.6 µmol/L) or UO of less than 0.3 mL/kg/hour for more than or equal to 24 hours, or anuria for more than or equal to 12 hours or the initiation of renal replacement therapy (RRT). In patients less than 18 years, decrease in estimated GFR to less than 35 mL/min per 1.73 m² body surface area also indicates stage 3.

CAUSES

Once AKI is established, it is important to find the cause and categorize it as prerenal, renal or postrenal for the purpose of management (Table 182.3).

In prerenal failure, the kidneys are structurally normal and the condition is due to ineffective renal

Table 182.3: Causes of acute kidney injury (AKI)

Prerenal	• Hypovolemia (hemorrhage, diarrhea, vomiting) • Sepsis • Cardiogenic shock • Drugs (ACEI/ARBs, NSAIDs) • Hepatorenal syndrome
Renal	• ATN (ischemia and toxins) • Interstitial nephritis • Glomerulonephritis (GN) • Malignant hypertension • TTP-HUS • Vasculitis • Rhabdomyolysis, tumor lysis syndrome • Atheroembolic disease
Postrenal	• Ureteric obstruction • Bladder neck obstruction • Urethral obstruction

Abbreviations: ACEI = Angiotensin-converting enzyme inhibitor; ARBs = Angiotensin-receptor blockers; NSAIDs = Nonsteroidal anti-inflammatory drugs; ATN = Acute tubular necrosis; TTP = Thrombotic thrombocytopenic purpura; HUS = Hemolytic uremic syndrome

perfusion. This can occur with hypovolemia or hypotension. In intrinsic renal causes, AKI results from structural damage to the glomeruli and renal tubules and postrenal causes are due to obstruction of the urinary tract. The relative frequency of the different causes of ARF varies with geographic region. Ninety five percent of hospital-acquired and 75% of community-acquired AKI is prerenal. The term **prerenal** is used when renal dysfunction is caused by decrease in renal perfusion. If renal perfusion is restored early and before irreversible changes develop, rapid recovery of renal function results. Since prerenal AKI is caused by underperfusion of an otherwise normal kidney it is quickly reversible with appropriate therapy. Prerenal AKI is often caused by volume depletion. The common causes are hemorrhage, gastrointestinal (GI) fluid loss, diuretic treatment, poor oral intake, 'third space' loss (e.g. pancreatitis), decreased cardiac output, systemic vasodilatation and drugs affecting renal perfusion [nonsteroidal anti-inflammatory drugs (NSAIDs), angiotensin-converting enzyme inhibitor (ACEI)/angiotensin-receptor blockers (ARBs), calcineurin inhibitors, amphotericin B, radiocontrast agents]. When there is systemic vasodilatation, the ratio of systemic to renal vascular resistance is altered and intrarenal vasoconstriction occurs. This is the probable mechanism for prerenal failure in sepsis, general anesthesia and anaphylaxis. The causes of prerenal AKI are often multifactorial and the potential causes have to be addressed while treating prerenal AKI. Early recognition and management of prerenal AKI is important because, delay may lead to development of intrinsic renal failure.

Disease of the renal parenchyma, due to involvement of the glomeruli, tubules or interstitium leads to intrinsic AKI. Acute tubular necrosis (ATN) is the most common cause and is due to untreated prerenal AKI resulting from ischemia, endogenous toxins (e.g. myoglobin, hemoglobin) or exogenous toxic substances and certain drugs. ATN is characterized by structural damage to the tubular cells. The tubular cells have the capacity to

regenerate and recovery of renal function is usual within 6 weeks. The clinical course of ATN is characterized by three phases:

1. **First phase** is the prodromal phase which starts from the period of initial exposure of the causative insult to the development of established AKI.
2. The prodromal phase is followed by the **second phase** which is usually the oliguric phase. In this phase, GFR is reduced resulting in metabolic consequences of AKI. Oliguric phase lasts for about 7–14 days but can be prolonged.
3. **Third phase** is the diuretic phase and indicates recovery of renal function. This phase is often characterized by uncontrollable diuresis (diuretic phase). The diuretic phase is due to:
   • Excretion of retained salt, water and other solutes
   • Continued use of diuretics
   • Delayed recovery of tubular cell function

If initial insult is reversed, 80% of patients with ATN will recover. Causes of **acute interstitial nephritis (AIN)** are:

- **Drugs:** Penicillins, cephalosporins, NSAIDs, proton-pump inhibitors, allopurinol, rifampin, indinavir, sulfonamides, etc.
- **Infection:** Pyelonephritis, viral nephritis, etc.
- **Systemic diseases:** Sjögren's syndrome, sarcoidosis, systemic lupus erythematosus (SLE), lymphoma, leukemia.

Glomerulonephritis (GN) is a very rare cause of AKI.

Postrenal AKI is caused by either intrinsic or extrinsic obstruction of the urinary tract. Common causes of intrinsic obstruction are blood clots, stones, sloughed papillae and of extrinsic obstruction are para-aortic nodes, tumors and retroperitoneal fibrosis. Type IV renal tubular acidosis (RTA) with hyperkalemia is the metabolic abnormality observed in postrenal AKI. The postrenal AKI can be corrected by relieving the obstruction. Relief of obstruction usually results in brisk diuresis. The cause of this is somewhat like the diuretic phase of ATN. Once the tubular functions return to normal, the diuresis subsides. The prognosis depends on the underlying cause and the promptness of relief of obstruction.

PATHOPHYSIOLOGY

Injury to endothelium is the hallmark of ATN. The injury occurs due to changes in the vascularity, direct effect of nephrotoxins, abolishment of renal autoregulation and release of inflammatory mediators.

The following are the mechanisms involved in the pathogenesis of renal failure in ATN:

- **Tubular obstruction:** Damaged tubular cells form intraluminal debris form cast and result in interstitial edema resulting in renal tubular obstruction. Tubular obstruction, in turn, raises the intraluminal pressure in the tubule which leads to reduction of GFR.
- **The back leak theory:** Due to the disruption of the renal tubular epithelium, the glomerular filtrate leaks back into the interstitium. This leads to increase in the hydrostatic pressure of the interstitium which in turn reduces glomerular filtration. This leads to retention of fluid and waste products.

- ***Hemodynamic theory:*** Relative or absolute hypovolemia and sustained renal vasoconstriction results in the reduction of GFR. Hypovolemia activates cardiovascular baroreceptors and the sympathetic nervous system. The vasopressor mechanisms, such as renin-angiotensin-aldosterone system (RAAS), vasopressin and endothelins are stimulated. These factors act together to sustain the blood pressure (BP), the cardiac output and cerebral perfusion. In the kidney, the vasopressors cause derangement of intrarenal hemodynamics leading to afferent arteriolar constriction, efferent arteriolar dilatation and decreased permeability of the glomerular membrane. These factors lead to reduction in GFR.
- ***Cellular mechanisms:*** Several cellular and subcellular mechanisms have been identified in the renal tubular cells. Cytoskeletal injury, loss of cell polarity, impaired cell-cell and cell-matrix interactions, necrosis and apoptosis lead to the development of ATN. In addition to ischemia, reperfusion injury results in free radical-induced oxidative stress, release of proinflammatory cytokines and reduction in nitric oxide, further perpetuating the injury. Recovery and repair mechanisms are also mediated by growth factors which are released locally.

CLINICAL FEATURES

Clinical features are often dominated by the underlying cause.

Prerenal Acute Kidney Injury

The common presenting symptom is oliguria. Patients should be assessed for volume status which is mainly clinical. Postural hypotension and postural tachycardia are very early signs of hypovolemia. In moderate degree of hypovolemia, patients develop persistent hypotension and tachycardia associated with signs of interstitial fluid volume deficit—loss of skin turgor is best elicited over skin overlying subcutaneous bone and in more severe cases, over the anterior abdominal wall. Decreased eyeball tension can be made out by gentle digital palpation of the eyeball. Patients with intracellular fluid deficit may present with thirst, dizziness, orthostatic hypotension or alteration of sensorium. Such patients often have evidence of hemorrhage, excessive fluid loss through gastrointestinal tract (GIT), kidneys or skin. Patients with advanced cardiac failure may present with signs of cardiac failure.

Intrinsic Acute Kidney Injury

ATN should be suspected in any patient presenting after a period of hypotension secondary to hemorrhage, sepsis, drug overdose or surgery. About 30% of patients with ATN may remain nonoliguric, especially if the initiating event is nephrotoxic injury, caused by drugs or radiocontrast agents. A careful search for exposure to nephrotoxins should include a detailed history of all current medications and any recent administration of radiocontrast agents. Allergic interstitial nephritis should be suspected in patients with history of recent drug ingestion, fever, rash and arthralgia. Presence of nephrotic syndrome or acute nephritic syndrome as evidenced by edema, hypertension and hematuria, points to glomerular etiology of AKI.

Table 182.4: Renal indices

Indices	Prerenal	Renal
Blood urea nitrogen to creatinine ratio	>20	<20
Fractional excretion of sodium (FENa)	<1%	>1%
Fractional excretion of urea	<35%	>35%
Urine osmolality (mOsm/L)	>500	<400
Urine sediment (cast type)	Bland, hyaline	Granular
Urine sodium (mEq/L)	<20	>40

Postrenal Failure

This usually occurs in older men with prostatic obstruction, main symptoms being urgency, frequency, hesitancy and obstruction to flow of urine. In women, the common causes include gynecologic conditions, like prolapse uterus, carcinoma cervix or irradiation of pelvic structures. Patients with renal calculi and papillary necrosis present with flank pain and hematuria. Serum and urinary indices can distinguish prerenal failure from established tubular necrosis (Table 182.4).

EVALUATION

History and examination should aim to distinguish between prerenal, intrinsic renal and postrenal causes. Weight gain and peripheral edema may be the only initial finding during the initial stages. Later, as nitrogenous products accumulate, the patient develops symptoms of uremia, such as anorexia, nausea and vomiting, weakness, confusion and coma. Urine output (UO) varies with the type and cause of AKI. AKI can be classified into oliguric and nonoliguric depending on urine volume. If the urine volume is less than 400–500 mL in 24 hours, it is classified as oliguric. Total anuria may suggest obstructive nephropathy, rapidly progressive GN or severe forms of ATN. If the urine volume is more than 500 mL/24 hours, it is classified as nonoliguric AKI. Nonoliguric AKI has a better prognosis. Patients who are predisposed for AKI should have their serum creatinine checked periodically.

Urinalysis

It is important in the initial evaluation of AKI and is considered as noninvasive biopsy of the kidney. Reddish-brown or cola-color urine may suggest acute GN, myoglobinuria or hemoglobinuria. Presence of red blood cell (RBC) casts is pathognomonic of active GN. White blood cell (WBC) casts may suggest pyelonephritis or AIN. Eosinophiluria suggests atheroembolic disease, or drug-induced interstitial nephritis. Granular muddy-brown cast is suggestive of tubular necrosis.

The fractional excretion of sodium (FENa) is commonly used as an indicator of tubular integrity.

$$FENa = (U_{Na}/P_{Na})/(U_{Cr}/P_{Cr}) \times 100$$

where U and P represent Urine and Plasma and Na = sodium and Cr = creatinine.

The FENa helps to differentiate oliguria caused by prerenal failure from that caused by ATN. In prerenal failure, the FENa is usually less than 1% whereas in ATN, it is greater than 1%. In patients exposed to diuretics or radiocontrast, this is not useful. In intrinsic renal disease like hepatorenal syndrome and postinfective GN, FENa is less than 1%.

Hemogram

Peripheral smear may show schistocytes in conditions associated with hemolysis as in hemolytic uremic syndrome (HUS) and thrombotic thrombocytopenic purpura (TTP).

Biochemical Investigation

Increase in the levels of serum urea and creatinine are the hallmarks of renal failure. The rate of rise of urea and creatinine is more important for confirming the diagnosis and follow-up than single values. In prerenal failure, the rate of rise of urea is higher than that of creatinine. The proportion of urea to creatinine is usually 20:1. Progressive daily rise in serum creatinine is diagnostic of AKI. However serum creatinine is not an ideal marker of GFR in AKI.

Ultrasound Examination

Normal-sized kidneys usually indicate AKI. Patients with diabetic nephropathy, autosomal-dominant polycystic kidney disease (ADPKD), bilateral hydronephrosis, infiltrative diseases like amyloidosis and lymphoma have normal-sized kidneys in spite of chronic kidney disease (CKD). Doppler studies can detect thromboembolic or renovascular disease.

Serologic Tests

These tests are very informative if ordered judiciously even though they are expensive. Tests such as antinuclear antibody, anti-neutrophil cytoplasmic antibody (ANCA), cryoglobulins and hepatitis serology, are helpful when AKI is suspected to be due to systemic vasculitis.

Renal Biopsy

Renal biopsy is considered in a patient with AKI:

- When renal recovery does not occur in a suspected case of ATN even after 6 weeks. The biopsy helps to exclude renal cortical necrosis.
- When glomerular disease is suspected.
- When the cause of AKI is unidentified (surprisingly, conditions like multiple myeloma, renal failure due to oxalate crystals or other rare etiologies and diagnosed only on the basis of renal biopsy).

NEWER MARKERS FOR AKI

The usual gold standard for assessment of GFR, like iothalamate or inulin clearance, is not feasible in clinical settings.

Cystatin is an alternative to serum creatinine as an endogenous marker for GFR. Cystatin C (Cys C) is a low-molecular-weight protein produced by all nucleated cells. Cys C is freely filtered by the glomerulus, reabsorbed and metabolized by the proximal tubule. If the tubule is damaged, Cys C is excreted in urine and is a superior marker compared to serum creatinine for the early diagnosis of AKI. Other serum and urinary biomarkers, which may have utility for early diagnosis of AKI, are neutrophil gelatinase-associated lipocalin (NGAL), interleukin-18 (IL-18), kidney injury molecule-1 (KIM-1) and N-acetyl-β-D-glucosaminidase (NAG). If validated, these molecules will offer substantial advantages over serum creatinine in the early detection of AKI.

MANAGEMENT

The management of AKI mainly involves identifying and treating the etiologic factor if identified. Life-threatening sequelae like hyperkalemia, pulmonary edema and severe acidosis, must be prevented and if they occur, should be managed till renal functions recover and take over the homeostasis.

Principles of Management of AKI

This include:

- Treatment of underlying cause
- Maintenance of fluid and electrolyte balance
- Maintenance of nutritional status
- Monitoring for life-threatening complications
- RRT when indicated.

Treatment of Underlying Cause

Treatment plan for AKI is mainly supportive. In the critical care setting, the causes of AKI are multifactorial. Early identification and treatment of these factors can reverse AKI. Appropriate modification of drugs, particularly in the elderly or in those with compromised renal function, will help to reduce the incidence of AKI in the intensive care units (ICUs).

Maintenance of Fluid and Electrolyte Balance

Maintenance of fluid and electrolyte balance is of paramount importance. Use of diuretics does not influence the final outcome in established AKI. Diuretics are used sometimes to convert oliguric to nonoliguric since the fluid administration can be more liberal in nonoliguric renal failure. It facilitates easier fluid management. Fluid restriction is crucial in the management of oliguric renal failure.

Correction of hypovolemia may be the only treatment required in the early stages of dehydration if renal injury is not established. Fluid replacement should be undertaken carefully to avoid fluid overload and pulmonary edema. Therefore, accurate determination of a patient's fluid volume status is essential. Assessment of fluid status is mainly clinical. Postural fall in BP and postural increase in pulse rate are very early indicators of hypovolemia and should be checked whenever possible. Loss of skin turgor and dryness of the mucous membranes are reliable clinical parameters of interstitial fluid volume depletion. Accurate fluid intake-output chart and daily weight monitoring are essential to detect changes in the fluid volume status promptly. Monitoring of central venous pressure (CVP) is indicated, especially when there is severe volume depletion, or if the clinical signs are equivocal. Patient has to be aggressively managed with isotonic saline preferably under CVP monitoring to attain a goal of 6–8 cm water in ventilated patients. Increase in urine volume to 0.5 mL/kg/hour indicates hypovolemia as the cause and fluids have to be given. If the urine volume fails to increase even after correction of hypovolemia, it suggests established ATN or other intrinsic renal diseases. CVP measurement has some pitfalls and it must be interpreted carefully.

In obstructive nephropathy as mentioned earlier, diuresis can occur following relief of obstruction. This is called ***postobstructive diuresis*** and the patient may develop dehydration, hyponatremia, hypokalemia and other abnormalities. Therefore, this should be looked for and promptly corrected. Once ATN is established, diuretics have no role.

Treatment of hyperkalemia depends on the degree of hyperkalemia and whether changes are seen in the electrocardiogram. Calcium gluconate 10 mL of 10% solution given slowly is cardioprotective and temporarily reverses the neuromuscular effects of hyperkalemia. Potassium can be temporarily shifted into the intracellular compartment by intravenous (IV) administration of 10 units of soluble insulin and 25 g of glucose, inhalation of β-agonists, such as salbutamol or IV administration of sodium bicarbonate ($NaHCO_3$). Bicarbonate infusions are given only if the patient is in acidosis. Elimination of potassium is achieved by using ion-exchange resins like calcium polystyrene sulfonate and diuretics. Calcium polystyrene sulfonate is given orally 15 g 6th hourly. This is dissolved in sorbitol to avoid constipation. Sorbitol can induce intestinal cell necrosis rarely. If these measures do not control the potassium level, dialysis should be initiated.

Metabolic acidosis is common in AKI. Correction of an anion gap metabolic acidosis with $NaHCO_3$ is controversial. But small amounts of $NaHCO_3$ can be given under close supervision if serum bicarbonate falls below 15 mmol/L. Uncontrolled severe metabolic acidosis is an indication for dialysis, especially if the patient is oligoanuric or fluid overloaded.

Maintenance of Nutritional Status

It is important because ARF is a catabolic state. The total daily caloric intake should be 30–45 kilocalories/kg bw. Most of this should be derived from a combination of carbohydrates and fats. In patients who are not on dialysis, protein intake should be restricted to 0.6 g/kg/day. Patients on dialysis need a daily protein intake of 1.0–1.5 g/kg bw. Fluid administration is based on the UO, body temperature and ambient temperature. Since the levels of potassium and phosphorus may go down in nonoliguric renal failure, they have to be monitored and supplemented.

Monitoring for Life-threatening Complications

Patients with AKI may develop life-threatening sequelae and complications. Most important complication is infection. Diligent search for source of infection should be done along with administration of appropriate antibiotic.

Renal Replacement Therapy (RRT) in AKI

Optimal timing of dialysis for AKI is not defined. In current practice, the decision to start RRT is based most often on clinical features (volume overload) and biochemical features (azotemia, hyperkalemia, severe acidosis). Whether risks outweigh the potential benefits of earlier initiation of RRT is still unclear.

Goals of RRT in AKI: They include the following:

- To maintain fluid and electrolyte, acid-base and homeostasis
- To prevent further insults to the kidney
- To permit renal recovery
- To allow other supportive measures (e.g. antibiotics, nutrition support) to proceed without limitation or complication.

Indications for dialysis can be clinical and biochemical. No fixed laboratory values can be applied. Clinical judgment and rate of rise in the biochemical markers are used to decide on dialysis. Hyperkalemia and fluid overload are indications for emergency dialysis.

Each modality has its own advantages and limitations and so the modality of RRT in AKI should be decided according to the clinical situation. Intermittent hemodialysis (IHD) is widely available and is the most efficient way to remove solutes and fluids. Dialysis-associated hypotension is an adverse factor, particularly in patients who are critically ill. Continuous venovenous hemofiltration (CVVH) is the technique of choice in patients who are hemodynamically unstable. In this, hypotension does not occur usually. It is more expensive and it is available only in a few centers. CVVH achieves better control of uremia and clearance of solutes. Since the procedure is continuous, patients on CVVH are able to remove larger fluid volumes. This is an added advantage for patients on parenteral nutrition and multiple infusions.

The principal methods of RRT are IHD, CVVH, sustained low-efficiency dialysis (SLED) and peritoneal dialysis (PD).

PD is a useful option in AKI in centers with limited facilities since no sophisticated machinery is required for the same. Indications for PD in AKI include hemodynamic instability and difficulty in obtaining a vascular access.

Once AKI is established, a precise diagnosis should be sought and further insults should be avoided. Newer criteria and biomarkers help in timely recognition of AKI and effective management. Attempts to prevent infection and further deterioration by modified dose of antibiotics and appropriate use of drugs will help to reduce the incidence of AKI.

CHAPTER
183

Chronic Kidney Disease

Ramdas Pisharody, Gomathy S

Chapter Summary
- Definition and Staging
- Causes–Clinico-Pathological Correlates
- Natural History and Progression
- Clinical Manifestations
- Diagnosis
- Management
- Conclusion

INTRODUCTION

Chronic kidney disease (CKD) has emerged as an important public health problem affecting more than 10% of the adult population at risk as per the new definition and classification of CKD by National Kidney Foundation–Kidney Disease Outcomes Quality Initiative (KDOQI), USA. CKD is now included in the list of non-communicable diseases and is an important risk factor for progression to end-stage renal disease (ESRD), cardiovascular disease and premature mortality. Diabetes mellitus, hypertension, metabolic syndrome and lifestyle diseases contribute to 60% of all CKD. It is a silent disease and if not detected and treated early, may progress to ESRD. Management of ESRD by renal replacement therapy (RRT) is expensive and hence, early detection and prevention of progression is the only answer to this public health problem.

DEFINITION AND STAGING

The present concept of CKD was put forth by the KDOQI in 2002. Over the years, there has been a shift in nomenclature from *chronic renal failure (CRF)* to *CKD*. CKD is defined as either kidney damage or glomerular filtration rate (GFR) less than 60 mL/min/1.73 m² for more than or equal to 3 months. Kidney damage is defined as structural, functional, or pathologic abnormalities characterized by abnormal tests or markers in blood, urine and imaging, irrespective of GFR. The various stages of CKD are given in Table 183.1. CRF now is defined as a condition where there is a permanent and irreversible impairment of renal function persisting over a period of 3 months or more. This represents stage 3 of CKD onwards. This definition in staging of CKD helps in identifying asymptomatic individuals at risk, who are likely to develop renal failure in future. These individuals are also at enhanced risk of cardiovascular disease and mortality. Thus, the new concept focuses on prevention of progression, morbidity and mortality.

GFR is the best measure of overall kidney function in health and disease. The normal GFR values in women are 8% lower from those of men at all ages. Agewise mean GFR

Table 183.1: Stages of chronic kidney disease

Stage description	GFR (mL/min/1.73 m²)	Remarks
1	Kidney damage with normal ≥ 90 kidney or increased GFR	Blood, urine with imaging markers of damage
2	Kidney damage with mild 60–89 decrease in GFR	Reduced renal reserve in earlier classification
3	Moderate decrease in GFR 30–59	Renal insufficiency in earlier classification
4	Severe decrease in GFR 15–29	CRF in earlier classification
5	Kidney failure < 15 or dialysis	ESRD in earlier classification (dialysis or transplantation)

Abbreviations: GFR = Glomerular filtration rate; ESRD = End-stage renal disease; CRF = Chronic renal failure

Table 183.2: Normal range and variability of GFR

Age (sex)	Mean GFR + SD (mL/min/1.73 m²)
1 week (males and females)	40.6 ± 14.8
2–8 weeks (males and females)	65.8 ± 24.8
>8 weeks (males and females)	95.7 ± 21.7
2–12 years (males and females)	133.0 ± 27.0
13–21 years (males)	140.0 ± 30.0
13–21 years (females)	126.0 ± 22.0

Abbreviations: GFR = Glomerular filteration rate; SD = Standard deviation

+ standard deviation (SD) is given in Table 183.2. Above the age of 30 years, GFR declines at the rate of approximately 0.6–0.8 mL/min/1.73 m²/year.

GFR can be estimated (eGFR) by several formulae which factor in serum creatinine, age, weight or body mass index (BMI) (*See* GFR formulae in www.nkf.org). The most widely used formula for adults which can be easily computed at the bedside is the Cockroft and Gault formula.

eGFR = [140 – age in years] × weight in kg/[72 × serum creatinine in mg/dL] for males

and

[140 – age in years] × weight in kg/[72 × serum creatinine in mg/dL] × 0.85 for females

CAUSES—CLINICO-PATHOLOGICAL CORRELATES

The cause of CKD is identified based on the morphological component of the nephron affected by disease, e.g. glomerular, tubulointerstitial or vascular. The etiology could be immune-mediated, degenerative, vascular, metabolic, heredofamilial or obstructive. Immune-mediated diseases are mostly idiopathic. However, autoimmune diseases such as systemic lupus erythematosus (SLE) and other collagen vascular disease can cause secondary glomerular diseases. Irrespective of the etiology, the end-stage kidney is contracted and granular which on microscopy shows glomerulosclerosis, tubular atrophy, interstitial fibrosis and vascular wall thickening. Table 183.3 shows the clinico-morphological and etiological categories of CKD.

Age, ethnicity and distribution of renal diseases may be different in various geographical regions. Diabetes and hypertension are the two most important causes of CKD worldwide. Primary glomerulonephritis (GN) such as focal segmental glomerulosclerosis (FSGS), immuno-globulin A (IgA) nephropathy, membrano-proliferative GN (MPGN), reflux nephropathy, secondary GN as in collagen vascular diseases and congenital anomalies of the urinary tract lead to CRF usually in the first 3 decades of life. Diabetes mellitus (DM), hypertensive nephrosclerosis, ischemic nephropathy, multiple myeloma, analgesic nephropathy and systemic vasculitis are more common above the age of 55 years. More than 50% of CKD is preventable, if detected early. Table 183.4 shows the distribution of causes of CKD in some studies.

NATURAL HISTORY AND PROGRESSION

Irrespective of the initial injury to the kidney by immune-mediated, metabolic, toxic or heredofamilial causes, the final common pathway of progressive renal damage and fall in GFR is mediated by nonimmune hemodynamic mechanisms. Damage to a critical mass of nephrons results in hypertrophy and hyperfiltration of the remaining nephrons. The functional changes like hyperfiltration are mediated by neurohumoral mechanism like sympathetic nervous system, renin-angiotensin system (RAS), and eicosanoids. The structural changes that follow hyperfiltration include hypertrophy, mesangial expansion, sclerosis and fibrosis. These changes are mediated by profibrotic chemokines like transforming growth factor β

Table 183.4: Distribution of CKD in different geographical regions in India and USA

	Distribution of CKD by cause (expressed in %)			
	Chandigarh	Chennai	Indian CKD registry	USA
Diabetes	24	30	27.5	33
Hypertension	13	11	15.5	21
Chronic glomerular disease	37	21	19.3	19
Chronic tubulointerstitial disease	14	31	8.6	4
Cystic (ADPKD) disease	3.5	2.3	2.0	6

Abbreviations: ADPKD = Autosomal dominant polycystic kidney disease; CKD = Chronic kidney disease

(TGF β). These consequences are influenced by various environmental and genetic factors (polygenic). Glomerular hyperfiltration initially maintains GFR but later, the overworked nephrons succumb to the increased workload and lead to proteinuria, which causes further damage to the glomeruli and the tubulointerstitium. The extent of tubulointerstitial damage is an important factor determining disease progression. Uncontrolled hypertension which is present in over 90% of cases of advanced CKD leads to further progression of the disease. Hyperglycemia also causes structural and functional changes in the glomeruli leading to progressive renal failure. Progressive destruction of nephrons leads to several adaptive mechanisms which enable the remaining nephrons to maintain body homeostasis. Though these adaptive changes are beneficial, later, they lead to maladaptive consequences. The hemodynamic changes that occur in remnant nephrons and hypertrophy are as shown below.

The nonimmune factors that facilitate progression can be categorized as:
- **Increased susceptibility to kidney damage:** Aging, family history of CKD, reduced renal mass, racial factors, low-birth weight.
- **Directly contributes to damage:** Diabetes, hyper-tension, infections, obstruction, drug toxicity, hyper-sensitivity.
- **Enhancing progression:** Proteinuria, uncontrolled hypertension, poor glycemic control, smoking, disorders of divalent ion metabolism, anemia and acidosis.
- **Newer factors:** Asymmetric dimethyl arginine (ADMA), adiponectin, kidney injury molecule (KIM), neutrophil gelatinase-associated lipocalin (NGAL).

CLINICAL MANIFESTATIONS

The early stages of CKD are usually asymptomatic and are detected only on estimation of GFR (stages 1–3). Renal failure is associated with a variety of signs and symptoms that are collectively referred to as the uremic state. The symptomatology may involve any system of the body. However, there is no correlation between the development of symptoms and severity of renal disease.

Edema

Most of the glomerular diseases are associated with edema. In chronic glomerular disorders, development

Table 183.3: Clinico-morphological and etiological classification

Chronic kidney diseases	Causes
Primary glomerular diseases	Focal segmental glomerulosclerosis (FSGS), IgA nephropathy, glomerulonephritis (GN) membranoproliferative GN (MPGN)
Secondary glomerular diseases	Diabetes, systemic lupus erythematosus (SLE) and autoimmune diseases, amyloidosis
Tubulointerstitial diseases	Reflux nephropathy, obstructive uropathy
Vascular diseases	Hypertensive nephrosclerosis, ischemic nephropathy
Cystic diseases	Autosomal dominant polycystic kidney disease (ADPKD) and autosomal recessive polycystic kidney disease (ARPKD)
Heredofamilial	Alport's syndrome
Miscellaneous	Vasculitis, microangiopathy, hemolytic anemia
Diseases in the transplant	Chronic allograft nephropathy

Abbreviation: IgA = Immunoglobulin A

of intermittent edema and hematuria indicates disease activity and may be an early manifestation. If the disorder is not primarily due to glomerular disease, but due to tubulointerstitial diseases, edema may appear late.

Hypertension

It is the most common manifestation. It may appear early during the course of renal disease in 90% of the glomerular diseases but occurs in more advanced stages of tubulointerstitial diseases in about 30% of cases. If untreated, hypertension leads to further renal damage. Rarely, uncontrolled hypertension can lead to precipitous and irreversible reduction in GFR. Hypertension is also an independent risk factor for cardiovascular morbidity.

Cardiovascular Manifestations

It include left ventricular hypertrophy (LVH) due to hypertension and anemia, ischemic heart disease (IHD), congestive cardiac failure (CCF) due to fluid overload and myocardial dysfunction due to uremia (uremic cardiomyopathy). Electrolyte disturbances, particularly hyperkalemia can lead to bradycardia, syncope and cardiac arrhythmias. Other manifestations include premature atherosclerosis, vascular calcification due to secondary hyperparathyroidism and pericarditis. Pericarditis presents with chest pain. Loud pericardial friction rub is audible on auscultation. Sometimes, fibrinous pericarditis may lead to pericardial effusion and cardiac tamponade. CKD is a major risk factor for cardiovascular disease and even mild impairment of renal function can lead to cardiovascular morbidity and mortality. Conversely, compromise in cardiac function worsens renal function too.

Gastrointestinal Manifestations

The gastrointestinal (GI) manifestations like anorexia, nausea, vomiting, dyspeptic symptoms, constipation or diarrhea usually appear in stage 4 CKD (GFR between 15 and 30 mL/min). The symptoms are mainly due to GI mucosal ulcerations. Uremic stomatitis with dry mucous membranes, multiple small oral ulcers and parotitis are seen in advanced uremia. Rarely, GI hemorrhage may occur. **Uremic fetor** describes the ammoniacal odor occurring in patients with advanced renal failure and it is due to the hydrolysis of urea in saliva by bacterial urease. Intractable hiccups may occur in advanced uremia. Severe abdominal pain and paralytic ileus may occur as a result of hypokalemia. Ascites may occur in advanced renal failure.

Neuropsychiatric Manifestations

Paresthesias, sensory or motor peripheral neuropathy, pruritus, restless legs syndrome and bladder dysfunction are the neurologic manifestations. Subtle to gross behavioral abnormalities such as anxiety, depression, personality changes and disturbances of sleep are the psychiatric manifestations. Flapping tremor (asterixis) and myoclonic jerks are features of uncontrolled uremia. Rarely, convulsions and coma may occur. When a patient is initiated on dialysis, abrupt and rapid removal of urea from the blood may lead to higher concentration of urea in the brain since it does not cross the blood-brain barrier rapidly. This leads to cerebral edema and transient neuropsychiatric manifestations, collectively called **dialysis disequilibrium syndrome**. This can be prevented by adjusting the initial few sessions of dialysis so as to achieve very gradual fall in blood urea. Patients on long-term dialysis may develop features of dementia and this is attributed to aluminum intoxication which may occur due to intake of aluminum containing antacids or through the water used for dialysis. This is no longer a major problem at present because of water treatment which involves removal of contaminants like aluminum in dialysis water and withdrawal of use of aluminum hydroxide as a phosphate binder.

Cutaneous Manifestations

The characteristic sallow complexion in renal failure is due to pallor and the deposition of yellowish-brown urochrome pigment. Recurrent skin infections, dry scaly skin with severe itching, rashes, erythema, vesicles, and ulcerations are common. Cutaneous calcification in association with secondary hyperparathyroidism contributes to severe itching. Pruritic hyperkeratotic papular eruptions or Kyrle's disease occurs in diabetics. In stage 5 CKD, precipitation of urea on the surface of the skin gives rise to **uremic frost**. Bleeding into the skin and mucosa may occur as a result of platelet dysfunction. Nail changes include pitting, burrowing and half and half nails. In half and half nail, the distal half of the nail is pink or brown and the proximal half is white or pale. The conjunctival deposition of calcium leads to redness and gritty feeling in the eye also called the **uremic red eye** while deposition of calcium as a horizontal band in the lamina propria of the cornea leads to **band keratopathy**.

Hematological Manifestations

Anemia is common in CKD. It appears when the GFR is below 50 mL/min (stage 3 CKD) and progressively worsens as GFR declines further. Symptoms appear much later (stage 4 CKD). Usually, the anemia is normocytic normochromic. The most important cause is decreased secretion of erythropoietin (EPO). Other factors, apart from EPO deficiency which contribute to renal anemia include the following:

- **Circulating uremic toxins:** Bone marrow resistance to the effect of EPO
- Reduced red blood cells (RBC) survival (from 120 days to 80 days) probably due to mild hemolysis
- **Platelet dysfunction:** Bleeding, including occult GI blood loss
- Iron deficiency
- **Hyperparathyroidism:** Bone marrow suppression or fibrosis
- Folic acid deficiency
- Chronic inflammation
- Aluminum toxicity (rare).

Prolonged anemia can lead to worsening of renal function and lead to LVH and increased myocardial oxygen demand. Disturbances in the coagulation system and platelet dysfunction are common in advanced uremia. Platelet dysfunction occurs due to factors like retention of uremic toxins, nitric oxide and hyperparathyroidism.

Skeletal Abnormalities-Renal Osteodystrophy

As renal failure progresses, hyperphosphatemia, hypocalcemia and secondary hyperparathyroidism develop leading to skeletal abnormalities. Renal tubular defects and altered vitamin D metabolism also contributes to skeletal changes of renal osteodystrophy. Stunting of growth, bone deformities and rickets occur due to end-organ resistance to hormones as a result of circulating uremic toxins. Adults with advanced CKD may manifest with high-turnover bone disease due to hyperparathyroidism, low-turnover bone disease due to vitamin D deficiency or aluminum toxicity or adynamic bone disease due to excessive suppression of parathyroid hormone (PTH). Skeletal deformities are more pronounced especially in children. These manifest even before there is significant reduction of GFR. This is called non-uremic renal osteodystrophy. This is caused by renal tubular acidosis (RTA) and disturbances in vitamin D metabolism. With advancing renal failure, bone disease and growth retardation become more evident. Short stature is an important feature of CKD of childhood. Uremic toxins and end-organ resistance to growth hormone or insulin-like growth factor (IGF) have been implicated. Prolonged use of corticosteroids may also contribute to growth retardation. Children with advanced CRF caused by chronic tubulointerstitial and glomerular diseases also develop severe rickets with deformities (*uremic renal osteodystrophy*). In adults, the most common skeletal disturbance is hyperparathyroid bone disease (*osteitis fibrosa*) characterized by increased osteoclastic bone resorption. This is known as high-turnover bone disease. Typical radiographic features include subperiosteal resorption in the phalanges, *salt and pepper* pattern in the skull. Vascular calcifications occur in the arteries. Osteosclerosis of the upper and lower parts of vertebral bodies give alternate bands of radiodensity and radiolucency in the X-ray spine resembling the jersey of rugby players (*rugger jersey spine*). Large osteoblastic tumors may be seen (brown tumors) in the skeleton around weight-bearing areas. A rare and unusual syndrome in patients with severe osteitis is calciphylaxis. This is due to extraosseous calcium deposition in soft tissues. It manifests as painful violaceous mottling of the skin followed by progressive gangrenous ulcerations at the fingers, toes and ankles. *Osteomalacia* is the second pattern of bone disease seen in CKD. Vitamin D deficiency and/or aluminum intoxication occurring in those receiving long-term hemodialysis aggravate this condition. It is characterized by severe bone pain, recurring fractures and proximal myopathy. In some cases, a mixed pattern of hyperparathyroidism and osteomalacia may be found. In addition, adynamic bone disease is being increasingly recognized. It is a histological diagnosis showing lack of bone formation and resorption. It is probably due to excessive suppression of PTH by calcium supplements and vitamin D therapy.

Respiratory Manifestations

Patients with advanced kidney disease may develop dyspnea due to pulmonary edema, pleural effusion or severe metabolic acidosis. Flash pulmonary edema occurs in patients with renovascular diseases due to accelerated hypertension. *Uremic lung* may be seen radiologically as a butterfly shadow in the area of the hilum and this is due to noncardiogenic pulmonary edema associated with increased pulmonary capillary permeability and exudation of proteinaceous fluid into the alveoli. Uremic serositis may present as pleurisy with associated pleural friction rub or underlying hemorrhagic pleural effusion.

Other Manifestations

In early CKD due to chronic tubulointerstitial diseases, hyperchloremic metabolic acidosis with a normal anion gap is common. As the renal failure advances, high anion gap metabolic acidosis supervenes. Chronic metabolic acidosis has deleterious effect on the bone and several organ functions. Chronic malnutrition is common and it is caused by anorexia, nausea and poor dietary intake and vomiting. Sexual dysfunction is also common in both sexes. In males, it manifests as decreased libido, erectile dysfunction and azoospermia. In females, reduction of libido and menstrual irregularities are common. Patients with CKD are more prone to develop infections due to immunocompromised state. Infection tends to persist longer.

DIAGNOSIS

Often CKD may go unnoticed until renal failure is advanced. Strong clinical suspicion and appropriate investigations are essential for early diagnosis. The diagnosis is established by demonstrating decreased GFR or markers of kidney damage. Serum creatinine is a poor marker of renal dysfunction as it rises only when GFR falls below 50%. Estimated GFR (eGFR) using Cockroft and Gault formula is a widely used and easy to compute formula which has been validated, markers of kidney damage include proteinuria, hematuria or abnormalities of urinary sediment. Detection of more than five erythrocytes per high-power field (HPF) in a freshly voided specimen of urine indicates significant microscopic hematuria if present on repeated examinations. Presence of dysmorphic RBCs and acanthocytes in urine usually indicates pathology in the glomerulus. Coexistence of proteinuria and cellular casts points to renal parenchymal disease. Urinary specific gravity and osmolality may be relatively fixed at around 1,010 and 290 respectively, signifying the inability of the kidneys to concentrate or dilute urine.

Low serum calcium, high phosphorus with high alkaline phosphatase (ALP) are seen when GFR falls below 25 mL/min. Serum bicarbonate is reduced as a result of metabolic acidosis. High anion gap metabolic acidosis is encountered in severe renal failure due to retention of unmeasured anions and failure of acid secretion by kidneys. Serum levels of sodium are usually normal until renal failure is very advanced. The ability of the kidney to maintain serum potassium homeostasis is preserved till the patient is in stage 4 CKD. Hyperkalemia may set in early in patients consuming excessive potassium in diet and those taking potassium sparing diuretics, angiotensin-converting enzyme inhibitors (ACEIs)or angiotensin receptor blockers (ARBs) and in patients with associated with distal tubular dysfunction (hyperkalemic RTA).

X-ray of the skeleton may show features of renal rickets in children or osteomalacia, osteitis fibrosa or osteosclerosis in adults. Presence of smaller kidneys detected by ultrasound imaging suggests long-standing kidney disease. The exceptions to this rule include DM, multiple myeloma, polycystic kidney disease and obstructive uropathy. Demonstration of scarring of the kidneys may be the earliest indicator of parenchymal damage in diseases like reflux nephropathy. Asymmetry of the kidneys on ultrasound examination may be an indicator of underlying renovascular disease. Calcification and stone disease may be demonstrated by plain X-ray kidney, ureters and bladder (KUB) or by ultrasound. Doppler imaging of the kidneys and renal blood vessels helps to detect renovascular disease early.

MANAGEMENT

All patients require conservative management in the early stages. When the patient approaches stage 5 CKD, RRT has to be adapted. The goals of conservative management are:

- Treatment of reversible causes of renal dysfunction.
- Preventing or slowing the progression of the renal disease.
- Treatment of the sequelae and complications of renal dysfunction.
- Identification of stage of CKD and adequate preparation for RRT.

Reversible Causes of Renal Dysfunction

The various reversible causes of renal dysfunction are as follows:

- Relapse or flare of original renal disease, e.g. crescentic transformation of primary GN, lupus flare
- Decrease in renal perfusion, e.g. hypotension, hypovolemia, hemorrhage, drugs
- Infections, e.g. urinary tract infection (UTI), other infections
- Use of drugs which reduce GFR, e.g. nonsteroidal antiinflammatory drugs (NSAIDs), ACEIs, radiocontrast agents, calcineurin inhibitors (immunosuppressive drug)
- Other nephrotoxic agents
- Urinary tract obstruction
- Accelerated hypertension
- Malnutrition, hypoalbuminemia, anemia
- CCF, hepatic failure
- Persistent metabolic abnormalities such as hyperuricemia, hypercalcemia and hypokalemia.

Preventing or Slowing the Progression of Disease

Hypertension, hyperfiltration, hypertrophy, proteinuria and dyslipidemia contribute to glomerulosclerosis and tubulointerstitial damage. The blood pressure (BP) should be maintained below 130/80 mm Hg by appropriate drug therapy and below 120/75 mm Hg in proteinuric patients. According to the latest recommendations of the Joint National Council (JNC 8), for control of BP, aggressive lowering of BP should be avoided in the elderly. Administration of ACEIs or ARBs slows the progression of CRF, particularly in those with proteinuria. This therapy is most effective if it is initiated early, before the serum creatinine level exceeds 1.5–2 mg/dL (132–176 μmol/L). ACEIs and ARBs should be used with caution since they can cause decline in renal function and hyperkalemia. Strict glycemic control is mandatory in diabetic nephropathy for slowing the rate of progression (target HbA1c < 6.5%). Statin should be used in patients with dyslipidemia as it reduces cardiovascular risk and also possesses pluripotent anti-inflammatory effects with potential renoprotective effects. Dietary measures include protein restriction 0.8 g/kg/day, sodium restriction 30–70 mEq/day, thereby minimizing accumulation of nitrogenous wastes and achieving better control of hypertension and preventing CCF. Similarly, salt wasting and depletion is to be avoided. Fluids need not be restricted if the patient is euvolemic, however, large quantities of water intake should be avoided especially in polycystic kidney disease. Other general measures include weight reduction, cessation of smoking, alcohol abuse and avoidance of potentially nephrotoxic drugs or agents such as NSAIDs and radiocontrast.

Treatment of the Complications of Renal Dysfunction

The complications include disorders of fluid and electrolyte balance, hyperkalemia, metabolic acidosis, hyperphosphatemia, anorexia, nausea, vomiting, fatigue, hypertension, anemia, malnutrition, hyperlipidemia, bone disease and pericarditis. The GI manifestations and symptoms like pruritus, insomnia are treated symptomatically. The major complications of CRF and their treatment strategies are summarized in Flowchart 183.1.

Treatment of Fluid and Salt Balance

Even though sodium and intravascular volume are usually maintained till the GFR falls below 15 mL/min, they are unable to cope up with rapid fluctuations in fluid and electrolytes. Treatment is by restriction of dietary sodium and fluids combined with administration of a loop diuretic. Salt intake is restricted to 2–4 g/day. Single large doses of furosemide (200–500 mg) or torsemide (30–100 mg) daily are necessary. Those with CKD and salt wasting state require additional salt intake.

Treatment of Hyperkalemia

Hyperkalemia develops in patients with CKD who are oliguric or those with increased dietary potassium intake. Use of potassium sparing diuretics, ACEIs, ARB's, NSAIDs or beta blockers tends to increase serum potassium. Patients with hyporeninemic hypoaldosteronism (especially diabetics) develop hyperkalemia early in the course of their disease. Hyperkalemia can be controlled by avoidance of the offending drugs, salt and K⁺ restriction, use of diuretics and potassium binding resins. Hyperkalemia above 6 mmol/L is an emergency warrant aggressive treatment.

Treatment of Metabolic Acidosis

Metabolic acidosis is common in stages 4 and 5 CKD. This is treated by administering sodium bicarbonate in doses of 0.5–1 mmol/kg/day so as to maintain serum HCO_3 above 22 mmol/L. As an alternative, **Shohl's solution** which contains a buffered pair of sodium citrate and citric acid can be used. One mL of Shohl's solution provides 1 mmol of bicarbonate. Severe metabolic acidosis is however, difficult to correct without dialysis.

Treatment of Mineral Bone Disease

The pivotal abnormality of mineral bone disease is hyperphosphatemia. Dietary restriction can reduce

Flowchart 183.1: Manifestations and treatment strategies

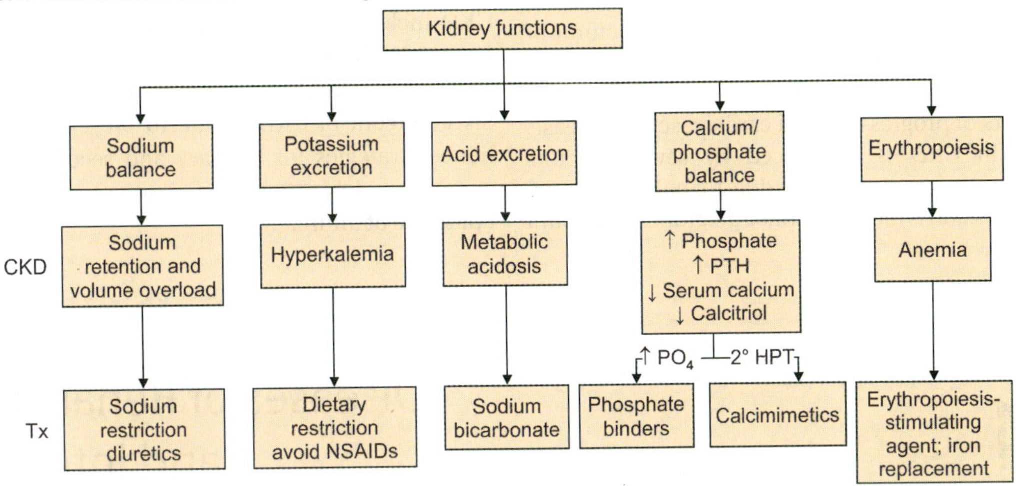

Abbreviations: CKD = Chronic kidney disease; PTH = Parathyroid hormone; NSAIDs = Nonsteroidal anti-inflammatory drugs; 2° HPT = Secondary hyperparathyroidism; Tx = Kidney transplantation

phosphate intake to less than 800 mg/day, oral phosphate binders that reduce phosphate absorption are therefore essential. Calcium-based phosphate binders such as calcium carbonate or acetate are the widely used binders. The dose required is 1–3 g/day. The risk of hypercalcemia is 10–20% and this can lead to vascular and metastatic calcification. The non-calcium binders available are *sevelamer hydrochloride, sevelamer carbonate* and *lanthanum carbonate*. They are expensive and not devoid of adverse effects. Aluminum hydroxide is the most potent phosphate binder, but not used due to risk of aluminum intoxication. In patients who have increased serum parathormone levels and/or hypocalcemia in spite of correction of hyperphosphatemia, 1,25-dihydroxyvitamin D (1,25,HD) supplementation is indicated. Vitamin D deficiency is not uncommon in South India and if suspected or detected is to be treated with mega doses of vitamin D_3 (60,000 units) weekly for a period of 4–12 weeks. Persistent hyperparathyroidism (tertiary) is treated with calcimimetic drugs like *cinacalcet*. However, the risk of hypocalcemia and hyperphosphatemia is high. Hence, it should be used only in dialysis patients for a limited period of time. In children, rickets is the manifestation of metabolic bone disease (MBD). Causes such as tubular acidosis should be evaluated for and treated. 1, 25 HD is indicated more often in children.

Treatment of Anemia

The main causes of anemia in CKD include a combination of poor dietary intake of iron, blood loss and erythropoietin (IEPO) deficiency. The initial step is detailed work-up to diagnose the cause. These include estimation of iron indices and body stores and for sources of blood loss. Patients with iron deficiency should be given parenteral iron preparation to correct iron deficiency. Parenteral iron is usually administered intravenous (IV) or intramascular (IM) as iron dextran, iron sucrose or iron polymaltose complexes. Once the iron levels are corrected, most patients with advanced CKD require erythropoietin in doses of 50–200 IU/kg/week. The hematocrit (HCT) has to be maintained at 36% [hemoglobin (Hb) 11–12 g/dL] by adjusting the dose. Correction of anemia improves the quality of life and improves functions of vital organs and possibly retards progression of CKD. EPO resistance is due to antibodies to EPO and hyperparathyroidism.

Treatment of Dyslipidemia

Hyperlipidemia causes progression of renal disease and therefore it should be managed aggressively. Early and judicious use of statins such as atorvastatin or simvastatin in doses 10–20 mg oral at bed time is necessary to maintain serum low-density lipoprotein (LDL) levels less than 100 mg/dL. Patients with elevated triglyceride levels need gemfibrozil in addition. Statins also have a pleuripotent anti-inflammatory and endothelial stabilizing effect which may prevent progression.

Treatment of Malnutrition

Patients with CKD are usually malnourished. This is due to poor intake of food, hypercatabolic state and the pro-inflammatory effects of uremia. In addition, protein restriction contributes to muscle wasting. The calorie intake should be 30–35 calories/kg bw/day in patients with no extra activity. The serum albumin levels should be maintained greater than 3.5 g/dL. Minimum protein intake of 0.6–0.8 g/kg/bw/day should be ensured to prevent negative nitrogen balance.

Treatment of Uremic Bleeding

Platelet dysfunction is the usual cause of bleeding in CKD. Usually, this is occult and no specific therapy is needed. In patients with overt manifestations or those undergoing invasive procedures, the administration of desmopressin (dDAVP), cryoprecipitate and/or dialysis is recommended to correct the bleeding manifestations.

Identification of Stage of CKD and Adequate Preparation for RRT

The term RRT is used to describe the life support or saving modalities of treatment, needed when the GFR falls below 15 mL/min and generally resorted to, when it is less than 5 mL/min. The options available are:

- Maintenance dialysis
- Kidney transplantation (Tx) (discussed in Ch 191).

CONCLUSION

In conclusion, CKD is now defined as any structural or functional abnormality of kidney with or without decrease in GFR. Five stages have been identified in order to stratify the risk factors of progression and cardiovascular disease. Progression in CKD is influenced by several factors including genetic predisposition due to polymorphism. Disease progression is inevitable once a significant amount of nephrons are damaged. The goals of management in CKD include retarding progression and reversing acute factors. Dialysis and Tx are options available to end stage renal disease (ESRD) patients, however they are expensive. Sixty percent of CKD is due to preventable factors and hence strategies for primary and secondary prevention are to be widely propagated in order to contain this major epidemic of future.

CHAPTER
184

Diseases of Renal Tubules and Interstitium

VN Unni, Manu G Krishna

Chapter Summary

- Tubulointerstitial Nephritis
  - Acute Interstitial Nephritis
  - Chronic Tubulointerstitial Nephritis
- Cystic Diseases of the Kidneys
- Functional Disorders of Renal Tubules

INTRODUCTION

This chapter deals with various diseases and disorders affecting the renal tubules and interstitium. These disorders have been divided into:

- Tubulointerstitial nephritis (TIN)
- Cystic diseases of the kidney
- Functional disorders of the renal tubules.

TUBULOINTERSTITIAL NEPHRITIS

The tubules and interstitium of the kidneys could be affected either primarily or the involvement could be secondary to glomerular diseases. Systemic diseases like diabetes mellitus (DM), hypertension and vascular disorders affect both the glomeruli and tubulointerstitium. The following description highlights the diseases where there is a primary involvement of tubules and interstitium. Acute tubular necrosis (ATN) (acute tubular injury) is described in the Chapter on Acute Kidney Injury; the involvement of the tubule-interstitium of the renal allograft is not touched upon here.

Acute Interstitial Nephritis (AIN)

It is often a reversible disease, characterized by inflammatory infiltrates within the interstitium of the kidneys. AIN is an important cause of AKI; it can be easily overlooked and the diagnosis can be missed. The causes of AIN are shown in Box 184.1.

Drug-induced Acute TIN

The pathogenesis of AKI is believed to be an idiosyncratic response to the drug.

Clinical features include fever, erythematous cutaneous rash, joint pains, eosinophilia and nonoliguric acute renal failure. A detailed questioning often reveals history of intake of the responsible drug. The injury to the kidney is usually idiosyncratic and not dose related.

Box 184.1: Common causes of acute tubulointerstitial nephritis

Drugs

Nonsteroidal anti-inflammatory drugs (NSAIDs)
- Nimesulide
- Ibuprofen
- Diclofenac
- Indomethacin

Antibiotics
- Rifampicin
- Penicillins
- Sulfa drugs

Diuretics
- Thiazides
- Furosemide

Anticonvulsants
- Phenytoin
- Valproate

Miscellaneous
- Indinavir
- Captopril
- Allopurinol

Infections

Spirochetes: Leptospira

Bacteria
- Gram-negative bacilli
- *Mycobacterium*

Virus
- Cytomegalovirus
- Hantavirus
- Human immunodeficiency virus (HIV)
- Epstein-Barr virus (EBV)
- Polyomavirus

Fungi: Histoplasma

Parasites: Microfilaria

Immunologic diseases
- Systemic lupus erythematosus (SLE)
- Goodpasture's syndrome
- Acute rejection in kidney transplants
- Sjögren's syndrome

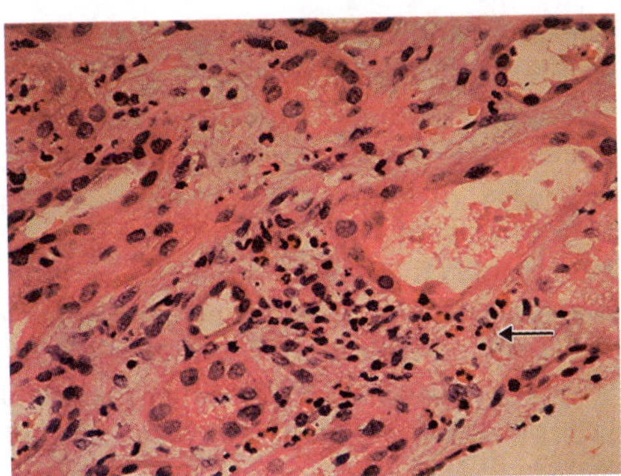

Fig. 184.1: Kidney biopsy (H&E × 400) showing mononuclear cell infiltration in the interstitium with plenty of eosinophils (arrow) in a case of drug-induced acute interstitial nephritis

Abbreviation: H&E = Hematoxylin and eosin

Urine examination shows a mild degree of proteinuria and eosinophiluria. Microscopic hematuria may be seen. AIN due to nonsteroidal anti-inflammatory drugs (NSAIDs) may present with proteinuria in the nephrotic range. Kidney biopsy, if performed, shows interstitial edema and infiltration with plenty of mononuclear cells and eosinophils (Fig. 184.1).

Treatment

Majority of patients recover when the offending drug is withdrawn. Hence, only supportive measures are needed in many cases. If renal functions do not show improvement within 7–10 days after stopping the drug, a short course of corticosteroids, usually prednisolone 1 mg/kg bw for 2–4 weeks, followed by tapering off at the rate of 10 mg every week would be necessary. If the patient has severe renal failure, short-term dialysis support will be necessary until the kidney function recovers.

Infection-induced Acute TIN

Acute TIN can is caused by various types of organisms.

Leptospirosis

Clinical disease caused by this spirochete is common in the tropics and presents with fever, acute renal failure (ARF), jaundice, subconjunctival hemorrhage and myalgia. ARF is due to acute TIN or ATN. ***Treatment*** of leptospirosis with antibiotics and other supportive measures would be essential.

Many viral infections can also cause acute TIN.

Acute Bacterial Nephritis

This condition, commonly caused by Gram-negative bacteria, is often termed acute bacterial pyelonephritis. The patient presents with high-grade fever with chills, loin pain and renal failure. Ultrasonogram or computed tomography (CT) scan shows enlarged kidneys; micro-abscesses or air in the kidney parenchyma or collecting system [emphysematous pyelonephritis (EPN)] can occur in severe cases. The treatment includes appropriate antibiotics and other supportive measures (*See* Chapter on Urinary Tract Infection).

Chronic Tubulointerstitial Nephritis

Long-standing insult or repeated injury to the tubules and interstitium results in chronic TIN (CTIN). The causes are given in Box 184.2.

Box 184.2: Common causes of chronic tubulointerstitial nephritis

- Analgesic nephropathy
- Drugs
  - Cyclosporin A
  - Tacrolimus
  - Lithium
- Heavy metals
  - Lead
  - Mercury
  - Cadmium
- Obstructive nephropathy
- Vesicoureteric reflux
- Renal calculus disease
- Immune-mediated disorders
  - Sarcoidosis
  - Sjögren's syndrome
  - Systemic lupus erythematosus (SLE)
  - Chronic graft rejection
- Infections
  - Tuberculosis
  - Viral infections (BK virus, HIV)
- Hematological diseases
  - Sickle-cell disease
  - Multiple myeloma
  - Light chain nephropathy
- Metabolic disorders
- Hyperuricemia
  - Hyperoxaluria
  - Hypercalcemia
  - Cystinosis
- Miscellaneous
  - Radiation nephropathy
  - Ischemia to the kidney

Pathology

Atrophy of tubular cells with flattened tubular epithelium, dilated tubules, loss of tubules, interstitial fibrosis with mononuclear cell infiltration are seen (Fig. 184.2). In advanced disease, periglomerular fibrosis and glomerulo-sclerosis is seen. Blood vessels in the interstitium show fibrointimal thickening.

Clinical Features

CTIN occurs only after prolonged and regular use of analgesics. In analgesic nephropathy, the degree of damage is related to the total dose of the drug consumed;

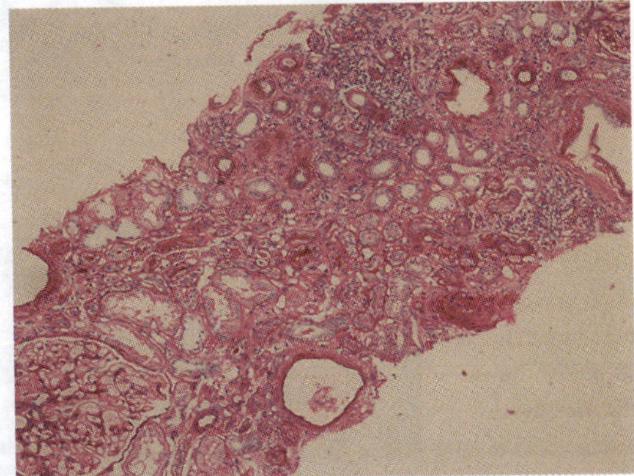

Fig. 184.2: Kidney biopsy (PAS stain × 100) showing simplification of tubular epithelium, tubular atrophy, loss of tubules and interstitial fibrosis in a case of CTIN

Abbreviation: PAS = Periodic acid–Schiff

combinations of drugs carry a higher risk. The total cumulative dose of acetaminophen combination needed to cause CTIN may be over 10–12 kg. Many patients remain asymptomatic until the renal functions worsen and patient is in cystic kidney disease stage 5. Hypertension and edema are usually absent or mild even with advanced renal failure. These subjects have normal urine output or have polyuria due to loss of concentrating ability of the kidneys. Nocturia occurs in some patients. Urine shows mild proteinuria with hematuria and leukocyturia. Defective urinary acidification and concentration may be present.

Management

Conservative management of chronic kidney disease (CKD) is advocated for all patients. In addition to withdrawing the offending drug or exposure to toxin, specific treatment should be given depending on the cause.

For example, obstruction to the urinary tract should be relieved. Infections should be treated with appropriate drugs, hematological and immunological diseases should be treated appropriately.

CYSTIC DISEASES OF THE KIDNEYS

Cysts are fluid-filled cavities lined by epithelium. They may be single or multiple, simple or complicated. Cystic diseases of the kidney can be either congenital or acquired.

Congenital Cystic Diseases

Polycystic Kidney Disease

It is an inherited disorder, characterized by the presence of innumerable cysts of varying sizes in both kidneys. This disorder is of two distinct types, which are clearly distinguishable by their mode of inheritance, pathological appearance and clinical presentation.

- Autosomal dominant polycystic kidney disease (ADPKD)
- Autosomal recessive polycystic kidney disease (ARPKD).

Autosomal dominant PKD

This disorder is characterized by the presence of numerous cysts in kidneys as well as other organs like liver, spleen, pancreas, arachnoid, epididymis and seminal vesicles. In the kidney, the cysts develop from different segments of the nephron. The two types of ADPKD are regulated by two different genes: PKD 1 gene on chromosome 16 and PKD 2 gene on chromosome 4. PKD 1 is associated with more severe disease and leads to end-stage renal disease (ESRD) earlier than PKD 2 (the mean age of occurrence of ESRD is 55 years in PKD 1, while it is 74 years in PKD 2).

Clinical features

These patients are often asymptomatic till the fourth or fifth decade of life. The usual presentation is with hypertension, abdominal discomfort, incidentally detected abdominal mass on ultrasonography (USG) or hematuria. Renal stones occur in 20% of cases. Complications known to occur in this disease include urinary tract infections (UTI), cyst infections, cyst hemorrhage, renal calculi (commonly uric acid) and malignancy. Saccular aneurysms of anterior cerebral circulation occur in 10% of patients and can cause subarachnoid hemorrhage. Colonic diverticulia, aortic root dilatation and mitral valve prolapse are the other associated abnormalities encountered in ADPKD. The renal cysts increase in size very slowly over many years, and the renal functions deteriorate gradually.

Pathologically, the kidneys are enlarged and can reach large sizes; the surface is riddled with innumerable cysts of varying sizes (Figs 184.3A and B).

The diagnosis is confirmed by ultrasonogram which shows enlarged kidneys with multiple cysts in both kidneys. The number of cysts increases with age of the patients. The presence of cysts in liver, pancreas and epididymis support the diagnosis of ADPKD. CT scan and magnetic resonance imaging (MRI) are more sensitive to identify small cysts but often not necessary for diagnosis if diagnosis can be confirmed by USG. A minimum of 6 cysts in each kidney should be visible on ultrasonogram.

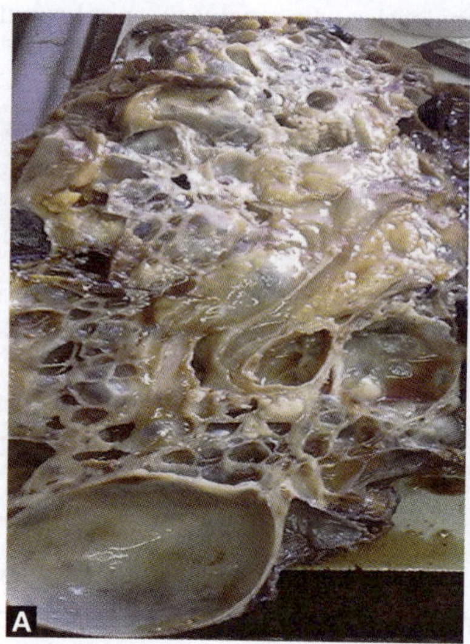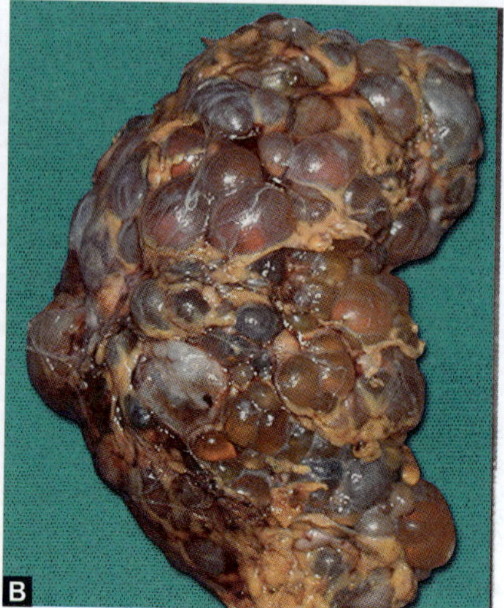

Figs 184.3A and B: A. Enlarged kidney with the surface showing multiple cysts of varying sizes [autosomal dominant polycystic kidney disease (ADPKD)]; **B.** Cut surface of the kidney (ADPKD) showing multiple cysts of varying sizes

Treatment

The treatment consists of good control of hypertension and regular monitoring of renal functions.

Urinary infections need to be treated promptly. Cyst infection is difficult to treat because of poor penetration of antibiotics into the cysts. Lipophilic drugs are more effective; quinolones and trimethoprim-sulfamethoxazole (TMP-SMX) can achieve good concentrations in the cyst fluid.

Pain may occur caused by stretching of the renal capsule by the enlarging cysts, cyst hemorrhage or cyst infection. Analgesics may be required to treat the pain. Cyst hemorrhage needs conservative management in most cases with bed rest, analgesics and good hydration. CT angiogram and segmental arterial embolization may be needed in severe cases.

Drugs like octreotide (somatostatin analogue), vasopressin receptor antagonist—tolvaptan and mammalian target of rapamycin (mTOR) inhibitor—sirolimus are being tried to retard growth of cysts and progression of the disease. V2 receptor antagonists reduce cyclic adenosine monophosphate (cAMP) in collecting ducts and reduce the enlargement of cysts. mTOR inhibitors are antiproliferative agents and decreases the enlargement of cysts. These drugs are in various phases of clinical trials only.

Autosomal recessive PKD

This condition is inherited as an autosomal recessive trait and is encoded by a gene on chromosome 6. This large gene is called PKHD 1 and codes for a protein called fibrocystin or polyductin. Varying degrees of renal collecting duct dilatation, biliary ductal atresia with hepatic fibrosis and pulmonary hypoplasia occur due to the defective gene.

Clinical features

The manifestations occur even during the neonatal period. The most severely affected fetuses have enlarged echogenic kidneys with pulmonary hypoplasia *in utero*. About 50% of affected neonates die very early due to pulmonary hypoplasia. Majority of those who do not have significant pulmonary involvement, develop hypertension and renal insufficiency in infancy or early childhood. Many develop hepatic fibrosis and liver failure. A few would reach early adult life and develop ESRD.

USG reveals enlarged echogenic kidneys. Cysts are not usually seen on ultrasonogram. Microscopic examination of kidneys show fusiform dilatation of collecting ducts seen perpendicular to the renal capsule. **Treatment** consists of treatment of hypertension and other supportive measures. Children who reach ESRD can be treated with renal replacement therapy (RRT). ARPKD has a very poor prognosis.

Medullary Cystic Kidney Disease (MCKD)

It is an autosomal dominant disorder which presents in adolescents and young adults with polyuria, polydypsia and urinary sodium wasting. Two types of MCKD have been identified by genetic analysis: MCKD1 and MCKD2. MCKD1 is genetically heterogenous disorder. In MCKD2, the mutated gene is called UMOD and it codes for uromodulin (Tamm-Horsfall protein). More than 30 UMOD mutations have been described.

Pathologically, kidneys show cysts at corticomedullary junction, irregular thickening of tubular basement membrane, tubular atrophy and interstitial fibrosis. Genetic testing for UMOD mutation is now available.

Clinical features include the presence of renal enlargement, hyperuricemia, gout and progressive renal failure during adulthood or old age. MCKD1 leads to ESRD by 60 years of age, whereas it leads to ESRD by 30 years in MCKD2.

Diagnosis can be made from family history with an autosomal dominant mode of inheritance, association of hyperuricemia and gout in a patient who has medullary cysts on ultrasonogram. There is no specific treatment for this condition, which progresses rather slowly. Conservative treatment and RRT at the appropriate time are undertaken.

Nephronophthisis

This autosomal recessive disorder can present in infancy, childhood or adolescence. It is genetically heterogenous and 10 genes [nephronophthisis (NPHP)] have been identified; NPHP 1 mutation accounts for about 21% of cases. NPHP 2 and NPHP 3 lead on to renal failure between birth and 3 years of age (infantile NPMP). In over 70% of patients, no mutation is identified indicating that many more genes remain to be discovered. The other mutations are associated with additional extrarenal manifestations.

Clinical features

Patients present with polyuria, polydypsia, volume depletion and metabolic acidosis. Hypertension is common in infantile form, but not in juvenile form. Sodium wasting is common; proteinuria is mild or absent and urine sediment is normal. Progressive kidney failure leading to growth retardation, anemia and ESRD occurs by 5 years of age in infantile form, by 13 years in juvenile form and by 19 years in adolescent form. The extrarenal manifestations reported are retinitis pigmentosa, amaurosis, oculomotor apraxia, cerebellar ataxia, mental retardation, hepatic fibrosis, situs inversus of the heart and ventricular septal defect (VSD).

The kidneys are small with a granular surface in the infantile form. On cut section, kidneys show thinning of the cortex and medulla with a variable number of small cysts of distal tubule and collecting tubule origin. Renal histopathology shows disintegrated tubular basement membranes, tubular atrophy, cyst formation and a sclerosing tubulointerstitial nephropathy. The kidneys are often enlarged and cystic in the infantile form.

Diagnosis

USG and excretory urography do not detect cysts in this condition, as the cysts are small. Even CT and MRI may fail to detect these corticomedullary and medullary cysts at times.

Treatment

No specific treatment is available. As they usually have sodium wasting, salt intake needs to be liberal. When they develop renal failure, conservative treatment followed by RRT may be undertaken at the appropriate time.

Multicystic Dysplastic Kidneys (MDK)

This is the most common cause of bilateral cystic disease in the neonate and presents as an abdominal mass in infancy. Often it is diagnosed *in utero* during antenatal screening by USG. The disease can be unilateral or bilateral; it is more often unilateral and is more common in males.

Bilateral multicystic dysplastic kidney results in oligohydramnios and is incompatible with life. Unilateral MDK may be diagnosed on evaluation of a renal mass in infancy or may go undetected until later in life; this condition is often associated with urinary tract malformation like pelviureteric junction obstruction and vesicoureteric reflux of the contralateral kidney. Gradually, the affected kidney involutes and becomes small.

Diagnosis is often made by ultrasonogram. There is no specific treatment for this condition.

Medullary Sponge Kidney (MSK)

It is characterized by dilatation of collecting ducts and cyst formation confined to medullary pyramids, which gives the renal medulla a spongy appearance. This condition has been reported with primary hyperparathyroidism, congenital hemihypertrophy and Ehlers-Danlos syndrome. A clear genetic basis has not been established in this condition.

It is a benign disorder and may be undetected in many subjects. The precalyceal parts of collecting ducts of one or more renal papillae in one or both kidneys are dilated. Small calculi can form in these dilated collecting ducts. Although many patients are asymptomatic, some present with hematuria, renal colic or mild form of renal tubular acidosis (RTA). These patients seldom progress to ESRD.

Diagnosis is made by finding of a cluster of tiny calculi in the papillary region on plain radiographs of the abdomen. Excretory urogram shows retention of the contrast dye in the dilated papillary collecting ducts giving a paint brush or bunch of grapes appearance.

There is no specific treatment for MSK. Liberal fluid intake reduces the risk of stone formation. *Treatment* of nephrolithiasis and UTI are indicated in patients who develop these problems.

Miscellaneous Cystic Disorders

Other inherited disorders associated with renal cysts: Renal cysts are seen in tuberous sclerosis, Von Hippel-Lindau syndrome, Orofacial digital syndrome, Joubert syndrome, Meckel-Gruber syndrome, Bardet-Biedl syndrome, Alstrom syndrome and some other disorders.

Acquired Renal Cystic Disorders

Acquired Cystic Kidney Disease (ACKD)

Cysts distributed in both cortex and medulla occur in patients with chronic kidney disease and is termed as ACKD. The incidence of these acquired cysts increase with severity of renal failure and the duration on dialysis; over 90% of patients who are on dialysis for more than 8 years have ACKD; it is not related to the cause of CKD, age, race or type of dialysis. These cysts can regress after renal transplantation and can appear in the grafts with chronic graft dysfunction.

Hyperplasia of the tubular epithelium induced by the uremic state seems to lead on to cyst formation. Although there are multiple cysts, the kidney size is usually small or normal (unlike ADPKD, where kidneys are invariably enlarged). Majority of these patients do not have symptoms related to the cysts; a few of them develop hematuria or rise in hematocrit and some develop renal tumors. The incidence of renal cell carcinoma is more in those who have ACKD.

Diagnosis can be made by ultrasonogram. CT scan or MRI would be needed to identify a renal tumor. There is no specific treatment for ACKD. If malignancy is considered or patient has severe hematuria, nephrectomy would have to be considered.

Simple Cysts of the Kidney

Single or multiple cysts filled with a fluid chemically similar to an ultrafiltrate of plasma is a common finding in older people. They are rare in children and increases in frequency with age (seen in 50% of persons by 50 years of age).

Simple cysts are thin walled, lined by one layer of epithelial cells and grow very slowly; some can be trabeculated. These are usually in the cortex, can distort renal contour and do not communicate with renal pelvis. Diverticula from distal convoluted and collecting tubules develop and subsequently, get detached leading on to formation of cysts. Calcification is uncommon in simple cysts.

Most patients are asymptomatic. Large cysts can cause abdominal discomfort or pain; rarely hematuria or infection of the cysts may occur. Ultrasonogram helps us to diagnose this condition; more details of the cyst can be ascertained by CT scan or MRI. These patients need only follow-up and no treatment is needed in most cases.

Renal Cystic Neoplasms

Tumors like cystic renal cell carcinoma, multilocular cystic neoplasms, cystic nephroblastomas and mixed epithelial and stromal tumors can also present as cysts in the kidneys.

Renal Cell Carcinoma (RCC)

It is more common in males than females. Factors which may predispose or increase the risk of RCC include ADPKD, blood group A, von Hippel Lindau's disease, exposure to toxins like N-nitroso compounds, asbestos, metals like cadmium and lead, tobacco smoking and phenacetin. The most frequent cytogenetic finding is deletion in the short arm of chromosome number 3. The most frequent renal neoplasm is the clear cell type with clear cytoplasm and small nuclei.

Renal adenocarcinoma is often referred to as *internist's tumor*, because the patients may present with some systemic symptoms. Hematuria, flank pain and palpable mass form the triad of manifestations, but all these three together are found only in 16% of patients. The other presenting features could be fever, hypertension, anemia, increased erythrocyte sedimentation rate (ESR), erythrocytosis and thrombocytosis.

Diagnosis is suspected by the finding of a solid mass or a cystic lesion with internal echoes and lack of acoustic enhancement of the back wall of the lesion. CT scan and MRI help in distinguishing simple cysts from RCC as well as in detecting extension of the tumor into the renal vein or presence of lymph nodes.

Treatment

Surgical removal of the kidney with the tumor with regional lymph nodes, perinephric fat and adrenal gland (radical nephrectomy) is considered to be the treatment of choice. In recent times, nephron sparing surgery in the form of partial nephrectomy has been advocated, if feasible, in order to retain as much kidney tissue as possible. Radiotherapy may be beneficial as an adjuvant to surgical treatment, in cases of solitary metastasis or for control of severe pain or hemorrhage due to tumor growth. Chemotherapy has a very limited role in treatment of RCC.

FUNCTIONAL DISORDERS OF RENAL TUBULES

The functional disorders of the renal tubules can be either inherited or acquired. These conditions could affect the proximal tubule, loop of Henle, distal tubule or collecting duct. The functional disorder could be either an isolated (single) transport defect in a particular part of the nephron or could be a part of a multiple transport disorder. These disorders can be classified as given in Box 184.3.

Some of the important, relatively more common disorders are described further.

Renal Fanconi's Syndrome

In this condition, there is a generalized dysfunction of the proximal renal tubule, resulting in phosphate,

---

Box 184.3: Functional disorders of renal tubules

Disorders affecting the proximal tubules

Disorders wherein multiple transport mechanisms are affected: Fanconi syndrome

Disorders primarily affecting a single transport mechanism
- **Aminoacidurias**
  - Cystinuria
  - Lysinuria
  - Hartnup's disease
  - Iminoglycinuria
  - Dicarboxylic aminoaciduria
- **Phosphate transport disorders**
  - X-linked hypophosphatemic rickets
  - Autosomal dominant hypophosphatemic rickets
  - Autosomal recessive hypophosphatemic rickets
  - Hypophosphatemic rickets with hypercalcemia
- **Urate transport disorders:** Familial renal hypouricemia
- **Glucose transport disorders:** Renal glycosuria
- **Acid-base transport disorders:** Proximal renal tubular acidosis (type 2 renal tubular acidosis)
- **Magnesium transport disorders:** Familial hypomagnesemia

Disorders affecting the loop of Henle

Ion transport disorders: Bartter syndrome

Disorders affecting the distal tubule

Acid base transport disorders: Distal renal tubular acidosis (type 1 renal tubular acidosis)
Ion transport disorders: Gitelman syndrome

Disorders affecting the collecting duct

Water transport disorders: Nephrogenic diabetes insipidus
Ion transport disorders
- Liddle syndrome
- Pseudohypoaldosteronism type 1 and type 2

Box 184.4: Causes of renal Fanconi syndrome

Inherited
- Idiopathic (autosomal dominant)
- Dent's disease
- Cystinosis
- Tyrosinemia
- Galactosemia
- Glycogen storage disease type 1
- Wilson's disease
- Lowe's syndrome
- Hereditary fructose intolerance

Acquired
- Multiple myeloma and other paraproteinemias
- **Heavy metals**
  - Mercury
  - Lead
  - Cadmium
  - Platinum

Drugs
- Cisplatin
- Ifosfamide
- 6-mercaptopurine
- Aminoglycosides
- Outdated tetracyclines
- Valproate

Chemicals
- Paraquat
- Toluene
- Lysol

---

glucose, amino acids, urate and bicarbonate wasting in the urine. Fanconi's syndrome in children is usually due to an inherited disorder, while it is acquired in adults. The causes are given in Box 184.4.

Clinical Features

Polyuria, growth retardation, rickets or osteomalacia and metabolic acidosis are the usual manifestations. In addition, the patient can have clinical features of the underlying cause of the Fanconi syndrome.

Diagnosis

Glycosuria, low molecular weight proteinuria, aminoaciduria, renal sodium, potassium, uric acid and phosphate wasting with hypokalemia, hypouricemia and hypophosphatemia and normal anion gap metabolic acidosis are the features.

The *treatment* includes treatment of the primary cause (if possible) and other supportive and symptomatic measures depending on the clinical features and the laboratory abnormalities. Alkali supplementation is the mainstay of treatment.

Renal Glycosuria

Familial renal glycosuria is an inherited benign condition, in which patient has glucosuria in the absence of hyperglycemia. It appears to be inherited as an autosomal recessive trait and has an incidence of 1 in 20,000 population. Mutations in the gene SLC5A2 on 16 chromosome, which codes for the glucose transporter in the proximal renal tubule, known as sodium-glucose co-transporter 2 (SGLT2) inhibitors is responsible for this condition. This can occur as an isolated condition or as part of Fanconi syndrome.

Diagnosis

Presence of excessive glucose in urine when the blood sugars are normal points to this diagnosis. No specific treatment is needed; these patients do not have a risk of developing DM.

Renal Tubular Acidosis (RTA)

A group of disorders characterized by hyperchloremic (normal anion gap) metabolic acidosis due to abnormal urine acidification; an inappropriately high urine pH, bicarbonaturia and reduced net acid excretion are the cardinal features.

Type 1 (Distal) RTA

Patients with distal RTA are unable to acidify their urine, either under basal conditions or in response to metabolic acidosis. The defect can be either in hydrogen ion secretion in the distal tubule or an increased back leak of secreted [H$^+$] ions in the distal tubule. The causes are shown in Box 184.5.

Clinical features

The hereditary form manifests in children and the acquired form can present in both adults and children. The dominant features are those involving bone and skeletal muscle. Impaired skeletal growth and rickets is common in children. Adults may have osteomalacia. Skeletal muscle weakness and paralysis (due to hypokalemia) are dominant symptoms. Nephrolithiasis, nephrocalcinosis and polyuria are common manifestations.

Diagnosis

Presence of hyperchloremic (normal anion gap) metabolic acidosis, urine pH more than 6.0, hypokalemia, nephrocalcinosis, nephrolithiasis and features of rickets strongly suggest the diagnosis of distal RTA.

Box 184.5: Causes of distal renal tubular acidosis

Hereditary
Acquired
- ***Disorders associated with hypercalcemia and nephrocalcinosis***
  - Hyperparathyroidism
  - Vitamin D intoxication
  - Hyperthyroidism
  - Idiopathic hypercalciuria
  - Milk-alkali syndrome
  - Medullary sponge kidney
  - Fabry's disease
  - Wilson's disease
- ***Drugs or toxins***
  - Amphotericin B
  - Ifosfamide
  - Foscarnet
  - Toluene
- ***Immune disorders***
  - Cryoglobulinemia
  - Sjogren's syndrome
  - Systemic lupus erythematosus (SLE)
  - Hypergammaglobulinemia
  - Primary biliary cirrhosis
  - Human immunodeficiency virus (HIV) nephropathy
- ***Genetically transmitted diseases***
  - Ehlers-Danlos syndrome
  - Sickle-cell anemia
  - Osteopetrosis
  - Medullary cystic disease

Treatment

In addition to treatment of any underlying disorder, alkali therapy with Shohl's solution containing sodium citrate with citric acid as buffer which gives 1 mmol of bicarbonate per mL can be used. Correction of the acidosis in patients with distal RTA restores normal growth in children and diminishes the occurrence of hypokalemia, nephrocalcinosis, calcium stones and possibly osteoporosis. The goal of bicarbonate therapy for patients with distal RTA is a relatively normal serum bicarbonate concentration (22–24 mEq/L). The dose and choice of the specific alkali salt depend upon the patient's age and the serum potassium concentration. Adults are treated with 1 to 2 mEq/kg of sodium bicarbonate or Shohl's solution. Children often require larger doses of alkali than adults; often doses of 4–8 mEq/kg/day, given as divided doses, may be required because bicarbonate losses may be higher than in adults. Moreover, the rapidly growing skeleton of children and adolescents generates an additional acid load.

If persistent hypokalemia is present, alkalinizing potassium salts, such as potassium citrate, alone or combined with sodium citrate (Polycitra) are used. They are contraindicated in the hyperkalemic form of type IV distal RTA.

Type 2 (Proximal) RTA

There is a defective reabsorption of bicarbonate in the proximal convoluted tubule, leading on to a large quantity of bicarbonate being delivered to the distal tubule. The high load delivered to distal tubule exceeds the capacity of the distal tubule to reabsorb bicarbonate and results in bicarbonate loss in the urine. This leads on to hyperchloremic metabolic acidosis with varying degrees of sodium and potassium wasting. This can occur as an isolated disorder of the proximal tubule or as part of a generalized proximal tubular dysfunction (Fanconi syndrome). The causes of type 2 RTA are given in Box 184.6.

Clinical features

The primary form occurs more in children while the secondary form is more in adults. The presentation in neonates includes failure to thrive, increased thirst, polyuria, vomiting and volume depletion. Rickets is often present if RTA is part of Fanconi's syndrome. In secondary forms of RTA, clinical features of the primary disease would also be present.

Diagnosis

Presence of hyperchloremic metabolic acidosis, hypokalemia, urine pH below 5.5, significant bicarbonaturia, absence of nephrocalcinosis or nephrolithiasis and features of Fanconi' syndrome point towards diagnosis

---

Box 184.6: Causes of type 2 renal tubular acidosis

Isolated proximal RTA
- Hereditary form
- Drugs
  - Acetazolamide
  - Sulfanilamide

As a part of Fanconi syndrome
(All causes mentioned under Fanconi syndrome in Box 184.4)

Table 184.1: Summary of findings in different types of renal tubular acidosis

Type	Renal defect	Plasma K+	Proximal acidification (HCO$_3^-$ reabsorption)	Distal acidification (minimum urinary pH)	Urinary ammonium plus titratable acid excretion	Daily bicarbonate needs
Classical distal RTA	Decreased distal pH gradient	Decreased	Normal	>5.5	Decreased	<4 mmol per kg
Proximal RTA	Decreased proximal acidification	Decreased	Decreased	<5.5	Normal	>4 mmol per kg
Generalized distal RTA	Decreased aldosterone action	Normal	Normal	<5.5	Decreased	<4 mmol per kg
Glomerular insufficiency	Decreased ammonia production when GFR 20–30 mL/min	Normal	Normal	<5.5	Decreased	1–3 mmol per kg

Abbreviations: RTA = Renal tubular acidosis; GFR = Glomerular filtration rate

of type 2 RTA. If renal phosphate loss is also significant, associated rickets will be present.

Treatment

Treatment of patients with proximal RTA includes correction of acidemia and in some patients, hypophosphatemia. Correction of the acidemia in patients with proximal RTA results in improvement of skeletal growth and healing of rickets and osteomalacia in children and adults. Treatment of acidemia is more difficult in proximal RTA because raising the serum bicarbonate concentration increases bicarbonate loss in urine. This is because the exogenous bicarbonate increases the filtered bicarbonate load above the reduced reabsorptive capacity. This results in bicarbonaturia and associated increase in urinary potassium losses. Patients with proximal RTA may require up to 10–15 mEq/kg/day of alkali to compensate for the increased urinary bicarbonate losses. Alkali replacement must be given preferably as the potassium salt (usually potassium citrate). If the patient cannot tolerate large doses of alkali supplements, use of a thiazide diuretic under careful monitoring may help to enhance sodium and bicarbonate reabsorption by causing mild volume depletion.

Type 3 RTA

It is a transient form which was reported in newborns. It is no longer considered to be a clear entity.

Type 4 RTA

It is a dysfunction of the distal nephron wherein the process of acidification is impaired due to mineralocorticoid deficiency or resistance. This is frequent in patients with diabetic nephropathy. Hyperchloremic metabolic acidosis, hyperkalemia, decreased ammonium excretion in the urine and a urine pH of less than 5.5 are the characteristic features (Table 184.1).

Bartter Syndrome

This disorder which usually occurs in childhood is characterized by hypokalemia, metabolic acidosis, low or normal blood pressure (BP) (caused by tubular wasting of sodium, chloride and potassium). The syndrome consists of a set of closely related disorders resulting from mutations affecting any one of the four transport proteins in the thick ascending limb of loop of Henle. The features closely mimic a state induced by chronic ingestion of a loop diuretic.

Polydypsia, craving for salt, vomiting, growth retardation, low BP and hypokalemia are the common manifestations. ***Treatment*** includes correction of fluid and electrolyte disturbances, potassium supplementation, use of potassium sparing diuretics and prostaglandin synthetase inhibitor like indomethacin.

Gitelman Syndrome

Gitelman syndrome, which usually presents in adolescents and young adults, is due to mutation in thiazide sensitive sodium chloride cotransporter in the distal convoluted tubule. Presence of hypomagnesemia and hypocalcemia distinguishes this from Bartter's syndrome. ***Treatment*** consists of potassium and magnesium supplementation with liberal salt intake.

Nephrogenic Diabetes Insipidus

Water conservation by the kidney is regulated by the hormone arginine vasopressin (AVP) released from neurohypophysis. AVP or the antidiuretic hormone (ADH) acts on the vasopressin receptor in the collecting ducts of the nephron; this leads on to exocytic insertion of specific water channels (aquaporins) into the luminal membrane of collecting duct cells, resulting in absorption of water from the tubular lumen. Thus, AVP conserves water.

In nephrogenic diabetes insipidus, an X-linked dominant condition, the collecting duct cells are unable to reabsorb water, even though serum AVP levels are normal or elevated. This occurs because of loss-of-function mutations in V2 receptors. The child presents with irritability, polyuria, dehydration, hypernatremia and often mental retardation. ***Complications*** can be prevented to a large extent by adequate water intake. Use of thiazides or indomethacin would reduce the urine output (UO) and give symptomatic relief.

Textbook of Medicine

CHAPTER
185

Urinary Tract Infection

Sreelatha M, Swaraj Sathyan

Chapter Summary

- Definitions
- Normal Host Defense Mechanisms of the Urinary Tract
- Clinical Syndromes of UTI
- Asymptomatic Bacteriuria
- Prostatitis
- UTI in Children
- Suppurative and Necrotizing Infections of Urinary Tract
- Genitourinary Tuberculosis
- Fungal Infections of the Urinary Tract

DEFINITIONS

Urinary tract infection (UTI) is defined as the presence and multiplication of bacteria or other microorganisms in the urine or genitourinary tissue which is normally sterile.

- ***Pyuria*** indicates presence of white blood cells (WBCs) in the urine, usually due to an inflammatory response of the urothelium to the bacteria, but does not always indicate UTI. More than one WBC per each high-power field (HPF) is considered abnormal.
- ***Bacteriuria*** is the presence of any bacteria in urine, and implies that these bacteria are from the urinary tract and are not contaminants (Normal urine is free of bacteria).
- ***Significant bacteriuria*** is defined as the presence of more than or equal to 10^5 colony forming units (CFU) of same organism per mL of urine (Kass criteria) in urine culture. It also depends on method of urine collection; explained later in this chapter.
- ***Asymptomatic bacteriuria*** is the presence of significant bacteriuria in the absence of urinary tract symptoms.
- ***Cystitis*** is a clinical syndrome of dysuria, urgency, frequency and sometimes suprapubic pain and often associated with pyuria.
- ***Acute pyelonephritis*** is a clinical syndrome of fever, chills and flank pain in the presence of pyuria and bacteriuria, specific for the acute bacterial infection of the kidney.
- ***Uncomplicated UTI*** is infection in an otherwise healthy person with a structurally and functionally normal urinary tract.
- ***Complicated UTI*** is infection occurring in a patient with a structurally or functionally abnormal urinary tract or in patients who are susceptible to infection like diabetics or immune-compromised individuals.
- ***Recurrent UTI*** is defined as at least 3 episodes of uncomplicated UTI in women, documented by urine culture over past 12 months.
- ***Relapse*** is recurrence of UTI with same organism within 3 weeks after treatment of previous episode.

Table 185.1: Differences between asymptomatic bacteriuria and symptomatic UTI

Asymptomatic bacteriuria	*Symptomatic (disease)*

• Presence of bacteriuria ($>10^5$/mL or two occasions in females and on one occasion in males) indicating UTI but without symptoms
• Common in pregnancy
• Occurs in the absence of symptoms
• Does not usually require treatment except in pregnant women
	• Includes
	  ▪ Acute urethritis
	  ▪ Acute cystitis
	  ▪ Acute prostatitis
	  ▪ Acute pyelonephritis
	  ▪ Septicemia with septic shock
	• Requires antimicrobial therapy

Both shows the presence of bacteria in the urinary tract, usually WBCs and inflammatory cytokines in the urine.

Abbreviation: UTI = Urinary tract infection

- ***Reinfection*** is recurrence of UTI with a different organism after 7–10 days.

Differences between asymptomatic bacteriuria and symptomatic UTI is shown in Table 185.1.

NORMAL HOST DEFENSE MECHANISMS OF THE URINARY TRACT

In spite of urine being a good nutrient medium for bacteria, normally the urinary tract is sterile due to the presence of various defense mechanisms (Table 185.2).

Role of Urine Culture

Urine culture is required for confirmation of diagnosis, identification of the organism and understanding the sensitivity to antibiotics, thereby guiding treatment. Urine specimen for culture should be obtained before initiation of antibiotic therapy by a clean catch midstream voided sample in both men and women and sent promptly to

Table 185.2: Normal defense mechanisms of the urinary tract

Anatomy of urinary tract	Unobstructed flow of urine avoids stasis
Normal microbial flora of distal urethra	
Physical properties of urine	Acidic pH, osmolality
Urine proteins	• Tamm-Horsfall protein, immunoglobulins • Lactoferrin, lipocalin, defensins
Inflammatory cells in urine	Polymorphs
Inflammatory molecules in urine	Cytokines, chemokines in prostatic secretions
Uroepithelium	Mucopolysaccharides, glycosaminoglycans

laboratory. If there is delay, refrigeration at 4°C is indicated to prevent multiplication of contaminants at room temperature. For those, in whom collection of clean catch voided sample is difficult, in-and-out catheterization for collection of urine or suprapubic aspiration (especially for infants) can be attempted. If the patient has a short term indwelling catheter, then urine should be collected by puncture of the catheter port and in case of long term indwelling catheter, sample needs to be collected through a new catheter after replacing the old one, to avoid contamination of urine sample by the organism from the biofilm on the chronic catheter. The connection between the catheter and collecting bag must not be disconnected frequently and the drainage system must be maintained as a ***closed system.***

For the diagnosis of significant bacteriuria, the colony count in urine culture varies depending on the method of collection and clinical scenario. In asymptomatic women, 10^5 CFU is considered significant, whereas in symptomatic women and males, a colony count of 10^3 CFU is sufficient for diagnosis. If the sample is taken through in-and-out urethral catheterization, even a count of 10^2 CFU is sufficient. If any growth occurs in a suprapubically aspirated urine sample, it is significant.

Microbial Virulence Factors

Certain strains of *Escherichia coli* have some characteristics which offer them advantage for colonization and infection of urinary tract. The most important of these is the presence of P-fimbriae, which enables the bacteria to adhere to the uroepithelium. Once they adhere to the uroepithelium, they attach to the toll-like receptors (TLRs) on the cell membrane and initiate an inflammatory response. Types 1, S and Dr fimbriae, adhesins and toxins like hemolysin are other virulence factors. These virulence factors have been associated with increased risk of acute pyelonephritis, but the association with cystitis and asymptomatic bacteria is less certain.

Host Factors

Determinants of host response to infection with virulent organism include genetic polymorphisms of TLRs, interleukin (IL)-8 receptor, chemokine (C-X-C motif) receptor 1 (CXCR-1) and tumor necrosis factor (TNF) promoter. Activation of TLRs on the uroepithelial cells by organisms result in production of cytokines, especially IL-6 and IL-8 and recruitment of inflammatory cells.

CLINICAL SYNDROMES OF UTI

Acute Uncomplicated Cystitis in Women

Epidemiology

Around 60% of women experience at least 1 episode of uncomplicated cystitis in their lifetime and at least 10% of sexually active women may develop one episode every year. Uncomplicated cystitis is uncommon in men, in whom the incidence is less than 0.1% per year.

Microbiology

E. coli is responsible for 80–85% of cases, *Staphylococcus saprophyticus* is the second most common organism, isolated in 5–10% of episodes and *Klebsiella, Entero-coccus* and group B *Streptococci* are responsible for a small number of cases. Organisms that are responsible for sexually transmitted infections (STIs) like *Ureaplasma urealyticum*, *Gardnerella vaginalis* and *Mycoplasma hominis* are responsible for the remaining cases.

Risk Factors

Factors which predispose to infection in young women are migration of bacteria from periurethral region to the bladder during sexual intercourse and use of spermicidal jellies which alter the normal vaginal flora. Attachment of the bacteria to the mucosa is necessary for establishing infection. Genetic factors determine the number of receptors for pathogenic strains of *E. coli* and these receptors mediate attachment of the bacteria to the mucosa. Therefore, incidence of UTI is higher in some families. The symptoms are more due to the body's response to the infection rather than the infection itself.

Clinical Features

Acute onset of severe irritative bladder symptoms such as urgency, frequency, hesitancy, dysuria, strangury with or without gross hematuria form the classical manifestation of acute cystitis.

Investigations

Pyuria is usually present with acute cystitis but its absence does not rule out UTI, if characteristic clinical symptoms are present. Urine dipstick for nitrite detects the presence of bacteria in urine, but false-negative tests are obtained in infections with organisms which do not produce nitrate (e.g. Enterobacter) or when urine is very dilute. False-positive tests in urine for blood or urobilinogen may occur in pyuria.

Treatment

Antimicrobial therapy results in prompt resolution of symptoms and cure rates of around 90% is expected with first-line empirical agents. First-line agents for treatment of acute uncomplicated cystitis are trimethoprim-sulfamethoxazole (TMP-SMX) (160/800 mg twice daily for 3 days) and nitrofurantoin (100 mg twice daily for 5 days). Treatment can be empirically started with any one of these antibiotics. Other first-line agents are fosfomycin (3 g single dose) and pivmecillinam (500 mg twice daily for 5 days), but they are not available in most countries. If the use of these first-line agents are contraindicated, then 3-day course of fluoroquinolone (norfloxacin 400 mg twice daily, ciprofloxacin 250 mg twice daily, levofloxacin 250–500 mg once daily) or 7 day course of amoxicillin (500 mg three times daily), cephalexin (250–500 mg four times daily), cefixime (400 mg once daily) or doxycycline (100 mg twice daily) can all be employed. Fluoroquinolones are not recommended as first-line agents as their widespread use can result in emergence of resistance. Amoxicillin or cephalosporins are the preferred first-line agents in pregnancy as they are not teratogenic.

No further investigation is required for young women with characteristic clinical features, especially when there is appropriate response to antibiotic therapy. Reinfection occurring within a month of treatment of episode of

Table 185.3: Antibiotics which are indicated for prophylactic therapy

Antibiotics	Long-term low-dose regimens—given at bedtime	Postcoital (single-dose) regimens (single-dose before or just after sexual intercourse)
Nitrofurantoin	100 mg daily	50 mg or 100 mg
TMP/SMX	40/200 mg daily or alternate day	40/200 mg
Trimethoprim	100 mg daily	100 mg
Norfloxacin	200 mg alternate day	200 mg
Cephalexin	500 mg daily	250 mg
Ciprofloxacin	125 mg daily	125 mg

Abbreviation: TMP-SMX = Trimethoprim sulfamethoxazole

cystitis, with organism of same strain as the previous episode, is usually due to failure of antibiotic therapy to eliminate the organism from gut or vaginal reservoir.

Recurrent Acute Cystitis

It is common in women. In women who experience more than 2 episodes in 6 months, prophylactic antibiotic therapy is indicated. It is administered either as long term low dose continuous regimen or as postcoital single dose regimen. Initially, prophylactic antibiotic is given for 6–12 months and in those who experience recurrence after stopping of antibiotic (~50%), it is continued for up to 2 years. Antibiotics which are indicated for prophylactic therapy are mentioned in (Table 185.3).

Nonantimicrobial interventions which may reduce the risk of recurrent UTI are avoidance of use of spermicidal jelly, oral or vaginal probiotics to restore normal vaginal flora and use of estrogen replacement for postmenopausal women. Rarely, postmenopausal women with estrogen deficiency develop urethral strictures and this has to be identified and corrected. Perineal and perianal cleaning should be explained clearly and it helps to reduce frequency of recurrence.

Acute Nonobstructive Pyelonephritis

Clinical Features

It is less common compared to acute cystitis but is often associated with more severe clinical manifestations. The classical clinical presentation is with fever, chills, flank pain and loin tenderness. Lower urinary symptoms similar to that seen with acute cystitis may or may not be present. Severe manifestations such as sepsis are uncommon in uncomplicated pyelonephritis. Highest incidence is seen in young, sexually active women. Pregnant women are at particularly high-risk for development of acute pyelonephritis.

Microbiology

E. coli is responsible for around 90% of acute nonobstructed pyelonephritis. The infecting strains of *E. coli* express P fimbriae, adhesion to upper urinary tract occurs and initiates the inflammatory damage.

Risk Factors

The genetic and behavioral risk factors are similar to that for acute cystitis. Acute pyelonephritis may occur by hematogenous spread of infection.

Investigations

Diagnosis is confirmed by a urine culture in the presence of characteristic clinical syndrome. Urine sample for culture should be obtained prior to initiation of antibiotic. Significant bacteriuria may be detected in up to 95% of cases. Blood culture may grow organisms in up to 25% of cases, but does not give additional information. In most of the cases, bacteremia is due to spread from the urinary tract. Rarely, hematogenous seeding of *Staphylococcus aureus* results in renal microabscesses as well as *Staphylococcal bacteriuria*. Improper drainage or squeezing of skin staphylococcal skin abscesses may lead to bacteremia and localization in tissues including kidney. Total leukocyte count (TLC), C-reactive protein (CRP) and procalcitonin levels are usually elevated and leukocyte count can be used to monitor response to therapy. Serum creatinine may be elevated in some cases.

Diagnostic imaging is not routinely indicated in cases of mild to moderately severe pyelonephritis, who respond promptly to antibiotic therapy. Indications for diagnostic imaging are severe clinical presentation, lack of improvement within 48–72 hours of starting parenteral antibiotic therapy, total resistance to initial treatment or early recurrence on stopping antibiotic treatment. The aim is to rule out the presence of obstruction, infected calculi or abscesses. Initial imaging modality of choice is ultrasonography (USG), which in cases of uncomplicated pyelonephritis reveals only bulky or edematous single or both kidneys. Computed tomography (CT) and magnetic resonance imaging (MRI) are more sensitive and specific, but reserved for complicated UTI where further intervention is planned.

Treatment

Uncomplicated pyelonephritis can be treated on an outpatient basis in a majority of women. Hospitalization is indicated in pyelonephritis complicating pregnancy, inability to take oral medications, poor gastrointestinal (GI) absorption, hemodynamic instability, when complicated by sepsis or when abscess formation is suspected. Treatment include symptomatic management for pain, fever, nausea and vomiting, supportive management to correct dehydration and hypotension, and definitive treatment in the form of antibiotic therapy. Empirical antibiotic should be promptly initiated after obtaining urine sample for culture and sensitivity study. In those patients, for whom administration of oral antibiotics is feasible, treatment should be started with oral ciprofloxacin (500 mg twice daily) or levofloxacin (750 mg once daily) and response assessed at 48–72 hours. If there is resolution of symptoms, then same is continued to complete course of 7 days for ciprofloxacin and 7 days for levofloxacin. If the response is unsatisfactory, then alternative antibiotics are chosen based on urine culture and sensitivity report. If the patient shows signs of toxicity, then parenteral antibiotic is indicated, ciprofloxacin or levofloxacin being the preferred initial antibiotic. Ceftriaxone is the preferred initial first-line agent for acute pyelonephritis in pregnant women. After 3–4 days of parenteral antibiotics, if response is satisfactory, then treatment can be continued

Table 185.4: Antibacterial drug regimen for pyelonephritis

Oral	Parenteral
• Ciprofloxacin: 500 mg twice daily × 7 days • Levofloxacin: 750 mg daily × 5 days	• Ciprofloxacin: 400 mg q12h × 7 days • Levofloxacin: 750 mg q24h × 5 days • Gentamicin: 3–5 mg/kg q24h ± • Ampicillin: 1 g q4–6h • Ceftriaxone: 1–2 g q24h • Cefotaxime: 1 g q8h

Table 185.5: Alternate agents used in pyelonephritis

Oral	Parenteral
• TMP/SMX: 160/800 mg bid × 7–14 days • Amoxicillin: 500 mg po tid × 14 days • Cephalexin: 500 mg qid × 14 days • Cefuroxime: 500 mg bid × 14 days • Cefixime: 400 mg od × 14 days	• Ertapenem: 1 g od • Meropenem: 500 mg q6h • Piperacillin/tazobactam: 3.375 g q6h

Abbreviation: TMP-SMX = Trimethoprim sulfamethoxazole

with oral antibiotic to complete the course of 7–14 days (Table 185.4). Alternate agents which can be used, are mentioned in (Table 185.5). Prophylactic antibiotic regimen to prevent recurrent uncomplicated pyelonephritis is similar to that for recurrent cystitis.

Complicated Urinary Tract Infection

Complicated UTI is infectious in a patient with a structurally or functionally abnormal urinary tract or in patients susceptible to infection such as diabetics or immunocompromised individuals.

Predisposing Factors

The abnormalities of urinary tract that predispose to complicated UTI are mentioned in (Table 185.6).

Clinical Features

The clinical presentation of complicated UTI can be varied. It may present as cystitis, pyelonephritis or as sepsis and septic shock. In patients with indwelling catheters, urologic devices and in those with neurogenic bladder, the symptoms and signs may not be classical. Compared to uncomplicated UTI, complicated UTI is associated with higher incidence not only of bacteremia, sepsis and renal function impairment, but also with suppurative complications like perinephric abscess.

Table 185.6: Predisposing factors lead to complicated UTI

Abnormalities	Complications
Obstruction	Stone, strictures, tumor, prostate, hypertrophy, pelviureteric junction (PUJ) obstruction
Neurologic	Neurogenic bladder
Urologic abnormalities	Cystocele, vesicoureterial reflux, urologic procedures
Urologic devices	Long indwelling catheter, ureteric stent, nephrostomy tube
Congenital abnormalities	Posterior urethral valves, nephrocalcinosis, polycystic kidneys
Metabolic abnormalities	Diabetes mellitus
Immunologic	Immunocompromised, postrenal transplantation

Microbiology

E. coli is the most common causative organism. The other organisms implicated are *klebsiella, Pseudomonas, Enterobacter,* proteus, acinetobacter and Gram positive organisms like coagulase negative staphylococci, enterococci and less commonly, *Staphylococcus aureus*. Higher incidence of candida UTI may be seen in diabetics, immunocompromised individuals, those on long-term indwelling catheters or urologic devices and those receiving broad spectrum antibiotic therapies. There is also higher incidence of antibiotic resistance in patients with complicated UTI.

Investigations

Urine culture is mandatory for all patients with suspected complicated UTI. Special care is taken for collecting urine particularly from catheters and drains. Persistent pyuria, but with negative culture may be due to fastidious organisms like chlamydia, ureaplasma or hemophilus. When pyuria persists and urine cultures are repeatedly negative, tuberculosis of urinary tract should be ruled out. TLC and serum creatinine should be done in all patients with complicated UTI.

Treatment

Treatment includes prompt initiation of antibiotic therapy after obtaining sample for urine culture and sensitivity. In patients with minimal or mild symptoms, antibiotic therapy may be delayed till results of urine culture are available so that a narrow spectrum antibiotic can be administered, thereby decreasing the incidence of antibiotic resistance. If severe symptoms are present, early empirical antibiotic therapy is indicated. Parenteral broad spectrum antibiotic to cover both Gram-positive and Gram-negative bacteria should be initiated, if the clinical picture is complicated by sepsis or septic shock. The common regimens used in these patients are:

- Aminoglycoside +/– ampicillin
- Piperacillin/tazobactam
- Cefoperazone/sulbactam
- Piperacillin + aminoglycoside
- Extended spectrum cephalosporins
- Carbapenems (meropenem, ertapenem, imipenem).

The choice of antibiotics in milder cases is similar to that for uncomplicated UTI (fluoroquinolones preferred first-line agents) and oral administration is appropriate. Nitrofurantoin is contraindicated in the presence of renal failure due to risk of peripheral neuropathy. It is also not effective with severe clinical presentation and there is high incidence of resistance with klebsiella, proteus and pseudomonas. Aminoglycosides should be used with caution and preferably avoided in patients with renal impairment. Clinical response to antibiotic is seen by 48–72 hours after initiation and initial therapy is modified based on urine culture reports to complete course of minimum of 14 days. Repeat urine culture after antibiotic therapy is not routinely recommended if patient remains asymptomatic.

In case of UTI complicating long indwelling catheter, it needs to be removed and replaced for appropriate response to antibiotics by removing the biofilm on the catheter. Relief of obstruction by cystoscopy and insertion of ureteric stent or percutaneous nephrostomy may be required to decrease the risk of complications and prevent recurrence. Appropriate supportive therapy should be initiated promptly for hemodynamic stabilization.

Other Investigations

The underlying urologic abnormality should be identified and corrected, if possible, to decrease the risk of complications and prevent recurrence. The choice of imaging modality and urologic investigation depends on the clinical presentation. Ultrasound is the usual first imaging modality utilized as it is the most accessible, but it is less sensitive than CT or MRI. Identification of hydroureteronephrosis in USG is helpful in identifying presence of obstruction and determines need for further evaluation. A plain X-ray of abdomen may reveal presence of radiopaque stones or emphysematous (collection of gaseous material) infection. Since plain or contrast CT scan provides more information, it is the imaging modality of choice as it can identify calculi, calcification, obstruction, abscesses, emphysematous infection and renal masses.

Recurrent Infection

Recurrent infection can be prevented in patients with indwelling catheter by appropriate catheter insertion and care, appropriate catheter use and limiting duration of use. Prophylactic antibiotic therapy is not recommended as it does not effectively reduce the incidence of symptomatic infection due to rapid reinfection with resistant organisms. For patients with persistent uncorrectable abnormality and recurrent infection, suppressive therapy, namely, continuation of antibiotic at half dose after 4–6 weeks of full dose therapy can be utilized to suppress bacterial growth.

ASYMPTOMATIC BACTERIURIA

Epidemiology and Risk Factors

Bacteriuria without lower urinary tract symptoms is common in the general population; the incidence is around 5% in sexually active young women. The incidence is about 10% in postmenopausal women less than 80 years and in men more than 80 years and about 20% in women more than 80 years age. It is rare in men less than 65 years. The incidence is very high in patients with persistent urologic abnormality, reaching around 100% in patients with chronic indwelling catheter. Even though patients with asymptomatic bacteriuria might be at a slightly higher risk for developing symptomatic UTI, they are not associated with negative long-term outcomes.

Only two groups of patients are at risk for poor short term outcome in the presence of asymptomatic bacteriuria. Pregnant women and those undergoing traumatic urologic surgical procedures are at higher risk of developing complications. Though the incidence of asymptomatic bacteriuria in pregnancy is similar to that of age matched nonpregnant women, they are at 20–30 fold higher risk of developing pyelonephritis. Hence, asymptomatic bacteriuria is treated as UTI with a view to avoid complications like premature delivery, pre-eclampsia or low-birth weight baby. Patients with untreated bacteriuria

undergoing traumatic urologic procedures are also at significantly higher risk of developing bacteremia.

Microbiology

The spectrum of organisms causing asymptomatic bacteriuria is similar to that causing uncomplicated UTI, with *E. coli* being responsible for more than 80% of cases. In men older than 65 years, coagulase negative staphylococci were found to be the most common causative organism followed by *E. coli* and *Enterococcus.*

Diagnosis

Growth of at least 10^5 CFU/mL of organisms should be present for diagnosis of asymptomatic bacteriuria. In women, this criterion should be satisfied in two consecutive urine samples, whereas in men, a single sample is enough.

Treatment

Since treatment of asymptomatic bacteriuria is indicated only in the two clinical situations mentioned above, screening to identify the presence of asymptomatic bacteriuria is reserved for these two situations only. In other patients, there is no short-term or long-term benefit and risk of reinfection with antibiotic resistant organisms increases with indiscriminate treatment.

Asymptomatic bacteriuria in pregnant women

Screening for bacteriuria is recommended by a urine culture in all pregnant women at the end of first trimester. Only 50% of pregnant women with significant bacteriuria have pyuria. If cultures are positive, a cephalosporin, amoxicillin or amoxicillin/clavulanic acid is recommended for 7 days, depending on the organism and sensitivity. Fluoroquinolones and TMP/SMX are contraindicated due to teratogenicity. Repeat urine cultures are recommended at least monthly after treatment for bacteriuria. In case of reinfection, repeat antibiotic therapy followed by prophylactic antibiotic continued till delivery, using either cephalexin or nitrofurantoin is recommended. Successful treatment of asymptomatic bacteriuria in pregnancy can decrease the risk of pyelonephritis to 1–2% and improves fetal outcome.

PROSTATITIS

Acute bacterial prostatitis is characterized by fever, severe dysuria, frequency and suprapubic pain with or without signs of bacteremia. *E.coli* is the most common organism responsible; klebsiella, proteus, pseudomonas, enterococcus and *Staphylococcus aureus* account for the rest. Per rectal digital examination of prostate or prostate massage should be avoided in cases where acute prostatitis is suspected. Immediate samples for urine and blood culture should be obtained, prompt initiation of empirical parenteral antibiotic therapy (ampicillin + aminoglycoside or a fluoroquinolone) and insertion of urethral or suprapubic catheter for bladder drainage forms the cornerstone of management. If prompt clinical response is obtained to parenteral antibiotics, continuation of appropriate oral antibiotic based on culture reports to complete 6 weeks course is considered adequate. If response to antibiotic is inadequate, prostatic abscess should be suspected. CT or MRI confirms the diagnosis and surgical drainage is indicated.

Chronic bacterial prostatitis is caused by persistent bacterial infection. It is one of the causes of recurrent acute cystitis in men, due to intermittent entry of bacteria into the bladder from the prostate. Diagnosis is confirmed by a negative culture in a midstream urine sample with a positive urine culture in a postprostatic massage sample. Organisms responsible are similar to that for acute prostatitis with addition of sexually transmitted organisms in younger men. Fluoroquinolones are the drugs of choice due to good penetration into prostatic tissue, macrolides and doxycycline being the second-line agents. Administration of antibiotics for a minimum of 4–6 weeks initially is indicated.

UTI IN CHILDREN

Clinical Features

The risk of UTI during the first decade of life is 1% in males and 3% in females. The clinical presentation of UTI in children is different from that of adults and varies with different age groups. UTI should be suspected in any infant or child presenting with unexplained fever beyond 3 days. Neonates may present with fever, vomiting, lethargy, jaundice, failure to thrive and seizures. In infants and young children, the presentation may be with recurrent fever, diarrhea, vomiting, abdominal pain and poor weight gain and in older children with burning, urgency, frequency, flank pain, turbid or foul smelling urine or a recent onset of enuresis.

Investigations

All children should undergo ultrasound imaging of kidney and urinary tract after first episode of UTI. Need for further evaluation depends on the age of the child at the time of first UTI, and presence of abnormality on USG. In children less than 2 years of age, a micturating cysto-urethrogram (MCU) and isotope scan with dimercaptosuccinal acid (DMSA) scan are indicated for detection of vesicoureteric reflux (VUR) and cortical scars, respectively, even if USG imaging is normal. In children between 2 and 5 years, DMSA scan is indicated even if USG is normal and MCU should be done, if either is abnormal. In children greater than 5 years of age, further evaluation with MCU and DMSA is indicated only, if USG is abnormal.

Treatment

Antibiotic therapy should be started after obtaining a urine culture. Parenteral antibiotics are indicated in children with complicated UTI and infants less than 3 months of age. Preferred antibiotics are combination of ampicillin + gentamicin or a third generation cephalosporin. Oral antibiotics are adequate for children above 3 months of age with a simple UTI. Duration of treatment is 7–10 days for simple infections and 10–14 days for infants and children with complicated UTI. Antibiotic prophylaxis is recommended in all children below 2 years of age following treatment of the first UTI and for complicated UTI in children below 5 years old, while awaiting imaging studies. Children with vesicoureteral reflux (VUR), those with frequent febrile UTI and those showing renal scars following a UTI even if reflux is not demonstrated should receive prophylactic antibiotics. Antibiotic prophylaxis is not recommended in patients with urinary tract obstruction (e.g. posterior urethral valves), urolithiasis or neurogenic bladder.

SUPPURATIVE AND NECROTIZING INFECTIONS OF URINARY TRACT

Renal and Perinephric Abscesses

These are suppurative complications. Renal abscess is limited to renal parenchyma and perinephric abscess involves the retroperitoneal fat and fascia surrounding the kidney. Such infections may occur by ascending infection of common organisms implicated in UTI in susceptible patients like diabetics with poorly controlled blood sugars, immunocompromised state or persistent obstruction. *Staphylococcus aureus* abscesses are often due to hematogenous spread. CT is the imaging modality of choice. ***Treatment*** consists of antibiotic therapy and surgical drainage for large and nonresolving abscesses.

Emphysematous Cystitis and Pyelonephritis

These are necrotizing infections with gas formation. *E. coli* and *klebsiella* are the usual organisms responsible, and obstruction and diabetes with poor glycemic control are the predisposing factors. CT is the imaging modality of choice, though in some cases the gas in the collecting system can be visualized in plain X-ray abdomen and during USG. Management involves glycemic control, relief of obstruction, bladder drainage and antibiotic therapy with or without surgical drainage. Nephrectomy may be required in refractory cases.

Xanthogranulomatous Pyelonephritis

It is a chronic suppurative complication where part or whole of kidney is replaced by histiocytes and foamy cells. Predisposing factors are chronic UTI in the presence of chronic obstruction, most commonly due to *E. coli* and proteus. Diagnostic imaging modality of choice is CT and usual management is nephrectomy.

GENITOURINARY TUBERCULOSIS

This accounts for 5% of extrapulmonary TB. Hematogenous dissemination is responsible for renal localization of *Mycobacterium tuberculosis*. Genitourinary tuberculosis clinically, manifests after a latent period of many years after primary pulmonary infection due to reactivation in the renal focus. Contiguous spread to ureter and bladder can occur and result in bacilluria. Involvement of prostate and epididymis in males and fallopian tube in females may also occur.

Clinical Features

Genitourinary tuberculosis can be asymptomatic or with mild dysuria, frequency or back pain. Systemic manifestations like low grade fever and weight loss may be present.

Investigations

Urinalysis reveals sterile pyuria with or without microscopic hematuria. Traditionally, intravenous urography (IVU) was considered the diagnostic imaging modality of choice, especially in the early stages, when renal calyx erosion may be the only finding. Later, it reveals cavitation and calcification of renal parenchyma, dilatation and clubbing of calyces, hydronephrosis and papillary necrosis. Total destruction of the kidney resulting in the characteristic **putty kidney** is a late feature. Thickened ureteric wall with strictures and areas of dilatation is seen as ureteric irregularity in the IVU. Thickening of bladder wall and ulceration followed by fibrosis and shrinking of bladder wall results in *thimble* bladder. The diagnosis is confirmed by growing *M. tuberculosis* in urine culture. This usually requires three sequential early morning voided urine collections. Urine examination by polymerase chain reaction (PCR) nucleic acid testing for *M. tuberculosis* antigen is more sensitive than culture techniques and enables more rapid diagnosis.

Treatment

Initial regimen consists of isoniazid, rifampicin, pyrazinamide and ethambutol for 2 months, followed by isoniazid and rifampicin for 4 months. Second-line agents are used in case of intolerance or resistance to first line agents (Table 185.7). *See* Section 6 Ch 49 for further details.

Modification of doses of antituberculosis drugs in renal failure is shown in Table 185.8.

FUNGAL INFECTIONS OF THE URINARY TRACT

Candida is responsible for most of the fungal UTIs with *Candida albicans* accounting for majority of the episodes and *C. glabrata*, *C. tropicalis* and *C. parapsilosis* for the rest. Manifestations can be as asymptomatic candiduria, cystitis and pyelonephritis or rarely as systemic fungemia.

Table 185.7: Recommended dosage for initial treatment of GUTB

Drugs	Thrice weekly dose	Daily dose
Isoniazid	15 mg/kg (max 900 mg)	5 mg/kg (max 300 mg)
Rifampicin	10 mg/kg (max 600 mg)	10 mg/kg (max 600 mg)
Pyrazinamide	30 mg/kg (max 3 g)	20 mg/kg (max 2 g)
Ethambutol	25–30 mg/kg	15–20 mg/kg

Table 185.8: Dose modifications of antituberculosis drugs in renal failure

Drug	Dose modification		
	GFR >50 mL/min	GFR 10–50 mL/min	GFR <10 mL/min
Isoniazid	100%	75–100%	75–100%
Rifampicin	100%	50–100%	50–100%
Pyrazinamide	100%	100%	50–100%
Ethambutol	q24h	q24–36h	q48h
Quinolones	100%	50–100%	50%
Capreomycin	q24h	q24h	q48h
Amikacin	q24h	q24–48h	q48h
Ethionamide	100%	100%	50%
Para-aminosalicylic acid (PAS)	100%	50–75%	50%
Cycloserine	q12h	q12–24h	q24h

Abbreviation: GFR = Glomerular filtration rate

Risk factors for candida UTI are diabetes mellitus (DM), immunocompromised state, exposure to broad spectrum antibiotics and prolonged presence of indwelling catheter or urologic devices. Demonstration of fungal hyphae in urine microscopy gives clue to the diagnosis, but definitive diagnosis requires growth of candida in urine culture. ***Treatment*** is not recommended for asymptomatic candiduria except, in patients having neutropenia and those awaiting traumatic urologic procedures. Antifungal agent of choice is fluconazole, given at a dose of 200–400 mg daily for 2 weeks. Alternative agents for fluconazole resistant non-albicans candida are amphotericin B and flucytosine. Echinocandins and azoles other than fluconazole are not indicated in UTI caused by fungi, as they are not adequately excreted in urine to be of therapeutic benefit. Indwelling catheter, if present should be removed to facilitate resolution. In patients with recurrent fungal UTI, imaging should be done to look for presence of fungal balls, which need surgical removal.

CHAPTER
186

Nephrolithiasis

Ramdas Pisharody, Vinu Thomas

Chapter Summary

- General Considerations
- Etiopathogenesis
- Types of Renal Stones
- Diagnosis of Renal Stones
- Obstructive Nephropathy
- Medical Management of Stone Disease

GENERAL CONSIDERATIONS

The term **nephrolithiasis** refers to stones in the kidneys, pelvicalyceal system, ureters, bladder and urethra. Renal stone disease affects 10% of the adult population and is 8 times more common in males than females. In children, nephrolithiasis is rare and generally, it is associated with a metabolic disease.

Nephrocalcinosis refers to renal parenchymal calcification and can be medullary or cortical. Medullary nephrocalcinosis occurs in metabolic diseases and can be associated with nephrolithiasis. Cortical nephro-calcinosis is rare and is often dystrophic.

Nephrolithiasis can be clinically categorized into surgically active and medically active varieties. *Surgically active stone disease* presents with severe pain, hematuria or complicated urinary tract infection (UTI) and may require endoscopic or surgical intervention. On the other hand, stones which are multiple, recurrent or growing are called *medically active stones*, often necessitating metabolic work up to elucidate an underlying cause, sometimes hereditary like hypercalciuria is always supersaturated.

ETIOPATHOGENESIS

An imbalance between water handling and solute clearance by the kidneys result in stone formation resulting from a metastable state which favors crystallization. Moreover, inhibitors of stone formation such as magnesium, citrate, pyrophosphates, glycoproteins, peptides and small proteins such as osteopontin help to maintain the solubility coefficient of the solutes at a low level. Increased excretion of solutes such as calcium (Ca), oxalate and uric acid increase the tendency to form stones. In metabolic disorders, like cystinosis, crystallization of substances such as cystine can be retarded by the inhibitors. Imbalances between the factors favoring and inhibiting crystallization result in stone formation. The other important factors leading to stone formation are summarized below:

- Reduction in water intake and excessive water conservation by the body in hot environment leads to reduced urine volume and concentration of urine
- *Excessive solute load:*
  - Ca and PO_4 intake may increase due to excessive consumption of milk
  - Purine gluttony (excessive red meat intake) results in excessive uric acid load
  - Food fads resulting in hyperoxaluria. Excessive consumption of some plant products rich in oxalate content may lead to hyperoxaluria, intratubular oxalate deposition leading to acute kidney injury (AKI) or oxalate stone formation.
- In vegetarians, alkaline urine combined with consumption of antacids favor calcium stone formation
- In nonvegetarians, acidic urinary pH following high meat intake result in crystallization of uric acid in the urine
- A nidus for crystallization and stone growth (epitaxy). Firstly, a nidus due to deposition of organic and inorganic matter deposition occurs. Crystallization and growth of stone occurs on the nidus, e.g. Randall's plaques of PO_4 deposits on tubules and uric acid crystal nidus for Ca precipitation
- Obstruction, cysts and stagnation of urine favor stone formation and growth
- *Infection-associated stone:* Struvite stones are the common infection-associated stones. They consist of magnesium, ammonium phosphate and Ca.

- *Metabolic and endocrine disorders:* Hyperparathyroidism, hyperthyroidism, hypercalcemic states—multiple myeloma, metastatic carcinoma, sarcoidosis, milk alkali syndrome, hyperuricemic states—tumor lysis syndrome, primary gout and primary hyperoxaluria
- *Inherited tubular disorders:* Idiopathic hypercalciuria, hyperoxaluria, cystinuria
- *Defects of renal tubular acidification:* Distal renal tubular acidosis (RTA), Fanconi's syndrome
- *Miscellaneous disorders:* Fat malabsorption syndromes, tumor lysis, hypercalcemic states, prolonged immobilization.

Despite innumerable causes of stone disease, up to 50% of stones are due to idiopathic or dietary causes. In Kerala, purine gluttony among expatriates in Gulf countries is a major cause of dietary uricosuria, acidic urine and calcium stone disease.

TYPES OF RENAL STONES (FIG. 186.1)

Types and features of different stones listed in Table 186.1.

Calcium Stones

Eighty percent of renal stones in the adult is composed of oxalate and phosphate. Oxalate stones are twice as common as phosphate. Phosphate stones are commonly seen in alkaline urine, vegetarians, RTA and primary hyperparathyroidism (phosphaturia). Calcium oxalate stones are seen in hypercalcemic states and malabsorption syndrome. Hyperuricosuria also leads to oxalate stones due to epitaxy. Mixed oxalate and phosphate stones are encountered in 30% of idiopathic calcium stone disease.

Uric Acid Stones

Pure uric acid stones are seen in severe hyperuricosuric states such as gout, tumor lysis and some rare disorders of purine metabolism associated with enzyme deficiencies.

Cystine Stones

Cystine stones are large radiopaque stones due to an inherited tubular transport defect of sulfur containing amino acids. They are often bilateral and can lead to stag horn calculus and obstructive nephropathy leading to renal failure.

Infection-associated Stones

These stones are usually associated with protease infection of the urinary tract, which results in formation of

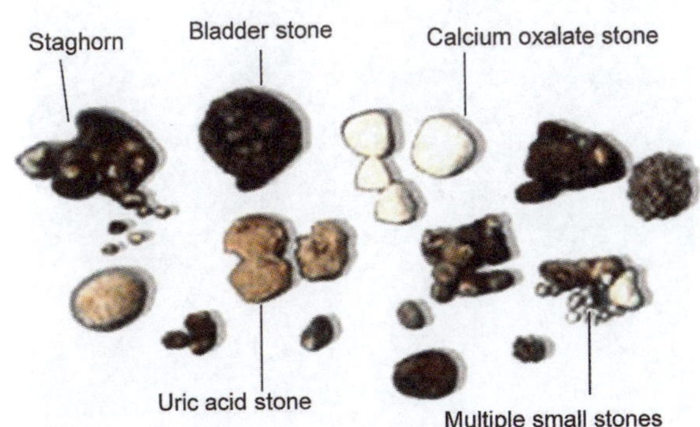

Fig. 186.1: Different types of renal stones

Table 186.1: Types and features of different stones

Types of renal stone	Shape of crystal	Radiologic findings	Clinical	Associated urinary findings	Incidence	Remarks
Calcium oxalate (with <50% calcium phosphate)	Envelope shaped	Rounded and radiopaque	Men 25–45 age group	Calcium oxalate uric acid ↑ Citrate volume ↓	80%	Most common among radiopaque stones
Mainly (>50%) calcium phosphate	Amorphous	Rounded and radiopaque	Primary hyperparathyroidism alkali treatment distal RTA	Calcium pH ↑	<5%	Purely calcium phosphate is rare
Struvite	Coffin lid	Radiopaque staghorn	Neurogenic bladder Other anatomic defects	Urease + UTI Alkaline pH	10%	Congenital anomalies, paraplegia
Uric acid	Diamond or rhomboid	Radiolucent staghorn	Gout/uremia diarrheas Diabetes metabolic syndrome	Uric acid ↑ pH (acid) ↓ Volume	10%	Commonly associated with other stones
Cystine	Hexagonal	Faintly radiopaque staghorn	Inherited	Cystine ↑	<1%	Very rare

Abbreviations: RTA = Renal tubular acidosis; UTI = Urinary tract infection

highly alkaline urine. This pH is favorable for the precipitation of Ca, NH_4, Mg and PO_4 (struvite) resulting in formation of staghorn calculus and urinary obstruction. Since the stones are also infected, it is difficult to eradicate and infection is intractable. Alkaline urine and struvite stone can also occur in chronic *Escherichia coli* and *Klebsiella* infections.

DIAGNOSIS OF RENAL STONES

Calcium oxalate stone typically, occurs in young adult males and is associated with passage of hard, brownish stone with spiked surface, following a renal colic and associated with hematuria. The urine examination would show abundance of envelope shaped crystals of calcium oxalate, dihydrate and dumb-bell shaped crystals of calcium oxalate monohydrate (Fig. 186.2). The urine is usually alkaline. Dietary causes include increased intake of calcium and oxalate in the form of green leafy vegetables and high-fiber. Excessive intake of animal protein leads to hypercalciuric calcium stone disease and acidic urine. Metabolic workup is essential for recurrent stone disease and/or passage. Common conditions include inherited hypercalciuria and hyperoxaluria. Primary hyperoxaluria may be inherited. Secondary hyperoxaluria may occur following fat malabsorption.

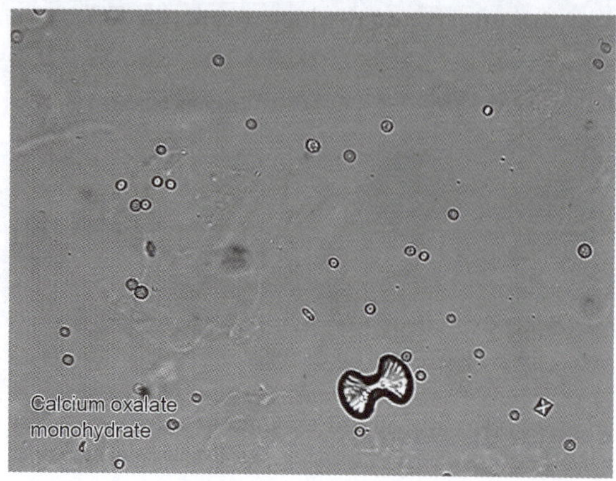

Fig. 186.2: Crystals in urine

Calcium Phosphate Stones

They are generally asymptomatic and are large. Generally, small stones cause more distressing symptoms compared to large ones. Stones have a chalky white color with smooth surface. Urine is usually alkaline and plenty of amorphous crystals of calcium phosphate are seen in the urine deposit. Most common metabolic cause is primary hyperparathyroidism. Others are milk alkali syndrome and renal acidification defects such as distal RTA and Fanconi's syndrome. Citrate is an inhibitor of stone formation. Hypocitraturia seen in these conditions cause precipitation of calcium phosphate.

Uric Acid Stones

They are not uncommon in a young meat eating individual who works in hot environments or outdoors. Excessive sweating and use of fresh or canned fruit juices rich in fructose and sucrose make them prone to stone formation. The common metabolic syndromes are tumor lysis syndrome and primary gout. The urine shows needle-shaped crystals and the pH is acidic (<6).

Struvite Stones

Struvite (triple phosphate) stones result from chronic UTI due to urea splitting organisms. Proteus group of organisms contain urease enzyme, which splits urea to generate ammonia and carbon dioxide. This results in mixed stones of calcium carbonate and magnesium ammonium phosphate. Urine is highly alkaline, with urine pH more than eight. The crystals have a ***coffin lid*** appearance.

Cystine Stones

They are very rare and can be seen in children with the inherited disorders associated with dibasic aminoaciduria (cysteine, ornithine, arginine and lysine). Urine microscopy is diagnostic which shows hexagonal cystine crystals.

Stone workup implies evaluation for metabolic stone disease. A practical outpatient protocol includes 24 hours urine volume, creatine, calcium, uric acid, oxalate, citrate and electrolytes along with urine pH and culture. Blood chemistry should include pH, electrolytes, creatinine, calcium and uric acid.

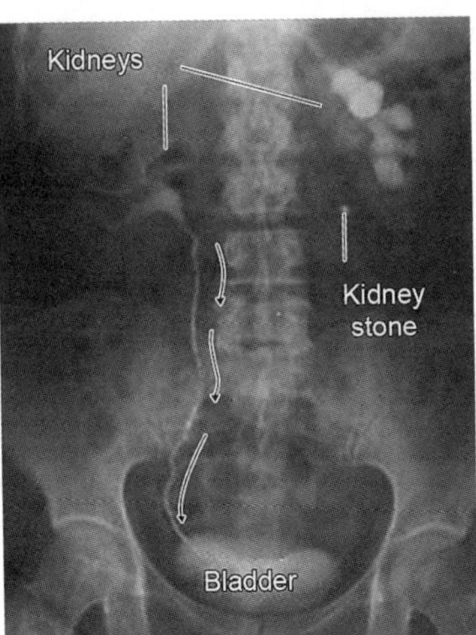

Fig. 186.3: Intravenous urogram (IVU) left ureteral stone with obstruction (arrows)

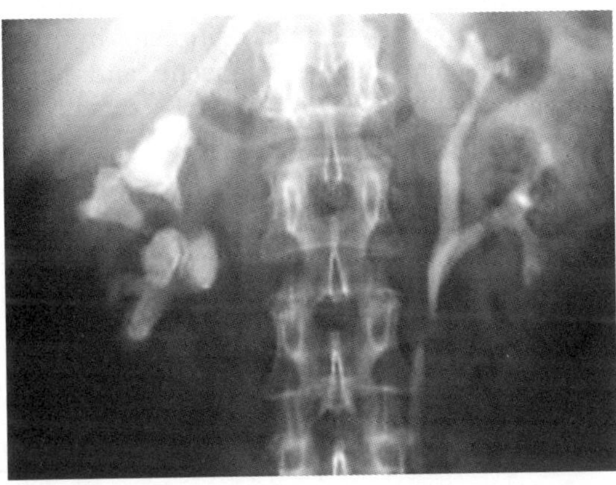

Fig. 186.4: Intravenous urogram (IVU) right staghorn calculus with nonfunction. ***Note:*** Normal functioning left kidney with bifid ureter

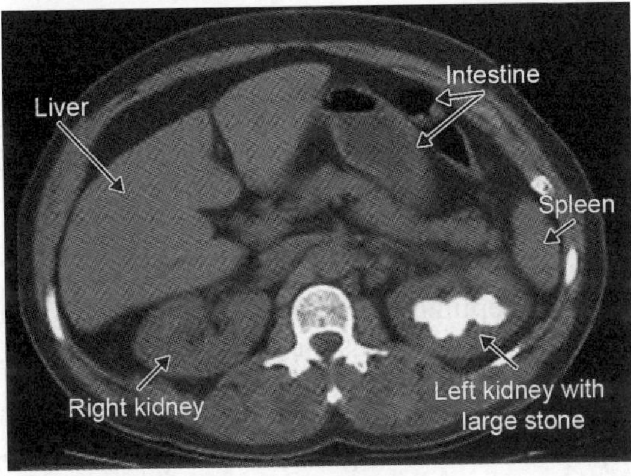

Fig. 186.5: Plain computed tomography (CT) scan showing large left renal pelvic calculus

Imaging studies include X-ray kidney, ureter and bladder (KUB) (urate stones are radiolucent), ultrasonography (USG), intravenous urogram (IVU) or intravenous pyelogram (IVP) (Figs 186.3 to 186.5).

OBSTRUCTIVE NEPHROPATHY

It refers to renal damage due to obstruction in the urinary tract. Nephrolithiasis is a leading cause of renal failure among young and middle aged. The importance lies in the potential for reversibility unlike many other forms of chronic kidney disease (CKD) even in advanced stages. The procedures usually employed are urethroscopy and removal for impacted urethral stone, cystoscopic removal for bladder stone, ureteroscopy for removal from lower ureter, ureterorenoscopy and ultrasonic or laser pulverization of stone for upper urinary tract stones, percutaneous nephrolithotomy (PCNL) (key hole procedure) for stones in pelvis and upper ureter. In most instances, temporary ureteric stenting may be necessary to enable passage of the pulverized stone particles. In extracorporeal shock wave lithotripsy (ESWL), sonic shock waves from outside the body are directed toward the stone which is powdered *in situ*, and eliminated per urethra. Such procedures may facilitate relief from obstructive nephropathy. Staghorn calculi require open surgery sometimes under hypothermia.

MEDICAL MANAGEMENT OF STONE DISEASE

Medical therapy, when promoted after adequate stone work up goes a long way in treatment. It helps to prevent further growth of stones avoiding urological intervention and obstructive nephropathy. Majority of the small stones (<6 mm) are easily passed by hydration and ureteric muscle relaxants such as tamsulosin, alfuzosin, prazosin. Large radiopaque stones are not dissolved easily. Radiolucent and pure uric acid calculi can be dissolved by long-term treatment with alkalinizing agents, maintaining good urine flow rate and use of drugs to facilitate elimination of uric acid.

Dietary advice may vary depending on the metabolic problem identified. Meat, particularly red meat and dairy products are avoided, if uric acid stone is present. Leafy vegetables are high in oxalate content and hence, avoided in oxalate stones. Generally, stone formation is favored by animal protein, alcohol, excess sodium, vitamin C and vitamin D. On the other hand, liberal fluid intake, magnesium, potassium and pyridoxine antagonizes stone formation. Generally, people with metabolic syndrome are more commonly detected to have stone disease. Lifestyle changes can help often much more than use of drugs.

General measures include making the urine dilute which can be achieved by increasing the fluid intake. If, the kidney functions are normal, the urine output will increase and urine becomes dilute. The concentration of stone forming ions can be reduced by dietary modifications or by specific drug therapy. Most stone formers may have a metabolic defect. Most fluids are safe in patients with stone forming tendency. Diet rich in animal protein and high sodium intake increase urinary calcium excretion and should be avoided. Patients with hyperuricemia should also avoid red meat. Since, citrate binds with calcium and decrease supersaturation of Ca, citrate containing fruit juices can be administered. But colas which are high in phosphoric acid, cranberry juice which is high in oxalate content and grapefruit juice are avoided since they increase stone forming tendency.

Patients with hypercalciuria are advised low Ca diet and given thiazide diuretics (trichloromethane—4 mg or hydrochlorothiazide 25 mg twice daily) combined with potassium citrate (20 mEq) twice daily to reduce hypercalciuria. Other drugs like indapamide 2.5 mg combined with sodium restriction are useful for some types of absorptive hypercalciuria. Hypocitraturia may be present in about 50% of stone formers. Citrate binds with the calcium in the tubule and prevents precipitation of calcium. Hence, potassium citrate is coadministered with the thiazides.

In hyperuricemia which occurs in those with very high red meat intake (purine gluttony), gout or during treatment of myeloproliferative disorders or tumors, uric acid and calcium stones may form in them. Solubility of uric acid can be increased markedly, if the urine pH is over 6.5–7.0. Use of Allopurinol 100 mg or Febuxostat 40 mg twice or thrice daily can be used. This should be combined with urinary alkalinizing solutions like buffered sodium or potassium citrate. Pure uric acid stones can be dissolved by alkali supplements, if treatment is given for many months.

Dietary hyperoxaluria is managed by restriction of high oxalate containing foods and use of oral calcium citrate which binds to oxalate and prevents the absorption. Hereditary hyperoxaluria is treated with low oxalate diet, vitamin B_6 supplements and oral orthophosphates. Enteric hyperoxaluria occurring in small bowel disorders can be treated by oral calcium citrate, gluten-free diet in sprue or cholestyramine in those with fat malabsorption.

The usual measures for management of cystine stones are:
- Diet (restriction of meat, dairy products)
- Alkalinize urine (pH > 7) using potassium citrate
- Restriction of dietary sodium (< 50 mEq/day)
- Maintain good urine flow rate (> 2,800 mL/day)
- Vitamin B_6 supplementation
- D-penicillamine may be used in specialized centers for dissolving cystine stones treatment has to be carefully monitored.

Infection-related stones consist of triple phosphate (magnesium, ammonium and Ca) in alkaline urine and often associated with infection with urea splitting organisms. *Treatment* consists of prolonged use of antibiotics and use of urease inhibitors. Acetohydroxamic acid in doses of 250 mg 3–4 times daily helps by inhibiting urease. *Side effects* include headache and hemolytic anemia.

CHAPTER

187

Kidney in Systemic Diseases

M Thomas Mathew

Chapter Summary

- Kidney in Diabetes (Diabetic Nephropathy)
- Systemic Lupus Erythematosus
- Rheumatoid Arthritis
- Sjögren's Syndrome
- Progressive Systemic Sclerosis
- Mixed Connective Tissue Disease
- Polyarteritis Nodosa
- Eosinophilic Granulomatosis with Polyangiitis (Churg-Strauss)
- Microscopic Polyarteritis Nodosa
- Granulomatosis with Polyangiitis (Wegener's Granulomatosis)
- Anaphylactoid Purpura (Henoch-Schonlein Purpura)
- Mixed Cryoglobulinemia
- Takayasu's Arteritis
- Amyloidosis
- Multiple Myeloma
- Renal Lesions Associated with Neoplasia
- Tumor Lysis Syndrome

KIDNEY IN DIABETES (DIABETIC NEPHROPATHY)

See also Section 10, Ch 92

Diabetes mellitus (DM) is the leading cause of end-stage renal disease (ESRD) universally. In most of the leading Nephrology and Transplant centers in India, it is the first or second leading cause of ESRD. Both type 1 insulin-dependent diabetes mellitus (IDDM) and type 2 noninsulin-dependent diabetes mellitus (NIDDM) will result in diabetic nephropathy (DN) leading to ESRD over the course of many years. Hyperglycemia is the most important factor for inducing injury to glomeruli and mesangium through overlapping pathways, like formation of advanced glycation end products (AGEs), activation of protein kinase-C (PKC), generation of reactive oxygen species (ROS) and altering the podocyte morphology and functions. However, other factors like genetic susceptibility, renin-angiotensin-aldosterone mechanisms, endothelin system, raised intraglomerular pressure, activation of cytokines and growth factors like insulin-like growth factor-1 (IGF-1), transforming growth factor-β, platelet-derived growth factor (PDGF) and vascular endothelial growth factor (VEGF) also play vital roles in the pathogenesis of diabetic kidney disease. The most common lesions involve the glomeruli and include thickening of capillary basement membrane, expansion of the glomerular mesangium and increased secretion of mesangial matrix leading to diffuse or nodular sclerosis of the glomeruli. The nodular glomerulosclerosis is also known as Kimmelstiel-Wilson (KW) lesion and is the hallmark of DN (Fig. 187.1). Exudative lesions like capsular drops and fibrin caps and hyalinosis and arteriolosclerosis of afferent arteriole are also seen. The podocyte become abnormal, foot processes get effaced and podocyte proteins becomes defective leading on to

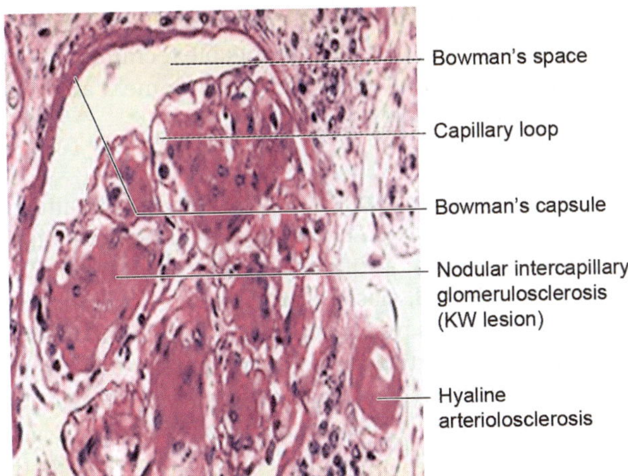

Fig. 187.1: Nodular sclerosis of the glomerulus

leakage of albumin through the glomerular filter. The slight increase in albumin excretion in urine is called *microalbuminuria*. This can be measured only by sensitive method and is the earliest clinical manifestation of involvement of the kidney in diabetes. In healthy normal adults, urinary albumin excretion in 24 hours is less than 30 milligram (20-30 µg/minute). Microalbuminuria is diagnosed when at least two out of three urine samples examined within a 6-week period is more than 30 mg/24 hours. Urinary albumin excretion of more than 300 mg or total protein excretion or more than 500 mg can be detected by conventional laboratory tests or by 'albustix', which are inexpensive tests. Microalbuminuria between 30 mg/day and 300 mg/day can be detected by special tests like radioimmunoassay. Microalbuminuria predicts the risks of developing overt DN, renal failure or cardiovascular complications in the future.

The natural history of DN is described as a series of stages in a relentlessly deteriorating course marked by increasing amounts of proteinuria, fall in glomerular filtration rate (GFR) and development of hypertension leading on to ESRD (Table 187.1). There are many risk factors for developing DN in an individual. Uncontrolled diabetes for a long duration, uncontrolled hypertension, and family history of DN, association of cardiovascular diseases, male gender, smoking and the presence of dyslipidemia are the important risk factors.

Stage I: Soon after the onset of diabetes, the kidney size enlarges (nephromegaly), renal blood flow increases, GFR increases and the blood pressure (BP) is normal at this stage. There is no albuminuria. This is the stage of hypertrophy and hyperfunction of the kidneys. Tight control of diabetic state can arrest further progression of the disease.

Stage II: Once diabetes has been present for more than 5 years or more, patient passes on to the silent stage of DN. In this clinical stage, there is thickening of glomerular and tubular basement membrane, expansion of mesangial matrix and mild increase in BP. If the diabetic state and hypertension are well-controlled, the illness will not progress further. If not, within 5–6 years, the disease will progress to stage III.

Stage III: This stage of incipient DN typically occurs 10–15 years after the onset of diabetes and is characterized by the presence of microalbuminuria of more than 30 mg/24 hours. GFR will begin to fall and the BP will gradually increase.

Stage IV: In the next 4–5 years, progression to advanced renal disease takes place. This stage is marked by overt proteinuria or macroalbuminuria. (**Note:** It is macroalbuminuria at this stage and not micro) in the nephrotic range (>3.5 g/24 hour), overt hypertension and rapid fall in GFR with elevated urea and creatinine leading on to the stage known as KW syndrome.

Stage V: In another 1–3 years time, disease progresses further to ESRD with severe hypertension and cardiac failure requiring dialysis or renal transplantation.

More than 60% of patients with DN will also have diabetic retinopathy and neuropathy—so called 'triopathy' of microvascular complications of diabetes. Patients may also have other renal and genitourinary manifestations of diabetes. These include tubular proteinuria, fluid and electrolyte disorders, hyperaldosteronism, hypercalciuria, hyperkalemia, type IV distal renal tubular acidosis (RTA), urinary tract infections (UTIs), papillary necrosis, emphysematous pyelonephritis or xanthogranulomatous pyelonephritis.

Treatment

Tight glycemic control with strict diet, insulin and/or antidiabetic drugs is the mainstay in the prevention

Kidney in Systemic Diseases

Table 187.1: Natural history and stages of diabetic nephropathy

Stages	Designation	Characteristics	GFR (minimum)	Albumin excretion	Blood pressure	Chronology
I	Hyperfunction and hypertrophy	Glomerular hyperfiltration	Increased in type 1 and type 2	May be increased	Type 1 normal Type 2 normal hypertension	Present at time of diagnosis
II	Silent stage	Thickend BM, expanded mesangium	Normal	Type 1 normal Type 2 may be <30–300 mg/d	Type 1 normal Type 2 normal hypertension	First 5 years
III	Incipient stage	Microalbuminuria	GFR begins to fall	30–300 mg/d	Type 1 increased Type 2 normal hypertension	6–15 years
IV	Overt diabetic nephropathy	Macroalbuminuria	GFR below N	>300 mg/d	Hypertension	15–25 years
V	Uremic	ESRD	0–10	Decreasing	Hypertension	25–30 years

Abbreviations: GFR = Glomerular filtration rate; ESRD = End-stage renal disease; BM = Basement membrane

and treatment of DN. Normalization of BP is equally important and is achieved by using a combination of angiotensin-converting enzyme inhibitors (ACE-I) and angiotensin-receptor blockers (ARBs). Lipid-lowering agents, diuretics and antioxidants also help in retarding the progression of nephropathy. Once patient develop ESRD, renal replacement therapy should be initiated. Kidney transplantation is preferable to dialysis because of risk of infection and frequent vascular access problems due to atherosclerotic vessels of the patients. Continuous ambulatory peritoneal dialysis (CAPD) is preferred in patients with vascular access problem or in those with associated severe congestive heart failure, angina or unstable BP.

Novel Therapies

A number of novel therapies have been demonstrated to reduce urine albumin excretion and prevent glomerulosclerosis. They have not yet been approved for clinical use.

Inhibitors of growth factors and vasopeptides:
- Biochemical—inhibitors of PKC
- Inhibitors of angiotensin-converting eyzyme (ACE)
- Angiotensin-converting enzyme blockers or ACE receptor blockers.

SYSTEMIC LUPUS ERYTHEMATOSUS

(Refer Section 12, Ch 108)

Renal disease is a common manifestation of systemic lupus erythematosus (SLE). Although the multiple immuno-logic abnormalities of lupus can virtually affect any organ system, renal involvement is a major cause for morbidity and mortality. Renal involvement is extremely diverse ranging from asymptomatic urinary findings to fulminant renal failure or florid nephrotic syndrome in over two-thirds of the patients.

The pathogenesis of SLE is complex and multifactorial. Immunologic dysregulation leads to production of autoantibodies to nuclear and other cellular antigens. The term 'lupus nephritis' and 'lupus glomerulonephritis' are commonly applied to the many patterns of glomerular involvement in SLE. This includes mesangial lesions, membranous patterns and proliferative lesions.

The clinical presentation may vary from mild-to-moderate proteinuria, microhematuria, telescoped urinary sediments, edema, hypertension or renal insufficiency. In telescoped urinary sediment, many cell types and different forms of casts will be seen in the same field under the micro-scope. Class III may present with nephrotic syndrome and moderate renal failure. Class IV is the most active form of lupus nephritis characterized by nephrotic syndrome, hematuria, hypertension and moderate-to-severe renal failure. Class V and VI also will present which nephrotic syndrome, hypertension and terminal renal failure.

Diagnosis

Apart from the clinical diagnostic criteria of SLE, the presence of LE cells, antinuclear antibody (ANA), anti-double standard deoxyribonucleic acid (anti-dsDNA) and hypocomplementemia and the renal histology as per the World Health Organization (WHO) classification are helpful in the diagnosis, treatment and for prognostication. LE cells can be demonstrated by suitable techniques even in laboratories without sophisticated equipment and than add to the diagnostic tests.

Treatment

A large number of controlled and uncontrolled treatment trials have been conducted in the treatment of lupus nephritis. However, a uniform regimen has still not emerged. In general, class I and most cases with class II do not require any treatment unless there is a specific indication for corticosteroids or nonsteroidal anti-inflammatory drugs (NSAIDs) for systemic manifestations. For class III and IV, prednisolone in a dose of 1–1.5 mg/kg/day alone is given for a period of 4–6 weeks or till remission is achieved following which the drug can be given on alternate days for 4–6 weeks. This can be combined with oral cyclophosphamide 2 mg/kg/day for about 3 months. Pulse therapy with cyclophosphamide in the dose of 0.5 g/m^2 as intravenous (IV) infusions every month for 6 months and then decreasing to once in 3 months for 18–24 months also has been found to be very effective. The leukocyte counts must be closely monitored and cyclophosphamide infusions must be administered after hydrating the patient and achieving good urine flow rate, so as to prevent development of hemorrhagic cystitis. Plasmapheresis has been tried in severe cases of lupus nephritis. Other therapies tried are cyclosporine, azathioprine, thromboxane antagonists and IV gammaglobulin. However, in spite of the treatment, 20–30% of patients particularly of class III and IV progress on to ESRD and require renal replacement therapy. SLE very often becomes quiescent with the development of ESRD and recurrence of nephritis is not common after renal transplantation.

RHEUMATOID ARTHRITIS

(*See* also Section 12, Ch 107)

Kidney involvement is uncommon in rheumatoid arthritis (RA). However in 10–20% of patients, there could be direct kidney involvement or the kidneys could be affected by the treatment given for RA. The changes resulting from RA per se are membranous glomerulonephritis, mesangial proliferative nephritis, diffuse proliferative nephritis or necrotizing vasculitis. Renal amyloidosis (AA type) can result from the chronic inflammatory state of RA. Drugs used in the treatment of RA like gold, penicillamine, NSAIDs, azathioprine or cyclosporine can indirectly produce kidney damage. ***Treatment*** is usually symptomatic, but in a rare patient with renal insufficiency, steroids or cyclophosphamide may be useful.

SJÖGREN'S SYNDROME

(Refer to Section 12, Ch 107)

Sjögren's syndrome (SS) is a chronic inflammatory disease characterized by lymphocyte and plasma cell infiltration of lacrimal and salivary glands with the resultant xerophthalmia and xerostomia known as sicca (dryness) complex. A spectrum of renal disorders including distal RTA, Fanconi's syndrome, impaired concentrating ability, interstitial nephritis, nephrogenic diabetes insipidus, hypercalciuria and nephrolithiasis may occur in 20–25% of patients. There is an increased incidence of UTIs in SS, especially in women who have vaginal sicca symptoms also. Some patients may progress to chronic renal failure (CRF) due to interstitial fibrosis or glomerular sclerosis. Steroids and immunosuppressive drugs or symptomatic treatment and renal replacement therapy when the patient is in ESRD are advocated.

PROGRESSIVE SYSTEMIC SCLEROSIS

Also refer to Section 12, Ch 109

Kidney involvement is the most common cause of death in progressive systemic sclerosis (PSS) and is found clinically in 40–70% of cases. There is a slowly progressive renal insufficiency accompanied by hypertension and moderate proteinuria. However, manifestation as acute renal failure (ARF) with or without malignant hypertension (scleroderma renal crisis) is not uncommon. The renal blood vessels are predominantly involved with marked intimal thickening, intimal cell proliferation and fibrinoid necrosis, which are indistinguishable from malignant hypertension. There is no specific treatment. However, energetic management of hypertension with ACE inhibitors and renal replacement therapy will be required in ARF or if patient goes on to ESRD. This is one of the exceptions for the use of ACE inhibitors in presence of advanced renal failure and the drug of choice for scleroderma renal crisis is ACE inhibitors.

MIXED CONNECTIVE TISSUE DISEASE

Also refer to Section 12, Ch 109

Kidney disease occurs in approximately 25% of patients with mixed connective tissue disease (MCTD). It may be clinically silent or mild with proteinuria or hematuria. Serious kidney involvement is common in children. Membranous or focal proliferative glomerulonephritis are common. Malignant hypertension can be a presentation with proliferative vasculopathy similar to the vasculopathy seen in systemic sclerosis. Some patients may end up with ESRD or may develop renal involvement due to treatment with NSAIDs. There is no specific treatment but patients with hypertension will require intense medication including ACE inhibitors.

POLYARTERITIS NODOSA

Refer to Section 12, Ch 110

Renal involvement occurs in more than 80% of patients and the glomerular lesions are those of ischemia with collapse of the glomeruli and fibrinoid necrosis. Renal infarctions may be seen because of the ischemia produced by vascular blocks and necrosis. Diagnosis is based on anemia, raised erythrocyte sedimentation rate (ESR), leukocytosis and positive test for hepatitis B virus. Antineutrophil cytoplasmic antibody (ANCA) is usually negative. Definite diagnosis can be made by angiography or tissue biopsy. *Treatment* consists of a combination of glucocorticoids 1 mg/kg bw and cyclophosphamide in doses of 1–2 mg/kg bw given for 4–6 weeks and tapered off gradually over 6–12

months. If hypertension is present, it has to be controlled adequately.

EOSINOPHILIC GRANULOMATOSIS WITH POLYANGIITIS (CHURG-STRAUSS)

Refer to Section 12, Ch 110

Renal involvement is less common than polyarteritis nodosa (PAN) and consists of granulomatous nephritis and focal-necrotizing granulomatosis. *Treatment* consists of corticosteroid therapy combined with cyclophosphamide.

MICROSCOPIC POLYARTERITIS NODOSA

Refer to Section 12, Ch 110

This is a variant of PAN and is a small vessel vasculitis. It differs from PAN because of the pathological features and association with perinuclear-ANCA. It involves small-size vessels like capillaries, venules and arterioles. But sometimes small and medium vessels are also involved and thus clinical pictures may overlap with PAN. *Clinical features* include constitutional symptoms and cutaneous involvement in the form of palpable purpura. Renal involvement is seen commonly and manifests with proteinuria, hematuria and red blood cell (RBC) casts. Hypertension is usually mild. The most striking feature is a rapidly progressive renal failure. In some cases, if the extrarenal features may be inconspicuous or missing, the condition is called renal-limited polyangiitis. Renal histology shows involvement of small vessels in the form of polymorphonuclear infiltration, fibrinoid necrosis and extravasation of erythrocytes. Glomeruli show focal-necrotizing lesions and there may be variable degree of crescent formation. Endocapillary proliferation is uncommon. Immunofluorescence shows occasional deposits of immunoglobulins (Ig) and complement (pauci-immune glomerulonephritis).

Treatment

Treatment is similar to PAN consisting of steroids and cyclophosphamide. Plasma exchange may be beneficial in some patients. IVIg and monoclonal antibodies directed against lymphocytes (CD4 or CD52) have been used in those who are resistant or intolerant to the conventional treatment.

GRANULOMATOSIS WITH POLYANGIITIS (WEGENER'S GRANULOMATOSIS)

Renal involvement is demonstrable in 85% and reduced GFR in about half of cases at the onset of the disease. The demonstration of positive cytoplasmic-ANCA is 90–95% sensitive and specific. *Prominent features* include hematuria, variable degree of proteinuria and progressive renal insufficiency. This is associated with ANCA. Two types of ANCA have been identified—(1) those with autoantibodies specific for myeloperoxidase (MPO-ANCA or cytoplasmic-ANCA) or proteinase 3 (perinuclear-ANCA).

Renal histology is that of diffuse or focal-necrotizing glomerulonephritis. Crescentic glomerulonephritis may be seen in patients presenting with rapidly progressive renal failure. Immunofluorescence shows a lack of immune deposits (pauci-immune) and electron microscopy may show scattered electron-dense deposits in capillary walls. The prognosis of untreated granulomatosis with polyangiitis is poor, with 1-year survival being of less than 20%. *Treatment* with prednisolone 1 mg/kg/day and cyclophosphamide 2 mg/kg/day is found to be effective. Steroid dose is reduced after 6 weeks and may be discontinued once clinical remission is achieved. Cyclophosphamide should be continued in the same dose for at least 1 year after achieving quiescence of disease activity. Plasma exchange and dialysis may be tried in patients who do not respond quickly to conventional therapy.

ANAPHYLACTOID PURPURA (HENOCH-SCHONLEIN PURPURA)

See Section 15, Ch 174

Renal involvement is seen in 50–80% of cases and is usually apparent within 4 weeks of diagnosis. The findings include gross or microscopic hematuria, proteinuria and rarely, rapidly progressive renal failure. Nephrotic syndrome is seen in 50% of cases. The most striking histopathological lesion in the kidney is segmental mesangial proliferation. The degree of proliferation is variable and may be associated with tuft necrosis and crescent formation. Exuberant crescent formation may be seen in some patients.

The renal lesion is generally nonprogressive. Adverse prognostic factors include older age, presentation with acute nephritic syndrome and persistent nephrotic-range proteinuria. *Treatment* is symptomatic. Steroids or immunosuppressive agents are unhelpful in altering the course of renal disease. Patients with rapidly progressive renal failure in association with crescentic glomerulonephritis may be benefited by intensive plasma exchange along with immunosuppressive drugs and dialysis.

MIXED CRYOGLOBULINEMIA

Refer to Section 12, Ch 110

This condition is characterized by presence of a mixture of monoclonal IgM and polyclonal IgG in the circulation, which precipitate in cold and give rise to clinical symptoms like purpura, necrotizing skin lesions, arthralgias, hepatosplenomegaly and Raynaud's phenomenon. Renal disease is seen in about 50% of cases and is especially common, if circulating cryoglobulin concentration exceeds 1 g/dL. *Clinical features* may be precipitated by dehydration or exposure to cold and include nephrotic syndrome (30%), asymptomatic proteinuria (30%), acute nephritic syndrome (20–30%) and ARF (5%). Light microscopy shows proliferative glomerulonephritis with endocapillary hypercellularity and infiltration by monocytes. Crescents may be seen in a few glomeruli. Large eosinophilic periodic acid-Schiff (PAS)—positive deposits are seen in the capillary lumina (intraluminal thrombi). There is uneven thickening of the glomerular basement membrane (GBM). Vasculitis is observed in 33% of cases. *Treatment* includes IV pulses of methylprednisolone (500–1,000 mg/day for 3 days) followed by a combination of oral prednisolone (30–60 mg/day) and cyclophosphamide (2 mg/kg/day). Plasma exchange may be required to bring down cryoglobulin levels in patients with crescentic glomerulonephritis with rapidly deteriorating renal function.

TAKAYASU'S ARTERITIS

Refer to Section 12, Ch 110

Various patterns of arterial lesions have been described. In India, the main seat of pathology is abdominal aorta and renal arteries as compared to Japan where aortic arch and its branches are involved more frequently. As a result, renovascular hypertension is the main presentation in India resulting in hypertension and its complications including CRF, congestive heart failure, stroke or limb ischemia. *General features* of toxemia like fever, malaise, arthralgias and anemia are not commonly seen in Indian patients. Occasionally, cases of renal amyloidosis have been described. *Treatment* consists of glucocorticoids or other immunosuppressive therapy for arterial inflammation during acute phase and strict control of hypertension. Stenotic lesions of almost all arteries can be treated by angioplasty, stenting and surgical correction.

AMYLOIDOSIS

Refer to Section 10, Ch 91

Amyloidosis frequently involves kidney and it is divided into amyloid light-chain (AL) amyloidosis in which the fibrils consists of Ig light chains and amyloid A (AA) variety in which the fibrils consist of serum AA. The amyloid associated with chronic hemodialysis and Alzheimer's disease usually does not involve the kidneys. The involvement of kidney is more common in AL amyloidosis as compared to AA variety. Kidney is involved in over 80% of the patients along with other organs like liver, spleen, lymph nodes, heart and other tissues. The renal presentation is of proteinuria going on to nephrotic syndrome. Relatively low frequency of hypertension and large kidney size are the hallmarks of amyloid renal disease. Renal failure is slow to progress. Usually the primary disease or the intervening complications decide the outcome. A few patients may present with amyloid deposition in the renal tubules and may result in various tubular syndromes like diabetes insipidus and RTA. *Diagnosis* can be made by renal biopsy. Abdominal fat biopsy and rectal biopsy are equally diagnostic. There is no satisfactory treatment of this condition except with the AL variety of amyloidosis, which may show regression with treatment of the primary disease. Therapy with colchicine, melphalan, prednisolone and other immunosuppressive agents have not been successful. Renal replacement therapy both with dialysis and transplantation is also not very encouraging because the involvement of extrarenal organs often decides the outcome of the disease.

MULTIPLE MYELOMA

Refer to Section 15, Ch 169

A variety of renal manifestations are encountered in multiple myeloma. Almost 50% of patients have overt renal insufficiency at sometime during the course of the disease. In many instances, renal disease may be the first indicator of multiple myeloma. Virtually, all areas of renal parenchyma can be damaged by the light chain deposition.

- Glomerulopathies
  - Amyloid, type AL
  - Granular light chain deposition disease
  - Fibrillary glomerulopathies
- Tubulointerstitial lesions
  - Fanconi's syndrome
  - Acute tubular necrosis or tubulopathy
  - Cast nephropathy (myeloma kidney)
  - Tubulointerstitial nephritis
- Vascular lesions
- Asymptomatic Bence-Jones proteinuria
- Hypercalcemic nephropathy
- Hyperviscosity syndrome
- Pyelonephritis
- Neoplastic cell infiltration
- Obstructive nephropathy.

The most common clinical manifestation is the detection of light-chain or Bence-Jones proteinuria, observed in 65–100% of patients. Proteinuria may rarely precede the development of myeloma by several months. The quantity of protein excreted often exceeds 3 g/day and if not carefully looked for, these patients may be diagnosed to have nephrotic syndrome. ARF occurs in about 7% of patients in the absence of pre-existing renal insufficiency. Precipitating factors include hypercalcemia, dehydration, increased plasma viscosity, hyperuricemia, contrast administration and infection. The pathogenetic mechanism is thought to be intratubular obstruction by casts due to precipitation of myeloma proteins. ARF in multiple myeloma is not always reversible.

A slowly progressive CRF occurs most frequently in light-chain and IgD myeloma. A highly significant relationship has been observed between the presence of Bence-Jones proteinuria and this complication. Hypertension and hematuria are rare and nonlight chain proteinuria is mild. Renal histology shows dilated tubules containing fractured glassy eosinophilic casts surrounded by multinucleated giant cells. There is widespread tubular atrophy, interstitial fibrosis and inflammation. On immunofluorescence, the casts exhibit κ or λ chains beside immunoglobulins, Tamm-Horsfall protein and complement. Tubular defects involving both proximal and/or distal segments may occur in myeloma and sometimes precede it. Secondary amyloidosis occurs in 6–15% of myeloma patients, leading to proteinuria and nephrotic syndrome.

The presence of renal insufficiency drastically shortens the survival of patients with multiple myeloma. The main principles of management and prevention of renal complications are maintenance of adequate hydration, vigorous control of hypercalcemia and hyperuricemia, and the cautious use of potentially nephrotoxic drugs. The standard chemotherapeutic regimen with melphalan and prednisolone ameliorates renal lesions in more than 50% of the patients. In those with severe renal failure, improvement in renal function has sometimes been observed with peritoneal dialysis or plasmapheresis, both of which can remove significant amounts of light chains. Survival rates of myeloma patients in maintenance dialysis average about 50% at 1 year. Although renal transplantation is not contraindicated, it should be done only after chemotherapy has induced prolonged remission and control of the tumor growth.

RENAL LESIONS ASSOCIATED WITH NEOPLASIA

Solid tumors of the lung, gastrointestinal tract (GIT), breast and ovary can lead to membranous nephropathy, minimal change disease or focal glomerular sclerosis manifesting clinically as proteinuria or nephrotic syndrome and in fact can antedate the diagnosis of the primary malignancy. The treatment is toward the primary tumor and symptomatic management for the nephrotic syndrome.

Lymphoreticular malignancies are associated with minimal change disease, focal segmental glomerulosclerosis, membranous or membranoproliferative glomerulonephritis. Minimal change disease is common in Hodgkin's lymphoma. Crescentic glomerulonephritis has been reported in non-Hodgkin's lymphoma. All these may present with significant proteinuria and/or nephrotic syndrome. Kidney may also be involved by direct infiltration in leukemias and lymphomas. The presentation could be with hematuria, proteinuria or might even manifest as ARF. Treatment is symptomatic and supportive. Dialysis may be required to tide over the crisis in ARF.

TUMOR LYSIS SYNDROME

This is a complication of cytoreductive therapy in rapidly growing radio/chemotherapy sensitive tumors. The blood concentrations of uric acid, xanthine, phosphate and potassium increase very rapidly while on treatment. The subsequent filtration and the intratubular precipitation of these substances will result in ARF. This condition can be prevented by vigorous hydration and urine alkalinization prior to, and during the treatment. Patients may require dialysis to tide over the crisis of ARF.

R Kasi Visweswaran, Reena Thomas

CHAPTER
188

The Kidney and Hypertension

Chapter Summary

- Classification of Hypertension
- The Kidney and Hypertension: Victim or Villain
- Resistant Hypertension
- Renal Causes of Hypertension

INTRODUCTION

Hypertension is the most common chronic noncommunicable disease in the world, affecting around 25% of the population. Hypertension can be either, primary when no cause is identified or secondary when an identifiable cause is present. Hypertension is due to multifactorial causes. The pathophysiology of hypertension is now better understood. It has been shown that the kidney plays a central role in the genesis of most forms of hypertension.

CLASSIFICATION OF HYPERTENSION

Based on the recommendations of the 7th report of Joint National Committee (JNC7) 2003, hypertension is diagnosed by the average of two or more properly measured readings during two or more visits.

- ***Normal blood pressure (BP):*** Systolic less than 120 mm Hg and diastolic less than 80 mm Hg
- ***Prehypertension:*** Systolic 120–139 mm Hg or diastolic 80–89 mm Hg
- ***Hypertension:***
  - ***Stage I:*** Systolic 140–159 mm Hg or diastolic 90–99 mm Hg
  - ***Stage II:*** Systolic greater than 160 mm Hg or diastolic greater than 100 mm Hg

The JNC8 guidelines which have been released in December 2013 have made minor modifications in the recommendations for management of hypertension. A summary of the guidelines are as follows.

Regulation of Blood Pressure

The major factors involved in the regulation of both normal and elevated arterial pressure are cardiac output and peripheral resistance. Cardiac output is determined by stroke volume and heart rate. Peripheral resistance is dependent on small vessels and arterioles and it is determined by functional and anatomic changes in them (Flowchart 188.1). Maintenance of a normal BP is dependent on the balance between the cardiac output and peripheral vascular resistance. Most patients with essential hypertension have a normal cardiac output, but a raised peripheral resistance.

Two major mediator systems, the renin-angiotensin system (RAS) and sympathetic nervous system (SNS) regulate the changes in the BP.

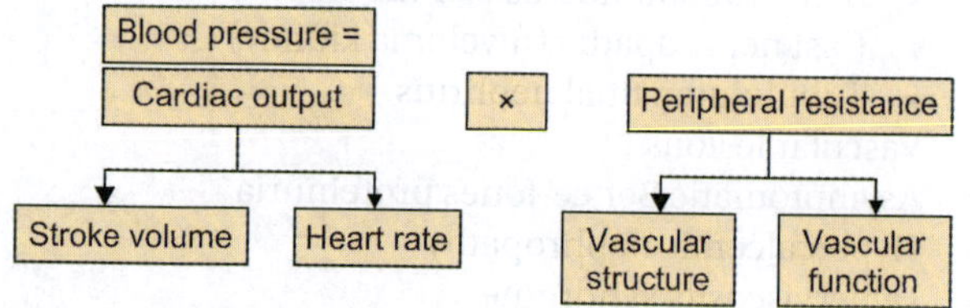

Flowchart 188.1: Components of blood pressure

Renin-Angiotensin System

It is the most important endocrine systems that affect the control of BP. Renin which is stored as granules in the modified smooth muscle cells of the afferent arteriole in the juxtaglomerular apparatus is released to the bloodstream in the kidney in response to:

- Glomerular underperfusion
- Reduced salt intake
- Stimulation from the SNS.

Renin converts angiotensinogen which is the renin substrate produced from the liver to angiotensin I (AT I). This is converted to angiotensin II (AT II) by the angiotensin-converting enzyme (ACE). AT II acts on AT I receptors and causes potent vasoconstriction. It also stimulates aldosterone release from the zona glomerulosa of the adrenal cortex. Aldosterone causes increase in BP by various mechanisms including:

- Renal sodium chloride (NaCl) retention
- Increased vasoconstriction
- Decreased nitric oxide-mediated vasodilatation
- Increased endothelin production

The RAS may not be directly responsible for the rise in BP in all cases of essential hypertension. Many hypertensive patients, especially elderly and black population may have low levels of renin and AT II. In such instances, drugs that block the RAS are not particularly effective (Flowchart 188.2).

Sympathetic Nervous System

Almost all of the blood vessels, except capillaries are innervated by SNS and its stimulation cause peripheral vasoconstriction and increase in heart rate. It also causes release of norepinephrine from adrenal medulla. All the above factors cause increase in the BP. Moreover, activation of sympathetic nervous system in the kidney causes decrease in renal blood flow and activation of RAS. There can be overactivity of the SNS due to various factors thus causing an increase in BP.

Factors stimulating sympathetic nervous system

- Stress and exercise
- Obesity, insulin resistance
- Drugs like nicotine, alcohol, cocaine, cyclosporine and
- Defective baroreceptor reflex.

Flowchart 188.2: Renin-angiotensin system—algorithm showing the varied functions and arrangements of renin, vasopressin and sympathetic activity

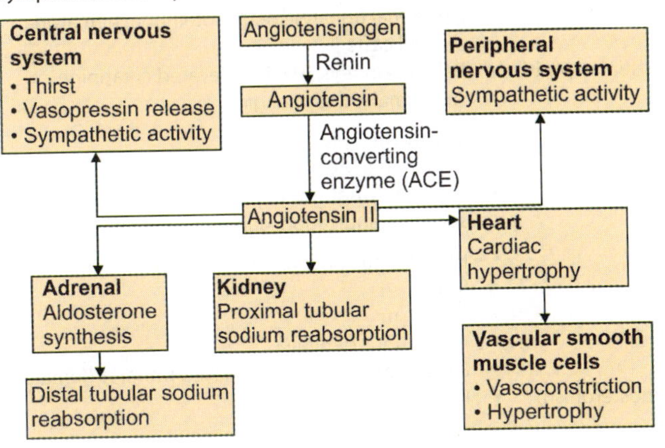

Primary or Essential Hypertension

It is the most common form of hypertension worldwide accounting for nearly 90% of all cases with elevated BP and is defined as BP greater than 140/90 mm Hg with no identifiable secondary cause.

Pathogenesis

The pathogenesis is polygenic and multifactorial. Genetic factors account for about 30% variation in BP. Other postulated causes include low-birth weight, reduced nephron mass or intrauterine developmental disturbances. Two candidate genes postulated for a genetic predisposition include aldosterone synthase gene and adducin gene. African, Americans and ethnic minorities like Hispanics have increased propensity due to genetic predisposition, obesity and others. Increased sodium retention by the kidneys and increased sympathetic activity has also been implicated for increasing BP.

With increasing age, thickening and stiffening of arterioles occur and this along with the other factors and diabetes if any, helps to establish persistent hypertension. After a variable, usually long asymptomatic period, persistent hypertension develops into complicated hypertension, in which target organ damage to the aorta and small arteries, heart, kidneys, retina and central nervous system (CNS) manifest.

Risk factors for essential hypertension include:

- Hypertension in parents
- Excessive sodium intake (more than 10 g NaCl per day)
- Obesity, metabolic syndrome
- Physical inactivity
- Dyslipidemia
- Personality traits.

Secondary Hypertension

This accounts for about 10% of all cases of hypertension. It results from an underlying, identifiable, often correctable cause. The causes of secondary hypertension include:

- ***Intrinsic renal disease:*** Glomerulonephritis (GN), polycystic kidney disease (PKD), acute interstitial nephritis
- ***Renovascular disease:*** Atherosclerotic and fibromuscular dysplasia (FMD)
- ***Mineralocorticoid excess:*** Primary hyperaldosteronism, congenital adrenal hyperplasia (CAH), apparent mineralocorticoid excess (AME), glucocorticoid remediable hypertension, liquorice ingestion
- ***Neuroendocrine:*** Pheochromocytoma, neurofibromatosis
- ***Endocrine:*** Cushing's disease, hypo- and hyperthyroidism and hyperparathyroidism, renin-producing tumors
- ***Genetic disorders:*** Liddle's syndrome, Gordon's syndrome
- ***Miscellaneous:*** Obesity, obstructive sleep apnea (OSA).

Any patient who has clinical clues suggestive of secondary hypertension needs a thorough extensive evaluation to rule out a primary cause.

Clues to Presence of Secondary Hypertension

- Severe or resistant hypertension
- Acute rise in BP in a previously normotensive aged less than 30 years
- Negative family history
- Malignant or accelerated hypertension
- Unexplained deterioration of kidney functions after starting ACE and angiotensin receptor blockers (ARB)
- Severe hypertension in patients with diffuse atherosclerosis
- Severe hypertension with asymmetric (>1.5 cm) size of kidneys
- Flash pulmonary edema
- Systolic–diastolic abdominal bruit.

Among the group of secondary hypertension renal lesions are the most common primary causes. The classification of renal lesions is given in Table 188.1.

Causes of Secondary Hypertension

A few of the secondary causes of hypertension are dealt with here:

Renovascular Disease

Renal artery stenosis: The mechanisms for development of renal artery disease are different from the other secondary causes, hence they are dealt with separately. Hypertension results from atherosclerotic or other causes of narrowing in the main or distal renal arteries.

Fibromuscular dysplasia is seen more often in females less than 40 years. Here, abnormal vascular modelling results in varying degrees of renal artery stenosis. It usually involves the distal two-thirds of the main renal artery. It is classified based on the vascular layer primarily involved into four different types.

1. Medial fibroplasia
2. Perimedial fibroplasia
3. Intimal fibroplasia
4. Adventitial fibroplasia.

A series of fibrotic bands occurs in distal renal artery with aneurysmal dilatation in between due to absence of internal elastic lamina giving a ***string of bead*** appearance in the angiogram. Conventional renal angiogram or digital subtraction angiogram is the ***gold standard*** confirmatory test. Other tests which may be useful are Doppler, magnetic resonance imaging (MRI), isotope renogram with captopril and renal vein renin assay.

Table 188.1: Secondary causes of hypertension, examples and clinical clues

Classification	Examples	Clinical Clues
Intrinsic kidney disease	• Glomerular disease, e.g. membranoproliferative GN, focal glomerulosclerosis, poststreptococcal GN • Tubulointerstitial disease, e.g. ADPKD, acute interstitial nephritis • Microvascular disease, e.g. TTP, PAN, scleroderma	• Abnormal urinalysis, e.g. proteinuria, hematuria, red cell casts • Palable kidneys, ADPKD, elevated creatinine • Abnormal kidney imaging
Renovascular Disease	• Fibromuscular hyperplasia • Atherosclerotic renovascular disease	• Young age (<40) • Abdominal bruit • Signs or symptoms of peripheral vascular disease such as claudication, gangrene, TIA, CVA
Mineralocorticoid excess	• Primary hyperaldosteronism • Cushing's syndrome • Congenital adrenal hyperplasia (11 or 17-hydroxylase deficiency) • Apparent mineralocorticoid excess • Glucocorticoid remediable hypertension (hyperaldosteronism Type I) • Familial hyperaldosteronism Type II	• Hypokalemia metabolic alkalosis • Striae • Hirsutism • Ambiguous genitalia • Early puberty (male) or delayed puberty (female) • Family history

Abbreviations: GN = Glomerulonephritis; ADPKD = Autosomal dominant polycystic kidney disease; TIA = Transient ischemic attack; CVA = Cerebrovascular accident; TTP = Thrombotic thrombocytopenic purpura; PAN = Polyarteritis nodosa

Symptoms depend on the degree of stenosis and whether it is unilateral or bilateral. Patients with bilateral renal artery stenosis are at increased risk of developing severe renal salt retention. In unilateral stenosis, the unaffected kidney can eliminate the salt and water by pressure natriuresis. However, if both kidneys have functional stenosis, recurrent episodes of ***flash pulmonary edema*** may occur and is due to fluid retention resulting from impaired pressure natriuresis.

Management: If the antihypertensive requirement is less, the condition may be managed by antihypertensive drugs. Procedures like percutaneous transluminal renal angioplasty (PTRA), renal artery stenting, aortorenal bypass or renal autotransplantation are other procedures undertaken in selected cases.

Atherosclerotic Renovascular Disease

Atherosclerosis involving the abdominal aorta near the origin of renal arteries extending to involve the proximal one-third of the main renal artery on one or both sides cause the typical finding in atherosclerotic renovascular disease. In advanced cases, segmental and diffuse intrarenal atherosclerosis is observed. When involvement is bilateral and diffuse within the kidneys, the condition is called ischemic nephropathy.

- Ischemic nephropathy is suspected when a patient has one or more of the following manifestations. Azotemia in the setting of coronary artery disease (CAD) or peripheral vascular disease
- Unexplained renal insufficiency in the setting of hypertension
- Progressive azotemia in the setting of hypertension
- ACEI-induced acute renal failure (ARF)
- Flash pulmonary edema.

Renal Parenchymal Hypertension

Renal parenchymal disease is the most common among the causes of secondary hypertension. In many instances, undetected renal parenchymal disease gets labeled as essential hypertension. The following are the common renal parenchymal causes:

- Diabetic nephropathy (40%)
- Hypertensive nephrosclerosis (20%)
- Primary glomerular disease (18%)
- Chronic tubulointerstitial disease (7%)
- Autosomal dominant polycystic kidney disease (ADPKD) and obstructive nephropathy (5%).

Hypertension can be commonly seen in primary glomerular diseases such as immunoglobulin A (IgA) nephropathy, focal segmental glomerulosclerosis (FSGS), membranoproliferative glomerulonephritis (MPGN) or other forms of GN. Hypertension results from activation or release of vasoconstrictors and retention of salt and water.

Reduction of proteinuria along with BP reduction can slow the progression of kidney disease.

Achieving a BP goal of less than 140/90 mm Hg is warranted and ACEI are the main stay of treatment with monitoring for hyperkalemia and worsening of glomerular filtration rate (GFR).

THE KIDNEY AND HYPERTENSION: VICTIM OR VILLAIN

The kidney plays a central role in almost all forms of hypertension. It not only causes certain forms of hypertension, it is also a target organ which is damaged by hypertension. The central role of the kidney in hypertension is highlighted by cross transplantation experiments in rats. When a normotensive rat undergoes bilateral nephrectomy followed by kidney transplantation from a hypertensive rat, it develops hypertension. However, when a hypertensive rat gets a kidney from a normotensive rat after the original kidneys have been removed, its hypertension is cured. This also occurs in humans. Transplantation of a kidney from a normotensive donor with no family history of hypertension to an individual with renal failure and resistant hypertension led to prolonged normalization of BP. Post-transplantation studies in experimental models of genetic hypertension have shown that inherited tendency to hypertension resides primarily in the kidney.

Multiple factors affect renal sodium excretion and therefore, the regulation of the effective circulating volume and BP. Aldosterone and possibly atrial natriuretic peptide (ANP) are responsible for day-to-day variations in sodium excretion, by their respective ability to augment and diminish sodium reabsorption in the collecting tubules. As sodium intake is reduced, for example, the ensuing decrease in volume enhances the activity of the renin-angiotensin-aldosterone system and reduces the secretion of ANP. The net effect is enhanced sodium reabsorption in the collecting tubules, which seems to account for the appropriate fall in sodium excretion in this setting.

This sequence is reversed with volume expansion, as an increase in the secretion of ANP and a reduction in that of aldosterone allow excretion of the excess sodium by diminishing collecting tubule sodium reabsorption. This *pressure natriuresis* phenomenon may be the *final defense* against changes in the effective circulating volume.

A reset pressure natriuresis due to multiple renal defects is postulated to have a role in hypertension.

The mechanisms of increased sodium reabsorption by the kidney in hypertension are not well-understood. Possibilities include increased activity of the proximal tubular Na-H exchanger, the thick ascending limb Na-K-Cl$_2$ co-transporter, the distal tubular NaCl co-transporter, and the collecting duct epithelial sodium channel (ENaC). Different ion channels may have a role in the genesis of hypertension as seen by the following few examples.

- Increased activity of the ENaC in the collecting tubule is responsible for the hypertension in Liddle's syndrome and genetic variants in this channel may explain salt sensitive hypertension in some populations.
- On the other hand, loss-of-function mutations in the distal tubule NaCl co-transporter in Gitelman's syndrome are associated with low to normal BP.

Examples of single or prohypertensive gene mutations are:
- Liddle's syndrome (gain-of-function mutation in the sodium channel gene)
- Pseudohypoaldosteronism type 2 (also called Gordon's syndrome or familial hyperkalemic hypertension). Due to mutations in with no lysine (WNK) kinases 1 and 4
- Glucocorticoid remediable aldosteronism (GRA) or familial hyperaldosteronism type I, due to a chimeric gene formed from portions of the 11β-hydroxylase gene and aldosterone synthase gene
- Familial hyperaldosteronism type II. The genetic defect appears to be on chromosome 7p22
- Syndrome of AME is due to defective 11β-dehydrogenase enzyme.

RESISTANT HYPERTENSION

Resistant hypertension may also be due to renal causes. It is defined as, inadequate BP control in a patient adhering to therapeutic doses of three antihypertensive agents including a diuretic.

A defective pressure natriuresis is postulated as a cause. Salt retention causes increase in extracellular fluid (ECF) causing hypertension. Drugs such as fludrocortisone and nonsteroidal anti-inflammatory drugs (NSAIDs) can also cause similar effects. Other causes of resistant hypertension may be due to increased RAS activity, sympathetic overactivity and excessive salt intake which also contribute to resistant hypertension both by increasing BP and by blunting the BP lowering effect of most classes of antihypertensives and diuretics. This effect was more pronounced in some patients who are labeled salt sensitive. Salt sensitivity is more common in elderly, and patients with chronic kidney disease (CKD).

Renal disease in essential hypertension: Most patients with well-controlled essential hypertension have a benign renal course. Proteinuria develops in 30–40% and 18% develop renal insufficiency. About 2–5% may progress to severe renal failure over 10–15 years.

HYPERTENSIVE NEPHROSCLEROSIS

It is a disorder, usually associated with chronic hypertension, more prevalent in African and Americans. It is characterized by long standing hypertension and progressive renal failure in the absence of other causes for renal failure. Benign nephrosclerosis is characterized histologically by vascular, glomerular and tubulointerstitial changes. The glomeruli may show both focal global and focal segmental sclerosis and glomerular enlargement Global sclerosis and nephron loss suggest ischemic injury and glomerular enlargement is due to compensatory hypertrophy of surviving nephrons.

RENAL COMPLICATIONS OF HYPERTENSION

CKD and end-stage renal disease (ESRD) progresses due to hypertensive nephrosclerosis and accelerating renal failure.

Hypertensive emergency is defined as a condition in which elevated BP results in target organ damage. The systems primarily include the CNS, i.e. the cardiovascular system (CVS) and renal system.

Malignant and ***accelerated hypertension*** are both hypertensive emergencies, with similar outcomes and therapies. Up to 1% of patients with essential hypertension may develop malignant hypertension. The characteristic vascular lesion is fibrinoid necrosis of arterioles and small arteries which causes the clinical manifestations of end-organ damage. Red blood cells (RBCs) are damaged as they flow through vessels obstructed by fibrin deposition, resulting in microangiopathic hemolytic anemia (MAHA). Causes of malignant hypertension include all causes of secondary hypertension.

Accelerated hypertension is defined as a recent significant increase over baseline BP that is associated with target organ damage. This is, usually seen as vascular damage on funduscopic examination, such as flame-shaped hemorrhages or soft exudates, but without papilledema.

Hypertensive emergencies require immediate therapy to decrease BP within minutes to hours. In contrast, there is no evidence to suggest any benefit from rapidly reducing BP in patients with hypertensive urgency. In fact, such aggressive therapy may harm the patient, resulting in cardiac, renal or cerebral hypoperfusion. For further details on the Management of Hypertension, refer to Section 13, Ch 126.

Renal Involvement in Systemic Diseases with Special Reference to Pregnancy

Jacob George, Usha Samuel

Chapter Summary

- Diabetes Mellitus and Pregnancy
- Hypertension and Pregnancy
- Pregnancy and Underlying Renal Disease
- Acute Kidney Injury in Pregnancy
- Urinary Tract Infections
- Systemic Lupus Erythematosus and Pregnancy

INTRODUCTION

Pregnancy is a physiological state and a safe outcome is often the rule. Medical problems in pregnancy can either be due to occurrence of pregnancy in a patient with a pre-existing illness or development of a new medical disease during pregnancy. The commonly encountered medical problems during pregnancy are diabetes mellitus (DM), hypertension, underlying renal disease, acute renal failure (ARF), chronic kidney disease (CKD), liver dysfunction, urinary tract infection (UTI) and systemic lupus erythematosus (SLE). These problems may cause miscarriage, preterm labor, intrauterine growth retardation, prematurity, perinatal mortality and worsening of the primary disorder in the mother. Hence, early diagnosis and appropriate management are essential.

DIABETES MELLITUS AND PREGNANCY

(*See* also Section 10, Chapters 91 and 92)

DM complicating pregnancy may either be due to pregnancy in a previously known type 1 or 2 diabetic patient (overt diabetes or pregestational diabetes) or first detection of an abnormal glucose tolerance during pregnancy. The latter is called gestational diabetes mellitus (GDM). This is due to an increased risk of insulin resistance and hyperinsulinemia during pregnancy. The diagnostic criteria for GDM include a fasting plasma glucose more than or equal to 92 mg/dL, but less than 126 mg/dL at any gestational age. Fasting plasma glucose more than or equal to 126 mg/dL is consistent with overt diabetes. The other criteria is 1 hour more than or equal to 180 mg/dL and 2 hours more than or equal to 153 mg/dL by 75 g oral glucose tolerance test (GTT) between 24 and 28 weeks of gestation.

Uncontrolled diabetes can affect both maternal and fetal health. Therefore, screening for diabetes in pregnancy is important. Hyperglycemia in first trimester is associated with fetal anomalies and miscarriages. In later pregnancy, hyperglycemia causes large for gestational age infants, macrosomia (birth weight >90th percentile), shoulder dystocia, birth injuries and neonatal hypoglycemia. There is also an increased risk of maternal hypertension and pre-eclampsia.

Risk Factors for Gestational Diabetes Mellitus

- Body mass index (BMI) more than 25 kg/m²
- Waist-hip ratio more than 1
- Family history of diabetes
- Age more than 25 years
- Multiparity
- Ethnic predisposition.

Management

Dietary management is on the same lines as for nonpregnant women. Extra calories and proteins should be provided to fulfill the needs of the fetus also. It is safer to start insulin early, when target glucose levels are exceeded despite nutritional therapy and exercise. Oral hypoglycemic agents are avoided as most of them can cross the placental barrier and affect the fetus. In those unwilling for insulin, Glyburide can be given. Metformin can also be given in the second and third trimesters.

Pregnancy is a state of relative insulin resistance. So, maternal nutrients are shunted to the developing fetus and the normal range of blood glucose is lower by approximately 20%. The target fasting blood sugar should be between 60 and 92 mg/dL, 1 hour post-prandial should be less than 140 mg/dL and 2 hours post-prandial should be less than 120 mg/dL. At fasting blood sugar levels of more than 95 mg/dL, the risk of macrosomia is more. Since blood sugar should be kept in the normal range, frequent self-monitoring is to be recommended.

Generally, spontaneous delivery is desirable. However, with the presence of maternal hypertension, history of previous stillbirth, poor metabolic control and macrosomia, delivery is planned around 37–38 weeks of gestation. If fetal weight is greater than 4 kg, cesarean section is done. The fetal loss and perinatal mortality are higher in diabetic compared to nondiabetic pregnancies. The infant of the diabetic mother has a risk of childhood obesity, impaired motor functions, higher rates of inattention and/or hyperactivity and diabetes in later life. Those with GDM have a sixfold to tenfold increased risk of developing type 2 DM subsequently.

HYPERTENSION AND PREGNANCY

The blood pressure (BP) falls from the prepregnant value from the time of conception, reaches the lowest value by the end of second trimester and gradually, rises to prepregnant levels by term. Hypertension is a common and important complication associated with pregnancy. The national high BP education program classifies hypertensive disorders of pregnancy as follows:

- Chronic hypertension
- Pre-eclampsia–eclampsia

- Pre-eclampsia superimposed on chronic hypertension
- Gestational hypertension.

Hypertension, defined as a BP higher than 140/90 mm Hg, is the most common medical complication of pregnancy, occurring in 6–8% of pregnancies. Hypertension is more common in young primiparous women and older multiparous women. The presence of a hypertensive disorder of pregnancy is associated with significant maternal and/or fetal mortality and morbidity and premature birth.

Chronic Hypertension

It is defined as a prepregnancy blood pressure of greater than 140/90 mm Hg or as hypertension occurring before 20 weeks gestation. The definition may also include some hypertensive women with minimal proteinuria diagnosed during pregnancy that does not resolve with delivery. However, some show nephrosclerosis on renal biopsy rather than pre-eclampsia.

Chronic hypertension increases the risk of pre-eclampsia, abruptio placentae, intrauterine growth retardation and second trimester fetal death. Methyldopa is the preferred treatment agent, but in mild cases, no therapy may be necessary. In women whose BP is well-controlled when they enter pregnancy, consideration should be given to continuing the same therapy. However, angiotensin II receptor blockers (ARBs) and angiotensin-converting enzyme inhibitors (ACEIs) are contraindicated in pregnancy due to the risk of fetal renal agenesis.

Pre-eclampsia and Eclampsia

Pre-eclampsia is defined as hypertension and proteinuria in previously normotensive pregnant women that typically develops after 20 weeks gestation and resolves with delivery. Clinically, pre-eclampsia usually begins after 32 weeks of pregnancy, although it may occur earlier in women with pre-existing renal disease of hypertension. Other disorders should be considered when hypertension and proteinuria occur before 20 weeks. Eclampsia is defined as the occurrence of seizures in women with pre-eclampsia.

The major features of pre-eclampsia are uteroplacental hypoperfusion and fetal ischemia due to inadequate embryonal trophoblast invasion of the uterine wall and of the spiral arteries into the placenta. *Treatment* of mild pre-eclampsia includes bed rest and antihypertensive therapy, but more severe disease is treated with aggressive measures to control hypertension and use of intravenous (IV) magnesium sulfate to prevent seizures and immediate or early delivery of fetus. Pre-eclampsia typically resolves within 10 days postpartum.

Risk Factors and Pathogenesis

Underlying essential hypertension, DM, renal disease, twin pregnancies, antiphospholipid syndrome (APS), fetal hydrops, insulin resistance and factor V Leiden deficiency are all risk factors. Low-dose aspirin can reduce the risk pre-eclampsia and its complications, primarily in high-risk patients.

In normal pregnancy, there is resistance to the action of angiotensin II. In pre-eclampsia, there is an increased sensitivity to the vasopressor effects of angiotensin II. In addition, there is increased synthesis of endothelin and thromboxane which predisposes to platelet aggregation and intravascular clotting. The synthesis of vasodilator factors, like prostacyclin and nitric acid decrease and result in uteroplacental insufficiency. Thus, impaired angiogenesis and placentation resulting in endothelial dysfunction, systemic vasoconstriction and coagulopathy are important pathogenetic factors.

HELLP Syndrome

The HELLP (hemolysis, elevated liver enzyme levels, low platelet count) syndrome, is a manifestation of severe pre-eclampsia, usually associated with severe hypertension and varying degrees of acute kidney injury (AKI). HELLP syndrome may also be associated with pulmonary edema, ascites and disseminated intravascular coagulation (DIC).

There is reduction in renal blood flow and glomerular filtration rate (GFR) with a decrease in urate clearance and increased calcium reabsorption. This leads to hyperuricemia and hypocalciuria. Hyperuricemia may correlate with severity. Histopathologically, there is swelling of the glomerular endothelial cells, referred to as glomerular capillary endotheliosis. These lesions resolve by 4 weeks after delivery.

Management of Pre-eclampsia

Initial therapy for mild pre-eclampsia (BP < 140/90 mm Hg, proteinuria < 500 mg/24 hours with normal renal function, serum urate < 4.5 mg/dL) is bed rest until fetal growth and maturation are adequate. It may be preferable to maintain the BP below 125/75 in the second trimester and 135/85 in the third trimester. To prevent seizures, magnesium sulfate should be used. After 32 weeks gestation, if the fetal maturity is achieved, delivery is the definitive treatment. If there is worsening disease, as evidenced by uncontrolled hypertension, headaches or hyperreflexia, eclampsia or HELLP syndrome, induction of labor should be immediate in view of the possible maternal risks.

Pre-eclampsia Superimposed on Chronic Hypertension

It is more likely in older women or those with underlying renal disease. This condition is difficult to distinguish from worsening hypertension in pregnancy, but should be suspected, if a woman who had hypertension before 20 weeks gestation develops any of the following in the second half of pregnancy:

- New-onset proteinuria
- A sudden increase in BP
- A sudden increase in pre-existing proteinuria
- Thrombocytopenia
- Liver function abnormalities.

Other clues to the diagnosis are hyperuricemia and increased serum creatinine.

Gestational Hypertension

It is defined as hypertension that appears after midterm, not associated with proteinuria, and resolves after delivery. Risk factors are a family history of hypertension, obesity and multiparity. Some progress to pre-eclampsia, especially when hypertension develops before 35 weeks gestation. Women who had gestational hypertension are at risk for developing chronic hypertension in later life. In addition, their children may have higher BP.

Drug Therapy for Hypertension in Pregnancy

The goal is to reduce fetal morbidity and mortality by preventing severe hypertension and/or pre-eclampsia. For mild hypertension, the centrally acting alpha adrenergic agonist methyldopa is the first-line therapy, based on a long record of effectiveness and safe fetal outcomes. Labetalol is an effective alternative. Calcium channel blockers (CCBs), like nifedipine is also a safe alternative. Hydralazine can be used for more severe hypertension, commonly in combination with methyldopa or beta-blockers. Beta-blockers, particularly atenolol, may cause fetal bradycardia in the first trimester, but these agents can be used safely later in pregnancy. Diuretic agents are, generally not recommended, but can be continued, if they are effectively controlling the hypertension. These drugs should not be used in superimposed pre-eclampsia because of associated hypovolemia. ACEIs and ARBs are contraindicated in pregnancy, because they have been associated with increased fetal loss in animal studies and have also been associated with fetal renal tubular dysplasia, oligohydramnios, perinatal ARF, and other congenital anomalies. First-trimester exposure to ACEIs has been associated with an increased risk of major congenital malformations. It is therefore, important to provide appropriate counseling to women of childbearing age who may be using ACEIs or ARBs for hypertension.

PREGNANCY AND UNDERLYING RENAL DISEASE

In general, patients with CKD have reduced fertility and carry higher risk depending on the nature and degree of kidney disease and presence of hypertension and proteinuria. Many can safely deliver healthy children with limited maternal risk, if they have only mild reductions in GFR. During pregnancy, most women with CKD who are not on dialysis experience hypertension (25%) and increased proteinuria (50%). Women with CKD are at increased risk of irreversible decline in GFR during pregnancy, fetal loss, intrauterine growth retardation, and early labor compared with women with normal renal function. High maternal blood urea levels can act as an osmotic diuretic in the fetal kidney and can cause early labor and fetal loss. Patients with less severe CKD, i.e. serum creatinine less than 1.4 mg/dL generally do well if they have no severe hypertension or significant proteinuria. One-third of women with moderate kidney disease (GFR < 70 mL/min or serum creatinine more than 1.4 mg/dL) are at risk for more rapid declines of renal function. Patients with a GFR less than 40 mL/min and proteinuria more than 1 g/day before conception are likely to have poor maternal and fetal outcomes.

Management

Pregnant women with kidney disease should be followed up more frequently. The obstetric follow-up includes careful BP monitoring, renal function and 24-hour urine protein assessments. If progressive renal failure occurs, either in early pregnancy or before fetal viability can be assured, dialysis may needed. Dialysis should be initiated when the serum creatinine level is 3.5–5.0 mg/dL or the GFR is below 20 mL/min. Fetal outcome is better with longer, more frequent hemodialysis sessions—about 20 hours per week. Daily dialysis is more likely to prevent hypotension and significant metabolic shifts. Dialysis should aim to keep blood urea nitrogen (BUN) levels below 50 mg/dL, because controlling uremia may avoid polyhydramnios, control hypertension and improve the mother's nutritional status. Peritoneal dialysis with smaller volumes and frequent exchanges can also be done to achieve these same goals. Anemia should be treated with erythropoietin (EPO) and careful attention to iron therapy. Nutritional support that allows weight gain of 0.3–0.5 kg/week should be maintained in the second and third trimesters. Although women on maintenance dialysis can conceive, the rate of spontaneous abortions is about 50%. The fetal survival is about 70% if the mother retains the pregnancy and goes on to third trimester.

Pregnancy Following Renal Transplantation

Transplantation restores fertility and women can conceive 2 years after successful renal transplantation. Pregnancy in kidney transplant recipients can be considered in the following:

- Good general health for 2 years post transplantation, with serum creatinine levels below 2.0 mg/dL (preferably < 1.5 mg/dL)
- No recent acute rejection or ongoing rejection
- Normotension, or hypertension controlled with minimal antihypertensive agents
- No minimal proteinuria
- No evidence of pelvicalyceal dilatation on renal ultrasonogram.

Recommended immunosuppression in kidney transplant recipients includes:

- ***Prednisone:*** Less than 15 mg per day (mg/day)
- ***Azathioprine:*** 2 mg/kg/day or less
- ***Calcineurin inhibitor***—based therapy at appropriate therapeutic levels
- Breastfeeding is not recommended, while on cyclosporine. Tacrolimus may be taken during breastfeeding, but monitoring of infant levels is recommended
- Mycophenolate mofetil and sirolimus should be discontinued 6 weeks prior to conception due to risk of fetal teratogenicity
- Methylprednisolone is the preferred agent for treatment of rejection should it occurs during pregnancy.

However, there are higher risks of miscarriage, abortion, stillbirth, ectopic pregnancy, preterm birth, low-birth-weight babies and neonatal death.

ACUTE KIDNEY INJURY IN PREGNANCY

AKI was a common complication of pregnancy during the mid to late part of the 20th century. The incidence has come down because of better antenatal care and awareness. While AKI may occur from any of the causes associated with the nongravid state, a number of disorders are specific to pregnancy. Pregnancy-specific renal disorders, generally can be classified into those occurring in early pregnancy and those occurring in late pregnancy. Disorders arising in early pregnancy include the following:

- Prerenal azotemia
- Acute tubular necrosis (ATN)
- Renal cortical necrosis
- Pyelonephritis
- Thrombotic thrombocytopenic purpura (TTP).

Disorders arising in late pregnancy, almost all of which are usually specific to pregnancy, include the following:

- Pre-eclampsia
- Acute fatty liver of pregnancy
- Hemolytic-uremic syndrome.

The following conditions should also be considered in evaluating AKI in pregnancy:

- Obstructive uropathy
- Nephrolithiasis
- APS.

Obstructive uropathy should be considered in the setting of moderate or severe dilatation of the collecting system in women with oliguria or anuria. Causes include compression by the gravid uterus, polyhydramnios, kidney stones and enlarged uterine fibroids. Obstructive uropathy usually resolves with delivery, although ureteral stenting may be required preterm. The most common cause of prerenal azotemia is hyperemesis gravidarum. Treatment consists of antiemetic therapy and volume replacement with IV normal saline and potassium. Less commonly, hemorrhage associated with spontaneous abortion can also result in prerenal azotemia.

Acute tubular necrosis (ATN) is often more severe and more likely to require temporary dialysis. In early trimester, this may be due to severe hyperemesis gravidarum, hemorrhage from spontaneous abortion or shock secondary to septic abortion. In late pregnancy, ATN may occur due to pre-eclampsia, HELLP syndrome or by uterine hemorrhage with abruptio placentae. ATN should be suspected from the clinical situation. Urine examination shows muddy-brown and granular casts under the microscope and elevated urinary sodium excretion. Renal cortical necrosis is a rare cause of severe AKI, although it is more commonly associated with pregnancy. It is more likely to occur following an obstetric catastrophe, such as abruptio placentae or septic abortion.

Unlike the nongravid condition, acute pyelonephritis in pregnancy may result in a reduced GFR that can be reversed, with treatment of the underlying infection. Acute pyelonephritis most commonly occurs during the second trimester, with the predominant pathogenic organism being *Escherichia coli*. Treatment often requires hospitalization, IV antibiotics and IV fluid administration. IV cephalosporin is an appropriate choice for initial therapy.

Postpartum AKI or TTP or Hemolytic-Uremic Syndrome (HUS)

This follows an apparently normal pregnancy and usually manifests 1 day to several weeks after delivery. The onset is a ***flu-like*** illness followed by rapidly developing renal failure. Congestive cardiac failure (CCF) and convulsions may occur. The cause is not clear. Retained placental fragments, oral contraceptives, oxytocin, ergot alkaloids, prostaglandin deficiency and immunologic basis have all been incriminated. Circulating large multimers of von Willebrand's factor (vWF) lead to platelet aggregation, and thrombosis in renal circulation, resulting in renal damage. Management consists of BP control and supportive measures. Renal functions may not recover fully. Specific measures include plasmapheresis done daily or on alternate days for the initial 2 weeks. Plasmapheresis helps to remove the toxins and vWF multimers.

URINARY TRACT INFECTIONS (UTIS)

Asymptomatic Bacteriuria

Because of the anatomical and functional changes in the urinary tract and increased urinary excretion of amino acids, protein, calcium, glucose and vitamins, asymptomatic bacteriuria may occur in 5–10% of all pregnancies. It is more common when pre-existing conditions like DM, sickle cell disease, renal diseases, multiparity, low, socioeconomic background or hypertension are present. Although asymptomatic bacteriuria may be a relatively benign disorder not requiring active treatment in nonpregnant subjects, 30–50% of pregnant women with asymptomatic bacteriuria develop symptomatic UTI. Asymptomatic bacteriuria may be associated with increased incidence of pre-eclampsia, premature delivery, anemia and low-birth weight. Therefore, routine screening during the first trimester for bacteriuria is advocated. If detected, any one of the following antibiotics should be administered orally for 14 days preferably based on the sensitivity. Amoxicillin 500 mg 8 hourly, ampicillin 500 mg 6 hourly, cephalexin 500 mg 6 hourly or cefixime 200 mg 12 hourly may be used safely during pregnancy. The patient should be followed up with urine cultures every month till delivery. In women in whom asymptomatic bacteriuria is difficult to eradicate, continuous antibiotic therapy during pregnancy and detailed investigations to rule out urinary tract obstruction in the postpartum period are warranted. Nitrofurantoin 100 mg, cephalexin 250 mg or trimethoprim 100 mg at bedtime can be given as low dose prophylaxis till term.

Acute Pyelonephritis

Symptomatic renal parenchymal infection with fever, rigor, chills, loin pain and pyuria may occur in about 1% of all pregnancies. Severe infections may lead to renal cortical abscess, renal carbuncle, sepsis, shock and fetal loss. Those with asymptomatic bacteriuria, having previous episodes of UTI or congenital abnormalities of the urinary tract are more prone to develop acute pyelonephritis. The patient should be hospitalized and prompt treatment instituted. Urine and blood samples should be sent for culture and treatment with IV fluids, antipyretics and antibiotics started. In severe infections, antibiotics which reach high concentrations in the renal parenchyma and which have no adverse effects on the fetus should be started immediately, e.g. amoxicillin 500 mg 8 hours or cefotaxime 1 g 6 hours or ceftazidime 1 g 6 hours IV. When the fever is controlled for 48–72 hours, antibiotics have to be continued orally for a total period of 3-weeks to ensure eradication of infection. During follow-up, urinalysis and cultures are essential. Tetracycline should be avoided during pregnancy.

Co-trimoxazole should not be given near term because of the risk of kernicterus in the newborn. Aminoglycosides may cause ototoxicity and hence they, should be avoided. Low dose antibiotic prophylaxis may be needed till term, especially if there is more than one episode.

Acute Fatty Liver of Pregnancy

This is characterized by the onset of abdominal pain and jaundice, typically occurring after 34 weeks of gestation. Pathogenesis involves microvesicular fatty infiltration of hepatocytes, which may be related to defective mitochondrial beta-oxidation of fatty acid. Diagnosis is established by the clinical presentation and laboratory studies. Hyperbilirubinemia is the predominant laboratory abnormality, with mild elevations of aspartate aminotransferase (AST) and alanine aminotransferase (ALT) levels. Severe cases may result in hypoglycemia, coagulation abnormalities and even fulminant hepatic failure. Most women with this disorder have AKI but only a small percentage requires dialysis. *Treatment* consists of immediate delivery and supportive care. While most patients recover completely, fulminant hepatic failure may require liver transplantation.

SYSTEMIC LUPUS ERYTHEMATOSUS AND PREGNANCY

(*See* also Section 12, Ch 108)

Pregnancy can affect the course of SLE and SLE can affect both the mother and fetus during pregnancy. In SLE, the best outcomes occur in those who have had stable, inactive lupus for 6 months or longer before conception. SLE can flare during pregnancy and usually presents as proteinuria, hypertension and falling GFR, making the distinction from pre-eclampsia very difficult. However, hematuria, low complement levels and elevated anti-double stranded deoxyribonucleic acid (anti-dsDNA) titers are more common with active lupus nephritis. SLE is also associated with an increased risk of abortions and prematurity. The fetus can also be affected because of the transplacental passage of autoantibodies. Congenital lupus can manifest as cutaneous lupus due to anti-La antibodies and congenital heart block due to anti-Ro antibodies. All pregnant patients with SLE should be screened for anti-SSA (Ro) antibodies, due to the risk of congenital heart-block. IV betametasone or dexameta-sones are preferred as they can cross the placental barrier. *Treatment of SLE* in pregnancy is problematic because cyclophosphamide and mycophenolate mofetil which are used in lupus therapy are potentially teratogenic in early pregnancy. Prednisolone and azathioprine are relatively safe in pregnancy.

Women with anticardiolipin antibodies and the lupus anticoagulant are at risk of fetal loss and worsening renal function. All pregnant women with lupus should be screened for antiphospholipid antibodies and lupus anticoagulant. Treatment with low-dose aspirin or heparin should be considered but depends on the antibody levels and previous obstetric history of early fetal loss and/or thrombosis.

CHAPTER

190

Urinary Tract Obstruction

Jayant Thomas Mathew, M Thomas Mathew

Chapter Summary

- General Considerations
- Causes
- Pathophysiology
- Clinical Features
- Diagnosis
- Management

GENERAL CONSIDERATIONS

Obstructive uropathy is defined as the structural and functional changes in the urinary tract that impede the normal flow of urine. Changes in the kidney secondary to the obstruction of urinary tract are termed ***obstructive nephropathy***. The terms ***hydronephrosis*** and ***hydroureterosis*** denote only dilatation of the drainage system and does not mean obstruction.

Obstruction of the urinary tract may occur anywhere between the renal tubule and urethral meatus. The impedance to the normal flow of urine results in complex structural and functional changes in the kidneys and urinary tract. Based on the site of obstruction, it can be classified as intrarenal or extrarenal. The extrarenal obstructions may be upper urinary tract obstruction or lower urinary tract obstruction. Urinary obstruction may be unilateral or bilateral, complete or partial, acute or chronic and may be caused by extraluminal or intraluminal causes.

CAUSES

Intrarenal
- Uric acid crystals
- Oxalate crystals
- Sulfonamide precipitates
- Acyclovir, indinavir precipitates
- Multiple myeloma (intratubular cast formation)

Extrarenal—upper urinary tract obstruction
- Causes in the lumen
  - Crystals and stones
  - Sloughed renal papillae

- Blood clots
- Fungus balls
- Causes in the wall
  - Functional
    - Pelviureteric junction obstruction
    - Vesicoureteric junction obstruction
  - Tumors (transitional cell carcinoma)
  - Infections (tuberculosis)
  - Strictures (tuberculosis, other granulomas, radiation)
- Causes outside the wall
  - Retroperitoneal fibrosis
  - Pelvic tumors—fibroid carcinoma of uterus, cervix, ovary, prostate
  - Radiation sequelae
  - Lymph nodes
  - Crohn's disease
  - Aneurysm of abdominal aorta
  - Aberrant arteries
  - Retrocaval ureter

Lower urinary tract infection

- Causes in the lumen
  - Stones
  - Blood clots
- Causes in the wall
  - Urethral stricture
  - Posterior urethral valve
  - Phimosis, meatal stenosis
  - Carcinoma of bladder
  - Trauma
  - Functional-neurogenic bladder
  - Anticholinergic drugs
- Causes outside the wall
  - Prostatic enlargement
  - Infiltrating pelvic malignancies.

PATHOPHYSIOLOGY

When the urinary system is obstructed, changes occur in both glomerular and tubular functions. The glomerular filtration rate (GFR) declines progressively depending whether the obstruction is complete or partial, unilateral or bilateral and acute or chronic. Abnormalities in tubular function include impairment of concentrating and acidifying functions. If the obstruction is relieved within 1–2 weeks, there is normalization of glomerular and tubular functions. Chronic obstruction for more than 12 weeks results in irreversible destruction of renal parenchyma. In such cases, functional recovery may be incomplete even after relief of obstruction. Eventually, the nephrons and renal parenchyma get replaced by extracellular matrix. When prolonged obstruction is relieved, there is temporary inability to concentrate urine or reabsorb solutes. This leads to polyuria, salt wasting and hypokalemia. This may last for variable periods. This referred to as ***postobstructive diuresis***. Pathologically, marked thinning of renal cortex occurs over many months with atrophy of tubular structures, obliteration of nephrons, progressive sclerosis and fibrosis of the renal parenchyma.

CLINICAL FEATURES

Clinical manifestations depend on the site, degree and duration of obstruction. Pain is a common presenting symptom and is due to distension of the bladder, collecting system or renal capsule. Pain is more severe in acute obstruction compared to chronic obstruction. The location and quality of pain often help to determine the site of obstruction. Obstruction at pelviureteric junction causes colicky pain in the loin. Mid-ureteric obstruction usually produces sudden lumbar pain with radiation from loin to groin. In lower ureteral obstruction, the pain radiates to the ipsilateral testicle, labia or inner part of the upper thigh. Distension of the bladder with stretching of the trigone leads to frequency, strangury and radiation of pain to the tip of the penis. In lower urinary obstruction, the patient often complains of poor stream of urine, intermittency, hesitancy, urgency, precipitancy, dribbling, nocturia or urinary incontinence. Urinary obstruction predisposes to resistant urinary infection. Infection can be eradicated only when the obstruction is cleared. If the urinary system is obstructed chronically, infection with *Proteus* group of organisms and secondary stone formation occur commonly. In neonates and children, obstruction by posterior urethral valve and secondary vesicoureteral reflux may lead to progressive renal damage. Obstruction due to calculi or neoplastic lesions may present with hematuria also. Complete lower urinary tract obstruction, bilateral ureteric obstruction or obstruction to a single functioning kidney may lead to total anuria. In partial obstruction, the urine output may be normal or even increased.

One or both kidneys may be enlarged and palpable depending on the site of obstruction. In the case of lower tract obstruction, the distended bladder may be palpable and tender. Enlarged prostate is identified by rectal examination. In females, pelvic examination is required to detect malignant lesions. Hypertension may occur in some cases due to salt and water retention or renin release.

Proteinuria, hematuria, pyuria and bacteriuria may be present. Rarely, urine examination may even be normal. In chronic obstruction, the specific gravity of urine is less than 1,010. Bilateral obstruction is associated with renal failure. There is impaired excretion of acid and potassium and this can lead to type IV renal tubular acidosis.

DIAGNOSIS

Diagnosis is often made by history and physical examination. Urinalysis, urine culture, hemogram, assessment of renal function, imaging studies such as X-ray procedures, ultrasound studies, computed tomography (CT) scans, magnetic resonance imaging (MRI) and isotope renography (as is indicated in each case) will help to detect the cause of the obstruction, functional state of the organs and in planning treatment.

MANAGEMENT

Management depends on the site and cause of obstruction and the degree of renal impairment. In acute obstruction, rapid intervention helps to salvage the kidney. Methods used for relief of obstruction include:

- Urethral catheters or suprapubic cystostomy for urethral or bladder neck obstructions. Relief of obstruction should be gradual in chronic obstructive lesions

- Cystoscopy and passage of retrograde ureteral catheter or the nephroscope
- Nephrostomy and nephroscopic examination for upper urinary obstruction.

These procedures will have to be undertaken with appropriate antibiotic cover under strict aseptic precautions. Specific therapy is decided depending on the cause of the obstruction and this is the realm of the urologists. In acute obstruction such as retention of urine careful catheterization of the bladder should be undertaken by the attending physician to relieve distress, before referring the patient to the specialist.

Renal Replacement Therapy

VN Unni, George Kurian

Chapter Summary

- Dialysis
  - Hemodialysis
  - Ultrafiltration
    - Artificial Kidney (Dialyzers)
  - Indications for Dialysis in Acute Kidney Injury
    - Hemodialysis in ESRD
    - Complications of Maintenance Hemodialysis
  - Continuous Renal Replacement Therapies
  - Peritoneal Dialysis
    - Continuous Ambulatory Peritoneal Dialysis
- Kidney Transplantation
  - Donor Selection
  - Recipient Selection
  - Immunusuppression in Kidney Transplantation
  - Complications of Renal Transplantation

INTRODUCTION

End-stage renal disease (ESRD) or chronic kidney disease (CKD) stage 5 is defined as CKD with a glomerular filtration rate (GFR) of less than 15 mL/min. Patients who have reached this stage of CKD cannot lead a comfortable life with conservative management alone and need some mode of renal replacement therapy (RRT), which may be long-term dialysis or kidney transplantation.

Options	Definition
• Dialysis	• Clearance of small molecules and toxins using diffusion occurring across a membrane
• Hemodialysis	• Dialysis with clearance occurring across a synthetic membrane
• Peritoneal dialysis	• Dialysis with clearance occurring across a native peritoneal membrane
Ultrafiltration	Fluid removal across a semipermeable membrane during dialysis by convection (solutes are moved under pressure across a membrane)
Hemofiltration	Continuous dialysis therapy which involves removal of plasma water and its dissolved constituents (e.g. K^+, Na^+, urea, phosphate) by convection flow across a high-flux semipermeable membrane and

	concurrent reinfusion of an electrolytic solution of the desired biochemical composition
Hemodiafiltration	Combination of hemodialysis and hemofiltration
Continuous renal replacement therapies	Include hemofiltration and hemodiafiltration

DIALYSIS

The word *dialysis* means *to remove from*. This treatment modality is essentially a process by which biochemical wastes and excess water, which are normally excreted by the kidney, are removed from the blood of a patient with ESRD. There are two forms of dialysis: (1) Hemodialysis and (2) Peritoneal dialysis (PD). Either of these techniques can be used as a short-term measure in patients with acute kidney injury (AKI) (acute dialysis) or as a long-term option in ESRD (chronic dialysis).

Hemodialysis (HD)

History: The first scientific description of the physical principle in HD (diffusion) was by the Scottish chemist Thomas Graham, who became known as the *Father of Dialysis*. First successful dialysis treatment in humans was done by Willheim Kolff in 1945 using a rotating drum device. Later a Norwegian doctor Fredrik Kiil developed a parallel plate dialyzer. A major step forward was the development of the hollow-fiber dialyzer by Richard Stewart in 1964.

Principles of HD: It is a process wherein the nitrogenous wastes and excess water that are normally excreted by the kidneys are removed, when the patient's blood passes through the artificial kidney. A solution known as *dialysate* or dialysis solution, which is a solution of specially treated water with appropriate levels of sodium, potassium, magnesium, calcium, chloride and dextrose and bicarbonate (as buffer) is also passed into the hollow fiber kidney. The constitution of dialysate is akin to plasma without proteins, except that potassium levels are usually kept low.

A semi-permeable membrane separates the blood compartment from the dialysate compartment. During the passage through the dialyzer, diffusion of solutes

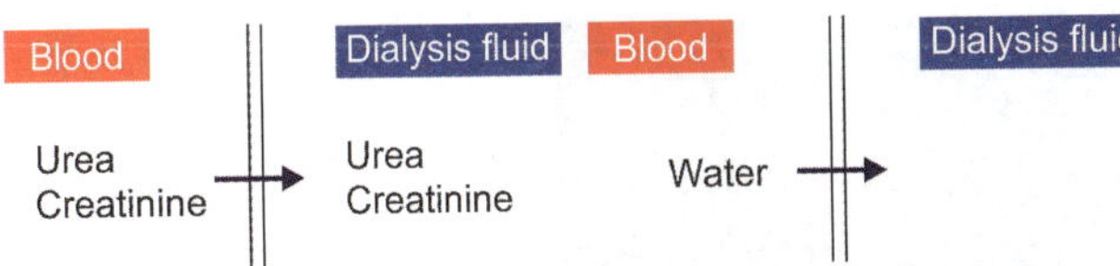

Figs 191.1A and B: A. Diffusion (movement of solutes based on concentration gradient); **B.** Ultrafiltration (movement of water based on hydrostatic pressure gradient)

like urea and creatinine (Fig. 191.1A) occurs across the membrane depending on the concentration gradient. Diffusion is maximized by maintaining high flow rates of blood and having the dialysate flow in a direction countercurrent to the direction of blood flow.

Ultrafiltration

The excess water from the patient's blood is removed by a process known as *ultrafiltration*, which denotes movement of water from the blood to the dialysate compartment based on hydrostatic pressure gradient (Fig. 191.1B). Three main requirements for dialysis are:

1. *Artificial kidney:* To facilitate excretion of waste products.
2. *Dialysis monitor (machine):* To prepare the dialysis fluid, circulate this fluid and blood through the artificial kidney, monitor the procedure and give alarms in case of malfunction.
3. *Vascular access:* To enable continuous removal and return of blood during hemodialysis.

Artificial Kidney (Dialyzers)

Hemodialysis is an extracorporeal method of purification of blood using a filter called as artificial kidney or dialyzer (Figs 191.2A and B). Patient's blood is drawn out with a pump and passed through bundles of hollow fibers in the dialyzer. Since the beginning of the hemodialysis in the last century, the dialyzer has undergone much modification so as to make it compact. At present, all dialyzers are cylindrical shaped with thousands of hollow fibers made of a semipermeable membrane inside the cylinders. The design has improved the efficiency of dialysis and re-duced the number of complications. There are four types of membranes which are currently used to make dialyzers. They are cellulose, substituted cellulose, cellulosynthetic and synthetic. Synthetic membrane materials include polyacrylonitrile, polyamide, polysulfone and polymethyl methacrylate. The synthetic membranes have higher permeability and they are more biocompatible compared to cellulose membranes. These dialyzers are available in various surface areas to cater to patients with different body surface areas.

Dialysis Monitor (Machine)

The modern dialysis machines are equipped with elec-tronic devices to monitor blood flow, dialysate flow, temperature and conductivity of dialysate, ultrafiltration rate (UFR) and sensors to detect blood leak into the dialysate or air in the blood circuit (Fig. 191.3).

Vascular Access for Hemodialysis

Blood is drawn into the extracorporeal circuit and is returned to the patient through the vascular access. The vascular access can be classified as temporary and permanent access. Arteriovenous (AV) shunt, which is not used anymore, was the form of vascular access in the olden days. Cannulation of major veins (femoral, internal jugular or subclavian) with a double lumen catheter is used as temporary vascular access at the present time (Figs 191.4A and B).

Tunneled double lumen dialysis catheters increase the longevity of the dialysis catheters, as they have a lower incidence of catheter related sepsis, which is the most important complication of temporary vascular access.

An anastomosis between the radial or brachial artery and the cephalic or basilic vein (AV fistula), or a synthetic graft between artery and vein either on the forearm or upper arm (AV graft) are the two types of permanent vas-cular access; AV fistulae (Fig. 191.5) are the most common permanent vascular access in patients on maintenance hemodialysis and are referred to as the *lifeline* of these patients. Tunneled catheters can be a suitable bridge till AV fistula matures (usually 6–8 weeks) or when dialysis is anticipated for a few weeks before renal transplantation. The AV fistula should be allowed to mature before it can be used. It may take up to 6–8 weeks. During this time, the high pressure of the blood and flow rate in the vein which has been anastomosed to the artery will cause hypertrophy of the muscles in the wall of the vein. The vein gets *arterialized* and dilated so that it can be easily cannulated using large bore needle and blood flow rate in the region of less than 300 mL/min can be achieved. The AV fistula is cannulated with two needles. One is directed

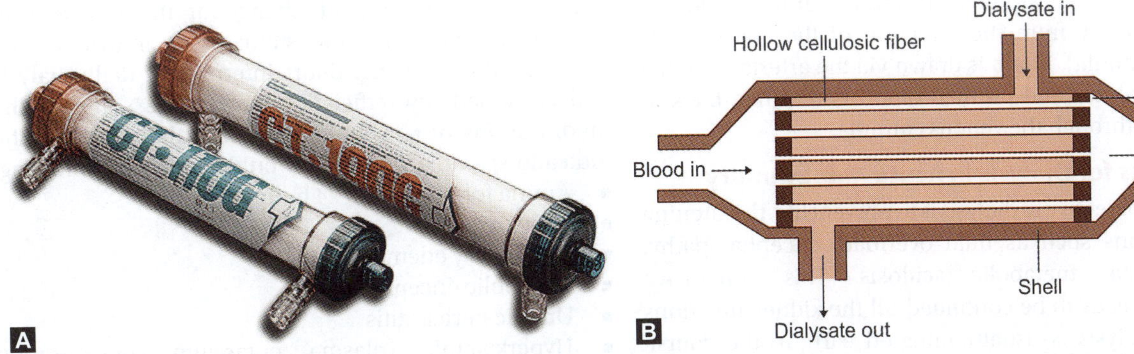

Figs 191.2A and B: A. Hollow fiber dialyzer; **B.** Hollow fiber artificial kidney (HFAK): 8,000–10,000 of hollow fibers encased within a cylindrical plastic outer coat, with ports for blood inlet and outlet, as well as inlet and outlet ports for dialysis fluid

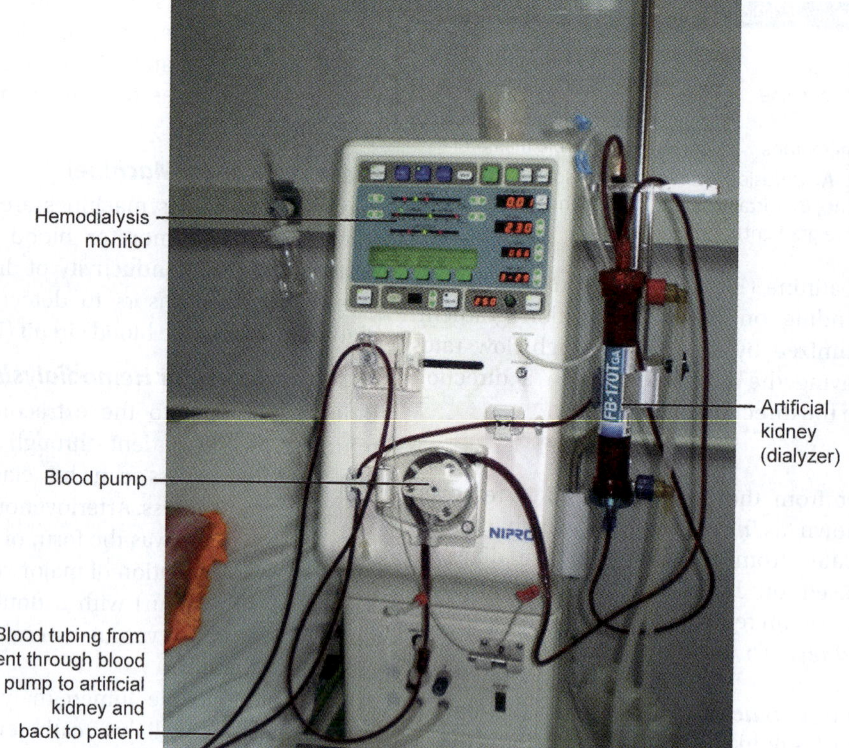

Fig. 191.3: Hemodialysis machine with the hollow fiber dialyzer and the blood tubings (extracorporeal circuit) which carry blood into and from the dialyzer (this machine is a monitor to ensure a dialysis prescription and to avoid complications during dialysis)

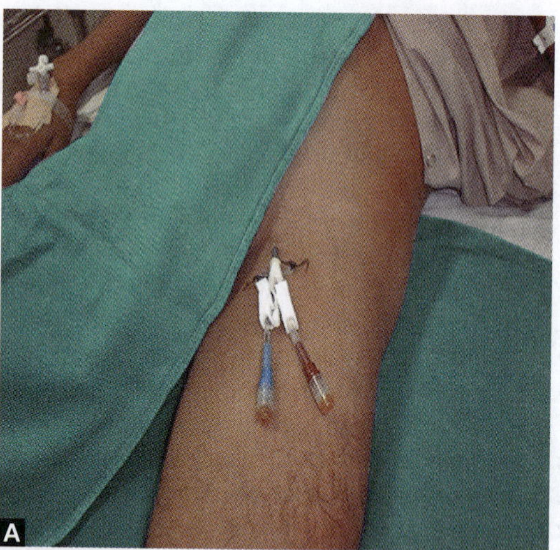

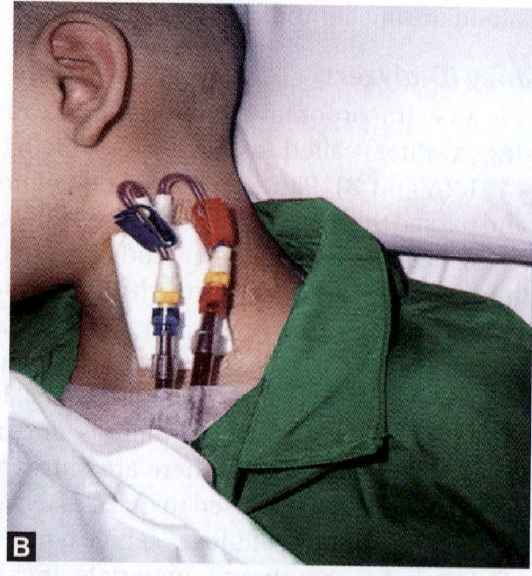

Figs 191.4A and B: Double lumen catheter. **A.** Left femoral vein; **B.** Left internal jugular vein

toward the AV anastomosis (arterial cannula) and the other one away from the direction of the anastomosis (venous cannula). Blood is drawn via the arterial cannula into the dialyzer and purified blood is returned back to the patient through the venous cannula.

Indications for Dialysis in Acute Kidney Injury

In AKI, the objective of dialysis is to prevent life-threatening complications such as fluid overload, encephalopathy, hyperkalemia, metabolic acidosis. This supportive treatment needs to be continued till the kidney functions recover. Dialysis is usually initiated early in the course of the illness. The duration and frequency of dialysis is determined by the catabolic state of the individual (reflected by the rate of change of the biochemical parameters), hemodynamic status of the individual and the general well-being. Short intermittent daily dialysis and sustained low efficiency dialysis are some of the modifications of conventional hemodialysis in AKI. The indications for dialysis in AKI would include the following:

- Anuria for more than 24 hours
- Fluid overload
- Pulmonary edema
- Metabolic encephalopathy
- Uremic pericarditis
- Hyperkalemia (plasma potassium concentration >6.5 mEq/L)
- Metabolic acidosis (pH less than 7.1).

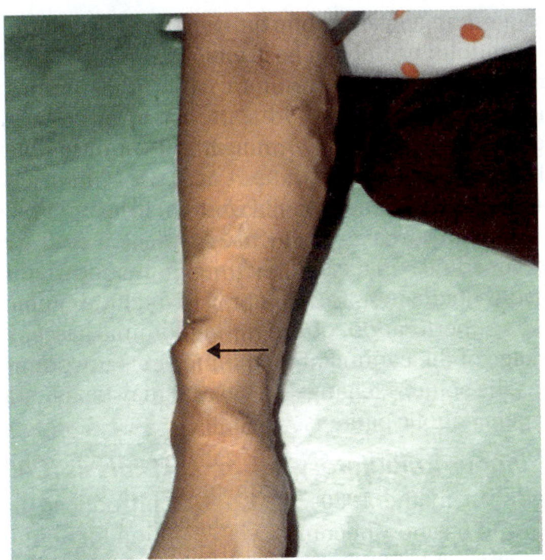

Fig. 191.5: Right radiocephalic arteriovenous fistula (the dilated veins on the forearm can be seen) (arrow)

Hemodialysis in ESRD

As patient approaches ESRD, the patient and family needs to be counseled regarding timely initiation of RRT. If the patient opts for maintenance HD and is clinically fit for the procedure, a permanent vascular access (AV fistula) is created and allowed to mature. Dialysis should be initiated when GFR falls below 15 mL/min or if the patient is symptomatic. Ideally, a patient with ESRD requires three sessions of hemodialysis a week, for duration of four hours each. The patient should be periodically evaluated for adequacy of dialysis, general well-being, bone disease, calcium-phosphorus balance, nutritional status and anemia. Most patients on dialysis require treatment with antihypertensive medications. Other supportive measures include erythropoietin (EPO) supplementation along with parenteral iron for correction of anemia, water soluble vitamin supplements, phosphate binders and active form of vitamin D_3 for treating bone disease.

Factors Determining Dialysis Efficacy

The efficacy of dialysis can be affected by many factors. The important ones are:

- Blood flow rate
- Dialysate flow rate
- Membrane permeability and surface area of dialyzers
- Duration and frequency of dialysis
- Rate of vascular access recirculation.

Increase in blood flow rate, dialysate flow rate, type of membrane and its surface area, duration and frequency of dialysis help to increase the efficacy of hemodialysis to a certain extent. No dialytic procedure can completely replace the kidney function fully. Only the excretory function of the kidney is performed by the dialysis. In conventional dialysis, blood flow is usually kept at 200–400 mL/min and dialysate flow at 500–800 mL/min. Dialyzer efficiency is usually measured by its ability to clear urea (urea clearance), remove water [ultrafiltration rate (UFR)] and clear larger molecules like vitamin B_{12} (B_{12} clearance). Conventional dialyzers have urea clearance of 300–500 mL/min and UFR of 5–10 mL/

mm Hg of transmembrane pressure. When the blood flow through the fistula is inadequate, the purified blood recirculates between arterial and venous limbs. Thus, the most of the purified blood recirculates within the dialyzer, thereby reducing the efficacy of dialysis. High efficiency and high flux dialyzers can achieve urea clearances of more than 700 mL/min. They have higher UFRs and they also clear larger molecular weight solutes. However, when using high flux dialyzers the machines need to be more sophisticated and the water used to prepare the dialysate needs to be ultrapure.

Dialysis Adequacy

Adequacy of dialysis is assessed by the clinical condition, including nutrition and objectively determined by biochemical indices. The most widely used index is the Kt/V, where K denotes the ability of a dialyzer to clear a substance, t is the duration of dialysis and V is volume of distribution of the substance in the body. The recommended Kt/V urea per dialysis session is 1.2–1.3. A 4-hour session of dialysis using a conventional dialyzer and blood and dialysate flow rates of 200 mL/min and 500 mL/min, respectively, often achieves this Kt/V in an average adult patient. Other measures of dialysis adequacy are urea reduction ratios (1-post dialysis serum urea/predialysis serum urea) and time average concentration of urea, which calculates the average urea between the beginnings of two successive dialysis sessions. Assessment of the quality of life (QOL) measured by specific questionnaire as well as nutritional indices are also important measures of adequacy.

Complications of Maintenance Hemodialysis

The common complications are hypotension, muscle cramps, nausea and vomiting, headache, chest pain, back pain, itching, pyrogen reactions, first use syndrome and dialysis disequilibrium. Rapid removal of urea during the initial dialysis sessions may cause symptoms due to brain edema as a result of concentration gradient of urea between brain and blood. This is referred to as ***disequilibrium syndrome***. This can be prevented by deliberately giving shorter and less efficient dialysis sessions initially. ***First use syndrome*** develops in some patients when a new dialyzer membrane is used. It does not occur during reuse. Vomiting, headache, muscle cramps, hemolysis and bleeding are less frequent adverse effects. Patients with cardiovascular disease may develop hemodynamic instability, angina, acute coronary events, arrhythmias and sudden death. Long-term complications of maintenance HD include metabolic bone disease, neuropathy, dialysis dementia, chronic subdural hematoma and amyloidosis.

Continuous Renal Replacement Therapies

In order to meet the high metabolic demands of acutely ill patients with AKI, who are hemodynamically unstable in the intensive care units (ICUs), newer forms of dialysis have come into vogue. They are collectively called as ***continuous renal replacement therapy*** (CRRT). Using the principles of ultrafiltration and convective transport through highly permeable and low resistance dialyzers, solute removal and fluid removal are achieved over a longer period of time compared to conventional hemodialysis. This slow procedure is likely to suit the hemodynamically unstable, hypercatabolic patients in the ICU. Vascular access is usually a double lumen venous catheter in a central vein. Various modes of CRRT include continuous hemofiltration (HF), slow continuous hemodialysis and hemodiafiltration (HDF) which combines the principles of both hemodialysis and HF.

The terminology depends on the physical process involved in solute removal and the type of vascular access used (i.e. AV or venovenous). Most common access used is venovenous access. Hence, the terminology for continuous hemodialysis using venovenous access is continuous venovenous hemodialysis (CVVHD). Likewise, the terms CVVH/CVVHF are used for HF and CVVHDF for HDF. Slow continuous ultrafiltration is used when a large volume of fluid removal alone is desired [patients with congestive cardiac failure (CCF)]. Advantages of CRRT include hemodynamic stability and removal of large volumes of fluid, thereby facilitating good nutritional supplementation. Disadvantages include continuous anticoagulation and its problems, increased manpower for close monitoring and increased cost compared to conventional hemodialysis.

Peritoneal Dialysis (PD)

This was first done in 1936 for a patient with ARF. The peritoneal membrane with its underlying capillary bed acts as the semipermeable membrane, and exchange of solutes occurs by diffusion between blood and dialysate. Water removal is by a process of osmosis, facilitated by adding glucose in the PD fluid. The peritoneal dialysate is a sterile solution of water with its solute concentration similar to that of plasma water. The buffer used is lactate and dextrose is used as an osmotic agent to facilitate ultrafiltration (Fig. 191.6).

Acute intermittent PD (IPD) is performed by introducing a stiff catheter into the peritoneal cavity.

Fluid exchanges of 30–40 mL/kg bw in children and 2 L in adults are given at a time. The fluid is allowed to remain in the peritoneal cavity for 30 minutes and drained off under strict sterile precautions. This exchange process is repeated. Each exchange takes about 1 hour and such exchanges can be continued for 24–48 hours. Acute PD is particularly effective in children, in whom the ratio of peritoneal surface area to body surface area is greater than in adults. PD can be done in hemodynamically unstable patients. Complications include infection, bleeding, perforation of hollow abdominal viscera and blockage of the cannula. Disequilibrium is uncommon in PD, as the solute exchange is slow. PD may be inadequate in hypercatabolic patients.

Continuous Ambulatory Peritoneal Dialysis (CAPD)

Introduced in the 1980s, CAPD was introduced in the 1980s and has now become a viable option for about 10% of patients with ESRD worldwide. The patient or a close family member is taught to do the procedure so that the procedure can be done at home and does not have to travel to dialysis center as in HD. The principles of CAPD are the same as that of IPD, except that the fluid is permitted to dwell for 3–4 hours during each exchange. A permanent soft silicon catheter with multiple small perforations at one end and 2 Dacron cuffs (Tenchkoff catheter) is usually used. The end with perforations is positioned inside the peritoneal cavity. The catheter is drawn out through a subcutaneous tunnel where the cuffs are positioned. One cuff is positioned just before the entry of the catheter into the peritoneum and the other cuff is positioned in the subcutaneous tissue about 2–3 cms deeper to the skin exit site of the catheter. The exit site is fashioned suitably below and lateral to the umbilicus on left or right side depending on the convenience of the patient. If the patient is right handed, it would be advantageous to position the exit site of the right side below the level of umbilicus. The PD fluid is available in fully collapsible bags, made of nonleachable plastic material. Single or double bags

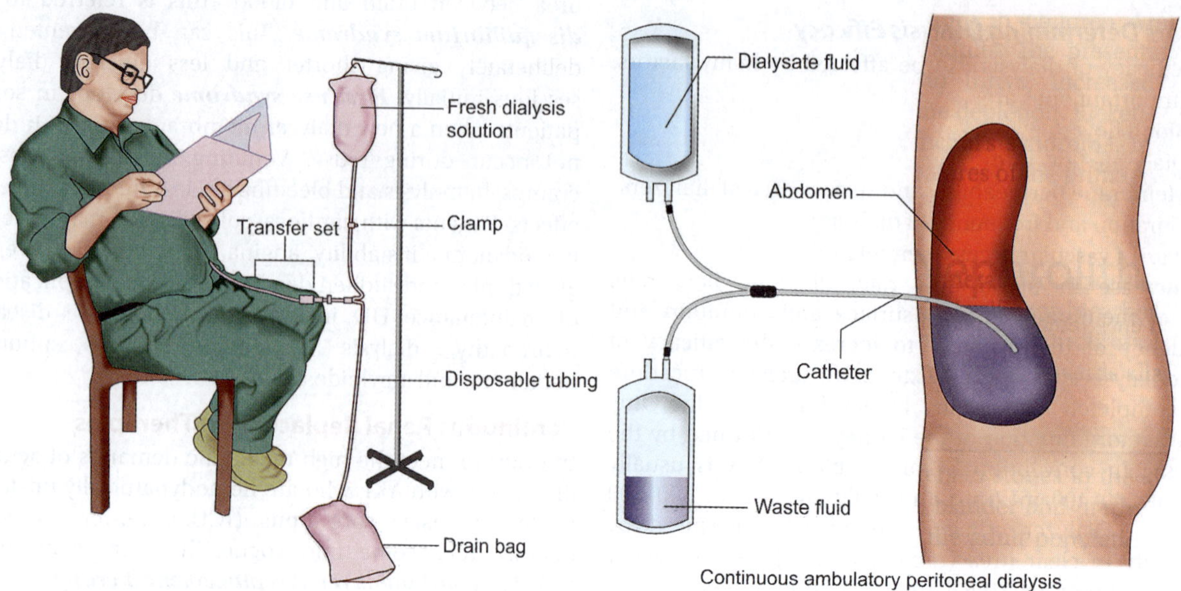

Fig. 191.6: Peritoneal dialysis fluid is infused into the peritoneal cavity through a catheter; the fluid is allowed to remain in the peritoneal cavity for a period of time normally 1–3 hours depending upon the condition and then drained out into a drain bag

with appropriate connecting and transfer sets are used. A titanium adapter is usually used to connect the catheter to the transfer set in order to minimize infection. Sufficient training of the patient or a bystander to the techniques is essential to avoid infection which is the most serious complication.

CAPD involves 3–4 exchanges per day for an average adult. Each exchange involves drainage of existing fluid in the peritoneum, refilling the peritoneum and disconnecting the set and securing the CAPD catheter. The steps may take about one hour for each exchange. If the steps are followed meticulously, the rate of infection will be considerably lower. Individual prescriptions vary depending upon the clinical condition of the patient, the transport characteristics of the peritoneal membrane and the type and concentration of PD fluid. Dialysis is considered to be adequate if the total Kt/V urea per week is 1.7 or more for adults (Fig. 191.7).

Indications

CAPD is a suitable option for patients with cardiovascular disease, poor vascular access, those living away from centers of hemodialysis facility and those who prefer home-dialysis. It is the preferred option for small children and elderly patients. The advantage of CAPD is the relative freedom of mobility, better rehabilitation and QOL, preservation of renal function and lesser need for EPO to manage anemia. Disadvantages include cost, need for clean and adequate space, self-reliance and likelihood of progressive ultrafiltration failure due to change in peritoneal permeability.

Complications

The complications of CAPD can be divided into infective complications and noninfective complications. The infective complications are peritonitis, tunnel infections and exit site infections. Infective complications are usually due to improper handling of the catheter and the transfer sets. Care givers of patients on CAPD need adequate training to do the procedure and to minimize the chances of infection. Signs of peritonitis may include one or more of the following: Abdominal pain and tenderness cloudy effluent dialysate fluid and fever. Peritonitis following CAPD is treated with intraperitoneal instillation of antibiotics. Occasionally, peritonitis can be fungal or tuberculous in etiology, in which case the PD catheter is removed and the patient is switched over to hemodialysis temporarily. The noninfectious complications of CAPD include blockage of catheter, abdominal hernias (umbilical, inguinal and incisional hernia), hydrothorax, gastroesophageal reflux (GER) and delayed gastric emptying, back and abdominal pain, hemoperitoneum, electrolyte imbalances like hypokalemia, hypocalcemia and hypermagnesemia, metabolic complications such as hyperglycemia and dyslipidemia. Other rare, but dreaded complications, include loculation of PD fluid and chronic sclerosing peritonitis.

Automated Peritoneal Dialysis (APD)

This modality has become popular in the recent years. The fluid exchanges in CAPD are done manually, while in APD, the exchanges are done by a machine called cycler; this avoids frequent human handling of the bags and transfer sets, thereby reducing the risk of peritonitis. Different modalities are available, few of them combining both manual and cycler exchanges. The different modalities are continuous cyclical peritoneal dialysis (CCPD), nocturnal intermittent peritoneal dialysis (NIPD) and tidal peritoneal dialysis (TPD). In CCPD, the cycler assisted exchanges are done during night and a long day dwells in order to attain improved adequacy of PD. In NIPD, the day time is kept dry and the cycler assisted exchanges are undertaken during night. In TPD, the APD is designed to optimize solute clearance by leaving a fixed volume of dialysis solution in the peritoneal cavity throughout the dialysis session (Fig. 191.8).

Adequacy of Peritoneal Dialysis

The adequacy of solute clearance is calculated by computing weekly Kt/V values. Studies have shown that a weekly Kt/V value of 1.7 or more is adequate. To make a PD prescription, the physician needs to assess the perito-

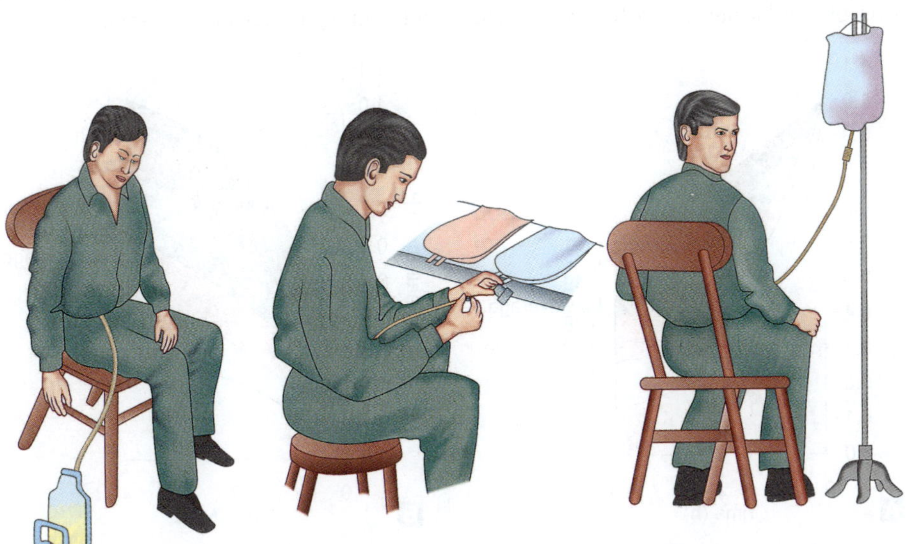

Fig. 191.7: Steps in continuous ambulatory peritoneal dialysis (CAPD) exchanges (the fluid in the peritoneal cavity is first drained out and then fresh fluid is infused into the peritoneal cavity). The patient can attend to his duties during the dialysis

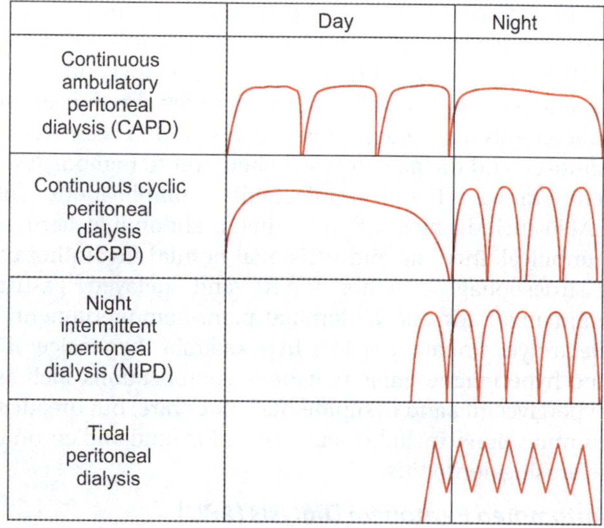

Fig. 191.8: Types of peritoneal dialysis

neal membrane transport characteristics. This is accomplished by doing peritoneal equilibration test (PET). In PET, after a 4-hour dwell of 2L of 2.5% dextrose CAPD fluid, the dialysate to plasma concentration of creatinine is measured at different time intervals and a graph is plotted. Likewise, CAPD fluid glucose concentration is measured and a graph is plotted and the membranes are classified into high transporters, high average, mean, low average and low transporters. The standard PET graph is shown in Figs 191.9A and B. According to the PET results, the PD prescription is modified. The low transporters are advised lower strength of dialysate fluid (1.5% dextrose) and longer dwells, while high transporters are benefited by higher strength (2.5 and 4.25% dextrose) of fluids and shorter dwells to achieve fluid removal.

KIDNEY TRANSPLANTATION

The best option for young patients with ESRD, who are fit to undergo surgery, is indeed kidney transplantation; this is because both hemodialysis and PD replace some of the excretory functions only and not the metabolic and endocrine functions of the kidneys. The first successful kidney transplantation was performed in 1955 by Joseph Murray at the Peter Bent Brigham Hospital, Boston, USA, using an identical twin as the kidney donor. Since then the growing understanding of the immunology of transplantation has led to the development of newer immunosuppressive drugs, which in turn led to improved survival of human allografts. The introduction of calcineurin inhibitors in the immunosuppressive armamentarium reduced the acute rejection episodes after transplantation. The patient survival rate at 5 years post-transplantation is 91% in live donor transplants and 84% in those who receive a deceased (cadaver) donor transplant. The median graft survival in live related donor kidney transplantation with matched donors is 24 years and in unmatched live donors it is 18 years; in cadaver transplantation the median survival is 14 years.

Donor Selection

Any healthy adult, aged 20–60 years, can be a kidney donor for his/her close or near relative, as defined in the Human Organs Transplantation Act. The donor should have two normally functioning kidneys and should not have any systemic illness known to affect the kidneys. The donor and recipient have to be ABO compatible and it is desirable that they are also matched to the best possible extent for the human leukocyte antigen (HLA). The recipient serum should not cross-react with donor lymphocytes (Lymphocytotoxic crossmatch should be negative). To reduce the widening gap between the demand and supply of donor kidneys, altruistic donors (genetically unrelated) and deceased donors (cadavers) also contribute significantly to the donor pool.

Recipient Selection

A patient with ESRD, who does not have any other organ disease, can be considered for kidney transplantation, if he/she is fit for surgery. Patients who have any active infection, malignancy or any other chronic or irreversible organ disease are not advised transplantation. Although there is no agreement on the age limits for this procedure, most centers would restrict transplantation to patients between ages of 5 and 65 years.

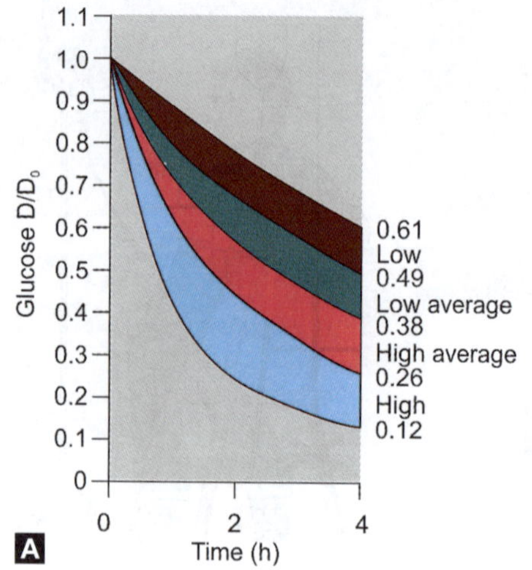
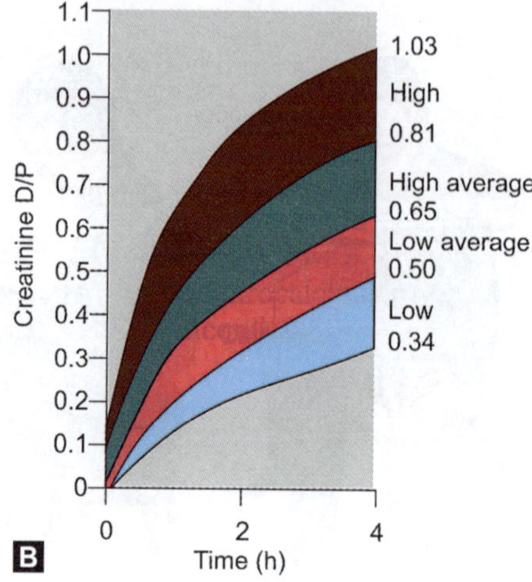

Figs 191.9A and B: Types of peritoneal membrane based on peritoneal equilibration test. **A.** Time is plotted on X-axis and the ratio of concentration of glucose at time 0 and at different intervals on the Y-axis; **B.** Time on X-axis and the ratio of creatinine in the dialysis fluid to creatinine in plasma on the Y axis

Box 191.1: Contraindications to renal transplantation

Absolute contraindications	Relative contraindications
• Renal causes • Reversible renal involvement • Active glomerulonephritis • Active vasculitis or recent anti-GBM disease • Previous sensitization to donor tissue • Nonrenal causes • Disseminated or active untreated cancer • Severe occlusive aortoiliac vascular disease • Severe psychiatric disease • Persistent substance abuse • Severe mental retardation • Severe heart disease/ refractory congestive heart failure • Active infection	• Age: Very young children (< 1 years) or older people (> 75 years) • Iliofemoral occlusive disease • Diabetes mellitus • Severe diseases of lower urinary tract: Bladder dysfunction or urethral abnormalities • Chronic liver disease • Treated malignancy • Significant comorbidity

Abbreviation: GBM = Glomerular basement membrane

The contraindications of renal transplantation are shown in Box 191.1.

Procedure

The donor kidney along with a portion of the ureter and the vascular pedicle is removed surgically and transplanted into the iliac fossa of the recipient. The donor renal artery is anastomosed to the internal iliac, external iliac or common iliac artery of recipient; donor renal vein to external iliac or common iliac vein of recipient, and donor ureter into the recipient's urinary bladder (Fig. 191.10). The vascular anastomosis is done after the kidney is perfused with cold isotonic solutions and the ureter is implanted into the native bladder. The native kidneys of the recipient are not removed, unless there are specific indications. Usually brisk diuresis

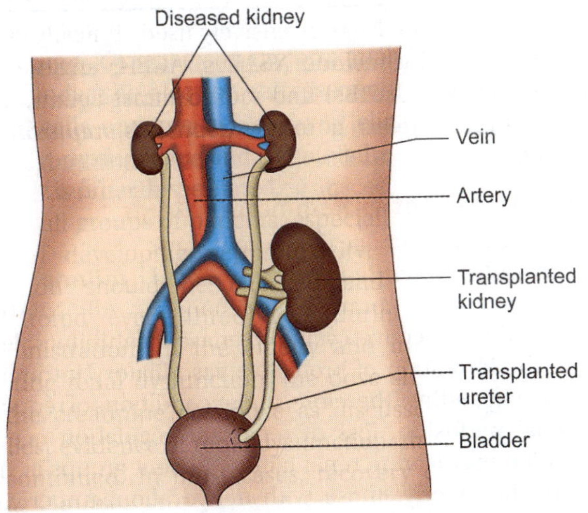

Fig. 191.10: Kidney transplantation. **Note:** Transplanted kidney in left iliac fossa, renal artery and renal vein anastomosed end to side with external iliac artery and external iliac vein, respectively, and the ureter anastomosed to the bladder. The native kidneys and ureter are left as such. The native kidneys are removed only if there are specific indications for removal

occurs after transplantation. Rarely graft function can be delayed due to acute tubular necrosis (ATN); this is more common with cadaver donors. Donor selection and recipient preparation goes a long way in ensuring a good outcome after transplantation.

Immunosuppression in Kidney Transplantation

The most important barrier to transplantation of human organs is the immune response mounted by the recipient against the donor organ. Lifelong immunosupression is required except in cases where the donor is an identical twin. Induction therapy is started either pre or intraoperatively and includes high dose corticosteroids, antilymphocyte antibodies like antithymocyte globulin (ATG) (thymoglobulin), interleukin-2 receptor (IL-2R) antagonists (basiliximab) or anti-CD20 antibodies (rituximab). Maintenance immunosuppression therapy include appropriate combination of 2 or more of the following drugs: Prednisolone, azathioprine, myco-phenolate mofetil, calcineurin inhibitors (cyclosporine, tacrolimus) or mammalian target of rapamycin (mTOR) inhibitors (everolimus and sirolimus). Regular use of these drugs and repeated follow-up visits involve heavy financial burden, which are being subsidized by public and private charities.

Complications of Renal Transplantation

Graft Rejection

Graft rejection occurs when the recipient's immune system mounts a destructive response against the donor kidney. Depending on the rapidity of the graft damage and the time of occurrence, there are three types of rejections: (1) Hyperacute rejection resulting from preformed lymphocytotoxic antibodies, occurring within the first 24 hours after transplant surgery, (2) Acute rejection due to sensitization to donor HLA antigens, commonly occurring in the first year after transplantation and (3) Chronic rejection due to low grade humoral and cell-mediated immune response against the graft, which takes a few months to years to damage the graft. Acute rejections are mostly reversible with treatment, but hyperacute rejection is irreversible, resulting in graft loss immediately after transplantation. Chronic rejection cannot be reversed, but the progression of CKD can be retarded with treatment. Current immunosuppressive therapy aims to minimize acute rejection episodes and to decrease chronic graft loss.

The other medical complications include side effects of the various drugs used for immunosuppression, increased incidence of certain malignancies in long-term survivors after organ transplantation, different types of bacterial, viral, fungal, protozoal and other infections which are more in people who are immunosuppressed. In countries with a high incidence of infective complications and economic constraints, the survival after successful transplantation is lower compared to developed economies with subsidized health care delivery.

Surgical complications include graft artery and vein thrombosis, ureteric obstruction or leaks, wound dehiscence, lymphoceles and urinomas. Current refinement in surgical technique has minimized these complications to a large extent.

CHAPTER
192

Drugs and the Kidney

Jacob George

> **Chapter Summary**
> - General Considerations
> - Vulnerability of Kidneys
> - Mechanisms of Drug-Induced Renal Damage
> - Common Drugs Implicated in Renal Damage
> - Adjustment of the Dosage of Drugs in Renal Failure
> - Drugs and Dialysis

GENERAL CONSIDERATIONS

Since the kidneys are involved in the excretion of several drugs or their metabolites, avoidance of certain drugs or modification of dosage may be needed in renal disease. In addition, as more and more drugs are introduced for various disorders, the risk of drug-induced kidney disease will increase. It is important to know why the kidneys are affected by some drugs, the mechanisms of injury and principles of modification of dosage in renal dysfunction.

VULNERABILITY OF KIDNEYS

The kidneys are highly vulnerable to the effect of drugs and toxins. The blood flow to the kidneys is nearly 20% of the cardiac output. Since the kidneys weigh about 300 g, the blood flow per gram of renal tissue is 3.5–4.0 mL/min/g. Thus, the kidneys are among the most vascular organs in the body. This results in drugs and toxins attaining high levels in the kidney. This load is exaggerated in the renal cortex, which gets 90% of renal blood flow. Substances that are filtered by the glomeruli reach the tubules and their concentration increases in the tubules because of selective water reabsorption. Some drugs such as gentamicin, which are reabsorbed by the proximal tubule reach the tubular cell in very high concentrations. Urinary concentration by countercurrent mechanism, high metabolic activity of the tubular cells, tubular secretion and precipitation of drugs in tubules depending on the concentration and pH are the other important reasons for the high vulnerability of the kidneys.

MECHANISMS OF DRUG-INDUCED RENAL DAMAGE

Drug-induced damage accounts for 5–20% of acute renal failure (ARF) and above 20% of chronic renal disease. In many instances, it may go off unrecognized. A high index of suspicion is necessary for early identification of drug-induced renal damage. The various mechanisms of cell injury due to drugs are:

- Direct interaction of drug with tubular cell membrane
- Insertion into the lipid components of the cell membrane
- Transportation into the cells
- Blockade of cytoplasmic metabolic events.

Renal damage due to drugs may be broadly classified as follows:

- ***Prerenal***
  - Volume depletion, e.g. diuretics
  - Increased catabolism, e.g. steroids
  - Vascular occlusion, e.g. oral contraceptives
  - Loss of renal autoregulation, e.g. nonsteroidal anti-inflammatory drugs (NSAIDs), angiotensin-converting enzyme inhibitors (ACEIs)
- ***Immune-mediated damage***
  - Acute interstitial nephritis, e.g. rifampicin, penicillin, allopurinol
  - Allergic vasculitis, e.g. thiazides, penicillamine
  - Glomerular damage, e.g. NSAIDs, gold salts and penicillamine
- ***Direct toxicity***
  - Acute tubular necrosis (ATN)
  - Papillary necrosis
- ***Obstructive uropathy***
  - Retroperitoneal fibrosis, e.g. practolol, methyldopa, methisergide, hydralazine
  - Urinary tract obstruction
  - Papillary necrosis, e.g. NSAIDs, acetaminophen
  - Tubular blockade due to crystalluria, e.g. sulfonamides, acyclovir.

COMMON DRUGS IMPLICATED IN RENAL DAMAGE

The most common drugs extensively used clinically causing nephrotoxicity include NSAIDs, ACEIs, angiotensin receptor blockers (ARBs) and radiocontrast agents. This combination is referred to as ***internist's nephrotoxic quartet***.

Nonsteroidal Anti-inflammatory Drugs

It produce renal damage in different ways.

- ***Hemodynamically-mediated renal failure:*** This is the most common mechanism. All NSAIDs, including selective cyclooxygenase-2 inhibitors, lead to the inhibition of protective vasodilatory intrarenal prostaglandins. Therefore, under conditions of reduced renal perfusion, loss of renal autoregulation occurs which may lead to renal failure. Patient groups at risk are the elderly, those with dehydration, underlying renal disease, decreased effective circulatory volume and use of other nephrotoxic drugs. Patients with hemodynamically-mediated renal failure present with oliguria, bland urine sediment and raised serum creatinine. Recovery usually occurs following timely withdrawal of the drug.

- ***Nephrotic syndrome:*** Nephrotic presentation may occur after several weeks to months of therapy particularly in elderly women. Renal biopsy reveals foot process fusion under electron microscopy along with interstitial edema and patchy infiltration with T lymphocytes. This may suggest a delayed hypersensitivity reaction to the drug. Recovery often occurs following withdrawal of the drug.
- ***Papillary necrosis:*** It follows the intake of large quantities of NSAIDs over a short period. Ingestion of 1–3 kg of paracetamol over a period of 3 years or the total ingestion of 2–8 kg of phenacetin over 8–10 years along with other analgesics can induce analgesic nephropathy. Papillary damage is due to the very high concentration of the drug established at the papillary tip.
- ***Hyperkalemia:*** This is secondary to hyporeninemic hypoaldosteronism and is seen usually when NSAIDs are used along with ACEIs, potassium sparing diuretics or potassium supplements.
- ***Salt and water retention:*** Edema occurs as a result of salt and water retention. This worsens pre-existing hypertension and congestive cardiac failure (CCF); and this can lead to resistance to the action of diuretics.

Aminoglycosides

Aminoglycoside-induced renal failure is commonly seen in clinical practice. The important risk factors for aminoglycoside nephrotoxicity include extremes of age, volume depletion, concurrent use of other nephrotoxic agents, hypokalemia, hypomagnesemia, sepsis and liver disease. The dose, duration and frequency of administration of the drug determine the pattern and severity of damage. Patients usually present with nonoliguric renal failure 7–10 days after the initiation of therapy. Sometimes, the manifestations of renal failure appear only after the completion of the course of antibiotic.

Aminoglycosides produce renal damage by acting as a direct tubulotoxins. They are freely filtered at the glomerulus and reabsorbed at the proximal convoluted tubule. The drug accumulates in the proximal tubule and can be seen under the electron microscope as ***myeloid bodies***. These cells undergo necrosis and clinically manifests as tubular dysfunction and renal failure. Aminoglycoside toxicity is often dose related.

In all groups of patients, especially in those at higher risk of developing nephrotoxicity, the baseline renal function should be checked and serum creatinine monitored every three days during and after drug administration. In the elderly and in those with pre-existing renal dysfunction, the dose should be adjusted to the creatinine clearance as discussed below. At the earliest evidence of renal dysfunction, the drug should be discontinued. In most cases, recovery occurs following drug withdrawal, but in those with established renal failure, dialysis support will be required.

Angiotensin-Converting Enzyme Inhibitors (ACEIs)

ACEIs are increasingly used now in the treatment of hypertension, congestive cardiac failure (CCF) and in the prevention of progression of diabetic nephropathy. ACEI can produce hemodynamically-mediated acute renal failure in a selected group of patients, e.g. bilateral renal artery stenosis, renal artery stenosis in a solitary kidney, moderate to severe congestive cardiac failure, volume depletion and pre-existing renal insufficiency. The efferent arteriolar tone, intraglomerular pressure and glomerular filtration rate (GFR) are modulated by angiotensin II. Administration of ACEI under these circumstances leads to relaxation of the efferent arterioles and a subsequent drop in the intraglomerular pressure and GFR. Although in most instances, the renal failure is reversible, ACEI can produce irreversible renal failure, especially when there is underlying renal parenchymal disease. ACEI can also produce hyperkalemia when used in conjunction with potassium sparing diuretics, beta-blockers or potassium supplements. Captopril can produce nephrotic syndrome (membranous nephropathy). Careful use of these drugs with monitoring of renal function and serum potassium levels and avoiding the use of these drugs in the high-risk group can prevent renal toxicity to a large extent.

Radiocontrast Agents

Renal failure associated with radiocontrast agents is reported as the third most common cause of in-hospital renal failure. Conventional contrast agents are hyperosmolar, a property contributing to their toxicity. Ionic contrast agents are especially toxic. Maximum reduction in renal function is usually noticed 48 hours after injection of the contrast. Patients can present with transient renal dysfunction or severe renal failure requiring dialysis. A persistent nephrogram 24 hours after contrast administration is another finding in radiocontrast related renal failure. Risk factors precipitating radiocontrast nephropathy are pre-existing renal insufficiency, dehydration, elderly age, severe congestive heart failure (CHF), multiple myeloma, concurrent use of other nephrotoxic agents, repeated exposure to radiocontrast agents and high dose of ionic contrast agents. Although uncomplicated diabetes as such is not a risk factor, those with diabetes and renal involvement are affected more.

Exact mechanism of contrast-mediated renal damage is not clear. The two proposed mechanisms are renal hypoperfusion and direct tubular toxicity. Urine osmolarity tends to be high with a low fractional excretion of sodium suggesting prerenal failure. This may be due to intense intrarenal vasoconstriction mediated by renin, angiotensin II, intracellular smooth muscle calcium, adenosine and endothelin.

There is no specific treatment. In most cases, it is reversible. The risk can be reduced by using minimum dose of nonionic contrast agent, avoiding multiple radiocontrast injections and avoiding dehydration prior to, and during the procedure. Administration of half normal saline starting 12 hours before and up to 12 hours after the dye injection is probably the most effective measure to reduce radiocontrast nephrotoxicity. N-acetylcysteine given in a dose of 600 mg twice daily before and after contrast has been shown to be useful in some cases. The urine output must be maintained at around 100 mL per hour before and after the procedure.

ADJUSTMENT OF THE DOSAGE OF DRUGS IN RENAL FAILURE

Renal disease can affect the absorption, bioavailability, distribution, metabolism and excretion of some drugs. Pharmacologically active metabolites of drugs may accumulate in renal failure causing adverse reactions, e.g. nitrofurantoin when administered in renal failure can cause peripheral neuropathy and anesthetic agents like morphine can cause respiratory depression. Drug excretion by the kidneys depends on glomerular filtration, tubular secretion and tubular reabsorption. These may be altered in renal failure. Thus, dose modification may be necessary in renal disease. The necessity and degree of dose reduction depends on the class of drug. The goal of drug modification would be to maintain efficacy while avoiding drug accumulation and adverse reactions. This is achieved by the following methods:

- ***Using dosage nomograms:*** This is based on knowledge of the creatinine clearance. This may either be estimated using 24 hours urine collection or calculated from serum creatinine using the Cockroft and Gault formula. For patients with ARF and/or end-stage renal disease (ESRD), the creatinine clearance must be assumed to be less than 10 mL/minute.

  The dose for the level of creatinine clearance for individual drugs can be read from the nomogram. Although the method is simple, the disadvantage is that different people behave differently and the nomogram may not be applicable to all individuals alike.

- ***Adjusting the loading dose and altering the maintenance dose:*** If extracellular fluid volume is normal, the loading dose in renal failure is usually the same as that for a normal person, except in the case of digoxin where only 50–75% of the normal loading dose is required. For aminoglycosides, 75–80% of the normal loading dose may be sufficient. In those with edema or ascites, a higher-loading dose may be required. The maintenance dose is adjusted either by decreasing the individual dose or by increasing the dosage interval. In the case of gentamicin, the daily maintenance dose can be roughly calculated by the formula:

  5 mg/kg bw
  serum creatinine
  or
  By the 'rule of 8'—i.e. frequency of administration may be 8-hourly if serum creatinine is 1 mg%, 16-hourly if serum creatinine is 2 mg% and 24-hourly if serum creatinine is 3 mg% and so on.

  It is prudent to monitor drug levels to ensure therapeutic levels while avoiding toxicity. Table 192.1 shows dose modification of commonly used drugs in renal failure.

Special Group of Drugs and Dose Modification in Renal Failure

- ***NSAIDs:*** Due to their inhibitory effects on vasodilatory prostaglandins, their use could result in a further fall in GFR and hyperkalemia. Of the NSAIDs, sulindac has less chances of renal failure.
- ***Diuretics:*** As most of the diuretics have to reach the lumen of the tubule for their action, efficacy may be affected in renal failure. Thiazide diuretics are generally ineffective when the creatinine clearance is less than 25 mL/minute. Loop diuretics are mainly secreted into the lumen in the proximal tubule through the organic anion transporter. In renal failure, high doses are required to overcome the competing action by other organic anions. So, high doses of oral loop diuretics are used. When parenteral administration is needed, high dose of furosemide IV or continuous infusion is more effective.
- ***ACEIs:*** Generally, it is better to be cautious in using ACEI in those with serum creatinine of more than 3.5 mg%. If ACEIs are used, periodic monitoring of renal functions and serum potassium are needed. Withdrawal of the drug may be necessary if serum creatinine or potassium increases steadily.
- ***Beta blockers:*** Dose reduction may be needed in advanced renal failure. They should be used cautiously as they can produce hyperkalemia particularly when used with ACEI and/or potassium sparing diuretics.
- ***Antibiotics:*** Aminoglycosides require significant dose reduction with renal failure as well as increased dose interval. Most of the cephalosporins also require dose reduction and/or increase in interval. Vancomycin has prolonged blood levels in renal failure and this needs to be given only once in five days for moderate renal failure and once a week in severe renal failure.
- ***Antituberculous drugs:*** Most of the antituberculous drugs with the exception of rifampin require dose reduction. Dose of ethambutol is reduced to 5 mg/kg in severe renal failure and isonicotinylhydrazide to 200 mg daily. Pyrazinamide is preferably avoided in severe renal failure. As rifampin is metabolized by the liver, dose reduction is not usually required.

Thus, knowledge of drug modification in renal failure is vital to the proper management of a patient with renal disease. At the same time, it is important to periodically monitor renal functions when drugs with potential deleterious effects are used in patients with renal disease.

DRUGS AND DIALYSIS

The dialyzability (dialytic clearance) of the drugs depends on its volume of distribution, molecular size and protein binding. Generally, protein-bound drugs are less dialyzable, e.g. secobarbitone, amylobarbitone and other short-acting barbiturates. The nonprotein-bound drugs such as phenobarbitone and other long-acting barbiturates are dialyzable. Drugs with lower molecular size and less protein binding are more dialyzable. Such drugs (barbiturates, certain antibiotics) should preferably be administered in the post-dialysis period to ensure therapeutic levels. In case of poisoning or overdose by nondialyzable drugs, their removal from the body is possible by charcoal hemoperfusion.

Some antibiotics are dialyzable and hence, a booster dose at the end of each dialysis will be required to achieve therapeutic blood levels, e.g. aminoglycosides. In patients who are on long-term dialysis, it is preferable to administer most drugs after dialysis. The property of

Table 192.1: Drug dose adjustment in renal failure

Drug	Normal dose	Mild renal failure (SCr 2–4 mg%)	Moderate renal failure (4–8 mg%)	Severe renal failure (>8 mg%)
Gentamicin	1.5 mg/kg q8h	1.5 mg/kg q12h	1 mg/kg q12h	1 mg/kg q24h
Amikacin	7.5 mg/kg q12h	7.5 mg/kg q24h	5 mg/kg q24h	5 mg/kg q24.4h
Cefazolin	1 g q6h	1 g q12h	1 g q24h	500 mg q24h
Cefotaxime	1–2 g q6h	1 g q8h	1 g q12h	500 mg–1 g q24h
Ceftazidime	1–2 g q6h	1 g q12h	1 g q24h	500 mg–1 g q24h
Crystalline penicillin	10–20 L q6h	10-20 L q6h	10–20 L q6h	10–20 L q8 h
Ampicillin	500 mg q6h	500 mg q6h	500 mg q6h	500 mg q12h
Ciprofloxacin	200 mg q12h	200 mg q12h	200 mg q12h	200 mg q24h
Vancomycin	500 mg q6h	500 mg once in 3 days	500 mg once in 5 days	500 mg once in 7 days
INH	300 mg od	300 mg od	200 mg od	200 mg od
Ethambutol	10 mg/kg od	10 mg/kg od	5 mg/kg od	5 mg/kg od
Rifampin	450–600 mg od	450–600 mg od	450 mg od	450 mg od
Methyldopa	250–600 mg orally 8 h	250–500 mg orally 8 h	250–500 mg orally 12 h	250–500 mg od 12 h
Enalapril	2.5–10 mg od	2.5–10 mg od	2.5–10 mg od	2.5–10 mg od
Digoxin	0.25 mg od	0.125 mg in 36 h	0.125 mg in 48 h	0.125 mg in 48 h

Abbreviations: SCr = Serum creatinine; INH = Isonicotinylhydrazide

dialyzability of drugs can be exploited in the management of poisoning or overdose with these drugs. Hemodialysis is more effective than peritoneal dialysis in drug elimination for most dialyzable drugs.

Since the kidneys are highly vulnerable and drugs can adversely affect the kidney function, the clinician must try to understand the basic pharmacology and pharmacokinetics of these drugs and use appropriate drugs with conventional or modified dose, depending on the level of renal function. This may help to reduce the incidence of drug-induced renal disease to a large extent.

CHAPTER 193

Nervous System: General Considerations

SR Chandra, Vidhya Annapoorni CS

Chapter Summary

- General Considerations
- The Adult Human Brain
- Functional Organization
- Sensory System
- Plasticity
- Good Clinical Practices and Ethics

"Asathoma satgamaya
Tamasoma Jyotirgamaya
Mirthyoma Amirthamgamaya"
—*O God Lead me*

GENERAL CONSIDERATIONS

Nervous system is the most differentiated system in the human body and is unique in several ways. Thirty three stem cells constitute the neuraxis by synapsing, inhibiting and interacting. Its main function is triaging (filtering off information) and not excitatory as commonly believed. Nearly 60,000 afferent sensory information is sent to the neuraxis every minute and normally only the desired information is sent to the neuraxis by the phenomena of *Gating* so that, the individual can attend to only what is needed. If this phenomenon does not exist, all of us will suffer from attention deficit. It controls all other systems and, therefore, its dysfunction can be a great imitator. It gives identity to the individual and links clinical neurology to philosophy. The appearance of mirror neurons in man started a fast pace of learning and creativity making man grow beyond evolutionary speed. In 1577, *Sat-chakra nirupana* described anatomy and physiology of the brain in astonishingly accurate detail, which was later elaborated by Charaka before the science of dissection, ablation and stimulation induced observations which came into existence.

THE ADULT HUMAN BRAIN

The adult brain weighs about 1.3–1.4 kg which becomes reduced to 50 g when floating in cerebrospinal fluid (CSF) and the spinal cord about 30 g. On the 19th day of gestation, the ectoderm organizes to form the neural tube with neural folds. By 4th week, the cephalic part organizes to form the brain and the caudal part to spinal cord. The processes of neuroblasts give rise to cranial and spinal nerves. The cell bodies are grouped in the periventricular region and migrate to outer zones. The prime functional unit of the nervous system is the neuron which consists of perikaryon, the cell body and processes which are axon and dendrites. Neuroglia is the connective tissue and microglia is the immunological cell. The greatest accumulation of nerve cells and their fiber tracts is seen in brain, spinal cord and first two cranial nerves which form part of the central nervous system (CNS), and the rest lower 10 cranial nerves and parts beyond anterior horn cells forms the peripheral nervous system. The cell bodies form the gray matter in brain, spinal cord and the ganglia whereas, axons form the white matter and nerves. Dendrites are the processes through which the nerve cell body receives information from neighboring cells. They are several in numbers and linked by dendrodendritic or axodendritic connections via the dendritic spines. Myelin is the insulation material for the fiber tracts secreted by oligodendroglia in the upper motor neuron (UMN) and Schwann cells in lower motor neurons (LMNs). The skull and vertebral canal offers protection to the CNS. The pia mater is a transparent membrane found on the surface of brain, in the sulci, cerebellum and invaginates into the ventricular surface via the rostral part of 3rd and 4th ventricle and it contributes to the formation of choroid plexus. Outside this is the subarachnoid space which is expanded in certain places to form the cisterns which are CSF containing spaces. Cerebellomedullary cistern located between cerebellum and medulla, is the largest, quadrigeminal cistern is located between splenium and superior part of cerebellum, pontine cistern in the anterior part of pons, interpeduncular, chiasmatic and suprasellar cisterns are rostral to this, cistern ambiens is in the dorsal midbrain. Arachnoid membrane is next to it and has fibrous pial extensions to pia and these two are derived from neural crest cells. Duramater is mesodermal in origin and is the outermost with a periosteal and a meningeal layer. The meningeal layer of it forms the falx cerebri in the interhemispheric region, falx cerebelli, tentorium cerebelli above cerebellum, diaphragma sellae and covering for the venous sinuses. CSF is produced by choroid plexus and from ventricles escapes to subarachnoid space. This offers buffering effect to brain, a sink for the products of brain metabolism and also nutritional support.

Parts of the Brain and Spinal Cord

The brain consists of prosencephalon which consists of cerebral hemispheres with frontal, temporal, parietal and occipital lobes and thalamus, mesencephalon consisting of midbrain and rhombencephalon composed of pons, medulla and cerebellum. The representation of man inside the brain is unique in the motor, sensory and cerebellar regions and is called the **homunculus**. The first two cranial nerves originate from brain, 3rd to 4th in midbrain, 5th to 8th in pons and 9th to 12th in medulla. Spinal cord is the continuation of medulla up to 2nd lumbar vertebra in adults and 3rd lumbar vertebra in children. It has 31 segments, 8 cervical, 12 thoracic, 5 lumbar, 5 sacral and 1 coccygeal segments. Each spinal segment has a pair of nerves roots, the dorsal sensory root with ganglion and ventral motor root. Spinal cord has a cervical and a lumbar enlargement, an anterior median fissure, posterior median sulcus and poster lateral sulci. It has white matter outside and gray matter inside. The gray matter is H-shaped with ventral horn, dorsal horn and an intermediolateral horn from 1st thoracic to 2nd lumbar segments.

Blood Supply and Venous Drainage

Two paired arterial sources supply the brain. The vertebral system arises from subclavian system, ascends through the transverse foramina of upper six cervical vertebrae, to enter foramen magnum. The two vertebral arteries unite to form basilar artery. The vertebral artery gives rise to posterior inferior cerebellar artery which supplies the lateral medulla and posterior cerebellum. Both vertebral arteries together give rise to anterior spinal artery to supply the spinal cord. The basilar artery gives rise to anterior inferior cerebellar artery which supplies pons and medial and lateral surfaces of cerebellum. There are short and long paramedian arteries including labyrinthine artery and superior cerebellar artery which supplies midbrain and superior surface of cerebellum. The terminal branches are posterior cerebral arteries which go around the brainstem and supplies occipital lobes. Through posterior communicating arteries, it communicates with internal carotid arteries. The internal carotids begin at C4 level at neck, enters skull via carotid canal, to reach the cavernous part and then gives ophthalmic artery, the supraclinoid part gives rise to middle and anterior cerebral arteries. The communication between the two major vascular systems formed by anterior cerebral artery (ACA), anterior communicating artery (ACoA), internal carotid artery, posterior cerebral and posterior communicating is called the **circle of Willis**. The spinal cord is supplied by anterior and posterior spinal arteries whose territories are maintained by reinforcing arteries. The veins accompany arteries and drain into venous sinuses. The middle cerebral vein drains to superior sagittal sinus via the **anastomotic vein of Trolard** and to transverse sinus via **inferior anastomotic vein of Labbe**. The thalamostriate veins, septal veins, internal cerebral veins and deep middle cerebral veins lead to **vein of Galen**. Superior sagittal sinus, inferior sagittal sinus and transverse sinus meet at the confluence of sinuses in the inner part of occipital bone, become straight sinus and sigmoid sinus and drain through internal jugular vein (IJV). Spinal venous channels are six in number and freely communicate with visceral veins since, they have no valves. Neurons can stand anoxia for 20 minutes and ischemia for 5 minutes.

FUNCTIONAL ORGANIZATION

Functionally, the neuraxis can be grouped as motor, sensory, extrapyramidal and cerebellar systems.

Motor Functions

For carrying out a motor activity, the schema has to be designed. Then, the right areas have to be instructed to recruit the right agonist, antagonist, synergist and fixators. The rate, range, rhythm and direction of action is to be decided and fine-tuned and executed through the LMN. A recordable potential called **Bereitschafts potential** appears in the supplementary motor and prefrontal areas before the person is consciously aware of initiating a movement. This is followed by **Readiness potential** in the parietal region. Idea to move is formed in the prefrontal lobe; motor schema is formulated in supplementary motor and premotor areas and executed by primary motor area. Motor activity is initiated by corticospinal tract which initiates and maintains dexterity by gracefully activating the agonist, inhibiting the antagonist and making the synergist and fixators to support. Fine programming is done by extrapyramidal system, rate range rhythm, amplitude and direction is determined by cerebellum. Autonomic system is concerned with involuntary motor activities and somatic system with voluntary ones. Basal ganglia and cerebellum have a feed forward role for anticipated movements and feed backward for unanticipated movements. The feed forward loops carry the action semantics for carrying out motor activity based on pre-existing motor plan. The feed backward loops formulate the plan based on the demands of the working environment as it does not follow a mathematical plan. Corticospinal, corticobulbar, cortico-cerebellar and corticostriate pathways carry out voluntary motor activity using the LMN. Brainstem pathways, which are the rubrospinal, tectospinal, reticulospinal and vestibulospinal, are concerned with posture and equilibrium.

Corticospinal tract is the longest connection between brain and spinal cord. About 25,000–35,000 Betz cells from areas 4 and 6 contribute 60% and areas 1, 2, 3, 5 and 7 contribute 40% of fibers to this tract. Fibers converge in the corona radiata and traverse through internal capsule, cerebral peduncle, pons, medulla and reach ventral horn of spinal cord. Eighty percent of these fibers decussate in the lower medulla and the rest is uncrossed. They descend as anterior and posterolateral columns. Lamination is the term applied to the pattern in which body parts are represented in various motor and sensory tracts. The sacral fibers are lateral most and cervical ones medial most in the pyramidal tract and spinothalamic tract, and it is reverse in the posterior column. The non-corticospinal motor fibers are vestibulospinal, reticulospinal, tectospinal, rubrospinal, propriospinal and olivospinal tracts. They act as adjuvants in posture maintenance, righting reflexes and maintenance of tone. When the UMN is paralyzed there is loss of dexterity, resulting in impairment of fine movements. There is movement of paralysis without muscle paralysis causing loss of voluntary movements with preserved reflex movements. There is hypertonia in the form of spasticity due to loss of cortical inhibition best appreciated in the flexors of upper limbs and extensors of

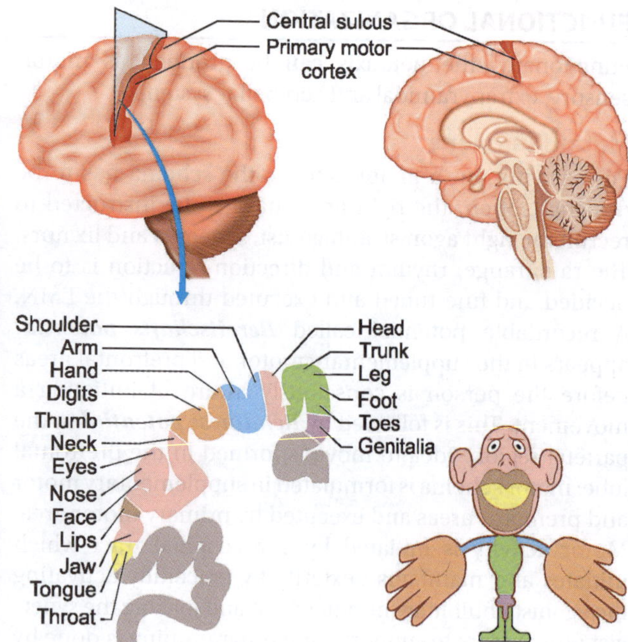

Fig. 193.1: Motor homunculus. **Note:** The disproportionate areas of representation of various parts of the body on the cerebral cortex depending on their functional importance

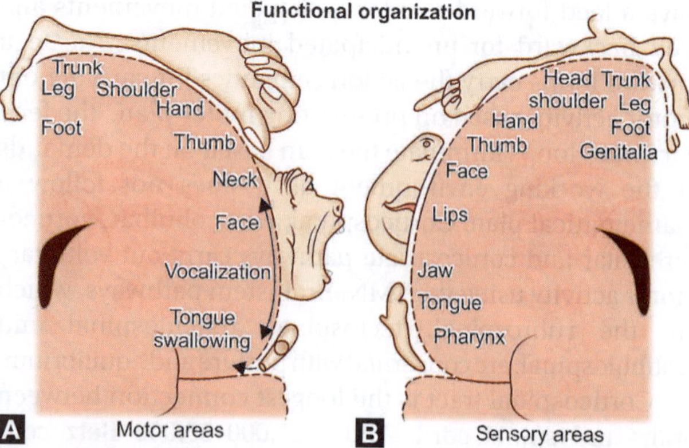

Figs 193.2A and B: **A.** Motor; **B.** Sensory homunculi showing proportional somatotopical representation in the main motor and sensory areas of the cortex

lower limbs. When voluntary control is lost this posture serves as reflex posture for feeding and locomotion (Figs 193.1 to 193.3).

Tone and its Abnormalities

Tone is defined as *the state of partial contraction always present in normal muscle for maintenance of posture with minimal expenditure of energy or resistance offered to passive movement*. It has a tonic component which is characterized by asynchronous contraction in response to slow sustained stretch for maintaining or changing posture. A phasic component in response to brief stretch contributes to *stretch reflex*. The abnormalities caused are spasticity, rigidity, hypotonia, paratonia, mitgehen and dystonia. Mitgehen is a state of excited or inhibited motor activity in the absence of a mood disorder or neurological disease. In mitgehen, there are exaggerated movements in response to light finger pressure, despite instructions to the contrary.

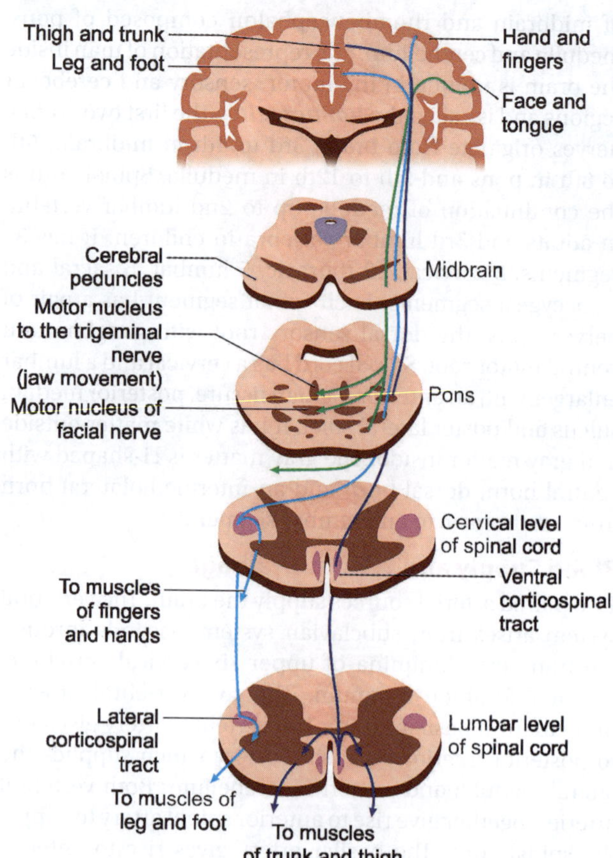

Fig. 193.3: Motor system showing the ventral and lateral corticospinal tracts

Tone is maintained by excitatory fibers from area 4 which descend to spinal motor neuron via tegmentum and medial vestibulospinal pathways. The inhibitory fibers arise from area 6 descend via lateral vestibulospinal, reticulospinal and dorsal reticulospinal pathways. The neurons in spinal cord, which are concerned with tone, are the alpha motor neurons which serve as efferent to extrafusal fibers, the gamma motor neurons which supply the spindles or the intrafusal fibers and beta motor fibers which supply both and called *skeleton-fusimotor fibers*. The muscle spindles contain nuclear bag fibers which are concerned with both dynamic and static stretch and nuclear chain fibers concerned with only static stretch. The bag fibers in addition to have annulospiral endings and the chain fibers have flower-spray endings. The intrafusal fiber is located parallel to extrafusal fiber so that, whenever, the skeletal muscle is stretched, the intrafusal also contracts. The gamma motor system is influenced by basal ganglia, cerebellum, motor and premotor cortex to decide the sensitivity of the muscle spindle to stretch.

Spasticity

It is a motor disorder with velocity and length-dependent changes in response to stretch resulting in a group of UMN features. It has static and phasic components causing hypertonia and exaggerated stretch reflexes. These features are due to loss of inhibition due to involvement of dorsal reticulospinal tract. If only corticospinal tract is involved which is excitatory there is weakness, loss of dexterity and extensor plantar responses. A series of 5–7 Hz contractions occurring in response to sustained stretch is called *clonus*. The spread of hyper-reflexia to neighboring zones is called irradiation and this is the cause of *crossed adductor reflex*. The superficial reflexes are lost and there is clasp knife effect. Measurement tools are used to assess severity of signs and symptoms. *Ashworth scale* is used to measure hypertonia.

Ashworth Scale

0 = No increase in muscle tone
1 = Slight increase in muscle tone, manifested by a catch and released by minimal resistance at the end of the range of motion when the affected limb is moved in flexion or extension
2 = More marked increase in muscle tone, throughout the range of motion, limb is easily moved
3 = Considerable increase in muscle tone, passive movement is difficult
4 = Affected limb is rigid in flexion and/or extension.

Spasticity is treated only when it is harmful as mostly it helps in ambulation in the presence of movement paralysis, usually when power is good, but patient is unable to walk due to spasticity, when there is adductor spasm interfering with personal hygiene, when appliances are to be fitted or when there is autonomic dysreflexia.

Autonomic Dysreflexia

This is due to aberrant somatomotor to sudomotor regeneration. This causes hypertension and bradycardia when bladder fills. *Treatment* options are 2% nitroglycerine applied 2–5 cm above the injury site, or administration of alpha-adrenergic blocker terazosin for normotensive patients and combined propranolol and prazosin in hypertensives.

Treatment Planning

Treatment of autonomous spasticity shown in Flowchart 193.1.

Rigidity

Uniform resistance throughout the range of passive movement is called *rigidity*. It lacks phasic component and is called lead pipe type, if only rigidity is present and cogwheel, if combined with tremor. This is seen in diseases of extrapyramidal system.

Hypotonia

Lack of resistance to passive stretch is called *hypotonia*. This is seen in LMN disease.

Flowchart 193.1: Management strategy—prevention of provocative factors

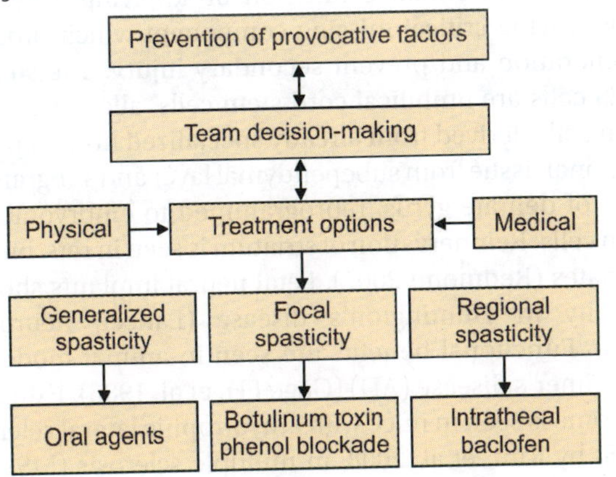

Table 193.1: Difference between upper motor neuron (UMN) and lower motor neuron (LMN)

UMN	LMN
Movement paralysis	Muscle paralysis
Tone increased	Decreased
Deep reflexes exaggerated	Depressed or absent
Superficial reflexes lost	Usually not affected
Plantar extensor	Flexor
Wasting absent	Wasting present
Fasciculation's absent	Fasciculation's present

Paratonia and Mitgehen

This is a situation characterized by inability of the patient to cooperate for passive examination inspite of good motivation. There is an increasing resistance with increasing stretch by examiner in paratonia and in mitgehen; the limb continues to stretch even after the examiner has stopped stretching.

Praxis

Ability to carry out a learned motor act on command in a non-paretic limb is called *praxis*, and it is a function of parietal lobe. Failure of this is called *apraxia*. They have problem in what to do and how to do, but are not easily evident and so do not complain. It is classified as ideational where patient does not know to use objects though he can identify, name and use the right object, but does not know the sequence of the motor activity (ideomotor).

Alien hand is a situation where left hand takes up seemingly complex movements in the absence of volition and opposes the right hand.

Lower Motor Neuron (LMN) (Table 193.1)

This is the final executor apparatus for the motor system. Damage causes muscle paralysis and therefore, both voluntary and reflex movements are lost. There is loss of trophic effect causing wasting. Both superficial and deep reflexes are lost as the end organ is damaged. There may be spontaneous contraction of denervated muscle fibers and motor units called *fibrillations* and *fasciculations*.

Extrapyramidal and cerebellar functions are dealt with separately.

Catatonia

This is a state where the person lies motionless without volition or reaction (inertia for action). This can be associated with depressive state causing withdrawal, dissociative, hallucinatory command asking patient not to move, panic state, etc. or organic disease of frontal lobe.

SENSORY SYSTEM

All sensations depend on information received from receptors. The receptors present in skin are called exteroceptors and constitute warmth, cold, touch and pain. The ones present deeper in somatic structures are called *proprioceptors*. They are Meissner's corpuscles for touch, Meckel's disk for pressure, Ruffini's plumes for warmth, Krause bulb for cold, Pacinian corpuscles for vibration, free nerve endings for pain, muscle spindles and

Golgi organs for position. Several receptors converge on a single cutaneous afferent fiber. A-delta fibers carry fast pain, C fibers slow pain and itch and A-alpha is for touch and pressure. These fibers enter posterior roots. The fibers concerned with position, vibration, touch and movement travel in posterior column, touch fibers travel in ventral spinothalamic tract, pain and temperature fibers in lateral spinothalamic tract and reach ventral posteromedial nucleus of thalamus and parietal lobe. Olfaction, vision, audition and gustatory sensations are called *special sensations*. Exteroceptive sensations are epicritic-like fine touch, tactile localization, discrimination, temperature in fine range or protopathic-like pressure, pain and temperature in wide range. Proprioceptive sensations are sense of position, tendon and muscle sensation, deep pressure and equilibrium. At the *substantia gelatinosa of Rolando,* there is gating of sensory inputs where all the unwanted sensory impulses are blocked (*Gate Control Theory of Melzack and Wall*). Pain, temperature and touch fibers ascend and descend one or two levels before they enter dorsal horn. They decussate in the anterior commissure and become contralateral spinothalamic tract. Dorsolaterally are the pain and temperature fibers, and ventromedially are the ones which carry touch. Posterior column is inhibitory to spinothalamic transmission which is the basis of dorsal column stimulation for intractable pain. Lateral spinothalamic carries pain and temperature, and anterior spinothalamic tract carries crude touch and pressure. Posterior columns carry vibration, movement and position. Lamination in posterior column is characterized by upper limb fibers being outer and sacral fibers being medial, they travel ipsilaterally to reach nucleus gracilis and nucleus cuneatus in caudal medulla. They form medial lemniscus and cross the midline in the medulla with fiber of gracilis ventromedial and cuneatus dorsomedial. In spinothalamic tract, the sacral fibers are outer and cervical fibers are medially placed. The pain fibers ascend and reach the thalamo-mesencephalic junction and organize into thalamic components which enter the ventral posteromedial and intralaminar thalamic nucleus—subthalamic and limbic components. The thalamic component enters the sensory cortex through the thalamocortical projections at post-central region for appreciation of sensations. The subthalamic component goes to the subthalamic nucleus and motor cortex for reflex withdrawal. The limbic component goes to the prefrontal regions for the affective element of pain appreciation which is responsible for pleasure or pain of a sensation. This is the basis of frontal leukotomy for intractable pain. As the affective component is removed, inspite of the pain, patient is able to carry out his daily activities.

There is endogenous pain control mechanism which is endorphin-mediated pathway from the frontal cortex, hypothalamus, periaqueductal gray matter, ventromedial medulla and lamina 1, 2 and 5 of spinal cord. This contains noradrenaline, serotonin and opiates. Sensations confer defense to the organism against potentially harmful stimuli and therefore, are protective. Abnormalities in these pathways result in bizarre sensory syndromes to perceptual interactions and phantom pains characterized by pain and paralysis of limbs lost long ago, but not forgotten by brain. Elaboration of these symptomatologies is beyond the scope of this chapter. Levels of principal dermatomes are described in Figure 193.4.

PLASTICITY

Neuronal Plasticity

Santiago Raman y Cajalin, 1913 opined that adult nervous system is fixed and nothing regenerates. Neuronal plasticity is the term applied to represent potential for alteration in function of adult as the brain develops. It may be activity-dependent, injury-induced following trauma or plasticity for learning and memory. Visual cortex develops only after eye opening in mice. If auditory inputs are cut out, the visual pathway wires into medial geniculate body (Mriganka Sur Massachusetts Institute). Plasticity takes place by changing synaptic efficacy, reducing or modifying protein synthesis, creation of new connections, elimination of existing connections and drop out by apoptosis. *Pruning* is the term by which unwanted synapses are eliminated and the right ones are preserved. Activity-dependent plasticity is described by Hebbs Law, i.e. nerves that fire together wire together. This is of great importance in understanding how much an adult brain can repair itself and how we can harness this for treatment. The enzymes involved in this activity are *Calpain family proteases*, brain derived neurotrophic factors, upregulated receptors, etc. Rapid stimulation of a neuron can lead to prolonged activation of cell body long after the stimulus stops by the phenomena called *long-term potentiation*. Specific genes called crest genes are involved in this process in rats. Several biochemical pathways including N-methyl-D-aspartate-related pathways are involved in plasticity. This is necessary for postnatal development, adaptability to change, gain new functions and recovery after injury. Abnormality of plasticity results in phantom pains, limb dystonias and dependence.

Stem Cells

Stem cells are cells capable of self-renewal. Embryonic stem (ES) cells can give rise to distinct glial and neuronal subtype cells in response to specific growth factors. They can be implanted by stereotactic surgery, injection to injury site, lumbar puncture, by intranasal and intraventricular routes (Hirokt 2007; Danielyan 2009). ES cells differentiate into dopamine neurons and glial cells, can be delivered via pumps to enhance function of surviving cells. This may provide critical missing component which promote regeneration and prevent secondary injury. The sources of ES cells are umbilical cord stem cells, allogeneic adult stem cells derived from already specialized human tissue, neuronal tissue from subependymal layer and subgranular zone of dentate gyrus, reprogrammed to embryonic-like stem cells. Reinnervation of striatum is seen in rats, but not primates (Redmond 2007). Fetal neural implants showed stability in Huntington's disease (Lancet, neurology 2006). Functional benefits are seen in animal models of Alzheimer's disease (AD) (Gage FH, et al. 1986). Extended outcome is seen in mice with amyotrophic lateral sclerosis (ALS) by Kim, et al. 2008, in multiple sclerosis (MS) and

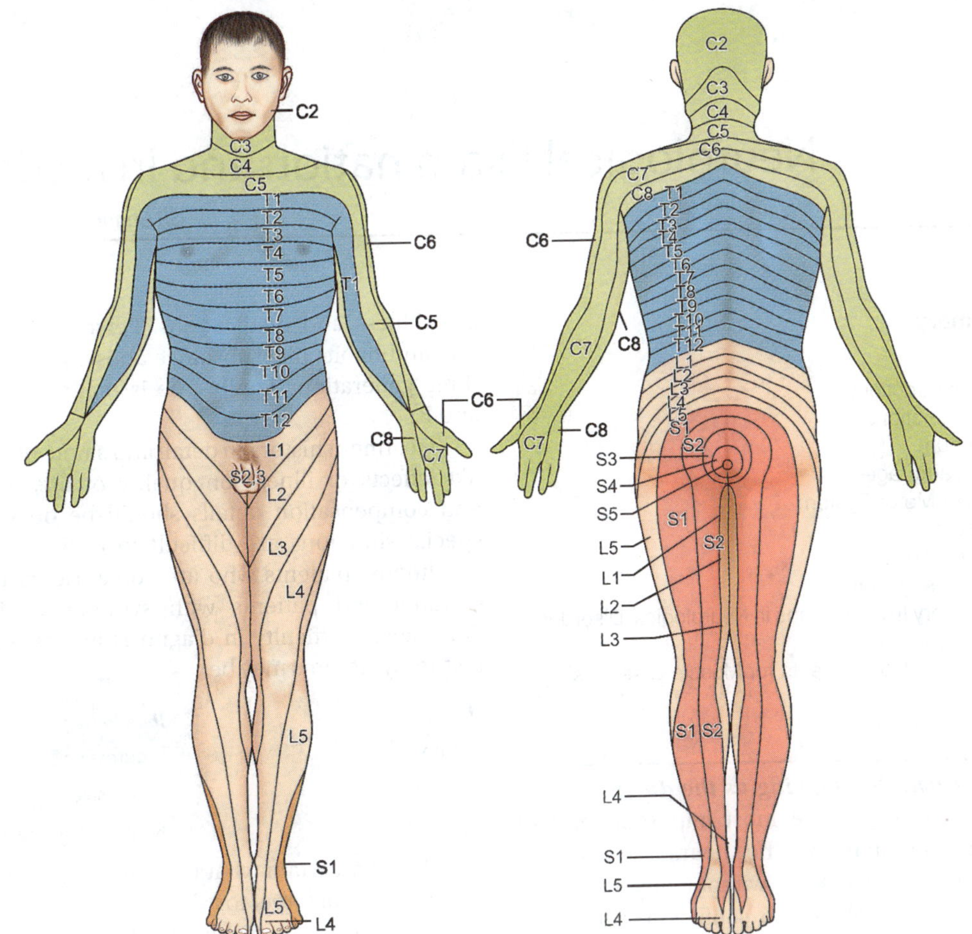

Levels of principal dermatomes

C5	Clavicles		T10	Level of umbilicus
C5, 6, 7	Lateral parts of upper limbs		T12	Inguinal or groin regions
C8, T1	Medical sides of upper limbs		L1, 2, 3, 4	Anterior and inner surfaces of lower limbs
C6	Thumb		L4, 5, S1	Foot
C6, 7, 8	Hand		L4	Medical side of great toe
C8	Ring and little fingers		S1, 2, L5	Posterior and outer surfaces of lower limbs
T4	Level of nipples		S1	Lateral margin of foot and little loe
			S2, 3, 4	Perineum

Fig. 193.4: Demarcation of dermatomes shown as distinct segments. There is actually considerable overlap between any two adjacent dermatomes

in epilepsy by Lee, et al. in 2007. Rat model of spinal cord injury improved (Karimi Abdolrezace, 2006). In tumors, tumoricidal proteins can be directly delivered to tumor by microsatellite (Aboody, 2000). Stem cells shows promise in Parkinson's disease, Alzheimer's, Huntington's disease, strokes, epilepsy, lysosomal storage diseases, tumors and injury, but a long way to go for human application.

GOOD CLINICAL PRACTICES AND ETHICS

CS Sindhu Krishnah

Word *ethics* is Greek meaning ethos; customs and character. Good clinical practice involves providing proper care to patients and in research following right rules and regulations, standard for the design, conduct, performance, monitoring and auditing, recording, analysis and reporting of clinical trials that provide assurance that the data and reported results are credible, accurate and that the rights, integrity and confidentiality of trial subjects are protected. Medical profession is unique and dedicated to healing, based on faith and allows the sick to claim their rights.

Charaka's oath was written in 300 BC, 2 centuries prior to Hippocrates oath. Geneva Convention 1949, Nuremberg Code following Second World War for human experimentation, Belmont Report 1979, Helsinki Declaration 1964, Indian Council of Medical Research (ICMR) guidelines 1980 and Revised Ethical Guidelines for broadened research have been formulated.

The foremost priority of medical profession is well being of patient, it needs commitment and dedication. However, with changing trends, ethical enforcement is important for safeguarding the right and safety of both parties.

Neurological Examination and Investigations

SR Chandra, SR Srinivasa Kannan

Chapter Summary

- History
- Higher Mental Functions
- Hemisphere Functions
- Corpus Callosum
- Speech and Language
- Examination of Motor System
- Sensory System
- Gait and Equilibrium
- Laboratory Investigations
- Clinical Laboratory Investigations in Neurological Disorders
- Chemical Analysis
- Muscle Biopsy and Other Tests for Muscle Diseases

HISTORY

Listen to the patient, he is giving us the diagnosis (Sir William Osler). History is the most important part of neurological examination. As the neuraxis is widely distributed, investigations done without any relevance to the patients history will add to confusion. Silent and incidental lesions which have got nothing to do with the patient's illness are very common in the neuraxis. Therefore, investigations without correlating with history are dangerous. History should be taken first from the patient and then from the active caregiver. It should contain complaints in order of duration and detailed description of the same. There should be details of

past illness and medications. Personal history includes diet and habits like substance abuse. Family history with three generations family tree is mandatory (Fig. 194.1A and B).

Treatment history in detail and a note of special factors like effects of illness on quality of life, any insurance and compensation details should be documented. The special situations are difficult to elicit in the following conditions; patients who are comatose, critically ill and children and patients with symptoms without signs. This causes difficulty in diagnosis in view of inadequate history symptoms may be:

I	II
Acute	Progressive
Subacute	Regressive
Chronic	Remitting and relapsing

Always ascertain what brought the patient to the hospital and do not forget to ask if he has anything more to say at the end. Clinical evaluation starts with general observations, documenting vital parameters, general examination including skin, hair, nail, tongue, teeth, tonsil and thorough neurological assessment. Neurological assessment starts with higher mental function examination, cranial nerves, motor systems, sensory system, reflexes, autonomic system, cerebellum, peripheral nerves, gait, spine and cranium.

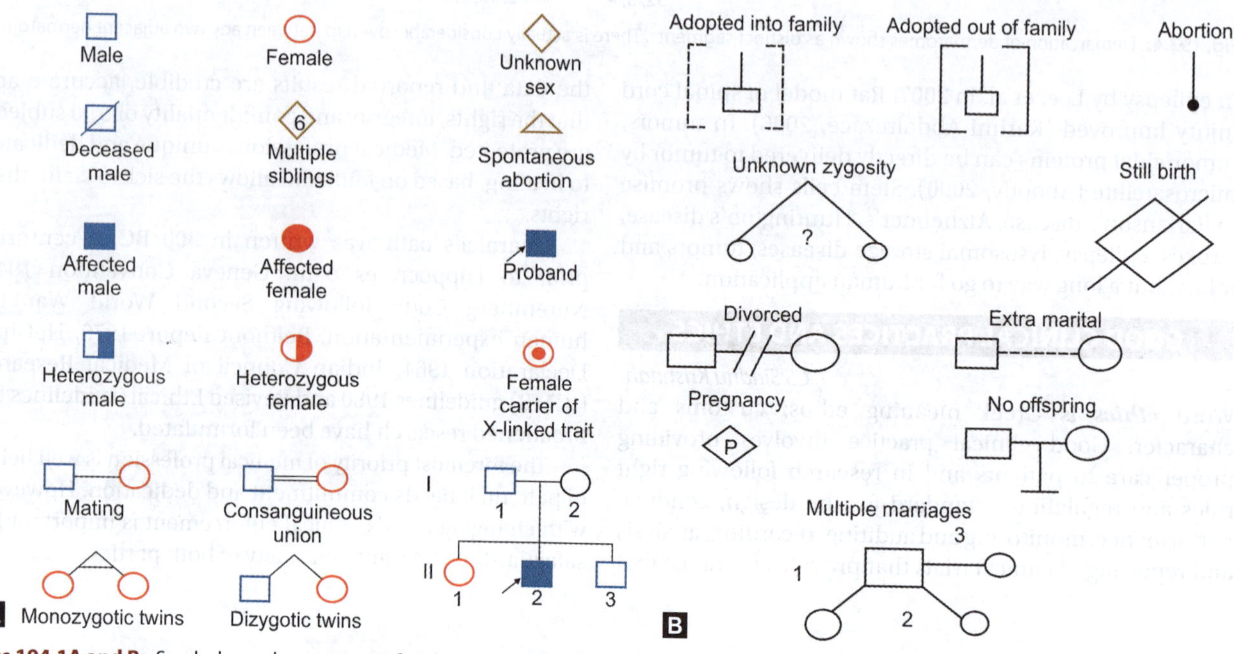

Figs 194.1A and B: Symbols used to represent family tree

HIGHER MENTAL FUNCTIONS

They are important because it makes human beings special, gives identity and links neurology to philosophy. It starts with basic information on educational status, sibling intelligence, occupation, premorbid personality, handedness (Edinburgh inventory, i.e. writing, drawing, throwing, using scissors, toothbrush, knife, spoon, striking a match, using a broom and opening a box). If eight out of these 10 activities is done with a hand, it becomes the dominant hand. Appearance and behavior includes information on personal cleanliness, dress, mood, affect like euphoric or depressed, friendly, irritable or showing mood swings, well or ill and any evidence for obvious neurological illness, whether cooperative and rapport can be established or not.

Consciousness

It is defined as wakeful awareness of self and environment and ability to interact effectively. Consciousness has depth, which is maintained by the ascending reticular activating system and content, which is maintained by the hemispheres (Fig. 194.2). Depth is measured using *Glasgow Coma Scale* (Table 194.1) and graded as wakefulness, stupor, drowsiness and coma. However, this score does not address properly aphasic and hemiplegic patients.

Orientation

It is the ability of the patient to relate himself to place, person and time. Time orientation is the function of temporal lobe, place is parietal lobe and person is temporo-parieto-occipital strip.

Attention and Intention

Attention is the process which permits humans to triage (filter off) afferent inputs based on set goals and biological goals-related requirements. Intention is the process by which brain triages action. Only the information which is essential for the organism is permitted to enter consciousness and all others are filtered out so that normal persons have the desired degree of attention without any distraction by unwanted stimuli.

Concentration

Selective attention is called *concentration* and alert attention is called *vigilance*.

Memory

It is defined as that mental process which enables the individual to store information for recall at a later date. Learning is modification of behavior by experience and memory is retention of that experience over time. One of the major functions of learning and memory is to adapt to environment. Memory involves encoding, storage and retrieval.

Different neural circuits are involved in different forms of memory. Memory can be grouped as follows through its various components (Table 194.2).

Working memory is attention related for brief storage of information and is a function of frontal lobe. Immediate memory is for hours, days or weeks and is a function of both hippocampi. Recent memory is a function of Papez circuit and remote memory is a function of whole brain (Fig. 194.3). Procedural memory is a function of cerebellum, basal ganglia and supplementary motor area.

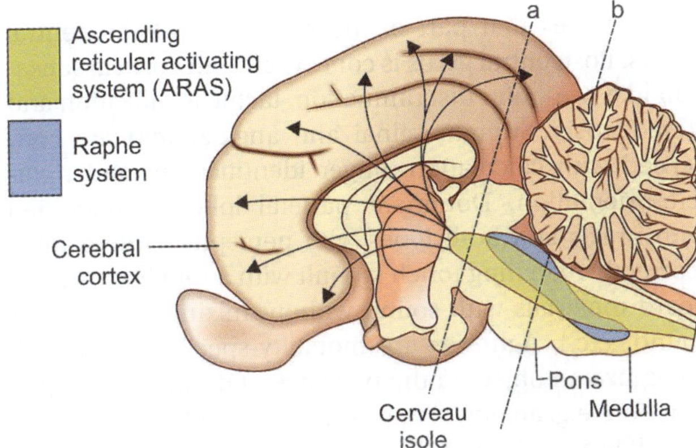

Fig. 194.2: Structures involved in consciousness

Table 194.1: Glasgow Coma Scale

Eye response	Verbal response	Motor response
–	–	6-obeys commands
–	5-oriented and converses normally	5-localizes to pain
4-spontaneous	4-disoriented and confused	4-withdraws in response to painful stimuli
3-opens in response to verbal stimulus	3-inappropriate words	3-decorticate rigidity
2-opens in response to painful stimuli	2-incomprehensible sounds	2-decerebrate rigidity
1-no response	1-no response	1-no response

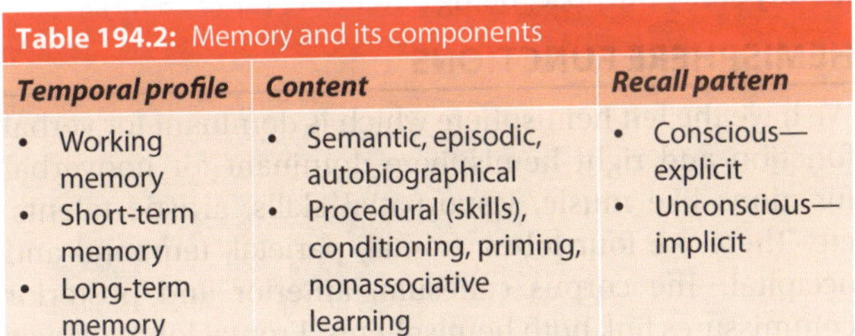

Table 194.2: Memory and its components

Temporal profile	Content	Recall pattern
• Working memory • Short-term memory • Long-term memory	• Semantic, episodic, autobiographical • Procedural (skills), conditioning, priming, nonassociative learning	• Conscious—explicit • Unconscious—implicit

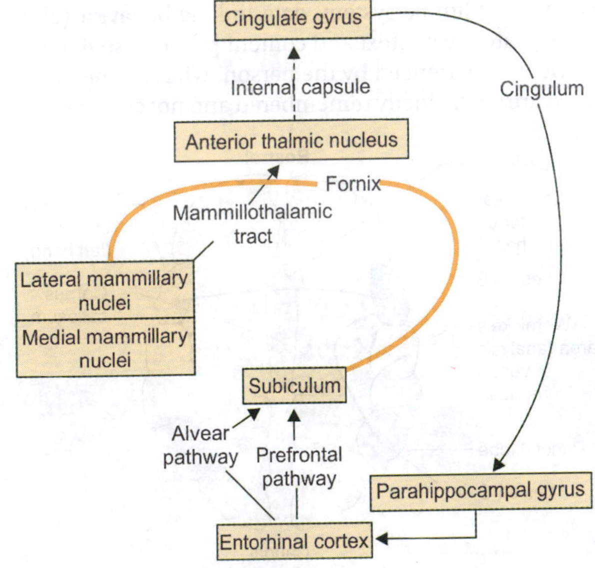

Fig. 194.3: Papez circuit for recent memory

Intelligence

It is ability to acquire knowledge and apply appropriately. It may be for verbal or performance-related activities and can be tested using the various intelligence scales.

Cognitive Functions

It is defined as the highest level of human intellectual functioning readily available for formal testing. It involves fund of knowledge, new learning, judgment, calculation and abstract thinking. Judgment is defined as construction of a behavior plan based on past experience, prefrontal anticipation, rules of socialization to optimize the satisfaction of the biological drives.

Praxis and Gnosis

Praxis: It is the ability to formulate skilled movements in a nonparetic limb by planning a schema-based on stored complex representations and previously learned movements on command (Fig. 194.4).

Gnosis: It is a modality-specific ability to access semantic information of an object or stimulus in the presence of normal perception.

Command is received by the language area and it is transferred to the ipsilateral supplementary motor area to prepare the motor plan. This is sent to the motor area to carry out the activity with the right-sided limbs. For left-sided limbs, this information is channeled through the anterior part of the corpus callosum to the right supplementary motor area and right motor area.

Hindi Mental State Examination (HMSE) has to be used for cognitive screening in India since the previous Mini-mental State Examination (MMSE) cannot be used for any study purpose, being patented (Table 194.3).

HEMISPHERE FUNCTIONS

We have the left hemisphere which is dominant for verbal function and right hemisphere dominant for nonverbal functions like music, visuospatial skills, artistic talents, etc. There are four lobes, frontal, parietal, temporal and occipital. The corpus callosum, anterior and posterior commissures link both hemispheres. Frontal lobe consists of orbitofrontal region which deals with neocortical functions of limbic system, data-linking behavior (ability to associate the context and content properly so that what has been experienced by the person, what has been read, heard are all distinctly remembered and not confused with

each other) and environmentally dictated behavior (even though the environment has a large number of stimuli, the individual seeks only what is needed for him and not just passively use everything in the environment). Disease of frontal lobe causes uninhibited, antisocial, cynical and maniacal personality who does well in standard tests but fails in life in addition to imitation (passively imitates what others are doing), utilization (uses everything in the environment), loss of insight, loss of error correction (does not learn from his own mistakes). Anterior frontal region is concerned with personality, ability to respond to pain, mugging up or nonsensical learning and insight. Dorsolateral frontal region dysfunction is concerned with loss of executive functions, frontal alexia characterized by ability to read whole words but not letters, frontal simultagnosia (where patient will identify a picture as representative of a temple festival but will not be able to say the individual components in the picture which made him draw that conclusion), construction defect characterized by normal outline lacking inner details, perseveration, working memory defect and distractibility.

Medial frontal region is concerned with alien hand where the left hand carries out independent activity unrelated to the will of the individual, loss of conditioned emotional learning (e.g. learning and unlearning associated with reward and punishment). Frontal eye field is concerned with ipsilateral and contralateral gaze deviation; supplementary motor area for motor schema formation and motor area for control of movement on the opposite side; Broca's area is for motor speech.

Parietal Lobe

It constitutes that part of the brain behind the central sulcus. Postcentral gyrus is concerned with cortical sensation like two-point discrimination, tactile localization and stereognosis. Supramarginal and angular gyri are concerned with calculation, finger identification and right-left orientation. Dominant parietal lobe is concerned with praxis and both lobes with perceptual interactions (correctly matching touch stimuli with a touch sensation, heard materials with sound without mixing up touch as sound, etc.). Agnosias are modality-specific inability to recognize an object in the presence of normal end-organ function (e.g. an object may be seen but not recognized as what it is even though vision is normal).

Parietal alexia is characterized by ability to read the letters but not the word. Superior parietal lobule is concerned with body schema dysfunction (inner unitary representational template of self) and inferior parietal lobule with polymodal association.

Neglect syndromes are characterized by a behavioral syndrome where a patient fails to represent, react, respond, report to meaningful stimuli to one-half of the body in the absence of sensory or motor defect due to defect in attention or intention characterized by failure to dress and shave in one-half of the body and behave as if one-half of the body and space do not exist. Deep parietal regions carry visual information from opposite lower quadrants. Nondominant parietal lobe deals with construction, dressing and visuospatial orientation (Fig. 194.5).

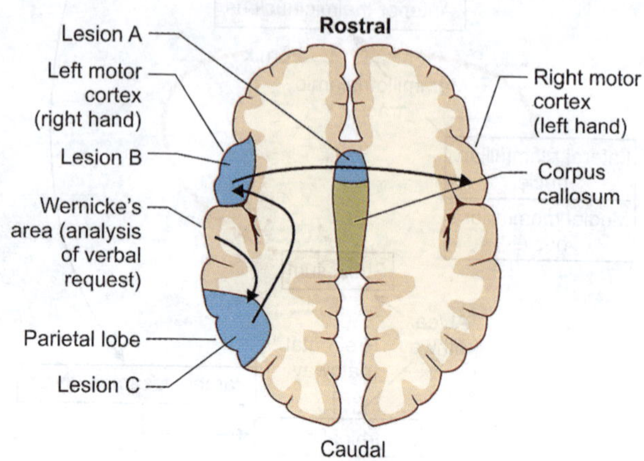

Fig. 194.4: Praxis circuit of Liepmann

Table 194.3: Mental state examination

S. no.	Areas	Corresponding items MMSE	Corresponding items HMSE
1	Orientation to time	Year	Time of day
2	Orientation to place	• Name of this place/building • Floor (storey) • Street address • City • Country	• Either 'which place is this', or 'whose house is this' depending on whether the testing was conducted in a home or health care center or other location in the village • Village • Post office • Block (or area of neighborhood), and • District
3	Registration	Apple, table, penny	Mango, chair, coin
4	Attention	• Serial subtractions of 7 starting at 100, or • Backwards spelling of WORLD	• A man has ₹ 20 for bus fare. Everyday he spends ₹ 3 on his bus fare. After spending the first day's bus fare he will be left with ₹ 17. How much money will be left after the next day's bus fare… and the next day's bus fare…, The first five consecutive responses are scored, or • To name the Days of the week backwards
5	Recall	Apple, table, penny	Mango, chair, coin
6	Naming	Wristwatch, pencil	Wristwatch, pen
7	Repetition	'No ifs, ands or buts'	'Neither this nor that'
8	Read and follow command	'Close your eyes'	Examiner says 'Look at me and do exactly what I do' and then closes his own eyes for three seconds
9	Sentence	Writing a sentence	'Tell me something about your house'
10	Copying	Two intersecting pentagons	Diamond

Abbreviations: MMSE = Mini-mental State Examination; HMSE = Hindi Mental State Examination

Temporal Lobe

This integrates olfaction (smell), vision, audition and gustatory [gastrointestinal (GI)] information. Wernicke's area concerned with sensory language is situated in the superior temporal gyrus. Deep temporal lobes carry visual fibers for opposite upper quadrants. Amygdala, a deep gray matter in the temporal lobe, controls behavior. Medial temporal regions process memory. Disease of the uncus produces olfactory hallucination characterized by spontaneous abnormal smells. Bilateral temporal lobe lesion cause *Klüver–Bucy syndrome* characterized by hyperorality (exploring everything with the mouth), hypersexuality, visual agnosia, hypomotile and tame behavior with hypermetamorphosis, characterized by compulsive tendency to observe and react to visual stimuli and failure to recognize familiar objects. Medial temporal lesion produces short-term verbal, visual and paired associate learning defect. With reference to hearing, there is defect in appreciation of rapidly spoken words and volume appreciation in the opposite ear during binaural hearing. There is *dysacusis,* i.e. normal intensity sounds are annoying. There can be pure word deafness, i.e. difficulty in identifying words, words selection anomia, transcortical sensory aphasia and Wernicke's aphasia. On the nondominant side, *amusia* (inability to appreciate music), *agnosia* and difficulty in spatially localizing sounds. There can be opposite upper quadrantanopia. Middle and inferior gyrus produce visual hallucination of formed nature including *heautoscopy* where self-images are perceived in the hallucinatory field. There can be micropsia (where all objects are seen small), macropsia (all objects are seen bigger than what they are), dejavu (feeling of familiarity in unfamiliar environment), dejavecu (feeling as if a particular statement has been heard before), jamaisvu (feeling of unfamiliarity in familiar environment), dejaetendu (feeling of having lived through a bygone era) and defective recognition of facial emotions. *The most common manifestation of temporal lobe disease is seizures of complex partial nature.*

Occipital Lobe

This is the region behind the parieto-occipital sulcus and above the calcarine sulcus. Main function is vision. Bilateral lesion produces cortical blindness with normal pupil, fundus and visual imagery. Unilateral lesion produces hemianopia with macular sparing and Wernicke's hemianopic pupillary reaction characterized by preserved pupillary reaction elicited through the seeing field. Partial lesions produce visual recognition fatigue called *asthenopia* where repeated exposure to visual stimuli results in failure of recognition. There can be visual *anosognosia* which manifests as *Anton's syndrome or denial of blindness*. This is due to blind sight through the superior colliculus where crude appreciation of vision

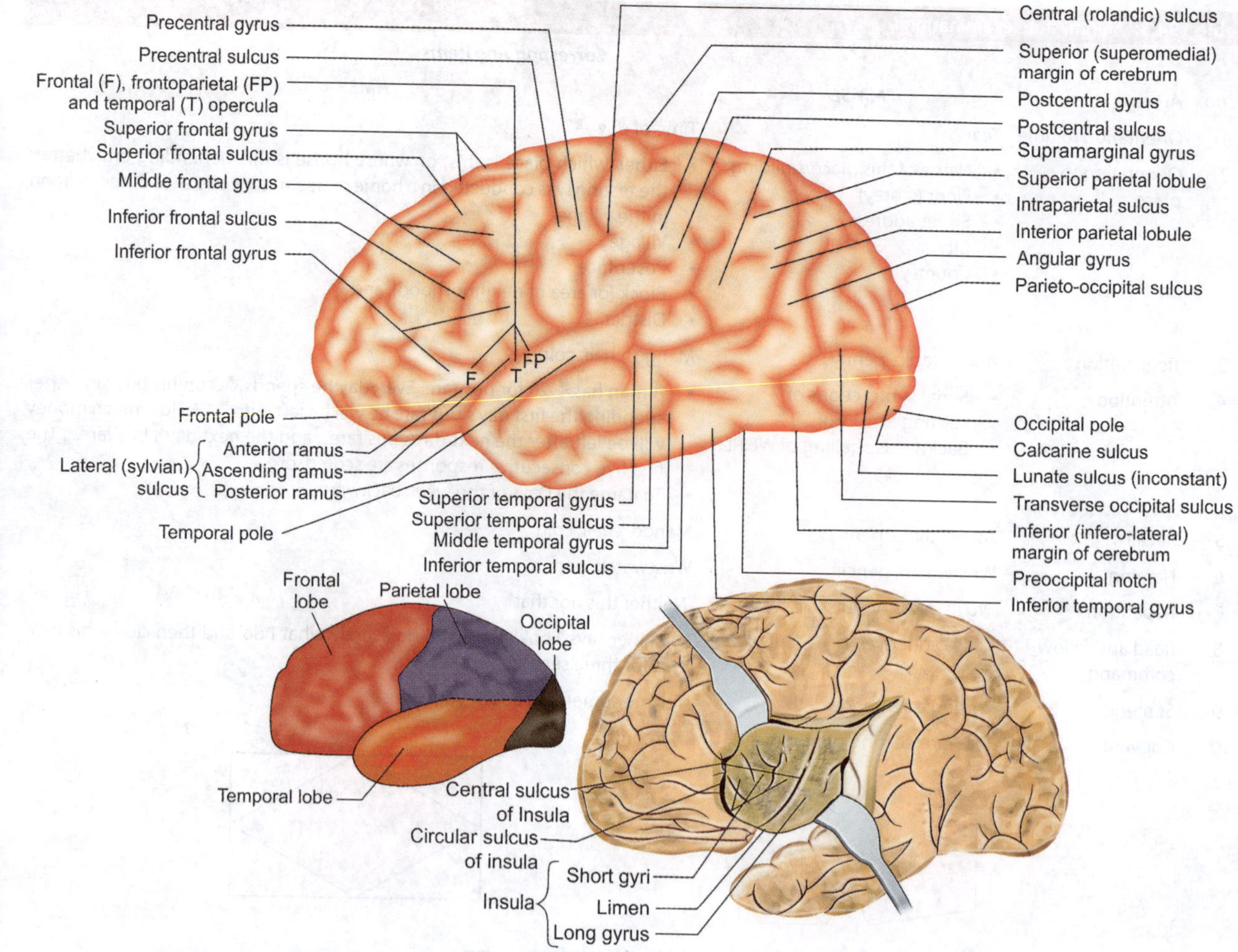

Fig. 194.5: Superolateral surface of the brain

takes place. There can be ***visual illusion*** in the form of distortion of form, shape, size, color, movement, ***polyopia*** (seeing several numbers of the same object), ***palinopsia*** or illusory persistence of object after it has been removed, alliesthesia or illusory displacement of the objects in the field and illusions of tilt, etc. (Fig. 194.6). There can be visual hallucinations involving elementary stimuli like light, color, geometric forms and movements or complex forms like objects, animals and persons. There can be hallucinations in the hemianopic field called ***Charles***

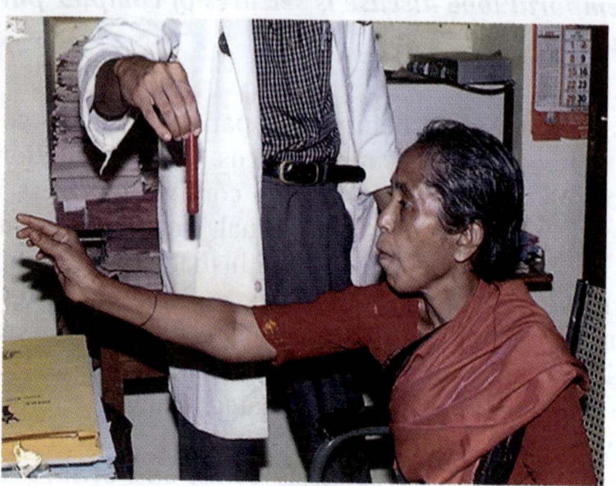

Fig. 194.6: Alliesthesia: Illusory displacement of the seen object in the space

Bonnet phenomena. There can be visual object agnosia (apperceptive) where patient does not even appreciate the size and shape of the seen object or associative nature, where the size and shape is appreciated but it is not synthesized into the object that it constitutes, parieto-occipital simultagnosia otherwise called ***piece meal vision*** or ***spelling dyslexia*** where patient sees the individual components of a scene or object but unable to derive the collective phenomena. There can be ***prosopagnosia*** for faces, environment agnosia for places, ***topographagnosia*** for maps and ***color agnosia***. There can be ***color anomia***.

CORPUS CALLOSUM

Disease of the corpus callosum presents with split-brain function abnormality in the form of inability to match words on one field with objects on other field as letter memory is in the dominant hemisphere and picture memory is in the nondominant hemisphere (right) and when corpus callosum is destroyed, these two functions cannot be linked. Left-arm apraxia is due to failure of transmission of movement-related information to the right motor cortex. In pure lesions of anterior part of the corpus callosum and sympathetic apraxia where patient has apraxia of the left hand and right hemiplegia due to lesion in the dominant motor cortex as we have seen in the praxis circuit above. Other features of corpus callosum involvement are ***dementia, double hemianopia***, where patient can localize objects in the right field with the right hand but not the left hand and vice versa. ***Color anomia*** is seen in the splenium of the corpus callosum lesion where patient can match the objects based on color but cannot name the color or point to the color when named.

Bedside Testing Methods
Memory Testing

Instantaneous	Identify objects by different modes
Immediate	Digit forward, digit backward, continue when interrupted
Recent memory	Breakfast, month, day, visitors, find five hidden objects
Recall	Three sentences to be reproduced
Registration, retention and recall	Pierre Marie's three paper test (cut a piece of paper into 3 unequal bits, tell the patient to keep the small bit with him, intermediate bit to the examiner and throw away the large bit).
Remote memory	Wedding day, school experiences

SPEECH AND LANGUAGE

Speech: This is the mechanical portion of one's ability to communicate with oral language which involves phonation and articulation (Fig. 194.7).

Language: It is the symbolization of ideas which converts thoughts into comprehensible modes of communication. Language has got five primary functions—seeing and reading, hearing and comprehending, writing, speaking and repeating. The structures concerned areas are in the dominant perisylvian region which includes Broca's area, arcuate fasciculus and Wernicke's area. The parasylvian areas are around the sylvian fissure which carry inputs to primary language areas. The subcortical areas include external capsule, internal capsule, thalamus, caudate and lentiform nucleus called ***Marie's quadrilateral space*** (Fig. 194.8). This area is concerned with preparation of the motor pattern to produce the correct language. Naming is a diffusely localized language function.

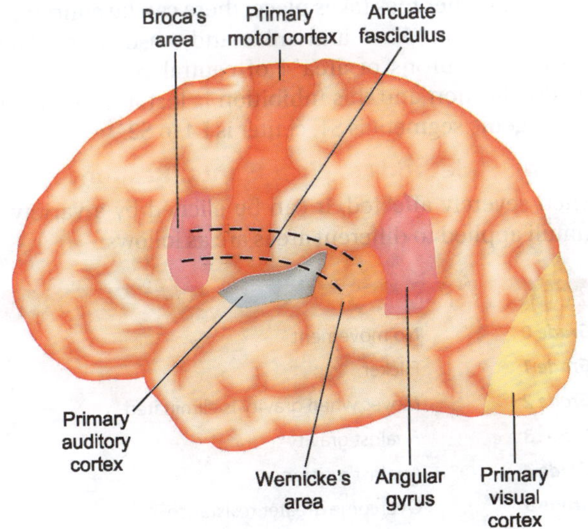

Fig. 194.7: Left cerebral hemisphere—cortical and subcortical areas of speech

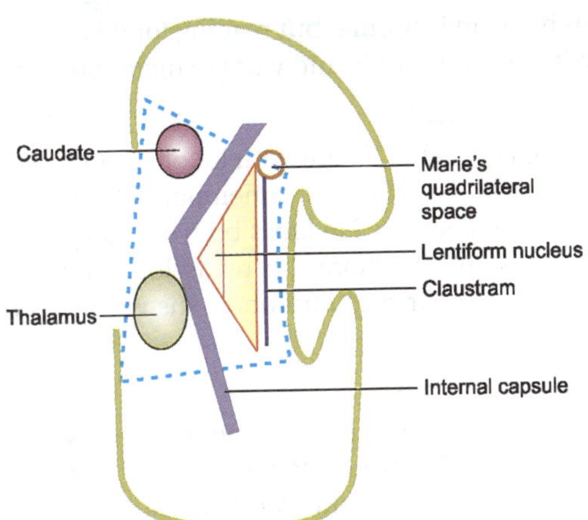

Fig. 194.8: Marie's quadrilateral space

Analysis of language at the bedside starts with assessment of a sample of spontaneous speech. This involves word output which is normally 100–150 words per minute. If less than 50, it is ***nonfluent*** and more than 150 it is ***fluent***. Check if the communication is effortful or effortless? Is there a dysarthric element? What is the phrase length? Is there dysprosody (alteration in the prosody), grammar, meaning, literal or verbal paraphasia (replacing letters in a word or words in a sentence with unrelated letters and words)? Is there any echoing (repeating a question asked indicating poor comprehension), echolalia (repeating like a parrot) or perseveration (repeating the same word)? What is the emotional state of the person? Does he have word finding difficulty? If so, does it improve with cues? or Can he select the correct words from the list?

This is followed by assessing the capacity to repeat words, simple sentences and complex sentences. Repetition involves registering through the Wernicke's area and transmitting to Broca's area through the arcuate fasciculus. Repetition is a unique function of perisylvian region and therefore of great help in localizing language defects at the bedside as perisylvian, where repetition is not possible or parasylvian where repetition is possible.

Writing involves sample of spontaneous writing analysis, which includes defects in the mechanics, syntax, content, spelling, meaning, looping, direction, size, shape, etc. Writing to dictation needs an auditory gnostic component and copying involves a visual gnostic component.

Assessment of two afferent limbs—audition and vision: This involves testing comprehension through auditory mode and visual mode, e.g. listen and obey, read and obey, read loud, write to dictation, copy write in addition to response to verbally presented commands, ability to differentiate different sounds and auditory attention.

In the laboratory, there are several testing methods including ***Porch Index of Communicative Ability (PICA) and PGI Aphasia Battery.*** These can be referred by the interested student.

Broca's Aphasia

This is a perisylvian aphasia; therefore repetition is affected. Patient is nonfluent effortful, emotional and speaks a telegraphic language with poor grammar, normal comprehension and no paraphasic errors. His reading for comprehension is normal but reading loud is affected. He can write telegraphically and write to dictation and copy.

Wernicke's Aphasia

Repetition is affected, fluent with lot of paraphasic errors. The language is effortless, unemotional with normal grammar, no meaning. He lacks both auditory and visual comprehension. Therefore, he reads loud nonsensically and cannot copy or read and obey. His writing is incomprehensible.

Conduction Aphasia

The pathology is in the arcuate fasciculus. There is disproportionately severe affection of repetition with mild features of both Broca's and Wernicke's aphasia.

Global Aphasia

It is nonfluent with poor comprehension, poor repetition and all five elements are affected.

Parasylvian and Subcortical Aphasia

As the perisylvian area is spared, repetition is normal. Transcortical motor aphasia otherwise Broca's aphasia with retained repetition and transcortical sensory aphasia is Wernicke's with normal repetition. Mixed transcortical aphasia is global aphasia with normal repetition. Subcortical aphasias are characterized by mute state, severe dysarthria, naming defect with or without paraphasic defects and rapid recovery.

Speech Disorders

These involve defects in converting language into audible sounds. The disorders may be spastic, flaccid, dyskinetic, ataxic and cortical, and dysphonias.

Spastic dysarthria occurs in lesions which involves the corticobulbar fibers. The speech is effortful; the syllables run into one another and are slurred. The ideal word used for testing this is by asking patient to repeat **British constitution**.

Flaccid dysarthria varies depending on the lower motor neuron (LMN) structure that is involved.

- If the tongue is involved patient has difficulty in pronouncing words which contains the linguals which need exclusive use of the tongue, e.g. L
- If lips are involved, the words which contain the labials, e.g. P and B
- If teeth are involved 'dentals', e.g. D and T
- If palatal muscles are involved, palatals or words containing NG, GG become affected.

Ataxic dysarthria is of two types—staccato, where there is undue stress and explosiveness and scanning, where the words are split into syllables. The common word used at bedside to test this is *Chakravarthi Rajagopalachari*. Dyskinetic speech may be hypokinetic in Parkinsonism. It is characterized by progressive decrease in voice volume. It can be hyperkinetic in chronic speech where there is a sudden unwarranted stop, voice tremor where speech is tremulous.

Lingual dystonia is a condition where the speech is arrested in its course by twisting of tongue which is task-specific. There are other speech disorders like stuttering, stammering and cluttering which do not carry serious neurological significance.

Phonation is the process by which voice is modulated by the vocal chords. Patient will be able to make syllables, gestures but has a husky quality with effortful speech.

Language Disorders

They are differentiated from global disorders of communication and psychogenic problems by the following parameters. Only spoken language is affected in psychogenic lesions whereas in organic lesions there is involvement of all the five limbs of language with retained gestural communication. In global disorder which affects language, significant impairment of other hemispheric functions will be noted. Power is the strength developed by voluntary actions.

EXAMINATION OF MOTOR SYSTEM

Motor system examination consists of examination of power, tone, reflexes, nutrition, coordination and abnormal movements.

Power testing is done using Medical Research Council (MRC) grading. Muscle strength is examined by asking the individual to oppose the examiner's power and it is graded as follows (Table 194.4).

Nutrition: It is considered as wasting when there is loss of power with loss of bulk. It is called thinning if bulk alone is lost and hypoplasia if there is uniform shrinking. Coordination is the maintenance of rate, range, rhythm and direction of a motor activity.

Reflexes

They are involuntary motor response to sensory stimuli. They are categorized as superficial, deep, organic and release reflex. Superficial reflexes are responses produced by stimulation of the cornea, mucous membranes or skin, e.g. corneal, conjunctival, pharyngeal, abdominal, cremasteric, anal bulbocavernosus and plantar response. When the lateral part of the sole of the foot is stroked, there is a slow tonic plantar flexion of great toe and flexion of other toes.

Babinski's reflex: This is a pathological response and signifies organic disease of pyramidal system. It is elicited by stroking the lateral part of the sole of the foot causing a nociceptive stimulus. Slow tonic dorsiflexion of big toe and fanning of other toes takes place; there can be contraction of flexors of hip, knee and ankle and tensor fascia latae. Normally, neurons of area 4 of central cortex suppress the dorsiflexion and this inhibition is lost in disease. The reflexogenic segment is S1, center is L4 to S2.

Alternate Methods to Elicit Plantar Response

When severely affected, it can be elicited by a variety of stimuli applied to different areas are as follows:

Table 194.4:	Grading power
Grade 0	No movement
Grade 1	Flicker
Grade 2	Moves when gravity is eliminated
Grade 3	Against gravity
Grade 4	Against resistance
Grade 5	Overcome greater resistance

Note: Gravity can be eliminated by changing the plane of testing, using a sling or testing under water.

Table 194.5: Neuroanatomy of the commonly elicited reflexes

Reflex	Afferent pathway	Center	Efferent pathway
Muscle stretch reflexes			
• Jaw jerk (masseter and temporalis muscles)	Cranial nerve V	Pons	Cranial nerve V
• Bicep reflex (biceps muscle)	Musculocutaneous nerve	C5–6	Musculocutaneous
• Triceps reflex (triceps muscle)	Radial nerve	C6–7	Radial nerve
• Supinator reflex (brachioradialis muscle, Syn: supinator longus)	Radial nerve	C5–6	Radial nerve
• Knee reflex (quadriceps femoris, mainly vastus medialis muscle)	Femoral nerve	L2, 3, 4	Femoral nerve
• Ankle reflex (calf muscles gastrocnemius, soleus, plantaris)	Tibial nerve	L5, S1–2	Tibial nerve
Superficial reflexes			
• Corneal reflex	Cranial nerve V	Pons	Cranial nerve VII
• Conjunctival reflex	Cranial nerve V	Pons	Cranial nerve VII
• Pharyngeal reflex	Cranial nerve IX	Medulla	Cranial nerve X
• Palatal reflex	Cranial nerve IX	Medulla	Cranial nerve X
• Abdominal reflexes:			
▪ Upper	T6–9 posterior roots	T6–9 cord segments	T6–9 anterior roots
▪ Middle	T9–11 posterior roots	T9–11 cord segments	T9–11 anterior roots
▪ Lower	T11–L1 posterior roots	T11–L1 cord segments	T11–L1 anterior
• Cremasteric reflex	Femoral nerve	L1, 2	Genitofemoral nerve
• Plantar reflex	Tibial nerve	L5, S1–2	Tibial nerve
• Anal reflex	Pudendal nerve	S3, 4, 5	Pudendal nerve
• Bulbocavernosus reflex	Pudendal nerve	S3, 4	Pudendal nerve

- ■ ***Chaddock's sign*** if elicited by stimuli below lateral malleolus
- ■ ***Oppenheim's sign*** if elicited by pressure along shin of the tibia
- ■ ***Stransky sign*** if there is little toe abduction
- ■ ***Gordon's sign*** squeezing calf
- ■ ***Gonda's sign*** pressing and releasing 4th toe downwards
- ■ ***Schaefer's sign*** by squeezing Achilles' tendon. Normally, extensor reflex is seen in newborns and in sleep.

Flexion pyramidal signs are flexion of toes caused by pressure on tips of toes called ***Rossolimo's sign***, flexion of toes caused by tapping of cuboid called ***Mendel-Bekhterev sign*** and flexion of toes caused by pin prick over dorsum of foot is called ***Bing's sign***.

Deep or Muscle Stretch Reflexes

It is the repeated contraction occurring on sustained stretch. The commonly elicited muscle stretch reflexes are jaw jerk, biceps jerk, triceps jerk, supinator jerk, quadriceps jerk, ankle jerk, internal and external hamstrings jerk and Hoffmann's reflex (Table 194.5). Whenever a muscle with intact nerve supply is sharply stretched, it contracts. Lesions of pyramidal tract by removal of suppression on final common pathway facilitate this reflex. Cerebellar and LMN disease inhibit it (Table 194.6). Clonus has the same significance as hyperactive tendon jerks.

Organic Reflexes

Bladder and bowel-related reflexes are called as organic reflexes. The reflexes which operate in the spinal stage of development for feeding and defense-related motor activity become suppressed during development to cortical stage. These reflexes get released during diseases which cause regression of cortical functions. They are ***palmomental reflex*** which helps to keep palm and chin approximated along with short latency flexor reflex

Table 194.6: Differences between upper and lower motor neuron

Upper motor neuron	Lower motor neuron
Movement paralysis	Muscle paralysis
Reflex movement present voluntary absent	Both absent
Hypertonia	Hypotonia
Disuse atrophy	Wasting, fasciculations
Superficial reflexes lost deep exaggerated	Both lost

Note: Refer basal ganglia, cerebellum in subsequent chapters.

Table 194.7: Grading of deep tendon reflexes

Grade	Response reaction
Grade 0	Absent
Grade 1	Present with reinforcement
Grade 2	Normal
Grade 3	Exaggerated
Grade 4	With clonus

Note: For reinforcement, the patient is made to clench the jaw or forcibly try to pull apart the flexed fingers. This increases the general muscle tone in the body and also helps to divert the attention of the person from the examiner which will suppress the normal reflex.

afferents which keep the child in universal flexion in intrauterine life. Others are the ***grasping*** and ***groping reflex, snout, rooting, sucking*** and ***corneomandibular reflex*** which help the newborn to grasp reflex and also seek feeds (Table 194.7).

Tone is resistance offered to passive movement or state of partial contraction always present in normal muscle for maintenance of posture with minimal expenditure of energy. This is dealt in detail in Ch 193.

SENSORY SYSTEM

Abnormal Appreciation of Sensations

Sensory symptoms may be positive or negative. Positive ones are ***paresthesias*** which are sensory perceptions in the absence of sensory stimuli due to uninhibited small fiber activity due to destructive disease of large fiber or irritative disease of small fiber.

Dysesthesias are altered perception of sensory stimuli due to neuronal crosstalk (when a particular fiber is destroyed, repair is carried out by functionally different fibers resulting in perceiving one kind of stimuli as another) and generally indicates faulty regeneration.

Hyperpathia is exaggerated threshold till a particular intensity stimuli and exaggerated perception beyond threshold. *Hyperalgesia* is lowered threshold for sensory perception due to sensitization which may be chemical (around areas of inflammation), neural (defective gating and endogenous analgesia) and psychic (limbic component of pain). Hypoesthesia or analgesia associated with pain is called *anesthesia dolorosa* and pain elicited by non-noxious stimuli is called *allodynia*.

Sensory Phenomena Produced by Lesions at Different Sites in the Sensory Pathways

Sensory abnormalities are considered as due to nerve lesion if they show a length-dependent distal symmetric pattern, individual nerve pattern, nonlength-dependent cranial or short nerve pattern. They may have Tinel's sign or dull nerve pain. Root pattern is radicular distribution, sharp shooting with aggravating and relieving factors. Lesions beyond dorsal root ganglion (proximal) are generally more ill-defined with severe sensory ataxia. In the spinal cord, tract pains are produced from posterior column and spinothalamic tract. Sacral sparing of spinothalamic sensations occurs in deep lesions and suspended and dissociated if only crossing spinothalamic fibers in few segments are affected. There can be tract pains, which present as a superficial burning paresthesia or feeling of coldness which is ill-localized and lack of precipitating or relieving factors when it comes from the spinothalamic tract. Posterior column presents with loss of vibration, position and sensory ataxia. The irritative symptoms may be Lhermitte's sign which is a shock-like pain on flexing neck, girdle sensation (a broad band like feeling), glove and stocking like sensory feeling, feeling that the limb is swollen, bizarre sensory feels and deep boring paresthesia as if the flesh is being pulled out of bone. Lesions of the lateral medulla presents with crossed dissociated anesthesia, medial medulla presents with opposite side posterior column and pyramidal features, pons can show perioral sensory loss due to quintothalamic tract involvement in the center or balaclava helmet like sensory loss due to involvement of outer quintothalamic fibers, sometimes bifacial sensory loss occurs as the fibers of spinal tract of trigeminal are crossed 60% and 40% is ipsilateral. Thalamus lesions produce hyperpathia and thalamic pain on the opposite half. Lesions of the posterior limb of internal capsule lead to a hemianesthesia with hemianopia. Lesions of sensory cortex usually produce patchy cortical sensory problems in the opposite side.

GAIT AND EQUILIBRIUM

Gait is a learned motor skill that is the most automatic of all automatic reflexes and can be performed without conscious effort in which the erect moving body is supported first by one leg and then the other. Posture, equilibrium and movement are controlled by a complex interaction of motor, sensory, cerebellar and extrapyramidal systems, delicately balanced in dynamic equilibrium between agonist-antagonist, synergist, flexor and extensor tone and channeled out to the muscles via the spinal motor neurons. *Equilibrium* is stable maintenance of posture during rest and activity

Movement is the ability of the organism to displace from one plane to another. It involves short phasic reactions mediated through several reflexes, postural righting reflexes, antigravity stretches, stepping, equilibrium and propulsion. *Posture* is ability to maintain body parts in desired alignment in balance with gravitational pull.

Gait involves the integrated functions of the postural and righting reflexes, integration and initiation by corticospinal tract, automatic movements and fine tuning by extrapyramidal system, coordination by cortico-cerebellar tracts and subjective awareness of posture via proprioceptive fibers. Normal gait starts with antigravity stretch when the limb opposes the pull of the gravity and clears, then the heel strikes the floor in the front followed by the toe. The opposite leg is flexed which is called *stepping*. Then the leg goes into the swing phase. This is followed by moving forward which involves stance (stance is the distance covered by two feet for stable standing), pace (distance covered between two feet for stable walking), balance, turns, etc. The last phase is propulsion. The two heels strike by one leg constitutes a *gait cycle*. Number of gait cycles per minute is called *cadence*. In lowest-level gait disorders, only one major afferent system is affected resulting in brief periods of disequilibrium. Middle-level disorders include myelopathy, spastic hemiparetic gait from unilateral impairment of the corticospinal tract; gaits associated with movement disorders and dystonic, choreic, hemiballistic and cerebellar ataxic gaits. The highest-level gait disorders include cautious gait, subcortical dysequilibrium, frontal dysequilibrium, isolated gait ignition failure, frontal gait, primary progressive freezing gait and psychogenic gait disorders.

Executory apparatus-related gait abnormalities involve dysfunction of the lower motor unit consisting of neurons and muscles resulting in waddling gait; paralysis of dorsiflexors of the ankle causing high-stepping gait, paralysis of plantar flexors causing slapping gait and diseases of bones and tendons causing shortening of limb and limping gait.

Spastic gait: It is characterized by poor antigravity stretch, dragging with tendency to scissoring. The stepping phenomena is not seen. This occurs due to the lesion of the corticospinal tract.

Stamping gait: Here, patient is unable to assess the relationship of his feet to the floor, so he will lift the leg too high and brings it down with a stamp. This is seen in large fiber neuropathy, tabes dorsalis, posterior column ataxias and diabetic pseudotabes.

Ataxic gait: Here, the stance is wide. The patient has tendency to sway to either side or one side based on the nature of the cerebellar involvement. If there is disease of anterior lobe of the cerebellum, there is gentle side-to-side swaying. Flocculonodular lobe and vestibular nucleus lesions produce wide arc reeling type of gait.

Waddling gait: When there is weakness of the opposite hip abductors during the phase of stepping, the hip sinks down resulting in a duck-like gait.

High stepping gait: It occurs in weakness of dorsiflexors where the patient lifts the legs too high to prevent injury to the toes.

Slapping gait: When plantar flexors are weak, after the heel strike the feet just falls to the floor.

Demodarans gait: This is seen in dystonia musculorum deformans where the pelvis tilts up and forward with each stepping action.

Armadillo gait: This is seen in patients with diffuse spasm of the muscle seen in conditions like Stiff-man's syndrome.

Apraxic gait: Where the antigravity stretch is not initiated and patient feels his feet glued to the floor. If helped, he will be able to move forward; seen in frontal lobe disease.

Festinating gait: Short pace and stance in diseases of frontal lobe and extrapyramidal system, especially parkinsonism.

LABORATORY INVESTIGATIONS

Electroencephalogram

A voltage versus time graph, which represents the sum total of the postsynaptic excitatory and inhibitory potentials of neurons, modified by the intralaminar nucleus of thalamus and picked up from scalp. Extracerebral potentials recorded by electroencephalogram (EEG) are called as artifacts (Fig. 194.9).

Recording is done with metal discs or cups with central hole attached to insulated lead wires. Placement of electrodes is done as per international 10–20 system of Jasper. This provides space for 21 electrodes and one-ground electrode modifications are done for brain death and pediatric use with fewer electrodes, and more electrodes for more sensitive records. The recording electrodes have a letter and a number. Even numbers pertain to right side and odd numbers to the left. The recording is done with a minimum of eight electrodes. Both bipolar and monopolar recordings are done. Bipolar is linking two active electrodes and the graph represents the potential difference between them and therefore good for focal pathology. Referential or monopolar recording is done using linking active electrode to an apparently inert one. This therefore is sensitive for picking generalized dysfunction. A minimum of 20 minutes recording is needed.

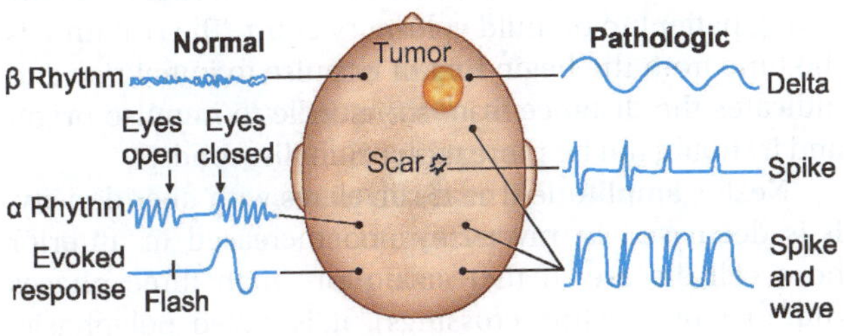

Fig. 194.9: Abnormal pattern in electroencephalogram (EEG)

EEG is the investigation of choice in functional brain disease like epilepsy. Activation procedures like sleep deprivation, starvation, hyperventilation at 20 respiration/min and photic stimulation is done to bring out abnormal discharges. Specific procedures are used in reflex epilepsies. Paper recording is now replaced by digital recordings which permit various combinations, changing paper speed, sensitivity and filter settings. Normally one page is 10 seconds and paper speed is 3 cm/second and 7 mm amplitude is 50 microvolts.

Normal adult wake record consists of alpha activity posteriorly which is 8–12 Hz, 15–50 microvolts, best seen with eye closure and beta activity anteriorly which is more than 13 Hz, 10–20 microvolts and increases by sedation. Sleep record shows slow waves called theta when 4–8 Hz, and delta when less than 4. Abnormal patterns are of a large number depending on the type of illness.

Special recordings are done with needle electrodes, sphenoidal, nasopharyngeal, esophageal and tympanic leads.

Video EEG

EEG and video recordings are simultaneously done for short-term or long-term especially in the study of seizures. This helps the physician to witness the attack so that true seizures can be distinguished from pseudoseizures. Semiology of seizures can be correctly studied. When structural changes are detected in brain whether it is an incidental one or is causative of epilepsy in the patient can be assessed. Event and discharge characterization are done.

Ambulatory Electroencephalogram

This serves as a mobile intensive monitoring system without hospitalization.

Electrocorticography

This is used during excision of epileptogenic foci to decide the extent of the pathology. Electrodes are either metal balls or saline cotton wicks mounted on springs.

Depth Electrodes Recording

Bundle of fine wires with uninsulated tips is used to define targets for surgical resection.

Magnetic Electroencephalogram

This is a technique for recording magnetic fields produced by electrical current occurring naturally in the brain. This method is sensitive spatiotemporal resolution, it is noninvasive. An artificial magnetic field is picked by superconducting quantum interference device (SQUID) and converted to voltage. Motor and language areas can be marked using special techniques. This method is especially useful in the assessment of nonlesional neocortical epilepsy. It is also useful in studying cortical organization in psychiatric disorders.

Polysomnography

It is a comprehensive recording of the biophysiological changes that occur during sleep, and it is done usually during night sleep. Sleep is staged using EEG, electro-oculogram and involuntary leg movements recorded using calf electrodes. ECG thermistors to assess airflow, chest wall and abdominal movement recording, pulse oximeter

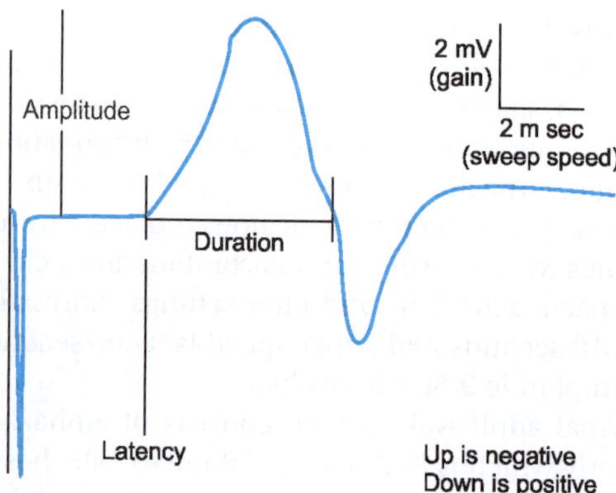

Fig. 194.10: Compound muscle action potential (CMAP)

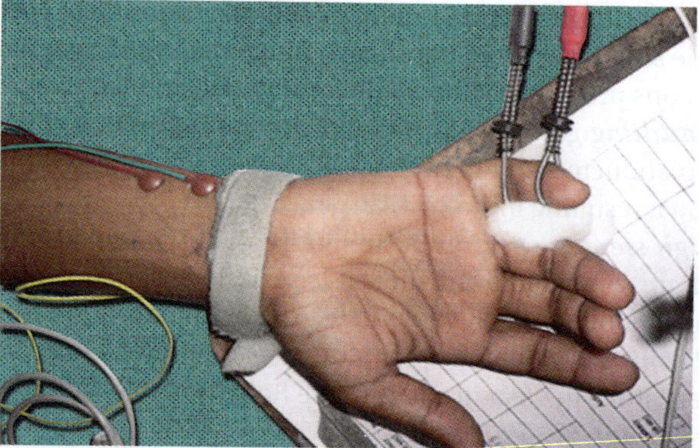

Fig. 194.11: Sensory conduction testing

and penile tumescence are recorded. Polysomnography is useful to record and quantify apneas, abnormal sleep patterns, leg movements, night terrors, abnormal arousals, cataplexy-narcolepsy syndrome and parasomnias.

Transcranial Magnetic Stimulation

This is a noninvasive method of stimulating the superficial cortical neurons using a powerful transient magnetic field which secondarily induces electric currents in the brain. It assesses central motor conduction and cortical inhibition and threshold of cortical excitation.

Nerve Conduction Studies and Electromyography

Nerve conduction studies are simple and reliable tests of peripheral nerve function. They help in determining the picture of the lesion and precisely localizing the site of maximal involvement. Basically, electrical stimulation of a nerve initiates an impulse that travels along motor, sensory or mixed nerves. This is recorded either as a *compound muscle action potential (CMAP)* in case of motor nerves or from the nerve itself in case of sensory nerves (Fig. 194.10). Surface or needle electrodes are used. Surface electrodes are silver plated, consisting of a cathode (–ve pole) and an anode (+ve pole). As the current flows between them, -ve charge from the cathode depolarizes the nerve, while +ve charge at the anode hyperpolarizes the nerve. For recording motor potentials, the recording electrodes are placed over a muscle supplied by the nerve being stimulated. This is called as *belly tendon method*.

The active electrode (G1) is placed on the center of the muscle belly (over the motor end-plate) and the reference electrode (G2) is placed distally over the tendon to the muscle.

Latency is the time from application of the stimulus to the initial CMAP deflection from the baseline. It represents nerve conduction from stimulus site to neuromuscular junction (NMJ). Delay across the NMJ and depolarization time across the muscle (latency) is a measure of the fastest conducting fibers. Amplitude is usually measured from baseline to the negative peak, less commonly from negative peak to the next positive peak. It reflects the number of muscle fibers that fire and are activated. Duration is usually measured from initial deflection to the first baseline crossing (i.e. negative peak duration). Area is electronically calculated. *Motor conduction velocity* measures of the fastest conducting motor axons. Two

stimulation sites are used. The difference in latency is recorded. The distance between the stimulating cathodes is measured (taking the midpoint of the cathodes as the two points) and entered. The nerve conduction velocity (NCV) is calculated as distance is divided by time, i.e. difference in latency.

Sensory conduction is studied as follows. Stimulation of the digital nerves using ring electrodes elicits an orthodromic potential at a more proximal site. Alternatively, stimulation of the nerve trunk proximally elicits antidromic digital potential distally. Sensory fibers with large diameters have lower thresholds and conduct 5–10% faster than motor fibers. Mixed nerve potentials allow determination of sensory conduction velocity in healthy nerves (Fig. 194.11).

Sensory Conduction Testing

Electromyography

Electromyography (EMG) records the electrical activity of the muscle when a needle is introduced into the muscle. Normal resting membrane potential is 70–80 mV and is negative inside. This needs an intact innervation. When a needle is introduced, acetylcholine is released causing focal depolarization which lasts for 5–10 seconds. This results in discharges which are called positive when the deflection is down and negative when they are up. The physiologically occurring discharges are end-plate noise and spike. Normal insertional activity lasts 5–10 seconds. It may be positive or negative. Then spontaneous activity starts at 50–100 microvolts. Physiological spontaneous activity is end-plate noise, end-plate spike (Fig. 194.12).

When the nerve supply to the muscle is disturbed the resting membrane is abnormal and so it will fire spontaneously and abnormally resulting in spontaneous and pathological discharges like fibrillation, positive sharp waves, complex repetitive discharges and myokymia. Motor unit action potentials are brought out by asking patient to do mild voluntary effort. The rise time is the time from the beginning of impulse to initial rise and indicates the distance from the needle to impulse origin and it should not be more than 0.5 milliseconds.

Next is amplitude which correlates with fiber density. It is decreased in myopathy and increased in anterior horn cell disease. If there are more than three phases (number of baseline crossings), it is called polyphasic. Recruitment pattern is the pattern of discharge obtained

Abnormalities		
Parameters	Myopathy	Denervation
Insertional activity	Normal	Increase
Spontaneous activity	Nil	+ve
MUAP duration	Decrease <5 Msec	Increase >16 Msec
Amplitude	<200 µv	>400 µv
Configuration	Polyphasic	Polyphasic

Fig. 194.12: Chart showing abnormalities of electromyography (EMG)

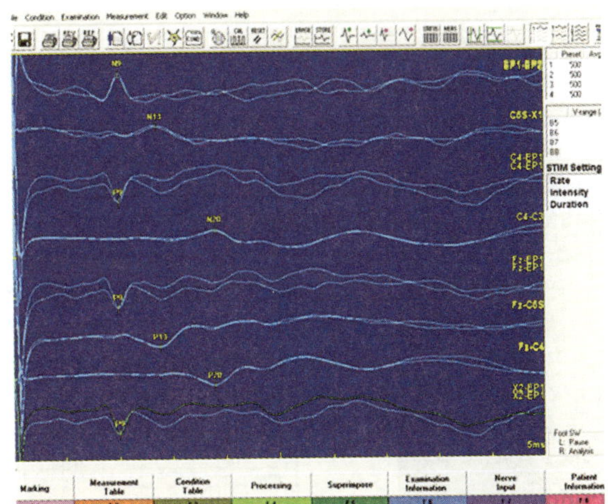

Fig. 194.13: Normal somatosensory evoked potential (SEP)

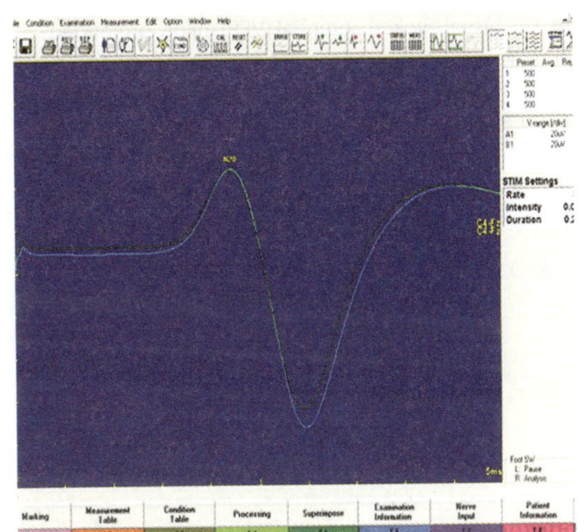

Fig. 194.14: Giant somatosensory evoked potential (SEP)

by maximum voluntary effort and it reflects the motor unit number. Based on these information, the site of disease (whether muscle belly or tendon, nerve or anterior horn cell) can be determined.

Macro electromyography: This gives information about one motor unit using special needles with a side pore exposing 2.5 mm diameter platinum electrode.

Single fiber electromyography: This is extracellular recording of single muscle fiber action potential by voluntarily contracting the muscle.

H reflex: This is named after Hoffman. It involves afferent conduction in large fast conducting 1a fibers, monosynaptic activation of motor neurons in the anterior horn of spinal cord, and efferent conduction in alpha motor nerves. This is a representation of monosynaptic reflex.

F reflex: This is produced by antidromic fixing of motor units and it involves only the motor pathways.

Repetitive N stimulation: This is a specialized test to study neuromuscular junction disease.

Blink reflex: This is a specified test to study 5th and 7th cranial nerves.

Evoked Responses

Somatosensory evoked responses [somatosensory evoked potential (SEP's)] are presynaptic and postsynaptic responses recorded over the limbs, spine and scalp following stimulation of peripheral nerves and nerve trunks (Fig. 194.13). The potentials are mainly generated by large diameter fibers in central and peripheral nervous system (PNS). They are closely associated with specific anatomical sites and they are not usually affected by physiological variations. The abnormalities are not specific to the etiological factor. They are useful to assess proximal segments of peripheral nerves and roots, and to evaluate large fiber sensory tracts in central nervous system (CNS). They are useful in the assessment of comatosed, brain dead and anesthetized individuals and at operation theaters during surgical procedures.

Giant SEP is seen in diseases like juvenile myoclonic epilepsy (JME), subacute sclerosing panencephalitis (SSPE), spinocerebellar ataxia (SCA), which directly or indirectly affect cerebellum resulting in reduced endogenous inhibition (Fig. 194.14).

Visual Evoked Potential (VEP)

It evoked electrophysiological potential in response to visual stimulation. This noninvasive method tests the function of the visual pathway from retina the occipital cortex. It is very useful in detecting an anterior visual conduction disturbance like multiple sclerosis, optic neuritis and optic atrophy, retrochiasmatic lesions, compressive lesions, hysteria and others. The stimulus used is reversal of a checkerboard pattern of black and white without change in luminance (Fig. 194.15).

Basis of VEP abnormalities

Each eye projects to the occipital lobes through the chiasma. Unilateral VEP abnormality obtained by full monocular stimulation is likely to be due to a prechiasmatic lesion. VEP abnormalities are detected by prolongation of latency.

- Demyelination of optic nerve pathways gives rise to reduction of amplitude.
- Ischemic optic neuropathy leads to combined abnormalities of latency and amplitude.
- Optic nerve compression leads to prolongation.

Brainstem Auditory Evoked Response (BAER)

This records electric waveforms of biologic origin elicited in response to sound stimuli that are recorded from ear

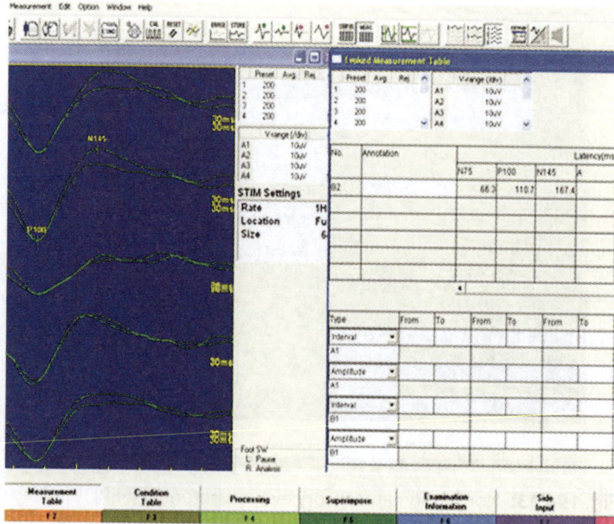

Fig. 194.15: Visual evoked potential (VEP) mildly prolonged

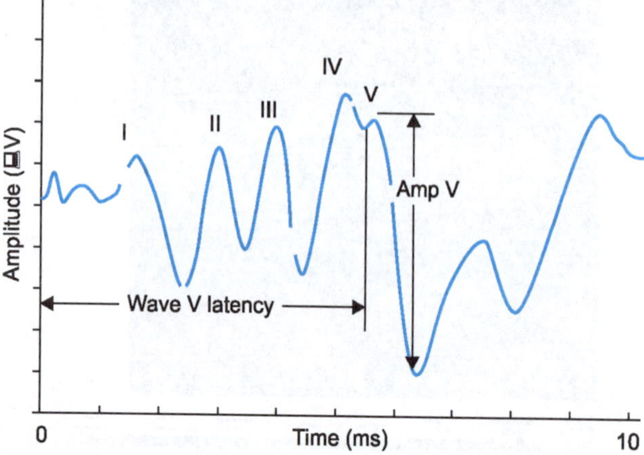

Fig. 194.16: Brainstem auditory evoked response (BAER)

and vertex to assess the conduction through auditory pathway up to midbrain. Normally, it consists of 1 to 7 waves, occurring during the first 10 milliseconds after the onset of stimulus with positive polarity at vertex of head. The stimulus consists of square wave pulse of 100 milliseconds with stimulus intensity 60 dB above hearing threshold. The other ear is masked with noise at 40 dB. Measurements are shown in Figure 194.16.

The parameters that are studied include absolute latency and amplitude, interpeak latencies, amplitude ratio of waves and innerear interpeak differences. Abnormalities include absence of waveforms, abnormal absolute or interpeak latencies, amplitude ratio abnormalities and significant right to left asymmetry.

EEG is useful in neonates and ***transcranial Doppler*** is used in assessing vascular patterns as well as other abnormalities of both CNS and PNS.

Brain mapping is used to map brain function. There are two brain mapping methods—electrical and functional.

- The techniques that are based on hemodynamic metabolic signals include functional magnetic resonance imaging (fMRI), positron emission tomography (PET) and single photon emission computed tomography (SPECT).

- The techniques that detect the electrical and electromagnetic activity of the brain include EEG and ERP (event-related potentials), magnetoencephalography (MEG) detects magnetic activity.

- fMRI refers to the use of the technology of magnetic resonance imaging (MRI) to detect the localized changes in blood flow and blood oxygenation that occur in the brain in response to neural activity.

- The blood oxygenation level dependent (BOLD) fMRI technique basically measures changes in the nonhomogeneity of the magnetic field, which are the result of changes in the level of oxygen present in blood (blood oxygenation).

Advantages: fMRI does not involve ionizing radiation, it can be used repeatedly on a single subject and even on child volunteers. It permits longitudinal studies and, improvement in signal-to-noise ratios if the task being used elicits the same general response when repeated. It is used for characterization of disease risk; for example, Alzheimer's disease. It is a diagnostic marker of disease; for example, schizophrenia. It is also possible to predict treatment response and potential for relapse after treatment. New paraclinical tests to support the diagnosis of functional disorders like conversion syndromes are being developed.

Positron Emission Tomography (PET)

Positron-emitting isotopes are generally produced by a cyclotron (Fig. 194.17) (Refer also Section 1, Ch 8).

Atoms from these positron-emitting isotopes are then used to tag molecules of a compound of interest, which are introduced into the human body, usually by intravenous (IV) injection. These labeled compounds are used to trace or probe biological processes and are therefore referred to as biological tracers or probes.

Advantages: PET over other nuclear medicine studies:
- Higher spatial resolution
- Higher signal to noise ratio
- Allows quantitative measurement
- Short half-lives of PET isotopes with high-specific activity permit high quality images and repeated measurements with tolerable radiation exposure to the patient.

SPECT: In this method, radiopharmaceuticals are administered IV or by inhalation to evaluate function in the human brain. These radiopharmaceuticals incorporate isotopes including xenon[133], iodine[123], technesium[99m] and others that emit gamma rays.

Magnetic Resonance Spectroscopy

This is based on chemical composition of the region of interest. N-acetylaspartate peak denotes cellularity, choline peak is indicative of cell membrane myelin and lactate indicates necrosis.

Plain X-rays

X-rays of the spine, skull, myelograms, angiograms, pneumoencephalograms, used to be the delights of the yesteryears, they are still very much in vogue. Skull X-ray should be systematically read, size and shape of cranium, thickness and density of bones, sutures, vascular

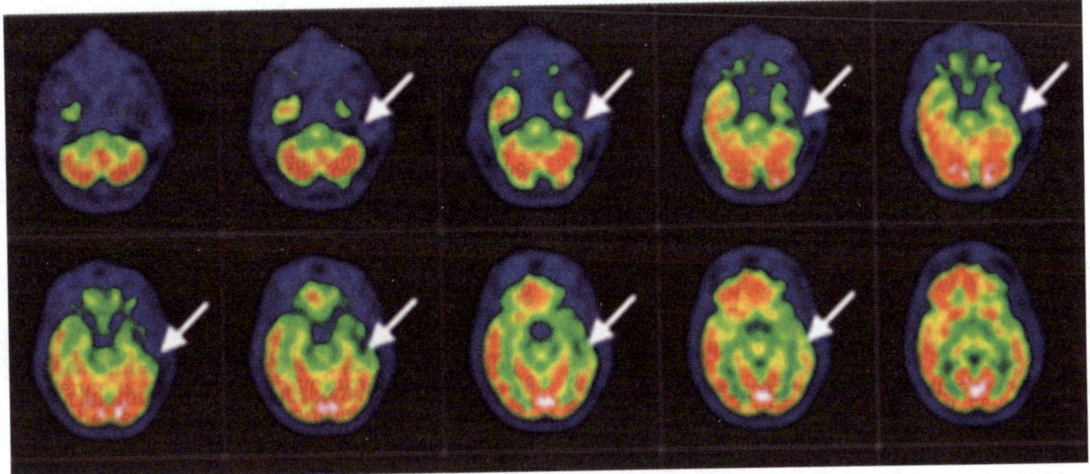

Fig. 194.17: Positron emission tomography images of the brain using F-18 FDG. ***Findings:*** Decreased FDG uptake in both temporal lobes, right worse and left (arrows)

markings, structures along base, sella surface, for normal and abnormal densities, calcifications, convolutional and digital impressions, and parietal foraminal and pacchionian impressions. Morphology is characterized by cephalic index, i.e. breadth/length × 100. Normal is 75–85.
Computerized axial tomography (Refer to Section 1, Ch 8 for description).
Magnetic resonance imaging (Refer Section 1, Ch 8 for description).

CLINICAL LABORATORY INVESTIGATIONS IN NEUROLOGICAL DISORDERS

Clinical investigations aid in the diagnosis of several neurological disorders in which investigations are mandatory.

As physicians, it is good to remember:

- The timing of any investigations is important. For example, creatine phosphokinase (CPK) value after an injection may be misleading; T3 values after exertion can mask minimal hypothyroidism. Before ordering for an investigation, we should have an idea about the physiological role of that particular parameter.
- The mode of collection and transport of samples is vital, as the result is as good as the sample. It is good to get a written policy regarding collection and transport of samples from the referring laboratory.
- No test is 100% infallible even in the best of hands. The quality maintained by the laboratory goes a long way in maintaining the reliability of the results. Always correlate the laboratory results in the background of clinical findings.
- The reference value given in the report may not be the universal normal range. In general, the reference values are 2 standard deviation (SD) from the mean of the population studied. That means there are still normal people in 3 SD and 4 SD zone who have apparently no abnormal values. Several national professional societies have published standard values applicable to their countries (including India).
- In serological investigations (and also in other investigations), sensitivity and specificity play vital role. Sensitivity is the ability of the test to pick up the disease when present and specificity is the ability to exclude a disease when not present. A test which is highly sensitive is usually chosen for screening purposes where we can expect a fair number of false positives and a test which is highly specific will miss out some real positives. A test which is 100% sensitive and specific is everybody's goal which unfortunately is hard to achieve.

- In general, return of an abnormal test to normal indicates recovery from the disease, e.g. blood glucose and hepatic enzymes. But sometimes, abnormal values may return to normal even when the disease process advances, e.g. in Duchene muscular dystrophy, in the final stages of the disease, CPK returns to normal because of total loss of the enzyme source—the muscle fibers.

Apart from general tests indicating the presence of illness nonspecifically, specific tests are of great value in neurological diagnosis. We will see a little more about those tests.

Examination of Cerebrospinal Fluid

Cerebrospinal fluid (CSF), the fluid in which the nervous system swims, to a metaphysicist is the seat of the soul; for a physician, is a simple fluid which gives complex information about a multitude of diseases if handled properly and studied meticulously.

Historical Landmarks

CSF is described in ***Vedas***. Even ancient physicians like Hippocrates and Galen have described about CSF. The modern ideas about CSF are the contribution of Emanuel Swedenborg. Thomas Willis noted that the consistency of the CSF is altered in meningitis. Heinrich Quincke popularized lumbar puncture (LP) for diagnostic and therapeutic purposes. William Mestrezat gave the first accurate description of the chemical composition of the CSF.

CSF for analysis is collected usually by LP, rarely cisternal puncture or even ventricular puncture at times. Other methods of collection include lateral cervical puncture or from surgical shunts and ventricular cannulas. Generally lumbar puncture is also used to measure pressure of CSF.

Indications for Cerebrospinal Fluid Examination

- Neurological infections
- Demyelinating conditions
- Subarachnoid hemorrhage (SAH)
- Malignancies in CNS.

As per American College of Physicians, examination of CSF has: *High sensitivity and specificity in diagnosing bacterial, tuberculous and fungal meningitis,* meaning, CSF examination is a highly dependable investigation for diagnosing as well as excluding the above conditions. *High sensitivity and moderate specificity in diagnosing viral meningitis, SAH, multiple sclerosis, CNS syphilis, infectious polyneuritis and paraspinal abscess, meaning, CSF examination is highly dependable in making a presumptive diagnosis in case of the above diseases. Moderate sensitivity and high specificity in meningeal malignancies,* meaning, CSF examination is highly dependable only confirming but not in ruling out the diseases. *Moderate sensitivity and moderate specificity in intracranial hemorrhage, viral encephalitis and subdural hematoma,* meaning, CSF examination is not so useful if considered in isolation.

Contraindications for LP

Absolute contraindications for LP are the presence of infection over the site of needle entry and the presence of unequal pressures between supratentorial and infratentorial compartments. Relative contraindications for LP are increased intracranial pressure, coagulopathy and brain abscess.

Wherever possible, a full clinical examination is a prerequisite to do a LP. If available, it is better to perform brain CT scanning before lumbar puncture in patients who are older than 60 years with known CNS lesions with focal findings on neurological examination and in patients with papilledema. Cranial CT is a must in patients with suspected SAH in order to diagnose obvious intracranial bleeding or any significant intracranial mass effect that might be present in awake and alert SAH patients with a normal neurological examination.

Procedure of Collection

The procedure should be done in a clean room with all aseptic precautions. Materials required for collection of CSF have been shown in Figures 194.18 and 194.19.

The procedure should be done under sterile conditions after instilling local anesthesia. CSF manometry should be done with the patient kept relaxed before withdrawing CSF.

- Labeled sterile plastic test tubes numbered 1–4 (glass tubes are better avoided as the cells will stick to the glass surface and will give falsely low values).
- ***LP needle (Quincke needle):*** A 22G needle will be good enough. Smaller needle, gradual withdrawal of CSF and minimal amount of withdrawn fluid are associated with less risk of postlumbar puncture headache. Use of the atraumatic Sprotte needle for LP will further reduce the incidence of post LP headaches, but flow rate may be compromised.
- Explain the whole procedure to the patient in detail in comfortable terms.

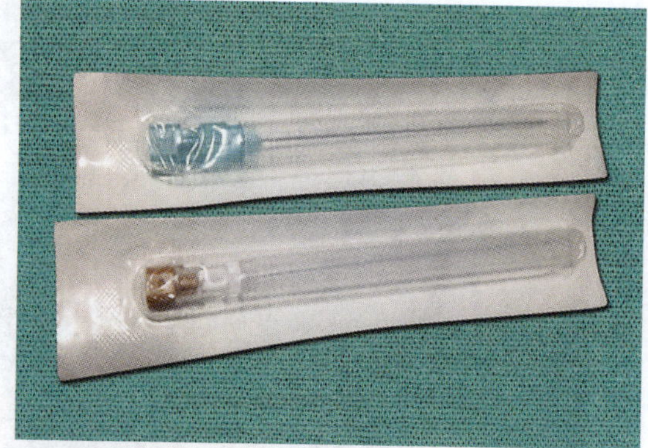

Fig. 194.18: Quincke needle

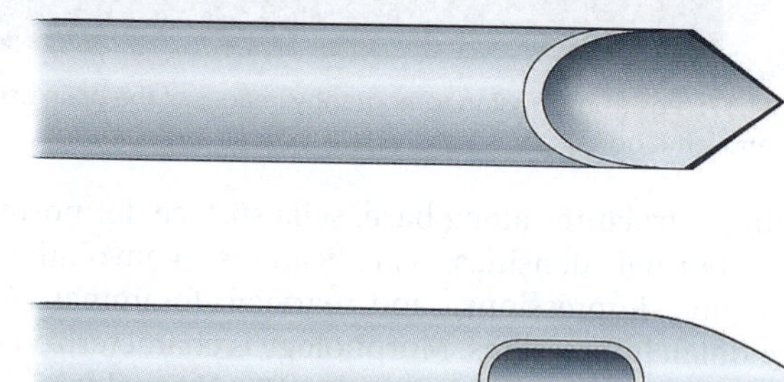

Fig. 194.19: Sprotte needle

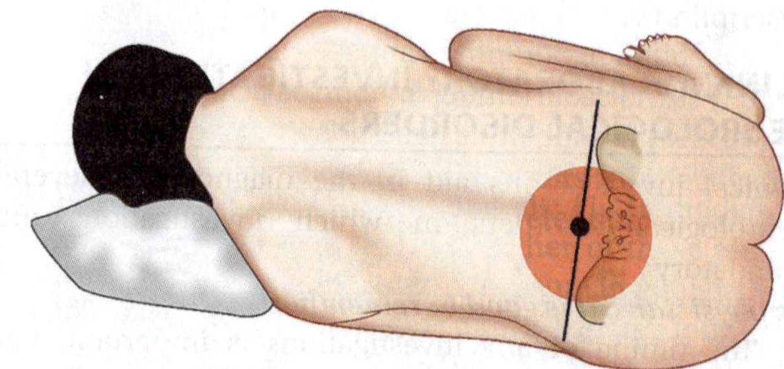

Fig. 194.20: Lateral recumbent position

The patient is placed in the lateral recumbent position with the hips, knees and chin flexed toward the chest so that the interlaminar spaces open to the maximum (Fig. 194.20). The sitting position is helpful in obese patients, but the patient should be leaning forward and be supported in front by a Mayo stand with a pillow on it, by the back of a stool or by another person.

- Look for the widest interspace among L2–3, L3–4 and L4–5. Mark that site as the entry site with a marker.
- Wear sterile gloves. Keep numbered plastic tubes ready for collection of CSF as required. Assemble the stopcock on the manometer.
- Use a sterile drape below the patient and a fenestrated drape on the patient over the site of puncture. Sterilize the site of puncture and administer local anesthetic over two intervertebral spaces so that repetition of anesthetic can be avoided even in case a change of site is required.
- Insert the spinal needle through the skin wheal. The bevel should be parallel to the longitudinal dural fibers so that the needle will separate the fibers rather than cut them, i.e. in the lateral recumbent position,

the bevel should face up, and in the sitting position it should face to one side or the other.

- A characteristic pop may be felt when the needle penetrates the dura. If not, withdraw the stylet after approximately 4–5 cm and observe for fluid return. If no fluid is returned, replace the stylet, advance or withdraw the needle a few millimeters, and recheck for fluid return. Continue this process until fluid comes out freely.
- Attach the manometer to the needle hub through the stopcock and note the height of the fluid column. The patient should be in lateral recumbent position with legs straightened; else a falsely elevated pressure may be noted. Disconnect the manometer.
- Collect at least 10 drops of CSF in each of the four containers, starting with tube one. The CSF that is in the manometer can be transferred to tube one and fresh CSF can be collected in subsequent tubes. If the CSF flow is too slow, ask the patient to cough or bear down (as in the Valsalva maneuver) or press intermittently on the patient's abdomen to increase the flow. Gentle compression of the jugular veins will increase the intracranial tension and this will speed up the flow of CSF this is known as Queckenstedt's test. Samples can be collected in additional tubes if required for repetition of tests.
- Replace the stylet and remove the needle. Apply a sterile dressing and place the patient in the supine position. No bed rest is necessary after the procedure. Fluid administration is neither required nor useful in reducing the incidence of postlumbar primary headache.
- Cisternal and ventricular punctures are better attempted by the anesthetists or neurologists.

Usually 2–5 mL of CSF is collected in most of the cases, even though up to 20 mL of CSF can be removed at a time in the absence of raised intracranial tension (ICT). In the presence of raised ICT, only minimal amount of fluid required for diagnosis should be removed. The specimen should be sent to the laboratory without delay since cells may start degenerating by 1 hour. It is better not to refrigerate the sample since fastidious organisms may die.

The most frequent complication in LP is post LP headache. Most patients present with pain in 3–7 days. Since the pain is postural, it impairs the patient's ability to perform activities of daily living. The incidence of post LP headache with

- 20 G cutting needle—40%
- 25 G cutting needle—5%
- 22 G atraumatic needle—4%.

Smaller atraumatic needle and replacing the stylet before removal of the needle will result in lesser incidence of post LP headache.

Laboratory Examination of Cerebrospinal Fluid and Interpretation of Results (Table 194.8)

Physical

Normal CSF is colorless.

Red color indicates a traumatic tap wherein the first tube is more colored than the subsequent tubes. Frank bleeding

Table 194.8: Normal CSF findings

Appearance: Colorless
pH: 7.4
Lumbar: 7.28–7.32
Cisternal: 7.32–7.34
Glucose: 50–80 mg/dL
Protein: 15–45 mg/dL
WBC: 0–5 in adult and 0–30 in children

Differential count	Adult	Neonates
Lymphocytes	38–96%	2–38%
Monocytes	16–56%	50–94%
Neutrophils	0–7%	0–8%

into the CSF space produces a uniformly red CSF in all the tubes. In case of doubt, presence of D-dimer indicates hemorrhage rather than traumatic tap.

Yellowish color (supernatant): Labeled as xanthochromia indicates red blood cell (RBC) lysis and hemoglobin breakdown products. Xanthochromia occurs when blood is present in CSF for more than 2–48 hours.

White and cloudy: Indicates presence of white blood cells (WBC) (>400 leukocytes/mm^3) or has very high protein content.

Yellow: Protein levels of more than 150 mg/100 mL and jaundice produces a faint yellowish color.

Microscopic examination

Cell count

CSF cell count is done in undiluted CSF using the age-old manual Neubauer counting chamber method. Normally, CSF contains up to 5 cells/mm^3, almost all of which are lymphocytes. In newborns, the reference limits are 0–30 cells/mm^3 with the majority being monocytes.

Differential count using cytocentrifuge (a special centrifuge used to prepare smears automatically from fluids using the principles of centrifugation and sedimentation) preparation if possible is highly useful as a direct smear or centrifuged deposit smear may not yield sufficient cells for accurate assessment.

Any irritation to meninges will lead to proportionate increase in CSF leukocytes, bacterial infections causing the maximal increase. Initially the counts may be normal, but it rapidly increases. Polymorphs predominate in bacterial infections. In viral infections, tuberculosis, listerial infections and tertiary syphilis, lymphocytes predominate. Eosinophils are rare in normal CSF. Increase in eosinophils is of diagnostic importance (Boxes 194.1 to 194.3).

In subarachnoid hemorrhage, initially CSF is clear and becomes xanthochromic in 2–48 hours. WBC count rises slowly to more than 1000/mm^3 because of meningeal irritation and subsequent inflammation due to blood. There is also concomitant increase in proteins. This does not signify infection. Usually by 3 weeks xanthochromia disappears and both protein and cell count return to normal.

In case of intracerebral hemorrhage close to the subarachnoid space, the findings resemble that of SAH. In other cases, the CSF will be relatively normal. Spec-

Box 194.1: Causes of increase in neutrophils

- Bacterial meningitis
- Early tuberculous and fungal meningitis
- Early viral meningoencephalitis
- Cerebral abscess
- CMV radiculopathy-AIDS associated
- Central nervous system infarct

Abbreviations: CMV = Cytomegalovirus; AIDS = Acquired immunodeficiency syndrome

Box 194.2: Causes of increase in lymphocytes

- Viral, tuberculous and fungal meningitis
- Aseptic meningitis
- Parasitic infestations
- Leptospiral meningitis
- Multiple sclerosis
- SSPE (subacute sclerosing panencephalitis)
- Guillain-Barre Syndrome
- Sarcoidosis

Box 194.3: Eosinophils in cerebrospinal fluid

- Parasitic infections especially *Coccidioides immitis*
- Idiopathic eosinophilic meningitis
- Acute polyneuritis

Table 194.9: Cerebrospinal fluid findings in meningitis

Features	Viral	Tuberculous and fungal	Pyogenic
Physical	Clear	Light yellow/viscous	Turbid yellow
Leukocytes	Normal or slightly increased	Moderate increase, mostly lymphocytes	Markedly increased, mostly polymorphs
Glucose	Normal	Normal or slightly decreased	Decreased markedly
Protein	Slightly increased or normal	Slightly increased	Increased

Box 194.4: Increase in cerebrospinal fluid (CSF) protein

- Bacterial, viral, fungal and tuberculous meningitis
- Hemorrhage
- Hypercalcemia
- Hypothyroidism
- Uremia
- Multiple sclerosis
- Guillain-Barre syndrome
- Collagen vascular disorders
- Mechanical obstruction to CSF Flow

trophotometry of the CSF for hemoglobin breakdown products, oxyhemoglobin and bilirubin are more reliable to confirm SAH than xanthochromia.

Examination of CSF in suspected cases of CNS metastasis is highly specific but lacks sensitivity. The highest yield of malignant cells is seen in leukemic infiltrates. Nevertheless, looking for malignant cells, preparation especially with cytospin is a rewarding exercise in all cases with a remote suspicion of metastatic deposit.

Chemical analysis

Glucose

CSF glucose values are about 60% of the plasma glucose values in normal adult subjects. In newborns, the usual CSF level is about 80% of the serum glucose level. It takes between 0.5 and 2 hours for maximum change to occur in CSF values after a change in serum values.

Reference values are 45 mg/100 mL or higher. Values of 40–45 mg/100 mL are equivocal, although in normal persons it is rare to find values below 45 mg/100 mL.

The most important and common change in the CSF glucose level is a decrease. The classic etiologies for CSF glucose decrease are meningitis due to bacteria, tuberculosis and fungi; the former being responsible for the maximum decrease. The decrease in glucose is because of consumption by leukocytes rather than by the bacteria which are usually low in number to account for the decrease. Occasionally in very early infection, the initial CSF glucose value may be normal, although later it begins to decrease. Studies have shown that only 60–80% of children and 50–90% of adults with acute bacterial meningitis have CSF glucose levels below the reference range. Hyperglycemia may mask a decrease in CSF values and so, concomitant measurement of blood glucose may be helpful. In the same lines, decrease in glucose may also be due to hypoglycemia (Table 194.9).

Protein

The normal adult CSF protein concentration is 15–45 mg/100 mL. In infants up to day 30, it is 75–150 mg/100 mL, 30–90 days, it is 20–100 mg/100 mL. The adult value is reached by the sixth month. After 60 years of age, upper limit increases to 60 mg/100 mL. Increased protein concentration usually parallels the degree of leukocytosis (Box 194.4). Increase in protein occurs due to:

- Leakage from blood brain barrier as in inflammation and hemorrhage
- Increase in intrathecal immunoglobulin (Ig) synthesis
- Due to mechanical obstruction to flow.

Decrease in CSF protein occurs due to increased CSF turnover, as in excess removal of CSF, CSF leakage due to head injury, hyperthyroidism and in case of increased intracranial tension.

An increase in proteins without increase in cells is known as albuminocytologic dissociation. Minor degrees of this dissociation is seen in many conditions like cerebral trauma, brain or spinal cord tumor, brain abscess, cerebral infarct or hemorrhage, sarcoidosis, systemic lupus erythematosus (SLE), lead encephalopathy, uremia, myxedema, multiple sclerosis and chronic CNS infections.

A marked degree of albuminocytologic dissociation is seen in Guillain-Barre syndrome (GBS) and temporal arteritis.

High-resolution agarose gel electrophoresis of CSF shows one or more discrete population of IgG known as the oligoclonal bands. More than one oligoclonal band is seen in multiple sclerosis in more than 80% of cases. It is also seen in SSPE, CNS infections, GBS, meningeal carcinomatosis, etc. Immunofixation electrophoresis picks up these bands more easily.

Cerebrospinal fluid—source of biomarkers in neurodegenerative disorders

The CSF is also a key source in the research for novel molecular biomarkers of neurodegenerative disorders.

Table 194.10: Different proteins in cerebrospinal fluid (CSF)

Protein	Disease
α_2 macroglobulin	Subdural hemorrhage, bacterial meningitis
β amyloid and τ protein*	Alzheimer's disease
β_2 microglobulin	Leukemia/lymphoma
C-reactive protein (CRP)	Bacterial/viral meningitis
Myelin basic protein	Multiple sclerosis
β_2 transferrin	To confirm CSF rhinorrhea

Note: *-τ protein also known as tau proteins. Tau proteins are proteins that stabilize microtubules. They are abundant in neurons of the central nervous system.

CSF is a rich source of neurosecreted biosynthesized and metabolized molecular products of the CNS. Advanced electrophoretic methods can differentiate various protein subunits which are specific for various diseases. More than 300 different proteins have been identified in CSF using two-dimensional electrophoresis. Some of the CSF proteins and their clinical importance listed in Table 194.10.

Culture

The exact diagnosis of bacterial meningitis requires culture to isolate the organism and also to determine the antibiotic sensitivity. Centrifuged spinal fluid sediment should be examined with Gram stain, so that the organisms can be seen, if present in sufficient amounts. If organisms are identified, depending upon the antibiotic policy, appropriate antibiotics can be started even before the culture results are ready. If there is a clinical suspicion of a specific type of organism, the same should be conveyed to the laboratory so that special media if required can be used. Previous or concurrent antibiotic therapy is reported to decrease culture detection rates by about 30%. As far as possible, do not start antibiotics before drawing CSF, except under emergencies like bacterial meningitis.

- *Latex agglutination tests* for different bacterial antigens are available. The tests are useful as a screening procedure.
- *Polymerase chain reaction (PCR)* analysis for various viruses is a highly specific test in the diagnosis of viral infections. Though costly, it is readily available and the results justify the cost.
- *CSF lactate is elevated* in acute bacterial, tuberculous and fungal meningitis. This can be used as a surrogate marker for infections. Hemorrhage and infarcts in brain and tumor necrosis may also raise lactate levels.
- *Vascular endothelial growth factor* is found elevated compared to serum in leptomeningeal malignancies. *Mass spectrometry-based quantitative proteomics* has emerged as a powerful approach for biomarker discovery, both for diagnostic as well as therapeutic purposes. Proteomics has traditionally been synonymous with 2D gels but is increasingly shifting to the use of gel-free systems and liquid chromatography coupled with tandem mass spectrometry (LC-MS/MS). Quantitative proteomic approaches have already been applied to investigate various neurological disorders, especially in the context of identifying biomarkers from CSF. They have been found useful in multiple sclerosis, motor neuron disease (MND), neoplasms and others.

Recently microwave analysis of CSF has been suggested as a useful procedure, but this has not come into routine practice. Application in clinical laboratory practices may take sometime.

MUSCLE BIOPSY AND OTHER TESTS FOR MUSCLE DISEASES

Muscles which give shape, strength and beauty to the body have always fascinated the neuropathologists because reading muscle biopsy is an interesting intellectual exercise as well as a rewarding experience in terms of contribution to the patient's positive outcome. Muscle biopsy, unlike other laboratory investigations, is a specialized procedure done only in selected laboratories, so most of the time the sample has to be shipped over long distances.

We briefly review the importance, procedure and key diagnostic findings in muscle biopsy. Muscle biopsy should be done only after full neurological examination and preliminary laboratory investigations. Since several muscle disorders can be diagnosed by genetic testing, muscle biopsy is required only in selected conditions. Site for muscle biopsy is determined by clinical assessment and aided electrodiagnostic studies in some cases.

Muscles with advanced disease and severe weakness may reveal only end-stage changes which may be similar in both myopathic and neurogenic atrophy, so they are better avoided. In chronic diseases, moderately affected muscles are selected for biopsy and in acute conditions, muscles with severe or moderate weakness are selected. Muscles subjected to any type of trauma should be avoided. If the symptoms are intermittent, biopsy is preferred during the active phase.

Usually biceps, deltoid, quadriceps (vastus lateralis) is selected for biopsy. In patchy disorders with widespread involvement, multiple biopsies may be needed.

Indications for Muscle Biopsy

- Common indication for muscle biopsy is to differentiate between myopathy and neuropathy.
- Symptomatic muscle diseases weakness, cramps, easy fatigability, and elevated creatine kinase. Though the classic presentation of myopathy and neuropathy is different, their clinical signs and symptoms may overlap and both conditions may also co-exist at times. Muscle biopsy can be performed by an open technique or by percutaneous needle biopsy.

Open Biopsy

This provides a bigger specimen and the muscle can be easily preserved in the noncontracted state by using either a special *Rayport clamp* or a simple wooden ice-cream stick.

Local anesthesia is induced by the anesthetic drug (without epinephrine) and avoiding direct infiltration into the muscle. Use of electrocautery should be avoided. Obtain two intact pieces of muscle approximately 1–2 cm in length and 0.5–0.8 cm thick. One specimen can be fixed in formalin and the other snap frozen in liquid nitrogen. If that is not possible, the tissue can be wrapped in saline moistened gauze and transported in a sealed container with dry ice. The tissue should not be immersed in sodium chloride as it will lead to formation of ice crystals. If required, an additional bit can be preserved in glutaraldehyde for electron microscopy (ultrastructural analysis of muscle biopsy reveals many abnormalities but it is still not a day-to-day practice in myology). In suspected metabolic myopathies, an additional piece of muscle can be frozen and preserved for biochemical assessment. Isometric muscle clamps are usually not needed and should be avoided in pediatric patient.

Percutaneous Biopsy

It can be done either by a needle or a conchotome. The percutaneous needle biopsy has the advantage of leaving a smaller scar and can be repeated if necessary for follow-up studies. But the specimen is small and orientation of the fibers for processing in the microtome may be difficult.

Needle Biopsy

It is performed using a Liverpool muscle biopsy needle (Fig. 194.21).

With all aseptic precautions under local anesthesia, the skin is pierced with a needle or passed through a skin incision. The needle is passed through the fascia up to the muscle with the aperture in the closed position. On entering the muscle, the aperture is opened by withdrawing the inner tube and it is then closed. The sample that is trapped in the barrel is taken for biopsy. Three or four samples can be obtained with a single penetration.

Conchotome Biopsy

Conchotome, an instrument used primarily in nasal surgeries, is also used for muscle biopsy. Under local anesthesia, a 5 mm skin incision is made. The conchotome is introduced through the incision with the jaws closed. When the muscle is entered the jaws are opened and the conchotome is advanced to 2–3 mm. The jaws are closed, twisted to 180 degrees and withdrawn. The procedure could be repeated three or four times.

The tissues are processed as for open biopsy. Some centers prefer percutaneous biopsy to open biopsy.

Basic Histology and Salient Diagnostic Findings in Muscle Biopsy

Histology

Basically, there are two types of muscle fibers, type 1 slow twitch fibers and type 2 fast twitch fibers. Type

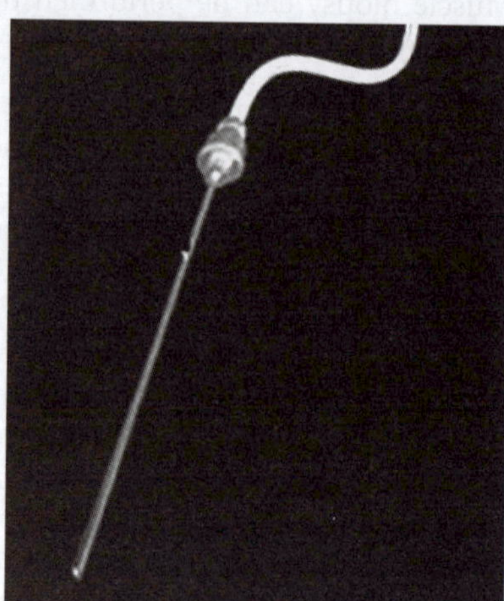

Fig. 194.21: Liverpool muscle biopsy needle

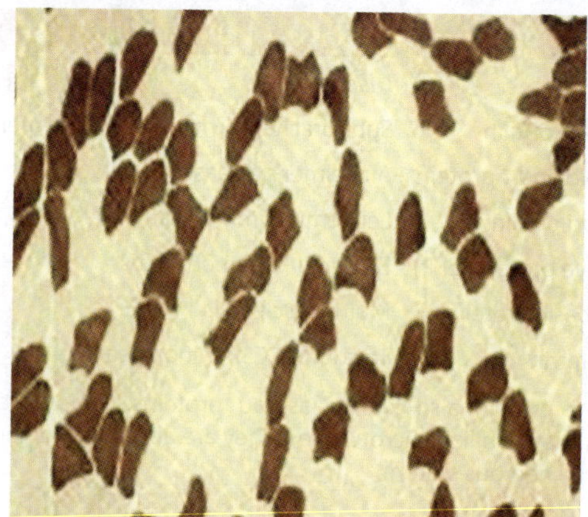

Fig. 194.22: Myosin ATPase at 10.5–type II fibers (4.3 for type I and 4.6 for types I and IIB)

1 fibers utilize aerobic pathways and type 2 fibers utilize anaerobic pathways for their energy needs. These two types of myofibers have their characteristic distribution in different muscles in a checkerboard fashion (Fig. 194.22). The checkerboard type of distribution is brought out nicely by enzyme histochemistry, though it can be visualized to some extent in routine stains.

In hematoxylin and eosin (H&E) stained sections, the muscle fibers show myofibers—the muscle cell surrounded by endomysium (connective tissue) bundled into fascicles which are in turn surrounded by perimysium (connective tissue). The muscle in turn is composed of fascicles and is covered by the epimysium (connective tissue) which extends into the tendon. The myofibers are of uniform size and shape and fit together in a mosaic pattern. The nuclei are placed at the periphery with less than 3% of the myofibers showing an internal nucleus. The cross striations can be easily visualized in H&E (Fig. 194.23).

Unlike other biopsies, muscle biopsy requires a battery of stains in the frozen sample like myosin ATPase, nicotinamide adenine dinucleotide dehydrogenase (NADH), periodic acid-schiff (PAS), Gomori's trichrome and Sudan black in addition to the routine H&E stain in the formalin fixed sample. Immunohistochemistry may be necessary especially for dystrophins in muscular dystrophy (Figs 194.24 and 194.25).

Pathological Findings

The different types of myofibers are differentially affected in various disease processes. Neuromuscular diseases presenting with weakness may have their pathology in the spinal cord, peripheral nerves or muscle fibers.

Important findings in myopathy are myofiber necrosis, myophagocytosis, rounded and atrophic fibers, myofiber atrophy and splitting, increase in internal nuclei, nuclear chain formation, endomysial thickening and others brought out by H&E and Gomori's trichrome stain (Figs 194.26 to 194.29).

- In parasitic diseases, such as cysticercosis and trichinosis, the parasites can be demonstrated by routine H&E stains.
- Immunohistochemistry for dystrophin shows decrease or absence of dystrophin in dystrophinopathies and there is increased expression of utrophin.

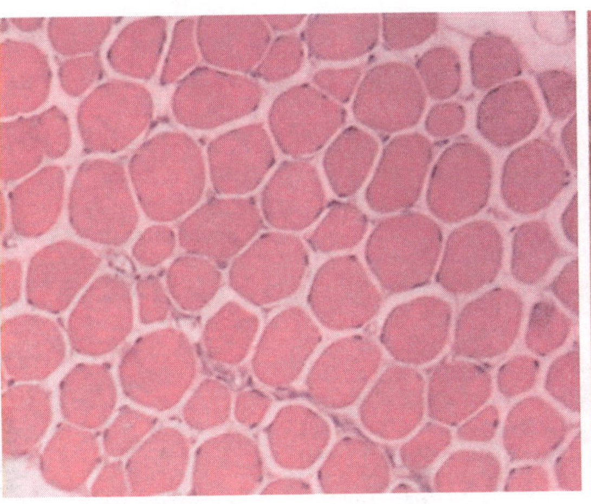
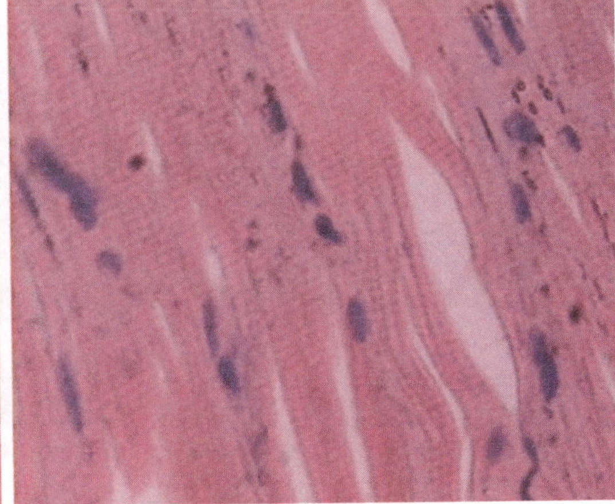

Fig. 194.23: Normal muscle hematoxylin and eosin (H&E)

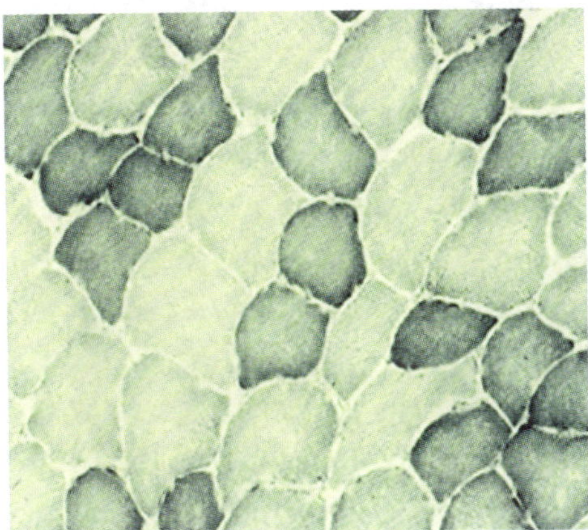

Fig. 194.24: Nicotinamide adenine dinucleotide-tetrazolium reductase (NADH-TR)—normal

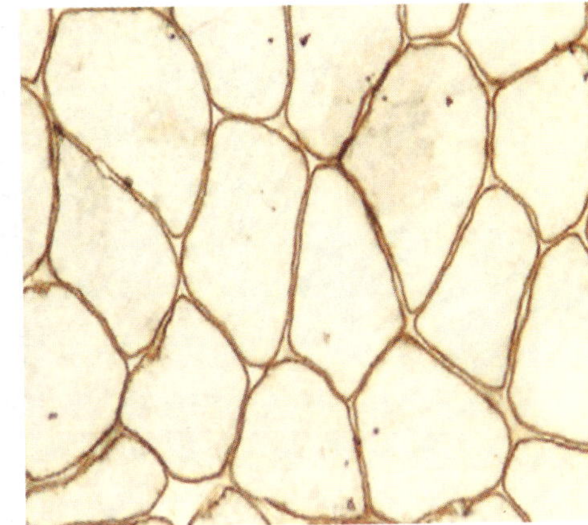

Fig. 194.25: Normal dystrophin—immunohistochemistry

- Immunofluorescence can demonstrate deposition of Igs in vasculitis.
- Storage disorders show vacuoles in the cytoplasm which can be characterized by histochemical stains and other biochemical investigations.

In neuropathy, there is evidence of atrophy of neurofibers in the form of angulated fibers. Because of regeneration of the myofibers by the adjacent viable nerve twig, there is fiber type grouping wherein a single type of myofibers are grouped together with loss of the normal checkerboard pattern clearly shown by histochemical stains (Figs 194.30 and 194.31).

Muscle biopsy studies have reached a high degree of development and are a subspeciality in myology. Further detailed information has to be obtained from monographs on the subject. No single finding is diagnostic of several muscle disorders. The constellation of findings including clinical presentation and specific laboratory findings can give accurate diagnosis.

Nerve Biopsy

Nerve biopsy can identify a variety of diseases like neuropathies, vasculitic disorders, granulomatous diseases-infective and noninfective, amyloidosis and others. However, nerve biopsy is recommended only when there is a progressive disorder of the nerve. Nerve biopsy is not recommended just to confirm the presence of neuropathy. In suspected vasculitic neuropathy, biopsy is the primary method of diagnosis. Combined muscle and nerve biopsy improves the accuracy. Nerve biopsy can be helpful in the diagnosis of chronic inflammatory demyelinating polyneuropathy (CIDP) in which the presence of inflammatory cells in the nerve fibers confirms the diagnosis.

Site of Biopsy

In cases where lower limbs are affected, the superficial peroneal nerve or the sural nerve is taken for biopsy. If only the upper limb is affected, superficial radial nerve or ulnar nerve or a branch of ulnar nerve in the dorsum of the hand can be biopsied.

Procedure for Sural Nerve Biopsy

The lesser saphenous vein runs lateral to the sural nerve. A short segment of the nerve is cut after infiltrating the proximal end of the nerve with local anesthetic. Wrap the biopsy in sterile gauze soaked in normal saline. About one-fourth of the excised nerve tissue is placed in 10% formalin, the second quarter is placed in isotonic glutaraldehyde fixative, the third quarter is fixed in special solution for RNA studies and the fourth piece is kept in Michel's medium and preserved in liquid nitrogen. It is better to perform nerve biopsy only if facilities for examining teased fiber and electron microscopic studies are available.

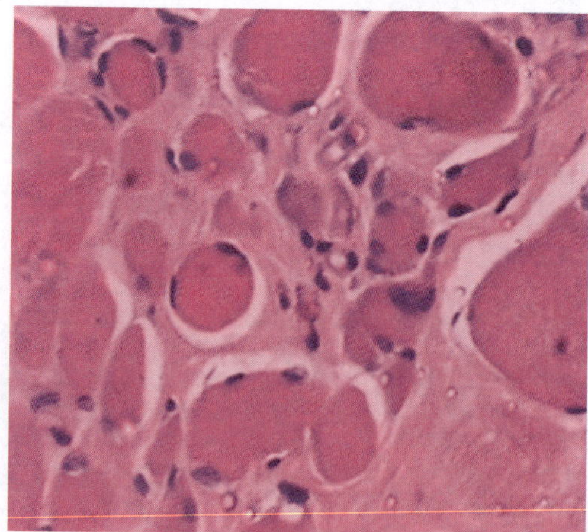

Fig. 194.26: Rounded and atrophic fibers—H&E

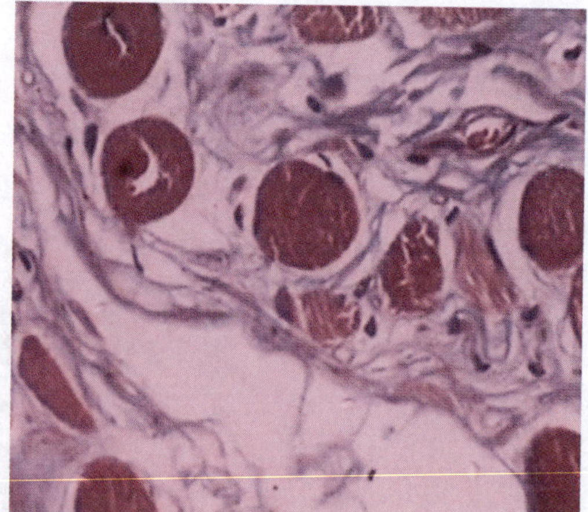

Fig. 194.27: Endomysial fibrosis—Gomori

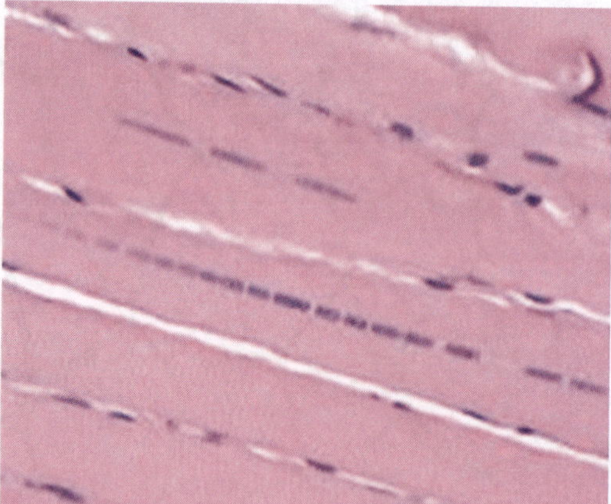

Fig. 194.28: Moth-eaten fibers and ring fibers are seen with NADH stain in myopathy

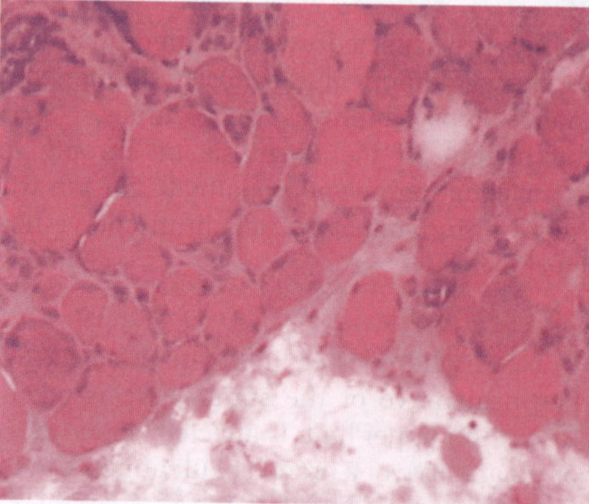

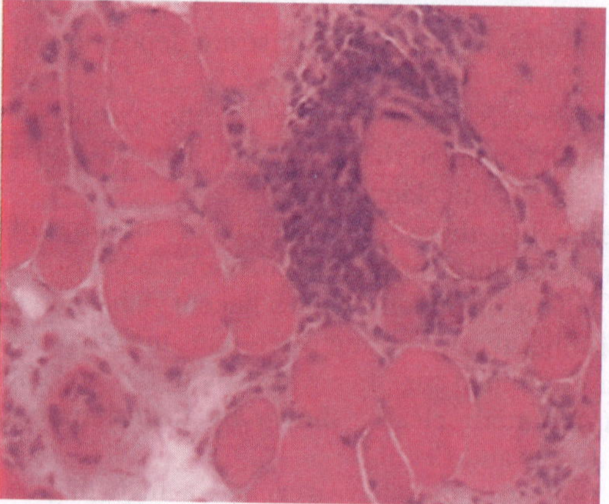

Fig. 194.29: Inflammatory myopathies show perifascicular atrophy (left) and lymphocytic infiltration (right)

Light microscopic examination of the formalin-fixed paraffin-embedded tissue is useful in diagnosing vasculitis, granulomatous disorders, amyloidosis and lymphoma. Semi-thin plastic embedded sections of nerve in glutaraldehyde fixed bits are useful for analysis of myelinated fibers in assessing demyelinating disorders.

Acute primary demyelination exhibits axons lacking myelin sheath surrounded by myelin debris-containing macrophages. This is followed by formation of concentric rings of myelin fibers known as onion bulbs (Fig. 194.32), demonstrable in transverse sections because of segmental remyelination. Demyelination, segmental remyelination and axonal changes can be better demonstrated in teased fiber preparations.

In contrast to muscle biopsy, nerve biopsy can have potential complications like pain, paresthesia for a prolonged period, neuroma formation and mild dysesthetic symptoms.

Of late, skin biopsy for examination of peripheral nerves (small fiber neuropathy) is gaining importance. The procedure is simple. It involves punch biopsy of the skin taken at standard size and sections are stained with varieties of immunostains (Figs 194.33 and 194.34).

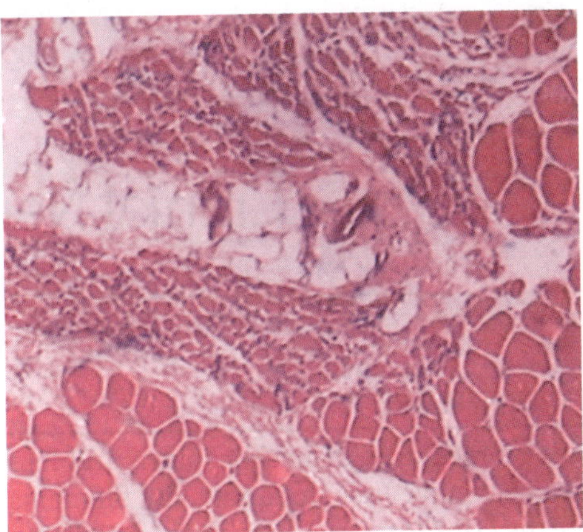

Fig. 194.30: Grouped atrophy

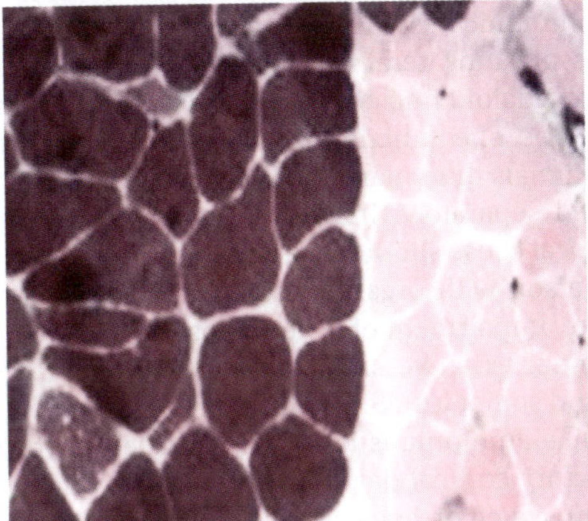

Fig. 194.31: Fiber type grouping—ATPase at 4.5 pH

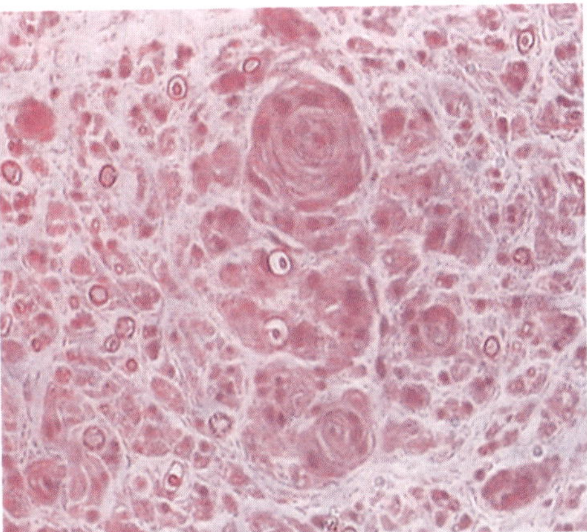

Fig. 194.32: Onion bulb formation

Two standardized techniques for morphometric analysis of nerve fibers are available:

1. Epidermal nerve fiber density (ENFD) test which measures the density of the small sensory nerve fibers in the skin.
2. Sweat gland nerve fiber density (SGFD) test which measures the density of the small autonomous nerve fibers in the sweat glands. Small fiber atrophy can be quantified and followed up in subsequent biopsies. The advantages of this technique are that the procedure is simple and that it can be repeated at regular intervals to assess the progress of the small fiber neuropathy.

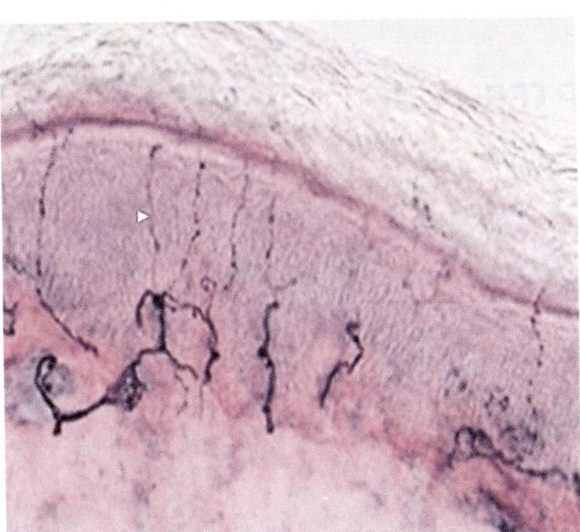

Fig. 194.33: Normal skin—immunostains

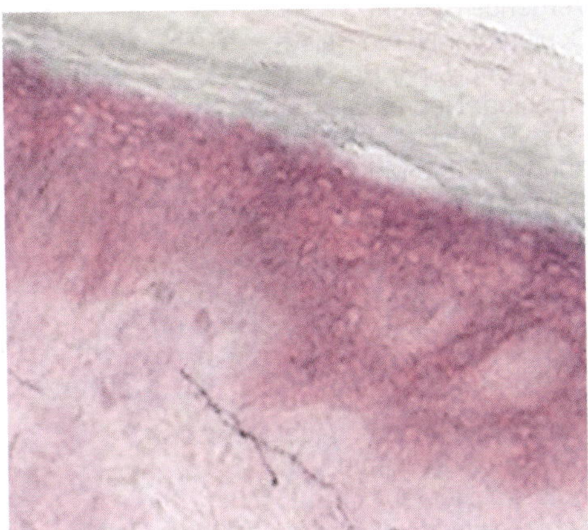

Fig. 194.34: Small fiber neuropathy

This has been shown to be useful in the early diagnosis of diabetic neuropathies.

Brain Biopsy

Stereotactic CT-guided or MRI-guided brain biopsy is used to diagnose neurodegenerative disorders, tumors, infections and inflammations. The risks associated with stereotactic brain biopsies are minimal except that the same may be inadequate at times. A small bit of lesional tissue is taken and is subjected to variety of examinations like routine histopathology with special stains for inclusions (of abnormal proteins), electron microscopic examination, biochemical analysis, culture, demonstration of viral genetic material using PCR techniques and *in-situ* hybridization techniques for viral genomes and genetic alterations, as the case may warrant. However, brain biopsy is not yet popular method of investigation except for diagnosis of tumors.

Recent Advances

Recent advances in genomics and proteomics has opened up a wild field of investigation based on mass spectrometry for the diagnosis of early biomarkers in neurodegenerative disorders. CSF and serum samples are used for the early and noninvasive diagnosis of CNS tumors, infections of CNS, neurodegenerative disorder and certain psychosis. They are also used for monitoring the progress of the disease. This particular branch of investigation modality may change the face of laboratory science in relation to CNS disorders in the near future.

CHAPTER

195

Cranial Nerves

SR Chandra, Karru Venkata Ravi Teja

Chapter Summary

- Olfactory Nerve
- Optic Nerves
- Oculomotor, Trochlear and Abducent (Abducens) Nerves and Eye Movement Control
  - Saccadic System
  - Vergence System
  - Oculomotor Nerve Palsy
  - Abducent Nerve Palsy
  - Trochlear Nerve Palsy
  - Gaze Paralysis
  - Abnormal Eye Movements
- Trigeminal Nerve
  - Trigeminal Neuralgia
- Facial Nerve
  - Bell's Palsy
- Vestibulocochlear Nerve
  - Vertigo
  - Ménière's Syndrome
- Glossopharyngeal and Vagal Nerves
- Spinal Accessory Nerve
- Hypoglossal Nerve
- General Points in Lower Cranial Nerve Palsies

INTRODUCTION

There are twelve pairs of cranial nerves of which, first two belongs to central nervous system (CNS), and rest belongs to peripheral nervous system (PNS). The first two cranial nerves become affected very early in several neurodegenerative diseases like Alzheimer's disease and serve as biomarkers for early diagnosis. The others help in localization of the site of disease and also the cause. We will deal with the key points which will help us in diagnosis as detailed discussion of all diseases it is beyond the scope of this chapter.

Questions to be asked:

- Is the symptom organic or functional?
- If organic, non-neurological or neurological?
- If neurological, the involvement at
  - Supranuclear
  - Nuclear
  - Intra-axial fascicular
  - Cisternal
  - Skull base
  - Foraminal
  - Soft tissue plane?
- What could be the cause and how to treat?

Note: Detailed description of all neural structures and the physical testing and investigations is given in 'Clinical Medicine', 4th edition edited by KV Krishna Das and others, published by Jaypee Brothers Medical Publishers which forms the companion volume for the Textbook of Medicine, hence these are not repeated here.

OLFACTORY NERVE

The olfactory receptors of nasal septum and lateral wall of nasal cavity give rise to about 20 filaments which penetrate the cribriform plate and enter the olfactory bulb, then course posteriorly as tract, divides into medial and lateral stria with olfactory trigone in between. The medial stria communicates with opposite side through anterior commissure and lateral stria to piriform cortex of temporal lobe, amygdaloid nucleus, septal area and hypothalamus. Olfaction is one function which is more developed in lower animals than man. While testing, each nose should be tested separately. Irritant substances should not be used. Local cause should be excluded.

A person with organic loss of smell loses flavor and therefore, impairment of taste is most often the complaint than smell. Irritative smell is carried out by trigeminal nerve and so not lost. Sneezing is preserved when irritant smells like ammonia is used. Supranuclear involvement, i.e. olfactory cortical pathology presents as olfactory aura of seizure which presents as episodes of stereotyped smell perceived for seconds. Thalamic and prefrontal lesions produce olfactory discrimination defect, i.e. patient will know some smell is there, but what it is, he will not know. *Parosmia* or perversion of smell, i.e. altered perception of smell and *cacosmia*, i.e. perceiving bad smell are seen after head injury and psychiatric illness. Neurodegenerative diseases like Parkinson's, Alzheimer's, ataxias, Refsum's syndrome, olfactogonadal dysgenesis like Kallmann's syndrome, Turner's syndrome and familial dysautonomias show defects in identification called **hyposmia** or loss of smell appreciation called **anosmia**. However, most common causes of bilateral loss of smell are local causes like head injury and local procedures. Olfactory groove meningioma cause optic atrophy and anosmia (loss of smell) on same side and papilledema on opposite side (***Foster Kennedy syndrome***).

Nasopharyngeal tumor producing anosmia with paralysis of trigeminal and oculomotor nerve is called as ***Jacobson's triad***. Tumors of frontal bone, sphenoidal wing, sella turcica aneurysm of anterior part of circle of Willis, esthesioneuroblastomas arising from nasal cavity are surgical conditions associated with anosmia. Zinc and vitamin A deficiency, Addison's disease, hypothyroidism, pseudohypoparathyroidism, sarcoidosis and cystic fibrosis are other medical conditions with loss of smell.

OPTIC NERVES

Rods and cones are located deep in retina, they react to visible light and are oriented to the pupils. Rods contain rhodopsin which reacts to light at 400–800 nm. They are not seen in optic disk and macula. Cones are of three types, each reacting maximally to red, green or blue. Fovea of macula is rich in cones, they convey information to ganglion cells—the M cells are concerned with stereopsis and project to magnocellular region of lateral geniculate body, P cells are more peripheral and deal with what is being seen.

Optic Nerve and Chiasm

The optic nerve is 5 cm long with intraocular, intraorbital, intracanalicular and intracranial parts. In the optic chiasm, the nasal fibers cross to opposite side and temporal fibers do not. The fibers from the inferior retina make a forward loop into the opposite optic nerve, and superior retina loop into ipsilateral optic tract and this is called as **Wilbrand's knee.** Because of this arrangement, patients can develop blindness in one eye and upper temporal field defect in opposite eye in pituitary adenomas. Understanding this loop is very important as a patient with this junctional scotoma due to a sellar mass can be mistaken as ipsilateral optic neuritis if we fail to look for the upper temporal field defect on the opposite side. Macular fibers form a chiasm (meaning = crossing) within the optic chiasma. Chiasm is prefixed or lies over anterior margin of sella in 5%, over diaphragm sella in 12%, above dorsum sella in 79% and behind dorsum sella or post-fixed in 4% which will decide the pattern of field defect a sellar lesion can produce. The classical bitemporal hemianopia which is a conventionally expected defect, is seen if the chiasm is suprasellar and compresses the nasal fibers which represent the temporal field.

Optic Tract and Lateral Geniculate Bodies

Optic tract is the part from dorsolateral chiasm to geniculate body. Lateral geniculate body is in the perimesencephalic cistern. Optic radiations sweep around the posterior part of lateral ventricle and form the external sagittal striatum. There are three bundles, upper one corresponding upper retina, central one macula, lower one retina. The lower one sweeps around temporal horn of lateral ventricle as **Meyer's loop**, the upper retinal fibers have an anterior extension to deep parietal lobe. Visual cortex is made up of Brodmann area 17 situated along superior and inferior lip of calcarine fissure.

Common problems in visual pathway disorders
• Acuity
• Field
• Color
• Pupil/fundus/eye movements
• Perceptual interaction.

Vision is a multidimensional function and acuity measures the ability of eye for spatial resolution of images.

It is important as it affords evaluation of optics of the eye which in many cases is correctable. It can be assessed by (1) high contrast Snellen's chart, (2) variable contrast, (3) color visual acuity, (4) stereoacuity, (5) Rosenbaum's cards (Fig. 195.1), (6) pinhole test, (7) photostress test and (8) Pulfrich phenomenon.

Pulfrich Phenomena

A small target oscillating in the frontal planes is viewed binocularly. When one eye is weakly stimulated due to

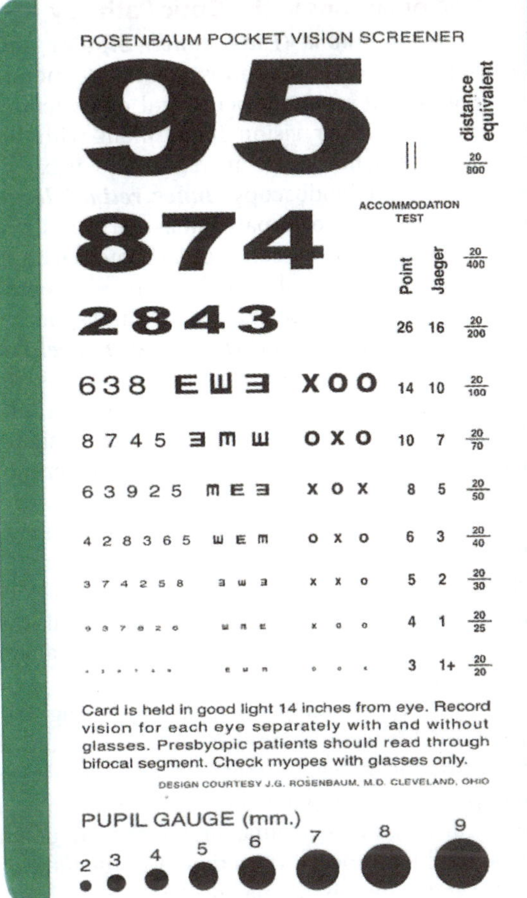

Fig. 195.1: Rosenbaum's pocket vision screener

optic nerve pathology, the delay in transmission makes it appear elliptic. Simple bedside test of optic nerve pathology.

Photostress Test

Visual acuity is assessed at base line. Then a powerful light is put on the eye so that patient becomes transiently blind. The time taken to recover the original acuity is less than 60 seconds, if the retina and macula are normal. This is a simple mandatory bedside test for all people who drive automobiles.

Visual Field

This is the sum total of objects perceived when the eye is fixed, and measures the extrafoveal retinal receptors and their intracranial projections. Visual field is tested as follows:

- **Confrontation method:** Goldmann perimetry
- Tangent screen
- Newer test—short wavelength automated test, etc.

The type of defect produced depends on the site of pathology in the visual pathway. For convenience, it can be grouped into those due to nerve bundle type which is anterior to optic tract, and non-nerve bundle type which is posterior. A scotoma is a blind area in the visual field. It is called positive, if it is perceived by the patient, called negative if detected during examination. Positive scotomas are commonly seen in retinal disease and negative in occipital lobe disease.

Textbook of Medicine

Localization of Lesions in the Optic Pathway

- ***Outer retinal lesions (rods, cones, bipolar cells):*** The most common condition is retinitis pigmentosa. It produces ring scotoma, peripheral constriction of field of vision, color vision impairment with bone corpuscle pigment change in retina and waxy pale disk evident on funduscopy. ***Inner retinal lesions***, e.g. those which involve papillomacular bundle and arcuate fibers causes of centrocecal scotoma, central scotoma, severe loss of visual acuity and arcuate defects with wedge shape attached to blind spot.
- ***Lesions at the chiasm (von Willebrand knee related):*** As lower nasal fibers from opposite side cross into ipsilateral optic nerve as we have seen earlier in this chapter, the patient presents with ipsilateral optic nerve type and contralateral upper temporal quadrantanopia. This binding is very important, as it localizes the lesion to a compressive pathology in sella. It can be mistaken as optic nerve demyelination. The upper nasal fibers loop into the ipsilateral optic tract before crossing, and can cause ipsilateral lower temporal field defect in addition to contralateral homonymous hemianopia.

  Bitemporal hemianopia occurs involving both temporal fields when there is a sellar tumor and the chiasm just above that. Binasal field defect is seen due to compression of temporal fibers due to atheromatous carotid artery, in glaucoma, and rarely in arsenic poisoning due to special vulnerability of the temporal fibers. Central hemiscotoma involving central fields alone occurs in central macular fibers involvement, mostly demyelinating disorders.
- ***Lateral geniculate body:*** Unique homonymous hemianopia sparing a horizontal sector or horizontal sector defects without hemianopia.
- ***Temporal lobe:*** Peripheral contralateral superior quadrantanopia (***pie in the sky***).

Table 195.1: Differences between hemianopia produced by optic tract lesions versus occipital lobe lesions

Optic tract	Occipital lobe
Incongruous	Congruous
Macular splitting	Macular sparing
Wernicke's hemianopic pupillary reaction absent	Present
Optic atrophy can be seen late due to retrograde trans-synaptic	Fundus changes do not occur as trans-synaptic
Wallerian degeneration	Wallerian degeneration does not occur

Note: Wernicke's hemianopic pupillary reaction is the phenomenon where light reflex is elicitable from the blind visual field.

- ***Parietal lobe:*** Contralateral inferior homonymous quadrantanopia (***pie in the floor***).
- ***Occipital lobe:*** Congruous contralateral homonymous hemianopia with macular sparing where macular vision is not affected. In lesions of ***optic tract***, macular vision also gets affected in half called ***macular splitting*** (Table 195.1 and Fig. 195.2).

Color Vision

Wavelength of human color range is from 400 (violet) to 700 (red) nm. Red-green defect incidence is 8% in male children. Testing is done with standardized light source and results are obtained after best refractory correction if present. Test at arm length, one eye at a time. ***Ishihara pseudoisochromatic plate, Holmgren's wool, Farnsworth-Munsell 100-hue test,*** contrast sensitivity test are commonly used methods.

Köllner's rule: This helps to identify the site of lesion.

- In patients with congenital color vision defect, discrimination between red and green is affected
- In acquired color blindness like toxic, diabetic and HIV-related situation, purple and blue-green are most affected

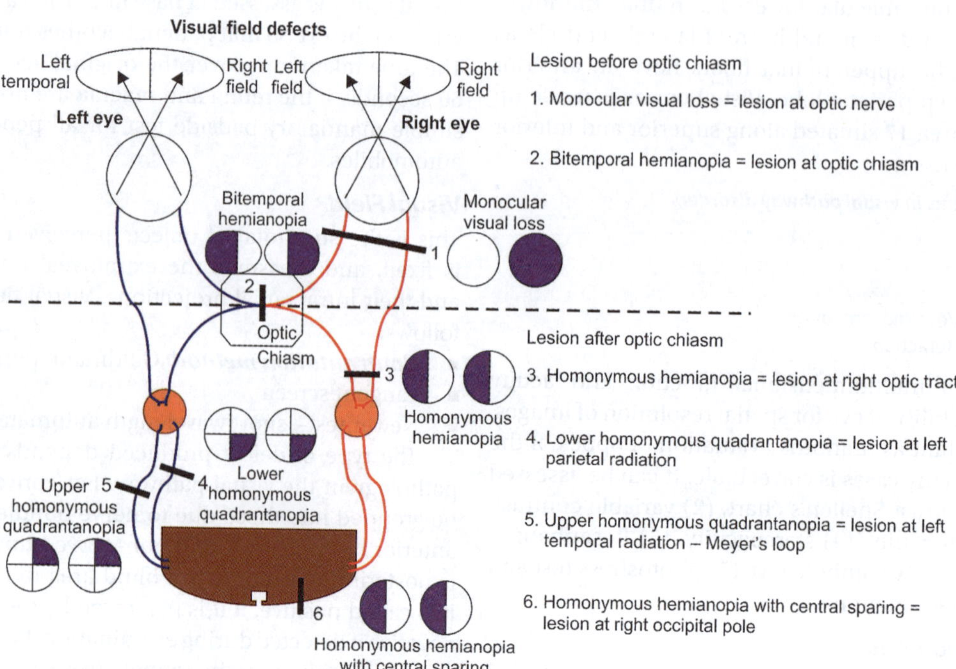

Fig. 195.2: Visual pathways and their lesions

- In optic nerve disease, defect of discrimination between red and green occurs
- In retinochoroidal disease, blue and yellow defect is seen unless proved otherwise.

Pupils

Eyes are considered as the windows to brain. Pupil is the door of the window. Its size is determined by the constrictor and dilator papillae muscles. Parasympathetic fibers are constrictor, sympathetic fibers are dilators. Parasympathetic fibers from *Edinger-Westphal nucleus* enter the ciliary ganglion, where they relay through ciliary nerves to the pupillary constrictor. Dilator fibers start at hypothalamus then go through the intermediolateral gray column of T1, T12 and C7, C8, D1, D2 ventral roots, and get relayed in stellate ganglion, superior cervical ganglion, carotid plexus, Gasserian ganglion and enter the long ciliary nerves on either side of optic nerve.

Testing

The following points must be tested—size, shape, regularity, equality, light reflex and near reflex (accommodation reflex). Size normal is 1.5–8 mm (1 mm difference between both sides is considered normal). Handheld pupil gauge, pupil camera, video pupillometry are used to record the pupillary size.

Light reflex: Simultaneous equal constriction of pupil occurs in response to light thrown into each eye (direct and consensual pupillary reaction).

Afferent pathway travels from optic nerve to chiasm, then cross nasal and uncrossed temporal fibers in the tract, reach superior colliculus then pretectal nucleus via posterior commissure, and ventral crossing around aqueduct to reach Edinger-Westphal nucleus. *Testing* is done with dim light, and patient fixing at distant object with open eyes. Oblique illumination for background and a bright light to pupil are used. Pupillary capture occurs in 0.2–0.28 seconds followed by pupillary escape, i.e. it starts dilating and the opposite side constricts (called consensual reflex).

Near reflex (accommodation reflex) has three components: (1) Accommodation, (2) pupil constriction and (3) convergence.

There are two types of vergence reactions: (1) Accommodative and (2) fusional.

Fusional vergence does not need vision. Proprioceptive fibers from medial rectus reach III nerve Edinger-Westphal nucleus and efferents come through the same muscle. Accommodative vergence involves the afferent visual pathway reaches occipital cortex, from there goes to frontal cortex via the long association fibers, and descends to Edinger-Westphal nucleus via the frontomesencephalic pathway and to the medial rectus and pupillocontrictors.

Ciliospinal reflex: Painful stimuli to skin of neck causes mydriasis due to inhibition of Edinger-Westphal nucleus. This is of importance in patients recovering from anesthesia, as it is the first to recover and failure to recover indicates hypoxic damage.

In darkness: Normally dilatation of the pupil is seen. If it is delayed or absent, it indicates sympathetic involvement.

Dissociation between light reflex and near reflex is tested in anyone with abnormal light reflex—both absence and sluggishness. A situation where accommodation reflex is present and light reflex is absent is seen in aberrant regeneration of nerve III, neurosyphilis, pineal tumors, hydrocephalus and tonic pupils.

A primarily constricted pupil with preservation of good vision, with retained accommodation reflex and absent light reflex and irregular reaction to mydriatics is called *Argyll Robertson pupil*. It may be interesting to know that Argyll Robertson died in India after adapting to Indian way of living and his last rights were done as per Indian customs.

Marcus Gunn Pupil

This is a test done to elicit minimal changes in pupillary response in patients with optic nerve disease. Pupil is tested with a bright light. When normal eye is covered, affected eye shows brief constriction followed by striking dilation. Kestenbaum's number can be used to record the difference in pupil size of both eyes.

Swinging Flashlight Test

Patient is examined in dark room and asked to fix at distant target. A bright light is shifted between both eyes, remaining in each eye for 3–5 seconds. The affected eye takes time to constrict, and it dilates slowly. Even when the swinging light has reached the opposite eye and the ipsilateral eye (the affected eye) will be found in the dilating phase after the initial constriction indicating slow transmission through optic nerve in that eye.

Relative Afferent Pupillary Dilatation

When light reflex is elicited, consensual response will be more than direct response. Direct response is graded as follows:

Grade 1: Weak constriction followed by strong dilatation
Grade 2: Slight stall (delay) then dilation
Grade 3: Immediate dilation
Grade 4: Pupil dilates then constricts
Grade 5: Pupil dilates without constriction.

Anisocoria

An isolated inequality in diameter of pupils of 0.5–1 mm is normal, greater inequality in a conscious patient is abnormal. The causes include drugs, trauma, Horner's syndrome, Adie's pupil, 3rd nerve palsy and ocular causes. In the unconscious patient, think of brainstem compression. Drug-induced mydriasis shows no reaction to 1% pilocarpine and absence of light and accommodation reflex.

Constricted pupil with decreased sweating in the forehead and mild drooping of eyelids is indicative of sympathetic involvement. It is called *Horner's syndrome*, and can be due to involvement of sympathetic pathways both preganglionic and postganglionic. The clinical points for localizing the site are shown in the Table 195.2.

Table 195.2: Distinguishing the site of lesion in Horner's syndrome

Horner	Central	Preganglionic	Postganglionic
2–5% cocaine	No response	No response	No response
1% hydroxy-amphetamine	++	++	No response
10% phenylephine	+	++	++++

Fundus Examination

Refractive error of the patient and examiner should be known, and appropriate lens of the ophthalmoscope should be used. Examiners right hand and right eye is used for examining the patient's right eye to avoid collision with the patient's nose. Three important structures need to be examined. They are the disk, macula and retina. Ask patient to fix at a distant object for seeing the disk, fix at the ophthalmoscopic light for macula, use green light for retina and pencil light for macula.

Order of Examination

Physiological cup, color of disk, contour of disk, peridiscal area, vessels crossing disk, macula and retina.

Opaque Nerve Fibers

In a small proportion of normal subjects, the optic nerve head (papilla) and its radiating fibers appear as opaque nerve fibers without compromise of vision. This is a benign nonprogressive condition, the importance is to distinguish it from several other pathological conditions (Fig. 195.3).

Optic neuritis: It is an inflammatory demyelinating condition of optic nerve head. This condition can involve one eye and present as acute painful visual loss in young adults. This can be the earliest manifestation of multiple sclerosis. In children, bilateral involvement can also occur. In adults, bilateral involvement indicates postinfectious demyelination described in acute disseminated encephalomyelitis (ADEM), toxic demyelination due to methyl alcohol, and paraneoplastic situations. The clinical and fundus changes are described in the Table 195.3. ***Investigations*** are done to confirm the cause of optic neuritis specially to rule out multiple sclerosis and treatment option is discussed in the chapter on demyelinating disorders.

Acute disseminated encephalomyelitis is a monophasic illness and treated with 3–5 g of methylprednisolone given intravenously over 3–5 days. Each 1 g is diluted in glucose saline and given over 4 hours as a drip. More than 80% patients recover, provided treatment is started early. Toxic and paraneoplastic conditions carry a poor prognosis.

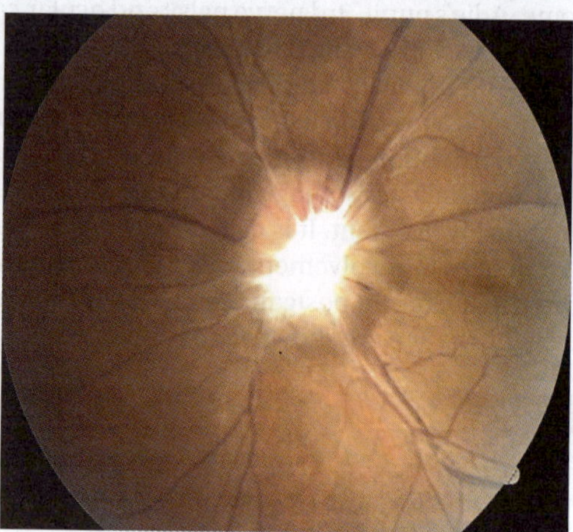

Fig. 195.3: Opaque optic nerve fibers (congenital persistence of myelin in the intraocular part of optic nerve not pathological). This is not a pathological condition

Table 195.3: Differences between optic neuritis and papilledema

Optic neuritis	Papilledema
Pupil abnormal	Normal
Vision poor	Good
Central scotoma	Field constriction + enlarged blind spot
< 3D swelling	> 3D swelling
Paton's lines –	+
Peripapillary h'gs –	+
Venous pulsation +	Absent
Retina macula	May or may not be

Papilledema: This is the term applied to optic nerve head swelling secondary to raised intracranial pressure (ICP). This can be due to space occupying lesions like tumors, granulomas, abscesses, subdural hematomas, intracerebral hematomas, hydrocephalus and tumor metastases. It can also occur due to medical conditions like malignant hypertension, vasculitis and renal diseases. Nonlocalizing rise in ICP occurs in as benign intracranial hypertension (BIH), chronic meningitis and cerebral venous thrombosis. ***Clinical features*** of ICP are dealt with in the chapter on tumors.

However, it is nice to remember that papilledema without macular edema is often surgical and papilledema with macular edema is due to medical causes. The macula is vascular and macular lesions reflect systemic changes.

Optic atrophy: This is the term applied to end-stage changes in optic nerve head. This is called primary optic atrophy when it is due to degenerative causes as a part of various neurodegenerative diseases, nutritional deficiency, drugs and toxins, and also compression on optic nerve. Here, physiological cup is deep, color of disk is chalky white, contour of disk is well cut out, sharp, peridiscal area is normal, vessels thin, retina and macula are normal. Pupillary reflexes are sluggish and acuity is grossly reduced. Irrespective of cause, treatment is ineffective.

Secondary optic atrophy: Indicates atrophy secondary to papilledema. Here, visual loss is less, there is constriction of peripheral fields of vision. Pupils are normal, fundus shows cup-filled, color is angry looking or dirty pallor, nasal more blurred than temporal as against postneuritic optic atrophy where temporal margin is more pale, contour of disk not very sharp, peridiscal area can show evidence of retinal edema in the form of folds called ***Paton's lines,*** vessels are sheathed and other areas are normal.

Consecutive optic atrophy: The term is applied to optic atrophy secondary to retinal disease. Here, the disk shows waxy pallor and its contours are not very sharp. The vessels are thin and the retina shows pigmentary degeneration. Ischemic optic atrophy is secondary to ischemia due to various causes. Here, the disk is pale and it may or may not show pale swelling called as ***pallid disk swelling***. The disk can show quadrantic pallor, altitudinal pallor of upper or lower half, bow-tie type pallor in the vertical or horizontal meridian, etc. At the crossings, the vessels appear amputated, ghost vessels appear like pale cords, corkscrew vessels and as new vessels. Different patterns of retinal pallor depend on the vessels affected. Macula can show degeneration, edema and dullness. Cherry red

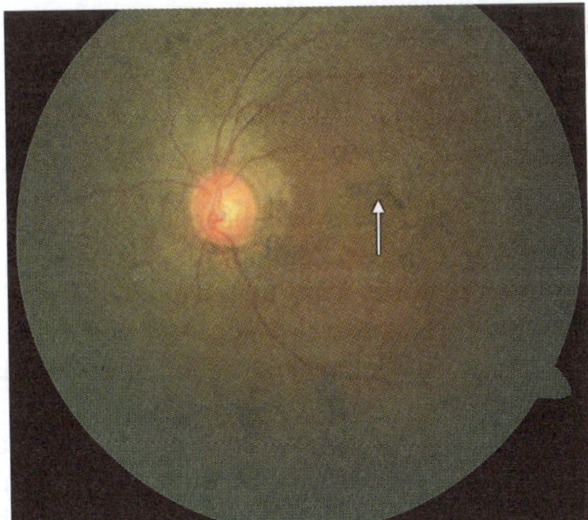

Fig. 195.4: Retinitis pigmentosa. **Note:** Pallor of the disk which appears punched out (primary optic atrophy) and pigment deposition along the periphery of the retina (arrow)

spots of the macula occur in retinitis pigmentosa and seen as bright red spots in the center of the macula (Fig. 195.4).

Treatment of the optic atrophy carries poor results for vision.

Psychogenic Blindness

It is diagnosed by clinical circumstances and observation of the patient when alone and by the following tests, when it is clubbed with partial organic features, it becomes very difficult to diagnose. The following points will help:

- Inconsistencies in acuity
- Role of compensation
- Normal menace reflex
- Normal optokinetic nystagmus and fundus appearance
- Normal photic drive in EEG, etc.

Visual evoked potential may be varied; even in the blind eye, visual evoked potential can be normal.

Occipital lobe dysfunctions are not discussed in this chapter.

OCULOMOTOR, TROCHLEAR AND ABDUCENT (ABDUCENS) NERVES AND EYE MOVEMENT CONTROL

Eyeball is supplied by superior, inferior, medial and lateral recti and superior and inferior oblique muscles. Abducent nerve supplies the lateral rectus, and trochlear nerve supplies the superior oblique, all others are supplied by oculomotor nerve.

The actions of the muscles are—the prime action of the superior rectus is to elevate, inferior rectus to depress, medial rectus to adduct, lateral rectus to abduct, superior oblique depresses and inferior oblique elevates. Recti acts better in the abducted eye, oblique acts better in adducted eye. Superior muscles that is superior rectus and inferior oblique intort, inferior muscles that is inferior rectus and superior oblique extort, vertical recti that is superior rectus and inferior rectus adduct, vertical obliques that is superior and inferior oblique abduct (Table 195.4).

The combined action of the intraocular muscles opposes the vicious drug of orbital contents and prevent the ocular imaging slipping on the retina. They also assist the rapid and coordinated movements of the eye balls rapidly.

Table 195.4: Combination of muscles moving the eyeball in different directions

Upward to the left	*Upward*	*Upward to the right*
Left superior rectus (SR)	Left and right SR	Right SR
Right inferior oblique (IO)	Left and right IO	Left IO
To the left	Straight ahead	To the right
Left lateral rectus (LR)	General contraction of all	Right LR
Right medial rectus (MR)	Extraocular muscles	Left MR
Downward to the left	Downward	Downward to the right
Left inferior rectus (IR)	Left and right IR	Right IR
Right superior oblique (SO)		Left SO

What are the movements taking place?
- Eye movements in response to head movements, e.g. vestibulo-ocular and optokinetic movements
- Spontaneous eye movements
  - Saccades
  - Pursuits
  - Vergence
- Infranuclear movements
- Abnormal movements.

What are the targets?
- Predicted or anticipated targets
- Dynamic or static targets
- Novel or unexpected targets.

Several neural structures participate in this intricate and highly precise eye movements. These include:

- Oculomotor nuclei, oculomotor muscles and oculomotor nerves
- Brainstem structures like neural integrator, i.e. parapontine reticular formation (PPRF) and cerebellum
- Neuronal arcs which are formed by several structures including PPRF, vestibular nucleus, perihypoglossal nucleus, medial longitudinal fasciculus (MLF), interstitial nucleus of MLF, interstitial nucleus of Cajal (INC), and nucleus of Darkschewitsch
- Mesencephalic reticular formation and superior colliculi
- Cortical structures concerned are frontal and occipital eye fields, frontomesencephalic pathway, occipitomesencephalic pathway and cerebellomesencephalic pathway.

The other structures involved are vestibular connection and cervico-ocular and cervico-colic systems.

Saccadic System

Saccade is the fastest eye movement with short refractory period. It reacts to one stimulus at a time. The initiation time is 200 ms. Saccadic pulse is carried out by burst neurons, saccadic step by tonic neurons and there is mathematical pulse/step match.

Pause neurons inhibit burst neurons tonically. Burst neurons are of three types. Medium head types are time locked to all fast eye movements, large head type inhibit and antagonist burst neurons.

Tonic neurons—discharge in relation to eye position and give step innervations.

Higher control for saccadic system is frontomesencephalic pathway.

Disorders of saccadic movements include saccadic inaccuracy (hypo- or hypermetric), slow velocity of movement, delay in initiation of saccadic pulse and oculomotor apraxia.

Defects in saccadic step causes gaze-evoked nystagmus.

Mismatch between pulse and step leads to opsoclonus, ocular flutter and macro- and microsquare wave jerks.

The ***pursuit system*** involves slow follow-up movements for continuous view of moving targets, and for continuous view of imagined targets. It is mediated through parieto-occipitomesencephalic pathway.

Abnormalities of the pursuit system: These include abnormalities in the amplitude, direction and balance.

Defects in amplitude lead to cogwheel pursuit where catch-up saccades compensate for defective pursuit.

Defects in direction lead to drift sign of Gay, where the eye keeps on drifting in the direction of the moving target without coming back to midline. Pursuit abnormality is involved in downbeat and upbeat nystagmus.

Defects in balance lead to abnormalities in balancing the plane of eye movement. Inverse pursuit is seen in patients with congenital nystagmus, where the fast component of optokinetic nystagmus is in the plane of the drum whereas it is reverse normally.

Note: Optokinetic nystagmus is assessed by focusing vision on a striped rotating drum.

Vergence System

This term refers to the slow, nonparallel eye movements. It serves to bring maximum focus on the visual target binocularly. This has been explained under the near reflex under optic nerves.

Novel target visualization is carried out by superior colliculus, and its connections. Medial temporo-occipital region perceives motion and depth, premotor area codes and motor area executes the movement.

Caloric test: It is a simple bedside test for assessing labyrinthine function, brainstem and its central connections.

Head of the patient is inclined resting on a pillow at 30°, to make the horizontal semicircular canal vertical. The impulse is transmitted as—semicircular canal to vestibular nucleus to ipsilateral gaze center then to contralateral gaze center.

Ice-cold water (0.4–1.0 mL) is injected into external ear. This lowers tonic firing at ipsilateral canal and excites ipsilateral PPRF and inhibits contralateral PPRF causing imbalance at gaze center. Eye is pushed to side of cold water injection, and corrective saccades take place to opposite side. In canal paresis, no movements are seen from the affected ear. Warm water produces the opposite effect. Absence of caloric response in a comatose patient indicates brainstem damage. In supranuclear eye movement disorder, reflex movements are elicited.

Questions to be asked:
- Is there an eye movement problem?
- If so, is it physiological or pathological?
- Is it congenital or acquired?
- Is it infranuclear or nuclear?
- Is it supranuclear or combined?
- What are the abnormal eye movements seen?
- Is it possible to localize them?
- Is it possible to treat them?

Patient with double vision elicit the following points:
- Uniocular or binocular, diplopia or polyopia
- Intermittent versus constant, sudden versus slow, horizontal versus vertical, other accompaniments
- Whether head tilt present or not, if so maximum separation at near or far vision.

Common symptoms in oculomotor imbalances include—squint, double vision (diplopia) restricted movements, head tilt, head thrust, head nod, blurring of vision, oscillopsia and presence of abnormal oscillations.

Oculomotor Nerve Palsy

This leads to drooping of the eyelid, dilated pupil, divergence when the eye is moved away from the direction of the paralyzed eye and downward due to paralysis of muscles supplied by the nerve III. Diplopia is worsened when the eye looks laterally, and downward due to normal activity of the lateral rectus and superior oblique muscles. In diplopia, the images from both eyes separate from each other. Diplopia may be in the horizontal, vertical or oblique planes depending on the action of the paralyzed muscle. Image arising from the paralyzed eye is fainter and it is termed as false images. The bright image arising from the normal eye is the true image.

Crossed diplopia is the term used when the false image is inner to the true image, and it occurs with medial rectus weakness. Drooping of eyelid which covers more than 3 mm of cornea is termed partial ptosis, and, if it covers the pupil fully it is called complete ptosis.

Patients may show different combinations of ptosis and abnormalities of the pupil due to paralysis of levator palpebrae superioris and the pupillary muscles respectively.

Assessment: Four different combinations of ptosis and pupillary abnormalities may occur, these include:
1. Ptosis with pupillary involvement
2. Ptosis without pupillary involvement
3. Unilateral versus bilateral
4. Persistent versus variable.

Common causes of third nerve palsy include nonspecific neuritis, vasculitis, diabetes mellitus, trauma, infectious and noninfectious granulomas, superior orbital fissure syndrome, cavernous sinus thrombosis, carotid artery aneurysm, caroticocavernous fistula, nasopharyngeal tumors, and lesions of the brainstem like posterior circulation stroke, demyelination and intrinsic tumors. Third nerve palsy in diabetes mellitus is painful and spares the pupil. The pupillary fibers are placed on the outer aspect of the third nerve, and receive nutrition from cerebrospinal fluid. The vessels supplying the third nerve traverse through the center of the nerve and therefore nerve infarction due to diabetes spares the pupillary fibers which are outer. This is treated by proper control of diabetes, drugs like pentoxifylline to

Table 195.5: Differentiating the various causes of drooping of eyelids

Orbital cellulitis	Superior orbital fissure syndrome	Cavernous sinus thrombosis
Orbital and conjunctival edema	Mild	Most severe
Eye movements restricted	Restricted	Restricted
Unilateral	Unilateral	Soon bilateral
Mastoid normal	Normal	Tender (Battle's sign)
Pupil normal	Affected	Affected
Ophthalmic 5th normal	Affected	Affected
Maxillary 5th normal	Normal	Often affected

improve microvascular circulation and sometimes even steroids may be needed. Nonspecific cranial neuritis is suspected when there is recurrent cranial nerve palsy on either side with a naturally remitting-relapsing course. If it is consistently on one side, investigations are needed to rule out lesions which involve the skull base such as basal meningitis, sclerosing lesions of the bone or malignancies (Table 195.5).

Features of superior orbital fissure syndrome associated with optic nerve involvement are seen in lesions of the orbital apex such as infiltrations involving the nerves passing through the superior orbital fissure.

Abducent Nerve Palsy (Sixth Cranial Nerve Palsy)

This nerve supplies the lateral rectus muscle of the eyeball, which is the main abductor. Paralysis produces convergent squint with ipsilateral head tilt, and diplopia worst while abducting and looking at distant objects.

The common causes are nonspecific neuritis, raised ICP, and lesions at the apex of the petrous temporal bone either due to inflammatory or neoplastic cause. When it is accompanied by involvement of the trigeminal nerve due to lesions at the apex of the orbit, it is called Gradenigo's syndrome. Sixth nerve palsy can occur in superior orbital fissure syndrome, orbital cellulitis, supraclinoid aneurysms of the internal carotid artery, basilar arteries, trauma, basal meningitis and cavernous sinus syndromes along with other cranial nerves. Abducent nerve palsy is common to occur in raised intracranial tension since the nerve has a long intracranial course and it is anchored at the base of the skull (Dolores canal). When intracranial tension increases, the brainstem is displaced downward resulting in tension on the nerve and paralysis. Abducent nerve palsy secondary to intracranial tension is a false localizing sign mimicking local pathology in the brainstem. The lesion often recovers completely with relief of the intracranial tension.

Trochlear Nerve Palsy

Trochlear nerve (fourth cranial nerve) supplies the superior oblique muscle which depresses, abducts and extorts the eye. Paralysis produces vertical squint with vertical oblique diplopia worst while looking down and in and head tilt to opposite side. The most common cause is trauma.

Bedside Assessment of Deviation

Hirschberg test, i.e. assessing the position of the reflected image by throwing light in each eye.

Cover Test and Alternate Cover Test

Cover test

Tests for detecting squint (abnormalities of version):

- Primary deviation—when a patient has a weak muscle, eye deviates in the plane of the normal antagonist.
- Secondary deviation—when patient fixes with defective eye and normal eye is covered, the normal eye deviates more as paretic muscle needs more energy to fixate and the normal muscle moves more. If the secondary deviation is more than the primary deviation, it indicates paralytic squint.

Alternate cover test

This is done due to detect subtle deviation. Patient has double vision but no squint. To know whether the double vision is due to subtle deviations of the eyeball and weakness of extraocular muscle, or due to nonorganic causes.

The test covers the nonparetic left eye, so the paralyzed right eye slightly moves out to fixate on the target. This movement of redress is the *primary deviation*. Then cover the paretic eye and fix with the normal left eye. Then the eye moves again to fixate on the target. This is the *secondary deviation*. Larger movement of redress will be seen in the paralyzed eye when it is done in a repeated way and thus the paralysis can be unmasked.

Assessment of Diplopia

The test should be done in bright light. Patient sits eye to eye with examiner. Observe resting eye position.

Duction movements: These are nonconjugate individual eye movements and are tested in six cardinal positions. In patients with horizontal diplopia, there is a horizontal squint. The muscles responsible are both medial rectus and lateral rectus. For lateral rectus, there is diplopia while looking at a distant object and false image is the outer one. For medial rectus, diplopia is more while looking at a near object and the diplopia is crossed (see above). Then assess the plane of maximum separation of images.

In a patient with vertical diplopia, if the resting eye position does not show vertical disconjugation, possibilities are—psychogenic, local cause and lesions of the occipital lobe.

Vertical disconjugation with uniform separation of images in all planes occurs in skew deviation. Skew deviation is vertical disconjugation of eye due to supranuclear cause. This is the only supranuclear cause for diplopia. Vertical disconjugation of resting eyes and variable diplopia, i.e. maximum separation of true and false image seen in the plane of action of the paralyzed muscle is unique feature in lower motor neuron (LMN) lesions. Let us look at resting eye position. If right eye is up and left eye is down—out of the eight vertical muscles, the culprits may be right inferior rectus and superior oblique or left superior rectus and inferior oblique. When we tell patient to look to the right and down based on principle of action of the muscles, muscles that are acting are right inferior rectus and left superior oblique. If our patient has maximum separation of eyes in this plane as we have already eliminated left superior oblique by looking at resting eye position, the culprit is right inferior rectus. That way moving in all cardinal planes and looking at maximum separation of images, the weak muscle can be identified. If the diplopia has a tilt, the oblique muscles are responsible.

Gaze Paralysis

Supranuclear conjugate eye movements are called gaze movements. There can be up, down or horizontal gaze deviation or paralysis based on whether the lesion is irritative or paralytic. The affected movement may be saccade, pursuit or both. There is no diplopia. Reflex movements are preserved. In brainstem, gaze palsy eye deviates away from side of pathology. Diplopia can be present and vestibulo-ocular reflex (VOR) can be impaired, both pursuit and saccade affected. When gaze and MLF are affected, one and half syndrome occurs, where there is no horizontal movement in one eye, and only abduction in the other eye. In bilateral MLF lesion, both eyes fail to adduct. Thalamic pathology is a common cause for vertical gaze palsy. When there is cortical gaze palsy due to involvement of frontal eye field, the eyes point towards the side of pathology, there is no double vision and VOR is preserved. There can be down gaze palsy in patients with progressive supranuclear paralysis, horizontal gaze abnormality in idiopathic Parkinsonism, horizontal gaze slowing to the opposite side in corticobasal ganglia degeneration syndromes, oblique gaze palsy in Whipple's disease and gaze up palsy in multisystem atrophy, kernicterus, neurodegenerative conditions like dystonia, Parkinsonism syndromes, neurolipidosis, dorsal midbrain tumors, etc. (Refer Chapter on Extrapyramidal Disorders).

Abnormal Eye Movements

Nystagmus

This term refers to involuntary rhythmic biphasic oscillations in which at least one phase is always slow and the other is fast. The slow phase indicates drifting of the eye due to the abnormality in neural mechanism whereas the fast phase is recovery to regain normal position.

Nystagmus may be:
- Congenital versus acquired
- Physiological versus pathological
- Pendular versus jerky.

Congenital nystagmus: It is horizontal and pendular, with no oscillopsia, worsens with fixation. There is good acuity of vision. There may be head tilt, since patient will have best vision in a particular head position in which he will keep his head tilted. This is called as null position. There is inverse pursuit on optokinetic testing. When asked to fix at the target moving in front of the eye with the optokinetic tape, instead of the fast correcting movement away from the side of movement of the tape, it follows the tape.

Physiological nystagmus: Symmetrical nystagmus may occur in extreme positions of gaze greater than 30° deviation. The nystagmus is of small amplitude, it is worse with fatigue, and often ill-sustained. Optokinetic nystagmus occurring while traveling in a moving vehicle is also a physiological nystagmus.

Pathological nystagmus may be of cerebellar, vestibular or brainstem origins.

Periodic alternating nystagmus is spontaneous, changes of the direction of the nystagmus every 3 seconds, slow phase affected and only fast phase remains. Pathology is disconnection between the visual optokinetic and vestibulo-ocular inputs.

Rebound nystagmus: This has to be elicited by the examiner in this, the eye rebound after reaching the end point. Usually it is cerebellar in origin.

Classical cerebellar nystagmus: This is gaze-evoked with the fast component in the direction of gaze. It does not lateralize but localize to cerebellum.

Other types of nystagmus include see-saw nystagmus seen in suprasellar lesions, down and upbeat nystagmus in brainstem lesions, and convergence and retraction nystagmus. Ocular flutter, opsoclonus and other involuntary movements should not be mistaken for nystagmus.

Nystagmoid Movements

This term refers to conditions in which eyeball undergoes a few oscillations on extreme movements of the eyeball, but spontaneously stopped after a while, this can occur in normal eyes especially on extreme positions of the eye and the eye muscles are fatigued.

Opsoclonus

This term refers to irregular, jerky conjugate movements of the eyes occurring in lesions of the brainstem such as multiple sclerosis, viral encephalitis and tumors, hyperosmolar nonketotic coma, as a paraneoplastic phenomenon and in poisonings. It consists of ocular saccades (brief rapid movements of eyeballs) occurring reflexly or voluntarily. These rapid eye movements are under control of several populations of neurones in the paramedian reticular formation. One group of neurons (burst neurons) are responsible for the production of saccades while another group (pause neurons) terminate them. Opsoclonus is the result of imbalance between these neuronal groups.

TRIGEMINAL NERVE (FIFTH CRANIAL NERVE AND ITS LESIONS)

The trigeminal nerve arises from pons and has a large sensory and small motor roots. It exits at the region where tentorium cerebelli attaches to temporal bone. **Gasserian ganglion** is located at the petrous part of temporal bone. The motor root is at its inferior part incorporated to mandibular division which leaves the skull through foramen ovale. This supplies the muscles of mastication, i.e. masseter, temporalis, medial and lateral pterygoids and other muscles—tensor tympani, tensor veli palatini, myelohyoid and the anterior belly of digastric.

The sensory root forms three divisions: (1) Ophthalmic, (2) maxillary and (3) mandibular. From the ganglion, the fibers course proximally and terminate in the spinal tract of trigeminal in the medulla, chief sensory nucleus at pons, and mesencephalic nucleus at midbrain. The spinal tract is concerned with appreciation of pain and temperature and the fibers from forehead are in the most ventral part, then the maxillary region and last the mandibular region. There is also another somatotopic representation—midline facial areas like nose and mouth are rostral, and lateral facial area is most caudal in representation. This is responsible for the onion peel pattern of facial sensory loss, i.e. sensory loss in the perioral region in intrinsic brainstem lesions of the trigeminal nerve. Chief sensory nucleus is concerned with touch, and the mesencephalic nucleus is concerned with proprioception from the muscles of mastication. The ventral crossed trigeminothalamic fibers (quintothalamic) and uncrossed dorsal trigeminothalamic fibers reach ventral posteromedial nucleus of thalamus, then by thalamocortical projections, they reach the sensory cortex and motor cortex, respectively.

1. ***Ophthalmic division*** lies in the lateral wall of cavernous sinus, it divides into tentorial, lacrimal, frontal and nasociliary branches. The frontal branch gives rise to supraorbital nerve for upper eyelid, conjunctival, frontal sinuses, forehead and scalp, supratrochlear branch supplies conjunctival, medial part of upper lid, forehead and side of nose. Lacrimal branch carries postganglionic parasympathetic fibers for reflex lacrimation. Nasociliary branch gives nasal branches for nasal sinuses and skin of tip of nose, infratrochlear branch supplies the medial canthus, lacrimal sac, caruncle and conjunctiva.

2. ***Maxillary division*** passes through the inferolateral part of cavernous sinus via foramen rotundum into the sphenopalatine fossa, enters the orbit through the inferior orbital fissure and it gives branches to the lower eyelids, side of nose, upper lip, cheeks and lower half of cornea, maxillary sinus, lower nasal cavity, palate, gum, teeth of upper jaw and dura of middle cranial fossa.

3. ***Mandibular division*** joins the motor root and leaves the skull through foramen ovale and enters the infratemporal fossa. Motor branch supplies all muscles supplied by this nerve and sensory division via lingual nerve supplies the anterior two-thirds of tongue, lower gum, teeth, mandible, chin, lower lip, tympanic membrane, auditory meatus and dura of posterior cranial fossa.

Common Diseases

Supranuclear problems do not affect the motor functions except that of masseter on the opposite side since there is bilateral representation for all other muscles. In nuclear lesions, sensory and motor parts dissociate. Sensory lesion can be only the type subserved by part of the brainstem affected. Combined sensorimotor trigeminal neuropathy is extra-axial, unless proved otherwise. The spinal tract, if involved at its lower part, will produce loss of pain and temperature in forehead. As the lesion becomes more proximal lower parts of the face are involved. Sometimes the involvement may be bilateral of the crossing fibers in the brainstem are affected as in the lateral medullary syndrome. In pontine lesion, there is midfacial sensory loss for touch with contralateral hemiparesis and at midbrain level, proprioception becomes impaired with tendency to bite the cheeks and depression of ipsilateral jaw jerk.

Testing

Sensory assessment for pain, light touch, heat and cold are checked on the cheeks and oral and nasal mucous membrane. Lesions proximal to Gasserian ganglia affect the whole cheek but distal ones spare the angle of mandible as it is supplied by C2 and C3. Motor testing—clenching the teeth tests masseter and temporalis. Medial and lateral pterygoids of one side move jaw to opposite side therefore when paralyzed jaw deviates to same side. Both medial pterygoids together close and retract jaw and both lateral pterygoids protrude and open the jaw. Tensor tympani paralysis produces difficulty in high tone hearing. The reflexes to be tested are glabellar tap, jaw jerk, corneal reflex and conjunctival reflex. For the corneal and conjunctival reflexes, the afferent nerve is provided by the fifth nerve which supplies these structures.

Corneomandibular reflex consists of brisk eye blink and anterolateral jaw deviation induced by corneal stimulation. This is seen in patients with lesions above the pons.

Trigeminal Neuralgia

Syn: Fothergill's disease, Tic douloureux

The patient experiences sudden lancinating pain lasting seconds to minutes which occurs several times a day. Pain may be triggered by exposure to cold, eating, touching, speaking, cold wind, etc. Women are more affected than men and older people are more affected than young. It can affect any one division or all divisions. It can occur with intrinsic brainstem disorders like multiple sclerosis, cerebrovascular accidents, tumors, aberrant vessels, or preganglionic lesions like infections and infiltrations of the nerve roots. Chronic aberrant circuits getting established due to metallic dental fillings and also chronic dental infections can lead on to trigeminal neuralgia.

A small proportion of patients have persistent trigeminal artery which is a branchial arch artery. Normally, this artery gets obliterated in postnatal life. If it persists and becomes arteriosclerotic, it may press on the trigeminal nerve at its point of exit from the brainstem and cause neuralgia. Such cases can be relieved by resection of this artery and release of the nerve.

Management

Initial treatment is medical. The condition responds satisfactorily in many cases to drug therapy. In secondary trigeminal neuralgia, treatment consists of attention to the cause and symptomatic measures with carbamazepine, gabapentin, botulinum toxin, and surgery on the sensory division.

Drug therapy consists of mainly the administration of antiepileptic drugs.

Gabapentin in a dose of 100–300 mg bd or tid is the drug of choice on account of its effectiveness and safety, but it is considerably more expensive compared to carbamazepine. Carbamazepine in a total dose of 600–800 mg/day is consistently effective in the majority of cases, at least initially. Toxic effects include hepatic damage, aplastic anemia and syndrome of inappropriate secretion of antidiuretic hormone (SIADH) and Stevens-Johnson syndrome. Phenytoin sodium and baclofen can be given as alternative or adjuvant drugs to carbamazepine. Pregabalin given in doses of 75 mg bd is also useful.

Percutaneous coagulation of the involved division of the nerve utilizing radiofrequency waves has been very useful in intractable cases. The advantage of this procedure is that, it selectively destroys the pain fibers without affecting other sensations over the face.

The major problem of the following surgery is severe dysesthesia over the face, which may be very disturbing. This complication is less with selective radiofrequency procedure. Modern treatment is to release the aberrant arterial loop compressing the nerve root by microvascular surgery.

Once the condition is relieved in the vast majority, it does not recur even though recurrence can occur rarely.

Bilateral trigeminal neuropathy is seen in Sjögren's disease, stilbamidine toxicity, systemic lupus erythematosus (SLE) and related disorders. Nasopharyngeal tumors present with facial sensory loss, nasal obstruction and opthalmoplegia **(Jacobson's triad)** or lower cranial nerve palsy, deafness and facial sensory loss **(Trotter's triad)**. Numbness of the chin is usually seen in patients with lymphoreticular malignancy **(Rogers sign)**. Numbness of cheek and weakness of lower lid are seen in squamous cell carcinoma. Intermittent numbness of tongue can occur due to pressure on lingual nerve due to sialolithiasis.

FACIAL NERVE

This nerve has a motor component which supplies the muscles of facial expression and stapedius, posterior belly of digastric, and stylohyoid and sensory component for the anterior two-thirds of tongue along with parasympathetic which travels in nervus intermedius of Wrisberg. The supranuclear motor fibers start from lower precentral gyrus, emotional fibers from frontal lobe anterior to precentral gyrus, supplementary motor area, medial temporal lobe, insula and thalamus. The nucleus of facial nerve is in the pons. Fibers from the nucleus wind round sixth nerve nucleus and forms **facial colliculus**. The nucleus is made up of four horizontal groups.

1. The first **dorsomedial group** supplies the auricular and occipital muscles
2. The **intermediate group** supplies frontalis and corrugator
3. **Ventromedial group** supplies the platysma
4. **Lateral group** supplies buccinator and facial muscles.

The fibers join the sensory division in the descending limb. Upper part of face has bilateral supranuclear motor control. The nervus intermedius of Wrisberg carries preganglionic parasympathetic fibers to submaxillary, pterygopalatine and sphenopalatine ganglia. Sensory fibers for anterior two-thirds of tongue, mucosa of nose, pharynx, palate and skin of pinna, mastoid and external auditory meatus arise from geniculate ganglion. Parasympathetic fibers arise from superior salivatory nucleus and the fibers for lacrimation from lacrimal nucleus in pontine tegmentum. Gustatory afferents end in the nucleus of the **tractus solitarius** in the medulla, and exteroceptive afferents in the nucleus of spinal tract of trigeminal.

The nerve escapes into petrous pyramid via cerebellopontine angle, traverses geniculate ganglion without synapse, and emerges from the temporal bone as greater superficial petrosal nerve. This passes under the Gasserian ganglion, enters the Vidian canal in the anterior part of foramen lacerum, where it joins the deep petrosal nerve to form the Vidian nerve, then enters the sphenopalatine ganglion in pterygopalatine fossa and via the maxillary division of 5th enters inferior orbital fissure, reaches lacrimal gland by an anastomosis with the lacrimal branch of trigeminal nerve.

The cisternal part of the nerve and the further course is—after leaving pons, the nerve enters the internal auditory meatus, together with 8th nerve. This is the meatal segment, next is labyrinthine segment, where the nerve travels at right angle to reach the geniculate ganglion, the first major branch is the greater superficial petrosal nerve, next is the horizontal segment, then the vertical mastoid segment which gives rise to the nerve to stapedius, and then the chorda tympani. It contains afferent taste fibers from anterior two-thirds of tongue and parasympathetic fibers to submandibular and sublingual glands. It comes out through the stylomastoid foramen, gives rise to posterior auricular nerve which supplies occipitalis posterior, transverse and oblique bellies of auricularis, digastric, and stylohyoid muscles. From there it enters the parotid gland and forms pes anserinus and divides into craniofacial and cervicofacial branches.

Paralysis of the facial nerve may be upper motor neuron (UMN) type as occurring in double hemiplegia, or LMN type as occurring in typical Bell's palsy which is the most common form of LMN facial palsy in clinical practice.

Bell's Palsy

This condition is named after Sir Charles Bell, a Scottish physiologist and surgeon (1774–1842). This is the most common cause of unilateral LMN facial palsy. It usually develops suddenly and spontaneously often starting with a mild pain in the ear. Sometimes, a history of exposure to cold or wind or a mild systemic infection is obtained. The lesion may be either compression of the nerve by edema or periostitis at the facial canal, ischemia of the nerve or a viral infection.

Facial nerve is involved distal to stylomastoid foramen, due to unidentified cause or viral infections like herpes simplex, Epstein-Barr virus, cytomegalovirus and varicella-zoster virus, Lyme disease, HIV and others. The Guidelines Development Group (GDG) defines it as unilateral facial palsy which reaches maximum disability within 72 hours, with no definite identifiable cause except inflammation and edema of multifactorial reason and is a diagnosis of exclusion. Pregnancy, diabetes, exposure to cold, use of influenza vaccine, cranial polyneuritis, pre-eclampsia, hypertension are other not uncommon causes. The incidence is 11.5–53.3/100,000 persons per year and 6.1/100,000 children between 1 and 16 years. LMN facial palsy can be easily differentiated from UMN facial palsy by the following features (Table 195.6).

Testing motor function: Normal rate of eye blinking is around 15/minute is reduced in weakness of 7th nerve,

Table 195.6: Clinical differences between UMN and LMN types of facial palsy

Upper motor neuron (UMN) facial palsy	Lower motor neuron (LMN) palsy
Upper part of the face is spared	Whole of one side of the face is affected
There can be dissociation between motor and emotional components	No dissociation
Facial reflexes are brisk and opposite to the side of hemiparesis	Reflexes are depressed and there is no hemiparesis
Bell's phenomena (i.e. rolling up of the eyeball when the patient attempts to close the eye) is absent	Present
Hyperacusis absent	Present
Taste in anterior two-thirds tongue and tears not affected	Affected based on level of lesion in the course of the nerve

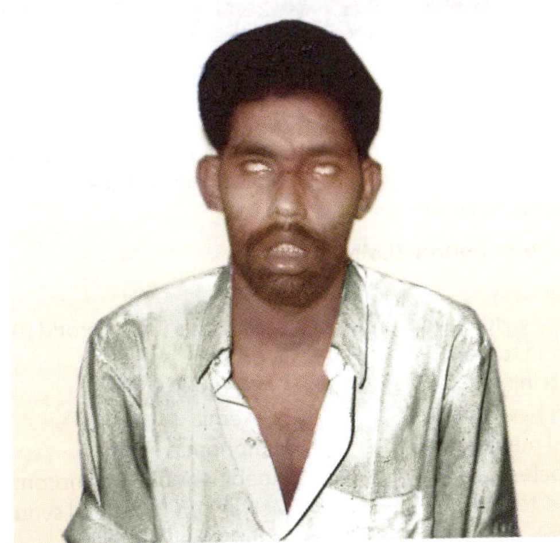

Fig. 195.6: Bilateral facial palsy. **Note:** Inability to close the eyes and Bell's phenomenon

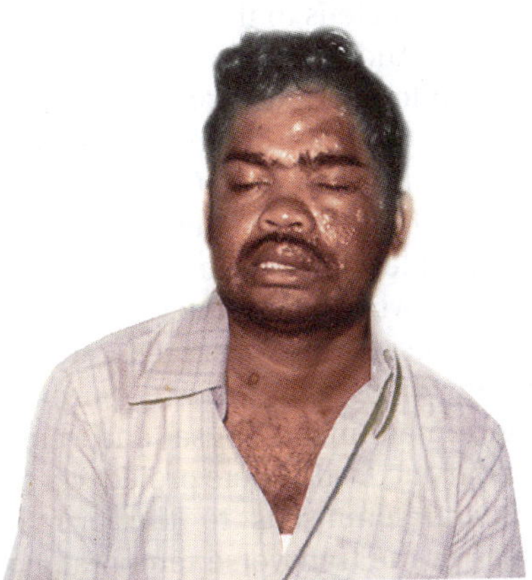

Fig. 195.5: Herpes zoster ophthalmicus left with facial palsy. **Note:** Vesicles and deviation of angle of mouth to the right

weakness of the facial muscles can be demonstrated by testing eye closure (orbicularis oculi), deviation of angle of mouth towards the normal side, inability to blow the cheeks and inability to contract the platysma which is attached to the skin of neck (Fig. 195.5).

Bell's phenomena is tested by asking the patient to close the eyes when examiner attempts to open the eyelids. Normally, there is symmetrical up and out rolling of eyes. This becomes exaggerated in the side of LMN type of 7th nerve palsy. This is because there is a physiological synkinesis between the orbicularis oculi supplied by 7th nerve and superior rectus supplied by 3rd nerve. As the 3rd nerve is normal, the balance is shifted in favor of superior rectus (Fig. 195.6).

Taste sensations which should be tested using sweet, salt, sour and bitter tested on each side of the protruded tongue separately. In LMN facial palsy, there is loss of taste. Parasympathetic function is tested by hanging a filter paper of 0.5 cm width on each eye for 5 minutes and quantifying the tear column in both eyes in 5 minutes. Usually it can reach 15 mm.

Course and Prognosis of Bell's Palsy

Usually, it has self-limited course and 70% recover at 6 months without any treatment. Electrophysiology testing can be done when there is complete paralysis in order to study the state of the nerve and assess the prognosis. More severe lesions which do not recover with time indicate poorer prognosis of recovery.

Management

The general recommendations of the US Centers for Disease Control and Prevention (CDC) are:

- Thorough examination to exclude other causes
- Antiviral therapy along with corticosteroids to be given within 72 hours
- Proper eye care to prevent damage to the cornea. This is usually, done by bandaging the eyes, antiseptic eye drops and in nonrecovering cases, occluding the palpable fissure by stitching the eyelids till recovery.

Drug Therapy

A short course of high-dose steroids (1 mg/kg) is started and given for 6 days, to be tapered fast. This can be clubbed with acyclovir 30 mg/kg/day in divided doses for 2 weeks. Surgical decompression of the stylomastoid foramen is not recommended.

Treatment of the disease depends on the cause. Symptom modifying treatment is needed to avoid dryness of the eyes and corneal ulceration with moisturizing agents and suturing of both eyelids, if required.

For chronic residual Bell's palsy, plastic surgical interventions can be undertaken and counseling done for psychological consequences of impaired smile. Some patients are left with hemifacial spasms, jaw winking (opening of eyes when jaw is opened), blepharospasm, facial contracture, involuntary tears or crocodile tears **(Bogorad's sign)** and **Gustatory sweating (Frey's sign)**, i.e. induction of generalized sweating on eating—due to faulty reinnervation during recovery. If left with sequelae, plastic surgery to correct facial deviations and injection botulinum toxin to control spasms (for varying periods) may be helpful.

Occurrence of bilateral UMN or LMN facial palsy may be seen at times.

Bilateral UMN and LMN are differentiated as follows:

The sparing of the upper part of the face and the Bell's phenomena will not be helpful. In UMN lesions,

Table 195.7: Common causes of unilateral and bilateral facial palsy

Unilateral	*Bilateral*
Upper motor neuron (UMN)	
• Vascular (stroke) • Tumor • Multiple sclerosis	• Vascular (multi-infarct dementia) • Motor neuron disease
Lower motor neuron (LMN)	
• Bell's palsy • Ramsay-Hunt syndrome • Parotid tumor • Head injury • Skull base tumor • Basal meningitis • Diabetes • Hypertension • CSOM	• GBS • Sarcoidosis (uveoparotid tumor) • Leprosy • Lyme disease • Leukemia • Lymphoma • Moebius (Möbius) syndrome • Melkersson-Rosenthal syndrome • Toxin—thalidomide • Bilateral Bell's palsy

Abbreviations: CSOM = Chronic suppurative otitis media; GBS = Guillain-Barré syndrome

patients have dissociation between emotional and motor fibers, so that emotional disturbances may be evident. Taste, hearing and lacrimation (tearing) are not affected. Corneal reflex, conjunctival reflex and jaw jerk are present.

In LMN lesions, both motor and emotional fibers are paralyzed, facial reflexes are depressed.

Ramsay-Hunt syndrome: This consists of severe facial palsy associated with vesicles in the pharynx, external auditory canal, and sometimes over the mastoid. The eighth cranial nerve may also be involved in many. The lesion is due to herpes zoster affecting the geniculate ganglion.

Common causes of unilateral and bilateral facial palsy have been shown in Table 195.7.

Chronic facial palsy: LMN facial palsy may become chronic and persistent in some situations. It is accompanied by the presence of hemifacial spasms on the side of paralysis, presence of features of faulty renervation like crocodile tears, jaw winking phenomena, prominent nasolabial fold, ipsilateral facial deviation with less power in the ipsilateral facial muscles and epiphora on chewing.

Subtle facial palsy: This is identified by reduced blink rate, wide palpebral fissure, incomplete burying of eyelashes and presence of ***von Graefe's sign***, where the obscure asymmetry in palpebral fissure diameter is unmasked by asking the patient to slowly lift the head and the eye from the flexed position of the neck. This movement has three components: (1) Eye on orbit, (2) orbit on head and (3) head on neck righting reflexes. ***Barbara Wartenberg's sign*** may be positive. This sign is elicited by palpating over the closed upper eyelid. Normally, quivering movements of the eyelid will be palpable. On the affected side, this is absent.

Melkersson-Rosanthal syndrome: It is characterized by recurrent orofacial swelling and fissuring of the tongue. It can be associated with a variety of autoimmune disorders.

Bilateral facial paralysis: It is commonly seen in Guillain-Barré syndrome (GBS), Hansen's disease, tick bite, poliomyelitis, vasculitis, infections such as borreliosis and others.

Brainstem lesions: It may be associated with LMN facial palsies. The most common cause is vascular occlusion.

Millard-Gubler syndrome: It is characterized by ipsilateral 6th and 7th palsy and contralateral hemiplegia.

Foville's syndrome: There is ipsilateral gaze palsy and LMN facial palsy along with contralateral hemiplegia.

Eight-and-a-half syndrome: It is the term given to patient having 7th nerve palsy with one-and-a-half syndrome due to PPRF and MLF involvement (see oculomotor nerve above).

Lesions at the cerebellopontine angle such as vascular lesions, tumors and inflammations of the meninges leads to the involvement of the facial nerve along with the trigeminal and auditory nerves. Cerebellar dysfunction may also occur.

VESTIBULOCOCHLEAR NERVE

Syn: Eighth cranial nerve, Auditory nerve

This nerve has its nucleus in the pons. It has two separate components: (1) Auditory (cochlear nerve) for hearing and (2) vestibular for equilibration and balance.

Cochlear system: The end-organs of the cochlear nerve are the hair cells in the organ of Corti, within the cochlea of the inner ear. The central fibers from the cell bodies pass as the cochlear nerve. It traverses the internal auditory meatus, where it is inferolateral to the facial nerve, and it crosses the subarachnoid space at the cerebellopontine angle and enters the upper part of the medulla to terminate in the dorsal and ventral cochlear nuclei. Secondary acoustic fibers project via the trapezoid body and lateral lemniscus to the primary auditory receptive areas in the transverse temporal gyri of Heschl through the auditory radiations. The cochlear nucleus crosses to the contralateral inferior colliculus. They in turn project to medial geniculate body and superior temporal cortex. There is dorsal cochlear nucleus which gives rise to dorsal acoustic striae and ventral cochlear nucleus whose dorsal part gives rise to intermediate, and ventral part gives rise to ventral striae. They decussate in trapezoid body, cross to the contralateral superior olivary complex, lateral leminiscus, inferior colliculus, and show a tonotopic arrangement (each fiber carries a different frequency sound), reach medial geniculate body, the geniculotemporal fibers enter transverse temporal gyri of Heschl. The direct auditory pathway with tonotopic arrangement is called ***core system*** and the secondary one as ***belt system***.

Vestibular system: This system consisting of the semicircular canals has the function of orienting the subject in space (all the three planes), and also maintaining the relative position between the head and the body. Changes in position set up electrical discharges in the neuroepithelium of the ampullae of the semicircular canals and the maculae of the utricle and saccule. Bipolar cells of the Scarpa's ganglion transmit these impulses to the vestibular nuclei of the same, and opposite sides in the upper part of the medulla. The vestibular nucleus has four components: (1) Superior or Bechterew, (2) lateral or Deiters, (3) medial or Schwalbe and (4) inferior or Roller. Their link with semicircular canals is unique. They are linked with medial and lateral vestibulospinal tract, cerebellum and reticular formation. Vestibular nuclei are connected to the cerebellum through the inferior cerebellar peduncle, to the spinal centers through the vestibulospinal tracts and to the motor nuclei of the eye muscles, through the MLF.

Disturbances of vestibular function lead to vertigo, inability to maintain posture, nystagmus and systemic disturbances such as nausea, vomiting, visual hallucination, feeling of rotation of the surroundings, sweating, tachycardia and hypotension. Vertigo, an illusion of movement, is the cardinal symptom of vestibular dysfunction. Rotational vertigo may indicate dysfunction of the semicircular canals or their central connections. A feeling of tilting or linear displacement may occur in disorders affecting otolith organs or their projections. In vertigo, there is a distinct sense of rotation. The objects may seem to revolve around the patient *(objective vertigo)* or the person may experience the sensation of spinning in the surroundings *(subjective vertigo)*.

Testing

In the evaluation of deafness, the term sensorineural deafness indicates lesion proximal to oval window, i.e. cochlea, nerve, nuclei and central pathways. Total deafness is always neural, high-pitched sounds are more difficult to decipher. Tinnitus occurs which varies in pitch and intensity.

At the bedside, the following tests are used to know organic from psychogenic deafness. Look for auditory startle, auditory localization, stethoscope test where a double tube stethoscope is used with the tube to the normal ear blocked. When tapped on diaphragm, if patient is able to hear, it means unilateral deafness may not be present. For bilateral deafness, we have to do swinging voice test where the time taken for the patient to read a passage loud is noted. Then again he is asked to read and the examiner starts reading after he has crossed the first sentence. If patient is truly deaf, he will go on as before but if he is not deaf, he will take longer time or will show intrusions from what the examiner is reading.

Then to type the deafness, tuning forks of 256 Hz or 512 Hz frequency are used.

Schwabach's test: Tuning fork is held in front of mastoid process as long as patient hears and after that placed over the doctor's mastoid process, to compare.

Weber's test: Useful for studying sensorineural or conduction deafness in unilateral disease. Tuning fork is kept over the forehead or nasal bone. In middle ear, deafness sound is localized to the affected ear due to the loss of the dampening effect of bones, it is localized to normal ear in nerve deafness.

Rinne's test: Here, air conduction and bone conduction are compared. When the patient stops hearing over mastoids, it is kept parallel to the sagittal plane of skull 1–2 cm from the ear and normally continues to be heard for twice the time. Bone conduction is better than air conduction in middle ear disease and both are impaired in nerve deafness.

Lesions of the vestibular division present with vertigo, vomiting, horizontal rotary nystagmus and imbalance in gait. It can be peripheral as in benign paroxysmal ver-

tigo, Ménière's disease viral vestibulopathy, middle ear disease, cerebellopontine angle lesions or central lesions due to involvement of the brainstem, vascular anomalies, demyelination, tumors, infections and others.

Caloric tests: Each ear is syringed with warm water (44°C) and cold water (30°C) with the patient resting supine and head flexed to 30° till a jerky nystagmus sets in the slow phase is due to local stimulation, and the fast phase is mediated through cortical connections. Irrigation with cold water produces nystagmus with fast component to the opposite side, nausea, vomiting, tendency to fall to the same side and pastpointing to the opposite side. The nystagmus persists for 90–140 seconds. Syringing with warm water produces nystagmus with the fast component to the same side. The time for onset of nystagmus and its duration are recorded. When there is perforation of the tympanic membrane, water should not be used for the test, instead jets of air at different temperatures can be used.

Significance of caloric tests: The caloric tests depend upon the integrity of the vestibular apparatus, its connections and the higher cortical influences. This test is used in assessing the integrity of these structures. In addition, since the fast phase of the nystagmus is mediated through the cortical connections, in conditions with deepening coma, loss of the fast phase indicates progressive loss of cortical function.

Vertigo

The word is derived from Latin meaning to turn (igo). Feeling of rotation is the classic manifestation of vertigo. Vertigo has to be distinguished from dizziness in which there is no real sense of rotation, but only unsteadiness and tendency to fall. In vertigo there is an illusion of body spinning when in fact it is stationary, this is due to mismatch between visual, vestibular and proprioceptive inputs. It is termed subjective when patient feels he is spinning or objective when the environment is spinning around him. The word dizziness is nonspecific, and indicates maladaptation of the individual with environment which can be light headedness, graying vision, transient ischemic attacks, poor cardiac function, hypotension or stress related.

Causes of Vertigo

Vertigo may be caused by central lesions in the neuraxis or peripheral lesions (cochlea and its connections to the brainstem) (Table 195.8).

Clinical Features

- Vertigo lasts for seconds in benign paroxysmal positional vertigo (BPPV)
- Persists for hours in disorders of the posterior circulation
- For several hours to days in Ménière's disease
- Days to weeks in vestibular neuronitis.

Accompaniments of vertigo include intense fright, nausea, vomiting, generalized sweating and autonomic disturbances.

Bedside evaluation consists of testing nystagmus, deafness, brainstem and cerebellar signs, positioning tests, Tullio phenomena (eye movement induced by loud noise), or eye movements induced by valsalva maneuver (forced expiration against closed glottis) or pressure on

Table 195.8: Causes of vertigo caused by central and peripheral cause

Parameters	Peripheral	Central
Vertigo	Severe	Mild
Autonomic nervous system (ANS)	Severe	Mild
Deafness	+/–	–
Duration	Long	Short
Nystagmus	Mixed	Uniplanar
Fixation	Reduces	No change
Latency	+	–
Fatigability	+	–
Adaptability	+	–
Environment spin	Towards fast phase	Variable
Past pointing	Towards fast phase	Variable
Falling	Towards fast phase	Variable
Head up to affected side	Better	No change
Brainstem signs	–	+

external auditory canal which indicates superior canal dehiscence. Change in head position triggers vertigo in BPPV. This is due to inappropriate detachment of calcium carbonate particles from utricle to one of the semicircular canal.

Management

Appropriate repositioning with Epley's maneuver for anterior and posterior canal and barbecue or Lempert maneuver for horizontal semicircular canal is the treatment of choice. Vestibular neuronitis is seen following respiratory infection, with vertigo and vomiting. Oral methylprednisolone 100 mg, decreased by 20 mg every fourth day for 3–4 weeks gives relief. If associated tinnitus and deafness are present, the diagnosis is Labyrinthitis. Long-term prognosis for complete remission is uncertain. Antihistamine and phenothiazine drugs such as prochlorperazine are helpful (see also treatment for Ménière's disease).

Ménière's Syndrome

Syn: Ménière's disease

It is a disorder of labyrinthine function characterized by recurrent attacks of vertigo associated with tinnitus and deafness. Prosper Ménière, a French physician described the disease. His name was given to the syndrome consisting of vertigo, tinnitus and deafness in 1870, 10 years after his death.

Pathophysiology

Semicircular canals sense linear acceleration and otolith organ senses angular acceleration. A disorder of semicircular canal or its connection will produce feeling of rotation and disease of otolith will produce tilt sensation. The diagnostic criteria include:

- At least two episodes of vertigo of 20 minutes or longer duration
- Hearing loss confirmed by audiometry at least on one occasion
- Tinnitus or aural fullness during the attacks.

It begins in the fifth decade. These attacks last for minutes to an hour. Nystagmus is present during the acute attack with a slow phase towards the affected ear. The

attacks, usually occur in clusters with progressive hearing loss. The pathologic change consists of dilatation of the endolymphatic system with destruction of the cochlear hair cells.

Treatment

It consists of salt restriction to 2.5 g salt/day and drugs.

- Acetazolamide 500–750 mg daily is divided doses which will reduce endolymphatic hydrops.
- Labyrinthine sedatives such as prochlorperazine or cyclizine. Paradoxically, histamine analogs such as betahistine 8 mg given in repeated doses may also help. High-dose long-term betahistine up to 48 mg three times a day for a year or more is recommended. Other mild diuretics, such as low-dose furosemide or amiloride may be tried in resistance cases. Salt restriction (below 4 g sodium chloride per day) and intermittent local instillation of 10–20 mg gentamicin (transtympanically) are useful.
- Anxiolytics such as alprazolam 0.25 mg/tds help to allay fear and insecurity.

Surgical measure used to be done to interrupt labyrinthine afferent impulses. These are not commonly done now. External appliances which counteract the tinnitus by neutralizing the frequencies from the labyrinth are helpful. These have to be made specifically for individual patients.

Labyrinthine adaptive exercises help to reduce the attacks.

GLOSSOPHARYNGEAL AND VAGAL NERVES (CRANIAL NERVES IX AND X)

These two cranial nerves are intimately connected and hence the dysfunction of these nerves overlap. The cranial nerves IX and X arise from medulla, dorsal to inferior olive. They have motor, sensory and autonomic components.

Anatomical Considerations

Glossopharyngeal Nerve

The motor fibers of IX nerve arise from **rostral part of nucleus ambiguous** and it innervates stylopharyngeus. The nuclei of the sensory fibers of the glossopharyngeal nerve are situated in the petrous ganglion which lies within the petrous bone below the jugular foramen and also the superior ganglion, which is small. The sensory fibers supply the faucial tonsils, posterior wall of the pharynx, part of the soft palate and taste sensations from the posterior third of the tongue. The sensory fibers carrying general and taste sensations reach petrous ganglia and tractus solitarius. The Jacobson's nerve supplies the tympanic membrane and parasympathetic which supplies the otic ganglion via lesser superficial petrosal nerve. The postganglionic fibers travel via the auriculotemporal branch of trigeminal nerve and supplies parotid gland. It carries the chemo- and baroreceptors of carotid body via **nerve of Hering**.

Vagus Nerve (Tenth Cranial Nerve)

This consists of several vagal rootlets which leave the skull by jugular foramen. Vagus consists of nerves to somatic organs as well as parasympathetic supply to various autonomic organs in different systems. The nerve has jugular ganglia for general somatic afferents and ganglion nodosa for special and visceral afferents. *Nerve of Arnold* is given off to the external ear in between the two ganglia. Then it gives meningeal branches to meninges of posterior cranial fossa and pharyngeal branches to form the pharyngeal plexus. The superior laryngeal branch gives external laryngeal nerve to cricothyroid and internal laryngeal nerve to larynx. In the neck the cardiac nerves, recurrent laryngeal nerve supply to all muscles of larynx except cricothyroid, then pulmonary, esophageal and abdominal branches to the appropriate organs arise and pass to the different organs.

Dysfunction

In disease of the cranial nerves IX and X, palatal arch becomes low, uvula is drawn to nonparalyzed side and the voice develops a nasal twang. The palate does not elevate on phonation. The vocal cord lies in the cadaveric position in between adduction and abduction. Coughing and respiration are affected more so in bilateral lesion. The cough is devoid of the explosive phase (it is called bovine cough). In nuclear lesions if only the upper part is affected palatopharyngeal paralysis occurs and if only the lower part is affected laryngeal palsy results. When involved with lesions of the nerve XI, it is called *Schmidt's syndrome*. Lesions of X, XI and XII is called *Hughlings Jackson syndrome*. Lesions of superior laryngeal nerve produce mild hoarseness and lesions of recurrent laryngeal nerve produce flaccid dysphonia and hoarseness.

Vagal paralysis leads to mild dysphagia lowering of palatal arch, and absence of gag reflex. Gag reflex is tested by stimulating posterior pharyngeal wall which causes tongue retraction, elevation and constriction of pharyngeal muscle. Supranuclear pathology produces dysphagia if bilateral. Brainstem lesion is identified by the presence of other accompaniments such as long tract signs. *Vernet syndrome* is caused by lesion at jugular foramen with IX, X, XI affected at the retroparotid space. In *Collet-Sicard syndrome*, the nerve XII is also involved.

Glossopharyngeal neuralgia refers to attacks of pain precipitated by cough or swallowing and causes paroxysms of pain, in the distribution of the nerve IX, syncope, salivation, hoarseness, bradycardia and others.

Autonomic disturbance caused by dysfunction of the vagus is described in Chapter 213.

SPINAL ACCESSORY NERVE

(Eleventh cranial nerve)

This has a cranial part starting from medulla and spinal part from spinal cord up to C6. The C1 and C2 innervate ipsilateral sternocleidomastoid and C4 and C5 innervate ipsilateral trapezius muscle. The spinal part enters the skull through foramen magnum and joins the cranial part. The cranial part joins vagus and supplies larynx and pharynx. Supranuclear fibers to trapezius are crossed, those to sternomastoid are mostly ipsilateral. The sternal head which turns the neck to opposite side has bilateral innervation. The clavicular head moves the head to same side.

Both sternomastoids together flex the neck and each one acting separately turns neck to opposite side.

The trapezius muscle elevates the shoulder, flex the neck laterally and acting with other muscles help to steady the shoulder during movements such as raising the arm, rotating the scapula and others.

Paralysis of trapezius produces drooping and squaring of shoulder, winging of the scapula in the upper part, with rotation which worsens with abduction of the arm. There is scapular hump at shoulder arch, and the arm hangs a little lower compared to the normal side. Due to the different patterns of innervation of trapezius and sternomastoid, different functional abnormalities occur in lesions such as hemiplegia. Weakness of trapezius is on the side opposite to pathology but weakness of the strernomastoid is on same side. This leads to head turning away from side of hemiplegia. Classic supranuclear lesion results in dissociated involvement of trapezius and sternomastoid accompanied by hemiplegia. In the brainstem, the nuclei for trapezius muscle are located below the nuclei for sternomastoid and peripherally the branches to both muscles are independent. Therefore in lesions at supranuclear, nuclear and infranuclear levels dissociated involvement of these two muscles can occur. Villaret's syndrome is caused by lesions of IX, X, XI and XII, cranial nerves and sympathetic involvement occurring in retroparotid or retropharyngeal lesions.

HYPOGLOSSAL NERVE

(Twelfth cranial nerve)

This is also a purely motor nerve which supplies the muscles of the tongue. This nerve arises from hypoglossal nucleus which lies in paramedian portion of the medulla in the floor of 4th ventricle. It emerges by a series of rootlets from the medulla between the pyramid and the inferior part of the olive and leaves the skull through the hypoglossal foramen, descends vertically in the neck to the angle of mandible, toward hyoid bone and then enter the tongue to supply the muscles.

Supranuclear fibers are in the lower precentral gyrus on the opposite side. The descending hypoglossal ramus and fibers of cervical C2, C3 nerves form *ansa hypoglossi*.

Testing the Function of the Hypoglossal Nerve

Observe tongue inside and outside mouth, note the movements, palpate the tongue to rule infiltrating lesions and the tone of the muscles, and the power through the cheek. The intrinsic muscles of tongue are superior and inferior longitudanalis, verticalis and transversalis. They are generally involved in degenerative diseases. This leads to difficulty in side to side movements, anteroposterior movements, rolling movements of the tongue both inside and outside the mouth. Supranuclear paralysis causes deviation of tongue to the side of hemiplegia irrespective of whether it is kept inside or outside the mouth.

In UMN disease, there is only movement paralysis. The tongue is shrunk and spastic.

In LMN palsy, the tongue deviates to side of paralysis when kept outside due to unopposed action of opposite genioglossus (which acts only when tongue is protruded) and to same side when tongue is kept inside the mouth due to weakness of ipsilateral hyoglossus (Figs 195.7A and B). In addition to paralysis, there is atrophy (manifested

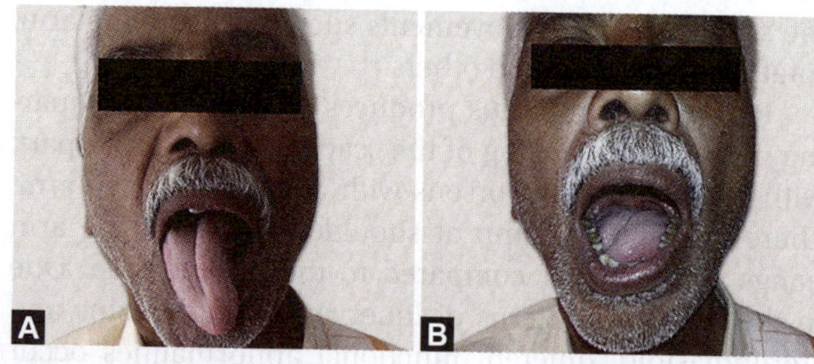

Figs 195.7A and B: Left lower motor neuron (LMN) hypoglossal nerve palsy with and without tongue protrusion

by loss of volume of the tongue and longitudinal folds of the mucous membrane), fibrillations, flaccidity and flaccid dysarthria of lingual type.

Note: Tongue deviates to the left when outside and to right when inside.

Medial medullary syndrome of Dejerine occurs due to occlusion of anterior spinal or vertebral artery causing ipsilateral LMN lesion of the cranial nerve XII, contralateral hemiplegia and loss of proprioceptive sensation.

Garcin syndrome (hemibasal syndrome) is the occurrence of paralysis of all the cranial nerves especially the lower ones in lesions in infiltrating the base of the skull such as secondaries and nasopharyngeal carcinoma, generally in carpeting skull base tumors such as advanced nasopharyngeal carcinomas.

Approach to cranial nerves is a subject by itself. We have just shown the outline and repeated and extended reading is required.

Recommended reading:
* Bing's Local Diagnosis in Neurology
* Adams and Victor's Principles of Neurology, 9th edition

GENERAL POINTS IN LOWER CRANIAL NERVE PALSIES

LMN paralysis of cranial nerves IX, X, XI and XII which arise from the medulla (bulb) occurring in various combinations, constitutes ***bulbar palsy***. UMN lesion affecting these cranial nerves leads to supranuclear bulbar palsy, also known as ***pseudobulbar palsy***. Clinically these two conditions have to be differentiated from each other (Table 195.9). Dysphagia, dysphonia, dysarthria and nasal regurgitation of fluids occur in bulbar as well as pseudo-

Table 195.9: Distinction between bulbar and pseudobulbar palsy

Clinical features	*Bulbar palsy*	*Pseudobulbar palsy*
Emotional lability	Nil	Present
Wasting of tongue and sternomastoid	+	Nil
Fasciculation of tongue and sternomastoid	+ +	Nil
Jaw reflex	Absent	Exaggerated
Type of lesion	LMN	UMN

Abbreviations: LMN = Lower motor neuron; UMN = Upper motor neuron

bulbar palsies. Emotional lability in the form of unprovoked and uncontrollable laughter or crying is an added feature in pseudobulbar palsy. Examination reveals marked wasting and fasciculations of the tongue and sternomastoid muscles in bulbar palsy, but not in pseudobulbar palsy. However in acute bulbar palsy as in diphtheria, poliomyelitis or GBS, there is no time for these muscles to undergo atrophy. The jaw reflex is usually absent in cases of bulbar palsy while it is brisk and exaggerated in pseudobulbar palsy.

LMN Lesions of the Lower Cranial Nerves

* ***Brainstem lesions:*** Vascular occlusions, tumors, motor neuron disease, poliomyelitis, demyelinating diseases including multiple sclerosis and syringobulbia.
* ***Lesions outside the brainstem:*** Fractures of the base of the skull, primary or secondary neoplasms affecting the base of the skull, basal meningitis, tonsilar herniation, coning of the brainstem, paralytic diphtheria, rabies, GBS and others.
* ***Lesions outside the cranial cavity:*** Left recurrent laryngeal nerve may be involved in upper thoracic lesions such as mediastinal tumors or other causes of thoracic outlet syndrome.

UMN Lesions of the Lower Cranial Nerves

These are due to bilateral lesions of the cerebral cortex or corticospinal tracts above the level of the medulla. Common causes include bilateral cerebrovascular accidents, motor neuron diseases, metastatic tumors and degenerative and demyelinating diseases.

Table 195.10 shows the characteristic of multiple cranial nerve palsies in different common intra- and extracranial syndromic lesions.

Table 195.10: Characteristic of multiple cranial nerve palsies in different common intra- and extracranial syndromic lesions

Cranial nerve	Cavernous sinus thrombosis	Superior orbital fissure syndrome	Orbital apex syndrome	Jacoud's (retrosphenoid space) syndrome	Petrous apex gradenigo syndrome	Tolosa-Hunt, lateral cavernous sinus syndrome	CP angle tumor	Vernet's jugular foramen syndrome	Villaret, post retroparotid syndrome	Collet-Sicard syn
II			✓	✓						
III	✓	✓	✓	✓		✓				
IV	✓	✓	✓	✓		✓				
V1	✓			✓	✓	✓				
V2	✓		✓	✓	✓					
V3				✓	✓					
VI		✓	✓	✓	✓	✓		✓		

Contd...

Contd...

Cranial nerve	Cavernous sinus thrombosis	Superior orbital fissure syndrome	Orbital apex syndrome	Jacoud's (retrosphenoid space) syndrome	Petrous apex gradenigo syndrome	Tolosa-Hunt, lateral cavernous sinus syndrome	CP angle tumor	Vernet's jugular foramen syndrome	Villaret, post retroparotid syndrome	Collet-Sicard syn
VII							✓			
VIII							✓			
IX								✓	✓	✓
X								✓	✓	✓
XI								✓	✓	✓
XII									✓	✓
Horner									✓	

Note: Collet-Sicard syndrome is a constellation of cranial nerve palsies due to a lesion at the jugular foramen such as a glomus jugulare tumor or schwannoma.

CHAPTER
196

Coma and Brain Death

SR Chandra, CV Soumya

Chapter Summary

- General Considerations
- Neural Substrates
- Coma
- Brain Death

GENERAL CONSIDERATIONS

Consciousness is such a fascinating elusive phenomenon that nothing worth reading has been written on it (Stuart Sutherland). Consciousness pervades the entire cosmos and is the highest plane of truth in various permutations and combinations and making no hard barriers between anything including the Devas and the other nonhuman neighbors of man (Rigveda). It is a state of normal awareness of the self and surroundings with ability to respond to various types of stimuli, both exogenous and endogenous. Coma is a state of sustained and unarousable state of unconsciousness.

Consciousness has two clinical aspects, namely level of consciousness and content of consciousness. Complete wakefulness is mediated by the reticular activating system and its connections to thalamus but content of consciousness which includes the cognitive and affective aspects is a global cortical function modulated through subcortical interactions.

Levels of Consciousness

The levels of consciousness are assessed using bedside testing and electrical as well as imaging methods.

NEURAL SUBSTRATES

The Ascending Reticular Activating System

This extends from medulla to midbrain, lateral reticular nucleus of thalamus and reaches the cortex as nonspe-cific afferent system. Serotoninergic neurons of midbrain raphe and norepinephric neurons of locus ceruleus (LC) carry excitatory inputs to limbic system. Cholinergic system is concerned with arousal, monoamine system with nonspecific modulating influence. For example, serotonin in sleep, dopamine for alerting, gamma-aminobutyric acid (GABA) for inhibition in neocortex.

Anatomically, coma is due to dysfunction of reticular activating system, bilateral cerebral hemispheres or both simultaneously. Patient remains with eyes closed unarousable and sleep wake cycles are absent, lacks both wakefulness and awareness. Vegetative state is wake-fulness without awareness.

COMA

It is defined as deep unconsciousness from which the patient cannot be aroused even by painful stimuli. When a patient gradually sinks into coma, the following stages are recognizable:

- ***Confusion:*** Inability to think with usual speed and clarity
- ***Drowsiness:*** Inability to sustain wakefulness without the application of external stimuli
- ***Stupor:*** Patient can be aroused only by vigorous and repeated external stimuli. Catatonic stupor refers to a state where patient lacks motor or verbal response with normal perception
- ***Turiya avastha:*** This Sanskrit term is used in philosophical discourses in which the person can attain this state by calm meditation and practice.

Fourth state: A state of awake, awareness but inactive externally and active internally. There is electrocerebral silence but highest intellectual activity is carried out.

Causes of Coma

The causes are herniations of brain structures, brainstem lesions, metabolic problems, drugs and toxins.

Herniations

Lateral herniation

Lateral temporal lobe masses push the uncus anteriorly and parahippocampal gyrus posteriorly against the free edge of the tentorium and the ipsilateral midbrain. Ipsilateral pupil becomes progressively dilated and sluggishly reacting to light. Midbrain is pressed against the opposite side of dura producing pressure on opposite temporal lobe causing hemiparesis ipsilateral to side of disease. This is called *Kernohan's phenomena*.

When there is increased intracranial pressure and the compliance of brain cannot compensate, the brain is squeezed through subfalcial, tentorial and transforaminal gaps in an upward plane resulting in compression of vital brainstem structures.

Central herniation

The frontal, parietal and occipital masses buckle on the midbrain causing a rostrocaudal deterioration starting with diencephalic stage and terminating at medullary stage.

Upward herniation

Transtentorial upward herniation occurs with infra-tentorial lesions causing midbrain and cerebellar features.

Neurological Causes

- Ischemia to the brain and brainstem, e.g. stroke, Stokes-Adam attacks, low cardiac output states and cardiac arrest
- Infections, e.g. meningitis, encephalitis
- Rise in intracranial tension due to various causes
- Physical agents, e.g. craniocerebral injuries, hyperpyrexia, hypothermia
- Degenerative disease, e.g. Tay-Sachs disease, Creutzfeldt-Jakob disease
- Demyelination—postvaccinal, infective and allergic causes
- Seizure disorders like status epilepticus.

Systemic Diseases

- **Metabolic causes:** Hyperglycemia, hypoglycemia, hyponatremia, hypernatremia, hypocalcemia, hypercalcemia, hypophosphatemia, acidosis, alkalosis hyperosmolar states, respiratory failure, hepatic failure, renal failure vitamin deficiencies and endocrine disorders such as hypothyroidism, Addison's disease and hypopituitarism.
- **Poisoning:** Alcohol, narcotics and other poisons like cobra and krait bites.
- **Infections:** Several infections affecting the brain or meninges directly as in meningitis and encephalitis lead to coma. Others give rise to toxic encephalopathy, e.g. septicemias, septic shock, salmonellosis.

Psychiatric Disorders

Though these are not comatose states, their presentation may very closely resemble that of coma from which they have to be distinguished, e.g. *catatonic stupor* and *hysterical coma*. Patients hold eyes forcibly closed. This is called *Rosenbach's sign*. The patient may keep eye fixed or make quick blinks in between, but lacks any other abnormality.

Source: Plum F, Posner JB. [The diagnosis of stupor and coma]. Brain Nerve. 2015;67(3):344-5.

In case of nontraumatic coma extending for at least 5–6 hours, the common causes are:

- Sedative drugs with or without alcohol—40%
- Cerebral hypoxic and ischemic damage caused by cardiac arrest and anesthetic accidents—25%
- Stroke and subarachnoid hemorrhage—15%
- Infections and metabolic derangements—15%.

Mechanisms of Coma

General mechanisms leading to coma are:

- Reduction in blood supply of brain
- Lesions affecting reticular formation
- Electrical disturbances as in seizure disorders
- Metabolic disturbances leading to dysfunction of cellular processes in neurons.

Examination of a Comatose Patient

History

The history given by immediate attendants and circumstances of the illness give valuable clue to the diagnosis. The onset, recent symptoms like headache, fever, depression and trauma are often helpful. Past medical history like diabetes mellitus (DM), liver disease, heart disease and others should be elicited.

General examination should be done after stabilizing the vital signs.

General appearance

- Look for evidence of trauma—bleeding from nose or ears which suggests fracture of skull base
- Tongue lacerations/urinary incontinence suggest seizures
- Cushingoid habitus may suggest Addisonian crisis due to withdrawal of oral steroids
- Emaciation may be a feature of carcinoma, Addison's disease, human immunodeficiency virus (HIV) infection or Wernicke's encephalopathy
- Features of chronic liver disease or chronic kidney disease (CKD).

Vital signs

- **Temperature:** Hypothermia in hypothyroidism, hypopituitarism, cold exposure, hyperthermia in sepsis, thyrotoxicosis and pontine or hypothalamic lesions.
- **Breathing pattern**
  - **Acidotic breathing**
    - Diabetic ketoacidosis
    - Cheyne-Stokes breathing in bihemispheric or diencephalic dysfunction, congestive cardiac failure (CCF)
    - Respiratory depression in metabolic or toxic causes
    - Central neurogenic hyperventilation (CNH) in upper pontine lesions.
  - **Heart rate:** Bradycardia occurs in raised intracranial tension, heart block occurs in organo-

phosphorus-poisoning, tachycardia occurs in hypovolemia and thyrotoxicosis

- ***Hypotension/hypertension:*** Hypotension occurs in hypovolemia, sepsis, Addison's disease and hypertension occurs in raised intracranial tension, hypertensive crisis secondary to subarachnoid hemorrhage (SAH), etc.
- ***Skin:*** Pallor, jaundice, cyanosis, purpuric rashes of meningococcemia, vesicles of Herpes simplex/varicella and bullous lesions in sepsis and barbiturate poisoning should be looked for. Signs of repeated venepunctures may be seen in intravenous (IV) drug abusers.

- ***Odor of breath:*** Smell of alcohol, fetor hepaticus of hepatic encephalopathy and poisons like organophosphorus, industrial chemicals and solvents should be looked for.

Signs of systemic or intracranial infection like neck stiffness should be elicited.

Cardiovascular examination to exclude cardiac lesions which may be the cause of cerebral emboli or infective endocarditis.

Detection of the Site of Pathology

To know the site of pathology, the following parameters are assessed—the status of the circulation, respiration, pupil reactions, eye movements and motor functions.

- ***Circulatory changes:*** Circulatory changes like Kocher-Cushing response, increasing blood pressure, decreasing heart rate, electrocardiography (ECG)-showing large upright T, long QT, ST, atrial fibrillation (AF), supraventricular tachycardia (SVT), bradycardia, atrioventricular block (AV block) and ventricular fibrillation (VF) should be looked for.
- ***Respiratory centers:*** These are apneustic center in pons and expiratory and inspiratory centers in the medulla. ***Posthyperventilation apnea*** is a test done in patients who can cooperate. The patient is asked to take five breaths which lower the PCO_2 by 10 mm Hg. This causes about 10 seconds of apnea in normal people. This is prolonged in patients with bihemispheric disease. Respiratory changes seen are:
  - Cheyne-Stokes respiration in forebrain insult
  - Hyperventilation is seen in patients with problems in pons and midbrain
  - Apneustic center lesions cause prolonged inspiratory pause seen in lateral tegmentum and lower pons lesions
  - Cluster breathing shows a cluster of breathing followed by an irregular sequence in ponto-medullary lesions
  - Ataxic breathing is irregular and indicates damage to dorsomedial medulla
  - Selective impairment of voluntary respiration seen in bilateral tegmental involvement is called ***Ondine's curse.***
    - ***Congenital central hypoventilation syndrome (Ondine's curse):*** Patient has failure of natural reflex respiration and patient survives only on voluntary respiration. When the patient sleeps, voluntary respiration may stop leading to fatal apnea. This is seen in lesions of the tegmentum.

- Examination of eyes and pupils
- Pupils light reflex is resistant to metabolic insult with a few exceptions.

Pupils

Inequality of the pupils suggest transtentorial herniation. The dilated nonreactive pupil is the result of oculomotor paralysis, which may be due to involvement of the nerve or its nuclei in the midbrain. Fixed dilated pupils can be a terminal phenomenon. Bilateral pinpoint pupils reacting to light are seen in pontine and thalamic hemorrhage. Pinpoint pupils not reacting to light are seen in organophosphorus compounds and narcotic poisoning, e.g. morphine.

Diencephalic pupil is a small reacting pupil. Unilateral hypothalamic damage causes small pupil and loss of sweating on the same side. Midbrain tectal lesions cause loss of light reflex and the pupils show hippus (alternate constriction and dilatation). The pupils dilate due to ciliospinal reflex elicited by pinching neck. Tegmental lesion produces irregular dilation of pupil causing pear-shaped pupil called ***corectopia***.

Examination of Optic Fundus

Look for papilledema and retinal abnormalities to exclude raised intracranial tension. This is absolutely necessary before lumbar puncture is attempted.

Movements of Eyes and Eyelids

Abnormalities in Resting Position

- ***Lateral conjugate deviation:*** It occurs in cerebral disease towards the side of pathology in cortical lesions and away from the site of pathology in pontine lesions. In tectal and thalamic lesions, the eyeballs are depressed and converged. Eyeballs deviate to the opposite side in cerebellar hemorrhage. Several combinations of eye movement abnormalities localize to various brainstem regions.
- ***Spontaneous eye movements:*** Subtle nystagmus may suggest ongoing seizure activity. Roving eye movements elicited by turning the head from side to side suggest intact brainstem function.

Oculocephalic Reflex (Reflex Eye Movements)

This is tested by turning the head of the patient firmly to either side by 90° and then passively flexing and extending the neck. The eyes move opposite to the movement of the head. These ***doll's eye movements*** depend on the intactness of the third, fourth and sixth cranial nerves and their nuclei, the labyrinth, otoliths and their central connections in the brainstem including the vestibular nuclei and medial longitudinal fasciculi. Unilateral absence of doll's eye movement suggests ipsilateral pontine lesion. The doll's eye movements are totally abolished in extensive structural damage to the brainstem and deep metabolic coma including drugs. ***However, this test should not be performed when injury to the cervical spine is suspected.***

The Caloric Tests

These tests give information of the integrity of the vestibular apparatus, its connections in the brainstem and with higher cortical centers. In deepening coma, when cortical function becomes progressively depressed, the fast phase of the nystagmus tends to disappear. Caloric test is done after excluding perforation of tympanic membrane. On irrigating the ear with 50 mL of cold water in normal persons, eyes deviate slowly toward the irrigated ear and then compensatory nystagmus with fast component opposite to the irrigated ear occurs. In comatose patients, eyes tonically deviate to irrigated side and nystagmus is not seen. Complete absence of ocular movement on caloric testing indicates irreversible damage to the brainstem. Cold water induces nystagmus to opposite ear and warm water to same side which can be remembered by the mnemonic **COWS**. Bilateral vestibular stimulation with cold water induces nystagmus with fast component upward and warm downward.

Posture

Coma with focal signs is often due to structural brain disease. Coma without focal signs is often due to drugs and metabolic problems and not due to structural damage.

In coma due to structural lesions in the brain such as tumor, hemorrhage, infarct and others the patient may assume certain postures unilaterally or bilaterally either spontaneously or in response to painful stimuli.

Decerebrate Posture

It is characterized by tonic extension and internal rotation of the upper extremity and tonic extension and plantar flexion of the lower extremity associated with jaw clenching and head retraction. It is important to recognize this grave sign because it indicates dysfunction of upper brainstem between the superior colliculus of the midbrain and vestibular nuclei in the pons. Decerebrate posture is caused by uninhibited vestibulospinal discharges indicating site of pathology above vestibular nucleus.

Decorticate Posture

It is characterized by tonic flexion of the forearms at the elbow, adduction and flexion of the arm at the shoulder and flexion of the fingers, with tonic extension of the lower extremity, either on one or both sides. This is seen in lesions above the brainstem, affecting the cortex or the corticospinal tracts. It indicates uninhibited rubrospinal discharges.

Diagnosis of Coma

In neurological disorders, localizing signs pointing to damage to parts of the nervous system may be present such as hemiplegia, cranial nerve palsies or focal seizures. Meningitis and subarachnoid hemorrhage are associated with signs of meningeal irritation such as neck rigidity, Kernig's sign and Brudzinski's signs. In metabolic coma, localizing signs may be absent. In poisoning, other effects of the poison may also be evident.

Differential Diagnosis of Coma

- Coma with focal or lateralizing neurological signs, e.g. cerebral tumor, cerebral hemorrhage, infarction, abscess
- Coma without focal-neurological signs, but with signs of meningeal irritation, e.g. meningitis, encephalitis, subarachnoid hemorrhage
- Coma without focal or lateralizing neurological signs is often anoxic—ischemic lesions, metabolic disorders, intoxications, systemic infections, seizures, physical agents such as heat or cold.

Investigations

- Complete urinalysis, estimation of blood sugar, urea, creatinine, blood counts, liver function tests (LFTs), electrolytes, chest X-ray, electrocardiogram (ECG), blood gases and pH
- In suspected poisoning, the gastric contents, blood, urine and other materials should be sent for chemical examination
- Cerebrospinal fluid (CSF) for meningitis, encephalitis, subarachnoid hemorrhage or meningeal leukemia
- Electroencephalogram (EEG), computed tomography (CT) scanning and magnetic resonance imaging (MRI)—based on need.

Glasgow Coma Scale

An objective method of evaluating the depth of coma is the Glasgow coma scale. Recording the progress of the patient by this method is extremely useful for initial assessment and follow-up in cases of coma due to head trauma and cardiorespiratory arrest (Table 196.1).

A conscious individual will have a score of 15. The score progressively diminishes as the coma deepens. The fallacy of this scale is that even a dead person will have a score of 3.

Four score (found unresponsive) is a recently validated score which assesses eye opening, motor response, respiration and brainstem reflexes with each item scored 0–4.

Electroencephalography-based Classification

Alpha coma is a condition in which the EEG tracing is replaced by alpha waves which are unresponsive. This occurs in brainstem pathology. Beta coma is often caused by drugs. ***Theta-delta coma*** occurs in structural disease or advanced metabolic disease. Spindle coma indicates that the brain is capable of generating spindles

Table 196.1: Glasgow coma scale

Test	Response	Scoring
Eye opening	Spontaneous	4
	To sound	3
	To pain	2
	Nil	1
Motor movements (M)	Obeys command	6
	Localizes pain	5
	Normal flexion withdrawal	4
	Abnormal flexion (decorticate rigidity)	3
	Extension (decerebrate rigidity)	2
	No response	1
Verbal response (V)	Well-oriented	5
	Disoriented and confused	4
	Inappropriate words	3
	Incomprehensible sound	2
	None	1

Table 196.2: Clinical conditions mimicking coma

Features	Awareness	Wakefulness	Brainstem respiratory cycles	Motor reflexes	EEG	Evoked potential
Coma	–	–	±	±	Abnormal	Abnormal
Brain death	–	–	–	–	Silence	Absent
Vegetative stage	–	Present, intact sleep wakefulness rhythm	+	±	Abnormal	Abnormal
Minimally conscious state	Intact but poor response	+	+	±	Nonspecific	Abnormal
Locked-in syndrome	Intact but communication poor	+	+	Quadriplegia Pseudobulbar palsy	Normal	Abnormal

Abbreviations: EEG = Electroencephalogram; + = Normal; – = Absent; ± = Variable

and therefore the lesion is above hypothalamus. The term *spindle coma* is used to denote coma in which the EEG pattern is similar to the spindles usually seen in normal non-rapid eye movement (NREM) second stage spindle sleep. Presence of spindles in EEG is a strong pointer to the localization of the cause. Burst suppression pattern and triphasic waves are seen in severe metabolic disease.

Conditions Mimicking Coma

Differential diagnosis of coma includes brain death, vegetative state, minimally conscious state *locked-in syndrome*, catatonic stupor and hysterical behavior.

Clinical conditions mimicking coma are shown in Table 196.2.

Locked-in Syndrome

The locked in syndrome is not a disorder of consciousness. This is a condition in which voluntary control of almost all body movements is abolished with intact consciousness and cognition. This state of profound paralysis may be mistaken for coma. In many cases, it is due to a disorder of the ventral pons. End-stage Parkinsonism and even some cases of lower motor disease like extensive radiculoneuropathy produce the locked-in state.

Akinetic Mutism

The patient is silent and inert due to lesions of anterior parts of frontal lobes. He is extremely apathetic but sensorimotor functions are not lost.

Minimally Conscious State

This is a state of severely impaired consciousness with minimal but definite awareness of self or environment. Here, patient responds in a rudimentary way like gesturing or producing simple words. Seen in patients with thalamic lesions.

Persistent Vegetative State

Vegetative state denotes a state of wakefulness without awareness. Sleep-wake cycles mediated by reticular system are preserved but higher functions are lost. Brainstem regulation of cardiopulmonary function and visceral autonomic regulation with crude sleep-wake cycling and some spontaneous limb, eye, swallowing, grimacing, grunting movements may be preserved. There is loss of sphincter control. All signs of conscious perception and deliberate action are abolished.

The *Multi-Society Task Force* on persistent vegetative state has concluded that vegetative state lasting for more than 12 months after traumatic brain injury and 3 months after anoxic brain injury are very unlikely to improve.

Management of a Comatose Patient

General Management

Comatose patient are very susceptible to develop several complications as a result of loss of protective reflexes and these have to be prevented.

Maintenance of the Airway

Maintenance of the airway is of utmost importance. The neck has to be kept extended to prevent *falling-back* of the tongue. If necessary, a patent airway should be introduced. Secretions have to be removed by postural drainage and suction. In cases with respiratory depression, assisted ventilation has to be instituted early. Tracheostomy may be required in some cases to facilitate ventilation and clearance of the airway. Ideally, all patients with Glasgow coma scale less than or equal to 8 should be intubated. Maintenance of nutrition, fluid and electrolyte balance, seizures, care of eyes and prevention of pressure palsies are all important. Adequate nutrition (at least 2,000 cal/day and 2 L of fluid) in the form of milk, sugar, eggs, cereals, salt and water are given through a nasogastric tube. Oral feeding carries the risk of aspiration into the respiratory tract and therefore, this should be avoided. Parenteral nutrition is started with aseptic precautions and position of the needle should be changed every 36–48 hours to avoid thrombophlebitis. This should be undertaken only by physicians conversant with the procedure since infections and other complications are common in such patients.

Care of the Skin

Bedsores develop due to continuous pressure on localized areas. This risk is avoided by turning the patient in bed every 2–4 hours, hand-keeping the skin clean and dry. Adequate intake of proteins and special beds are useful.

Care of Bladder and Bowel

Institution of a closed drainage system for the bladder helps to avoid soiling of the clothes and prevents infection. Bowels are moved by enemas or suppositories at regular intervals.

Positioning of the Limbs and Physiotherapy

The limbs should be maintained in optimal position to avoid fixed deformities. Regular passive movements of the limbs and pneumatic compression devices help to prevent venous thrombosis (VT) and subsequent pulmonary embolism (PE). Heparin 5,000 units 12th hourly can be given in special cases depending upon the indications.

Specific therapy and prognosis depends on the cause. If the reflexes and corneal responses do not recover, persistent atonia, absent cortical component of somatosensory evoked potential for several hours useful recovery is less likely.

BRAIN DEATH

It is defined as the irreversible loss of all functions of the brain, including the brainstem. *The three essential findings in brain death are coma, absence of brainstem reflexes including apnea and irreversibility.* Most common cause is cardiac arrest persisting for over three minutes. Other causes include traumatic damage to the brainstem, extensive infarction and others.

Brain death has become an important issue since removal of organs for transplantation is done from comatose patients who are unlikely to recover. Patients who are on supportive measures including artificial ventilation may pass into a stage where the cerebral and brainstem functions are irreversibly lost, still the patient may continue to have circulation on account of the supportive measures. Withdrawal of these supports will lead to physical death. The decision to withdraw these supports is a medicolegal one.

Prerequisites Before Diagnosing Brain Death

History and Examination to Find Out the Clear Etiology of Unresponsiveness

Exclusion of reversible causes—rule out hypothermia, hypovolemic shock, anesthetics, neuromuscular blockade, alcohol and central nervous system (CNS) depressants, metabolic causes like hepatic failure, renal failure, hypophosphatemia, hyperosmolar state and others.

Complete neurological examination—absence of motor or verbal response to pain, absence of seizures and brainstem reflexes like pupillary, oculocephalic, corneal, cough, gag reflex and oculovestibular reflexes. Reflexes mediated by cranial nerves are absent whereas spinal reflexes may be present. *Two assessments should be done at least 6 hours apart.*

Apnea test is usually performed after the second examination. It is positive if there is no respiratory effort even with hypercarbia. Euthermia and euvolemia should be ensured before proceeding to apnea test and preoxygenation is done with 100% oxygen delivered through a nasal cannula to keep the arterial PO_2 more

than 200. Watch for respiratory efforts closely. Connect ventilator back if pulse oximeter shows hypoxemia or patient develops hypotension or arrhythmias. If arterial PCO_2 is more than 60 mm Hg or rises more than 20 mm Hg from the baseline and even then there is no discernible respiratory effort, apnea test is declared positive.

In some patients, cervical spine injuries or cardiovascular instability may limit the clinical declaration of brain death. In that case, confirmatory tests are useful. These are:

- *Transcranial Doppler test:* This shows small systolic peaks without diastolic flow, or reverberating flow in the basal vessels indicating very high vascular resistance associated with greatly increased intracranial pressure (ICP).
- *Electroencephalography (EEG):* Absence of electrical activity of more than 2 mV for at least 30 minutes with EEG meeting the technical criteria set by the American Electroencephalographic Society, with at least 16 electrodes
- *Angiography:* Angiography is performed by conventional, CT, MRI or radionuclide methods. There will be no intracerebral filling at the level of the carotid bifurcation or circle of Willis whereas external carotid circulation may be normal
- *Single-photon emission CT:* Absence of uptake of Tc-99m hexamethylpropylene amine oxime (HMPAO) isotope in brain parenchyma and/or vasculature, described as *hollow skull phenomenon*
- *Somatosensory evoked potentials:* Brain death confirmed by bilateral absence of N20–P22 response with median nerve stimulation.

As per the Transplantation of Human Organs Act (THOA), brain death should be declared and form number 8 should be signed by 4 doctors before withdrawing life support measures—(1) Registered Medical Practitioner (RMP) in-charge of the hospital in which the event has occurred; (2) an independent RMP nominated from the panel of names approved by the appropriate authority; (3) neurologist/neurosurgeon and (4) RMP and the treating doctor.

In children, brain death should be declared only after the 7th postnatal day and period of observation should be at least 48 hours in neonates and 24 hours in infants. Adverse prognostic factors include:

- Absence of pupillary, occulovestibular and corneal reflexes
- Persistent atonia
- Absence of the cortical component of the sensory evolved potentials for several hours.

These indicate that the chances for recovery are unlikely.

CHAPTER
197

Headache

AS Girija

Chapter Summary

- General Considerations
- Classification
- Migraine
- Other Common Secondary Headaches
- Diagnosis
- Management

GENERAL CONSIDERATIONS

Headache is one of the most common and yet the most difficult clinical problem encountered by the physician. Though the term **headache** can mean pain anywhere in the head, it is usually confined to pain arising in the region of the cranial vault. Most often headache is a symptomatic expression of some minor ailment, mental tension or fatigue and in vast majority of cases, the cause is non-neurological. Occasionally, it is of sinister significance, indicative of serious intracranial disease.

Pain in the head may arise from different structures, which include:

- The cranial vault consisting of skin, subcutaneous tissue, muscles, arteries and periosteum of skull
- Intracranial venous sinuses and their tributaries
- Intracranial arteries before they penetrate brain parenchyma
- Meninges at the base of the brain
- Trigeminal, glossopharyngeal, vagal and the first three cervical nerves
- Structures of eye, ear and nasal cavity.

CLASSIFICATION

The third international classification of headache is into three major categories—(1) Primary headache, (2) Secondary headache and (3) Painful cranial neuropathies and other headache disorders (Table 197.1).

Primary Headache Syndromes

- Migraine and related disorders
- Tension type headache
- Trigeminal autonomic cephalalgias
- Other primary headache disorders.

Secondary Headache

- Headache attributed to trauma or injury to the head
- Headache attributed to cranial or cervical vascular disorders
- Headache attributed to nonvascular intracranial disorder
- Headache attributed to a substance or its withdrawal
- Headache attributed to infection
- Headache attributed to disorders of homeostasis
- Headache or facial pain attributed to disorder of the cranium, neck, eyes, ears, nose, sinuses, teeth, mouth, or other facial or cervical region
- Headache attributed to psychiatric disorders.

Other Headache Syndromes

Painful cranial neuropathies and other facial pains. Headaches not elsewhere classified (Table 197.2).

Headache as a symptom constitutes 30% cases attending the neurology out-patient (OP) and about 10–15% in a medical OP. It is important to take a detailed history to arrive at a proper diagnosis and to decide if patient needs detailed investigations. The important primary headache syndromes are one of the most common cause of headache and among this, migraine tops the list followed by tension headache. The rare varieties of the primary headache syndromes like coital, hypnic headache are dealt with. The secondary headaches are mentioned in the respective chapters and are not discussed in this section except drug-induced headache and that associated with psychiatric disorders. The readers can refer monographs for detailed accounts.

MIGRAINE

The most common form of vascular headache is migraine (megrim means hemicranial). Migraine is characterized by episodic, throbbing hemicranial headache, beginning

Table 197.1: Types of primary and secondary headache

Primary headache		Secondary headache	
Type	**%**	**Type**	**%**
Tension-type	69	Systemic infection	63
Migraine	16	Head injury	4
Idiopathic stabbing	2	Vascular disorders	1
Exertional	1	Subarachnoid hemorrhage	< 1
Cluster	0.1	Brain tumor	0.1

Table 197.2: Extracranial and intracranial pain sensitive structures

Extracranial pain sensitive structures	Intracranial pain sensitive structures
• Sinuses • Eyes/orbits • Ears • Teeth • Temporomandibular joints (TMJ) • Blood vessels • 5, 7, 9 and 10 cranial nerves carry pain from these structures	• Arteries of circle of Willis and proximal dural arteries • Dural venous sinuses, veins • Meninges • Dura

in childhood, adolescence or early adult life with a tendency to decrease in intensity and frequency as age advances. It is estimated that 5% of the population suffers from migraine. Women are slightly more affected. In many cases, a positive family history is elicitable.

Mechanism of Migraine

Current thinking has moved away from vascular dysregulation as a primary cause of migraine. It is now believed that vasodilation and vasoconstriction are probably epiphenomena and that neuronal dysfunction is the possible primary driver in the pathophysiology of the disorder. Specifically, activation of the trigeminovascular system, cortical spreading depression and neuronal sensitization are seen as playing important roles in migraine pathophysiology. Sensory neurons from the trigeminal ganglion and upper cervical dorsal roots innervate dural-vascular structures (e.g. pial vessels, dura mater and large cerebral vessels). Input from dural-vascular structures and from cervical structures through the upper cervical dorsal root ganglia project to second order neurons in the trigeminocervical complex (TCC), then to the thalamus and then to the sensory cortex. Distribution of headache pain to regions of the upper neck and head can be attributed to the convergence of projections from the trigeminal nerve at the trigeminal nucleus caudalis and upper cervical nerve root. Sensory modulation can occur via both direct and indirect projection, by descending influences such as those from the hypothalamus, midbrain periaqueductal gray (PAG), pontine locus coeruleus (LC) and nucleus raphe magnus onto the TCC.

Cortical spreading depression, a self-propagating wave of cellular depolarization that slowly spreads across the cerebral cortex, has been linked to migraine aura and headache. Cortical spreading depression is thought to activate neurons in the trigeminal nucleus caudalis, leading to inflammatory changes in pain-sensitive meningeal vascular structures, which produces headache via central and peripheral reflex mechanisms.

Neuronal sensitization in the primary afferent neuron and central sensitization of higher-order neurons of the spinal cord and brain have been shown to play an important role in somatic pain. It is likely that many of the symptoms of migraine, including throbbing headache pain, exacerbation of headache by physical activity and allodynia are linked to sensitization.

Migraine with aura or classic migraine: Here, the episode begins with prominent neurologic symptoms *(auras)* such as visual disturbances like dazzling zig-zag lines, spreading scotoma, homonymous hemianopia, field defects or rarely total blindness, sensory disturbances affecting one-half of the body, disturbances of speech or hemiparesis. These neurologic symptoms last for 15–30 minutes and usually merge into a hemicranial or generalized throbbing headache with nausea and vomiting, all of which may last even for 1–2 days. In the majority of cases, the duration is much shorter. Many complain of photophobia and phonophobia during the attacks.

Migraine without aura or common migraine: Here, there is no preceding neurological symptom, but there is unheralded onset of headache, nausea and vomiting following the same sequence.

Diagnosis of both classic and common types of migraine is made mainly from history. Long duration of illness, onset during childhood, positive family history and relief with ergot derivatives are in favor of migraine. Migraine has to be differentiated from other organic disorders such as raised intracranial tension, subarachnoid hemorrhage (SAH) and arteriovenous malformations (AVM).

Course and prognosis: In the majority of patients, migraine tends to be chronic with periods of exacerbation and remission. With increasing age, the attacks tend to come down. Complications may occur rarely in some cases. These include cerebrovascular accidents, ocular and other cranial nerve palsies.

Treatment

The physician should give full explanation of the nature and phenomena of migraine to the patient and this often relieves the patient's anxiety and helps to restore his morale. All known precipitating factors such as emotional tension, exposure to cold, foods such as cheese and chocolates should be avoided. Hypoglycemia is a common precipitating factor and this should be avoided by proper timing of meals.

Many cases are made symptom-free by simple analgesics such as aspirin in a dose of 900 mg or paracetamol 0.5–1 g given at suitable intervals. Non-steroidal anti-inflammatory drugs (NSAIDs) such as ibuprofen, naproxen and mefenamic acid are good alternatives. If nausea and vomiting are troublesome, metoclopramide 10 mg or domperidone 30 mg may be helpful. These drugs often help to abort an attack if given early. The specific drug which helps to abort an attack if taken at the earliest symptom is *ergotamine* which is a nonselective 5-hydroxytryptamine agonist, in a dose of 1 mg. Available preparations include sublingual tablets of 1 mg, chewable tablets, subcutaneous (SC) injection (0.25 mg) or aerosols. If the drug is taken after the headache has set in, higher doses and repeated medication may be needed. In any case, the weekly dose should not exceed 12 mg. Ergotamine preparations are contraindicated during pregnancy and in patients with ischemic heart disease, hypertension and peripheral occlusive vascular disease.

Adverse side effects include nausea, muscle cramps and peripheral vasoconstriction. Other drugs which can terminate an attack are metoclopramide 10 mg intravenous (IV) and prochlorperazine 10 mg IV.

Selective Serotonin Receptor Modifying Drugs in Migraine

The serotonin receptors $5HT_1$, $5HT_2$ and $5HT_3$ are relevant to migraine. $5HT_1$ inhibitory receptors produce vasoconstriction. $5HT_2$ receptors are excitatory. Drugs such as cyproheptadine, propranolol and methysergide are $5HT_2$ antagonists.

$5HT_1$ receptors are subclassified into $5HT_{1A}$, $5HT_{1B}$, $5HT_{1D}$ and $5HT_{1F}$. Most of the triptan drugs which act in acute migraine act as agonists on $5HT_{1B}$ or $5HT_{1D}$.

Sumatriptan was the first drug of this class introduced to stop acute migraine attacks.

It is effective in the treatment of acute attacks of migraine, complicated migraine and cluster headache (CH). The dose is 50–100 mg to be taken soon after the onset of migraine. For the same attack, a second dose should not be given. If migraine attacks recur, doses up to 300 mg can be given in 24 hours.

A parenteral preparation of sumatriptan is available for SC injection in a dose of 6 mg as soon as possible after the onset. Peak plasma levels are reached in 20 minutes. For the same attack of migraine, the drug should not be repeated.

A second dose can be given for subsequent attacks up to a total dose of 12 mg in 24 hours.

Side effects include tingling, feeling of tightness of the different parts of the body, flushing, transient rise in blood pressure, hypotension, brady- or tachycardia and seizures. A nasal spray preparation has also been introduced.

Newer analogs are available for treatment of acute attacks of migraine. These include zolmitriptan, naratriptan, rizatriptan, almotriptan and others. Side effects, especially cardiac side effects are less for the newer analogs.

Rizatriptan is available in India. It is given in a dose of 5–10 mg at the onset of the attack.

Drug prophylaxis: This is employed to prevent migraine attacks and allay their severity. The commonly used drugs include:

- Propranolol 10–40 mg/day bd or tid. It can produce night terrors in children.
- Cyproheptadine 4 mg hs.
- ***Calcium channel blockers (CCBs):*** Verapamil 40–60 mg bd. Flunarizine 5–10 mg hs and is of particular use in children.

These drugs have to be continued at first for 6 months after which the case has to be reviewed for continuation of therapy. In asthmatic subjects, propranolol may have to be replaced by more selective beta-adrenergic blockers.

Topiramate 25 mg starting with 12.5 mg bd may be stepped up to 50 mg bd or less in cases which are resistant to propranolol or in whom it cannot be tolerated due to side effects.

Divalproex sodium in doses up to 500 mg bd may also be useful.

General measures such as regulated life, physical exercise, avoidance of smoking and leisure activities are important to prevent relapse.

Chronic Daily Headache

This term denotes presence of headache for more than 15 days in a month for longer than 3 months. The term ***transformed migraine*** is used to denote a condition where classic migraine is altered, to assume the character of chronic daily headache, often due to overuse of drugs. The term ***medication overuse headache*** is given to conditions where headache is present at least for 15 days a month, associated with worsening of the headache during medication overuse and reversion to previous episodic pattern (<15 days per month) within 2 months after withdrawal of the medication.

Transformed migraine is an iatrogenic condition in which head pain occurs daily or almost daily (>15 days per month), each attack lasting for 4 hours or more and worsening over the previous 3 months. At some point of time, features of episodic migraine meeting the International Headache Society (IHS) criteria, may be elicitable. The reason for this transformation is not clear. The IHS criteria for migraine without an aura include the following:

- At least five attacks that last for 4–72 hours—untreated or successfully treated.
- Headache must have at least two of the characteristics: Unilateral location, pulsating quality and moderate or severe pain intensity, avoidance of usual physical activities such as walking or climbing stairs.
- These attacks themselves should be accompanied by at least one of the features such as nausea, vomiting, phonophobia not accountable by other conditions. Most patients with transformed migraine and medication overuse headache are women and they have a history of episodic migraine from adolescence or early adulthood.

The transformation from ***migraine*** to ***transformed migraine*** occurs over a period of months or years and the clinical picture is a mixture of tension type headache and migraine.

The overuse of acute-headache medications such as aspirin, acetaminophen, caffeine, ergot, opioids or triptans by patients with frequent headache gives rise to medication overuse headache which occurs almost daily (at least more than 15 days a month) and maintained by the same medications used to relieve pain. Withdrawal of medication relieves the headache dramatically. Once the drugs are withdrawn, the headache reverts to the original pretreatment pattern within months.

Management of Transformed Migraine and Medication Overuse Headache

- Withdrawal of the offending medications
- Lifestyle changes including regular exercise, leisure activities
- Yoga and meditation
- Reintroduction of drugs should be based on trial and observations. In addition to regulated use of the common analgesics, drugs like amitriptyline 10 mg HS, corticosteroids (prednisolone 20–40 mg/day for 5 days) and NSAIDs have been used with benefit. Physical measures such as injections of botulinum toxin into specific points over the forehead and neck 25–75 units once in 4–6 weeks allays the frequency and severity of the headache in many cases.

Trigeminal autonomic cephalalgias (TACs) are a group of headache syndromes that includes cluster headache (CH), paroxysmal hemicrania and short-lasting unilateral neuralgiform headache attacks with conjunctival injection and tearing (SUNCT). They are recognized clinically by their episodic, stereotypic attack profile and very often prominent cranial autonomic symptoms, such as lacrimation, conjunctival injection or rhinorrhea. They involve afferent activation of the trigeminal innervation of intracranial pain-producing structures, or the perception of that activation, and reflex activation of the facial, seventh cranial nerve outflow pathway.

CLUSTER HEADACHE

Syn: Histamine Headache

Horton's Syndrome

This is a migrainous variant. The name *cluster headache* refers to its occurrence in bouts. Men are more affected than women in the ratio of 4:1. The headache starts within 3 hours of falling asleep and it is nonthrobbing, unilateral and orbital in location. Along with pain, there may be lacrimation, nasal obstruction, rhinorrhea and sometimes miosis, ptosis and flushing and edema of cheek—all lasting approximately for an hour or two. It tends to occur every night for weeks or months followed by complete freedom for years. Such clusters of headache may recur over the years. Periods of headache are brought on by stress, prolonged strain, overwork and emotional disturbances. Alcohol, nitroglycerine or tyramine-containing foods may precipitate the headache. The hypothalamus is probably at fault. Diagnosis is clinical.

Treatment

This may respond to antihistamine drugs. In resistant cases, drugs used in migraine may be necessary. Acute attacks respond to oxygen inhalation at a rate of 7 L/min. Sumatriptan is given in doses of 6 mg by SC injection. It controls 75% of attacks. Ergot preparations given oral or by aerosol inhalation (1–2 mg) are effective. Nasal instillation of 1% lidocaine solution on the side of headache helps to arrest the attack. A short course of setroids starting with 1 mg/kg of prednisolone for 10 days to 2 weeks and tapered after that may help to decrease the clusters.

Prevention of recurrence: Verapamil in doses of 240–320 mg or lithium in doses of 600–1,500 mg a day is effective. In intractable cases, surgical treatment by greater occipital nerve block, occipital nerve and deep brain stimulation of hypothalamus have been employed.

Chronic paroxysmal hemicrania (PH) and SUNCT/ SUNA (satirical unconventional naive able): PH and SUNCT/SUNA are characterized by multiple daily attacks of unilateral head pain with cranial autonomic features. As with cluster, PH comes in two forms—(1) an episodic form, in which attacks occur in periods lasting 1–3 months followed by times of remission and recurrence and (2) a chronic form without a month of remission during a year. Chronic PH is more common. PH unlike CH is a disease mostly of women.

Attacks of PH last 2–30 minutes and occur more than five times per day at least half the time. Attacks can be differentiated from CH in that they are shorter, 50% of patients will not experience the restlessness that comes along with CH and the patients may not be awakened from sleep. PH occurs more often in women; CH in men.

The best diagnostic marker for PH is the excellent response to indomethacin. Treatment is with 25 mg of indomethacin three times a day and stepping up every 2–3 days until 75 mg tid is reached (if needed). This should be tapered often to see if remission has occurred, as the natural progression of PH is largely unknown. Other medications reported with occasional success include verapamil, acetazolamide, lithium, oxygen, ergotamine and prednisone.

SUNCT/SUNA is similar to PH but attacks last only 5–240 seconds (average 10–60 seconds) with up to 200 attacks per day. Because the attacks are so short, therapy must be preventive. Lamotrigine (especially for SUNCT) and gabapentin (especially for SUNA) are the two most efficacious medications reported, but topiramate, intranasal lidocaine, corticosteroids and IV phenytoin have been used as well.

TENSION HEADACHES

They may be either episodic or chronic are the most common headaches and include muscle contraction, headache, stress headache and psychogenic headache. The sensation is often described as the pressure exerted by a tight hat. The pain is mild to moderate, bilateral and does not worsen with normal physical activity. This group can be further subdivided into two:

1. Those with abnormalities of the pericranial muscles, detected by palpation or demonstrating overactivity by electromyographic studies
2. Those without such abnormalities.

Muscle contraction headaches may also be secondary to localized disease of the head, temporomandibular joint (TMJ) dysfunction, cervical spondylosis, eye muscle disorders and sinus diseases. Treatment of such headaches consists of attention to any removable underlying cause, use of sedatives, altering the lifestyle and relaxing techniques such as biofeedback, meditation and leisure activities.

Coital headache occurs at the time of sexual intercourse and may cause severe anxiety. This is a benign condition in the vast majority of cases, but if it is of recent onset, SAH has to be excluded by suitable investigations before reassuring the patient. Exercise induced headache also comes under the same category.

HYPNIC HEADACHE

This occurs in the older population, usually after 60 years. Patient wakes up with sudden severe headache at night which tends to recur. Lithium prophylaxia is found to be of use.

Headache is one of the most common nonspecific symptoms occurring in several systemic illnesses such as infections, fever, digestive disturbances, fatigue and others. It is also a very common adverse side effect of several drugs.

OTHER COMMON SECONDARY HEADACHES

Headache following an alcoholic bout ('hangover' headache) is thought to be due to vascular mechanisms. Vascular dilatation and headache may be a feature of hypercapnia in patients with respiratory failure. Severe arterial hypertension may cause headache. In the elderly, localized temporal headache may be due to cranial arteritis (temporal arteritis).

Headache due to Traction on Intracranial Structures

An intracranial lesion such as a growing tumor or subdural hematoma may press upon pain sensitive structures situated intracranially and produce headache. This may occur even if there is no generalized rise in intracranial pressure (ICP).

Rise in ICP almost invariably produces headache which is often diffuse and aggravated by maneuvers which increase ICP further, such as straining at stools, stooping forward or coughing. Headache of raised ICP tends to be troublesome on waking up in the morning and when the patient is lying flat. When he assumes the erect posture, there is a slight fall in pressure and this relieves the headache to some extent in early cases. Headache is an important symptom in benign intracranial hypertension.

Post-lumbar puncture headache: Following lumbar puncture (LP), if there is excessive leak of cerebrospinal fluid (CSF) through the puncture site, the CSF pressure falls and this leads to traction on intracranial structures. This produces postlumbar puncture headache. Other mechanisms also operate to perpetuate this symptom.

This can be avoided by doing LP with a small-bore needle, withdrawing only small quantities of CSF (<2 mL) and administering drugs like caffeine (50–100 mg) and theophylline 100 mg orally and plenty of parenteral fluids. Creation of an epidural blood patch may be necessary if the headache is persistent.

Spontaneous hypotension headache or low tension headache: It can occur due to rupture of diverticula from subarachnoid space which is located mostly in thoracic regions. Bout of cough may produce the rupture at times. The clinical manifestations are like postlumbar puncture headache. There will be diffuse headache, neck pain and neck stiffness improved on lying down and worsened by sitting and walking. Magnetic resonance imaging (MRI) picture is diagnostic showing gadolinium enhancement and thickening of patchy meninges, tonsillar herniation and enlargement of enhancement of pituitary. Treatment is as for postlumbar puncture headache. Surgical repair of defects in dura can be done or they may get blocked with epidural patch.

Referred headache: This includes pain arising from the eyes, ears, nose, air sinuses, teeth, cervical spine and other structures which may be referred as headache. Iridocyclitis and glaucoma produce headache which is referred to the frontal region. Nasal and paranasal sinus diseases may cause pain over the frontal or malar region. ***Cervical spondylosis*** may cause severe occipital headache. In some people, a cold stimulus in the soft palate may produce referred headache which is spoken of as an ***ice-cream headache***, which has been included under primary headache.

Neuralgic headache: Trigeminal neuralgia is a typical example of cranial neuralgia. The pain is episodic and lancinating in character. This occurs within the distribution of the fifth cranial nerve. In postherpetic neuralgia, pain is continuous and burning in character. In glossopharyngeal neuralgia, a pain of stabbing character is felt in the pharynx and deep in the ear. Loss of teeth or ill-fitting dentures cause malalignment of the bite and secondary to this, changes occur in the TMJ resulting in temporomandibular neuralgia. Here, the pain varies from dull ache to intense agonizing stabbing pain. The pain may radiate from the region of the affected joint to temporal and frontal areas and to the cheek or neck.

Meningeal irritation: Headache is almost always a symptom of meningitis and encephalitis. This results from meningeal inflammation which lowers the threshold of pain-sensitive structures at the base of the brain and hence, minimal mechanical stimuli produce headache. This headache may be generalized or sometimes more severe in the occipital region. It is aggravated even by minimal movements of the head. The diagnosis is suggested by the associated fever, photophobia and neck stiffness.

Headache of SAH is often abrupt in onset, sometimes precipitated by exertion and felt at particular regions depending on the vessel involved. The patient is afebrile. Many become unconscious. At times, incontinence may develop. It is important to recognize the extremely severe headache of SAH which demands immediate referral to a center where neurosurgical intervention can be undertaken.

Drug-induced headache: Many drugs can induce acute headache mainly cardiovascular agents; nitroglycerine, angiotensin-converting enzyme inhibitors (ACEIs), dipyridamole, erectile dysfunction agents like sildenafil, gastrointestinal (GI) medications namely histamine receptor antagonists cimetidine, ranitidine, proton pump inhibitors (PPIs) like omeprazole and lansoprazole, oncologic agents; anagrelide, cyclosporine, tacrolimus and oral contraceptives, antibiotics, amphotericin and griseofulvin.

Thunderclap headache: The term refers to first or worst severe headache of a type the patient has never experienced before. A sudden severe headache with maximal onset within 1 minute without evidence of SAH is termed as ***thunderclap headache***.

Psychogenic headache and other cranial pains occurring in psychiatric diseases: Headache is a common symptom in psychiatric disorders. Such headache involves the whole head or may be confined to the front or vertex. Though the sensation is usually described as pain, further scrutiny reveals it as a sort of pressure or tightness felt by the patients. Tension headache tends to occur following emotional excitement or other stresses. Constant tension developing in the muscles of the forehead and upper part of the face leads to this symptom. This type of headache may persist continuously for days or weeks. Common analgesics like salicylates and paracetamol are ineffective. Patients with tension headache reveal prominent symptoms of depression, anxiety and hypochondriasis. Majority of patients with anxiety neurosis, hysteria, obsessive compulsive neurosis and schizophrenia with prominent anxiety, exhibit this type of headache.

DIAGNOSIS

Majority of headaches encountered in clinical practice are nonrecurrent and occur as manifestations of systemic illnesses. Recurrent headaches present a common diagnostic problem since one has to differentiate conditions like migraine and tension headache from more serious causes like intracranial structural lesions. Presence of accompanying signs like neurological deficits simplifies the problem, but usually history is the only clinical guide for diagnosis and further management. Some general points help to assess the severity of the disorder (Box 197.1).

Headache described as throbbing or burning is more significant than tension headaches. Localized headaches are often indicative of serious underlying disease than diffuse pain. Headache situated over the occipital or frontal region is more important than that situated over the vertex. Headaches which disturb sleep usually arise from organic lesions. Headache of recent onset is more sinister than that of long-standing. Presence of phenomena like double vision or epilepsy indicates the presence of an intracranial lesion. *Late onset headache and recent change in pattern in chronic headaches are indications for brain imaging studies*.

MANAGEMENT

The investigation and treatment depend upon the clinical setting. Detailed history serves to sort out the cause in the majority of cases. Investigative procedures such as chest X-ray, electroencephalogram (EEG) and computed tomography (CT) of the brain are done before embarking upon more advanced procedures like MRI

Box 197.1: Red flags of headache which demand detailed investigations and care

- 'Worst' headache ever
- First severe headache
- Subacute worsening over days or weeks
- Altered level of consciousness
- Abnormal neurologic findings
- Fever or unexplained systemic signs
- Weight loss
- Vomiting that precedes headache
- Pain induced by bending, lifting, cough, worsens with Valsalva maneuvers
- Pain that disturbs sleep or presents immediately upon awakening
- Known systemic illness, history of trauma, cancer or human immunodeficiency virus (HIV)
- New onset headache in a patient older than 50 years of age
- Focal neurologic deficits, jaw claudication
- Morning headache associated with nausea and vomiting
- Pain associated with local tenderness, e.g. region of temporal artery.

and angiography. In those cases in which no serious underlying lesion is detected, reassurance and periodic follow-up is all that is required. It is important to avoid unnecessary medication and life-long invalidism.

CHAPTER 198

Nutritional Disorders of the Nervous System

Thomas Gregor Issac, SR Chandra

Chapter Summary

- Vitamin B$_1$ Deficiency (Thiamine)
- Other Nutritional Deficiencies
- Protein-energy Malnutrition
- Nutritional Amblyopias
- Alcohol and the Nervous System

Note: The general aspects of the topics in this chapter are given in Section 5, which may also be referred to as appropriate.

INTRODUCTION

On the basis of the amount required by the human body, nutrients are classified into two categories: macronutrients and micronutrients. *Macronutrients* include carbohydrates, proteins and fat, whereas vitamins, minerals and trace elements constitute *micronutrients*. Vitamins and minerals are required in optimal quantities for proper maturation and functioning of the central nervous system (CNS) and peripheral nervous system (PNS). Nutritional disorders of the nervous system are contributed by the deficiency of vitamins and minerals and often result due to insufficient intake, especially in developing countries in addition to specific disorders which involve absorption, transportation defects and

disorders of metabolism. This can manifest with involvement of CNS, PNS or both with or without features of other system involvement. As these are potentially treatable conditions, adequate supplementation of the deficient nutrient will reverse the disease process.

VITAMIN B$_1$ DEFICIENCY (THIAMINE)

Thiamine deficiency occurs due to poor intake, alcoholism, pregnancy, hyperemesis, malabsorption or increased requirements, such as postoperative states including bariatric procedures strenuous exercise, systemic infections and malignancy and use of polished rice. Also seen acutely in conditions where a large amount of glucose is given parenterally without concurrent thiamine administration due to utilization of thiamine stores for glucose metabolism. Deficiency results in CNS and PNS features. The spectrum of thiamine deficiency involves wet beriberi (cardiovascular involvement) with concurrent edema, dry beriberi (without edema) and Wernicke-Korsakoff syndrome.

Clinical Features

Beriberi is a Sinhalese word, meaning 'weak-weak'. Polyneuropathy in beriberi manifests as stocking-glove (length dependent) symmetric sensorimotor neuropathy affecting mainly the lower limbs. The neuropathy can be acute, subacute or chronic with patients having pain and tingling paresthesias, bilateral foot and wrist drop. Deep tendon reflexes in ankle are lost in majority of patients. Cranial nerve deficits are unusual although laryngeal nerve paralysis resulting in hoarseness and weakness of voice may be seen. Calf tenderness is a prominent feature and rarely may develop an autonomic neuropathy with orthostatic hypotension. When cardiac dysfunction is present, patients also experience tachycardia, palpitations, dyspnea, fatigue and ankle edema.

Wernicke-Korsakoff Syndrome

First described in 1881 by Carl Wernicke as a triad of mental confusion, ophthalmoplegia and gait ataxia seen in alcoholic patients, later, Korsakoff described the amnesic syndrome and came to be called as *Wernicke-Korsakoff syndrome*. Pathologically, there is congestion, petechial hemorrhages, atrophy and discoloration seen adjacent to the fourth ventricle and aqueduct.

Wernicke's Encephalopathy

This presents with a clinical triad of confusion, ophthalmoplegia and ataxia. The confusional state develops after days or weeks and is associated with poor attention, disorientation, apathy and memory loss. Oculomotor abnormalities seen include nystagmus, lateral rectus palsy, conjugate gaze palsy, sluggishly reacting pupil in addition to truncal ataxia, hypothermia and postural hypotension. Magnetic resonance imaging (MRI) shows involvement of the periaqueductal regions (Fig. 198.1A), medial thalamus and bilateral mammillary bodies (Fig. 198.1B). Lesions usually resolve following prompt treatment but those in mammillary bodies take longer. The cerebrospinal fluid (CSF) is usually normal or shows mild elevation of protein. Serum thiamine and red blood cell (RBC) transketolase levels may be decreased and pyruvate levels are usually elevated. Clinical suspicion is the indication to treat. Treatment consists of parenteral thiamine 200 mg given intravenous (IV) in 5% glucose solution slowly after test dose followed by 100 mg 8th hourly for 48 hours then weekly for 4 weeks and monthly for 3 months with adequate care for nutrition. Ocular defects are usually reversible even though behavior and gait difficulties take longer time to resolve. As soon as the global confusional state recedes, some may be left with impaired memory and learning, which are features of Korsakoff's syndrome.

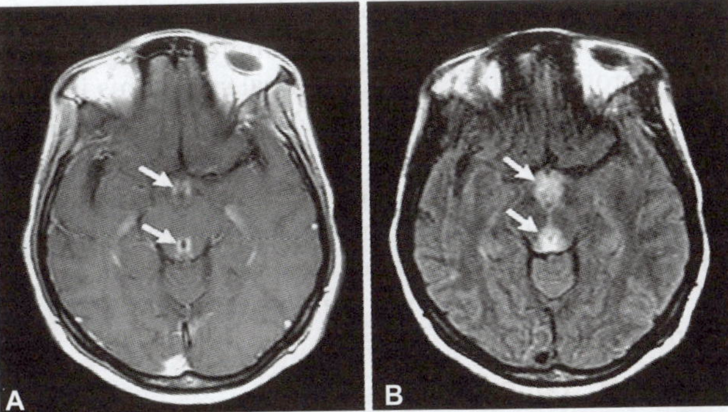

Figs 198.1A and B: Wernicke's encephalopathy: MRI features. **A.** Periaqueductal regions (arrows); **B.** Demyelination of medial thalamus (arrows)
Abbreviation: MRI = Magnetic resonance imaging

Korsakoff's Syndrome

Memory is more impaired than other cognitive functions characterized by both anterograde and retrograde amnesias. This is due to selective localization of the lesion in the diencephalon and temporal lobes. Some patients may be disoriented to place and time. Affected patients have severe difficulty in establishing new memories, along with retrieval deficit which precedes the onset of illness by several years but executive functions like alertness and attention are usually well-preserved. Confabulation to fill up gaps in memory is also seen in majority of the patients (*See* also Section 5, Ch 31).

Pathology in Korsakoff's syndrome is complementary to that of Wernicke's encephalopathy, but in addition has involvement of the dorsal medial nucleus of thalamus. *Treatment* includes thiamine administration along with supervised care and guarded prognosis with respect to cognitive functions which may take longer (more than 1 year) with possibility of residual deficits. Abstinence of alcohol and smoking and nutritional improvement serve to prevent relapse.

OTHER NUTRITIONAL DEFICIENCIES

Riboflavin (Vitamin B₂)

It is a part of the oxygen transport chain in mitochondria, acting as a coenzyme in oxidation-reduction reactions. Mainly deficiency occurs along with thiamine and pyridoxine deficiencies. It clinically manifests as glossitis, angular stomatitis, conjunctivitis, keratitis cheilosis and genito-facial dyssebacia manifested as skin lesions. Rapid recovery follows oral administration of riboflavin 10 mg daily.

Niacin and Nicotinic Acid (Vitamin B₃)

Niacin includes both nicotinic acid and nicotinamide, which forms the metabolically active nicotinamide adenine dinucleotide (NAD) and NAD phosphate (NADP), an end product of tryptophan metabolism. More than 200 enzymes are dependent on NAD and NADP to carry out oxidation-reduction reactions which are involved in synthesis and breakdown of all carbohydrates, lipids and amino acids. The classic advanced disease caused by deficiency of niacin is pellagra which used to be common in those consuming large quantities of maize with deficiency of proteins and vitamins.

Pellagra

Pellagra affects three organ systems in the body; the gastrointestinal tract (GIT), skin and nervous system (hence the mnemonic of three D's—diarrhea, dermatitis and dementia).

In alcoholics, niacin deficiency presents with encephalopathy, altered sensorium, limb rigidity, grasping and sucking reflexes (*Jellife's syndrome*), dementia and confusion, followed by diarrhea and dermatitis. Deficiency usually coexists with thiamine and pyridoxine deficiency. Spinal cord and peripheral nerve defects have also been reported, particularly in prisoners of war. Hartnup disease, an autosomal recessive defect in tryptophan absorption, and carcinoid syndrome, due to excessive tryptophan consumption can predispose to niacin deficiency. Excess of amino acid leucine (a niacin inhibitor) has also been postulated to play a role in causing niacin deficiency.

Electroencephalogram (EEG) shows absence of alpha (α) rhythm and excess of theta (θ) and occasional delta (δ) activity, which reverts with niacin supplementation.

Recommended daily allowance for nicotinic acid is 6.6 mg/1,000 cal dietary intake. Doses of niacin 40–250 mg reverses majority of the symptoms. Doses of 1.5–3 g daily have been successfully used in treatment of dyslipidemia and decreases mortality due to coronary diseases. **Side effects** of high dose niacin include flushing, hyperuricemia, hyperglycemia and elevation of liver enzymes. Laropiprant is a newly introduced drug which prevents flushing after administration of large doses of niacin. The dose of laropiprant is 20 mg along with 1 g of niacin.

Vitamin B₅ (Pantothenic Acid)

It is a part of coenzyme-A and plays an important role in the secretion of hormones, such as cortisone because of the role it plays in supporting the adrenal gland. These hormones assist the metabolism, help to fight allergies and are beneficial in the maintenance of healthy skin, muscles and nerves. Pantothenic acid plays a role in the metabolism of fat, protein, carbohydrates and adenosine triphosphate (ATP) production. It is used in synthesis of lipids, neurotransmitters, steroid hormones and hemoglobin. Biochemical changes include increased insulin sensitivity, lowered blood cholesterol, decreased serum potassium and failure of adrenocorticotropin to induce eosinopenia. Daily requirement is 10 mg.

Deficiency results in fatigue, headache, nausea, tingling in the hands and feet (*Gopalan's syndrome*), muscle weakness, depression, personality changes, cardiac arrhythmias, frequent infections, abdominal pains and sleep disturbances. Examination may reveal pallor, cyanosis, excessive sweating and areas of capillary dilatation over both feet. Diminished sensations along with hyperalgesia are usually seen. Coexistent deficiency along with other B vitamins is considered as the etiological factor. Most of them respond well to parenteral pantothenic acid.

Vitamin B₆ (Pyridoxine)

Pyridoxal phosphate is the active form of the vitamin which plays an important role as coenzyme in converting tryptophan to methionine. This produces secondary niacin deficiency with features similar to pellagra. It is also involved in lipid and neurotransmitter synthesis. Dopamine, serotonin, epinephrine, norepinephrine and gamma-aminobutyric acid (GABA) require pyridoxine for their synthesis.

Congenital pyridoxine dependency presents with a very unique situation where the child is born convulsive and responds only to life-long pyridoxine treatment. Development of dependency on the vitamin by the newborn due to prenatal use of the vitamin as antiemetic in the mother causes neonatal seizures which needs short-duration therapy with pyridoxine.

Pyridoxine is also unique in the fact that both deficiency and toxic states result in peripheral neuropathy and myelopathy. Deficiency also produces sideroblastic anemia and pellagra-like rash. Recommended daily dose is 2 mg/day.

Therapy with isoniazid and hydralazine can induce peripheral neuropathy by competition with pyridoxine and this can be prevented by supplementation with pyridoxine 6 mg/day. Administration of daily doses of more than 200 mg/day can result in paresthesias and ataxias over a period of 1–3 years. Nerve biopsies demonstrate reduction of myelin fiber density and presence of myelin debris, suggesting axonal degeneration.

Vitamin B₇ (Biotin)

Biotin, also known as **vitamin H** or **coenzyme R,** is a water-soluble B vitamin (vitamin B₇) and is necessary for cell growth, production of fatty acids and metabolism of fats and amino acids. Biotin assists in various metabolic reactions involving the transfer of carbon dioxide (CO_2). It may also be helpful in maintaining a steady blood sugar level and is often recommended as a dietary supplement for strengthening hair and nails.

Symptoms of biotin deficiency include hair loss (alopecia), conjunctivitis, dermatitis in the form of a scaly red rash around the eyes, nose, mouth and genital area, depression, lethargy, hallucination and numbness and tingling of the extremities. The characteristic facial rash, together with an unusual facial fat distribution, has been termed the **biotin-deficient face.** Individuals with hereditary disorders of biotin deficiency have evidence of immunodeficiencies leading to increased susceptibility to bacterial and fungal infections. Pregnant women tend to have a high-risk of biotin deficiency. Nearly half of pregnant women have abnormal increase of 3-hydroxyisovaleric acid, which reflects reduced status of biotin. Biotin deficiency during pregnancy causes congenital malformations, such as cleft palate. Excess consumption of dried raw egg processes during gestation induces biotin deficiency.

Inherited metabolic disorders involving biotin and characterized by deficient activities of biotin-dependent carboxylases. These are termed as **multiple carboxylase deficiency**. These include deficiencies in the enzyme biotinidase. Its deficiency prevents the body's cells from using biotin effectively, and this interferes with multiple carboxylase reactions. Biochemical and clinical manifestations include—ketolactic acidosis, organic aciduria, hyperammonemia, skin rash, feeding problems, hypotonia, seizures, developmental delay, alopecia and coma.

Biotinidase deficiency is due to deficiency in the enzymes that process it. Biotinidase catalyzes the cleavage of biotin from biocytin and biotinyl-peptides and thereby recycles biotin. It is also important in freeing biotin from dietary protein-bound biotin. General symptoms include decreased appetite and growth. Dermatologic symptoms include dermatitis, alopecia and achromotrichia (absence or loss of pigment in the hair). Perosis (shortening and thickening of bones) is seen in the skeleton. Fatty liver and kidney syndrome and hepatic steatosis also can occur.

Treatment involves oral administration of 30 µg/day for adults over 18 years of age.

Vitamin B₉ (Folic Acid)
(Refer also to Section 15, Ch 160)

Folic acid is crucial for proper brain function and plays an important role in mental and emotional health. It aids in the production of deoxyribonucleic acid (DNA) and ribonucleic acid (RNA), the body's genetic material, and is especially important when cells and tissues are growing rapidly, such as in infancy, adolescence and pregnancy. Folic acid and vitamin B_{12} have crucial roles in hematopoiesis and metabolism of homocysteine. High levels of homocysteine are associated with heart disease and cerebral atherosclerosis. People with high levels of homocysteine are about 1.7 times more likely to develop coronary artery disease (CAD) and 2.5 times more likely to have a stroke than those with normal levels. Other B complex vitamins, especially vitamins B_9, B_6 and B_{12} also help lower homocysteine levels. Alcoholism, inflammatory bowel disease (IBD) and celiac disease can lead to folic acid deficiency. Drugs like phenytoin, carbamazepine, sulfa drugs, chemotherapy, proton pump inhibitors (PPIs) and others may lower the levels of folic acid in the body. Folic acid deficiency leads to poor growth, glossitis, gingivitis, loss of appetite, shortness of breath, diarrhea, irritability, forgetfulness and mental sluggishness. Pregnant women need more folic acid to lower the risk of neural tube birth defects, including cleft palate, spina bifida and brain damage.

Birth Defects

Pregnant women should get 400–600 µg of folates per day. Women who plan to become pregnant should make sure to get the recommended 400 µg/day, as the damage occurs in the period of organogenesis.

Age-related Hearing Loss

One study suggests that folic acid supplements help slow the progression of age-related hearing loss in elderly people with high homocysteine levels and low folate in their diet. It is doubtful whether healthy seniors would benefit by routine supplementation.

Age-related Macular Degeneration

One large study found that women who took 2,500 µg of folic acid along with 500 mg of vitamin B_6 and 1,000 µg of cyanocobalamin (vitamin B_{12}) daily reduced their risk of developing age-related macular degeneration (AMD) that can cause loss of vision.

Folate deficiency may be associated with depression. Folates also protect against malignancies of colon and breast.

Vitamin B_{12} (Cyanocobalamin)

It is an important vitamin for maintaining integrity of the neuraxis. *Charaka Samhita* reports of a disease with the triad of diarrhea, weight loss and neurocognitive disturbances resembling the clinical picture of vitamin B_{12} deficiency. The reader may refer to Section 5, Ch 31 and Section 15, Ch 160 for general information about vitamin B_{12}.

Neuropathology

The term subacute combined degeneration (SACD) of the spinal cord is commonly used. Microscopically, spongiform changes and foci of myelin and axonal destruction are seen in the white matter of the cervical and upper thoracic levels of the cord. Changes may be also seen in the lateral columns. Affected peripheral nerves show axonal degeneration and rarely demyelination. Optic nerve and deep cerebral white matter is also involved.

Clinical Features

Symptoms are insidious in onset with paresthesias in the distal limbs most commonly seen. Weakness and unsteadiness are the next most frequent symptoms. Lhermitte's sign, mental slowing, depression, confusion, delusions and hallucinations are common. About one-third of these patients have hematological abnormalities like megaloblastic anemia and hypersegmented neutrophils. Loss of vibration sense and joint position sense is common. Romberg's sign is also seen in later stages. Deep tendon reflexes are variably affected depending on the degree of pyramidal and peripheral nerve involvement. Visual impairment is seen occasionally and examination reveals bilateral visual loss, optic atrophy and centrocecal scotoma. Brainstem and cerebellar involvement may also be seen in severe cases.

Imaging Studies

As many patients present with myelopathy and encephalopathy, imaging is pertinent to rule out other structural causes. MRI will show signal changes in the lateral or posterior columns in cervical and thoracic cord. Contrast enhancement and spinal cord swelling also have been described. Patients with encephalopathy will have multiple deep cerebral white matter signal changes.

Nerve conduction studies show small or absent sural nerve sensory potentials in 50% of the patients with evidence for axonal polyneuropathy.

Laboratory Features

Laboratory features of vitamin B_{12} (normal 200–900 pg/mL) and cobalamin-dependent metabolites provide a direct measure. Levels of metabolites which accumulate in deficiency states, like serum homocysteine and methylmalonic acid, also provide an indirect estimate of vitamin B_{12} deficiency.

Treatment and Prognosis

Typical regimen includes daily muscular injections of cobalamin 1,000 µg for 1 week, followed by cobalamin 1,000 µg injection once weekly for a month and then on monthly basis for life. Megadoses of oral supplementation up to 2 g/day have also been tried with beneficial effect. With proper treatment, partial improvement is seen within 6–12 months of treatment. As remission correlates inversely with time lapse between onset of symptoms and initiation of treatment, early detection of this deficiency state is important.

Vitamin C (Ascorbic Acid)

This vitamin plays many roles. Its presence is required for the transformation of dopamine into noradrenaline, the biosynthesis of catecholamines and has a role in cognition apart from its well-known function in maintaining tissue integrity, cell-mediated immunity and oxygen transport and antioxidant effect. A regular intake of vitamin C reduces the risk of cataract.

Vitamin E (Tocopherol)

It is a fat-soluble vitamin which is a free radical scavenger and an antioxidant. Vitamin E depends on the activity of pancreatic esterases and bile salts for its solubilization and absorption in the intestinal lumen. Neurological symptoms of deficiency occur most commonly in patients with significant malabsorption syndromes.

Clinical Features

Patients develop areflexia, cerebellar ataxia, cutaneous sensory impairment, loss of position and vibration sense, less commonly ophthalmoplegia, muscle weakness, nystagmus, extensor plantar responses, ptosis and dysarthria. Acanthocytosis and pigmentary retinopathy are seen primarily in patients with abetalipoproteinemia. Adults with acquired malabsorption usually presents with progressive ataxia with areflexia in addition to muscle, cranial nerve and peripheral nerve involvement.

Laboratory Studies

Low serum vitamin E and carotene levels along with increased stool fat are highly suggestive of the deficiency state. CSF is normal. Nerve conduction studies usually reveal sensory polyneuropathy. Somatosensory and visual evoked responses are frequently abnormal and there may be hyperintensities in the posterior column on T2-weighted MRI.

The recommended daily dose is 10 mg for men and 8 mg for women and found in abundance in vegetable oils and wheat germ. Supplementation of water-miscible tocopherol at doses of 200–600 mg/day is found to be effective. Increased doses of up to 100 mg/kg/day may be required in hereditary familial deficiency of vitamin E.

Vitamin A

It [recommended daily allowance (RDA)] 2,000–3,000 IU) is derived from β-carotene, is fat soluble and is necessary for normal vision and reproduction. Retinol-rich products are liver, milk, butter, eggs, some cheeses and fish; while green vegetables, carrots, colored tubers, yellow fruit and oranges are rich sources of carotenoids. The addition of vegetable oil increases the bioavailability of β-carotene in the intestine by at least six-fold. Deficiency will lead to ocular symptoms, like night blindness and corneal liquefaction, and ulceration and skin changes called *phrynoderma* over the extensor aspect of the elbows and dry skin. Ingestion of 25,000 IU daily for 1–2 years leads to hypervitaminosis A. This manifests as pseudotumor cerebri causing raised intracranial pressure (ICP), visual disturbances and painful bony swellings. In pregnant women, hypervitaminosis A can lead to birth defects and learning disabilities in the offspring.

Strachan's Syndrome

First described by Dr Henry Strachan in Jamaica, this consists of painful peripheral neuropathy, ataxia, optic neuropathy and stomatitis. Patients may also develop sensorineural deafness, spasticity, dizziness and confusion due to mixed nutritional deficiency among prisoners of war. Infections usually exacerbate this syndrome. Nerve biopsies show axonal degeneration of large myelinated fibers. *Treatment* consists of re-establishing a balanced diet with B-complex vitamin and vitamin A supplementation.

Vitamin D

It is necessary for calcium absorption in the gut, and deficiency results in osteomalacia, hypocalcemia, hypophosphatemia, neuropsychiatric disorders including dementia, Parkinson's disease, multiple sclerosis, epilepsy and schizophrenia. There are several proposed mechanisms by which vitamin D deficiency may affect these disorders. One of these mechanisms is through neuronal apoptosis. Neuronal apoptosis is the programmed death of the neurons. Hypovitaminosis D causes this specific apoptosis by decreasing the expression of cytochrome C and decreasing the cell cycle of neurons. Cytochrome C is a protein that promotes the activation of proapoptotic factors. A second mechanism is through the association of neurotrophic factors like nerve growth factor (NGF), brain-derived neurotrophic factor (BDNF) and glial cell line-derived neurotrophic factor (GDNF). These neurotrophic factors are proteins that are involved in the growth and survival of developing neurons. In addition, they are also involved in the maintenance of mature neurons. Deficiency of vitamin D impairs these beneficial effects.

Iron

Many symptoms such as apathy, somnolence, irritability, decreased attention, inability to concentrate and memory loss have been reported to be clinical signs of iron deficiency, even in the absence of anemia. But these symptoms are difficult to interpret because of their subjective nature. It is known that iron plays an important role in growth and development of children, including neurological and cognitive performance. The relationship between iron status and cognitive performance is currently attracting interest. The deficit in iron acts globally at two different levels: on the one hand by less efficient supply of oxygen to the brain; and on the other by decreasing brain energy production, as iron deficiency decreases the activity of the enzyme cytochrome c oxidase in certain cerebral regions. Even though the exact molecular roles played by iron deficiency on brain structure and function, it is a common finding that massive iron supplementation in marginated communities have led to reduction in several functional impairment in children and adolescence including neurological impairment.

Effect of iron deficiency in the dopaminergic system is probably related to attention-deficit/hyperactivity disorder, developmental delay, stroke, breath-holding episodes, pseudotumor cerebri and cranial nerve palsies.

Copper

In the aging process of the brain, oxidative stress is aggravated by abnormal interactions of iron and copper with metal-binding proteins, such as neuromelanin or amyloid-beta (Abeta) peptide. Copper deficiency and iron accumulation have a role in augmenting dementing diseases and accelerating aging process of the brain.

In humans, copper deficiency presents with axonal peripheral neuropathy with mixed sensorimotor involvement, myelopathy or less commonly encephalopathy and optic neuropathy. Microcytic anemia with normal iron studies will give a clue with regard to the same. Serum copper, ceruloplasmin and 24-hour urinary copper are all reduced. MRI shows nonspecific white matter changes and posterolateral hyperintensities in spinal cord. Treatment includes oral elemental copper supplements 2–4 mg once daily.

Zinc

Elemental zinc plays a role in cognitive development, taste and smell. Deficit induces anosmia and ageusia by its association with gustin. Deficiency of zinc can result in cognitive and behavioral problems by its mechanism through accumulation of polyunsaturated fatty acids. However, excess of zinc leads to formation of amyloid plaques. Oysters and cheese contains zinc, whereas green vegetables, fruit, sugar, fats and drinks are low in zinc.

Iodine

The human body contains 15–20 mg of iodine as one of the trace elements. Iodine is an essential component of thyroxine (T4) and tri-iodothyronine (T3) which are the main hormones of the thyroid. They play great roles in the growth metamorphosis and metabolism of almost all tissues in the body including neural structures during intrauterine and postnatal life. Deficiency leads to several neurological disorders depending on the severity and the time of development of the disorder. Cretinism, myxedema and various shades of hypothyroidism are important causes of retardation of growth and child development. Neurological cretinism presents with severe mental retardation, characteristic facies, spastic diplegia with greater proximal weakness, bradykinesia, shuffling gait, hyporeactive tendon jerks short stature, dysarthria and an often palpable goiter.

In the myxedematous variety, signs of hypothyroidism are most obvious and motor disability and deaf mutism minimal. There is stunting, evident cretinoid facies with macroglossia, abdominal distension, umbilical hernia, severe cognitive disability, cerebellar disturbances, delayed bone age and slow tendon reflexes. Thyroid gland is rarely prominent. Therefore, all pregnant women and children should undergo screening for thyroid disease. For detailed description refer to Section 5, Ch 32.

Magnesium

Its deficiency is usually linked to spasmophilia, a state characterized by tetany not caused by calcium deficiency. About 22 g of magnesium is stored in the body in the adult mainly in bone (+50%) and in skeletal muscle (25%). The rest is distributed throughout the organism, especially in the nervous system. Magnesium has two roles— (1) structural and (2) metabolic. It is a stabilizer of the different compartments of the cell (organelles, such as the nucleus, or the mitochondria that produce energy). Magnesium plays a role in all the major metabolisms— oxidation-reduction and ionic regulation. It activates about 300 enzymes. In animals, brain from magnesium deficient rats is more susceptible to permanent focal ischemia.

Magnesium participates in the formation and use of chemical links rich in energy that are the basis of all biological activity in the cell. About 18% of men and 23% of women have intakes lower than two-thirds of the RDA (for details refer to Section 5, Ch 32). Milk is an easily available source of magnesium.

Selenium

In the brain, about 15% of this important trace element is metabolized in association with glutathione peroxidase (GPx), Along with vitamin E, it is having a membrane protective role, as a crucial enzyme for protection against peroxidation. Deficiency results in **Keshan disease** due to myocardial necrosis in addition to delay in neuronal development.

PROTEIN-ENERGY MALNUTRITION

(Refer to Section 5, Ch 29)

The human brain shows development spurt from the 13th week of gestation and shows maturation, myelination and synaptogenesis up to 8 years after birth. These processes are mainly dependent on proper nutrition of the infant and mother and deficiency can result in severe and permanent neuronal damage. Children manifest with apathy, irritability, delayed acquisition of mental and fine motor skills, clumsiness, generalized muscle weakness, hypotonia and hyporeflexia. Neuropsychological deficits are more prominent in **kwashiorkor**. About 25% of the children with protein energy malnutrition (PEM) show cerebral atrophy. During the first few weeks of restarting protein refeeding, some children with kwashiorkor may develop encephalopathy ranging from drowsiness to rigidity, myoclonus, coarse tremors and rarely coma, known as **nutritional recovery syndrome**. It is of utmost public health importance to ensure proper nutrition during pregnancy and infancy.

NUTRITIONAL AMBLYOPIAS

Visual disturbances may develop due to deficiency of multiple nutrients, including B-complex vitamins. This sets in insidiously with dimness of vision, photophobia and retrobulbar discomfort on moving the eyes. Visual acuity is reduced. Central or paracentral scotomas may develop, but the peripheral fields of vision may remain intact.

ALCOHOL AND THE NERVOUS SYSTEM

(Refer to Section 4, Ch 23 and Section 19, Ch 244)

In acute intoxication, alcohol acts as a CNS depressant, and small doses lead to disinhibition or a slight euphoria which is the basis of dependence. Alcohol affects the neuraxis in multiple ways by its direct effect as well as by the secondary complications of chronic alcoholism. We here report a very interesting patient who had all the neurological complications of alcoholism during management of his comatose condition.

A 40-year-old male who was a daily drinker for 20 years was found unresponsive in the house and left without treatment for about 2 weeks. As he did not wake up, he was brought to the hospital. Examination showed a stuporose patient who was hallucinating and was disoriented. He had gaze-evoked nystagmus and slowing of horizontal eye movements and bipyramidal signs. His MRI showed features of chronic alcoholism in the form of diffuse cerebellar atrophy, osmotic demyelination evidenced by signal changes in the transverse pontine fibers, hypoglycemic insult seen as hyperintensities in putamen, hepatic derangement seen as signal changes in globus pallidus and Wernicke's encephalopathy seen as thalamic and periaqueductal hyperintensities (Figs 198.2A to C). The adverse effects are due to the following:

- Direct toxicity
- Complications due to adulterants

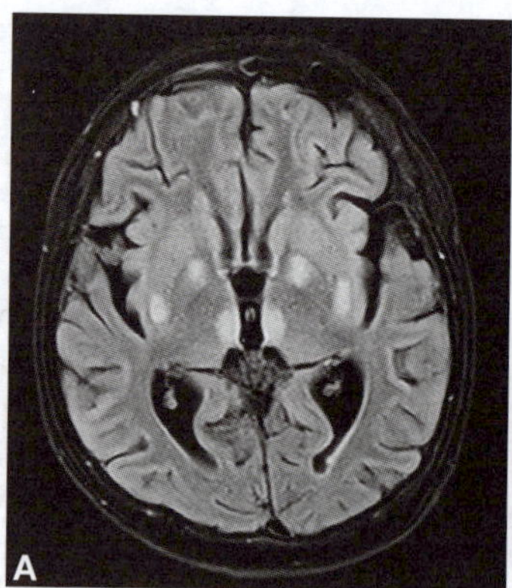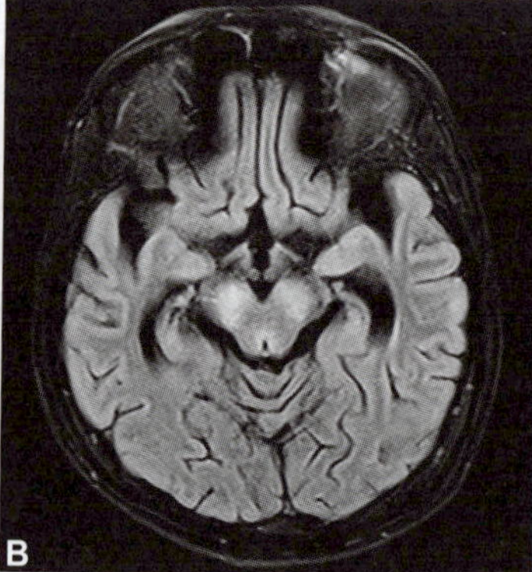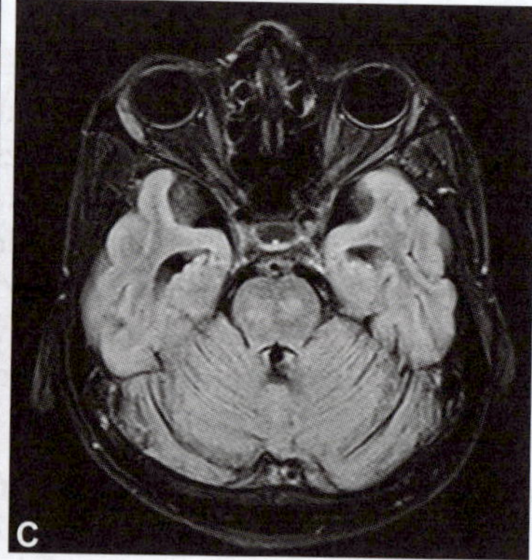

Figs 198.2A to C: A. Bilateral putaminal and pallidal necrosis in MRI; **B.** Bilateral midbrain and periaqueductal signal changes with cerebellar vermis atrophy; **C.** Osmotic demyelination seen in bilateral pons along with prominent cerebellar folia

Abbreviation: MRI = Magnetic resonance imaging

- Nutritional deprivation
- Withdrawal

Acute toxicity results in ataxia, due to involvement of archicerebellum, encephalopathy and delirium. Adulterants like methyl alcohol lead to acidosis, blindness and encephalopathy. Nutritional deprivation results in peripheral neuropathy, myopathy and encephalopathy. Alcoholics are also prone for hyponatremia, hypoglycemia with their effects on the neuraxis. Chronic intoxication results in nonreversible paleocerebellar atrophy and partly reversible conditions like dementia and the classical *Marchiafava-Bignami disease*. The psychiatric complications of alcoholism lead to antisocial and criminal activities in addition to severe manpower and material loss.

Withdrawal Syndromes

Withdrawal syndromes occur when a person decreases or stops a high level of alcohol intake, either after a binge lasting a matter of days or after the regular ingestion of alcohol sustained over many months. It is postulated due to the overactivity of various portions of the nervous system resembling a rebound phenomenon after profound suppression and may relate to alterations in the status of GABA and N-methyl-D-aspartate receptor (NMDA) receptor systems and seen as early as 6 hours after last drink. This is characterized by tremulousness, seizures, delirium and hallucinations in addition to hyper-reflexia, hypervigilance, anxiety, tachycardia, hypertension and insomnia.

Delirium Tremens

It comprises a combination of psychic and autonomic hyperactivity, occurring usually after 3–5 days of alcohol abstinence but may be seen as late as 2 weeks. Patients are agitated, tremulous, hallucinating (mostly visual) and confused. Fever, tachycardia, diaphoresis, hypertension and confusion are typically seen. They are also more prone for complications in neuraxis secondary to end-organ damage like hepatic encephalopathy, increased platelet adhesiveness and cardiomyopathy resulting in cerebral venous and arterial thrombosis, subarachnoid hemorrhage (SAH) and accidents.

Alcoholic Dementia

This is a partially reversible dementia of multifactorial origin like toxic, nutritional and degenerative factors.

Other complications are toxic and deficiency amblyopias and cerebellar degeneration.

Marchiafava-Bignami Disease

This is seen in long-standing alcohol abuse. It causes degeneration of middle lamina of the corpus callosum resulting in dementia of frontal lobe type, behavioral problems and split brain dysfunction in addition to personality changes, incontinence, dysarthria, seizures and hemiparesis.

Alcoholic Myopathy

It can be acute as a toxic myopathy with all the features of muscle necrosis or chronic due to nutritional deficiencies and systemic complications of alcohol.

Alcoholism and Movement Disorders

Alcohol presents with classical delirium tremens, essential tremor, ataxia, chorea and asterexis.

Fetal Alcohol Syndrome

It is postulated to be due to direct teratogenic effect of alcohol. It results in low birth weight and microcephaly, poor feeding, tremors and cranial and joint abnormalities. The infant mortality in this condition is quite high with survivors having increased incidence of mental subnormality. There is no direct treatment for this condition although proper postnatal nutrition and care may help. Approximately, one in six babies born with this disease die. Preventive measures should target married women planning to conceive along with appropriate psychosocial interventions and education.

Source:

1. Kinsella LJ, Riley DE. Nutritional deficiencies and syndromes associated with alcoholism. In: Goetz Christopher G. (Ed). Textbook of Clinical Neurology, 3rd edition. Philadelphia: Saunders; 2007. pp. 897-918.

2. So YT, Simon RP. Deficiency diseases of the nervous system. In: Daroff RB, Fenichel Gerald M, Jankovic Joseph, Mazziotta John C (Eds). Bradley's Neurology in Clinical Practice, 5th edition. Philadelphia: Elsevier; 2012. pp. 1643-57.

3. Polívka J, Peterka M, Rohan V, et al. Vitamin D and neurological diseases. 2012; 58(5): 393-95.

Infections of the Central Nervous System

SR Chandra, Nethravathi M, Thomas Gregor Issac

Chapter Summary

- CNS Tuberculosis
- Neurosyphilis
  - General Paralysis of the Insane
  - Tabes Dorsalis
- Brucellosis
- Parasitic Infections
  - Echinococcosis or Hydatid Cyst
  - Cysticercosis
  - Cerebral Malaria
  - Toxoplasmosis
  - Amoebic Meningoencephalitis
- Viral and Fungal Infections
- Central Nervous System Viral Infections
  - Herpes Viruses
    - Enterovirus (EV)
    - Poliovirus
    - Nonpolio Enteroviruses
  - Arboviruses
    - Japanese Encephalitis
    - Rabies
    - Kyasanur Forest Disease
    - St. Louis Encephalitis virus and West Nile Encephalitis
  - Measles
  - Rubella
  - Mumps
  - Dengue
  - Progressive Multifocal Leukoencephalopathy (PML)
  - Retroviruses
  - Other Viruses
- Fungal Infections of the CNS
  - Cryptococcus
  - Histoplasmosis
  - Blastomyces
  - Candida
  - Mucormycosis
  - Aspergillus
- Pyogenic Meningitis

Note: All these infections have been dealt with in detail in Section 6, which may be referred to for further details.

INTRODUCTION

Infections of the nervous system are global problems. Once infection is suspected, it is an emergency as ***time is brain*** in all situations. Suspicion by a physician who has examined and assessed the patient is an indication to initiate treatment based on the prevalence pattern in that region. Cerebrospinal fluid (CSF) examination is done to determine the cause and schedule treatment appropriately. Infections may reach the brain by:

- Hematogenous spread
- Extension from nearby structures, e.g. paranasal sinuses, mastoid, etc.
- Iatrogenic during surgical and medical procedures.

In the adult, the most common acute bacterial infection of the nervous system is caused *Streptococcus pneumoniae*. Chronic infections are caused by tuberculosis, brucellosis, borreliosis, leptospira, syphilis and the like.

CENTRAL NERVOUS SYSTEM TUBERCULOSIS (TB)

(*See* Section 6, Ch 49)

TB is still prevalent in the community, though its incidence and prevalence are coming down. Recently, it is found that certain polymorphisms in the human NRAMP1 gene affects susceptibility to TB. Protective effect of Bacillus Calmette-Guerin (BCG) in preventing TB is less than 60%.

Infection starts in the lungs and from the lungs it spreads to the draining lymph node forming Ghon's complex. This phase is called ***tuberculous exposure***. A variable percentage of these patients progress to active ***tuberculous disease***. Hematogenous seeding occurs to highly oxygenated regions including the brain. This leads to small foci called ***Rich foci***. Rupture into subarachnoid space leads to development of meningitis which is the most common form of tuberculous affection of the central nervous system (CNS). Less commonly, encephalitis, tuberculoma and abscess can occur. Local production of tumor necrosis factor-alpha (TNF-α) leads to altered permeability of the blood-brain barrier (BBB) and pleocytosis in the CSF. The microglial cells become the principal targets in the CNS. They produce good amount of cytokines and also attempt intracellular killing of the bacilli which might restrict the infection locally resulting in granuloma formation. Progressive course results in complication due to adhesions causing hydrocephalus, obliterative vasculitis, encephalitis, myelitis, arachnoiditis and others. The exudate contains lymphocytes, plasma cells, fibrin and macrophages. Adhesions around the region of the sella turcica affect the optic chiasm leads to blindness. Adhesions due to basal meningitis affect other cranial nerves. Increase in the intracranial pressure (ICP) leads to global cognitive dysfunction and infarcts in the brain caused by vasculitis lead to focal functional deficits and seizures. Hyponatremia and consequent encephalopathy is very common. TB is an acquired immune deficiency syndrome (AIDS) defining condition and therefore coexistence of human immunodeficiency virus (HIV) should be ruled out in all patients.

Clinical Features of Tuberculous Meningitis

Common features are fever, headache, neck stiffness, focal neurological deficits, behavioral changes and alteration of consciousness. Nonspecific symptoms like malaise, anorexia, fatigue, fever and myalgia. Fundus examination might show optic neuritis, papilledema and choroid tubercles. These are seen as yellow lesions with indistinct borders present singly or in clusters, and they are diagnostic of miliary TB. Children have higher tendency to develop encephalopathy and seizures.

Diagnosis

CSF examination shows lymphocytic pleocytosis, elevated protein (200–1,000 mg/dL) and low glucose values (20–30% of the corresponding blood glucose). Identification of acid-fast bacilli (AFB) in CSF by smear or culture is indicative of definite TB (positive in ± 30%). Examination of the cobweb formed in the CSF on standing gives higher positivity for AFB. Molecular diagnosis is much more rapid than culture, it includes nucleic acid amplification, polymerase chain reaction (PCR), adenosine deaminase, measurement of tuberculostearic acid and interferon (IFN) release assays. Antibody detection is suggestive of tuberculous infection. Even though it is fast, it does not differentiate past and present infection and it gives false-negative results in immunocompromised patients. Antigen detection involves dot immunobinding assay for the specific 14 KDa antigen. Tuberculin skin testing is an adjunct in the diagnosis in 10–20% of patients. QuantiFERON-TB Gold In-Tube test is very fast and results are obtained in 16–24 hours. Computed tomography (CT) and magnetic resonance imaging (MRI) reveal basal meningeal thickening, infarcts, tuberculomas, edema and hydrocephalus. Gadolinium enhanced T1 weighted images highlight exudates and show parenchymal infarcts better. Magnetic resonance spectroscopy (MRS) is other features may reveal T2 shortening and lipid peak.

Diagnostic Criteria

Definite tuberculous meningitis: Patients to fulfill criteria A or B:

A. AFB seen in CSF and cultured.
B. AFB seen in histology.

Probable tuberculous meningitis: Features of meningitis and exclusion of alternative diagnosis.

Possible tuberculous meningitis: Features of meningitis and exclusion of alternative—

- Not tuberculous meningitis
- Alternative diagnosis established.

MRI in TB are shown in Figures 199.1 to 199.5.

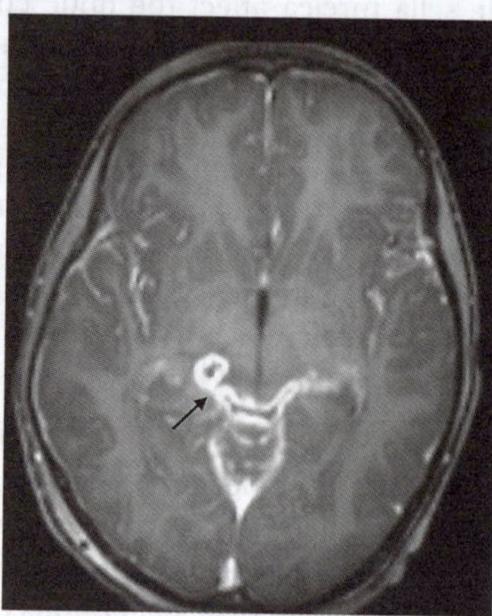

Fig. 199.1: Tuberculoma and exudates (arrow)

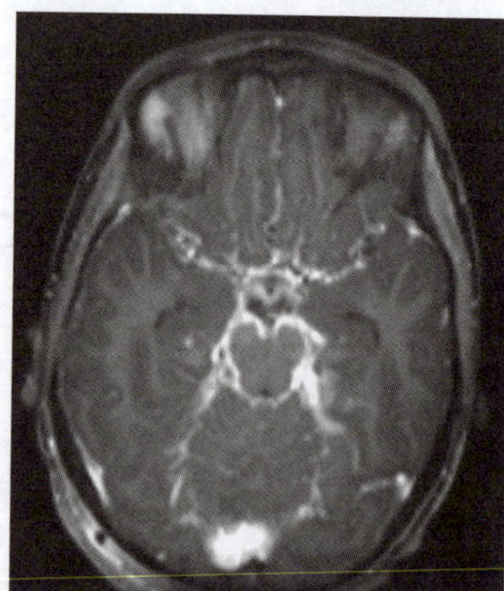

Fig. 199.2: Exudates

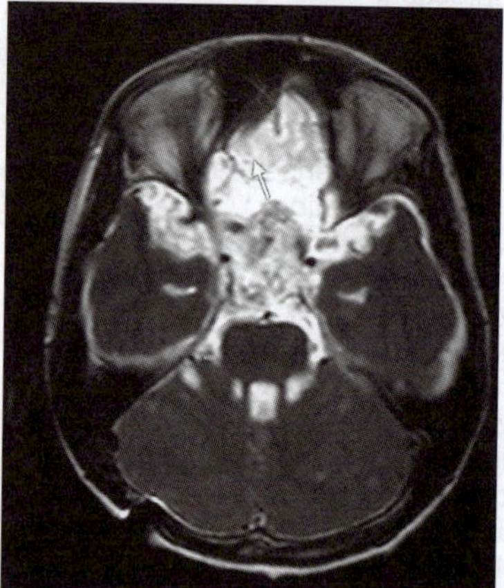

Fig. 199.3: Massive exudates (arrow)

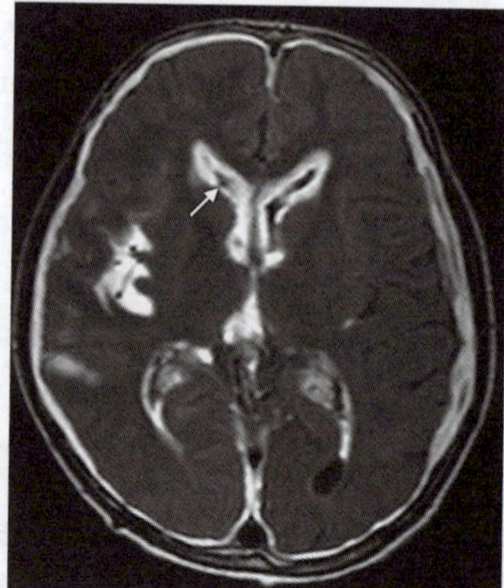

Fig. 199.4: Ventriculitis (arrow)

Treatment

Treatment should be started as early as possible and continued fully. Pyrazinamide and isoniazid cross BBB effectively. The usual regime is to start with 4 drugs (isoniazid, rifampicin, pyrazinamide and streptomycin) in the intensive phase, following which a continuation phase containing isonicotinylhydrazide (INH) and rifampicin should be started.

Doses of Drugs

INH 10 mg/kg in children and 5 mg/kg in adults; rifampicin 10–20 mg/kg/day in children and 450 mg

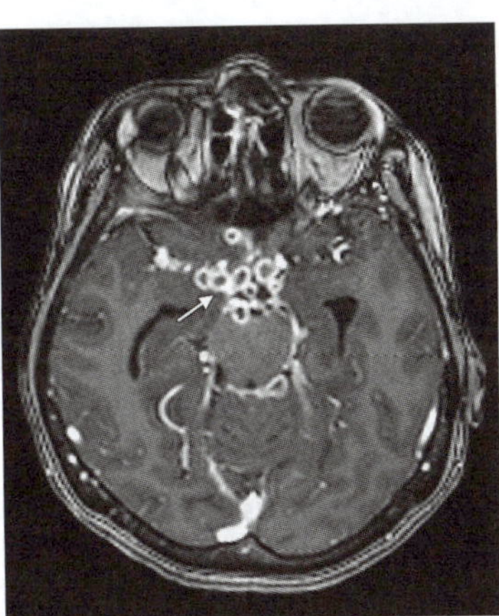

Fig. 199.5: Optochiasmal tuberculomas. *Note:* The ring lesions (arrow)

in adults less than 50 kg bw and 600 mg in adults more than 50 kg bw. Rifampicin crosses the BBB only during inflammatory phase. The dose of pyrazinamide is 30–35 mg/kg bw in children and 1.5 g in adults less than 50 kg and 2 g if more than 50 kg. Ethambutol is given in doses of 15–20 mg/kg in children and 15 mg/kg in adults. It is bacteriostatic and carries the risk of optic nerve toxicity in the presence of inflammation and therefore should be used only when absolutely indicated. World Health Organization (WHO) recommends 2 months intensive phase and 4 months continuation phase. British Thoracic Society recommends 9–12 months of continuation phase. However, our experience suggest that it is safe to use daily regime with 2 months of intensive therapy using four drugs followed by 12–18 months of continuation therapy with two drugs. Steroids are used as adjunct in doses of 1–2 mg/kg in children and 60 mg/day in adults during the acute phase and gradually tapered over 3–4 weeks monitoring the clinical response.

Surgery may be required in hydrocephalus and tuberculous abscess. Patients need regular monitoring of liver function during treatment. If there is three-fold elevation of liver enzymes serum glutamic oxaloacetic transaminase (SGOT) and serum glutamic-pyruvic transaminase (SGPT), pyrazinamide, INH and rifampicin are withdrawn and the patient should be maintained on ethambutol, ofloxacin and streptomycin. After the liver enzymes normalize, the drugs are reintroduced one by one closely monitoring the liver function tests (LFT), and till the full dose is reached. If culture or systemic infection shows resistance to drugs, treatment recommended for multidrug-resistant tuberculosis (MDRTB) or extensively drug-resistant tuberculosis (XDRTB) should be instituted.

NEUROSYPHILIS

Involvement of the nervous system in syphilis used to be common before 1950s, but now it is distinctly uncommon to see fresh cases. Neurological involvement occurs in 4% of untreated cases of syphilis. Men are affected 4–5 times more commonly than women. Along with the AIDS pandemic, syphilis has assumed greater importance since it predisposes to AIDS infection and the two diseases influence each other to causes greater severity. Neurological lesions are caused by direct invasion of the tissues by *Treponema pallidum*. Meningovascular involvement is more common in India, constituting 60–70% of cases (Box 199.1).

Syphilis involves CNS in 3–18 months of inoculation during the secondary stage of syphilis and later. If the CSF is negative at the end of 5 years, chances of CNS invasion becomes remote. Usually, meningitis is asymptomatic but it can present with cranial nerve palsies, seizures, stroke and increased ICP. The earliest CNS manifestation is meningitis and the late ones are meningovascular syphilis, general paralysis of the insane, tabes dorsalis, optic atrophy, meningomyelitis and gumma. They usually occur in combination.

Congenital syphilis presents as blindness due interstitial keratitis and deafness due to cochlear damage. Epiphysitis may lead to gait abnormalities. Congenital syphilis can go through all the features seen in adult neurosyphilis, but the parenchymal lesions develop at younger age groups compared to the acquired form [juvenile general paralysis of the insane (GPI) and tabes].

Meningovascular syphilis may present with stroke like episodes in the young due to occlusion and fibrosis of Heubner's artery and small asymptomatic infarcts. Presence of meningeal enhancements in MRI suggests the diagnosis of meningitis.

General Paralysis of the Insane

GPI develops 15–20 years after primary infections, men are affected more. GPI develops 15–20 years after the primary infection. Men above 40 years are more affected. The frontal and temporal lobes of the brain show cortical atrophy with gliosis. The meninges show thickening and lymphocytic infiltration. Ventricles show dilation and ependymitis. In about 50% of cases, the organism (*T. pallidum*) can be demonstrated in brain biopsy. Clinical picture is characterized by dementia, dysarthria, myoclonus, action tremor, seizures, hyper-reflexia and Argyll Robertson pupil which is strongly suggestive of neurosyphilis. Limbs, lips and tongue may be tremulous and the to and fro movements of the tongue are described as *trombone tremor* since it bears similarity to the movements of the musical instrument trombone. Later, patient becomes unsteady with aphasia hemianopia, and cranial nerve palsies, psychiatric manifestations in the form of delirium, depression and schizoid psychosis.

Vascular episodes occur from time-to-time. These manifest as focal neurological deficits such as hemiparesis, dysphasia or hemianopia. These recover spontaneously. The course of the disease is one of gradual progression with fluctuations, finally proceeding to incapacitation. Prognosis is good if treated early. If untreated, they develop extrapyramidal features as well and become bed bound.

Tabes Dorsalis

This form of parenchymal neurosyphilis is less common than GPI. It develops 25–30 years. Pathologically, primary damage is in the dorsal root ganglia and is characterized by inflammation. Later, posterior roots and columns of spinal cord undergo atrophy. Clinical features consists of paresthesias, predominant spinal cord features in the form of posterior column ataxia, stamping gait, areflexia, loss of deep sensations manifested as failure to elicit pain by squeezing the tendo-Achilles (Abadie's sign) Lhermitte's sign, lightning pains which may be distressing, optic atrophy, Argyll Robertson pupil, sensory denervated bladder and constipation. They develop painless swelling of large joints known as Charcot's joints. Other complications are syphilitic optic atrophy, deafness and vestibulopathy.

Tabetic Crises

The course of the disease is often disturbed by the occurrence of **lightning pains**, which are unique for tabes dorsalis. These are lancinating pains occurring in transverse directions in the limbs, chest and face. Lightning pains differ from neuralgic pains in that the former do not follow the direction of nerve roots. Visceral crises develop frequently. Gastric crisis is characterized by severe epigastric pain and vomiting. Rectal crises give rise to tenesmus. Stridor develops as a result of laryngeal crisis. Early treatment arrests the progress of lesion and physiotherapy may improve functional disability. Once the lesions become established, functional disabilities tend to persist.

Spinal Cord Involvement

Spinal cord can be involved by hypertrophic pachymeningitis, arachnoiditis, acute myelitis and Erb's spinal syphilis. Pachymeningitis and arachnoiditis may present with slowly progressive compressive lesions of the spinal cord giving rise to segmental and long tract signs. These have to be differentiated from other causes of patchy or total compression.

Optic Atrophy

Optic nerve involvement may result from meningovascular or parenchymal involvement. Former leads to arachnoiditis, optic neuritis or retrobulbar neuritis. Changes occur early during the tertiary stage of syphilis. At this stage, specific treatment may help to reverse the condition. Optic atrophy due to parenchymal involvement occurs during the late stages.

Syphilitic Deafness

Deafness may result from several mechanisms in the different stages of syphilis. It may result from affection of cochlea, acoustic nerve, basal meninges or damage to the middle ear.

Gumma of the Central Nervous System

Gumma occurs in tertiary syphilis. Pathologically, the gumma consists of collagen deposition forming an amorphous matrix with lymphocytes and plasma cells at the periphery and multinucleated giant cells in the center. Later, lesions undergo fibrosis. *T. pallidum* is not demonstrable in these lesions. Gumma may be seen in the cranial, dura, leptomeninges, cerebrum and spinal cord where they behave as space occupying lesions. Response to treatment is poor.

Diagnosis of Neurosyphilis

CSF shows lymphocytic pleocytosis with up to 100 cells (lymphocytes/mm^3). Moderate elevation of protein (200–300 mg/dL), increased gamma globulin including oligoclonal bands and positive serological test are seen. Venereal disease research laboratory (VDRL) test, if positive in the CSF is diagnostic. Other tests used *T. pallidum* immobilization (TPI) test and fluorescent treponemal antibody-absorption (FTA-ABS) test.

Treatment of Neurosyphilis

Treatment consists of penicillin G intravenous (IV) 8–24 million units daily in 3–4 divided doses for 14 days. Erythromycin and tetracycline in doses of 500 mg four times a day for 20–30 days can be tried. Lightning pains respond partially to gabapentin or carbamazepine. The affected joints (Charcot's joints) need bracing and support. Atropine and phenothiazines are useful in the treatment of crisis. CSF should be examined every 6 months and if the cells remain increased treatment should be repeated.

Gumma is a rare complication when tumor like masses attached to the dura is seen.

BRUCELLOSIS

Early phase is nonspecific with constitutional symptoms and later can present with cranial nerve palsy, meningitis, meningoencephalitis, optic neuritis, brain abscess and peripheral neuropathy. Diagnosis is made by positive *Brucella* agglutinating antibody in CSF. **Treatment** consists of doxycycline given along with an aminoglycoside like streptomycin or gentamicin. When there is significant neurological involvement, triple therapy with addition of cotrimoxazole is recommended for prolonged periods.

PARASITIC INFECTIONS

(**See Section 6, Ch 68/70 for full details of the parasites**)

A parasite is an organism that lives on or in an organism of another species, known as the host, from the body of which it obtains all its metabolic requirements and is able to multiply and develop.

Several parasites can affect humans and lead to general and organ-based lesions. Details of these are given in Section 6 Ch 68/70. Central and peripheral nervous systems (PNS) may be focal points of infection in many and therefore such cases may present themselves to the neurologist initially. Such cases of cysticercosis, echinococcosis, toxoplasmosis have become more common in recent times. Their neurological manifestations are described in this chapter.

Echinococcosis or Hydatid Cyst (Dog Tapeworm)

(*See* Section 6, Ch 68)

This is caused by the dog tapeworm *Echinococcous granulosus* transmitted to man feco-orally from dogs. Cattle and other mammals are the natural definitive hosts. Humans are accidentally infected. Hydatid cysts are mostly seen in the liver, lungs and other viscera and body cavities. Cysts in the nervous tissues are rarely seen. They give rise to symptoms and signs of intracranial or spinal space occupying lesions. Diagnosis can be established by imaging studies in addition to serological tests which are positive in 60–90% of cases. Biopsy of the lesion should be avoided due to rupture of the cysts and fatal anaphylaxis. A major complication is the development of seizures in addition to focal neurological deficits (Figs 199.6 and 199.7).

Treatment

Drug treatment consists of albendazole given in doses of 400 mg tds or bd for 6–8 weeks. In many cases, the scolex dies and lesion resolves. It also reduces the size of the cyst and partially sterilizes it. Early cases respond fully to oral therapy, but larger ones may have to be removed surgically. Intra and perioperative complications of surgery include anaphylaxis and spread of the lesion. Antiepilepsy drugs may have to be continued for long periods before and after the surgery.

Cysticercosis

(*See* Section 6, Ch 68)

It is the larval form of the pork tapeworm, *Taenia solium* seen in the intermediate host (pigs). Humans are definitive

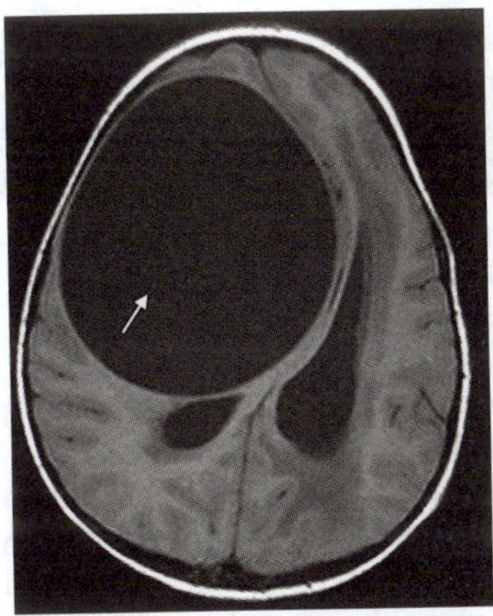

Fig. 199.6: CT scan hydatid cyst. *Note:* The large cysts (arrow) causing displacement of midline structures

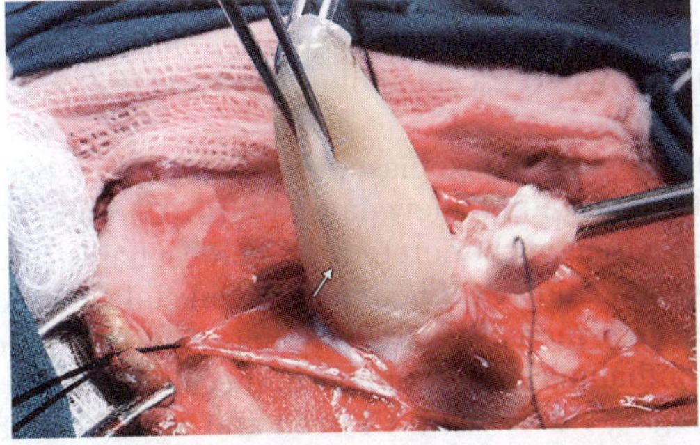

Fig. 199.7: Intraoperative picture removing the hydatid cyst (arrow) from the brain

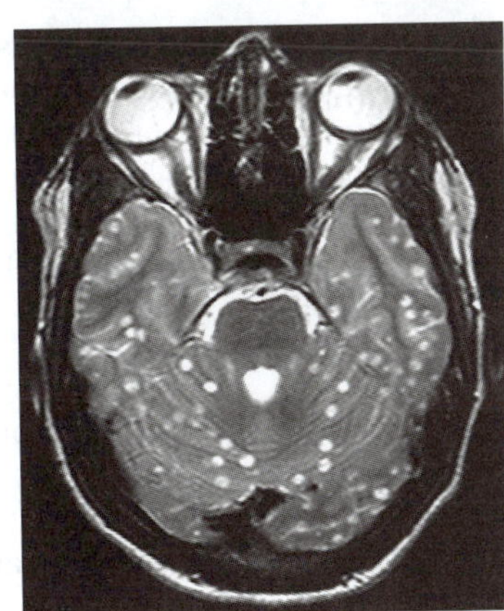

Fig. 199.8: Neurocysticercosis—starry sky appearance

hosts in whom adults develop. Common source of infection is by eating partially cooked or uncooked pork which contain cysticerci. Infection can also occur by ingesting the eggs of the adultworm passed out in feces of man. Uncooked foods like salads, chutneys, pickles and others which are contaminated by the tapeworm eggs hatch out in the intestine and the bladder worms reach the tissues where they grow and mature. Accidently, the larval forms can develop in humans as well. Vegetarians also get infections frequently. They develop into bladder worms with a hollow vesicle and an invaginated scolex, commonly seen in muscles, and in the brain and spinal cord as well.

Less commonly, retrograde peristalsis in the intestines carry the gravid proglottids of the adultworm to the digestive parts of the small intestine leading to digestion of the proglottides and release of the eggs. This is auto-infection. These eggs also hatch out and the larvae reach the tissues. Cysticerci can reach the nervous tissues and develop. The symptoms present with seizures, dementia and obstructive features. It secretes a host of immunomodulatory compounds which suppresses host inflammation but over a period of time triggers inflammation through cytokines, especially when the cysts die 1–2 years after infection. Finally they get calcified (Fig. 199.8).

Clinical features include vague allergic manifestations, various types of seizures, obstructive lesions in the CSF pathway and signs of raised intracranial tension. Epilepsy due to cysticercosis has become a very common cause of seizure disorder in several parts of India and the neighboring countries.

Diagnosis

Del-Brutto Criteria

Clinically, a definite, if absolute criterion is satisfied with one major or with two minor and epidemiological areas. ***Probable:*** One major history of exposure or three minor and exposure.

- Absolute criteria major
  - Direct visualization of the cyst on fundoscopy
  - Scolex in CT or biopsy
  - Suggestive MRI cysts size less than 20 mm without midline shift or lesion spontaneously disappearing.
- ***Minor criteria:*** Radiologically consistent findings but need not be pathognomonic.

Note: Rajasekhar and Chandy in 1997 introduced clinical criteria.

The immunological tests consist of passive hemagglutination, immunofluorescence, complement fixation, enzyme-linked immunosorbent assay (ELISA) and enzyme-linked immunoelectrotransfer blot (EITB).

Diagnosis is readily confined by MRI, which shows multiple or single ring lesions or cysts which may show scolices.

Treatment

Symptomatic treatment is for seizures and brain edema. Fundus examination is done to rule out intraocular lesions which will precipitate endophthalmitis when the cysts die especially under treatment with albendazole. The popular drug which is easily available is albendazole given in doses of 5 mg/kg bw td for 15–30 days or longer depending upon the repeat MRI and clinical features. Presence of intraocular cysts or other lesions due to cysticerci may develop endophthalmitis in addition to encephalopathy on starting specific anthelmintic drug. This is prevented by concurrent or prior administration of glucocorticoids. An alternative is praziquantel given in doses of 50 mg/kg bw for 15–30 days.

Antiepileptic drugs in full dosage (*See* Ch 202) should be started early and continued along with the anthelmintic therapy and for varying periods thereafter to prevent the onset of seizures which are the major long-term complications of the condition.

Glucocorticoids are given along with antiepileptic drugs on a short-term basis (months). If the lesions are less than 5 and ocular lesions are not present albendazole can be safely initiated. If the number is 10 or more the risk of encephalopathy should be kept in mind and might need prolonged steroid therapy. In patients with more than 10 lesions disease modifying treatment can sometimes result in fatal complications due to toxic encephalopathy which is rare. Such situations demand careful modulation of specific therapy and concurrent use of immunosuppressant drugs.

Cerebral Malaria
(*See* Section 6, Ch 64)

Plasmodium falciparum malaria has predilection to stick to vascular endothelium and produce microvascular occlusion in several organs including the brain, which is commonly affected. Diagnosis of cerebral malaria can be made by the presence of *Plasmodium falciparum* in the blood smear along with increase in CSF pressure, xanthochromia, mild lymphocytosis and mild rise of proteins with normal sugar levels in the CSF. Low density lesions can be seen in thalamus on MRI studies (Table 199.1 and Fig. 199.9).

Treatment consists of symptomatic treatment in addition to IV artesunate derivations or quinine hydrochloride along with other antimalarial drugs. Early and intensive treatment saves life, otherwise cerebral malaria is associated with high mortality and residual morbidity.

Toxoplasmosis
(*See* Section 6, Ch 65)

Toxoplasma gondii is an obligate intracellular protozoan which can affect the CNS. Clinical manifestations are generally due to recurrence of latent infection. *Toxoplasmosis* is

Table 199.1: Neurological manifestations and neuroimaging findings of cerebral malaria	
Neurological manifestations	**Neuroimaging findings**
• Coma • Seizures • Ataxia • Hemiplegia • Language disturbance • Cognitive dysfunction, etc.	• MR findings are nonspecific • **Most common:** Cerebral edema • Thalamus, cerebellum, centrum semiovale, corpus callosum, cortex • Contrast may show enhancement • Gradient–blooming • Diffusion weighted imaging (DWI)–restriction • Decreased signal on attenuation diffusion coefficient (ADC)

Note:
- Contrast enhancement indicates increase in the signal intensity after gadolinium contrast
- Blooming: This term is used to denote hypointense shadows in gradient images indicative of bleeding
- Restriction is the term applied to hyperintensity in diffusion weighted images and hypointensity in ADC
- ADC (attenuation diffusion coefficient 3 and 4 if present indicate ischemia).

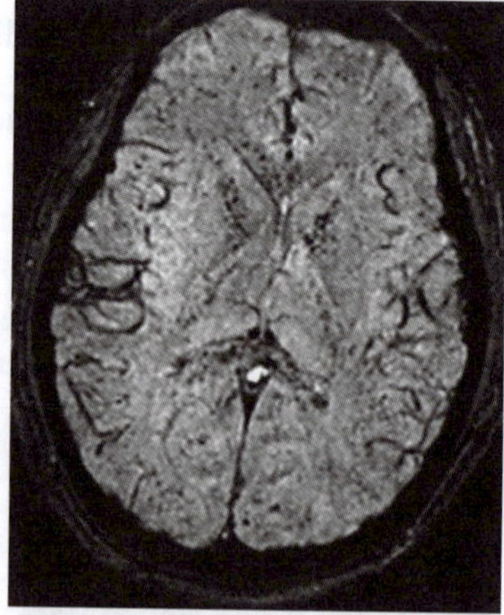

Fig. 199.9: MRI scan in cerebral malaria showing petechial hemorrhages and gradient sequences indicative of bleeding

Abbreviation: MRI = Magnetic resonance imaging

the most common cause of brain space-occupying lesions in AIDS patients. Acquired primary infection presents with chorioretinitis, abscess and encephalitis with areas of hemorrhage. The preferred site is basal ganglia. Human infection is transmitted by cat feces contamination. Patients present with general constitutional symptoms, drowsiness, delirium and seizures with features of meningitis and encephalopathy.

Diagnosis: CSF shows normal glucose with increased pressure, leukocytes and proteins. Immunoglobulin M (IgM) ELISA, fluorescent antibody test and PCR in CSF are diagnostic.

In congenital toxoplasmosis, the infants becomes symptomatic within a few days of birth. Cerebral lesions include a triad of chorioretinitis, hydrocephalus, and cerebral calcifications. ***Clinical features*** include microcephaly, seizures, mental retardation, spasticity, opisthotonus, microphthalmia and hepatosplenomegaly.

Imaging studies both CT scan and MRI show abnormalities which should suggest the lesions (Figs 199.10 and 199.11).

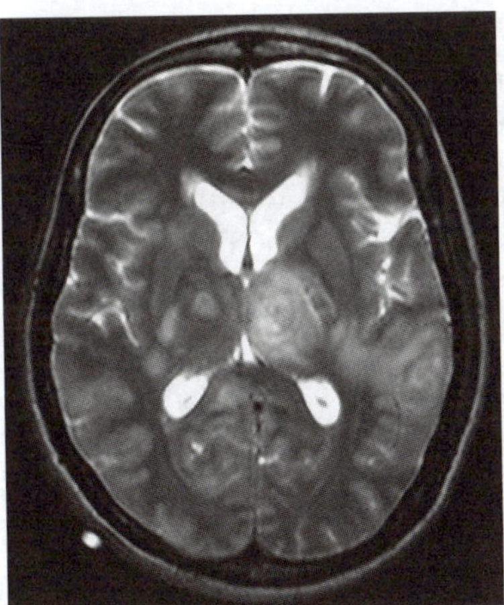

Fig. 199.10: Acquired toxoplasmosis—MRI scan showing nonspecific multiple lesions in both hemispheres

Abbreviation: MRI = Magnetic resonance imaging

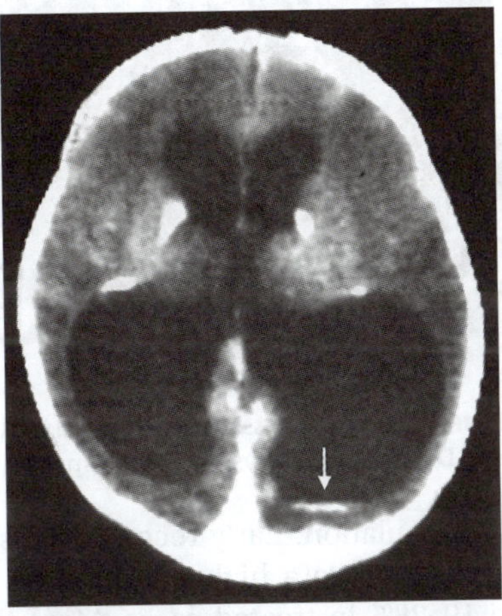

Fig. 199.11: Congenital toxoplasmosis with hydrocephalus (arrow)

Treatment: It consists of a combination of pyrimethamine 25–200 mg/day depending on severity and sulfadiazine 1 g 6th hourly for 14 days. Clindamycin and azithromycin are reserve drugs to be used in resistant cases.

Amoebic Meningoencephalitis

This is caused by *Naegleria gruberi* obtained from contaminated water sources during swimming or immersion. ***Clinical features*** and CSF resemble those of pyogenic meningitis and the condition rapidly fatal if not treated aggressively. In many cases the diagnosis is made at postmortem. CSF may contain motile amoebae with ingested erythrocytes. The recommended treatment is amphotericin B, rifampicin, ketoconazole, azithromycin, and chloramphenicol (Table 199.2).

Gross appearance and histology in amoebic meningoencephalitis are given in Figures 199.12A to D.

Source:

1. Rajshekhar V, Chandy MJ. Validation of diagnostic criteria for solitary cerebral cysticercus granuloma in patients presenting with seizures. Acta Neurol Scand. 1997;96(2):76-81.
2. Chandra SR, Adwani S, Mahadevan A. Acanthamoeba meningoencephalitis. Ann Indian Acad Neurol. 2014;17(1):108-12.

Table 199.2: Differentiating features between GAE and PAM

Parameters	GAE	PAM
Agent	*Acanthamoeba/ Balamuthia*	*Naegleria fowleri*
Victim	Immunodeficient individual	Healthy individual
Entry	Lung, skin/olfactory epithelium	Olfactory neuroepithelium
Clinical	Mass lesion	Pyogenic meningitis
Pathology	Chronic, granulomatous lesions	Acute, fulminant inflammation
CSF	Mononuclear cells, ameba rare	Polymorphs, trophozoites
Gross	Multiple necrotic foci-cortex, posterior fossa	Necrosis orbitofrontal, olfactory bulbs, base of the skull

Abbreviations: GAE = Granulomatous amoebic encephalitis; PAM = Primary amoebic meningoencephalitis; CSF = Cerebrospinal fluid

VIRAL AND FUNGAL INFECTIONS

Nethravathy

CNS VIRAL INFECTIONS

Many of the viruses are neurotropic; resulting in both acute and chronic conditions (Table 199.3). Diagnosis of these disorders is assisted by use of diagnostic tests like electroencephalography (EEG) and imaging modalities (CT or MRI), viral serology and culture. They present with varied features ranging from aseptic meningitis to fatal encephalitis. Though, there are many viruses affecting the CNS, only a few viruses like herpes virus, HIV, Epstein-Barr (EB) virus and cytomegalovirus have specific therapy. For the others supportive care and immunomodulating therapy are useful at times.

Herpes Viruses
(*See* Section 6, Ch 53)

The human herpes viruses (HHV) are a group of deoxyribonucleic acid (DNA) viruses that includes herpes simplex virus (HSV)-type I, HSV-type II, varicella-zoster virus (VZV), cytomegalovirus (CMV or HHV-5), EBV or HHV-4, HHV-6, HHV-7, HHV-8. These are double-stranded DNA viruses, with ability to reactivate resulting in acute and chronic infection of the CNS. The primary entry sites are skin, conjunctiva and mucosa of oropharynx or genitalia. Following replication in these primary sites they show neurotropism either by hematogenous spread or neuronal transmission. The most pathognomonic feature of these HHV is their ability to remain latent in the neuronal tissue and they get reactivated following physical or emotional stress, fever, ultraviolet light and other stimuli resulting in CNS disease.

Herpes Simplex Virus-Type 1 (HSV-1)
(*See* Section 6, Ch 53)

Herpes simplex encephalitis (HSE) is the most common necrotizing encephalitis. HSV encephalitis is caused by HSV-1 in 90% of the immunocompetent adults, while HSV-2 accounts for neonatal and immunocompromised individuals. HSV encephalitis occurs with a frequency of

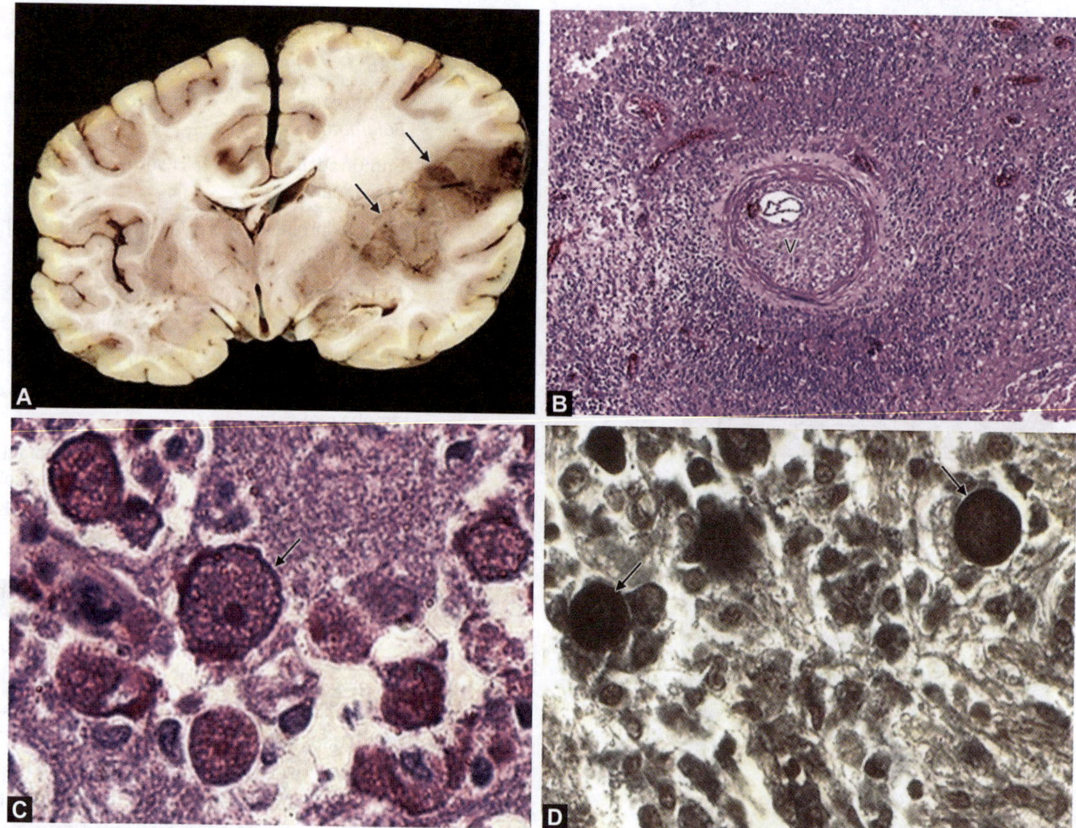

[B: H&E 10X, C: Periodic acid Schiff stain 40X, D: H&E 20X] Amoebic meningoencephalitis

Figs 199.12A to D: A. Large coalescing necrotizing hemorrhagic lesion with perilesional edema and compression of ipsilateral ventricle (arrows); **B.** Dense vasculitis and inflammation; **C.** Large trophozoites with prominent nuclei (arrow); **D.** Thick walled cyst of acanthamoeba (arrows)

Table 199.3: Physical examination findings in viral infections of the central nervous system (CNS)

Physical findings	Viral agents
Vesicular rash	Herpes simplex virus, varicella-zoster virus
Hand-foot-and-mouth disease—vesicles in palms, soles, buttocks	Enterovirus
Maculopapular rash after ampicillin	Epstein-Barr virus (EBV)
Roseola	Human herpes virus (HHV)-6, Colorado tick fever
Pharyngitis	Adenovirus, enterovirus
Conjunctivitis	Adenovirus, enterovirus, St. Louis encephalitis virus
Retinitis	Cytomegalovirus (CMV), West Nile virus, measles, rubella
Parotitis	Mumps, lymphocytic choriomeningitis virus (LCMV)
Orchitis	Mumps, LCMV, EBV
Lymphadenopathy	Mumps, LCMV
Pneumonia	Influenza, parainfluenza
Myocarditis	Enterovirus
Gastroenteritis	Rotavirus
Arthritis	LCMV, parvovirus, chikungunya

Source: Solbrig MV, Koob GF. Epilepsy, CNS viral injury and dynorphin. Trends Pharmacol Sci. 2004;25(2):98-104.

1 per 250,000 population. Early recognition is important as untreated cases have a high mortality of 70% which decreases to 19–28% in treated cases. More than half of the treated cases survive with severe neuropsychiatric sequelae. The virus spreads from the olfactory mucosa to the anterior cranial fossa or from the latent virus in the trigeminal ganglia. Patients present with nonspecific flu-like illness followed by neurological symptoms. The clinical features noted in HSV encephalitis includes fever (90%), headache (80%), behavioral changes, disorientation, visual hallucinations (70–85%), seizures (40–67%), memory disturbances (25–45%), motor deficit (30–40%). MRI is more sensitive in detecting changes than CT. MRI brain shows high signal intensity changes on T2 and fluid attenuation inversion recovery (FLAIR) images in temporal lobes, orbitofrontal lobe, insular cortex and angular gyrus. CSF shows evidence of red blood cells (RBCs) or xanthochromia with lymphocytic pleocytosis [10–1000 white blood cell (WBC)/μL] with moderate elevation of protein and normal sugar levels. CSF and PCR testing have a high sensitivity of 98%, specificity of 94%, and have become a diagnostic gold standard in the diagnosis of HSV encephalitis. EEG may show slowing of background in the initial stages or focal spike and slow wave or periodic lateralized epileptiform discharges (PLEDs) in temporal lobes. Specificity of the EEG is 32.5% and sensitivity is approximately 84%.

Empirical acyclovir therapy has to be started as soon as there is a clinical suspicion at a dose of 10 mg/kg every

8 hours IV in adults for 14–21 days (20 mg/kg is preferred in neonates and children).

Herpes Simplex Virus-Type 2 (HSV-2)
(*See* Section 6, Ch 53)

HSV-2 causes genital herpes and remains dormant in the sacral dorsal root ganglia. The most common cause of neonatal encephalitis is HSV-2 acquired by the child as it passes through the maternal birth canal. Other types of CNS involvement include frontotemporal or diffuse encephalitis, aseptic meningitis, benign recurrent lymphocytic meningitis and myelitis. Neonatal meningitis is treated with acyclovir in doses of 20 mg/kg bw given IV.

Varicella-Zoster Virus (VZV)
(*See* Section 6, Ch 53)

Primary infection with VZV results in acute varicella or chickenpox. The virus remains latent after primary infection in the cranial nerve ganglia (trigeminal, geniculate), dorsal root ganglia (often in the thoracic ganglia) or autonomic ganglia. It gets reactivated after injury, trauma, immunosuppression (HIV, cancer, cytotoxic drugs, systemic illness) and results in various CNS complications that includes cerebellar ataxia, meningoencephalitis, transverse myelitis, aseptic meningitis, herpes zoster (shingles), acute retinal necrosis, retrobulbar optic neuritis, zoster sine herpete (pain without rash), granulomatous arteritis resulting in stroke, multifocal infarcts and small vessel vasculopathy. Drug treatment of encephalitis and myelitis consists of acyclovir given IV in repeated high doses along with glucocorticoids given to prevent complications and sequelae.

Cytomegalovirus (CMV)
(*See* Section 6, Ch 61)

CMV causes both acute and latent infection and persists in asymptomatic phase in the population. It is more common in immunosuppressed individuals and neonates. *Congenital CMV:* Infants acquire this infection while passage through the birth canal or in perinatal period resulting in severe neonatal encephalitis, ependymitis and retinitis. It is fatal in 10% of the patients and severe neurological disability occurs in 80% of survivors. Affected children have developmental delay, hepatosplenomegaly, retinitis and sensorineural hearing loss. Imaging of the brain shows periventricular calcification, polymicrogyria and hydrocephalus.

Immunocompetent individuals: The infection may be inapparent or flu-like illness, aseptic meningitis, Guillain-Barre syndrome (GBS) or chorioretinitis may develop. *Immunosuppressed hosts:* CMV encephalitis presents as nonspecific febrile encephalopathy with or without focal features, microglial nodular encephalitis or ventricular encephalitis characterized by confusion, delirium and multiple cranial nerve palsies. It may also lead on to chorioretinitis, transverse myelitis, myelitis and myeloradiculitis.

CMV encephalitis is generally underdiagnosed. PCR testing has 82% sensitivity and 99% specificity. Treatment consists of IV ganciclovir given as 5 mg/kg twice a day for 2 weeks as induction therapy followed by maintenance therapy with 5 mg/kg/day, 5 days a week. The peripheral and retinal involvement show better response to antiviral agents than cerebral involvement. Other antiviral agents that can be used are valganciclovir, foscarnet and cidofovir.

Epstein-Barr Virus (EBV)
(*See* Section 6, Ch 61)

EBV is the frequent etiological diagnosis in acute infectious mononucleosis. CNS complications occurs in less than 1% of the individuals and results in chronic active EBV infection, nasopharyngeal carcinoma, Burkitt's lymphoma, Hodgkin's disease, lymphoproliferative disorders, acute encephalitis, meningitis, meningoencephalitis, cerebellitis, acute disseminating encephalomyelitis, cranial neuropathy, myelitis, myeloradiculitis, GBS, chronic fatigue syndrome and small fiber sensory or autonomic neuropathy. Immunomodulation with intravenous immunoglobulin (IVIG) may be helpful in EBV-associated neuropathies. None of the antiviral agents have been helpful in acute EBV infection.

Human Herpes Virus-Types 6 and 7 (HHV-6, HHV-7)
(*See* Section 6, Ch 53)

HHV-6 and occasionally HHV-7 results in *exanthema subitum (roseola infantum)* as primary infection in children. HHV-6 is associated with febrile seizures, subacute encephalitis, meningoencephalitis, myelitis, chronic fatigue syndrome and multiple sclerosis. It is also implicated in causing acute encephalitis similar to HSV encephalitis. HHV-7 is implicated in febrile seizures and meningoencephalitis.

Human Herpes Virus-Types 7 and 8 (HHV-7, HHV-8)
(*See* Section 6, Ch 53)

HHV-7 has been detected in CSF and sera of patients with primary or metastatic brain tumors, in children with roseola and encephalopathy. But it is not clear whether this represents reactivation in an immunosuppressed individual or is primarily involved in the pathogenesis. HHV-8 has been associated with Kaposi's sarcoma, lymphoma and multicentric Castleman's disease.

Enterovirus
(*See* Section 6, Ch 56)

The enterovirus family consists of polioviruses, coxsackieviruses A and B, echovirus and enteroviruses. They are the most common cause of viral meningitis.

Poliovirus
(*See* Section 6, Ch 56)

The infection begins as nonspecific flu-like illness and is followed by acute anterior poliomyelitis. Asymmetric flaccid weakness of the limbs, diaphragm or cranial nerves develops within a few days. The other clinical features reported are cerebellitis and transverse myelitis. *Diagnosis* is established by the clinical picture, and CSF pleocytosis, serology and virus isolation. *Treatment* is mainly supportive. Generally, the mortality is less than 10% but it may rise to 50% in bulbar-onset cases. Post-polio syndrome can develop 30–40 years after acute attack of polio and is characterized by progressive lower motor neuron (LMN) weakness.

Non-polio Enteroviruses

These have become more in the limelight after the eradication of poliomyelitis.

The non-polio enteroviruses cause a wide spectrum of diseases in the CNS and PNS.

These include:

- *Meningitis:* Strains most commonly implicated are coxsackie A9, B3–5 and echovirus 4, 6, 7, 8, 11, 18 and 30. The infection spreads by feco-oral or respiratory route. Exanthem of herpangina or the rash of hand-foot-and-mouth disease suggests the possibility of enteroviral infection.
- *Meningoencephalitis:* This is more common in immunodeficient patients with hypogammaglobulinemia, and neonates.
- Epidemic conjunctivitis and acute motor neuron disease. The eye symptoms consist of eye pain, photophobia, blurred vision and subconjunctival hemorrhage. Two weeks later a few patients develop neurological involvement, polio-like illness. The causative viral agents etiological viral agents implicated are EV-70, EV-71 and coxsackie A24.

Most of these patients would require supportive care, especially ventilator support. IVIG may be beneficial in chronic progressive meningoencephalitis.

Pleconaril may be useful in cases of EV-70.

This is a drug specifically used against enteroviruses meningitis in new born nurseries. It was an investigational drug till recently. Maximum effectiveness is at 0.03 µmol concentration. It blocks the viral uncoating in the host cytoplasm. It is not available in India for general use.

Arboviruses

(*See* Section 6, Ch 60)

Among the arboviruses, Japanese encephalitis virus, rabies virus, Kyasanur forest disease and St. Louis encephalitis virus and West Nile encephalitis are rarely reported from some parts of India. They are the etiological agents in causation of different forms of encephalitis.

Japanese Encephalitis

Following an incubation period of 6–16 days, patients develop abdominal complaints followed by headache, seizures, altered sensorium. Signs of extrapyramidal, cerebellar and bulbar features may be present. The mortality rate is 30–40% and survivors are left with severe extrapyramidal impairment, seizures and cognitive and behavioral changes. MRI brain shows T2 and FLAIR hyperintensities in thalami, basal ganglia, substantia nigra, brainstem, cerebellum and cerebral cortical and white matter areas. There is no specific antiviral therapy available; corticosteroids have been used with benefit in many instances. Preventive vaccination is available.

Rabies

(*See* Section 6, Ch 59)

Rabies form an important public health problem in India and neighboring countries with almost 100% mortality. Following a bite, incubation period varies from few days to months (sometimes years), followed by prodromal illness with headache, fever, paraesthesias, pruritus, pain at the bite site (due to involvement of local dorsal root ganglia) and then the neurological symptoms and coma. Nearly 80% of them develop furious (encephalitic) rabies characterized by aerophobia or hydrophobia, spasms of nuchal and pharyngeal muscles. Agitation, hallucinations, autonomic hyperactivity and seizures develop. Paralytic or dumb rabies mimicking Guillain–Barré syndrome (GBS) develops in 20% patients. Rapid diagnosis is established by nuchal biopsy or corneal smear for the presence of rabies antigen. Presence of neutralizing antibodies is diagnostic in unimmunized persons. Once the disease occurs treatment is supportive. Survival in rabies victims is at present remote. Postexposure treatment includes proper cleansing of the wound and administration of rabies vaccine and in specific cases rabies immunoglobulin. Postexposure vaccination, if done properly prevents the development of the disease.

Kyasanur Forest Disease

(*See* Section 6, Ch 60)

It is endemic in Mysore district of Karnataka. It is a tick-borne biphasic illness with initial hemorrhagic fever followed by meningoencephalitis. No specific treatment is available, treatment is supportive.

St. Louis Encephalitis Virus and West Nile Encephalitis

It may be transmitted by *Culex* mosquitoes from birds to humans. They may produce encephalitis, meningitis and neuropathy.

Measles

(*See* Section 6, Ch 53)

Measles is a highly contagious respiratory borne disease caused by measles virus. It may cause four types CNS lesions:

1. *Acute encephalitis:* It develops along with the systemic features of fever, coryza, cough, Koplik's spots
2. Postviral encephalomyelitis
3. Measles inclusion body encephalitis develops 1–6 months after the acute measles infection in immunosuppressed individuals. It is characterized by acute change in cognition, mentation, behavioral changes, myoclonus and seizures. IVIG may be helpful.
4. *Subacute sclerosing panencephalitis (SSPE):* It is a rare fatal disease of the CNS due to persistent infection of mutant measles virus infection. Annual incidence ranges from 0.1 to 5 cases per million populations. Median interval between the acute infection and development of SSPE ranges from 2 to 12 years with median interval of 8 years. Early stages are characterized by cognitive changes, decline in scholastic performance, behavioral changes. Second stage is characterized by myoclonus, ataxia, extrapyramidal involvement, spasticity, optic atrophy or chorioretinitis. This is followed by quadriparesis, autonomic instability, mutism and vegetative state.

Dyken Criteria for Diagnosis

1. *Clinical:* Progressive cognitive impairment with myoclonus
2. *EEG:* Periodic, stereotyped high amplitude slow wave discharges
3. *CSF:* Raised gamma globulin or oligoclonal bands

4. ***Measles antibodies:*** Raised titers in serum ($\geq$ 1:256) or CSF ($\geq$ 1:4)
5. Brain biopsy suggestive of panencephalitis. No adequate therapy is available, combination of intraventricular IFN-α plus oral isoprinosine is the best available treatment option.

SSPE is diagnosed when three of the five features proposed by Dyken are satisfied.

Rubella

(*See* Section 6, Ch 53)

Rubella or German measles can cause these different types of syndromes:
- Asymptomatic stage or mild fever with maculopapular rash and lymphadenopathy
- Postinfectious encephalomyelitis
- ***Congenital rubella:*** Child appears irritable, lethargic, with abnormal muscle tone, bulging fontanelle. Survivors develop sequelae in the form of mental retardation, sensorineural hearing loss, cataract, pigmentary retinopathy and congenital heart disease (CHD).
- ***Late-onset rubella encephalitis:*** Symptoms are similar to SSPE except for the absence of myoclonus, with more protracted course and affecting older children or adults. EEG abnormalities may occur but are not diagnostic.

Mumps

(*See* Section 6, Ch 54)

Mumps virus results in parotitis and meningoencephalitis. Parotitis precedes meningitis by 5 days in 30–40% cases. Active immunization with measles, mumps and rubella (MMR) vaccine has reduced the incidence of these disorders.

Dengue

(*See* Section 6, Ch 60)

Neurological complications of dengue include encephalitis, mononeuritis multiplex, cranial neuropathy, GBS and Reye's syndrome. There is no specific antiviral therapy available, care is supportive. Permanent neurological sequelae are rare.

Progressive Multifocal Leukoencephalopathy (PML)

PML is a subacute demyelinating disease of the CNS as a result of oligodendrocyte infection by JC virus (John Cunningham virus). The virus persists in humans in a latent form. It gets activated with decreasing immunity of the host (e.g. from corticoid use, HIV, lymphoproliferative disorders, tuberculosis and treatment with monoclonal antibodies). There is subacute onset of focal neurological deficits in the form of limb weakness, visual deficit, behavioral changes and ataxia.

MRI brain shows nonenhancing (less than 10% enhancement) white matter changes. No specific therapy is available, though a few beneficial reports on treatment with cidofovir and cytarabine have been reported. Antiretroviral therapy with high active antiretroviral therapy (HAART) improves the cell-mediated immunity and thus helps to improve the patient.

Retroviruses

Human Immunodeficiency Virus

(*See* Section 6, Ch 48)

HIV infection leads to various neurological manifestations either as part of the primary disease process or secondary to opportunistic infection. Various disorders include: aseptic meningitis, dementia, vacuolar myelopathy, various opportunistic infections that includes tuberculosis, cryptococcal meningitis, toxoplasmosis, PML etc.

Human T-Cell Lymphocytotropic Virus (I and II)

Human T-cell lymphocytotropic virus (HTLV) infection is more common in IV drug abuse and homosexuals. It develops as a progressive spastic paraparesis or myeloneuropathy. Patients develop gradually progressive spastic weakness of lower limbs with sphincter dysfunction. Diagnosis of HTLV infection is by ELISA or western blot tests of the serum.

Other Viruses

Nipah virus encephalitis (See Section 6, Ch 52): It is an emerging zoonotic disease first identified in 1998 in Malaysia and Singapore among those working in pig farms. It causes severe encephalitis with mortality rate of 40–75%. It is transmitted to humans by infected pigs.

Chikungunya virus (CHIKV) (See Section 6, Ch 60): It is a togavirus transmitted to man by aedes (*Aedes aegypti*) mosquito. It was first reported in 1952 in Africa and first reported in India from 1963–1973. The virus then re-emerged in 2005 in India. Neurological manifestations include meningoencephalitis, encephalitis, GBS, acute flaccid paralysis, myelopathy and neuropathy. MRI brain is either normal or shows restricted diffusion in white matter with no signal changes in T1 or T2. No specific antiviral agent or vaccine available for this virus.

Chandipura (CHP) virus (See Section 6, Ch 58): It is a rhabdovirus transmitted by sandflies and mosquito. This was reported in South India in 2003 and in West India in 2004. It causes symptoms of brainstem encephalitis.

FUNGAL INFECTIONS OF CNS

Fungi may be saprophytic and pathogenic fungi. Saprophytic fungi infect immunocompromised hosts and they include *Candida*, *Aspergillus* and *Mucor*. Pathogenic fungi infect normal hosts as well. They include blastomyces, histoplasma and coccidioides. Fungal infection is rare in immunocompetent individuals. It is more common in immunocompromised individuals such as patients with AIDS, usage of immunosuppressants, transplant recipients, diabetics and so on. The sites of lesions of different fungi are different due to areas of predilection in the CNS, which is dependent on their size, virulence and type of fungus.

Broadly, fungi are classified into dimorphic fungi and filamentous fungi. Filamentous fungi include *Aspergillus* and *Mucor*. These are larger fungi which cause occlusion of large major arteries resulting in infarction and parenchymal lesions. *Candida* and *Cryptococci* belong to the group of yeasts. These are smaller fungi which reach through the cerebral microcirculation to the meninges and CSF resulting in meningitis and microabscesses.

Dimorphic fungi include *Blastomyces*, *Histoplasma*, *Coccidioides* and *Paracoccidioides*.

General Features

The type and incidence of fungal infections depend and on the geographical distribution of the organism. Histoplasmosis is common in Central United States (Ohio River Valley) and areas infected with bats. Cryptococcosis and histoplasmosis are common in patients exposed to birds. Coccidioidomycosis is common in Central America and Southwestern United States. *Cryptococcosis, Mucor, Aspergillus* and *Candida* species have more universal distribution. Even though there is no clear geographical map of fungal infections in India, it is the clinical experience that almost all fungal infections (both superficial and systemic) are encountered in all parts of India in different specialties.

Cryptococcus

(*See* Section 6, Ch 62)

Cryptococcus neoformans is present in the soil and pigeon excreta in the encapsulated yeast form. Infection is acquired by inhalation. It results in asymptomatic phase of infection with or without mild pulmonary symptoms. Pulmonary involvement occurs in 30–45% cases.

Various forms of CNS involvement include meningitis, cryptococcomas, granulomas and abscesses. Cryptococcal meningitis presents with subacute (1–31 days) onset of fever, headache (65–90%), photophobia, neck stiffness (30%), alteration of mental status (20%) and seizures (10%).

Recommended treatment regimen includes amphotericin-B 0.7 mg/kg bw/day IV and flucytosine 100 mg/kg/day for two weeks. At the end of two weeks, repeat lumbar puncture with fungal culture is done to look for response. Once, response appears, patient continues fluconazole 400 mg oral for prolonged periods. Renal functions (for amphotericin toxicity) and cell count (for flucytosine toxicity) have to be monitored. In cases, where *Cryptococcus* complicates AIDS, treatment has to be continued till the CD4+ count rises about 200/mm³ with antiretroviral therapy (ART).

Histoplasmosis

(*See* Section 6, Ch 62)

Histoplasmosis, which is one of the common mycoses in AIDS patients, is a dimorphic fungus present in soil. Inhalation of infected spores in soil contaminated with bird excreta results in histoplasmosis. It leads to disseminated infection in 95% cases. Patients present with fever, weight loss, dyspnea, hepatosplenomegaly and lymphadenopathy in 25% cases. Meningitis, encephalitis, or focal parenchymal lesions occurs in a proportion of them. Meningitis patients present with fever, headache, altered mental status, seizures and focal neurological deficits. Induction treatment is with amphotericin followed by maintenance therapy with oral itraconazole 200 mg bd for 6 months or more.

Blastomyces

(*See* Section 6, Ch 62)

Blastomyces dermatitidis is a dimorphic fungus that produces mycelia with or without conidia and yeasts. It causes two patterns of illness in immunocompromised hosts but is uncommon in AIDS. It presents as either localized pulmonary involvement or disseminated disease. Intracranial involvement is in the form of meningitis or localized abscesses. Amphotericin-B is used initially for induction therapy followed by maintenance therapy with itraconazole.

Candida

(*See* Section 6, Ch 62)

Candida albicans is the most important pathogenic fungus causing neurological involvement in immunodeficient individuals. Intracranial abscess, small vessel thrombus, microinfarcts occur most commonly in middle cerebral artery (MCA) distribution.

Mucormycosis (Zygomycetes)

(*See* Section 6, Ch 62)

It is a saprophytic fungus that grows on decaying vegetables or food with high carbohydrate content. Individuals with diabetic acidosis, malignancy, transplant recipients and treatment with high-dose corticosteroids are predisposed to develop mucormycosis. Rhino-orbito-cerebral syndrome occurs by vascular invasion producing ischemic lesions. Hence, cavernous sinus involvement and internal cerebral artery thrombus are common. A black discharge from nose due to underlying necrosis suggests the diagnosis of mucormycosis.

Aspergillus

(*See* Section 6, Ch 62)

It has a predilection to stored grains and decaying vegetation. It affects paranasal sinuses and causes pneumonitis. Dissemination occurs due to embolization or direct extension and invasion from pulmonary focus resulting in CNS involvement. Posterior circulation is more vulnerable resulting in vertebrobasilar stroke. Parenchymal involvement occurs in the form of vasculitis, granuloma or abscess. Pulmonary infection may cause direct extension towards thoracic vertebrae resulting in compressive myelopathy (Fig. 199.13).

Take Home Message

Viral and fungal infections of the CNS are difficult to diagnose clinically and they can be catastrophic and

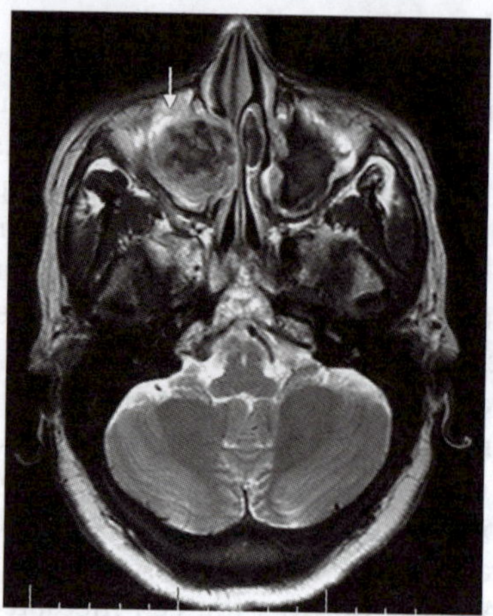

Fig. 199.13: Aspergilloma of maxillary sinus (arrow)

fatal with high mortality and morbidity. Knowledge of the geographical distribution plays a major part in diagnosis. Early investigations with radiological studies, CFS examination and imaging of the brain with CT, MRI and EEG may help to reach specific diagnosis early. The organism can be detected in the CSF by microscopy, culture and molecular methods like PCR. In all atypical infections where bacteria or viruses are excluded, fungal infections should be specially sought for and appropriate treatment instituted early.

Source: Big C, Reineck LA, Aronoff DM. Viral infections of the central nervous system: A case-based review. Clin Med Res. 2009;7(4):142–6.

PYOGENIC MENINGITIS

Thomas Gregor Isaac

(*See* **Section 6, Ch 37**)

Bacterial meningitis presents as an acute purulent infection within the subarachnoid space affecting the leptomeninges and the underlying brain tissue. Clinically it is associated with impaired consciousness, seizures, raised ICP and stroke.

Etiology of Meningitis

This depends on the age of the patient and prevalence of the organism. Infection is through close contact and droplet spread (Table 199.4).

Pathogenesis and Pathophysiology

The common bacteria which cause pyogenic meningitis include *Streptococcus pneumonia, Hemophilus influenza,* and *Neisseria meningitides* which initially colonize the nasopharynx and secrete immunoglobulin A (IgA) proteases that breakdown the mucous barrier and attaches to the receptors on the epithelial cell surface. They are then carried inside by either membrane bound vacuoles to intravascular space or as in case of *H. influenza* by making changes in the apical tight junctions and invading through inside.

Once inside, pathogens avoid phagocytosis by neutrophils because of the presence of the polysaccharide capsule, which also helps the organisms to avoid the complement pathway. Once bacteria have entered the bloodstream, they enter the subarachnoid space in places where the BBB is vulnerable, such as the choroid plexus and other areas of disruption of the BBB. Cells in the choroid plexus and cerebral capillaries possess receptors for adherence of specific bacterial cell surface structures,

favoring the attachment and adherence of meningeal pathogens. Decreased levels of complement lead to defects in opsonization. Low levels of circulating immunoglobulins (Igs) in CSF impair the phagocytosis of pathogens, leading to interference with the clearance mechanisms of the CSF. Group B *Streptococci* cause meningitis in 25% of newborns with bloodstream infections with the organism.

The wide spread inflammation that occurs in the subarachnoid space due to meningitis is not totally the direct result of bacterial infection. This is largely being attributable to the immune response to bacterial infection. Components of the bacterial cell membrane are identified by astrocytes and microglia which are the immunocytes of the brain and they respond by releasing large amounts of cytokines, hormone-like mediators that recruit other immune cells and also stimulate other tissues to participate in the immune response. The BBB becomes more permeable, leading to *vasogenic cerebral edema*. Large numbers of WBCs enter the CSF, causing inflammation of the meninges and also leading to *interstitial edema* of tissues. In addition, the walls of the blood vessels themselves become inflamed (cerebral vasculitis), which leads to decreased blood flow and a third type of edema—*cytotoxic edema*. The three forms of cerebral edema combine to result in increased ICP. Lowering of blood pressure (BP) in the brain caused by acute infection further reduces cerebral blood flow which deprives brain cells of oxygen and lead to apoptosis (programmed cell death) (Fig. 199.14).

It is recognized that administration of antibiotics may initially worsen the process outlined above, by increasing the amount of bacterial cell membrane products released through the destruction of bacteria. Use of corticosteroids is aimed at dampening the immune systems response to this phenomenon.

Clinical Presentation

Seizures can occur in 20–40% of the patients. Focal seizures are due to focal arterial ischemia, focal edema or cotical venous thrombosis with hemorrhage. Generalized seizure activity or status epilepticus may be due to hyponatremia, cerebral anoxia or even as a side effect of high dose antibiotics. Raised ICP is a common feature and evidenced by altered level of consciousness, papilloedema, presence

Table 199.4: Etiology of bacterial meningitis	
Age group	**Causes**
Newborns	Group B *Streptococcus, Escherichia coli, Listeria monocytogenes*
Infants and children	*Streptococcus pneumoniae, Neisseria meningitidis, Haemophilus influenza* type B
Adolescents and young adults	*Neisseria meningitidis, Streptococcus pneumoniae*
Older adults	*Streptococcus pneumoniae, Neisseria meningitidis, Listeria monocytogenes*

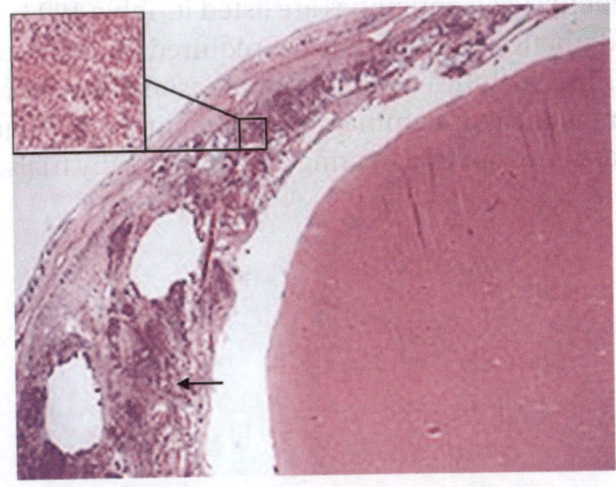

Fig. 199.14: Biopsy specimen showing dense neutrophilic infiltration of the meninges especially in the subarachnoid space (arrow)

Table 199.5: CSF abnormalities in bacterial meningitis

Opening pressure	>180 mm H$_2$O
White blood cells	10 to 10,000/μL; neutrophils predominate
Red blood cells	Absent in nontraumatic tap
Glucose	<2.2 mmol/L (<40 mg/dL)
CSF/serum glucose	<0.4
Protein	>0.45 g/L (>45 mg/dL)
Gram's stain	Positive in >60%
Culture	Positive in >80%
Latex agglutination	May be positive in patients with meningitis due to *S. pneumoniae*, *N. meningitidis*, *H. influenzae* type b, *E. coli*, group B *Streptococci*
Limulus lysate	Positive in cases of Gram-negative meningitis
PCR	Defects bacterial DNA

Abbreviations: CSF = Cerebrospinal fluid; PCR = Polymerase chain reaction; DNA = Deoxyribonucleic acid

Table 199.6: Empirical antibodies to start treatment in acute bacterial meningitis

Indication	*Antibiotic*
Preterm infants to infants < 1 month	Ampicillin + cefotaxime
Infants 1–3 months	Ampicillin + cefotaxime/ceftriaxone
Immunocompetent children >3 months and adults <55 years	Cefotaxime or ceftriaxone + vancomycin
Adults >55 years and adults of any age with alcoholism or other debilitating illnesses	Ampicillin + cefotaxime or ceftriaxone + vancomycin
Hospital acquired meningitis, post-traumatic or postneurosurgery meningitis or patients with impaired cell mediated immunity	Ampicillin + ceftazidime + vancomycin

Note: The dosage and therapeutic details of antibiotics are given in Section 1, Ch 5.

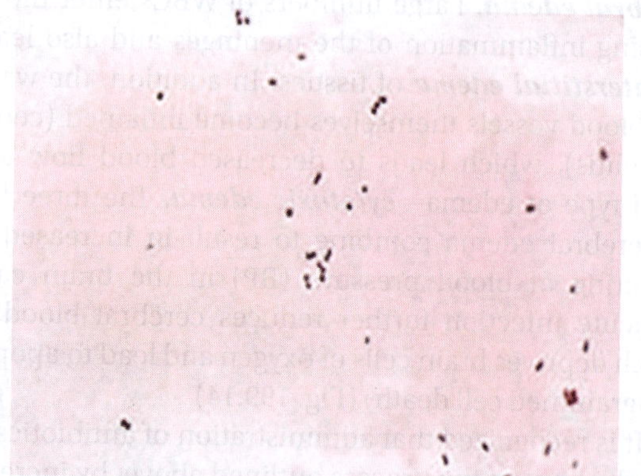

Fig. 199.15: Gram staining showing meningococci from culture. This helps in starting specific antibiotics early

of dilated poorly reactive pupils, sixth nerve palsies, decerebrate posturing and Cushing's reflex bradycardia, hypertension and irregular respirations. The disastrous complication of raised ICP is herniation of intracranial structures which may occur in up to 8% of the cases. Specific clinical features like rash are highly suggestive of meningococcemia.

Diagnosis: Clinical suspicion should be confirmed by CSF findings are diagnostic (Table 199.5 and Fig. 199.15).

Treatment

Commonly used antibiotics are listed in Table 199.6.

Adjunctive therapy is also required in most of the cases. This includes use of dexamethasone as it decreases the meningeal inflammation and neurologic sequelae such as sensorineural hearing loss as per many trials.

Management of raised ICP with supportive measures and agents which lower ICP are also useful to prevent brainstem herniation and mortality.

Anti-*H. influenzae* type B vaccines are now advocated in India and are preventive for meningitis due to *H. influenzae* especially in children.

In a culture proved case of pyogenic meningitis in immunocompetent person, duration of treatment is 2 weeks for Gram-positive organisms and 3 weeks for Gram-negative organisms. The medicines should be continued in the same dose and by parenteral route. As the disease improves, BBB closes and CSF penetration of the drug decreases and therefore to maintain optimum level in the CSF, it should be continued in the same dose parenterally. Repeat lumbar puncture is not indicated unless there is a suspicion of a neighborhood septic focus.

Prognosis

Mortality rate is 3–7% for meningitis caused by *H. influenzae*, *N. meningitidis* or group B *Streptococci* and 20% for *S. pneumoniae*. In general the risk of mortality increases with:

- Decreased level of consciousness at time of presentation
- Early onset of seizures before 24 hours
- Raised ICP
- Extremes of age
- Presence of comorbid conditions including shock or need for mechanical ventilation
- Delay in initiation of treatment.

Common sequelae which are seen in survivors include mental subnormality, seizure disorder, memory impairment, hearing loss, dizziness and gait disturbances.

Dementias and Metabolic Encephalopathy

AS Girija

Chapter Summary

- Types of Memory
- Taking History and Examination of Memory Impaired Patient
- Conditions Mimicking Dementia
- Cortical and Subcortical Dementias
- Reversible Dementias—How to Identify Them?
- Alzheimer's Disease (AD)
- Adjunctive Therapies for Behavioral Symptoms
- Subcortical Dementia
- Mixed Cortical Subcortical Dementia
- Dementia with lewy bodies
- Corticobasal Degeneration

INTRODUCTION

Dementia is a clinical state characterized by loss of function in at least two cognitive domains. When making a diagnosis of dementia, features to look for include memory impairment and at least one of the following— aphasia, apraxia, agnosia and/or disturbances in executive functioning. To be significant, the impairments should be severe enough to cause problems with social and occupational functioning and the decline must have occurred from a previously higher level. It is important to exclude delirium when considering such a diagnosis. Delirium can be distinguished by the following features:

- Sudden onset
- Altered consciousness
- Disproportionately impaired attention and concentration
- Fluctuation in cognitive function with lucid intervals
- Psychomotor and autonomic overactivity
- Hallucinations.

An understanding of cognitive function and its anatomical correlates is necessary in order to ascertain which brain areas are affected. This in turn, aids diagnosis. A discussion of the localization of all cognitive processes is beyond the scope of this review. It is however, particularly important to have an understanding of memory and its subdivisions, which is necessary to aid in differential diagnosis. We shall then illustrate how the history and examination, including bedside cognitive testing are used in diagnosis.

TYPES OF MEMORY

Memory can be thought of in terms of working memory, episodic memory (anterograde and retrograde), semantic memory, remote memory and implicit memory (Box 200.1). Classically, early Alzheimer's disease (AD) causes defects in anterograde episodic memory (e.g. the ability to remember an address after 5 minutes or longer).

Box 200.1: Classification of memory

Working memory: Immediate retention of new information for a few seconds.
Episodic memory: Personally experienced events that rely on temporal and contextual clues for retrieval.
- ***Anterograde:*** Newly encountered information.
- ***Retrograde:*** Past events.
Semantic memory: Word meaning and general knowledge.
Implicit Memory: Learned responses not available for conscious reflection, e.g. driving, playing music, etc.

TAKING HISTORY AND EXAMINATION OF MEMORY IMPAIRED PATIENT

It is vital to obtain a corroborating history from a relative or close friend in addition to the patient's account if they can provide one. The need to physically examine the patient, looking for signs pointing to a particular cause, is discussed below.

History Taking

It is useful to interview the patient and the accompanying person separately. The absence of a concerned relative or friend at the appointment may lessen the likelihood of dementia in a patient complaining of memory problems. Interviewing the patient separately enables the cooperation and language skills to be assessed without them being masked by interruptions or assistance from a third party. It also allows an assessment into the degree of insight of the affected individual. Conversation with the patient may be as important as any formal cognitive assessment. The presence of word finding difficulties, paraphasic errors, and inappropriate behavior is helpful in determining the likely cause of the dementia. Documentation of specific examples is a useful way of providing information that can be utilized by subsequent clinicians. Difficulties with specific aspects of memory are suggested by certain problems encountered in day to day activities. Anterograde memory deficiencies are suggested by losing of objects, repetitive questioning, difficulty taking messages, an increasing reliance on lists, failure to follow plots of films or television programs and getting lost (navigation). Semantic memory breakdown may manifest as a diminution of vocabulary with words being substituted by 'thing'. The meaning of unusual or infrequently used words may be lost. The level of alertness and cooperation during the interview should be assessed. If alertness is decreased, causes of this should be sought, e.g. by a careful scrutiny of the drug history. Delirium as opposed to dementia should be considered if the patient appears poorly responsive.

Important features to note in the history include

- Symptoms at onset
- The tempo of evolution of symptoms
- The impact on work and family life
- Issues of safety, e.g. driving
- A family history of dementia
- Risk factors, e.g. vascular
- Past medical history.

The age of the patient is important as dementia in the young has a different etiological profile than that seen in the elderly. AD, however, remains the most common dementia even in younger people, followed by vascular dementia and frontotemporal lobar degenerations (FTLDs). Genetic and metabolic disorders are more common in this age group and other diagnoses to consider include vasculitis, infections [e.g. acquired immunodeficiency syndrome (AIDS), tuberculous meningoencephalitis, Lyme disease, subacute sclerosing panencephalitis (SSPE)] and Creutzfeldt-Jakob disease (CJD).

Formal Cognitive Assessment

A more detailed assessment of memory is necessary and performed by using several specific bedside cognitive tests. During a thorough cognitive assessment, it is useful to examine the following:

- *Orientation*—in time and place.
- *Attention*—e.g. serial sevens, months of the year or 'WORLD backwards'.
- *Memory*—e.g. address recall, name of prime minister and others.
- *Language*—e.g. naming of items, reading, writing, comprehension and repetition.
- *Executive function*—e.g. letter and category fluency.
- *Praxis*—e.g. alternating hand movements, imitation of gestures.
- *Visuospatial function*—e.g. drawing a clock face, overlapping pentagons.

Rating Scales

The widely used mini-mental state examination (MMSE) provides useful information in grading established dementia but does have limitations, particularly in detecting early disease. It contains a crude test of delayed recall, with only three items being employed and not enough time allowed between registration and recall. It lacks a timed test to detect problems with verbal fluency. The language items are also very easy, with all but significantly aphasic patients tending to perform at ceiling on these items. The Addenbrooke's cognitive examination (ACE) has been developed to address the deficiencies of the MMSE. It also has the advantage of being brief enough to allow a clinician to use it within the time constraints of a new patient appointment. It should be noted that even ACE is no match for formal neuropsychology assessment. Such services are, however, patchy and in some services are nonexistent, so the clinician must remain competent at assessing cognition.

Neurological System

Aside from the mental state examination and specific tests of cognitive function, it is important to examine the neurological system in any patient with possible cognitive impairment. Neurological examination is, however, often normal in the early stages of many neurodegenerative dementias and specific abnormalities may point to rarer or potentially treatable causes of dementia. It is important to assess the patient at rest for any involuntary movements, including chorea, tremor, dystonia and myoclonus (which may be spontaneous or stimulus sensitive). The muscles should be observed for fasciculations. The presence or absence of primitive reflexes (frontal release signs) should be determined. An ocular examination should involve careful assessment of visual acuity, pupillary responses, eye movements, optic disks and visual fields. Assessment of speech and swallowing may reveal the presence of bulbar features. Examination for pyramidal or extrapyramidal signs is important and gait should be assessed wherever possible. Ataxia is unusual in AD, dementia with Lewy bodies (DLB) and frontotemporal dementia (FTD); its presence should raise the possibility of a different cause. The presence or absence of apraxia should be assessed by asking the patient to perform alternating hand movements or copy gestures. A peripheral neuropathy may be present and when cooperation allows signs of this should be sought. The significance of these findings in relation to specific potential diagnoses is outlined in Table 200.1.

Ataxia

Ataxia includes paraneoplastic disease, cerebellar tumor, Whipple's disease, CJD, AIDS, dementia complex, spinocerebellar ataxia (SCA), Wernicke-Korsakoff syndrome, Hallervorden-Spatz syndrome, ornithine transcarbamylase deficiency, Niemann-Pick disease, mitochondrial disorders, adrenoleukodystrophy, neurodegeneration with brain iron accumulation (NBIA), lead poisoning. Hallervorden-Spatz syndrome is caused by pantothenate kinase-associated neurodegeneration (PKAN), which is an autosomal recessive disorder characterized by involuntary spasticity and progressive dementia. It is included in the disorders of neurodegeneration associated with iron accumulation in the brain.

Involuntary Movements

Involuntary movements include Huntington's disease (HD), inherited metabolic disorders including Wilson's disease, CJD, corticobasal degeneration (CBD), systemic lupus erythematosus (SLE), Whipple's disease, Hallervorden-Spatz and Lesch-Nyhan syndrome. This syndrome is inherited as an X-linked or sex-linked trait and the disease occurs mostly in boys. Main pathology is the absence or severe deficiency of hypoxanthine-guanine phosphoribosyltransferase 1 (HPRT1) which is needed for purine metabolism. They show abnormally high levels of uric acid with the deposition of urate crystals, may abnormally accumulate in the joints and kidneys. They also show neurological disabilities.

Myoclonus

Myoclonus include postanoxia, CJD, AD, SSPE, myoclonic epilepsies, Hashimoto's encephalopathy, DLB and CBD.

Extrapyramidal Signs

Extrapyramidal signs include DLB, Parkinson's disease (PD), progressive supranuclear palsy (PSP), vascular

Table 200.1: Abnormal neurological signs and their significance in dementia

Physical sign	Seen in
Ataxia	Paraneoplastic disease, cerebellar tumour, Whipple's disease, Creutzfeldt-Jakob disease (CJD), AIDS dementia complex, spinocerebellar ataxia (SCA), Wernicke-Korsakoff syndrome, Hallervorden-Spatz, ornithine transcarbamylase deficiency, Niemann-Pick disease, mitochondrial disorders, adrenoleucodystrophy, neurodegeneration with brain iron accumulation (NBIA), lead poisoning
Involuntary movements	Huntington's disease (HD), inherited metabolic disorders including Wilson's disease, CJD, corticobasal degeneration (CBD), systemic lupus erythematosus (SLE), Whipple's disease, Hallervorden-Spatz, Lesch-Nyhan syndrome
Myoclonus	Post-anoxia, CJD, Alzheimer's disease (AD), subacute sclerosing panencephalitis (SSPE), myoclonic epilepsies, Hashimoto's encephalopathy, dementia with Lewy bodies, CBD
Extrapyramidal signs	Dementia with Lewy bodies, Parkinson's disease (PD), progressive supranuclear palsy (PSP), vascular dementia, frontotemporal dementia (FTD), CJD, Wilson's disease, HD, dentato-rubro-pallido-luysian atrophy (DRPLA), neuroacanthocytosis, cerebral autosomal dominant arteriopathy with subcortical infarcts and leucoencephalopathy (CADASIL), Niemann-Pick, mitochondrial disorders, NBIA
Pyramidal signs	Motor neuron disease, CJD, B_{12} deficiency, multiple sclerosis (MS), SCA, multisystem atrophy, hydrocephalus, AD, Hallervorden Spatz, CADASIL, mitochondrial disorders, adrenoleucodystrophy, FTD
Optic disc pallor	MS, B_{12} deficiency
Papilloedema	Tumor, subdural hematoma, hydrocephalus
Cortical blindness	Vascular disease, AD, CJD
Anosmia	Subfrontal meningioma, head injury, AD, PD, HD
Abnormal eye movements	Progressive supranuclear palsy, Wernicke-Korsakoff, Whipple's disease, CBD, mitochondrial cytopathies, cerebellar tumors, causes of raised intracranial pressure, CJD, mitochondrial disorders, HD, Niemann-Pick type C
Other cranial nerve signs	Sarcoidosis, tumors, neoplasia, tuberculous meningitis
Alien hand	CBD
Visual field defect	Tumor, vascular disease, CJD
Pupillary abnormalities (Argyll Robertson pupil)	Neurosyphilis
Peripheral neuropathy	Vitamin B_{12} deficiency, paraneoplastic disorders, neuroacanthocytosis, spinocerebellar ataxia, Hallervorden Spatz, adrenoleucodystrophy, NBIA, lead poisoning, SLE
Early onset incontinence	Tumor, hydrocephalus, PSP
Bulbar features	Frontal dementia (motor neuron disease)
Fasciculations	Frontal dementia (motor neuron disease), rarely CJD
Seizures	Vasculitis, neoplasia, primary angiitis of the nervous system, limbic encephalitis, acquired immunodeficiency syndrome (AIDS) dementia complex, neurosyphilis, SSPE, Hashimoto's encephalopathy
Grimacing facial expression	Wilson's disease

dementia, FTD, CJD, Wilson's disease, HD, dentatorubro-pallidoluysian atrophy (DRPLA), neuroacanthocytosis, cerebral autosomal dominant arteriopathy with subcortical infarcts and leukoencephalopathy (CADASIL), Niemann-Pick, mitochondrial disorders, NBIA.

Pyramidal Signs

Pyramidal signs include motor neuron disease, CJD, LCBD, vitamin B_{12} deficiency, multiple sclerosis (MS), SCA, multisystem atrophy, hydrocephalus, AD, Hallervorden-Spatz, CADASIL, mitochondrial disorders, adrenoleukodystrophy and FTD.

Optic Disk Pallor

It include vitamin B_{12} deficiency and MS.

Papilledema

Papilledema include tumor, subdural hematoma and hydrocephalus.

Cortical Blindness

Cortical blindness include tumor, subdural hematoma and hydrocephalus.

Anosmia

Anosmia include subfrontal meningioma, head injury, AD, PD and HD.

Abnormal Eye Movements

Abnormal eye movements include progressive supranuclear palsy, Wernicke-Korsakoff, Whipple's disease, CBD, mitochondrial cytopathies, cerebellar tumors, causes of raised intracranial pressure, CJD, mitochondrial disorders, HD and Niemann-Pick type C.

Other Cranial Nerve Signs

Other cranial nerve signs include sarcoidosis, tumors, neoplasia and tuberculous meningitis.

Alien Hand

Alien hand includes CBD.

Visual Field Defect

Visual field defect include tumor, vascular disease and CJD.

Argyll Robertson Pupil

Argyll Robertson pupil include neurosyphilis.

Peripheral Neuropathy

Peripheral neuropathy include vitamin B_{12} deficiency, paraneoplastic disorders, neuroacanthocytosis, SCA, Hallervorden-Spatz, adrenoleukodystrophy, NBIA, lead poisoning and SLE.

Bulbar Features

Bulbar features include frontal dementia (motor neuron disease).

Fasciculations

Fasciculations include frontal dementia (motor neuron disease), rarely CJD.

Seizures

Seizures include vasculitis, neoplasia, primary angiitis of the nervous system, limbic encephalitis, AIDS dementia complex, neurosyphilis, SSPE and Hashimoto's encephalo-pathy.

Examination of Other Systems

It is also useful in looking for evidence of multisystem disease. In addition to the neurological examination, patients should be assessed for signs of immuno-compromise predisposing to opportunistic infections such as progressive multifocal leukoencephalopathy (PML), toxoplasmosis or primary cerebral lymphoma possibly indicating human immunodeficiency virus (HIV)/AIDS. Features of systemic disease may indicate an underlying neoplasm, vasculitis, infection, or a metabolic disorder. Uveitis may indicate sarcoidosis, Behçet's disease or MS. The presence of cardiac disease, hypertension or a previous transient ischemic attack (TIA) or stroke may suggest cerebrovascular disease.

Armed with the above theoretical knowledge regarding memory and its subdivisions along with how to elicit information from history taking and examination, we can now return to trying to achieve a diagnosis in a patient with possible dementia.

CONDITIONS MIMICKING DEMENTIA

The first and most important question to be asked when assessing the memory impaired patient is 'Is this dementia?'. Conditions mimicking dementia are considered under the term *pseudodementia* and often relate to affective disorders that represent treatable psychiatric pathology, such as anxiety or depression.

Certain features may point to an early pseudodementia rather than a dementia, but often it is the clinical assess-ment overtime that enables a distinction between the two to be made. Biological features of depression should be enquired about in all cases (anorexia, weight loss, sleep disturbance and motor retardation) although none of these are exclusive to pseudodementia. Emotional blunting, loss of interest, pessimism, guilt and negative ruminations may be present. An identifiable emotional precipitant may be present in pseudodementia, along with a relatively abrupt onset and lack of progression. Some organic dementias, however, present with anxiety and depression and may be mistaken initially for a pure psychiatric illness.

If it is dementia, what sort of dementia is it?

The whole brain is not affected equally in dementia. Psychological processes are organized into specific brain areas and therefore different diseases reflect the distribution of pathology within the anterior, medial and posterior cortex by producing distinct neuropsychological syndromes.

CORTICAL AND SUBCORTICAL DEMENTIAS

Deficits in certain areas, especially relatively early in the disease may point to a specific dementia. One of the more widely used categorizations of dementia is into cortical (predominantly involving the cerebral cortex) and subcortical forms (primarily affecting the basal ganglia, thalamus and deep white matter) (Table 200.2). Examples of cortical dementias include AD and CJD. The clinical manifestations of cortical dementias include agnosia, spatial disorientation, language problems, apraxia, amnesia and problems with visuospatial functioning depending on the location of the pathology.

Examples of subcortical dementias include PD, HD, vascular dementia, PSP, Wilson's disease and AIDS dementia complex. Patients with a subcortical dementia show slowness and rigidity of thinking (bradyphrenia) often with perseveration. Although forgetful, they do not have a severe amnesia. There is difficulty in planning and sequencing of events and the pattern of cognitive impairment may be similar to that seen in frontal lobe dysfunction.

Some disorders display signs of both a cortical and subcortical dysfunction relatively early in the disease. Examples of cortico-subcortical conditions include cortical DLB and CBD.

INVESTIGATIONS

Recommended investigations in all patients with dementia include full blood count, erythrocyte sedimentation rate (ESR), urea and electrolytes, liver function tests (LFTs), vitamin B_{12}, red cell folate, thyroid function, chest X-ray, and computed tomographic (CT) brain scan. In some circumstances, it may be considered appropriate to perform immunological tests for vasculitis, serum angiotensin-

Table 200.2: A comparison of cortical and subcortical dementia according to neuropsychological profile

Characteristic	Cortical	Subcortical
Speed of cognitive processing	Normal	Slowed
Planning, problem solving, initiative (frontal 'executive' abilities)	Preserved in early stages	Impaired from onset
Personality	Intact until late, unless frontal type	Apathetic, withdrawn
Memory	Severely amnesic	Forgetful
Language	Aphasia	Normal except for dysarthria and reduced output
Visuospatial and perceptual difficulties	Impaired	Impaired
Mood	Depression not uncommon in early Alzheimer's disease	Depression common
Agnosia/prosopagnosia	Often present	Not usually seen

converting enzyme (ACE), HIV testing, paraneoplastic antibodies and screening for inborn errors of metabolism. Additional investigations are recommended in specific circumstances and include brain magnetic resonance imaging (MRI), functional imaging [single-photon emission computed tomography (SPECT)], cerebrospinal fluid (CSF) analysis and electroencephalography (EEG). Further specialized investigations to be considered include a slit lamp examination (looking for the Kaiser-Fleischer rings of Wilson's disease), cardiac screening for emboli and further specific genetic screening for individual disorders. Cerebral biopsy should be considered if a treatable cause is thought possible (e.g. a cerebral vasculitis) in the absence of an alternative diagnosis.

REVERSIBLE DEMENTIAS—HOW TO IDENTIFY THEM?

Reversible dementias represent a minority of dementias but the importance of identifying them is obvious. Clinicians should have an understanding of what may differentiate reversible dementias from the progressive, largely untreatable neurodegenerative conditions. Some 'treatable' dementias may not be cured, but the disease course may be modified by addressing the underlying cause (e.g. vascular disease and modification of risk factors). Causes of dementia amenable to treatment are outlined in Box 200.2. Examples of non-neurological

---

Box 200.2: Illnesses associated with treatable dementia

Depressive pseudodementia
Space occupying lesions
- Benign tumors, especially subfrontal meningiomas
- Subdural hematoma

Hydrocephalus
Deficiency states
- Vitamins B_{12}, B_1 (Wernicke-Korsakoff), B_6
- Niacin (pellagra)

Endocrine disease and metabolic disorders
- Hypothyroidism
- Chronic hypocalcemia
- Recurrent hypoglycemia
- Cushing's disease
- Addison's disease
- Uremia
- Hepatic encephalopathy
- Hashimoto's encephalopathy
- Wilson's disease

Infections
- Acquired immunodeficiency syndrome (AIDS) dementia complex
- Lyme disease
- Tuberculosis (TB)
- Syphilis
- Whipple's disease

Inflammatory and vasculitides
- Systemic lupus erythematosus (SLE)
- Giant cell arteritis (GCA)
- Polyarteritis nodosa (PAN)
- Behçet's disease
- Neurosarcoidosis

Alcoholic dementia
Chronic intoxications
- Heavy metals
- Drugs
- Carbon monoxide poisoning

Immune mediated: Limbic encephalitis (paraneoplastic or associated with voltage gated potassium channel antibodies)

Box 200.3: Examples of non-neurological clinical features associated with potentially treatable causes of dementia

Clinical signs	Diseases
Lymphadenopathy	HIV/AIDS, malignancy, sarcoidosis, tuberculosis (TB)
Signs of immunocompromise • Herpes simplex ("cold sores") • Herpes zoster • Oral candida • Hairy leucoplakia • Kaposi's sarcoma	HIV/AIDS, malignancy
Hepatomegaly	Malignancy
Cachexia	• Nutritional deficiency • Alcoholism • Malignancy • AIDS
Hypertension	Vascular disease
Kaiser-Fleischer rings	Wilson's disease
Uveitis	Sarcoid, TB, multiple sclerosis
Rash • Erythema nodosum • Vasculitic purpura • 'Butterfly' rash • Erythema chronicum migrans • 'Casel's necklace'	• Sarcoid, TB • Systemic vasculitides • Systemic lupus erythematosus • Lyme disease • Niacin deficiency
Non-pulsatile, tender temporal arteries	Giant cell arteritis
Hyperpigmentation of skin	Addison's disease
Cushingoid appearance	Cushing's syndrome
Pretibial myxoedema	Hypothyroidism
Loss of eyebrows	Hypothyroidism
Oral/genital ulceration	Behçet's disease
Blue gums (a 'lead line')	Lead poisoning
Arthritis	Whipple's disease, SLE, Lyme disease, Behçet's disease

---

clinical features associated with specific, potentially treatable causes of dementia are shown in Box 200.3.

Imaging can contribute to making a positive diagnosis of dementia, such as MRI showing hippocampal atrophy in early AD. It is, however, also of use in excluding some reversible causes of dementia, such as a benign tumor. Claims that clinical prediction rules can allow the clinician to differentiate between, say, early AD and space occupying lesions have not been borne out by the evidence and we feel that, at the least, a brain CT is mandatory for investigating the dementing patient.

Benign Tumors

Change in personality may be the only manifestation of a slow growing frontal tumor such as a meningioma. Deeper tumors, around the pituitary or third ventricle, may present solely with cognitive impairment.

Chronic Subdural Hematoma

This can present with subacute dementia, often with fluctuations. There may be no obvious history of head trauma, especially in alcoholics or in patients on anticoagulants. It is eminently surgically treatable and must not be missed.

Normal Pressure Hydrocephalus

Traditionally, it was claimed that this disorder should be suspected if the clinical triad of gait apraxia, subcortical dementia and urinary dysfunction are present. The feet are said to show the 'glued to the floor' sign when the patient tries to walk. Imaging shows ventricular dilatation out of proportion to the degree of sulcal enlargement. Subsequent pressure monitoring may show B waves or a therapeutic trial of lumbar puncture may significantly improve gait, in which case shunting is indicated.

Metabolic and Endocrine Causes

Metabolic disorders tend to produce delirium rather than dementia, but hypocalcemia and recurrent hypoglycemia can present with dementia, usually with a movement disorder.

Hypothyroidism must obviously be excluded in any patient with cognitive impairment. Addison's and hypopituitarism may occasionally present with cognitive impairment.

In any young patient with dementia, especially if showing a subcortical pattern with a movement disorder, Wilson's disease must be excluded. This is a disorder of copper metabolism and treatment becomes less effective if the diagnosis is delayed.

Infections

HIV may cause a direct infection of the brain, resulting in a subcortical dementia. White matter changes are seen on MRI and CSF shows a pleocytosis with oligoclonal bands. A more rapidly progressive dementia can occur in AIDS due to opportunistic infections, such as cerebral toxoplasmosis, cryptococcal meningitis or PML.

Syphilis, although rare, is becoming less uncommon, and should be considered in the dementing patient, especially if accompanied by supportive neurological signs such as Argyll Robertson pupils.

Whipple's disease should be considered if there is oculomasticatory myorhythmia, ocular palsies or ataxia.

Whipple's disease is caused by infection by *Tropheryma whipplei* primarily affecting the gastrointestinal tract (GIT). Neurological features may occur in a few. These include supranuclear ophthalmoplegia, disorders of vergence movements of the eyes, myorhythmia, ocular palsies, ptosis (23%) and pupillary abnormalities such as anisocoria or unreactive pupil in 18% of patients (*See* also Whipple's disease in Ch 201).

Cerebral Vasculitis

When considering a diagnosis of vasculitis, it is important to remember that vasculitis may occur as a primary condition (i.e. Wegener's granulomatosis, temporal arteritis, polyarteritis nodosa (PAN), Churg-Strauss syndrome, primary angiitis of the nervous system) or as part of a multisystem disorder that may cause a vasculitis (e.g. systemic lupus, sarcoid, Behçet's disease, lymphoma and cryoglobulinemia). Vasculitis affecting the central nervous system (CNS) in isolation is rare.

Autoimmune Encephalopathies

Paraneoplastic limbic encephalitis (PLE) may present with subacute onset cognitive impairment, often with seizures, and is associated with paraneoplastic antibodies. This disorder gives the clinician the opportunity to identify an occult primary cancer at an early stage, with the possibility of early treatment.

Certain other antibodies have been identified in the context of cognitive impairment, e.g. thyroid antibodies in Hashimoto's encephalopathy. Whether such antibodies are implicated in the pathogenesis is, however, less clear.

More recently, a voltage gated potassium antibody mediated limbic encephalitis has been described, which appears to respond well to immunosuppression if diagnosed and treated early.

ALZHEIMER'S DISEASE

It is the most common cause of dementia, accounting for approximately two-thirds of all cases. One in nine people aged 65 years and older (11%) has AD. About one-third of people aged 85 years and older (32%) have AD. Of those with AD, an estimated 4% are under age 65 years, 13% are 65–74 years, 44% are 75–84 years and 35% are 85 years and older. The prevalence of AD is more in females which is explained by the longevity in females. Other possible risk factors for the development of AD include gender, education and head trauma. Several studies indicate that lack of education is also a risk factor for AD. Although some have hypothesized that individuals with increased levels of education are better equipped to compensate for cognitive decline, thereby decreasing ease of clinical detection, others suggest that higher educational attainment imparts a 'cognitive reserve' that delays the onset of clinical manifestations.

Although there is currently no laboratory test to confirm AD, several promising avenues of biologic markers are being pursued. For example, markers related to the histopathologic hallmarks of AD, neuritic plaques and the neurofibrillary tangles, are being investigated. There is general consensus that $A\beta1$-42, the important constituent of the neuritic plaques, is significantly reduced in CSF of AD patients compared with normal older adult controls. CSF tau, on the other hand, the important component of the neurofibrillary tangles, is significantly increased in patients with AD compared with normal controls. Combining the findings for $A\beta1$-42 with tau appears to improve diagnostic accuracy slightly. *In vivo* imaging of amyloid plaques using positron emission tomography (PET) with a radiolabeled specific A ligand, such as Pittsburgh Compound-B (PIB), is a promising potential biomarker that is currently under investigation.

Pathology

At autopsy, the brain is atrophied. The atrophy is most prominent in the frontal and temporal lobes. Microscopically, there are deposits of amorphous material scattered throughout the cerebral cortex, best seen by silver staining methods **(senile plaques)**. Presence of fiber like strands of silver staining material in the form of loops and coils within the nerve cell cytoplasm (Alzheimer neurofibrillary tangles) and granulovacuolar degeneration of the neurons are other remarkable pathological features. Extracellular amyloid fibrils consisting of 4-KD peptide, designated as β-amyloid protein (A4 protein) accumulate in cerebral and meningeal microvasculature. Other proteins involved in the plaques are presenilin 1 and 2, α-1 antichymotrypsin, apolipoprotein E (ApoE), α-2 macroglobulin and ubiquitin. Hyperphosphorylated tau protein and ubiquitin are found in the neurofibrillary tangles.

Genetic Facts in Alzheimer's Disease

Alzheimer's disease is associated with age and Down syndrome. Abnormalities in chromosomes 1 and 14 are also incriminated in familial, early onset AD. The genes for presenilin 1 and 2 are located on these chromosomes, respectively. Three to five percent of Alzheimer's dementia cases show autosomal dominant inheritance. Familial Alzheimer's disease also shows abnormality in chromosome 21 and the gene for β-amyloid protein is situated on this chromosome.

The gene for ApoE is situated on chromosome 19. ApoE can be used as a marker for AD since it is absent in other dementias. The importance of an individual's ApoE gene status on chromosome 19 has received significant attention as an important genetic susceptibility risk factor for the development of the more typical, or 'sporadic' AD. ApoE, a protein involved in cholesterol transport and probably neuronal repair, alters risk for AD but does not in itself cause the disease. This gene has three possible alleles: ε2, ε3 and ε4. The ε3 allele is the most common and the ε2 allele the least common in the general population. The ε4 allele increases the risk of developing AD in a dose-dependent manner, and the ε2 allele appears to decrease the risk. Among Caucasians, the ε4/ε4 genotype has been associated with ~15 times the risk of AD compared with the ε3/ε3 genotype. The ε4/ε3 genotype has been associated with about three times the risk. The increased risk of the ε4 allele was found across all ages between 40 and 90 years in both men and women, with a diminished effect after age 70 years. The ε4 allele represents a major risk factor for AD in all ethnic groups studied to date, including Caucasians, African-Americans, Hispanics and Japanese. The mechanism by which an individual's ApoE gene status affects the risk of AD is not known.

Clinical Features

Alzheimer's disease does not exhibit a global decline from onset but rather a relatively predictable pattern through various stages. By far the most common presentation is with amnesia, in particular a failure of anterograde episodic memory. Delayed recall (e.g. a name and address after 5 minutes) is the most sensitive measure of early AD. Typically patients with AD perform well on test of working memory, including digit span. Although focal features have been reported at onset in AD, these represent the very small minority. Depression is relatively common early in the disease and this may cause problems with diagnosis.

A progressive disturbance of semantic memory is seen as the disease advances and verbal fluency becomes impaired. Category fluency is more severely affected than letter based verbal fluency. Remote memory for famous faces and events is impaired and shows a gentle temporal gradient (i.e. more distant memories are relatively well-preserved compared with more recently acquired ones). In the middle stages of the disease, it is common to find visual and perceptual difficulties emerging. Ideomotor apraxia occurs rendering tasks such as dressing and eating difficult. Language skills decline as the illness progresses and paucity of speech is evident. Comprehension is impaired and reading, writing and calculation all become affected.

In notable contrast to FTLD, basic aspects of personality, demeanor, social interaction and behavior are strikingly preserved well into the disease. Most patients retain at least partial insight for sometime.

Clinical diagnostic criteria have been developed that may be about 80% sensitive; National Institute of Neurological and Communicative Disorders and Stroke (NINCDS)–Alzheimer's Disease and Related Disorder Association (ADRDA) criteria, although these are not widely used in the clinic in the authors' experience.

In AD, as the disease progresses, akinesia, rigidity and myoclonus may all develop, reflecting the more widespread involvement of cortical and subcortical structures. Both extrapyramidal and pyramidal signs may be observed.

By this stage, cognition is often severely impaired with a disintegration of personality and incontinence. Death often occurs when immobility or poor nutrition predispose to bronchopneumonia.

It is worth stressing that it is not uncommon for a combination of pathologies to exist—that is AD and cerebrovascular disease.

Management

Tacrine was the earliest drug introduced for the treatment of AD. It is an active noncompetitive inhibitor of actylcholinesterase. Positive benefit occurs in 40% of cases. The drug is expensive and toxic. Main adverse effect is hepatotoxicity.

The less toxic anticholinesterase drug donepezil is effective, when given orally in doses of 5 mg daily for 6 weeks and followed-up with 5 mg bd thereafter. This drug does not produce hepatotoxicity.

Other drugs include rivastigmine which can be given in all stages of the disease. It is an inhibitor of cholinesterase action. It gives good symptomatic control of AD. Galantamine hydrobromide (galantamine) which acts on acetylcholine and nicotine receptors is beneficial in early cases.

Memantine N-methyl-D-aspartate (NMDA) receptor blocking agent is of use, in later stages, when given along with rivastigmine. NMDA is an excitotoxin.

Several other drugs such as dihydroergotoxine mesylate, nicergoline and piribedil have been tried with varying results.

ADJUNCTIVE THERAPIES FOR BEHAVIORAL SYMPTOMS

The principal treatable behavioral disturbances in AD are agitation, psychosis, depression, anxiety and insomnia. Agitation and psychosis are common, especially in the later stages of AD. As cognitive function becomes increasing impaired, small changes in a patient's internal (e.g. infection) or external (e.g. change in environment) homeostasis produce agitation. Identification and treatment of any possible underlying cause of agitation is therefore important. Workup should be directed at common causes of delirium in the elderly such as infections, electrolyte imbalances, medications and pain.

Extrapyramidal adverse effects are more common with typical than with atypical antipsychotics, which appear to be better tolerated than traditional agents. Atypical antipsychotics are, therefore, the *treatment of choice* for patients with psychotic symptoms; sedation is the most common adverse effect. The initial antipsychotic dose in AD patients should be low, about one quarter of that used in young adults, and the total daily dose should be gradually increased as needed, titrating against adverse effects such as cognitive deterioration, low blood pressure (BP) and parkinsonism. Thus, need for these drugs for the treatment of behavioral disorders in patients with dementia should be continually reassessed. Trazodone and divalproex (sodium valproate) may be useful in the management of agitation especially when the response to an atypical antipsychotic is inadequate. *Treatment* of depressive symptoms in AD commonly includes selective serotonin reuptake inhibitors. Alternatives include tricyclic antidepressants with low anticholinergic adverse effects such as desipramine or nortriptyline, or the combined noradrenergic and serotonergic reuptake inhibitor venlafaxine. Most AD patients with anxiety do not require pharmacological treatment; however, for those that do, benzodiazepines should be avoided if possible given their potential deleterious effects on cognition. Nonbenzodiazepine anxiolytics such as buspirone are preferred. Insomnia is best treated with nonpharmacological sleep hygiene measures. If medications are necessary, sedating antidepressants such as trazodone may be effective choices for promoting sleep, and anticholinergic hypnotics should be avoided.

On account of the worldwide increase in the incidence of AD in the aging population, there is worldwide interest in the study of the disease and its management. Caregivers have an important role. Nongovernmental organizations (NGOs) like Alzheimer's society are active in different countries including India. In late stages, patients may need institutional care.

Mild Cognitive Impairment

This term refers to slight but noticeable and measurable decline in cognitive abilities including memory and thinking skills. It is of two types, amnesic and nonamnesic. It does not interfere with daily life or action. MCI may progress to AD usually by 2–3 years.

SUBCORTICAL DEMENTIA

The classical examples in this category include progressive supranuclear palsy (PSP), dementia-associated with Parkinsonism [Parkinson's disease dementia (PDD)] and Huntington's disease (HD). Details of these are discussed under extrapyramidal disorders.

MIXED CORTICAL AND SUBCORTICAL DEMENTIA

Frontotemporal degeneration is associated with a focal degeneration of the frontal and temporal lobes. Several variants exist within this group including dementia of frontal type, progressive aphasia and semantic dementia.

The etiology of the condition is unknown although it may be seen after the development of motor neuron disease when the neuronopathy is of amyotrophic form displaying bulbar palsy, weakness, wasting and fasciculations.

The pathological changes seen in FTD are varied. Many cases are associated with tau inclusions but mild spongiform change with neuronal loss and gliosis may occur in the absence of inclusions. The clinical phenotype reflects the anatomical distribution of the pathology, rather than the particular pathological process.

The Frontal Variant of Frontotemporal Lobar Degeneration

In contrast to patients with AD, those with frontal dementia often remain utterly unaware of the changes brought to their personality. The initial presentation may be subtle but is characterized by personality change, emotional problems and behavioral disturbances. Patients may appear apathetic, withdrawn, inappropriately jocular, socially disinhibited, facetious (marked by pleasantry or joking), or unmotivated. There is a reduced capacity to demonstrate appropriate emotional responses such as happiness, fear and surprise. Sympathy, empathy and embarrassment are often lacking and may be replaced by impulsivity and carelessness.

The presentation is quite distinct from that seen in AD. Memory is typically unaffected early in the course of the disease with problems largely secondary to poor concentration and usually relating to difficulties with working (immediate) memory. The severe amnesic presentation of AD is not the pattern seen here.

Verbal perseveration and echolalia frequently occur. Speech is factually empty and reduced in quantity and has been described as 'concrete'. In advanced cases, comprehension becomes impaired and muteness ensues. Sparing of the posterior cortices means that visuospatial problems are absent until the terminal stages. Neurological signs are minimal and consist of primitive reflexes, with akinesia and rigidity observed in the terminal stages.

Semantic Dementia: Progressive Fluent Aphasia

This variant of FTD reflects selective atrophy of the left anterior temporal lobe. Patients display increasingly empty, circumlocutory speech reflecting the profound loss of semantic knowledge. Presenting complaints may relate to forgetting of names of things with an unawareness of the parallel decline in word comprehension. The fluent dysphasia observed in such patients is coupled with a severe anomia, reduced vocabulary and a pronounced impairment of single word comprehension. Patients exhibit a surface dyslexia—that is, an inability to read words with irregular spelling such as dough, pint or island.

Progressive Nonfluent Aphasia

This variant of FTD reflects focal left perisylvian atrophy. Here, a progressive decline in language output occurs with a relative absence of other psychological deficits. Speech is nonfluent, effortful and lacking in prosody. Articulation is disturbed, word finding pauses occur, and syntactic errors are prominent. The communication difficulties are evident to both the patient and the observer. Repetition and reading aloud are impaired and there is pronounced anomia.

Patients have difficulties reciting the days of the week or similar well-rehearsed series. With disease progression, speech becomes unintelligible. Comprehension is, by contrast, relatively preserved.

Vascular Dementia

The term 'vascular dementia' is hampered by lack of agreement regarding definition. It comprises several different entities, such as multi-infarct disease, large cortical infarcts and diffuse small vessel ischemia.

The clinical picture in vascular dementia depends on the site and number of the infarcts. Diagnosis depends on:

- The clinical picture
- Brain imaging findings
- The presence of predisposing factors.

There is commonly an accumulation of neurological and psychological deficits. There may be multiple cortical infarcts causing a 'step-wise' deterioration in function. Dysarthria, dysphagia, rigidity, visuospatial deficits, ataxia and pyramidal or extrapyramidal signs may occur depending on the site of the pathology. Alternatively, subcortical deficits may occur exclusively, with infarcts involving the thalamus, basal ganglia or internal capsule. These may present without any sudden deteriorations, rather manifesting as impaired attention and poor executive function. It is important to differentiate this syndrome from other causes of subcortical dementia and it may coexist with other dementias (e.g. AD). Small vessel disease is associated with a syndrome of gait apraxia, urinary incontinence and pseudobulbar palsy. Urinary and gait disturbances typically occur relatively early in the disease course and sometimes before there are overt signs of cognitive impairment. This pattern of disease is associated with brain imaging findings of lacunes in the deep gray matter nuclei with associated ischemic demyelination histopathologically (known as Binswanger's disease). A combination of cortical and subcortical pathology is not uncommonly seen leading to a mixture of cognitive impairments.

DEMENTIA WITH LEWY BODIES

Lewy bodies are neuronal inclusions composed of abnormally phosphorylated neurofilament proteins aggregated with ubiquitin and α-synuclein that are deposited in brainstem nuclei, paralimbic and neocortical areas. The clinical phenotype often involves visual hallucinations, parkinsonism and fluctuating attention and alertness with intervals of lucidity. Delusions also are a feature. The cognitive profile reflects a combination of cortical and subcortical disease. There is cognitive slowing with impairment of frontal executive functions and attention. In addition, there are pronounced visuospatial and memory problems implicating parieto-occipital regions. The presence of aphasia, agnosia and apraxia may lead to confusion with AD. Along with the cognitive effects, DLB is associated with repeated falls and episodes of transient loss of consciousness. These cognitive impairments may develop before or after Parkinsonism symptoms and signs including akinesia, rigidity and tremor.

CORTICOBASAL DEGENERATION

It usually presents with an asymmetric akinetic-rigid syndrome, progressing to death within 4–6 years. Ideomotor limb apraxia is often observed and there are associated visuospatial and constructional difficulties. The alien hand sign (spontaneous, coordinated hand movements outside of the patient's control) may develop in one limb. This may be associated with cortical sensory loss, dysarthria, ataxia, chorea, pyramidal signs, dysarthria and/or buccofacial apraxia. Dyscalculia and a nonfluent aphasia may be observed and frontal dysfunction may also occur.

Memory impairment is typically less pronounced than that observed in AD.

Prion Disease and Related Encephalitis

SR Chandra, Thomas Gregor Issac

Chapter Summary

- Prion Protein Disease
  - Creutzfeldt-Jakob Disease (CJD)
  - Gerstmann-Straussler-Scheinker (GSS) Syndrome
  - Fatal Insomnia
  - Kuru
- Differential Diagnosis of Prion Transmitted Diseases
  - Whipple's Disease
  - Autoimmune Encephalitis
  - Anti-VGKC Syndrome
  - Anti-NMDA Syndrome
  - Limbic Encephalitis
  - Hashimoto's Encephalopathy

INTRODUCTION

Prion disease consists of a group of disorders which includes Creutzfeldt-Jakob disease (CJD) and others which are degenerative, infectious and fatal, rapidly progressive dementing diseases. These are peculiar disorders arising from pathological protein folding of a normal cellular prion protein (PrP^c) to create a pathological form (PrP^{Sc}, 'Sc refers to scrapie'). This can be sporadic, when it occurs spontaneously or familial when a mutation occurs in the PrP gene. The familial variety is generally autosomal dominant with a wide range of phenotypes including fatal familial insomnia (FFI) and Gerstmann-Straussler-

Scheinker (GSS) disease. The infectious one occurs by exposure of the normal protein to the abnormal isoform which usually occurs iatrogenically through the use of human growth hormone (HGH), corneal and dural grafts and exposure to contaminated neurosurgical and electro-physiological equipments. Based on their phenotypic variation, different proper names are used. When it present with dominant cerebellar ataxia it is called as Brownell–Oppenheimer variant, when there is dominant blindness it is called *Heidenhain variant*. This spectrum of acquisition of this disease makes it special as it is genetic, infectious and degenerative. Other diseases in this category are *Kuru* due to cannibalism, *variant CJD (vCJD)* transmitted from bovine spongiform encephalopathy (BSE) by exposure to pathogenic bovine PrP—(currently rare except in United Kingdom).

Other rapidly progressive dementing syndromes which can closely mimic prion disease are *autoimmune encephalitis* related to N-methyl D-aspartate (NMDA) antibody, *Voltage gated potassium channel (VGKC) antibody, Glutamate decarboxylase (GAD) antibody, Thyroid peroxidase (TPO) antibody* and *a spectrum of Paraneoplastic limbic encephalitis (PLE)* which needs to be remembered in view of their potential for treatment.

PRION PROTEIN (PrP) DISEASE

This class of diseases are caused by neither viruses nor a viroid agent but its transmissible nature was discovered by Gajdusek and Gibbs, in people who practiced ritual cannibalism. These patients could transmit the disease to chimpanzees establishing their potential risk of infection. The infective agent is called as *proteinaceous infectious particle* which does not contain nucleic acid. Therefore, it resists enzymes that destroy nucleic acids and it does not elicit an immune response. It does not have the structure of any known infectious agent. This protein PrP is encoded by a gene in the short arm of chromosome 20 in humans and a mutation of this is seen in patients who suffer familial CJD and GSS. The formation of the sporadic disease involves the conformational change in the protein structure based on an abnormally folded PrP which acts as a template for the conversion of normal PrP to PrP^{sc}, as postulated by Prusiner in 2001. Eighty percent of this disease is sporadic and the rest is genetic or acquired. CJD constitutes less than 1% of human prion disease.

Creutzfeldt-Jakob Disease (CJD)

Epidemiology

The annual incidence is 1–2 per million. It is higher in people of Libyan origin. An outbreak of prion disease among cows in the British Isles labelled as *mad cow disease* was reported in 1986 and this can be symptomatic in humans within 24 hours of exposure to the infected meat and it manifests with psychiatric features and it is called as new *variant CJD (vCJD)*.

Pathogenesis

The sporadic forms probably have access through nasal mucosa as reported by Zanusso and colleagues and all forms of spongiform encephalopathies involve conversion of the PrP^c to PrP^{sc}. Several isoforms of the prion which causes sporadic type is devised based on the presence

of methionine (M) or valine (V) at codon 129 of PrP^c. The most common is MM and the least common is VV. Approximately, two thirds of the cases are related to MM_1 mutation. These MM_1 patients show the classical electroencephalogram (EEG) changes and MV_2 show the MR_1 changes. The pathogenesis of the relationship between the genotypic variation and the phenotypic expression is not very clear.

Pathology

The disease affects cerebrum, cerebellum and occipito-parietal region in some cases. There is astroglial proliferation with microscopic vacuoles within the cytoplasm giving the spongy appearance. Involvement of the thalamic nuclei results in myoclonus. Characteristically, inflammation is absent, though the disease was considered as an infective disease previously.

Clinical Features

Sporadic CJD manifests between 55 and 75 years with rapidly progressing dementia (RPD) and behavioral symptoms in the form of delusions, hallucinations, delirium and pyramidal, extrapyramidal and cerebellar features with myoclonus. The myoclonus is typically generalized, non-epileptic and occurs at a frequency of 1 Hz. The myoclonus can be elicited by sound, light and touch. Patients also have severe asthenia, anxiety, weight loss, altered sleep-wake cycle and some patients show features of anterior horn cell involvement. Both sexes are equally affected. Ataxia and abnormalities of vision occur in some cases. The visual symptoms may be loss of acuity or distortion of seen objects. Headache, vertigo and sensory symptoms can be seen in some patients. Patients can develop eye signs in the form of paralysis of convergence and upgaze. The disease progresses very rapidly on a week to week basis resulting in a mute state, contractures and leading to death in 1–3 years. Very rarely patients have survived up to 10 years.

Diagnosis

Definite diagnosis requires demonstration of neuro-pathological features of neuronal loss, gliosis, vacuolation with evidence of prions on immunohistochemistry (IHC) or Western blot. The EEG pattern is very characteristic in at least two-thirds of the patients during the course of the disease showing periodic epileptiform discharges or triphasic waves of 1–2 Hz (Fig. 201.1). However, this pattern can also be seen with toxic, hypoxic, ischemic and Hashimoto's encephalopathies. This pattern is not seen in the vCJD. Cerebrospinal fluid (CSF) is usually normal with <100 mg of proteins. Rarely oligoclonal bands may be seen. When there is elevated immunoglobulin G (IgG) index or pleocytosis (more than 10 cells), other differential diagnosis of infectious and autoimmune nature should be ruled out. Marker proteins that are present in CSF help in diahnosis include 14-3-3 Tau S 100 and neuron specific enolase (NSE).

Imaging Features

Imaging carries high sensitivity and specificity. Diffusion-weighted images show changes earlier than the usual fluid attenuated inversion recovery (FLAIR) images. Long

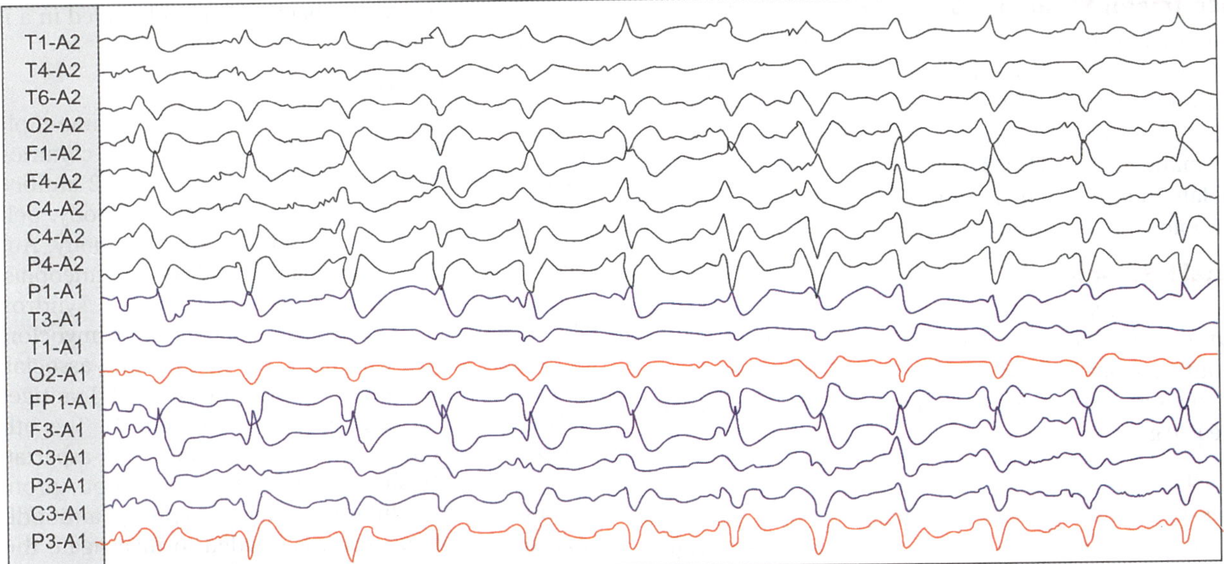

Fig. 201.1: EEG in CJD. ***Note:*** The periodic 1Hz complexes

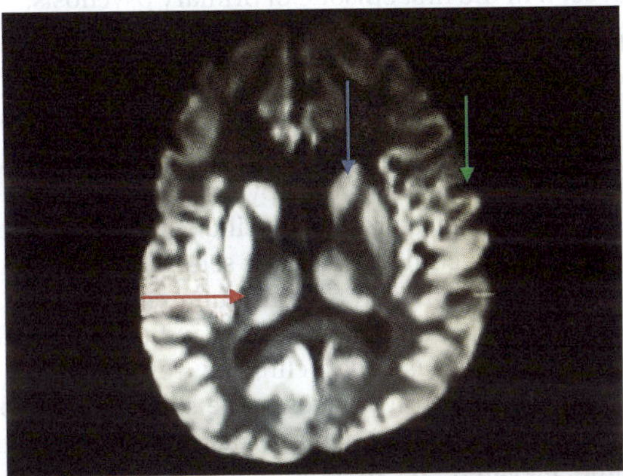

Fig. 201.2: Pulvinar sign in CJD. Pulvinar of thalamus, caudate and putamen (blue arrow); also called as ***Hockey stick sign*** (red arrow) as well as cortical ribboning (green arrow)

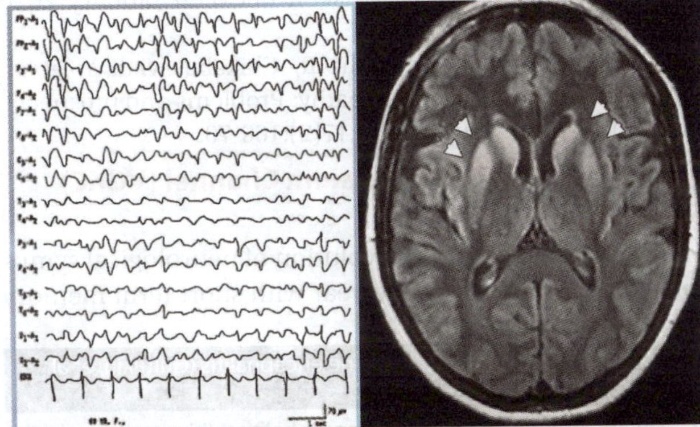

Fig. 201.3: Characteristic EEG with hyperintensities in caudate and putamen (white arrowheads)

contiguous segments of cortex show hyperintensity which is described as cortical ribboning as well as hyperintensity in the lentiform nucleus, pulvinar of thalamus and cortex which are called as ***Hockey stick sign*** as well as ***Pulvinar sign***. The term pulvinar sign is used when the pulvinar part of the thalamus is more hyperintense than other basal ganglia structures (Figs 201.2 and 201.3). However, these changes can also be seen in hypoxia, vasculitis, following seizures, immune-mediated disorders, hepatic encephalopathy, hyperglycemia, paraneoplastic syndromes, extra pontine myelinolysis and in Wilson's disease.

Differential Diagnosis

- ***Lithium toxicity:*** Lithium produces depletion of sodium resulting in mini polymyoclonus, confusion and hyponatremia-induced basal ganglia demyelination causing extrapyramidal features. If history of lithium intake is missed, the syndrome may be totally misdiagnosed. Lithium toxicity generally reverses with sodium chloride (NaCl) administration.
- ***Other differential diagnoses*** include autoimmune encephalopathies, Whipple's disease, paraneoplastic and neoplastic syndromes and rarely, end-stage of Alzheimer's disease and Lewy body dementia (LBD) which can resemble clinical CJD. These should be differentiated based on history of onset and other laboratory features.

Treatment

Treatment consists of symptom modifying medications for myoclonus using sodium valproate and benzodiazepine group of drugs like clonazepam. Behavioral complications are managed with antipsychotics and anti-anxiety agents based on individual requirements. Recently, flupiritine in dose of 100 mg two times daily is tried. It acts as a selective neuronal potassium channel opener that also has NMDA receptor antagonist properties. However, its efficacy is not known.

Prevention of Transmission

Instruments used on the patient should preferably be not reused. The agent (prion) can be deactivated only by autoclaving at 132°C at 1 kg/cm² for at least one hour or by immersion in 5% sodium hypochlorite solution for 1 hour. Other methods of disinfection are ineffective. Patient should not be a candidate for organ donation. People who are exposed to the body fluids of a patient should wash thoroughly with ordinary soap.

Gerstmann-Straussler-Scheinker (GSS) Syndrome

This an autosomal dominant disease which presents with cerebellar ataxia, pyramidal signs and mild dementia. It runs a chronic course and rarely muscle weakness can be seen in the proximal muscles of the leg. Magnetic resonance imaging (MRI) is normal except diffuse atrophy in late stages. There is mutation in the PrP gene and pathology shows spongiform change.

Fatal Insomnia

This is characterized by severe insomnia, dementia, autonomic overactivity and progression to death in 7–15 months. It may be both sporadic and familial. Pathological changes are seen in the thalamus and there is mutation in the PrP gene.

Kuru

This is exclusively seen in the natives of New Guinea Islands where ritualistic cannibalism used to be practiced after death of relatives. It presents as eye movement abnormality, cerebellar ataxia, contractures, incontinence and death within 3–6 months. This disease is transmissible by consuming infective tissues from affected subjects. Pathology shows spongiform change and also amyloid like plaques called *Kuru plaques*. This is seen mostly in females and children in view of the unique ritual cannibalism.

DIFFERENTIAL DIAGNOSIS OF PRION TRANSMITTED DISEASES

Whereas the prion transmitted diseases are not amenable to curative treatment at present, there are diseases which mimic the former, but are readily treatable if properly diagnosed. These include Whipple's Disease, autoimmune encephalitis, anti-VGKC syndrome, anti-NMDA syndrome, limbic encephalitis and Hashimoto's encephalopathy. A short description of these entities are as follows.

Whipple's Disease

It is a very rare multisystemic granulomatous disease caused by *Tropheryma whipplei*. Patients manifest with gastrointestinal (GI) symptoms in the form of diarrhea, skin changes in the form of alopecia, large flushed scleroderma like lesions in the nape of the neck, chin and other parts. Other manifestations include rheumatological symptoms, endocarditis, pneumonia, lymphadenopathy and eventually neurological features including cognitive disturbance, headache, papilledema. They develop peculiar oculomasticatory or oculo-skeletal myorhythmia. They have progressive dementia and extrapyramidal manifestations, myoclonus and seizures. There are less than 100 cases reported in the world literature. *Diagnosis* is confirmed by the typical clinical picture, jejunal biopsy or demonstration of polymerase chain reaction (PCR) positive test for the organism in brain and CSF. MRI shows demonstrable abnormalities. High degree of suspicion in patients who have traveled to endemic areas will help in planning the appropriate test. It is eminently treatable with ceftriaxone for two weeks in doses of 2 g twice daily followed by maintenance with sulfadiazine or sulfamethoxazole and trimethoprim for 1–2 years.

(Though rare, a case has been recently identified in a Haj pilgrim by the author).

Autoimmune Encephalitis

It usually manifests as limbic encephalitis, paraneoplastic or nonparaneoplastic. Paraneoplastic is commonly seen with testicular tumors showing anti-Ma2 antibody, bronchogenic malignancy with anti-Hu antibody, pelvic malignancy in females with anti-NMDA antibody. Autoimmune encephalitis associated with nonparaneoplastic conditions are VGKC antibodies-related syndrome which presents with faciobrachial dystonic myoclonus and seizures. This can be of two types, either associated with LGI1 (Leucine-rich glioma inactivated 1 antigen), or CASPR2 (Contactin-associated protein 2). The other groups of antibodies are NMDA-R (N-methyl D-aspartate), CV2/CRMP5 (Collapsin response mediator protein 5) and GAD (Glutamate decarboxylase) antibodies. High degree of suspicion is needed to investigate these patients appropriately. They are differentiated from pure psychiatric illness by the presence of EEG changes which is not seen in the first episode of primary psychosis.

Clinical Features

They can present in any age and diagnostic criteria of Gultekin, et al. is applied for diagnosis (Box 201.1). They closely resemble PrP disease, evidenced by RPD, myoclonus, psychosis, extrapyramidal features and others. EEG changes are nonspecific. The typical one per second periodic complex is never seen. CSF markers can be seen in both CJD and autoimmune encephalitis. MRI will show nonspecific changes or may be normal. Great caution is needed as it can clinically resemble CJD and by CSF examination it can resemble subacute sclerosing panencephalitis (SSPE) where measles antibody titers become elevated as an epiphenomena. If this is not realized, patients will be labelled as either of the above two conditions resulting in denial of the required treatment and mortality from a treatable disease. Authors have recently published 26 cases seen between January 2010 and 2011.

Source: Chandra SR, Seshadri R, Chikabasaviah Y, et al. Progressive limbic encephalopathy: Problems and prospects. Ann Indian Acad Neurol. 2014;17(2):166-70.

Anti-voltage Gated Potassium Channel (VGKC) Syndrome

The patients present with evolution of neurological symptoms over 5 months to one year with short term memory

---

Box 201.1: Criteria for autoimmune encephalitis (Gultekin, et al. criteria)

- Demonstration of limbic encephalitis (histopathologically whenever possible)
- All four of the following:
  - Short term memory loss, seizures, psychiatric symptoms
  - Less than 4 years duration in patients with malignancy
  - Exclusion of other disorders
  - CSF showing inflammatory changes, MRI of FLAIR images showing temporal lobe features, EEG showing slowing in the temporal region.

Abbreviations: CSF = Cerebrospinal fluid; MRI =Magnetic resonance imaging; FLAIR = Fluid attenuated inversion recovery; EEG = Electroencephalogram

Revised WHO Definition of CJD Subtypes (Incorporating the new definition of probable sporadic CJD as per Section 3.1)

Sporadic CJD

- **Definite:** Diagnosed by standard neuropathological techniques; and/or immunocytochemically and/or Western blot confirmed protease resistant PrP and/or presence of scrapie-associated fibrils
- **Probable:** Progressive dementia and at least two out of the following four clinical features:
  - Myoclonus
  - Visual or cerebellar disturbance
  - Pyramidal/extrapyramidal dysfunction
  - Akinetic mutism
    Or
  - A typical EEG during an illness of any duration and/or
  - A positive 14-3-3 CSF assay and a clinical duration to death <2 years
  - Routine investigations should not suggest an alternative diagnosis
- **Possible:** Progressive dementia and at least two out of the following four clinical features:
  - Myoclonus
  - Visual or cerebellar disturbance
  - Pyramidal/extrapyramidal dysfunction
  - Akinetic mutism
    Or
  - No EEG or atypical EEG
  - Duration <2 years

Iatrogenic CJD: Progressive cerebellar syndrome in a recipient of human cadaveric-derived pituitary hormone; or sporadic CJD with a recognized exposure risk, e.g. antecedent neurosurgery with dura mater graft.

Familial CJD: Definite or probable CJD plus definite or probable CJD in a first degree relative; and/or Neuropsychiatric disorder plus disease-specific PrP gene mutation.

Abbreviations: CJD = Creutzfeldt-Jakob disease; PrP = Prion protein; EEG = Electroencephalogram = CSF = Cerebrospinal fluid

loss, myoclonus, seizures, behavioral changes, dyssomnias, extrapyramidal features, autonomic dysfunction, hallucinations and ataxia. Sixty percent of the patients might qualify the WHO criteria for CJD (Box 201.2). They often show hyponatremia and hyperphagia. They often have evidence of diabetes mellitus (DM), thyroiditis, vitiligo and rarely malignancies. CSF shows elevated VGKC antibody 0.16 nmol/L and striated muscle autoantibody up to 1:30720 (reference range <1:60).

Treatment consists of immunomodulation in the same way as NMDA antibody syndrome (discuss further) and treatment of secondary complications like hyponatremia, seizures and myoclonus. They should be regularly followed up for malignancies which have to be removed when detected.

Anti-N-methyl-D aspartate (NMDA) Syndrome

This syndrome is an autoimmune disorder due to IgG antibodies directed against NR1-subunit of NMDA-receptor. New onset psychosis in the form of delusions, mood changes, aggression, young age, female more than male, encephalitis like symptoms with no definite etiological clue should raise the suspicion of the above syndrome. Mild neurological abnormalities in the form of transient facial twitching, cognitive dysfunction and nonspecific EEG changes are seen. Suspicion and recognition is important in all new onset psychosis with

cognitive features as it is eminently treatable. *Treatment* consists of pulses of methylprednisolone 3–5 g or intravenous (IV) Ig 2g/kg bw or plasmapharesis monthly for a minimum of 6 months. Additional drugs which can be used are mycophenolate mofetil, rituximab, cyclophosphamide and azathioprine. In addition, seizures and psychosis are treated with anticonvulsants and anti-psychotics. The duration of treatment varies from 6 to 23 months. Relapses are not uncommon. *Diagnosis* is confirmed by clinical features supported by elevated NMDA-receptor antibodies in CSF.

Limbic Encephalitis due to Less Common Infections

Infections with cytomegalovirus (CMV),varicella, chronic herpes can manifest with progressive dementia with seizures and radiological changes in the limbic structures like cingulum, insula and medial temporal regions. They can have varying duration of the disease from few months to 2–3 years. *Diagnosis* is based on suspicion, clinical features, radiological features (Figs 201.4A to F) supported by CSF and serum evidence of viral markers and histopathology when possible.

Treatment consists of symptomatic treatment for psychosis and seizures in addition to antiviral agents like acyclovir 30 mg/kg for 2–3 weeks for chronic herpes and varicella and gancyclovir and steroids for CMV encephalitis.

Hashimoto's Encephalopathy

This presents with confusion, myoclonus and cognitive dysfunction in patients with Hashimoto's disease. They can also manifest with hemiparesis, ataxia, palatal tremor or features suggestive of essential tremor. It is not uncommon for some of these patients to be labelled as CJD. They can have a steadily progressive or relapsing remitting course over years.

Investigations

General thyroid functions may be normal or deranged but the titres of anti-thyroid antibody specially against thyroid peroxidase (TPO) and thyroglobulin are high. Minimum of two fold elevation in symptomatic patients is necessary to make a diagnosis as moderate elevation of these antibodies may be seen even in normal people. CSF shows mild pleocytosis. MRI shows white matter lesions (Figs 201.5A and B).

Treatment: Patients can be treated with plasmapharesis or steroids in the form of repeated pulses as in other autoimmune encephalitis.

CONCLUSION

RPDs form a challenging group of disorders involving a wide spectrum of syndromes with similar phenotypic characters distinguishable by biochemical, electrophysiological and radiological features. The PrP-related disorders carry a very poor prognosis with no specific treatment whereas the close mimics are eminently treatable with near normal life expectancy. Good number of them are mistaken as CJD and denied treatment. Many of them are diagnosed as psychiatric disorders and treated with potentially contraindicated treatment options like electroconvulsive therapy (ECT). Therefore, every patient

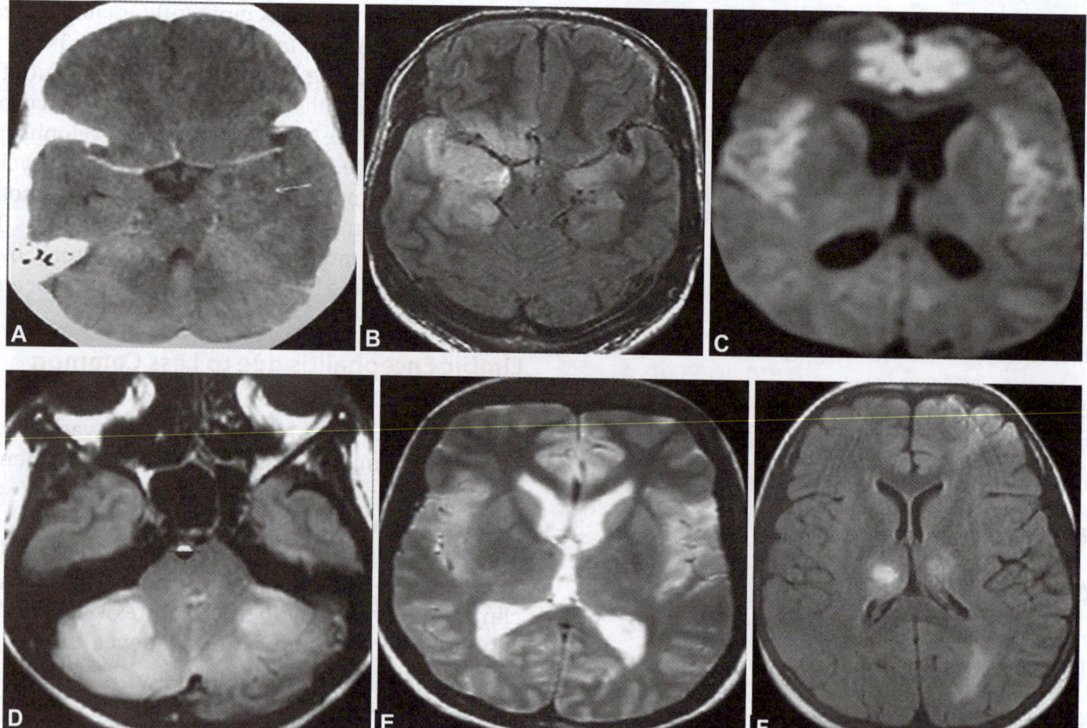

Figs 201.4A to F: **A.** CT—hypodensity in the left medial temporal lobe—paraneoplastic; **B.** FLAIR hyperintensity both hippocampi, parahippocampi, adjacent anterior temporal lobes—herpes simplex; **C.** Autoimmune limbic encephalitis; **D.** Autoimmune limbic encephalitis: Axial DWI reveals bilateral symmetrical foci of diffusion restriction involving cingulate, medial superior frontal gyri and insula; **E.** Case of varicella encephalitis: Axial T2WI shows abnormal bilaterally symmetrical hyperintensities involving cingula, insula and thalami; **F.** Axial FLAIR images
Abbreviations: DWI = Diffusion-weighted imaging; FLAIR = Fluid attenuated inversion recovery

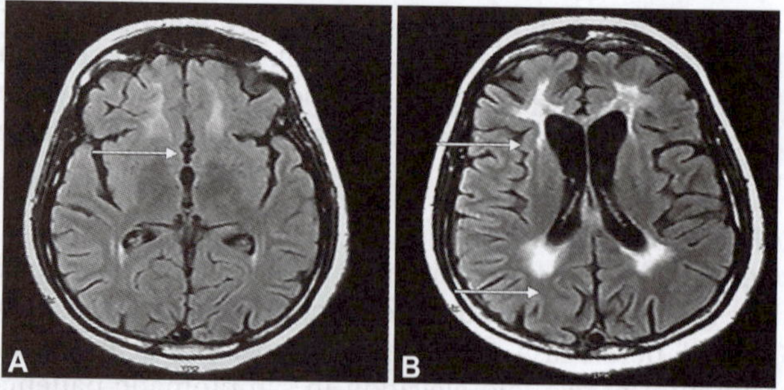

Figs 201.5A and B: White matter changes in a patient with Hashimoto's encephalopathy (arrows)

with new onset psychosis with scanty changes in the usual laboratory investigations should receive special attention to exclude treatable conditions. EEG is a simple, cheap and sensitive screening tool showing both specific and nonspecific changes based on which appropriate investigations and treatment options can be chosen for confirmation of diagnosis.

Histological patterns in different forms of encephalopathies (Figs 201.6A to C).

Source: Rooper AH, Sanwels MA, Klein JP. Adams and Victor's Principles of Neurology. 10th ed. McGraw-Hill education Medical Publisher; 2014.

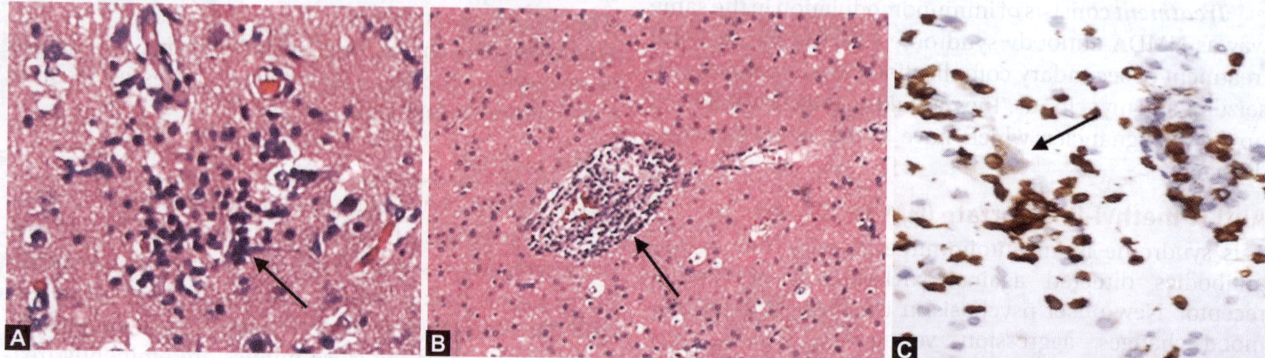

Figs 201.6A to C: **A.** Microglial nodule in the gray matter marking a focus of neuronophagia (arrow); **B.** White matter with perivascular inflammation (arrow); **C.** CD3 immunostaining shows mainly T lymphocytes in the microglial nodule with neuronophagia (arrow)

Epilepsies

AS Girija

Chapter Summary

- General Considerations
- Prevalence
- Etiology
- Pathogenesis
- Molecular Genetics of Epilepsy
- Classification of Epilepsies
- Partial Seizures
- Primary Generalized Epilepsies
- Common Epileptic Syndromes
- Febrile Convulsions
- Progressive Myoclonic Epilepsies
- Epilepsy and Pregnancy
- Diagnosis
- Prognosis
- Management of Epilepsy
- Status Epilepticus

GENERAL CONSIDERATIONS

An epileptic seizure is electrophysiologically characterized by abnormal transient and excessive electrical discharge of cerebral neurons and clinically characterized by paroxysmal episodes of excess of motor, sensory, autonomic or psychic functions with or without alteration in consciousness. Very rarely, it can be loss of these functions. The abnormal electrical discharges (epileptic or seizure discharges) may involve only a small part of the brain or a much wider area in both cerebral hemispheres. The clinical manifestations of epilepsy correspond to the activation of the brain area(s) affected by the electrical discharges. This explains the wide diversity of clinical forms that a seizure might take. The term *epilepsy* denotes the peripheral events resulting from the abnormal electrical discharges from the brain, recurring on two or more occasions.

In other words, seizure is a symptom and epilepsy is a syndrome. Though epilepsy begins first with a seizure, not all first seizures lead to epilepsy. Seizures may often occur in acute systemic conditions, such as metabolic disturbances (hypoglycemia), drug toxicity (chloroquine) and drug withdrawal (diazepam), but usually they do not constitute epilepsy.

PREVALENCE

One in 20 persons in the general population would have had seizures at some point in their lives. One in 200 among the general population has epilepsy at any one period of time. A house-to-house study done on 25,000 persons in Central Travancore gave the prevalence rate as 5/1,000 persons. The International League against Epilepsy gives the incidence as 50–100/100,000 population. Epilepsy is one of the common neurological abnormalities seen in general practice. Although eminently treatable in the majority of cases, in a minority, it leads to poor long-term outcome with loss of employment and productivity, adverse psychosocial effects and poor quality of life. The family physician whom an epileptic patient first contacts has to suspect the diagnosis, initiate the appropriate treatment and arrange for further specialist advice.

Source: Radhakrishnan K, Nayak SD, Kumar SP, et al. Profile of Antiepileptic Pharmacotherapy in a Tertiary Referral Center in South India: A Pharmacoepidemiologic and Pharmacoeconomic Study. Epilepsia. 1999;40(2):179-85.

ETIOLOGY

In about 70% of cases of epilepsy, no cause can be determined even after extensive investigations (primary or idiopathic epilepsy). In the remaining group, etiology varies and is multifactorial depending upon age of onset and the type of epilepsy. The causes include a large variety of genetically determined, congenital and acquired conditions. Among the acquired causes, central nervous system (CNS) infections (encephalitis, meningitis and brain abscess), cerebrovascular diseases [cerebral arteriovenous malformation (AVM), cerebral hemorrhage and infarction], perinatal hypoxic ischemic cerebral damage, head trauma and brain tumors predominate. Drug-induced seizures are common. Most of the centrally-acting drugs cause generalized convulsions following parenteral administration at high doses. Likewise, withdrawal of drugs, like phenobarbitone, benzodiazepines and also alcohol, may precipitate generalized convulsions. The onset of epilepsy due to hereditary, metabolic or genetic disorders like hypocalcemia and aminoaciduria is in childhood. Sturge-Weber syndrome and tuberous sclerosis usually lead to epilepsy in early life. Seizures in the first few days after birth are most commonly due to birth anoxia or neonatal intracerebral hemorrhage. Seizures in the first few weeks of life are due to CNS infections, hypocalcemia or other metabolic disturbances. Onset of seizures after the 2nd week of life usually indicates developmental abnormalities of the brain. Epilepsy due to birth trauma manifests in childhood but occasionally the first attack may occur in adult life. Cerebral tumors, head trauma, neurotuberculomas, neurocysticercosis, cerebrovascular disease (overt or salient) and presenile dementia are the common causes of late-onset epilepsy.

Simple partial seizures starting in adult life should suggest a newly developed focal structural lesion in the brain (e.g. tumor, tuberculoma or cysticercosis). Complex partial seizures are most frequently due to unilateral temporal lobe damage, such as mesial temporal sclerosis or hamartomas. Typical absence seizures and generalized tonic-clonic seizures without aura are almost exclusively manifestations of primary generalized epilepsy. Atypical absence and atonic, tonic or clonic seizures usually occur in children with mental retardation and brain damage due to a variety of causes. Myoclonic seizures can be a manifestation of primary generalized epilepsy as well as several other symptomatic epilepsies.

PATHOGENESIS

The cortical neurons become abnormally excitable due to differentiation. The cytoplasm and cell membrane of such cells have increased permeability rendering them susceptible to activation by hyperthermia, hypoxia, hypoglycemia and hyponatremia. Deficiency of the inhibitory neurotransmitter gamma (γ)-aminobutyric acid (GABA) and disturbance of local regulation of extracellular K^+, Na^+, Ca^{2+} or Mg^{2+} are probably responsible for the membrane instability which leads to abnormal electrical discharge. Transition from normal to epileptiform behavior of the brain is caused by greater spread and neuronal recruitment secondary to a combination of enhanced connectivity, enhanced excitatory transmission, failure of inhibitory mechanisms and changes in intrinsic neuronal properties. Generalized epilepsies are due to electrical activity occurring throughout the cerebral cortex, because of lowering of seizure threshold. Often this is genetically determined. If unchecked, this electrical discharge spreads to the ipsilateral and contralateral hemisphere across intra- and interhemispheric pathways and also to the subcortical structures, like basal ganglia and brainstem reticular nuclei, from where the excitatory activity is fed back to the rest of the cortex.

MOLECULAR GENETICS OF EPILEPSY

Epilepsies have both simple and complex inheritance pattern. Most idiopathic epilepsy syndromes have a complex inheritance. In these cases, more than one gene with or without the influence of acquired factors leads to a particular epilepsy syndrome. A number of syndromes with simple inheritance are also known. To site examples, benign familial neonatal convulsions are linked to 20q, the abnormal gene being KCNQ2. That for autosomal dominant nocturnal frontal lobe epilepsy is linked to 20q, the abnormal gene being CHRNA4. Juvenile myoclonic epilepsy (JME) is linked to 6p and 15q. The readers can refer to 'Monographs on Epilepsy' for details.

CLASSIFICATION OF EPILEPTIC SEIZURES

The classification of epilepsy has undergone several changes from time to time and it is likely that further changes may follow. To standardize the classification, the International League against Epilepsy has suggested the following two classifications:

1. *Classification of epileptic seizures:* This is largely based on the seizure type and to a lesser extent on electroencephalogram (EEG) findings. In this classification, seizures are divided into two main categories depending upon the location of the initial epileptic discharge in the brain, i.e. localized to a small area (partial seizures) or larger areas in both hemispheres (generalized seizures).

2. *Classifications of epilepsies and epileptic syndromes:* This is based on clinical manifestations, age of onset, genetic predisposition, associated neurological and other abnormalities, response to specific antiepileptic drugs (AEDs) and overall prognosis.

Classification of Epileptic Seizures

Partial Seizures
- Simple partial seizures with:
  - Motor manifestations
  - Somatosensory or special sensory manifestations
  - Autonomic manifestations
  - Psychic manifestations
- Complex partial seizures with:
  - Simple partial features at onset followed by impairment of consciousness
  - Impairment of consciousness at onset
- Partial seizures evolving to secondarily generalized seizures:
  - *Simple partial seizure:* Generalized seizure
  - *Complex partial seizure:* Generalized seizure

Generalized Seizures
- Absence seizures
- Myoclonic seizures
- Clonic seizures
- Tonic seizures
- Tonic-clonic seizures
- Atonic seizures.

Unclassified Seizures

Classification of Epilepsies and Epileptic Syndrome

Localization related (focal, local, partial) epilepsies and syndromes
- Idiopathic with age-related onset
  - Benign childhood epilepsy with centrotemporal spikes
  - Childhood epilepsy with occipital paroxysms
  - Primary reading epilepsy
- Symptomatic seizures
  - Chronic progressive *epilepsia partialis continua* of childhood
  - Syndromes characterized by seizures with specific mode of precipitation
  - Temporal lobe epilepsies
  - Frontal lobe epilepsies
  - Parietal lobe epilepsies
  - Occipital lobe epilepsies
- Cryptogenic

Generalized epilepsies and syndromes
- Idiopathic with age-related onset
  - Benign neonatal familial convulsions
  - Benign myoclonic epilepsy of infancy
  - Childhood absence epilepsy (pyknolepsy)
  - Juvenile absence epilepsy
  - Juvenile myoclonic epilepsy (impulsive petit mal)
  - Epilepsy with grand mal seizures on awakening
  - Other generalized idiopathic epilepsies not defined above
  - Epilepsies with seizures precipitated by specific modes of activation

- Cryptogenic
  - West syndrome (infantile spasms, Salam seizures)
  - Lennox-Gastaut syndrome (LGS)
  - Epilepsy with myoclonic/astatic seizures
  - Epilepsy with myoclonic absences
- Symptomatic
  - Nonspecific etiology
    - Early myoclonic encephalopathy
    - Early infantile epileptic encephalopathy with suppression burst
    - Other symptomatic generalized epilepsies
  - Specific syndromes: Epilepsies, which form part of the clinical profile of certain neurological disorders

Epilepsies and syndromes, undetermined whether focal or generalized

- With both generalized and focal seizures:
  - Neonatal seizures
  - Severe myoclonic epilepsy of infancy
  - Epilepsy with continuous spike and wave during slow wave sleep
  - Acquired epileptic aphasia
  - Other undetermined epilepsies not included above.

Special syndromes

- Situation-related seizures
  - Febrile convulsions
  - Isolated seizures or status epilepticus (SE)
  - Seizures occurring only when there is an acute metabolic or toxic event caused by factors, such as alcohol, drugs, eclampsia and nonketotic hyperglycemia.

PARTIAL SEIZURES

Partial or focal seizures are due to a small epileptic focus in the brain. They are divided into two main categories:

1. **Simple partial seizure** in which the seizure starts as a focal discharge and remains focal throughout without alteration of consciousness
2. **Complex partial seizure** when a seizure starts as a focal discharge, but consciousness is also altered or lost.

Simple Partial Seizures

These seizures may have motor, sensory, autonomic or psychic manifestations.

Simple focal or partial motor seizures are due to a discharging epileptic focus in the opposite frontal lobe (motor cortex). These consist of clonic movements of the hand, foot or angle of mouth or turning of the head or eyes. These movements may constitute the entire motor component of the seizure or may be followed by generalized clonic movements and loss of consciousness. The term **Jacksonian motor seizures** (Jacksonian epilepsy) is applied to the type where clonic contractions start in the fingers of one hand, one side of the face or the foot and slowly spread (march) to the other muscles on the same side of the body. This may or may not be followed by involvement of the opposite side and loss of consciousness. The presence of the characteristic march distinguishes Jacksonian seizures from partial motor seizures. However, both have the same localizing significance.

Complex Partial Seizures

These are defined as focal or partial seizures in which consciousness is impaired or lost. They are frequently due to epileptic discharges in the temporal or frontal lobes. Less commonly, they may arise from discharges in other parts of the brain. This forms the single most common type of seizure in adults. The seizure usually consists of complex hallucination of perceptual illusions, indicating its origin from the temporal lobe. The hallucinations are usually auditory and visual but sometimes they may be olfactory or gustatory. The subjects may show increased familiarity (***déjà vu***) or unfamiliarity (***jamais vu***) with the surroundings. In some cases, these subjective experiences may constitute the entire seizure. Often, this is followed by a period of unresponsiveness, during which the patient exhibits certain automatic behavior like smacking of the lips or chewing movements (automatism). The patient may walk about or repeat a habitual act. However, when asked a question, the unresponsiveness becomes evident. Sometimes unprovoked aggression or laughter may be the striking feature. The automatism usually lasts for a few minutes, but may sometimes be prolonged. The patient is totally amnesic for the whole period of automatism. The EEG recorded during sleep or hyperventilation may demonstrate the temporal lobe focus. Rarely, other areas of brain, like the orbital surface of the frontal lobe or limbic system, may be seat of epileptic discharge.

Partial Seizures Evolving to Secondarily Generalized Seizures

In many cases, the generalized seizures are not generalized from their onset. They start as partial seizures, either simple or complex and then soon spread to become generalized, usually as tonic-clonic convulsions. These are called partial seizures becoming secondarily generalized. In such cases, the initial manifestations of partial seizures are called ***aura*** or ***warning symptoms***.

PRIMARY GENERALIZED EPILEPSIES

These are seizures in which there is no evidence of an epileptic focus, either clinically or on EEG, as opposed to secondary generalized seizures. The epileptic discharge involves both cerebral hemispheres simultaneously from the onset of the seizures. Hence, consciousness is almost invariably impaired or lost at the onset of the attack. Generalized seizures are divided into several clinical types and some patients may suffer from more than one seizure type. Atypical seizure patterns may also occur, especially if the patient is on treatment.

Tonic-clonic Seizures

These are also called ***grand mal epilepsy***. The seizure attack occurs in different stages sequentially. The stages may be subdivided into the prodromal phase, tonic phase, clonic phase and postictal phase. The ***prodromal phase*** may start several hours before the ictus (fit). It consists of several subjective phenomena, like depressed or apathetic mood, irritability, vague abdominal cramps or other funny sensations, which are easily recognized by the patient. In many instances, there is no aura and the patient gets the attack without any forewarning. Presence of aura suggests the nature of the seizure as of focal onset, i.e. partial seizure.

The ***tonic phase*** consists of rolling up of the eyes associated with stiffening of the limbs followed by clenching of the jaws, often resulting in injury to the tongue. The attack may be heralded by an epileptic cry as the entire musculature goes into spasm forcing air through the closed vocal cords. The patient becomes cyanosed due to spasm of respiratory muscles. This phase lasts for about 10–30 seconds.

The tonic phase is followed by ***clonic phase*** characterized by alternate flexion-extension movements of all the four limbs (convulsions), strenuous breathing, sweating, frothing of the mouth and excess salivation. Urine and feces may be voided. The clonic phase usually lasts for 1–2 minutes. This is followed by a ***deep comatose state***, which lasts for about 5 minutes. The pupils slowly begin to react and the patient then resumes speech, but still remains confused. If left undisturbed, he goes into sleep for several hours and often wakes up with severe headache and at times, vomiting. This is the ***postictal phase*** and patient does not remember anything that had happened.

EEG taken during the attack or sometimes even during the intervals shows generalized seizure discharges. The EEG is often normal in the interictal period.

Absence Seizures (Petit Mal)

These are seen mostly in children. These are distinguished by brevity and absence of motor phenomena. The child does not fall. The attacks come on without any warning and consciousness is impaired only for a brief period often less than 10 seconds. The child abruptly stops all ongoing motor activity and speech. There is a vacant stare. External stimuli fail to evoke any response from the patient at that period. These attacks usually last for 2–10 seconds after which the patient resumes the pre-seizure activity. At times, there may be clonic movements of the eyelids or occasionally automatisms like smacking of lips or chewing movements. The attacks can be precipitated by hyperventilation. The attacks occur several times during the day, but they become less frequent or may even disappear in adolescence. Sometimes, these may be replaced by tonic-clonic seizures.

The EEG abnormality in petit mal epilepsy is diagnostic. It shows classic ***three per second*** spike and wave generalized discharges.

Juvenile Myoclonic Epilepsy (JME)

This is a primary generalized epilepsy which starts in early adolescence. The cardinal feature of this type of epilepsy is myoclonic jerks. This term refers to brisk, brief contractions of one or several muscle groups or a single muscle. The movements are jerky, generally abrupt and uncontrollable and render the patient momentarily helpless. The attacks may occur as a single jerk or may recur every few seconds. Recovery from the attacks is immediate and the subject does not lose consciousness. Myoclonic jerks occur with or without generalized tonic-clonic seizures. Attacks occur early in the morning on waking up. A small proportion of childhood absence seizures may evolve into JME. Often the myoclonus may be missed or misinterpreted as focal seizure activity. It is

important to make a proper diagnosis since AEDs, such as phenytoin and carbamazepine, used in partial epilepsy may worsen the myoclonus.

Myoclonic Jerks

They are not always ***epileptic*** in origin, and may occur in many other nonepileptic neurological conditions. The abnormal electrical discharges may arise from the cerebral cortex, brainstem or spinal cord. Myoclonus is seen in a variety of conditions *viz* different types of metabolic encephalopathies, like hepatic failure, renal failure and electrolyte disturbances. It is an important feature of progressive myoclonic encephalopathy (PME). At times, it is precipitated by light, sound and touch stimuli. Physiological myoclonus may occur in many normal persons during sleep or in other disease states.

Atonic Seizures

These are less common generalized seizures characterized by sudden loss of postural tone and consciousness without any other motor phenomena. This may lead to sudden ***drop*** of the individual to the floor without any warning. Atonic seizures have to be distinguished from cataplexy in which the drop attacks are not accompanied by loss of consciousness and syncope.

COMMON EPILEPTIC SYNDROMES

Infantile Spasms

Syn: Salaam spasm (Hypsarrhythmia)

This condition is seen in infants below 1 year of age. This is characterized by brief sudden jerky flexion or less commonly extension movements of both arms, neck and torso. Usually, these jerks or spasms occur in clusters, precipitated by sudden noise or tactile stimulus and may occur several times in a day. Usually, there is evidence of other neurological disorders, secondary cerebral anoxia or birth injury. As the infant grows, the frequency of spasms comes down but other forms of seizures may supervene. The characteristic EEG pattern is called ***hypsarrhythmia***.

Lennox-Gastaut Syndrome (LGS)

This is an epileptic syndrome with onset between 1 and 6 years of age. It is characterized by mental retardation and intractable seizures with mixture of tonic, atonic, tonic-clonic and atypical absence seizures. EEG shows diffuse slow spike wave disturbances at 2 Hz. The syndrome may occur without any definite cause or may be associated with a variety of neurodevelopmental or metabolic abnormalities in which case the prognosis is poor.

Benign Rolandic Epilepsy

This is a common form of partial epilepsy in childhood with onset between 3 and 11 years. It is characterized by attacks of hemifacial twitches sometimes with involuntary vocalizations which may progress to a generalized or unilateral convulsion. These seizures usually or exclusively occur in sleep. The family history suggestive of autosomal-dominant inheritance may be available. The EEG abnormality is highly characteristic showing frequent spike discharge in the Rolandic area, especially during non-rapid eye movement (REM) sleep. The prognosis is excellent as it is not associated with any other neurological, psychiatric or behavioral disorder and seizures respond well to anticonvulsant drugs. In some, they may remit spontaneously around puberty.

FEBRILE CONVULSIONS

A febrile convulsion may be defined as a brief generalized convulsion occurring during fever in a child in the age group of 6 months to 5 years without pre-existing or concurrent neurological abnormalities or intracranial infection. About 70% of febrile convulsions occur in the age of 6–18 months. The convulsions usually last for a few seconds but may extend up to 15 minutes. At least 5% of children have one febrile fit before the age of 5 years and nearly 25–50% of them have recurrent attacks, but the risk progressively diminishes with age. A strong family history of febrile fits is evident in many cases. The fits usually occur when the rectal temperature rises above 39°C.

Generally, the body temperature normalizes after the fit. About 4–20% cases may develop convulsions even without noticeable fever. Though the risk of developing chronic epilepsy in such children is only about 2%, it is however, higher than in the general population. The risk of developing epilepsy in later life is higher in the following groups:

- When the first febrile convulsion is complicated, i.e. prolonged (>30 minutes) or localized or is followed by multiple seizures in 24 hours
- Presence of neurological abnormalities before or after the onset of convulsion.

In general, the intellectual performance of children who had febrile convulsions does not differ from normals but prolonged or recurrent frequent febrile convulsions lead to brain damage and medial temporal sclerosis, which in later life, causes *epilepsy*.

Management

Rectal diazepam in a dose of 0.08–0.3 mg/kg or buccal midazolam can be given to abort an acute attack. Intramuscular (IM) administration of diazepam should be avoided since absorption is erratic.

The temperature should be brought down by administration of paracetamol in a dose of 30 mg/kg bw and tepid sponging.

Further convulsions can be prevented by administration of phenobarbitone in a dose of 15 mg/kg given IM or 30 mg orally repeated 6 hourly. In children, below the age of 18 months, since fever and convulsions may be a presenting feature of meningitis, lumbar puncture (LP) is indicated; so also in children showing prolonged or lateralized seizures. Prophylactic administration of clobazam 5–10 mg oral is useful in preventing fits.

Prolonged prophylaxis is indicated for children who show:

- Complicated and prolonged convulsions or focal seizures
- Frequent recurrence
- Abnormal birth history or neurodevelopmental abnormalities
- Onset after 5 years of age
- Presence of interictal EEG abnormality.

Sodium valproate given in doses of 20 mg/kg/day oral is a good and safe for prophylactic and prolonged use. Cognitive impairment has been described if sodium valproate is used as AED on long-term basis. Levetiracetam is preferred.

PROGRESSIVE MYOCLONIC EPILEPSIES (PMEs)

They are rare, distinctive epileptic disorders with myoclonic seizures, tonic-clonic seizures and progressive neurologic dysfunction, particularly ataxia and dementia. A heterogeneous group of disorders may give rise to PME:

- ***Biochemical disorders:*** Unverricht-Lundborg disease (ULD), Lafora body disease, neuronal ceroid lipofuscinosis (NCL), sialidosis, mitochondrial encephalomyopathy, noninfantile neuronopathic Gaucher's disease and others.
- ***Clinically-defined groups:*** They may give rise to seizures, West's syndrome, Ramsay-Hunt syndrome (dyssynergia cerebellaris myoclonica) and others.

Diagnosis of these groups of disorders depends on the clinical patterns, characteristic fundal changes and biopsy studies of the skin, skeletal muscle, liver, rectal mucosa or brain. Study of these diseases is the realm of the specialist.

Management consists of accurate diagnosis, genetic counseling and control of myoclonus by sodium valproate or clonazepam.

Reflex Epilepsy

Epilepsy precipitated by external stimuli has been designated as reflex epilepsy. The common stimuli, which precipitate reflex epilepsy in susceptible people, are hot water bath of the head, photic stimulation, such as flickering light and TV watching, exposure to sunlight, reading, hearing music, startle and eating. Avoidance of precipitating factors and prophylactic anticonvulsants serve to prevent the attacks.

EPILEPSY AND PREGNANCY

One-fourth to one-third of pregnant women with epilepsy get aggravation of seizure tendency during pregnancy. Status epilepticus may complicate 1–2% of epileptics who are in labor. Since drug levels of AEDs are lower in many pregnant women, it is better to monitor-free drug levels every month during pregnancy. Risks of AED during pregnancy include the following:

- ***First trimester of pregnancy:*** Congenital malformation in child 12.3%
- ***Status epilepticus:*** Generalized convulsions during labor:
  - Risk of hypoxia and acidosis for mother and fetus is high
  - Increased rate of neonatal hypoxia, low APGAR scores in the baby
  - Pregnant women with epilepsy have higher risks of hyperemesis gravidarum, pre-eclampsia, abruptio placentae and premature labor. Serum AED levels rise after delivery and therefore, monitoring is required.

Complication in the Offspring

These include fetal congenital malformations and developmental delay. Teratogenicity has been established for valproate, carbamazepine, phenytoin and phenobarbitone. Minor congenital malformations occur in 6–20% and major abnormalities occur in 4–6% of infants exposed to these drugs *in utero*, compared to 3% in babies of epileptic mothers not exposed to drugs.

Major malformations are particularly seen in babies exposed to phenytoin and phenobarbitone. These include cleft lip, cleft palate and congenital heart disease (CHD). Neural tube defects (NTDs) increase from a general rate of 0.2 to 1–2% in pregnancies exposed to valproate and carbamazepine. Administration of 5 mg folate daily early in pregnancy may reduce this risk. Perinatal death rates of the baby may rise from 1 to 3.9% in controls to 1.3–7.8% in the case of epileptic mothers. Low-birth-weight (7–10%) and prematurity (4–11%) may occur. Risk of epilepsy is higher in children of parents with epilepsy, especially so if the mother is epileptic. Mental retardation is more frequent in children of epileptic parents—8% if only mother is affected, 4% if only father is affected and 25% if both are affected.

Management of Women with Epilepsy

- Preconception counseling
- Lamotrigine and levetiracetam may be less teratogenic and hence, they should be preferred
- If patient is on other AEDs or on multiple AEDs, it should be changed to monotherapy and that too in the minimum effective dose well in advance of conception
- Use of folic acid 4 mg/day along with AED when planning pregnancy may help to decrease the incidence of teratogenicity
- Monitoring of serum α-fetoprotein (AFP) in the mother for NTDs if feasible
- Ultrasonographic (USG) examination with vaginal probe for demonstration of NTDs—USG at 18 weeks should be able to detect most of the abnormalities. Serum level of AEDs may be monitored
- AEDs may impair the metabolism of vitamin K and lead to bleeding tendencies. Oral supplementation of vitamin K 20 mg/day throughout pregnancy reduces this risk. The baby should be given vitamin K 1–2 mg IM at birth
- *Delivery:* Elective lower segment cesarean delivery is done in those with risk of status epilepticus. If seizures occur lorazepam is the drug of choice. Pethidine should be avoided since it can exacerbate seizures
- Concurrent administration of oral contraceptives along with AEDs may lower serum levels of AED and precipitate seizures

Menopause: Usually, the seizure tendency subsides, but hormone replacement therapy increases seizure tendency.

DIAGNOSIS

Diagnosis of epilepsy is essentially clinical. History is most important in making the diagnosis. Careful interrogation of witnesses of an attack is essential to determine the nature of the diagnosis. Epilepsy should be differentiated from simple faint and syncopal attacks. The epileptic attack can occur during day or night regardless of the position of the patient. Syncopal attacks usually do not occur in the

Table 202.1: Distinction between epilepsy and syncope

Features	Seizures	Syncope
Immediate precipitating factor	Usually none	Emotional stress, Valsalva, orthostatic hypotension, cardiac etiologies
Premonitory symptoms	None or aura (e.g. odd odor)	Tiredness, nausea, diaphoresis, tunneling of vision
Posture at onset		Usually erect; gradual over seconds
Transition to unconsciousness	Variable	Seconds
Duration of unconsciousness	Often immediate	Never > 15 seconds
Duration of tonic or clonic movements	Minutes 30–60 seconds	<5 min
Facial appearance during event		Pallor
Disorientation and sleepiness after event	Cyanosis, frothing at mouth	Rarely
Headache, muscle pain, tongue bite incontinence	Many minutes to hours	Short duration

recumbent posture. Also, the occurrence of pallor at the onset, gradual loss of consciousness and prompt return of consciousness on adopting recumbent posture are diagnostic of syncope. In epilepsy, loss of consciousness is abrupt and consciousness returns only slowly. Occurrence of postictal headache and vomiting should suggest the possibility of epilepsy. So also occurrence of seizure during deep sleep is a strong point in favor of epilepsy. Occurrence of injuries, such as biting the tongue or due to falls, should suggest seizure disorder since these are practically absent in hysterical convulsions.

Epilepsy has to be distinguished from syncope. The clinical features of both are listed in Table 202.1.

Hysterical Attacks (Nonepileptic Seizure)

They should be differentiated by the lack of aura, absence of injuries and incontinence, presence of peculiar variables grimacing or squirming movements and the retention of consciousness during a motor seizure, which involves both sides of the body. They are bizarre and they continue for long periods, as long as the patient is being observed. They can be induced by suggestion.

Diagnosis of the type of epilepsy depends upon proper clinical examination and if possible witnessing an attack. The epileptic focus and pattern of epilepsy are determined by investigations.

The *EEG* is the most useful investigation to establish the diagnosis of epilepsy. It gives positive records in 60–90% of cases, if the records are repeated during or after an attack and after 24 hours of sleep deprivation. Refinements in EEG procedure include the use of special electrodes, such as sphenoidal, nasoethmoidal, nasopharyngeal and in selected cases, intracerebral electrodes. Photic stimulation, sleep and hyperventilation are measures used to elicit abnormalities in the EEG (Figs 202.1A and B).

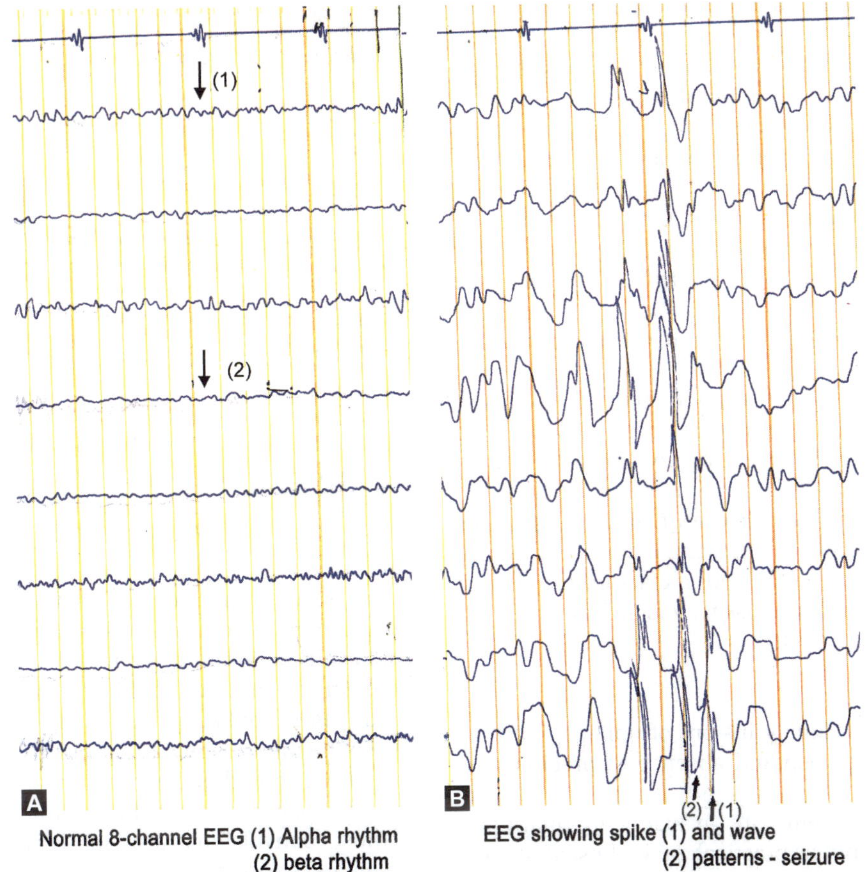

Figs 202.1A and B: **A.** Normal electroencephalogram (EEG); **B.** EEG in seizure

However, normal EEG does not exclude the diagnosis of epilepsy. Conversely, a small number of normal persons may show paroxysmal EEG abnormalities. Thus, EEG can be used only as an additional evidence to the clinical diagnosis of epilepsy. So, also its role in predicting remission or selection of AEDs is also limited. But in confirmed epileptics with EEG abnormalities, the decision to stop drug therapy can be based on the persistence of the abnormality.

Video EEG

Video EEG monitoring refers to continuous EEG recorded for a prolonged period with simultaneous video recording of the clinical manifestations. This permits having correlation of the recorded behavior and the EEG activity. The indications for video EEG include:

- Confirmation of the epileptic nature of attack
- To characterize seizure semiology and thus the seizure type, particularly in children
- Diagnostic evaluation of patients with drug-resistant seizures
- Presurgical evaluation of potential surgical candidate.

Invasive EEG

Intracranial EEG and electrocorticography are used in special situations as part of pre-surgical evaluation of resistant epilepsy, the former in nonlesional, extratemporal, bitemporal or dual pathology and the latter during surgery or interictally to define the extent of irritative cortex.

Magnetic Resonance Imaging (MRI)

It is done in all cases of intractable epilepsy as it detects:

- Mesial temporal sclerosis (MTS)
- Lesions and abnormalities of cortical development
- ***Focal abnormalities of any type:*** Magnetic resonance spectroscopy (MRS), functional MRI (fMRI) and diffusion tensor imaging (DTI) are the other adjunctive MRI techniques used in the pre-surgical evaluation.

Ictal Single Photon Emission Computed Tomography and Interictal Positron Emission Tomography

Ictal single photon emission computed tomography (SPECT) and interictal positron emission tomography (PET) are at times used in presurgical evaluation. These tests help in the functional assessment of the epileptic and nonepileptic areas.

In epilepsy occurring for the first time after 20 years of age, partial epilepsy, presence of focal neurological deficit and in those where the disease is resistant to conventional treatment, further investigations to exclude anatomical abnormalities and space-occupying lesions in the brain are indicated. These include computed tomography (CT) and MRI scans of brain.

PROGNOSIS

Over 60% of patients attain remission, which is defined as freedom from seizures for 2–3 years after stopping their antiepileptic treatment. About a third does not achieve this state.

Chances for achieving remission are greater within the first few years after diagnosis and treatment. In those in whom remission does not occur within 1–2 years of starting therapy, the chances of remission are low and these patients may require lifelong anticonvulsant therapy. As a practical guide to long-term management, epileptics can be categorized into four groups:

1. Mild cases which may even be self-limiting or remit after short course of treatment: 30%
2. Easily controlled with drugs and go into remission early: 30%
3. Chronic epilepsy, which responds partially to drugs, but relapses on withdrawal of the drugs: 20%
4. Response to drugs is unsatisfactory and remission is unusual (intractable): 20%.

Factor which predicts recurrence of seizures after the first attack: If risk factors are present, recurrence is more likely. In those with more than two risk factors, the chance of recurrence is about 100%. Risk factors include:

- Prior neurological insult
- Partial seizure
- Abnormal EEG
- ***Todd's paralysis,*** family history of epilepsy, seizure occurring during sleep and absence of precipitating factors.

Various rating systems are available to quantitate intractable seizures but as practical guide those that have one or more seizures per month despite regular, adequate and appropriate trial of minimum of two AEDs in different combinations for minimum of 2 years may be considered as intractable epilepsy.

Epilepsy and its treatment can have deleterious cognitive and behavioral consequences. Affected individuals have a higher prevalence of neuropsychological dysfunction compared to the nonepileptic population. Convulsive status is consistently associated with neuronal necrosis in vulnerable parts of the brain, especially the hippocampus, amygdala, cerebellar cortex, thalami and cerebral cortex.

Sudden death in epilepsy is due to trauma, aspiration, and continued status leading to hyperthermia, aspiration pneumonia and cardiac asystole or rarely due to SUDEP (sudden unexpected death in epilepsy); symptomatic epilepsy reduces life expectancy by 18 years.

Table 202.2 shows major causes of onset of epilepsy in relation to age.

MANAGEMENT OF EPILEPSY

Management of epilepsy consists of:
- Treatment of acute convulsions
- Prophylactic management of convulsive and nonconvulsive seizures.

The latter consists of:
- Removal of precipitating or causative factors
- Antiepileptic medication
- Social rehabilitation.

Management of an Acute Convulsion

Convulsion is a medical emergency, especially if prolonged, which should be arrested without delay. The patient is put on his side on a soft bed to avoid injuries, tight clothing is loosened and airway is protected so as to avoid asphyxiation and aspiration. Dentures and foreign bodies in the mouth should be removed and a suitable mouth gag is applied in the position of the molar teeth, to keep the mouth open and prevent injury to the tongue. The patient should be kept with head low, so as to avoid aspiration of vomitus into the respiratory tract.

Most convulsions are self-limited and need no immediate treatment. However, slow intravenous (IV) injection of 4 mg of lorazepam has to be given, especially in a case of convulsive seizure for immediate effect. An alternate anticonvulsant drug is diazepam 10 mg IV given slowly over 5–10 minutes. The risk of respiratory depression is high for the latter. Other drug that must be given parenterally is phenytoin sodium 100–200 mg IV. This helps to prevent recurrence as well.

The physician may encounter the patient with convulsions in the most embarrassing situations and therefore, the first injection of anticonvulsant medication may have to be given IV in order to terminate the convulsion forthwith, fully realizing the risk involved. Adverse drug effects include anaphylaxis, respiratory depression, hypotension and allergic manifestations.

Once the convulsions are controlled, further management has to be carefully planned. All cases of convulsions should be investigated for the presence of primary or secondary neurological conditions giving rise to symptomatic seizure. Conditions like meningitis, encephalitis, neurosyphilis, neurocysticercosis, fluid and electrolyte imbalance, hypocalcemia, abnormal glucose levels and intracranial space-occupying lesions have to be excluded.

Prophylactic Management
Antiepileptic Drugs (AEDs)

Treatment of epilepsy is primarily medical and the mainstay is the use of AEDs. Though AEDs are not curative in epilepsy, they help to control seizures and give symptomatic relief. In many instances, prolonged administration results in abolition of the epileptic tendency. The response varies in the different types of seizures and hence, it is

Table 202.2: Major causes of onset of epilepsy in relation to age

Parameters (age)	Major causes
Neonates (< 1 month)	• Perinatal hypoxia and ischemia • Intracranial hemorrhage and trauma • Central nervous system (CNS) infections • Metabolic
Infants and children (> 1 month and < 12 years)	• Febrile seizures • **Genetic disorders:** Metabolic, degenerative, primary epilepsy syndromes • CNS infections
Adolescents (12–18 years)	• Trauma • Genetic disorders • Infection
Young adults (18–35 years)	• Trauma • Alcohol withdrawal
Older adults (> 35 years)	• Cerebrovascular disease • Brain tumor • Alcohol withdrawal

necessary to administer the appropriate AED in optimum dosage. The present consensus is to start with a single drug and add others later on, only when absolutely necessary. The first-line AEDs are the time tested drugs, such as phenytoin, carbamazepine, ethosuximide, sodium valproate, phenobarbitone and primidone. The last two drugs are sparingly used now-a-days. *Oxcarbazepine, topiramate* and *lamotrigine* are increasingly used as first-line drugs (Table 202.3).

If the response to a single drug is not adequate, another drug should be added. In some, the combination produces better effect. A stable drug regimen should not, however, be frequently changed. Sudden withdrawal of AED should be avoided since this is the most common cause for precipitation of status epilepticus.

Indications for starting antiepileptic therapy: When more than one unprovoked seizure has occurred in the preceding 1 year or when the risk of recurrent convulsion is high as in head injury or intracranial infections, AEDs should be started. Since the medication has to be prolonged and the drugs are potentially toxic and expensive, patients with single attack without demonstrable focal abnormalities either clinically or on investigations, such as EEG, CT or MRI, the patient should be observed and therapy started only if seizures recur.

Guidelines for AED Therapy

- Start with a single drug in minimum dose and adjust its dosage gradually to achieve maximal clinical benefit without side effects.
- If seizures occur even after achieving tolerable dose of the single drug, a second drug should be introduced and the first one slowly withdrawn.
- Different combinations of two drugs may be tried, each trial lasting for a maximum of 6 months, till the ideal combination is arrived at. There is no role for combining more than two drugs.
- ***Therapy should continue till at least 2–3 year seizure-free period*** is completed after which the drugs can be gradually withdrawn. Nearly, 50% of the patients may not require any further treatment. The rest may relapse and this usually occurs within 5 years. Children who develop primary epilepsy in early life and who show prompt response to AED have greater chance for permanent remission.
- Twenty-five percent of cases may develop chronic epilepsy and require lifelong medication. Risk of chronicity is high in patients with neurological and psychological abnormalities and social handicaps. Partial seizures are more refractory to medical treatment in up to 20% of cases. These may require surgery.

When confronted with intractable seizures, newer drugs should be considered. Before doing so it is wise to verify the following:

- Is the diagnosis correct?
- Is the epilepsy secondary to other disease processes?
- Are the appropriate drugs taken regularly and in full doses?
- Are there any adverse psychosocial factors?
- Associated nonepileptic seizure (pseudoseizure).

Newer AEDs (Table 202.4)

Several newer AEDs are on the anvil. Many of these are now freely available in India. At present, these newer drugs are recommended as add-on drugs along with conventional drugs to treat intractable cases, although some of them are found effective as initial monotherapy.

- ***Oxcarbazepine:*** This is chemically-related to carbamazepine. Its action is similar to carbamazepine but this drug is better tolerated. Side effects including Steven-Johnson syndrome encountered with carbamazepine are only occasionally seen. Ataxia is the main adverse effect. ***Dose:*** 1,200–2,400 mg/day.
- ***Levetiracetam:*** It is an add-on drug for refractory partial and generalized seizures in adults in a dose of 500 mg bd. It has the least drug interactions. It is useful in the presence of hepatic and renal insufficiency. It is being used increasingly as monotherapy in generalized as well as partial epilepsies in children and adults.
- ***Topiramate:*** Topiramate (100–500 mg) is useful in partial seizures with secondary generalization and primary generalized seizures. It is used in children as monotherapy and as add-on in adults. The side effects include paresthesia of hands. Renal stones have been described as a complication.

Table 202.3: Details of the commonly used anticonvulsant drugs

Name of the dose	Children dose (mg/kg)	Adult dose (mg)	Toxic effects	Serum half-life (in hours)
Phenytoin (dilantin) (Fig. 202.2)	4–7	300–400	Gingival hypertrophy, ataxia, chorea, dyskinesia lymphadenopathy peripheral neuropathy, anemia hirsutism	24 ± 12
Carbamazepine (tegretol)	20–30	600–1,200	Diplopia, giddiness, Stevens-Johnson syndrome hyponatremia, weight gain	12 ± 3
Oxcarbazepine	20–30	600–2,400	Less toxic, toxicity similar	12 ± 3
Ethosuximide (zarontin)	20–30	750–1,500	Hepatotoxicity, blood dyscrasias, nephrotoxicity	30 ± 6
Valproic acid (sodium-valproate)	30–60	1,000–3,000	Transient hair loss, tremors, obesity, thrombocytopenia	8 ± 2
Levetiracetam	Broad spectrum, mainly partial	1,000–3,000	Broad spectrum, few somnolence, drug L-interactions ataxia behavioral	
Phenobarbitone	3–5	60–200	Sedation, cognitive decline, ataxia	96 ± 12

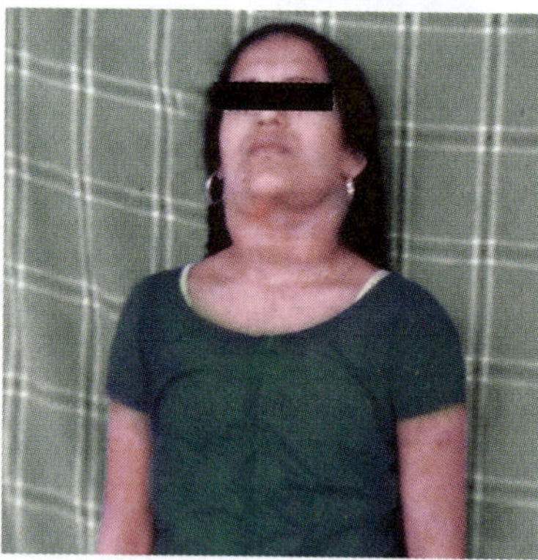

Fig. 202.2: Phenytoin-induced pseudolymphoma

- *Lamotrigine:* This drug inhibits the release of the excitatory amino acid glutamate. The effective dose is 200–300 mg/day. The drug is started at 50 mg/day and gradually increased till the full dose is reached over 3–6 weeks. Further increase in dosage should be done only very cautiously, when combined with sodium valproate, it should be used in smaller doses. It is indicated in intractable partial seizures with secondary generalization, infantile status and LGS. Adverse effects include dystonia, ataxia, severe hepatotoxicity and skin rash.
- *Clobazam:* Its antiepileptic activity is related to its binding to one or more specific GABA receptors increasing GABA-mediated inhibition. It is effective in complex partial seizures with or without secondarily generalization as add-on. The adult daily dose is 20–30 mg. Sedation, irritability and weight gain are the main side effects.
- *Tiagabine:* Tiagabine (30–60 mg) may be of use in partial epilepsies with secondary generalization.
- *Vigabatrin:* It is also called gamma-vinyl-GABA (GVG). This drug irreversibly inhibits GABA amino-transferase.
  Dose: 50–100 mg/kg/day. It is not available in India.

Indications: Complex partial seizures with secondary generalization, infantile spasms. Adverse effects include defects in the visual fields, sedation and behavioral disturbances.

- *Zonisamide:* This is a benzisoxazole derivative.
  Dose: 6–10 mg/kg/day. The initial dose is 100 mg/day.
  Indications: Partial seizures with secondary generalization, primary generalized tonic-clonic, atonic and myoclonic seizures. Adverse effects include feverishness, ataxia, leukopenia and urinary calculi.
- *Gabapentin (neurontin):* This is a GABA-related amino acid with broad-spectrum antiepileptic activity.
  Dose: The initial daily dose is 300 mg increased to 600–1,300 mg over a few days. Even doses as high as 3,600 mg/day are safe. This drug is well-tolerated and the full dose can be attained within 3–4 days. It can be safely combined with any other AEDs. Gabapentin is an add-on drug for resistant partial and secondarily generalized seizures. Main adverse effects are somnolence, ataxia, fatigue, nystagmus, gastrointestinal (GI) upset and weight gain.
- *Felbamate:* This drug raises the seizure threshold. Adult dose may vary from 1,800 to 4,800 mg/day. Daily dose for children is 15–45 mg/kg given in 3–4 doses.
  Indications: Felbamate is used as add-on therapy for partial seizures with generalization resistant to other drugs and for LGS. When used as an add-on drug, the dosage of the original drug should be reduced progressively and withdrawn, when the full dose of felbamate is reached.
  Side effects include insomnia, weight loss, nausea, anorexia and aplastic anemia. Due to serious toxic effects this drug is not licensed in many countries.
- *Rufinamide:* It acts by prolonging the time spent in inactive state in the sodium channel. It has been found to be of use in atonic seizures in LGS.
- *Retigabine (ezogabine):* It acts in potassium channels and is of use as add-on treatment in partial epilepsy.

Table 202.4: Details of newer antiepileptic drugs (AEDs)

Drug	Indications	Daily dose (mg)	Benefits	Toxicity
Lamotrigine	Intractable partial enzymes with secondary generalization	100–500	Broad spectrum, wide experience, once	Skin rash, ataxia, tremor, gastrointestinal (GI)
Topiramate	Partial seizures	100–500	Broad spectrum, wide experience, twice daily dosing	Ataxia, confusion, loss of weight, renal stones, word finding difficulty
Clobazam	Complex partial, secondary and primary generalized sizures	20–50	Less side effects and few drug interactions, Twice-daily dosing	Sedation, irritability, weight gain disturbances
Vigabatrin	do + secondary generalized	1,000–2,000	Broad spectrum	Psychosis, visual field defect weight gain, depression
Gabapentin	-do-	1,800–3,600	No drug interactions, rapid titration	Somnolence, fatigue, ataxia
Felbamate	-do- + Lennox-Gastaut syndrome (LGS)	2,400–3,600	—	Aplastic anemia, hepatic failure
Tiagabine	Partial and secondary generalized	32–56	Only a few drug interactions	GI disturbances, confusion
Zonisamide	-do- and also generalized epilepsy	100–600	Broad spectrum, few drug interactions, once-daily dosing	Somnolence, renal calculi, ataxia
Lacosamide	Add-on in partial	200–500	Of use in status epilepticus	Caution in using in heart disease
Eslicarbazine	-do-		Alternate for carbamazepine	Sedation, ataxia

Table 202.5: Drug interaction with AED

	Serum drug levels	
	Phenytoin	**Carbamazepine**
Concurrent drug therapy		
Isoniazid	↑	↑
Rifampicin	↓ι	↓
Erythromycin	↑ρ	↑
Lithium	–	↑
Antacids	↓ν	↓
Cimetidine	↑ι	–
Warfarin	↑α	–
Pyridoxine	↓ψ	↓
Oral contraception	↓ρ	↓ρ

↑ serum levels increase; ↓ serum levels decrease

Table 202.6: Drug of choice in various types of epilepsy

Types of epilepsy	Drugs of choice
Generalized tonic-clonic seizures with partial onset, simple partial and complex partial seizures	Phenytoin sodium Carbamazepine, oxcarbazepine Levetiracetam, clobazam, lamotrigine, topiramate Sodium valproate and rest of newer AEDs
Primary generalized epilepsy	Levetiracetam, sodium valproate, lamotrigine, topiramate, zonisamide, phenobarbitone
Absence seizures with 'three per second' spike and waves on EEG	Sodium valproate, ethosuximide, clonazepam
Myoclonic seizures	Sodium valproate, nitrazepam, clonazepam
Infantile spasms	ACTH/corticosteroids, Vigabatrin, nitrazepam, sodium valproate, clonazepam
Neonatal seizures	Phenobarbitone: Febrile seizures: Clobazam
LGS	Felbamate, Lamotrigine, sodium valproate

Abbreviations: AED = Antiepileptic drugs; LGS = Lennox-Gastaut syndrome; EEG = Electroencephalogram; ACTH = Adrenocorticotropic hormone

These three drugs just mentioned are not available in India.
- ***Acetazolamide:*** Acetazolamide, which is a carbonic anhydrase inhibitor, can be used as a second-line drug along with other AEDs to potentiate their action. It also reduces intracranial tension.
   Dose: 0.25–1.00 g in divided doses daily.

A serious problem on long-term AED therapy is the occurrence of drug interactions when other drugs are given concurrently. These may lead to rise or fall in blood levels of the AED, resulting in occurrence of toxic effects of the drug or the development of seizures (Tables 202.5 and 202.6).

STATUS EPILEPTICUS

When recurrent seizures occur at a frequency which does not allow consciousness to be regained in the interval between seizures, it is called status epilepticus. More than one seizure within 30 minutes without gain in consciousness is the definition given by the World Health Organization (WHO). For practical purposes, a duration of 5 minutes as proposed by Lowenstein, et al. may be better adopted for adults and children aged above 5 years.

Classification

Status epilepticus is classified into convulsive and nonconvulsive types:
- ***Convulsive status*** is the most dangerous type. It is subdivided into tonic/clonic/myoclonic/tonic-clonic types.
- ***Nonconvulsive:*** It is a state of electromechanical dissociation where the epileptiform discharges evident on the EEG are not accompanied by clinical manifestations other than hardly discernible motor manifestations or coma. It is subdivided into absence status and complex partial status. Patients with this type of status need to be managed as convulsive status using EEG as a guide rather than clinical observation as the determinant of response to treatment. Cases of complex partial status have to be suspected in cases of altered state of consciousness or coma of undetermined origin in an intensive care unit (ICU) setup in old age group with septicemia.

Pathophysiology and Complications

Recurrent seizures exhibit the tendency to become self sustaining even after removal of epileptogenic stimulus. This is the rationale for treating status epilepticus at the earliest instance. The initial phases of status epilepticus can be terminated by drugs which augment inhibition or depress excitation of the membrane potential. But once it becomes established, only drugs specifically those inhibiting glutaminergic transmission are found to be effective. Permanent damage to hippocampus and cerebellum are inevitable in uncontrolled status epilepticus.

Etiology

- Acute symptomatic related to acute medical or neurological illness, e.g. herpes simplex encephalitis (HSE)
- Remote symptomatic status epilepticus owing to static encephalopathy, such as stroke
- Cryptogenic where the cause is unclear
- On the background of established epilepsy, usually due to abrupt stoppage of AEDs.

Management

Time is a critical factor in the management of status epilepticus. There are many therapeutic regimes but none is totally satisfactory. Parenteral benzodiazepines are all potent fast acting AEDs preferred for terminating the attack immediately. Lorazepam is preferable to diazepam because of its longer duration of action of more than 4 hours and less respiratory depression. Simultaneously, a loading dose of IV phenytoin 0.5–1 g (18 mg/kg) in saline is given over 20 minutes at the rate of 50 mg/min. Fosphenytoin (FOS) (150 mg equivalent to 100 mg of phenytoin) is given in dose of 15–20 mg/kg phenytoin equivalents (PE) at a rate of 75–150 mg/min. Side effects of IV phenytoin like cardiac arrhythmias and hypotension and extravasation at injection site can be avoided if FOS (which is water soluble) is used though the latter is costlier. If seizures still persist 20

Box 202.1: Algorithm for management of status epilepticus

0 min: Diagnose status epilepticus
0–2 min: Airway, breathing, circulation, capillary glucose level
- **First-line:** 1–3 min IV thiamine with 50% glucose 3–10 min: IV lorazepam. Prepare loading dose of phenytoin/FOS phenytoin
- **Second-line:** 5–30 min phenytoin/FOS phenytoin infusion
- **Third-line:** 30–60 min valproate/levetiracetam/phenobarbitone/lacosamide. Initiate EEG monitoring. If EEG shows persistent seizure activity after third-line agent, initiate infusion therapy
- **Fourth-line:** >60 min IV: Midazolam/thiopentone sodium/propofol
  - **Coma induction:** Bolus and infusion. Assess after every 5 min for clinical or EEG seizure control
  - **Coma phase:** Pharmacologic coma for 24 hours after last seizure; continue EEG for 24 hours after end of infusion to evaluate for recurrence. Titration goals EEG seizure control-midazolam
  - **Burst suppression:** Thiopentone
  - **Weaning:** Slow reduction of infusion with frequent EEG review
  - Gradual replacement of parenteral drugs by oral substitution.

Abbreviations: IV = Intravenous; FOS = Fosphenytoin; EEG = Electroencephalogram

minutes after the injection of loading dose of phenytoin, it can be repeated at a dose of 5 mg/kg till a maximal total dose of 30 mg/kg is given. Phenobarbitone given IV in doses of 0.8–1 g/kg in 24 hours (20 mg/kg at 100 mg/min) is effective if further seizures occur. In intractable cases, thiopental anesthesia is given with IV injection of 0.3–0.6 g. Assisted ventilation is mandatory when phenobarbitone or thiopentone is given. Levetiracetam (third-line) is given in dose of 20–30 mg/kg as bolus IV over 15 minutes followed by maintenance of 1,500 mg bd orally or IV. Sodium valproate (third-line) is given as 15–30 mg/kg as loading dose and maintained as 500 mg tds.

Lacosamide is a functionalized amino acid that has activity, used for the adjunctive treatment of partial-onset seizures and status epilepticus. It is given orally bd and also it can be given IV as infusion in doses of 50 mg/min to control status epilepticus. Lacosamide in doses of (50 mg/min) is repeated bd. Algorithm for management of status epilepticus is given in Box 202.1. There are trials which have shown that IV sodium valproate is superior if used as second-line drug instead of phenytoin. On many occasions, status epilepticus may be encountered outside hospital setting. Management of such cases becomes more difficult due to problems of IV medication in a convulsing patient. In such patients, drugs such as midazolam in a dose of 0.07–0.08 mg/kg given IM may be effective. The seizure stops in 10 minutes. Buccal application or intra-osseous injection can be tried in children. Another safe but less effective method is to give rectally any parenteral preparation of diazepam in a dose of 0.5 mg/kg to a maximum of 20 mg in adults.

Source: Misra UK, Kalita J, Patel R. Sodium valproate vs phenytoin in status epilepticus: a pilot study. Neurology. 2006;67(2):340-2.

Emergency Measures

The maintenance of airway, breathing and circulation is the priority in patients presenting with status epilepticus. The reversible factors which should be kept in mind that include hyponatremia, hypoglycemia, hypocalcemia, hypomagnesemia, acidosis, hyperthermia and hypoxia. Hypoxia may not manifest clinically and oxygen supplementation is recommended in all patients in status epilepticus. Emergency investigations include blood gases, glucose, renal and hepatic functions, calcium, magnesium, full blood count, clotting screen. Toxicology screening may be done in suspected cases. Electrocardiogram (ECG) has to be done as soon as patient arrives.

Prognosis

Mortality in status epilepticus in various studies is up to 20%. Major determinants of outcome in status epilepticus are the underlying etiology, age and the time lapsed for initiating treatment. Acute symptomatic status epilepticus has the worse prognosis. A duration of less than 10 hours was associated with a better outcome. Lack of response to first-line drugs had also been noticed to be a bad prognostic indicator. A good percentage develops permanent neurological sequelae.

Surgical and Other Physical Interventions in Resistant Case

Surgery for Drug-resistant Epilepsy

There is class I evidence that epilepsy surgery is more efficacious than continued medical treatment in people with drug-resistant epilepsy. The pre-surgical evaluation for this includes in addition to the tests sited, detailed neuropsychological assessment. Concordance of data obtained from these tests may be adequate to perform surgery with good results in the classical mesial temporal epilepsy syndrome with mesial temporal sclerosis. Anterior temporal lobectomy along with amygdalohippocampectomy is the surgery done for this. For extra-temporal lesions, surgery has been found to be of benefit. The results for non-lesional cases in this group are less impressive. The other surgical procedures include cortical excision, hemispherectomy and stereotaxic surgery.

Vagal Nerve Stimulation in Epilepsy

Stimulation of the left vagus by an implantable electrical device might result in extensive activation or deactivation of the brain circuits thought to be involved with epileptic seizures. It is in vogue for past 1 decade and has been approved by United States Federation of Drug Administration (USFDA). It is best suited for nonlocalized uncontrolled epilepsy where respective surgery is not feasible. It has been found to produce 50% reduction in seizure frequency. Compared to surgery, it is expensive.

Deep Brain Stimulation in Epilepsy

Stimulation of cerebellum, anterior and centromedian nucleus of thalamus have been tried in controlling epilepsy where respective surgery is nonfeasible with variable results.

Ketogenic Diet

Induction of mild ketosis by instituting ketogenic diet has been found to decrease the frequency of seizures in children. Diet that constitutes 80% of energy by fat is used to produce ketosis. The effect of ketosis is mediated by stimulating the inhibitory GABA pathways.

Parkinson's Disease and Related Disorders

SR Chandra, R Jeyachandran

Chapter Summary

- Anatomy
- Physiology of the Basal Ganglia
- Parkinson's Disease
- Other Parkinsonian Syndromes
  - Diffuse Lewy Body Dementia
  - Other Causes of Parkinsonism
- Wilson's Disease

INTRODUCTION

James Parkinson defined this condition as a disease characterized by involuntary tremulous motion in parts not in action with lessened muscular power even when supported and propensity for running than walking, stooped posture, mind and intellect remaining unaltered. *Charaka* the great Indian physician called it as *Kampavata*, described all features in detail and classified, so beautifully into *karokampam, shirokampam, padakampam* and *sarvankakampam* (tremors of hands, head, legs and all parts respectively) based on phenotypic characteristics and used the leaves of 'Naikurunai' which is the source of levodopa which is still the most effective treatment. Diagnosis is clinical as it is a syndrome characterized by a constellation of signs of varying etiology consisting of (1) tremor, (2) rigidity, (3) bradykinesia and (4) postural disturbance. Two or more of these features must be present for making the diagnosis.

The term 'parkinsonism plus' or syndrome is used if there is, in addition, evidence for involvement of other parts of nervous system. Secondary parkinsonism is secondary to drugs, infections, trauma or metabolic disorders. This diagnosis is of prognostic and therapeutic importance.

ANATOMY

The basal ganglia are a group of subcortical nuclei. They are comprised of the neostriatum (caudate nucleus and putamen), the ventral striatum, the globus pallidus (externa and interna), the subthalamic nucleus (STN) and the substantia nigra pars reticularis (SNR) and pars compacta and red nucleus. Basal ganglia receive inputs and send efferents to the cerebral cortex and brainstem. These form circuits which are responsible for maintaining and smoothening out various movements that are carried out by the body. Although traditionally, defects in the basal ganglia and its circuits were believed to cause only movement disorders, in view of their extensive connections with cortical structures, they are also now known to cause a combination of movement, affective and cognitive disorders.

PHYSIOLOGY OF THE BASAL GANGLIA

The basal ganglia receive inputs from predominantly the cerebral cortex. The principal nucleus receiving the inputs is the striatum. The inputs are mainly excitatory. The output of the basal ganglia is from the globus pallidus interna (GPi), the ventral striatum and SNR. The output from the striatum and the globus pallidi is inhibitory with gamma-aminobutyric acid (GABA) being the chief neurotransmitter. The output from the STN is excitatory, with glutamate as the neurotransmitter. The efferents from the GPi and SNR project to pedunculopontine nuclei and to the thalamus. In addition, the SNR also projects to the superior colliculi.

The basal ganglia are connected to frontal lobe by five circuits:

1. Motor
2. Oculomotor
3. Dorsolateral prefrontal
4. Lateral orbitofrontal
5. Limbic.

The circuits are further divided into five pathways depending on the connections between the basal ganglia. These are the direct and indirect pathways, hyperdirect pathway, nigrostriatal pathway and connections of SNR to pedunculopontine nucleus.

In the direct pathway, the outflow from the striatum projects directly to the GPi, whereas in the indirect pathway, the projection is through the globus pallidus externa (GPe) and SNR. As a result, the actions of these pathways are different. The direct motor pathway facilitates movement, while the indirect pathway inhibits movement. Disorders affecting the direct pathway result in parkinsonian features like bradykinesia while disorders of the indirect pathway results in hyperkinetic disorders (choreic disorders) discussed in chapter on Movement Disorders. The direct and indirect pathways appears to be an over simplification. These pathways cannot explain the coexistence of bradykinetic and hyperkinetic features seen in disorders like Huntington's disease.

The increasing knowledge of the functional anatomy and neurochemistry of the basal ganglia has enabled the discovery of newer and more effective modalities of treatment for movement disorders.

PARKINSON'S DISEASE

This is one of the common neurodegenerative diseases seen all over the world, including India. In other countries such as the USA, Parkinson's disease (PD) is the second most common neurodegenerative disease after Alzheimer's disease. Clinically, parkinsonism is a generic term that is characterized by a triad of bradykinesia, rest tremor and rigidity. PD refers specifically to idiopathic PD where there is no definite identifiable precipitating cause.

Idiopathic PD is characterized by asymmetric onset of symptoms. In addition to the above mentioned cardinal features of PD, there are several other manifestations. These include postural instability, freezing of gait, sensory disturbances, autonomic disturbances, and psychiatric manifestations. The cardinal symptoms of PD respond to dopamine therapy, while the other symptoms may not respond.

Pathology

Pathologically, the hallmark of PD is degeneration of the dopaminergic neurons of the substantia nigra (SN). Nondopaminergic regions like the brainstem such as nucleus basalis of Meynert and locus coeruleus (LC) may also be implicated, and it is possible that the additional clinical features that do not respond to dopaminergic drugs are possibly due to these areas also being affected. As previously mentioned, the underlying pathology in PD appears to be the involvement of the direct pathway which leads to bradykinesia.

Etiology

Most cases of PD are sporadic and cause cannot be ascertained in many. Genetic factors have been implicated in young onset PD. Based on genetic studies, familial PD has been found to occur in 10–15% of the cases and multiple genetic loci have been implicated. Sixteen genetic loci for familial PD have been isolated labeled as Park genes mutations.

In addition, twin studies have also shown that there may be several environmental factors that could play a role in the pathogenesis of PD. Some of these are enumerated below:

- **Toxins**
  - 1-methyl-4-phenyl-1,2,5,6-tetrahydropyridine (MPTP)—found in heroin addicts
  - Manganese
  - Carbon monoxide
- Vascular
- Drug-induced
  - Antipsychotics
  - Antiepileptics, e.g. sodium valproate
  - Antiemetics, e.g. metoclopramide
- Tumors
- Caffeine and smoking are found to have an inverse (protective) relation with PD.

Clinical Features

PD typically occurs in the sixth or seventh decade. Familial PD occurs at a younger age. Although PD was previously considered to involve only the motor system, it is now known to affect the nervous system across multiple axes.

- **Motor:** The motor manifestations of PD are characterized by the cardinal features of bradykinesia, tremor and rigidity. Additionally, there may also be postural instability and freezing of gait. The parkinsonian features typically are asymmetrical in onset; tremor is usually a dominant feature. The tremor in PD is a rest tremor, which is coarse and reduces on assuming posture or on action. The tremor is also

referred to as 're-emergent' tremor, as after assuming a posture for sometime, the tremor reappears. In certain cases, PD may be of the akinetic-rigid variety, which is characterized by absence of tremor. The core features of PD appear to be the asymmetrical in onset. Dopaminergic medication gives good response to the motor symptoms. Bradykinesia is one among the earliest manifestations in PD. In early PD, the manifestations are subtle and often the patient and relatives do not notice the manifestations. The patient may manifest with reduced facial expression (hypomimia) and reduced blink rate. As the limbs are involved, the patient may develop reduced arm swing on the affected side and the affected lower limb may lag behind the normal limb while walking. With progression of the disease, manifestations become more overt and the patient becomes slower in all activities. There is loss of dexterity in finer movements. Handwriting becomes smaller (micrographia). Speech is affected with low volume, monotonous speech. The gait is characterized by a slow, shuffling nature and there may be occasions when the patient is unable to control the speed of walking and tends to walk more rapidly with smaller steps (festination). Sudden freezing of activity is observed in advanced stages of the disease. Falls due to postural instability also occur later during the disease.

- **Nonmotor manifestations**
  - **Sensory:** PD patients may complain of positive sensory phenomena like paresthesiae and pain. The sensory manifestations can precede the motor manifestations.
  - **Autonomic:** Autonomic dysfunction is known to occur in PD. This manifests as postural giddiness, sphincter disturbances and erectile dysfunction.
  - **Neuropsychiatric manifestations:** PD patients present with slowness of cognition and thought. This is referred to as **bradyphrenia**. Depression is a common among PD patients. The patient may also develop disorders of impulse control in the form of tendency to gamble excessively or spend money excessively. Later stages of PD may manifest with cognitive decline and dementia. In PD, dementia usually follows the motor manifestations at least by 1 year (Table 203.1).

Some clinical features suggest parkinsonism may not be due to Parkinson disease (Table 203.2). These features are:

- Falls within the first year of onset
- Symmetrical onset
- Involvement of the trunk more than the limbs
- Poor response of motor symptoms to dopaminergic medication
- Early onset of dementia
- Early and prominent autonomic disturbances
- Prominent cerebellar signs
- Downward gaze palsy
- High frequency tremor
- Onset before the age of 40 years.

Table 203.1: Signs and symptoms of Parkinsonism

Autonomic dysfunction	Neuropsychiatric symptoms	Sensory problems
• Orthostatic hypotension • Urinary incontinence • Impotence • Constipation • Sialorrhea • Anhidrosis	• Depression • Psychosis • Dementia • Anxiety • Panic attacks	• Reduces smell • Pain

Sleep disorders	Rheumatologically
• Restless legs • Insomnia • Daytime somnolence	• Frozen shoulder • Periarthritis • Swan neck deformity of fingers

Symptoms/signs	Diagnosis to consider
Early speech and gait impairment (lack of tremor, lack of motor asymmetry)	Atypical parkinsonism
Exposure to neuroleptics	Drug-induced parkinsonism
Onset prior to age of 40 years	Genetic form of Parkinson's disease
Liver disease	Wilson's disease
Early hallucinations and dementia with later development of PD feature	Dementia with Lewy bodies
Diplopia, impaired downgaze	Progressive supranuclear palsy (PSP)
Poor or no response to an adequate trail of levodopa	Atypical or secondary parkinsonism

Physical examination	
Dementia as first or early feature	Dementia with Lewy bodies
Prominent orthostatic hypotension	Multiple system atrophy-p (MSA-P)
Prominent cerebellar signs	MSA-C
Slow saccades with impaired downgaze	PSP
High frequency (6–10 Hz) symmetric postural tremor with a prominent kinetic component	Essential tremor

Table 203.2: Clinical features of Parkinson's disease

- Age < 50 years
  - Symmetric bradykinesia and rigidity
  - Absence of tremor
  - Prominent myoclonus
  - Limb apraxia
  - Alien limb phenomena
  - Impaired downaze
  - Facial dystonia
  - Early loss of postural reflexes
  - L-dopa-induced facial dyskinesias
  - Ataxia
  - Stridor
  - Spasticity
  - Early dementia or hallucinations
  - Early and prominent dysautonomia
- Sudden onset or fast progression
- Early falls
- Early dementia
- Unusual tremor or myoclonus
- Early autonomic disturbances
- Poor levodopa response
- Gaze palsies
- Marked dysarthria or dysphagia
- Family history

Investigations

PD is a clinical diagnosis that has to be confirmed by careful history and clinical examination. There are several clinical scales available to assess the severity of symptoms and serially assess the response to treatment. The scales that are used commonly include the Unified Parkinson's Disease Rating Scale (UPDRS), Modified Hoehn and Yahr Scale and Schwab-England Scale.

Clinical staging (Hoehn and Yahr and Schwab-England Scales)

Stage 0	=	No signs of disease
Stage 1	=	Unilateral disease
Stage 1.5	=	Unilateral plus axial involvement
Stage 2	=	Bilateral disease, without impairment of balance
Stage 2.5	=	Mild bilateral disease, with recovery on pull test
Stage 3	=	Mild to moderate bilateral disease; some postural instability; physically independent
Stage 4	=	Severe disability; still able to walk or stand unassisted
Stage 5	=	Wheelchair bound or bedridden unless aided.

Imaging is unremarkable and is done to rule out other causes of parkinsonism. Other investigations are directed toward suspected complications and nonmotor manifestations of the disease. These include autonomic function tests, neuropsychological assessments to evaluate cognition and more recently genetic analysis to rule out familial causes of PD.

Treatment

PD differs from other forms of parkinsonism in that there is good response to dopaminergic agents.

Levodopa

This forms the mainstay in the pharmacological management of PD. Dose of levodopa is 100–200 mg bd or tid. Levodopa is a precursor of dopamine that is converted to dopamine *in vivo* by dopa-decarboxylase. While dopamine cannot cross the blood brain barrier, levodopa can do so. Levodopa is combined with a peripheral decarboxylase inhibitor (carbidopa). This ensures that the conversion to dopamine occurs only in the central nervous system (CNS). This ensures better availability of dopamine in the brain and also prevents unwanted side effects of dopamine like nausea and vomiting which can occur as a result of stimulation of the area postrema. It also avoids orthostatic hypotension.

Presently, there are no available modalities of treatment that give better response than levodopa. However, there are limitations to treatment of levodopa. The effect of levodopa begins to reduce after a period of a few years. There are fluctuations in motor response. The duration of effect of levodopa reduces progressively. There may be a sudden *wearing off* of levodopa effect (on-off phenomenon). This can be partially offset by using levodopa in combination with other drugs like monoamine oxidase-B (MAO-B) inhibitors and catechol-O-methyltransferase (COMT) inhibitors (discussed further). Other motor complications include levodopa induced dyskinesias. These usually begin 4–5 years after starting therapy. It is more likely to occur among patients with early onset of disease and those with severe disease, taking higher doses of levodopa. Behavioral alterations are encountered in patients on levodopa in the form of impulse control disorders, purposelessness, stereotyped behavior (pounding). Patients may also develop craving for levodopa. In addition, levodopa does not modify other symptoms of parkinsonism like postural instability and freezing. It also does not have satisfactory effect on nonmotor manifestations of PD. There are a lot of controversies with reference to when and how to start levodopa; however, after confirmation of diagnosis it is better to maintain the patient with other drugs and keep levodopa as a reserve. If the patient is in the late decades of life, treatment can be initiated with levodopa. This therapy which has been introduced about four decades ago has changed the lifestyle and quality of parkinsonism patient substantially.

Dopamine Agonists

These drugs act directly on dopamine receptors. They are classified into ergot derivatives (bromocriptine, cabergoline and pergolide) and nonergot derivatives (pramipexole, ropinirole and rotigotine). The ergot derivatives are associated with cardiovascular side effects such as vasospasms and angina.

The dose of ergot derivatives and nonergot derivatives are as follows:

- Dose of bromocriptine is 2.5 mg hs to start with and increased up to 5 mg to a maximum of 40 mg/day
- Dose of cabergoline is 0.5–1 mg twice a week oral
- Dose of pergolide is 50 µg to start with and gradually worked up once a day up to 3,000 µg
- Dose of pramipexole is 0.25–1 mg tid oral
- Dose of ropinirole is 6–24 mg/day oral given as three doses
- Dose of rotigotine is applied as a transdermal patch 10 mg/day, patches of 2, 4 and 6 mg are available.

In general, dopamine agonists are not as efficacious as levodopa. However, initial use of dopamine agonists is advocated in early PD as it avoids early onset of dyskinesias. In most patients, supplemental levodopa is required as the response to dopamine agonists tends to be wane off.

The side effects of dopamine agonists include nausea, vomiting, orthostatic giddiness, behavioral disturbances, hallucinations and excessive somnolence.

MAO-B Inhibitors

Monoamine oxidases are a group of enzymes involved in the degradation of catecholamines, including dopamine. The two predominant subtypes are termed MAO-A and MAO-B. MAO-B is the subtype that is found in the CNS. MAO-B inhibitors avoid the peripheral side effects associated with nonselective MAO inhibitors.

The drugs in this group are selegiline and rasagiline. They are moderately effective. They are used primarily as monotherapy in early disease or more commonly as an adjunct to levodopa therapy especially when the 'wearing off' to levodopa starts or when there are unexpected 'off' periods. There is increased incidence of dyskinesias among patients on MAO-B inhibitors. Dose of selegiline is 5 mg bd with breakfast and lunch. **Side effects** include nausea, headache, insomnia and hallucinations. Dose of rasagiline is 1 mg given in the morning.

COMT Inhibitors

Catechol-O-methyltransferase is another enzyme involved in catecholamine metabolism. COMT inhibitors also serve to increase the availability of dopamine. The drugs in this group include entacapone and tolcapone. These drugs also serve to reduce the 'off' periods while on levodopa and also serve to reduce the dose of levodopa by 20–25%. Hepatotoxicity has been reported, especially with tolcapone and frequent monitoring of liver enzymes is recommended. The doses are as follows:

- *Dose of tolcapone:* 100–200 mg tid
- *Dose of entacapone:* 200 mg with each L-dopa tablet.

Amantadine

It is used as an adjunctive therapy. It is believed to be an inhibitor of N-methyl-D-aspartate (NMDA) pathway. Predominant action appears to be to reduce dyskinesias. The major side effects include neuropsychiatric disturbances, hypotension, flushing and livedo reticularis. Dose of amantadine is 100 mg tid; side effects include mental confusion, disorientation and leg edema.

Central Anticholinergic Agents

Trihexyphenidyl, benzearside and benztropine are used predominantly for their effect on tremor. **Side effects** include cognitive deficits, especially in the elderly; urinary retention and glaucoma. Dose of this drug is 2 mg three times a day; side effects include dryness of the mouth, constipation, urinary retention, impairment of memory, confusion and hallucinations.

Surgical Treatments

Cases not fully responding to medical therapy should be considered for surgery. Surgical modalities in PD treatment are broadly divided into lesional surgeries and deep brain stimulation (DBS). The pioneers of surgical treatment in India are professor VB Alasubramaniam, S Kalyanaraman and TS Kanaka of Chennai as early as the 1980s.

In lesional surgeries, *pallidotomy* (lesion placed in GPi) provides the most significant benefit as in addition to improvement of bradykinesia and rigidity. It also helps to reduce contralateral dyskinesia. Other lesional surgeries include 'thalamotomy', which reduces contralateral tremor (lesion is placed in ventral anteromedial nucleus of thalamus).

Deep brain stimulation (DBS) is the most commonly used surgical modality presently. An electrode is placed into target area in the brain and stimulator is placed subcutaneously in chest wall. The stimulation parameters can be adjusted using an external apparatus. The targets in the brain include GPi and STN. STN stimulation is more commonly used. DBS provides improvement in dyskinesias and also reduces the off periods. However, the efficacy of DBS never exceeds that of levodopa and DBS does not improve symptoms that are not affected by levodopa, like postural instability, drooling, autonomic disturbances, etc. Complications associated with DBS include infection, bleeds, breaking of electrodes, suicidal tendencies and later development of other newer movement disorders.

Treatment of Nonmotor Manifestations

Psychiatric manifestations are common in PD, with depression being the most common (Refer Section 19, Ch 246). Antidepressants should not be withheld when indicated. Selective serotonin reuptake inhibitors are preferred although they should be used with caution when the patient is on MAO-B inhibitors. Psychosis is treated with antipsychotics, with either quetiapine or clozapine being preferred. The medication used to treat PD may also present with psychosis and cognitive problems. In this situation, it may be necessary to withdraw one or more medication. Usually, amantadine and anticholinergics are stopped first, followed by MAO-B and COMT inhibitors. Dopamine agonists may also need to be reduced. Levodopa is the last drug to be reduced. Cognitive symptoms and dementia in PD is known to occur. This may require judicious treatment with acetylcholinesterase inhibitors. Autonomic disturbances require supportive measures such as judicious intake of fluid and salt. Pharmacological treatment includes fludrocortisone and midodrine. Mild laxatives may help to relieve constipation. Sleep disturbances, in particular rapid-eye-movement (REM) sleep behavior disorders, are common among PD patients. Apart from maintaining sleep hygiene, clonazepam may help in controlling the symptoms.

OTHER PARKINSONIAN SYNDROMES

Parkinsonian syndromes should be considered when symptoms are symmetrical to start with, axial more than appendicular and there is evidence for involvement of parts of the neuraxis other than the basal ganglia.

The parkinsonian syndromes are pathologically classified, based on the pathological inclusions found in the brain, into alpha-synucleinopathies and tauopathies.

Alpha-synucleinopathies include idiopathic PD, diffuse Lewy body dementia (DLBD) and multiple systems atrophy (MSA).

Tauopathies are a broad group of disorders, with clinical overlap. The main parkinsonian syndromes in this group include progressive supranuclear palsy (PSP), corticobasal degeneration and variants of frontotemporal lobar degeneration.

Diffuse Lewy Body Dementia

It is considered the second most common cause of dementia according to western literature. Pathologically, DLBD is characterized by presence of Lewy bodies in the neocortical regions. Clinically, it is characterized by the triad of fluctuating cognition, visual hallucinations and spontaneous parkinsonian motor features (2 of the 3 features). Although, cognitive decline is known to occur in PD; in DLBD the cognitive symptoms begin either before or within a year of the onset of the motor symptoms. There is significant neuroleptic sensitivity in patients with DLBD. The parkinsonian features worsen on administration of neuroleptics. In addition, there is worsening of symptoms on administration of levodopa which was previously used to differentiate between PD and DLBD.

Although, the dementia syndrome in DLBD is similar to PD, there is early onset of visual hallucinations, visuo-spatial disorientation, REM sleep behavior disorders and extrapyramidal motor manifestations.

Functional brain imaging shows early involvement of the occipital lobe in the form of hypometabolism and hypoperfusion.

The mainstay of pharmacological treatment is acetylcholinesterase inhibitors, like donepezil and rivastigmine. In view of the prominent neuropsychiatric manifestations, antipsychotics are frequently required. Atypical antipsychotics like quetiapine and clozapine are used. Dopaminergic agents should be used with caution.

Dose of Drugs

- **Donepezil:** 10 mg/day
- **Rivastigmine:** 6 mg bd or 9.5 mg as a cutaneous patch
- **Quetiapine:** 25–50 mg bd
- **Clozapine:** 25–50 mg bd.

Multiple Systems Atrophy

It is a parkinsonian syndrome that manifests with prominent autonomic symptoms with cerebellar signs and pyramidal tract dysfunction. Cognitive functions remain unaffected. Previously, three clinical variants of MSA were recognized—Shy-Drager syndrome, striatonigral degeneration and olivopontocerebellar atrophy (OPCA). However, based on newer consensus criteria, two main subtypes are proposed—those with predominant cerebellar manifestations (MSA-C), and those with predominant parkinsonian (MSA-P) symptoms. Thus, Shy-Drager syndrome and striatonigral degeneration are now classified under MSA-P and OPCA is classified under MSA-C.

MSA-P is characterized by absence of rest tremor, with severe autonomic dysfunction and pyramidal features. Cognition is usually well-preserved.

OPCA manifests with cerebellar and pyramidal features with relative absence of extrapyramidal manifestations. Other features in MSA include nocturnal stridor, sleep apnea and dysarthria.

Neuroimaging is characterized by mineralization of the striatum and brainstem (due to iron accumulation) (Fig. 203.1) and cerebellar atrophy. Signal changes occur in the pons in the form of 'hot cross bun' sign. Pathologically, degeneration is noted in the substantia nigra pars compacta, striatum, cerebellum and inferior

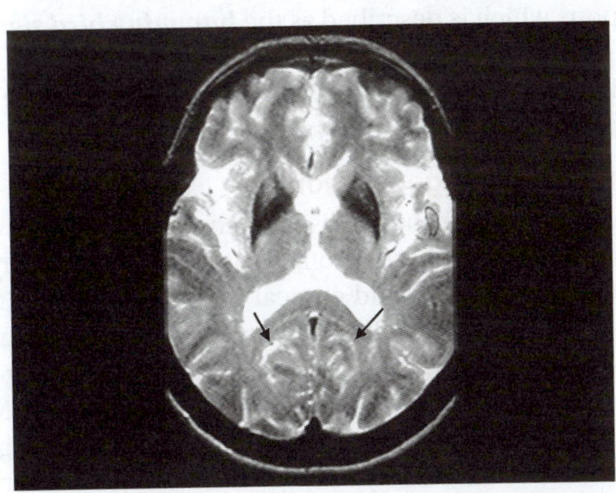

Fig. 203.1: Magnetic resonance imaging (MRI) mineralization of striatum due to iron accumulation (arrows)

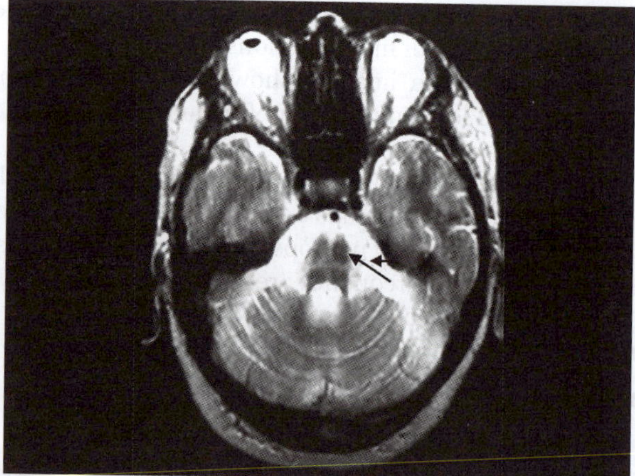

Fig. 203.2: Magnetic resonance imaging (MRI) mineralization iron accumulation 'hot cross bun sign' in pons (arrows)

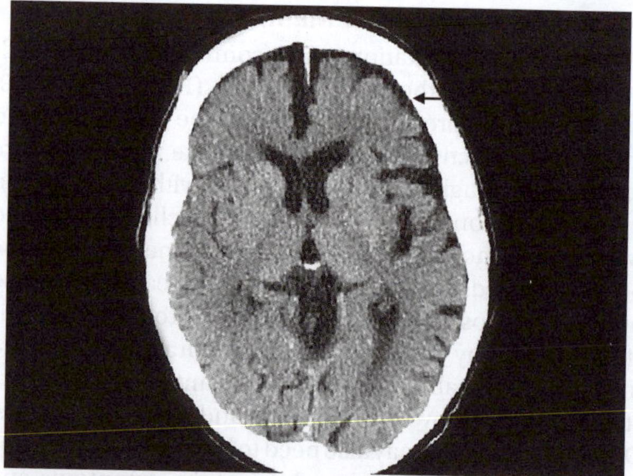

Fig. 203.3: CT scan (corticobasal degeneration) showing asymmetrical atrophy of right frontoparietal regions (arrow)

olivary nucleus with glial cytoplasmic inclusions staining for alpha-synuclein hot cross bun sign (Fig. 203.2).

Response to treatment is poor. A trial with dopaminergic agents is given usually. Supportive treatment for autonomic symptoms is given in the form of compression stockings and intermittent self-catheterization. Pharmacological treatment in the form of α-agonists like midodrine is tried. For bladder disturbances, anticholinergic agents like oxybutynin may be tried.

Progressive Supranuclear Palsy

This is a form of atypical parkinsonism that is characterized by symmetrical onset of parkinsonian symptoms. The salient features include absence of tremor, axial more than appendicular rigidity and impairment of vertical gaze (including downward gaze). Patients are typically found to have hyperextension of neck with early gait disturbances and falls. They have greater difficulty in coming down steps rather than climbing up. In later stages, the patient may develop speech disturbances and difficulty in swallowing. PSP has been recently subclassified into various types. One of these subtypes, PSP-P is characterized by response to dopaminergic therapy, although PSP largely is a form of parkinsonism that does not respond to therapy.

Diagnosis is primarily clinical, with imaging studies supporting the diagnosis. Magnetic resonance imaging (MRI) shows atrophy of the midbrain with preservation of the pons which is described as the ***humming bird sign*** on midsagittal section.

Response to treatment is poor. Frequent falls are the major problem which have to be guarded against.

Corticobasal Degeneration

This is a rare parkinsonian disorder characterized by asymmetrical signs, with additional features of asymmetrical dystonia, myoclonus and cortical sensory loss. Cognition is frequently involved. The patients may characteristically present with 'alien limb' phenomenon, wherein they are unable to control the movements of the affected limb. MRI shows asymmetrical cortical atrophy. Functional imaging shows asymmetrical hypometabolism of the thalamus and cortex (Fig. 203.3). ***Treatment*** is supportive with poor response to drugs.

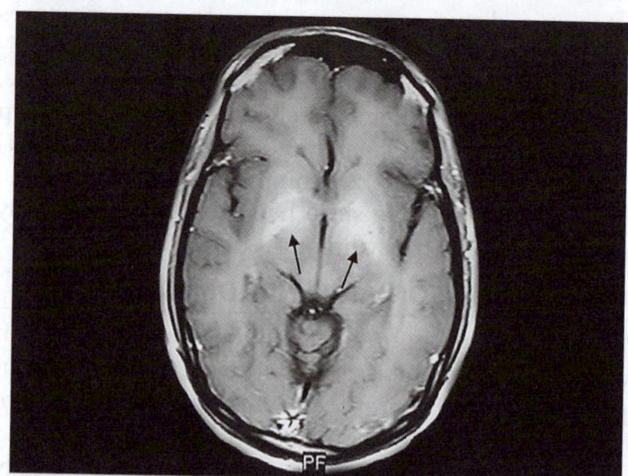

Fig. 203.4: Hypointensity in lentiform nucleus in T1. Manganese toxicity (T1 hyperintensity in lentiform nucleus in manganese poisoning) (arrows)

Other Causes of Parkinsonism

Drug like the previous generation antipsychotics, antiemetics like metoclopramide and metals like manganese (Fig. 203.4) can cause parkinsonism by blocking D2 receptors. Vascular parkinsonism is characterized by small vessel ischemic disease in the presence of vascular risk factors. This manifests with symptoms in the lower limbs (lower body parkinsonism). Parkinsonian features are also seen in the Westphal variant of Huntington's disease, Wilson's disease and in neurodegeneration with brain iron accumulation.

WILSON'S DISEASE

(Refer Section 10, Ch 94)

Wilson's disease affects about 1–2 persons/100,000 population. It is an autosomal recessive disorder of copper transport due to mutations in the ATP7B gene. Clusters of Wilson's disease occur among communities where consanguineous marriages are common. The copper transport proteins, apoceruloplasmin and ceruloplasmin are low or absent. This leads to defect of excretion of copper into the bile from hepatocytes. Excessive accumulation of copper occurs and it gets deposited in the liver, brain, cornea, kidneys, heart and muscles leading to

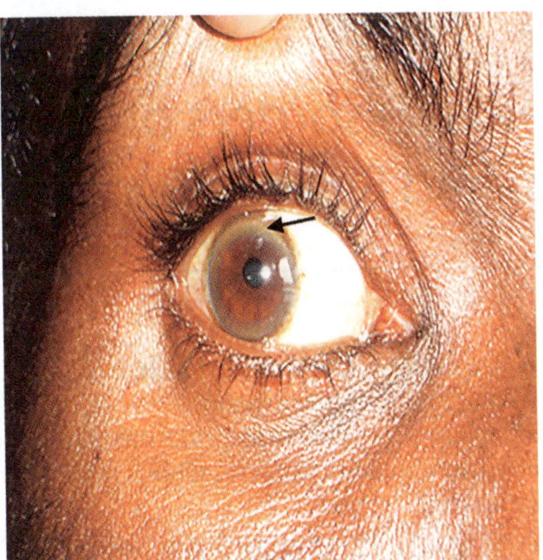

Fig. 203.5: Wilson's diseases Kayser-Fleischer ring (arrow)

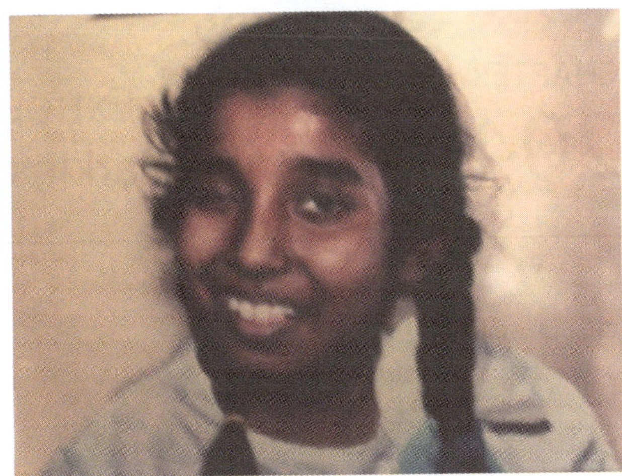

Fig. 203.6: Mitochondrial (Leigh extrapyramidal sequelae) torticollis, blepharospasm right eye and dystonic smile

damage of these organs. Children present with prominent hepatic abnormalities. With passage of time, the brain, eye, kidneys and blood abnormalities develop. Hemolytic anemia due to hypersplenism develops later. Neurological features include mental retardation, parkinsonian features, cerebellar features, movement disorders like chorea and titubation, seizures, dystonia, tremors and psychosis. They also show a characteristic silly smile.

Osteodystrophic: Wilson's disease is the Asian form with bone and muscle changes. By the time neurological manifestations start, the characteristic diagnostic Kayser-Fleischer ring in the Descemet's membrane (due to copper deposition) is seen (Fig. 203.5). Sunflower cataract and brownish staining of teeth may also occur.

Imaging features: MRI shows decreased signal intensity in the striatum, superior colliculi and increased density in the tegmentum except red nucleus (called giant panda sign). (For diagnosis and treatment Refer to Section 10, Ch 94).

MPTP-induced Parkinsonism

This may develop in animals consuming the toxin MPTP in plants like yellow star thistle and Russian star weed. Animals eating them would become rigid and die.

MPTP is a product found in Heroin and its metabolic product, 1-methyl-4-phenylpyridinium (MPP+), is toxic to the basal ganglia. This is also used in producing animal models of parkinsonism. Generally carries a poor prognosis. MPTP is a simple molecule. It could spontaneously form from methylstyrene, formaldehyde and methylamine. MPTP is metabolized to MPP+. MPP+ is considered to be directly responsible for MPTP-induced PD-like symptoms by inhibiting NADH—ubiquinone oxidoreductase (complex I) in the mitochondrial respiratory chain.

The first case of MPTP causing parkinsonism was diagnosed in 1976. He responded to sinemet, 2 years later he committed suicide and the autopsy showed cell destruction in the SN. In 1982, it was again manufactured as ***street heroin***.

Postencephalitic Parkinsonism

This may occur as a complication of Japanese encephalitis (Refer Section 6, Ch 60 and Section 17, Ch 199).

Mitochondrial Diseases

Leigh's disease has a special predilection to basal ganglia and leaves sequelae with movement disorders. It is characterized by torticollis, blepharospasm eyes and dystonic smile (Fig. 203.6).

CONCLUSION

The ability to maintain body parts in desired alignment against gravitational pull is a very exciting phenomena and is never realized until it becomes disturbed in disease.

Source: Wolters E Ch, van Laar T, Berendse HW (Eds). Parkinson's Disease and Movement Disorders, 3rd edition. Association of Parkinsons disease and related disorders. Amsterdam; VU university press, 2010.

CHAPTER 204

Extrapyramidal Disorders other than Parkinsonism and Related Syndromes

SR Chandra, Thomas Iype

Chapter Summary

- Basal Ganglia Circuits
- Pathogenesis
- Approach to Common Hyperkinetic Movement Disorders
- Dystonias
  - Management of Dystonias
- Athetosis
- Ballistic Movements (Ballism)
- Chorea
  - Sydenham's Chorea
- Huntington's like Diseases
- Huntington's Disease
- Ballism
- Tics
- Myoclonus
- Tremors
- Dyskinesias
  - Neuroacanthocytosis
  - Fragile X Associated Tremor Ataxia
  - Restless Leg Syndrome
  - Rett syndrome
- Miscellaneous Conditions
  - Stiff Person Syndrome

INTRODUCTION

Equilibrium is a state of balance of body parts under dynamic conditions in the plane and direction of locomotion, dual or multitasking at any angle to it. There are continuous adjustments taking place for these shifts in equilibrium. Anticipatory postural reflexes ensure adjustments prior to intended movements, reactive reflexes adjust to sudden change. Abnormal movements are a heterogeneous group of disorders characterized by involuntary movements without loss of consciousness.

Alpha motor neuron and its connection to muscles form the final pathway in executing movement. It is controlled by segmental and suprasegmental inputs. At segmental level, Renshaw cell is inhibitory using glycine as transmitter. Type Ia afferents give a sensitive measure of muscle stretch, type Ib via Golgi tendons responds to muscle tension, type Ia from antagonist muscle links to inhibitory interneuron. Polysynaptic excitation is provided by polysynaptic afferents of flexor reflex afferents. Supraspinal control comes from corticospinal tract, reticulospinal pathways, rubrospinal tract and other basal ganglia circuits.

BASAL GANGLIA CIRCUITS

The direct pathway, indirect pathway, hyperdirect pathway and striatonigral pathway, and striatum to pedunculopontine oscillator complex are the clinically important circuits apart from five circuits linking the various parts of the frontal lobe.

- Direct pathway links motor cortex, striatum, palladium interna, thalamus and cortex.
- Indirect pathway links cortex, striatum, globus pallidus externa, subthalamic nucleus, globus pallidus interna, thalamus and cortex.
- Hyperdirect pathway is cortico-subthalamo-pallidal connection.

Disease of direct pathway produces hypokinetic movement disorder like parkinsonism and indirect pathway disease produces hyperkinetic movement disorders. Frontal lobe circuits are motor circuit, oculomotor circuit, dorsolateral prefrontal circuits, medial orbitofrontal circuits and cingulate circuits which terminate in the pallido-thalamo-cortical projection system.

PATHOGENESIS

A common pathogenic mechanism is described for most neurodegenerative movement disorders. Misfolded proteins accumulate in the cytosol, nuclei of neurons and/or glial cells. These have neurotoxic properties causing cell death.

Abnormal protein—protein interaction or fatal attraction hypothesis states that soluble filamentous polymers are converted to beta-pleated insoluble sheets. Amyloidogenic proteins are formed by improper folding, misbinding, due to mutations, local conditions, post-translational modifications and other molecular mechanisms. There are inbuilt cell saving systems which are incorporated to keep the integrity of neurological cells. These cells save quality control systems acting through chaperons, promote proper protein folding and prevent the accumulation of non-native proteins. Ubiquitin proteasome system and phagosome lysosome system remove proteins that remain unfolded which lead to proteinopathies.

The second mechanism is accumulation of microtubule-associated protein-hyperphosphorylated tau and alpha synuclein. Tau is normally associated with axon transport and when hyperphosphorylated, it causes filamentous inclusions which are enhanced by oxidative stress, metals, insecticides and herbicides causing loss of function and gain of toxic function (*tauopathies*). Alpha-synuclein acquires an alpha-pleated sheet, and helps the formation of amyloid fibrils (*synucleinopathies*).

The ill effects of proteinopathy caused by defective repair process and by stander effects (passive) caused by other factors lead to damage to neural structures.

Conditions Causing Abnormal Movements

- Inherited disorders
- Acquired causes—demyelination, ischemia, infections, trauma, metabolic disorders, neoplasms and drugs and toxins.

APPROACH TO COMMON HYPERKINETIC MOVEMENT DISORDERS

All movements can be categorized as voluntary (i.e. planned), semivoluntary (planned by an inner sensory stimulus, e.g. need to stretch), involuntary (e.g. seizures), or automatic (e.g. learned behavior, like walking, speaking, etc.).

- Whenever a patient presents with a movement disorder, we need to answer a few questions.
- Is it organic or psychogenic?
- If organic, is it early onset or late onset? (childhood < 13 years, adolescent 13–20, adult > 20) paroxysmal or persistent? Ask is it specific or not?
- Is it familial or sporadic? If familial, X-linked, autosomal dominant, autosomal recessive?
- Is it focal, segmental or generalized?

Psychogenic movements are bizarre, unpatterned, nonstereotyped, disappearing during sleep, improving by distracting the attention and also by asking the patient to initiate a voluntary movement of another frequency.

If the abnormal movements are organic, the following aspects have to be noted: Rate, range, rhythm, direction, amplitude; effect of sleep, stress, distraction and effect of alcohol; any specific triggers and/or sensory tricks which ameliorate the movement disorder.

Commonly seen abnormal movements are fast movements (ballistic), which include tremors, tics, chorea, myoclonus, dyskinesias, ballismus and others or ramp movements like athetosis and dystonias. They may be fluctuating or constant in course.

Ramp Movements

Movements performed slowly are called ramp movements. They are more efficiently controlled by sensory afferents.

DYSTONIAS

They are involuntary movements which at peak remain stationary for 30 seconds to 1 minute (dystonic movement) and lasting more than 1 minute (dystonic posture) due to abnormal muscle spasm as a consequence of distorted motor control and cause undesired postures. It is a sustained patterned and can be painful.

The postulated mechanisms include an imbalance between direct and indirect pathways at striatum causing decreased cortical inhibition, decreased gamma-aminobutyric acid (GABA)-A receptors, D2 receptors, as well as defective surround inhibition which suppresses unwanted movements, abnormal plasticity in motor cortex, and abnormalities in inhibitory integration of afferent proprioceptive sensory inputs.

Clinical classification of dystonias
• Primary dystonias
• Dystonia-plus syndrome
• Part of paroxysmal dyskinesias
• Dystonia as a part of other degenerative diseases
• Dystonia due to specific causes
• Pseudodystonia.

Primary Dystonias

In primary dystonias, the only abnormality seen is dystonia with occasional tremors. It may be familial or sporadic.

The identified genetic defects involve DYT1, 2, 4, 6, 7 and 13 genes.

Oppenheim's dystonia or dystonia musculorum deformans is autosomal dominant disorder, with onset before 40 years, in which the limbs are affected most. The DYT1 gene is involved.

Autosomal dominant, childhood onset craniocervical dystonia is due to defect of DYT6 gene.

Autosomal dominant, adult onset, limited to neck is due to defect of DYT7 gene.

Dystonia-plus Syndromes

Dystonia-plus syndromes or secondary dystonias are disorders where dystonia is associated with myoclonus, parkinsonism or other abnormalities. These may be sporadic or due to inherited causes, these include dopa-responsive dystonia (DRD), dopa-agonist responsive dystonia, and dystonia myoclonus syndrome. Since there is biochemical abnormality, these are called neurochemical disorders. The common abnormalities include cyclohydrolase 1 deficiency, tyrosine hydroxylase deficiency and pterin synthesis deficiency.

Dopa-responsive Dystonia

Dopa-responsive dystonia have childhood onset with disorder of gait. Girls are more affected than boys. Following sleep, the patient's involuntary movements reduce. This is called sleep benefit. At the end of the day patient shows worsening of the dystonia. This is the clinical clue to the etiology. Parkinsonian signs may be present and they respond well to a very small doses of L-dopa.

Dopa-agonist Responsive Dystonia

Dopa-agonist responsive dystonia can be autosomal recessive due to aromatic amino acid deficiency, and also autosomal dominant with mutation in Na/K ATPase. They occur in adolescence, rapidly progresses over hours or weeks and tend to plateau.

Dystonia with Myoclonus

Dystonia with myoclonus is autosomal dominant and alcohol responsive. The upper part of the body is affected sparing the legs. The disability tends to plateau with time.

Dystonia as Part of Paroxysmal Dyskinesia

This may be kinesigenic and precipitated by sudden unexpected movements or nonkinesigenic. Dystonia may be hypnagogic (occurring with sleep onset) or exertional.

Heredodegenerative Dystonias

This includes X-linked, disorders like Lubag dystonia-parkinsonism, Pelizaeus-Merzbacher disease, dystonia-deafness syndromes and others.

Autosomal dominant disorders include Huntington's disease, rapid onset dystonia-parkinsonism, spinocerebellar degenerations, dentatorubral-pallidoluysian atrophy, hereditary spastic paraplegia with dystonia and others. Autosomal recessive disorders include Wilson's disease, and neurodegeneration with brain iron accumulation.

Several other inherited movement disorders occur. The clinical classification of genetic pattern has been shown in Table 204.1.

Table 204.1: Clinical classification of genetic pattern

Genetic pattern	Clinical condition
X-linked dominant	Rett syndrome
Autosomal dominant	Huntington's disease, neuroferritinopathy, Machado-Joseph disease, dentatorubro-pallidoluysian atrophy and Creutzfeldt-Jakob disease
Autosomal recessive	Wilson's disease, Niemann-Pick disease, metachromatic leukodystrophy, Lesch-Nyhan's syndrome, GM2 gangliosidosis, glutaric acidemia, ataxia telangiectasia, hartnup disease, neuroacanthocytosis, Sjögren-Larsson, mitochondrial disorders and other parkinsonism plus syndromes

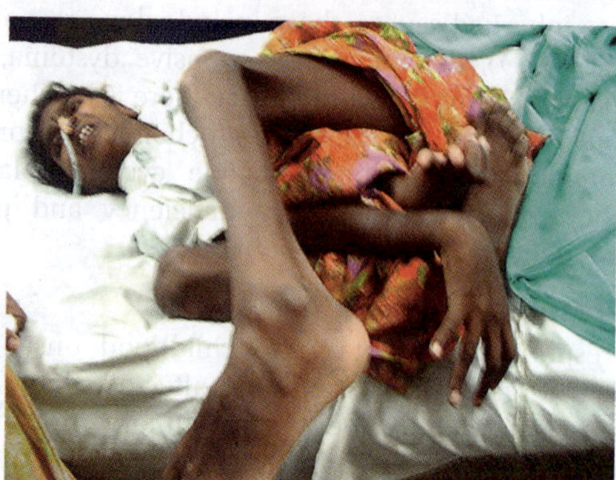

Fig. 204.1: Dystonic storm. ***Note:*** The complex grotesque postures which undergo constant movement and change

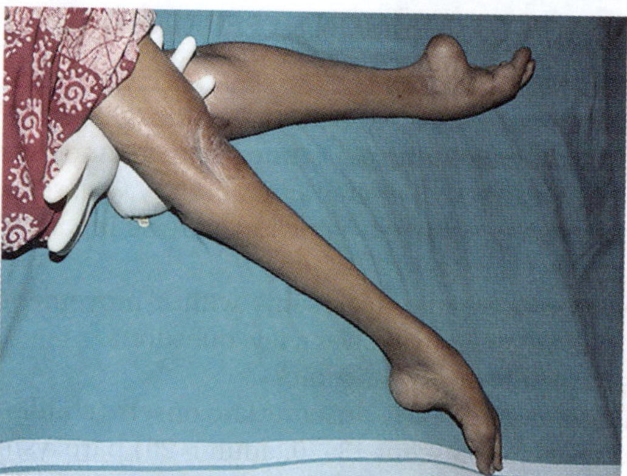

Fig. 204.2: Pseudodystonia due to hip dislocation

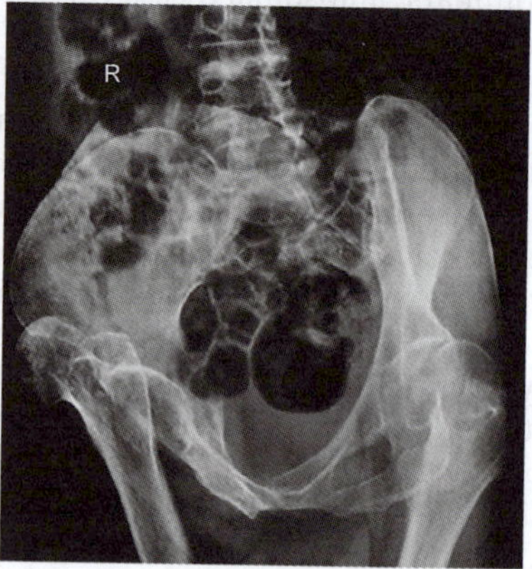

Fig. 204.3: X-ray of the same patient showing bilateral hip dislocation

Dystonia due to Specific Causes

In these conditions, the dystonia is sequela or an acute complication of other specific causes. These include perinatal injury, infections, trauma, surgical sections, intracranial arteriovenous malformations (AVMs) spinal disorders, adverse effects of drugs and immune-mediated encephalopathies.

Dystonic storm: Severe dystonia occurring suddenly and requiring special intensive management is termed dystonic storm (Fig. 204.1).

Pseudodystonias

These include conditions where the abnormal postures are not due to dystonia, e.g. malingering due to trauma, psychogenic causes, 'stiff person' syndrome, muscle disease orthopedic deformities (Figs 204.2 and 204.3).

Management of Dystonias

If there is a treatable cause, it should be identified and treated. If there is a known neurochemical imbalance, it should be corrected. If not, the mainstay of management is symptom alleviation. Always must try to look for DOPA or DOPA agonist-responsive syndromes and use them for relief. If not, anticholinergics and muscle relaxants are given and titrated to get optimum response. Surgical options like myotomy, rhizotomy, cordotomy and thalamotomy are tried at times. Botulinum toxin (BTX) injection is a temporary but effective option and lifesaving in conditions like laryngeal dystonia. The effect of BTX wanes off with time, with recurrence of symptoms. Repeat injections give further periods of relief.

ATHETOSIS

Slow, sinuous, writhing movements which flows from one joint to another are termed athetosis. Some consider it as dystonia affecting distal muscles. It differs from dystonia by not being persistent and from chorea by being writhing. It can coexist with chorea when it is called choreoathetosis. It is commonly seen in children with neonatal injury. Deafness, upgaze palsy and athetosis are known as the triad of kernicterus. Organic acidurias, Lesch-Nyhan's syndrome, lipidosis are other causes.

BALLISTIC MOVEMENTS (BALLISM)

They are very rapid movements with triphasic pattern agonist, antagonist, agonist burst. Basal ganglia and cerebellum set the pattern.

CHOREA

It is an involuntary movement characterized by sudden jerky, nonrepetitive, quasi-purposive movements which are distal more than proximal and absent during sleep. The patient often introduce the involuntary movement into some voluntary movements and therefore, the abnormality is often missed in the early phase (***parakinesia***). There is inability to maintain voluntary contraction, this is called ***motor impersistence***, e.g. milkmaid's grip (the grip tightens and loosens alternatively), lizard's tongue (the tongue quivers in the mouth to and fro), quick pronation of outstretched hand (choreic hand), etc. There may be hypotonia with pendular muscle stretch reflexes or hung

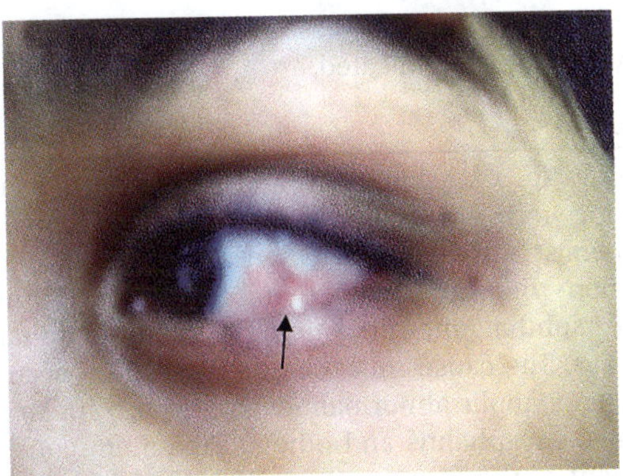

Fig. 204.4: Telangiectasia of the eyeball in ataxia telangiectasia (arrow)

up reflex when a choreic movement intervenes in the reflex. They may have a clumsy *dancing gait*.

Pathogenesis

Caudate is site of involvement. Intracortical inhibition is normal. Thalamus shows increase in activity which may be due to loss of inhibition.

Causes

Several causes have been known to lead to chorea. These include developmental disorders, like cerebral palsy, kernicterus, senile chorea, hereditary early onset disorders like aminoacidurias, lipid and glycogen storage disorders, Lesch-Nyhan syndrome, neurodegeneration with brain iron accumulation, ataxia telangiectasia (Fig. 204.4), mitochondrial disorder. Deoxyribonucleic acid (DNA) repair disorders, Wilson's disease, Huntington's disease, dentatorubropallidoluysian atrophy, non-Huntington chorea, Behr syndrome, Fahr syndrome, porphyria, neuro-acanthocytosis, drugs, toxins, thyroid disease, nutritional, infective, postinfective, immune-mediated, hematological and other causes like AVMs and mass lesions in basal ganglia.

Sydenham's Chorea

(Refer to Section 6, Ch 37)

Described by Thomas Sydenham, it is also called St. Vitus dance. It is a delayed manifestation of rheumatic fever. Children present with all features of halting gait, jerky movements, attention deficit and obsessive compulsive behavior. Tics are common. Now the incidence is drastically falling all over the world. It affects children of 5–15 years or women who are older. There is predilection for chorea to occur during pregnancy (chorea gravidarum). Cardiac involvement is common (about 20%). Molecular mimicry between central nervous system (CNS) antigens and group A beta hemolytic streptococci and formation of antibasal ganglia antibody [demonstrable by enzyme-linked immunosorbent assay (ELISA)] account for the pathogenesis.

Apart from chorea, pediatric autoimmune neuro-psychiatric disorders associated with streptococcal infection (PANDAS) may develop. Diagnosis is made by history of acute onset chorea with or without recent or remote history of streptococcal infection. Antistreptolysin O (ASO) titer may be normal or elevated at times. Magnetic resonance imaging (MRI) is normal. Positron emission tomography (PET) scan may show striatal hypermetabolism which returns to normal when the condition subsides.

Prognosis

The course is benign, and recovery occurs in 3–6 months in almost all cases, occasionally course may be prolonged to several months.

Treatment

Chorea can be controlled by using valproic acid 20–25 mg/kg in 3 doses, carbamazepine 15 mg/kg, dopamine receptor blockers-risperidone 1 mg/day to be titrated based on the response; haloperidol, pimozide, tetrabenazine, and chlorpromazine can be used as alternate drugs. In resistant cases, prednisolone 2 mg/kg given orally accelerates recovery. For patients with refractory chorea, methyl prednisolone 1 g/day given for 5 days intravenous (IV) followed by 1 mg/kg for a month orally can be tried. Plasmapheresis and intravenous immunoglobulin (IVIG) may have to be used in an unusually resistant cases.

HUNTINGTON'S LIKE DISEASES

These may be encountered rarely.

Dentatorubral-pallidoluysian atrophy (DRPLA): The early onset type is due to DRPLA which presents with myoclonus, epilepsy and mental retardation before the age of 20 years. Late onset type has ataxia, dystonia, tremor, dementia and parkinsonism. Diffuse atrophy with white matter changes and unstable cytosine adenine guanine (CAG) expansion in chromosome 12 are seen.

- ***HDL1 (Huntington's disease like-1):*** Phenotype is like Huntington's disease chromosome 20p
- ***HDL2:*** It shows CTG or CAG trinucleotide expansion
- ***HDL3:*** Autosomal recessive linked to chromosome 4p15.3.

HUNTINGTON'S DISEASE

George Huntington described this disease in 1872 presenting with hallucination, sleep disturbance, lack of motivation, poor memory, speech difficulty, depression, paranoia, weight loss, sexual disturbance, unsteadiness and chorea. Typical age of onset is 4th to 5th decade. Rarely onset may be before 20 years.

Pathogenesis

This is inherited in an autosomal dominant disorder. There is decrease in choline acetyltransferase, gamma-aminobutyric acid, glutamic acid dehydrogenase, encephalin, met-enkephalin, substance P, angiotensin and cholecystokinin.

There is increase in somatostatin, thyrotropin-releasing hormone (TRH), neurotensin, neuropeptide Y, etc. There is down regulation of N-methyl-D-aspartate (NMDA) receptors and upregulation of DA, GABA, benzodiazepine and cholinergic muscarinic receptors. The mutation causing disease is an unstable CAG repeat, at the 5' end of IT15 gene at 4p16.3. Trinucleotides are three base sequences within a specific gene. Normal individuals have a range of trinucleotides which are stable during meiosis and the person in the next generation inherits it as a simple stable Mendelian trait. In disease state, their copy number is increased-more than 35 for Huntington's disease. They code for polyglutamine trait. This expanded glutamine residue causes toxicity to the neuraxis. The trinucleotide is stable in lymphocyte DNA, but not so in sperms. So paternally inherited patients (offsprings of affected fathers) have large repeat size and they develop the disease at younger age. Cell-death occurs, mechanism of which is toxic gain of function. Impairment of proteasomal degradation of mutant Huntingtin leads to caspase-mediated apoptosis. There is excitotoxicity by interfering with vesicular glutamate uptake. Mitochondrial energy deprived state and decrease in chaperones cause N terminal fragment accumulation and disruption of axoplasmic flow.

Clinical Features

Juvenile onset type presents with akinetic-rigid state. Less common features are myoclonus, bruxism, dysarthria, dysphagia, aerophagia, dystonia and tourettism or tics. On testing the eye movements, increased saccadic latency, errors and variable latency may be observed. Myoclonus is more commonly seen in patients with juvenile Huntington's. Unified Huntington's disease rating scale (UHDRS) is used to grade the severity of the various symptoms. Breakdown of frontal cortical circuits is responsible for the behavioral features. Impulse control defect can present as criminal behavior.

Imaging shows caudate atrophy. Striatal volume loss is found to correlate with the size of CAG repeats. Hypometabolism and reduced regional blood flow can be demonstrated in these regions. Pathologically caudate and putamen shows cell loss, specially the medium spiny neurons.

Treatment

Treatment is mainly symptomatic for chorea. General treatment consists of care of nutrition, speech, prevention of complications like aspiration. Drug treatment includes anxiolytics, antidepressants, antiexcitotoxins like riluzole, remacemide, mitochondrial electron transport enhancers, caspase inhibitors and trophic factors.

Dosages of Drugs

- Anxiolytic like benzodiazepines (2.5 mg onward titrated based on need)
- Antidepressants like escitalopram (5 mg–20 mg)
- Antiexcitotoxins like riluzole (100 mg/day), memantine (20 mg/day) and remacemide (150–600 mg/day)
- Mitochondrial electron transport enhancers like carnitine, coenzyme Q10 and the mitochondrial cocktail
- Mitochondrial cocktail consists of coenzyme Q10, levocarnitine, vitamin B_1, E, C, alpha-lipoic acid, vitamin B_6 and K
- Caspase inhibitors are antiapoptotic agents which include; Z-VAD-FMK, Z-VAD (OH)-FMK, necrostatin-5, Biotin-FMK, used in 0.5–2 mL dosage
- ***Trophic factors:*** This includes brain derived neurotrophic factor (BDNF) and insulin like growth factors (IGF).

Surgical treatment includes transplant of fetal striatum tissue. There have been reports from a few centers about the benefit of this procedure but this is not universally accepted due to ethical reasons. Genetic counseling of family members is indicated.

BALLISM

These are forceful, flinging, high amplitude movement, involving both proximal and distal parts of limbs. They may persist during sleep. Often they involve one-half and then they are called hemiballismus. Lesions are at the subthalamic nucleus and pallid subthalamic pathways. The causes may be vascular, space occupying lesions, metabolic abnormalities like hyperosmolar states diabetes, encephalitis and others. Treatment consists of treatment of the cause and specific drug therapy which includes:

- Dopamine receptor blocking drugs like perphenazine, haloperidol, chlorpromazine, and pimozide
- Dopamine depleting drugs like reserpine and tetrabenazine
- GABA agonists like valproate and clonazepam, and as last resort ventrolateral thalamotomy.

These drugs have to be started in low doses which have to be worked up to optimum levels by observations.

Surgical Options

When the patient does not respond to pharmacotherapy, there are two interventional options:

- One is deep brain stimulation (DBS) involving the various basal ganglia structures. This is expensive as it involves implantation of electrodes and pulse generator which have to be implanted under MRI control. They work for several years. Since no permanent lesion is made, the condition is reversible. DBS is an expensive procedure requiring ₹ 5–10 lakhs.
- The other surgical procedure is thalamotomy in which a surgical lesion in the thalamus is made by stereotactic surgery. It does not involve implantation of the electrodes and pulse generator, therefore it is cheap. The lesions remain permanent.

TICS

These are compulsive automatisms-motor and/or vocal, repetitive, stereotypic, sudden brief, and can be voluntarily suppressed to an extent. They are simple tics if it involves only one muscle group, e.g. clonic causing sudden jerks, dystonic like blepharospasm, oculogyric spasm, bruxism, mouth opening, torticollis, shoulder rotation and, tonic like tensing abdominal or chest muscles. Dystonic tics can interfere with ongoing motor activity and these are called ***blocking tics***.

Rarely, patients get premonitory sensations which can involve other people such as being relieved by touching; these are called extracorporeal phantom tics.

Complex motor tics consist of inappropriately timed and inappropriately intense coordinated sequenced movements. They can be gesturing with fingers, copropraxia, exposing genitalia, echopraxia, (imitating gestures), burping, vomiting, retching, and ear dyskinesia or moving ear forward and backward.

Simple phonic tics like sniffing, throat clearing, grunting, squeaking, screaming, sucking, coughing, blowing, etc. occur in many. Shouting obscenities are coprolalia, repeating others words are echolalia, repeating last syllable is palilalia. Some varieties of tics occur during sleep as well. Tourette syndrome is a situation where patient has motor and phonic tics, many times a day for at least 1 year, age less than 21, and other movement disorders excluded. Whiplash injuries can occur with violent cervical tics. Truncal bending tics can produce degenerative spine changes. Attention deficit hyperactivity disorders (ADHD) and obsessive compulsive disorders (OCD) are common.

Secondary tics occur as a result of degenerative diseases, drugs, infections, metabolic disorders and others. Abnormal motor excitability and decreased cortical inhibition are evident. Dopamine hyperinnervation of striatum and limbic system is postulated as the mechanism. There is association with frame shift mutation on Slit and Trk-like 1 (SLITRK1) gene in chromosome 13q31.1.

Slit and Trk-like 1 (SLITRK1) are candidate genes on chromosome 13q31.1. This is the name of the genetic locus found to be pathogenic in tics. Frame shift mutation is the term applied to the situation where there is insertion or deletion of a number of nucleotides in a DNA sequence which is not divisible by three. The gene expression codons are normally triplets by nature. Therefore, this change leads to change in the reading frame at the level of transcription and post-transcription edition of proteins resulting in the formation of a totally unwanted protein.

Treatment

Most important step is to educate acquaintances regarding nature of illness. Decide if pharmacotherapy is needed or not. Behavioral therapy (habit reversal training) is needed.

Drug Therapy

Most troublesome symptom should be targeted for treatment with minimal drugs. Haloperidol, fluphenazine, aripiprazole, pergolide, clonazepam, clonidine, tetrabenazine, transdermal nicotine patch, baclofen, and BTX have been tried.

Deep brain stimulation of ventrolateral and ventral medial thalamus has found to be useful.

MYOCLONUS

Myoclonus causes sudden shock like contraction of a single muscle, a group of muscles or whole body producing a focal jerk or throws patient to ground. It may be physiological, essential, epileptic, or symptomatic. It can be cortical, subcortical, or spinal, epileptic or nonepileptic; focal, segmental or generalized. Physiologically myoclonus can be a hiccup, hypnic jerks, exercise or anxiety-induced jerks. Essential myoclonus is a situation where myoclonus is the only problem of the patient. It may be sporadic or inherited. Epileptic myoclonus may be part of childhood epilepsy or progressive myoclonic epilepsy. It may be symptomatic as part of neurometabolic diseases, infections, paraneoplastic conditions and degenerations.

Cortical myoclonus may be focal, multifocal, irregular or rhythmic, and stimulus sensitive. It lasts for 55–75 ms and comes after the electroencephalography (EEG) discharges.

Subcortical myoclonus is slow, periodic, axial or segmental in head and neck, not stimulus sensitive, and lasts 50–100 ms. It precedes EEG discharge.

Spinal myoclonus is periodic, rhythmic, axial, and can be stimulus sensitive.

Propriospinal myoclonus usually starts in thoracic region and spreads caudally and rostrally.

Peripheral myoclonus is irregular and focal.

EEG-electromyogram (EMG) jerk locked back averaging helps to localize the lesion. Simultaneous recording of the EEG and EMG is done and studying the temporal sequence of the EEG discharge and the EMG discharge helps to localize the origin of the myoclonic focus. This method is known as 'EEG-EMG jerk locked back averaging study'. Characterization is the most important step toward providing proper treatment. Unified myoclonus rating scale (UMRS) is used to assess severity.

Treatment

Gamma-amino butyric acid agonists like valproic acid and clonazepam, high dose piracetam, clobazam, ethosuximide, levetiracetam, and primidone are all useful. DBS at globus pallidus internal (GPI), and BTX injection are tried at times.

Epileptic myoclonus of Janz is seen in children in 2nd decade and presents as early morning jerks and seizures. Myoclonus dystonia is due to chromosomal mutation in 7q 21–31. Sodium oxybutyrate is found to be moderately useful.

Symptomatic myoclonus is the term applied to myoclonic attacks secondary to some other underlying disease. Lafora body disease which is associated with myoclonus is characterized by accumulation of specific abnormal glycogen called ***polyglucosans***. These starch-like polyglucosans are insoluble and hence precipitate inside cells. Lipidosis and sialidosis are storage diseases where myoclonus is one of the features. Unverricht-Lundborg disease is a genetic disease with severe myoclonus, mental retardation and ataxia. Among spinocerebellar ataxias (SCAs), some are associated with myoclonus.

TREMORS

Tremors are rhythmic repetitive, oscillatory movement around a fixed point.

Physiological and Enhanced Physiological Tremor

The body is put in a subtle vibratory mode by the ballistocardiographic effect at 8–13 Hz. This is also influenced by natural resonating frequencies of muscles, spindle input, and group firing rate (critical fusion frequency) of motor neurons. When this has a larger amplitude it becomes perceptible. This type of tremor is seen in hyperdynamic states like anxiety, thyrotoxicosis, hypoglycemia, Cushing's disease, pheochromocytoma, tremorgenic drugs and this is described as ***enhanced physiological tremor***.

Pathological Tremors

Ventral intermediolateral nucleus of thalamus, medial pallidum, and subthalamic nucleus are shown to discharge in the same frequency as tremor. Reduction in tremor following thalamotomy can be explained by interruption of pallidothalamic and dentatothalamic projections. Release of an oscillatory mechanism in the inferior olivo-dentato-rubro-thalamo cortical circuit is also pro-

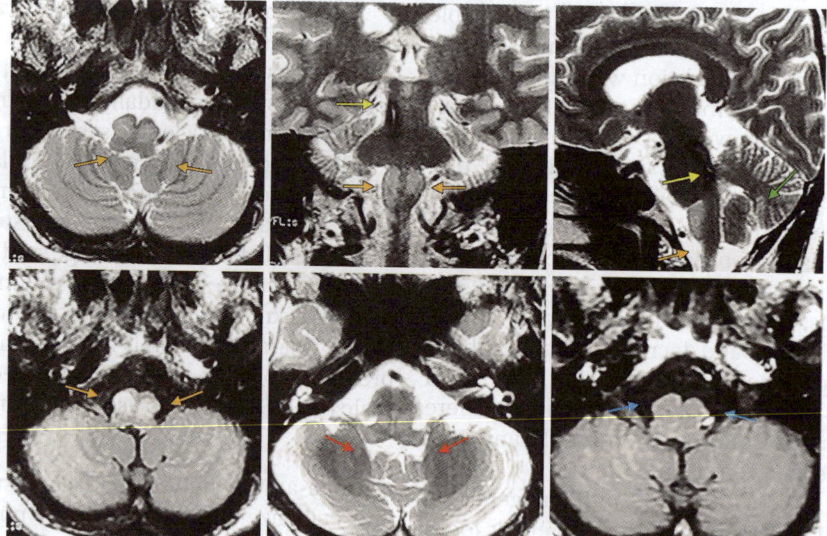

Fig. 204.5: Hypertrophic degeneration of olive (arrows) in pathological tremor, sections at different levels

bably causal. In patients with tremors, the olive shows hypertrophic degeneration (Fig. 204.5).

Psychogenic Tremors

These are often dramatic in onset, restricted to one limb, and they improve when attention is distracted. The tremor may move to other areas if the affected part is restrained, this is called 'chasing tremor'. The tremor improves when the patient is asked to do a movement in the unaffected limb in another frequency.

Essential Tremors

Tremor is the primary abnormality without a demonstrable underlying cause. It may be familial or senile. Frequency is 4–8 Hz. Hands, head and vocal cords are involved. Head tremor disappears when supported. Voice gets a quivering quality. The tremor starts usually in the 2nd decade but it can be earlier or later. There is marked postural component and invariably starts in the upper limbs. Alcohol, propranolol, primidone are helpful in treatment. There is a subgroup with kinetic predominant essential tremor of alternate beat, slow high amplitude type which is less responsive to treatment. Thalamic stimulation and botulinum toxin may have to be used. Treatment consists of administration of botulinum toxin parenterally. The total dose is 155 units injected in different sites, at each site 0.1 mL (5 units).

Parkinsonian Tremors

This is coarse, rhythmic, 3–5 Hz tremors, starts in one hand generally rarely bilateral, jaw, tongue, feet, lips and other parts are tremulous. Tremor occurs during repose and abolished during action, therefore called resting tremor. When the limb is fully supported, the tremor disappears. Flexion-extension, adduction-abduction, and alternating movements causes drum-beating and pill-rolling movements. It may become obvious during walking and when patient is asked to count backward from 100 with eyes closed. Palpable tremor superimposed on rigidity is called Negros sign. Usually, the tremor does not interfere much with activities. It responds to treatment

with anticholinergics, phenothiazines like ethopropazine and dopa.

Intention Tremors

These are tremors which occur in the most demanding phase of an active performance which involves a precise projecting movement. It is interrupted by oscillations in more than one plane at 2–4 Hz. This is seen in cerebellar disease involving the tremor loop. This can involve head and then is called *titubation*. Wing beating tremor involves even movements like lifting arm over a wide range at 2–5 Hz. Usually, the lesion involves tremor loop close to midbrain. Interruption of dentatothalamic fibers traversing the red nucleus, at superior cerebellar peduncle may abolish the tremor. It is therefore kinetic or action-related, pharmacotherapy is less effective, and thalamic stimulation may be beneficial. Lesions of nucleus interpositus produces ipsilateral ataxic tremor.

Primary Orthostatic Tremors

This occurs only during quiet standing in the legs at 14–16 Hz probably spinal in origin and disappears while walking. Patients experience imbalance. This tremor is treated with clonazepam, gabapentin, primidone and sodium valproate. Spinal cord stimulators can also be implanted with benefit.

Dystonic Tremors

Often this is superimposed on torticollis or focal dystonia of hand.

Geniospasm

This is chin tremor which is episodic with onset in early childhood.

Palatal Tremor

The tremor is characterized by rhythmic palatal movement, produces an audible click, and which persists during sleep. There can be enlargement of olivary nucleus unilaterally or bilaterally. The triangle of Guillain and Mollaret-consisting of dentate nucleus, brachium conjunctivum, olivary nucleus, central tegmental tract and red nucleus is affected.

Asterixis

Asterixis consists of rhythmic lapses of sustained posture resulting in a gravity-assisted movement which the patient corrects, better elicited in outstretched hand, dorsiflexed. It is seen in metabolic and toxic encephalopathy. Unilateral asterixis is seen in thalamic disease.

Tremor in Peripheral Nerve Disease

Chronic peripheral neuropathy produces tremors, worsening during action, with variability in amplitude. The tremor consists of side to side movements. Faulty reinnervation in peripheral nerve disease leads to mismatch between agonist, antagonist and synergist resulting in the production of tremors.

Complex Tremor

This term is used to describe situation where a particular type of tremor shows characters not fitting with it, e.g. parkinsonian tremor getting worse with action, etc.

Stereotypies

These are repetitive seemingly purposeless actions or utterances probably in response to inner urge.

Drug-induced Movement Disorders

Acute reactions like movements involving the tongue, neck, lips following prochlorperazine and phenothiazine administration this is called akathisia.

- Toxic syndromes like drug-induced parkinsonism.
- Unexplained reactions like neuroleptic malignant syndromes.
- Tardive reactions come after a minimum period of 3 months of phenothiazine use even though there are exceptions to this rule.
- Use of L-dopa induces a set of movements like peak dose dyskinesia, end of dose dyskinesia, and random dyskinesias called 'yo-yoing' and also episodes of sudden arrest of movements called 'freezing'.

DYSKINESIAS

These are randomly occurring involuntary movements with pathology in indirect pathways and may be uncharacterized.

Neuroacanthocytosis

This syndrome is characterized by spiky deformation of erythrocytes and neurological features. The conditions included are chorea-acanthocytosis (chAc) syndromes, McLeod syndrome (MLS), Huntington's disease like-2 (HDL-2), pantothenate kinase associated neurodegeneration (PKAN). Second group of conditions are associated with atypical Wolman's disease familial hypobetalipoproteinemia, abetalipoproteinemia (Bassen Kornzweig's) malignancy, malnutrition, mitochondrial disease and others. Basic pathology is abnormality of membrane protein band three and erythrocyte transporter enzyme. Wolman's disease belongs to the group of lysosomal storage disorders which has hematological, endocrine, gastrointestinal and muscle manifestations. Familial hypobetalipoproteinemia is another condition associated with acanthocytes, ataxia and peripheral neuropathy.

Symptom management is like other hyperkinetic movement disorders, and psychiatric syndromes.

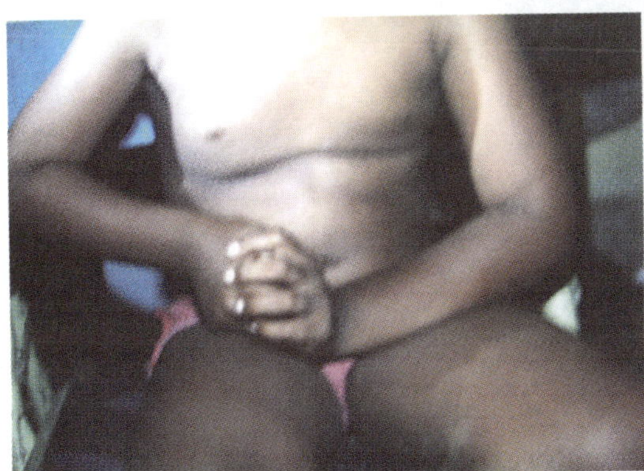

Fig. 204.6: Hand wiggling posture in Rett syndrome

Fragile X-associated Tremor Ataxia

It is a multisystem neurological disorder associated with 55–200 CGG repeats. Clinical features include defects in executive function ataxia, memory problems, parkinsonism, and tremor. Other associated findings are marfanoid body proportions, arachnodactyly, dysmorphic features, macro genitalia and others. MRI shows changes in middle cerebellar peduncle and brainstem.

Restless Leg Syndrome

This syndrome is characterized by urge to move legs, symptoms occurring more at rest. The patient gets relief with movement. The conditions worsen at night. Abnormality in iron metabolism, alteration in dopamine metabolism, and endocrine dysfunction are all reported.

Rett Syndrome

Rett syndrome is an autistic disorder affecting only girls. It manifests between 9 months and 3 years. It is characterized by language and cognitive regression, tremor, breath holding, myoclonus, athetosis, dystonia and repetitive hand wiggling (Fig. 204.6). There is loss of function mutation of X-linked gene encoding methyl-CpG binding protein 2.

MISCELLANEOUS CONDITIONS

There are several other movement disorders which are seen occasionally. These include:

Painful legs and moving toes, periodic movements during sleep, rapid eye movement (REM) sleep-associated syndromes, hemifacial spasms, myokymia of extraocular muscles, jumpy stumps, belly dancer's dyskinesia and spasms of reflex sympathetic dystrophy are other movement disorders.

Stiff Person Syndrome

Spasm of proximal lower limb and paraspinal muscles are seen in stiff person syndrome. It disappears in sleep, with general anesthesia, and nerve block. Painful spasms can be precipitated by touch, sound and other stimuli. Treatment consists of administration of diazepam (which may be required in high doses) increased in gradually in gradual steps, some cases may require IVIG for relief.

Source: Anthony H, Schapira V, Anthony ET, et al. Movement Disorders 4: Blue Books of Neurology Series. Volume 35, 1st edition. Philadelphia, USA: WB Saunders Elsevier publications; 2010.

CHAPTER
205

Cerebrovascular Diseases

SR Chandra, Ranjit Sanu Watson

Chapter Summary

- Reversible Ischemic Neurological Deficit
- Classification of Strokes
- Risk Factors for Cerebral Thrombosis
- Risk Factors for Ischemic Stroke in the Young
- Causes of Intracranial Hemorrhagic Stroke in Young
- Causes of Cardioembolic Stroke
- Pathogenesis of Ischemic Stroke
- Clinical Evaluation of a Patient with Stroke
- Common Stroke Syndromes
  - Anterior Circulation
  - Posterior Circulation Stroke
  - Lacunar Stroke Syndromes
- Ischemic Stroke Syndromes
- Lateral Medullary Syndrome of Wallenberg
- Medial Medullary Syndrome of Dejerine
- Lacunar Syndromes
- Crossed Hemiplegic Syndromes due to Brainstem Lesions
- Cryptogenic Stroke
- Guidelines for Early Management of Patients with Ischemic Stroke
- Criteria to Institute Thrombolytic Therapy
- Treatment of Stroke-related Complications
- Adverse Prognostic Indicators in Stroke
- Cerebral Venous Thrombosis (CVT)
  - Treatment of CVT
- Subarachnoid Hemorrhage (SAH)
  - Hess and Hunt Scale for Assessment of SAH
  - Complications of SAH
  - Investigations
  - Treatment of SAH
- Intracerebral Hemorrhage
- Lobar Hemorrhage
- Putaminal Hemorrhage
- Thalamic Hemorrhage
- Cerebellar Hemorrhage
- Pontine Hemorrhage
- Prevention of Stroke
- Vascular Cognitive Impairment

INTRODUCTION

The term cerebrovascular disease is an all-embracing term that includes any disease of the brain caused by an abnormality of blood supply. It may be symptomatic or asymptomatic. It can be transient or permanent. It can occur acutely or insidiously.

Stroke is the third most common cause of death in developed countries after cardiovascular diseases (CVD) and cancer.

WORLD HEALTH ORGANIZATION (WHO) DEFINITION OF STROKE

Stroke is defined as rapidly developing signs of focal or global disturbance of cerebral function, with symptoms lasting for 24 hours or longer or leading to death, due to cerebrovascular cause.

Transient Ischemic Attack

This is acute onset of a focal neurological deficit due to a focal cerebrovascular disease with full recovery in 24 hours.

But in practice, transient ischemic attacks (TIAs) last for less than 30 minutes. If the deficit has not started to recover in 60 minutes, majority of patients will still have a major deficit the next day also. Longer lasting TIAs show evidence of acute infarct in imaging also. So, the newer proposed definition of TIA has suggested a time cut off of 1 hour and should not show any evidence of acute infarction in imaging. Magnetic resonance imaging (MRI) is more likely to show an abnormality in TIAs lasting more than 1 hour than computed tomography (CT). The causes of TIAs are same as that of ischemic stroke. TIAs are neurological emergencies, which need urgent evaluation and treatment of risk factors predisposing to the impending stroke.

REVERSIBLE ISCHEMIC NEUROLOGICAL DEFICIT

This term is used for stroke lasting for 24 hours or more, but recovering completely within 72 hours.

Progressive intellectual and neurological deterioration or prolonged ischemic neurological deficit is the term applied for deficits, which last more than 72 hours but recover.

CLASSIFICATION OF STROKES

Strokes are broadly classified as:
- Arterial strokes
- Venous strokes.

Arterial Strokes

Arterial strokes are further classified into ischemic (80%) and hemorrhagic (20%) subtypes. Ischemic strokes are of two types—(1) thrombosis and (2) embolism; thrombotic strokes are of two types—(1) large vessel thrombosis and (2) lacunar (small vessel) strokes. Embolic strokes are of two types—(1) cardioembolism and (2) low-flow or artery-to-artery embolism. Ischemic strokes, therefore, form the most common type of stroke (Table 205.1 and Box 205.1).

Hemorrhagic strokes are subdivided into intracerebral (15%) and subarachnoid (5%) hemorrhage.

All these types can be in the anterior or carotid circulation or in the posterior or vertebrobasilar system.

The distinction between ischemic stroke and hemorrhagic stroke is crucial; early, appropriate use of thrombolytic therapy reduces the risk of moderate-to-severe disability by 30% in ischemic strokes, but is absolutely contraindicated in hemorrhagic stroke.

Table 205.1: Clinical features of the major categories of stroke

Clinical feature	Thrombosis	Embolism	Hemorrhage
Age	Old	Younger	Younger
Onset	Mostly at sleep	Active	Active
Course	Subacute	Hyperacute	Hyperacute
Condition on waking up	Wakes up with weakness	-----	Wakes up if occurring in sleep
Vomiting	Often absent	Rarely occurs	Vomiting common
Headache	Precedes the attack	Variable	Often severe
Seizures	Late to occur	Single at onset	Repetitive and sometime continuous
Progress	Can progress for 72 hours	Peak at onset and recovery starts	Progress up to 6 hours
Mortality	Less or moderate	Less	More

Box 205.1: Etiology of ischemic stroke

Thrombosis
- Lacunar stroke (small vessel)
- Large vessel thrombosis

Embolic occlusion
- Artery-to-artery
- Carotid bifurcation
- Aortic arch
- Arterial dissection
- Cardioembolic
- Atrial fibrillation (AF)
- Mural thrombus
- Myocardial infarction (MI)
- Dilated cardiomyopathy
- Valvular lesions
- Mitral stenosis
- Mechanical valve
- Bacterial endocarditis
- Paradoxical embolus
- Atrial septal defect (ASD)
- Patent foramen ovale
- Hypercoagulable disorders
- Protein C deficiency
- Protein S deficiency
- Antithrombin III deficiency
- Antiphospholipid syndrome (APS)
- Factor V Leiden mutation
- Prothrombin G20210A mutation
- Systemic malignancy
- Sickle-cell anemia
- B-thalassemia
- Polycythemia vera (PV)
- Systemic lupus erythematosus (SLE)
- Homocysteinemia
- Thrombotic thrombocytopenic purpura (TTP)
- Disseminated intravascular coagulation (DIC)
- Dysproteinemias
- Nephritic syndrome
- Inflammatory bowel disease (IBD)
- Oral contraceptives
- Venous sinus thrombosis
- Fibromuscular dysplasia of arteries, e.g. renal
- Vasculitis
- Systemic vasculitis—polyarteritis nodosa, granulomatosis with polyangiitis (Wegener's)
- Primary central nervous system vasculitis
- Meningitis (syphilis, tuberculosis, fungal, bacterial, zoster)
- Subarachnoid hemorrhage vasospasm
- Drugs—cocaine and amphetamine
- Moyamoya disease

Risk Factors for Embolic Stroke

Cardiogenic embolism: Atrial fibrillation (AF) due to any cause mitral stenosis, atrial myxoma, prosthetic heart valves, vegetation from infective endocarditis (IE), mural thrombus postmyocardial infarction and cardiomyopathies and calcified valves.

Artery-to-artery embolism:
- Atherosclerosis plaques in larger vessels
- Arterial dissection
- Vasculitis
- Arterial trauma
- Fibromuscular dysplasia.

Paradoxical embolism: Systemic embolism from venous thrombi passes through a cardiac septal defect to reach the aorta and its branches without passing through the lungs.

RISK FACTORS FOR CEREBRAL THROMBOSIS

Nonmodifiable risk factors include increasing age, male sex, family history and past history of stroke.

Modifiable risk factors include systemic hypertension, DM, dyslipidemia, smoking, obesity, TIA, high fat, low-fiber diet and peripheral occlusive vascular disease.

Risk factors for hemorrhagic stroke include increasing age, male sex, systemic hypertension, cerebral amyloid angiopathy, alcoholism, bleeding disorders, vascular tumors (primary or secondary), aneurysms, cavernous angiomas, arteriovenous fistulas, drug abuse, especially cocaine, and hemorrhagic infarcts as in venous strokes.

Young stroke is the term given to stroke developing before the age of 40 years. The risk factors differ from elderly persons developing stroke.

RISK FACTORS FOR ISCHEMIC STROKE IN THE YOUNG

These include several conditions such as: Cardioembolism, especially AF (sustained or paroxysmal) aortoarteritis, meningovascular syphilis arteritis due to meningitis, especially tuberculosis meningitis, postpartum cerebral venous thrombosis (CVT) (venous stroke), hyper-homocysteinemia, thrombophilia such as protein C and protein S deficiency, factor V Leiden and prothrombin gene mutation, various forms of vasculitis, polyarteritis nodosa, systemic lupus erythematosus (SLE), antiphospholipid antibody syndrome, sickle-cell disease, polycythemia, thrombocytosis, drug abuse (especially cocaine), oral contraceptive use, migraine and vasospastic drugs like ergot given for migraine and triptans.

CAUSES OF INTRACRANIAL HEMORRHAGIC STROKE IN YOUNG

Vasculitis, ruptured berry aneurysms, hemophilia and other bleeding diathesis, Marfan's syndrome, Ehlers-Danlos syndrome, polycystic kidney disease, drugs—amphetamine and cocaine.

CAUSES OF CARDIOEMBOLIC STROKE

These include valvular diseases, IE, ischemic heart disease (IHD) and arrhythmias such as AF, congenital heart disease and cardiomyopathies.

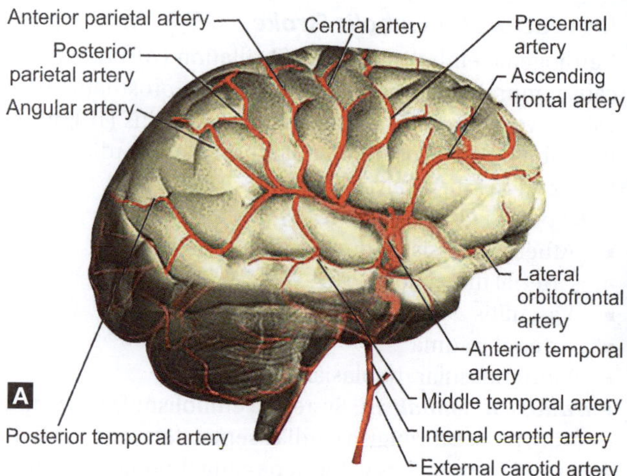

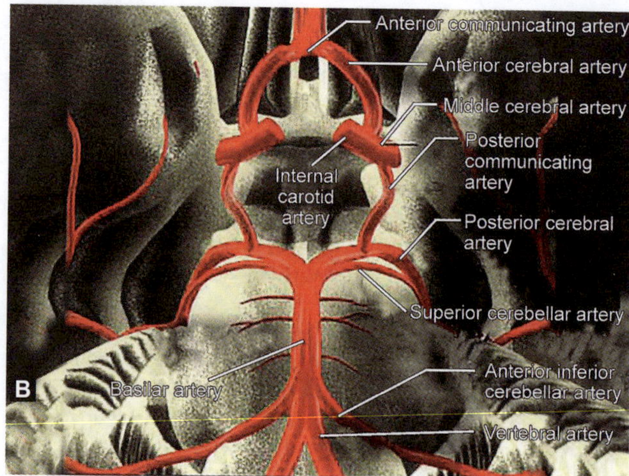

Figs 205.1A and B: A. The distribution of middle cerebral artery and its branches; **B.** Formation of the circle of Willis and its branches

Vascular accidents can occur in any of the major arteries of their branches. Figures 205.1A and B give the formation and distribution of the major arterial trunks and their branches.

PATHOGENESIS OF ISCHEMIC STROKE

Even though the human brain constitutes 2% of bw, it accounts for 20% of oxygen consumption. Glucose is the main nutrient substrate for the brain. Aerobic oxidation yields 36 adenosine triphosphate (ATP)/mol of glucose while anaerobic glycolysis yields 2 ATP. Stores of fuel (glycogen, plasma creatine) support neuronal function for 1–3 minutes after cessation of blood flow. Normal cerebral blood flow (CBF) is 55 mL/100 g/min, i.e. (750–1,000 mL/min). Gray matter gets 70 mL of arterial blood/100 g/min while white matter has only 30 mL amount of glucose in blood far exceeds extractable oxygen and leads to anaerobic glycolysis and lactic acidosis under ischemic conditions.

There are no changes in cerebral metabolism as long as CBF is above approximately 20 mL/100 g/min. Below this level, electrical activity of brain fails and symptoms appear. Normal cellular biochemistry is disrupted as energy supply becomes insufficient due to inadequate supply of oxygen. Depletion of high-energy phosphate stores (ATP and phosphocreatine) occurs and lactic acidosis ensues locally. Anaerobic metabolism of small amounts of residual glucose occurs. At CBF of 8–10 mL/100 g/min, there is loss of integrity of cell membrane and leakage of intracellular K^+ to the extracellular space. Ca^{++} influx into the cells occurs. Cell death occurs if reperfusion is not restored. The irreversibly dead central zone of infarct is called the ***core of infarct*** and the dying vulnerable peripheral region is called the ***ischemic penumbra***. Reperfusion strategies during treatment of stroke are aimed at salvaging the ischemic penumbra.

With the progression of cerebral ischemia, the ischemic area becomes edematous. The cells in the ischemic area swell up due to failure of Na^+–K^+ ATPase pump leading to accumulation of sodium and water in the cells. This is called cytotoxic edema, which contributes to the raised intracranial tension (ICT) and cerebral herniation. Rise of ICT is more pronounced with hemorrhagic strokes.

CLINICAL EVALUATION OF A PATIENT WITH STROKE

Is it a Stroke?

Acute onset and the characteristic pattern of the stroke syndrome respecting arterial territory give the clinical impression of a stroke as the patient is brought in. Steady progression beyond 72 hours, drowsiness out of proportion to neurological deficit and rapid improvement with antiedema suggest a stroke mimic.

Accurate time of onset has to be asked specifically. That is important to plan treatment. If history is unavailable, attempt to establish the time the patient was seen in full health. Activity at the time of onset has to be enquired into.

Thrombosis occurs when the patient is resting, whereas embolism and hemorrhage are more common during activity. In many cases, this may not be so. Temporal progression of symptoms such as 'whether maximal at onset', gradual worsening and worsening in a step-like fashion should be asked for. The clinical diagnosis has to be confirmed by imaging before starting on specific management.

Differential Diagnosis of Stroke

Sudden catastrophic lesions in the central nervous system (CNS) other than vascular accidents may occur, which have to be distinguished from strokes. These include seizures, migraine, complications of intracranial tumors, hypoglycemia, hyperglycemic coma, toxic and infective encephalopathies, syncopal attacks, hysterical phenomena, acute demyelination mitochondrial encephalopathy with lactic acidosis and stroke-like episodes (MELAS).

What is the Stroke Type Clinically? Is it Hemorrhage or Infarct?

Clinical presentation of subarachnoid hemorrhage (SAH):
- Sudden onset, worst ever headache as if patient feels being banged on head called as ***thunderclap headache*** which peaks within moments of onset
- Typically during exertion
- Prior warning headache (sentinel leak) in 15–30%
- Focal deficits uncommon (may have mild hemiparesis or third nerve palsy)

- Recurrent vomiting
- Transient or persistent impairment in level of consciousness (in such patients history may not reveal the headache)
- Neck rigidity
- Photophobia
- Agitation and restlessness.

Sites of hemorrhage in spontaneous hypertensive intracerebral hemorrhage (ICH):

- Putamen
- Thalamus
- Lobar white matter
- Cerebellum pons.

COMMON STROKE SYNDROMES

Anterior Circulation Stroke

This involves the middle cerebral, anterior cerebral, internal carotid, lenticulostriate and anterior choroidal territories.

Posterior Circulation Stroke

This involves the basilar, superior cerebellar, anterior inferior cerebellar, posterior inferior cerebellar, short- and long-paramedian arteries, top of basilar artery, posterior cerebral artery (PCA) and other branches.

Lacunar Stroke Syndromes

They are caused by small ischemic infarcts in the deep regions of brain or brainstem (lacunes) that range in size from 0.5 to 15 mm and which result from occlusion of the penetrating arteries. Their presentations include in Table 205.2:

- Pure motor—hemiplegia
- Hemianesthesia (pure sensory stroke)
- Motor-sensory (hemiplegia-hemianesthesia)
- Ataxic hemiparesis
- Dysarthria with clumsy hand syndrome (lesion in ventral pons).

Site of lesion in faciobrachial monoplegia (paralysis of the ipsilateral face and upper limb):

- Lateral part of the cortex at the cortical branch territory of the middle cerebral artery (MCA)
- Corona radiata (affecting the arm and face fibers)

- Genu of internal capsule—recurrent branch of anterior cerebral artery (ACA) (Heubner's artery). Paralysis in Heubner's artery occlusion is characterized by higher degree of weakness proximally compared to the weakness distally and absence of aphasia.

ISCHEMIC STROKE SYNDROMES

Carotid Artery Stroke Syndrome

The internal carotid artery (ICA) supplies the eye and anterior two-thirds of the cerebral hemisphere via the anterior and middle cerebral arteries through the deep perforators and the superficial cortical branches. The cervical segment of ICA has no branches. Intracranial part of the ICA gives off the ophthalmic artery after emerging out of cavernous sinus. Transient monocular blindness called amaurosis fugax is a common form of TIA involving this vessel. It is a pointer to ipsilateral carotid artery thromboembolism.

The posterior communicating artery and anterior choroidal artery arise before the ICA divides into the terminal ACA and MCA. The difference between a classic MCA stroke syndrome and ICA syndrome is the additional involvement of the eye opposite to the hemiplegic limbs. Palpation for asymmetry of carotid pulse and auscultation of carotids for a systolic bruit are valuable clinical signs pointing to this condition. Doppler studies and angiography can detect the lesions.

Middle Cerebral Artery Stroke

The MCA is the most common site for an ischemic stroke: MCA is the largest branch of ICA supplying most of the lateral surface of cerebrum, the perisylvian area and through the deep-penetrating vessels—(lenticulostriate branches) supply the deep white matter consisting of internal capsule and corona radiata, and deep-gray matter structures like the putamen and globus pallidus.

The clinical picture varies whether occlusion is at the stem of MCA or the deep-penetrating lenticulostriate branches or at the superficial cortical divisions. Occlusion of the stem of MCA leads to a massive infarct involving the cortex, the deeper parts of corona radiata, basal ganglia and the internal capsule. The cytotoxic edema which

Table 205.2: Clinical syndromes, features, site of lesions and obstructed blood vessels

Syndrome	Signs/symptoms	Localization	Vascular supply
Pure motor	Contralesional hemiparesis	• Internal capsule—posterior limb • Corona radiata • Basis pontis	Lenticulostriate branches of the MCA perforating arteries from basilar artery
Pure sensory	Contralesional hemisensory loss	VPL nucleus of thalamus	Lenticulostriate branches of MCA; Small thalamoperforators of PCA
Sensorimotor	Contralesional weakness and numbness	Thalamus and adjacent posterior limb of internal capsule	Lenticulostriate branches of MCA
Dysarthria-clumsy hand	Slurred speech and weakness of contralateral hand (fine motor)	Basis pontis (between rostral one-third and caudal two-thirds)	Basilar artery perforators
Ataxia-hemiparesis	Contralesional hemiparesis and ataxia out of proportion to weakness	Internal capsule-posterior limb; basis pontis	Lenticulostriate branches of MCA; perforating arteries of basilar artery
Hemiballismus/hemichorea	Contralesional limb flailing/dyskinesis	Subthalamic nucleus	Perforating arteries of anterior choroidal or posterior communicating artery

Abbreviations: MCA = Middle cerebral artery; VPL = Ventral posterolateral; PCA = Posterior cerebral artery

follows can produce mass effect, midline shift, uncal herniation and death. But if the occlusion is at the distal cortical branches, it leads to faciobrachial weakness. It may be associated with aphasia and paresis of conjugate gaze to the side of lesion, hemianopia, and upper limb weakness more than that of the lower limb. If the deep-lenticulostriate branches alone are involved, it results in dense hemiplegia due to involvement of posterior limb of internal capsule.

Anterior Cerebral Artery Syndrome

Supplies mainly the medial anterior three-fourths of the cerebral hemisphere, anterior four-fifths of the corpus callosum and anterior limb of the internal capsule. If the occlusion is distal to the communicating artery, predominant finding is weakness of the contralateral leg with lesser degree of weakness of arm and shoulder movements. Patients may display lack of initiative or *abulia*. With bilateral ACA territory damage to the mesiofrontal region patients develop paraplegia, incontinence and amnesia with apathy.

Anterior Choroidal Artery Syndrome

It is the branch of the ICA. Infarction leads to a triad of contralateral hemiplegia, hemianesthesia and homonymous hemianopia. Sensory symptoms are prominent.

Posterior Cerebral Artery Syndrome

Infarction in the hemispheric branches of PCA leads to contralateral congruous homonymous hemianopia with macular sparing. Bilateral disease leads to cortical blindness with preservation of pupillary reflexes. Thalamus can be involved at times.

Basilar Artery Syndrome

The basilar artery is formed from the union of two vertebral arteries (VAs) and it supplies the pons, middle and superior cerebellar peduncles and the cerebellum via the cerebellar arteries. Total occlusion is nearly fatal due to damage to the vital centers. More frequently, only the branches are occluded. Often the deficits include bilateral long-tract signs with variable abnormalities of cranial nerves and cerebellum. Total basilar artery occlusion is fatal (Table 205.3).

Table 205.3: Common sites of infraction giving rise to characteristic neurological findings

Syndrome	Clinical features	Localization
Claude's syndrome	Third nerve palsy + contralateral ataxia	Red nucleus/cerebral peduncle
Weber's syndrome	Third nerve palsy + hemiplegia	Medial midbrain/cerebral peduncle
Benedikt's syndrome	Third nerve palsy + hemiplegia + ataxia	Red nucleus/medial midbrain
Hemiballismus	Contralateral hemiballismus	Subthalamic nucleus
Thalamic Déjerine-Roussy syndrome	Contralateral hemisensory loss and agonizing pain	Thalamus
Top of the basilar artery syndrome (Kaplan's syndrome)	Variable findings in gaze and pupils somnolence, delirium and visual field defects	Embolic occlusion of basilar artery tip

Usually embolic occlusion occurs at the basilar tip. Infarction occurs in the midbrain, thalamus, occipital lobe and medial parts of the temporal lobes. This syndrome results in variable vertical gaze palsy, disorder of convergence of the eye, skew deviation, pupillary abnormalities, somnolence, agitated delirium, visual field defects and amnesia and less commonly long-tract signs. This is also called Kaplan's syndrome.

LATERAL MEDULLARY SYNDROME OF WALLENBERG

This is the result of occlusion of branches or stem of the VAs. In occlusion of the VA or posterior inferior cerebellar artery supplying the dorsolateral medulla, this *syndrome of Wallenberg occurs*. This is characterized by vertigo, ipsilateral ataxia, ipsilateral Horner's syndrome, ipsilateral facial hemianesthesia, ipsilateral palatal palsy and contralateral hemianesthesia of the body. Hoarseness of voice and hiccups are usual accompaniments. Pyramidal tract dysfunction may not be present.

MEDIAL MEDULLARY SYNDROME OF DEJERINE

There is ipsilateral paralysis of the tongue along with contralateral hemiparesis, the face is spared; in addition there is impaired proprioception contralaterally and this is due to occlusion of the anterior spinal artery.

LACUNAR SYNDROMES

Lacunes are small ischemic infarcts in the deep regions of brain or brainstem that range in size from 0.5 to 15 mm and resulting from occlusion of the penetrating arteries. Lacunes more than 15 mm diameter are called *giant lacunes*. Lacunes usually occur in patients with long-standing arterial hypertension. The most frequent sites of involvement are the putamen, basis pontis, thalamus, posterior limb of internal capsule and caudate nucleus. Multiple lacunes may lead to pseudobulbar palsy or dementia.

CROSSED HEMIPLEGIC SYNDROMES DUE TO BRAINSTEM LESIONS

Lesions in the brainstem leads to crossed hemiplegia syndromes, which include lower motor neuron (LMN) cranial nerve palsy (nuclear) on the ipsilateral side and hemiplegia (upper motor neuron) on the contralateral side. Midbrain lesions lead to ipsilateral LMN palsy of oculomotor nerve and contralateral hemiplegia—*Weber's syndrome*. Pontine lesions give rise to ipsilateral LMN facial and abducens palsy and contralateral hemiplegia—known as *Millard-Gubler syndrome*. Medial medullary lesions lead to ipsilateral LMN hypoglossal palsy with contralateral hemiplegia (Tables 205.4 to 205.6).

CRYPTOGENIC STROKE

Cryptogenic strokes are symptomatic cerebral infarctions for which no adequate cause is identifiable even after detailed evaluation. Cryptogenic mechanisms account for 10–40% of all ischemic strokes. In practice, 20–30% ischemic strokes remain cryptogenic after standard diagnostic investigations.

Table 205.4: Lateral pontine syndrome (Marie-Foix syndrome)

Tracts	Manifestation	Side
Cerebellar—middle cerebellar peduncle	Ataxia—arm and leg	Ipsilateral
Corticospinal tracts	Hemiparesis	Contralateral
Spinothalamic tract	Hemisensory loss	Contralateral

Table 205.5: Ventral pontine syndrome (Raymond-Cestan syndrome)

Tracts	Manifestation	Side
Cranial nerve VI	Lateral gaze palsy	Ipsilateral
Corticospinal tracts	Hemiparesis	Contralateral

Table 205.6: Ventral pontine syndrome (Millard-Gubler syndrome)

Tracts	Manifestation	Side
Cranial nerve VII	Facial palsy	Ipsilateral
Cranial nerve VI	Lateral gaze palsy	Ipsilateral
Corticospinal tracts (basis pontis)	Hemiparesis	Contralateral

The most common causes of ischemic strokes identified in clinical practice include large artery atherosclerosis, cardioembolism and small-vessel disease

The age-wise frequency of stroke is caused by the following causes:

- Age between 18 and 30 years—dissection of arteries, thrombophilias and congenital heart disease
- Age between 31 and 60 years—early onset atherosclerosis, acquired structural cardiac disease
- Age more than 60 years—occult atrial fibrillation.

In practice, among patients aged 18–55 years of age, cryptogenic strokes were milder and when treated with aspirin, the recurrence rate was 1.9% in the first year and 0.8% in the subsequent 3 years.

Cryptogenic stroke is at present a diagnosis of exclusion having excluded all known causes and possible investigations. Transthoracic echocardiography is better at ventricular imaging whereas as transesophageal echocardiography (TEE) is better at locating aortic arch lesions. In 50–75% of young patients, TEE may reveal potentially salient abnormalities such as patent foramen ovale (PFO), atrial septal aneurysm, endocarditis, aortic atherosclerosis, regional myocardial dysfunction, dilated left atrium and atrial appendage thrombi.

In the usual sequence of standard investigations, common causes can be excluded. If there are negative specialized investigations like catheter angiography of blood vessels, studies of vasculitis, monitoring cardiac rhythms for prolonged periods to detect paroxysmal atrial fibrillation (4 weeks or more) and hematological tests for thrombophilia are undertaken.

If the cause is elusive even after these advanced tests, specialized investigations such as genetic testing, detailed autoimmune evaluation, CT and MR imaging for cardiac structural changes, long-term cardiac rhythm monitoring (1–3 years) and hematological testing for occult cancer are undertaken. As little as single 1-hour episode of atrial fibrillation during 2 years of monitoring has been associated with a doubling in the risk of ischemic stroke.

Patient foramen ovale which normally closes at 3 years of age may remain patent throughout life in a small proportion of people and this facilitates cryptogenic stroke by paradoxical embolism from right to left. Mean diameter of PFO is 4.9 mm, which can allow passage of thrombi which can occlude MCA trunk which is usually 3 mm and arterial branches which are 1 mm in diameter.

Atrial septal aneurysm, which leads to hypermobile interatrial septum, which protrudes alternately into the right and left atria is an abnormality associated with increased risk of stroke in patients with PFO.

Patent foramen ovale is seen in 25% of general population but in those with cryptogenic stroke it is present in 50% and it is casually related to stroke in approximately 50%. Factors that increase the risk include Valsalva maneuver, extended airplane or car travel, concomitant deep venous thrombosis (DVT), coexisting atrial septal aneurysm and migraine with aura.

Antiplatelet therapy is the first-line in cryptogenic stroke with PFO, warfarin is equally effective. Occlusion of the PFO by the disk occluder significantly reduces the risk of ischemic stroke from six to two in 100 patients followed up for 5 years.

Source: Saver JL. Cryptogenic stroke (clinical practice). N Engl J Med. 2016;374(21):2065–73.

GUIDELINES FOR EARLY MANAGEMENT OF PATIENTS WITH ISCHEMIC STROKE

CT remains the most widely used neuroimaging technique for the evaluation of patients with suspected acute ischemic stroke. CT brain may not show the infarct in the early hours of stroke but helps to rule out hemorrhage even in the early hours. CT brain also helps to rule out stroke mimics like space occupying lesions and subdural hematoma. The infarct appears hypodense and bleed appears hyperdense in CT brain (Figs 205.2A and B). MRI also may be used to detect acute infarcts and ICH and that it could be an alternative to CT. Diffusion-weighted MRI is helpful in diagnosing and treating patients with acute stroke. However, MRI is more costly and imaging is time consuming. Recombinant tissue plasminogen activator (rtPA) should be given. In ideal cases of non-

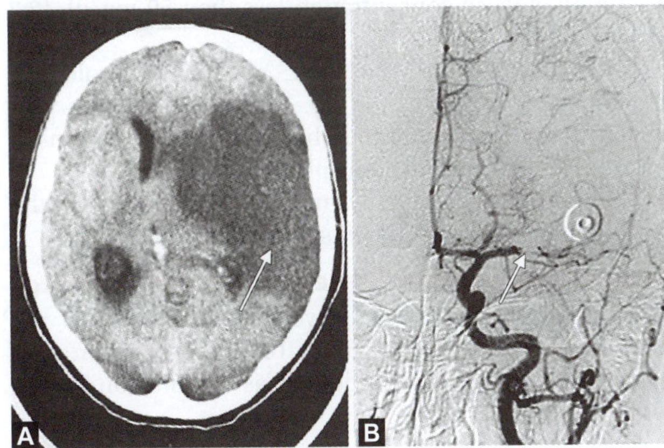

Figs 205.2A and B: A. Middle cerebral artery infarct—computed tomography brain (arrow); **B.** Computed tomography—angiogram digital subtraction angiography. **Note:** Occlusion (arrow)

hemorrhagic stroke, in the absence of contraindications, intravenous (IV) administration of rtPA as a thrombolytic is the ideal treatment to restore functional recovery if given within 3 hours (this time has been extended to 4.5 hours at present) from the onset of stroke to be maximally effective.

Early imaging signs of MCA territory infarction (<6 hours):

- Dense MCA sign—indicates thrombus/embolus in first part of MCA much before infarction becomes visible on CT loss of gray-white differentiation (especially in cortical ribbon of the insula)
- Effacement of sulci and sylvian fissure obscuration of lentiform nucleus.

CRITERIA TO INSTITUTE THROMBOLYTIC THERAPY

Criteria with recombinant tissue plasminogen activator: Clinical and radiologic diagnosis of ischemic stroke causing measurable neurological deficit in patients more than 18 years:

- The neurological signs should not be clearing spontaneously
- The neurological signs should not be minor and isolated
- The symptoms of stroke should not be suggestive of SAH. Onset of symptoms less than 3 hours before beginning treatment
- No evidence of head trauma, stroke or myocardial infarction (MI) in previous 3 months
- No gastrointestinal or urinary tract hemorrhage in previous 21 days
- No major surgery in the previous 14 days
- No arterial puncture at a noncompressible site in the previous 7 days
- No history of previous intracranial hemorrhage
- Blood pressure (BP) not elevated above systolic 185 mm Hg and diastolic above 110 mm Hg
- Patient is not on oral anticoagulant therapy or if anticoagulant therapy is being taken, international normalized ratio (INR) less than 1.7
- If receiving heparin in previous 48 hours, activated partial thromboplastin time (aPTT) must be in normal range
- Platelet count more than 100,000 mm³
- Blood glucose concentration less than 50 mg/dL (2.7 mmol/L)
- No seizure with postictal residual neurological impairment
- CT does not show a multilobar infarction (hypodensity >one-third cerebral hemisphere)
- The patient or family members understand the potential risks and benefits from treatment.

Dose of Recombinant Tissue Plasminogen Activator

Total dose 0.9 mg/kg body weight—maximum 90 mg infused over 60 minutes. About 10% of dose given over 1 minute as a bolus and the rest as an infusion to run within an hour.

Antiplatelet Drugs in Stroke

All patients with ischemic strokes who are not candidates for thrombolytic therapy should be treated with aspirin as early as possible at stroke onset. Once imaging studies rule out a hemorrhage or a nonstroke pathology, loading dose of aspirin 300 mg is given to be followed by 75–150 mg given orally daily. If aspirin intolerance occurs, clopidogrel 75 mg once daily is given. In patients, who develop stroke while on aspirin, combination of aspirin and dipyridamole is instituted.

Heparin in Ischemic Stroke

Indications include cardioembolic strokes and dissection of neck vessels, venous strokes and procoagulant state. Heparin is also used in venous thrombosis. A large brain infarct is a relative contraindication for heparin use. Unfractionated heparin is given as an IV infusion at 1,000 units per hour to maintain the aPTT at 1.5–2.5 times the control.

Endovascular intervention is a therapeutic adjunct to thrombolytic therapy in the management of acute ischemic stroke, in particular, mechanical thrombectomy is recommended for patients with large proximal intracranial artery occlusions due to emboli from the heart or artery-to-artery embolism. The procedure is done using endovascular tools for removing thrombi from occluded vessels. This procedure of thrombectomy done in the ideal time (which is being debated) completely relieves the ischemia and restores normal function. This procedure is becoming more and more popular in tertiary care neurosurgical centers. Many hospitals in India perform this procedure.

TREATMENT OF STROKE-RELATED COMPLICATIONS

Increased Intracranial Pressure

Usually this develops 1–4 days after the onset of stroke. Manifestations include headache, decreased consciousness, papilledema, vomiting, bilateral extensor plantar and features of brainstem compression. Imaging shows brain edema, midline shift and tonsillar herniation.

Therapeutic measures include elevation of the head of the bed (25–40 cm), modest fluid restriction and avoidance of hypotonic fluids like 5% dextrose. Control of pain and agitation is by sedatives and analgesics. Osmotic agents like mannitol and glycerol help to maintain lower intracranial pressure (ICP). Mannitol is given as 0.5 g/kg as first dose over 20 minutes. Maximum cumulative dose is 2 g/kg/day. About 20% mannitol is available as 100 mL bottles for IV infusion. Steroids are not useful in stroke. Intubation and hyperventilation to induce hypocapnia (pCO_2 25–30 mm Hg) is useful as a temporary measure to reduce ICP.

Seizures in Stroke

Embolic strokes and venous strokes have the highest propensity to produce seizures. About 5–20% of strokes are complicated by seizures. Phenytoin or fosphenytoin is given as IV bolus 100 mg followed by oral phenytoin at 300 mg night dose.

Deep Vein Thrombosis (DVT)

Prevention is the key with early ambulation, bedside physiotherapy and compression stockings. In the absence of brain hemorrhage, heparin or enoxaparin is used to prevent DVT.

Pulmonary Embolism

Prevention should be instituted as soon as the patient is admitted with tight stockings over the legs and active physiotherapy to lower limbs. Treatment with IV heparin is administered, if there is no history of recent brain hemorrhage. If there is history of intracranial hemorrhage, inferior vena cava filters have to be used (surgically or by intervention) to prevent migration of emboli from the lower limb to the central circulation.

Depression

This is difficult to diagnose in stroke patients. Antidepressants are given to those with slower than expected recovery, poor cooperation to therapy or emotional lability.

Blood Pressure

It should not be lowered in the acute stages of stroke unless it is above 220/120 mm Hg or more than 185/110 mm Hg after thrombolytic therapy since higher than normal BP is needed to maintain perfusion to the ischemic brain. Aggressive lowering of BP increases the risk of cerebral ischemia.

Myocardial Ischemia and Arrhythmias

This occurs during stroke and is an important cause of mortality. It is possibly due to the high catecholamine levels. This should be anticipated and at the earliest evidence of myocardial ischemic or infarctions, appropriate emergency treatment has to be instituted (Refer Section 13, Ch 127).

Infections and Sepsis

Urinary infections and pneumonia are the most common causes of sepsis in stroke. A high index of suspicion is needed to detect sepsis and institute early treatment.

Upper Gastrointestinal Bleed

This may occur in cerebrovascular accidents especially the hemorrhagic ones (cerebral subarachnoid). Most episodes are caused by stress-related gastric mucosal damage (*Cushing's ulcers*). Lesions develop rapidly and hemorrhage may be massive. Prevention is by giving oral proton pump inhibitor like pantoprazole or H_2-receptor blockers like cimetidine or ranitidine. If hemorrhage occurs, emergency measures have to be instituted (Refer Section 8, Ch 78).

Hyponatremia

Serum-sodium levels below 120 mmol/L constitute an adverse prognostic factor in stroke. It is often due to syndrome of inappropriate antidiuretic hormone (SIADH). Ensure euvolemia and correct the electrolyte imbalance early.

Decubitus Ulcers

Meticulous attention to skin care is mandatory. Keep skin clean and dry. Turn the patient frequently and use water beds or air beds. Wound debridement and skin grafting in severe cases.

Fever

Fever is an adverse prognostic factor. Search for infective causes. Administer antipyretics frequently to maintain euthermia. Hyperthermia and hyperglycemia are very deleterious for the ischemic penumbra.

ADVERSE PROGNOSTIC INDICATORS IN STROKE

- Prior stroke
- Older age
- Multi-infarct
- Pseudobulbar palsy
- Persistent urinary and fecal incontinence
- Unconsciousness at onset
- Severity of paralysis
- Persisting neuronal shock
- Right hemispheric stroke*
- Anterior cerebral artery infarct
- Level of social support

Note: *It is realized that patients with right hemisphere lesions do worse than left hemisphere lesions in the long run. Left hemispheric strokes are apparently alarming because of the loss of language. But right hemisphere is altruistic and takes over the functions of left hemisphere at the cost of its own function. This is evident in a large number of children with right hemiplegia who have no aphasia and recover based on the degree of insult. But patients with right hemispheric damage have elements of neglects and denial which interferes with their voluntary cooperation for rehabilitatory methods used and the left hemisphere unlike the right does not take over the functions of the right hemisphere. Therefore, long-term outcome is poor in right hemispheric strokes compared to left.

CEREBRAL VENOUS THROMBOSIS

The incidence of CVT is uncertain. It is a cause of stroke in the young where the dural venous sinuses (like superior sagittal sinus, lateral sinus, cavernous sinus, etc.) get occluded partly or completely by thrombosis.

Clinical Features

These include headache, papilledema, vomiting, hemiparesis, seizures, cranial nerve palsies depending on the location of the thrombus. The presentation is more slow and subacute than in arterial strokes. Sometimes the onset may be much slower and chronic so that the lesion may mimic the onset of tumor.

Cerebral venous thrombosis may of two types:

1. Septic CVT
2. Nonseptic CVT—due to thrombophilic states (diseases predisposing for thrombosis).

Septic Cerebral Venous Thrombosis

Cavernous sinus thrombosis and lateral sinus thrombosis are usually due to infection in the areas of their drainage. Septic cavernous sinus thrombosis is often due to the hematogenous spread of infection from the medial parts of the face, nose, orbit or paranasal sinuses. Most common organism—*Staphylococcus* followed by *Streptococci*. In sinusitis and dental abscess, anaerobes are more common. The thrombosis can spread to other venous sinuses also by contiguity.

Another frequent site of extracranial infections leading to cerebral venous thrombosis is the mastoid air cells and infections of the middle ear, which may spread up to the lateral sinus and other veins in the posterior fossa. At present, there is a dramatic decrease in incidence of infective thrombophlebitis over the years.

Nonseptic Cerebral Venous Thrombosis

It occurs secondary to:

- Hematological disorders and thrombophilias (Section 15, Ch 158 and 178)
- Oral contraceptive pills
- Pregnancy and puerperium
- Systemic connective tissue disorders and vasculitis
- Behçet's disease
- Homocystinuria
- Nephrotic syndrome (mechanism being loss of protein C and protein S lost in the urine)
- Dehydration due to gastroenteritis (sluggish flow predisposes to CVT)
- Congestive cardiac failure
- Diabetic ketoacidosis
- Local compression due to meningiomas.

The most important inherited defect for systemic venous thrombosis is resistance to activated protein C and polymorphism of factor V Leiden.

Imaging Studies in Cerebral Venous Thrombosis

- *Delta sign* is the term applied to the dense triangular shape of the superior sagittal sinus in plain CT due to the thrombus inside. *Cord sign* is used to describe the long segment of hyperdensity inside a vein due to thrombus in plain CT commonly seen in the region of the straight sinus. *Empty delta sign* is the term applied in contrast images when the contrast goes to the margins, but cannot penetrate inside causing an empty space like appearance in the region of the clot.
- Magnetic resonance imaging (MRI) brain with MR venography is the investigation of choice. It is more sensitive than CT in detecting the thrombus and cerebral changes. Venogram demonstrates absence or poor *flow* in the sinuses. Figures 205.3A to C show mixed density lesion in MRI (blue and red arrows).
- Investigations for the cause of CVT; for diagnosis of thrombophila (*See*, Section 15, Ch 178).

Treatment of Cerebral Venous Thrombosis

Anticoagulation with IV heparin 5,000 units 6th hourly even in the presence of hemorrhagic infarction followed by warfarin for 3–6 months, which have to be continued for longer periods in patients with underlying prothrombotic states.

Anticonvulsants are given prophylactically or therapeutically as identicated. Antibiotics are given in septic CVT at meningitic doses with good coverage for *Staphylococcus* and other suspected organisms. Local thrombolytic therapy has been given in patients who deteriorate in spite of heparin treatment with variable results.

SUBARACHNOID HEMORRHAGE (SAH)

Bleeding into subarachnoid space constitutes SAH. It may be traumatic (head trauma and others) or spontaneous. About 85% of spontaneous SAH are secondary to ruptured berry (saccular) aneurysms most frequently seen in the circle of Willis and vertebrobasilar vessels. Other causes include arteriovenous malformations (AVMs), dural AV fistulas, vasculitis and bleeding disorders. Hypertension, smoking and alcoholism increase the risk of development of berry aneurysms and SAH. Polycystic kidney disease, Marfan syndrome and Ehlers-Danlos syndrome are also associated with increased frequencies of berry aneurysms.

Berry Aneurysms

These are saccular dilatation of medium- and large-sized arteries, mostly developing at branching points 40% at anterior-communicating artery, 30% at junction of ICA and posterior communicating, 20% in the MCA and 10% in posterior circulation including basilar tip aneurysm. Aneurysms arising from the anterior communicating artery can produce visual field defects, impaired visual acuity, endocrine defects and localized frontal headache. Aneurysms of ICA in cavernous sinus, if of sufficient size, can cause cavernous sinus syndrome. In the substance of the cavernous sinus, carotid artery along with sympathetic and sixth nerve are embedded. The third, fourth and fifth cranial nerves run along its lateral wall. There will be extensive lid edema, conjunctival and corneal edema as well as mastoid edema called *Battle's sign*. In addition, there will be palsy of three, four, five and sixth cranial nerve palsy. This is referred as *cavernous sinus syndrome*. Cavernous vein thrombosis is a serious complication occurring due to thrombosis of the sinus, secondary to

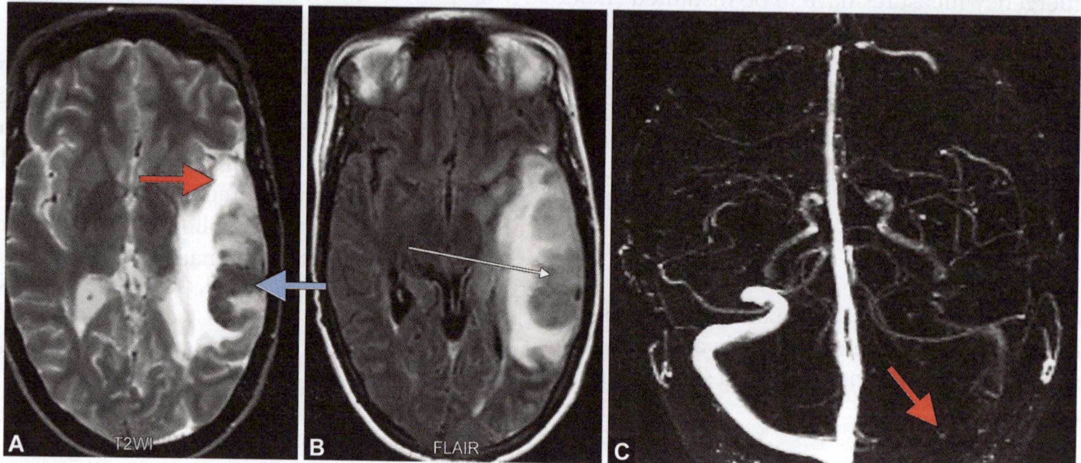

Figs 205.3A to C: Cerebral venous thrombosis—magnetic resonance imaging scan: **A.** Mixed density lesion (blue and red arrows); **B.** Magnetic resonance imaging filling defect seen of left transverse sinus due to thrombi (arrows); **C.** Occulsion of the transverse sinus (red arrow)

spread of infection from the 'dangerous area' of the face, especially in diabetics.

Posterior communicating artery aneurysms produce third nerve palsy by pressure effects on the third nerve, which manifests as pupillary abnormalities dilatation.

Sentinel Headache

Previous episodes of warning headaches occur in some patients with SAH as a result of minor leak from the aneurysm. It lasts for hours-to-days. This occurs in about one-half of patients before rupture.

Spinal Subarachnoid Hemorrhage

This occurs from a spinal AVM or aneurysm of anterior spinal artery. Headache is usually absent or less prominent. Neck pain or back pain of acute onset may be the presenting symptom.

Focal Signs to Look for in SAH

- Hemiparesis with dysphasia—in MCA aneurysmal bleed
- Third nerve palsy from aneurysm of posterior communicating artery
- Bulbar cranial nerve palsies from posterior fossa aneurysms
- Papilledema and subhyaloid (preretinal) hemorrhage—Terson syndrome.

Terson's syndrome is characterized by vitreous hemorrhage in association with SAH. The classic presentation is in the subhyaloidal space, which is beneath the posterior vitreous space and in front of the retina. In SAH, 13% of patients have Terson's syndrome, which is associated with more severe SAH (higher Hess-Hunt score, a marker of severity) and risk of death is significantly increased.

Hess and Hunt Scale for Assessment of SAH

- Grade 0—asymptomatic
- Grade 1—mild headache alone
- Grade 2—severe headache
- Grade 3—severe headache and drowsiness
- Grade 4—stupor and hemiparesis
- Grade 5—deep coma and decerebrate rigidity.

World Federation of Neurological Surgeons Scale

- Grade 1—Glasgow coma scale (GCS) 15. No motor deficits
- Grade 2—GCS 13 or 14, motor deficits absent
- Grade 3—GCS 13 or 14, motor deficits present
- Grade 4—GCS 7–12, motor deficits present or absent
- Grade 5—GCS 3–6, motor deficits present or absent.

Complications of SAH

- Rebleeding—most major risk in first 4 weeks
- Vasospasm—blood irritates the distal vessels leading to cerebral infarction. The delayed cerebral ischemia starts at 48 hours, peaks at 7–10 days and wanes off in 2 weeks
- Hydrocephalus
- Frontal neuropsychological damage and abulia (complete lack of initiative and drive), especially due to anterior communicating artery aneurysm
- Intraparenchymal or intraventricular extension of bleed

- Seizures in 10%
- Brain edema, raised ICT and coning
- Neurogenic pulmonary edema due to excessive sympathetic drive
- Syndrome of inappropriate antidiuretic hormone
- Electrocardiogram changes and acute coronary syndromes.

Investigations

- *CT brain* is the most sensitive test. It detects SAH in 80–90% cases, if done within 24 hours. Location of the densest part of hemorrhage provides a clue to the site of hemorrhage.
- *MRI brain*—this is less sensitive than CT in early stages, but later in the course is more diagnostic. It also reveals parenchymal pathology like AVMs or cavernomas in better detail.
- *Magnetic resonance angiography*, CT angiography and digital subtraction angiography help to locate the aneurysm precisely.
- *Lumbar puncture*—if the CT brain is normal, but the clinical suspicion of SAH is high, lumbar puncture should be done. In SAH, it is uniformly blood stained if samples are collected in different bottles successively. Hemolysis occurs if blood is present in the subarachnoid space for more than a few hours and xanthochromia (yellow tinge in the supernatant if left to stand), which can be identified by naked eye examination. If in doubt, spectrophotometry will help. Xanthochromia developing after a single episode of bleeding may persist for about 2 weeks.

Treatment of SAH

Early treatment of the aneurysm is taken up in the majority of patients with aneurysmal SAH. The definitive method is to prevent rebleeding by securing the aneurysm with microsurgical clipping or endovascular coiling (platinum coils in the aneurysmal sac). Vasospasm occurs by second to seventh day, leading to cerebral ischemia and delayed deterioration. The amount of blood in the subarachnoid space is an important predictor of vasospasm. Optimization of volume status and cardiac output prevents vasospasm to some extent. Nimodipine, a selective cerebral vasodilator in doses of 60 mg every 4 hourly is efficacious in preventing vasospasm.

Other CNS complications of SAH include hydrocephalus and convulsions. Systemic complications include neurogenic pulmonary edema and SIADH.

INTRACEREBRAL HEMORRHAGE

Deep hemorrhages in hypertensive patients are often due to hypertension, whereas lobar hemorrhages in nonhypertensive and in elderly patients often due to cerebral amyloid angiopathy.

The classic clinical presentation includes the onset of a sudden focal neurological deficit while the patient is active, which progresses over minutes-to-hours. This smooth symptomatic progression of a focal deficit over a few hours is uncommon in ischemic stroke and rare in SAH. Headache is more common with ICH than with ischemic stroke, although less common than in SAH.

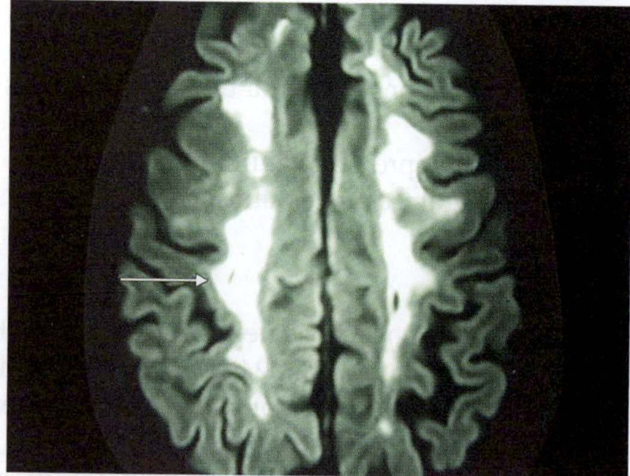

Fig. 205.4: Small vessel disease (arrow)

Vomiting is more common with ICH than with either ischemic stroke or SAH. Increased BP and impaired level of consciousness are more common. However, clinical presentation alone, although helpful, is insufficient to reliably differentiate ICH from other stroke subtypes. The early risk of neurological deterioration and cardiopulmonary instability in ICH is high (Fig. 205.4).

The volume of ICH and grade on the GCS on admission are the most powerful predictors of death by 30 days. Patients with ICH often have greater neurological instability and risk of very early neurological deterioration than do patients with ischemic stroke and will have a greater need for neurocritical care, monitoring of increased ICP and even neurosurgical intervention.

LOBAR HEMORRHAGE

Frontal lobe hemorrhage leads to contralateral hemiparesis, aphasia (dominant lobe), abulia, contralateral gaze palsy (frontal eye field).

Parietal lobe hemorrhage may cause contralateral hemianesthesia, anosognosia (unawareness of neurological deficit) and neglect of contralateral visual field. Dominant temporal lobe hemorrhage may lead to Wernicke's aphasia. Occipital lobe hemorrhage leads to contralateral homonymous hemianopia.

PUTAMINAL HEMORRHAGE

It is the most common site for hypertensive intracerebral hemorrhage. It may remain localized to the putamen or extend to nearby internal capsule, corona radiate or temporal lobe. There is contralateral hemiplegia with conjugate gaze preference to the side of hematoma.

THALAMIC HEMORRHAGE

This is second most common site of hypertensive bleed. It may be confined to thalamus or extend to internal capsule, third ventricles or into midbrain. Physical signs include contralateral pan-sensory loss, hemiparesis, decreased level of consciousness, restriction of vertical gaze. The eyes may show a tonic downward deviation or tonic deviation away from the bleed (wrong way eyes).

CEREBELLAR HEMORRHAGE

It presents with acute frontal or occipital pain, vertigo, nausea, vomiting and ataxia. They have truncal or limb ataxia, small-reactive pupils, nystagmus, dysarthria and skew deviation of eyes.

PONTINE HEMORRHAGE

Large bleed presents with coma, decerebrate rigidity, pinpoint pupils, hyperthermia, quadriparesis and absence of horizontal eye movements.

PREVENTION OF STROKE

Systemic hypertension is the most important modifiable risk factor for stroke. About 30–40% reduction of stroke risk can be achieved with BP lowering. Proper and sustained maintenance of normal BP should be achieved by adequate therapy (*See* Section 13, Ch 126).

Control of diabetes, dyslipidemias, chronic renal disease and systemic vasculitis can all lead to prevention of vascular occlusion or rupture. All these are given in appropriate chapters in Sections 10, 12, 13 and 17.

VASCULAR COGNITIVE IMPAIRMENT

Vascular cognitive impairment (VCI), this term encompasses all instances where cognitive impairment is attributable to cerebrovascular disease and is greater than expected for normal aging. VCI results when vascular risk factors lead to cerebrovascular disease and subsequently to vascular brain injury that disrupts brain networks for memory and thinking.

Vascular Dementia

Vascular dementia (VaD) is a subset of VCI. VaD is a subset of VCI where cognitive impairment is sufficiently severe to interfere with everyday social and occupational function. VaD is the second most common cause of dementia after Alzheimer's disease (AD).

Features

Vascular dementia starts abruptly within 3 months of stroke. Specific features are lacking as features are defined by the site of involvement. Patterns of cognitive impairment are patchy. Memory loss is not prominent. Although the term dementia implies progressive irreversible disease, VaD follows a stepwise course and can stabilize or recover.

Artery of Percheron is the name of the branch of the basilar artery, which supplies both thalamus and occlusion of which results in severe cognitive impairment with other thalamic signs (Fig. 205.5). Such lesions are common to produce vascular cognitive impairment.

Classification

Causes of vascular cognitive impairment
• VCI without dementia
• Vascular dementia
• Alzheimer with vascular component
Vascular dementia
• Cortical VaD
• Subcortical VaD
• Strategic infarct
• Hemorrhagic dementia
• Hypoperfusion dementia
• Dementia due to specific vasculopathy

Abbreviations: VCI = Vascular cognitive impairment; VaD = Vascular dementia

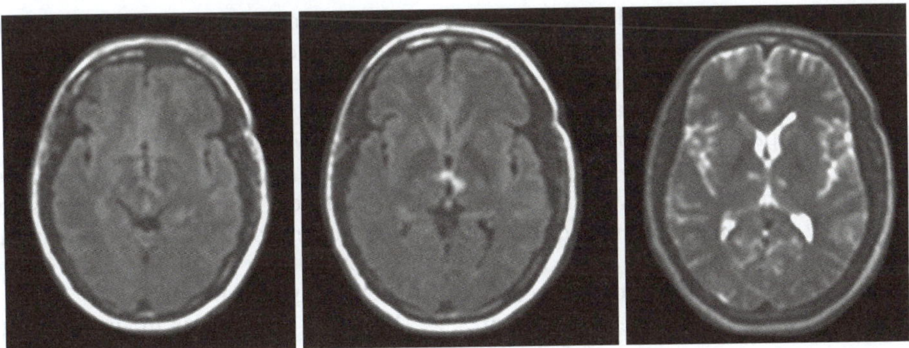

Fig. 205.5: Strategic infarcts of the artery of Percheron

Hachinski Ischemic Score

Symptoms qualifying for 2 points

Abrupt onset, fluctuating course, history of stroke, focal neurologic symptoms and focal neurologic signs.

Symptoms qualifying for 1 point

Stepwise progression, nocturnal confusion, relative preservation of personality, depression, somatic complaints, emotional incontinence, hypertension and atherosclerosis.

Total: 0–18 points

- Hachinski ischemic score 7 suggests multi-infarct dementia
- Hachinski ischemic score 5–6 suggests mixed AD/VaD
- Hachinski ischemic score 4 suggests AD.

Treatment

Attention to the predisposing causes and normalization of the diabetic state, hypertension and dyslipidemia may prevent or alleviate the development of VCI. Once VCI has developed, in addition to management of the primary causes, specific treatment includes cholinesterase inhibitors, such as donepezil, antiplatelet drugs such as aspirin and mood elevators have been tried with variable results.

Prevention

- **Primary prevention:** Identify and manage vascular risk factors from early life including childhood.
- **Secondary prevention:** Prevent recurrent stroke or TIA.
- **Tertiary amelioration:** Treatment of symptomatic cases.

Source: Stein J, Harvey R, Winstein C, et al. Stroke Recovery and Rehabilitation, 2nd edition. USA: Demos Medical Publisher; 2014.

CHAPTER
206

Intracranial Space-Occupying Lesions

Anand Kumar, Arun N Babu

Chapter Summary

- General Considerations
- Clinical Presentation
- Diagnostic Evaluation
- Complications
  - Herniation
- Imaging Studies
- Management
- Intracranial Neoplasms
  - Primary Intracranial Neoplasms
- Gliomas
  - Glioblastoma Multiforme
  - Astrocytomas
  - Oligodendrogliomas
  - Ependymomas
  - Medulloblastoma
- Extra-axial Tumors
  - Meningiomas
- Cerebellopontine Angle Tumors
  - Schwannoma
  - Acoustic Neuromas
- Pituitary Fossa Tumors
- Tumors that Invade the Base of the Skull from Below
- Metastatic Tumors
- Differential Diagnosis
- Management
- Intracranial Hematomas
- Extradural Hematomas
- Subdural Hematoma
- Hydrocephalus
- Idiopathic Intracranial Hypertension

GENERAL CONSIDERATIONS

The term intracranial space-occupying lesion (SOL) refers to any type of pathology or lesion that has the dangerous characteristic of occupying space within the narrow confines of the closed cranial cavity. Such lesions can increase intracranial tension and produce severe pressure effects on brain structures resulting in a failure of neural function and often rapidly progressing to death.

Intracranial SOLs encompass tumors, parasitic cysts, abscesses, granulomas, lymphoma, large infarcts with edema and hematomas in the cranial cavity. All these conditions are commonly seen in India and constitute around 5–6% of our neurological disorders.

Hydrocephalus is another cause of increased intracranial pressure (ICP) and will also be discussed in this chapter.

CLINICAL PRESENTATION

The clinical symptomatology of SOLs depends on the degree of pressure, the rapidity with which it develops and the area of the brain affected. Rapidly growing lesions produce more symptoms as the surrounding neural structures have less time to adapt to the pressure effects.

Acute lesions such as an epidural hematoma may produce sudden, severe symptoms like an acute hemiparesis. Chronic lesions such as a meningioma, growing over a period of years, may produce only subtle clinical symptoms even after it has grown large enough to cause midline shift of the cerebral hemispheres because the cerebral tissue has had time to adapt to the pressure.

In general, the symptoms produced by an intracranial tumor are progressive over a period of weeks to months but occasionally they may appear more rapidly or even abruptly due to:

- Acute development of vasogenic edema around the tumor
- Hemorrhage into the tumor causing increased mass effect
- Displacement causing dysfunction of critical brain structures.

Lesions that occur within the brain parenchyma will initially cause symptoms by direct pressure effects on the surrounding neural tissue producing a breakdown of neural activity. The pattern of deficit will be based on the neural pathways affected by the lesion. Lesions that involve the cerebral cortex may also give rise to seizures, when the lesion disturbs normal function and produces hyperexcitability. Focal or generalized seizures are seen in about 25–30% of brain tumors.

Frontal lobe lesions may cause symptoms of memory loss, dementia, poor judgment, personality changes, confusion and gait dysfunction. Focal seizures may occur with simple motor seizures in a contralateral extremity or progressing as a Jacksonian march to involve the entire contralateral side prior to becoming a generalized seizure.

Parietal lobe involvement can lead to sensory loss, behavioral changes and confusion. Focal seizures may initially present as recurrent episodes of paresthesia or abnormal sensation.

Occipital lobe lesions commonly cause a contralateral visual field deficit that is homonymous, almost identical in the visual fields of both eyes. Seizures may initially present as flashing lights or visual phenomena.

Temporal lobe lesions can cause memory loss and behavioral changes. Language deficits can occur with lesions on the dominant side. Seizures are frequent with temporal lobe lesions. Typically, they may be complex partial seizures, consisting of staring spells and automatic movements with amnesia for the event.

Infratentorial lesions usually cause symptoms more quickly due to smaller space available for expansion and the critical brainstem structures in the area. Even mild brainstem compression can compress the cerebral aqueduct in the midbrain and soon produce life-threatening hydrocephalus.

Vomiting may occur in up to one-third of cases of tumor and is more common in infratentorial lesions. When this occurs due to brainstem compression, vomiting may be very forceful and is termed ***projectile vomiting***. Nausea is often absent. Like headache, vomiting also occurs most frequently upon waking from sleep.

Extra-axial lesions occurring outside the brain parenchyma such as an extradural or subdural hemorrhage or a meningioma, produce focal neurological deficits by direct compression of the adjacent neural structures. Supratentorial lesions will put pressure on the adjacent cerebral cortex and cortical irritation may give rise to seizures. Other focal deficits are less frequent compared to parenchymal lesions, but may occur if the extra-axial lesions is acute and rapidly evolving or very large with significant pressure effects.

The brain is largely pain insensitive but the meninges are pain sensitive. SOLs may often cause headache, due to increased ICP with meningeal traction or direct meningeal irritation. Even when the ICP is in the normal range, headache may result from traction or pressure on the dura mater, major cerebral blood vessels or pain-sensitive cranial nerves. Again, acute, rapidly-developing lesions produce more significant headache than chronic, slowly-evolving lesions.

Papilledema is a common but sinister finding in intracranial tumors. It usually occurs when the cerebrospinal fluid (CSF) pressure is over 200 mm of CSF. It is usually bilateral but occasionally unilateral or asymmetric. Blurred of vision and loss of peripheral vision are early symptoms. Objective examination can reveal an enlarged blind spot.

In addition to these general features, different lesions may produce symptoms specific to their nature. For example, brain abscess may be associated with fever and other signs of infection. Secondary subarachnoid hemorrhage may be associated with signs of meningeal irritation. Box 206.1 gives the common intracranial SOLs.

DIAGNOSTIC EVALUATION

In about one-third of cases, headache may occur as an early symptom. However, it should also be remembered that out of all the cases of headache seen in clinical practice, only a small number turnout to be due to a tumor. Neither location nor intensity correlates directly with the level of ICP.

Headache from an SOL may start as a dull, episodic headache, either diffuse or unilateral on the side of the lesion. It may gradually progress to be more severe and constant. Headache due to increased ICP is increased with coughing, laughing, during Valsalva or when bending. In

Box 206.1: Common intracranial space-occupying lesions

- **Congenital:** Dermoid, epidermoid, hamartoma and teratoma
- **Traumatic:** Subdural and extradural hematomas
- **Inflammatory:** Abscesses (acute and chronic), tuberculomas, syphilitic gumma, fungal granulomas
- **Parasitic causes:** Cysticercosis, hydatid cyst, amebic abscess, *Schistosoma japonicum*
- **Neoplasms:**
    - **Tumors arising from neural structures:** Gliomas, astrocytoma, ependymoma, oligodendroglioma, mixed glioma, medulloblastoma, medulloepithelioma, sarcoma, pinealoma
    - **Tumors arising from appendages:** Meningioma, neurilemmoma (Schwannoma, e.g. acoustic neuroma), chordoma, osteoma
    - **Pituitary tumors:** Adenomas of the pituitary which are intracellular and craniopharyngiomas which arise from remnants of the Rathke's pouch—which are suprasellar
- **Vascular lesions:** Angioma, hemangioblastoma, hemangiopericytoma and papilloma of the choroid plexus
- **Secondary neoplasms:** The brain is a common site of secondaries from carcinoma of the lung, kidney, breast and alimentary tract. In addition, acute leukemias and lymphomas cause infiltration and tumor formation in the central nervous system leading to rise in intracranial tension.

children, constipation can result from the avoidance of defecation as it causes rapid worsening of the headache. Headache is also often present on waking from sleep in the mornings. This is due to the fact that ICP is normally increased in the mornings even at baseline, due to increased intracranial blood flow as a response to hypercapnia from nocturnal hypoventilation during sleep. Early morning headaches seldom occur in common benign headaches such as migraines or tension headaches. Therefore, early morning or waking headaches can be ominous signs that require further investigation.

Any new-onset headache that is severe or sudden in onset or headaches that are confined only to one-side or early-morning or waking headaches should be evaluated carefully. Any complaint of unexplained focal sensory or motor loss or a visual field deficit or the presence of any focal deficits on neurological examination should lead to prompt imaging studies. Papilledema on funduscopy should prompt emergent evaluation. Even subtle symptoms of personality or behavioral change need further evaluation. The new onset of a seizure after the age of 15 years should also prompt the search to rule out any focal mass lesion.

In more advanced cases, constellation of headache, vomiting and papilledema may present as the classic clinical features of an established intracranial tumor.

Increased ICP may also produce a unilateral or less commonly bilateral sixth nerve palsy (referred to as a *false localizing sign*).

Rise in intracranial tension also leads to disturbances of hypothalamic vasomotor regulatory mechanisms. These lead to the development of bradycardia with systolic hypertension (*Cushing's vasomotor phenomena*).

Chronic elevated intracranial tension can produce hypothalamic or pituitary dysfunction resulting in amenorrhea, precocious puberty, obesity, gigantism, somnolence or hyperphagia. Behavioral changes can include apathy, abnormal behavior and lack of attention to personal details.

COMPLICATIONS

Herniation

It occurs when the lesion and resultant edema reach a critical size where it displaces the normal brain tissue out of its normal anatomical position. When the lesion is in either cerebral hemisphere, increasing mass effect and edema can push the hemisphere under the falx cerebri and across the midline. Further mass effect can push inferomedial aspect of hemisphere, the uncus of the temporal lobe, downward through the narrow opening of tentorium cerebelli and force it against lateral aspect of midbrain.

- Compression of ipsilateral third cranial nerve results in ipsilateral pupillary dilatation and ptosis. These can be the first signs of the catastrophe that is to follow.
- Compression of the ipsilateral posterior cerebral artery can result in ischemia of the occipital cortex, producing a contralateral hemianopia.
- Compression of the contralateral cerebral peduncle against the tentorial edge can cause an *ipsilateral* hemiparesis (*false localizing sign*), in addition to the contralateral hemiparesis that may already be present from the primary lesion. This can result in bilateral upper motor neuron signs.

Infratentorial lesions can herniate downwards forcing the cerebellar tonsils through the narrow opening of the foramen magnum (tonsillar herniation).

If untreated, both types of herniation rapidly lead to destruction of the brainstem and death.

IMAGING STUDIES

Computed tomography (CT) also called computerized axial tomography (CAT) scanning is the optimal test for initial screening. CT scan essentially is able to noninvasively detect the density of intracranial structures.

Acute blood is more dense than brain due to high protein content and so epidural, subdural, subarachnoid or intraparenchymal blood is usually readily visible on a CT scan as hyperdense (or white).

Almost all other types of acute brain pathology produce cerebral edema. This swelling of the brain makes the brain less dense and it therefore appears hypodense or darker than normal brain tissue. Tumors can be difficult to detect in early stages because they are often the same density (isodense) as normal brain. Here, we make use of CT scanning with contrast. The contrast is a radiodense substance that does not cross the normal blood-brain barrier (BBB). A CT scan of normal brain will only show the hyperdense contrast in the blood vessels. If there is a tumor or abscess, most tumors or the cell walls of abscesses do not have a functioning BBB and these structures will appear hyperdense or white on CT scan with contrast.

Magnetic resonance imaging (MRI) is superior to CT in detecting the presence of multiple lesions including very small lesions. This is particularly important as the finding of multiple lesions may influence the decision of whether to attempt a full surgical resection of the main lesion. MRI is also more effective at detecting lesions near the skull base and in the posterior fossa as CT has difficulty accurately imaging areas adjacent to high-density bone.

MANAGEMENT

Anti-edema agents: Administration of 20% mannitol solution 200 mL as an intravenous (IV) drip within 30 minutes helps to draw fluid from the brain and transfer it to the vascular compartment. This leads to a temporary fall in intracranial tension. Other hyperosmotic solutions such as 3% saline and glycerol act by the same principle but they are less efficient.

In tumors or abscesses with vasogenic edema, dexamethasone in a dose of 4–12 mg given IV every 6 hours can dramatically decrease the edema and lower the intracranial tension.

While these measures serve to buy time, specific treatment may be instituted to address the causative lesion. Surgical measures may be required in many cases.

INTRACRANIAL NEOPLASMS

Intracranial tumors may be primary or secondary. ***Primary tumors*** arise from the brain parenchyma, intracranial blood vessels, cranial nerves, meninges, pituitary gland and skull. They may be benign or malignant.

Secondary tumors are due to hematogenous spread from malignant tumors at distant sites, to produce intracranial metastases. These metastases may develop in the brain parenchyma, meninges or the skull vault.

Primary Intracranial Neoplasms

The most abundant cell type in the brain are glial cells. They are 10 times more numerous than the neurons. The main glial cells are astrocytes that surround neurons and their processes, and oligodendrocytes that generate the myelin sheaths that cover axons. Most intracranial primary tumors are derived from glial cells and called ***gliomas***. Astrocytomas are most common, followed by oligodendrogliomas. Among astrocytomas, high-grade tumors called ***glioblastoma*** multiforme are the most common, followed by lower-grade astrocytomas. After gliomas, meningiomas are common. These are slow growing, extra-axial benign tumors arising from the meningeal coverings of the brain.

Depending on the age of patient, clinical history and the location of tumor on CT or MRI, nature of tumor can be accurately inferred in many cases.

GLIOMAS

Glioblastoma multiforme (high-grade astrocytoma): Astrocytomas are graded-based on their pathological characteristics. Grade I is the least malignant and grade IV is the worst. Grade IV astrocytomas are known as ***glioblastoma multiforme*** (due to their varied morphology with areas of necrosis). Unfortunately, they comprise vast majority of all gliomas. In some cases, tumors are multicentric or bilateral. The common locations for gliomas are cerebral hemispheres but they can occur anywhere. Median survival is less than 6 months. Surgery, radiation and chemotherapy with temozolomide can increase survival to just over a year.

Astrocytomas (low-grade): These are slow-growing tumors, seen more commonly in the cerebrum, cerebellum, thalamus, pons and optic chiasm. Young adults sometimes have cerebellar astrocytomas that have a good prognosis with surgical resection. Other astrocytomas are also amenable to surgery and radiation therapy but prognosis is not as favorable. Cavitation and/or calcification may develop in many cases and occasionally malignant transformation can occur. The mean survival is 5–6 years.

Oligodendrogliomas: These are rare, slow-growing tumors, usually seen in the cerebrum. Like other chronic lesions, they are often calcified and appear hyperdense on CT. They have an indolent course and may remain stable for many years.

Ependymomas: These grow inside the fourth ventricle and less commonly in other sites. They are more frequent in children. They often spread by seeding through the CSF to other areas and it is important to image the entire brain and spine to identify all lesions.

Medulloblastoma: This term is a misnomer which has been handed down by common usage, because medulloblasts are not identified in these lesions. These are rapidly-growing primitive neuroectodermal tumors affecting the vermis of the cerebellum and giving rise to widespread metastases in ventricles, spinal cord, and meninges. Children are more often affected. The course and progress are so rapid that these tumors may clinically resemble inflammatory lesions.

EXTRA-AXIAL TUMORS

Meningiomas (Endotheliomas)

These benign tumors arise from the dural covering of the brain particularly seen in sites having arachnoid granulations. The sites of predilection are parasagittal regions, olfactory groove, turberculum sellae, sylvian fissure, sphenoidal wing, occipital region and spinal cord. Older age groups are affected more. More than 90% of meningiomas are associated with abnormalities of chromosomes 22. Meningiomas are more common in women and may be associated with breast cancer.

The tumors are firm, lobulated, highly vascular and adherent to the dura. They usually indent adjacent brain tissue without actual invasion. They are often calcified. The overlying bone may show hyperostosis or sometimes erosion. An arterial bruit may be heard over highly vascular meningiomas. Surgical removal often gives excellent results.

CEREBELLOPONTINE ANGLE TUMORS

Schwannoma

Syn: Neurofibroma, Neuroma, Neurinoma, Neurilemmoma

These are benign, slow-growing tumors arising from nerve sheaths with maximum incidence in the fourth and fifth decade. The commonly affected nerve is the auditory nerve in the extramedullary area and the auditory neuroma is located in the cerebellopontine (CP) angle. Bilateral acoustic neuromas are seen to be strongly associated with neurofibromatosis type 2. Less commonly, the neuroma may arise from the trigeminal nerve.

Acoustic Neuromas

They produce a characteristic progression of symptoms as a result of the anatomy of this region. The onset is with tinnitus, vertigo or deafness. Later on, there is rise in intracranial tension. As the lesion extends, there is progressive compression of the VII, V, IX and X cranial nerves sequentially. Compression of the brainstem may cause contralateral hemiplegia and hemianesthesia. As the compression progresses, countercoup pressure on the side opposite to the brainstem give rise to the development of hemiplegia and sensory disturbances on the ipsilateral side as well. The tumor is highly vascular. The internal auditory meatus is often eroded and this can be demonstrated by X-ray of the base of the skull (Towne's view). Isolated tenth nerve palsy, raised intracranial tension and even postpapilledematous optic atrophy can be presenting features of acoustic neuroma. This occurs as it is a slow-growing tumor and compensatory mechanisms mask the localizing features and even the symptoms of raised intracranial tension. CT or MRI scan visualizes the lesion. Treatment is surgical removal.

Other tumors in the CP angle region include meningiomas, trigeminal schwannomas, cholesteatomas, arachnoidal cysts and aneurysms.

Meningiomas and acoustic neuromas can be removed by surgery completely. However, if the surgical resection is incomplete, eventual recurrence is likely.

PITUITARY FOSSA TUMORS

Pituitary adenoma: Tumors arising from the pituitary start within the sella turcica. These may be chromophobe or chromophil adenomas. They produce enlargement of sella turcica and as they enlarge, the diaphragm sella is eroded and the tumor presses on the anterior aspect of the optic chiasm. This compresses the optic nerve fibers from the inferonasal aspect of retina, leading to a bitemporal hemianopia that progresses from upper quadrant downwards. Endocrine manifestations are also seen. Depending on the cell type that gave rise to adenoma, there may be overproduction of a particular pituitary hormone, most commonly of prolactin, leading to hyperprolactinemia. If the tumor consists of growth hormone-secreting cells, there may be acromegaly or gigantism. Eventually, pressure of the tumor on the normal pituitary tissue leads to hypopituitarism.

Craniopharyngioma: Suprasellar tumors and cysts commonly arise from the remnants of the pituitary stalk, called Rathke's pouch. These are midline tumors occurring at variable distances near the diaphragm sellae. Pressure on the posterior aspect of the optic chiasm leads to compression of the optic nerve fibers from the superonasal aspect of the retina, leading to a bitemporal hemianopia that typically progresses from the lower quadrant and progresses upwards. Eventually, it can progress to total blindness and optic atrophy. Pressure on the region of the hypothalamus gives rise to somnolence, hyperphagia, obesity and diabetes insipidus.

Stunted growth with papilledema in a child should make one suspect craniopharyngioma.

It can also present later on in the fifth decade with features of dementia and vision loss.

Suprasellar tumors are generally very slow growing. Many show calcification in skull radiographs. CT and/or MRI will delineate the lesion.

Pineal tumors: *See* Section 11, Ch 98.

TUMORS THAT INVADE THE BASE OF THE SKULL FROM BELOW

Nasopharyngeal carcinoma can infiltrate several cranial nerves arising from medulla and pons.

Glomus jugulare tumors arise from glomus tissue embedded in the external coat of the jugular vein. These tumors may grow into the jugular foramen leading to pressure effects on the VIII, XII, IX, X and VII cranial nerves and can cause intense pain. Erosion of the jugular foramen can be demonstrated on CT scan.

METASTATIC TUMORS

The tumors that more commonly give rise to intracranial metastases are tumors of the lung, breast, thyroid and abdominal and pelvic viscera. Neoplastic cells from the abdominal and pelvic viscera such as kidney and alimentary tract can also reach intracranial structures directly through the vertebral venous plexus called Batson's system of veins. Most of the intracranial metastatic lesions are solid. Some tumors may be cystic or hemorrhagic. Some tumors are more prone to hemorrhage, especially renal cell, melanoma and choriocarcinoma.

Acute lymphocytic leukemia (ALL) and less often acute myeloid leukemia (AML) may produce lesions in the central nervous system (CNS). Lymphomas also may produce neurological manifestation by infiltration (*See* Section 15, Ch 170).

The cerebral cortex is richly vascularized and the majority of arteries are end arteries that terminate at the junction of the cortex with the subcortical white matter. Since metastases to the brain are commonly bloodborne, they may often lodge at the end of one of these end arteries. A mass lesion on CT or MRI that appears to have its epicenter at the gray-white junction should raise suspicion of a metastatic lesion.

A thorough search for the primary should be made when intracranial metastases are suspected. A radiograph of the chest should always be obtained in order to exclude carcinoma of the lung which is a common source of intracranial metastases.

Computed tomography angiography (CTA) and magnetic resonance angiography (MRA) are noninvasive tests that can help delineate the vascular structures to aid in the evaluation of a tumor and to exclude the rare giant aneurysm masquerading as a tumor.

Lumbar puncture (LP) is contraindicated with any SOL because of the risk of precipitating fatal brain herniation by withdrawing CSF and decreasing pressure below the lesion while there is high pressure above. If MRI shows there is no focal mass and therefore no risk of a pressure differential, LP may be performed to evaluate for meningeal carcinomatosis or lymphoma. In these cases, CSF glucose is very low (even below 10 mg/dL) and protein is elevated. A variable leukocytosis may be present. Cytology may be positive but there are false negatives.

Electron microscopy and immunocytochemistry and specific markers for glial cells, neurons and epithelial cells can now help make the histopathological diagnosis in otherwise equivocal cases. There are also methods to identify gene structure and gene localization by molecular probes.

DIFFERENTIAL DIAGNOSIS

Whenever a brain tumor is suspected, other intracranial SOLs such as subdural hematomas, brain abscess, tuberculoma, cysticercosis, fungal granulomas, large demyelinating plaques, large cerebral infarcts and cerebral hematomas should be considered in the differential diagnosis. Sometimes, conditions like hydrocephalus and benign intracranial hypertension (BIH) may masquerade as tumors.

MANAGEMENT

Symptomatic medical therapy aims at reducing intracranial tension with IV steroids (dexamethasone), mannitol and furosemide. Antiepileptic drugs should be given to control seizures and given prophylactically prior to seizures in patients with large or cortical lesions that are more likely to cause seizures.

The present day management of brain tumor is not uniformly ideal. Recent advances in refined microsurgical techniques, radiation therapy and chemotherapy have made the therapeutic regimen more acceptable and effective. In recent years, conventional surgery is being replaced by destruction of the tumor using gamma knife, wherever it is available. Radiation is damaging to all dividing tissue, and therefore tumors are more susceptible. However, the dose required to destroy a tumor would severely damage normal brain tissue. The gamma knife is essentially a method of applying radiation from different directions, all focused on the site of the tumor in such a way that maximal dose is applied to the tumor but surrounding tissues get away with a less damaging dose. This is accomplished by using stereotactic frames applied to the patient's head and using imaging (CT/MRI) data to direct the radiation beam to the target area. This is only available in few places and only patients with few lesions that are small in size are usually candidates for the procedure.

Gene therapy, gene transfer therapy and immunotherapy with monoclonal antibodies are exciting areas of current research that may hold promise for the future.

INTRACRANIAL HEMATOMAS

Hematomas are common complications following injury to the skull. Blood may collect in the extradural space or subdural space or there may be a cerebral contusion.

EXTRADURAL HEMATOMAS

Extradural (or epidural) hematoma is hemorrhage between dura and skull. This is seen in up to 2% of cases of head injuries and occur most often in the temporal fossa. They usually result from an arterial bleed following head trauma, typically due to a skull fracture with damage to an adjacent artery. It may also occur from damage to an adjacent vein but this is likely to be far less severe as it is under low (venous) pressure. The bleeding from a torn artery is under high (arterial) pressure and it can evolve quickly, over minutes to an hour. Clinically significant hematomas exceed 25 mL in volume. It is uncommon in children below 3 years of age. It is also uncommon in the elderly where there is close adherence of the dura to the skull.

Typically, head trauma that is severe enough to cause an extradural hematoma will also produce an initial concussion, with loss of consciousness. If the concussion is not too severe, the patient will become conscious after the initial trauma and may even appear neurologically intact. This is referred to as *lucid interval*. Then, the evolving epidural hematoma expands and starts compressing the adjacent brain, causing unilateral findings like hemiparesis, followed by midline shift with pressure on the third cranial nerve producing dilation of the ipsilateral pupil as a prelude to uncal herniation. If this is not recognized and treated emergently with immediate surgery, death will soon follow.

Note that in cases where the concussion is severe or expansion of hematoma is rapid, there may not be any lucid interval. Sometimes pupil on the side of the hematoma is noted to initially constrict, followed by dilatation and this sequence is referred to as *Hutchinson's pupillary reaction*.

Epidural hematoma should always be ruled out first in cases of skull fractures.

Imaging: On a CT scan, epidural hematoma appears hyperdense along the inner table of the skull, compressing the adjacent brain. It typically has a convex inner border where it abuts the brain, due to the high pressure which is responsible for dissecting out the dura from the inner table of the skull.

Treatment: Management of a significant extradural hematoma and most subdural hematomas is surgical evacuation. If the hematoma appears small, it can be observed in a critical care setting such as a neurointensive care unit with serial CT scans to make sure there is no expansion. Any increase in focal neurological symptoms or the development of papillary asymmetry should prompt repeat CT scanning. Medical management involves management of intracranial tension, prophylactic anticonvulsant medication and maintenance of hemostasis. If the patient was on any antiplatelet or anticoagulant medications, these should be stopped immediately. If the patient was on warfarin, vitamin K should be given as well as fresh frozen plasma (FFP) in life-threatening cases. If the patient was on aspirin, platelet transfusion can be given.

Prognosis: Prompt diagnosis and management can lead to full recovery. Seizures may develop as a long-term sequela.

SUBDURAL HEMATOMA

Subdural hemorrhage is bleeding into the space between the dura and the arachnoid mater. This usually occurs from rupture of the bridging veins that run from the cortical surface across the subdural space to drain into the dural venous sinuses. These veins are particularly susceptible to injury in the elderly, presumably because age-related cerebral atrophy leads to increased stretching of these veins. Evolution may be acute (within 3 days), subacute (within 2 weeks) or chronic (within months).

Subdural hematomas may occur even after relatively mild head trauma, and sometimes patient and family are unable to recall any antecedent head trauma. The elderly, dehydrated children, alcoholics and people on anticoagulant medications are most susceptible.

They sometimes occur as a complication of cerebral hemorrhage or cortical tumors. Subdural hematoma may also arise following sudden reduction in ICP following shunting and has rarely occurred following LP.

Subdurals occur in about 60% of cases of skull fracture. Subdurals can be bilateral in about 10% of cases. The hematoma can consist of blood and clotted blood products and sometimes may be mixed with CSF. When they appear less dense on imaging, they are called *subdural hygroma*.

The symptoms of a subdural are similar to an epidural but less dramatic and often atypical. Chronic subdurals may present with subtle symptoms such as memory loss or mild gait dysfunction. A high degree of clinical suspicion is necessary to make the diagnosis in elderly patients, specially if a history of head trauma is not forthcoming. The diagnosis should always be considered in patients with head trauma on anticoagulation even with minimal or subtle symptoms.

Imaging: On a CT scan, subdural hematoma, like an extradural hematoma, has a hyperdense appearance along the inner table of the skull. If it is chronic, it may appear less dense. Unlike an extradural, however, subdural hematoma has a concave inner border where it abuts the brain, as it is under lower pressure and more passively extends along the convexity of the cerebral hemisphere.

The hematoma consists of fluid blood covered on the inner and outer aspects by layers of fibrin. The high protein content of the fluid makes it hyperosmotic, it absorbs fluid from the surroundings and it may enlarge. Subdural hematoma may occur along with extradural or intracerebral hemorrhage and edema.

Treatment: Same as the treatment of an extradural hematoma (see previous topic).

Prognosis: Prompt diagnosis and management can lead to full recovery.

Intracerebral hemorrhage: See Ch 205.

Infectious space-occupying lesions: See Ch 199.

CAUSES OF INCREASED INTRACRANIAL TENSION OTHER THAN SPACE-OCCUPYING LESIONS

- *Infection or inflammatory conditions:* Meningitis,, encephalitis, cerebral edema.
- *Vascular accidents:* Subarachnoid hemorrhage, cerebral infarctions with edema, cerebral venous thrombosis.
- *Obstruction to flow of cerebrospinal fluid:* Hydrocephalus.
- *Miscellaneous causes:* Systemic hypertension (specially malignant hypertension), idiopathic intracranial hypertension (IIH), chronic respiratory failure, water intoxication, high altitude cerebral edema.

HYDROCEPHALUS

Syn: Hydroencephalus

Dilatation of the ventricular system of the brain due to accumulation of CSF is called hydrocephalus. This may be congenital or acquired. CSF is produced by the choroid plexus in the ventricles. The CSF passes through the ventricular system and into the subarachnoid space and drains via arachnoid granulations into the dural

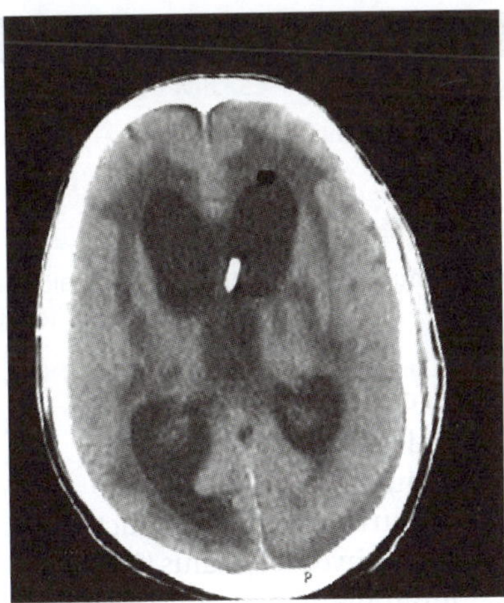

Fig. 206.1: CT scan showing hydrocephalus. *Note:* The dilated ventricles and thinned cortex

venous sinuses. If there is a blockage to the flow of CSF in the ventricular system at a vulnerable spot such as the cerebral aqueduct, or at the foramina of Munro, Luschka or Magendie, this will lead to a dilatation of the ventricular system proximal to the lesion. This is called an obstructive (or noncommunicating) hydrocephalus. If the communication between ventricular system and subarachnoid space remains patent, it is called communicating (or nonobstructive) hydrocephalus. When ventricular dilation is simply due to surrounding tissue loss from cerebral atrophy or old infarcts, this is called *hydrocephalus ex vacuo* (Fig. 206.1).

In congenital hydrocephalus and those developing in early infancy, the fontanelle and skull sutures separate and the head is enlarged. The eyeballs are depressed and optic atrophy may develop. The brain and skull are thinned out. Percussion over the skull may give a cracked-pot note.

Causes of Hydrocephalus Developing in Infancy

- Bleeding into the brain during delivery and subsequent adhesions
- Congenital absence of arachnoid granulations
- Stenosis of the aqueduct
- Improper development of the mantle layer of the brain. In the early stages of embryonal development, the ventricular system is relatively larger. As the mantle layer develops and the brain grows, this relative disparity disappears. In conditions, where the mantle layer does not develop normally, hydrocephalus persists
- Arnold-Chiari malformation
- Obstruction to the foramina of Magendie and Luschka.

Course and Prognosis

If the obstruction is not relieved, the condition progresses. Mental deficiency, optic atrophy and convulsions may develop in many.

Treatment

Surgical procedure are available to divert CSF from the ventricles and relieve tension using suitable valves, in case of obstructive hydrocephalus (Box 206.2). Endoscopic third ventriculostomy is another surgical method employed.

Box 206.2: Surgical procedures and their principles

Type of surgery	CSF diverted into
Ventriculo-peritoneal shunt	Peritoneum
Ventriculo-atrial shunt	Right atrium
Ventriculo-sinus shunt	Sagittal sinus
Theco-peritoneal shunt	Draining the spinal subarachnoid space into the peritoneum

Causes of Hydrocephalus in Adults

- Subarachnoid hemorrhage
- Basal meningitis
- Neoplasms obstructing the aqueduct
- Normal pressure hydrocephalus (NPH).

The basal foramina may be obstructed in meningitis and subarachnoid hemorrhage. The skull is not enlarged if hydrocephalus occurs after closure of the fontanelle. Chronic rise of intracranial tension can lead to radiological features such as resorption of the clinoid processes and thinning of the skull vault giving rise to a ***silver beaten appearance***.

Normal Pressure Hydrocephalus

It is one type of communicating hydrocephalus. Pressure may appear normal during a LP but studies have shown that patients may have elevated pressures intermittently. The condition appears to be due to inefficient drainage of the CSF into the dural venous sinuses via the arachnoid granulations. Since CSF drainage cannot keep up with CSF production, CSF tends to accumulate and hydrocephalus gradually develops. Patients with a history of meningeal insults in the remote past, such as meningitis, subarachnoid hemorrhage or head trauma with hemorrhage, appear susceptible to developing this condition, usually 6 months to several years later.

It occurs in elderly patients and is characterized by clinical triad of gait dysfunction, memory loss and urinary incontinence. Gait dysfunction is usually the first to appear. Gait consists of short steps and appears to have a magnetic quality (like an astronaut wearing magnetic boots in space) and is referred to as a magnetic gait. It may be easily mistaken for a parkinsonian gait. The presence of concomitant memory loss and occasional incontinence should prompt imaging to exclude NPH. On a CT or MRI, elderly patients may often have enlarged ventricles due to cerebral atrophy, which also results in widening of the cortical sulci. In NPH, ventricles typically appear enlarged out of proportion to the cortical sulci, thereby suggesting the diagnosis.

Once the diagnosis is considered, a diagnostic LP with removal of at least 40 cc of CSF can be performed. If gait symptoms improve immediately following the tap, this suggests that the patient indeed has NPH and may respond favorably to a shunting procedure with a ventriculoperitoneal shunt. If gait does not improve, patient either does not have NPH or may have NPH that is less likely to respond to shunting.

IDIOPATHIC INTRACRANIAL HYPERTENSION (IIH)

Syn: Benign intracranial hypertension, Pseudotumor cerebri

In IIH, there is greater production of CSF than resorption into the venous system, due to dysfunction of the arachnoid granulations, leading to sustained increased ICP, often above 200–250 mm of water. It is most common in obese young women. Most cases are idiopathic. Secondary IIH has been associated with both steroid use as well as withdrawal of steroid therapy and also hypoparathyroidism, cerebral venous sinus thrombosis, hypervitaminosis A and use of drugs such as outdated tetracycline, phenytoin and oral contraceptive pills.

Patient's typically present with headache, often with blurred vision that may be related to change in posture. Funduscopy reveals papilledema sometimes with retinal hemorrhages. Occasionally, sixth nerve palsy may be present. CT or MRI scan is normal but may show small, slit-like lateral ventricles. Papilledema with negative imaging studies should prompt consideration of IIH. LP with measurement of opening pressure is diagnostic, with pressures usually between 200 and 250 mm CSF. The patient should be recumbent and the abdominal musculature should be relaxed during manometry to avoid falsely elevated results. MRI venogram can also be performed to exclude cerebral venous sinus thrombosis.

Treatment

Some cases are self-limited and may regress. CSF production can be inhibited by acetazolamide 250–500 mg tid or prednisolone 1 mg/kg bw. Repeated LP can drain CSF when symptoms worsen. With persistent or recurrent symptoms with risk of permanent vision loss from pressure on the optic nerve, optic nerve sheath fenestration procedure or CSF shunting may need to be performed.

Acknowledgment: The authors gratefully acknowledge the contribution of late Dr PK Mohan, who co-authored this chapter previously.

Multiple Sclerosis and other Demyelinating Lesions

Anand Kumar, Arun N Babu

Chapter Summary

- General Considerations
  - Role of Myelin
- Classification of Diseases Affecting Myelin
- Multiple Sclerosis (MS)
- Treatment
  - Treatment of Exacerbations
  - Disease Modifying Therapy
  - Symptomatic Treatment
- Neuromyelitis Optica (NMO)
- Acute Disseminated Encephalomyelitis (ADEM)

GENERAL CONSIDERATIONS

Role of Myelin

Most axons are covered by a membrane called *myelin*. The myelin is divided into segments along the axon. In between the segments, the axon membrane is exposed (nodes of Ranvier) and has ion channels that allow depolarization and generation of action potentials. The myelin segments allow action potentials to jump from node-to-node, thereby increasing the conduction velocity. Myelinated axons can conduct action potentials faster than unmyelinated axons. But when a myelinated axon suffers damage to its myelin, action potentials may be unable to propagate at all past the site of the lesion.

Axons are myelinated in the central nervous system (CNS) by oligodendrocytes and in the peripheral nervous system by Schwann cells. The term *demyelinating* diseases refers to acquired disorders where the myelin is destroyed with relative sparing of the axon. This should not be confused with congenital disorders where normal myelination does not occur, referred to as *dysmyelinating diseases*.

CLASSIFICATION OF DISEASES AFFECTING MYELIN

Autoimmune

- *Multiple sclerosis*
  - Relapsing-remitting form
  - Progressive form
- Isolated demyelinating syndromes

Neuromyelitis Optica (NMO) Spectrum Disorders

- NMO (Devic's disease)
- Asian opticospinal multiple sclerosis (MS)
- Others.

Acute Disseminated Encephalomyelitis (ADEM)

- *Postinfections:* Following viral, bacterial, mycoplasma and rickettsia infections.
- *Postvaccinal:* Following rabies, smallpox vaccinations.
- Idiopathic.

Others

Acute hemorrhagic leukoencephalopathy (AHLE), Schilder's disease, concentric sclerosis of Balo.

Infections

Progressive multifocal leukoencephalopathy (PML).

Toxic/Metabolic

- Carbon monoxide
- Vitamin B_{12} deficiency
- Mercury intoxication (Minamata disease)
- Alcohol/tobacco amblyopia
- Central pontine myelinolysis (due to rapid correction of hyponatremia)
- Marchiafava-Bignami syndrome
- Hypoxia
- Radiation.

Vascular

- Binswanger's disease
- Reversible posterior leukoencephalopathy (due to hypertensive crisis).

Hereditary Disorders (Dysmyelination)

- Adrenoleukodystrophy due to defect in metabolism of long chain fatty acids. Metachromatic leukodystrophy due to deficiency of arylsulfatase enzyme
- Krabbe's globoid leukodystrophy
- Alexander's disease
- Canavan's disease
- Phenylketonuria (PKU).

MULTIPLE SCLEROSIS (MS)

It is the most common demyelinating disease, especially in countries in the higher latitudes (closer to the poles). It is less common in India and other Asian countries. In India, MS constitutes about 1.5% of all diseases seen in neurology services in the northern parts, but only about 0.05% in the southern parts of the country. Women are affected twice as much as men. Peak incidence is at the age of 20–35 years in women and 35–45 years in men. It is rare before the age of 14 years or after the age of 60 years.

Etiology

The disease is much more prevalent with increasing latitude from the equator. The prevalence per 100,000 people is less than 1 in equatorial areas, 6–14 in the Southern United States of America (USA) and 30–80 further North in Canada. Interestingly, when people from equatorial countries migrate to places such as Northern USA, if they migrate before the age of 16 years, they develop about the same risk as people born in USA, whereas if they migrate after the age of 16 years, they retain lower risk level of their equatorial homeland. Genetically, there is no definite inheritance pattern for the disease, but first-degree relatives of patients with MS have a significantly higher risk of developing the disease. It is therefore clear that both genetic and environmental factors play a role.

Immunopathogenesis

The presence of T- and B-lymphocytes, macrophages and activated microglia in MS lesions is proof to the fact that immune mechanisms play a role in the genesis of MS lesions (plaques). What induces the immune system to launch this ill-conceived attack on the body's own myelin is still largely unclear.

Pathological hallmarks are the breach in the integrity of the blood-brain barrier and upregulation of adhesion molecules on the endothelium of the brain and spinal cord further the pathological processes. Leukocytes enter the normally immunologically privileged CNS. If lymphocytes reactive to myelin antigens enter the tissues, acute inflammatory demyelinating lesions ensue. These lesions primarily involve white matter and the primary targets are the myelin sheath and oligodendrocytes.

Presentation

MS is characterized by recurrent attacks of neurological deficits due to recurrent episodes of focal demyelination in different places, anywhere throughout the white matter of the cerebrum, cerebellum, brainstem, optic nerves and spinal cord. It does not affect the peripheral nerves. Since any pathway in the CNS can be so afflicted, symptoms can be almost anything including hemiparesis or unilateral sensory loss from cerebral white matter lesions, paraparesis from segmental spinal cord lesions (transverse myelitis), monocular or binocular vision loss from unilateral or bilateral optic neuritis, etc. (it may be noted here that the term optic nerve is a misnomer—embryonically and histologically, it is not a nerve, but actually a tract of the brain, surrounded by meninges and myelinated by oligodendrocytes).

The inflammation may subside after several days to a few weeks. The inflammatory damage to the nerve results in demyelination, and once severe enough, it can lead to a conduction block. Symptoms typically evolve over one to several days. A course of steroids may help cut-short the period of inflammation and ameliorate the extent of damage.

Once the inflammation subsides, the brain's remarkable capacity to repair itself swings into action. Sodium (Na) channels migrate from the nodes into the demyelinated regions. This allows action potentials to be conducted across the damaged area, even if it is slower than usual. More channels may be manufactured and the nerve can also gradually remyelinate over a few months. Symptoms may start to improve in several days and continue to improve for up to 6 months. However, if the inflammatory damage was very severe, it may have also caused axonal damage leading to permanent deficits.

Patients may also present with transient symptoms. This usually occurs when there is a subclinical lesion which is not severe enough to cause a significant conduction block under normal circumstances. However, under special circumstances, such as during exposure to heat (a hot shower or very warm weather), conduction block may develop. This is because at increased temperature, depolarization and repolarization of the action potential occur more quickly and the action potential itself is of shorter duration. As a result, there may be insufficient time to generate enough local ion flow to depolarize the next segment of the axon to allow the action potential to pass through the affected area. Thus, when exposed to heat, the patient may become symptomatic. The classical example is a young lady developing transient monocular vision loss (due to a subclinical optic neuritis) while taking a hot shower, which improves after cooling off.

Clinical Course

Based on the clinical course, MS is classified into the following subtypes:

- ***Relapsing-remitting type (R-R type):*** Most common (85%).
- ***Progressive type:*** Deterioration continues for at least 1 year.
    - ***Primary progressive MS:*** In this type, the neurological deficit is progressive from the onset without acute exacerbation, plateau or remissions.
    - ***Progressive-relapsing MS:*** Consists of patients with primary progressive disease who later in their course develop acute relapses with or without full recovery.
    - ***Secondary progressive MS:*** Illness starts as a R-R MS, but later assumes a progressive course.

Imaging

Computed tomography (CT) scanning is usually normal but magnetic resonance imaging (MRI) can show MS lesions in almost all cases (Fig. 207.1).

Acute MS plaques may enhance with contrast due to local disturbance of the blood-brain barrier as part of the inflammatory response. They may also show increased signal on diffusion-weighted imaging, an MRI sequence that is usually indicative of acute ischemia. Enhancing lesions are confined to the white matter, although edema from the lesions may involve subjacent gray matter. ***Juxtacortical lesions***, where the lesion ends abruptly at the

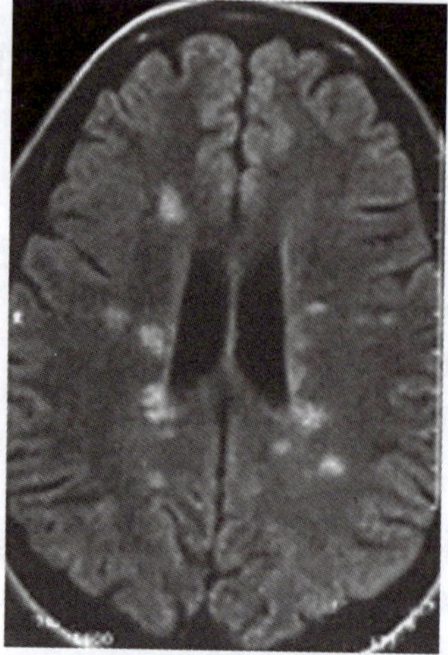

Fig. 207.1: Magnetic resonance imaging (MRI) showing periventricular lesions in multiple sclerosis (MS). ***Note:*** The demyelinated plaques

gray-white junction is highly suggestive of a demyelinating lesion.

Cerebrospinal fluid (CSF) may show a mild lymphocytosis and protein elevation, but is often normal. Electrophoresis of CSF in MS can show bands indicating the presence of monoclonal antibodies called *oligoclonal bands*. This is compared with the bands on electrophoresis of the patient's blood. If there are two or more oligoclonal bands present in CSF that are not present in blood, this is taken as evidence of immunoglobulin (Ig) synthesis in the CNS and supports a diagnosis of MS. In general, if a patient has an isolated demyelinating syndrome, the risk of later turning out to be MS may be about 50%. If oligoclonal bands are positive in the CSF, the risk goes up to 67%. If negative, the risk goes down to 33%.

Diagnosis

A single attack of demyelination may represent an isolated demyelinating syndrome that may be idiopathic or postinfectious. When there are at least two separate attacks in the same patient, the odds of this happening by chance or so low, this indicates that the patient indeed has MS and further attacks can be expected. The main principle behind making this diagnosis is to be certain that there have been at least two separate (unrelated) attacks. To be certain, there are two separate attacks; by convention, the attacks should be at least 1 month apart and in two different sites.

When a patient presents with a demyelinating syndrome, careful elicitation of the history may reveal previous transient neurological deficits that may have been deemed unimportant by the patient, but may now help establish the diagnosis. Sometimes, even if MRI only shows one lesion, evoked potential testing of somatosensory, auditory or visual responses may show evidence of other subclinical demyelinating lesions. There are additional criteria such as McDonald criteria, to assist in making a diagnosis of MS even with one clinical attack based on supportive data from MRI, lumbar potential or evoked potential studies. However, once a patient has a definite second attack, the diagnosis is confirmed in any case.

In patients with only one attack, they should be educated about potential symptoms and advised to seek follow-up promptly, should these occur. MRI with contrast should be repeated in 4–6 months (or sooner if there are additional symptoms) to determine if any new lesions develop—this may then confirm a diagnosis of MS.

In the progressive type, the duration of illness should be more than 1 year. In both types, there should be no other evident reasons to account for the neurological deficit.

Last but not least, it is important to exclude other conditions before the diagnosis of MS is established. In India, it still remains a diagnosis of exclusion.

Prognosis

It is very variable. Some patients may have only few attacks over periods of years and continue their normal careers and daily activities. Other patients may go on to have more progressive symptoms and disability.

Clinical features suggestive of MS or not suggestive of multiple sclerosis are shown in Table 207.1.

Table 207.1: Clinical features of multiple sclerosis (MS)

Clinical features suggestive of MS	Clinical features not suggestive of MS
Onset between the ages of 15 and 50 years	Onset before the age of 10 years or after the age of 60 years
Involvement of multiple areas of the CNS	Involvement of the PNS
Optic neuritis	Hemianopias
Lhermitte's sign	Rigidity, sustained dystonia
Internuclear ophthalmoplegia	Cortical deficits such as aphasia, apraxia, alexia and neglect
Fatigue	Deficit developing within minutes
Worsening with elevated body temperature	Early dementia

Abbreviations: CNS = Central nervous system; PNS = Peripheral nervous system

Treatment

There are three main categories in the treatment of MS:
1. Treatment of exacerbations
2. Disease modifying therapy
3. Symptomatic treatment.

Treatment of Exacerbations

Acute exacerbations are treated with a course of intravenous (IV) methylprednisolone, 1 g over at least 4 hours, daily for 3–5 days. This can be tapered off over 2 weeks with a course of oral prednisone.

Occasionally, in patients with severe symptoms who cannot tolerate or fail to respond to steroids, a course of IV immunoglobulin or plasmapheresis can be used.

When patients present with increased symptoms, it is necessary to exclude concurrent systemic infections such as urinary tract infection (UTI) as these can cause transient worsening of chronic or subclinical MS symptoms without being a true MS exacerbation. This probably happens due to the systemic inflammatory response or due to fever. Treatment and resolution of the systemic infection produces full resolution of the MS symptoms and steroids are not necessary.

Disease Modifying Therapy

These agents are medications that have been shown to reduce the risk of subsequent exacerbations when taken on a regular basis. The older established agents are available only as injections and need to be taken on a daily to weekly basis.

- Interferon β1b (IFN-β1b) can be self-administered every other day or three times weekly. IFN-β1a can be self-administered intramuscularly (IM) just once weekly making it more popular with some patients. Both agents have been shown to decrease future exacerbations by about one-third. MRI data has shown less new lesions and decrease in the size of the lesion burden compared to patients not on disease-modifying regimens. Common side effects are flu-like symptoms and injection-site reactions. Elevation of liver enzymes can occur and these should be checked every 6 months. Some patients eventually develop neutralizing antibodies against the medication leading to loss of efficacy.

- ***Glatiramer acetate:*** This is a novel medication not related to the IFNs. It is self-administered subcutaneously (SC) on a daily basis. Efficacy data is not as extensive as with the IFNs but it appears to be almost as effective. The agent is better tolerated and is often used first-line in patients with less aggressive disease.
- ***Natalizumab***, a recombinant monoclonal antibody against α4 integrins is a more recent addition for the treatment of relapsing MS. It appears to work by preventing activated T-lymphocytes from entering the CNS. In trials, it appeared to have even greater risk reduction of future exacerbation than the IFNs, but later 1–2% of patients developed PML from John Cunningham (JC) virus reactivation. Nowadays, it is used in patients who have failed other conventional therapy, only after being confirmed negative for JC virus antibody titers.
- ***Fingolimod*** is the first oral immunomodulating agent to be approved for preventing relapses in MS. In studies, it was able to decrease the incidence of relapses by about half. Due to a risk of bradycardia, the first dose requires hospital observation for 6 hours. Common side effects are cold-like symptoms, headache and fatigue. Recently, however, a case of PML has been reported.
- ***Daclizumab high-yield process (DAC HYP):*** This is a humanized monoclonal antibody that binds to CD25 [alpha subunit to the interleukin 2 (IL2) receptor] and modulates IL2-signalling. It is given by SC injection 150 mg every 4 weeks. It was superior in efficiency to IFN β1a given IM 30 μg weekly up to 144 weeks. Daclizumab reduced the frequency of exacerbations and clearance of MRI findings. The incidence of rashes, infection and abnormal liver functions were higher with daclizumab.

Source: Kappos L, Wiendl H, Selmaj K, et al. Daclizumab HYP versus Interferon Beta-1a in Relapsing Multiple Sclerosis. N Engl J Med. 2015;373(15):1418-28.

- ***Mitoxantrone*** is a cytotoxic anthracenedione, a chemotherapeutic agent which is reserved for refractory cases. It is given IV once in 3 months. Major toxicity is cardiac.
- ***Repeated courses of steroids:*** A single dose of IV methylprednisolone may be administered on a monthly basis to select patients whose symptoms appear to improve with this regimen.
- ***IV immunoglobulin (IVIG),*** as a monthly dose sometimes provides benefit for patients not responding to other therapy.
- ***Bone marrow/stem cell transplantation:*** Only anecdotal reports are available on the use of this mode of therapy for MS. This is likely to be put to use in the future.

Symptomatic Treatment

MS patients often complain of fatigue. Some patients may respond to ***amantadine*** 10 mg given once or twice daily during waking hours, other patients may respond to ***4-aminopyridine*** (fampridine) is a potassium channel blocker and can help improve visual function and motor skills, particularly in patients with chronic symptoms. It can increase the risk of seizures. Dose needs to be adjusted in renal failure. Renal function should be checked prior to therapy and at least annually thereafter.

Patients with paresis of one or more extremities often have severely disabling spasticity. ***Baclofen*** (lioresal), a central acting muscle relaxant, is usually effective at doses of 5–10 mg, three to four times a day. High doses may sometimes worsen the degree of weakness. Patients who have disabling spasticity sometimes have an implanted baclofen pump for intrathecal administration for greater efficacy.

Tizanidine, diazepam and ***gabapentin*** may benefit some patients.

Oxybutinin and ***propantheline*** can help with urinary frequency and urgency.

NEUROMYELITIS OPTICA (NMO)

Syn: Devic's disease

This is a variant of MS that predominantly affects the optic nerves and spinal cord, causing recurrent bouts of optic neuritis and/or transverse myelitis. Spinal lesions may sometimes show significant inflammation with cord enlargement due to edema, typically extending over multiple spinal segments. MRI of the brain often reveals no lesions except sometimes in the optic nerves (these can be hard to visualize even on MRI). Blood may show positive titers to antiaquaporin-4 (also called anti-NMO) antibody.

Management starts with IV methylprednisolone for acute exacerbations for 5–10 days. If there is no improvement, plasmapheresis or IVIG therapy for 5 days should be promptly instituted as some patients respond more to these. Recent studies have suggested that monoclonal antibody therapy using rituximab can be beneficial and this may become a more common option in the future.

NMO Spectrum Disorders

The development of the NMO-antibody test has led to the detection of positive NMO titers in other variants of MS that do not have all the typical features of NMO. These are now considered related conditions and referred to as ***NMO spectrum disorders***. They include the following:

- ***Asian opticospinal multiple sclerosis:*** This condition is more common in India and other parts of Asia. The opticospinal MS differs from western type MS in the following aspects:
  - A higher frequency of female patients
  - Older age of onset
  - More frequent exacerbations
  - Fewer number of lesions in the cerebrum on MRI
  - Higher cell counts and total proteins in the CSF
  - Low frequency of oligoclonal bands or increased immunoglobulin G index in the CSF
  - A benign course.

Some NMO spectrum variants have lesions in the brainstem or hypothalamus in addition to optic neuritis and myelitis.

The NMO-antibody test has also resulted in another variant of the condition that of patients who are seronegative for the NMO-antibody but have obvious clinical features of the disease. This is referred to simply as seronegative NMO.

ACUTE DISSEMINATED ENCEPHALOMYELITIS (ADEM)

It is an autoimmune, monophasic, demyelinating disease generally associated with a preceding viral infection. The disease has an immunological basis and is thought to be secondary to molecular mimicry and formation of T-cell and B-cell response to endogenous proteins in the myelin layer. Although most cases begin within a few days of a preceding infection or vaccination, at times there is no history of any antecedent event. It may be difficult to differentiate ADEM from the first attack of MS and the two may have a similar underlying pathophysiology.

ADEM has been reported following infections with measles, rubella, varicella, corona virus, mycoplasma, influenza, parainfluenza, cytomegalovirus (CMV), Epstein-Barr virus (EBV), human herpesvirus 6 and nonspecific upper respiratory pathogens. It has also followed vaccinations for smallpox, rabies, mumps, rubella and influenza.

The clinical course is highly variable, ranging from a slow progression over weeks to a fulminant course over hours to days. Unlike MS, however, it is a *monophasic* illness without recurrences.

Headache, meningismus and altered mental status with confusion progressing to lethargy and coma are common and these also distinguish it from MS. Any neural system can be affected and there can be any combination of motor or sensory deficits and visual and cerebellar dysfunction.

Laboratory evaluation typically shows a CSF pleocytosis with up to 150–200 white blood cells (WBCs), generally with a lymphocytic predominance. Sometimes polymorphonuclear cells, predominate in the CSF (a finding that may initially suggest meningitis rather than ADEM). The protein level is usually elevated, but generally not higher than 180 mg/dL. CSF electrophoresis typically shows no additional bands in the CSF when compared to serum.

Diagnostic Criteria for ADEM

- First clinical attack of inflammatory or demyelinating disease in the CNS
- Acute or subacute onset
- Affects multifocal areas of the CNS
- Polysymptomatic presentation
- Must include encephalopathy with behavioral changes, confusion or altered consciousness
- Attack should be followed by some degree of improvement, clinically or radiologically (MRI)

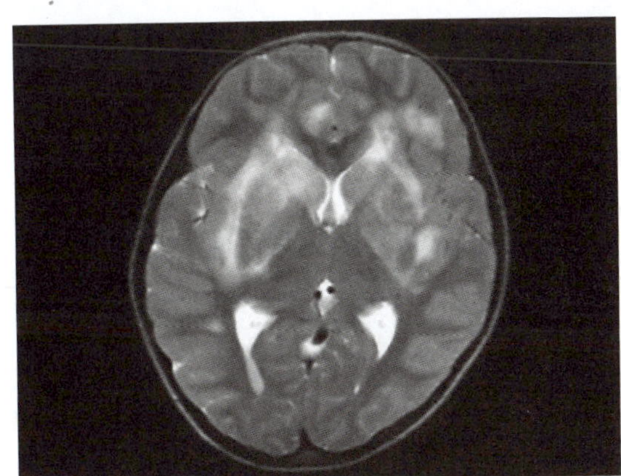

Fig. 207.2: White matter and basal ganglia lesions in acute disseminated encephalomyelitis (ADEM)

- Sequelae may include residual deficits
- No other etiology to explain the event
- Relapses within 3 months are considered part of the original event.

Magnetic resonance images show multiple white matter lesions on T2 and flair sequences with gadolinium enhancement on T1, similar to acute MS lesions. They are however, frequently more confluent and larger in size than typical MS plaques. Lesions may occur in gray matter such as the basal ganglia, thalamus and cortex which are not seen in MS. The posterior fossa and spinal cord are frequently involved. Acute inflammatory demyelinating lesions often involve breakdown dysfunction of the blood-brain barrier and these lesions will therefore, enhance with contrast. This does not occur with old, chronic lesions. In ADEM, there is usually uniform enhancement of lesions (suggesting they are all acute) unlike MS in which there are also old lesions which will be nonenhancing (Fig. 207.2).

Prognosis

In milder cases, 90% of patients recover completely. In more severe cases, mortality may be as high as 5–20% and 50% of patients so affected are left with permanent neurological disability.

Treatment

Treatment is with high dose corticosteroids such as IV methylprednisolone 1 g daily for 3–5 days. Plasma exchange and IVIG are used if there is only partial benefit with steroids.

Acknowledgment: The authors gratefully acknowledge the contribution of Late Dr PK Mohan, who co-authored this chapter previously.

Source:

1. Multiple sclerosis. Neurol Clin North Am. 2011;29(2).
2. Chandra SR, Kumar BS. A disease modifying treatment protocol in patients with RRM. KMJ. 2009;9(3): 111-4.

CHAPTER

208

Motor Neuron Disease

SR Chandra, KA Kabeer

Chapter Summary

- Classification of Sporadic Motor System Disorders
- Classification of Genetic causes of Motor System Disease
- Amyotrophic Lateral Sclerosis (ALS)
- Progressive Muscular Atrophy
- Progressive Bulbar Palsy
- Primary Lateral Sclerosis
- Vulpian-Bernhart Syndrome
- Pseudopolyneuritic Form of ALS
- Familial ALS
- Madras Motor Neuron Disease
- Monomelic Atrophy
- Brown-Vialetto-Van-Laere Syndrome
- Fazio-Londe Syndrome
- ALS Plus Syndrome-FTLD Complex
- ALS-Parkinsonism Dementia Complex
- Spinal Muscular Atrophy

INTRODUCTION

Motor system consists of corticospinal tracts of the upper motor neuron (UMN) system and brainstem motor nuclei and anterior horn cells of spinal cord belonging to lower motor neuron (LMN). A group of disorders are capable of affecting this system and also diseases can be imitators. Therefore, careful evaluation is needed before diagnosis of a neurodegenerative disease is made. Usually, the patient presents with functional disability referable to one or more of the above structures (refer previous chapters). Careful drawing of family tree, detailed evaluation of the course as relapsing course might point to early phase demyelination, minor symptoms referable to bladder and sensory system will help in looking for compressions, pattern in nerve or root distribution will indicate motor neuropathy and radiculopathy, acute nonprogressive course will point to static insults caused by viruses, signs restricted to entrapment sites indicate entrapment neuropathy, involvement of other parts of neuraxis and other systems points to more extensive neuro-degenerative or neurometabolic disorders. Therefore, even if at first site provisional diagnosis may be glaring, detailed history and evaluation is of utmost importance so that better proper diagnostic options are not missed. The common features clinically seen in motor neuron disease (MND) are as follows:

- Emotional lability with tendency to laugh or cry
- Presence of release reflexes like pouting, snout, facial reflexes, jaw jerk, point to UMN lesions
- Frontal lobe and basal ganglia features occur in some in selected patients.

Spastic tongue with dysarthria, swallowing defect, spastic limbs, exaggeration of deep reflexes including Hoffman's, finger jerks, crossed adductor reflex, with or without involvement of abdominal and plantar reflexes, point to UMNs lesion. Pure motor syndromes with upper motor alone, lower motor alone or combined involvement without sensory features is suggestive of MND. Fasciculations which are widespread, well seen over the tongue, thigh and other muscles, combined with wasting of muscles and normal sensory and autonomic system is very characteristic of MND. Selective involvement of some muscles severely and sparing of others within the territory of a root or nerve apart from being purely motor is the point in favor of disease of anterior horn cells. Extraocular muscles and lower cervical segments do not generally get involved in the process. Pure motor syndromes may be caused by a wide range of conditions. Among these, degenerative lesions are responsible for MND.

CLASSIFICATION OF SPORADIC MOTOR SYSTEM DISORDERS

- **_Chronic_**
  - **_UMN and LMN:_** Amyotrophic lateral sclerosis (ALS)
  - **_UMN:_** Primary lateral sclerosis
  - **_LMN:_** Multifocal motor neuropathy
  - Motor neuropathy with paraproteinemia
  - Motor predominant neuropathies, motor neuro-nopathy
- **_Acute:_** Poliomyelitis, herpes zoster, coxsackie viruses and other enteroviruses.
- **_Others:_** Secondary causes of MND

CLASSIFICATION OF GENETIC CAUSES OF MOTOR SYSTEM DISEASE

- **_UMN and LMN:_** Familial ALS; autosomal dominant, recessive or mixed (AD/AR/M)
- **_LMN:_** Spinal muscular atrophy
  - X-linked spinobulbar muscular atrophy (Kennedy's)
  - **_GM2 gangliosidoses:_** Tay-Sachs and Sandhoff are disorders under the group of GM2 gangliosidosis. They are due to deficiency of hexosaminidase A and B, respectively. Type A presents with pure neurological features and Type B with neurological and systemic features. Both of them involve anterior horn cells.
- **_UMN:_** Familial spastic paraparesis, adrenomyeloneu-ropathy (AMN).

AMN is a form of X-linked adrenoleukodystrophy due to abnormality in very long chain fatty acids (a peroxisomal storage disorder also called glutaric aciduria type 3). AMN patients generally have spinal cord dysfunction with LMN features.

ALS plus syndromes: Sometimes features of ALS may be coexisting with other conditions which have to be distinguished from ALS. Differential diagnosis include following conditions—chronic inflammatory demyelinating neuropathy, inclusion body myosistis, cervical myeloradiculopathy, multi-infarct syndromes, progressive supranuclear palsy (PSP), multisystem atrophy, corticobasal degeneration, Machado-Joseph disease (MJD), parkinsonism ALS, dementia ALS and others.

MJD, also known as Machado-Joseph Azorean disease or Joseph's disease or spinocerebellar ataxia type 3 (SCA3) is a rare autosomal dominantly inherited neurodegenerative disease that causes progressive cerebellar ataxia, which results in a lack of muscle control and coordination of the upper and lower extremities. The symptoms are caused by a genetic mutation that results in an expansion of abnormal ***CAG*** trinucleotide repeats in the ATXN3 gene that results in an abnormal form of the protein ataxia which causes degeneration of cells in the hind brain. This can be associated with motor neuron involvement of the bulbar and limb muscles.

There are five subtypes of MJD that are characterized by the age of onset and range of symptoms.

AMYOTROPHIC LATERAL SCLEROSIS (ALS)

This is the most frequent form of MND seen in adults in India. It is a progressive disorder characterized by degeneration of motor neurons of the primary motor cortex, brainstem and spinal cord. Incidence varies from 1 to 3/100,000 person years with point prevalence rates of 4–6/100,000 person years, it increases with age up to 75 years. The disease sets in insidiously by the age of 50–55 years, men are more frequently affected than women with a ratio of 1.5:1 in sporadic ALS. Average age of onset is 45 years in India, a decade younger than in the West. It is not uncommon to find several members of a family affected.

Pathogenesis

This is largely unknown.

Genetic Factors

Twenty percent of patients with familial ALS and 2% with sporadic ALS have the superoxide dismutase (SOD) gene mutation. Other genes like alsin, senataxin and TAR DNA-binding protein-43 (TDP-43) induce toxic gain of function and glutamate induced excitotoxicity. This leads to calcium influx and neuronal cell death.

Oxidative stress, mitochondrial dysfunction, impaired axonal transport (slowing of anterograde and retrograde transport) have all been found in mouse models. Abnormal assembly with accumulation of neurofilaments, protein aggregation and intracytoplasmic inclusions are a hallmark of both sporadic and familial ALS. Inflammatory dysfunction and microglial, and dendritic cell activation produce inflammatory cytokines like interleukins (ILs) and tumor necrosis factor-alpha (TNF-α) along with deficits in neurotrophic factors and these lead to apoptosis.

Pathological Features

There is degeneration and loss of motor neurons with astrocytic gliosis and formation of intraneuronal inclusions which include Bunina bodies, which are small eosinophilic, hyaline intracytoplasmic inclusions that stain positive for cystatin and are present in 70–100% of cases. Ubiquitinated inclusions can be divided into skein-like inclusions which have a filamentous profile and presence of spherical bodies. TDP-43 is the major protein constituent in these inclusions. Hyaline conglomerate (neurofilament inclusions) is seen with familial ALS. These are argyrophilic inclusions seen in spinal cord with phosphorylated and non-phosphorylated neurofilaments.

Histopathology shows group atrophy denervation and reinnervation has been illustrated in Figure 208.1.

Clinical Features

The clinical pattern may follow the classical description in most of the cases, but some may show atypical features. Variant forms of the disease have been described depending upon the genetics and geographical distribution. The mean age of onset in sporadic ALS varies between 60

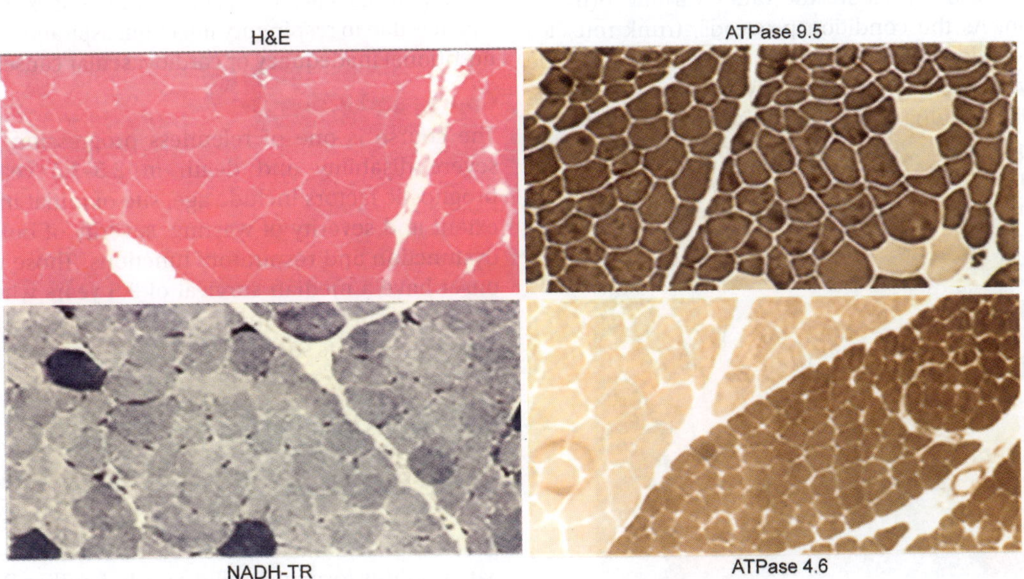

Fig. 208.1: Denervation atrophy and reinnervation type of grouping
Abbreviations: H&E = Hematoxylin and Eosin; NADH-TR = Nicotinamide adenine dinucleotide tetrazolium reductase

and 65 years. In 5%, onset is in the limbs. In those cases where the onset is in the lower limbs, ALS starts with unexplained tripping during walking, in those with onset in the hands there is difficulty handling buttons, stiffness with cramping, fasciculations, which later progresses to other uninvolved sites as well. Muscle strength and bulk decrease over a period of time, but reflexes remain well-elicitable. Gross asymmetry in involvement with either upper limb, lower limb or head or neck with difficulty to hold the head erect may develop. The unique feature of ALS is the combination of UMN lesion in the form of spasticity and exaggeration of deep tendon reflexes, and also evidence of LMN lesion in the form of fasciculations and atrophy.

The classic form starts with wasting of the small muscles of the hand, deltoid and shoulder girdle muscles and then progresses to involve the other muscles of the limb. In the majority of cases, the affection is bilateral though asymmetrical. Rarely, the manifestations may remain unilateral for considerable periods of time. Still minor manifestations such as fasciculations can be observed over more extensive areas. Bulbar muscles are affected later. Bulbar onset is more common in older patients, especially older women. Finally, all muscles of the body may be involved. Camptocormia (kyphotic defect) is common. Diaphragmatic weakness and girdle type weakness may develop. The wasted muscles show fasciculations readily, whereas they are less prominent in the apparently unaffected muscles. *Fasciculations* can be made more prominent by exerting the muscle, exposure to cold air or subcutaneous (SC) injection of 0.5 mg neostigmine. Atrophy of small muscles of the hand gives rise to claw hand (Fig. 208.2) in which there is extension of the metacarpophalangeal joints and flexion of the interphalangeal joints. In the feet, atrophy of the intrinsic muscles gives rise to pes cavus (exaggeration of the arch of the foot), when the feet are in the resting position.

ALS with onset early in life may resemble muscle disease (Wohlfahrt-Kugelberg-Welander). Hemiplegic types (Mills) and spastic types are the other variant forms of presentation. As the condition proceeds, trunk muscles and other major muscles of the limbs may also be affected giving rise to considerable wasting and paralysis. Affection of the bulbar muscles gives rise to LMN lesion of the tongue (Fig. 208.3), leading to its atrophy and UMN lesion of the soft palate and pharynx, giving rise to exaggeration of gag reflex and dysphagia. The jaw jerk is

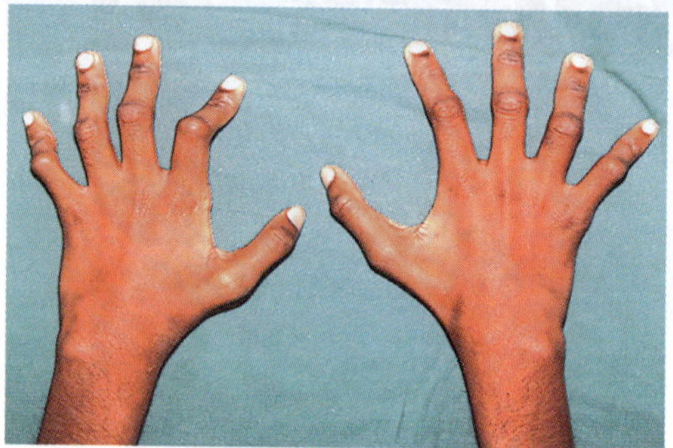

Fig. 208.2: Complete claw hand. ***Note:*** Wasting of the small muscles of the hand and clawing due to affection of the C8T1 motor neurons

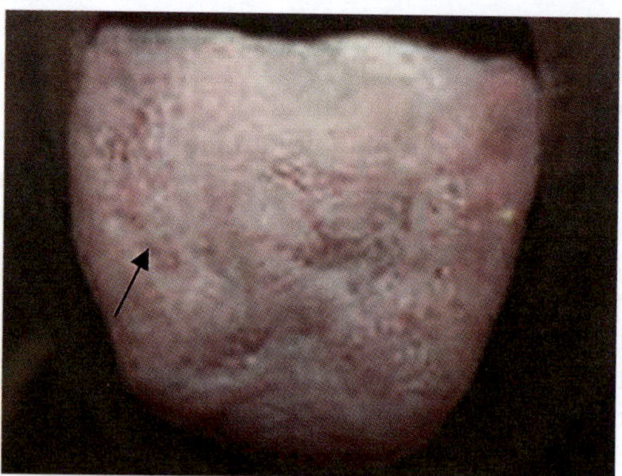

Fig. 208.3: Atrophy of the tongue in ALS due to involvement of hypoglossal nucleus. ***Note:*** The furrows on the mucous membrane due to loss of bulk of the muscle (arrow)

Box 208.1: The El Escorial research diagnostic criteria is used for diagnosis of ALS

Revised El Escorial Criteria 2000
To make diagnosis of ALS, there should be clinical or electrophysiologic evidence of progression within the region or other regions as well as exclusion of ALS-mimics by EMG, appropriate imaging and laboratory studies
Definite ALS: UMN and LMN signs in three regions
Probable ALS: UMN and LMN signs in two regions with some UMN signs rostral to LMN signs
Probable laboratory supported ALS: UMN and LMN signs or only UMN signs in one region with evidence by EMG of degeneration in two regions
Possible ALS: UMN and LMN signs in one region or UMN signs in at least two regions.

Abbreviations: ALS = Amyotrophic lateral sclerosis; EMG = Electromyogram; UMN = Upper motor neuron; LMN = Lower motor neuron

---

exaggerated. The plantar responses are bilaterally extensor indicating UMN lesion. Sensations and mental functions are unaffected. Oculomotor nuclei are spared for some unknown reason. Autonomic functions such as micturition and defecation remain intact, for considerable periods. Speech is affected early. Spastic dysarthria develops with time. In the advanced case, the picture is of extreme wasting. Death is due to respiratory infection, aspiration pneumonia, nutritional inadequacy or cardiovascular causes.

Course and Prognosis

The course is one of relentless progression to produce severe disability and death in 2.5–3.5 years. Known prognostic factors include age, site of initial involvement, extent and severity of wasting, severity of bulbar muscle dysfunction and respiratory functions. Those with bulbar onset have a median survival of 2.5 years whereas those with onset in the limbs have a lifespan of 3.5–13 years. Younger patients survive longer.

Diagnostic Criteria in ALS

ALS remains a clinical diagnosis (Box 208.1).

PROGRESSIVE MUSCULAR ATROPHY (PMA)

This is the purely LMN type of MND, males are more affected than females. Five-year survival is seen in 72% patients. This form generally runs in families. Mutation in SOD gene is commonly associated. Lesions may or may not be symmetrical. Initial disease starts in proximal arms with twitching and cramp like pains. There is selective LMN degeneration leading to weakness and wasting in one upper extremity (75%) or one lower extremity (25%) and this becomes generalized over a period of 3–5 years. Fasciculations are present but less common. Despite the marked wasting, reflexes are preserved normally or they may even be brisk, even though there will be no other signs of UMN involvement.

PROGRESSIVE BULBAR PALSY (PBP)

This is the most serious form of MND since it terminates life within a period of 1 year. There is LMN affection of the lower cranial muscles as evidenced by wasting of the muscles and fasciculation of the tongue, muscles of mastication and face. Patient presents with difficulty in pronouncing linguals, labials, dentals and palatals, which progressively deteriorates to anarthria. Later, pharyngeal muscles, masticatory muscles, phonatory and deglutatory muscles become involved. Lower facial muscles become involved. There is no emotional lability. Emaciation develops rapidly. The jaw reflex is normal or absent. Eventually, respiratory muscles become involved. A purely heredofamilial form of trinucleotide repeat expansion-related type is called ***Kennedy's syndrome***.

PRIMARY LATERAL SCLEROSIS (PLS)

It is an uncommon form of MND in which signs of UMN lesion develop over the limbs. Usually, it starts in the 5th or 6th decade in the lower limbs without any sensory symptoms. Corticospinal tract symptoms dominate. These signs may persist for many years before the development of bulbar or LMN signs. Disease progression varies between patients. Fifty percent die within 3 years of onset of symptoms. Majority of deaths is due to respiratory failure.

PLS has to be differentiated from primary progressive multiple sclerosis, tropical spastic paraplegia, human immunodeficiency virus (HIV) myelopathy, B_{12} deficiency and others.

VULPIAN-BERNHARDT SYNDROME OR PROGRESSIVE AMYOTROPHIC BRACHIAL DIPLEGIA

This affects males more; the male:female ratio is 9:1. This presents with localized wasting and weakness of one arm which gradually evolves into bilateral upper limb weakness and wasting. Usually, UMN signs develop in the legs in about 70% of the patients (Table 208.1).

PSEUDOPOLYNEURITIC FORM OF ALS

Usually, this presents with unilateral LMN foot drop, and progresses proximally and spreads to the other leg.

Table 208.1: Operational definition of flail arm and flail leg syndrome		
Features	**Flail arm syndrome**	**Flail leg syndrome**
Inclusion criteria	• Proximal upper limb • Brisk jerks	• Distal lower limb • Brisk jerks
Exclusion criteria	• Bulbar involvement in 12 months	• Upper limbs, respiratory and bulbar in 12 months
	• Hypertonia	• Hypertonia, clonus
	• Distal without proximal	• Proximal without distal

- Electromyography shows fibrillation potentials, positive sharp waves and abnormal recruitment.
- Magnetic resonance imaging (MRI) may show hyperintensities of bilateral corticospinal tracts, bilaterally extending from internal capsule to brainstem wine glass appearance on coronal T2/FLAIR images.
- Serial MRIs show progressive atrophy of premotor, parietal and primary sensorimotor cortex with sparing of temporal and occipital lobes and cerebellum.

FAMILIAL ALS

- Clinical phenotype indistinguishable from sporadic ALS, clinically it resembles sporadic ALS
- Symptoms include progressive muscular weakness and stiffness with sparing of eye movements and sphincters
- Sensory symptoms occurring without physical signs are not uncommon. Several types are distinguishable.

Type 1

ALS 1: Copper/zinc (Cu/Zn) SOD1 mutation seen in 2% of cases SOD mutations may be found in absence of family history. They are associated with predominantly LMN pattern of ALS. Nearly, all are associated with poor prognosis with survival less than 3 years. Extra motor symptoms such as paresthesiae, shooting pains, bladder disturbance or autonomic failure may occur.

Type 2

This is a form of juvenile onset autosomal recessive motor neuron disorder first identified in Tunisian families, linkage has been demonstrated to chromosome 2q33. The gene gives rise to a novel protein alsin. These patients had predominantly upper MND. Onset is in the 1st or 2nd decade of life.

Type 3

The phenotype is that of classic ALS without any atypical features. Onset is at around 45 years of age with mean survival for 5 years. Lower limbs are affected more. There is linkage to chromosome 18.

Type 4

This is linked to chromosome 9q34 with senataxin gene mutation. It is an autosomal dominant juvenile onset slowly progressive disorder. Onset is before 25 years with distal weakness and amyotrophy with UMN signs. Bulbar muscles are spared; life expectancy is normal.

Type 5

This is an autosomal recessive disease, linked to chromosome 15. Onset is between 8 and 18 years of age with progressive gait disturbance. Significant amyotrophy occurs with exaggerated reflexes. The patient presents with LMN features. After 3–4 years, they develop dysarthria and bulbar involvement. Survival is between 10 and 25 years from symptom onset.

Types 6 and 7

This is autosomal dominant adult onset ALS, linked to chromosome 16q12. Clinical phenotype is that of classic limb onset ALS with rapid progression. ALS 7 is typical ALS, linked to chromosome 20p13.

Type 8

Linkage with chromosome 20q13, vesicle-associated membrane protein-associated protein B/C (VAPB) mutation. Age of onset is between 31 and 45 years. Presentation is with LMN disorder with very slow rate of progression.

MADRAS MND

This was first recognized in South India in 1970 by Jegannathan and Arjundhas at Government General Hospital Madras (presently Chennai). Patients presented with bulbar and limb involvement, brisk jerks, extensor plantar response and deafness. Males are more affected and the disease starts around the 2nd or 3rd decade. Weakness and wasting may be uni- or bilateral, proximal or distal and asymmetrical. Bulbar muscles may be involved in 60% of cases. Unilateral or bilateral sensorineural deafness, younger age of onset with ALS-like features and a benign course are characteristic of this condition. Indian workers have incriminated defects of glucose utilization by spinal motor neurons to have a causative role (Valmikinathan). Although this condition was initially described in patients from Madras in South India, similar cases are now encountered in many parts of India.

MONOMELIC ATROPHY

This condition tends to remain confined to one limb. Males are more affected than females and distal muscles are more affected than proximal. This is a nonfamilial, insidiously progressive condition, usually affecting adolescents and adults. It is characterized by weakness, wasting and fasciculations restricted only to one extremity, either upper or lower. In some cases, the involvement may be only focal or segmental in one extremity, focal or segmental MND. UMN signs are usually absent. The course is benign. Although clinically one limb is affected, electromyographically subclinical involvement of LMNs in other limb muscles may be evident. A small percentage may become generalized.

BROWN-VIALETTO-VAN-LAERE (BVVL) SYNDROME

This has a variable onset and course. Deafness and pontobulbar features are seen.

FAZIO-LONDE SYNDROME

This has early onset with rapidly progressive course. Bulbar involvement with respiratory manifestations predominates.

ALS FRONTO-TEMPORAL LOBAR DEGENERATION (FLTD) COMPLEX AND ALS-PARKINSONISM DEMENTIA-COMPLEX-OF-GUAM

ALS type of MND can be associated with involvement of other parts of the neuraxis. These are called ALS plus syndromes. When it shows features of frontal lobe dysfunction, it is called fronto-temporal lobar degeneration (FTLD). When it is associated with Parkinson's disease it is called ALS-PD. When features of both ALS-PD and FTLD occur together it is called ALS dementia complex.

The overlap between dementia and ALS is demonstrable. FTLD with ubiquitinated inclusions occurs in 50% of cases.

Several genes, chromosome 9p, chromosome 17 (progranulin) and others have been linked to FTLD-U (ubiquitinated inclusions). TARDBP mutations are found in some cases of autosomal dominant ALS, causing TDP 43 proteinopathy.

ALS-PARKINSONISM DEMENTIA COMPLEX

There is a significant concentration of ALS and related Parkinsonism-dementia (PD) features among the Chamorro people on Guam. The age of onset 20–72 years. The findings in a series of 1,153 patients with ALS (Nalini, et al.) are as follows

Male:female ratio 3:1. Mean age of onset was 46.2 ± 14.1 years, limb onset group (43.7 ± 14.1 years) and bulbar onset group was 52.8 ± 11.6 years. 33.7% had onset of illness below 40 years. The mean time from onset of symptom to diagnosis was 17.7 ± 20.7 months. The site of onset was limbs in 72.9% (2/3 in the upper limb and 1/3 in the lower limb) and bulbar muscles in 27%. Median survival duration 114.83 ± 25.9 months in both sexes (55.9 ± 2.9 for bulbar onset disease and 177.9 ± 3.2 months for limb onset type). Younger patients who developed the disease lived longer. The mean age at death was 52.95 years (range 25.7–82.6).

Spinal Muscular Atrophy

These are motor neuronopathies with a definite pattern of inheritance. These are pure anterior horn cell degenerations with a definite genetic pattern of inheritance and hence, can be considered as hereditary motor neuronopathies. They are subdivided into various types depending on the pattern of muscle involvement, age of onset and mode of genetic transmission (Table 208.2).

Investigations

These are mainly aimed at excluding treatable causes. Nerve conduction studies and electromyography (EMG) are essential in all patients. Infections, toxins, paraproteinemia, paraneoplastic, endocrine, nutritional, inherited, metabolic, vascular and compressive problems have to be excluded when ever indicated.

Management

At present, none of the known modalities arrest the progress of the disease. Palliative measures include physiotherapy, use of orthotic devices to help functioning of the limbs and treatment of intercurrent illness and ventilatory support.

Table 208.2: Spinal muscular atrophy (SMA) classification based on age of onset and maximum motor function achieved

SMA 0–AR	Onset *in utero*; needs respiratory support at birth; fatal at birth if not given respiratory support
SMA 1–AR	Werdnig-Hoffmann disease; onset from birth to 6 months; sits with support; death by 2 years
SMA 2–AR	Intermediate SMA; onset between 6 and 18 months; sits independently; no walking; survives till adulthood
SMA 3–AR	Kugelberg-Welander syndrome; onset above 18 months; walks independently; survives into adulthood
SMA 4–AR/ AD	Adult onset SMA; onset after 5 years; mostly after 30 years; walks normally; slow progression; proximal and distal

Abbreviations: AR = Autosomal recessive; AD = Autosomal dominant

Disease modifying treatments have been tried to give symptoms relief. These include—antiexcitotoxins (riluzole), antioxidants, antiviral agents and immuno-modulation based on some observational studies, but none is found to be effective.

Symptom Management

Sialorrhea: Drooling of saliva which may be distressing.

Anticholinergic medications are generally tried. These include—atropine, hyoscine, amitriptyline and glycopyr-rolate. Botulinum toxin injection into parotid gland, low-dose radiation and posterior transposition of parotid glands are other options.

Pseudobulbar Features

They can be partly relieved by a combination of dextro-methorphan/quinidine, or fluoxetine 200 mg bd, with some benefit.

Fatigue

This may respond to modafinil in a dose of 200–400 mg once a day can be tried. Cramps can be reduced by admini-stration of antiepileptic drugs like gabapentin, carbama-zepine, phenytoin vitamin E (400 mg bd) and riluzole.

Spasticity

Exercise or medication is poorly effective. Baclofen, tiza-nidine and dantrolene are some drugs used for spasticity depression, anxiety, insomnia also need care.

Doses of Drugs

The recommended dose of provigil (modafinil) is 200–400 mg given once a day. Usual adult dose for ALS are:

- ***Riluzole:*** 50 mg orally every 12 hours before food
- ***Tizanidine:*** Usual adult dose for muscle spasm
- ***Initial dose:*** 4 mg orally every 6–8 hours (maximum of 3 doses in 24 hours). Dose may be increased in 2–4 mg steps to optimum effect and tolerance
- ***Maintenance dose:*** 8 mg orally every 6–8 hours (maximum of 3 doses in 24 hours)
- ***Maximum dose:*** 3 doses in 24 hours; 12 mg per dose; 36 mg per day
- ***Approved indication:*** For the acute and intermittent management of increased muscle tone associated with spasticity.

Dantrolene

For use in controlling the manifestations of clinical spas-ticity resulting from UMN disorders:

- 25 mg orally once daily for 7 days, then
- 25 mg three times a day for 7 days, then
- 50 mg three times a day for 7 days, then
- 100 mg three times a day.

Nutrition needs special care with percutaneous endoscopic gastrostomy. Noninvasive ventilation to avoid nocturnal hypoventilation and mechanical removal and suction for pooling of saliva are temporarily useful.

CHAPTER
209

Diseases of the Cerebellum

Anand Kumar, Arun N Babu

Chapter Summary

- General Considerations
- Heredofamilial Ataxias
- Hereditary Ataxias
- Spinocerebellar Ataxia (SCA)
- Friedreich's Ataxia
- Cerebellar Ataxias Responsive to Specific Therapy
  - Acute Recurrent Ataxia
  - Chronic Progressive Ataxia
  - Cerebrotendinous Xanthamatosis
  - Von Hippel-Lindau Syndrome
  - Ataxia Telangiectasia
  - Hereditary Spastic Paraplegia
  - Cerebellar Tumors
  - Inflammatory Lesions of the Cerebellum
  - Vascular Lesions of the Cerebellum
- Other Causes of Cerebellar Dysfunction

GENERAL CONSIDERATIONS

The cerebellum is a part of the brain posterior to the brainstem. It lies in the posterior cranial fossa, separated from the cerebrum by a fold of dura called the ***tentorium cerebelli***. The cerebellum has two hemisphere connected by the vermis in the midline. The major function is motor coordination. The outer gray matter, the cerebellar cortex contains the nerve cell bodies. The cortex has many small sulci and gyri that increase the total surface area. There are also four collections of deep nuclei in each hemisphere—dentate, emboliform, globose and fastigial.

The cerebellum is connected to the brainstem by three peduncles (superior, middle and inferior) through which afferent and efferent fibers connect to various parts of the brain and spinal cord. Histologically, the cerebellar cortex consists of the;

- Outermost molecular layer
- Middle Purkinje cell layer
- Inner granular layer.

Functionally, the cerebellum is the great comparator of the brain. A predominant function appears to be to constantly monitor peripheral activity and compare this to the intended activity by the cerebral motor cortices. For this, the cerebellum has extensive connections both from

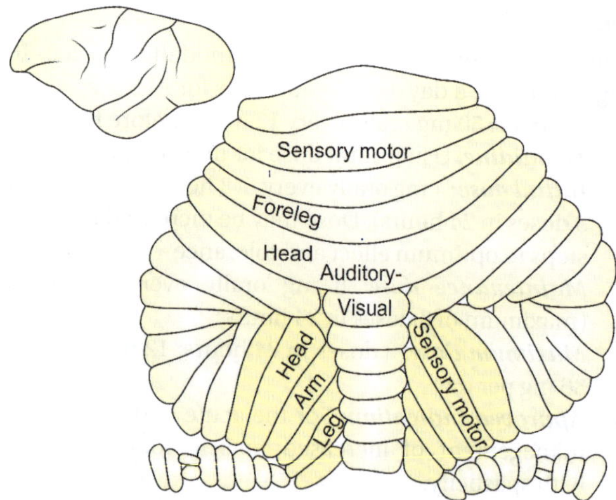

Fig. 209.1: Representation of the body on cerebellar cortex

peripheral sensory pathways as well as to and from motor areas in the cerebral cortex (Fig. 209.1). Functions include:

- Coordination of voluntary and reflex movements
- Modulation of muscle tone
- Maintenance of body posture.

The *vermis* controls the midline structures of the body and trunk, whereas the lateral hemispheres control the limbs of the same side. The hemispheres are functionally and anatomically divided into three lobes:

1. *Anterior lobe*—functionally related to the gross movements of heads and neck
2. *Middle lobe*—related to fine voluntary movements
3. *Flocculonodular lobe*—related to equilibration.

Cerebellar Homunculus

Blood supply is derived from three pairs of arteries:

1. Superior cerebellar arteries (from basilar artery)
2. Anterior inferior cerebellar arteries (from the basilar artery)
3. Posterior inferior cerebellar arteries (from vertebral arteries).

The clinical features of cerebellar disease and testing for cerebellar function are described in Ch 193 and 194.

Acute lesions of the cerebellar system produce sudden, severe and disabling symptoms. Chronic lesions lead to insidious deterioration of function.

HEREDOFAMILIAL ATAXIAS

These include a wide spectrum of degenerative diseases which are progressive, familial and manifesting early in life, with their main brunt on the cerebellar pathways. Variable degrees of involvement of the spinal cord, brainstem and cranial nerves also occur. The exact etiology is not known but recent evidence points to defects in mitochondrial energy systems and pyruvate metabolism as probably important factors. Hereditary ataxias are of many types, the most common being Friedreich's ataxia.

HEREDITARY ATAXIAS

They are broadly defined by mode of inheritance—autosomal dominant, autosomal recessive or X-linked. With better understanding of the molecular basis and pathogenesis of these diseases, other classification schemes

Table 209.1: Autosomal dominant ataxias—Harding's classification

Type	Clinical phenotype	Common genotype
ADCA I	Cerebellar ataxia plus other symptoms: Extrapyramidal symptoms, neuropathy	SCA 1, 2, 3, 4, 12, 17, 21, 23 and 25
ADCA II	Cerebellar ataxia plus retinal degeneration	SCA 7
ADCA III	Cerebellar ataxia—pure	SCA 5, 6, 8, 10, 11, 14, 15, 16 and 22

Abbreviations: ADCA = Autosomal dominant cerebellar ataxias; SCA = Spinocerebellar ataxia

have been suggested. These classifications are based on the disorders of trinucleotide repeat expansions or toxic *gain of function* due to abnormal proteins and accumulation of polyglutamine inclusions, channelopathies, mitochondrial dysfunction, defective deoxyribonucleic acid (DNA) repair and metabolic disorders. Autosomal dominant cerebellar ataxias (ADCA) were initially classified according to phenotype and accompanying signs by Harding, as given in Table 209.1. Genetic advances have led to modification of these criteria as specific genes and mutations responsible for cerebellar ataxias have been discovered.

SPINOCEREBELLAR ATAXIA (SCA)

It is characterized by cerebellar ataxia, manifesting with gait ataxia, dysarthria, slow saccades, nystagmus, corticospinal tract signs, neuropathy and later on opthalmoplegia and bulbar dysfunction (dysphagia and tongue fasciculations). Extrapyramidal signs may be seen but cognitive deficits are not typically present. Age of onset varies from adolescence to late adulthood with the average age of onset around the 3rd and 4th decades. SCA1 is due to an expansion of an unstable CAG trinucleotide repeat on chromosome 6p23.

FRIEDREICH'S ATAXIA

This is an autosomal recessive disorder. Prevalence in European population is 1/50,000. The locus of genetic defect is on chromosome 9. There is a mutation on the gene encoding a protein called *frataxin*.

Frataxin is a mitochondrial protein taking part in energy metabolism. The defect in frataxin leads to abnormal accumulation of iron in the mitochondria followed by cell death. There is neuronal loss in the motor and sensory systems.

Pathology

There is degeneration of the spinocerebellar tracts, posterior columns, Clarke's columns and pyramidal tracts. Cardiac involvement occurs in many, taking the form of interstitial myocarditis and conduction defects.

Clinical Features

The onset is in the 1st or 2nd decade of life. Cardinal features of Friedreich's ataxia include ataxia of all four limbs, cerebellar dysarthria, areflexia in the lower limbs, sensory loss and pyramidal signs. Earliest manifestations are ankle areflexia and gait ataxia due to loss of posterior column sensations and cerebellar dysfunction. Later, other signs of cerebellar disease and posterior column dysfunction are evident. Ankle jerks are lost earlier than the knee jerks. Loss of vibration and proprioceptive sensations are more evident in the lower limbs. Skeletal deformities such as kyphoscoliosis and pes cavus (increased convexity of the arch of the foot) are common. Optic atrophy and muscle wasting may develop in some cases. Diabetes develops in 10% of cases. Features of cardiomyopathy may develop in those with cardiac involvement.

Diagnosis

Diagnosis has been mainly clinical. Nowadays, specific blood tests are commercially available, but often expensive. Insidious onset of ataxia with signs of cerebellar and posterior column dysfunction, absence of ankle jerks, and presence of Babinski's sign in the first 2 decades of life should suggest this diagnosis. Associated congenital defects such as kyphoscoliosis and pes cavus are further suggestive. Presence of the disease or other stigmata in family members strengthens the diagnosis. Relatives of the patient may show abnormalities such as pes cavus, kyphoscoliosis, loss of ankle jerks, nystagmus or upper motor neuron signs.

Several neurological disorders may resemble Friedreich's ataxia superficially. These include multiple sclerosis, other forms of ataxias, craniovertebral junction anomalies, intracranial tumors, tabes dorsalis and diabetic neuropathy.

Course and Prognosis

The diseases progresses steadily over several years, but rate of progression may vary widely between cases. In many cases considerable disability in gait, speech and daily activities develop though lifespan is not shortened. In some case, interstitial myocardial fibrosis and cardiac conduction defects may occur and account for premature death.

Treatment

Idebenone is a new agent that has recently been found to be beneficial to some extent. Physiotherapy to improve coordination is beneficial. Occupational therapy to rehabilitate these patients is to be instituted early.

CEREBELLAR ATAXIAS RESPONSIVE TO SPECIFIC THERAPY

Most of these have a metabolic abnormality caused by congenital or acquired defect of enzymes which take part in the metabolism of amino acids.

These disorders usually present in early life but can also manifest in later life. The presentation can be acute or recurrent and static or progressive.

Acute Recurrent Ataxia

Familial episodic ataxia is an autosomal dominant disorder of uncertain etiology.

Clinical features include paroxysmal ataxia, nausea and vertigo. There are two types—type 2 is more common. Attacks begin in late childhood or adolescence and are precipitated by stress, exertion and fatigue. Duration is from hours to days. The acute episodes may be superimposed on a mild form of chronic progressive truncal ataxia. The disease predominantly affects the vestibulocerebellum. Diagnosis is made by the episodic nature of attacks, positive family history and magnetic resonance imaging (MRI) evidence of cerebellar vermis atrophy. Therapy is with acetazolamide which reduces the frequency and severity of episodic ataxia. Type 1 is earlier in onset with briefer attacks and absence of signs between attacks. Myokymia of the hands and face can occur.

Maple Syrup Urine Disease (MSUD)

It is an autosomal recessive disorder due to a deficiency of branched chain ketoacid dehydrogenase. The intermittent form of MSUD can present with episodic ataxia and encephalopathy. Infection and excess dietary protein precipitate attacks and diagnosis is established by finding increased levels of branched chain aminoacids and ketoacids in plasma and urine. Dietary restriction of branched chain amino acids and use of thiamine are the modes of treatment.

Hartnup Disease

It is an autosomal recessive disorder resulting from defective transfer of neutral amino acids. Affected individuals present with episodic ataxia, personality change and pellagra-like skin rashes. There is an increased excretion of neutral amino acids and indole products in the urine. **Treatment** is by giving a high protein diet and nicotinamide.

Multiple Carboxylase Deficiency

It is an autosomal recessive disorder due to deficiency of biotinidase (biotine recycling enzyme) or biotin containing carboxylase. The disorder often presents in the first 6 months of life with seizures, alopecia and decreased hearing. Milder forms may present in later life. **Diagnosis** is by finding reduced levels of biotin in serum and urine and lactic acidemia. **Treatment** is oral biotin 10 mg/day.

Urea Cycle Disorders

They are present in infancy with ataxia, seizures, vomiting and varying levels of altered sensorium. They are autosomal recessive disorders with the exception of ornithine transcarbamylase deficiency which is X-linked. Altered function of several enzymes involved in the urea cycle can present with increased levels of ammonia and abnormality in levels of specific amino acids. Insulin-glucose regimen, sodium benzoate and sodium phenylacetate are used to bring down ammonia. Severe cases may require dialysis.

Chronic Progressive Ataxia
Abetalipoproteinemia

It is an autosomal recessive disorder presenting with steatorrhea in infancy followed a few years later by ataxia, peripheral neuropathy and retinitis pigmentosa. There is absence of apolipoprotein B resulting in fat malabsorption and deficiency of vitamins A, E and K. Investigations reveal acanthocytes in the peripheral smear, low serum cholesterol and triglycerides, and absence of apolipoprotein in serum. **Treatment** is by giving vitamins A, E and K. Diet should be low in long chain fatty acids.

Ataxia due to Vitamin E Deficiency

This is an autosomal recessive disorder presenting in the 2nd decade of life with progressive ataxia, areflexia and proprioceptive loss. **Diagnosis** is made by finding low serum levels of vitamin E and treatment is vitamin E supplementation.

Refsum's disease is an autosomal recessive disorder due to deficiency of the enzyme phytanic acid alpha hydroxylase. Ataxia, polyneuropathy, retinitis pigmentosa and deafness are the common clinical manifestations. Phytanic acids levels are increased in blood and urine. **Treatment** is by giving a diet low in phytanic acid. During acute exacerbations, plasmapheresis may be required.

Cerebrotendinous Xanthamatosis

This is an autosomal recessive disorder due to deficiency of chenodeoxycholic acid which is necessary for the synthesis of bile acids. Presentation is in adolescence or early childhood with ataxia, spasticity, neuropathy and dementia. **Diagnosis** is suggested by the typical association of tendinous xanthomas and cataract. Serum cholesterol level is increased and treatment is by giving chenodeoxycholic acid.

Wilson's Disease

Wilson's disease, an abnormality of copper metabolism, may be present with cerebellar ataxia (*See* Section 10, Ch 94). This is a treatable condition that is fatal if undiagnosed, so it should always be suspected in any case of ataxia and tremors.

Von Hippel-Lindau Syndrome

It is an autosomal dominant disorder presenting with hemangioblastoma of the cerebellum and angioma of the retina. Other associations include renal cell carcinoma, renal and pancreatic cysts, phenochromocytomas and polycythemia.

Ataxia Telangiectasia

Syn: Madame-Louis-Bar syndrome

This is an autosomal recessive condition occurring in children and manifesting by the age of 10 years. The features are cerebellar ataxia, wasting of leg muscles and areflexia. The bulbar conjunctiva shows telangiectasia. There is deficiency of immunoglobulins and this leads to repeated sinopulmonary infections. The condition is associated with a poor prognosis.

Hereditary Spastic Paraplegia

In this form, the predominant lesion is degeneration of the pyramidal tracts with minor involvement of the spinocerebellar tracts and posterior columns. It is inherited as autosomal dominant disorder and the disease manifests clinically between 3 and 15 years of age. In the fully evolved form, the picture is one of spastic paraplegia with less weakness of the upper limbs, dysarthria and pseudobulbar palsy.

Cerebellar Tumors

The cerebellum may be seated of the tumors such as medulloblastoma, cystic astrocytoma, and oligoden-droglioma, which are all more common in children. Usually, medulloblastoma affects the midline structures and astrocytoma usually affects the lateral hemispheres. Hemangioblastoma and metastatic tumors usually occur in adults.

Inflammatory Lesions of the Cerebellum

The cerebellum may be involved in viral and bacterial meningoencephalitis, chickenpox and postvaccinial, postinfectious or idiopathic inflammatory cerebellitis. Cerebellar abscess may occur as a complication of otitis media. Tuberculomas are not uncommon in the cerebellum, especially in children.

Vascular Lesions of the Cerebellum

Cerebellum is the seat of hemorrhage in 5–10% of all hemorrhagic strokes occurring in hypertension. The patient presents with headache, neck rigidity, nystagmus, vomiting and ataxia. If the bleeding increases or edema develops, other features such as ocular palsy, loss of sensation in the trigeminal territory, facial palsy and coma may set in surgical evacuation of the clot is life-saving. If left untreated, 50% die within a week.

Occlusive lesions of the vertebrobasilar system can lead to cerebellar infarction with edema.

OTHER CAUSES OF CEREBELLAR DYSFUNCTION

Alcoholism: Acute alcoholic bouts may lead to ataxia, nystagmus and dysarthria. Cerebellar degeneration as a complication of chronic alcoholism results in ataxia of gait and stance, often without nystagmus and dysarthria.

Multiple sclerosis: The cerebellum and its connections are affected in multiple sclerosis.

Subacute cerebellar cortical degeneration: This may occur as a paraneoplastic complication of malignancy, especially bronchogenic carcinoma. Anti-Hu antibodies may be detected in blood. The cerebellar lesion manifests as ataxia, dysarthria, rarely nystagmus, depression of tendon reflexes and Babinski's sign.

Metabolic disturbance: Cerebellar ataxia may occur in hypoglycemia, hypothyroidism, hypoxia and hyper-thermia. In the early stages, it is reversible.

Drugs: Drugs like phenytoin and most anticonvulsants may lead to reversible cerebellar disturbances such as dysarthria, ataxia and nystagmus. In advanced cases, the Purkinje cells may show degeneration and the condition becomes irreversible.

Nutritional deficiencies: Thiamine and niacin deficiency (pellagra) produce cerebellar deficits similar to chronic alcoholism.

Developmental anomalies: Arnold-Chiari malformation, basilar invagination, Dandy-Walker cysts and cerebellar aplasia cause cerebellar dysfunction along with other deficits.

CHAPTER
210 Diseases of Spinal Cord, Nerve Roots and Plexuses

SR Chandra, CS Vidhya Annapoorni, Thomas Gregor Issac, KV Krishna Das

Chapter Summary

- General Considerations
- Blood Supply and Venous Drainage
- Diseases and Symptomatology of Affection of Particular Structures
  - Lesions of Conus Medullaris and Cauda Equina
- Compressive Myelopathy
- Spinal Cord Syndromes
  - Anterior Spinal Artery Syndrome
- Spinal Arteriovenous Malformations
- Infectious and Inflammatory Myelopathies
  - Transverse Myelitis
- Necrotizing Myelopathy
  - Hereditary Myelopathies
  - Myelopathy due to Contrast Agents
  - Spinal Epidural Abscess
  - Hematomyelia
  - Craniovertebral Junction Anomalies
  - Interpretation of Spine X-ray
  - Syringomyelia
  - Spinal Shock
  - Paraplegia in Flexion
  - Paraplegia in Extension
    - Cerebral Paraplegia
  - Radiculopathies and Plexopathies
  - Brachial Plexus
  - Lumbosacral Plexus

GENERAL CONSIDERATIONS

Spinal cord starts from the end of medulla and stops at conus medullaris. At birth, conus is at L3 level and at L1 level in adult. The cord is 45 cm in length, weighs 30 g and has 31 segments. There are 8 cervical, 12 thoracic, 5 lumbar, 5 sacral and 1 coccygeal segments. There is one anteromedian, one posteromedian and two anterolateral and posterolateral fissures. It is covered by pia mater which is fibrous. Close septae penetrate into the substance of spinal cord. On either side, thick pia forms the ligamentum denticulatum suspending it in the dural sheath.

Arachnoid mater of the spinal cord continues with the arachnoid mater of the brain and ends at filum terminale at the lower end of S2. Subarachnoid space contains cerebrospinal fluid (CSF). Dura is outermost, double layered, except at foramen magnum. It ends at S2. The extradural space contains external vertebral venous plexus. The spinal cord contains gray matter inside and white matter outside. The size of the gray matter depends on the number of muscles it supplies, e.g. cervical and lumbar enlargements. Ventral root comes out of the anterolateral sulcus and dorsal root from the dorsolateral sulcus. The gray column consists of Rexed laminae I–X. *Rexed laminae* comprise a system of 10 layers of gray

matter (I-X), identified in the early 1950s by **Bror Rexed** to label portions of the gray columns of the spinal cord. Anterior gray column has a medial group for neck and trunk muscles, central group for diaphragm at C3 to C5, lateromedial group for limb muscles. Posterior group has substantia gelatinosa of Rolandi which is seen throughout spinal cord and subserves pain, touch and temperature. Next is nucleus proprius, seen throughout and it is concerned with proprioception. There is the Clarke's column which extends from C8 to L3 which is the site of origin of spinocerebellar pathways. Next is the visceral afferent nucleus. Then, the intermediolateral gray column which contains preganglionic sympathetic fibers from D1 to L2 and parasympathetic fibers from S2 to S4. The white matter consists of anterior column, lateral column and posterior column. The muscles supplied by a spinal segment are called *myotome* and the skin supplied is called *dermatome*.

The sensory and motor tracts passing through spinal cord are shown in Table 210.1 and Figure 210.1. The

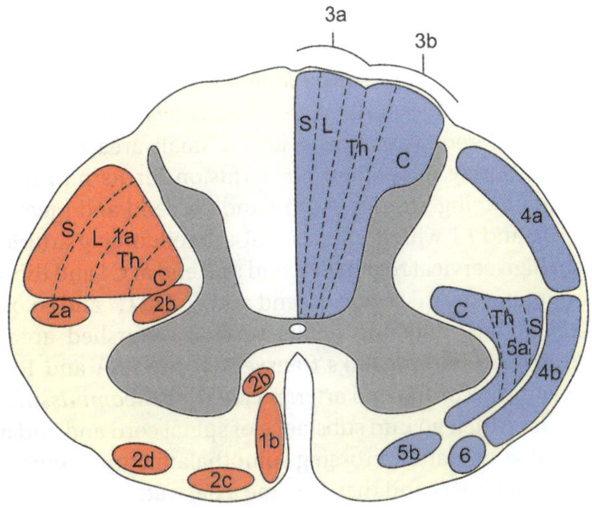

Fig. 210.1: Section of spinal cord

Motor and decending (efferent) pathways (left, red)
1. Pyramidal Tracts
1a. Lateral corticospinal tract
1b. Anterior Corticospinal tract
2. Extrapyramidal Tracts
2a. Rubrospinal tract
2b. Reticulospinal tract
2c. Vestibulospinal tract
2d. Olivospinal tract

Sensory and ascending (afferent) pathways (right, red)
3. Dorsal column Medical Lemniscus System
3a. Gracile fasciculus
3b. Cuneate fasciculus
4. Spinocerebellar Tracts
4a. Posterior spinocerebellar tract
4b. Anterior spinocerebellar tract
5. Anterolateral system
5a. Lateral spinothalamic tract
5b. Anterior spinothalamic tract
6. Spino-olivary fibers

Abbreviations: C = Cervical; L = Lumbar; Th = Thoracic; S = Sacral

Table 210.1: Tracts of the spinal cord

Tract	Location in spinal cord	Function
Fasciculus gracilis	Dorsal column	Proprioception, vibration sense, touch
Fasciculus cuneatus	Posterior column	Rotation, touch, vibration
Pyramidal	Lateral column deep and anteromedial	Voluntary muscle contraction
Lateral spinothalamic	Ventrolateral column	Pain and temperature
Anterior spinothalamic	Anterior column	Touch
Spinocerebellar	Lateral column -superficial	Muscle position, tone

pathway for bladder and bowel control is located in lateral column.

Fibers in the spinal cord tracts are arranged in a specific pattern called laminations. In dorsal columns, sacral fibers are medially placed while thoracic and cervical fibers are arranged more laterally. In lateral spinothalamic and pyramidal tracts, arrangement of fibers is reverse, sacral fibers being more lateral and cervical fibers medial.

BLOOD SUPPLY AND VENOUS DRAINAGE

The anterior and posterior spinal arteries (ASA and PSA) arise from vertebral artery and reinforced after C4 by ascending cervical, inferior thyroid, intercostals, lumbar, iliolumbar, lateral sacral arteries and others. ASA supplies the whole cord except the posterior column which is supplied by PSA. The *arteria* cervicalis magna at cervical level and *Adam kiewies artery* at D10 to L3 supply the whole cord. Watershed zones are the areas where different vessels end and a small area of spinal cord is purely dependent on perfusion for its nutrition. The reinforcing arteries ascend and descend and meet at C4, D4 and L1 which implies that the reinforcing arteries from high cervical region descend and end at C4 and those from upper dorsal region ascend and end at C4 and so on, making these meeting points vertical watershed areas. The *arteria corona* links transversely the ASA and PSA from arteria corona end arteries called *sulcocommissural arteries* which go into substance of spinal cord and end at ventral gray matter, crossing spinothalamic tract, medial pyramidal fibers and they become axial watershed zones.

There are six venous channels which have no valves and which are a low-pressure system. They have close access to systemic veins like azygos, hemiazygos and pelvic veins. They ascend to join the intracranial venous sinuses.

As there are seven cervical vertebrae but eight spinal segments in the cervical region and spinal cord stops at L1 vertebral level; vertebral number and spinal segments do not correspond to each other. They have a special relationship which is given below.

For getting the corresponding spinal segment add 1 to cervical vertebrae, add 2 to upper 6 thoracic, add 3 to T7 to T9 vertebrae, D10 corresponds to L1 and 2; D11 corresponds to L3 and 4; D12 corresponds to L5 and L1 to sacral and coccygeal segments.

DISEASES AND SYMPTOMATOLOGY OF AFFECTION OF PARTICULAR STRUCTURES

Lesions can be compressive, degenerative, vascular, toxic, demyelinative, infective, nutritional and others. The common features of spinal cord disease are due to involvement of various structures indirectly or directly. Corticospinal tract involvement produces spasticity, exaggerated deep tendon reflexes and diminished superficial reflexes below the lesion, extensor plantar response and dragging type of gait. Involvement of bladder fibers which travels along this tract can produce:

- Precipitancy or inability to control if inhibitory fibers are involved
- Hesitancy characterized by difficulty in initiating micturition if facilitatory fibers are involved
- *Automatic bladder:* If both are involved in which the patient has no control over initiation of micturition and bladder starts emptying when about 300 mL of urine accumulates. Patient cannot stop the act at will. At the end, patient has incomplete emptying causing tendency to double void and also has postvoiding dribbling.

Posterior column involvement presents with irritative features like **Lhermitte's, sign** characterized by shock-like sensation down the spine on flexion of vertebrae, tight band-like sensation in trunk called *girdle sensation*, asymmetrical or bizarre sensory symptoms in upper and lower limbs, lightning pains and deep boring paresthesia as if flesh is being pulled out from bones. There can be tingling, numbness, loss of sense of vibration, position and movement. Patient will have sensory ataxia with sense of imbalance felt more at night (due to abolition of visual sensation) and stamping gait due to inability to assess depth of floor.

Spinothalamic tract involvement can present with irritative features like superficial ill-defined burning paresthesia and subjective coldness; or paralytic features like loss of pain and temperature.

In lesions of crossing sensory tracts, pattern of sensory loss is described as descending suspended pattern. The spinothalamic pathways ascend and cross carrying sensations from 2 or 3 dermatomes. Therefore, when this crossing fibers are involved, only the dermatomes represented by them will show sensory loss. Therefore, it will be with respect to that segment alone and this gives a suspended appearance with normal areas above and below. As the disease advances, more crossing tracts will be involved causing descend of the sensory loss.

Anterior horn cells and their roots can be involved in various combinations giving rise to motor paralysis and fasciculations.

False Localizing Signs

These may confuse picture of spinal cord disease and they have to be distinguished from involvement of multiple sites of lesions in the neuraxis. For example, Horner's syndrome in lesions at C8 level due to involvement of the sympathetic, lower cranial nerve (LCN) palsy at lesions of the craniovertebral junction (CVJ), and loss of sensation of the forehead (sensory distribution of the ophthalmic division of 5th cranial nerve) due to involvement of spinal tract of trigeminal which comes down to C4 vertebral level. Papilledema may occur due to high protein content in the CSF. Other findings such as phrenic nerve palsy and optic atrophy may occur along with primary spinal cord disease.

The pattern of involvement may be pan-cord, anterior-cord, posterior-cord, central-cord and hemicord. Progressive lesions may show different patterns of development of symptoms.

Z pattern is seen in encircling lesions at foramen magnum, i.e. lower motor involvement of one upper limb, the next upper limb, ipsilateral upper motor involvement of lower limb and then other lower limb.

Elsberg pattern, there is onset of upper motor involvement of one upper limb, ipsilateral lower limb, then opposite lower limb and finally opposite upper limb. This indicates that the heralding event is ischemia of medial pyramidal fibers and not compression. Therefore, decompression treatment may not give satisfactory relief for the limb.

Cervical foot drop is seen in spinal canal stenosis. Myeloradiculopathy occurring at C7 level gives rise to Jolly sign in which upper arm is held in abduction, forearm in flexion and wrist and fingers are in flexion. When same occurs bilaterally, it is called ***Thorborn's sign***.

Beevor's sign is elicited in lesions of the cord D10 in which umbilicus is pulled up, when neck is flexed with patient lying supine.

In lesions of conus medullaris, patient has incontinence of urine and stools, sexual dysfunction and perianal anesthesia, but patient is walking and ambulant (walking, leaking patient).

In lesions below L3 level, patient develops asymmetric, atrophic, areflexic weakness of lower limbs with late bladder involvement. In lesions of cauda equina (spinal segments from L3 to S1 called conus medullaris) and lesions of L1 to L3 (called epiconus), bladder involvement is late.

Lesions of Conus Medullaris and Cauda Equina

They cause similar symptoms and it is often not possible to differentiate between the two. When the cauda equina is affected, symptoms and signs are attributed to root involvement. Common conditions include neoplasms, prolapsed intervertebral disks and spinal arachnoiditis. Lumbar canal stenosis may lead to additional symptom of intermittent neurogenic claudication. Lesions of ***conus medullaris*** (S3, 4, 5, coccygeal spinal segments) are characterized by early loss of sphincter functions. Common conditions include neoplasms such as ependymoma and demyelination. Lesions of the ***epiconus*** affect the L4, 5, S1 and S2 spinal segments. Table 210.2 enlists the points useful to differentiate between conus medullaris and cauda equina lesions.

COMPRESSIVE MYELOPATHY

Compressive myelopathies differ from noncompressive ones by being of relatively of shorter duration, asymmetrical, having a definite upper level bladder involvement, flexor spasms being more common and absence of distant signs like peripheral or cranial nerve involvement (Tables 210.3

Table 210.2: Clinical features which help differentiate conus medullaris and cauda equina lesions

Clinical feature	Conus medullaris	Cauda equina
Onset	Sudden, bilateral	Usually gradual, unilateral
Motor weakness	Symmetric, minimal	Asymmetric, may be severe, fasciculations common
Sensory loss	Saddle anesthesia, symmetric	Asymmetric
Spontaneous pain	Unusual, not severe	Prominent, severe, asymmetric
Neurogenic claudication	Absent	May be present
Dissociated sensory loss	Present	Absent
Sphincter incontinence	Early and marked	Late, less severe
Erectile dysfunction	Early	Late, less severe
Loss of anal and bulbocavernosus	Early	Late reflexes
Ankle jerk	Preserved	May be lost

Table 210.3: Differences between compressive and noncompressive lesions of spinal cord

Compressive pathology	Noncompressive pathology
Short duration	Long duration
Asymmetry	Symmetry
Definite upper level present	Absent
Distant features like affection of 2nd and 8th cranial nerve, peripheral nerves absent	May be present
Early bladder involvement	Late involvement of urinary bladder
Flexor spasms common	Rare
Vertebral changes can be present	Absent

and 210.4). Compressive lesions may be due to congenital conditions like bony and soft tissue anomalies, traumatic, inflammatory, infective, degenerative problems of vertebrae, disks, ligaments, meninges neoplasms or others (Table 210.5 and Fig. 210.2).

SPINAL CORD SYNDROMES

Myelopathies can be approached syndromically based on constellation of symptoms and signs. The common spinal cord syndromes include:

- ***Complete transverse section:*** Syndrome of complete transverse section at a particular level of the spinal cord results in symmetric upper motor neuron (UMN) paralysis, sensory loss and autonomic disturbance below the level. This syndrome is classically seen in transverse myelitis, but can occur in post-traumatic spinal cord injury (SCI) and acute spinal cord compression (SCC).
- ***Unilateral transverse section [Syn: Brown-Sequard syndrome (BSS)]:*** This syndrome of hemisection of spinal cord results in ipsilateral UMN paralysis and loss of sensation for vibration and proprioception

Table 210.4: Clinical distinction between spinal cord compressions at different locations

Extradural compression	Intradural compression	Intramedullary compression
Gibbus tenderness and spinal tenderness may be present	No gibbus, no tenderness	No gibbus, no tenderness
Paraspinal muscle spasm present	Nil	Nil
Root signs are more than pains	Root pains are more	Tract pains are present
Symmetrical weakness present	Asymmetry	Asymmetry
Sensory loss—ascending radicular pattern	Sensory loss—ascending radicular pattern	Descending dissociated, suspended sensory loss
Bladder—involvement variable	Bladder involvement—late Scalloped	Bladder involvement is early if lesion is intrinsic and symmetrical; if asymmetrical—it may be late
Vertebral pathology—often present	Intervertebral foramen on imaging	Cord enlargement demonstrable
Trophic changes—late	Late	Early

Table 210.5: Features of compression of spinal cord at different locations

Extradural compression	Intradural compression	Intramedullary	Noncompressive
Vertebral anomaly	Scalloping of intervertebral foramen	Interpedicular distance may widen	–
Tuberculosis	Pachymeningitis	Intramedullary tumor syrinx	Infective myelitis
Metastases	Meningioma, neurofibroma	Ependymoma, astrocytoma,	Metastases, lymphoma
Trauma	–	–	Inherited problems
Disk disease	–	–	
Degeneration of ligaments	–	Syringomyelia	Demyelination, degeneration, toxic and nutritional lesions
Osteomyelitis	–	–	

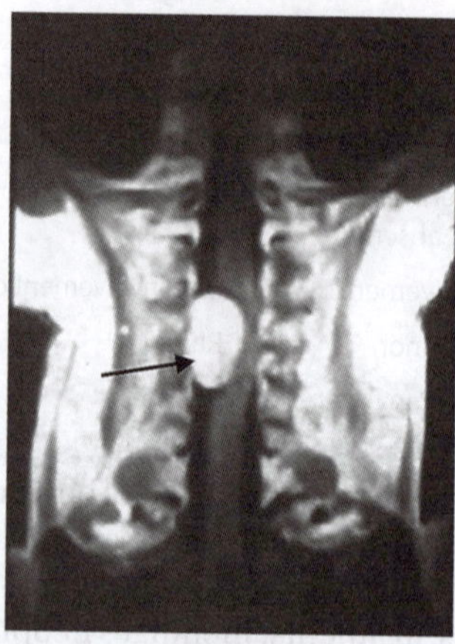

Fig. 210.2: Neurofibroma—intradural compression (arrow)

and contralateral loss of appreciation of pain and temperature. Otherwise known as the **BSS**, it most commonly occurs following spinal cord trauma or compression due to tumur.

- **Central cord syndrome (CCS):** Intramedullary lesions damage the decussating fibers of the spinothalamic tract that carry sensations of pain and temperature at that level, resulting in dissociated sensory loss. This is characterized by loss of pain and temperature sensations and preserved appreciation of joint and proprioception sensations. Because of the arrangement of fibers in the spinothalamic tract, sacral sensations are usually preserved resulting in a **suspended pattern** of sensory loss. Common causes include syringomyelia, intramedullary tumors and post-traumatic hematomyelia or contusion.

- **Anterior spinal artery (ASA) syndrome:** ASA supplies the anterior two-third of cord. Artery may be occluded by thrombosis or embolism leading to ischemia and infarction in vascular territory. Arterial occlusion may be due to vascular disease of aorta, generalized atherosclerosis, vasculitis, cardiac arrest and global hypoperfusion, diseases of the vertebral artery such as dissection, aortoarteritis or descending aorta aneurysm repair. Embolism may occur as a complication of infective endocarditis or ischemic heart disease (IHD). **Clinical features** depend on level of arterial occlusion. Recovery may start within a few days of onset and improvement may occur with time.

  Occlusion of ASA results in a characteristic constellation of signs due to infarction of spinal cord parenchyma supplied by it. It is characterized by involvement of anterior horn cells and anterolateral tracts leading to motor paralysis, loss of bowel, bladder and sexual functions and sensory disturbances characterized by loss of appreciation of pain and temperature sensations and preservation of joint and proprioception sensations. This can occur following vascular and thoracic-abdominal surgeries.

- **Anterior horn and pyramidal tract syndrome:** Disturbance of anterior horn and pyramidal tract function with preservation of sensory and autonomic nervous system function can occur in motor neuron disease (MND).

- **Combined posterior and lateral column disease:** Syndrome of loss of joint and proprioception sense with UMN pattern of weakness leads to spastic ataxic gait and is seen in vitamin B_{12} deficiency (subacute combined degeneration). Friedreich's ataxia, neurosyphilis and human immunodeficiency virus (HIV) myelopathy may show signs of loss of pyramidal tract, posterior columns, lateral columns and spinocerebellar tract functions.

SPINAL ARTERIOVENOUS MALFORMATIONS

Dural arteriovenous malformations (AVMs) are the most common. Others are glomus tumors which present like cord compression. Intramedullary lesions may present like recurrent and acute syringomyelia causing long dorsal tract like symptoms. Bleeding from AVMs causes arachnoiditis or gravitational paraplegia due to accumulation of blood in lower parts of the spinal subarachnoid space. Bleeding from AVMs may cause myeloradiculopathy. Large AVMs may present with arteriovenous (AV) bruit which can be detected by auscultation over the spine. Imaging studies with computed tomography (CT) or magnetic resonance imaging (MRI) reveal nature of the disease.

INFECTIONS AND INFLAMMATORY MYELOPATHY

Transverse Myelitis

Inflammatory disease affecting gray and white matter of cord is called *myelitis*. Involvement of anterior horn is called *poliomyelitis.* Selective involvement of white matter is called *leukomyelitis*. When disease is localized over several segments of cord, it is called *transverse myelitis*. The cord lesion may occur alone or as part of a more extensive disease such as meningitis or encephalitis (encephalomyelitis).

Table 210.6 enlists cause for transverse myelitis. However, in nearly 40% of cases, no specific cause may be detectable even after investigations.

Pathology

The affected segment of cord becomes hyperemic and edematous. Histologically, there is perivascular inflammation, edema, vascular thrombosis and in chronic stage, neuroglial proliferation.

Clinical Features

Transverse myelitis usually affects thoracic segments of spinal cord. Initial symptoms may be nonspecific such as fever, malaise, backache and root pains. Spinal cord involvement results in a syndrome of complete or partial transection of the cord. Patient presents with sudden weakness and sensory loss involving the lower limbs extending up to the trunk and upper limbs, depending upon upper level of involvement. Neurological deficits are often asymmetric. Bladder and bowel disturbances

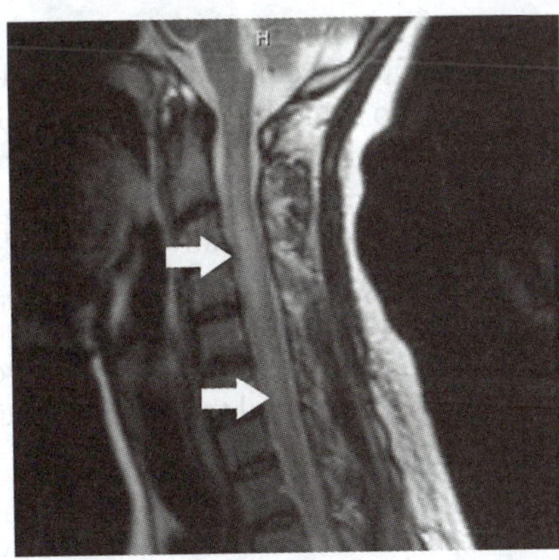

Fig. 210.3: MRI cervical spine showing demyelinating lesions in a patient with transverse myelitis. ***Note:*** (1) General swelling of the cord and (2) Hyperintense (whitish) lesions

occur early. Within 2–48 hours, paralysis and sensory loss are fully manifest and a clear upper level of sensory and reflex loss is definable which indicates the level of lesion. The initial phase is one of spinal shock in which there is flaccidity and areflexia. The spinal shock period extends for a few days to weeks and is followed by hyper-reflexia and spasticity.

CSF shows moderate lymphocytic pleocytosis and rise in proteins (up to 400 mg/dL). CSF sugar remains normal. MRI is the investigation of choice and confirms diagnosis and facilitates identification of etiology (Fig. 210.3). MRI shows hyperintense lesions in spinal cord, representing myelitis and demyelination.

Course and prognosis: Improvement occurs with time and complete or near complete recovery occurs in most cases.

Differential diagnosis: Transverse myelitis should be considered when syndrome of complete cord transection develops within hours or a few days. Acute cord compression can present similarly. This may be seen in conditions such as epidural abscess, tuberculosis, metastasis, bleeding or edema into spinal cord tumur, bleeding from a vascular malformation or occlusion of the ASA. MRI is useful to distinguish these conditions. Occasionally, Guillain-Barré syndrome (GBS) may mimic acute myelopathy.

Occasionally, postinfectious/postvaccinal demyelination may affect other regions of nervous system as well and patient may have encephalopathy, ataxia or brainstem signs in addition. This condition is called as ***acute disseminated encephalomyelitis (ADEM).***

Management

Investigations (blood and CSF) should be done to exclude conditions such as multiple sclerosis, vasculitis or any infections such as herpes zoster, HIV, human T-lymphotropic virus (HTLV-1), tuberculosis, syphilis, etc. If a specific cause is identified, appropriate treatment can be initiated. When no specific cause is detectable or when immune-mediated disease is suspected, trial of high dose corticosteroids such as intravenous (IV) methylprednisolone may be given. Plasma exchange and intravenous immunoglobulin (IVIG) have also been used in refractory cases. General management of

Table 210.6: Causes for transverse myelitis

• ***Demyelinating illnesses***
   ▪ ***Post-infectious/post-vaccinal myelitis:*** Allergic response to infection or vaccination, e.g. antirabies vaccine, smallpox vaccine
   ▪ Multiple sclerosis
   ▪ Neuromyelitis optica
 • ***Direct infections***
   ▪ ***Virus:*** Enterovirus, herpes zoster, rabies
   ▪ ***Bacteria:*** Syphilis, pyogenic infection, tuberculosis
 • ***Vasculitis:*** Systemic lupus erythematosus (SLE), Sjögren's disease, antiphospholipid antibody syndrome

paraplegia consists of attention to nutrition, frequent change of position and skin care to avoid bedsores, proper positioning of limbs to avoid contractures, physiotherapy to prevent venous thrombosis and to improve muscle tone and drainage of urine using an indwelling catheter. Constipation is treated using laxatives or small enemas. Flexor spasms can be controlled by avoiding stimuli to lower limbs and administering medications such as diazepam 5 mg or baclofen. As patient improves, active physiotherapy and occupational therapy are instituted.

Multiple sclerosis and neuromyelitis optica (NMO) (Devic's disease) are primary demyelinating diseases. ADE and postvaccinal encephalomyelitis are secondary to other causes.

Common infections are herpes virus-6, rabies, HIV, HTLV-1, hepatitis A and B, Ebstein-Barr virus (EBV), coxsackie virus, cytomegalovirus (CMV), measles, mumps, varicella and polio viruses. Bacterial infections are syphilis, tuberculosis, campylobacter, pertussis, mycoplasma, streptococcus. Parasitic infections like schistosomiasis, echinococcus, *Taenia solium*, toxoplasma and fungal infections like aspergillosis is blastomycosis and cryptococcosis can also lead to myelopathy multiple sclerosis have been described in Ch 207. Sarcoidosis can produce inflammatory myelopathy which is diagnosed by evidence of nodular enhancement of meninges in addition to cord changes.

NECROTIZING MYELOPATHY (FOIX-ALAJOUANINE SYNDROME)

This affects young males with a pan-cord syndrome involving several segments; occasionally, it can be relapsing and carries a poor prognosis, it is considered to be a veno-occlusive disease (VOD).

Hereditary Myelopathies

Wide varieties of noncompressive myelopathies can be inherited. Common among them is **hereditary spastic paraplegias (HSPs)**. They are characterized by severe spasticity which starts in lower limbs with relatively less weakness, very late bladder involvement and mild proprioceptive dysfunction.

Based on pattern of inheritance, they are classified into autosomal dominant, autosomal recessive and X-linked. They are called simple **hereditary myelopathies,** if the lesions are confined to the spinal cord and **complex,** if other parts of neuraxis are involved. These conditions are associated with thickness of corpus callosum (CC). Other inherited mimics are leukodystrophies MND and spinocerebellar ataxia-associated myelopathies. The less common ones are mitochondrial myelopathy, arginase deficiency, biotinidase deficiency, **Sjögren-Larsson syndrome (SLS)** and myelopathies accompanied by abnormalities in zinc and copper.

Non-compressive Myelopathies

They may be manifestations of nutritional deficiency, ischemic myelopathy, radiation-related sequelae, lathyrism, fluorosis, tropical myeloneuropathies, chemotherapy-induced myelopathies, chronic hepatic failure-associated myelopathies, organophosphorus poisoning, siderosis

Table 210.7:	Fundus changes in myelopathy
Papilledema	High protein in cerebrospinal fluid (CSF)—tumors, arachnoiditis
Optic neuritis	Devics/spinoptic multiple sclerosis toxins
Optic atrophy	Nutritional, toxic, degenerative
Vasculitic fundus	Sjögrens, vasculitic myelopathy
**Gyrate atrophy	Metabolic myelopathy—ornithine transcarbamase deficiency

** Gyrate atrophy of the choroid and retina, is an inherited disorder characterized by progressive vision loss. Due to loss of cells in the retina (Fig. 210.4), additional features of this disorder include hyperammonemia and myelopathy.

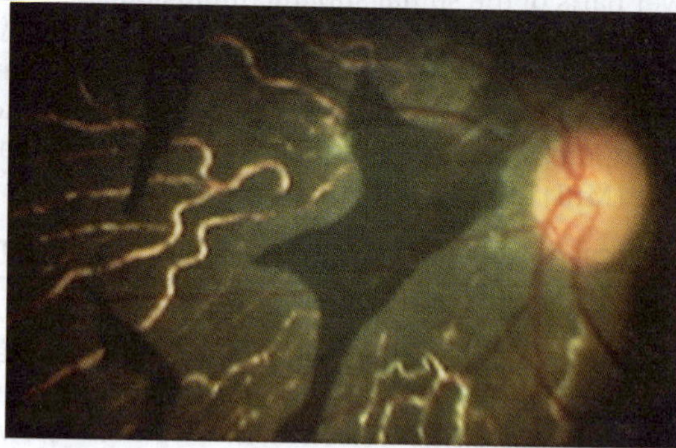

Fig. 210.4: Gyrate atrophy of retina

and heroin-related myelopathies. Less common causes are exposure to toxins such as Konzo due to cassava ingestion, triorthocresyl phosphate, adult polyglucosan body disease and paraneoplastic myelopathies (Table 210.7).

Myelopathy due to Contrast Agents

Following aortic and brachial angiography, flaccid paraparesis is reported. Believed to be due to vasoconstriction. Myelographic non-water soluble contrast agents like metrizamide which were used in yester years were associated with complication of myelopathy and arachnoiditis. Nitric oxide used by dental surgeons for dental anesthesia also used to cause subacute myeloneuropathy. Intrathecal chemotherapy with methotrexate, cytosine arabinoside and others may be accompanied by necrotizing myelopathy. Spinal anesthesia, both epidural and intradural, can produce myelopathy due to direct toxicity. **Diagnosis** is made on the basis of history and investigations including CSF examination. **Treatment** includes symptomatic measures, supportive treatment, antidotes if available and corticosteroids. In a few cases, recovery may be only partial.

Spinal Epidural Abscess

It commonly presents as subacute progressive compressive myelopathy associated with fever. However, it may occasionally present as acute paraplegia. Epidural abscess develops as a result of septic emboli reaching the epidural space during systemic infection. Root pains may develop. Fever is highly variable and some patients may have mild fever while others may have hectic fever and appear toxic. *Staphylococcus aureus* is the causative organism in 50% of cases. **Diagnosis** is established by MRI and confirmed by evacuation of pus and culture/

sensitivity. At times, the condition will be diagnosed when pus is aspirated during a lumbar puncture for other indications.

Hematomyelia

Bleeding into the substance of the spinal cord is termed *hematomyelia,* though bleeding into the cord may follow injuries. The term *hematomyelia* is reserved for those conditions where there is no obvious precipitating factor.

Etiology

- Transmitted violence
- Intramedullary telangiectasia or angioma
- Spontaneous hemorrhage into the cavity of syringomyelia
- Hemorrhagic disorders, especially purpura.

Common site is the cervical cord enlargement. Bleeding is primarily into the central gray matter and long tracts are compressed by hematoma.

Clinical features

The onset may be sudden or gradual and progressive. The condition is clinically characterized by syndrome of partial or complete transection of cord, depending on extent of hematoma. Usually, patients gradually improve as hematoma resolves. Rarely, condition may be fatal if hematoma extends to cervical cord leading to diaphragmatic paralysis.

Treatment

This consists of complete rest and immobilization of neck in a collar or suitably made splints. The underlying cause should receive appropriate treatment.

The spinal cord and roots, blood supply, meninges, surrounding bony structures all are individually and collectively capable of developing disease processes which may be acquired or congenital. Disease of any of these structures mainly reflex on the neural tissue by several mechanisms such as trauma, pressure effects, vascular occlusions, inflammation, or neoplasia. In this group, several primary lesions of the vertebral column and its other structures are common.

Collectively known as craniovertebral junction (CVJ), anomalies they may involve the foramen magnum, atlas, axis, odontoid, base of skull or soft tissues including the transverse ligament of odontoid, alar ligament, apical ligament, cruciate ligament and tectorial membrane. The joints are atlanto-occipital joint which is involved in nodding movement, atlantoaxial joint, a double synovial joint involved in side to side head rotation and upper cervical spine joints for flexion and extension movements. Herniation of normal intracranial structures through the foramen magnum is not uncommon. Cavities such as syringomyelia develop in cord more frequently in association with craniovertebral anomalies. The bony anomalies include platybasia, basilar invagination, atlantoaxial dislocation, os odontoideum, occipitalization of atlas, Klippel-Feil syndrome (KFS) which consists of basilar invagination, KFS and deafness. Acquired diseases in this region include osteomalacia, Paget's disease of bone and abnormalities associated with Down syndrome, Morquio syndrome and traumatic lesions. Tumors, metastases, degenerations, infective causes like tuberculosis, pyogenic osteomyelitis, and soft tissue abnormalities such as Arnold-Chiari malformations, arachnoid and other cysts and Dandy-Walker anomaly are discussed in Ch 211.

Interpretation of Spine X-ray

Both lateral and anteroposterior as well as oblique views are taken. Start with counting the number of vertebrae. Lesser number of cervical vertebrae are seen in Klippel-Feil abnormality in which there is fusion of two or more cervical vertebrae (Fig. 210.5). Supernumerary cervical vertebrae occur in giraffism. Carefully examine the body, pedicle, spinous process for change in shape, density and destruction. Locate the odontoid and measure the atlanto-odontal distance. If it is more than 3 mm in adult and 5 mm in children it indicates atlantoaxial dislocation.

Draw the anterior spinal line along the anterior part of body of vertebrae, posterior spinal line along the posterior and spinolaminar line along lamina. If they are not parallel, it indicates subluxation of vertebrae. The distance between posterior spinal line and spinolaminar line gives diameter of spinal canal. Unusually, large foramen magnum and upper cervical canal is seen in Arnold-Chiari malformation (Fig. 210.6). If canal diameter is less than 16 mm in a patient with SCC symptom, it indicates canal stenosis. Spinal canal diameter less than

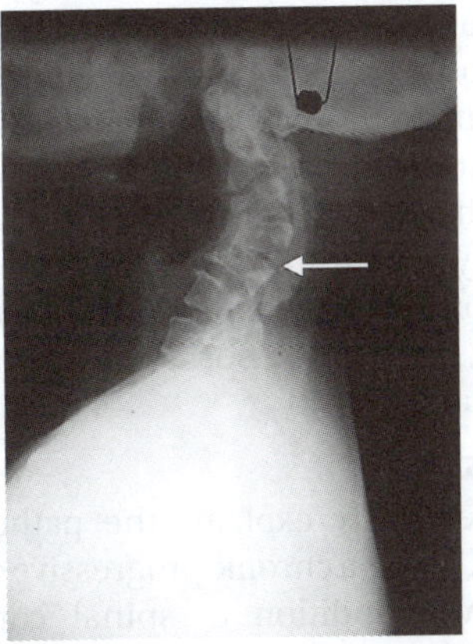

Fig. 210.5: Klippel-Feil anomaly. *Note:* The fusion of C3, 4, 5 spinous process (arrow)

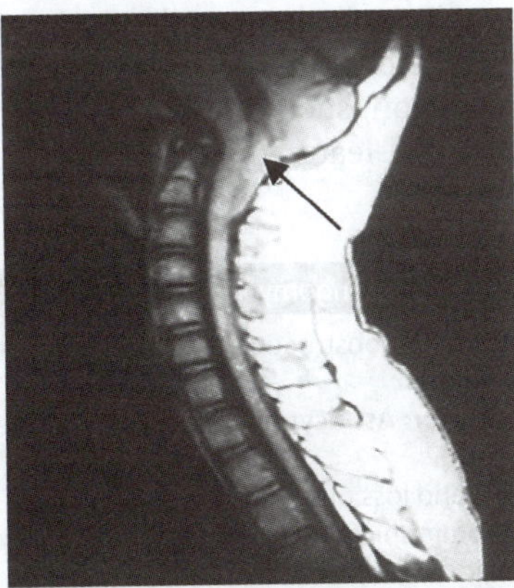

Fig. 210.6: Arnold-Chiari malformation. *Note:* The cerebellar tonsils herniating into cervical spinal cord (arrow)

13 mm is significant and if it is less than 10 mm, is critical stenosis. Pedicle erosion and vertebral lesions are seen in malignant metastases, myeloma, tuberculosis, osteo-myelitis and others. CVJ is studied in the lateral view of the skull and cervical vertebrae. A line drawn from hard palate to region of confluence of sinuses is called *McGregor's line*. A line drawn from hard palate to the posterior lip of foramen magnum is *Chamberlain's line*. Tip of odontoid should be well below these lines.

In anteroposterior view, *digastric line* is between both digastric grooves. *Fishgold's line* is between both tips of mastoid process and this should be above odontoid. *Boogards angle* is the angle between plane of anterior cranial fossa and middle cranial fossa, should not be more than 145°.

Lateral view in flexion reveals occipitalization of atlas and extension reveals atlantoaxial dislocation.

Treatment

Treatable causes should be always looked for and treated appropriately. Surgery is indicated in compressive syndromes as early as possible. Symptom management consists of treatment of pain, spasms, bladder, bowel, back care and occupational rehabilitation.

Syringomyelia

This is a chronic disorder pathologically characterized by progressive cavitation *(syrinx)* and gliosis of central portions of spinal cord. Usually, the syringomyelic cavity is longitudinal and extends over a few segments and rarely entire length of the cord. Transversely, it tends to extend irregularly into anterior horns and lateral columns. Dorsal columns are late to be involved. The contours of cavity are irregular and its walls are formed by gliosis. When lesion extends into the medulla, it is called *syringobulbia*. The condition may be primary (congenital) or secondary (acquired) (Box 210.1). In about 50% of cases of primary syringomyelia, there are associated bony and soft tissue abnormalities at the CVJ.

Pathogenesis

No theory adequately explains the pathophysiology of syringomyelia. This is a chronic progressive developmental or degenerative condition of spinal cord. Disruption of CSF circulation at the level of foramen magnum is seen in many cases of syrinx. Pressure waves develop at the foramen magnum due to periodic downward displacement of cerebellar tonsils during systole and results in compression and elongation of syrinx. Following trauma and infection, such as tuberculous arachnoiditis, scarring results and leads to altered CSF dynamics and tethering of cord.

Box 210.1: Causes for syringomyelia

- Foramen magnum obstruction—Arnold-Chiari malformation, basilar invagination
- *Spinal cord tumor:* Astrocytoma, ependymoma, hemangioblastoma
- Myelomalacia and loss of spinal cord parenchyma
- Intracranial communicating hydrocephalus
- Post-traumatic
- Postinfectious, postinflammatory
- Idiopathic

Pathology

The site of predilection of primary or congenital syringomyelia is the lower cervical region, but cavity may extend for several segments down into thoracic region or up into the medulla. Lumbosacral cord may be affected either by extension of cavity or by independent cavities. Usually, cavity starts as enlargement of central canal of spinal cord, which extends forward and laterally to involve anterior commissure, anterior horns and lateral columns. The anterior horn cells and the segmental fibers carrying pain and temperature, which cross in anterior commissure, are affected early. The corticospinal and lateral spinothalamic tracts are involved subsequently. The posterior columns get involved only late in disease or not at all. Slowly, lesion extends down to spinal cord. Usually, associated abnormalities like CVJ abnormalities, Arnold-Chiari malformation, Dandy-Walker cyst may be present.

Classification by Barnett and colleagues

Type 1: With obstruction to foramen magnum: (A) With Arnold-Chiari; (B) other obstructions
Type 2: Without obstruction at foramen magnum
Type 3: With other diseases
Type 4: Hydromyelia

Clinical Features

The age of onset is usually between 25 and 40 years in the primary form. Initial symptoms in cervicothoracic syringomyelia consists of loss of pain and thermal sensation in cervicothoracic segments (especially C8, T1) associated with weakness, wasting and even fasciculations of small muscles of hands. Loss of pain and temperature sensation with preservation of touch *(dissociated anesthesia)* in an irregular distribution is hallmark of syringomyelia. The patient may not appreciate burns and injuries. Depending upon the level of interruption of crossing fibers and lateral spinothalamic tracts, distribution of dissociated sensory loss varies. In high cervical lesions, spinal tract of trigeminal nerve is affected and this also gives rise to dissociated anesthesia over face. Trophic changes develop as a result of loss of pain sensation. These include painless perforating ulcers and neuropathic joint *(Charcot's joints)*. Destructive changes in joints induced by denervation were described by Jean Martin Charcot (French physician) in 1868. The affected joints undergo degenerative changes due to hypermobility and laxity of capsule and ligaments and articular surfaces may disintegrate. Commonly, elbow and shoulder joints are also affected. Radiological changes of destruction are demonstrable in these joints. Patients may complain of vague pains and paresthesias over affected parts. In some, sensory symptoms may be most troublesome presenting symptom.

Horner's syndrome occurs due to involvement of sympathetic fibers in cervical cord or medulla. Function of bladder and rectum is generally not affected. When cavity extends into brainstem, patients develop multiple cranial nerve palsies.

Course and Prognosis

The condition is slowly progressive and causes significant disability over several years. Some cases are self-limiting. In a few, rapid worsening may be due to bleeding into syrinx.

Diagnosis

The combination of lower motor neuron paralysis, dissociated sensory loss at the level of lesion and UMN features below level of lesion should raise possibility of syringomyelia. Intramedullary tumors, vascular lesions and hematomyelia have to be excluded. Syringomyelia and CV anomalies may coexist in some cases. MRI is investigation of choice. In all cases, therefore, it is necessary to investigate CV region with X-ray and CT scan or MRI.

Treatment

It depends upon the cause. There is need for great caution in decision-making. Treat the cause whenever present. Protection against trophic change and related complication is mainstay of treatment. Syrinx due to Arnold-Chiari malformation is managed by foramen magnum decompression. Syrinx associated with hydrocephalus is managed with ventricular shunt. Tumor removal is treatment of choice for tumor-related syrinx. Syrinx related to trauma and infection is managed by adhesiolysis and duraplasty. Second-line treatment for syringomyelia includes syringostomy, which drains syrinx cavity into spinal subarachnoid space or peritoneal space. Laminectomy with dural grafting have all been tried.

Spinal Shock

It is a clinical state characterized by loss of all functions below level of lesion in acute spinal cord injury (SCI) due to sudden withdrawal of regular corticospinal impulse transmission. Patient presents with flaccid symmetrical weakness, areflexia, with dribbling incontinence as both the body of bladder and the sphincter is atonic, bladder is also unable to store. The factors which determine duration of shock are:

- **Species:** Humans have a longer period of shock than lower animals as there is very little autonomy in human spinal cord
- Location of the lesion, i.e. as the lesion moves away from brain shock is longer and
- If there are secondary complications like infections, bedsores, etc. Generally, within 24 hours, effect of shock improves with respect to sensory and motor functions. Then, sphincters recover resulting in retention of urine and motion. Then, proximal reflexes like knee jerk recover earlier than ankle jerk and tone recovers last.

Paraplegia in Flexion

The reticulospinal and vestibulospinal pathways which are concerned with spinal extensor tone are resistant to compressive and destructive pathology until late. When these tracts are destroyed, the short latency flexor reflex afferents are released resulting in universally flexed posture. This is a sign of almost irreversible spinal cord damage. This is commonly associated with mass reflex in the form of sudden sweating, tachycardia, hypertension which can sometimes lead to intracranial bleed, with emptying of bowel and bladder. In this posture, it becomes very difficult to nurse patient and secondary complications come early. It is recommended that these patients be nursed in prone position so that patient may develop extensor contracture making rehabilitation little more easy.

Paraplegia in Extension

An incomplete cord lesion with sparing of structures concerned with spinal extensor tone results in paraplegia in extension.

Differential diagnosis of spinal cord disorders include pseudospinal presentation of lateral medullary syndrome, parasagittal meningioma, unpaired anterior cerebral artery (ACA) syndrome, hyperparathyroidism cerebral diplegias, leukodystrophy and other cerebral white matter disorders in children.

Cerebral Paraplegia

Lesions occurring over vertex affecting leg areas of cerebral cortex bilaterally lead to bilateral UMN lesions of both lower limbs. Compressive lesions such as midline meningiomas lead to this condition. Cerebral paraplegias are characterized by extensor hypertonia in all groups. Sometimes convulsions may be seen in the lower limbs. Depending on extent of lesion of cerebral cortex, cortical sensory impairment in lower limbs sparing other sensations may develop. In most cases, a clear cut upper margin may not be definable. Micturition may be involved, and cortical type of incontinence may be present.

Radiculopathies and Plexopathies

Radiculopathies are characterized by irritative or paralytic symptoms referable to sensory, motor, autonomic and reflex functions referable to the distribution of roots. Root pains are sudden shock like pains which have precipitating and relieving factors like movement of the spine, weight lifting and pain may be relieved by rest. However, in destructive disorders like metastases and osteomyelitis, rest can precipitate root pain. Motor symptoms can be fibrillations, fasciculation and weakness involving muscles supplied by particular root with or without involvement of sweating and thermoregulation.

Brachial Plexus

It is formed by C4-T1 roots. There are three trunks— (1) upper trunk formed by C5 and C6, (2) middle trunk by C7 and (3) lower trunk by C8, T1. They divide into anterior and posterior divisions. All posterior divisions together form posterior cord. Upper trunk and anterior division of the middle trunk forms lateral cord. The anterior division of lower trunk forms medial cord. The roots give rise to dorsal scapular nerve and long thoracic nerve. The upper trunk gives rise to suprascapular nerve, nerve to subclavius and rhomboids. The lateral cord gives rise to lateral pectoral nerve, lateral root of median nerve, musculocutaneous nerve, lateral cutaneous nerve of arm and forearm; posterior cord gives rise to subscapular nerve, thoracodorsal nerve, axillary nerve and radial nerve. The medial cord gives rise to medial pectoral nerve, medial root of median nerve, medial cutaneous nerve of the arm and forearm and ulnar nerve. In children, most common cause of partial or pan-plexopathy is due to trauma, hemorrhage in bleeding disorders as well as the manifestation of hereditary neuropathy with pressure palsy. In adults, demyelination with infection, vaccination and radiation, diabetes, malignant infiltrations are common causes. Plexopathy is suspected when patient experiences severe pain in location of plexus which radiates along distribution of nerves. Motor signs are more than sensory signs.

Lumbosacral Plexus

It is formed by T12–S4 roots. It gives rise to iliohypogastric, ilioinguinal and genitofemoral nerves from L1 to L2. L2 and L3 give rise to lateral cutaneous nerve of the thigh. Anterior division of L2, L3 and L4 gives rise to femoral nerve, nerve to iliacus and psoas major. The medial division gives rise to obturator nerve. L4, L5, S1, S2, S3 give rise to sciatic nerve and its branches. L5 gives rise to superior and inferior gluteal nerve. S1, S2 and S3 give rise to posterior cutaneous nerve of thigh and pudendal nerve.

Common causes for lumbosacral plexopathy are diabetes in addition to bleeding in hematological disorders and infiltration from pelvic malignancies.

Evaluation consists of thorough history, examination, electrophysiological examination and imaging. ***Treatment*** depends on etiology. Supportive management is needed for pain and weakness. When there is avulsion of roots, occupational therapy and tendon transplant may improve function. When continuity of nerve is lost, immediate primary repair, internal neurolysis, resection and anastamosis, nerve grafting, joint stabilization and other treatments have to be given.

Source:

1. Continuum, Lifelong learning in Neurology, American academy of Neurology; 60th Anniversary series, Volume 14 NO. 3 June 2008.
2. Textbook of Neurology by Raymond Adams.

CHAPTER
211

Diseases of the Vertebral Column Causing Neurological Lesions

Anand Kumar, KV Krishna Das

Chapter Summary

- Craniovertebral Anomalies
- Basilar Invagination (Basilar Impression)
- Platybasia
- Occipitalization of Atlas
- Klippel-Feil Syndrome
- Arnold-Chiari Malformation
- Dandy-Walker Malformation
- Cervical Spondylosis
- Lumbar Disc Lesions
- Lumbar Canal Stenosis

CRANIOVERTEBRAL ANOMALIES

Craniovertebral anomalies are developmental defects involving the bony and/or neural structures at the occipitocervical transition zone. These defects manifest clinically in a variable manner as craniospinal deformities and/or neurological deficits. Secondary changes such as repeated trauma, pressure effects and vascular occlusion aggravate the neurological disability and lead to its progression. Several major and minor abnormalities have been described. Common features which should draw attention to the presence of craniovertebral anomalies are short neck (total body height/neck length ratio > 13.86), low hairline (posterior hairline below C4 spine level) and facial asymmetry. Neck movements may also be abnormal.

Classification

The more important anomalies have been classified in Table 211.1.

Table 211.1: Classification of craniovertebral anomalies

Skeletal anomalies
- Basilar invagination—primary or secondary
- Platybasia
- Occipitalization of atlas
- Atlantoaxial dislocation—congenital or acquired
- Klippel-Feil anomaly

Neuraxial anomalies
- Arnold-Chiari malformation
- Dandy-Walker syndrome, i.e. failure of the foramina of Magendie and Luschka to open, associated with cerebellar hypoplasia
- Occipitocervical meningomyelocele
- Cysts in the posterior fossa

Combined neural and skeletal anomalies

Basilar Invagination (Basilar Impression)

In this condition, there is invagination of whole or part of the margins of the foramen magnum into the posterior cranial fossa. Although most often it is a developmental anomaly, it may also be acquired because of softening of the bones as in osteomalacia, Paget's disease of the bone, osteogenesis imperfecta, achondroplasia and gargoylism.

Clinical Features

Primary basilar invagination may present at any age and may be symptomatic or asymptomatic. In symptomatic cases, occipital headache and hyperalgesia in the distribution of the second cervical nerve roots are common features. Episodic vertigo, diplopia and drop attacks reflect circulatory disturbances in the vertebrobasilar territory. Drop attacks are sudden episodes of loss of tone in the limbs leading to falls. Motor weakness with pain and paresthesiae in the limbs may progress gradually or in a stepwise manner. Dysphagia, dysarthria, dysphonia, and ataxia are the other well-recognized symptoms. Nystagmus, ataxia and intention tremors occur due to cerebellar involvement. Paralysis of the lower cranial nerves occurs due to compression along their course. Among the pressure effects on the cervicomedullary region of the cord, pyramidal tract involvement is the most common. This manifests as spastic quadriparesis or rarely hemi- or monoparesis. Weakness and wasting of the small muscles of the hands may develop in some and this has been attributed to ischemic myelopathy. Posterior column disturbances are maximum in the distal aspects of the limbs. Dissociated sensory disturbances may occur in some cases which may suggest coexisting *syringomyelia* or *secondary* hydromyelia. This association is seen in about 30% of cases. Sphincter disturbances are uncommon but they may develop late in the disease.

Diagnosis

The clinical diagnosis is confirmed by radiological studies of the craniovertebral region and magnetic resonance imaging (MRI).

Lateral view of skull and cervical spine in the skiagram

McGregor's line: This imaginary line joins the posterior tip of the hard palate and most caudal point (inferior tip) on the occipital squama. Normally, the tip of the odontoid is below or up to 3 mm above this line. In basilar impression, the tip of the odontoid lies at a higher level than normal (Fig. 211.1).

Bull's angle: The line drawn extending the hard palate backwards and the line drawn through the plane of the atlas subtend an angle less than 13°. Increase in this angle is suggestive of basilar invagination (Fig. 211.2).

Anteroposterior view of skull and craniovertebral junction

The tip of the odontoid lies at or below a line joining the tip of both mastoid processes in normal individuals. If it lies above this line it suggests basilar impression (Fig. 211.3).

Platybasia

It is defined as flattening of the base of the skull. As a result, there is an increase in the angle subtended by lines.

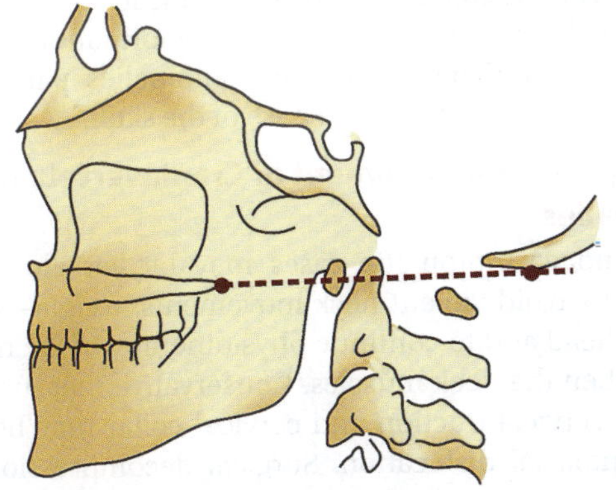

Fig. 211.1: McGregor's line from posterosuperior margin of hard palate to the lowermost point of the occipital bone in the midline. Tip of odontoid does not project more than 3 mm above this line in normal individuals

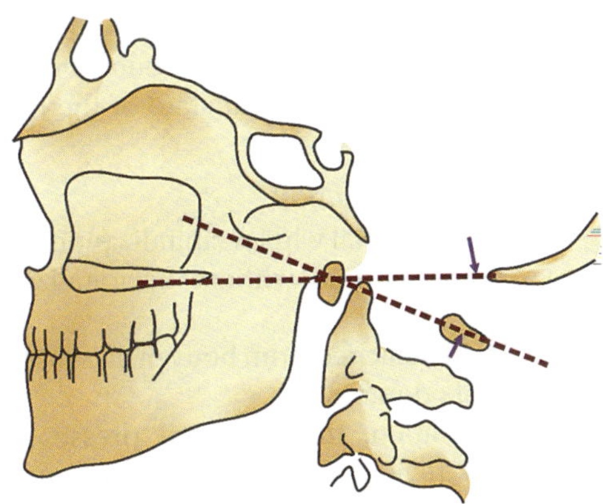

Fig. 211.2: Bull's angle formed between—1. Line drawn along the plane of the hard palate and 2. Along the plane of the atlas. If this angle (indicated by asterick) exceeds 13°, the position of the odontoid is abnormal

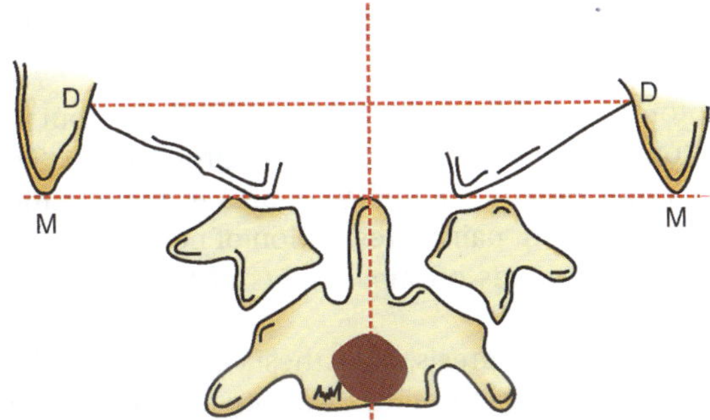

Fig. 211.3: Intermastoid (MM) and digastric (DD) lines. The intermastoid line (MM) joins the tips of the mastoid processes. The digastric line joins the two digastric grooves lying medial to the bases of the mastoid processes. Tip of odontoid should always be below these lines

- Joining the nasion to the tuberculum sellae
- From the tuberculum sellae to the anterior lip of the foramen magnum. (In normal, this angle ranges between 115° and 140°).

Values above 148° are abnormal. This angle can be measured in a true lateral X-ray of skull. This condition per se is asymptomatic. It may be associated with other craniovertebral anomalies.

Occipitalization of Atlas

This refers to the bony fusion of whole or part of the atlas to the occipital bone. This may occur as an isolated lesion or as part of multiple anomalies. It is often accompanied by congenital atlantoaxial dislocation.

Atlantoaxial Dislocation

The transverse ligament of the atlas holds the dens (odontoid) of the axis against the anterior arch of the atlas and prevents posterior subluxation in normal subjects. The apical and two alar ligaments fix the tip of the dens to the occiput. They limit the degrees of rotation and lateral flexion. Abnormal mobility of the atlas on the axis may be due to congenital or acquired causes. Congenital anomalies include non-fusion of the odontoid with the axis, agenesis of part of the odontoid or agenesis of the transverse ligament of the atlas. Acquired causes may be traumatic or may follow vertebral tuberculosis, rheumatoid arthritis (RA) and ankylosing spondylitis. Atlantoaxial dislocation has been classified radiologically depending on the presence or absence of occipitalization of the atlas and state of the odontoid process.

Types of atlantoaxial dislocation

Type IA—Odontoid normal with occipitalization of atlas
Type IB—Odontoid normal without occipitalization of atlas
Type II—Odontoid detached from body of axis or agenesis of part or whole of odontoid.

Due to subluxation, the odontoid presses on the cervicomedullary region of the spinal cord in certain positions of the head. This gives rise to pressure effects, secondary vascular changes and progressive degenerative changes in the lower part of the medulla and upper part of the spinal cord. Neurological symptoms may be abrupt such as drop attacks and quadriparesis, or slowly progressive due to degenerative changes in this region.

Clinical features

Symptoms may begin abruptly or gradually, but once symptoms start, they show stepwise progression. Trivial trauma may precipitate the symptoms in many patients. Suboccipital pain, painful restriction of neck movements, and clicking sounds on movements of the neck are the local symptoms.

Spastic quadriparesis, paresthesia and sensory disturbances in the extremities and wasting and fasciculations of the small muscles of hands constitute the other manifestations. Lower cranial nerve palsies and cerebellar disturbances are less common than in basilar impression. Horner's syndrome may be present.

Diagnosis

Once atlantoaxial dislocation is suspected, violent movements of the head over the neck, with a view to elicit the ***click***, should not be attempted. Diagnosis is confirmed by radiology. Lateral view pictures are taken with the neck in full flexion and extension to visualize the atlantoaxial joint. In atlantoaxial dislocation, the distance between the posterior surface of the anterior arch of atlas and the anterior surface of the dens is increased (normal distance is less than 3 mm in adults). In addition, the morphology of the odontoid can also be studied. An open mouth view in an anteroposterior projection gives a good picture of the odontoid process. MRI gives a clear picture of the whole abnormality.

Klippel-Feil Syndrome

Syn: Block vertebrae syndrome

Fusion of two or several of the cervical vertebral bodies or their spines occurs in Klippel-Feil syndrome. This may be associated with congenital hemivertebrae, kyphoscoliosis, limitation of neck movements, short-neck, low hairline and facial asymmetry. ***Mirror movements*** of the upper limbs may be seen in this condition, i.e. any movement initiated by one hand is involuntarily initiated by the other. The exact pathogenesis of this remains unclear, though anomalous decussation of the corticospinal tracts is a possible explanation in some cases. Various other congenital abnormalities involving the nervous,

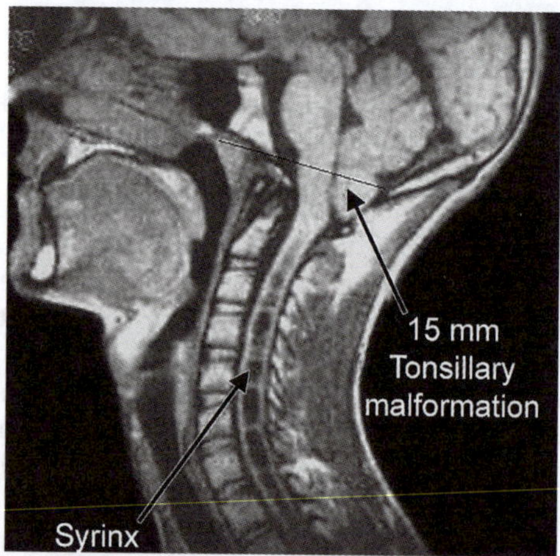

Fig. 211.4: MRI showing Arnold-Chiari malformation (arrow) herniation of the cerebellar tonsils through the foramen magnum and syrinx in the substance of the cord (arrow)

musculoskeletal, cardiopulmonary, gastrointestinal (GI) and excretory systems may be associated with Klippel-Feil syndrome.

Arnold-Chiari Malformation

This is characterized by herniation of the cerebellar tonsils with or without the medulla and fourth ventricle into the cervical spinal canal. In some patients, this is associated with cervical meningomyelocele and syringomyelia. This is one of the causes of hydrocephalus in infancy. Other features are cerebellar and lower cranial nerve involvement which may develop in older patients. Contrast myelography done with the patient in the supine position demonstrates obstruction to the flow of dye and kinking of the cord in the cervical region due to the herniated cerebellar tonsil. Computed tomography (CT) scan studies give details about the neurological and vertebral abnormalities. MRI gives a more vivid picture of the total abnormality (Fig. 211.4).

Dandy-Walker Malformation

In this condition, the midline portions of the cerebellum fails to develop normally and the vermis shows partial or complete agenesis. This leads to formation of cysts in the posterior fossa as a result of dilation of the posterior half of the fourth ventricle. This cyst may obstruct the flow of cerebrospinal fluid (CSF) and lead to obstructive hydrocephalus. Dandy-Walker malformation shows association with craniovertebral anomalies particularly the upper cervical spine and base of the skull.

Principles of Management of Craniovertebral Anomalies

Mild and asymptomatic cases may be left alone with advice to avoid violent neck movements, weight-bearing on the head and to continue physiotherapy of the neck to strengthen the neck muscles. Conservative measures like graded cervical traction and cervical collar may be used in atlantoaxial dislocation. Surgical decompression and fixation is required only when the above measures fail. Surgical treatment has to be undertaken in symptomatic patients. The surgical procedures include methods to reduce the compressive effects on the neural structures and measures to limit abnormal mobility. Surgical treatment of Arnold-Chiari malformation is accompanied by good clinical improvement.

CERVICAL SPONDYLOSIS

Degenerative changes develop in the vertebral column with advancing age. The nucleus pulposus of the intervertebral discs undergoes degeneration with reduction in its fluid content and this result in their collapse and narrowing of the intervertebral spaces. The annulus fibrosus also shows degenerative changes and they protrude backwards behind the vertebral bodies to form ridges. Osteophytes develop from the vertebral bodies and laminae resulting in compression of the nerve roots in the intervertebral foramina.

The cord may be compressed by osteophytic bars formed in the midline behind the vertebral bodies or the roots may be compressed by osteophytes growing into the intervertebral foramina. Degenerative changes are seen most markedly and symptoms are more frequent in the cervical and lumbar regions of the vertebral column. In addition to the higher mobility of the spine in these regions, which accounts for greater predilection to degenerative changes, it is also likely that subjects who develop cervical spondylotic myelopathy have congenitally narrower spinal canal.

In addition to the bony changes, soft tissue changes also develop. The ligamenta flava loses its elasticity and tends to buckle forwards when the cervical spine is extended. This leads to compression of the posterior aspect of the cord. In the intervertebral foramina, fibrosis of the dural sheaths contributes to further pressure on the spinal nerves and their roots. Pressure on the spinal arteries and vertebral arteries occurs during their course in the bony structures of cervical vertebrae. This leads to secondary vascular changes which cause vascular occlusion and ischemic damage to the cord and lower brainstem. The clinical presentation may vary widely from that of a myelopathy, radiculopathy or both. The site of cord dysfunction may be at the actual level of compression, or even distant from that, on account of vascular occlusion.

Neurological Complications: Clinical Features

Cervical radiculopathy: This condition develops when the intervertebral foramina are grossly narrowed. In the cervical region, maximal degenerative changes are seen between the fifth, sixth and seventh cervical vertebrae and these nerve roots are most frequently affected.

Cervical spondylosis: This is a common condition seen in day-to-day practice. Though the older age groups are more affected by osteoarthritis, many patients even in the 4th and 5th decades of life may suffer from this disease and this fact should be borne in mind in all cases presenting with painful symptoms in the neck and around the pectoral girdle. Initial symptoms consist of paresthesia and pain in the distribution of fifth to the eighth cervical dermatomes, pain being felt most frequently over the shoulder, arm, scapular region, forearm and hands. Movements of the neck, travel and adoption of certain postures aggravate the pain, which may be intermittent or even constant. In the majority of patients, objective sensory loss to pin-prick may be demonstrable. Motor phenomena consist of weakness and wasting of the deltoid, triceps, biceps or forearm muscles. Wasting of small muscles of the hand is rare in pure cervical spondylosis. Involvement of the C5 segment gives rise to ***inversion of the supinator jerks.*** Fasciculations may be seen over the affected muscles. Tendon reflexes of the affected roots are diminished. The lesion may be unilateral or asymmetrically bilateral.

Compressive myelopathy: This develops as a result of compression of the spinal cord by the osteophytic bars in front and ligamentum flavum behind. Most frequent site of compression is the C5–C6 region. Ischemia further enhances the damage.

The clinical picture is one of insidious onset of spastic paraparesis with motor and sensory symptoms. Pressure on the posterior columns is more common than the spinothalamic tract and this gives rise to sensory ataxia. Bladder and bowel dysfunction is less common.

Vertebrobasilar ischemia: The vertebral artery which ascends through the foramina in the transverse processes of the cervical vertebrae and passes over the atlas to enter the foramen magnum is kinked, compressed and stretched, when the vertebral column loses height and spondylotic changes occur. In addition, atherosclerotic changes develop early. These changes result in vertebrobasilar ischemia.

Diagnosis

Cervical spondylosis has to be suspected in all cases presenting with cervical cord or root symptoms in persons above the age of 40 years. Differential diagnosis includes other causes of cord compression, syphilitic pachymeningitis, arachnoiditis, syringomyelia and motor neuron disease. In some cases of cervical spondylosis, flexion or extension of the cervical spine causes ***electric shock-like sensation*** over the segments affected. This is called Lhermitte's sign. This may occur in other causes of cervical cord compression as well.

The clinical diagnosis should be confirmed by radiological studies of the spine. X-ray taken in the lateral view with the neck in straight, flexed and extended positions and oblique views reveal the abnormalities well. Radiological changes include narrowing and irregularity of the intervertebral spaces, osteophytes and encroachment of the intervertebral foramina. In young subjects, bony outgrowths may not be evident, but alteration in the alignment of cervical vertebrae, especially loss of the cervical curvature caused by spasm of neck muscles should be taken as a suggestive sign (Fig. 211.5).

Myelography reveals the narrowing of the spinal canal and compression of the cord. Anteroposterior (AP) diameter of the spinal cord in the cervical region is 9–10 mm. If the spinal canal is less than 10 mm in the lateral view, X-ray cord compression is likely. MRI clearly brings out the total picture of vertebral changes and compression of the neural structures. Somatosensory evoked potentials help to evaluate physiological and anatomical malfunction of the posterior column of spinal cord.

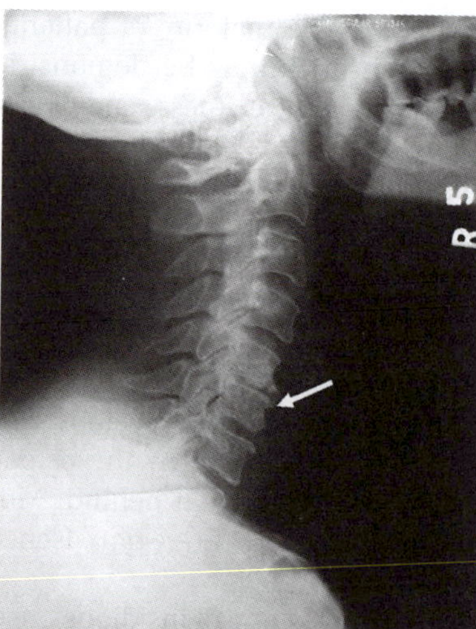

Fig. 211.5: X-ray cervical spine or cervical spondylosis. **Note:** Irregularity of vertebral margins diminution of intervertebral space, osteophytes on the vertebral borders (arrow)

It has to be borne in mind that radiological changes in the cervical spine are seen in a high proportion of elderly subjects without neurological damage and the mere presence of such changes is not adequate to establish the diagnosis of cord compression as due to vertebral disease. Cervical spondylosis may coexist with other disorders involving the spinal cord such as motor neuron disease (MND), tumors and syringomyelia.

Treatment

In the early stages of spondylotic radiculopathy, proper positioning of the neck, physiotherapy and use of a cervical collar to restrict neck movements help to relieve root pains. Exercises designed to strengthen the shoulder girdle muscles, especially elevators of the scapula help to relieve traction on the nerve roots and prevent recurrence of symptoms. Persons who have had symptoms should be advised to wear cervical collar during long journeys, so as to prevent recurrence of the symptoms. Graded cervical traction may help to relieve pressure on the nerve roots. Nonsteroidal anti-inflammatory drugs (NSAIDs) are of some benefit. If definite bony ridges are demonstrable causing root or cord compression, surgery is indicated to relieve pressure and to prevent further neurological deterioration. Presence of motor phenomena such as paresis, or muscle wasting is an indication for early surgery. Before surgery, all cases should be fully investigated to exclude other causes of myelopathy which may also present with similar clinical picture.

Treatment has to be based on individual considerations. There is no general agreement on any standard therapy.

LUMBAR DISC LESIONS

The lumbar intervertebral discs are particularly vulnerable to injury and degenerative damage, irrespective of age. Males engaged in heavy manual work and weight-lifting are particularly affected. Sudden jerky movements, unaccustomed lifting of heavy weights and heavy falls on the gluteal region or back may lead to sudden rupture of the annulus fibrosus even in otherwise normal persons. The nucleus pulposus herniates through ruptured annulus fibrosus to impinge upon the nerve roots. The L4–5 or L5–SI discs are more often affected. The onset is generally abrupt with severe radicular pain in the lumbosacral dermatomes in the sciatic distribution *(sciatica).* The pain is aggravated by flexion of the spine, coughing, sneezing or jolting movements. Motor weakness of spinal root distribution will occur if the anterior roots are impinged upon.

Flexion of the spine is more restricted than extension. Objective neurological findings of root compression may be evident. In acute cases, the normal lumbar lordosis is obliterated. Local tenderness may be elicited over the affected region and the paraspinal muscles may exhibit spasm. Straight *leg raising test* is positive—*Lasegue's sign.* This sign is elicited by passively lifting up the lower limb held straight by the examiner when the patient is in supine position. In normal subjects, the limb can be brought to near-vertical position without discomfort. In lumbosacral root due to irritation due to disc prolapse, this movement is restricted by severe pain.

Diagnosis

Low back pain, especially aggravated by coughing or sneezing, should suggest the possibility of lumbar disc prolapse. X-ray spine may reveal narrowing of intervertebral spaces. CT scan, MRI and myelography bring out the actual pathology distinctly.

Course and Prognosis

This is variable. In mild cases, the condition may improve with rest and conservative measures. Progressive neurological disability may develop in some cases. In many, sudden onset of sciatica may be very disabling.

Management

Conservative measures include uninterrupted rest in bed with slight extension of the back on a hard non-sagging bed for periods of 2–3 weeks, traction on the legs, exercises to strengthen the paraspinal muscles and to prevent wasting of the affected muscles and use of spinal braces to limit spinal movement. Analgesics and muscle relaxants like diazepam help in the acute stage or intractable pain.

Presence of progressive neurological damage or intractable pain is an indication for surgical treatment which consists of laminectomy and removal of the prolapsed disc.

Modern surgical techniques employ keyhole procedures to remove the damaged disc without conventional laminectomy.

LUMBAR CANAL STENOSIS

The term *spinal canal stenosis* covers any type of narrowing of the spinal canal, but it usually affects the lumbar spinal canal. Most often it is congenital, but the patient becomes symptomatic later in life due to the development of other pathological changes that result in the compression of neurovascular tissues. The compression may be due to any of the following causes:

- Prolapse of the intervertebral disc
- Hypertrophic changes of the ligaments within the narrowed spinal canal

- Angulation of vertebrae due to loss of disc height
- Spondylolisthesis
- Paget's disease of bone
- Neural arch degeneration (spondylolysis)
- Bony and ligamentous compression at the exit foramina.

In addition to mechanical compression, the arterial supply of the cord may also be compressed. Multiple factors may operate in the same case. Males are generally affected more than females, except in case of spondylolisthesis. L5 and S1 roots, which run a long oblique course within the spinal canal before changing direction to emerge through the exit foramina, are most affected.

Clinical features

Symptoms fall into three categories. These are:
- Lumbago (backache) in almost all cases
- Lumbosacral radicular symptoms in a third
- Neurogenic claudication in another third of cases.

Cases with neurogenic claudication get pain when bending backwards or on walking. Such patients assume a stooping posture to avoid pain. Both postural and exertional claudication results in transient root pain, paresthesia, weakness or numbness. Dermatomal sensory loss, muscle weakness and other motor deficits may be present. All these symptoms temporarily subside following rest. Straight leg raising test is positive in a third of the cases, especially if tested after exertion.

Diagnosis

Clinical diagnosis should be supported by radiography. The narrowed lumbar canal may be demonstrable in lateral and AP view skiagrams. MRI demonstrates the narrowing precisely. Electromyographic demonstration of segmental muscle denervation in the legs gives diagnostic localization and this procedure is done routinely before surgical decompression.

Treatment is preferably surgical decompression by a partial undercutting facetectomy with decompression of nerve root canal by removal of the hypertrophied bony fragments, ligamentum flavum and degenerated disc. The results are excellent in majority of cases.

CHAPTER
212

Diseases of the Peripheral Nervous System

Anand Kumar, Arun N Babu

Chapter Summary

- General Considerations
- Peripheral Neuropathy
- Guillain-Barré syndrome
- Chronic Inflammatory Demyelinating Polyneuropathy (CIDP)
- Neuropathy in Systemic Diseases
- Neuralgic Amyotrophy
- Entrapment Neuropathies
- Hereditary Motor Sensory Neuropathies
- Neurofibromatosis
- Diagnostic Approach to Peripheral Neuropathy

GENERAL CONSIDERATIONS

The peripheral nervous system (PNS) consists of:
- Sensory receptors and the first-order sensory neuron with its axon coursing into the spinal cord
- The last-order alpha motor neuron that sends its axon out from each level of the spinal cord to innervate specific muscle fibers via the neuromuscular junction—this is collectively referred to as the lower motor neuron (LMN).

The sensory and/or motor axons from different spinal levels come together in the brachial and lumbosacral plexii and then particular sensory and/or motor axons headed for a particular part of the body travel together bundled into a ***peripheral nerve***. Damage to the PNS can result in:

- Sensory loss, ***hypesthesia*** to one or more modalities (***negative phenomena***)
  - Pain and temperature (mediated by small-diameter fibers)—patients may have unexplained painless injuries and burns
  - Light touch, vibration and proprioception (mediated by large-diameter fibers)—patients may feel like they are walking on cotton wool. Loss of position sense causes loss of balance and falls in darkness or if patients are visually distracted when walking.
- Abnormal sensory phenomena (***positive phenomena***)
  - ***Hyperesthesias or hyperpathia:*** Exaggeration of normal painful stimuli
  - ***Dysesthesias:*** Severe pain provoked even by light touch
  - ***Parestheshias:*** Spontaneous pain, burning or tingling
  - ***Neuralgia:*** Provoked or unprovoked, brief but severe, ***lightning stabs*** of lancinating pain.
- Weakness and motor symptoms
  - Weakness can affect one or more muscles depending on the site of nerve dysfunction (***negative phenomena***). Axonal degeneration can lead to atrophy of related muscle fibers
  - ***Fasciculation, cramps, spasms and neuromyotonia (positive phenomena)***
  - Reflexes tend to be lost early in most neuropathies.

- Autonomic dysfunction
  - Postural hypotension, loss of sweating and trophic changes
  - ***Causalgia***—severe dysesthesias with autonomic features (edema) confined to one extremity.

Depending on the site of the lesion, the above symptoms may occur in the distribution of:

- One or more spinal nerve roots (discussed in Ch 210)
- Brachial or lumbosacral plexus
- One or more particular peripheral nerves
- Diseases of muscle or neuromuscular junction.

PERIPHERAL NEUROPATHY

This refers to any disease of the peripheral nerve. Damage to a peripheral nerve can be of two types:

1. ***Axonal:*** Most neuropathies are axonal in nature
2. ***Demyelinating:*** Most demyelinating neuropathies are usually autoimmune.

Axonal as well as demyelinating damage may coexist in some etiologies.

Clinical Approach to a Patient with Peripheral Nerve Disease

The clinical features of peripheral nerve disease depend upon a number of factors.

Onset and Rate of Progression

Acute: Less than 1 week—Guillain-Barré syndrome (GBS), porphria, toxins.

Subacute: Less than 1 month—GBS, toxins, metastatic lesions.

Chronic: More than 1 month duration—toxic neuropathies, metabolic neuropathies, chronic inflammatory demyelinating polyneuropathies (CIDP), hereditary neuropathies, diabetic neuropathy, paraproteinemic neuropathy. They may continue to exist over several years.

Relapsing: Multiple episodes occur as in CIDP or repeated exposure to toxins.

Clinical Pattern

Mononeuropathy: Involvement of one nerve, such as nerve entrapments and nerve injuries.

Mononeuritis multiplex: Asymmetrical simultaneous or sequential affliction of more than one nerve, as in systemic vasculitis or cryoglobulinemia.

Polyneuropathy: Symmetric involvement of multiple nerves as in diabetic polyneuropathy.

Radiculopathy: Involvement of multiple spinal nerve roots.

Polyradiculopathy: Involvement of several isolated spinal nerve roots.

Plexopathy: Involvement of the brachial or lumbosacral plexii.

Clinical Deficit

Sensorimotor: Many of the common neuropathies show involvement of sensory and motor functions.

Motor predominant: Lead, porphyria, GBS, diphtheritic neuropathy, dapsone-induced neuropathy.

Sensory: Paraneoplastic neuropathy, leprosy, Sjögren's disease.

Autonomic predominant: Diabetes, demyelinating neuropathies.

Initial Distribution in the Limbs

Distal: Common pattern of most of the neuropathies.
Proximal: Plexopathy, diabetic amyotrophy.

Causes of Peripheral Neuropathy

Causes	Diseases
Hereditary	Hereditary sensory motor neuropathies
Metabolic	Diabetes mellitus (DM), hepatic failure, renal failure porphyria
Endocrine	Hypothyroidism
Toxic	Alcohol, organophosphates, arsenic, lead, gold, thallium, lithium
Drugs	Vincristine, isonicotinylhydrazide (INH)
Immune-mediated	Guillain-Barré syndrome (GBS), chronic inflammatory demyelinating polyneuropathy (CIDP)
Infections	Leprosy, diphtheria
Vasculitis	Polyarteritis nodosa (PAN), other forms of vasculitis in sarcoidosis, Wegener's granulomatosis, Behcet's syndrome
Nutritional	Vitamin deficiencies: B_{12}, B_1, B_6, folic acid
Miscellaneous	Lymphomas, paraneoplastic syndromes, critical illness neuropathy.

GUILLAIN-BARRÉ SYNDROME (GBS)

Syn: Acute idiopathic polyneuropathy, Acute inflammatory demyelinating polyneuropathy (AIDP), Postinfective polyneuropathy

It is an acute inflammatory demyelinating polyneuropathy (AIDP). It is symmetrical, predominantly motor, frequently involving facial and bulbar muscles, almost always with absent reflexes. The weakness develops over a few days and reaches its peak within a few weeks of onset. Most patients recover within six months. Many cases follow a systemic infection, usually a viral respiratory or diarrheal. It is believed that as the immune system attacks the foreign organism, the immune attack also mistakenly gets directed against myelin structures. Immunological reactions involving T cells, antibodies and complement-directed against peptides from myelin proteins take place leading to demyelination and sometimes axonal degeneration. GBS has been associated with herpes virus, cytomegalovirus (CMV), Epstein-Barr virus (EBV), mycoplasma and *Campylobacter jejuni* infections are present in some cases (14–18%). Vaccinations for rabies, typhoid and tetanus may be followed by this syndrome. All age groups and both sexes are affected. Male to female ratio is 1:1.25. Most of the cases are sporadic but small epidemics have been reported. Infection leads to activation of antigen specific T and B cells. Antibody reaction and cell-mediated immune process lead to toxic damage to Schwann cells resulting in demyelination and axonal degeneration. Anterior nerve roots are most commonly affected.

The clinical syndromes in GBS include at least four subtypes of acute peripheral neuropathy:

1. AIDP
2. Acute motor axonal neuropathy (AMAN)
3. Acute motor and sensory axonal neuropathy (AMSAN)
4. Miller-Fisher syndrome.

The distribution of gangliosides may explain the distribution of lesions and symptoms in GBS.

Clinical Features

The disability may progress steadily to reach its peak within three weeks, by which time 60% of patients are unable to walk. Respiratory function is impaired in about 50% of patients of which about 15–20% will require assisted ventilation. Almost 80% make a good recovery. Some (10–20%) may be left with residual paralysis.

Diagnosis

GBS should be suspected in every case of acute onset of symmetric sensory or motor systems involving bilateral lower or all extremities. In Guillain-Barré, reflexes will be diminished or already absent (areflexia) at presentation. Tone is decreased. Preserved or brisk reflexes or spasticity would be inconsistent with GBS and suggests an upper motor neuron (UMN) process such as a myelopathy. Sometimes, patients may be found to have one or more reflexes that are diminished the first day that disappear and become absent in the following one to two days. This disappearing reflex is almost pathognomonic for GBS and should prompt emergent monitoring and treatment.

Patients with GBS may present initially at the general medical clinic with somewhat vague complaints of tingling in the feet or difficulty walking that they attribute to fatigue. They may appear weak but comfortable, without much complaint and may give no overt indication of the fact that without the attentive intervention of an astute physician, death will follow in a matter of days. It is imperative to consider GBS in every patient who presents with any acute sensory or motor symptoms. If reflexes appear even slightly diminished, further work-up or at the very least, close observation for progression is required.

If reflexes are still present despite significant motor or sensory loss, this is a reassuring indication of some alternate diagnosis. Pure sensory syndrome, preserved reflexes, a definite sensory level over the trunk, severe and persistent sphincteric disturbance and more than 50 cells/mm^3 in the cerebrospinal fluid (CSF) make the diagnosis of GBS unlikely.

Differential diagnosis often includes toxic polyneuritis, poliomyelitis, transverse myelitis, demyelinating diseases and acute myopathies associated with polymyositis, hypokalemic paralysis, botulism and myasthenia. Neurotoxic snake bite particularly krait may give rise to diagnostic difficulties, especially if the bite occurs during sleep.

Investigations

CSF shows elevated proteins after the first week and no leukocytosis. This is referred to as albuminocytological dissociation (as in most other pathology both are elevated together). Blood tests are usually normal. Electromyogram (EMG) and nerve conduction studies help to distinguish the condition from myopathies and poliomyelitis.

Treatment

Treatment is two-pronged—(1) to reduce the inflammatory attack on the nerves as much as possible and (2) to provide adequate supportive care such as ventilator support as needed.

Plasmapheresis or intravenous immunoglobulin (IVIG) for 5 days have both been found to be equally efficacious. In severe cases, treatment with either may be increased to 10 days based on anecdotal data. Further prolongation of treatment or combining the two treatments have not been shown to be of any added benefit.

The forced vital capacity (FVC) should be measured at least every 8 hours. Any drop should prompt closer monitoring. If the FVC drops below 1 L, the patient should be electively intubated without waiting for further decline. Patients with neuromuscular respiratory dysfunction generally do not complain as their gas exchange system is intact and they do not experience subjective dyspnea since the PO$_2$ is well-maintained. Once decompensation sets in, it is very rapid and may occur during sleep, with the unmonitored patient being found dead the next morning.

Since patients may be paralyzed for prolonged periods, careful nursing care with regular turning in bed, attention to pressure areas, proper care of the eyes when there is facial palsy, care of the oral cavity and attention to bowel and bladder are of great importance. Lung and urinary tract infections (UTIs) should be treated promptly. As deep vein thrombosis (DVT) and pulmonary emboli are recognized complications, prophylaxis with heparin 5,000 units subcutaneously (SC) twice daily should be given.

Autonomic disturbances are complications demanding emergency intervention. Continuous electrocardiogram (ECG) and blood pressure (BP) monitoring in an intensive care unit (ICU) is essential in such cases. On recovery, physiotherapy and rehabilitation should be started.

Prognosis

In about 10% of cases with rapid onset and progress, respiratory failure may threaten life. Mortality is around 5%. The vast majority of patients start improving after a week or so of onset and recovery may be complete within 6 weeks. In about 25% of cases resolution is slower, taking up to six months. In a smaller number, severe paralysis may persist and the patient may be crippled for life. Presence of axonal degeneration and occurrence of the disease at the extremes of age are associated with a bad prognosis. About 3% of cases will have a relapse or second episode.

Miller-Fisher Syndrome

This is a descending variant of GBS characterized by the triad of acute ophthalmoplegia, ataxia and areflexia. Systemic weakness and sensory loss are uncommon at presentation. This is more frequently associated with *C. jejuni* infection. Course is generally more benign with good recovery.

CHRONIC INFLAMMATORY DEMYELINATING POLYNEUROPATHY (CIDP)

The presentation of CIDP is with signs of motor and sensory polyneuropathy that evolves subacutely over more than eight weeks or chronically over many months. There is weakness in proximal and distal muscles and involvement is usually symmetrical, accompanied by sensory deficits and paresthesias. Pain is a rare symptom. CIDP can begin at any age and the course is progressive, stepwise progressive or relapsing. Patients can become

Table 212.1: Salient features of the common types of peripheral neuropathy

Disease	Type of onset	Distribution	Pattern	Fiber affected	Pathology
Guillain-Barré syndrome	Acute	Proximal or diffuse	Polyneuropathy	Small and large	Demyelinating
Porphyria	Acute	Proximal/diffuse	Polyneuropathy	-do-	Axonal
Diphtheria	Acute	Distal, proximal or diffuse	Poly or mononeuropathy	-do-	Demyelinating
Connective tissue disorders and vasculitis	Acute or chronic	Distal	Poly or mononeuropathy	-do-	Demyelinating
Diabetes mellitus	Acute or chronic	Proximal or distal	Poly or mononeuropathy	-do-	Axonal and demyelinating
Lead poisoning	Subacute	Distal	Mononeuropathy	-do-	Axonal
Arsenic poisoning	Subacute	Distal	Polyneuropathy	-do-	Axonal
Leprosy	Subacute or chronic	Mononeutritis or distal symmetrical	Mono or polyneuropathy	Small	Axonal and demyelinating
Vitamin B$_{12}$ deficiency	Chronic	Distal	Polyneuropathy	Small and large	Axonal
Hereditary motor sensory neuropathy	Chronic	Distal	Polyneuropathy	-do-	Axonal
Paraneoplastic	Chronic	Distal	Poly or mononeuropathy	-do-	Axonal

considerably disabled. Spontaneous remissions are rare. CIDP can also occur in the presymptomatic phase of human immunodeficiency virus (HIV) infection.

Diagnosis

Diagnostic testing for CIDP include detailed electrophysiological examination of all four limbs, lumbar puncture (LP) to look for CSF protein elevation and pleocytosis (in HIV related CIDP), serum and urine protein electrophoresis to rule out monoclonal gammopathy and skeletal survey to exclude myeloma. A nerve biopsy and teased fiber analysis will be confirmative. If required, a genomic deoxyribonucleic acid (DNA) testing can be done for exclusion of hereditary demyelinating neuropathy.

Treatment

IVIG at a dose of 0.4 g/kg bw is given daily for 5 days. Plasma exchange or plasmapheresis, 5 treatments over several days is equally effective. They are both safe but expensive. These help to produce improvement acutely. Chronically, steroid therapy is the mainstay of treatment, with prednisolone at a dose of 60–80 mg per day for 6–8 weeks with subsequent tapering by 10 mg per month and then switching to an alternate day regimen. Prednisolone although cheap, takes time to act and long-term complications are to be anticipated. Current practice is to recommend IVIG or plasma exchange as primary treatment.

NEUROPATHY IN SYSTEMIC DISEASES

Diabetic Neuropathy

This manifests as four main types:

1. ***Distal symmetrical neuropathy:*** Sensory, motor, autonomic or mixed—most common
2. ***Proximal neuropathy:***
   - Symmetrical proximal sensorimotor neuropathy
   - Asymmetrical proximal neuropathy
3. ***Mononeuritis and mononeuritis multiplex, affecting:***
   - Cranial nerves
   - Peripheral limb and trunk nerves
4. ***Entrapment neuropathies.***

Several of these neuropathic manifestations and autonomic neuropathy may coexist in the same patient. Sometimes small fibers or large fibers may be selectively affected producing predominant pain/temperature loss or vibration/proprioception loss respectively. Proximal neuropathy in the lower extremities is usually subacute and painful, followed by proximal weakness and muscle wasting and may be bilateral. Symptoms may improve over a few months.

The major pathological finding is axonal degeneration. Optimal control of diabetes with careful maintenance of euglycemia helps to reduce the frequency and severity of diabetic neuropathies (*See* also Section 10, Ch 92).

Other systemic diseases like hypothyroidism, chronic liver failure, porphyria, uremia, connective tissue disorders, malignancy and paraproteinemia may be associated with peripheral nerve involvement (Table 212.1).

Several disorders of the peripheral nervous system termed ***paraproteinemic neuropathies*** are closely connected with the presence of excessive amounts of abnormal immunoglobulins in blood which can be detected by immunoelectrophoresis or more sensitive immunofixation tests. The neuropathies may precede or occur concurrently along with benign monoclonal gammapathies or conditions like multiple myeloma, primary amyloidosis, Castleman's disease, other lymphatic diseases and chronic leukemia. The polyneuropathy of cryoglobulinemia is due to vasculitis in numerous nerve fascicles. The final picture is the sum total of multiple incomplete mononeuropathies. Sensorimotor polyneuropathy also develops. ***Treatment*** of the primary condition halts the progress of the neuropathy also.

Toxic and Drug-induced Neuropathies

Exposure to several toxins like alcohol, lead, arsenic, triorthocresyl phosphate (TCP) and organophosphorus compounds and drugs like dilantin, INH, nitrofurantoin, methotrexate and vincristine can cause polyneuropathies.

Vasculitic Neuropathy

Many forms of vasculitis cause widespread destruction of epineural arterioles with resultant ischemic damage to peripheral nerves. Peripheral neuropathy can be an early manifestation of vasculitis and diagnosis can be established by nerve biopsy. The three major categories of diseases that cause vasculitic neuropathy are:

- Systemic lupus erythematosus (SLE) and rheumatoid arthritis (RA).
- Systemic necrotizing vasculitis (SNV), such as polyarteritis nodosa (PAN).
- Nonsystemic vasculitic neuropathy.

Clinically, the most common presentation is mononeuritis multiplex caused by segmental nerve trunk infarction. Radiculopathies, distal sensorimotor neuropathy and cutaneous neuropathy are other manifestations of vasculitic neuropathy. Cranial neuropathies are common in Wegener's granulomatosis and sarcoidosis. Painful paresthesias can be severe and disturbing and difficult to treat. Specific treatment is directed at the vasculitis itself.

Critical Illness Neuropathy

It is an acute symmetric axonal sensorimotor polyneuropathy that is seen in patients with a prolonged critical illness. It is typically seen in patients in the ICU setting requiring mechanical ventilation for one week or more. The condition may progress to flaccid quadriplegia. With resolution of the critical illness, the condition plateaus and usually improves over about 6 months.

Related conditions include critical illness myopathy (CIM) with predominant myopathic features or a combination of both neuropathy and myopathy which has been termed critical illness neuromyopathy. One of these conditions occur to a significant degree in about 25% of ICU patients and subtle degrees of weakness may occur in even more, up to 50%.

Risk Factors

Factors associated with critical illness neuropathy/myopathy include:

- Severity of underlying critical illness and systemic inflammatory response syndrome
- Prolonged mechanical ventilation
- Use of IV steroids
- Low-albumin level
- Hyperglycemia and diabetes
- Use of neuromuscular paralytic agents with mechanical ventilation.

Etiology of this condition is believed to be due to microvascular ischemia to the peripheral nerves associated with the systemic inflammatory response and hypoperfusion related to hemodynamic compromise from the critical illness.

Diagnosis

Clinical presentation is a flaccid quadriparesis with diminished or absent reflexes and decreased distal sensations. Since ventilated patients are usually sedated, it requires regular, methodical physical examinations to detect worsening weakness as in decreased withdrawal to noxious stimuli. Reflexes are diminished or absent. If the cause of the initial respiratory failure is unclear, one should consider the possibility of an evolving GBS as the primary diagnosis that may have caused the initial respiratory failure and is now manifesting as a full-blown quadriplegic neuropathy. Guillain-Barré may be distinguished from a critical illness neuropathy in two ways. On nerve conduction studies, critical illness neuropathy is an axonal neuropathy whereas Guillain-Barré is usually a demyelinating neuropathy. If a LP has been performed, CSF protein is normal in critical illness neuropathy but elevated in Guillain-Barré.

If a patient in the critical care setting has an evolving flaccid quadriparesis but with intact reflexes and intact sensation, one should consider a CIM. An elevated creatine phosphokinase (CPK) would also support the diagnosis but in some patients it may be normal. If such a patient has been treated with steroids, one must also consider an acute steroid myopathy. Since it is difficult to accurately distinguish between these conditions and given that steroid use has been implicated in both, it would be wise to taper the steroids as soon as clinically feasible to do so.

Management

One cannot predict the occurrence of critical illness neuropathy and there is no specific treatment, since by the time of manifestation, the nerve damage is already done and one has to give the nerves 6 months or so to recover. The mainstay of medical care is to prevent further damage once the condition is recognized and also to prevent secondary complications.

Patients in the critical care setting should be monitored for signs of increased weakness, such as decreased withdrawal to pain even in the absence of increased sedation. If there is any such evidence, efforts should be redoubled to:

- Taper steroid use
- Avoid paralytic agents
- Correct hyperglycemia
- Continue management of critical illness and maintain hemodynamic stability.

One should be alert to increased risk of decubitus ulcers in these patients due to quadriparesis and preventive care should be provided accordingly. Furthermore, such patients may have increased difficulty in weaning off the ventilator and coughing up secretions and this should be kept in mind during pulmonary management.

Bedside physiotherapy should be instituted as soon as the patient is hemodynamically stable and increased once he is off the ventilator and out of the ICU.

Finally, when the patient who has just battled a life-threatening illness awakens to find that he is paralyzed and debilitated, he should be emphatically reassured that the condition is often temporary and the chances are that he will be back on his feet within 6 months.

NEURALGIC AMYOTROPHY

Syn: Brachial neuralgia, Brachial plexitis

This disorder is thought to be caused by demyelination occurring secondary to several causes such as infection, immunization and surgery. The patients complain of sudden severe pain in the shoulder region. This is followed by weakness and wasting of muscles around the shoulder joint. Most commonly muscles supplied by the axillary nerve (circumflex nerve) or long thoracic nerve (nerve to serratus anterior) are affected. Sensory loss can occasionally be found at the lateral aspect of the shoulder in an axillary nerve distribution. Recovery occurs within 6 months to one year.

ENTRAPMENT NEUROPATHIES

These result from compression of a nerve by normal anatomical structures at certain sites. Common examples are Carpal Tunnel Syndrome (CTS) caused by compression of the median nerve under the flexor retinaculum at the wrist and meralgia paresthetica caused by compression of the lateral cutaneous nerve of thigh between anterior superior iliac spine and inguinal ligament.

Carpal Tunnel Syndrome

It presents as pain and paraesthesia in the lateral three-and-a-half fingers, worsened at night. The pain may spread proximally. Shaking the hand in the air gives relief (flick test). Sensations over the median nerve distribution are dulled. This may be accompanied by weakness of the thenar muscles. Weakness of thumb opposition may result in sudden loosening of grip and dropping things. Caution needs to be exercised when holding things like cups of hot tea or coffee to avoid injury. In about half the cases the condition is primary. In the others some underlying cause is evident. CTS may occur in acromegaly, myxedema, multiple myeloma, RA, and in pregnancy. Phalen's sign is pain caused upon flexion of the wrist for 60 seconds. Tinnel's sign is the occurrence of sharp shooting pain along the distribution of the median nerve when the flexor retinaculum is tapped gently. Electrophysiological studies facilitate the diagnosis but are sometimes inconclusive.

Treatment: When the condition is curable with medical treatment as in pregnancy or myxedema, splinting of the band, use of diuretics and local instillation of hydrocortisone acetate may give temporary relief. Decompression of the nerve by surgical splitting of the flexor retinaculum gives permanent relief.

Meralgia Paresthetica

Present as pain and paresthesia in the lateral aspect of the thigh often following exertion or with wearing of tight belts. There are no motor signs in this disorder. It is usually self-limited. Severe cases respond to surgical decompression. Other nerves likely to be compressed in other sites are the radial, suprascapular, femoral, obturator, posterior tibial, plantar and intercostal nerves.

HEREDITARY MOTOR SENSORY NEUROPATHY (HMSN)

They are clinically complex and genetically heterogeneous group of disorders that cause slowly, progressive degeneration of peripheral nerves. Recent advances in the understanding of the molecular basis of hereditary neuropathies have resulted in a new genetic classification of HMSN. This is important for genetic counseling and planning future research for effective therapy. Type I and II are known as Charcot-Marie-Tooth disease 1 and 2 (CMT-1 and CMT-2). Genetic studies have revealed four subtypes of CMT-1 and six subtypes of CMT-2 depending on the chromosomes affected. CMT-1 is the more common demyelinating form with loss of muscle stretch reflexes, hypertrophy of nerves and a markedly slow conduction velocity on nerve conduction velocity (NCV). CMT-2 is the less common neuronal form where there is no nerve hypertrophy or delayed conductions. Muscle stretch reflexes are usually preserved. Most forms are transmitted as autosomal dominant. A few subtypes are autosomal recessive or sex-linked.

Neuropathy of Dejerine and *Sotta* is an autosomal recessive demyelinating sensory neuropathy in which the onset is much earlier and the disease progress to make the patient bed-ridden by the age of 20–30 years. The nerves are thickened. Sensory impairment is more marked. It may be associated with other neurological abnormalities such as optic atrophy, deafness, retinitis pigmentosa and spastic paralysis.

Clinical Features

The symptoms of CMT-1 appear in the first decade or early second decade. Toe walking, gait abnormalities, loss of balance and foot deformities are common presentations. Weakness of peroneal and anterior tibial muscles results in foot drop with a high-stepping gait. Pes cavus deformity and hammer toes are late manifestations. Atrophy of legs gives the classical inverted champagne bottle appearance. Vibratory sense is the usual sensory modality affected. *Diagnosis* is made based on the family pedigree, neurological examination, electrophysiological studies and DNA analysis. As of now there is no effective treatment. Steroid responsive forms of CMT-1 and hereditary neuropathy with liability to pressure palsy have been described.

NEUROFIBROMATOSIS

This entity consists of two distinct subgroups designated as von Recklinghausen's neurofibromatosis (VRN or type-1) and bilateral acoustic neurofibromatosis (BANF or type-2). The former used to be called peripheral neurofibromatosis and latter central. Both entities are genetically and clinically distinct.

Peripheral Neurofibromatosis

Syn: Type-1 or VRN

Peripheral neurofibromatosis has a prevalence of one in 3,000 adults. It is inherited as an autosomal dominant condition with 100% penetrance. The abnormal gene is located on chromosome 17. About 50% of cases arise as new mutations without family history. Clinical picture is varied. This includes dermatological features such as *café au lait* patches (Fig. 212.1) which grow with age, Lisch nodules (brown hamartomas seen in the iris) and dermal

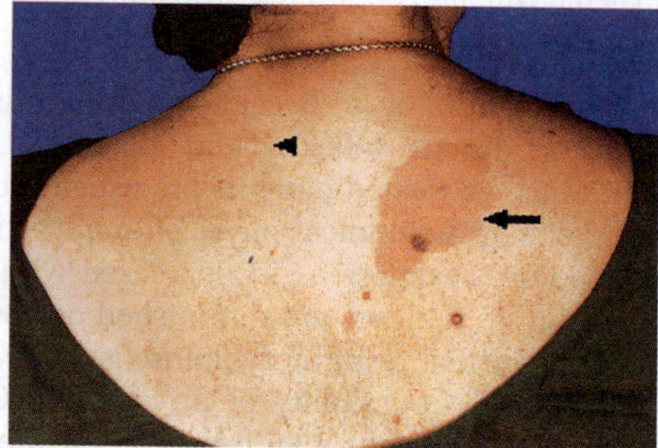

Fig. 212.1: Café au lait lesions in VRN type-I (arrow)

Table 212.2: Diagnostic criteria in neurofibromatosis

Type 1: Two or more of the following must be present	Type 2: At least, one criterion must be present for diagnosis
• Café au lait macules with the greatest diameter 5 mm in prepubertal and 15 mm in postpubertal patients, at least six in number • Two or more neurofibromas of any type or one plexiform neuroma • Presence of optic glioma • Two or more Lisch nodules • Bony lesion in sphenoid or long bones • Parent, sibling or child with neurofibromatosis	• Bilateral eighth nerve tumors seen by imaging techniques • Parent, sibling or child with neurofibromatosis Type-2 showing neurological tumors or juvenile posterior lenticular opacity

neurofibromas which appear during puberty and continue to grow throughout life. Plexiform neurofibromas may produce local hypertrophy and physical disfigurement. Rare associations include congenital defects in the posterior orbital wall, proptosis due to orbital neurofibroma, pseudoarthoses of the tibia and ulna and vertebral lesions giving rise to kyphoscoliosis. Neurofibromas of the spinal roots or in the intracranial structures and gliomas and meningiomas may occur but the risk is much less than in the central type.

Acoustic neuromas are extremely rare, but optic nerve or chiasmal gliomas may occur. Plexiform neurofibromas may develop malignancy, but not dermal neurofibromas. Two rare associations include pheochromocytoma and renal artery stenosis.

Central Neurofibromatosis

Syn: Type-2 or BANF

This is much rarer than type-1 (1 in 100,000) transmitted by a different autosomal dominant gene located on chromosome 22 with a 95% penetrance so that 50% of offspring develop the diseases. There is a very high prevalence of bilateral acoustic neuromas (schwannomas). The early symptoms manifest in the second or third decades of life with eighth nerve dysfunction. Rarely, the condition may be unilateral.

Other central nervous system tumors such schwannomas in other sites, gliomas and meningiomas may occur simultaneously. Management consists of surgical removal of the tumors and genetic counseling. Patients with BANF and their relatives should avoid underwater swimming.

Diagnostic criteria for type-1 and type-2 neurofibromatosis are described in Table 212.2.

DIAGNOSTIC APPROACH TO PERIPHERAL NEUROPATHY

The first step is to confirm that the patient indeed has a peripheral neuropathy. There should be no evidence of spasticity or hyperreflexia to suggest a myelopathy or other UMN process. There should be no definite sensory level to suggest a myelopathic process. Back or neck pain associated with radicular pain suggests a focal radiculopathy. Proximal weakness with muscle tenderness should prompt workup with blood CPK and EMG to exclude a myopathy.

If symptoms are isolated to a single extremity, the patient should be evaluated for an entrapment neuropathy

or plexopathy or radiculopathy. Radiculopathy usually is associated with radicular pain. Plexopathy is relatively less common, may also be painful and may not conform to any particular radicular or peripheral nerve distribution. Neuralgic amyotrophy has already been discussed. Lumbosacral plexopathy can occur from a pelvic mass or retroperitoneal hematoma in patients with a history of surgery or who are on anticoagulants. If the pain, paresthesias, numbness or motor deficit conforms to the distribution of a particular peripheral nerve, entrapment should be considered. Examples include wrist drop from a radial neuropathy or paresthesias over the thenar aspect with wrist pain at night suggesting CTS affecting the median nerve. If no evidence of entrapment is apparent, the patient should be worked up for a mononeuritis, which can be secondary to diabetes or vasculitis.

Nonhealing painless ulcers and neuropathic joints develop due to loss of pain and temperature sensation and loss of protective reflexes. When the protective influence of pain is lost, the joints undergo minor and major trauma due to overuse and injuries. Degenerative and destructive changes of joint structures develop, leading to disorganization of the joint (Charcot's joints). Such joints may occur in severe peripheral neuropathy and also in tabes dorsalis and syringomyelia.

The tendon reflexes are lost early in peripheral neuropathies which affect the large fibers. The reflexes may be spared in neuropathies which affect the small fibers alone, e.g. leprosy.

Peripheral nerves may be palpably hypertrophic in conditions such as leprosy, amyloidosis, acromegaly, neurofibromatosis and Refsum's disease.

Burning feet is a frequent symptom but its mechanism is not clear. It may occur in neuropathies, accompanying alcoholism, diabetes and beriberi.

Pupillary changes, bladder and bowel dysfunction and impotence point to central lesions; these do not occur in pure peripheral neuropathy.

EMG/NCV is helpful to differentiate an axonal versus demyelinating neuropathy, helping to narrow the differential. If it is demyelinating, it may raise the possibility of CIDP that may otherwise not have been suspected. LP may also help here to confirm that there is elevated protein. EMG/NCV is also helpful to determine if there is subclinical disease elsewhere, such as making a diagnosis of a mononeuritis multiplex in case that may clinically have appeared as just a single monoeuropathy. It may also help exclude a myopathy if there is any doubt. It can also help distinguish between a radiculopathy and neuropathy, such as in a patient with wrist drop and chronic neck pain, to differentiate between a true cervical radiculopathy versus simple cervical strain with unrelated radial nerve palsy.

Acknowledgement: The authors gratefully acknowledge the contribution of late Dr PK Mohan, who co-authored this chapter previously.

Source:

1. Disorders of peripheral nervous system by dick and lambert.
2. Continuum series American Academy of neurology.
3. Coir workers Neuropathy KMJ, July 1999 recommended reading.

CHAPTER
213

Disorders of the Autonomic Nervous System

SR Chandra

Chapter Summary

- Anatomy
- General Considerations
- Autonomic Disorders
- Common Clinical Features of Autonomic Disturbances
- Examination of the Patient
- Classification by Krane
- Treatment

INTRODUCTION

This term autonomic nervous system (ANS) is applied to the part of the neuraxis which predominantly functions autonomically and fully controllable voluntarily (Fig. 213.1). This is a critical component of the neural network important for homeostasis including control of blood pressure (BP), blood flow, thermoregulation and gastro-intestinal (GI), respiratory, genitourinary and sexual functions. It has three major components—(1) sympathetic, (2) parasympathetic and (3) the enteric nervous system. Langley in 1921 coined the term, Claude Bernard said that *nature thought it prudent to remove important organs from the ignorant will and created autonomic system.* It becomes affected in several systemic diseases as well as the primary diseases of the ANS. In this chapter, we shall deal with the anatomy, physiology and diseases primarily and secondarily affecting the ANS.

ANATOMY

Sympathetic System

Sympathetic nervous system has a central component in the hypothalamus which is connected to orbitofrontal cortex, cingulum, amygdala and bulbar reticular formation. The descending fibers reach the nucleus tractus solitarius, serotonergic raphe nuclei, cells of A5 catecholamine group and synapse with intermediolateral columns of the spinal cord which extends from T1 to L2.

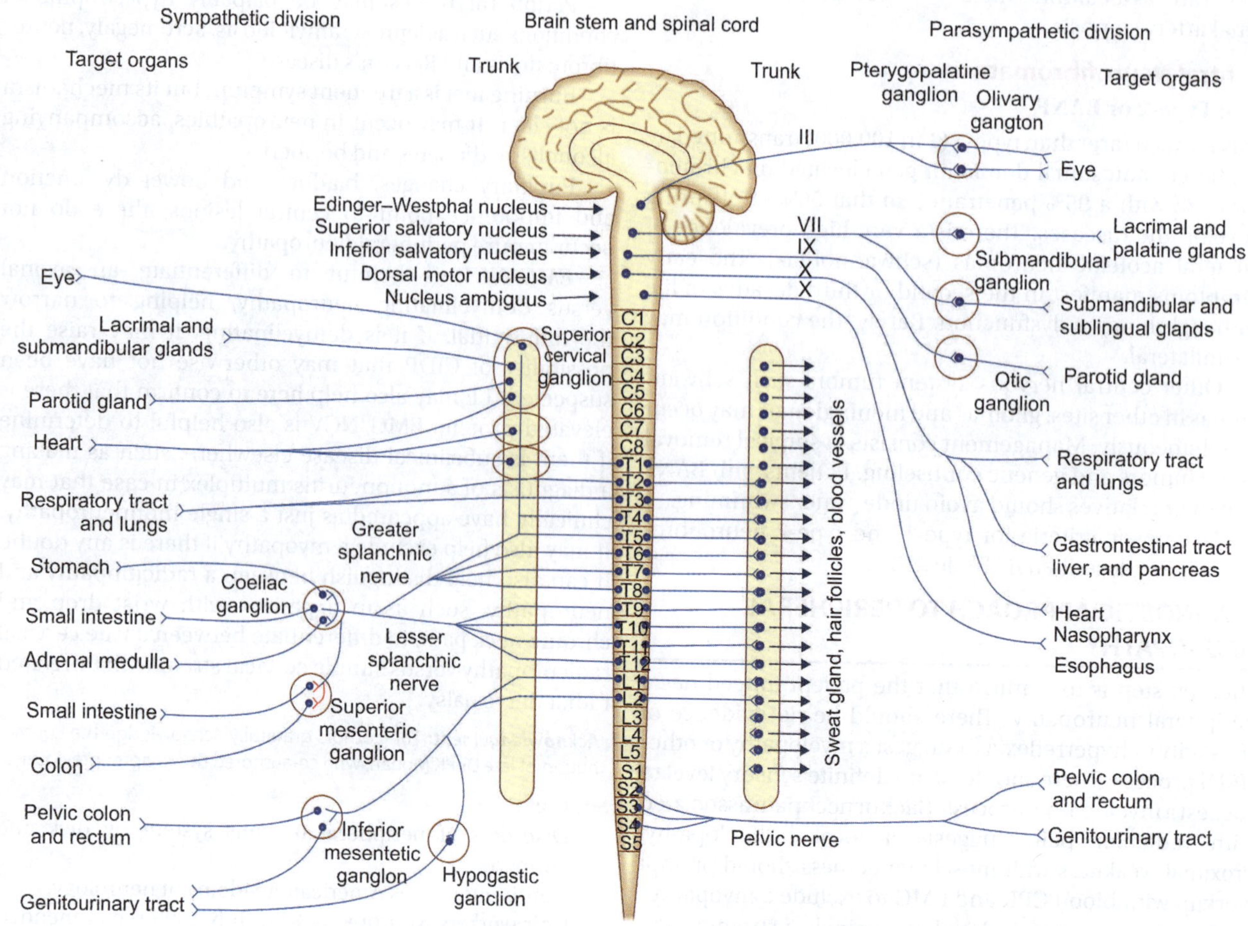

Fig. 213.1: Schematic representation of autonomic nervous system

The axons emerge through the ventral roots as the small myelinated preganglionic white rami communicantes and enter ganglia, to form the gray communicating rami communicantes which along the spinal nerves supply visceral structures, peripheral nerves, blood vessels, muscle, skin and sweat glands. There are plexuses which supply heart, lungs, kidneys, intestines, pancreas, urinary bladder and sex organs. The preganglionic fibers are cholinergic and postganglionic fibers are noradrenergic except at sweat glands where both are cholinergic. There are purinergic fibers which are important for regulation of blood flow.

Parasympathetic System

The suprabulbar connections are the same as the sympathetic system. Fibers leave the brainstem via 3rd, 7th, 9th and 10th cranial nerves and sacral spinal cord in the 2nd, 3rd and 4th sacral nerves. The ganglia lie close to the innervated structures. Unlike the sympathetic both pre and postganglionic fibers are cholinergic. Vagal fibers from aortic arch baroreceptors and glossopharyngeal fibers from the carotid sinus and their efferents to the heart are unmyelinated.

GENERAL CONSIDERATIONS

General sympathetic functions are ***fight*** or ***flight reaction***, increased heart rate, rise in BP, bronchodilation, increase in GI motility and sphincter tone, ejaculation and pupillary dilatation. Parasympathetic functions are to rest, digest and store energy, reduce heart rate, BP, GI motility and sphincter tone, bronchoconstriction, pupillary constriction, tearing, salivation and penile erection.

Control of BP

Cardiac output and vascular resistance determine BP. The sympathetic neurons in the intermediolateral column control vascular resistance. Cardiac output is a function of heart rate and stroke volume. The heart rate is determined by vagus and the sympathetic nerves. Stroke volume which is dependent on venous return is influenced by the sympathetic system in the abdominal viscera. The baroreceptors in the carotid sinus and aortic arch sense changes and maintain constancy.

Sweat Glands and Skin Blood Vessels

The sudomotor fibers are fast conducting fibers belonging to postganglionic sympathetic cholinergic system as well as those containing vasoactive intestinal peptide (VIP).

The blood vessels are innervated by sympathetic noradrenergic fibers. Postganglionic cholinergic sympathetic fibers supply sweat gland and sympathetic noradrenergic fibers supply blood vessels of skin. Skin sympathetic activities are directly affected by mental and emotional stress.

Thermoregulation

The medial preoptic hypothalamus is the thermostat containing warm sensitive neurons that dissipate heat by vasodilatation and sweating and cold sensitive neurons that trigger shivering, brown fat metabolism and vasoconstriction. This system receives afferents from periaqueductal gray matter and rostral medullary raphe.

Emotions and Stress

Anterior part of the cingulum, ventromedial prefrontal cortex, amygdala, hypothalamus and periaqueductal gray matter provide affective value to incoming sensory information which initiates visceral and endocrine responses of defense reaction.

Control of Urinary Bladder

Bladder contains both efferent and afferent innervation from sympathetic and parasympathetic in addition to somatic innervation. Parasympathetic afferents have volume and pressure sensors in the bladder which enter the spinal cord through the posterior root and column and from the detrusor nucleus through lateral column. The efferents enter sacral plexus through the spinal nerves and travel via nervi erigentes, pudendal nerve, pelvic nerve and vesical plexus to the base of the bladder. They are mainly concerned with emptying.

Sympathetic nerves start from the beta-receptors of the body of the bladder and alpha-receptors of the sphincter and enter the afferent pathway. The efferents from the intermediolateral column in the spinal cord leave along the ventral roots, enter the spinal nerve, white rami communicantes, paravertebral chain, hypogastric and mesenteric ganglia, to emerge as the hypogastric nerve to form the pelvic plexus and enter the bladder. Higher control is influenced by Bradley's circuit 1, 2, 3 and 4 (for further information refer to monographs on this topic).

Source: Autonomic disorders continuum. Am Acad Neurology. 2007;13(6):1-280.

Gastrointestinal System

The ANS in the gastrointestinal tract (GIT) can be called mini-brain because the enteric interneuronal circuitry processes information and generates output signals for the muscles, secretory apparatus and vasculature. The afferent inputs are received from wall tension, pH, osmolarity of the luminal content and these are coordinated with the programmed digestive behavior to decide the motility pattern. The circuits involved are chemical, mechanical and receptor-mediated, sensory neurons and motor neurons. Reproducible automatic and purposeful contractions of circular muscles and relaxation of longitudinal muscles produce peristalsis. There is a migrating motor complex which times the pattern generation which is called ***enteric driver circuit*** and a gating mechanism to prevent unwanted peristalsis. The enteric motor neurons are noradrenergic noncholinergic. The excitatory neurons contain substance-P. The secretomotor neurons contain VIP and vasculature contains VIP, substance-P and acetylcholine.

AUTONOMIC DISORDERS

Disorders can be classified into diseases affecting the central autonomic system and those affecting the peripheral autonomic system.

Central autonomic system

- ***Progressive autonomic failure (PAF)***
  - Pure PAF
  - PAF with Parkinson's disease (PD)
  - PAF with multiple system atrophy (MSA) (Shy-Drager syndrome)

- **Parkinson's disease (PD)**
- **Spinal cord disease**
- **Wernicke's encephalopathy**
- **Miscellaneous**
  - Cerebrovascular accident (CVA)
  - Brainstem tumors
  - Multiple sclerosis (MS)
  - Adie's syndrome
  - Tabes dorsalis.

Peripheral autonomic system

- **Pure autonomic dysfunction**
  - Pandysautonomia
  - Cholinergic dysautonomia
  - Botulism
- **Associated with peripheral neuropathy**
  - Diabetes
  - Amyloidosis
  - Acute inflammatory neuropathy
  - Porphyria
  - Riley day syndrome (familial dysautonomia)
  - Chronic inflammatory demyelinating polyneuropathy (CIDP)
- **Peripheral neuropathy with mild autonomic dysfunction**
  - Alcoholic neuropathy
  - Toxic neuropathy
  - Hereditary motor sensory neuropathy (HMSN)
  - Paraneoplastic neuropathy
  - Vitamin B_{12} neuropathy
  - Neuropathy associated with autoimmune disorders
  - Fabry's disease.

COMMON CLINICAL FEATURES OF AUTONOMIC DISTURBANCES

Orthostatic Intolerance

Fall of BP exceeding 20 mm Hg when the person assumes erect posture or stands for 5 minutes is called *orthostatic hypotension*.

The most common symptom in orthostatic intolerance is light headedness or presyncope on standing. Retrocolic heaviness and headache can occur, these are called *coat hanger phenomena*. They may be unsteady and later develop cognitive dysfunction. The symptoms are worst in the morning and can be provoked by exercise, heat and heavy meal.

Grading

Grade 0: Normal

Grade 1
- Symptoms precipitated by severe orthostatic stress
- Symptoms after 15 minutes of standing
- Activities of daily living unaffected but mild symptoms

Grade 2
- Frequent symptoms
- Can stand up to 5 minutes
- Mild limitation of activities of daily living

Grade 3
- Symptoms are present most of the time
- Can stand up to 1 minute
- Marked limitation of activities of daily living

Grade 4
- Constant orthostatic symptoms—cannot stand
- Can stand less than 1 minute
- Wheel chair bound
- Syncope on standing.

Treatment consists of treating the cause. Whenever possible, look for drugs like beta and alpha blockers,

vincristine, alcohol and others. Symptomatic treatment of orthostatic hypotension includes increasing the salt intake, 4–10 g day, administration of fludrocortisone 0.1–0.5 mg day or indomethacin, ibuprofen or aspirin. Nonpharmacological measures include the assumption of head tilt (up to position 15–25 cm), exercises and reconditioning.

- **Vasomotor symptoms:** These include coldness, changes in skin color and trophic changes and development of wrinkles on immersion in water. Noradrenergic dysfunction results in absence of wrinkling.
- **Sweating:** Generalized or focal loss of sweating is manifested as dryness of the eyes, dry mouth, dry skin, heat intolerance, hot feeling, flushing, dyspnea and weakness.
- **Digestive symptoms:** These include anorexia, early satiety, feeling of fullness, nausea, regurgitation of undigested food, weight loss and constipation alternating with diarrhea.
- **Eye signs:** These include pupillary abnormalities and defective dark adaptations.
- **Genitourinary symptoms:** Bladder, bowel and sexual dysfunctions. Retention incontinence inadequate emptying of bladder and bowel, precipitancy, hesitancy, nonrecognition of distended bladder and bowel.

Sexual Dysfunction

Sexual response consists of libido, penile erection, ejaculation and detumescence. Erection is mediated by cholinergic parasympathetic pathways and nonadrenergic-noncholinergic pathways which release acetylcholine and cause vascular smooth muscle relaxation. This increases the blood flow and facilitates erection. Detumescence is by norepinephrine mediated sympathetic pathway causing contraction of smooth muscles.

Ten to twenty percent of middle-aged men and women suffer from sexual dysfunction. Both males and females develop sexual dysfunction due to autonomic disorders. Both sexes may suffer from loss of libido, frigidity, absence of lubrication and consummation of the intercourse. Males suffer more frequently from erectile inadequacy, failure of insertion, premature ejaculation, absence of ejaculation and retrograde ejaculation. Women suffer more from frigidity, dryness of the vagina, dyspareunia, vaginismus and loss of libido.

Sexual dysfunction may be psychogenic, endocrinological, neurogenic, arteriogenic, adverse effects of drugs or due to debilitating systemic diseases. The most common endocrine diseases causing impotence are diabetes and hypogonadism. Medications including diuretics, antihypertensives, cardiac drugs, tranquilizers, hormones, anticancer drugs, anticholinergics, H_2-receptor antagonists and substance abuse. *Treatment* involves looking for correctible factors, psychoeducation, specialized testing, looking for nocturnal penile tumescence, Doppler, penile angiography, neurological testing including evoked responses and psychological testing. Treatment consists of attention to the underlying cause. Drug therapy is given to stimulate erection and libido in both sexes (Refer to Section 11, Ch 102).

EXAMINATION OF THE PATIENT

General Assessment

General examination involves looking for features of manifestations of other parts of the neuraxis and other systemic signs like dysfunction of cognition, posture, facial expression, eyes, hair and features of hypothalamic involvement like dwarfism, sexual immaturity, pallor and hypothermia. Paroxysmal autonomic symptoms include paroxysmal hyperhydrosis, orthostatic tachycardia, presyncope, sympathetically mediated pain and reflex syncope related to cough, micturition and defecation. Rarely, ANS symptoms can be manifestations of seizure activity presenting as paroxysmal piloerection, sweating and arrhythmias. Acral vasomotor changes include cyanosis, pallor, mottling and redness, sweating, swelling, trophic changes, dryness, features of hyperalgesia and allodynia.

Nails may be thick, distorted and discolored. Joints may show disorganization resulting in Charcot's or Clutton's joints. Charcot's joints are painless joints with destructive changes caused by denervation of the sensory fibers. Clutton's joints are large painless joints with fluid and abnormal mobility. Pupils may vary in shape, size, light reflex and accommodation reflex. The patient may complain of orthostatic symptoms such as syncope. Stigmata of systemic diseases may be present if the autonomic dysfunction is secondary to systemic disease.

Testing the Autonomic System

Aim of evaluation is to identify the presence and distribution and severity of autonomic dysfunction.

BP and Heart Rate Related Tests

Cold pressor test, isometric hand grip and orthostatic hypotension are tests of sympathetic function. Valsalva maneuver and deep breathing are tests of parasympathetic.

BP and heart rate are recorded at supine posture standing for 5 minutes, 10 minutes and 15 minutes, repeated after 12 squats. In sympathetic adrenergic dysfunction, there is decrease in BP and increase in heart rate. Fall in systolic BP of at least 20 mm Hg or diastolic BP 10 mm Hg during the first 3 minutes of standing constitutes orthostatic hypertension. Paroxysmal orthostatic tachycardia on minimal exertion is often associated with *chronic fatigue syndrome*.

Deep breathing techniques: In the supine position with the patient breathing, at the rate of six breaths per minute taking 5 seconds for inhalation and 5 seconds for exhalation with continuous electrocardiogram (ECG) monitoring. The difference between the maximum average R-R interval in inspiration (I) and minimum R-R interval in expiration (E) is calculated, the E:I ratio. A heart rate variation of more than 15 beats/min or measurement of (E:I) ratio is an accurate test of vagal function. E:I ratio less than 1.2 is abnormal. This can be repeated six times. The ratio decreases with age and markedly so beyond the age of 60 years (at which time it approaches 1.04 or less).

Sinus arrhythmia: There is normally a beat to beat variation in heart rate during deep inspiration of about 10 beats/minute. An absence of this indicates vagal denervation.

Valsalva test: It is performed by making the patient blow into a mouth piece connected to a mercury column. A column of mercury is maintained at 40–50 mm Hg for 10–15 seconds. Heart rate is recorded using ECG before, during and 10 seconds after the maneuver.

- In phase 1, there is increase in the BP due to intra-thoracic pressure
- In phase II, there is gradual decrease in BP and then plateaus and heart rate increases
- During phase III, i.e. 2 seconds after the release of blowing, there is sudden drop in intrathoracic pressure and decrease in BP
- In phase IV, systolic BP and mean arterial pressure (MAP) increases and returns to normal in 90 seconds.

Then, the ratio of longest R-R to the shortest R-R interval is calculated. Normal is 1.5 or more. It is a screening test for baroreceptor function. This is called *Valsalva ratio*. Other abnormalities are absence of systolic BP over shoot in phase IV, lower heart rate in phase II than phase IV, decreases in MAP in phase II below 50% of the resting state.

The Pressor Stimuli

- The *cold pressor test* is performed by immersing a subject's hand in water at 4°C for 2–3 minutes. BP and heart rate measured while the hand is still immersed and blood flow assessed using plethysmography in the opposite limb.

  Immersing the hand in hot water produces vasodilatation in the opposite hand due to central temperature regulation mechanism. Mental arithmetic or sudden noise or isometric handgrip for 5 minutes, increases the heart rate and diastolic BP.
- *Isometric handgrip test:* First patient has to exert maximum effort and squeeze a handgrip dynamometer to assess maximum voluntary capacity and later maintained at 30% of that for 2 minutes and BP is measured before and after contraction at 2 minutes in the contralateral arm.

  Absence of increase in heart rate and BP is indicative of sympathetic dysfunction. Lower body vacuum suction, radiant heating of the trunk and measuring BP and heart rate are other tests of sympathetic function.
- *Cortical arousal:* Sudden sound or mental arithmetic produce heart rate and BP changes which are lost in central sympathetic dysfunction.

Axon Reflex

About 5–10 mg intradermal acetylcholine produces local piloerection and sweating. Absence of this indicates ganglionic and postganglionic sympathetic lesion. It is normal in preganglionic disease.

Sweat Test

Patient is administered a hot cup of tea with aspirin. He/she is smeared with starch iodate powder and areas of sweating turn blue (iodine solution and starch powder can be used).

Sympathetic skin response can be assessed in the electrophysiology laboratory using sound, electrical stimulation or mental arithmetic as stimuli and picking up sympathetic changes using electrodes fixed on the dorsal and palmar aspect of the hand or feet.

Quantitative Sudomotor Axon Reflex Test (QSART)

Physiologic basis: It is used to evaluate postganglionic sympathetic cholinergic sudomotor function by measuring the axon reflex-mediated sweat response. Innervation of human eccrine sweat gland is mainly by sympathetic postganglionic cholinergic fibers. The regulation of sweating is cholinergic and muscarinic because it is completely inhibited by atropine. The neural pathway consists of an axon reflex-mediated by the postganglionic sympathetic sudomotor axon. The axon terminal is activated by acetylcholine. The impulse travels antidromically, reaches a branch-point, then travels orthodromically to release acetylcholine from nerve terminals. Acetylcholine traverses the neuroglandular junction and binds to M3 muscarinic receptors on eccrine sweat glands to evoke the sweat response. The stimulus is a constant current of 2 mA applied for 5 minutes and the sweat response is recorded during the stimulus and also for the subsequent 5 minutes.

QSART is done using a multicompartmental sweat capsule. The capsule is placed on the skin and the outer ring is filled with 10% acetylcholine. The inner ring has nitrogen gas. Iontophoresis of the acetylcholine is started with a 2 mA current for 5 minutes. Humidity produced is used as a measure of the quantity of the sweat. The test is sensitive and reproducible in controls and in patients with neuropathy (Box 213.1).

Schirmer's Test

By tucking a 5 mm filter paper into the lower eyelid the tear column generated in 5 minutes should be at least 15 mm. Reduction in tear secretion suggests xerophthalmia which may be due to autonomic dysfunction or other causes such as Sjögren's syndrome.

Other Tests of Autonomic Function

Sweat imprint test, microneurography, gastric motility studies, penile plethysmography and sphincter electromyography (EMG).

Box 213.1: Tests employed to detect atrial natriuretic peptide (ANP)

- ***Tests for parasympathetic functions:***
  - Recording of sinus arrhythmia and BP
    - Heart rate response to Valsalva maneuver
- ***Tests for sympathetic adrenergic and cholinergic functions:***
  - Heart rate and BP responses to standing
  - BP response to Valsalva maneuver
  - Cold pressor test—BP rises
  - ***Isometric exercise test—BP rises:*** BP response to drugs such as noradrenaline, angiotensin II, atropine and neostigmine
- ***Tests for sympathetic cholinergic functions:***
  - Thermoregulatory sweat test
  - Quantitative sudomotor axon test
  - Sympathetic skin response
  - Sweat imprint methods
- ***Test for lacrimal secretion (parasympathetic):***
  - Schirmer's test
  - Test for cutaneous flare response: Subcutaneous histamine injection or scratch test
  - Tests for pupillary responses: Instillation of drugs such as homatropine, cocaine, pilocarpine—response depends on the type of drug instilled.

Note: For practical details, monographs on clinical neurology may be consulted.

- ***Pupil*** becomes small in sympathetic and large in parasympathetic denervation
- ***Adie's pupil:*** It is primarily large pupil but shows good constriction to 2.5% methacholine due to denervation supersensitivity which is not seen in normal pupil
- ***Horner's syndrome:*** Constricted pupil which will not dilate with 4% cocaine, but 0.1% adrenaline shows dilatation if the lesion is postganglionic.

Biochemical Tests

Plasma noradrenaline is checked both in supine and standing positions. Normally, nonadrenaline levels increase on standing. This response is absent in sympathetic disease.

Vasopressin levels normally increases on head tilt but this response is defective in central autonomic disease. When noradrenaline is infused slowly, the BP and heart rate increase indicating denervation super sensitivity of alpha-1 receptors. Isoprenaline-β produces transient BP fall if there is beta-2 supersensitivity. Clonidine causes increase in growth hormone and decrease in plasma adrenaline normally. If this response does not happen, it indicates failure of central sympathetic.

URINARY BLADDER

The bladder has dual innervations. Urine is secreted at a rate of 0.1 mL/min but emptying takes place only intermittently. It has to store urine at low pressure so that reflux into the kidney does not take place. After emptying, there should not be residual urine. Parasympathetic innervations are motor for emptying. Sympathetic innervations are for storage with β-receptors in the body and α-receptors in the sphincters. Accumulation of up to about 100 mL of urine in the bladder does not evoke any neural activities and takes place. But, after that bladder wall receptors get activated. The β-receptors relax the body and α-receptors contract the sphincter. After about 300 mL, the afferents carrying volume and pressure sensation enter the spinal cord through the posterior column and spinothalamic to tract reach the brainstem and basal ganglia. The efferents descend and exit through the ventral root, paravertebral chain, hypogastric nerve and receptors in the bladder and facilitate storage beyond 300 mL based on the necessity. The parasympathetic is inhibited via the pelvic nerve. The external sphincter is kept tightly closed by the pudendal nerve. When the urine volume is more than 350 mL it trickles into the proximal urethra. Parasympathetic and sympathetic impulses are carried to the cortical centers and a voluntary element is added from the frontal lobe and these information are transferred to the autonomic system through corticospinal tract for facilitating or preventing emptying based on learned social behavior.

When a person comes with a bladder symptom, we have to rule out a urological cause and type the neurological dysfunction if present. This is done by ascertaining the frequency and volume of urine passed each time in 24 hours, presence of dysuria, hematuria and intermittent stream indicating obstructive uropathy. Features associated with prevoiding phase like ability to appreciate fullness and ability to appreciate pain, ability to initiate and terminate micturition at will. During the voiding phase, features such as the volume of urine passed, capacity to stop the stream at will and in the postvoiding phase feeling of incomplete emptying and presence of postvoiding dribbling are ascertained. The old Lapide's classification is still useful to understand grossly the bladder dysfunction at the bedside and this can be objectively characterized by urodynamic studies later.

Uninhibited Bladder

Patient does not have any dysuria, hematuria or intermittent stream. All phases of voiding are normal. But, he passes urine in socially inappropriate places due to loss of learned social inhibitions.

Automatic Bladder

It is seen in spinal cord disease. The prevoiding phase may be totally or partly lost depending on type of spinal cord damage. In the voiding phase, patient can neither initiate nor stop urine at will. When urine volume in the bladder reaches about 300 mL, it automatically empties. There is lack of synergy between the body and sphincters resulting in incomplete emptying and tendency to void again and postvoiding dribbling persists. Incomplete lesions can present with urinary hesitancy or retention if only the facilitatory fibers are damaged, precipitancy if only the inhibitory fibers are damaged.

Sensory denervated bladder: This develops when sensory roots or the sensory tracts are affected as in tabes dorsalis or diabetes where the patient develops a large bladder with painless retention of urine. Therefore, he does not initiate micturition but can voluntarily or by suprapubic pressure can initiate micturition but empties incompletely and leads to postvoiding dribbling.

Motor denervated bladder: This is seen in conditions like acute poliomyelitis and Guillain-Barré syndrome (GBS). There is painful retention which needs temporary catheterization.

Autonomous Bladder

This occurs when the sacral centers are also destroyed like in Cauda equina syndrome. Patient has a large bladder and all three phases of emptying are affected. When urine accumulates and the volume exceeds 1.5 L, weight of the urine opens up the internal sphincters resulting in continuous dribbling.

Detrusor-external Sphincter Dyssynergia

Here, the autonomic control of micturition is alright. The somatic innervation is affected due to usually painful perianal conditions or irritative disease of the pudendal nerve. All phases of micturition are normal except emptying. A clue can be obtained by attempting a pudendal block which will facilitate micturition and the patient can be treated with pudendal neurectomy or external sphincter resection.

Transformed Bladder

Any neurological bladder over a period of time gets transformed by infection, calculus formation and trabeculation and its characters become difficult to assess. Such a bladder is called *transformed bladder* and is very difficult to treat.

Classification by Krane

Type I: Detrusor hyper-reflexia
- With coordinated sphincter
- With striated muscle sphincter dyssynergia
- With smooth muscle sphincter dyssynergia

Type II: Detrusor hyporeflexia
- With coordinate sphincter
- Nonrelaxing striated muscle sphincter
- Denervated striated muscle sphincter
- Nonrelaxing smooth muscle sphincter

Functional classification
- Continent bladder
- Incontinent bladder
- Bladder which is both continent and incontinent.

Treatment

Pharmacotherapy to facilitate emptying includes bethanechol 25 mg to be titrated up to the effective dose, intravesical prostaglandins, botulinum toxin injection and surgically sphincterotomy or training for intermittent clean self-catheterization based on the clinical parameters. To decrease outlet resistance diazepam, dantrolene sodium, nicergoline, prazosin, phenoxybenzamine are used. To facilitate storage oxybutynin, propantheline, dicyclomine hydrochloride, imipramine can be used. However, the best option to prevent reflex and infection is intermittent self-catheterization.

CONCLUSION

Apart from the well-known manifestations, autonomic dysfunctions are elusive. High degree of suspicion is required to detect obscure autonomic derangements. This will serve to relieve distressing autonomic symptoms in patients who may mimic non-organic disease.

CHAPTER
214

Myasthenia Gravis

SR Chandra, KA Kabeer

Chapter Summary

- General Considerations
- Pathogenesis and Pathology
- Double Seronegative Myasthenia Gravis
- Congenital Myasthenias Syndrome
- Neonatal Myasthenia Gravis
  - Pathophysiological Classification
  - Lambert-Eaton Myasthenic Syndrome
- Diagnosis of Myasthenia Gravis
- Complications of Myasthenia Gravis
- Course and Prognosis
- Treatment
- Myasthenic Reactions

GENERAL CONSIDERATIONS

The word 'myasthenia gravis' (MG) is a combination of Greek word 'muscle weakness' and Latin word 'grave' severe. MG is an acquired disease of neuromuscular junction (NMJ) characterized by pathological fatigability and weakness. They present with fluctuating weakness with special predilection for muscles innervated by motor nuclei of brainstem. Young females are more affected than males and its incidence is around 1.7–21.3 per million per year. Thomas Willis in 17th century first described this condition. In 1935, Mary Walker identified beneficial use of physostigmine and neostigmine in therapy. Jon Lindstrom and Simpson postulated autoimmune nature and Daniel Drachman in 1973 localized its pathology to postsynaptic membrane.

PATHOGENESIS AND PATHOLOGY

Function of Neuromuscular Junction

The pathology is in postsynaptic NMJ (Fig. 214.1) which links efferent nerve fibers and muscles via axon terminals. When action potentials arrive at motor endplate, voltage-dependent calcium channels open, calcium binds to sensor proteins and transmitter acetylcholine (ACh) is released to synaptic cleft; this binds to nicotinic ACh receptor (AChR) of the muscle fiber. This results in depolarization of muscle fiber and sets in a cascade of events which lead to muscle contraction.

About 80% of patients with MG have circulating antibody (Ab) which leads to the following effects: Block AChRs which cause destruction of AChR receptor and cause complement-mediated destruction of folds, accelerated degradation of AChR, and in some cases, they block ACh-AChR binding.

Note: Family members of MG are 1,000 times more susceptible to develop MG than the general population.

Thymus gland may act as source of antigen through thymic myoid cells sharing common antigen with NMJ. Thymosin produced by thymus also inhibits neuromuscular transmission. Anti-MuSK or muscle-specific kinase antibody (MuSKAb) can be detected in patients who are AChR—Ab positive in up to 30–40%. The typical picture is neck, bulbar and respiratory symptoms without ocular involvement causing diagnostic confusion. During development, MuSK is needed for clustering of

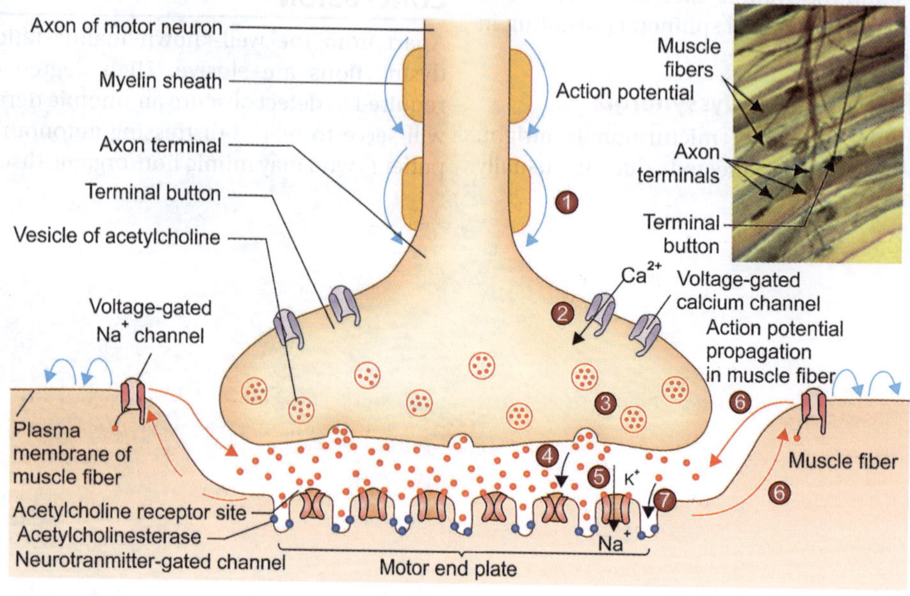

Fig. 214.1: Neuromuscular junction (NMJ)

AChR at NMJ and deficiency causes loss of structure of NMJ and declustering of AChRs. Atrophy of facial and tongue muscles may develop and poor response to conventional treatment may necessitate alternate therapy and need for second-line management. In anti-MuSKAb positive cases, weakness of eye closure may result in inability to close eye. Wasting and fasciculations of the tongue may occur in MuSKAb positive disease and this may give diagnostic problem unless condition is kept in mind. In addition to AChR Ab, several other Abs are also present in varying amounts in MG.

DOUBLE SERONEGATIVE MYASTHENIA GRAVIS

In this condition, antibodies (Abs) may not be readily demonstrable by ordinary methods. It is believed that Ab may be very low that they are not picked up, but probably they bind *in situ* and it is found that ACh currents are inhibited by plasma or serum of such patients. Undetected Abs may be a possibility.

Clinical Features in Adults

Most prominent feature of myasthenia is early fatigability of striated muscles on repetition of voluntary activity. The affection may be generalized or confined to groups of muscles, e.g. ocular myasthenia. With rest, fatigued muscle recovers to resume activity.

Repeated activity of a muscle produces weakness and fatigability of voluntary muscles which can be demonstrated by a decrease in muscle power grade and recovery after rest. Usually eye muscles, then face, neck and later limbs show signs. Ninety percent patients develop generalized myasthenia during course of their disease. Pregnancy, puerperium, drugs like quinine infections, surgery and anesthesia can unmask first symptom. Fifty percent of patients present with ocular symptoms in form of variable ptosis (Fig. 214.2), double vision, squint, etc. Eighty percent progress within first year and 90% within 3 years. About 10% have spontaneous remission.

The disease can run in families as an autoimmune disease, congenital ones are also seen. MG is associated with thymoma in 15% of patients and thymus hyperplasia in 65%. Other autoimmune diseases, like thyroiditis and diabetes mellitus, can coexist. Complement regulatory genes are differently expressed and this makes the tissues more vulnerable for complement-induced injury. Only

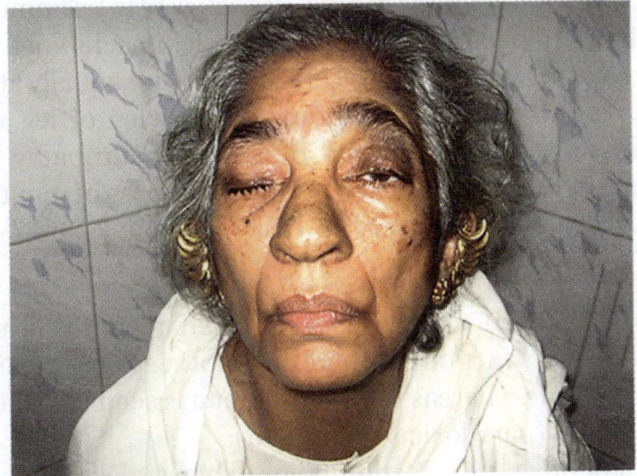

Fig. 214.2: Myasthenia gravis—asymmetric ptosis

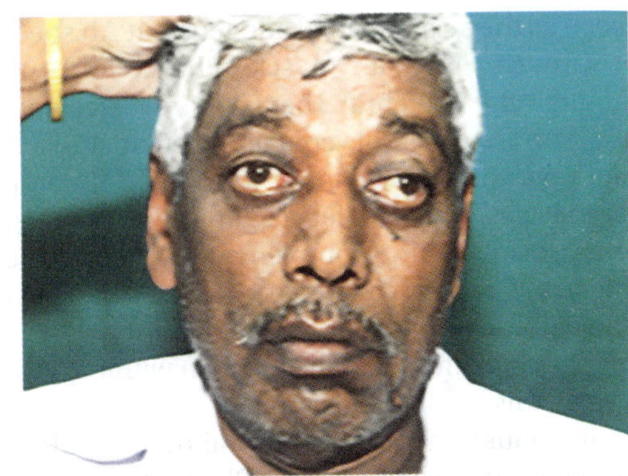

Fig. 214.3: Curtain sign: Development of ptosis when patient looks up for 30 seconds

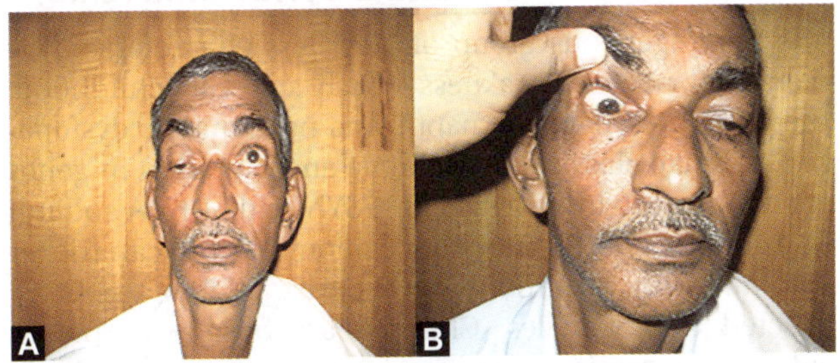

Figs 214.4A and B: Plus minus sign: Opening one eye causes other one to close

one-third of cases become generalized. The conversion into generalized form is maximum within 1 year and it does not occur after 3 years.

The common eye signs are ***curtain sign*** (Fig. 214.3) where patient develops ptosis on sustained upgaze for 30 seconds or more. ***Peep sign*** or ***yawning sign*** is spontaneous opening of eye after sustained closure. ***Plus minus sign*** is opening of one eye causes other to close and vice versa due to supranuclear mechanisms (Figs 214.4A and B). Within available range of eye movements, saccades can be elicited as against myopathy where saccades are not possible. Continuous chewing of food weakens muscles of mastication and jaw drops.

Cogan's twitch sign is elicited by asking patient to slowly open eyes at speed of examiner's moving finger held in front. The holding back muscle is orbicularis oculi and levator of lid is levator palpebrae superioris. Orbicularis weakens earlier than levator and therefore half way through opening of eyelid levator is unopposed and patient suddenly stares at doctor due to pull of levator.

Icepack test is a simple bedside test where application of icepack improves the symptoms in 5 minutes. Early involvement of flexors and extensors of neck, shoulder girdle, hip flexors and tongue muscles is seen in anti-skeletal muscle antibody (anti-MuSKAb) associated myasthenia. Usually patient is weak in evening but if patient does not take medication at night paradoxically more weakness is seen in morning.

Smile becomes a snarl and chewing becomes difficult early in disease even when no other muscles show myasthenic reactions. Later proximal muscles, respiratory muscles, all get affected.

Ocular myasthenia is a situation where signs and symptoms are confined to ocular muscles. Ocular muscles are special as they express fetal antigens but Ab specificity is not proven. Normal muscles have fold pattern (resembling the cerebral hemisphere) designed to increase surface area of contact. Ocular muscles in localized myasthenia have fewer folds in NMJ compared to other muscles. Hence, safety factor is less. Seronegative state may also occur. Complement regulatory genes are differently expressed and this makes tissues more vulnerable for complement induced injury. Only one-third of cases become generalized, often within 1 year and after 3 years this tendency disappears.

Spontaneous remission occurs in about 10%. Morbidity and mortality are relatively less. Phenotypic prognostic markers are not known.

CONGENITAL MYASTHENIAS SYNDROME (CMS)

It is heterogeneous group of disorders characterized by exertional muscle weakness which starts in childhood. There are presynaptic, synaptic and postsynaptic dysfunctions. Unlike classical myasthenia and mutation in genes of choline acetyltransferase, RAPSYN and SCN4A sodium channels are found. The genetic anomaly itself can trigger autoimmunity and both can coexist. Males are more affected than females. Children are born with ptosis, ophthalmoparesis, facial weakness and fatigue. Limb weakness is mild and respiratory distress is unusual. The presence of dysmorphic features, muscle wasting, absence of deep tendon reflexes (DTR) and arthrogryposis should give clue that it is not classical MG. In such cases, it is difficult to predict the prognosis.

Clinical Classification and Features of Congenital Myasthenia

Congenital Myasthenic Syndrome (CMS) with Episodic Apnea

Child presents with hypotonia, life-threatening apnea and arthrogryposis with feeding difficulty. Ocular muscles are spared. Edrophonium test is positive and repetitive nerve stimulation (RNS) shows decremental response. Abnormal resynthesis and repackaging of ACh is the underlying cause.

Slow Channel Syndrome

This manifests in early adult life with slowly progressive weakness of arm, leg, neck and face. RNS shows decremental response. Repetitive discharges suggest congenital deficiency of endplate acetylcholine esterase (AChE) and prolongation of opening time of ACh channels. Quinidine sulfate and fluoxetine are useful in management of such cases.

NEONATAL MYASTHENIA GRAVIS

Transient neonatal MG may be present in 10–20% (15%) of babies born to mothers with MG due to transplacental transfer of Abs. Usually condition clears in a few days to weeks. This should be anticipated and treated.

Pathophysiological Classification

Presynaptic
- Defect in ACh resynthesis
- Paucity of synaptic vesicle
- Lambert-Eaton, like CMS

Myasthenia Gravis Foundation of America Scale

Myasthenia Gravis Foundation of America (MGFA) clinical classification has been described in Box 214.1.

Lambert-Eaton Myasthenic Syndrome (LEMS)

It is described as a paraneoplastic syndrome in patients with oat cell carcinoma of lung. It is believed to be immune-mediated defect in voltage-gated calcium channel and defect is presynaptic. Males and females are equally affected; painful weakness of proximal muscles of leg with depression of reflexes, mild peripheral neuropathy and autonomic dysfunction in the form of dryness of mouth in 50%.

Nerve Stimulation Studies

Normally when a nerve is stimulated repetitively with current, motor action potential does not keep on increasing in amplitude whereas this phenomena is seen in patients with LEMS (paradoxical increment).

Repetitive nerve stimulation shows decrement of the compound muscle action potential (CMAP) at low-stimulation rate and increase at high-stimulation rates. In LEMS, presynaptic release of ACh does not occur but postsynaptic release of ACh can occur.

DIAGNOSIS OF MYASTHENIA GRAVIS

Diagnosis of myasthenia is clinical. It can be confirmed by investigations.

Pharmacological Tests

When undertaking pharmacological tests, special precaution should be taken in those who pose special risks, such as coronary artery disease, obstructive airway disease and active peptic ulcer.

Tensilon Test

Tensilon or edrophonium chloride is given intravenously. Inject an initial test dose of 2 mg and monitor response for 60 seconds. Subsequent injections of 3 mg and 5 mg may then be given, but if clear improvement is seen within 60 seconds after any dose, test is positive, and no further injections are necessary. Complications include bradycardia, syncope and respiratory distress. Atropine should be available (at hand) for intravenous (IV) injections to terminate complications. Though this test is of theoretical interest, it is not done since tensilon test is not available at present.

Neostigmine Injection Test

Improvement [recovery of muscle strength within 15–30 minutes on injecting 0.04 mg/kg bw of neostigmine subcutaneously (SC)] is most practical method to diagnose the disease.

Injecting 0.5 mg IM or SC has a longer duration of action. Onset of action after IM injection is 5–15 minutes. Neostigmine methylsulfate is injected IM in a dose of 1.5 mg. Atropine sulfate (0.8 mg) should be given several minutes in advance to counteract muscarinic effects (neostigmine may be given IV in a dose of 0.5 mg, but its effect is too brief to be very useful). After IM injection of neostigmine, objective improvement occurs within 10–15 minutes, reaches its peak at 20 minutes and lasts up to 1 hour.

Icepack Test

Icepack test in which cooling of drooped eyelid improves within 2 minutes.

Acetylcholine Receptor Antibodies (AchRAbs)

It can be detected in the serum by radioimmunoassay. Presence of Abs in serum confirms diagnosis, but their levels do not always correlate with clinical severity. Their absence does not exclude the diagnosis. Other Abs found are anti-MuSK and anti-striated muscle antibodies.

Electrodiagnostic Tests

Repetitive Nerve Stimulation

This involves supramaximal stimulation given to the motor nerve at 3–5 Hz keeping the arm temperature at 34°C. Increasing response, which tends to decrease with increasing stimulus rate, is suggestive (Fig. 214.5). Maximum decrement is seen at fourth or fifth response followed by tendency to repair. More than 10% decrement is considered abnormal.

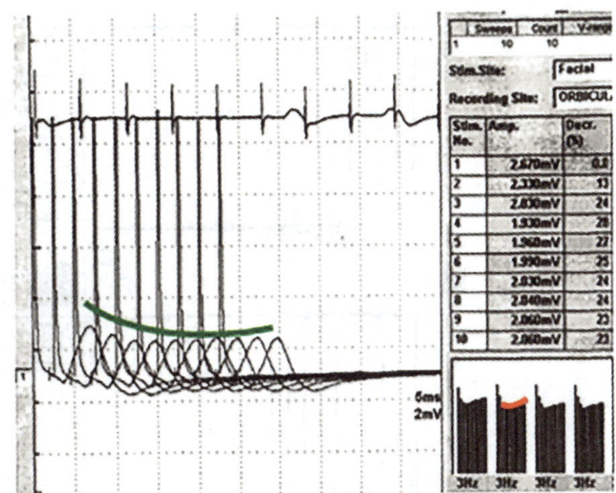

Fig. 214.5: Repetitive nerve stimulation (RNS) in myasthenia gravis (MG)—typical U-shaped curve in MG

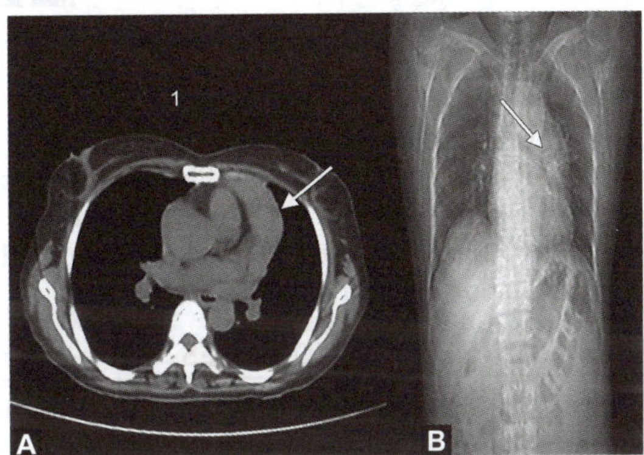

Figs 214.6A and B: A. Computed tomography (CT) of thorax showing thymoma (arrow); **B.** X-ray of chest showing thymoma (arrow)

Imaging Studies

X-ray, computed tomography (CT) scan and magnetic resonance imaging (MRI) of chest help to demonstrate enlargement of thymus (Figs 214.6A and B and 214.7A to D).

Single-fiber Electromyography (SFEMG)

There will be increased jitter and blocking with normal fiber density on SFEMG examination. This measures neuromuscular transmission time between two endplates innervated by same fiber.

Differential Diagnosis

Most important differential diagnosis is ocular and oculopharyngeal myopathy. Clinically in myopathy there is no diplopia due to symmetrical involvement on both sides as against myasthenia. Both progressive fatigability and sleep benefit are absent in myopathy. In addition, fast movements within available range of mobility cannot be elicited and this point strongly favors myopathy.

Botulism (also *Refer* to Section 4, Ch 24) has to be differentiated from acute myasthenic crisis. In a typical case with history of food poisoning, diagnosis is easy, but, in an obscure case diagnostic difficulties may rise. Botulinum toxin blocks release of ACh from motor nerve terminals. Symptoms begin within 12–36 hours of food poisoning with nausea, vomiting, blurring of vision, dysphagia, dysarthria, impairment of pupillary reactions

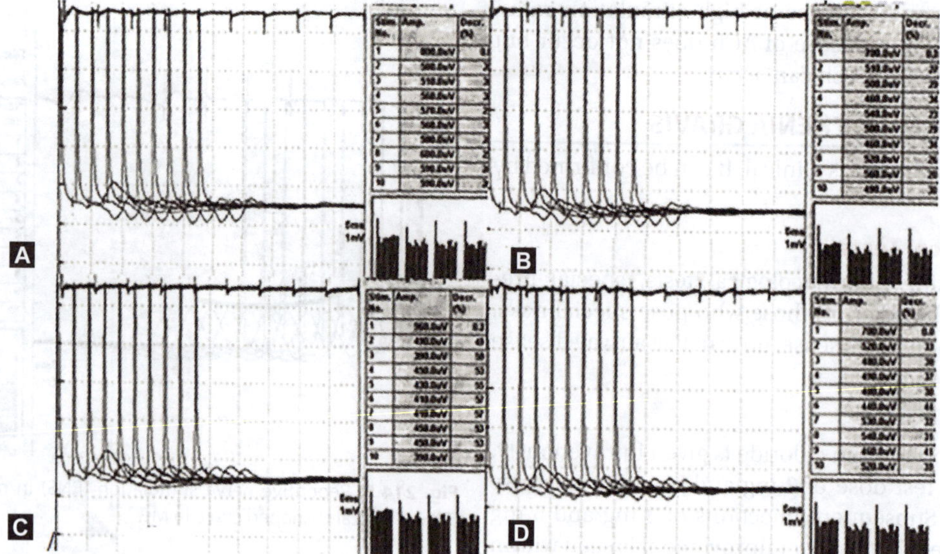

Figs 214.7A to D: Decremental response: repetitive nerve stimulation (RNS) in myasthenia gravis (MG): **A.** Orbicularis at rest; **B.** Immediate postexercise; **C.** 1-minute postexercise; **D.** 3-minute postexercise

and reduction of tendon jerks. Respiratory paralysis and autonomic dysfunction can occur. Electrophysiological assessment shows reduced CMAP amplitude and facilitation by at least 20% after tetanic stimulation. There is no postactivation exhaustion.

OTHER MYASTHENIC SYNDROMES

Acute myasthenic reaction may develop as a complication of cobra bites (*Refer* to Section 2, Ch 11).

Myasthenic crisis and *cholinergic crisis* are two acute complications. These are characterized by sudden occurrence of severe degree of paralysis affecting several muscles in body including respiratory paralysis with increase in secretions. Infections, drugs, surgery and unaccustomed exertions precipitate myasthenic crisis. Cholinergic crisis is usually seen in patients undergoing plasmapheresis and on cholinergic drugs. They have fasciculations. Unless emergency measures are instituted to tide over paralytic episode, condition may prove fatal. A simple test which was used to distinguish the types was IV administration of 2 mg edrophonium which rapidly relieved myasthenic crisis, but not cholinergic crisis.

COURSE AND PROGNOSIS

In about 10% of cases, spontaneous remission may occur during first few years. Purely ocular myasthenia, which is double seronegative, usually does not progress after a steady period of 1 year. Prognosis is worse for acute fulminant and late-onset cases. Cases associated with thyrotoxicosis show a seesaw relationship with severity of latter. Crisis developing in myasthenia can be fatal unless attended to as emergency.

TREATMENT

Drugs contraindicated in myasthenia are fluoroquinolones, macrolides, especially telithromycin, polymyxin, procainamide, penicillamine, oral contraceptives, opiate analgesics, β-blockers (propranolol), calcium-channel blockers, diazepam, muscle relaxants, antiepileptic drugs, chloroquine, colistin and sulfonamides.

Symptom Management

Cholinesterase Inhibitors

These prevent the breakdown of ACh at the NMJ and thus help to improve neuromuscular transmission. The commonly used anticholinesterase drugs are:

- **Neostigmine:** 7.5–45 mg every 2–6 hours (15 mg tablet)
- **Pyridostigmine:** 30–60 mg given every 4–8 hours (30 mg and 60 mg tablet).

The dose and frequency of administration of these drugs have to be tailored to patient's requirement. Common gastrointestinal (GI) side effects include nausea, vomiting, abdominal cramps, loose stools and diarrhea. Increased bronchial and oral secretions may be a serious problem in patients with swallowing or respiratory insufficiency.

Short-term (Rapid-onset) Immune Therapies

Plasma Exchange

Plasma exchange temporarily reduces levels of circulating antibodies and produces improvement in a matter of days in vast majority of patients with acquired severe myasthenia, myasthenic crisis, preoperative preparation and corticosteroid-induced exacerbations.

Intravenous Immunoglobulin (IVIG)

Improvement in MG occurs in 50–100% of MG patients after infusion of high-dose IVIG, given at a total dose of 2 g/kg given over 3–5 days. Improvement usually begins within 1 week and lasts for several weeks or months.

Long-term Immune Therapies

Steroids (Glucocorticoids)

All seropositive patients with generalized myasthenia need long-term immunomodulation. Common drugs used for this purpose are corticosteroids. In some cases, at initial phase of therapy steroids suppress suppressor β-cells leading to a surge of prepared Abs and worsening

Table 214.1: Clinical distinction between myasthenia gravis (MG) and Lambert-Eaton myasthenic syndrome (LEMS)

MG	LEMS
Postsynaptic disorder	Presynaptic disorder
Autoantibodies directed against AChR in postsynaptic membrane	Autoantibodies directed against P/Q calcium channels in presynaptic membrane
Normal release of ACh from presynaptic nerve terminals	Impaired release of ACh from presynaptic terminals
Starts with ocular weakness and then spreads craniocaudally	Starts with limb weakness
Preserved DTRs	Depressed or absent reflexes
No autonomic changes	Autonomic changes (+)
Decremental response in RNS test (Figs 214.7A to D)	Incremental response
Most commonly associated with thymoma	Most commonly associated with small cell lung cancer

Abbreviations: AChR = Acetylcholine receptor; ACh = Acetylcholine; DTRs = Deep tendon reflexes; RNS = Repetitive nerve stimulation

of disease. Therefore, caution is required if high-dose (0.75–1.00 mg/kg/day of prednisone) is started. As an alternative, small-dose is started (0.5 mg/kg bw) and built up to maximum as required. Once sustained improvement occurs, dosage can be reduced. Addition of other immunosuppressants, such as azathioprine will have steroid-sparing effect.

- Azathioprine is started in a dose of 50 mg/day, increased by 50 mg/day every week to a total of 150–200 mg/day (2–3 mg/kg/day). An alternate is to give cyclophosphamide pulses (0.5–1.0 g) at weekly or at longer intervals as required.
- Cyclosporine given in two divided doses daily, to a total of 6 mg/kg is effective. Adverse side effects include mainly hypertension and 3Q nephrotoxicity.
- Mycophenolate mofetil is currently being used as an adjunct to corticosteroids in doses of 1,000–3,000 mg/day for varying periods.

More than 50% of cases can be managed by medical treatment if compliance with drugs is adequate. In those in whom drugs are in effective or drug compliance is not perfect, surgical measures have to be considered. The most preferred surgical procedure is thymectomy which helps to remove site of antibody production, at least partially.

Thyroid function tests (TFTs) and tuberculin skin test for tuberculosis are required before starting therapy with immunosuppressive drugs.

Thymectomy: Best outcome is seen in young females with short duration (< 1 year) and in those who have thymic hyperplasia and seropositivity. Removal of thymic lymphoid tissue is associated with complete remission of disease. In presence of thymomas, surgical removal has to be undertaken irrespective of age. Among 35–50% patients improve long-term outcome depends on nature of thymic mass. Endoscopic thymectomy carries fewer complications.

The previous practice of advocating thymectomy even in patients with normal thymus is not universally accepted at present.

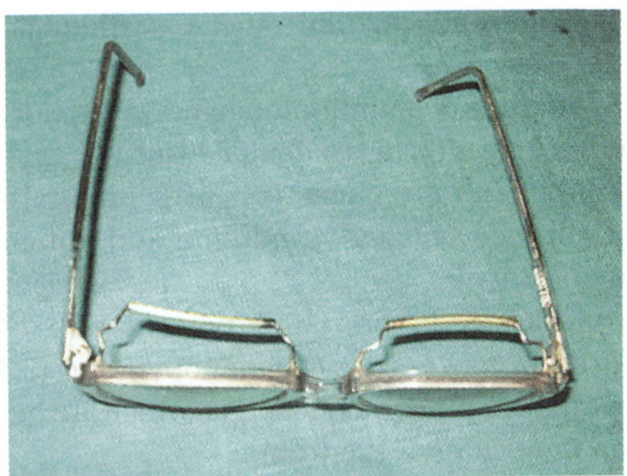

Fig. 214. 8: Clip glass

Table 214.1 showing the clinical distinction between myasthenia gravis and Lambert-Eaton myasthenic syndrome.

Management of Ocular Myasthenia

Question often asked are following:
- Could symptoms improve with a safer form of therapy?
- Will steroid treatment lead to resolution of symptoms?
- Does severity of symptoms warrant risk of steroid-induced adverse effects?
- Do steroids reduce chances of generalization?

Purely ocular double seronegative myasthenics without thymus changes do not generally progress after 1 year. In such cases, anticholinesterases clubbed with glass and tendon-shortening surgery for levator is sufficient. But in seropositive patients, risk of generalization is high and immunomodulation is indicated. At doses required in these cases (~50–60 mg prednisolone per day), adverse effects almost always occur. Shorter courses of 3–6 months might be safer. But once introduced weaning is difficult.

Do Steroids Reduce Chances of Generalization?

Studies show variable results. Risk of generalization is highest in first 2 years. About 11–30% of cases do not become generalized. Ten percent of patients go into remission spontaneously without any treatment.

In patients with ptosis, better vision can be obtained by use of clip glasses (Fig. 214.8), which keep upper eyelid elevated.

Treatment of Myasthenic Crisis

Timely and careful intubation followed by mechanical ventilation in a critical care unit saves life. PLEX therapy and IVIG are equally effective in disease stabilization. Once respiratory support is established, discontinuing neostigmine is safe and recommended. This eliminates the possibility of cholinergic crisis and permits determination of disease severity. *Treatment* of underlying cause should be instituted simultaneously.

Myasthenia in Pregnancy

Pregnancy is usually uncomplicated and when pregnancy occurs myasthenia abates. AChE-I (neostigmine) is quite safe during pregnancy. Cytotoxic drugs should be avoided. Caution is needed to avoid muscle relaxants if lower segment cesarean surgery (LSCS) is planned.

Treatment of Congenital Myasthenia Syndromes

- Treatment of respiratory distress, infections, nutrition and spinal deformities is mandatory.

- Drugs contraindicated for other myasthenias should not be used.
- Thymectomy and immunomodulation are not recommended unless there is a double insult.
- Anticholinesterases (such as neostigmine) are useful except in slow-channel syndrome and anticholinesterase deficiency.
- The weakness in pre- and postsynaptic types in children responds to 3,4-diaminopyridine (3,4-DAP) drugs, like quinine and fluoxetine, which are beneficial in the slow-channel syndrome.
- Fluoxetine, salbutamol and ephedrine are useful in fast-channel syndromes.

CHAPTER
215

MYASTHENIC REACTIONS

Syn: Secondary myasthenia

Thyrotoxicosis, snake bites (especially cobra and krait), black widow spider bite, drugs like aminoglycosides, penicillamine and several other drugs produce NMJ dysfunction.

Source:

1. Puneeth CS, Chandra SR, Yadav R, et al. Heart rate and blood pressure variability in patients with myasthenia gravis. Ann Indian Acad Neurol. 2013;16(3):329-32.
2. Meriggioli MN, Sanders DB. Autoimmune myasthenia gravis: emerging clinical and biological heterogeneity. Lancet Neurol. 2009;8(5):475-90.

Diseases of Muscles

SR Chandra

Textbook of Medicine

Chapter Summary

- Symptomatology of Muscle Disease
  - Role of Genetics
  - Genetic Constitution
- Diagnosis of Muscular Dystrophies
  - Role of Brain Imaging
  - Muscle Imaging
  - Electron Microscopy
- Clinical Features
  - Congenital Myopathy
  - Congenital Muscular Dystrophy
- Classification of Muscular Dystrophy
  - Duchenne/Becker Muscular Dystrophy
  - Facioscapulohumeral Muscular Dystrophy
  - Emery-Dreifuss Muscular Dystrophy
  - Limb Girdle Muscular Dystrophy
- Myotonic Disorders
  - Distal Muscular Dystrophy
  - General Treatment Options
- Metabolic Muscle Diseases
  - Mitochondrial Diseases
  - Inflammatory Muscle Diseases
  - Endocrine Myopathy
  - Statin Myopathy

INTRODUCTION

Around 40% of body weight is constituted by approximately 600 muscles. Each muscle fiber consists of outer basement membrane and inner sarcolemma membrane and several subsarcolemmal nuclei. Cytoplasm contains myofibrils in the form of sarcoplasmic reticulum which communicates through T tubules with plasma membrane. Myofibrils contain actin, myosin, titin, nebulin, tropomyosin, troponin and others, in addition to mitochondria, ribosomes, droplets of fat, glycogen, proteins, enzymes and myoglobin.

Neuromuscular junction and neurotransmitters: Type 1 fibers are rich in oxidative enzymes and are slow twitch fibers and type 2a is fast twitch fibers with oxidative glycolytic metabolism, type 2b is fast twitch glycolytic and type c is embryonic type fibers called *satellite fibers*. The fiber type is determined by innervation and if innervation changes, fiber type also changes. Soleus is an example of purely type 1 fiber muscle.

Diseases can involve one or all of these components due to congenital, degenerative, inflammatory, metabolic and genetic causes. Type 1 fiber atrophy is seen in dystrophy, type 2b fiber atrophy in cachexia and disuse, type 2b fibers are absent in myotonia. Muscle fibers as such are not pain sensitive. Any progressive muscle disease is called myopathy and genetically determined progressive primary muscle diseases characterized clinically by progressive weakness and degeneration pathologically, are called *dystrophies*. Patients presenting without a family history of disease but with pain as a presenting feature generally indicates involvement of endomysium, perimysium and intramuscular (IM) nerves or vessels which are pain sensitive and involvement of nonmuscle systems as well. They show fatigability, i.e. change in power with exertion, this is mostly seen in myositis. This requires careful evaluation for a treatable cause. They should be assessed as follows:

- Clinical history and examination
- Computed quantitative muscle testing
- *Biochemical tests*: The usual tests done include blood and urine analyses which estimate serum creatine kinase (CK), screening for metabolic diseases and enzyme assays, which help to arrive at the diagnosis. Exercise tests done include forearm exercise test and treadmill or bicycle ergometry. Neurophysiological studies include nerve conduction,

electromyography (EMG)—single fiber EMG and repetitive nerve stimulation tests. Histological studies of muscles include muscle biopsy, routine histology and histochemistry, immunohistochemistry (IHC), specific enzyme assays, molecular genetic tests and muscle imaging and others.

SYMPTOMATOLOGY OF MUSCLE DISEASE

Symptoms are as follows—pain and weakness are the most frequent symptoms. Other common symptoms include abnormal gait, fatigue, wasting, spontaneous movements, local or diffuse swelling of muscles and contractures. Clinical history and examination are invaluable and will point to the differential diagnosis and also enable to choose the muscle for EMG and biopsy. All important investigations may be inconclusive if the disease is too advanced or too early. Patient should be assessed during activity and rest. Phenotypic markers of several diseases like specific selectivity of muscle weakness, distribution of the lesion, symmetry, fatigability atrophy/hypertrophy involvement of cranial nerves like 7, 2, 3 and 10, winging of scapula and dysmorphic features give reliable clues to diagnosis (Table 215.1).

A Patient with Limb Girdle Weakness

Questions asked are:

- Is it organic or functional?
- Is it myelopathy, anterior horn cell disease, myositis, dystrophy, myotonia or myasthenia?

Myotonia and myasthenia are picked up only clinically.

For proper diagnosis of muscle diseases, careful history including genetic and family history, evolution of the disease and assessment of the state of the muscles are all important. Clinically, myopathy is classified into various types based on several parameters. The involvement of muscle groups in different types of myopathies gives clue to diagnose various different myopathies and dystrophies affecting different selective groups of muscles and this distribution is a valuable clue.

Useful Early Clues for Clinical Diagnosis Depending Upon the Selective Muscle Involvement

Sarcoglycanopathy: This is characterized by early selective involvement of the adductors of the upper limb and winging of the scapula.

- In *muscle dystrophy*, the brachioradialis is weak and wasted. Winging of scapula is seen in sarcoglycanopathy.
- In *facioscapulohumeral dystrophy (FSHD), scapuloperoneal dystrophy* and others winging of the scapula occur. In FSHD, the deltoid is spared till late in the disease and asymmetry occurs. *Popeyes sign* is characterized by sudden tapering of middle part of upper arm due to wasting of the biceps is seen in FSHD.
- In *calpainopathy*, the rectus abdominis is weak.
- In *inclusion body myositis*, flexor muscles of the forearm, ocular muscles and quadriceps are weak.
- In *myositis, myotonia* and *motor neuron disease (MND)*, swallowing muscles and neck muscles are affected. Among the ocular muscles, levator palpebrae superioris is most affected in myotonia. Cadaveric facies is seen in myotonia.
- In *myasthenia, mitochondrial diseases* and *oculopharyngeal dystrophy,* ocular and pharyngeal muscle involvement occur. Superior rectus muscle is most affected in myasthenia.
- In *thyrotoxic ophthalmopathy,* medial rectus and inferior oblique are most affected.
- In *cretinism,* paraspinal muscles are hypertrophied and this is called as *Kocher-Debre-Semielaigne* (Fig. 215.1) and calf muscle hypertrophy with *myxedema,* this is called *Hoffman's syndrome*.
- Paraspinal muscles are involved in *Emery-Dreifuss myopathy* and *Bethlem myopathy*.
- Early involvement of the diaphragm occurs in acid maltase deficiency and superoxide dismutase deficient type of MND.
- Rippling muscles are seen in *caveolinopathy*.
- *Cupids bow sign* where the upper lip is flat and *tapir's mouth* where the mouth is kept in whistling posture indicate facial muscle involvement.
- *Valley sign* is seen in Duchenne muscular dystrophy (DMD) due to the prominent deltoid, medial scapular border and wasting of latissimus dorsi.
- *Poly hill sign* with six hills formed by enlarged infraspinatus, winged inferior angle of scapula, superior angle of scapula making a dent in the wasted trapezius, prominent acromioclavicular joint, inferolateral fibers of deltoid, preserved biceps and brachioradialis.

Table 215.1: Differentiating features between different lesions

Dystrophic muscle disease	Anterior horn cell disease with muscle atrophy—neurogenic	Secondary muscle disease
Weakness more than wasting; pain is absent	Proportional; absent	Weakness more; present
Pseudohypertrophy, segmental atrophy, selectivity, extensor digitorum brevis (EDB) hypertrophy	Rarely pseudohypertrophy. Others never	No
Brachioradialis, quadriceps weak	Generally, triceps is the last to be involved. Hamstrings affected earlier than quadriceps	No such features
Ankle jerk retained till late; Achilles tendon contracture	All usually absent; flat foot	All present; normal
Fasciculations generally absent	Present	Absent
Cardiac involvement is common	Does not occur. Tremor hands are common	Other systems involvement is common
EMG, enzymes studies and histopathology reveals myopathic features	Nerve conduction studies diagnostic	Myopathic features are present

Abbreviation: EMG = Electromyography

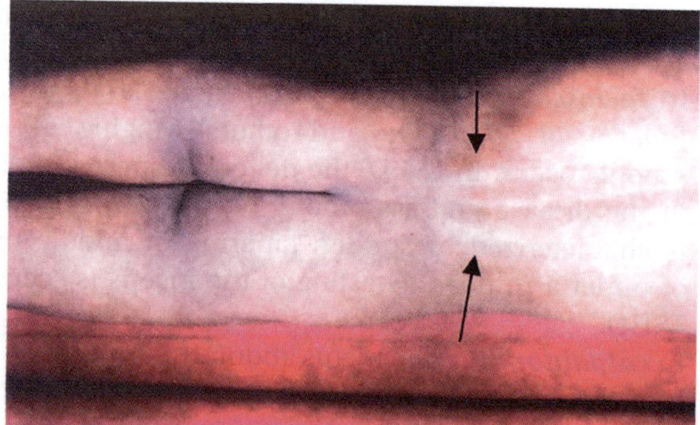

Fig. 215.1: Paraspinal muscle hypertrophy in cretinism (arrows)

- ***Calf head on trophy sign*** is seen in ***Miyoshi myopathy*** due to prominence of the deltoid, wasting of lateral head of triceps and infraspinatus (head), cord like upper border of trapezius (horn), prominent infraspinatus (downward directed ear), prominent spinous process of scapula (which becomes neck) and levator scapulae and rhomboids (subnuchal hump).
- ***Diamond on quadriceps sign*** due to asymmetric diamond-shaped bulges is seen when patients with Miyoshi myopathy and limb girdle muscular dystrophy (LGMD) 2B are asked to stand with slightly flexed knee (***Pradhan's sign***).
- ***Shank sign*** is seen in myotonic dystrophy when patients are asked to keep the shoulder abducted and arm flexed, the wasting of biceps, triceps and forearm muscles produced the appearance of shank of animals.
- ***Aldermoniac posture*** (which is characterized by exaggerated lumbar lordosis, shoulder thrown forward, arms thrown backward and belly protruding to the front) is usually seen in ***central core disease*** in children (Fig. 215. 2).

A patient with weakness of hip extensors and well-preserved paraspinal muscles will use the paraspinal muscles to elevate the hip temporarily without acting to erect the spine while getting up from sitting posture. This is called the ***Hip-up sign*** in which the hip is raised and the trunk is bent, then she slowly erects herself (Fig. 215.3).

- The ***Gowers sign*** is characteristic of DMD, the condition in which the patient starts slowly climbing on his own legs while getting up from sitting or lying.

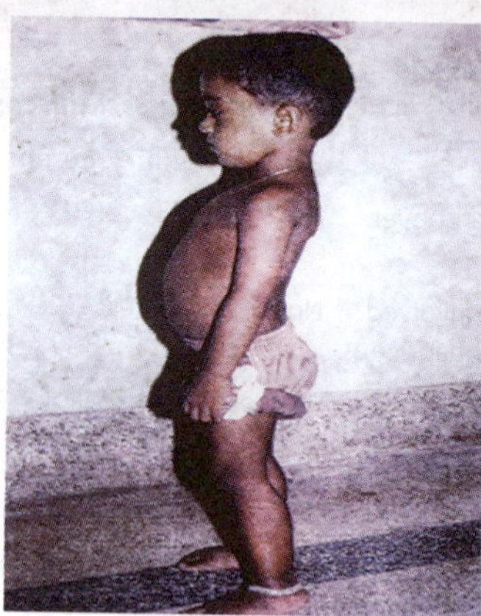

Fig. 215.2: Aldermoniac posturing

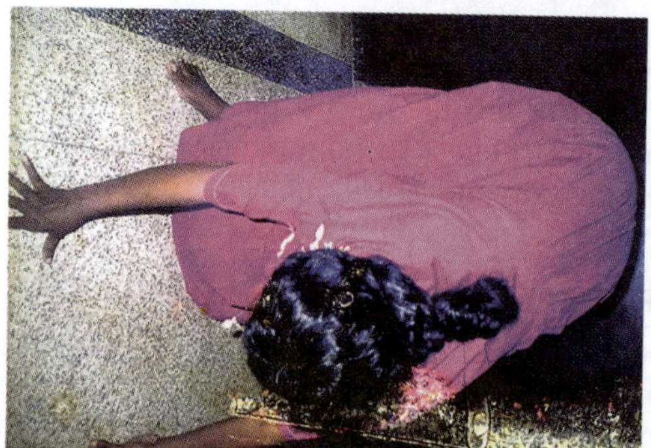

Fig. 215.3: Hip-up sign

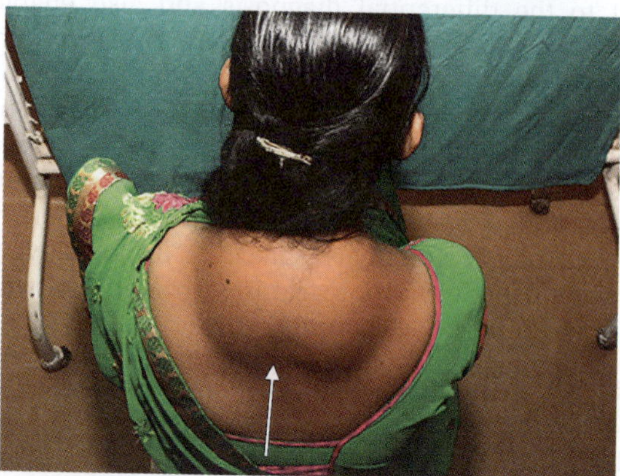

Fig. 215.4: Large midline lipoma (arrow) is typically seen in MELAS (Mitochondrial disorders)

Abbreviation: MELAS = Mitochondrial myopathy, encephalopathy, lactic acidosis and stroke

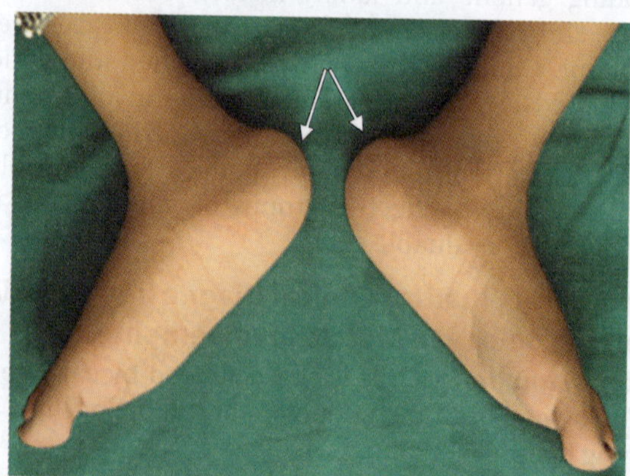

Fig. 215.5: Ullrich congenital muscular dystrophy. ***Note:*** Prominent calcaneum (arrows)

- Finger contractures and keloids suggest ***Bethlem myopathy***.
- Lipomas at the back of the neck suggests mitochondrial myopathy (Fig. 215. 4).
- Prominence of heels occurs in ***Ullrich congenital myopathy*** (Fig. 215. 5). Contractures in unusual sites occur in ***rigid spine syndrome***.

Emery-Dreifuss myopathy and others: Contractures of the elbow occur in congenital muscular dystrophy (CMD). Early toe-walking is seen in calpainopathy. Calf pseudo-hypertrophy is seen in DMD, hypothyroidism (***Hoffman's syndrome***), carnitine deficiency, Woolman's disease, parasitic myopathy, amyloidosis and storage diseases.

Table 215.2: Diagnosis of muscular dystrophies—recessive limb girdle muscular dystrophy (LGMD)

Recessive LGMD	Gene locus	Defective protein
LGMD 2A	15q15.1	Calpain -3
LGMD 2B/Miyoshi	2p13	Dysferlin
LGMD 2C	13q12	Gamma-sarcoglycan
LGMD 2D	17q12-q21.33	Alpha-sarcoglycan
LGMD 2E	4q12	Beta-sarcoglycan
LGMD 2F	5q33-q334	Delta-sarcoglycan
LGMD 2G	17q11-q12	Telethonin
LGMD 2H	9q31-q34	Trim 32
LGMD 2I	19q13.3	FKRP
LGMD 2J	2q31	Titin
LGMD 2K	9q34	POMT 1

Abbreviations: FKRP = Fukutin-related protein; POMT1 = Protein o-mannosyltransferase 1

Table 215.3: Limb girdle muscular dystrophy (LGMD)

Dominant LGMD	Gene locus	Defective protein
LGMD 1A	5q31	Myotilin
LGMD 1B	1q11—q21	Laminin A/C
LGMD 1C	3p25	Caveolin
LGMD 1D	6p23	?
LGMD 1E	7q	?
LGMD 1F	7q32.1—q32.2	?
LGMD 1G	4q21	?

Preservation of deep reflexes which are brisk points to inflammatory, hypo or hyperthyroid and hypo or hypercalcemic muscle disease.

At times, unexpected elevation of biochemical parameters during routine investigation points to specific muscle diseases, e.g. high values of CK should suggest the following conditions:

- Intense physical exercise
- Frequent trauma
- Sustained alcohol use
- Hypothyroidism
- Myopathies/muscular dystrophies
- Female carriers of the Duchenne/Becker muscular dystrophy gene
- Asymptomatic McArdle's disease
- Malignant hyperthermia
- Neuroleptic malignant syndrome
- Drugs causing subclinical myopathy (e.g. lovastatins)
- Hereditary persistent high CK levels in flow
- Inflammatory muscle disease.

Role of Genetics

Genetic studies help to identify defective genes and gene products and helps in the prenatal diagnosis, carrier detection and genetic counseling. Samples used for testing include peripheral blood leukocyte buffy coat, amniotic fluid, chorionic villi and placental tissue. Common genetic abnormalities which point to disease include deletion, duplication, insertion, base substitution, splice site and frame shift mutations.

Genetic Constitution

Muscular dystrophies show varied genetic constitution and different genetic loci. Based on these genetic characteristics they can be classified into different distinct entities (Table 215.2). The important genetic abnormalities seen in the main and subvarieties of various muscle dystrophies.

DIAGNOSIS OF MUSCULAR DYSTROPHIES

Genetic variants in limb LGMD have been shown in Table 215.3.

Role of Brain Imaging

Some of the muscular dystrophies are associated with morphological changes in the brain and therefore, magnetic resonance imaging (MRI) studies on the brain give good evidence for the nature of the disease (Figs 215.6A to C).

Muscle Imaging

It helps to pinpoint the diagnosis in muscle diseases in all cases results of muscle histology and electrical activities (combined) give almost certain diagnosis in most cases (Table 215.4). Points to elicited by muscle imaging studies:

- Selection of appropriate site for biopsy/needle EMG
- Evaluation of distribution of muscle involvement
- To monitor disease progression
- To monitor response to treatment
- To determine force generating capacity of muscle.

Muscle biopsy (*See* Ch 194 on Laboratory Investigation).

Electron Microscopy

When cryosections and enzyme histochemistry are not available, electron microscopy can be used. It is used as confirmatory tool in mitochondrial diseases, storage diseases, congenital myopathies and diagnostic tool in other metabolic disorders, neuronal ceroid lipofuscinosis (NCLs).

CLINICAL FEATURES

Congenital Myopathy

This presents with very early onset with generalized symptoms. Other systems are not involved in a good majority. Congenital myopathy is classified as given below. The disease gets arrested on its own.

- Protein surplus type which includes desminopathy, actinopathy, alpha-beta crystallinopathy
- Nemalin 1, 2, 3, 4 types (Fig. 215.7)
- Central core, myotubular and vacuolar types.

Congenital Muscular Dystrophy (CMD)

These are potentially fatal and show multisystem involvement. They are classic CMD which may be merosin negative or positive. The merosin negative ones may be primary or secondary. Merosin-positive cases may be classic CMD, rigid spine syndrome, CMD with distal hyperextensiblity (Ullrich congenital myopathy), CMD with sensory abnormalities and others (Table 215.5).

CMD with central nervous system (CNS) abnormalities includes Fukuyama in which muscle, eye and brain are

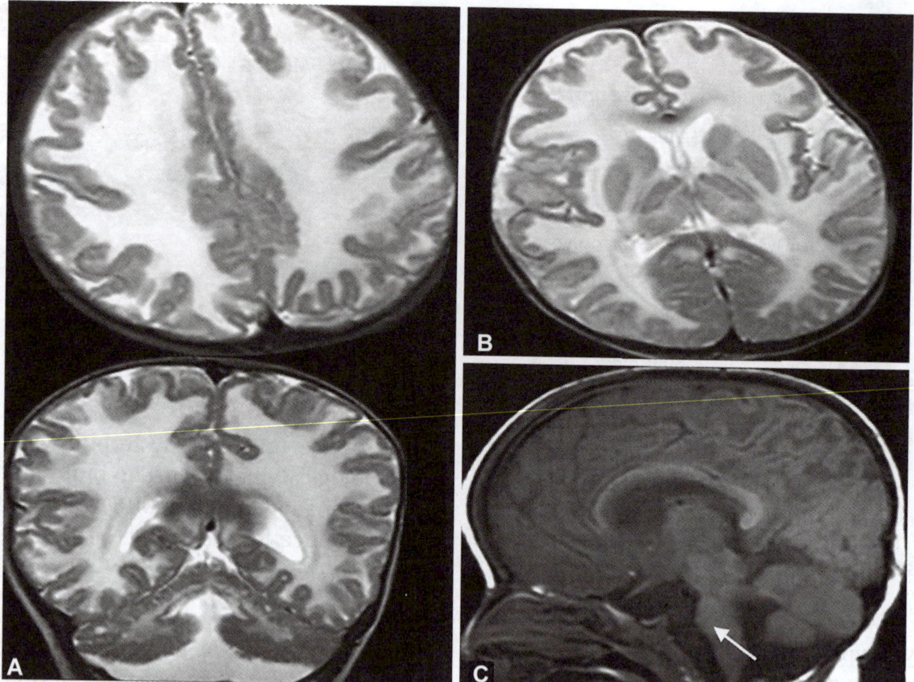

Figs 215.6A to C: Brain changes detected on MRI in patients with muscular dystrophy **A.** MRI polymicrogyria; **B.** Pontine hypoplasia; **C.** White matter changes (arrow)

Table 215.4:	Advantages and disadvantages of muscle imaging techniques			
	Scintigraphy	*USG*	*CT*	*MRI*
Availability	Available	Readily available	Readily available	Increasing
Cost	Expensive	Inexpensive	Expensive	Very expensive
Portability	Fixed	Portable	Fixed	Fixed
Resolution	Poor	Fair	Good	Excellent
Muscle detail	Poor	Fair	Good	Very good
Safety	Radiation	Excellent	Radiation	Excellent
Repeatability	Limited	Yes	Limited	Yes
Preparation	Sedation	None	Sedation	Sedation
Quantification	Yes	Possible	Yes	Yes

Abbreviations: USG = Ultrasonography; CT = Computed tomography; MRI = Magnetic resonance imaging

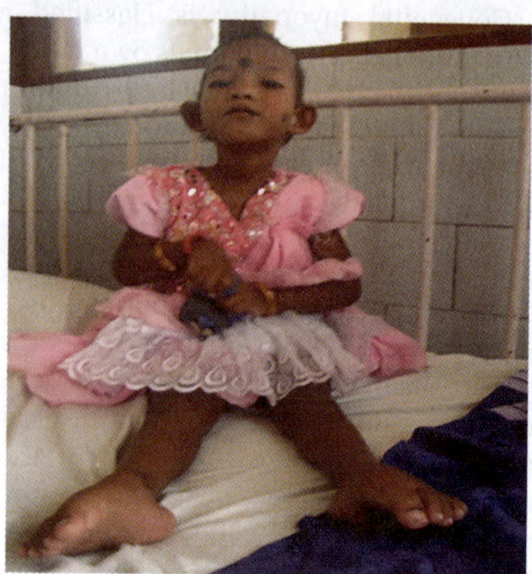

Fig. 215. 7: Nemalin myopathy

affected and also Walker-Warburg disease (Table 215.6 and Fig. 215.8).

CLASSIFICATION OF MUSCULAR DYSTROPHY

An important criterion taken for classification is the genetic constitution which points to the clinical course, outcome of treatment and symptom relief.

X-linked recessive: DMD, Becker muscular dystrophy (BMD), Emery-Dreifuss and scapuloperoneal muscular dystrophies

Autosomal dominant: LGMD A, B, C, D, E

Autosomal recessive: LGMD-2 A, B, C-F, G, H, I, J, M (*See* Tables 215.2 and 215.3).

Duchenne/Becker Muscular Dystrophy (DMD/BMD)

Epidemiology

These two muscular dystrophies occur more frequently in clinical practice. These follow X-linked recessive pattern of inheritance. Male children are affected, females are carriers. DMD affects 1 in 3,300 male births with a prevalence of 3 per 100,000. BMD is a milder form of the disease and incidence varies from 1/18,000 to 1 in 31,000 male births. There is also an intermediate type with moderate severity called *outliers*.

Genetic Changes

They are caused by mutation in Xp21 chromosome and deficiency of its gene product dystrophin. This leads to disruption of dystroglycan protein complex. There is muscle necrosis, mild inflammatory cell accumulation and split fibers with rounding and variation in fiber size.

Clinical Features

DMD patients become symptomatic by 3–6 years. Motor milestones are delayed or they regress later. The child presents with difficulty in running, climbing, jumping

Table 215.5: Clinical features of congenital muscular dystrophies based on normal presence or deficiencies in merosin

Clinical feature	Congenital muscular dystrophy (CMD) with normal merosin	Merosin-deficient CMD
Weakness	Mild-to-moderate weakness	Correlates with level of residual laminin alpha (α) 2 protein; absent laminin alpha (α) 2 protein—severe weakness
Course	Nonprogressive course; mild disability	Nonprogressive
Contractures and disability	Present	Progressively severe contractures at multiple joints
Intelligence	Normal	Intelligence often normal Perceptual-motor dysfunction in some
Seizures	Absent	Present in 12–20%
Creatine phosphokinase (CPK)	Normal-to-moderately elevated	Moderately high
MRI brain	Normal CNS	White matter changes (increased signal on t2) cortex usually normal

Abbreviations: MRI = Magnetic resonance imaging ; CNS = central nervous system

Table 215.6: Congenital muscular dystrophy (CMD) and its gene defects

Disease	Gene	Gene locus	Defective protein
Merosin-deficient CMD (MDC1A)	LAMA2	6q	Laminin alpha (A) A2 (Merosin)
• -MDC1B	?	1q42	?
• MDC1C	FKRP	19q1	Fukutin-related protein
• MDC1D	LARGE	22q12	Large
Fukuyama CMD (FCMD)	FCMD	19q31-q33	Fukutin
Integrin alpha (a) 7 deficiency	ITGA	12q13	Integrin 7
Muscle eye brain disease (MEB)	POMGNT1	1p3	Glycotransferase
Walker-Warburg syndrome (WWS)	POMT1 POMT2	9q34 14q24.3	Glycotransferase
Ullrich syndrome			
UCMD 1	COL6A1	21q22	Collagen V1
UCMD 2	COL6A2	21q22	Collagen V1
UCMD 3	COL6A3	2q37	Collagen V1
Rigid spine syndrome (RSMD1)	SEPN1	1q36	Selenoprotein

Abbreviations: LAMA = Laminin Subunit Alpha 2; FKRP = fukutin-related protein; FCMD = Fukuyama congenital muscular dystrophy; ITGA = Integrin alpha subunit; POMGNT1 = Protein o-linked mannose N-acetylglucosamin trandferase1; POMT = Protein o-mannosyltransferase ; COLGA1 = Callagen type VI alpga 1; SEPN1 = Selenoprotein N, 1

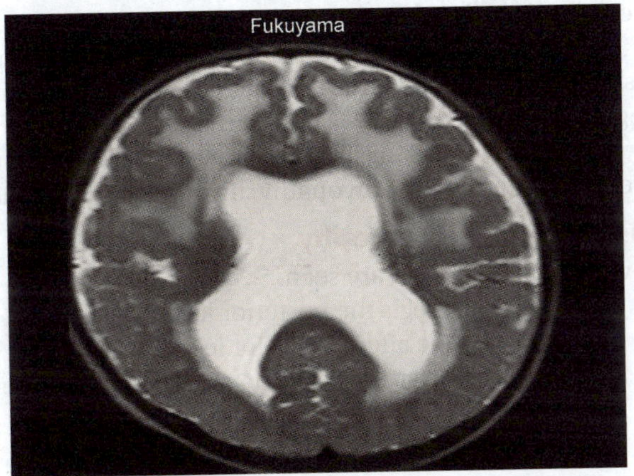

Fig. 215.8: MRI in Fukuyama myopathy. *Note:* The ventricular dilation

and other activities. Examination reveals waddling gait, exaggerated lumbar lordosis and ***Gower's sign*** (described earlier). Muscle weakness is symmetrical and lower limbs are affected earlier with tendo-Achilles contracture. Neck muscles are involved in all stages of DMD. Ileopsoas, glutei, quadriceps are involved early. Calf muscles, quadriceps, deltoid, infraspinatus and other muscles become pseudohypertrophic and rubbery on feel. Pseudohypertrophy is enlargement of the region of the muscle due to deposition of non-muscle tissue such as fibrous tissue, fat and infiltrations. Despite the enlargement, the action is weak. Tibialis anterior and peroneal muscles are generally not involved. Upper limbs and abdominal muscles get involved later in the disease and the ***valley sign*** (described earlier) is seen. Mild mental retardation and cardiac involvement are common. After about a decade of onset, the child becomes wheelchair-bound (by 13–16 years) and further expectation of life is generally not more than 25 years.

BMD, which is a clinically milder disease, becomes symptomatic between 5 and 15 years. Cardiac and cognitive involvement is uncommon. Their survival is between 30 and 60 years. Diagnosis is based on clinical features and genetics.

Laboratory features: CK values are grossly elevated in the order of 10,000–50 000 IU/mL.

Treatment

Nonpharmacological treatment involves continued maintenance of function, prevention of contracture and psychological support. Lightweight foot orthosis to prevent contractures and long leg braces to assist walking can be

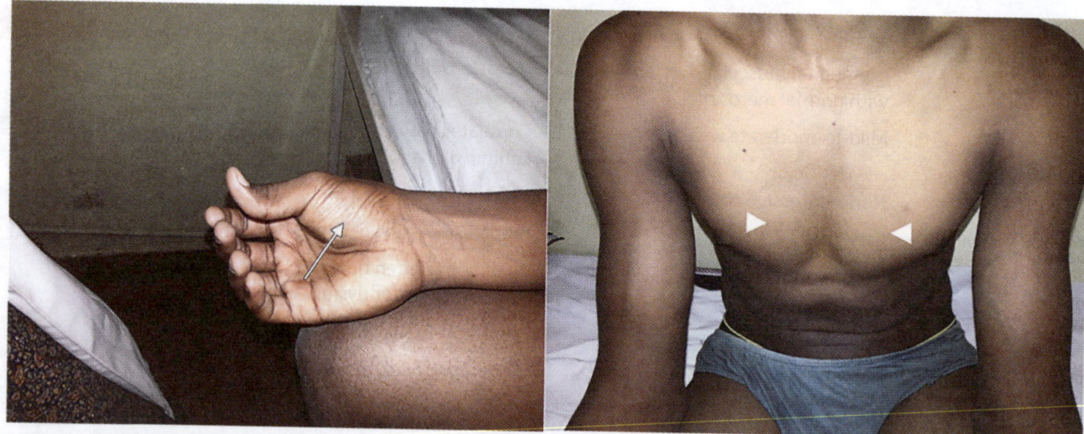

Fig. 215.9: Thomsen's disease with precocious development of the muscles (arrowheads). **Note:** The occurrence of myotonia after tapping the thenar eminence of the right hand (arrow)

used. Pulmonary function and cardiac assessment should be done annually and external ventilators can be used for nocturnal hypoventilation.

Pharmacological treatment: Prednisolone 0.75–1.5 mg/kg/day improves muscle strength and reduces the rate of progression. Prednisolone should be continued as long as patient is ambulant. Steroids delay progression by 3–5 years to wheelchair-bound stage.

Other options under trial are dystrophin and its related protein replacement, myoblast transfer and exon skipping. A newer drug eteplirsen is under active trial. Results are awaited.

Other dystrophinopathies include myalgic cramps, myoglobinuric syndromes, X-linked cardiomyopathy and isolated quadriceps myopathy.

Facioscapulohumeral Muscular Dystrophy

This is an autosomal dominant 4q deletion, muscle dystrophy with predominant involvement of face and shoulder muscles. Deltoid appears large, Beevor's sign is positive (Beevor's sign is upward traction of the umbilicus when the supine patient tries to sit up), the EMG picture is mixed and mild-to-normal elevation of CK occurs.

Emery-Dreifuss Muscular Dystrophy

This is genetically X-linked, but can be genotypically variable. Muscular contractures at elbow, neck extensors, and tendo-Achilles develop with severe cardiomyopathy.

Limb Girdle Muscular Dystrophy (LGMD)

A heterogeneous group of muscle diseases which spare facial muscles and lack hypertrophy of the calf. EMG is myopathic, there is only moderate elevation of CK and cardiac involvement is rare. Mental functions remain normal. The autosomal dominant variety is called LGMD1 and the recessive LGMD2. Subclassification is based on genotype.

MYOTONIC DISORDERS

Myotonia is a state of persistence of contraction of the muscles after cessation of the stimulus for voluntary contraction. Myotonia is most pronounced after a period of rest. ***Myotonia congenta (Syn. Thomsen's disease)*** is an autosomal dominant disorder leading to hypertrophy of the muscles, muscle spasm, cramping, stiffness and myotonia (Fig. 215.9). Myotonia can be demonstrated by watching the muscle contraction produced by direct tapping on the muscle. Normal muscle quickly relaxes whereas the myotonic muscle remains in the contracted stage for much longer (several seconds). The same phenomenon can be assessed by making the patient to do a handshake and noting the time his grip remains tight without relaxation. EMG shows myotonic pattern which is characterized by continued after discharges even after cessation of the voluntary (or external) stimulus. When recorded phonographically, the sounds produced by these after discharges resemble that of a dive bomber.

Eulenberg's myotonia is called ***paramyotonia*** since the myotonia is more obvious after exercise. Becker's type is the autosomal recessive form.

Myotonic dystrophy (dystrophia myotonica): This condition presents with CMD with evidence of myotonia. Type 1 is called ***Steinert's dystrophy***. It is autosomal recessive. Facial and neck muscles are involved giving rise to the cadaveric facies. Involvement of the ocular lens, testes, heart, skin and endocrine glands occurs in varying degrees.

Type 2 myotonic dystrophy is autosomal dominant, presents with proximal myopathy, myotonia and cataract.

Distal Muscular Dystrophy

Several types of LGMD are seen.
- Miyoshi type affects the posterior leg muscles
- The Nonaka type affects anterior leg muscles
- Laing muscle dystrophy affects anterior leg and neck flexors
- Welander type affects the fingers and wrist flexors.

General Treatment Options

Myotonia can be allied by administration of drugs like quinine in doses of 400–600 mg oral twice or thrice a day. Other muscle relaxants such as carbromol and small doses of librium may help in some cases.

Deflazacort 0.9 mg/kg or prednisolone 0.75 mg/kg is useful in maintaining muscle strength in the ambulant stage of DMD. Passive stretching, splinting at night and application of serial casts to prevent contractures are useful.

Correction of scoliosis, scapular fixation for winging, cardiac surveillance and use of angiotensin-converting enzyme inhibitors (ACEIs) are useful in DMD.

In laminopathy, treatment for myotonia and evaluation for cardiac arrhythmias and use of cardiac pacemakers are indicated. Respiratory management includes prompt treatment of infections, immunization and cough augmentation techniques. Nocturnal ventilation, diaphragmatic pacing, etc. help to improve ventilation.

Pain can occur due to postural problems, contractures and osteoporosis and this needs individualized care. Patients need precautions against gastroesophageal reflux. Dietary counseling, management of gastroparesis with prokinetics like cisapride, motilin agonist like erythromycin, cholestyramine for diarrhea due to bile acid malabsorption and also measures to prevent obesity are required from time-to-time. During any surgery, many patients are at risk of ventilatory inadequacy and therefore, they need special care.

METABOLIC MUSCLE DISEASES

These are disorders due to defects in glycogen, lipids, mitochondrial metabolites, adenine nucleotide and endocrine disorders. They present with early multisystem features, myoglobinuria, exercise intolerance and reversible weakness. Early recognition reduces morbidity and mortality. Forearm exercise test is a simple bedside test of great validity. It normally shows 3–4 times increase in ammonia, lactate and pyruvate.

- *Glycolysis and glycogenolysis defects* show normal ammonia, no rise or less than two times rise in lactate and pyruvate.
- *In defects of fatty acid oxidation*, there is no rise in ammonia, lactate or pyruvate.
- *In mitochondrial disease* increase in lactate and pyruvate occurs with no rise in ammonia.
- *Myoadenylate deficiency*, no rise in ammonia and normal lactate and pyruvate.
- *In acid maltase deficiency*, all these parameters are normal.
- *In phosphorylase B deficiency*, ammonia is normal, but there is decrease in lactate and pyruvate.
- *Lactate dehydrogenase deficiency*, ammonia levels are normal and there is no rise in lactate and pyruvate.
- *Glycogen storage diseases* associated myopathies include Pompe, Cori-Forbes, Anderson, McArdle's, Tauri, etc.
- *Lipid storage-related disorders* include carnitine deficiency, carnitine palmitoyltransferase deficiency, and acyl co-enzyme A dehydrogenase deficiency.

Mitochondrial Diseases

These include a group of disorders which involve the function of the mitochondria. Krebs cycle takes place inside the mitochondria and electrons are transported to respiratory chain. This forms the essential process in muscle function. Mitochondrial myopathies are classified as those due to oxygen transport defect, substrate utilization defect, Krebs cycle defect, oxidation phosphorylation coupling defect and respiratory chain disorders.

Patients may have varying presentations from normal to severe muscle weakness. Usual symptoms are exertion-induced muscle pain and weakness. They will have episodes of encephalopathy due to lactic acidosis. Symptoms can also be precipitated by systemic infection, starvation and unaccustomed exertion or use of mitochondrial toxic drugs like chloramphenicol, sodium valproate, phenobarbitone, anticancer drugs and antiviral drugs. In addition, there may be bad obstetric history with multiple abortions, short stature, lipomas (*See* Fig. 215.4), deafness, blindness, seizures and encephalopathy. Multiple abnormalities in siblings, which are phenotypically not similar, are important clue. High degree of suspicion is necessary for diagnosis. Mitochondrial cocktail is useful in reducing the morbidity. Muscle biopsy, electron microscopy and mitochondrial genetics confirm the diagnosis. Mitochondrial disorders may show ragged red fibers on biopsy (Fig. 215.10). Mitochondrial cocktail consisting of co-enzyme Q10, levo carnitine, α-lipoic acid and vitamins B_1, E, C, B_6 and K may give relief.

Inflammatory Muscle Diseases

These belong to three major categories—dermatomyositis, polymyositis and inclusion body myositis.

Dermatomyositis affects females more than children though adults are also affected (Fig. 215.11). Proximal muscle weakness with involvement of skin, heart, lungs, joints, blood vessels and systemic malignancy are associations. CK may be elevated up to 50 times the normal value (Table 215.7).

Polymyositis also affects females more, usually adults. There are no skin changes, proximal muscles, neck and swallowing muscles are involved, cardiac and pulmonary changes can occur.

Inclusion body myositis is seen mostly in males, usually above the age of 50 years. There is predilection for finger, wrist flexors and knee extensors. They may have associated sensory neuropathy, Sjögren-like vasculitis including vasculitic skin ulcers (Fig. 215.12). They are responsive to immune-modulation. General treatment options include steroids, IVIG, immunesuppressive drugs, monoclonal antibodies, plasmapheresis, thymectomy and total body radiation.

Endocrine Myopathy

Several endocrine disorders give rise to secondary effects on muscle structure, function and morphological changes. These may be primary as in gigantism, acromegaly, hypothyroidism, hypogonadism and others. Electrolyte disturbances such as hypocalcemia and hypercalcemia, hyponatremia, hypernatremia and hypokalemia can all lead to secondary dysfunction of nerves and muscles (Refer to Section 11 for further details).

Statin Myopathy

This is a classic example of muscle disease secondary to therapeutic intervention, which includes several types of muscle disorders. Muscle pain and weakness with mild-to-moderate CK elevation is reported in several small series. Whether patients had pre-existing disease is a question, but remission on stopping and relapse

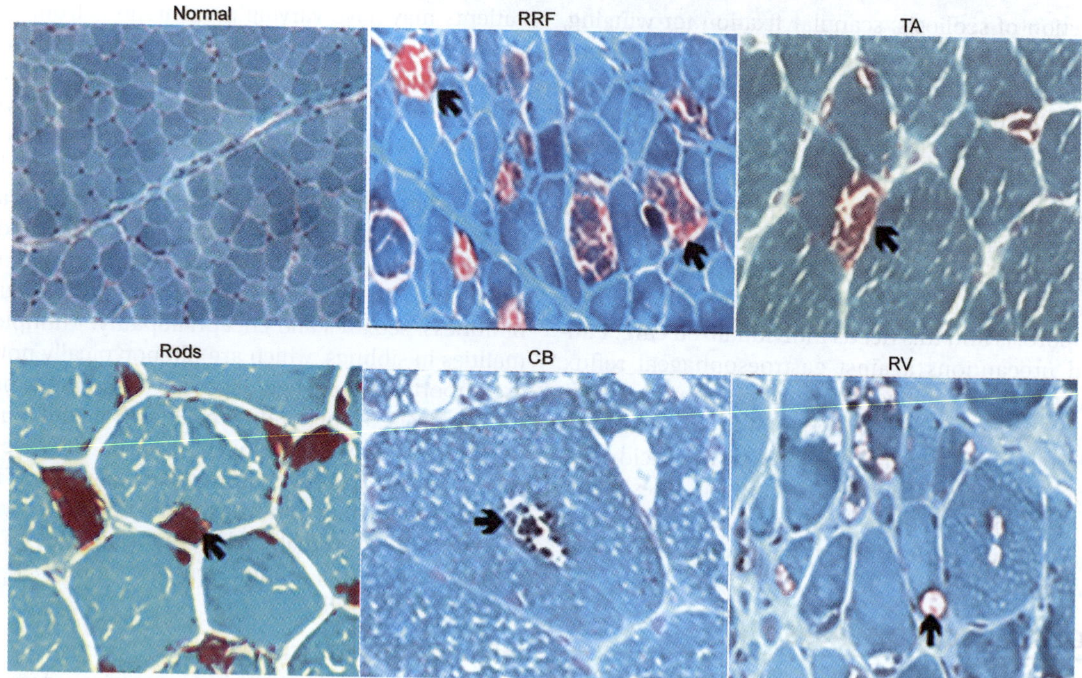

Fig. 215.10: Mitochondrial disease modified Gomori's trichrome stain (MGT) showing ragged red fibers (arrowheads)
Abbreviations: RRF = Ragged-red fibers; TA = Tubular aggregates; CB = Cytoplasmic bodies; RV = Rimmed vacuoles

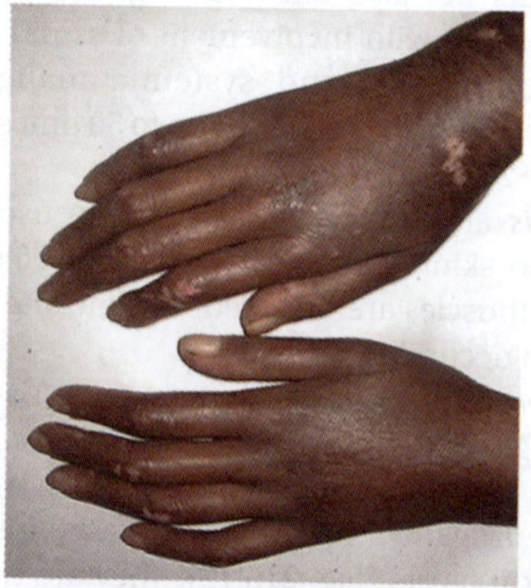

Fig. 215.11: Dermatomyositis. ***Note:*** Skin changes (erythema and shining). Swellings of finger joints and wrist and scars of ulcerations

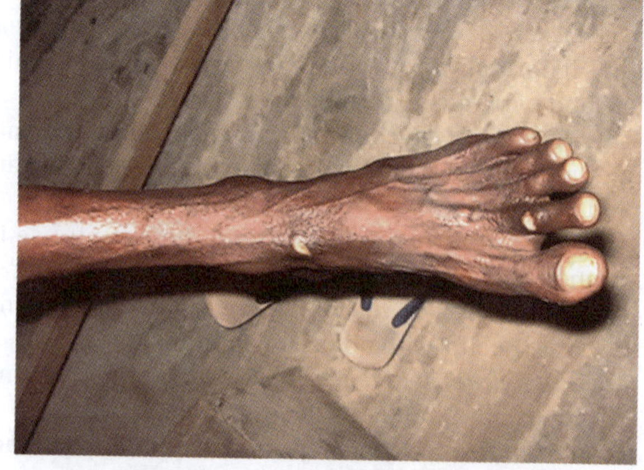

Fig. 215.12: Punched out ulcers typical of vasculitis

Table 215.7: Distinguishing features and its common forms of inflammatory myopathies

Disease	Dermatomyositis	Polymyositis	Inclusion body myositis
Gender	Female	Female	Male
Age	Child	Adult	Old
Skin changes	Yes	No	No
Weakness pattern	Proximal	Proximal	Both
Creatine kinase	Increased up to 50 times	Increased up to 50 times	Normal
Biopsy	Perivascular, perimysial, endomysial inflammation	Perivascular, perimysial, endomysial inflammation	Amyloid deposit (tubulofilament inclusions)
Neuropathy	Absent	Absent	Present
Response to treatment	Good	Good	Poor

on reintroduction is observed. Possible mechanisms are impaired mitochondrial function, cholesterol loss interfering with membrane integrity, impairment of laminin A, disruption of actin cytoskeleton, impairment of extracellular matrix, abnormalities of nitric acid metabolism and others have being implicated. Both acute rhabdomyolysis and chronic immune-mediated muscle disease have been reported.

Among the statins, the earlier ones (e.g. simvastatin, lovastatin) have being reported to be more prone to produce myopathy especially when given in higher doses (more than 40 mg/day). Even though none of the available statins are totally free from this risk. The newer ones (atorvastatin and rosuvastatin) are probably less harmful. ***Diagnosis*** is based on circumstantial evidence and supported by improvement on withdrawal of the drug.

Source: Disease of Muscle by George Karpadi, et al.

CHAPTER

216

Rehabilitation in Neurology

SR Chandra

Chapter Summary

- Burden of Disease in India
- Cerebrovascular Accidents
- Management of Aphasia
- Cognitive Rehabilitation
- Movement Disorders
- Spinal Cord Injury
- Muscle and Nerve Problems
- Neurogenic Dysphagia
- Other Methods
- Chronic Pain Management and Palliation
- Indian Concept

INTRODUCTION

Disease-modifying treatments depend on etiopathology of the disease while symptom-modifying treatments aim at reducing disability and improving activities of daily living and quality of life, irrespective of its causation. Treatment planning needs thorough assessment of the disability and needs of patient. At basic level, these modalities aim at preventing bedsores, contractures, muscle wasting, aspiration pneumonia, bladder and bowel associated complications. But there is a greater dimension to this aspect of neurology which is psychological well-being by rendering a shoulder to lean and thus remove problems of helplessness, improving actual pathology by enhancing plasticity, robot-based improvements in function, specific treatments to allay disabilities and improve occupational skills.

BURDEN OF DISEASE IN INDIA

The term DALY indicates disability-adjusted life years (*See* also Section 1, Ch 1). The burden of communicable and perinatal diseases is 47% in the world community whereas 50.5% in India while that of noncommunicable diseases is 52.7 in the world and 40.3% in India and injuries, 9.2% in India (Rao SN, et al.). A sample survey described disability as any restriction or lack of ability to perform an activity in manner or within the range considered normal for human beings. Quantification should be done in all cases as per recommendations laid down by task force to develop a uniform data system for rehabilitation.

Common neurological problems which need some kind of rehabilitation are dementias, mental retardation, epilepsy, cerebrovascular accidents (CVAs), disorders of spinal cord, nerve and muscle.

CEREBROVASCULAR ACCIDENTS

Rehabilitation should start as early as possible. In mildly affected patients, the needs are less but others need care with special reference to skin, heel and scapula. The position should be changed 2 hourly, body should be cleaned and antiseptic applied and kept dry. Food should contain optimum calories, proteins, vitamins, minerals, fluids and adequate fiber to facilitate bowel movements. To prevent contractures and pain in shoulders and other joints, passive exercises are started, this also helps to prevent venous thrombosis (VT) and pulmonary embolism (PE). Bladder and bowel care and measures to prevent deep vein thrombosis (DVT) are instituted. As patient starts stabilizing, a team-approach is needed to take care of mood, language, cognition, seizures, neglects, motor, sensory, psychosocial and financial matters.

Physical therapy aims to improve ambulation through a sit-up phase to set-out stage. Speech and language training using gestures, typewriters, computers, cued speech, cognitive retraining with simple household work-related tools to computer-assisted tools all yield modest result. For patients with agnosias, apraxias and other defects of communication, specifically trained teams with experience of handling such cases are required. For long-term self-help devices, modification of environment and continuation of daily exercises are needed. Mirror therapy, treadmill training and functional electrical stimulation can all be tried.

MANAGEMENT OF APHASIA

Therapy is individualized and need-based to deficit. It may be facilitatory or compensatory. Constraint-induced movement therapy insists on communicating without any gestures. Sensory input enhanced through auditory, visual, tactile modes and also computer-assisted auditory perceptual training hastens recovery.

COGNITIVE REHABILITATION

It is a comprehensive, holistic approach to improve and restore impairment of mental, psychomotor and behavioral functioning and it also enhances ability to compensate for lasting deficits which can be assessed through various neuropsychological tests. Relearning does occur by reorganization of functional connectivity. Passive participation, limitation of interest and catastrophic reactions must all be anticipated. Therefore, competent patient management strategies should be adopted. Mechanism of expected improvement is restitution, reorganization and compensation through plasticity.

Brain has several data linking circuits and improvement of one domain in circuit might make connectivity complete and improve the related domains. Thus, rehabilitation is attempted through retained areas of circuit. The approach can be basic function-based or domain-specific. Improvement of focused attention and reaction time can be done with computer-based tests or tasks which require paper and pencil or based on simple household tasks. Sorting of grains improves information processing speed and focused attention. Crossing out target letters in newspapers increases sustained attention. More than one task given simultaneously, e.g. listening to music and sorting grains, improves divided attention. It should not combine the same stimulus and modality of response.

Memory improvement can be achieved by following techniques:

- *Frequency encoding:* If association of information was impaired then improving contextual cues of recall will improve memory.
- *Temporal encoding*: Asking patient to identify words at beginning, middle or in the end of list.
- *Spatial encoding:* To remember the location of individual objects which were arranged on a table. Compensatory strategies using external tools like tape recorders, alarm watch and pictures and maps, improve orientation by using anchor points, organize work environment, one task at a time. Pictorial task plans for the day, demanding increasing goals help to hasten functional competence. For new learning, rehearsals, imagery and mnemonic technique are used.

Verbalize visual-spatial information (e.g. X is to left of Y), visualize verbal information in graphs, pictures, cartoons or action-based imagery, keep items in designated places. Executive functions can improve by use of a problem-solving guide. Use self-questioning for alternatives or consequences (What else could I do?, What would happen if I did that?). Verbalize a plan of action prior to and during execution of task. Look at possible solutions from at least two different perspectives. For retrieval, search your memory according to various categories and subcategories (e.g. person: family). Describe the concept; circumlocute freely (talk about or around subject). The commonly targeted domains are mental speed, attention, executing function, visuospatial function and learning and memory. It certainly provides coping skills and greater independence in daily life. Reduce restrictions caused by cognitive impairments. Help reintegration into society. Improve emotional adjustment. Develop social skills and improve motivation. Task-specific training based on needs of the patient is done in individual basis.

MOVEMENT DISORDERS

Patients with Parkinson's disease (PD) experience dysfunction due to loss of dexterity, slowness, falls, postural problems and like. Gait training, mobility exercises and supportive instruments like walking stick are recommended. Disorders of balance such as unsteadiness and ataxias may be related to ear, basal ganglia, cerebellum, spinal cord or lower motor neuron (LMN). The exact cause should be sorted out. Timing, sequencing, preparatory strategy scaling can be trained to a great extent by comprehensive *balance rehabilitation.*

SPINAL CORD INJURY (SCI)

The degree of completeness of injury decides the outcome. Patients with lesion above C3 will need varying degrees of ventilator support and phrenic nerve pacing. Electric wheel chair mobility and control over environment is possible in patients with C4 level. In injuries at C5 level, shoulder control may be possible and they can benefit with feeding straps. Patients with injuries at C6 can be trained to transfer objects. They may benefit with arm reconstruction methods such as tendon transplant and others. In patients with injuries at thoracic level will need trunk balancing to use long leg calipers. Apart from the usual complications, spasms need special care. These may have to be controlled using intrathecal baclofen and pumps. Postural hypotension, sexual functions, depression, all need care to improve quality of life.

MUSCLE AND NERVE PROBLEMS

They need passive stretching exercises, active exercises, respiratory muscle strengthening exercises, orthosis and surgery for contractures. Pain management, weight reduction and bracing weak muscles will minimize suffering to a great extent.

NEUROGENIC DYSPHAGIA

This is a common symptom which leads to pneumonia and death. There are several approaches based on type and extent of mechanism of swallowing. Management should take into consideration whether one of three phases of swallowing or all phases are involved. The assessment should yield information on whether it is oral, pharyngeal, esophageal or a combination. Rehabilitation starts with simple methods like altering consistency of food, posture and position of swallowing, chin-tuck neck extension, side lying and head rotation which help in unilateral disease. Bolus control can be done with lingual manipulation, size adjustment, position of placement and use of prosthetic devices with palatal lifts and tracheostomy valves.

OTHER METHODS

There are other techniques which help rehabilitation: *Biofeedback:* This is based on using one's own ability in altering one's function and training to detect errors and correct them. This uses visual, auditory and tactile modes of feedback. Electromyography-based feedbacks, temperature feedback, electroencephalogram (EEG) feedback, heart rate, respiration-based feedback and others are available. However, good cognitive capacity and endurance from patient are mandatory. Alternative methods like meditation and yoga, acupuncture, pranic healing, etc. are also helpful.

CHRONIC PAIN MANAGEMENT AND PALLIATION

Pain is defined as the psychic adjunct of an imperative protective reflex or anything patient feels hurting. In the context of neurological illness, thorough assessment of illness and expected outcome have to be assessed with professionalism, humanistic qualities and compliance to ethical practices. Nonpharmacological approaches are important. Transdermal patch containing analgesics, oral or parenteral anti-inflammatory agents, analgesic mood stabilizers, oral opioids, parenteral and other invasive analgesics have all to be tried if indicated.

The World Health Organization (WHO) defines palliative care as an approach that improves quality of life of patients and their families facing problems with life-threatening illness, through prevention and relief of suffering by means of early identification and impeccable assessment and treatment of pain and other problems, physical, psychological and spiritual.

End-of-life care: A methodology by which dignity of patient and caregiver is maintained should be sensitive and respectful. Use appropriate choices consistent with patient's desire, alleviate pain, address psychological, social and religious problems, continue to provide care, respect the right of patient to refuse treatment, and optimize therapeutic decisions. The question remains: Could I have done something more, is life and death in my hands?

INDIAN CONCEPT

The chariot of body, how to make it carry you where you really want to go?

Tamas is inertia and must be overcome by *Rajas* and *Rajas* be conquered by *Sattva,* i.e. tranquil joy.

Editor's Note: The terms *Tamas, Rajas* and *Sattva* are described and frequently mentioned in the Hindu philosophical literature pertaining to basic characteristic nature of humans—Tamas (dull in nature), Rajas (very active and positive) and Sattva (tranquil, firm and equanimous).

Source: Regeneration, Repair and Rehabilitation: Redefined by Prof AB Taly and team. 2 Tidy's Physiotherapy.

CHAPTER 217

Investigation of a Child with a Suspected Neurometabolic Disorder

Rita Christopher

Chapter Summary

- General Considerations
- Chronic Encephalopathy
- Acute Encephalopathy
- Ataxia and Extrapyramidal Movement Disorders
- Myopathy
- Psychiatric Problems
- Biochemical Investigations
  - Glucose
  - Blood gases and Acid-base Profile
  - Ketones
  - Ammonium
  - Amino Acids
  - Organic Acids
  - Mucopolysaccharides (MPS)
  - Oligosaccharides
  - Acylcarnitine and Acylglycines
  - Very Long Chain Fatty Acids (VLCFA)
- Red Cell Plasmalogens
- Pipecolic Acid
- Enzyme Studies
- Tandem Mass Spectrometry

GENERAL CONSIDERATIONS

Inherited disorders of metabolism encompass a spectrum of conditions that have been defined on a biochemical, clinical and radiological basis. A single gene defect causes a deficiency in an enzyme or transport protein, which results in a block in a metabolic pathway leading to an accumulation of substrate behind block or a deficiency of product. Broad categories include disorders of carbohydrate metabolism, disorders of amino acid metabolism, organic acidemias, lysosomal storage diseases, fatty acid oxidation disorders, peroxisomal and mitochondrial disorders. Though individually rare, they are collectively numerous and significant cause of morbidity and mortality worldwide. The reported cumulative incidence varies between 1 in 1,500 and 1 in 5,000 live births. Prevention of death or permanent neurologic sequelae in patients with these disorders is dependent on early diagnosis and institution of appropriate therapy. In addition to comprehensive clinical assessment, imaging studies, electrophysiologic investigations and histopathologic information from biopsies which help to establish distribution and type of abnormality, biochemical studies are required in many cases to confirm diagnosis.

Over one-third of inherited metabolic disorders present with central nervous system (CNS) features which can be grouped into chronic encephalopathy, acute encephalopathy, movement disorder, myopathy, psychiatric or behavioral abnormalities and combinations of one or more of these.

CHRONIC ENCEPHALOPATHY

Chronic encephalopathy presents as progressive global psychomotor retardation, hypotonia, impairment of special senses, seizures, pyramidal, extrapyramidal and cranial nerve deficits.

The disorders include GM$_2$ gangliosidosis, GM$_1$ gangliosidosis, neuronal ceroid lipofuscinosis (NCL), mitochondrial encephalopathy lactic acidosis syndrome (MELAS), X-adrenoleukodystrophy (X-ALD), metachromatic leukodystrophy (MLD), mucopolysaccharidosis (MPS) and multiple sulfatase deficiency (MSD) (adapted from Clarke JTR, 2002).

ACUTE ENCEPHALOPATHY

It is seen in disorders of amino acid metabolism [maple syrup urine disease (MSUD), urea cycle disorders (UCD), nonketotic hyperglycinemia] (Table 217.1).

- Organic acidemias
- Fatty acid oxidation defects (FAOD)
- Mitochondrial respiratory chain defects.

Table 217.1: Differential diagnosis of neurometabolic disorders presenting as acute encephalopathy

Biochemical investigation	Urea cycle disorders (USD)	Maple syrup urine disease (MSUD)	Organic acidurias	Fatty acid oxidation defects (FAOD)	Nonketotic hyperglycinemia (NKH)
Metabolic acidosis	Not present	Maybe present	Present +++	Maybe present	Not present
Plasma glucose	Normal	Normal or decreased ↓	Decreased ↓↓	Decreased ↓↓↓	Normal
Plasma ammonium	Elevated ↑↑	Normal	Elevated ↑	Elevated	Normal
Plasma lactate	Normal	Normal	Elevated ↑	Maybe elevated	Normal
Liver function tests (LFT)	Normal	Normal	Normal	Liver enzymes elevated	Normal
Plasma amino acids	Abnormal	Increased leucine, isoleucine, valine	Increased glycine	Normal	Increased glycine
Plasma carnitine	Normal	Normal	Decreased	Decreased	Normal
Urinary ketones	Normal	Elevated	Urinary ketones	Normal	Elevated
Urinary organic acids	Normal	Abnormal	Abnormal	Abnormal	Normal

ATAXIA AND EXTRAPYRAMIDAL MOVEMENT DISORDERS

Diseases included are progressive ataxia in many late-onset lysosomal storage disorders (late-onset MLD, Krabbe's disease, galactosialidosis, GM_2 gangliosidosis and Niemann-Pick type C), abetalipoproteinemia, mitochondrial electron transport chain (mtETC) defects, NCL, Refsum's disease and Hartnup disease. L-2-hydroxyglutaric aciduria (L-2-HGA) is a newly identified metabolic disorder which can present with ataxia and macrocephaly in adulthood. Degenerative ataxias do not involve other systems and present with steady progression (Table 217.2). Extrapyramidal signs are seen in the following conditions:

- Glutaric aciduria (GA)
- Methylmalonic and propionic acidemias (MMA/PA)
- Lesch-Nyhan syndrome (LNS) and
- Wilson's disease.

Lysosomal storage disorders which can present with dystonia include Niemann-Pick's disease type C, Gaucher's disease type 3, GM_2 and GM_1 gangliosidosis.

Table 217.2: Diagnostic approach for inherited neurometabolic disorders presenting as recurrent attacks of ataxia

Biochemical feature associated with ataxia	Most frequent diagnosis	Differential diagnosis
Ketoacidosis	Late-onset MSUD, Methylmalonic aciduria, Propionic aciduria, Isovaleric aciduria	Diabetes mellitus
Hyperammonemia	UCD (ornithine transcarbamylase deficiency, argininosuccinic aciduria)	Intoxications, encephalitis
Hyperlactacidemia Normal lactate/ pyruvate No ketosis High lactate/ pyruvate Ketosis	Pyruvate dehydrogenase deficiency Multiple carboxylase defect Mitochondrial respiratory chain defects	Migraine, cerebellitis Acetazolamide-responsive ataxia Polymyoclonia
Generalized aminocidura	Hartnup disease	–

Abbreviations: MSUD = Maple syrup urine disease; UCD = Urea cycle defects

MYOPATHY

Inherited metabolic disorders presenting as myopathy are commonly result of defects in energy metabolism (Table 217.3). They consist of three categories:

1. Progressive muscle weakness
2. Exercise intolerance with cramps and myoglobinuria
3. Myopathy as a manifestation of multisystem disease.

PSYCHIATRIC PROBLEMS

Some of the neurometabolic disorders presenting with behavioral problems and their diagnostic tests are given in Table 217.4.

BIOCHEMICAL INVESTIGATIONS

The initial biochemical investigation of a suspected inherited neurometabolic disease should include following tests (Table 217.5):

- Blood glucose
- Liver function tests (LFT)
- Serum creatine phosphokinase (CPK), lactate dehydrogenase (LDH)
- Blood gases and electrolytes
- Blood lactate
- Plasma ammonium
- Plasma and urine amino acid analysis (screening by thin-layer chromatogram and quantitative amino acid analysis if abnormalities are found).
- Urine reducing substances, ketones
- Urinary mucopolysaccharide (MPS) screening test
- Urinary oligosaccharide screening test.

Glucose

Hypoglycemia (blood glucose < 45 mg/dL, < 30 mg/dL in neonates) is a common nonspecific problem in severely ill neonates and young children regardless of illness (Box 217.1).

Blood Gases and Acid-base Profile

The second most important laboratory feature of many inherited neurometabolic disorders during episodes of illness is metabolic acidosis demonstrable by measurement of arterial blood gases and bicarbonate. An increased anion gap (> 16) is observed in many of these disorders due to accumulation of fixed acids such lactic acid, ketoacids and other organic acids (Flowchart 217.1).

Table 217.3: Biochemical differentiation of inherited metabolic disorders presenting as muscle cramping

Disorder	Results of ischemic forearm exercise test	Other biochemical features	Confirmatory test
McArdle's disease (GSD V)	Normal pretest lactate and no increase post test	Elevated CPK myoglobinuria	Deficiency of phosphorylase in muscle
Phosphofructokinase (PFK) deficiency	Excessive increase of ammonium	Myoglobinuria, hyperuricemia, elevated CPK	Deficiency of PFK in muscle
Phosphoglycerate kinase (PGK) deficiency	Normal response	–	Deficiency of PGK in erythrocytes
Phosphoglycerate mutase (PGAM) deficiency	Excessive increase of ammonium	Myoglobinuria, hyperuricemia, elevated CPK	Deficiency of PGAM in muscle
Lactate dehydrogenase (LDH) defect	No lactic acidosis, but marked hyperpyruvic acidemia during test	Myoglobinuria, hyperuricemia, elevated CPK	Deficiency of LDH-M subunit in erythrocytes
Carnitine palmitoyltransferase II (CPT II) deficiency	Normal lactate and ammonium response, but increased CPK	Increased CPK during fasting, myoglobinuria	Deficiency of CPT II in fibroblasts
Long-chain acyl-CoA dehydrogenase defect (LCAD)	Normal lactate and ammonium response, but increased CPK	Decreased plasma carnitine	Characteristic acylcarnitine profile, deficiency of LCAD in fibroblasts
Short-chain hydroxyacyl-CoA dehydrogenase (SCHAD) defect	Normal response	Myoglobinuria	Characteristic acylcarnitine profile Deficiency of SCHAD in fibroblasts
Myoadenylate deaminase deficiency	Normal lactate response, no increase in ammonium	Elevated CPK in 50%	Deficiency of myoadenylate deaminase in muscle

Abbreviations: GSD-V = Glycogen storage disease type V; CPK = Creatine phosphokinase; CoA = Coenzyme A

Table 217.4: Inherited metabolic disorders characterized by psychiatric or behavioral abnormalities

Disorder	Associated psychiatric/behavioral abnormality	Diagnostic laboratory tests
Late-onset MLD	Anxiety, emotional lability, disorganized thinking, poor memory, psychosis	Leukocyte arylsulfatase A ↓ mutation studies
Late-onset GM$_2$ gangliosidoses	Acute psychosis, agitation hallucinations	Leukocyte β-hexosaminidase A ↓
X-linked adrenoleukodystrophy	Social withdrawal, irritability, obsessional behavior, rigidity	Plasma VLCFA ↑
Lesch-Nyhan syndrome	Self-mutilatory behavior	Serum uric acid ↑, urine uric acid/creatinine ratio ↑
Wilson's disease	Anxiety, depression, mania schizophrenia, antisocial behavior	Serum copper ↓, Serum ceruloplasmin ↓ Urine copper ↑, hepatic copper ↑
Acute porphyrias	Anxiety, depression, paranoia, restlessness	Urine porphobilinogen ↑
Sanfilippo's disease (MPS III)	Hyperactivity, impulsivity, aggressiveness, sleeplessness	Urine MPS↑ heparan sulfates present Assay of relevant enzymes
Hunter's disease (MPS II)	Hyperactivity, impulsivity, aggressiveness, sleeplessness	Urine MPS ↑ heparan sulfate, dermatan sulfate present
Urea cycle disorders	Periodic acute agitation, hallucination, anxiety	Plasma ammonium ↑, abnormal plasma amino acids

Abbreviations: MLD = Metachrometic leukodystrophy; MPS = Mucopolysaccharides; VLCFA = Very long-chain fatty acids

Lactic Acidosis

The inherited metabolic causes of lactic acidosis include:

- **Defects of pyruvate metabolism**
  - Pyruvate dehydrogenase deficiency
  - Pyruvate carboxylase deficiency
  - **Defects of NADH oxidation:** Mitochondrial electron transfer chain (mETC) defects
- **Disorders of gluconeogenesis/glycogen storage disorders**
  - Glucose-6-phosphatase (G6P) deficiency
  - Fructose 1,6-bisphosphatase deficiency
  - Phosphoenolpyruvate carboxykinase (PEPCK) deficiency
  - Glycogen debrancher deficiency glycogen storage disease III (GSD III)
  - Glycogen synthase deficiency (GSD 0)
- **Fatty acid oxidation defects (FAOD)**
- **Defects of biotin metabolism**
  - Biotinidase deficiency
  - Holocarboxylase synthase deficiency
- **Defects of organic acid metabolism**
  - Propionic acidemia
  - Methylmalonic acidemia, etc.
- **Others:** Hereditary fructose intolerance

Ketones

Ketonuria is a physiological finding due to nutritional defects but metabolic acidosis is not physiologic. Ketolytic defects [succinyl coenzyme A (CoA): oxoacid transferase and 3-ketothiolase deficiencies] can present as moderate ketonuria occurring mainly in fed state at end of day. Severe fasting ketonuria without acidosis is often observed

Table 217.5: Biochemical clues to differential diagnosis of elevated lactate

Lactate (fasting)	Lactate (after meal)	Lactate/pyruvate (fasting)	Ketones	Blood glucose (fasting)	Disorder
(N–) ↑↑↑	(Rise)	(N–) ↑↑	(↑)- ↑↑	N	Respiratory chain defect
(N–) ↑↑↑	Rise	N	N	N	Pyruvate dehydrogenase deficiency
(N–) ↑↑↑	Fall	(N–) ↑	↑↑	(↓)	Pyruvate carboxylase defect
(N–) ↑↑↑	Rise	N	(N–)↑	↓↓	Gluconeogenesis, GSD I
N	Rise	N	↑↑↑	↓↓	Glycogen storage disease types III, 0
N– ↑	(Fall)	N	↓↓	↓↓	FAOD
(N–) ↑↑	(Rise)	(N–) ↑↑	↑↑↑	↓↑	Organic acidurias

Abbreviations: N = Normal; ( ) = Inconstant; ↑= Increased; ↓ = Reduced; GSD = Glycogen storage disorder

- Blood gases and electrolytes
- Blood lactate, ammonia
- Ketones in urine
- Plasma free fatty acids
- Organic acids (in first urine sample after hypoglycemia)
- Serum carnitine and acylcarnitines
- Amino acids in plasma
- **Hormone studies:** Insulin, C-peptide, glucagon, cortisol, IGF-1
- Isoelectric focusing for transferrin (if indicated)

Abbreviations: HFI = Hereditary fructose intolerance; FAO = Fatty acid oxidation; GSD = Glycogen storage disease; FBP = Fructose-1, 6-bisphosphatase; GH = Growth hormone, IGF-1 = Insulin-like growth factor-1

Flowchart 217.1: Evaluation of metabolic acidosis

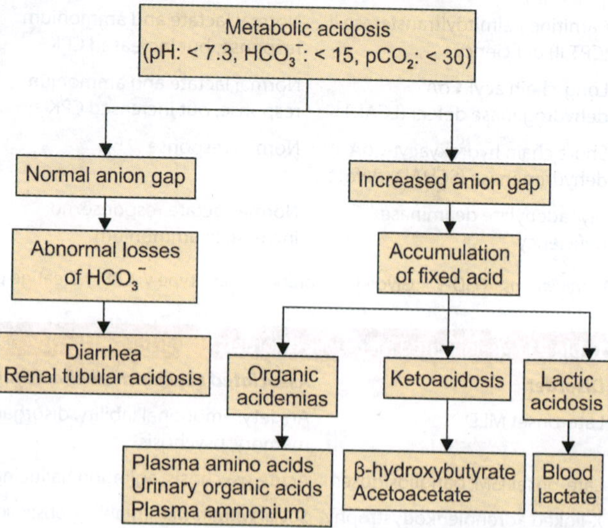

Box 217.1: Etiology of genetic hypoglycemia

Immediate postprandial hypoglycemia (within several minutes after feeding)

- Hyperinsulinism (plasma insulin > 3 mU/L when glucose is < 40 mg/dL)
  - Sulfonylurea receptor (SUR 1) defect
  - Inward-rectifying potassium channel (Kir.2) defect
  - Glutamate dehydrogenase (GLUD 1) deficiency
  - Glucokinase (GK) gene defects
    - Short-chain 3-hydroxyacyl CoA dehydrogenase (SCHAD)
    - Congenital disorders of glycosylation (CDG), types I a, b
  - Usher syndrome (contiguous gene syndrome)
  - Beckwith-Wiedemann syndrome (BWS)
  - Sotos' syndrome
  - Perlman's syndrome (PS)

Hypoglycemia a few hours after meal (3–4 hours)

- Glycogenosis I and III
- Glycogen synthase deficiency
- Respiratory chain disorders

Fasting period

- Fatty acid oxidation disorders (FAOD)
- Fructose-1,6-bisphosphatase deficiency
- Ketogenesis and ketolytic defects
- Respiratory chain disorders
- Fanconi-Bickel syndrome (FBS)
- Endocrinological causes
  - Growth hormone (GH) deficiency
- Insulin-like growth factor-1 (IGF-1) defects
  - Glucagon deficiency
  - Adrenal steroid disorders

Others

- Hereditary fructose intolerance (provoked by fructose ingestion)
- Galactosemia (provoked by galactose ingestion)
- Tyrosinemia, type I
- Glucose transporter 1 (GLUT1) defect (↓ CSF glucose only)

The laboratory investigations during symptomatic hypoglycemia should include

- Blood counts, C-reactive protein (CRP)
- Liver function test (LFT), creatine kinase (CK), uric acid, triglycerides

Contd…

in debrancher and glygogen synthase deficiencies. In both disorders there is hepatomegaly, fasting hypoglycemia and post-prandial hyperlactacidemia. Ketosis without acidosis is also observed in ketotic hypoglycemia due to adrenal insufficiency, hyperinsulinemic states at any age and growth hormone deficiency in infancy.

Ammonium

Normally plasma ammonium is less than 50 μmol/L (reference range: 15–35 μmol/L). It may be elevated in patients with severe hepatocellular dysfunction regardless of the cause. Other causes include viral infection and intoxications, infection with urease-positive bacteria particularly with stasis in urinary tract, Reye's syndrome, valproate therapy and leukemia therapy including treatment with asparaginase.

Inherited metabolic disorders presenting with hyper-ammonemia include:

- Urea cycle defects:
  - N-acetylglutamate synthetase (NAGS) deficiency
  - Carbamoyl phosphate synthetase I (CPS I) deficiency
  - Ornithine transcarbamylase (OTC) deficiency
  - Argininosuccinate synthetase (ASS) deficiency
  - Argininosuccinate lyase (ASL) deficiency
  - Arginase deficiency.
- Organic acidemia:
  - Isovaleric acidemia (IVA)
  - Propionic acidemia (PA)

Table 217.6: Biochemical abnormalities in some of peroxisomal disorders

Disorder	Plasma VLFCA	Urinary pipecolic acid	Plasma phytanic acid	RBC plasmalogens	Plasma bile acid metabolites
Zellweger syndrome	↑↑↑	↑↑↑	↑	↓↓↓	↑↑↑
Neonatal adrenoleukodystrophy	↑↑↑	↑↑	↑	↓↓	↑↑↑
Ketoacyl-CoA thiolase deficiency	↑↑↑	↑↑↑	–	–	↑↑↑
Rhizomelic chondro dysplasia punctata	–	–	↑↑	↓↓↓	–
X-linked adrenoleukodystrophy	↑↑	–	–	–	–
Adult Refsum disease	–	–	↑↑↑	–	–

Abbreviations: VLFCA = Very long-chain fatty acids; RBC = Red blood cell

- Methylmalonic acidemia (MMA)
- Glutaric aciduria, type II (GA II)
- Multiple carboxylase deficiency (MCD)
- 3-ketothiolase deficiency.
- Congenital lactic acidosis:
  - Pyruvate dehydrogenase deficiency
  - Pyruvate carboxylase deficiency
  - Mitochondrial respiratory chain defects.
- Fatty acid oxidation defects:
  - Medium chain acyl-CoA dehydrogenase (MCAD) deficiency
  - Long-chain acyl-CoA dehydrogenase (LCAD) deficiency
  - Systemic carnitine deficiency.
- Dibasic amino acid transport defects (SCD):
  - Lysinuric protein intolerance
  - Hyperornithinemia-hyperammonemia-homoc-itrullinuria (HHH) syndrome.
- Hyperammonemia secondary to hepatic dysfunction:
  - Tyrosinemia type I
  - α_1-antitrypsin deficiency
  - Galactosemia
  - Bile acid synthesis defects
  - Respiratory chain defects.
- ***Others:*** Glutamate dehydrogenase (GDH) deficiency (hyperinsulinemia-hyperammonemia syndrome).

Amino Acids

Analysis of amino acids in various physiological fluids like plasma, urine and cerebrospinal fluid (CSF) is central to the investigation of a possible neurometabolic disorder.

Organic Acids

Organic acids comprise key metabolites of virtually all pathways of intermediary metabolism as well as exogenous compounds. They are generally estimated in urine by gas chromatography-mass spectrometry (GC-MS).

Mucopolysaccharides (MPS)

Urinary excretion of MPS is typically increased in the mucopolysaccharidoses (MPSs), GM_1 gangliosidosis and MSD.

Excess acidic MPS in urine can be detected and quantified by measuring change in color of a metachromatic dye such as Alcian blue, dimethylmethylene blue or toluidine blue.

Oligosaccharides

The oligosaccharides in urine are derived from incomplete breakdown of carbohydrate side-chains of complex glycoproteins. Analysis of urine oligosaccharides and thin layer chromatography of unconcentrated urine are screening tests for glycoproteinoses. Free sialic acid can be determined in urine by spectrophotometry.

Acylcarnitine and Acylglycines

Analysis of carnitine and glycine esters has become an important part of investigation of organic acidopathies and disorders of mitochondrial β-oxidation.

Very Long-chain Fatty Acids

The quantitative analysis of very long-chain fatty acids (VLCFA) is required for differential diagnosis of various peroxisomal disorders (Table 217.6).

RED CELL PLASMALOGENS

Plasmalogens are major components of phospholipids of myelin and other membranes including the red blood corpuscles. In peroxisomal biogenesis disorders, there is a deficiency of plasmalogen biosynthesis, which results in decreased concentrations in myelin and other membranes including red cell membranes. Plasmalogens are measured by extraction of membrane lipids and measurement of lipid phosphorus after saponification to remove phosphoglycerides.

PIPECOLIC ACID

Elevated levels of pipecolic acid, which is an intermediate in lysine metabolism. It is a characteristic finding of inherited defects of peroxisomal biogenesis in plasma and urine.

ENZYME STUDIES

The final diagnosis of many neurometabolic disorders rests on ability to demonstrate a specific enzyme deficiency to account for disease (Appendix 217.1).

TANDEM MASS SPECTROMETRY

Tandem mass spectrometry (MS-MS or tandem MS), a technique of identifying and quantifying analysis based on their molecular mass and charge, is a major technological advantage in screening inborn errors of metabolism.

Appendix 217.1: Enzymes useful in investigation of lysosomal storage disorders (Refer also to Section 10, Ch 94)

Disorder	Enzyme	Enzyme source
Sphingolipidoses		
GM₁ gangliosidosis	β-galactosidase	S, L, F
GM₂ gangliosidoses	β-hexosaminidase	S, L, F
Tay Sach's disease	β-hexosaminidase A	S, L, F
Sandhoff disease	β-hexosaminidase A and B	S, L, F
Metachromatic leukodystrophy	Arylsulfatase A	L, F
Krabbe globoid cell leukodystrophy	Galactocerebrosidase	L, F
Fabry disease	α-galactosidase A	L, F
Gaucher disease	Glucocerebrosidase (β-glucosidase)	S, L, F
Niemann-Pick disease, types A and B	Sphingomyelinase	L, F
Farber lipogranulomatosis	Ceramidase	L, F
Mucopolysaccharidoses		
Hurler disease (MPS I-H)	α-L-iduronidase	S, L, F
Scheie disease (MPS I-S)	α-L-iduronidase	L, F
MPS I variants (MPS IH/S)	α-L-iduronidase	L, F
Hunter disease (MPS II)	Iduronate 2-sulfatase	L, F
Sanfilippo disease, type A (MPS IIIA)	Heparan N-sulfatase	L, F
Sanfilippo disease, type B (MPS IIIB)	α-N-acetylglucosaminidase	L, F
Sanfilippo disease, type C (MPS IIIC)	Acetyl CoA: α-glucosaminide acetyl-transferase	L, F
Sanfilippo disease, type D (MPS IIID)	N-acetylglucosamine-6-sulfatase	L, F
Morquio disease, type A (MPS IVA)	N-acetylgalactosamine-6-sulfatase	L, F
Morquio disease, type B (MPS IVB)	β-galactosidase	L, F
Maroteaux-Lamy disease (MPS VI)	N-acetylgalactosamine-4-sulfatase	L, F
Sly syndrome (MPS VII)	β-glucuronidase	S, L, F
Mucopolysaccharidosis type IX (MPS IX)	Hyaluronidase	S
Glycoproteinoses		
α-fucosidosis	α-fucosidase	S, L, F
α-mannosidosis	α-mannosidase	L, F
β-mannosidosis	β-mannosidase	L, F
Sialidosis, type I	α-neuraminidase	L, F
Galactosialidosis	α-neuraminidase and β-galactosidase	L, F
Schindler disease	α-N-acetylgalactosaminidase	L, F
Aspartylglucosaminuria	Aspartylglucosaminidase	L, F

Contd...

Contd...

I-cell disease and Pseudo-Hurler	All lysosomal enzymes elevated in	S, F
Polydystrophy (mucolipidosis, II and III)	Plasma except β-glucosidase	
Other storage disorders		
Wolman disease	Acid esterase	L, F
NCL 1	Palmitoyl protein thioesterase	L, F
NCL 2	Tripeptidyl peptidase I	L, F
Pompe disease	Acid maltase	Muscle

Abbreviations: S = Serum; L = Leukocytes; F = Fibroblasts; NCL = Neuronal ceroid lipofuscinosis

It has potential for simultaneous and robust multi-disease screening using a single analytical technique. Generally a set of amino acids, free carnitines and acylcarnitines are measured in a spot of blood collected on a S and S 903 filter paper to identify disorders of organic and amino acid metabolism and fatty acid oxidation disorders. The utility and application of tandem MS for newborn screening has been demonstrated in many countries worldwide (Appendix 217.2).

Molecular Genetic Studies

Molecular genetic studies are increasingly relied upon to confirm the diagnosis of many neurometabolic diseases.

CONCLUSION

Diagnosis of neurometabolic disorders always poses difficulty to physicians. This is mainly due to fact that these disorders are rare and most of them share common clinical manifestations. The main obstacle to making a correct diagnosis is failure to think of possibility. Definitive long-term treatment usually requires that a specific diagnosis is made. With progress of basic science and technology over past century, pathogenesis of these disorders has been better understood. This knowledge has opened up possibility of therapeutic intervention for many of these disorders.

Appendix 217.2: Some disorders detectable by tandem mass spectrometry

Disorder	Primary abnormal metabolite(s)
Amino acidemias	
Phenylketonuria	Phenylalanine
Maple syrup urine disease	Leucine/isoleucine, valine
Homocystinuria (cystathionine b-synthase deficiency)	Methionine
Hypermethioninemia	Methionine
Citrullinemia	Citrulline
Argininosuccinic aciduria	Citrulline
Tyrosinemia, types I, II	Tyrosine
Hyperornithinemia	Ornithine
Hyperammonemia, hyperornithinemia, homocitrullinuria (HHH) syndrome	Ornithine

Contd...

Contd...

Argininemia	Arginine
Hyperglycinemia	Glycine
Organic acidemias	
Propionic acidemia	C3
Methylmalonic acidemia	C3
Malonic acidemia	C3DC
Isobutyryl-CoA dehydrogenase deficiency	C4
Isovaleric acidemia	C5
2-methylbutyryl-CoA dehydrogenase deficiency	C5
Glutaric acidemia, type I	C5DC
3-Methylcrotonyl-CoA carboxylase deficiency	C5OH
Multiple carboxylase deficiency (MCD)	C5OH, C3
3-hydroxy-3-methylglutaryl-CoA lyase deficiency	C5OH, C6DC
Mitochondrial acetoacetyl-CoA thiolase deficiency	C5OH, C5:1

Contd...

Contd...

Fatty acid oxidation disorders	
Short-chain acyl-CoA dehydrogenase (SCAD) deficiency	C4
Medium-chain acyl-CoA dehydrogenase (MCAD) deficiency	C8, C6, C10, C10:1
Very long-chain acyl-CoA dehydrogenase (VLCAD) deficiency	C14:1, C14, C16
Long-chain 3-hydroxyacyl-CoA dehydrogenase (LCHAD)	C16OH C18:1OH, C18OH
Trifunctional protein deficiency	C16OH, C18:1OH, C18OH
Carnitine palmitoyltransferase I (CPT I) deficiency	C16, C18:1, C18, free carnitine
Carnitine palmitoyltransferase II (CPT II) deficiency	C16, C18, C18:1
Carnitine-acylcarnitine translocase (CACT)	C16, C18:1, C18
Multiple acyl-CoA dehydrogenase deficiency (Glutaric acidemia type II)	C4, C5, C8:1, C8, C12, C14, C16, C5DC
Primary carnitine deficiency	Free carnitine, all acylcarnitines

CHAPTER
218

Central Nervous System Manifestations in Systemic Disorders

SR Chandra, Mirza Masoom Abbas

SR Chandra, Mirza Masoom Abbas

Chapter Summary

- Gastrointestinal Disease and Central Nervous System Manifestations
- Neurological Manifestations of Liver Disease
- Central Nervous System Manifestations in Respiratory Disease
- Neurological Symptoms in Obstructive Sleep Apnea
- Neurological Complications of Renal Disease
- Neurological Manifestations of Endocrine Disorders
- Neurological Manifestations of Hematological Disorders
- Neurological Complications of Cardiac Disease
- Neurological Complications of Malignancy
- Neurological Involvement in Pregnancy-Associated Diseases
- Mobile Phone Radiation and Related Complications

INTRODUCTION

Nervous system disorders secondary to derangement of other organ systems constitute a major proportion of illness seen in general practice and they form a link between general medicine and neurology.

In this chapter, we discuss diseases pertaining to dysfunction of gastrointestinal (GI), respiratory, renal and endocrine diseases. Brief mention is made regarding neurological complications arising from pregnancy.

GASTROINTESTINAL DISEASE AND CENTRAL NERVOUS SYSTEM MANIFESTATIONS

GI diseases produce central nervous system (CNS) dysfunction either as a part of disease process or secondary to nutrient malabsorption.

Malabsorption Syndromes

Celiac Disease (See Section 8, Ch 79)

Neurologic involvement is seen in 10% of cases. These include peripheral neuropathy (sensory motor or sensorimotor) ataxia, chorea, seizures, myoclonus inflammatory myositis cognitive decline, psychiatric symptoms. Magnetic resonance imaging (MRI) brain may show cerebellar atrophy and white matter signal changes. The neurological symptoms are attributed to nutrient deficiency and immune-mediated CNS damage resulting from antigliadin autoantibodies (AGA).

Diagnosis is by small intestinal biopsy and demonstration of immunoglobulin A (IgA) antiendomysial and IgG transglutaminase antibodies. IgA and IgG AGA has less specificity, being found in 10–20% of normal population.

Treatment is mainly directed against the primary disease which clears the neurological features as well. Residual neurological manifestations are treated depending upon their cause.

Tropical Sprue (Refer Section 8, Ch 79)

Neurological manifestations include subacute combined degeneration of cord due to vitamin B_{12} deficiency, peripheral neuropathy, myopathy, night blindness and cognitive decline.

Diagnosis is by small intestinal biopsy which reveals inflammatory changes. *Treatment* comprise of dietary therapy, prolonged administration of oral antibiotics, along with supplementation of deficient nutrients especially folate and vitamin B_{12}.

Whipple's Disease (Refer Section 17, Ch 201)

CNS involvement is seen in 15% of patients and characterized by cognitive changes leading to dementia, psychiatric features like depression, supranuclear gaze palsy, hypothalamic dysfunction, cranial nerve palsies, seizures, myoclonus and ataxia.

Oculomasticatory dysrhythmia (slow pendular vergence oscillations occurring with slow rhythmic mouth and palatal movements) and oculofacial-skeletal myorhythmia (slow pendular vergence oscillations synchronous with rhythmic movements of mouth, face and extremities) are pathognomonic of Whipple's disease being found in 20% of patients. These movements often persist during sleep.

Diagnosis is by demonstration of periodic acid–Schiff (PAS) positive macrophages in biopsy specimen obtained from small intestine or extraintestinal sites (liver, lymph nodes, heart, eyes, CNS or synovial membranes).

Treatment is with injectable ceftriaxone or streptomycin. Penicillin G combination for 2 weeks followed by oral trimethoprim or sulfamethoxazole for 1–2 years.

Presence of CNS features especially dementia is a poor prognostic sign. One-fourth of patients with CNS involvement die within 4 years and one-fourth have major sequelae.

Inflammatory Bowel Disease (IBD)

It includes ulcerative colitis and Crohn's disease. Extraintestinal manifestations are seen in up to one-third patients. Neurological manifestations are often poorly characterized and under reported in IBD. Their incidence range from 0.5–19% in various studies. They can be part of the primary disease, its complications or due to therapy.

Peripheral neuropathy can be focal (mononeuropathy, cranial neuropathy and brachial plexopathy), multifocal (mononeuritis multiplex, multifocal motor neuropathy), or generalized (acute or chronic inflammatory demyelinating neuropathy, small or large fiber axonal sensorimotor neuropathy). Axonal loss is more common than demyelination. Both demyelinating and axonal neuropathies show good response to immunomodulatory therapy. Other contributory factors for neuropathy include nutritional deficiencies (e.g. vitamin B_{12}) and medications (e.g. metronidazole).

Other CNS manifestations of IBD include arterial and venous thrombosis resulting from hypercoagulable state and vasculitis, seizures, cranial nerve palsies (Bell's palsy, optic neuritis and sensorineural hearing loss), cerebellar ataxia, extrapyramidal features, myelopathy and inflammatory myopathy.

Gastric Surgery

Gastric surgery for peptic ulcer, bariatric surgery includes gastric restriction procedures (gastric stapling and laparoscopic banding) and gastric bypass procedures (Roux-en-Y gastric bypass).

Postsurgery neurological dysfunction is commonly due to nutrient deficiencies of vitamin B_1, B_6, B_{12}, folate, copper and vitamin E. Chronic sensorimotor neuropathy, acute inflammatory demyelinating polyneuropathy (AIDP), chronic immune-mediated polyneuropathy, mononeuropathy like median, ulnar and common peroneal nerve are often seen. Encephalopathy in postoperative period is due to thiamine deficiency caused by recurrent vomiting. Myelopathy is a sequelae of gastric surgery occurring after many years. Potentially treatable causes include deficiency of vitamin B_{12}, copper and in some cases vitamin E.

NEUROLOGIC MANIFESTATIONS OF LIVER DISEASE

(Refer to Section 9, Ch 85)

Hepatic encephalopathy may complicate either acute or chronic liver disease. Cognitive decline has been noted even in mild liver disease in recent studies.

Hepatic Encephalopathy

It is characterized by development of cognitive decline and loss of other higher functions.

Pathophysiology

Hyperammonemia is linked to hepatic encephalopathy and therapies aimed at reducing ammonia level are often beneficial. There is increase in benzodiazepine receptors in encephalopathy patients on which gamma-aminobutyric acid (GABA) might act to increase CNS inhibitory tone. Free fatty acids (FFA) and mercaptan levels are elevated. These might act synergistically with ammonia to produce CNS dysfunction. There is production of false neurotransmitters which competitively inhibit normal neurotransmission.

Clinical Features

Initial changes of encephalopathy need neuropsychological analysis and they show decreased attention, concentration, visual perception, motor speed and accuracy in up to 60% of cases even without clinical signs of encephalopathy. In later stages, there is progressive decline in sensorium alteration in sleep rhythm and progresses to coma. Motor symptoms include asterixis (flapping tremor), dysarthria, rigidity and gait ataxia. Psychiatric features include paranoid delusions, visual hallucinations and mood changes. Neuropsychological analysis may be required to unravel these symptoms (Table 218.1). Hepatic encephalopathy is often precipitated by sedatives, GI hemorrhage, azotemia, electrolyte disturbances, high protein diet, infections and creation of *transjugular intrahepatic portosystemic shunt (TIPS)* as a treatment to reduce portal hypertension.

Laboratory Evaluation

Diagnosis of hepatic encephalopathy is mainly clinical with laboratory tests providing supportive evidence. Serum ammonia is an early sensitive indicator of hepatic encephalopathy, provided arterial samples are analyzed

Table 218.1: West-Haven grading of hepatic encephalopathy

Grade	Clinical symptoms
0	No personality or behavioral abnormality
1	Trivial lack of awareness, euphoria or anxiety, shortened attention span or impairment of the ability to add or subtract
2	Lethargy, disorientation, personality change
3	Somnolence, respond to verbal stimuli with confusion or gross disorientation
4	Coma

immediately. Electroencephalogram (EEG) can show characteristic intermittent burst of high amplitude low frequency waves in the range of 1.5–2.5 Hz and triphasic waves (Fig. 218.1).

MRI brain can show T1 hyperintensities in globus pallidus resulting from manganese deposition. T2 hyperintensities can be seen in cerebral white matter. MR spectroscopy reveals decreased choline with normal N-acetyl aspartate.

Acute Liver Failure

Acute liver failures occur with rapid progression, patients lapsing from drowsiness to comatose state in a few hours to days. Cerebral edema and seizures are more frequent.

Non-Wilsonian Cerebral Degeneration

This is a less recognized entity but a common disease resulting from long-standing liver disease with portosystemic shunting.

Onset is in 4th to 5th decade but can be seen in young adults with metabolic liver disease. Orofacial dyskinesia is a characteristic clinical feature. Others include extrapyramidal features like, dysarthria, generalized bradykine-

sia rigidity and cognitive dysfunction involving executive function and attention. Slowly progressive ataxia and myelopathy can develop.

This is postulated to be due to excess manganese deposition in basal ganglia and hyperammonemia altering chemical balance of dopaminergic neurons in basal ganglia.

MRI showing T1 hyperintensity in bilateral globus pallidus and subthalamic nuclei resulting from manganese deposition (Figs 218.2A and B). Other diseases like hyperglycemia, carbon monoxide poisoning and hypoxic ischemic injury can produce similar picture.

Treatment is correction of underlying liver disease. Liver transplantation can produce gradual improvement over many months. Symptomatic relief of chorea and dystonia can be obtained with medications like tetrabenazine which is a presynaptic dopamine depleting agent. Dopamine agonists and anticholinergics are minimally useful.

CENTRAL NERVOUS SYSTEM MANIFESTATIONS IN RESPIRATORY DISEASE

Respiratory function is intimately related to CNS, with CNS regulating ventilation through peripheral and central chemoreceptors. Cerebral tissue is highly sensitive to change in blood oxygen levels, carbon dioxide and pH.

Acute Respiratory Failure

It is defined as blood partial pressure of oxygen (PaO_2) below 50 mm Hg and partial pressure of carbon dioxide ($PaCO_2$) above 50 mm Hg. Neurological symptoms depend on rate of onset, duration and severity of hypoxia. These include delirium, somnolence, anxiety, tremor, myoclonus, headaches and coma in the terminal stages. Prolonged hypoxia can produce irreversible hypoxic

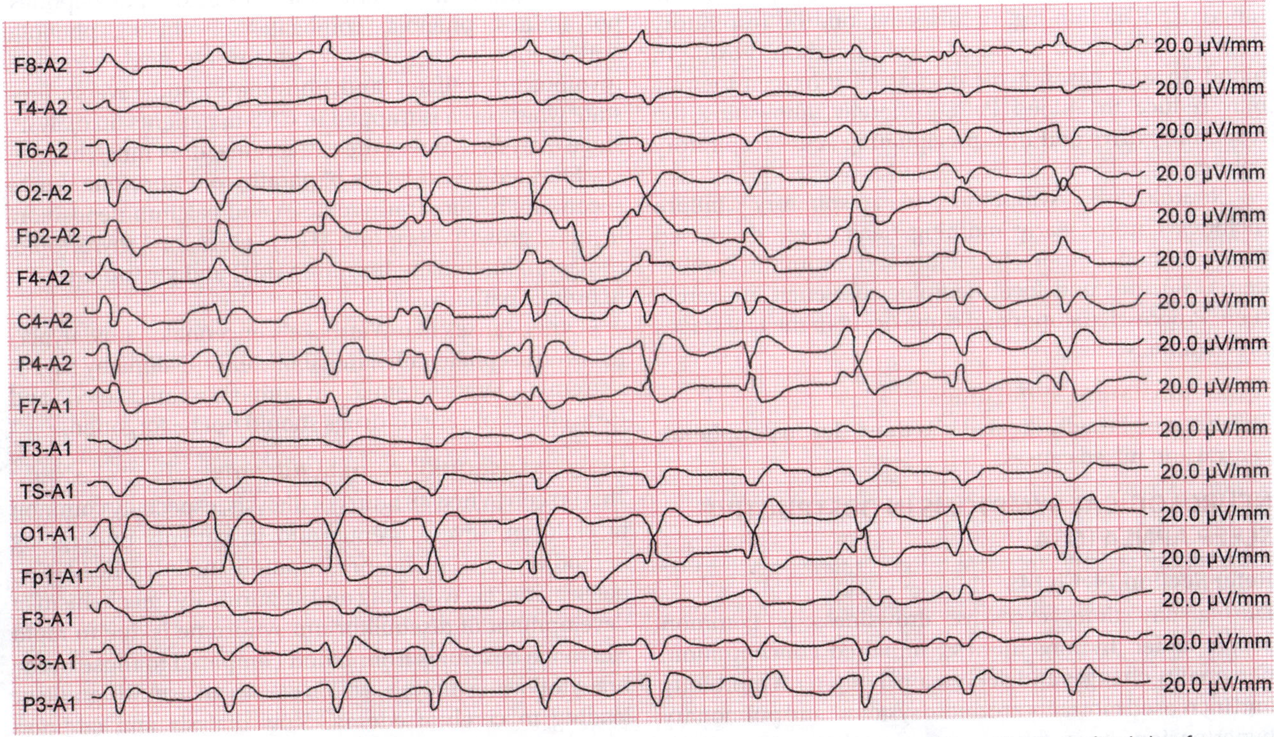

Fig. 218.1: Hepatic encephalopathy—electroencephalogram (EEG) can show characteristic intermittent burst of high amplitude low frequency waves in the range of 1.5–2.5 Hz and triphasic waves

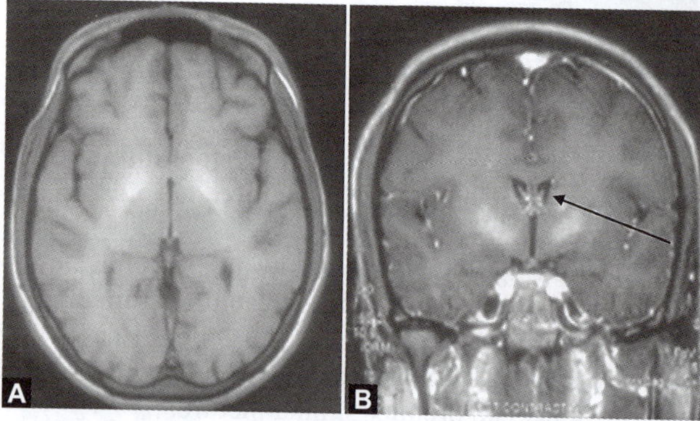

Figs 218.2A and B: Magnetic resonance imaging (MRI) T1 axial and coronal showing T1 hyperintensity in bilateral globus pallidus (arrow) manganese deposition of Wilson's disease cerebral degeneration

ischemic damage of brain with prolonged coma, pupillary and brainstem abnormalities and death in severe cases. Cognitive impairment, extrapyramidal features, action myoclonus and ataxia can develop in surviving individuals. Level of consciousness and pupillary reflexes provide most important prognostic clues for recovery. Structures like cerebral cortex, hippocampus and Purkinje cells of cerebellum, occipital cortex and basal ganglia are sensitive to hypoxic changes.

MRI can show T2 and fluid-attenuated inversion recovery (FLAIR) hyperintensities in cortex suggestive of laminar necrosis.

Chronic Respiratory Failure

Chronic obstructive pulmonary disease (COPD) is the most common cause of chronic respiratory failure, others being fibrosis infiltrations, interstitial lung disease (ILD), sleep apnea syndrome and cardiac disorders. Compensatory mechanisms involving central chemoreceptors can maintain normal function even with elevated $PaCO_2$ in the range of 55–60 mm Hg. In this situation, the respiratory drive is maintained by raised level of carbon dioxide in blood. In such cases, acute uncontrolled oxygen therapy may reduce the blood $PaCO_2$, thereby, abolishing the respiratory drive and thus precipitating acute respiratory failure.

Neurological symptoms in respiratory failure include—chronic early morning headaches, decreased concentration, tremors, irritability and insomnia. Papilledema, seizures and focal neurological deficit are rarely seen. Progressive stupor and coma occur in the late stages preterminally.

Hypoventilation Syndromes

These can be broadly divided into those due to peripheral, central and mixed causes.

NEUROLOGICAL SYMPTOMS IN OBSTRUCTIVE SLEEP APNEA (OSA)

Refer Section 14, Ch 149

During day time, excessive drowsiness is common accompanied by forgetfulness, impaired concentration, personality changes and depression. Long-term morbidity and increased mortality are due to systemic and pulmonary hypertension, heart failure, myocardial infarction (MI), cardiac arrhythmia and stroke.

Management comprises of lifestyle modification, smoking cessation and weight reduction and continuous positive-pressure ventilation during sleep.

NEUROLOGICAL COMPLICATIONS OF RENAL DISEASE

Renal disease can produce a variety of neurological complications depending on rapidity of onset (acute vs chronic renal failure), severity and rate of progression of renal failure, associated metabolic and infective complications and therapeutic interventions (dialysis, transplantation).

Neurological complications along with vascular events are major cause of mortality and morbidity and are usually apparent once glomerular filtration rate (GFR) falls below 10% of normal.

Uremic Encephalopathy

It is seen in both acute and chronic renal failure. Its course is more fulminant in acute renal failure (ARF). Symptoms include fluctuating alertness and attention span, fatigue and restlessness and progressive drowsiness culminating in coma.

Focal deficits are rare but motor weakness, visual abnormalities, focal muscle twitching and seizures can be present. Confusion, hallucinations and frank psychosis, movement disorders including chorea, asterixis, myoclonic jerks and restless leg syndrome may develop. The level of encephalopathy correlates weakly with the degree of azotemia even though dialysis can produce significant improvement in symptoms. EEG shows slowing and triphasic waves. EEG recording is useful to exclude other causes of confusional state.

Accumulation of urea, guanidino compounds, uric acid, hippuric acid, various amino acids, polypeptides, polyamines, phenols, conjugates of phenol, phenolic and indolic acids, acetone, glucuronic acid, carnitine, myoinositol, sulfates and phosphates and reverse urea state where urea is trapped in CNS in patients on dialysis, since dialysis removes the extracranial urea much better.

Elevated blood levels of parathyroid hormone due to secondary hyperparathyroidism and calcium deposition, insulin, growth hormone (GH), glucagon, thyrotropin, prolactin, luteinizing hormone (LH) and gastrin are seen in uremic patients.

Other causes like Wernicke's encephalopathy, hypertensive encephalopathy, metabolic encephalopathy (hyponatremia, hypocalcemia, hypomagnesemia, etc.) and toxic effects of various drugs should not be forgotten.

Dialysis Disequilibrium Syndrome

This is seen in first 48 hours of dialysis, especially common in children, severe uremia and in patients undergoing hemodialysis. Clinical presentation includes headache, nausea, muscle twitching and seizures. The mechanism of development of disequilibrium syndrome is due to rapid clearance of solutes from blood compared to those in the brain following dialysis, which causes an osmotic gradient leading to cerebral edema. Slow dialysis and addition of osmotically active solute to the dialysate can prevent this condition. This is one of the rare metabolic situation which presents with headache as the main symptom. Urea present in extraneural tissues is removed better by dialysis than the urea trapped in neural tissue.

Dialysis Dementia

Multi-infarct dementia due to hypertension and accelerated atherosclerosis is seen in these patients. Rapidly progressive dementia (RPD) should arise a suspicion of progressive multifocal encephalopathy and dialysis dementia.

Cerebrovascular Disease and Ischemic Heart Disease (IHD)

Renal failure patients are at risk of accelerated atherosclerosis and ischemic stroke due to hypertension, diabetes, dyslipidemias, increase in inflammatory cytokines and oxidative stress. Hyperhomocysteinemia and disorders of calcium phosphate metabolism predispose to vascular calcification. Arterial hypotension seen with hemodialysis, clubbed with the presence of dysautonomia can predispose to cerebral ischemia.

Peripheral Neuropathy

It is seen in around 60% of patients with uremia. Most common presentation being distal symmetric sensory polyneuropathy. Motor neuropathy, autonomic and cranial nerve involvement may also be seen. Renal transplantation can arrest progression in some cases. Other causes of polyneuropathy in renal failure include diabetes, vasculitis and graft-versus-host reaction in transplant patients.

Myopathy

This is common when glomerular filtration falls below 25 mL/min. Myopathy is seen in around 50% of uremic patients. Proximal muscle weakness, decreased endurance and easy fatigability are the presenting features. Muscle enzyme levels remain normal. Muscle biopsy can show predominant type 2 muscle atrophy.

Accumulation of uremic toxins, vitamin D deficiency, anemia and protein malnutrition contributes to uremic myopathy. Other causes of myopathy in renal failure include ischemia resulting from atherosclerosis, hypokalemia, hypo/hypercalcemia and hypo/hypermagnesemia and steroid induce myopathy. Renal transplantation can produce significant improvement in symptoms.

NEUROLOGICAL MANIFESTATIONS OF ENDOCRINE DISORDERS

Diabetes constitutes the most frequent entity. Diabetes along with electrolyte disturbances seen with endocrine dysfunction constitute the major chunk of neurological features. These entities are covered elsewhere in the book (*See* Sections 10 and 11).

- ■ ***Hypopituitarism secondary to pituitary tumors***: In addition to specific hormone deficiencies, patients with pituitary adenoma may present with headache, visual field defects, diplopia and hydrocephalus due to local mass effect. Patients with hypopituitarism are also at risk for development of cardiovascular and cerebrovascular events.
- ■ ***Pituitary apoplexy:*** It is a life-threatening condition resulting from acute intrapituitary hemorrhage. Patient presents with signs of meningeal irritation, visual field defects, ophthalmoplegia and coma. If untreated, the patient dies of shock due to acute adrenal cortical insufficiency.
- ■ ***Hypothyroidism:*** It can present with apathy, fatigue, impaired concentration and cognitive decline. Myxedema coma occurs in severe hypothyroidism and it is characterized by hypotension, hypothermia, bradycardia and progressive decrease in consciousness. It carries a high mortality unless rapid correction is undertaken.

Hypothyroidism is associated with muscle stiffness, myalgia and proximal muscle weakness with are flexia and in some cases muscle enlargement is seen. Slowly progressive proximal myopathy is seen in long-standing hypothyroidism. Serum creatine phosphokinase (CPK) is elevated in hypothyroid patients even without myopathy and it is nonspecific, very high values can be encountered in severe cases signifying rhabdomyolysis. Prognosis is good with early thyroid replacement.

Entrapment neuropathy like carpal tunnel syndrome (CTS) is commonly seen in hypothyroid in addition to sensorimotor axonal neuropathy is also seen in hypothyroid as well as hyperthyroid patients.

Hyperthyroidism: It is associated with irritability, hyperactivity and generalized fatigue. Stress (infection, stroke and trauma) or radioiodine intake can precipitate fatal thyrotoxic crisis or thyroid storm characterized by hyperthermia, delirium, seizures and coma. Enhanced physiological tremor is seen in hyperthyroidism; chorea is a rare feature.

Hyperthyroidism produces muscle weakness in more than 50% of patients. Deep tendon reflexes are retained and this condition is called ***Basedow's paraplegia***. Periodic paralysis due to disturbances in potassium metabolism may alternate with features of hyperthyroidism in some patients.

Hyperparathyroidism: It leads to hypercalcemia clinically characterized by lethargy, drowsiness, confusion, generalized muscle weakness, autonomic dysfunction such as anorexia, vomiting and constipation, severe cases go into coma. Unless attended to urgently, condition is fatal.

Hypoparathyroidism: It leads to hypocalcemia and tetany. It also increases the risk of seizures in predisposed individuals.

Pseudohypoparathyroidism: Parkinsonian signs (bradykinesia and rest tremor) as well as basal ganglia calcification may occur.

Hyperadrenocorticism: Cushing syndrome has been associated with irritability, depression, mania and even frank psychosis. Cushing's syndrome, insidious onset of progressive painless proximal muscle weakness with normal CPK levels may develop. In massive glucocorticoid therapy in acute care patient, steroid-induced myopathy may develop as flaccid paralysis. This may also occur in ***critical illness neuromyopathy***.

Hypoadrenocorticism: Common neurological features include fatigue, anorexia, nausea, recurrent vomiting, giddiness and syncope. In severe cases, coma can result from hyponatremia.

NEUROLOGICAL MANIFESTATIONS OF HEMATOLOGICAL DISORDERS

Iron deficiency anemia (IDA): It causes generalized weakness and fatigue. Children develop impairment of faculties in higher functions such as cognition, learning efficiency and intellectual skills. Poor academic performance is common. Nutritional anemia predisposes to stroke and cerebral venous thrombosis.

Sickle cell anemia: It is associated with neurological complications in 25% of patients. These include transient ischemic attacks (TIAs), thrombotic strokes, intracerebral hemorrhage (ICH), seizures, coma, sensorineural hearing loss, spinal cord infarction, infections of the CNS.

Leukemias: Acute lymphatic leukemia (ALL) is invariably complicated by the development of neuroleukemia (Refer Section 15, Ch 165). Acute nonlymphatic leukemia may also lead to neuroleukemia, less frequently. The pathological manifestations include infiltration of the meninges with CSF pleocytosis involvement of neural tissues (diffuse or localized), rise in intracranial tension, thrombocytopenia, hemorrhage and disseminated intravascular coagulation (DIC).

Polycythemia vera (PV): Primary polycythemia and to a lesser extent, secondary polycythemia cause headache, dizziness and visual blurring and thrombotic occlusion of arteries and veins leading to stroke.

Thrombocytopenia: It may result from several causes such as immune thrombocytopenic purpura (ITP), aplastic anemia, acute leukemias, drug toxicity and others. Moderate and severe thrombocytopenia ($<20,000/mm^3$) may lead to purpura and spontaneous or minimal trauma induced intracranial bleeding which resolves with improvement in platelet number.

In severe thrombocytopathies, intracranial bleeding is a major risk.

In ***thrombotic thrombocytopenic purpura (TTP)*** neurological manifestations are due to microvascular thrombosis. It presents with headache, confusion, seizures and coma. Focal neurological deficits can be seen rarely.

Thrombocytosis

Platelet counts above $600,000/mm^3$ may lead to vascular thrombosis in several parts of the body including intracranial structures resulting in various forms of stroke. Clinical symptoms include headache, paresthesia and TIAs.

Lymphoproliferative Malignancies

Tumor formation in the neuraxis, demyelination, compression of normal neural structures by lymphomatous tissue in closed spaces such as the cranium and the spinal cord give rise to various manifestations.

Multiple myeloma, leads to polyneuropathy, organomegaly, endocrinopathy, monoclonal gammopathy and skin (POEMS) syndrome consisting of peripheral neuropathy, organomegaly, endocrine changes, monoclonal gammopathy. Chemotherapy with vincristine, cisplatin and others may lead to peripheral neuropathy.

Compressive myelopathy due to plasmacytomas or myelomatous deposits may present as tumors. Vertebral compression occurring in myeloma may lead to compression of the spinal cord.

NEUROLOGICAL COMPLICATIONS OF CARDIAC DISEASE

Endocarditis: Noninfective endocarditis presents as strokes and infective ones with meningitis, abscess, strokes and hemorrhage. Seizures, headaches and toxic encephalopathy can occur. Roths spots detected on fundus examination give very valuable clue to embolization in bacterial endocarditis.

Cardiopulmonary bypass surgery; cerebral microemboli may occur intra and postoperatively and cause encephalopathy, confusion, cognitive, impairment strokes and coma.

Aortic and aortic valve surgery done under hypoerythemia and circulatory arrest, may be followed by impaired coagulation activity leading to neurological complications.

Low output cardiac failure is accompanied by obtundation and drowsiness which clear up only when the cardiac output improves.

NEUROLOGICAL COMPLICATIONS OF MALIGNANCY

Refer also Section 1, Ch 2

Nervous system can be affected by metastases, non-metastatic paraneoplastic mechanisms and iatrogenic complications. In many cases, the metastases may remain silent probably due to a symbiosis established between the malignancy and normal tissue. The common paraneoplastic complications are seen tumors of the lung, thymus, lymphoreticular tissue, gastrointestinal tract (GIT), kidneys and ovaries, renal and ovarian malignancy.

One of the mechanism for paraneoplastic syndromes is molecular mimicry by which antibodies to cross reacting onconeural antigens develop. These cause lesions in several tissues other than the tissue bearing the tumor. T cells play an important role. Common manifestations in the CNS include encephalitis (limbic encephalitis and brainstem encephalitis), cerebellar degeneration, and opsoclonus myoclonus. Dorsal roots and peripheral nerves may be involved. Dermatomyositis, myasthenia gravis (MG), polymyositis and Lambert-Eaton myasthenic syndrome may develop. Optic neuritis and retinopathy are not uncommon. Other less common presentation include stiff person syndrome, necrotizing myelitis, motor neuron disease (MND), subacute and chronic neuropathy, vasculitis and neuromyotonia. Affection of the VGCC (voltage-gated calcium channel) and VGKC (voltage-gated potassium channel) present as limbic encephalitis, and neuromyotonia, (Morvan's disease). Antibody to ganglionic acetylcholine receptors (AChRs) leads to pan autonomic dysfunction.

Well-known antibodies developing in individual having carcinomas:

- Hu (Anna-1), Zic4, PCA-2, Anna-3, amphiphysin in small cell carcinoma of lung
- Yo in ovary and breast
- CV2 and CRMP5 in thymus and lung
- Ri breast and pelvic tissue
- Ma2 in testis and lung.

The manifestations of these antibody interaction include encephalomyelitis, cerebellar ataxia and stiff person syndrome.

Diagnostic Criteria for Nonmetastatic Syndrome

Definite Criteria

- A classic syndrome and cancer
- Nonclassic syndrome which improves with cancer treatment
- Nonclassical syndrome, antibody and cancer
- A neurological syndrome and antibody, cancer not identified

Possible Criteria

- Classic syndrome, no antibody or cancer
- Classic or nonclassic syndrome and partially characterized antibody
- Nonclassic syndrome and cancer without antibody.

NEUROLOGICAL INVOLVEMENT IN PREGNANCY-ASSOCIATED DISEASES

Involvement of the Nervous System in Pregnancy

Common diseases which involve the nervous system in pregnancy include eclampsia, CTS, headache and worsening of pre-existing sellar tumors, meningiomas and arteriovenous malformations (AVM). Injury to the pelvic nerve may occur in difficult deliveries.

Pre-eclampsia and Eclampsia

Generalized seizures develop in eclampsia which is common in the third trimester of pregnancy or during and after labor. Management comprises of immediate control of seizures and reducing blood pressure (BP).

Wernicke's encephalopathy may be seen in cases with hyperemesis gravidarum during 14–20 weeks of gestation. (*See* Section 5, Ch 31).

Strokes

Twenty percent of cerebral venous thrombosis is associated with pregnancy, in third trimester and postpartum period. Amniotic fluid embolism and paradoxical embolism are more common during labor (*See* Section 13, Ch 130).

Idiopathic intracranial hypertension (IIH): It is seen in obese women who rapidly gain weight during pregnancy. It manifests around 14th week and disappear by 1–3 months following delivery.

Cranial nerve palsy: The incidence of Bell's palsy is increased during pregnancy compared to normal population (38–45 women per 100,000 pregnancies vs 17 per 100,000 women-years in nonpregnant women of child bearing age).

Movement disorders: Restless leg syndrome is seen in up to 20% of pregnant women. It has been attributed to folate deficiency, although IDA might also play a role. Levodopa is helpful in management.

Chorea gravidarum refers to chorea seen during pregnancy. It is a long-term complication of rheumatic fever.

Prevalence of CTS is increased during pregnancy. Usually, it resolves after pregnancy. Other entrapment neuropathies like meralgia paresthetica are also more frequent.

Lumbosacral plexopathy can occur during prolonged vaginal delivery. It may lead to foot drop if it involves L5 radicle. Postpartum plexopathy can produce autonomic and perineal manifestations, like urinary difficulty, anorectal incontinence, sexual dysfunction such as vaginismus and dyspareunia if the lesion involves only S2–S4 spinal roots. Other nerves like obturator nerve and pudendal nerve may be injured during labor. Most of these neuropathies resolve by 6 weeks.

MOBILE PHONE RADIATION AND RELATED COMPLICATIONS

Mobile phone base stations produce high-energy electromagnetic fields and mobile phones form a source of radiofrequency nonionizing radiation. Long-term exposure may cause headache, poor concentration, tiredness, sleep related problems, mood swings, memory loss, and migraine. There are reports of fourfold increase in all cancers on 7 years exposure to mobile tower radiations within 300 m radius. Other reported adverse effects on mobile phones include in risk of tumors by 10–20% and decreased pregnancy rates (29%). Mobile phones are reported to heat up the semicircular canals and alter the orientation of hair cells in the organ of corti. ***Ringxiety*** is the term introduced for the phantom phone rings experienced by persons after prolonged use of mobile phones.

Editor's Note: Mobile phones have been in the use all over the world for over 20 years. Several studies have reported absence of ill-effects on human health from mobile phones. Till now, no governmental actions have been taken to limit the production or use of mobile phones.

Source: American Academy of Neurology. Continuum series annals of the American Academy of Neurology. Neurological complications of systemic disease.

CHAPTER 219

Skin: General Considerations

Usha Vaidhyanathan

Chapter Summary

- General Considerations
- Structure of the Skin
- Glands of the Skin
- Hair
- Nails
- Functions of the Skin
- Clinical Examination
- Principles of Therapy

GENERAL CONSIDERATIONS

Skin covered by terminal hair is an identifying feature of terrestrial mammals. Further evolution of human brain necessitated a better thermoregulatory system, transforming the skin to a functionally naked skin in a range of colors. Thus, majority of the skin, except over the scalp, is covered by vellus hair. The body is insulated by a good layer of subcutaneous fat and provision for appropriate degree of sweating for dissipating heat.

Loss of terminal body hair facilitated the evolution of epidermis with specialized stratum corneum and permanent protective melanin pigmentation. Sun exposure reduces the photosensitive blood folate level, by half and facilitates photogeneration of 25-hydroxycholecalciferol (vitamin D).

Increased demands of folate for cell division and repair during phases of growth and reproduction facilitated the evolution of dark skin. Increased melanin pigmentation protects the skin from damage as well as reduction of blood folate levels, at the expense of vitamin D synthesis in tropical climate.

On the contrary, the evolution of fair skin facilitated the migration of man to temperate climate maintaining adequate vitamin D and folate levels. Fair skin with its lower melanin content allows better penetration of ultraviolet (UV) rays and thus facilitates the conversion of precursors into vitamin D. Folate levels are maintained because the intensity of UV radiation declines as one move away from the equator.

Melanin pigments are capable of absorbing visible light, UV light, ionizing radiations and also neutralizing the reactive oxygen species. Dark pigmentation protects from skin cancers in the tropical regions. Due to their lower melanin pigment, fair skinned people have to adopt sun protection recommendations while moving to tropical regions.

STRUCTURE OF THE SKIN

The skin is a major organ in the body with a surface area of 1.8 m² in an adult, constituting up to 16% of the total body weight. Skin is composed of three layers—(1) epidermis (2) dermis and (3) subcutaneous tissue. Normal skin of man is relatively water resistant and also resistant to abrasion.

Epidermis

The epidermis which originates from ectoderm is the most superficial layer of the skin. It is a stratified squamous epithelium about 0.1 mm thick. The thickness varies in different parts of the body. Its main function is to act as a protective barrier. Epidermis is mainly composed of keratinocytes, which produce a protein called **keratin**. It is devoid of blood vessels and lymphatics. It gets its nutrition from the underlying dermis. Histologically, the epidermis consists of four layers—stratum basale, stratum spinosum, stratum granulosum and stratum corneum.

Stratum basale (basal cell layer): It is composed of columnar cells. This layer rests on a basement membrane, which attaches it to the dermis. These cells are attached to the basement membrane by attachment plaques called ***hemidesmosomes***. Thirty percent of basal cells divide. One of the daughter cells moves into the suprabasal layer and differentiates and synthesizes keratin. This process of daughter cells maturing and migrating to the superficial layer is called ***keratinization***. Stem cells reside amongst the basal cells and divide in response to injury.

Melanocytes, seen as clear cells in between the basal keratinocytes, constitute about 5–10% of the basal cells. They arise from the neural crest. Melanocytes synthesize melanin and transfer it to neighboring keratinocytes via dendritic processes. Melanin granules are uniformly distributed in the stratum corneum and they reduce the UV radiation penetrating the skin. In the deeper layers of the epidermis, the melanin granules form a protective cap over the outer part of the nucleus of the keratinocyte.

Stratum spinosum (prickle cell layer): It is composed of 5–8 layers of polygonal cells called ***keratinocytes***. These keratinocytes are interconnected by desmosomes which are seen as prickles on light microscopy. These desmosomes are specialized attachment plaques that contain certain proteins like desmoplakins, desmogleins and desmocollins. Autoantibodies to these proteins are responsible for the various autoimmune blistering disorders. Tonofilaments are small fibers running from the cytoplasm to the desmosomes. Bundles of tonofilaments are called *tonofibrils*. In the superficial spinous layer, *lamellar granules* or *Odland bodies* which are derived from the Golgi apparatus appear. They contain phospholipids, cholesterol and glucosylceramides, which are discharged into the intercellular space of the granular cell layer. These are the precursors for lipids in the superficial layers which are very important for barrier function of the skin.

Langerhans cells are found mostly in this layer. These dendritic cells, derived from the bone marrow are the outermost sentinels of the cellular immune system. These cells are characterized by unique cytoplasmic organelles known as *Birbeck granules,* on electron microscopy.

Stratum granulosum (granular layer): It is composed of 2–3 layers of flattened cells containing coarse basophilic keratohyalin granules which merge with the tonofibrils. These keratohyalin granules contain proteins like involucrin, loricrin and profilaggrin. In the outer layers, these granules break up and their contents are dispersed throughout the cytoplasm, leading to keratinization. This tough peripheral protein coating is called *the horny envelope*.

Stratum corneum (horny layer): It is composed of sheets of overlapping, flattened, non-nucleated, cornified and dead cells. The barrier function of the skin is due to the special properties of the horny layer. The cytoplasm is packed with keratin filaments embedded in a matrix with a peripheral tough protein coat inside the cell. These proteins bind to lipids in the intercellular space by transglutaminases. These protein rich corneocytes are embedded in a bilayer lipid matrix. They have a brick and mortar appearance. These bricks are the keratinocytes and the mortar is made up of lipids discharged into the intercellular space by lamellar granules. This envelope gives the corneocytes its toughness to withstand all the chemical and mechanical insults.

Another important protective function of the stratum corneum is prevention of transepidermal water loss. The protein filaggrin (filament aggregating protein) is formed from its precursor profilaggrin. The break down products of filaggrin comprises a substance known as natural moisturizing factor (NMF). These intercellular NMF and extracellular lipids maintain skin hydration.

Keratinization

The epidermal keratinocytes undergo characteristic changes as they ascend and transform from undifferentiated columnar basal cells to fully differentiated horizontally aligned corneal cells. As the basal keratinocytes mature toward cornified cells, they lose their nuclei and cytoplasmic organelles and become filled with tonofilaments. This process is called *cornification* or *keratinization*.

Dermoepidermal Junction

It is a highly specialized attachment between the epidermis and papillary dermis. The various structures of the dermoepidermal junction such as tonofilaments, hemidesmosomes, trilaminar plasma membrane, lamina lucida, anchoring filaments, basement membrane, anchoring fibrils, type III collagen and microfibrils provide attachment and support between the dermis and epidermis and also regulate the permeability across the junction.

Dermis

The dermis is a tough supportive connective tissue matrix found immediately below the epidermis. Its thickness varies from 0.6 mm on the eyelids to about 3 mm on the palms and soles. It is made up of connective tissue fibers like collagen (70%) and elastin in a ground substance of glycosaminoglycans.

The thin upper layer of the dermis is called *papillary dermis* which interdigitates with the epidermal rete ridges. The deeper thick layer is called *reticular dermis* with coarse bundles of collagen. The dermis also contains fibroblasts (which synthesize collagen, elastin and the ground substance), dendritic cells, mast cells, macrophages and lymphocytes. The dermis shows epidermal down growths of hair follicles, the sebaceous glands and sweat glands. It also contains an extensive network of blood vessels and nerves. The caliber of the dermal blood vessels can be controlled by arteriovenous (AV) anastomoses that act as shunts. The blood vessels are under neural and hormonal control as in other parts of the body. This mechanism ensures a proper supply of blood to the cutaneous appendages like hair bulbs, sweat glands and sebaceous glands and also plays a major role in temperature regulation.

The cutaneous nerves in the dermis are both autonomic and sensory. The arterioles are supplied by adrenergic sympathetic nerves that mediate vasoconstriction. The adrenergic sympathetic fibers also supply arrectores pilorum muscles. The myoepithelial cells of the apocrine and eccrine sweat glands are cholinergic sympathetic. The skin is devoid of any demonstrable vasodilator nerves. Free sensory nerve endings are seen in the dermis, also extending to the epidermis. There are specialized receptors called Pacinian corpuscles to detect pressure and vibration and Meissner's corpuscles in the skin of hands and feet, which detect touch. The free nerve endings that transmit pain also subserve the sensation of pruritus, the intensity of the stimulus being low.

GLANDS OF THE SKIN

Sebaceous glands: These are of epidermal origin seen in close proximity of the hair follicles at the upper part of the dermis. They are most numerous on the scalp, face, front of the chest and back and they are absent on the palms and soles. Their secretion sebum is formed by disintegration of the lining cells (holocrine secretion) and this is not under neural control. The sebum is discharged to the surface through the hair follicle. The major components of sebum are triglycerides, wax esters, squalene, cholesterol esters and cholesterol. Sebum that is present on the skin surface inhibits microbial proliferation. The sebaceous glands hypertrophy occurs during puberty under hormonal influences.

Apocrine glands: They are large coiled tubular glands opening into the hair follicles and their function is not clearly known. They are seen in the axillae, around the nipples, perineum and genital regions. Specialized apocrine glands are seen in the eyelids and in the ear canal. Apocrine glands are surrounded by contractile myoepithelial cells that help to expel their contents (apocrine secretion). These myoepithelial cells derive their innervation from adrenergic twigs that respond to emotional stimuli.

Eccrine glands: Eccrine sweat glands are small coiled glands in the dermis whose ducts empty directly on to the cutaneous surface. Eccrine sweat produced in the gland by merocrine secretion (only the contents of the secretory vesicles are discharged, unlike in a holocrine secretion, the cells disintegrate to liberate their secretion) is colorless and odorless. They are more numerous over the forehead, axillae, palms and soles though they are widely distributed throughout the body.

Heat and emotional stress are the main stimuli for sweat secretion. The temperature control center in the hypothalamus is able to detect minute changes in temperature and when excited, stimulates the number and activity of sweat glands via sympathetic nonmyelinated class C nerve fibers. Excessive body heat is dissipated by evaporation of sweat. Aldosterone prevents the loss of electrolytes in sweat by inducing re-absorption of sodium in the sweat ducts. Sweat moistens the skin of palms and soles and provides grip. Substances like griseofulvin, lead, mercury, ethanol and ketoconazole are excreted by eccrine glands. In healthy persons, sweat contains all the electrolytes found in the plasma or interstitial fluid but to a lesser extent.

HAIR

Hairs are found over the entire surface of the skin with the exception of the glabrous skin of the palms, soles, glans penis and vulval introitus. The density of the follicles is greatest on the face. Embryologically, hair is developed from the primordial epithelial germ cells formed from the ectoderm. Hair follicle is formed by an invagination of the epidermis into the dermis.

In longitudinal sections, a mature hair follicle consists of an infundibulum, isthmus, stem and bulb. The germinative cells are in the hair bulb, interspersed with melanocytes. The bulb encloses the follicular papilla which organizes and maintains the function of the hair follicle. Cut section of the hair shaft shows an outer cortex and an inner medulla.

The growth of hair is cyclical and different phases of follicle are—growing phase (anagen) which lasts for 3–10 years, involuting phase (catagen) which lasts for 2–3 weeks and resting phase (telogen) which lasts for 3–4 months. The stem and bulb shrink to form a thin column of epithelial cells in the catagen phase. When a new cycle of anagen phase begins, these residual undifferentiated epithelial cells proliferate and generate a new follicular matrix. At least, 85% of hair follicles are in anagen phase at any one time. There are three types of hair:

1. ***Lanugo hairs*** are fine and long and are formed in the fetus at 20 weeks of gestation. They are normally shed before birth, but may be seen in premature babies.
2. ***Vellus hairs*** are short, fine light colored hairs that cover most body surfaces.
3. ***Terminal hairs*** are long, thick and dark and are found on the scalp, pubic and axillary regions, beard area, upper trunk and limbs. They originate as vellus hair and change into terminal hair at puberty under the influence of androgens.

NAILS

The nail is a phylogenetic remnant of the mammalian claw and consists of hardened and densely packed keratin. It protects the finger tip, facilitates grasping and tactile sensitivity in the finger pulp. The nail matrix contains dividing cells which mature, keratinize and form the nail plate. The pink color of the nail is due to dermal capillaries and white lunula is the visible distal part of the matrix. The nail plate rests on the nail bed. The nail plate grows at a rate of 0.1 mm/day for finger nail and the toe nails at a rate of 0.03 mm/day.

FUNCTIONS OF THE SKIN

The skin has many vital functions:

- The skin acts as a mechanical barrier to protect the deeper structures from external injury and invasion by microbes
- The eccrine sweat glands and the blood vessels of the skin, play a major role in temperature regulation
- The skin regulates the loss of body fluids by altering the rate of perspiration
- Melanin pigment protects the skin from the harmful effects of UV rays
- Skin acts as a major sensory organ receiving all superficial sensations
- Vitamin D synthesis occurs in the skin on exposure to sunlight. Twenty minutes of exposure can supply the day's need of vitamin D
- Dendritic cells in the skin play a major role in immune surveillance
- Sebum has antimicrobial properties
- Several drugs and chemicals are absorbed through the skin when applied in suitable vehicles. This property has been made use of therapeutics.

CLINICAL EXAMINATION

Skin disorders are widespread in India contributing to 20–25% of the total attendance in any general hospital. The skin closely reflects the disorders occurring in the internal organ systems and several cutaneous disorders have systemic manifestations. Therefore, clinical examination of the skin is not complete without a full systemic examination. Examination should be done under conditions of proper lighting, preferably natural light.

Descriptive Terms

The initial lesions that herald the onset of any dermatological disorder are called ***primary lesions***. ***Secondary lesions*** are those that develop during the course of disease.

Primary Lesions

- Macule is an alteration of color of the skin up to 1 cm in diameter and is flush with the surrounding normal skin. A macule more than 1 cm is called a ***patch***.

- Papule is a solid elevated lesion up to 1 cm in diameter. A papule more than 1 cm is called a ***plaque***.
- Vesicle is a clear fluid filled lesion up to 1 cm. A vesicle more than 1 cm is called a ***bulla***.
- Pustule is a small vesicle containing pus. An abscess is a deeper and localized collection of pus in a cavity more than 1 cm in diameter.
- Nodule is a solid elevated mass, more than 1 cm in diameter and depth, better palpated than seen.
- Wheal is an evanescent edematous skin lesion. It may be erythematous, skin colored or pale.
- Purpura is a hemorrhagic macule or papule that does not blanch on pressure. Larger lesions are called ***ecchymoses*** and pinpoint lesions are called ***petechiae***.
- Burrow is a tunnel produced by the movement of a parasite within the tissue. It is seen as a straight or zigzag line that may be grayish.
- Comedones are dark plugs seen inside the opening of a hair follicle.
- Telangiectasia is the visible dilatation of the small cutaneous blood vessels.

Secondary Lesions

- ***Scales:*** Visible dry exfoliation of the horny layer.
- ***Crust:*** Dried up discharges such as serum, pus or blood.
- ***Erosion:*** An area of denuded skin due to a complete or partial loss of the epidermis.
- ***Ulcer:*** Discontinuity in the skin due to a loss of epidermis as well as part or whole of the dermis.
- ***Excoriation:*** Superficial denudation of the skin due to scratching.
- ***Atrophy:*** Thinning of the skin (epidermis, dermis or subcutaneous fat). With epidermal atrophy, the skin becomes shiny, translucent and wrinkled. Atrophy of the deeper tissues leads to depression in the skin.
- ***Fissure:*** A slit or linear tear in the epidermis.
- ***Scar:*** The replacement of normal structures by fibrous tissue when a tissue heals at the site of injury.
- ***Lichenification:*** Visible and palpable thickening of the epidermis with accentuated skin markings.
- ***Induration:*** Thickening of the dermis that makes the skin feel more thick and firm.

PRINCIPLES OF THERAPY

Locally applied drugs as well as systemic drugs are employed for the treatment of dermatological diseases. The fact that locally applied drugs exert their action in addition to systemic drugs is an added advantage. Many disorders respond to local therapy, some require a combination of local and systemic therapy, while a third group requires only systemic therapy. In a limited number of cases, surgical as well as electrosurgical measures may also be necessary.

Local Therapy

The advantages of local therapy are—achievement of a high concentration of the drug at the site of lesion, which is not generally obtainable by systemic therapy; freedom from serious adverse side effects; and even drugs which cannot be administered systemically can be given locally.

Though drugs applied over the skin are not absorbed significantly, systemic toxicity becomes a problem with many drugs, especially if applied over extensive raw areas for prolonged periods.

Modes of Local Therapy

Compresses, soaks and ***baths:*** These help in mechanically removing the exudates, poorly formed crusts, tissue debris, remnants of previously applied medicines, etc. The absorption of a drug from the local site is facilitated if it is administered after applying compresses, soaks or baths. Compresses and soaks are given for localized lesions, whereas baths are given for more extensive and generalized disorders.

Potassium permanganate ($KMnO_4$), sodium chloride (NaCl), liquor picis carbonis, ichthyol or sodium bicarbonate ($NaHCO_3$) is added to the compresses, soaks and baths to enhance their therapeutic value.

Vehicle or base: For local applications, the active ingredients are dissolved or suspended in a vehicle called the base, the main function of which is to keep ingredients in contact with the lesion. The base is selected according to the type and location of lesion and also solubility and compatibility of the active ingredients with the base. Commonly used vehicles are water, glycerine, alcohol, cream, petrolatum and talcum.

Astringents: These are agents which when applied on raw areas of the skin, react with tissue proteins to form a protective covering on the surface. They help to reduce the pain. Liquor aluminum acetate, liquor plumbi subacetate and silver nitrate are commonly used astringents.

Soothing agents: These are applied to relieve pain, burning, and pruritus, generally associated with inflammation of the skin. Alleviation of these symptoms is achieved by the evaporation of the water component of the medication which produces a cooling effect and vasoconstriction. All aqueous preparations can act as soothing agents, e.g. calamine lotion and cream.

Emollients: These form a thin greasy layer over the surface of the skin and prevent evaporation of water from the stratum corneum. Vaseline, oils, cream and glycerine are commonly used emollients.

Antipruritic agents: Itching is the most common and troublesome complaint in dermatological disorders. No doubt, specific therapy is the ideal way to abolish this symptom, but when this is not possible or immediate relief is to be provided, symptomatic therapy is indicated. Chloretone (butyl chloral) which is an analogue of chloral hydrate is a safe antipruritic agent in a concentration of 3–5%. Menthol, camphor and phenol in acceptable concentrations are also effective.

Keratolytic agents: These are employed for promoting desquamation of scales or removal of thickened stratum corneum. They are useful in the treatment of disorders like palmoplantar keratoderma (PPK), ichthyosiform dermatoses, psoriasis and dermatitis associated with lichenification. Salicylic acid, urea and resorcin are commonly used keratolytic agents.

Anti-inflammatory agents: These agents reduce the severity of inflammation and minimize tissue damage when employed with other specific therapy. Though mild inflammatory processes can be controlled with soothing agents, severe inflammatory responses demand the use of drugs like corticosteroids, gentian violet and ichthyol. The commonly used corticosteroid preparations include betamethasone valerate (0.12%), fluocinolone acetonide (0.025%), fluticasone propionate 0.05%, hydrocortisone 1%, clobetasol propionate 0.05% and others.

Antibacterial agents: Topical antibacterial agents play an important role in the treatment and prophylaxis of microbial infections of the skin, especially infections of the epidermis and dermis. The commonly used topical antibacterial agents are neomycin, polymyxin, framycetin, gentamicin, silver sulfadiazine, fusidic acid and mupirocin.

Hexachlorophene, povidone iodine, benzalkonium chloride and chlorhexidine have been used as antiseptics, particularly in the context of disinfection of skin prior to surgical procedures. Topical antibacterial agents are used prophylactically in trauma, cuts, wounds and burns.

Sunscreens: These are used to protect the skin from sunlight. These may act as reflectors or absorbers of light. Reflectors help to prevent the rays from entering the skin whereas chemical absorbers absorb sunlight. Agents like para-aminobenzoic acid, benzophenones, avobenzones tannic acid, titanium dioxide and zinc oxide are usually employed as sunscreens.

Occlusive dressings: These are employed when a drug is to be applied in close contact with the skin and it is to be kept in position to favor absorption and prolonged action. Moreover, the moisture released by the skin helps to soften the lesions and favor resolution, e.g. psoriasis.

Systemic therapy: It is often included in many cases depending upon the condition. Several classes of drug may be needed according to the conditions. Commonly used drugs include antibiotics, anti-histaminis, antiprurites, vitamins sedatives and analgesia. These are discussed in their respective sections.

Textbook of Medicine

CHAPTER
220

Infections of the Skin and Appendages

Usha Vaidhyanathan

Chapter Summary

- Normal Microbial Flora
- Bacterial Infections
  - Pyoderma
- Viral infections
  - Verrucae
  - Molluscum Contagiosum
  - Herpes Simplex
- Superficial Fungal Infections
  - Dermatophytosis
  - Candidiasis
- Pityriasis Versicolor

NORMAL MICROBIAL FLORA

A healthy normal skin is colonized by a variety of nonpathogenic microorganisms. This constitutes the normal flora of the skin. It is classified into resident flora and transient flora. **Resident flora** includes bacteriae that grow on skin and are relatively stable in number and composition. Some organisms linger briefly on the skin in small numbers before disappearing, unable to multiply and thrive in the relatively inhospitable environment. These are labeled as temporary residents or transients. Most of the organisms reside on the surface of the stratum corneum in the crevices between squames in the loose outermost layers. The hair follicles are inhabited by anaerobes like *Propionibacterium* species. Streptococci are usually absent, but may be found as transient residents on perioral skin, from the mouth. Coagulase positive *Staphylococcus aureus* should not be considered as a resident on healthy skin, although it is frequently found

in the anterior nares and perineum and on damaged skin in eczema or psoriasis. Of the coagulase negative *Staphylococcus* species, *S. epidermidis* and *S. hominis* are the most important. Other resident flora are *Micrococcus* (intertriginous areas and scalp), *Corynebacterium* species (axilla), *Propionibacterium* species (face, scalp, axilla), Gram-negative organisms (axilla, toe webs, nose) and fungi like *Pityrosporum* (scalp) and *Candida* species (intertriginous areas). The resident flora prevents colonization by pathogenic organisms and also other commensal flora.

An intact stratum corneum is the most important defense against invasion by pathogenic bacteriae. Skin infection results when the skin defenses are compromised due to physical factors such as excessive hydration, occlusion and systemic factors like immunosuppression.

BACTERIAL INFECTIONS

Pyoderma

It is an infection of the skin caused by pyogenic organisms. *S. aureus* and group A beta hemolytic *Streptococcus* are the most common. Less commonly *Pseudomonas*, *Escherichia coli* and other organisms can also invade the skin. Pyoderma may be primary or secondary.

- **Primary pyoderma** occurs in previously normal skin. It is caused by a single group of organisms and has a characteristic morphology.
- **Secondary pyoderma** occurs in skin previously damaged by other diseases such as scabies, fungal infection, eczema and others.

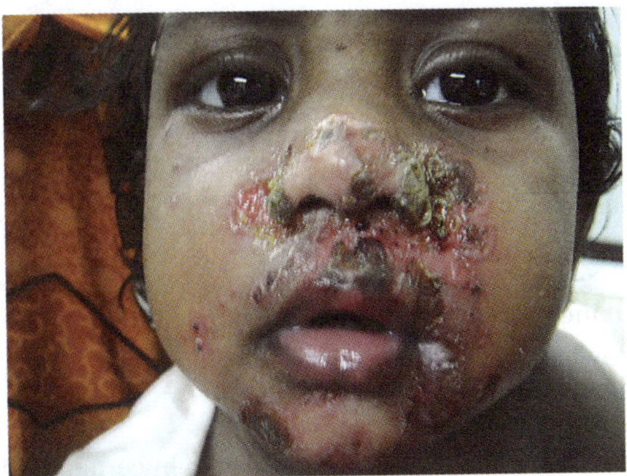

Fig. 220.1: Impetigo on the face

Primary Pyoderma

Impetigo: It is a superficial infection of the epidermis due to *S. aureus* and occasionally group A beta hemolytic streptococci. There are two types:

1. ***Impetigo contagiosa*** commonly affects the face of small children, but any site can be involved. It begins as transient superficial small vesicles or pustules on an erythematous base that soon rupture and form erosions and crusting (golden yellow crusts) (Fig. 220.1). If the lesions persist, central clearing can occur and may become confluent. Complications include cellulitis and post-streptococcal glomerulonephritis.

2. ***Bullous impetigo*** is common in neonates and infants, but can occur at any age. Eighty percent are caused by *S. aureus*, phage group 2, type 71 and 55. Vesicles and bullae containing yellow fluid arise on normal appearing skin without surrounding erythema and persist for a few days. Lesions rupture and varnish like yellow crusts are formed. Lesions can occur anywhere and commonly involves intertriginous areas.

Ecthyma: Commonly, it affects the distal extremities. The infection extends up to the dermis. It presents as a purulent tender indurated ulcer with adherent crust and surrounding erythema. Healing occurs with scarring.

Folliculitis: It is infection of the hair follicle mostly due to *S. aureus* and appears as pustules with a hair or follicular orifice at the center. Chronic folliculitis of the legs is a common problem in India. Mostly, it affects the shin of young males. The pustules are chronic, recalcitrant and cause atrophy on healing. A deep folliculitis involving the whole depth of the hair follicle, affecting the beard (*sycosis barbae*) and nape of the neck (*sycosis nuchae*) is also described. It appears as discrete erythematous, edematous, follicular papules or pustules.

Furuncle: Infection of the hair follicle and perifollicular region caused by *S. aureus* is called ***furuncle*** or ***boil***. It is an extremely painful follicular nodule that may suppurate and become an abscess. Common sites are neck, face, scalp, axilla, perineum, buttocks and thighs.

Carbuncle: It is a deep infection caused by *S. aureus*, extending up to the subcutaneous tissue, involving a group of contiguous follicles, with multiple discharging points on the surface. The common sites are the back of the neck, shoulders, hips and thighs. It is frequently associated with diabetes mellitus (DM) and immunocompromised states.

Erysipelas: It is an acute streptococcal infection of the dermis. Streptococci can enter only through a damaged skin. It presents as an erythematous, edematous, elevated, indurated and well-demarcated lesion, commonly on the face and the legs. There may be vesiculation at the periphery in acute cases.

Cellulitis: It is an acute, subacute or chronic streptococcal infection affecting the deeper subcutaneous tissue. The margins are indistinct and not elevated unlike as in erysipelas. Common sites are the legs but any area can be involved. Cellulitis of face can occur in children due to *Haemophilus influenzae* type b. Cheeks and periorbital region are indurated, violaceous and is typically unilateral. The common source of infection is an otitis media on the same side. Systemic symptoms are common.

Treatment

Majority of cases need systemic antibiotics. Cloxacillin 500 mg qid or first generation cephalosporins like cephalexin 500 mg qid are preferred. Severe cellulitis or erysipelas needs in-patient care with intravenous (IV) cloxacillin and IV benzyl penicillin. Clindamycin 600 mg tid or clarithromycin 500 mg bid are alternatives. Supportive therapy includes improvement of local hygiene, elimination of any predisposing factors, saline compresses for crusted lesions and topical antibiotics like mupirocin, fusidic acid and retapamulin.

Points to Remember
- Intact stratum corneum is the most important defense against invasion by pathogenic bacteriae.
- Staphylococcal infections include impetigo, ecthyma and folliculitis.
- Streptococcal infections are erysipelas and cellulitis.
- Staphylococci and streptococci cause secondary infection of eczema or leg ulceration.
- Cloxacillin and first generation cephalosporins are preferable.

VIRAL INFECTIONS

Verrucae

Syn: Warts

Warts are common benign epithelial hyperplasia due to infection with human papillomavirus (HPV). Papilloma viruses are double-stranded deoxyribonucleic acid (dsDNA) viruses of the papova class with host and tissue specificity. They infect squamous epithelia of the skin and mucous membrane causing cell proliferation. The virus infects the basal layer of the epithelium, but viral replication takes place in fully differentiated cells of upper stratum spinosum and stratum granulosum. After initial infection, HPV may persist in a latent form and may be reactivated later leading to recurrence of lesion. More than 150 types of HPV have been identified and some types have a role in the oncogenesis of cutaneous malignancies. The virus infects by direct inoculation and spreads by skin-to-skin contact. Common clinical patterns are:

- ***Common warts*** (HPV-2) present as dome-shaped papules with verrucous surface commonly on the hands (Fig. 220.2) and feet, but can affect any site.

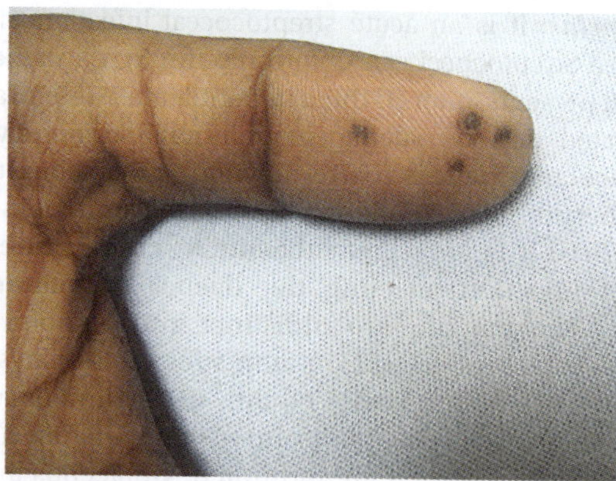

Fig. 220.2: Verrucae on the thumb

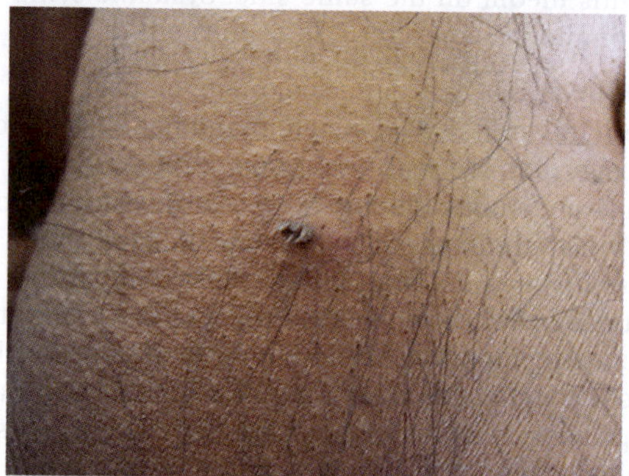

Fig. 220.3: Filiform wart on the thigh

Some warts are *filiform* with fine digit like projections (Fig. 220.3).

- *Verruca plana* (HPV-3 and 10) are smooth flat topped papules, often multiple, commonly seen on the face and dorsa of the hands and these resolve spontaneously. *Koebner's phenomenon* is seen frequently, i.e. new warts forming over sites of trauma.
- *Plantar warts* (HPV-1) are seen on the pressure points of the soles of the feet. They are painful. When pared, reveals dark punctate spots due to thrombosed capillaries. Multiple warts can coalesce to form a *mosaic wart*.

Genital warts (HPV-6 and 11) are sexually transmitted, but sometimes the transmission may be nonvenereal. Genital warts have a high infectivity. In one study, around two-thirds of sexual contacts of patients with genital warts developed lesions within 9 months. They affect the penis in males, perianal area in homosexuals and the vulva, perineum and vagina in females. The warts may be small or may be large cauliflower like *condylomata acuminata*. Rectal and cervical warts have to be identified and followed up because of the risk of malignant change. Sexual partners should be examined.

Management

In children, 30–50% of common warts resolve spontaneously within 6 months. The common modalities of treatment for different types of warts are as follows:

Hand and foot warts: Salicylic and lactic acid in a liquid formulation is applied daily till resolution. Other modal-ities of treatment include cryotherapy (liquid nitrogen at −196°C) sprayed on to the lesions and intralesional bleomycin for resistant warts. Periungual and subungual warts are difficult to treat and relapses are common.

Genital warts: Podophyllin (25%) applied under super-vision weekly till resolution or podophyllotoxin (0.5%) self-application, twice daily for 3 days/week for 4 weeks yields good results. Podophyllin should not be used in pregnancy. Cryotherapy is very effective and may need to be repeated till clearance of lesions.

Filiform and large perineal warts: Curettage and electrodesiccation are effective.

Carbon dioxide (CO_2) laser is useful in certain difficult sites like periungual and subungual warts. Pulsed dye lasers, erbium YAG and Nd:YAG lasers are also used.

Points to Remember

- Hand and foot warts are common and often resolve spontaneously. Duofilm application and cryotherapy are effective treatments.
- Plane warts on the face are treated by electrosurgery.
- Plantar warts are painful and when pared reveals dark punctate spots.
- Genital warts are transmitted sexually. Treated by podophyllin or cryotherapy.

Note: Liquid formulation containing salicylic and lactic acids is available.

Molluscum Contagiosum

It is a self-limiting epidermal viral infection caused by *Molluscum contagiosum* virus, a DNA poxvirus. Two types are identified—MCV-1 and 2. **MCV 1** is associated with most infections. **MCV 2** is associated with adult infections and human immunodeficiency virus (HIV). It mainly affects children or young adults. Spread is by contact, fomites or sexual route. Incubation period varies between 2 weeks and 6 months.

It presents as discrete, multiple, grouped, umbilicated, pearly, dome-shaped papules with a central punctum and if squeezed, releases a cheesy material (Fig. 220.4). Lesions are most common on the face, neck and trunk.

Diagnosis is usually by typical clinical features. It can be confirmed by incising one of the papules, smearing the contents between two slides and staining with Gram's stain. **Molluscum bodies** or **Henderson Patterson bodies**, which are cytoplasmic masses of virions, appear as ovoid,

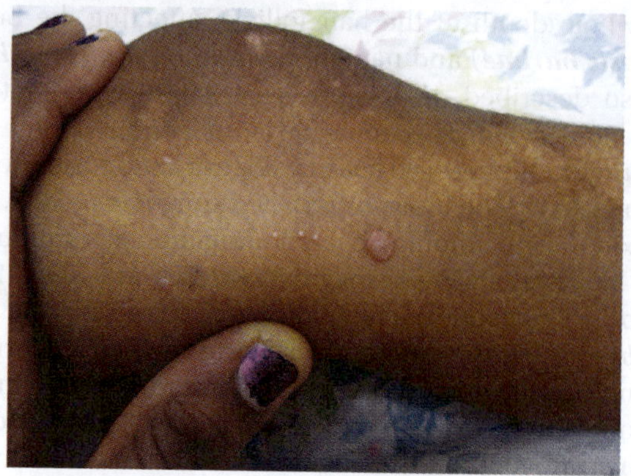

Fig. 220.4: Molluscum contagiosum on the left knee. **Note:** Central umbilication on the papule

homogenous inclusion bodies. The host cell is pushed to the periphery giving a signet ring appearance to the cell.

In healthy individuals, molluscum lesions persist for 6 months to 2 years and then undergo spontaneous regression. Such lesions undergoing spontaneous regression have an inflammatory erythematous halo. In HIV infected individuals, lesions persist and proliferate even after aggressive therapy. Lesions resolve with highly active anti-retroviral therapy (HAART). Painful aggressive therapy is not indicated. Lesions spread by autoinoculation and cause cosmetic disfigurement. *Treatment* includes curettage, phenol cautery, cryotherapy, salicylic and lactic acid combination (avoided on the face lesions) and electrodesiccation. In resistant cases, an antiviral agent, cidofovir is found to be effective, topically as 1–3% ointment and also intravenously (IV).

Herpes Simplex

See **also Section 6, Ch 53**

It is a primary or recurrent mucocutaneous disease caused by herpes simplex virus (HSV), a DNA virus that infects only humans. There are two serotypes—HSV 1 and HSV 2. *HSV 1* is the primary agent in orofacial herpes and *HSV 2* is involved in genital infections. Overlap does occur. Infection spreads by direct contact. After the primary mucocutaneous infection, the virus enters the sensory ganglia and remains dormant until reactivation. Precipitating factors for recurrence include ultraviolet (UV) radiation, menstruation, fever, common cold and altered immune states.

Clinical Features

Primary infections are preceded by a prodrome of local tenderness for a day or two. *Gingivostomatitis* is the most frequent manifestation and presents as vesicles, erosion and maceration over the entire buccal mucosa. There is marked erythema and edema of the gums. There is often severe pain and tender lymphadenopathy making it difficult to eat or drink. The lesions usually heal in 2 weeks. *Recurrent lesions (cold sores)* are usually preceded by a burning or tingling sensation for several hours. Multiple grouped vesicles on a normal or erythematous skin appear at the site of premonitory symptoms. The lesions heal within 7–10 days. The most common sites are the lips, perioral area, cheeks and nose, though it can occur anywhere. Intraoral lesions are extremely rare in recurrence, except in immunocompromised hosts.

Inoculation herpes occurs when secretions containing the virus come in contact with abraded skin anywhere on the body. In wrestlers, rugby and football players, transmission occurs during contact sports. This is known as *herpes gladiatorum*. Painful vesicles, erythema and edema associated with lymphadenopathy on the fingers and hands, called *herpetic whitlow* is commonly an occupational hazard in health care professionals especially dental personnel. This is uncommon after the universal precautions are followed.

Cutaneous HSV infection in immunodeficiency causes significant morbidity. Lesions may persist for months. Dissemination can lead to esophagitis, hepatitis and pneumonia. Pre-existing skin conditions such as atopic dermatitis predispose patients to develop widespread cutaneous disease called *eczema herpeticum* or *Kaposi's varicelliform eruption*. The infection spreads via the damaged skin surface and so complications from viremia are rare. It is associated with fever and lymphadenopathy. The eruption lasts for 2–6 weeks.

Neonatal HSV infection occurs when the mother has an acute primary genital herpes infection at the time of delivery. Infection may be limited to skin, eyes and mouth or disseminated. If untreated, neonates have a risk of visceral and CNS involvement and a mortality rate of over 50%.

Genital herpes in a pregnant woman at the time of delivery is an indication for cesarean section (CS), as neonatal infection can be fatal. Genital herpes is covered under the section sexually transmitted diseases (STDs).

Treatment

General measures: The area should be kept dry and clean. Secondary infection, if present should be treated.

Specific therapy: Acyclovir in a dose of 200 mg five times daily or 400 mg thrice daily for 10 days in primary infections and for 5 days in recurrent infections is the preferred drug. To prevent frequent attacks, prophylactic treatment with 400 mg twice daily for 4–6 months may be required. Except for transient renal dysfunction following rapid IV infusion, side effects are uncommon. Valacyclovir has greater bioavailability than acyclovir. Recommended doses are 1 g bid for 10 days for primary infection, 500 mg bid for 5 days for recurrent infection and 500 mg once daily for suppressive therapy. Famciclovir 250 mg tid for 5–7 days is an effective alternative. *Treatment* should be started as early as possible after the onset of symptoms. Early treatment shortens the duration and intensity of an episode.

Points to Remember

- Type 1 HSV infection has usually orofacial lesions—childhood onset.
- Type 2 HSV infection occurs in genitalia—adult onset.
- Characterized by recurrent grouped vesicles that leave superficial erosions at the same site.
- Acyclovir is effective.

Orf: This is primarily a disease of sheep. This virus can infect human beings by contamination. It manifests as painful purplish nodules on the exposed parts of the body like hands, arms, legs and face. It heals spontaneously in 4–6 weeks.

Milker's nodule: It is caused by pseudocowpox or parapox virus which normally infects cattle (papular lesions occur on the oral cavity and on teats of cows) and only accidentally cause infection in humans. The manifestation is similar to orf.

Cowpox: This is a zoonotic infection accidentally transferred to humans from cattle. Cowpox is caused by vaccinia virus *(cowpox virus).* In humans, lesions start as painful papules which evolve into vesicles and then to umbilicated pustules surrounded by erythema, finally developing into an eschar or ulcer. Fever and local lymphadenopathy are common. Multiple lesions occur on the face or hands, which resolve in 3–4 weeks.

Dermatophytosis

Dermatophytoses are caused by a group of filamentous fungi known as dermatophytes or ringworm fungi. There are three genera of dermatophytes—(1) trichophyton (T), (2) microsporum (M) and (3) epidermophyton (E). The dermatophytes are termed geophilic, zoophilic or anthropophilic depending upon whether their normal habitat is the soil, animal or man respectively.

Dermatophytosis is commonly classified depending upon the site of infection as tinea capitis (head), corporis (body), cruris (crural region), pedis (feet), manuum (hands), faciale (face), barbae (beard region) and tinea unguium (nails).

Tinea Capitis

It is dermatophyte infection of the scalp hair and skin. It is common in Asia, Africa and Southern and Eastern Europe. It is primarily a disease of the prepubertal children between 6 and 10 years of age and is more common in males. It spreads by direct contact from infected humans or animals such as dogs, cattle, horses, rodents and others. *Microsporum audouinii*, *Trichophyton tonsurans* and *Trichophyton violaceum* are commonly associated with tinea capitis. There are four distinct clinical types.

1. *Gray patch type:* This presents as circular scaly patches of alopecia. Hairs are broken off 2–3 mm above the scalp surface. The infected hairs show green fluorescence under Wood's light.
2. *Inflammatory type (kerion):* It presents as a painful inflammatory mass or a boggy swelling with crusting, oozing of pus and matting of adjacent hairs (Fig. 220.5). Hairs that remain are easily detachable. This is often caused by zoophilic species like *T. verrucosum* or *T. mentagrophytes*.
3. *Black dot type:* There are irregular scaly patches of alopecia with a black dot appearance due to the breaking of affected hairs at the scalp surface.
4. *Favus:* It is uncommon. Yellowish crusts (scutula) around follicular openings with a fetid odor are characteristic.

Treatment

The recommended treatment in children is oral griseofulvin in a dose of 10–15 mg/kg/day for 6–8 weeks. Treatment is to be continued till hair regrows. Alternative treatments include: (1) Terbinafine in a dose of 62.5 mg/day for children less than 20 kg, 125 mg/day for those of 20–40 kg and for those more than 40 kg, 250 mg/day is recommended for 4 weeks. (2) Itraconazole in a dose of 3–5 mg/kg for 4–6 weeks is also effective. Topical azole creams can be adjunctive to oral therapy, but not by themselves curative.

Prevention

- Avoid sharing of combs and brushes.
- Asymptomatic carriers should be traced and treated.
- Family contacts should be screened.
- Source of infection like pets should be identified and treated.

Tinea Corporis

It is the dermatophyte infection of the trunk, legs and arms. It presents as annular polycyclic lesions with erythematous raised vesicular and scaly border and a central clearing (Fig. 220.6). The frequent misuse of combination creams with steroids modifies this picture (tinea incognito). Lesions on the face are called *tinea faciale* (Fig. 220.7).

Tinea Barbae

It is the involvement of the beard hair. Clinical features are perifollicular pustules, papules, erythema, crusting and easy pluckability of hair.

Tinea Cruris

It is the involvement of crural regions like axillae and groins and inframammary, abdominal and intergluteal folds

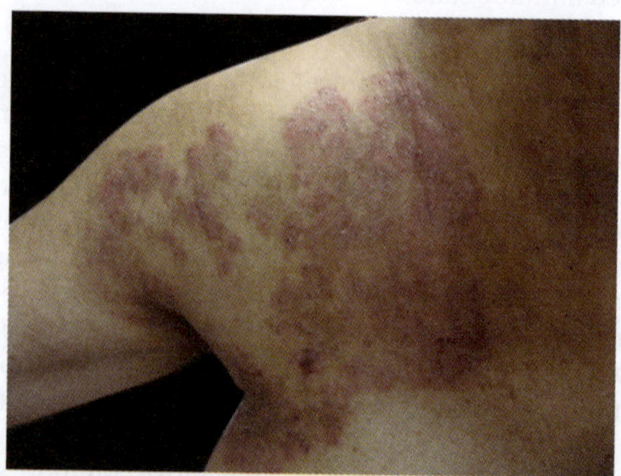

Fig. 220.6: Erythematous annular plaques of tinea corporis on the upper chest

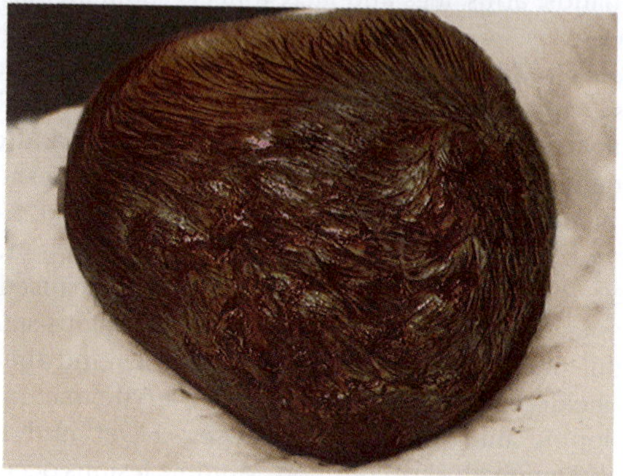

Fig. 220.5: Inflammatory tinea capitis. ***Note:*** Inflammation and crusting

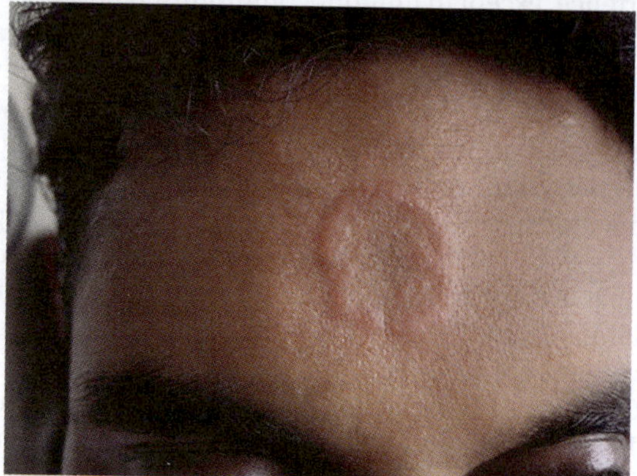

Fig. 220.7: Tinea faciale on the forehead

which are warm and moist. Lesions are usually bilateral but asymmetrical. Prevention is by keeping the area dry and avoiding occlusive and synthetic undergarments. Other sites of infection should be identified and treated.

Tinea Pedis

It presents as scaling, fissuring or maceration of the interdigital spaces of the feet, commonly the lateral two web spaces or as dry hyperkeratotic scaling of the soles and rarely as vesicular type involving the instep of soles. This is commonly acquired from communal bathing places and showers.

Prevention: Maintaining the feet dry, use of antifungal powders, cotton socks and avoidance of occlusive foot wear prevents recurrence.

Tinea Manuum

It is the dermatophyte infection of the palms. Diffuse hyperkeratosis of palms and fingers is the common type. Unilateral involvement with accentuation of creases is characteristic. It is commonly associated with tinea pedis.

Tinea Unguium

It is the dermatophyte infection of the nails commonly due to *T. rubrum* and *T. mentagrophytes*. The nails become discolored, thickened and friable. There is onycholysis (separation of nail plate from nail beds). Nail involvement usually starts from the distal end. Onychomycosis is a general term that includes infection of nails due to dermatophytes, nondermatophytes and yeasts. Onychomycosis accounts for more than 50% of nail diseases.

Laboratory Diagnosis of Superficial Fungal Infections

Direct microscopic examination of fungal scrapings provides immediate confirmation of fungal infection. Scrape the active edge of a lesion with a scalpel and collect the scales on a glass slide. Add a drop of 10% potassium hydroxide and cover with a cover slip and heat gently, but not to boiling. Examine under low power of microscope (x10 magnification) after the slide cools. Dermatophytes appear as long septate and branched hyphal filaments without constriction at the branching points. Fungal species can be identified by culture in Sabouraud's medium.

Treatment

Dermatophyte infection of the skin usually responds to topical: (1) Azoles like clotrimazole 1%, ketoconazole 2%, miconazole 2%, oxiconazole 1%, or terconazole cream, (2) allylamines like terbinafine 1% and butenafine 1%, (3) tolnaftate 1% or (4) ciclopirox olamine 0.77%. Topical creams should be used at least 3 cm beyond the advancing margin of the lesion, twice daily for 2–4 weeks. Treatment should be continued for at least 1 week after the lesions have cleared.

Oral treatment is indicated for extensive lesions and for failure of response to topical therapy. Tinea capitis, pedis and manuum requires oral treatment. The drug of choice is terbinafine 250 mg/day for 2 weeks and for scalp infection 4–6 weeks, for nail infection 3–4 months.

Itraconazole 200 mg/day for 2 weeks and griseofulvin 250 mg bd for 4–6 weeks are also effective.

Candidiasis

Superficial candidiasis is caused mostly by *Candida albicans*, though occasionally other species of candida may be responsible. This organism is found as a commensal on the skin, oral cavity and the gastrointestinal tract (GIT). Under favorable conditions of growth such as excessive moisture and maceration, immune deficiency, diabetes mellitus (DM) or treatment with tetracyclines or immunosuppressive drugs, this fungus multiplies and becomes invasive to cause disease. In its natural habitat, the organism is found in the spore or yeast form but when it invades the skin or the mucous membrane, it grows to form pseudomycelium and the filaments can be demonstrated microscopically in skin scrapings. The source of infection is usually from the individual's own endogenous reservoir. In some cases, person to person transmission can occur.

Candida affects the skin, mucous membranes of the mouth and genitalia, base of the nails and nail plates.

Oropharyngeal candidiasis can be classified into pseudomembranous (thrush), erythematous (atrophic) and hyperplastic.

Thrush is an acute infection and can be recurrent in immunocompromised patients. It is also seen in neonates and among terminally ill-patients. It is characterized by white plaques often painless, on the surfaces of the buccal mucosa, tongue, hard and soft palate and tonsils (Fig. 220.8). The white pseudomembrane can be dislodged to reveal an eroded erythematous base. Involvement of the throat causes severe dysphagia. It is the most common form of candidiasis in patients with acquired immunodeficiency syndrome (AIDS). In human immunodeficiency virus (HIV) infected individuals, the lesions are persistent and often spread to all parts of the mouth.

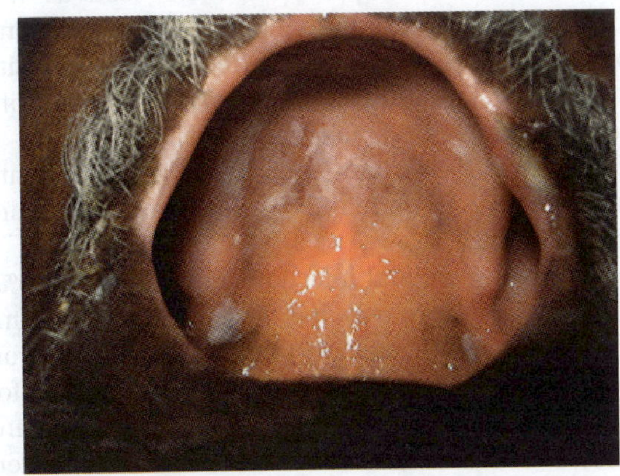

Fig. 220.8: *Oral thrush*. White plaques on the hard palate

Erythematous (atrophic): This type is often associated with broad spectrum antibiotic treatment, chronic corticosteroid use and HIV infection. It manifests as a flat red lesion, usually on the palate or dorsum of the tongue. The dorsum of the tongue is depapillated, shiny and smooth with restriction of tongue movement. The mouth is often tender.

Hyperplastic type (candida leukoplakia): This condition is important because 15–20% can undergo malignant transformation. It presents as dense opaque plaques, usually asymptomatic, on the inner side of the cheeks or less commonly on the tongue. It is often associated with smoking or local trauma. The lesions cannot be removed from surface in contrast to the pseudomembranous type.

Chronic atrophic candidiasis (denture stomatitis) occurs in up to 60% of denture wearers. The characteristic presenting signs are chronic mucosal erythema and edema of the portion of the hard palate that comes in contact with the denture. It is often associated with angular chelitis.

Angular chelitis (perleche) is most common in patients with moist, deep folds at the corners of the mouth. It has been reported in up to 20% of HIV infected persons. It presents as soreness, erythema and fissuring at the corners of the mouth.

Vulvovaginal candidiasis: The condition is often abrupt in onset, with intense pruritus and burning of the vulva and vagina with or without vaginal discharge. Vulval erythema and fissuring can spread to labia majora (Fig. 220.9). Perineal intertrigo with vesicopustular lesions may be present. The discharge is often thick and curdy, but may be thin or even purulent. Dyspareunia and dysuria are common.

Balanoposthitis: In men, genital candidiasis presents as soreness, edema, fissuring, papules and diffuse erythema of the glans penis and prepuce. Patients should be investigated for DM.

Cutaneous candidiasis: The lesions tend to occur in the folds of the skin, such as the groins and the intergluteal folds, where the environment is warm and moist due to maceration and occlusion. Interdigital spaces can be involved. Predisposing factors include overweight and DM.

It presents as erythematous lesions with papules or vesicopustules and an irregular margin. The main lesion is surrounded by numerous small pustules called ***satellite lesions***. Severe itching and burning sensation are common. Lesions on the interdigital spaces are seen as white fissures with surrounding erythema and maceration. It is common in individuals whose occupation necessitate frequent immersion of hands in water. This is often associated with paronychia of the same hand.

Diaper dermatitis in infants and chronically ill-patients is primarily an irritant dermatitis with superadded candidal infection (Fig. 220.10).

Nail infection: Candidal infection accounts for 5–10% of all cases of onychomycosis. It is more common in women than men and in finger nails than in toe nails. Chronic paronychia usually begins in the proximal nail fold. Periungual skin is erythematous edematous and painful with absence of cuticle. Nails become discolored. Bacterial superinfection is common.

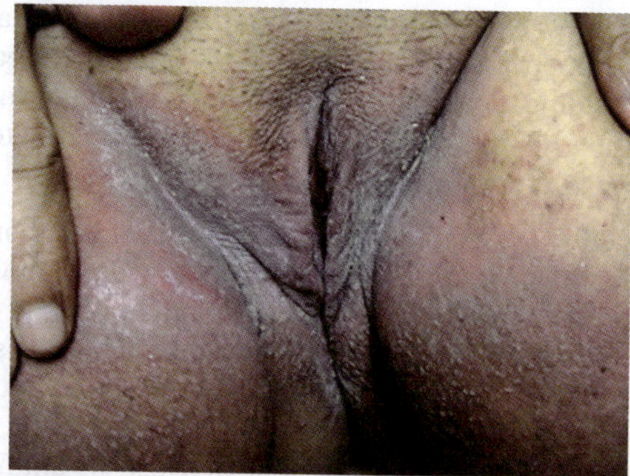

Fig. 220.9: Vulvovaginal candidiasis—whitish sodden appearance with erythema and fissuring

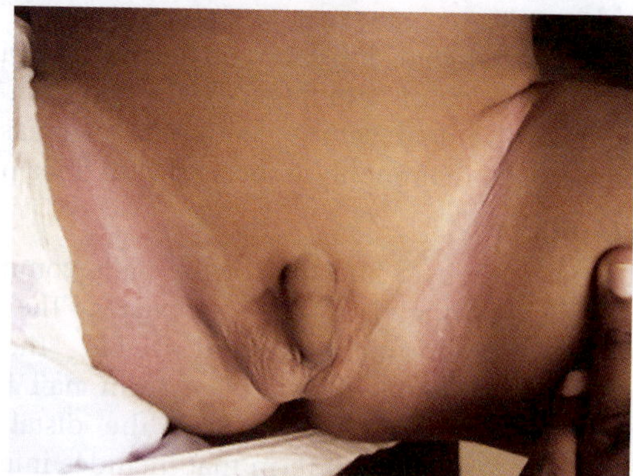

Fig. 220.10: Diaper dermatitis

Diagnosis: It is confirmed by the microscopic demonstration in 10% potassium hydroxide mount, of oval thin-walled yeasts that bud on a narrow base and filaments which are either true hyphae or pseudohyphae.

Treatment: Oral candidiasis is treated with nystatin oral suspension 100,000 units/mL at 4–6 hours interval or clotrimazole mouth paints. The medication should be retained in the mouth for as long as possible. In HIV infected persons and other immunocompromised individuals, systemic drugs are preferred. Oral fluconazole 200 mg first dose, followed by 100 mg/day for 7–14 days is more effective than itraconazole or ketoconazole 200–400 mg/day for 14 days.

Vaginal candidiasis: Imidazole compounds like clotrimazole, miconazole or terconazole cream topically twice daily for 2–3 weeks and intravaginal clotrimazole pessaries daily for 6 nights are effective in vaginal candidiasis. Oral fluconazole 150 mg as a single dose or itraconazole 200 mg bid for 1 day is as effective as topical therapy. In recurrent candidiasis, ensure that the patient avoids the potential precipitating factors. The partner should also be treated. Oral fluconazole 150 mg/week for 3–6 months is also effective. Penile and cutaneous candidiasis responds to topical imidazole creams like clotrimazole or ketoconazole, applied twice daily for 2–3 weeks.

Candidal paronychia responds to antifungal cream or lotion applied twice daily for 6 months. Nail damage should be managed with oral drugs. Itraconazole 200–400 mg/day for 6 weeks or pulse therapy (3 pulses of 200 mg bd/day for 1 week/month) is the treatment of choice.

Terbinafine is less effective in candidal infections. Amorolfine nail lacquer applied once or twice weekly for 3–6 months is also useful.

PITYRIASIS VERSICOLOR

Syn: Tinea versicolor

It is a common, mild but often recurrent infection of the stratum corneum due to lipophilic yeasts of the genus *Malassezia*. These organisms can cause serious systemic infection in immunocompromised and debilitated individuals. *Malassezia* species form part of the normal microbial flora of the human skin where it exists in the yeast form. Most infections are endogenous in origin, but human-to-human transmission is possible. Pityriasis versicolor, pityrosporum folliculitis and seborrheic dermatitis are associated with *Malassezia* species. It is most prevalent in hot, humid tropical climates, where 30–40% of the adult population may be affected.

Clinical Features

It presents as hypopigmented or fine brown well-defined scaly patches, particularly on the face, trunk, neck and upper arms. The lesions become confluent and have a polycyclic border. Different shades of lesions can be present in the same patient and so named as *versicolor* (Fig. 220.11). It is usually asymptomatic but some patients may have itching, especially on sweating. Pityrosporum folliculitis is characterized by multiple itchy papules and pustules on the shoulders and back.

Diagnosis

Scrapings for direct microscopic examination in 10% potassium hydroxide shows a mixture of spherical thick-walled yeast cells and a coarse mycelium fragmented to short filaments, having a classical **spaghetti and meat**

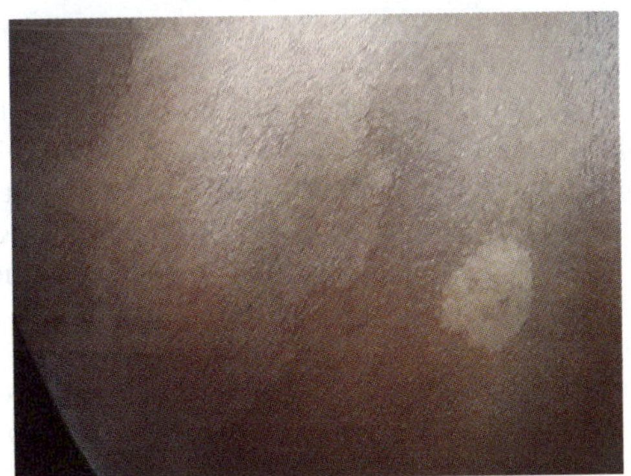

Fig. 220.11: Pityriasis versicolor on the trunk. **Note:** The classical wrinkled appearance

balls appearance. Their isolation in culture does not contribute to diagnosis because they form a part of normal cutaneous flora. The hyphae are diagnostic and demonstrated only in its pathogenic phase.

Differential diagnosis: Pityriasis versicolor is at times difficult to differentiate from **pityriasis alba**. The borders are ill-defined, lesions are mostly on the face and the initial lesions may be erythematous in **pityriasis alba**. In pityriasis versicolor, the borders are usually distinct, the surface is wrinkled and scaly and the lesions may involve the chest and back.

Treatment

Selenium sulfide shampoo or ketoconazole shampoo applied to the affected areas for 10–15 minutes before bath for 1–2 weeks is effective. Topical imidazole creams such as clotrimazole, oxiconazole, miconazole and ketoconazole applied twice daily for 2–3 weeks are effective. Topical terbinafine and butenafine are also useful. Oral terbinafine and griseofulvin are not effective in tinea versicolor. Oral therapy is reserved for patients with extensive lesions or recalcitrant infection unresponsive to topical therapy. Itraconazole and ketoconazole in doses of 200 mg/day for 1 week and fluconazole 400 mg, two doses, 2 weeks apart are effective. It is very important to explain to the patient that the hypopigmentation may take a long time to clear and it is not necessary to continue the treatment till hypopigmentation clears.

CHAPTER
221

Skin Infestations

Usha Vaidhyanathan

SCABIES

It is an intensely pruritic disease of the skin caused by the ectoparasitic mite *Sarcoptes scabiei var hominis*. The adult female mite measures approximately 0.4 mm long and 0.3 mm broad. Around 40–50 eggs are laid by each female mite. The average life span is 4–6 weeks. The mite can survive for only 24–36 hours in the environment at room temperature, away from the host. Transmission to a new host is by contact and through infested clothes and linen.

Pathogenesis: Infection of a new host is initiated by the pregnant female mite that burrows into the superficial layers of the skin to lay eggs. The pruritic lesions develop about four weeks after the initial infection. Immediate and delayed hypersensitivity reactions play a role in the development of symptoms and skin lesions.

Clinical features: Scabies is most common in children and young adults. Overcrowding, poor hygiene and poverty predisposes to scabies. The patient presents with pruritus that is worse at night, but in warm humid conditions it may occur throughout the day. Itching in the early states is confined to the sites of lesion, but it becomes generalized later on. The pathognomonic lesion is the burrow which is a curvilinear track made by the mite. Papules, pustules, vesicles and excoriations are seen in the webs of the fingers (Fig. 221.1), flexor aspects of the wrist (Fig. 221.2), extensor aspects of the elbow, anterior axillary fold, nipple and areola in the female, umbilicus and periumbilical regions, genitalia, upper thighs, knees and ankles. Burrows and inflammatory papules are characteristically seen on male genitalia, which should always be examined. The lower part of the gluteal region is affected, but rest of the back is spared. In general the scalp, face, palms and soles are spared. In children, these areas can also be affected.

The lesions soon get secondarily infected with nephritogenic strains of group A streptococci and ***Staphylococcus aureus*** and infection converts them into pustules. In some cases, the lesions are crusted and scaly. This type is called ***crusted scabies*** or ***Norwegian scabies***. In this type, in addition to classical areas of involvement, the scalp, face, ear lobes and back may also be affected. Millions of organisms are present in these cases and it usually occurs in people with poor nutrition or immunosuppression.

When scabies affects infants and children, it tends to involve the scalp, palms and soles as well. Vesiculation, secondary pyoderma and eczematization are common. Whenever an infant presents with a suggestive lesion, examination of the mother is mandatory. The diagnosis of infantile scabies may be strengthened by the presence of lesions in the mother as well.

Persistent itchy nodular lesions (nodular scabies) on male genitalia, especially scrotum (Fig. 221.3) can be very troublesome.

Complications: Complications occur frequently. These include pyoderma, eczematization and development of acute glomerulonephritis. One-third of the cases of acute glomerulonephritis (AGN) in India, Africa and many other tropical countries are attributable to infected scabies.

Diagnosis: It is based on the classical clinical features like characteristic distribution, nocturnal aggravation of itching and a positive family history of similar disease. Diagnosis is confirmed by demonstration of mite or its products, larva, egg or fecal matter (scybala). Scrapings are obtained from the burrows and examined under low power of the microscope under a drop of mineral oil or 10% potassium hydroxide solution. Wait for a few minutes

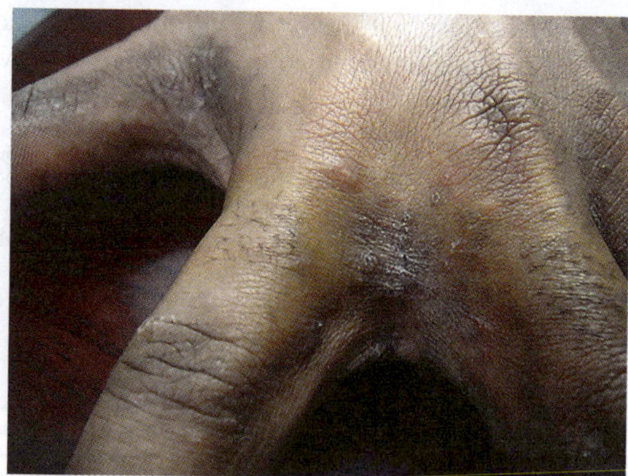

Fig. 221.1: Classic scabies on the interdigital space

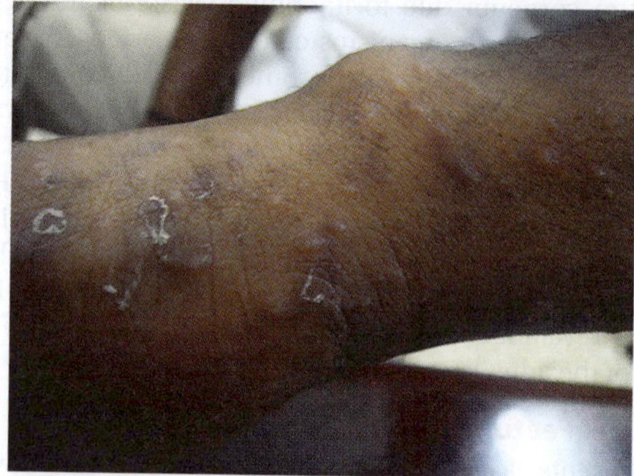

Fig. 221.2: Scabies papules and burrows on the wrist

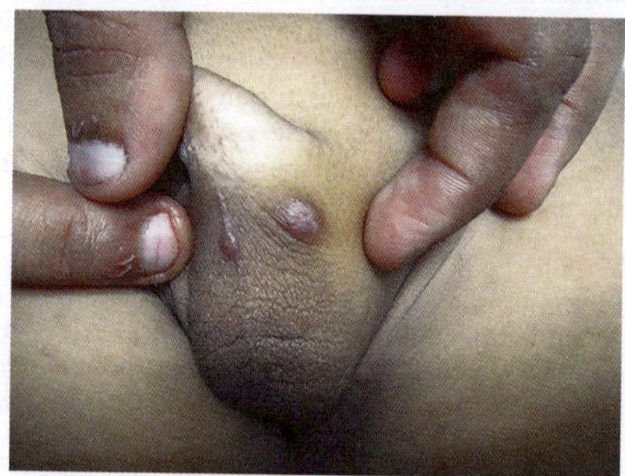

Fig. 221.3: Nodular scabies on the scrotum

for the keratinous material to be cleared and the mite and its products will be clearly visible.

Treatment

General measures: It is mandatory to treat all family members and close contacts simultaneously. All clothes and bed linen are disinfected by laundering or hot ironing. Secondary infection should be treated with antibiotics before the initiation of topical antiscabietic treatment. Erythromycin 500 mg qid for 5 days or cephalexin 500 mg qid for 5 days or amoxicillin plus cloxacillin 250 mg each tid for 5 days are effective.

Specific treatment: Permethrin 5% cream is the drug of choice. Gamma benzene hexachloride 1% (GBHC) is also effective. Permethrin and GBHC are to be applied overnight over the entire body below the neck. In infants and pregnant women, permethrin is safe. Benzyl benzoate 25% applied all over the body after a scrub bath, three applications 12 hour apart is an effective and freely available alternative. Ivermectin, a macrocyclic lactone, is a safe oral drug available for the treatment of scabies. 200 µg/kg bw as a single dose on empty stomach is recommended in crusted scabies and in immunocompromised hosts in addition to topical therapy. A second dose 7–10 days later gives better results. It is also effective in classical scabies. It is available as 3 and 6 mg tablets.

Nodules on the genitalia or other sites cause persistent itching for prolonged periods. Crotamiton with hydrocortisone cream applied twice daily for 2 weeks will relieve the itch. Crusted scabies is treated with 2 doses of ivermectin and multiple applications of topical scabicides is 200 µg/kg oral (dose of ivermectin adult dose 12 µg).

Points to Remember
- Scabies is spread by direct contact.
- Intensely itchy papules in the classical sites—interdigital spaces of fingers, genitalia.
- Severe crusted lesions occur in immunosuppression.
- Common predisposing factor for glomerulonephritis in India.
- Mites and its products can be demonstrated by microscopy on scraping the burrows.
- Overnight application of permethrin is the treatment of choice.

PEDICULOSIS

Pediculosis or louse infestation is a worldwide problem. Poor living conditions and poor personal hygiene contribute to infestation. There are two species of blood sucking lice—*Pediculus humanus capitis* and corporis (head and body louse respectively) and *Phthirus pubis* (crab louse).

Pediculosis Capitis (Head Louse Infestation)

Adult head lice are 1–3 mm long, flattened dorsoventrally, have three pairs of legs that end in powerful claws. The female louse lives for about one month and lays up to 300 eggs (nits) during her lifetime. Eggs hatch in 6–10 days. Empty egg cases remain on hair shaft. Head louse is not a vector of infectious disease. The louse is transmitted through direct contact or through fomites. It commonly affects young girls with long hair.

Itching is the main symptom. As the lice feed, they inject their digestive juices and fecal material into the skin and this causes severe pruritus. Secondary infection and occipital lymphadenopathy are common. Crawling lice or nits that are firmly attached to the hair can be seen with naked eyes.

Treatment

Permethrin 1% is applied for 10–15 minutes and then washed off. One percent GBHC applied for 5 minutes and malathion 0.5% applied for 8–12 hours are also effective pediculicides. Most of the pediculicides are not effective ovicides. A second application 7–10 days later is more effective. After treatment, the hair is wet-combed with a fine-toothed comb to remove nits.

Pediculosis Corporis

Body lice are present on the clothes of a person and causes severe itching, excoriations and crusting when they come in contact with the body for a blood meal. Body louse transmits many infectious agents while feeding and spread diseases like epidemic typhus, louse borne relapsing fever and trench fever. *Treatment* includes maintaining good personal hygiene, application of insecticides to clothing and permethrin or GBHC to body hair.

Pediculosis Pubis

Crab louse spreads commonly by sexual contact. It is mainly seen attached to the pubic hair, but may spread to axillary hair, eyebrows and eyelashes. Patients will have severe itching and blue grey macules *(maculae cerulae)* on the lower abdomen and thighs. Secondary infection and regional lymphadenopathy are common. Oral Ivermectin 200 µg/kg bw, 2 doses, 7–10 days apart is effective for all types of pediculosis.

Points to Remember
- Head lice infestation is transmitted by direct contact especially between school children.
- Secondary infection is common.
- Body lice transmits diseases like epidemic typus, trench fever and relapsing fever.
- Body lice are present on the clothes of the infected persons.
- Crab lice spread by sexual contact and are seen attached to the pubic hair.
- Topical permethrin 1% and oral ivermectin are effective.

CHAPTER
222

Acne and Rosacea

Usha Vaidhyanathan

Chapter Summary
- Acne Vulgaris
  - Variants of Acne
- Rosacea

ACNE VULGARIS

Acne vulgaris, a chronic inflammation of the pilosebaceous units, is an extremely common disorder with peak prevalence during adolescence. Acne begins early in females, but is more severe in males. Acne usually persists until early 20s, although in a few patients, it may even continue into the fifth decade.

Etiopathogenesis

Acne is multifactorial in origin. Major pathogenic factors include:

- Defective keratinization of the follicular infundibulum above the opening of the sebaceous duct initiates acne. Keratinocytes multiply and show enhanced cohesiveness thereby obstructing follicular channels. Cellular debris and sebum collect behind and forms a solid mass known as *comedo*.
- There is increased sebum production, which is primarily controlled by androgenic hormones. In some patients, elevated androgen levels have been documented. In others with normal androgen levels, the affected skin has increased sensitivity to androgenic stimulation.
- Inflammation due to the proliferation of *Propionibacterium acnes* within the follicles.

Clinical Features

The pathognomonic lesion is the comedo. Comedones are small papules that are either open with a dilated follicular ostium with black plugs of keratin (black head) or closed (white head). The comedones develop into inflammatory papules or pustules (Fig. 222.1) and sometimes nodules or cysts. Face is the most common site of involvement, but back, shoulders and upper chest may also be involved. Lesions may leave behind postinflammatory hyperpigmentation and scars. Severely inflamed lesions heal with small but deeper scars known as *ice-pick scars*.

Variants of Acne

- ***Acne excoriée:*** It is seen in depressed or obsessional young women who often squeeze the lesion. Picking and scratching the lesions lead to exacerbation of lesions.
- ***Infantile acne:*** It is seen on the face of some infants, mostly males and disappears spontaneously.
- Drugs like systemic/topical steroids and androgens induce acne.
- ***Acne conglobata:*** It presents as severe acne with abscesses, burrowing sinuses and scarring.

- ***Occupational acne:*** Exposure to cutting oils and lubricating oils causes acne due to occlusion at the site of contact. Oily cosmetics can also cause acne.

Management

General measures: Gentle washing of the face with soap and water without vigorous scrubbing is recommended. Cosmetics should be noncomedogenic. Diet has no effect on acne.

Specific therapy: In the early stages with comedones and papules, a topical retinoid such as tretinoin 0.025%–0.1%, adapalene 0.1% or tazarotene 2.5% at night and benzoyl peroxide 5% in the morning would suffice. Topical retinoids cause dryness, scaling, redness and an initial flare of acne. Benzoyl peroxide (BPO) may produce a mild burning sensation for a short period of time. Topical retinoid and BPO should not be mixed. It may take a few weeks for the response to begin. The patients should be adequately warned about these problems. Otherwise, the patient may discontinue treatment due to irritation and lack of response. Recently, techniques have evolved to mix adapalene and BPO without causing irritation and improving patient compliance. BPO and clindamycin combinations are also available. Avoidance of sun exposure and use of sun block lotions diminish the side effects.

In the pustular stage, a topical antibiotic like clindamycin or erythromycin should be added. If no response, systemic antibiotics like tetracycline, doxycycline and minocycline for 2–3 months are very effective. Erythromycin is also useful. Long-term treatment for at least 3 months is required. In severe recalcitrant cases, oral retinoids (isotretinoin) and hormonal therapy may be needed.

Management of Complications

Pigmentation and scarring can have profound psychological effects. Postacne pigmentation can be reduced to some extent by chemical peeling, e.g. 20–70% glycolic acid peels (Fig. 222.2). In Indian patients, lower concentrations are preferred due to postinflammatory hyperpigmentation. Multiple sittings are needed.

Superficial scars (Fig. 222.3) improve with multiple sittings of microdermabrasion. Erythema and edema may develop immediately after dermabrasion. Aluminum oxide crystals are used to abrade the skin superficially. Many other cosmetic procedures like intralesional injection of triamcinolone into the cysts, subcision, punch

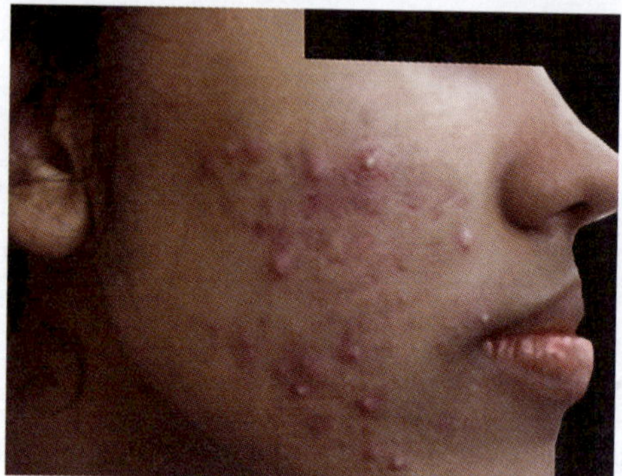

Fig. 222.1: Acne vulgaris showing inflammatory papules and pustules

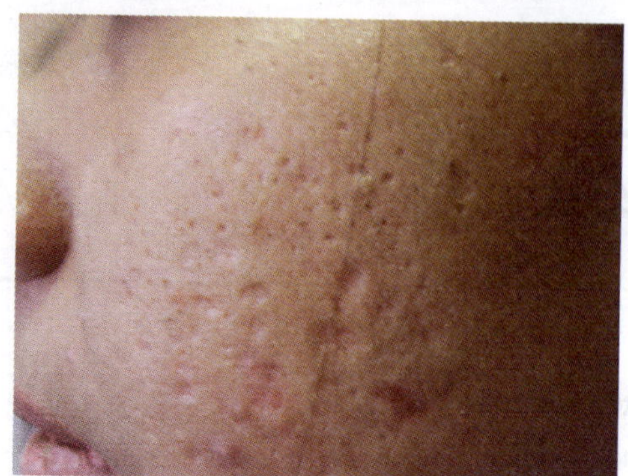

Fig. 222.2: Postacne scars

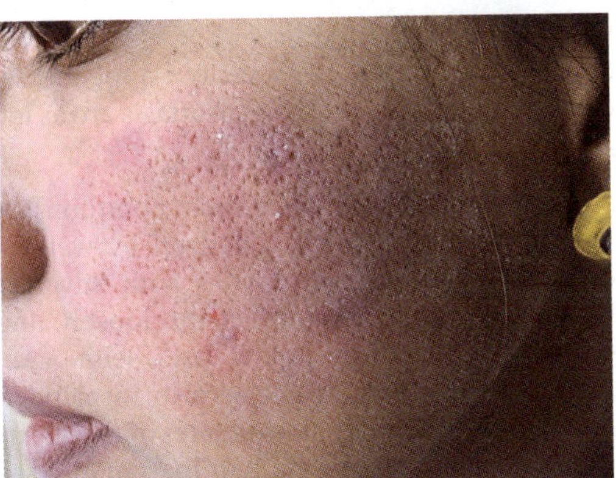

Fig. 222.3: Superficial scars improved after six sittings of microdermabrasion

elevation and grafting and laser surgery are also useful. Laser resurfacing using carbon dioxide or erbium YAG lasers give very good cosmetic results.

Points to Remember

- Peak prevalence in adolescence.
- Abnormal keratinization of the follicular epithelium, increased sebum production and proliferation of *Propionibacterium acnes* are the main causes.
- Characterized by comedones, erythematous papules, pustules, cysts and nodules on the face, chest and back.
- Topical benzoyl peroxide, tretinoin, clindamycin and oral tetracycline, minocycline or erythromycin are used to control the lesions.
- Severe cases need oral antiandrogens or isotretinoin.

ROSACEA

It is a chronic inflammatory facial dermatosis characterized by erythema and pustules. The cause is unknown. There is an abnormal vascular reactivity. Rosacea commonly affects fair-skinned middle-aged females. The earliest symptoms are the intermittent episodes of flushing that resolve with increasingly permanent erythema and telangiectasia. Papules, pustules and occasionally lymphedema involve the cheeks, nose, forehead and chin. Sunlight and topical steroids exacerbate the condition.

Rosacea is different from acne by the absence of comedones, occurrence in middle-age group, presence of flushing and telangiectasia. Other differential diagnoses include seborrheic dermatitis, lupus erythematosus and photosensitive dermatoses.

Complications include rhinophyma (hyperplasia of the sebaceous gland and connective tissue of the nose and ocular rosacea (blepharitis, conjunctivitis).

Treatment: Irritants like strong soaps and alcohol-based cleansers should be avoided. Oral tetracycline 250 mg bid, erythromycin 250 mg bid, doxycycline 100 mg daily (effective in even low doses), oral metronidazole, azithromycin pulse dose of 250 mg/day for 3 days in a week, alternate days, are all effective. Topical metronidazole 1%, clindamycin 1%, BPO 5% are all effective. Topical tacrolimus and pimecrolimus have also been tried. Treatment should be continued for a minimum of 3 months and may need to be continued for longer periods. Sun protection with sunscreens helps to allay the condition.

CHAPTER 223

Papulosquamous Disorders

Usha Vaidhyanathan

Chapter Summary

- Psoriasis
- Lichen Planus
- Pityriasis Rosea
- Reiter's Syndrome
- Exfoliative Dermatitis

PSORIASIS

It is a chronic recurrent, papulosquamous disorder of the skin. It affects 2% of the world population. The sex incidence is equal. The disease can start at any age but the peak onset is in the second or third decades.

Etiopathogenesis

Genetics

Psoriasis is a multifactorial genetic disease that requires both polygenic and environmental factors for its clinical expression. About 35% of patients have a family history. There are strong correlations with the human leukocyte antigen (HLA) Cw6 and B57.

Immunopathogenesis

Psoriasis has a T cell-mediated immunopathogenesis. There is an interaction between environmental, genetic and immunologic factors. Antigens may be environmental antigens, super antigens or autoantigens. These antigens are taken up by the antigen presenting cells (APCs) in the skin. These APCs migrate from the skin to the lymph nodes, where they encounter naïve T cells. These T cells become activated through a series of interactions with APCs. Once activated, T cells migrate back to the skin where they secrete proinflammatory cytokines such as interleukin-2 (IL-2) and interferon-gamma (IFN-γ). This induces further production of cytokines including tumor necrosis factor-alpha (TNF-α). These cytokines induce epidermal and vascular changes that lead to psoriatic plaques. TNF-α is involved in many important cellular functions such as proliferation, activation, migration and apoptosis. The actions of TNF-α initiate and maintain the inflammatory process.

Pathophysiology

Psoriasis is characterized by erythematous scaly plaques. The characteristic pathophysiological events that occur in lesional skin are:

- **Epidermal proliferation:** There is an increase in the number of proliferating keratinocytes in the basal layer of the epidermis and there is loss of differentiation. This causes the thick silvery scale. The growth rate of psoriatic epidermis is up to 10 times that of normal epidermis.
- **Expansion of the dermal vasculature:** The blood vessels in the upper dermis become dilated and hyper-permeable and increased in number. This accounts for erythema of lesions.
- Accumulation of inflammatory cells like neutrophils and T lymphocytes in the dermis and epidermis.

The lymphocytes play a key role in the disease process and epidermal changes are secondary and a consequence of the release of mediators from infiltrating lymphocytes.

Points to Remember
- Affects 2% of the population
- Peak onset in the second or third decades
- Polygenic inheritance. Thirty five percent have a family history of psoriasis
- Epidermal cell proliferation rate is increased
- Mainly T cell-mediated immunopathogenesis.

Precipitating Factors

- Physical trauma to the skin can precipitate psoriasis in the damaged skin. This is known as **Koebner phenomenon**. Rubbing and scratching stimulate the proliferative process.
- **Infection:** Streptococcal infection precipitates guttate psoriasis.
- **Drugs:** Beta-blockers, lithium, antimalarials and withdrawal of systemic steroids aggravate psoriasis.
- Exposure to sunlight can aggravate psoriasis in about 10% of patients, although in the majority, it has a beneficial effect.
- Psychological stress can exacerbate psoriasis.

Pathology

The characteristic histologic picture of a fully developed skin lesion shows:

- Regular elongation of rete ridges with thickening in their lower portion
- Papillae are edematous with dilated capillaries
- Suprapapillary thinning of stratum malpighii with the occasional spongiform pustule
- Absence of stratum granulosum
- Parakeratosis (nucleated stratum corneum cells)
- Collection of neutrophils (**Munro microabscess**) in the parakeratotic mounds
- Systemic involvement includes inflammation of joint structures leading to psoriatic arthropathy.

Clinical Features

Psoriasis widely varies in severity, appearance and behavior. Presentation patterns of psoriasis are as follows:

Psoriasis Vulgaris

Psoriasis vulgaris ('vulgaris' means common) is the most common type. It is characterized by well-defined erythematous papules and plaques with silvery white scales (Fig. 223.1). On removal of the loosely attached scales, minute bleeding points are seen (**Auspitz' sign**). Papules and plaques coalesce to form polycyclic (Fig. 223.2) or serpiginous patterns. Sites of predilection of lesions are elbows, knees, scalp hair margin and sacrum. Lesions are bilateral and often symmetrical. Differential diagnosis includes seborrheic dermatitis, hypertrophic lichen planus, psoriasiform drug eruption (beta-blockers, gold and methyldopa), tinea corporis, secondary syphilis, lichen simplex chronicus and mycosis fungoides.

Guttate Psoriasis (latin-gutta, 'drop')

Guttate psoriasis is an acute symmetrical eruption of a shower of small papular lesions usually on the trunk (Fig. 223.3). Adolescents or young adults are commonly affected. It often follows a streptococcal sore throat. It should be differentiated from pityriasis rosea, which has a classical morphology of oval papules with peripheral scaling and central wrinkling. The prognosis is good with spontaneous resolution but may evolve into chronic plaque psoriasis.

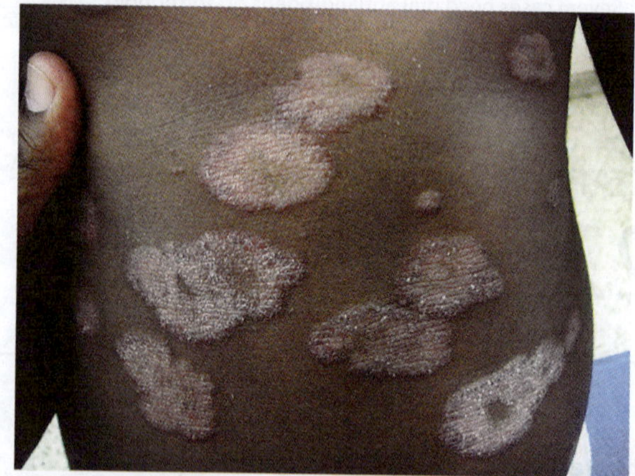

Fig. 223.1: Psoriasis vulgaris

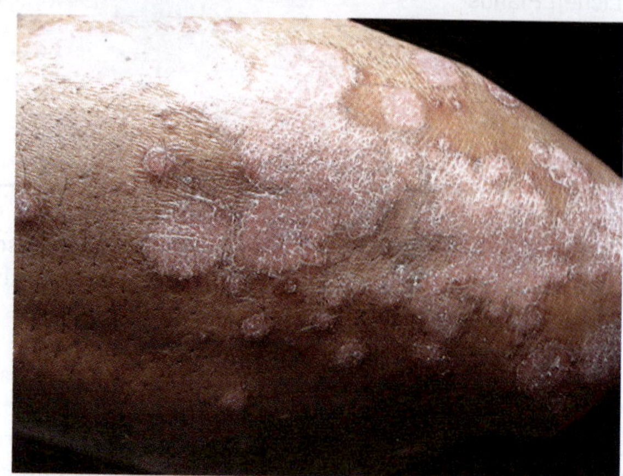

Fig. 223.2: Multiple psoriatic lesions coalesced together

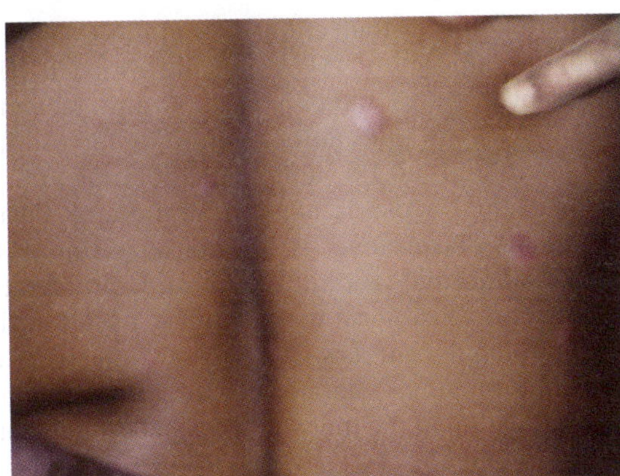

Fig. 223.3: Guttate psoriasis—drop like lesions

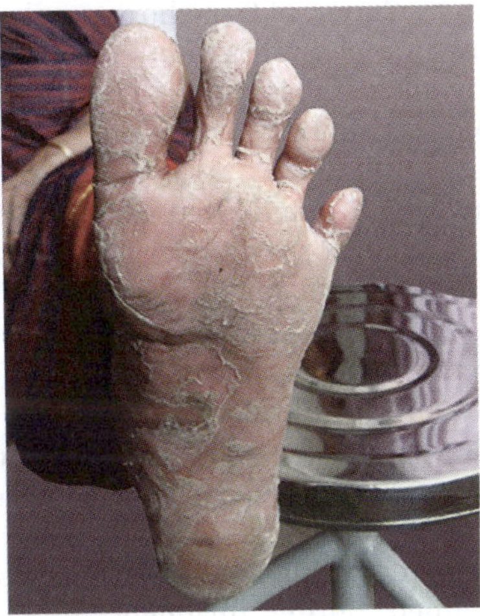

Fig. 223.4: Plantar psoriasis

Flexural Psoriasis

It affects the axillae, groins, submammary areas and natal cleft. Due to the moist and warm environment in these regions, psoriatic plaques are usually not scaly, but erythematous and fissured. It is commonly seen in the elderly. The sharp demarcation permits distinction from intertrigo, candidiasis, contact dermatitis, seborrheic dermatitis and tinea cruris.

Localized Forms

Palmoplantar psoriasis: Palms and soles may be the only areas involved. There is hyperkeratosis and scaling which is not easily removed. There may be painful fissures and bleeding (Fig. 223.4).

Scalp psoriasis: It is characterized by sharply marginated pruritic plaques especially at the occiput with thick adherent scales. Lesions may be discrete or the entire scalp is involved. There is no hair loss. Scalp may be the only site involved or may be a part of generalized psoriasis. Scalp psoriasis has to be differentiated from seborrheic dermatitis. Seborrheic dermatitis is diffuse in distribution, whereas psoriatic lesions are patchy and have well-defined edges. Silvery scales, if present are typical of psoriasis.

Psoriasis of the nails: Psoriasis affects the matrix or nail bed in up to 50% of cases. Thimble pitting is the most common change, followed by onycholysis (separation of nail plate from the nail bed). Discoloration of the nail bed resembling an oil drop (***oil drop sign***) is seen adjacent to onycholysis. Subungual hyperkeratosis affects mainly the toe nails. Nail changes are frequently associated with psoriatic arthropathy. ***Treatment*** is often difficult, but the condition responds to oral methotrexate.

Pustular Psoriasis

It is characterized by sterile pustules, not papules, arising on a normal or inflamed skin. It is classified into two types.

1. Localized pustular psoriasis
   - Chronic palmoplantar
   - Acrodermatitis continua
2. Generalized pustular psoriasis (GPP)
   - Acute GPP of von Zumbusch
   - GPP of pregnancy.

Chronic palmoplantar pustular psoriasis: It is most common in females in the fifth or sixth decades. It presents as symmetrical well-defined erythematous plaques studded with pustules. The lesions cause a burning sensation and itching is variable. The thenar eminence of palm, instep, heel and borders of the feet are the common sites involved. Digital lesions are uncommon. It has a prolonged course and is refractory to treatment.

Acrodermatitis continua of Hallopeau: It is a chronic sterile, pustular form of psoriasis affecting the tips of fingers or toes which tends to extend proximally. There is erythema, scaling and pustules. When the pustules dry up, they leave behind glazed, red and painful digits. The nails become dystrophic. It is common in children. It often evolves into GPP in elderly patients.

Acute GPP of von Zumbusch: It is a serious life-threatening form of psoriasis. It may develop from a pre-existing typical psoriasis, often after provocation by steroid withdrawal or other factors. It can begin later in life as an atypical acral or flexural psoriasis and rapidly progress to GPP. The eruption may begin with a sensation of burning with a dry tender skin and an abrupt onset of high fever and severe malaise. Generalized sheets of erythema and pustulation occur in crops and dries up into exfoliation. The configuration of lesions can be annular, circinate, plaques of erythema with pustular collarettes, isolated pustules, lakes of pus or erythroderma. Nails are dystrophic. Buccal mucosa and tongue may be involved (geographic tongue). ***Complications*** include hypoalbuminemia, hypocalcemia, renal and liver damage and deep vein thrombosis (DVT).

Generalized pustular psoriasis of pregnancy (impetigo herpetiformis): It is very rare and usually begins in the third trimester of pregnancy (Fig. 223.5). ***Clinical features*** are similar to von Zumbusch type of GPP. Constitutional

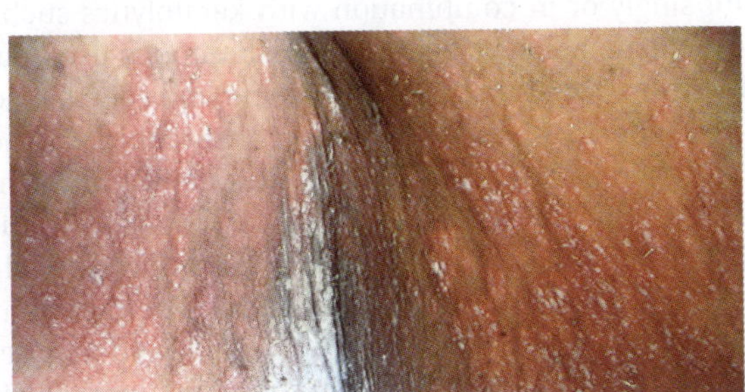

Fig. 223.5: Generalized pustular psoriasis—pustules on an erythematous base on the chest and right arm

symptoms are severe and may be fatal. Severe and long-standing disease may cause placental insufficiency leading to still birth, neonatal death or fetal abnormalities. Fulminating disease is best treated with prednisolone. Methotrexate, retinoids or photochemotherapy (PUVA) may be needed after delivery to wean off the steroid.

Erythrodermic Psoriasis

It is characterized by generalized (> 90% body surface area involved) erythema, scaling and itching. It is a medical emergency requiring hospitalization (Refer erythroderma).

Psoriatic arthropathy (Also Refer to Section 12, Ch 113) is a common seronegative polyarthritis. If not managed properly, the arthropathy progresses leading to considerable morbidity. It is seen in about 5% of psoriatic patients. Four types are described: (1) Distal arthritis involving the distal interphalangeal joints, (2) rheumatoid like arthritis, (3) ankylosing spondylitis or sacroiliitis and (4) mutilating arthritis (arthritis mutilans).

Course and Prognosis

The course is prolonged, but unpredictable. It may remain as discrete plaques or may become generalized. Relapse is the rule. Guttate psoriasis has a better prognosis.

Points to Remember

- Extremes of presentation from a few lesions to erythroderma or generalized pustular psoriasis.
- Chronic plaques with silvery scales over the elbows, knees and scalp are the most common lesions. Remissions and relapses are common.
- Nails show pitting, onycholysis and oil drop sign. Associated with psoriatic arthropathy.
- Pustular psoriasis is characterized by sterile pustules. It may affect the palms and soles or may be a generalized disease.

Management

Psoriatic lesions can be cleared considerably but recurrence is the rule. The need for long-term treatment and the noninfectious nature of psoriasis should be explained. *Treatment* depends upon the type and extent of the disease, age, social factors and general health of the patient.

Topical therapy: Topical corticosteroids and bland emollients are the mainstay of treatment in localized psoriasis. The preparations include betamethasone dipropionate, fluocinolone acetonide and clobetasol propionate for lesions on the limbs and trunk and fluticasone, mometasone or clobetasone for lesions on the face and flexures.

In chronic plaque psoriasis, coal tar preparations are useful singly or in combination with keratolytics such as salicylic acid. Salicylic acid and tar shampoos used daily and lotions containing betamethasone and salicylic acid are very effective in scalp psoriasis. Dithranol as a short contact therapy applied for 30 minutes daily and washed off is very effective. Dithranol can cause local irritation and staining and so less commonly used now, though it is safe and effective. Topical formulations of natural and active metabolite of vitamin D_3, calcitriol and synthetic analogues like calcipotriol, tacalcitol and maxacalcitol are widely prescribed preparations for plaque psoriasis. Calcipotriol when combined with a topical corticosteroid

has a superior efficacy than either drug alone. Calcipotriol enhances the efficacy of PUVA and ultraviolet B (UVB) phototherapy. Topical tacrolimus 0.1% and tazarotene 0.05% and 0.1% are alternative treatments for psoriasis. Topical tacrolimus 0.1% and pimecrolimus 1% are especially useful for psoriasis affecting the face, flexures and genitalia. Tazarotene is a topical retinoid that modulates abnormal keratinization and proliferation. Tazarotene can cause local irritation. It is useful in thick recalcitrant plaque psoriasis. Start with 0.05% cream and increase the strength as tolerated. Apply at night. A topical steroid application in the morning decreases the irritation due to tazarotene.

Topical psoralen soaks and exposure to sunlight is very effective in chronic plaque psoriasis. Hands and feet are immersed in a solution of 8-methoxypsoralen (10 mg/L) of warm water for 15 minutes and then exposed to UVA phototherapy units. If these equipment are not available, exposure to direct sunlight for not more than 5 minutes would suffice.

Systemic therapy: It is indicated when psoriasis is life-threatening as in GPP or erythroderma, extensive and not responding to topical treatment. The common drugs used are:

- Methotrexate, a folate antagonist is a well-established treatment for severe psoriasis. It is given orally once a week as a single dose (7.5–15 mg) or in 3 divided doses per week, 12 hours apart in succession. Blood counts, liver and renal function tests should be normal before starting methotrexate and should also be monitored during treatment. Improvement is seen within 2–4 weeks. The major side effects include hepatotoxicity, upper gastrointestinal symptoms, leukopenia, thrombocytopenia, megaloblastic anemia, oligospermia in men and teratogenesis.

- *Photochemotherapy:* 8-methoxypsoralen is given orally 2 hours prior to ultraviolet exposure from PUVA chambers or natural sunlight (PUVA–SOL). Psoralen cross-links with cellular deoxyribonucleic acid (DNA) inhibiting cell division. PUVA is usually given 2–3 times a week and there is progressive clearance in about 6 weeks. It is continued for 2 months after the skin lesions have resolved.

- Narrowband UVB therapy (311 nm) is a safe and useful therapy in plaque psoriasis. Philips TL-01 fluorescent lamps emit a narrow UVB band at 311 nm. This is found to be superior to conventional broadband UVB, producing longer remissions. UVB therapy 3 times per week is sufficient. This therapy is particularly useful in plaque psoriasis, guttate psoriasis, sebopsoriasis and psoriasis in a pregnant woman. It is not effective in erythroderma or generalized pustular psoriasis.

- Retinoids are vitamin A derivatives, particularly useful in pustular psoriasis and plaque psoriasis. Acitretin (25-50 mg/day) is useful either alone or in combination with retinoid psoralen and ultraviolet A (Re-PUVA). Acitretin is started in a daily dose of 25 mg and gradually increased to 50 mg for 3–4 months, depending on the response and side effects. After good clearance of lesions is achieved, dose is gradually tapered and stopped. Etretinate is not used nowadays due to its longer half-life.

- Cyclosporine is an immunosuppressant used in doses of 3–5 mg/kg/day orally and it is highly effective. The drug is continued till lesions resolve and the dose is slowly tapered. It can cause hypertension and renal toxicity and so monitoring is mandatory.

Recent Advances in the Treatment of Psoriasis

Biological response modifiers (biologics) are a new class of drugs and are likely to revolutionize the treatment of moderate to severe psoriasis. Biologics are proteins derived from recombinant DNA technology, hybridomas and blood and whole human cells. Three main types are used to treat psoriasis and other immune mediated diseases like rheumatoid arthritis or Crohn's disease. They are:

1. Recombinant cytokines
2. Monoclonal antibodies
3. Fusion proteins.

They interfere with T cell activation and effector function and prevent the inflammatory effects. Biologics are large molecules and administration is via injection or infusion. Biologics available to treat moderate to severe psoriasis or psoriatic arthritis are:

- ***Etanercept*** is a fusion protein which blocks the TNF-α. It is given subcutaneously (SC) in a dose of 50 mg twice a week for 12 weeks and then tapered to 25 mg. Injection site reactions and multiple sclerosis like syndrome are the main side effects.
- ***Alefacept*** is a fusion protein and acts by eliminating the pathogenic T cells. Dose is 7.5 mg intravenous (IV) or 15 mg intramuscular (IM) weekly for 12 weeks. CD4 suppression is the main side effect and should be monitored.
- ***Efalizumab*** is a monoclonal antibody that blocks the T cell activation, co-stimulation and migration. Dose is 1 mg/kg SC every week. Headache, nausea and chills are the side effects noted.
- ***Infliximab*** is a monoclonal antibody that blocks TNF-α. Side effects include infusion reactions and reactivation of tuberculosis. It is undertrial.
- ***Adalimumab*** and ***onercept*** are undertrial.
- ***Ustekinumab*** is a fully human recombinant antibody to the p 40 component of IL-12/IL-23.

Their major advantage is the low-risk for end organ toxicity and drug–drug interactions. Some of these may offer long-term remissions. For stable disease, if not very severe, etanercept or adalimumab are the first options. For rapid onset of action, adalimumab and infliximab are effective. Infliximab is useful in generalized pustular psoriasis and severe nail disease. Long-term safety of biologics is yet to be determined.

Points to Remember
- Topical corticosteroids, coal tar, salicylic acid, dithranol, tacrolimus and tazarotene are used for localized lesions.
- Generalized involvement necessitates systemic treatment with methotrexate, PUVA or retinoids.
- Newer biological are now approved for the treatment of psoriasis.

LICHEN PLANUS (LP)

It is an immunologically mediated acute or chronic inflammatory dermatosis involving skin and/or mucous membrane. LP is most common between 30 and 60 years of age.

Etiology

It is idiopathic in most cases, but it is evident that cell-mediated immunity (CMI) plays a major role. It is probably directed at self-antigens expressed on keratinocytes. Majority of the infiltrate contains CD8+ and CD45 RO+ memory cells. Proinflammatory cytokines are produced by both cytotoxic cells and by lesional keratinocytes, ultimately leading to apoptosis of keratinocytes. Drugs such as beta-blockers, antimalarials, thiazides, gold and mercury salts and infection with hepatitis C virus result in altered CMI. All these have been implicated as triggering factors for LP.

Pathology

It is quite characteristic. There is epidermal hyperkeratosis, hypergranulosis, acanthosis, basal cell degeneration and a band-like lymphohistiocytic infiltrate in the upper dermis.

Clinical Features

The onset is usually insidious with the classical violaceous, polygonal, flat topped extremely pruritic shiny papules (Fig. 223.6) distributed symmetrically over the flexor aspect of forearms, wrists, lower parts of legs and genitalia. The initial lesions may be erythematous. Some lesions show a white lacy network (***Wickham's striae***) on the surface. Koebner phenomenon (spread of lesions along the lines of trauma) is seen. In two-thirds of cases, the buccal mucosa is involved.

Sometimes the onset may be acute and generalized. Scalp involvement leads to scarring alopecia. Nails become dystrophic with longitudinal splintering.

Several clinical variants may occur. These include hypertrophic LP that presents as hyperkeratotic verrucous plaques especially on the lower parts of legs. ***Annular*** lesions occur commonly on the glans penis. Linear violaceous papules of LP occur on the limbs and trunk and ***follicular*** lesions on the scalp (Fig. 223.7). ***Graham Little syndrome*** is the occurrence of follicular lesions and scarring alopecia of scalp with classical LP. In ***LP***

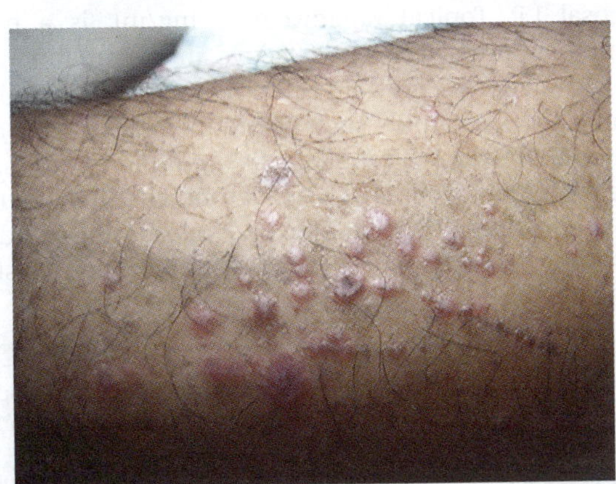

Fig. 223.6: Classical lichen planus. ***Note:*** The flat topped polygonal papules with Koebner phenomenon

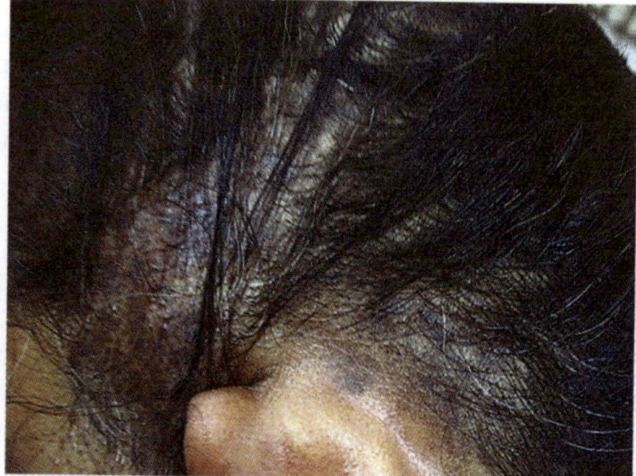

Fig. 223.7: Follicular lichen planus with scarring alopecia

actinicus, the lesions are on the sites exposed to sunlight. *Ulcerative lesions* are common on the soles and are resistant to therapy.

Diagnosis: Diagnosis is usually clinical. It can be confirmed by histopathology.

Differential diagnosis: It includes pityriasis rosea, psoriasis, cutaneous lupus erythematosus and contact dermatitis. Hypertrophic LP should be differentiated from lichen simples chronicus and prurigo nodularis. Lichenoid drug eruption is generalized and often spares the classical sites of LP. Wickham striae are absent. Lesions are more scaly, psoriasiform or eczematous on the trunk or on a photodistribution. Rash may develop after several weeks or months of drug intake. Nail or mucosal involvement is not seen. Common drugs causing lichenoid drug eruption are angiotensin converting enzyme (ACE) inhibitors, chloroquine, hydrochlorothiazide, isoniazid, hydroxychloroquine and quinidine.

Course: The lesions usually subside within 9–18 months. Remissions and relapses are common. Resolving plaques may leave a postinflammatory hyperpigmentation.

Treatment: Classic LP can be treated with potent topical steroids such as clobetasol propionate 0.05% twice daily for 2–3 weeks, if there are few lesions. Emollients should be applied 4–5 times daily in one direction, from above downwards on the limbs in order to avoid folliculitis. Moisturizers are used as soothing and steroid sparing agents. Topical calcineurin inhibitors like 0.1% tacrolimus or 1% pimecrolimus are useful adjuncts to topical corticosteroids. They are also effective in mucosal LP. Topical rapamycin, 1 mg/mL is a novel immunosuppressive agent effective in the treatment of recalcitrant erosive oral and vulvar LP. In acute generalized LP, oral corticosteroids such as prednisolone 30–40 mg/day tapered over 1–3 months halt the rapid progression. Intralesional injection of 0.1 mL of triamcinolone (10 mg/mL) is effective in hypertrophic LP. Cyclosporine in a dose of 3–5 mg/kg orally for chronic LP induces long-lasting remission.

Points to Remember

- Characterized clinically by pruritic violaceous flat topped papules with flexor distribution. Resolves mostly within 18 months.
- Lichenoid reactions occur due to drugs like gold, chloroquine and chlorothiazide.
- Responds to topical steroids and emollients.

PITYRIASIS ROSEA (PR)

It is an acute self limiting disorder of unknown etiology, probably infective in origin, affecting mainly children and young adults. Recently, herpes virus types 6 and 7 has been incriminated to play a role in the pathogenesis.

Clinical Features

PR is characterized by the onset of herald patch in 80% of patients. 'Herald patch' is an oval plaque, 2–5 cm in size, erythematous, with fine collarette of scales at the periphery. The scales are attached at the periphery and free towards the center of the lesion. After an interval of 1–2 weeks, a generalized eruption appears in crops, mainly over the trunk and proximal limbs. The characteristic lesion is a small oval papule with a crinky surface and a rim of fine scales (Fig. 223.8). The long axis of the lesions are oriented in the planes of cleavage, running parallel to the ribs and classically form a *fir tree* or *Christmas tree* like pattern. PR is asymptomatic in 50% of patients. The others get pruritus of varying severity.

Atypical presentations may occur. This includes—(1) lesions occurring only on the face and neck, (2) localized, (3) unilateral, (4) vesicular, (5) inverse PR (PR occurring in the flexures of the axillae and groins) and (6) erythroderma. The lesions undergo spontaneous remission in 6–12 weeks. Recurrence is uncommon.

Treatment is mainly symptomatic with oral antihistamines such as cetirizine 10 mg or levocetirizine 5 mg once at night for 2–3 weeks depending on the severity of itching. If asymptomatic, emollients like petrolatum alone would suffice. Topical steroid creams like fluticasone 0.05%, mometasone 0.1% or betamethasone dipropionate 0.05% applied once at night over severely pruritic lesions alleviate the itching. However, topical steroids should not be applied over large areas.

REITER'S SYNDROME

***See** also Section 12, Ch 113*

Reiter's syndrome consists of polyarthropathy, urethritis, iritis and a psoriasiform eruption. It invariably affects males and is preceded by genitourinary (GU) or gastrointestinal infection. There is a strong association with HLA-B27.

The main skin lesions are *keratoderma blennorrhagica* which are brownish-red papules or macules,

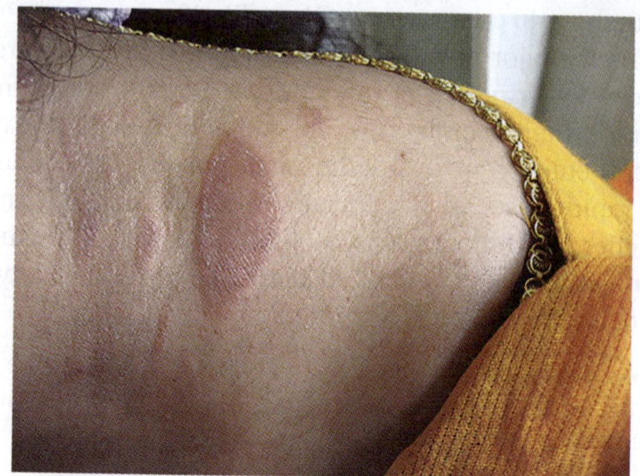

Fig. 223.8: Pityriasis rosea—oval papules with a collarette of scales. The larger one is the *herald patch*

sometimes with a central vesicle seen mainly on the palms and soles. Center of lesions become pustular or hyperkeratotic and crusted. Circinate balanitis is another classic feature of Reiter's and presents as shallow erosions with serpiginous micropustular borders on the glans, if uncircumcised. Only 30% develop the complete triad of arthritis, urethritis and conjunctivitis. Majority have a self limited course and resolves in 3–12 months. *Treatment* is similar to psoriasis. Methotrexate and retinoids are needed in severe cases (*See* Section 12, Ch 113).

EXFOLIATIVE DERMATITIS (ERYTHRODERMA)

It includes any inflammatory dermatosis which involves more than 90% of the body surface area. It is a dermatological emergency as the systemic side effects are potentially fatal. Exfoliative dermatitis is a secondary process and represents the generalized spread of a dermatosis or a systemic disease.

Common causes are eczemas (atopic, contact, photo dermatitis), psoriasis, lymphoma or Sézary syndrome, drug eruption [sulfonamides, barbiturates, non-steroidal anti-inflammataory drugs (NSAIDs) and phenytoin are the common drugs], pityriasis rubra pilaris and ichthyosis. In about 23% of cases the cause is unknown.

Clinical features: It is commonly seen in middle-aged and elderly males. The onset is often acute. It is characterized by generalized erythema and scaling. Temperature regulation is altered. Large amounts of warm blood are present in the skin due to dilatation of capillaries and there is considerable heat dissipation through insensible fluid loss and by convection. So the patient shivers. Scalp and body hair is lost and nails may be thickened or shed. Generalized lymphadenopathy which is a secondary response to severe skin inflammation is common.

Complications: In exfoliative dermatitis, there is skin failure, and so all the normal functions of the skin are affected. Edema, cutaneous and respiratory infection, cardiac failure, hypoalbuminemia due to protein loss through scales, dehydration and metabolic derangement, impaired temperature regulation and dermatopathic lymphadenopathy are the major complications.

Diagnosis: History, pathognomonic signs and symptoms of the pre-existing dermatosis, if present, help in the diagnosis.

Course and prognosis: It depends upon the underlying cause. In most patients, the problem subsides in weeks to months though recurrence is possible. Death rate ranges from 11 to 30%. *Common causes of death* are pneumonia, sepsis, high output cardiac failure and other cardiac complications and lymphoma.

Management: Patient needs to be hospitalized. A warm environment and good nursing care are needed. Pulse, blood pressure (BP), temperature and fluid balance are monitored. Emollients and topical steroids are the mainstay of treatment. Antibiotics against *Staphylococcus aureus* will be required as they colonize the skin. Adequate nutrition is maintained. The primary cause is treated. Cardiac failure and infections should be corrected.

Points to Remember
- Exfoliative dermatitis is a dermatological emergency.
- Uncommon, but potentially fatal, often sudden in onset.
- Psoriasis and eczema are the common causes.
- Characterized by generalized erythema, edema and scaling.
- Skin failure leads to complications such as cardiac failure, hypothermia, infection and lymphadenopathy.
- Inpatient management is needed to correct the nutrition, electrolyte imbalance, secondary infection and other complications.
- Treatment of the underlying cause and emollients are essential.

CHAPTER
224

Eczema

Usha Vaidhyanathan

Chapter Summary
- General Considerations
  - General Principles in the Management of Eczema
- Endogenous Eczema
  - Atopic Dermatitis
  - Seborrheic Dermatitis
  - Nummular Eczema
  - Stasis Eczema
  - Pompholyx
- Exogenous Eczema
  - Contact Dermatitis
  - Photosensitive Dermatitis
- Asteatotic Eczema (Eczema Craquele)
- Lichen Simplex Chronicus (LSC)
- Infective Eczema

GENERAL CONSIDERATIONS

Eczema is a polymorphic inflammatory reaction pattern of the skin involving the epidermis and dermis. The term *eczema* literally means to **boil over** (Greek). The terms eczema and dermatitis are used interchangeably. Dermatosis is a general term which denotes any skin disorder.

The etiology of most eczema is not known. It is classified into endogenous (due to internal or constitutional factors) and exogenous (due to external agents). However, in clinical practice these distinctions are often blurred.

Depending on the morphology of eruption, eczema can be divided into—(1) acute eczema characterized by pruritus, erythema, edema, vesiculation, oozing, crusting and scaling, (2) chronic eczema characterized by pruritus, lichenification (thickened with prominent skin markings), excoriation and either hypo- or hyperpigmentation.

Microscopic changes in the early stages (acute eczema) show intercellular and intracellular edema with resultant vesicle formation and associated dermal vasodilatation and infiltration with chronic inflammatory cells.

In chronic eczema, there is thickening of the epidermis (acanthosis, hyperkeratosis) and retention of nuclei by some corneocytes (parakeratosis). Rete ridges are elongated, dermal vessels dilated and inflammatory mononuclear cells infiltrate the skin.

Classification of eczema is given below.

Endogenous	*Exogenous*	*Unclassified*
• Atopic dermatitis • Seborrheic dermatitis • Nummular eczema • Stasis eczema • Pompholyx	• Allergic contact dermatitis • Irritant contact • Photosensitive • Infective eczema	• Asteatotic eczema • Lichen simplex chronicus

General Principles in the Management of Eczema

- Acute eczema is managed with wet dressings or compresses. Normal saline, 1 in 8,000 dilution of potassium permanganate solution or 1% boric acid can be used. This removes the crusts, stops oozing and provides comfort
- Topical creams, particularly combination of gluco-corticoid and antibiotic creams, e.g. fusidic acid and betamethasone/hydrocortisone, or mupirocin and fluticasone, are preferred
- Severe secondary infection needs treatment with systemic antibiotics. Erythromycin 250 mg qid for 5 days is cheap and effective
- Ointments should not be used over oozing eczema as it would cause occlusion and worsen the oozing
- Creams are preferred in acute and subacute stage and ointments in chronic stage.

ENDOGENOUS ECZEMA

Atopic Dermatitis (AD)

It is an intensively pruritic acute, subacute or chronic relapsing skin disorder that usually begins within the first 6 months of life, though it can begin at any age. Approximately, 70% of patients have a family history of atopy like asthma allergic rhinitis.

Etiopathogenesis

There is a complex interaction between skin barrier, genetic, environmental, pharmacologic and immunologic factors. Triggering factors include:

- *Inhalants:* Dust mites, pollens
- *Microbial agents:* Exotoxins of *Staphylococcus aureus* act as super antigens and stimulate T-cells and macrophages
- Autoallergens are released from damaged tissue
- *Foods:* Eggs, milk, peanuts, fish, wheat.

These allergens are taken up by the antigen presenting cells in skin and processed and presented to the CD4+ T-cells along with class II major histocompatibility complex (MHC) antigens. The activated T-cells secrete many cytokines, especially interleukin-4 (IL-4), (Th-2 type of response). There is a relative reduction in the number of CD4+ T-cells that secrete IL-2 and γ-interferon and also a decrease in CD8+ T-cells. IL-4 activates the B-lymphocyte to produce excess of immunoglobulin E (IgE). IgE interacts with the antigen and sensitizes mast cells and basophils and causes degranulation. Inflammatory mediators are liberated and cause intense itching and eczema. The damaged skin provides a good environment for the *S. aureus* population to grow and exotoxins further worsen the eczema, by acting as superantigens.

Exacerbating Factors

- Skin barrier function is disrupted causing dehydration. Xerosis of skin is the most important aggravating factor
- Infection with *S. aureus*
- *Seasonal variation:* AD usually improves in hot season and flares in cold season
- *Clothing:* Wool and fur aggravate the condition
- Emotional stress.

Clinical Features

Pruritus is the main symptom. It is the itch that rashes rather than the rash that itches. The constant scratch leads to a vicious cycle of itch → scratch → rash → itch. Itching is severe and often interferes with sleep. The skin becomes very dry.

The clinical picture of eczema varies with age:

Infantile phase: Lesions of acute eczema first occur on the cheeks, forehead and scalp and later the trunk and extremities. When infant begins to crawl, the extensor aspects of knees are involved (Fig. 224.1). Secondary infection with *S. aureus* is common. In patients with active AD, extensive and widespread infection by *herpes simplex* virus may occur (eczema herpeticum). In more than half patients, the eczema resolves by 18 months.

Childhood phase: Papules, lichenified plaques, erosions and crusts are seen mainly on the antecubital and popliteal fossa (Fig. 224.2) neck, wrists and ankles. There is erythema on face with infraorbital folds (Dennie-Morgan folds). Periorbital pigmentation and loss of eyebrows on the lateral one-third may occur due to rubbing Hertoghe's sign. Palmar markings may be exaggerated (hyperlinearity of palms. At times, periorbital and perinasal pallor can occur due to vascular changes and is called head light sign).

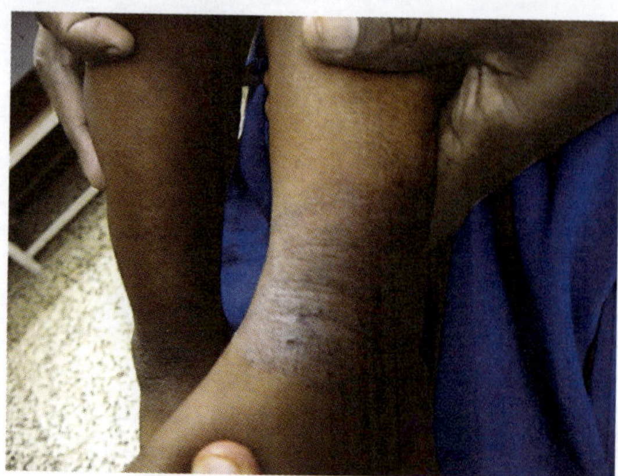

Fig. 224.1: Atopic dermatitis in an infant

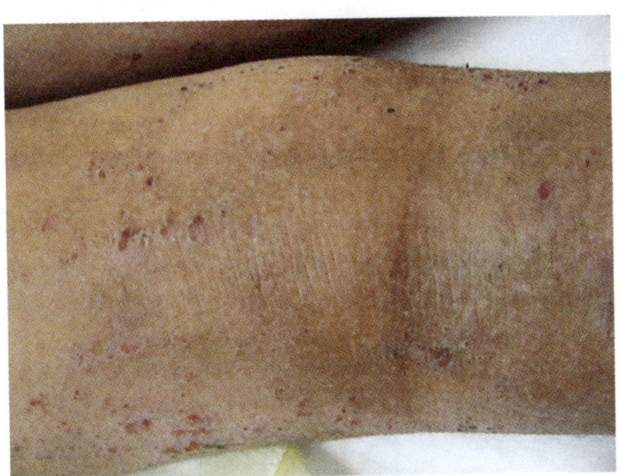

Fig. 224.2: Atopic dermatitis in a child

Adult phase: Lichenification and excoriations in a flexor distribution is characteristic feature in this phase. Irritant dermatitis of the hands is common. Eyelid dermatitis, retroauricular dermatitis and hand eczema are the common residuals of childhood atopy in adults. The disease tends to wax and wane. Acute flares can occur on a chronic eczema.

Other features

- Stroking leads to blanching and not redness as in normal skin. This unique feature of AD is called **white dermographism**.
- Cheilitis, conjunctivitis, facial pallor, ichthyosis and nipple eczema are the minor features of AD. Pitted keratolysis of palmar creases, geographic tongue, pityriasis alba are other associated conditions.
- Extensive skin involvement may cause exfoliative dermatitis.

Diagnosis: It is based on clinical findings such as onset in infancy, severe pruritus, typical distribution, morphology of lesions, personal or family history of AD, allergic rhinitis or asthma.

Differential diagnosis: Seborrheic dermatitis (SD), irritant and allergic contact dermatitis (ACD), psoriasis, nummular eczema and dermatophytosis should be differentiated from AD.

Prognosis: Spontaneous and complete remission occurs during childhood. Thirty to fifty percent of patients may develop asthma or hay fever later in life. Adult onset AD often runs a severe course.

Management

The patient is advised to avoid any predisposing factors like dust, infection or any particular food which aggravates the condition. Dry skin management is the most important. The child should be given a quick bath with lukewarm water. Soap substitutes like cleansers containing cetyl and stearyl alcohol or superfatted soaps used for bathing to prevent drying skin. Moisturizers and emollients should be applied immediately after bath and repeated many times to prevent drying. Moisturizers should be applied along the direction of hair follicles to avoid folliculitis. Creams are preferred in an acute eczema and petrolatum for dry eczema. Wet compresses with saline or dilute potassium permanganate solution reduce the oozing associated with acute eczema. Oral and topical antibiotics to eliminate the *S. aureus* infection promote healing. Cotton clothes are preferred. Cool and comfortable environment prevents itching. Antihistamines such as hydroxyzine should be used without hesitation because it is the *itch that rashes*.

Topical steroids like fluticasone, desonide or mometasone applied once or twice daily till the lesions resolve, reduces inflammation and itching. Tacrolimus (0.03%, 0.1%) and pimecrolimus creams are also widely used now. Severe and resistant forms are managed by phototherapy and systemic steroids like prednisolone 1 mg/kg bw till the acute symptoms are controlled. Oral cyclosporine is very effective but the side effects and cost restricts its use.

Points to Remember
- Usually begins in infancy
- Immunologically mediated, environmental factors also play a role
- ***Clinical features*** include acute eczema in infancy affecting face and hands, subacute eczema in childhood affecting antecubital fossa and popliteal fossa, neck, wrists and ankles and chronic lichenified eczema in flexor distribution in adults.
- Itch scratch cycle is predominant
- Infection, heat, wool, stress, inhalants (dust) and certain foods are the exacerbating factors
  Treatment includes emollients, topical steroids, antihistamines and antibiotics.

Seborrheic Dermatitis (SD)

It is a very common, chronic inflammatory dermatosis characterized by erythema and scaling in regions where the sebaceous glands are most active. Mild scalp SD causes flaking (dandruff). SD is more common in males and occurs after puberty and incidence increases with age. Onset in infancy is also common due to maternal androgens (cradle cap). Human immunodeficiency virus (HIV) infected individuals have an increased incidence of SD that is often severe and intractable.

Etiology

It is unknown. **Malassezia furfur** is said to play a role. Abnormalities in sebaceous gland activity and zinc, niacin and pyridoxine deficiencies are also implicated.

Clinical Features

The common clinical patterns are:

- **Scalp and face involvement:** Greasy or dry scaling, erythematous macules and papules often cause a diffuse involvement of the scalp (Fig. 224.3). Other classical sites are eyebrows, eyelashes, beard, malar region, scalp hairline (corona seborrheica), nasolabial folds, retroauricular and meatal region (Fig. 224.4).
- **Petaloid:** Lesions simulating pityriasis rosea, occur over the presternal area.
- **Flexural:** In the axillae, groins, anogenital and submammary areas, SD presents as diffuse, sharply marginated erythema with erosions and fissuring. It is common in elderly.
- **Pityrosporum folliculitis (PF):** It is an erythematous follicular eruption with papules or pustules over the back.

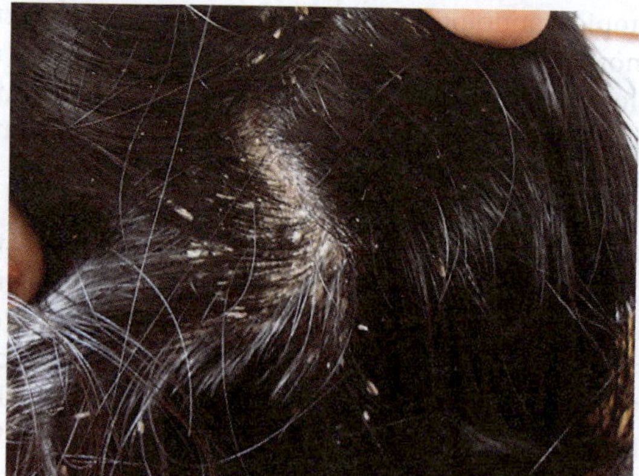

Fig. 224.3: Seborrheic dermatitis of the scalp

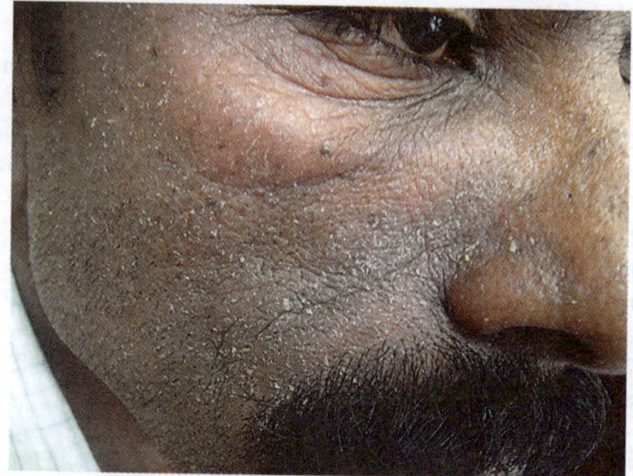

Fig. 224.4: Seborrheic dermatitis of the face

Course and Prognosis

It affects majority of individuals at sometime during life. Recurrences and remissions are common. Infantile and adolescents SD disappears with age.

Management

As the condition is chronic, initial therapy followed by long-term maintenance therapy is required.

Scalp: Shampoos containing selenium sulfide (2.5%), zinc pyrithione (1–2%), ketoconazole 2%, fluocinolone acetonide, applied twice a week (the frequency can be reduced later) are effective. Salicylic acid and coal tar shampoos are useful in reducing thick greasy scales.

Face and trunk: Topical glucocorticoid creams (1–2.5% hydrocortisone), ketoconazole 2% cream, tacrolimus 0.03%, pimecrolimus 1% are all effective.

Cradle cap: Removal of crusts with warm oil (olive), followed by creams or shampoos are useful in infantile seborrhea.

Nummular Eczema (Discoid Eczema)

It is a chronic pruritic inflammatory dermatitis, typically affects middle-aged or elderly, clinically characterized by coin-shaped erythematous plaques with exudation and crusting (Fig. 224.5). It is severely pruritic, with excoriations. Sometimes dry scaly lichenified plaque may be seen. Lesions may be clustered on the lower parts of legs or trunk in males and hands or fingers in females. It may be generalized and scattered. It has a chronic course from weeks to months and tends to recur. Secondary bacterial infection is common.

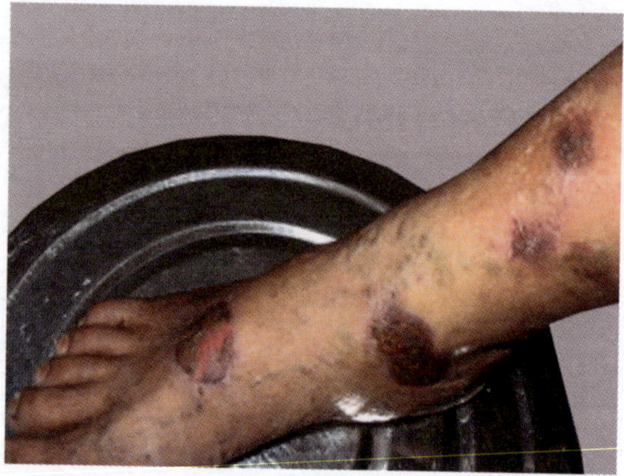

Fig. 224.5: Coin-shaped lesions of nummular eczema on the leg

Management

Moderate to high potency topical steroid combined with antibiotics (fusidic acid and betamethasone), moisturizers and antihistamines like hydroxyzine or cetirizine are the mainstay of treatment. Systemic antibiotics may be needed if secondary infection is severe. Photochemotherapy (PUVA) or narrowband ultraviolet B (UVB) (311 nm) are very effective in severe cases with extensive involvement.

Stasis Eczema

Chronic venous insufficiency leads to stasis eczema (varicose eczema) in the lower parts of legs and feet.

Pathogenesis

Incompetence of deep perforating veins increases the hydrostatic pressure in dermal capillaries. This widens the endothelial pores of capillary bed, allowing the leakage of fibrinogen into the interstitial fluid. Pericapillary fibrin deposition impedes the oxygen diffusion and other nutrients into the skin. This leads to the pathological and clinical changes. Increased sequestration of white cells in the venules causes cutaneous inflammation.

Clinical Features

Inflammatory edema, papules, scaling, crusting, erosions, pigmentation stippled with recent and old hemorrhages and dermal sclerosis are the characteristic features. There may be concomitant irritant contact dermatitis (ICD) due to secretion from stasis ulcer and ACD secondary to topical medications and bacterial colonization.

Management

Emollients and topical steroids are needed. Venous insufficiency should be managed. Foot end elevation at bed time and elastic stockings during day time will prevent the worsening of varicose complications.

Pompholyx

It is an acute, chronic or recurrent dermatosis of the lateral aspects of fingers, palms and soles characterized by symmetrical deep-seated pruritic, clear vesicles (Fig. 224.6) and later by scaling, fissures and lichenification. Spontaneous remissions can occur in 2–3 weeks. Recurrence is the rule. Secondary infection may occur. Hyperhidrosis is common.

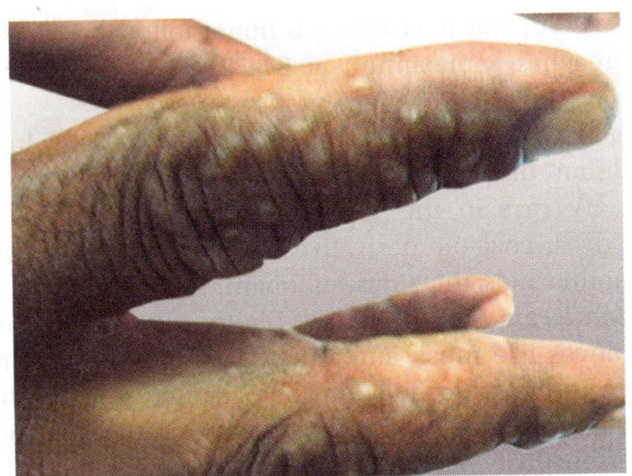

Fig. 224.6: Pompholyx. **_Note:_** Vesicles on the sides of fingers

Management

Wet compresses with saline, topical steroids and in severe cases, a short course of systemic steroids are needed. Topical PUVA (as soaks) are also useful in severe cases.

Points to Remember
- SD affects the scalp and face. Treated with combination creams of steroids and antifungals.
- Nummular eczema presents as coin-shaped lesions on the limbs of elderly.
- Stasis eczema, associated with venous insufficiency is treated with emollients and low or moderate potency topical steroids.

EXOGENOUS ECZEMA

Contact Dermatitis (CD)

It is a term applied to acute or chronic inflammatory reaction to substances that come in contact with the skin. There are two types of CD. ICD caused by a chemical irritant and ACD caused by an allergen (antigen), which elicits a type IV hypersensitivity reaction.

Irritant Contact Dermatitis

It is caused by exposure of skin to chemical or physical agents that are capable of producing cell damage, acutely or chronically. It is dependent on the concentration of offending agent and occurs in all those who are exposed, depending on the penetrability and thickness of stratum corneum. There is a threshold concentration for these substances above which they cause acute dermatitis and below which they do not.

ICD may occur minutes after exposure or may be delayed up to 24 hours. Acute ICD can occur due to strong irritants like acids, chloroform, methanol, phenol or propylene glycol and cause toxic reactions after a short exposure. The spectrum of changes ranges from erythema to vesiculation. Erosion, crusting and scaling follows. Papules are not seen. In chemical burns, necrosis of tissues leads to ulceration. Lesions are sharply demarcated to the site of contact with irritant. Configuration is often bizarre.

Most cases however, are caused by cumulative exposure to one or more mild irritants like water, soaps and detergents. This causes a chronic disturbance of barrier function that allows even subtoxic concentrations of the offending agents to penetrate into the skin and elicit a chronic inflammatory response. Hands are most commonly affected. There is dryness, chapping, erythema, scaling, fissuring, and crusting. Stinging and itching are the main symptoms.

Allergic Contact Dermatitis

It is dependent on sensitization and thus occurs only in sensitized individuals. Depending on the degree of sensitization, even minute amounts of allergen may elicit a reaction.

The eruption starts in a sensitized individual 48 hours or a few days after contact with the allergen. The eruption worsens on repeated exposures (crescendo reaction). There is intense pruritus. Lesions are initially confined to the area of contact with the allergen and later spread to the surrounding areas. Generalized involvement can also occur, if sensitization is strong. In the acute stage, there is erythema, papules, vesicles, erosions, scaling and crusting and in the chronic stage (Figs 224.7 and 224.8), there is lichenification, fissuring, scaling and crusting.

Patch test: It is done to identify the specific allergen. In ACD, sensitization is present on all parts of the skin as it is immunologically mediated. Therefore, application of allergen to any area of normal skin provokes an eczematous reaction. It should be performed on a previously uninvolved skin after the dermatitis has subsided. The upper back is preferred site (Fig. 224.9). Finn chambers are used commonly and fixed to the skin using adhesive tapes. The allergens are applied on to the chambers. If patient is sensitized to the allergen, a reaction develops at contact site within 48 hours. Readings are taken from one hour after removal on day 2 and day 4 of applying the patch.

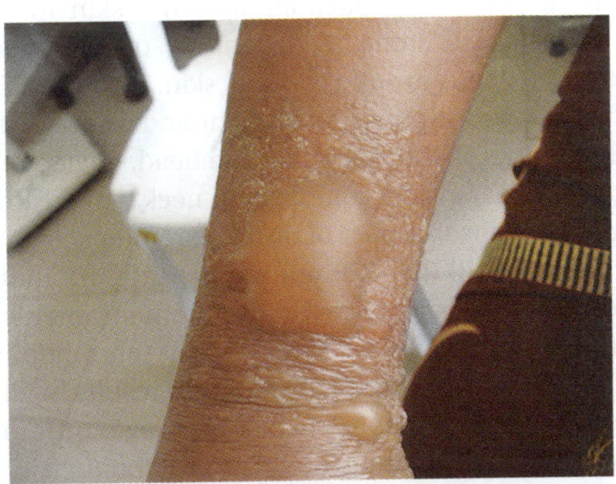

Fig. 224.7: Allergic contact dermatitis to diclofenac spray

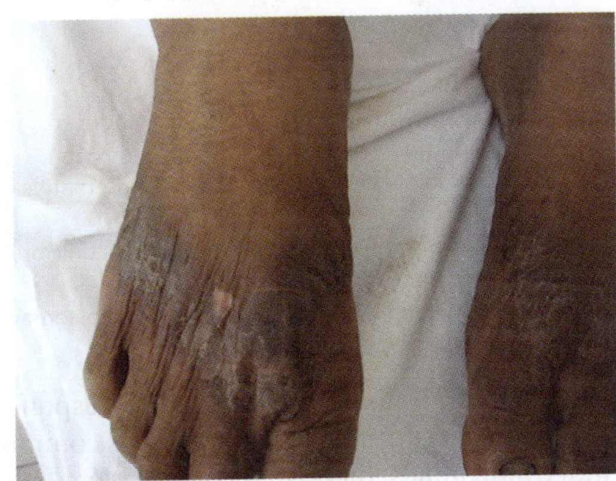

Fig. 224.8: Allergic contact dermatitis to rubber

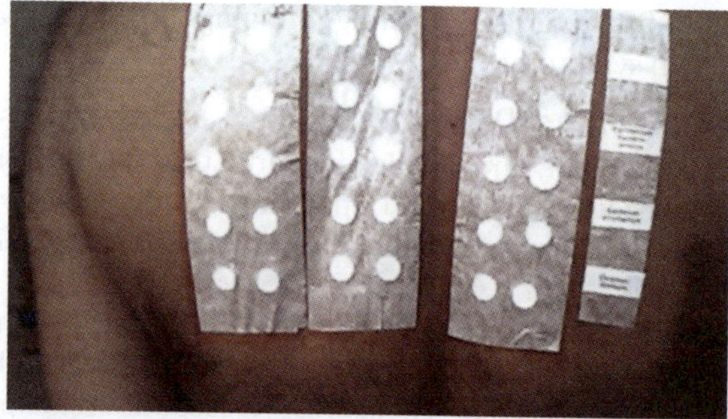

Fig. 224.9: Patch test allergens pasted on the back

Management of Contact Dermatitis

- Avoidance of irritants or allergens
- Wet dressings and topical steroids for acute reaction and if severe, systemic glucocorticoids are indicated
- In chronic CD, protective or lubricating creams and high potency topical steroids are necessary.

Points to Remember
- ICD is more common than ACD. Atopics are more susceptible to irritants
- Common irritants are water, abrasives, chemicals (alkalis) and detergents
- Common allergens are nickel (jewelry, zips, instruments), chromates (cement, primer), cobalt (paint, ink), colophony (glue, adhesive tape), preservatives, perfumes and paraphenylene-diamine (dye).
- Avoidance of allergens and irritants are important in the prevention of CD.

Photosensitive Dermatitis

In normal persons, pigmentation of the skin increases with exposure to sunlight, depending on its intensity, duration of exposure and type of skin. Photosensitivity is an abnormal response to sunlight and affects the sun exposed parts of the body like forehead, malar region, nose, rim of ears, sides and back of neck, 'V' area of the chest and extensor aspect of distal extremities. UVA 320–400 nm and UVB 290–320 nm are the primary inducers of most photosensitivity reactions. The photon energy is absorbed by molecules such as skin cells (chromophores) and then either dispersed harmlessly or results in clinical disease. The chromophore can be—(1) exogenous (topical or systemic), (2) endogenous [deoxyribonucleic acid (DNA) is the most important skin chromophore], (3) endogenous or exogenous allergen causing an immune reaction activated by photoradiation.

Photodermatosis is broadly classified into:
- **Phototoxicity:** Sunburn, drug or chemical-induced, plant-induced (phytophotodermatitis)
- **Photoallergy:** Drug or chemical, chronic actinic dermatitis, solar urticarial
- **Idiopathic:** Polymorphous light eruption (PMLE), actinic prurigo, hydroa vacciniforme
- **Miscellaneous:** Metabolic, nutritional, genetic, photo aggravated dermatosis, chronic photo damage.

Sunburn: It is a transient inflammatory response of normal skin due to exposure to UVB rays. It is common in fair skinned individuals. There is uniform erythema, edema, vesicles and bullae strictly confined to the sun exposed areas. Erythema is visible 2–6 hours following exposure and reaches a maximum at 24–72 hours and fades in 3–5 days, followed by pigmentation.

Drug or chemical-induced phototoxic reactions: In this condition interaction occurs between drugs/chemical with UV rays in the skin and manifests like an ICD (e.g. dyes, coal tar derivatives, psoralens, tetracyclines, phenothiazines, thiazides, sulfonamides and others).

Photoallergic reactions: A photo allergen such as fragrances like musk ambrette, para-aminobenzoic acid (PABA), phenothiazines and halogenated salicylanilides in deodorant soaps, formed in the skin initiates a type IV hypersensitivity reaction and manifests like an ACD.

Idiopathic: Polymorphous light eruption (PMLE) is the most common photodermatosis. This is common in women. UVA and UVB can evoke PMLE, UVA being more common. Lesions are papular, papulovesicular or urticarial plaques that begin within 24 hours of exposure. In the individual patient, usually one type of lesion predominates. Recurrences are common. Spontaneous improvement occurs after years.

Management: Strict avoidance of sunlight is necessary. Sun block creams like zinc oxide or titanium dioxide, broad spectrum sunscreens, topical glucocorticoids and antihistamines are used in treatment of PMLE. Severe eruption may necessitate systemic steroids.

Points to Remember
- Sunlight can cause tanning, sunburn and photoageing in normal skin.
- Important idiopathic photodermatoses are PMLE and chronic actinic dermatitis.
- Some conditions like lupus erythematosus, porphyria and rosacea are worsened by sunlight.
- Treatment includes avoidance of sun exposure, irritants and allergens, use of sunscreens and topical steroids.

ASTEATOTIC ECZEMA (ECZEMA CRAQUELE)

It is a dry eczema with fissuring and cracking of the skin, often affecting the limbs in the elderly. The skin is dry, erythematous and itchy that shows a crazy-paving pattern of fissuring (Fig. 224.10). Dry winter climate, over washing and hypothyroidism exacerbates the condition. Extensive or generalized forms are rare but found to be associated with internal malignancy like lymphoma or carcinoma breast or gastric carcinoma. Topical emollients

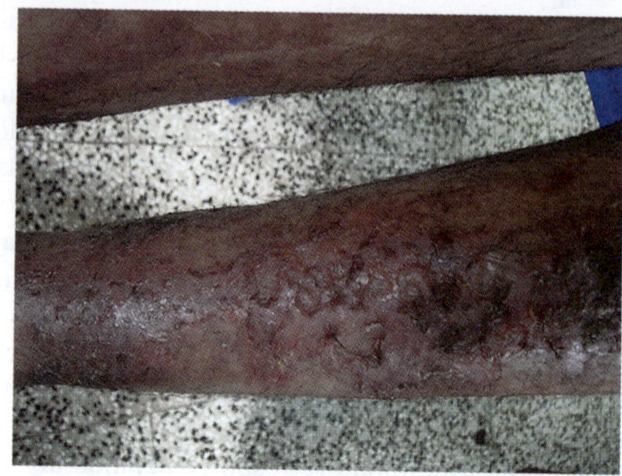

Fig. 224.10: Asteatotic eczema of the legs. Crazy pavement appearance

and bath emollients should be used regularly. Sometimes a mild topical steroid is necessary.

LICHEN SIMPLEX CHRONICUS (LSC)

It is a localized form of lichenification due to rubbing or scratching as a habit or due to stress. The skin becomes highly sensitive and hyperexcitable in response to minimal external stimuli. LSC is common in elderly females. It usually occurs as a single plaque of lichenification with exaggerated skin markings and hyper pigmentation (Fig. 224.11), associated with paroxysms of pruritus. Common sites are the lower parts of legs and back of neck. Sometimes a nodular lichenification known as prurigo nodularis develops on the shins and forearms.

It should be explained to patient that the rubbing and scratching must be stopped. Potent topical steroids, coal tar and intralesional triamcinolone are effective.

INFECTIVE ECZEMA

Infectious eczematoid dermatitis (IED) or infective eczema is an eczema that occurs secondary to an infection in the skin. It can occur around discharging wounds, sinuses or ulcers as an acute eczema (Fig. 224.12). This should be differentiated from infected eczema where a primary eczema is complicated by secondary bacterial infection. Systemic antibiotics are essential. Potassium permanganate soaks twice daily till the oozing clears and application of a topical steroid and antibiotic cream, effectively reduces the eczema.

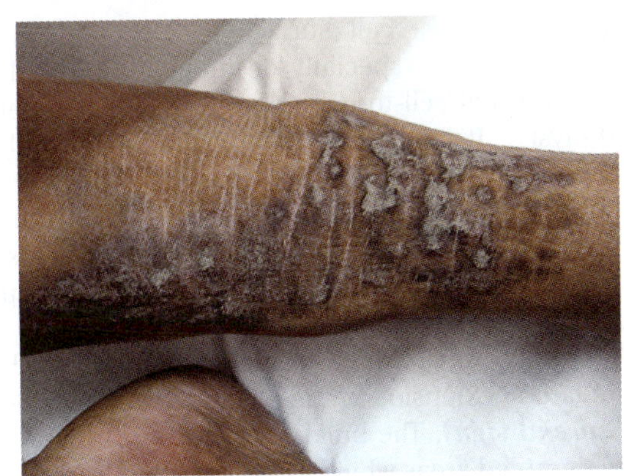

Fig. 224.11: Lichenified plaques of lichen simplex chronicus (LSC)

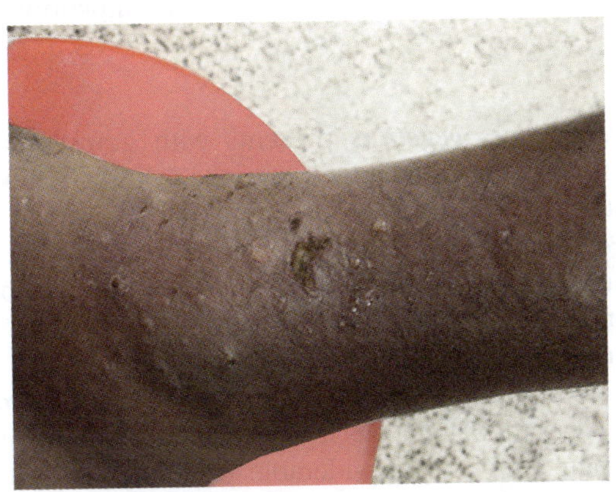

Fig. 224.12: Infective eczema—edema vesiculation oozing and crusting

CHAPTER 225

Vesiculobullous Disorders

S Pradeep Nair

Chapter Summary

- General Considerations
- Pemphigus Vulgaris
- Bullous Pemphigoid
- Dermatitis Herpetiformis
- Linear Immunoglobulin A Disease
- Investigations and Treatment

GENERAL CONSIDERATIONS

Blistering disorders are a heterogeneous group of diseases presenting with vesicles and bullae on the skin and mucous membrane. These groups of disorders cause great morbidity and even mortality in dermatological practice. The basic classification of blistering disorders is given in Table 225.1.

The genetically transmitted group of blistering disorders like epidermolysis bullosa is mechanobullous disorder where friction and trauma contribute to the

Table 225.1: Classification of blistering disorders

Genetic	*Immunobullous*
- Epidermolysis bullosa - Simplex, junctional - Dystrophic type	- Pemphigus vulgaris - Bullous pemphigoid - Dermatitis herpetiformis - Linear IgA disease

Abbreviation: IgA = Immunoglobulin A

formation of blisters. In immunobullous disorders, autoimmune mechanisms contribute to the formation of blisters. Autoimmune blistering disorders account for 0.49% of the skin disorders in Kerala, pemphigus vulgaris being the most common.

PEMPHIGUS VULGARIS

The word pemphigus is derived from the Greek word **pemphix** meaning **bubble**. The usual age group is 40–60 years. Autoantibodies [Immunoglobulin G (IgG)] are directed against cell surface glycoproteins called pemphigus antigens, specially desmoglein-3. This leads to loss of normal cell-to-cell adhesion in the epidermis (acantholysis). It is clinically characterized by multiple flaccid vesicles and bullae, arising on normal skin, distributed on the flexures, scalp and oral mucous membrane (Figs 225.1 and 225.2). Thick crusted erosions are seen on the scalp. A tangential pressure applied adjacent to a bulla or vesicle will cause the skin to peel away *(Nikolsky sign)*, while vertical pressure on the bulla leads to lateral extension of the blister *(Asboe-Hansen or bulla spread sign)*. The bulla on rupture leads to large, painful denuded areas which extend without healing. The oral mucosa shows erosions and ulcers. It is invariably fatal if not treated aggressively with immunosuppressive agents.

Variants

- ***Pemphigus vegetans*** presents with granulomatous vegetative purulent plaques on the flexures, trunk and other areas.
- ***Pemphigus foliaceus*** presents with superficial pustules, erythema, scaling and crusting distributed on the face, scalp, upper chest and abdomen, may present as exfoliative dermatitis.
- ***Pemphigus erythematosus (Senear-Usher syndrome)*** is a variant of foliaceus where there is erythema on the malar area and considerable overlap with systemic lupus erythematosus (SLE).
- ***Paraneoplastic pemphigus*** may be associated with internal malignancies like non-Hodgkin's lymphoma, chronic lymphatic leukemia and Castleman's tumor.
- ***Drug-induced pemphigus:*** Drugs like D-penicillamine, captopril and piroxicam can induce ***pemphigus foliaceus*** types. Some drugs like penicillin, rifampicin, phenytoin and phenobarbitone trigger pemphigus vulgaris either directly or indirectly.

BULLOUS PEMPHIGOID

It occurs after 60 years of age. Autoantibodies interact with bullous pemphigoid antigen in the hemidesmosomes of basal keratinocytes and there is complementary activation and attraction of neutrophils and eosinophils. These inflammatory cells release various bioactive molecules causing bullous lesions.

Clinical Features

It includes multiple large, tense bullae and vesicles distributed on the flexures, mainly lower abdomen, thighs and axilla (Fig. 225.3). The bulla heals after rupture with no peripheral extension. Nikolsky and bulla spread sign are negative. Oral and scalp lesions are rare (Table 225.2).

DERMATITIS HERPETIFORMIS

The age of onset is 20–40 years. It is associated with gluten-sensitive enteropathy and immunoglobulin A (IgA) deposits in the skin. Autoantibodies to epidermal transglutaminases probably cross-react and bind to transglutaminases in the gut and circulate as immune complexes and deposits in the skin. IgA activates complement leading to chemotaxis of neutrophils and

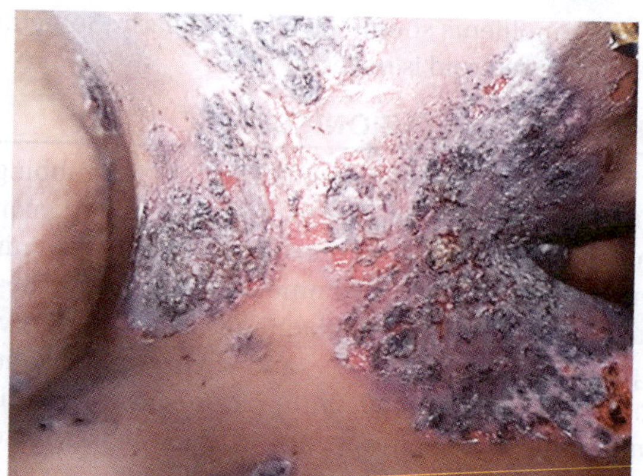

Fig. 225.1: Crusted erosions and plaques of pemphigus vulgaris, back of neck

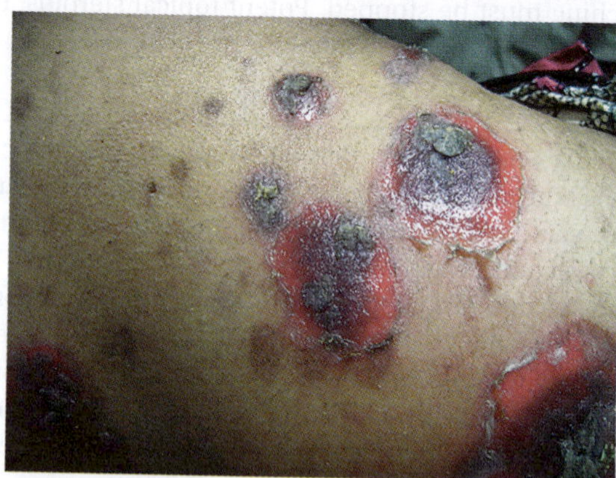

Fig. 225.2: Large superficial erosions due to rupture of flaccid bullae on the trunk

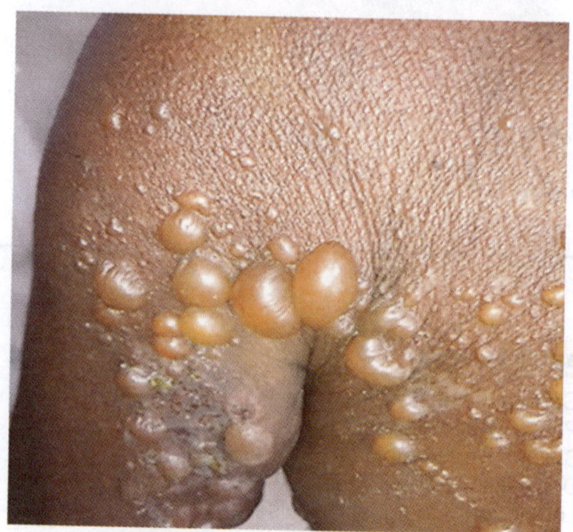

Fig. 225.3: Large tense bulla of bullous pemphigoid

Table 225.2: Clinical differences between pemphigus and pemphigoid	
Pemphigus	**Pemphigoid**
Usually affects middle age (40–60 years)	Older age (60–75 years)
Mucosal involvement is common	Rare
Blisters are common on trunk, scalp and seborrheic sites	Flexures, extremities
Itching is less common	Common
Nikolsky's sign and bulla spread sign are positive	Negative

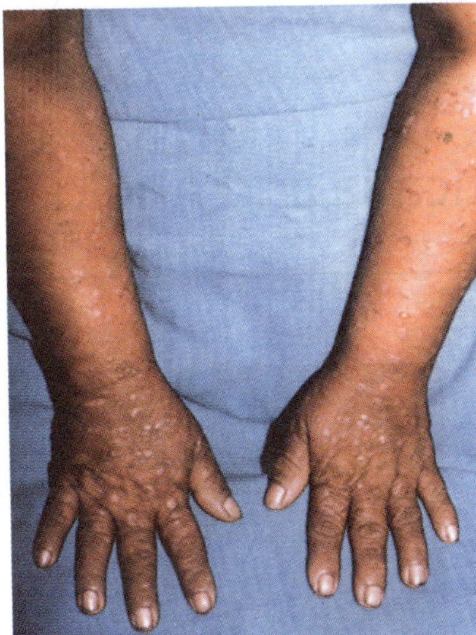

Fig. 225.4: Grouped vesicles of dermatitis herpetiformis

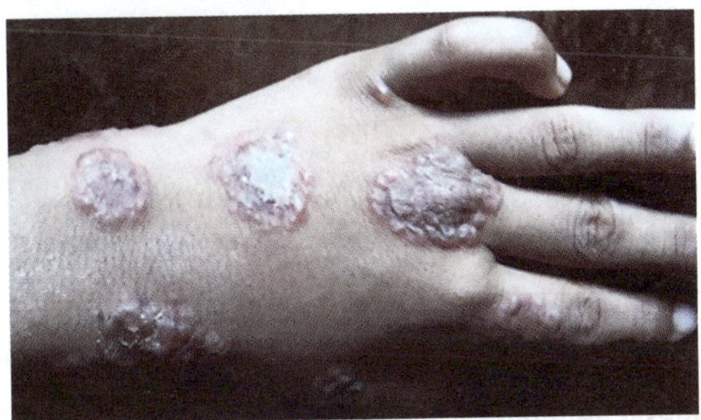

Fig. 225.5: Chronic bullous disease of childhood—annular plaques with peripheral vesicles give a *string of pearl appearance*

produces tissue injury. The patient presents with severely pruritic multiple grouped vesicles, papules and urticarial plaques distributed on the upper shoulder, lower back and extremities (Fig. 225.4). Nikolsky's sign and bulla spread sign are negative. Oral lesions are uncommon. Seventy percent of the patients may give history of exacerbation of lesions and diarrhea while taking gluten-containing food such as wheat, barley and oats.

LINEAR IMMUNOGLOBULIN A DISEASE

Linear IgA disease presents with multiple pruritic tense subepidermal bullae on the extensor surfaces of elbows, knees, buttocks and trunk. Oral erosions and ulceration are common.

A similar disease occurring in children is known as *chronic bullous disease of childhood (CBDC)*. Here, the lesions are confined to the perineum, lower abdomen, eyelids and scalp. Annular lesions with vesicles along the edge give a *string of pearl* appearance (Fig. 225.5). Homogenous linear deposits of IgA are present at the basement membrane zone. Fresh vesicles appear in cluster around the margin of resolving lesions forming a *cluster of jewels* pattern. Mucous membranes can be involved. Histopathology shows a subepidermal blister with eosinophils. CBDC responds to dapsone and sulfapyridine. Steroids can be used in unresponsive cases.

INVESTIGATIONS AND TREATMENT

Tzanck test, skin biopsy and immunofluorescence are the investigations done to diagnose vesiculobullous disorders. Tzanck test is a cytodiagnostic technique where a smear is taken from the floor of a deroofed bulla and stained with Giemsa and Leishman stain. Specific cells are seen in each condition (Table 225.3). Immunofluorescence is the gold standard for diagnosing these disorders.

Treatment consists of oral corticosteroids, dapsone, cyclophosphamide, azathioprine, mycophenolate mofetil (MMF), dexamethasone-cyclophosphamide pulse therapy (DCP therapy) in severe cases and also plasmapheresis in life-threatening cases. The investigatory findings and treatment are summarized in Table 225.3.

RECENT ADVANCES

Immune electron microscopy can be used to determine the exact deposition of immunoreactants at various parts of the dermoepidermal junction. Rituximab, a monoclonal anti-CD20 biologic is used for treating resistant and recalcitrant pemphigus.

Table 225.3: Investigatory findings and treatment of vesiculobullous disorders

Description	Pemphigus vulgaris	Bullous pemphigoid	Dermatitis herpetiformis
Tzanck test	Acantholytic cells*	Eosinophils	Neutrophils
Skin biopsy	Suprabasal intraepidermal bullae with acantholytic cells	Subepidermal bullae containing eosinophils	Subepidermal bullae containing neutrophils
Immunofluorescence	IgG against intercellular cement substance	IgG against basement membrane zone	Granular IgA against upper papillary dermis
Electron microscopy	Antibody against desmoglein-3	Antibody against bullous pemphigoid antigen in hemidesmosomes	Antibody against epidermal transglutaminases
Treatment	Steroids, dapsone, cyclophosphamide, gold therapy, DCP therapy, plasmapheresis	Steroids	Dapsone

*Acantholytic cell is a rounded epidermal keratinocyte with hyperchromatic nuclei and perinuclear halo

Abbreviations: Ig = Immunoglobulin; DCP = Dexamethasone cyclophophamide pulse

CHAPTER
226

Urticaria and Angioedema

S Pradeep Nair

Chapter Summary

- History and Definition
- Clinical Features
  - Physical and Cholinergic Urticaria
  - Urticarial Vasculitis
  - Contact Urticaria
- Treatment of Urticaria
  - Recent advances
- Hereditary Angioedema
  - Other Forms of Treatment

HISTORY AND DEFINITION

Hippocrates first described urticarial pruritic lesions caused by nettles and mosquitoes which he named *knidosis*. It was in 1769 that William Cullen coined the term *urticaria*. Urticaria (*syn:* wheals, hives) is defined as transient erythematous papules and plaques occurring in the skin due to plasma leakage. Angioedema (*syn:* angioneurotic edema) is transient erythematous swelling of the dermis, subcutaneous and submucosal layers. Angioedema usually affects eyelids, lips, larynx and rarely genital mucosa. Laryngeal edema can be life-threatening. Urticaria and angioedema can coexist and occur as part of immunological and inflammatory reactions on the skin. Urticaria occurring on and off, for less than 6 weeks duration is acute urticaria and more than 6 weeks duration is called *chronic urticaria*. Dermatographism is an exaggerated axonal triple response, where urticarial lesions occur when a blunt object is drawn over the skin surface taking the pattern of the drawing. The classification and etiological factors for urticaria/angioedema are given in Table 226.1.

CLINICAL FEATURES

Urticaria presents as severely pruritic, superficial, well-defined, erythematous transient papules and plaques on any part of the skin (Fig. 226.1). The lesions can be round, oval, arciform, annular or serpiginous. These lesions are

Table 226.1: Classification and etiology of urticaria	
Classification	**Etiology**
• Acute and chronic urticaria • Physical and cholinergic urticaria • Urticarial vasculitis • Contact urticaria	• Infection • Infestation • Injections • Ingestion (food and drugs) • Inhalation (pollen grains, dust and smoke) • Insect bite (mosquitoes, wasp and bee stings) • Implants (dental and orthopedic)

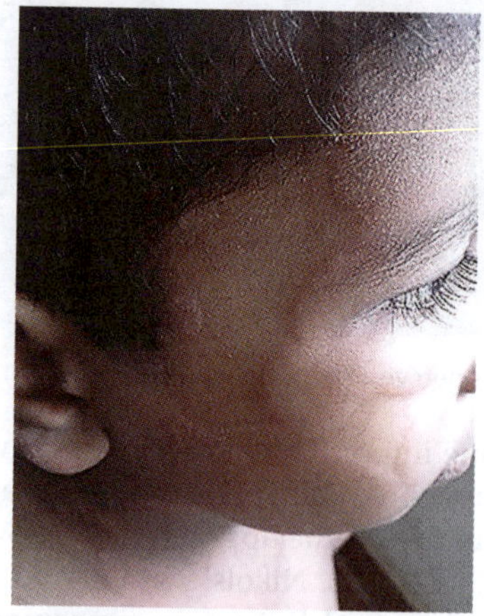

Fig. 226.1: Urticaria in a child due to food allergy

transient lasting not more than 24 hours and then fresh crops of lesions occur. Angioedema presents with ill-defined edema involving the dermis and subcutaneous tissue, commonly of the lips and eyelids. It may involve the upper respiratory tract and the patient may present with dyspnea and runs the risk of impending life-threatening laryngeal edema which is a medical emergency. Meticulous history-taking is very important keeping the etiological factors in mind. *Acute urticaria* is commonly due to drugs, food or infections. In children, foci of infection specially dental caries, helminthiasis and food are important factors. In most cases of chronic urticaria, the cause may be obscure (idiopathic).

Physical and Cholinergic Urticaria

Physical urticaria is caused by external stimuli. *Dermographism* is a type of physical urticaria where stroking the skin elicits the triple response.

Cholinergic urticaria (heat urticaria) is characterized by the presence of wheals when the patient sweats or does exercise. The wheals are very small and sometimes perifollicular.

Cold urticaria: The lesions are confined to the sites exposed to cold and occur within minutes after rewarming.

Aquagenic urticaria: It occurs when the patient comes in contact with water, irrespective of its temperature.

Solar urticaria: It occurs on exposure to sunlight (290–400 nm of the electromagnetic spectrum).

Urticarial Vasculitis

This type of urticaria is a type III hypersensitivity reaction and occurs in autoimmune disorders. Here, the wheals will persist for more than 24 hours and may be painful. Bullous lesions may also occur and investigations

Flowchart 226.1: Treatment protocol of urticaria

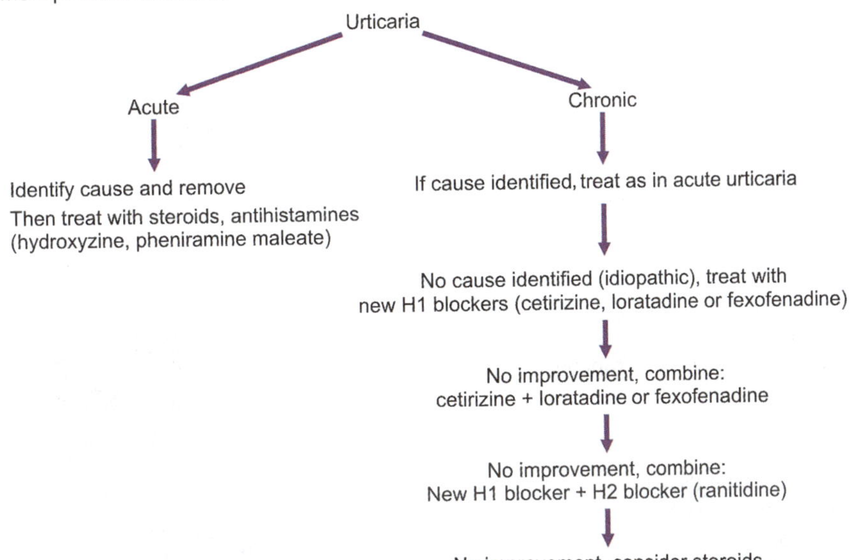

have to be done to find out systemic disorders. Collagen vascular disorders should be ruled out in this type of urticaria.

Contact Urticaria

It may be immune-mediated or nonimmune-mediated. Immunologic contact urticaria occurs in individuals sensitized to contact with external allergens like latex rubber gloves. This is also commonly seen in atopic children. Nonimmunologic contact urticaria is due to the direct effects of exogenous urticants penetrating into the skin or blood vessels, e.g. benzoic acid in eye solutions and foods, cinnamic aldehyde in cosmetics and serotonin in nettle stings. The wheals may occur within 2 hours of contact.

TREATMENT OF URTICARIA

In most cases, if the cause is identified and removed the urticaria subsides. The treatment protocol of urticaria is given in Flowchart 226.1.

Angioedema with impending laryngeal edema is a medical emergency as it is life-threatening. The treatment protocol is given below.

Treatment of angioedema with airway obstruction
• Injection adrenaline 0.5 mL SC or IM
• Injection hydrocortisone 100 mg IV
• Injection pheniramine maleate 22.75 mg IM
If no improvement: Endotracheal intubation/tracheostomy

Recent Advances

Omalizumab, a biologic, an anti-immunoglobulin E (IgE) monoclonal antibody is now used for treating recalcitrant chronic idiopathic urticaria.

HEREDITARY ANGIOEDEMA

It is a rare genetic disorder with autosomal dominant inheritance caused by complement (C1) esterase inhibitor deficiency characterized by recurrent attacks of swelling of the lips, usually precipitated by trauma, which may be painful and even life-threatening. It is nonpruritic and urticarial lesions are usually not present. Involvement of the respiratory tract and genitourinary tract has also been noted. Acquired C1 esterase inhibitor deficiency has been observed in systemic lupus erythematosus (SLE) and B-cell lymphomas.

Treatment of hereditary angioedema: Acute attack; fresh-frozen plasma (FFP) contains C1 esterase inhibitor, hence, 2–3 units of FFP are effective when specific drugs are not available. Anxiety, trauma, surgery, etc. aggravate angioedema and these situations have to be covered with C1 inhibitor. *Ruconest*® is a protein harvested from the milk of genetically modified rabbits and it is effective as a C1 esterase inhibitor.

Other Forms of Treatment

- The 17-alpha-alkylated attenuated androgens such as danazol and unattenuated androgens such as methyltestosterone reduce frequency and severity of attacks. Dose 200 mg danazol/day or 2 mg stanozolol/day. Dose of methyltestosterone 10–50 mg orally once a day or 5–25 mg buccal tablet once a day.
- Fibrinolytics like tranexamic are good prophylactics against acute attacks.
- Icatibant which is a 10 amino acid peptide inhibitor of bradykinin B2 receptor is effective in 30 mg doses given subcutaneously (SC) once a day.
- Nanofiltered C1 esterase inhibitor concentrate in a dose of 1,000 units IV once or twice reduced the frequency and duration of angioedema acute attacks.
- Ecallantide for treatment of acute attacks of hereditary angioedema. This is a recombinant protein specifically inhibiting kallikrein. *Dose:* 30 mg SC injection.

Source: Cicardi M, Levy RJ, McNeil DL, et al. Ecallantide for the treatment of acute attacks in hereditary angioedema. N Engl J Med. 2010;363:523-31.

Cutaneous Drug Reactions

S Pradeep Nair

Chapter Summary

- Common Drug Eruptions
- Clinical Features of Different Types of Eruptions
  - Maculopapular
  - Vesiculobullous
  - Erythema Multiforme
  - Stevens Johnson Syndrome (SJS)
  - Toxic Epidermal Necrolysis (TEN)
  - Exfoliative Drug Eruption
  - Fixed Drug Eruption (FDE)
  - Urticarial Drug Reactions
  - Acneiform Eruptions
  - Lichenoid Eruptions
  - Photosensitive Drug Reaction
  - Hyperpigmentation

INTRODUCTION

A drug reaction is defined as an undesirable clinical manifestation resulting from administration of a particular drug. Cutaneous drug reactions constitute 2.85% of the dermatological conditions seen in Kerala. The clinical manifestations of drug reactions are protein and can mimic many dermatoses. The classification of drug reactions as follows.

Common drug eruptions

- Maculopapular
- Vesiculobullous
- Exfoliative dermatitis
- Fixed drug reaction
- Urticarial
- Acneiform
- Lichenoid
- Photosensitive
- Hyperpigmentation

CLINICAL FEATURES OF DIFFERENT TYPES OF ERUPTIONS

Maculopapular

Maculopapular reaction (*syn.* exanthematous drug reaction) is the most common type of drug reaction. They are usually caused by penicillin and related antibiotics, allopurinol, gold salts and carbamazepine. Initial reaction usually occurs less than 14 days after drug intake. These eruptions present with symmetrical, pruritic erythematous macules and papules on the trunk and limbs (Fig. 227.1). Buccal mucosa may be involved. The *treatment* is to stop the incriminated drug. Antihistamines and topical calamine lotion relieve the symptoms. This type of drug reaction may mimic viral exanthems.

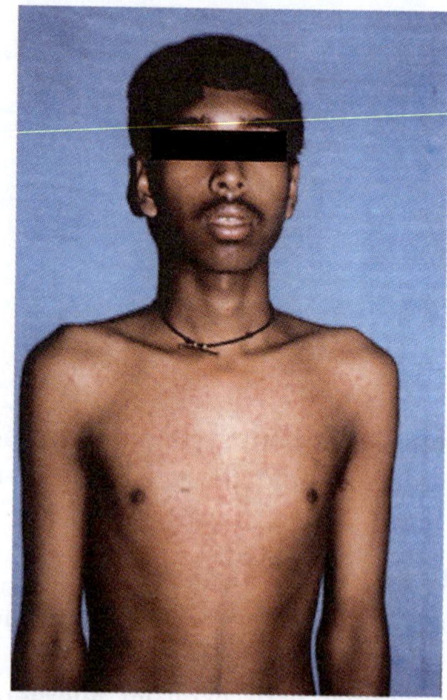

Fig. 227.1: Maculopapular rash due to ampicillin

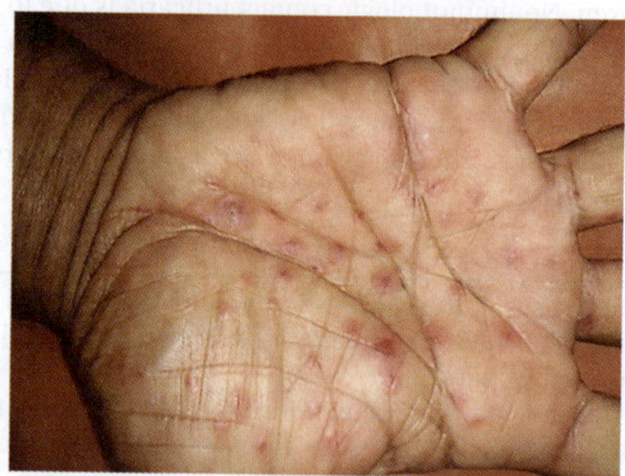

Fig. 227.2: Iris lesions of erythema multiforme

Vesiculobullous

Vesiculobullous drug reactions are commonly due to drugs like naproxen, nalidixic acid, furosemide and piroxicam. They can mimic pemphigus, pemphigoid, porphyria or linear immunoglobulin (Ig) A disease.

Erythema Multiforme

It is an acute self-limiting inflammatory disorder characterized by vesicles or bullae, papules, plaques, urticaria and the distinctive lesion is called *iris* or *target* lesion. The iris lesion presents with a central area of vesicle or purpura, a mid zone of edema and an outer ring of erythema (Fig. 227.2). The lesions are usually distributed on the dorsum of the hands, palms and extensor aspect of extremities. The oral mucous membrane and eyes can also be affected. Penicillins, sulfonamides, anticonvulsants and nonsteroidal anti-inflammatory drugs (NSAIDs) are the usual culprits. Other than drugs, a wide variety of etiological factors can cause erythema multiforme, specially infections like herpes simplex and mycoplasma. Recurrent erythema mutiforme is associated with herpes simplex infection.

Erythema multiforme is classified as minor and major (Table 227.1).

Stevens-Johnson Syndrome (SJS)

This is a serious drug reaction characterized by constitutional symptoms like fever followed by maculopapular rash, vesicles and bullae involving the trunk and limbs. The bullae rupture to form areas of extensive erosions. In contrast to erythema multiforme, atypical target lesions with only two zones and a poorly defined border characterize SJS. Atypical targets in SJS are flat with a central purpura with or without a vesicle, which may become confluent. Skin detachment is limited to less than 10% of body surface area, but with severe mucosal involvement. The eyes, oral cavity and genitals are invariably involved. The lips and oral cavity shows erosions and ulcers covered by hemorrhagic crusts (Fig. 227.3). The eyes may show purulent conjunctivitis and later corneal ulcers. The drugs commonly causing SJS in the state of Kerala is given in Box 227.1. Treatment is with high-dose prednisolone (40–60 mg/day), antibiotics and antihistamines. Intravenous immunoglobulin (IVIG) in doses of 0.4 g/kg/day given for 3–4 days is life-saving and therefore should be considered in severe cases. The care of the eye is very important. Frequent sterile saline irrigation for the eyes, topical eye antibiotics like tobramycin or quinolones, topical betamethasone or prednisolone eye drops are necessary. Eye should be managed by the ophthalmologists. Frequent rinsing of the oral cavity with chlorhexidine or dilute potassium permanganate mouthwashes is essential.

Management

Most of the milder cases resolve spontaneously in 2–3 weeks.

Aims of management
- Elimination of precipitating factors
- Treatment of underlying infection:
  - Erythromycin or azithromycin for mycoplasma infection.
  - Acyclovir for herpes simplex infection.
- Antihistamines
- Care of the eyes and mucous membranes
- Severe cases need hospitalization and administration of intravenous fluids and supportive care. Including acute care attention. Systemic glucocorticoids and immunosuppressants including human Ig may be necessary.

Toxic Epidermal Necrolysis (TEN)

It is a dermatological emergency with a very high mortality. Recently, some anti-human immunodeficiency virus (HIV) drugs are also known to cause TEN.

Table 227.1: Comparison between minor and major erythema multiforme	
Minor	**Major**
Typical target lesions are seen	Typical target lesions are seen
Acral distribution	Acral or widespread
Mucosal involvement is absent or few	Severe and often multiple mucosal involvement

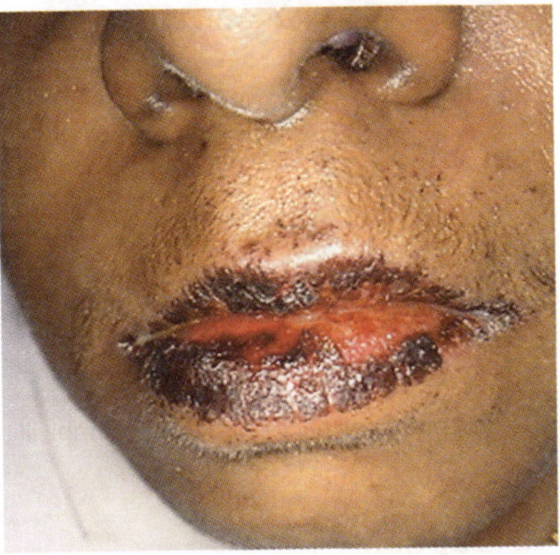

Fig. 227.3: Stevens-Johnson syndrome showing ulceration and crusting of lips

Box 227.1: Drugs causing Stevens-Johnson syndrome and toxic epidermal necrolysis

- Carbamazepine—abacavir
- Phenytoin—nevirapine
- Phenobarbitone
- Penicillins
- Sulfonamides
- Isonicotinylhydrazide (INH)
- Piroxicam
- Allopurinol

The patient first presents with high-grade fever and severe toxemia followed by purpuric macules on the trunk and limbs with a ***charred*** appearance involving more than 30% of the body area (Fig. 227.4). These lesions are soon followed by blistering and large areas of the skin sloughs off leading to extensive areas of erosions. When blisters and erosions involve 10–30% of the body surface area, it is termed as SJS-TEN overlap. There is severe oral, eye and genital mucosal involvement. Hepatitis and acute renal tubular necrosis are the systemic complications. Loss of large areas of skin leads to electrolyte imbalance, septicemia, bronchopneumonia and temperature dysregulation, which may lead to death. High-dose systemic steroids, antibiotics and IVIG have to be given. The use of systemic steroids in TEN is controversial and some have found an increased morbidity due to use of steroids. Barrier nursing, proper skin and eye care is essential for the patient.

Exfoliative Drug Eruption

Heavy metals like gold, phenytoin, isonicotinylhydrazide (INH), ayurvedic and homeopathic preparations are notorious to cause exfoliative type of drug reaction. Emollients like liquid paraffin, systemic steroids and antihistamines have to be given (Refer erythroderma).

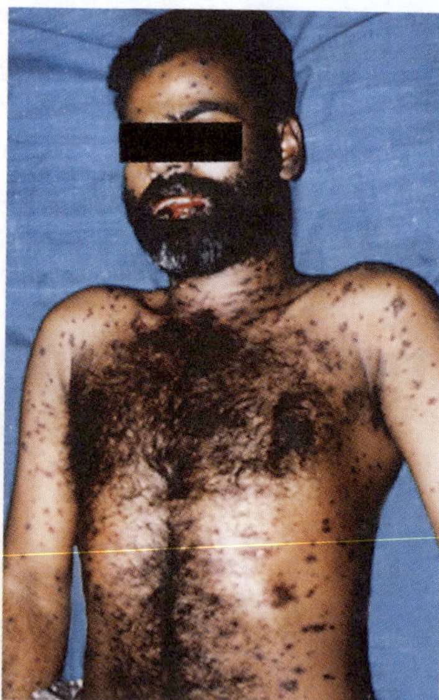

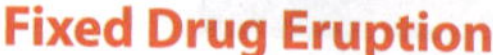

Fig. 227.4: Toxic epidermal necrolysis due to ampicillin carbamazepine

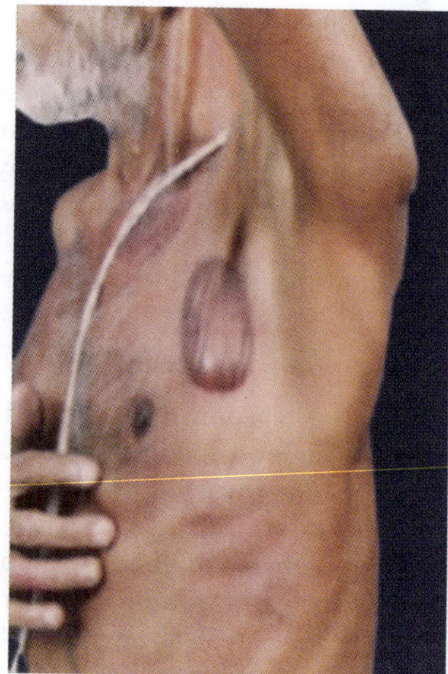

Fig. 227.5: Bullous lesion of fixed drug eruption caused by antituberculosis drugs

Fixed Drug Eruption

This is a localized type of drug reaction caused by paracetamol, sulfonamides, dapsone and tetracyclines. About 30 minutes to 8 hours after taking the drug, the patient may develop sharply demarcated macules, initially erythematous, then dusky red to violaceous and then become edematous, which may evolve to a bulla and erosion (Fig. 227.5). Common sites are the limbs, face or trunk. Sometimes there may be painful blisters and erosions on the oral or genital mucosa. The lesions heal by themselves with postinflammatory hyperpigmentation, but on subsequent exposure to the same drug the lesions recur at the same sites or other sites (Fig. 227.6).

Urticarial Drug Reactions

Urticaria and angioedema are usually caused by penicillins, cephalosporins and sulfonamides. Urticarial drug reactions can also occur as a part of anaphylaxis where the patient will have bronchospasm and vasomotor collapse. Adrenaline (0.5 mL SC), hydrocortisone (100 mg) and pheniramine maleate (10–20 mg) injections are life-saving.

Acneiform Eruptions

Steroids, INH and phenytoin are the drugs causing acneiform eruptions. It is characterized by monomorphic, acne-like lesions distributed on the face, limbs and trunk. Comedones are absent. Stopping drug will clear the lesions.

Lichenoid Eruptions

It presents as pruritic violaceous papules resembling lichen planus on the trunk and upper limbs. Oral lesions are absent. Gold salts, captopril, antimalarials and beta-blockers may produce lichenoid eruption.

Photosensitive Drug Reaction

Photosensitizing drugs like psoralens, sulfonamides, tetracyclines, retinoids, chlorpromazine and thiazide diuretics cause this type of reaction. Erythema, papules

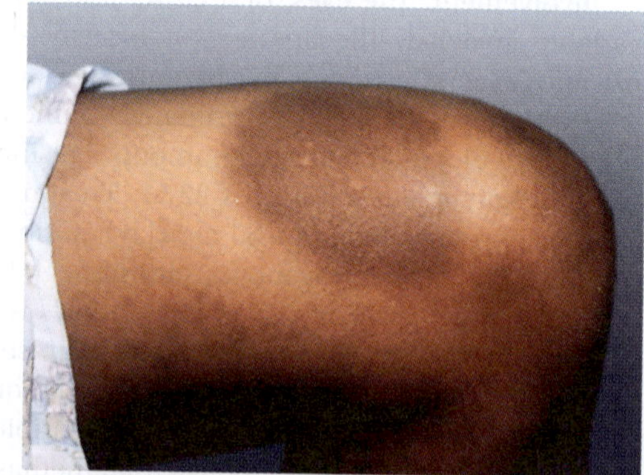

Fig. 227.6: Fixed drug eruption due to sulfonamide. **Note:** The post-inflammatory hyperpigmentation

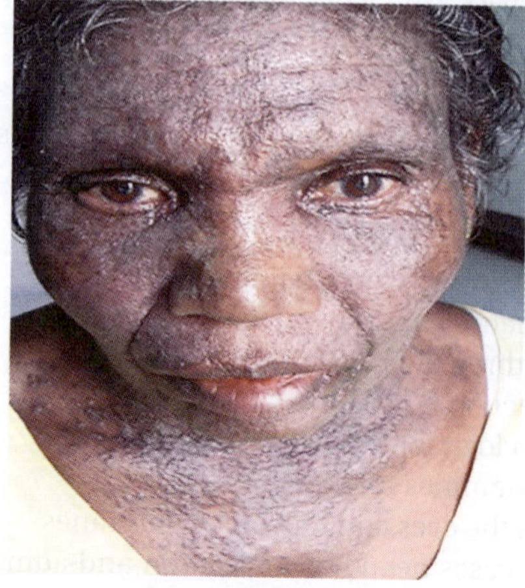

Fig. 227.7: Psoralen-induced photosensitive hyperpigmentation

and sometimes vesiculation occurs on the face and extensor aspect of upper limbs (sun-exposed areas).

Hyperpigmentation

Clofazimine, chlorpromazine, minocycline, psoralens and antimalarials are the common drugs which cause diffuse hyperpigmentation of the face and trunk (Fig. 227.7).

CHAPTER
228

Disorders of Blood Vessels and Lymphatics

S Pradeep Nair

Chapter Summary

- Disorders of Blood Vessels
  - Vasculitis
  - Stasis Ulcer (Varicose Ulcer)
  - Neuropathic Ulcers
- Disorders of Lymphatics
  - Lymphedema
  - Lymphangioma Circumscriptum

DISORDERS OF BLOOD VESSELS

Diseases of arteries and veins contribute to a large variety of dermatoses, leg ulcers being the most common. The common causes of leg ulcers in India are given in Box 228.1.

Vasculitis

It is the inflammation of small- and large-blood vessels. The blood vessel is infiltrated by polymorphonuclear cells, lymphocytes or granulomas. It presents with well-defined painful punched out ulcers on the lower aspect of the legs (Fig. 228.1). It can also be a manifestation of systemic disorders like systemic lupus erythematosus (SLE). ***Pyoderma gangrenosum*** is a type of vasculitis that presents with single or multiple well-defined painful ulcers with undermined edges and a violaceous border on the trunk and lower extremities (Fig. 228.2). It may be associated with systemic disorders, especially inflammatory bowel disease (IBD). Treatment of the primary cause leads to healing of ulcers.

Stasis Ulcer (Varicose Ulcer)

Chronic venous insufficiency of the deep veins of the legs leads to edema and later ulceration. It presents as chronic nonhealing ulcers on the lower-medial aspect of the legs along with stasis eczema with surrounding hyperpigmentation due to stasis of blood (Fig. 228.3). The lesions in the veins can be demonstrated by Doppler studies of the venous system. Foot-end elevation, pressure stockings and management of eczema by regular use of emollients and topical steroids and antibiotics are

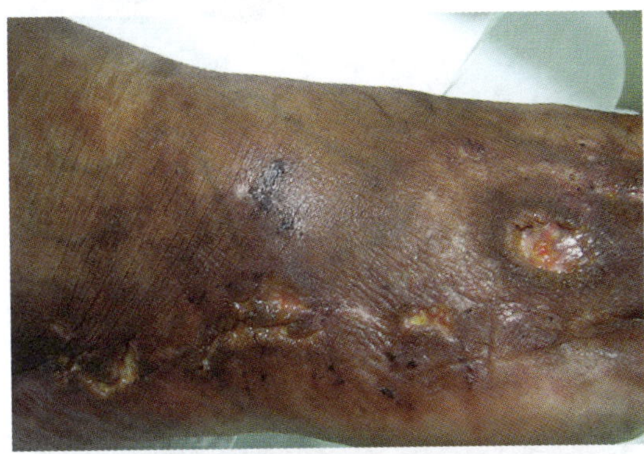

Fig. 228.1: Vasculitic ulcers. ***Note:*** The deep punched out ulcers

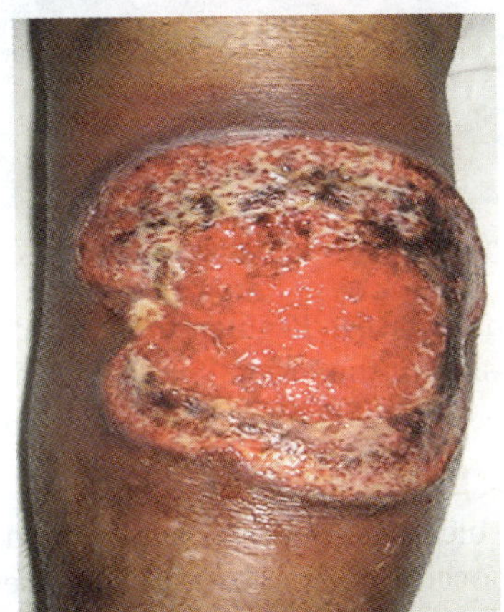

Fig. 228.2: Pyoderma gangrenosum

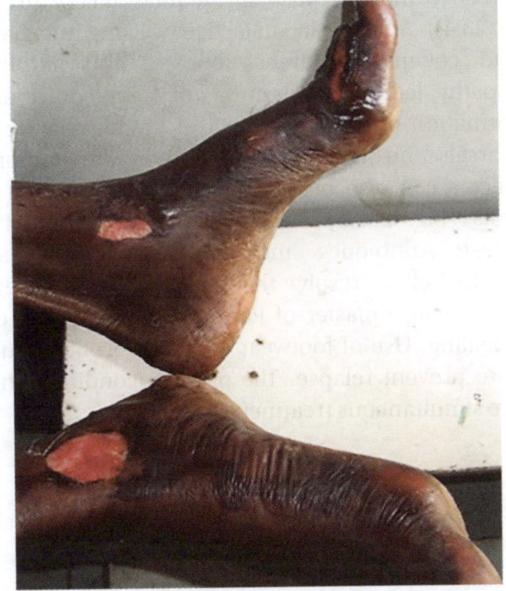

Fig. 228.3: Stasis ulcer. ***Note:*** The surrounding pigmentation

---

Box 228.1: Common causes of leg ulcers

- Traumatic
- Arterial occlusion—atherosclerosis, thromboembolism and thromboangiitis obliterans
- Vasculitis—SLE, rheumatoid arthritis, pyoderma gangrenosum
- Venous—stasis ulcers
- Infections—fungal and parasitic
- Neuropathic—leprosy, diabetes mellitus, tabes dorsalis
- Malignancies—squamous cell carcinoma and Kaposi's sarcoma

Abbreviation: SLE = Systemic lupus erythematosus

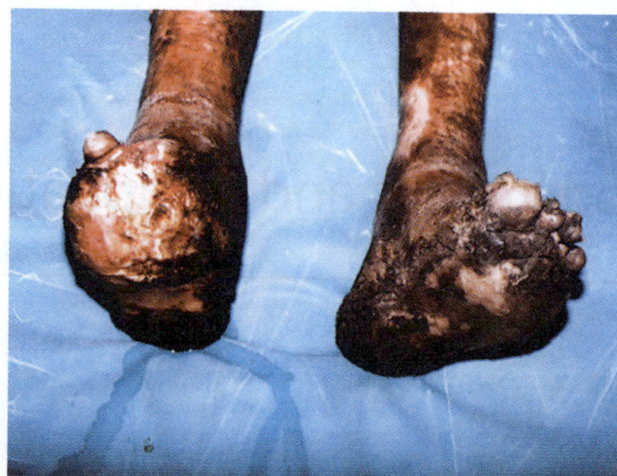

Fig. 228.4: Leprosy with neuropathic ulcer

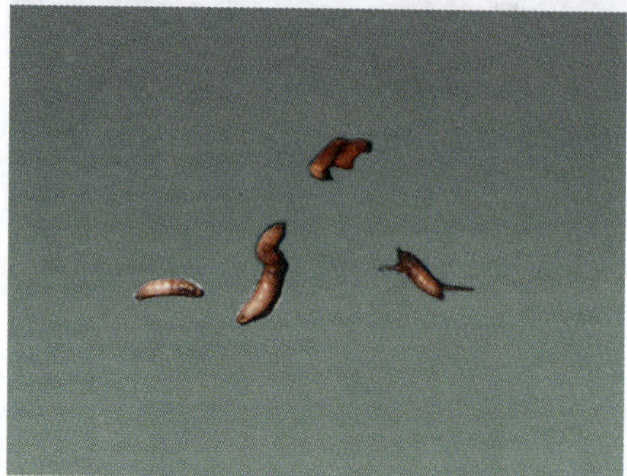

Fig. 228.5: Maggots in the neuropathic ulcer

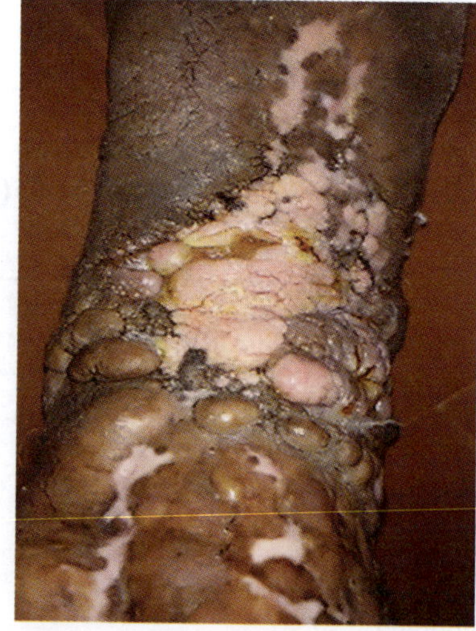

Fig. 228.6: Elephantiasis verrucosa nostra

helpful in mild cases. Regular foot exercises help to allay progression of the lesion. Surgical treatment of the varicose veins may be required in intractable cases.

Neuropathic Ulcers

Neuropathic ulcers complicate sensory and autonomic neuropathy occurring in several diseases such as diabetes mellitus (DM), leprosy and other forms of sensory neuropathies, syringomyelia and others. Leprosy is a very common cause for plantar ulcers in India (Fig. 228.4). Anesthesia, defective walking mechanism due to collapse of arches of feet and autonomic neuropathy leading to fissuring of soles contribute to the formation of the ulcers. Ball of the big toe, head of metatarsals and heel are the common sites for ulcers. The ulcers can also be complicated by infestation with maggots (Fig. 228.5). The patient should be advised bed rest. Antibiotics and potassium permanganate foot baths help to resolve the ulcers. Once the ulcer has become clean a plaster of Paris cast may be applied to help healing. Use of footwear with microcellular rubber helps to prevent relapse. The primary condition should receive simultaneous treatment.

DISORDERS OF LYMPHATICS

Lymphedema

Accumulation of lymph in the soft tissues due to obstruction leads to lymphedema. The common causes of lymphedema are given below.

Causes of lymphedema
• Congenital—Milroy's disease, rare
• Acquired
▪ Filariasis
▪ Chronic cellulitis
▪ Lymphangitis
▪ Proximal lymphatic obstruction

Lymphedema presents with erythema and edema of the lower limbs, upper limbs or external genitals depending upon the cause. In chronic cases, the edema becomes nonpitting. Recurrent fever with rigor and chills and streptococcal cellulitis complicates lymphedema caused by filariasis. Chronic lymphatic obstruction is common in malignant metastasis in the lymph nodes, in surgical removal and irradiation of the lymphatic system. Chronic lymphedema may be complicated by verrucous nodules and plaques on the skin surface known as *elephantiasis verrucosa nostra* (Fig. 228.6). This may be rarely complicated by lymphangiosarcoma. There is no specific treatment. Cellulitis and lymphangitis should be treated with penicillin. Surgery may be required in some cases (*See* also Section 6, Ch 70).

Lymphangioma Circumscriptum

This is a localized congenital lymphatic malformation characterized by confluent vesicles resembling frog spawn, distributed on the axillary folds, proximal part of limbs, perineum and tongue. ***Treatment*** is by surgical excision or ablation by CO_2 laser.

CHAPTER
229

Disorders of Pigmentation

S Pradeep Nair

Chapter Summary

- Disorders of Hypermelanosis
- Freckles
- Lentigines
- Melasma (Chloasma)
- Incontinentia Pigmenti
- Disorders of Hypomelanosis
- Vitiligo

Normal skin color is determined by the amount and distribution of melanin in the skin. Increase or decrease of melanin in the epidermis results in hyper- or hypomelanosis respectively.

DISORDERS OF HYPERMELANOSIS

Dermatoses and systemic disorders that present with hypermelanosis are given in Table 229.1.

FRECKLES

Also known as ephelides, this autosomal dominant condition presents with hyperpigmented macules on the face and other sun-exposed areas (Fig. 229.1). This disorder is more common on the white Caucasian skin. There is no increase in the number of melanocytes. ***Treatment*** is by applying sunblocks like zinc oxide or sunscreens containing avobenzones, oxybenzone, anthranilates, cinnamates or octyl salicylates, avoiding excessive sunlight and cosmetic chemical peeling by phenol, solid CO_2 and glycolic acid.

Table 229.1: Disorders of hypermelanosis

Dermatoses	Systemic disorders
• Freckles	• Incontinentia pigmenti
• Lentigines	• Peutz-Jeghers syndrome
• Melasma	• Albright syndrome
• Café-au-lait macules	• Fanconi's anemia
	• Endocrine disorders

LENTIGINES

Lentigines are hyperpigmented macules arising due to increased melanocytes at the dermoepidermal junction. They may be single, segmental or multiple. Lentigines can be differentiated from freckles by the persistence of lesions even in the absence of sun exposure. Freckles become conspicuous on sun exposure and lighten when not exposed. Multiple lentigines can occur as part of syndromes like ***LEOPARD syndrome*** consisting of ***L***-lentigines, ***E***-electrocardiogram (ECG) abnormalities, ***O***-ocular hypertelorism, ***P***-pulmonary stenosis, ***A***-abnormal genitalia (infantilism, cryptorchidism), ***R***-retardation of growth, ***D***-deafness. Lentigines can affect any area of the skin and mucous membrane. There is no specific treatment.

MELASMA (CHLOASMA)

This disorder mainly affects women and presents with hyperpigmented macules and patches on the cheeks and forehead (Fig. 229.2). It results from exposure to sunlight. Pregnancy and use of oral contraceptives predispose to the condition, indicating a hormonal relationship. Treatment is by a combination of topical depigmenting agents like hydroquinone 2–4%, tretinoin 0.025–0.05% and hydrocortisone 1%. Chemical peeling with trichloroacetic acid or glycolic acid is useful. Sun block creams such as zinc oxide are essential in the prevention of melasma.

INCONTINENTIA PIGMENTI

This X-linked dominant genodermatoses present with bullous lesions at birth evolving into warty plaques

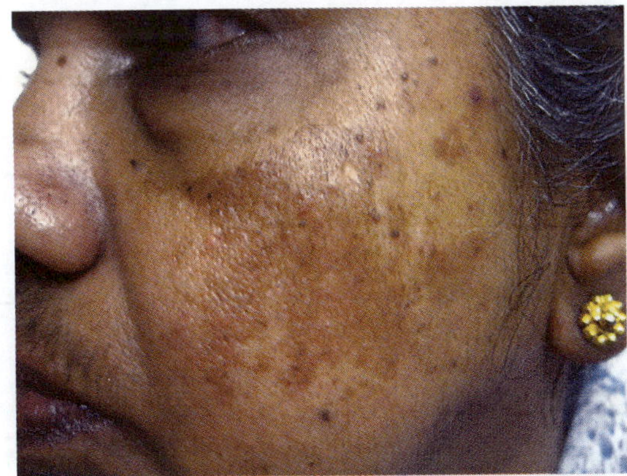

Fig. 229.1: Freckles on the face

Fig. 229.2: Hyperpigmented macules of melasma on the malar region

and later healing with hyperpigmented macules and patches with a bizarre pattern resembling Chinese figures distributed on the trunk and limbs. There may be associated ocular defects like cataracts, papillitis, congenital retinal folds and optic atrophy and dental defects like delayed dentition, impacted and missing teeth, pegged teeth and malformed crowns. There is no definite treatment. Genetic counseling is a must.

Peutz-Jeghers Syndrome (PJS)

It is characterized by intestinal polyposis with periorificial lentigines. They are prone to develop intestinal malignancy (Refer Section 8, Ch 79).

DISORDERS OF HYPOMELANOSIS

Disorders presenting with hypopigmentation and depigmentation are given in Table 229.2.

VITILIGO

This is a primary autoimmune depigmentary disorder. Vitiligo accounts for 3.12% of the skin disorders in Kerala. Secondary postinflammatory depigmentation is called leukoderma. In a vitiligo patch, melanocytes are absent and hence no melanin production. Vitiligo presents with multiple depigmented macules and patches on any area of the skin including oral and genital mucosa (Fig. 229.3). They may be localized, segmental or generalized. Sometimes the hair on a vitiligo patch may also be depigmented known as leukotrichia. Vitiligo may be associated with other autoimmune disorders.

Vitiligo Subtypes

- Localized
  - Focal—one more depigmented macules
  - Segmental
  - Mucosal

Table 229.2: Disorders of hypomelanosis		
Genetic	**Systemic disorders**	**Dermatoses**
- Albinism - Piebaldism - Tuberous sclerosis - Vitiligo	- Hypopituitarism - Thyroid diseases - Pernicious anemia - Other autoimmune diseases	- Leprosy - Pityriasis alba - Pityriasis versicolor - Syphilis - Sarcoidosis

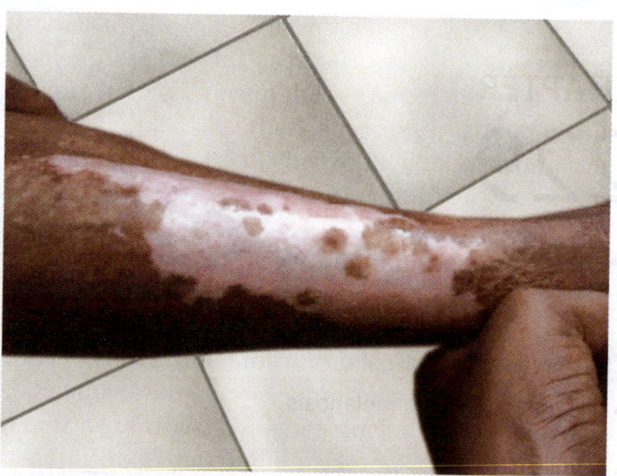

Fig. 229.3: Vitiligo—depigmented patches on the shin

- Generalized
  - Vitiligo vulgaris—multiple bilateral macules and patches
  - Lip-Tip vitiligo—tips of digits and lips only
  - Acrofacial—hands, feet and face are involved

Universal: Complete or near complete depigmentation of the body.

Treatment: Psoralens + ultraviolet A (PUVA) is very effective in extensive vitiligo. 8-methoxy psoralen is given in a dose of 0.6 mg/kg (20 mg for an adult) orally. Two hours later, the lesions are exposed to UV light repeatedly for increasing duration till repigmentation, which usually occurs in 12–18 months. Alternatively, sunlight can be employed as the source of ultraviolet light (PUVA-SOL) for 15–30 minutes. This procedure is done 2–3 times/week. Eye protection with UVA blocking glasses is necessary during and after treatment. Extensive and acutely occurring vitiligo responds satisfactorily to systemic steroids and these drugs have to be used with caution. Localized vitiligo with a few patches, especially on the face, responds to topical steroids and tacrolimus or pimecrolimus. Topical PUVA can also be added.

RECENT ADVANCES

Advances in cosmetic and dermatosurgery for vitiligo has now greatly helped vitiligo patients. Punch grafting, suction blister grafting and autologous melanocyte transfer are some of new procedures. These should be done in stable vitiligo.

CHAPTER
230

Disorders of Hair and Nails

S Pradeep Nair

Chapter Summary

- Disorders of Hair
  - General Considerations
  - Alopecia Areata
- Hypertrichosis
- Hirsutism
- Pseudopelade of Brocq
- Folliculitis Decalvans (FD)

- Acne Keloidalis Nuchae (AKN)
- Canities
- Diseases of Nails
  - Paronychia
  - Onychomycosis
  - Nail Psoriasis
- Miscellaneous Conditions Affecting the Nails
  - Leukonychia
  - Longitudinal Melanonychia
  - Ingrowing Toenail

DISORDERS OF HAIR

General Considerations

The hair is a skin appendage unique to mammals. It develops from the primary epithelial germ layer at the third month of gestation. Hair is a vestigial structure with no vital function, though it has immense psychological importance.

The hair growth is cyclic. The growing phase is known as *anagen* and lasts for an average 3 years. The involutionary stage, *catagen* is driven by apoptosis. It lasts for a few weeks. *Telogen* is the quiescent resting phase which lasts for a few months, normally 10% of follicles are in telogen. The active process of hair shaft shedding is called *exogen*.

The human scalp has approximately 100,000 hair follicles. Normally an average of 100 hairs are shed daily. Scalp hair grows at a rate of 0.3 mm/day.

Hair disorders account for 1.89% of skin diseases seen in Kerala. The common hair disorders are:

- *Alopecia*—loss of hair (Flowchart 230.1)
- *Hypertrichosis*—excessive hair growth
- *Hirsutism*—male pattern hair growth in a female—androgen dependent
- *Hair shaft abnormalities*—trichorrhexis (breaking of the hair), pili torti, trichorrhexis invaginata, monilethrix (beaded hair), woolly hair
- *Congenital*—hypohidrotic ectodermal dysplasia
- *Variation in hair pigmentation*—canities.

Flowchart 230.1: Classification of alopecia

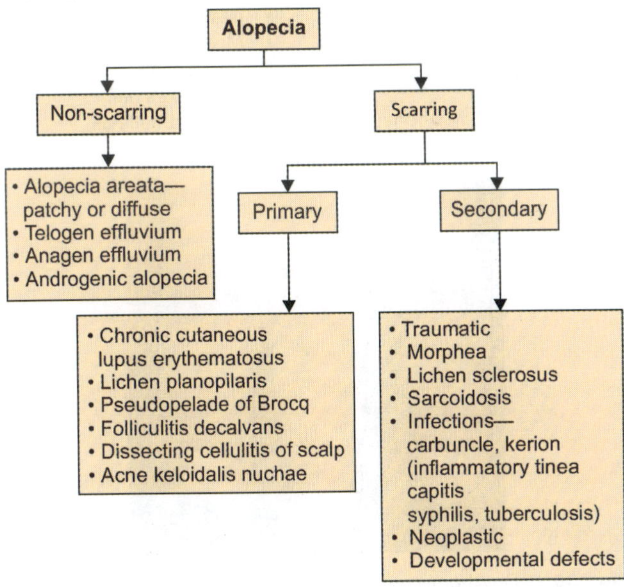

Alopecia Areata

This is an autoimmune disease characterized by localized reversible loss of hair usually involving the scalp, moustache and beard area, even though any hair bearing area can be affected. The involved area will resemble a bald patch and at the periphery typical 'exclamatory' hairs can be seen (Fig. 230.1). Exclamation mark hairs are broken off stubby hairs where the distal ends are broader than the proximal ends. *Alopecia totalis* is denoted when the entire scalp hair is lost and *alopecia universalis (AU)*, when the entire body hair is lost (Fig. 230.2). Treatment is by topical irritants like salicylic acid, topical steroids and intralesional triamcinolone. Tacrolimus, a calcineurin inhibitor, is a new topical preparation for alopecia areata. The patient should be reassured of its benign nature and spontaneous recovery.

AT and AU have poor prognosis and may require PUVA (psoralen and ultraviolet A radiation) therapy and systemic steroids.

Cicatricial Alopecia

This is a scarring alopecia and the hair does not regrow. Scarring alopecia is caused by trauma, infections, follicular lichen planus of scalp, discoid lupus erythematosus (DLE) and malignancies. Hair transplantation or the use of artificial hair is indicated to relieve psychological distress and social disability.

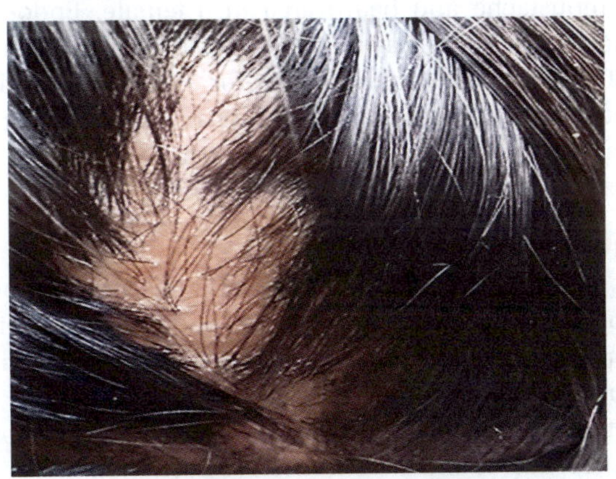

Fig. 230.1: Alopecia areata

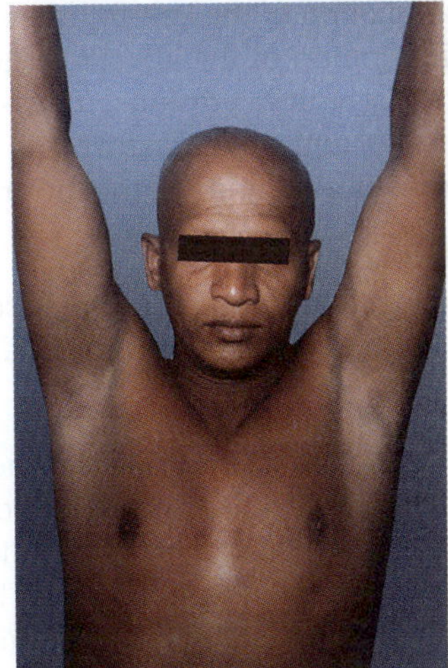

Fig. 230.2: Alopecia universalis (AU)

Androgenic Alopecia

This is male pattern baldness and is an androgen-dependent condition with a strong familial background. The most common type of clinical presentation is frontoparietal hair recession. Hamilton's scale is used for grading the degree of hair loss. Treatment is with topical minoxidil 2–5% and/or systemic antiandrogen drugs like finasteride (1 mg/day). Female pattern alopecia may have to be treated with antiandrogens like cyproterone acetate (100 mg/day), flutamide (250 mg/day) and spironolactone (200 mg/day). Unresponsive patients may require hair transplantation.

Hypertrichosis

Increased hair growth in areas of normal growth is called hypertrichosis. It can be congenital, acquired or iatrogenic. *Congenital hypertrichosis lanuginosa (CHL)* is a condition where the infant's skin is covered by lanugo hair. The hair will be silky and the entire body, except the palms and soles will be affected. *Acquired hypertrichosis lanuginosa (AHL)* is a paraneoplastic manifestation. Steroids, phenytoin, minoxidil and diazoxide are the drugs causing hypertrichosis.

Hirsutism

This is male pattern hair occurring in females. Terminal hairs develop on the androgen-dependent areas like the moustache and beard area in a female. Endocrine abnormalities may play a role. Polycystic ovary syndrome (PCOS) is an important cause for hirsutism. Medical treatment includes antiandrogens like finasteride, flutamide and spironolactone. Electrolysis and laser epilation are the new modalities of therapy.

Pseudopelade of Brocq

This is a unique form of cicatricial alopecia resembling alopecia areata; commonly it affects middle age. It is a rare idiopathic self-limiting hair disorder leading to cicatricial alopecia involving the parietal and other regions. No treatment is fully satisfactory. Even though topical glucocorticoids and tacrolimus have been tried.

Folliculitis Decalvans (FD)

This is an inflammation of the hair follicle which leads to bogginess or induration of the affected regions of scalp. This may show pustules, erosions, crusts and scales. Treatment consists anti-inflammatory and antibacterial local applications, local steroid creams and oral antibiotics.

Acne Keloidalis Nuchae (AKN)

This is acne with pustules running a chronic course leading to keloid formation, especially over the neck.

Canities

Graying of hair is known as canities and premature graying of hair is denoted when graying occurs below 20 years of age. Genetics may play a role in premature graying. Calcium pantothenate may be beneficial in some patients. Premature graying may also occur in some congenital premature aging syndromes like Werner's syndrome (WS).

DISEASES OF NAILS

The fingernails grow approximately 0.1 mm/day and toenails one-third of this rate. The nail lesions may at times reflect serious systemic disorders. The common nail disorders are given in Box 230.1.

Paronychia

Acute paronychia is a staphylococcal infection of the nail folds. The patient presents with painful swelling and erythema of the nail folds. Compression helps to extrude pus. *Chronic paronychia* is seen in domestic workers, fishmongers and canteen workers who frequently come into contact with water. Chronic paronychia is caused by a combination of *Staphylococcus* and *Candida albicans*. There is separation of cuticle from nail plate and retraction of the proximal nail fold. It may be associated with swelling, redness and mild tenderness of the proximal nail fold.

Acute paronychia may need incision and drainage, and systemic antibiotics like cloxacillin or cephalosporins. Chronic paronychia is managed by topical antifungal agents like clotrimazole lotion or a combination with topical steroids like betamethasone twice daily for 3–6 months. Topical amorolfine nail lacquer applied twice weekly is effective in localized distal nail infection. If proximal nail damage occurs, oral antifungal therapy with itraconazole 200–400 mg/day for 6 weeks or pulse therapy with 400 mg/day for 1 week/month, for 3 months, is required. Prevention is by stopping wet work and use of gloves to protect hands.

Onychomycosis

Fungal infection of the nails is called onychomycosis and caused by dermatophyte species or by *Candida albicans* (Fig. 230.3). One or more nails may be affected. The nails will be discolored, brittle and sometimes total dystrophy may occur. The condition is generally resistant to treatment. Systemic therapy with griseofulvin (500 mg/day) for 3 months for fingernails and 6 months for toenails is required. Pulsed doses of itraconazole, 200 mg bd for 7 days a month, repeated twice for

Box 230.1: Common nail disorders	
• Paronychia	• Beau's nail
• Onychomycosis	• Mee's nail
• Nail psoriasis	• Terry's nail
• Leukonychia	• Muehrcke's nail
• Twenty-nail dystrophy	• Half-and-half nail

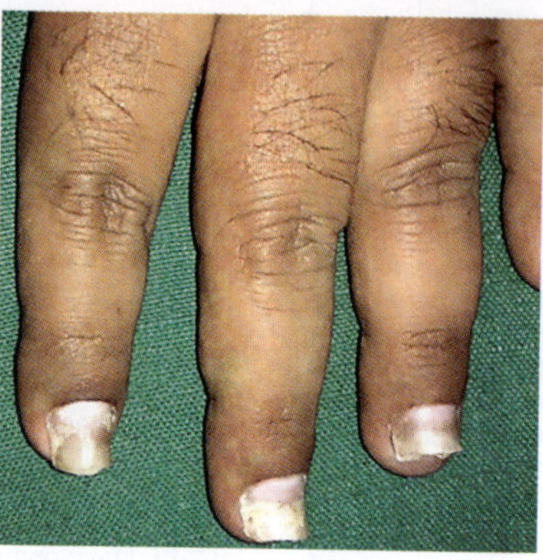

Fig. 230.3: Onychomycosis of the finger nails

fingernails and thrice for toenails are effective. Terbinafine 250 mg/day for 6 weeks is the treatment for dermatophyte infections of nails. Amorolfine, a nail lacquer applied once or twice a week is effective.

Nail Psoriasis

Psoriasis is the most common dermatosis affecting the nails. Fine pitting is the hallmark of psoriasis. Pitting of nail can also occur in alopecia areata. ***Oil spot macule*** is the most specific nail change seen as a yellowish brown macule on nail plate. Subungual hyperkeratosis is thickening of distal end of the nail with retained keratin underneath. Onycholysis is lateral or distal separation of the nail plate from nail bed which can be seen in fungal infections and eczemas also. Sometimes dystrophy of all the nails can occur (Fig. 230.4).

MISCELLANEOUS CONDITIONS AFFECTING THE NAILS

Leukonychia is whitish discoloration of the nails as a consequence of hypoproteinemia and renal or hepatic disease. *Longitudinal melanonychia* is a hyperpigmented streak seen in the nail plate which may be congenital, drug induced (zidovudine) and due to lichen planus (Fig. 230.5).

- ***Twenty-nail dystrophy*** is considered to be a manifestation of lichen planus where all the 20 nails are dystrophic.
- ***Beau's nails*** are transverse grooves seen on the nail plate sometimes involving all the nails. They may

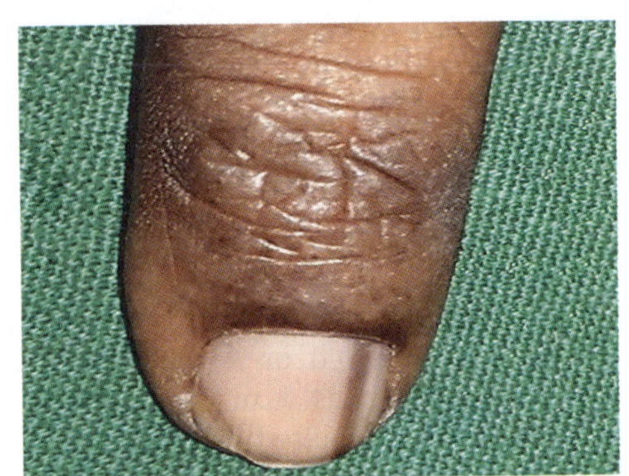

Fig. 230.5: Longitudinal melanonychia due to zidovudine

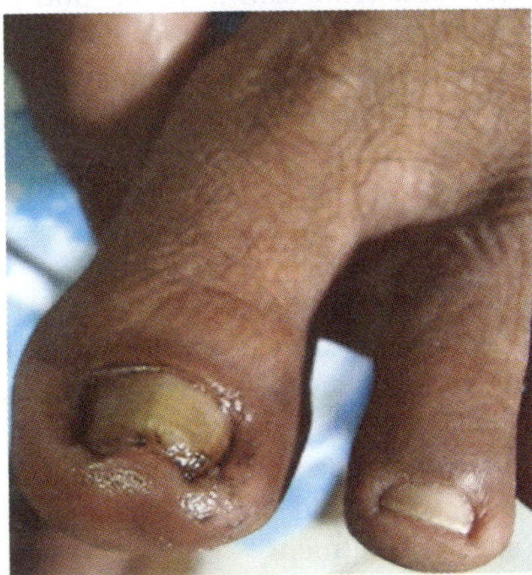

Fig. 230.6: Ingrowing toenail

follow severe systemic illnesses like pneumonia and is due to a temporary arrest of nail growth.

- ***Mee's nails*** are white transverse bands seen on the nail plate and may be a manifestation of chronic arsenic poisoning or chemotherapy.

Ingrowing toenail is where the distal lateral part of the nail penetrates the skin and grows downward causing severe inflammation and pain (Fig. 230.6). This occurs due to poor nail cutting technique and tight fitting shoes. The nail has to be avulsed and lateral matrix cauterized by phenol.

The other nail disorders shown in the Box 230.1 are described in the cutaneous manifestations of systemic disorders.

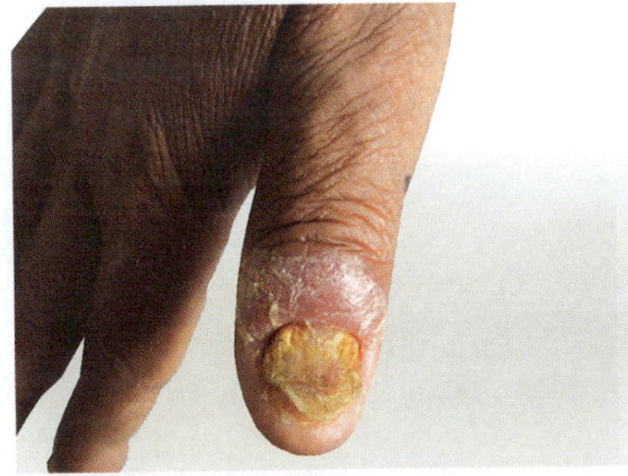

Fig. 230.4: Nails show onychodystrophy, onycholysis and subungual hyperkeratosis with psoriasis of the adjacent skin

CHAPTER
231

Disorders of Elastin and Collagen Fibers

S Pradeep Nair

Chapter Summary

- Elastin and Collagen Fibers
  - Cutis Laxa
  - Pseudoxanthoma Elasticum

- Striae Distensae
- Anetoderma (Macular Atrophy)
- Ehlers-Danlos Syndrome
- Keloid and Hypertrophic Scar

ELASTIN AND COLLAGEN FIBERS

The elastin and collagen fibers of the skin give strength and elasticity to the skin. The disorders affecting these fibers are given in Table 231.1.

Cutis Laxa

It is a heterogeneous group of elastic tissue disorders characterized by skin laxity and involvement of internal organs. It may be inherited or acquired, localized or generalized. Inherited cutis laxa may be autosomal dominant or recessive. Acquired cutis laxa is seen as a sequel of recurrent urticaria, angioedema and systemic lupus erythematosus (SLE) in a few cases. Abnormalities of elastic fibers cause the skin to be lax and pendulous, hanging in folds especially on the face and axilla giving the patient a **blood hound** or **old man** facies (Fig. 231.1). The skin loses its elasticity. Pinching the skin causes slow recoiling. Plastic surgery procedures like **face lift** operations may benefit the patient.

Pseudoxanthoma Elasticum

This autosomal dominant disorder affects the elastic fibers of the skin, blood vessels and eyes. The skin is soft, lax and wrinkled involving the sides of neck, flexures and abdomen. The skin on the neck may have a **chicken skin** or **cobblestone** appearance. The patient may have cardiac and ocular defects. Angioid streaks of the retina are seen. There is no specific treatment.

Striae Distensae

These are linear scars occurring due to skin stretching in pregnancy, weight lifters and sometimes in Cushing's syndrome. These present as linear hypopigmented or depigmented scars on the breast, axilla, lower abdomen and thighs. Prolonged topical therapy with potent corticosteroids may also cause striae (Fig. 231.2) in the area of application. Topical retinoids may help to resolve the condition in some patients.

Anetoderma (Macular Atrophy)

This represents a localized area of slack skin due to elastic fiber damage. It may be primary or secondary to syphilis, leprosy or SLE. They present as outpouchings of the skin on the trunk, upper arms and thighs. The surface of the skin is wrinkled. A finger can be insinuated into the lesions. There is no effective treatment.

Ehlers-Danlos Syndrome

This is an inherited disorder of collagen fibers. There are eleven subtypes of this syndrome. Abnormalities of collagen fibers cause increased fragility of the skin and blood vessels. The skin is hyperextensible and rebounds quickly after pinching in contrast to cutis laxa. There is

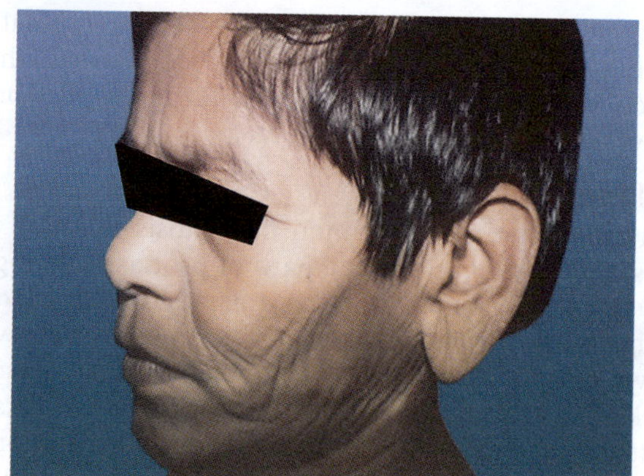

Fig. 231.1: Acquired cutis laxa

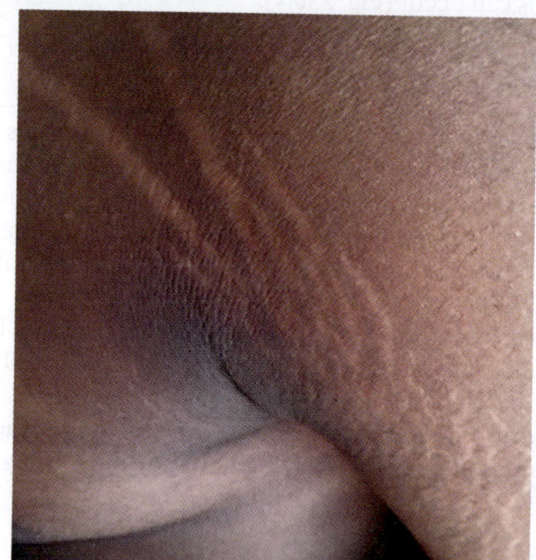

Fig. 231.2: Striae distensae on the axilla

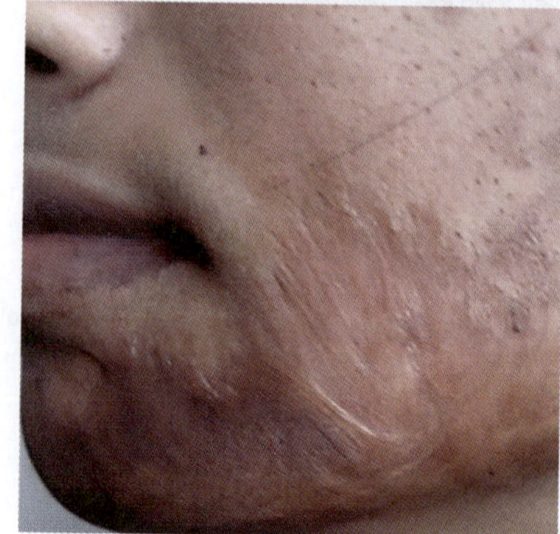

Fig. 231.3: Postburn keloid on the face

hypermobility of the joints resulting in joint damage. Ecchymosis is seen in type V and ocular involvement in type VI (*See* Section 10, Ch 95).

Keloid and Hypertrophic Scar

These are localized areas of excessive collagen tissue response following injury. Keloids may occur *de novo* or following injury, burns or acne (Fig. 231.3). It presents as firm skin colored or hyperpigmented plaques with

Table 231.1: Disorders of elastin and collagen fibers	
Elastin	**Collagen**
• Cutis laxa	• Ehlers-Danlos syndrome
• Pseudoxanthoma elasticum	• Pachydermoperiostosis
• Striae distensae	• Keloid/hypertrophic scars
• Anetoderma	
• Marfan's syndrome	

peripheral pseudopodia like extensions. The most common site is over the sternum. Extensive keloids are seen following burns. Keloid has to be distinguished from hypertrophic scar. The latter is confined to the original site of injury unlike keloid and it usually undergoes resolution. *Treatment* is recommended for both conditions. Intralesional triamcinolone up to a maximum of 10 mg per sitting is helpful to favor resolution. Simultaneous use of cryotherapy with liquid nitrogen hastens resolution. Results are better for hypertrophic scars. Carbon dioxide (CO_2) laser ablation therapy is helpful in resistant cases.

Cutaneous Manifestations of Systemic Disorders

CHAPTER 232
Cutaneous Manifestations of Systemic Disorders

S Pradeep Nair

Chapter Summary

- General Considerations
- Generalized Pruritus
- Thyroid Disorders
- Diabetes Mellitus
- Liver and Kidney Disorders
- Internal Malignancy
- Erythema Nodosum

GENERAL CONSIDERATIONS

Several systemic diseases produce cutaneous manifestations which may be the first indication of the disease. Skin is considered to be the mirror of the body.

GENERALIZED PRURITUS

This is a very common manifestation of systemic disorders. The systemic conditions causing generalized pruritus are given in Box 232.1. Common dermatological causes of generalized pruritus are given in Box 232.2.

Generalized pruritus associated with systemic disorders is worsened during night. In diabetes mellitus (DM), hepatic disorders and chronic renal failure (CRF) the dryness (xerosis) of the skin may worsen the pruritus.

Box 232.1: Systemic causes of pruritus

- Diabetes mellitus (DM)
- Liver disorders, obstructive biliary disease hepatitis C
- Chronic renal failure (CRF)
- Hyperthyroidism, hypothyroidism
- Iron-deficiency anemia (IDA)
- Polycythemia
- Chronic leukemias
- Lymphomas
- Drug reactions

Box 232.2: Common dermatological causes of generalized pruritus

- Atopic dermatitis, contact dermatitis, seborrheic dermatitis, asteatotic eczema
- Dermatitis herpetiformis, bullous pemphigoid
- Urticaria
- Xerosis
- Scabies
- Psoriasis, lichen planus
- Pregnancy specific dermatitis

Management: Emollients like liquid paraffin, white soft paraffin and antihistamines like hydroxyzine (10–25 mg thrice daily) alleviate pruritus. The underlying systemic disorder should be treated appropriately.

THYROID DISORDERS

The skin manifestations of thyroid disorders are given in Table 232.1.

Thyroid disorders may also be associated with diabetes and vitiligo. Pretibial myxedema presents with skin colored or yellowish waxy nodules and plaques on the anterolateral aspect of lower limbs. *Treatment* is with topical potent steroids or with intralesional triamcinolone. Treatment of the basic thyroid problem may alleviate some of the skin manifestations.

DIABETES MELLITUS (DM)

Diabetes is associated with a large number of skin manifestations (Box 232.3). Some of the manifestations

Table 232.1: Skin manifestations of thyroid disorders

Hyperthyroidism	Hypothyroidism
Generalized pruritus	Xerosis
Warm skin	Cold skin
Palmar erythema	Palmoplantar keratoderma (Fig. 232.1)
Hyperpigmentation	Decreased sweating
Increased sweating	Edema of hands, face and eyelids
Pretibial myxedema	Xanthelasmas (Fig. 232.2)
Chronic urticaria	Sparse and coarse hair

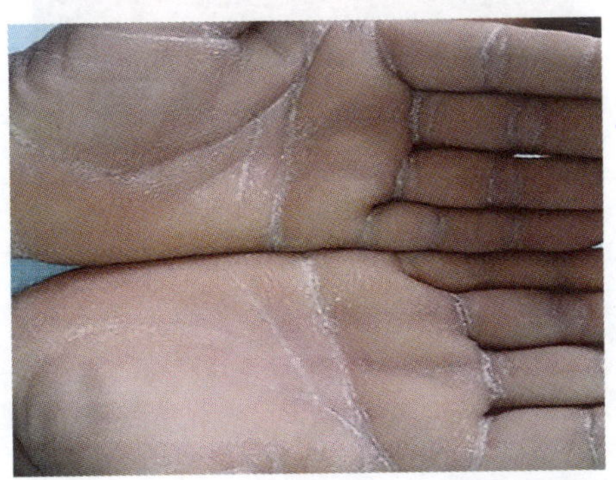

Fig. 232.1: Palmoplantar keratoderma in a hypothyroid patient

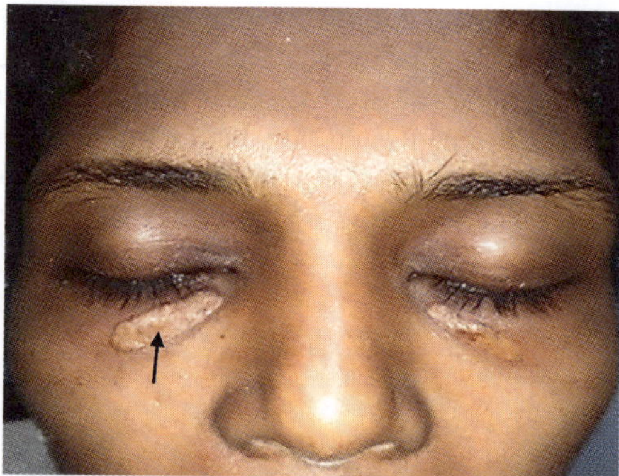

Fig. 232.2: Xanthelasma palpebrarum in a hypothyroid patient (arrow)

Box 232.3: Skin manifestations of diabetes

- Generalized pruritus
- Xeroderma or ichthyosis
- Granuloma annulare
- Necrobiosis lipoidica diabeticorum
- Infections—bacterial, fungal
- Diabeticorum bullosum
- Scleroderma diabeticorum
- Eruptive xanthomas
- Diabetic dermopathy
- Acanthosis nigricans
- Diabetic ulcers

may be related to poor diabetic control. The autonomic neuropathy of diabetes leads to xeroderma and ichthyosis which in turn leads to generalized pruritus.

Granuloma annulare: It presents with multiple discrete annular plaques with peripheral pebbling. ***Treatment*** is with topical steroids.

Candidal intertrigo: It is a very common fungal infection seen in diabetes.

Bacterial infections: These are like furuncles and carbuncles caused by *Staphylococcus aureus* are very common in diabetics (Fig. 232.3).

Necrobiosis lipoidica diabeticorum: It is a very specific skin lesion associated with diabetes. The patient presents with erythematous plaques on the shin which later ulcerates and becomes yellowish brown and undergoes central atrophy (Fig. 232.4). The lesions have a glazed appearance and may ulcerate and then heal with scarring.

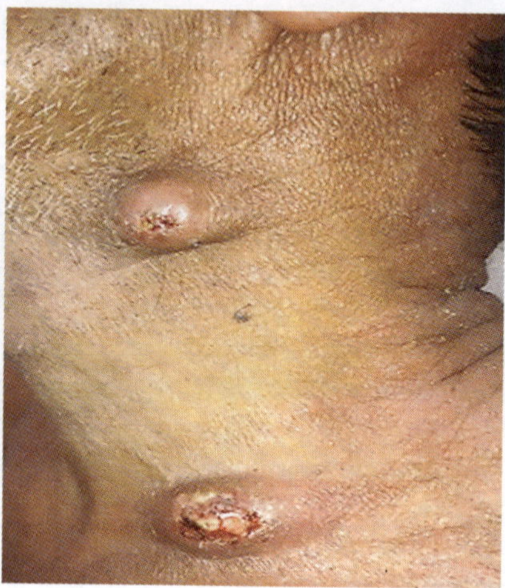

Fig. 232.3: Multiple furuncles in a diabetic patient

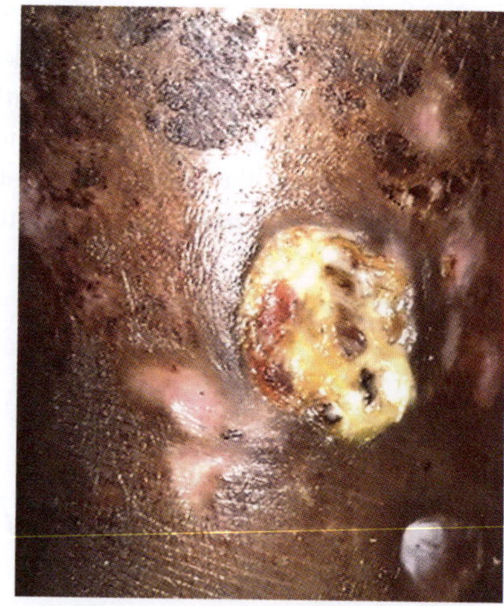

Fig. 232.4: Necrobiosis lipoidica in a diabetic patient

Local treatment consists of application of a potent glucocorticoid like clobetasol propionate 0.05% ointment.
Diabeticorum bullosum: It is the presence of large hemorrhagic bullae on the lower limbs.
Scleroderma: It presents with edema and sclerosis of the skin of the upper back.
Diabetic dermopathy (shin spots): It presents with multiple hyperpigmented atrophic macules on the lower limbs.
Eruptive xanthomas: The hyperlipidemia seen in diabetes may cause eruptive xanthomas presenting with skin-colored to yellow papules on extensor surfaces and buttocks.
Acanthosis nigricans: It presents as velvety plaques on the nape of the neck and flexures.
Diabetic ulcers: These are common complications of long-standing diabetes (*See* Section on Diabetes).

LIVER AND KIDNEY DISORDERS

Liver and kidney disorders present with a wide variety of skin manifestations (Table 232.2).
Liver disorders: Hepatitis B and C infection can present with chronic urticaria. Palmar erythema and spider angiomas occur in liver failure. Spider angiomas are usually seen on the upper half of the body. ***Terry's nails*** present with proximal white color and distal pink color. They occur in cirrhosis liver. ***Muehrcke's nails*** present with white bands and may be due to hypoalbuminemia.
CRF: The skin signs are seen in advanced cases and are of limited diagnostic value.

Half and half nail presents with proximal white color and distal pink, red or brown color and is seen in 10% of patients with CRF.

Table 232.2: Skin manifestations of liver and kidney disorders	
Liver disorders	**Kidney disorders**
• Generalized pruritus	• Generalized pruritus
• Xeroderma	• Xeroderma
• Jaundice	• Hyperpigmentation
• Hyperpigmentation	• Kyrle's disease
• Palmar erythema	• Half and half nail
• Spider angiomas	• Calcinosis cutis
• Terry's nails	
• Muehrcke's nails	

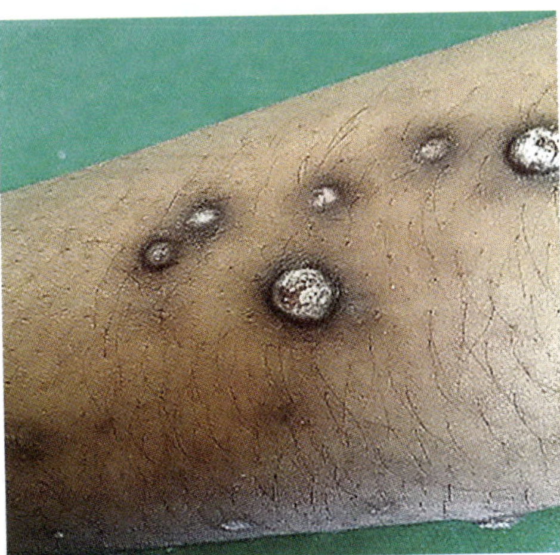

Fig. 232.5: Kyrle's disease in a patient with chronic renal failure

Kyrle's disease is a perforating dermatosis of the skin and is often associated with diabetic nephropathy and/or retinopathy. It presents with multiple discrete hyperpigmented keratotic papules on the limbs and trunks (Fig. 232.5). The lesions may even precede the renal failure.

Metastatic calcification in the form of *calcinosis cutis* over the joints and flexures may occur.

INTERNAL MALIGNANCY

The skin manifestations of internal malignancy may be either in the form of secondaries or as paraneoplastic syndromes. The abdominal skin is the most common site of cutaneous secondaries in intra-abdominal malignancies and occur in the form of papules, plaques or nodules (Fig. 232.6), a classic example being 'Sister Joseph's nodules' which are periumbilical cutaneous secondaries. Secondaries may be seen on the trunk and scalp in lung cancers and on the scalp or operative scars in hypernephroma. The skin manifestations of paraneoplastic syndromes are given in Table 232.3.

Malignant acanthosis nigricans presents with diffuse hyperpigmentation of face and flexures. The palms of the hands show increased rugosity and hyperkeratosis (tripe palms). The usual malignancy is carcinoma stomach.

Leser-Trélat sign is the occurrence of multiple pruritic seborrheic keratoses in a short duration, on the trunk.

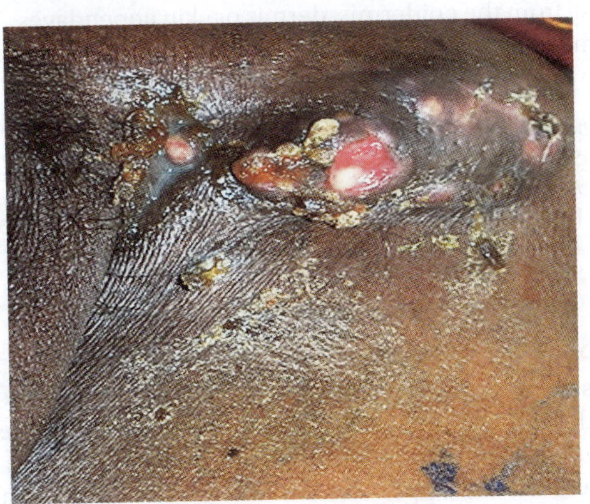

Fig. 232.6: Plaques, nodules and ulcers due to non-Hodgkin's lymphoma in inguinal region

Table 232.3: Skin manifestations of paraneoplastic syndromes

Skin manifestation	Malignancy
Generalized pruritus	Leukemia, lymphomas
Exfoliative dermatitis	Leukemia, lymphoma, rectum, colon and prostate cancer
Acquired ichthyosis (Fig. 232.7)	Leukemia, lymphomas
Bullous eruptions	GIT, breast, lung, thymoma and Castleman's tumor cancer
Acanthosis nigricans	Adenocarcinoma of GIT
Leser-Trélat sign	Adenocarcinoma of GIT
Pityriasis rotunda	Hepatocellular carcinoma
Erythema gyratum repens	Lung cancer
Erythema annulare centrifugum	Leukemia, lymphomas
Erythema multiforme	Leukemia, lymphomas
Erythema nodosum	Leukemia, lymphomas
Necrolytic migrating erythema	α-cell tumor of pancreas
Migratory thrombophlebitis	Pancreas, stomach and lungs cancer
Acquired hypertrichosis lanuginosa	Colon, rectum and bladder cancer

Abbreviation: GIT = Gastrointestinal tract

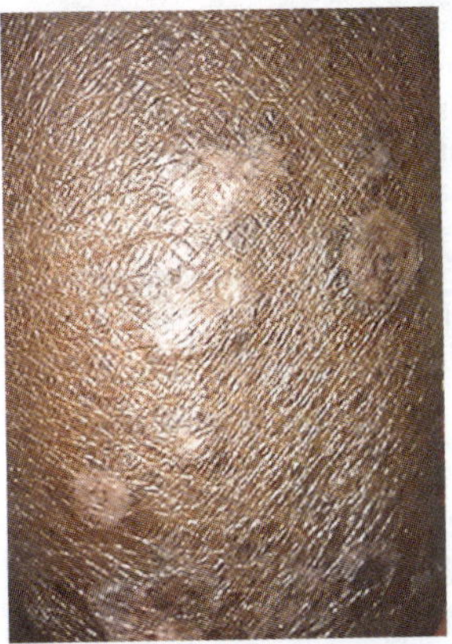

Fig. 232.7: Acquired ichthyosis due to Hodgkin's lymphoma

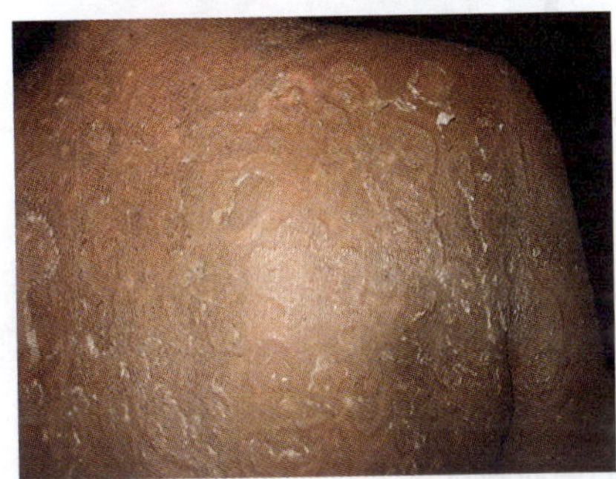

Fig. 232.8: Erythema gyratum repens. ***Note:*** The concentric plaques with wood-grain appearance

Erythema gyratum repens (Fig. 232.8) is characterized by multiple confluent erythematous scaly concentric and whorled patches on the trunk resembling 'wood-grain' pattern. These patients have a high incidence of lung carcinoma.

Erythema annulare centrifugum presents with multiple erythematous annular patches on the trunk with peripheral trailing scales.

Necrolytic migratory erythema (glucagonoma syndrome) presents with superficial eroding areas of erythema and scaling distributed on the lower abdomen, buttocks and thighs.

Migrating thrombophlebitis (Trousseau's sign) involves the veins of the upper limbs and trunk.

Acquired hypertrichosis lanuginosa presents with excess lanugo or vellus hairs on the face and ears and later other hair bearing areas. This cutaneous manifestation has a very strong relation with internal malignancy.

ERYTHEMA NODOSUM

It is a reaction pattern of skin, a hypersensitivity to an often, unknown antigen. It presents as tender red nodules on legs and is associated with a variety of underlying diseases (Box 232.4).

Erythema nodosum is the most common form of panniculitis (inflammation of the subcutaneous fat). It is common in young age, 20–30 years women are 3–6 times more commonly affected than men.

Clinical Features

The onset can be abrupt or preceded by a prodrome of fever, malaise and arthralgia, frequently of the ankle joints.

Box 232.4: Causes of erythema nodosum

- **Infections:** Streptococcal, tuberculosis, yersinia coccidioidomycosis, histoplasmosis infectious mononucleosis, hepatitis B, herpes simplex infection.
- **Drugs:** Sulfonamides, halides, oral contraceptives, minocycline, penicillin and salicylates.
- **Malignancies:** Lymphoma, leukemia, renal cell carcinoma.
- **Others:** Sarcoidosis, pregnancy, inflammatory bowel diseases and Behcet's diseases.

The lesions occur as crops of tender, erythematous, deep nodules that are better palpable, with ill-defined margins. Their size varies between 3 and 20 cm. Lesions are bilateral but not symmetrical.

The most common site is the anterior part of the shin, occasionally they occur on the arms and knees. The lesion evolves from red to purple to brown and eventually fade in 3–6 weeks without scarring. Nodules do not ulcerate.

Histologically, erythema nodosum is a septal panniculitis with vasculitis.

Laboratory Investigations

Complete blood count (CBC), erythrocyte sedimentation rate (ESR), urine analysis, tuberculosis test, chest X-ray, antistreptolysin O (ASO) titer, throat culture, other tests, relevant for underlying diseases.

Treatment

- Treatment of underlying diseases.
- Bed rest with foot end elevation.
- Analgesics and anti-inflammatory drugs.
- In symptomatic patients a saturated solution of potassium iodide 6–15 days daily in fruit juice for 3–4 weeks, decrease the pain and swelling. The dose is 300 mg (5–6 drops) 3 times daily initially, increased by 1 drop/dose/day to resolution. The result is often dramatically beneficial.
- Some respond to colchicine (0.5–1 mg twice daily).
- Intralesional triamcinolone or oral steroids are needed in resistant cases.

CHAPTER

233

Skin Tumors

S Pradeep Nair

Chapter Summary

- Benign Skin Tumors
  - Seborrheic Keratoses
  - Acrochordon
  - Keratoacanthoma
  - Trichoepithelioma
  - Syringoma
  - Cylindroma
- Premalignant Skin Conditions
  - Actinic Keratoses
  - Arsenical Keratoses
  - Bowen's Disease
  - Bowenoid Papulosis
  - Cutaneous Horn
  - Erythroplasia of Queyrat

BENIGN SKIN TUMORS

This chapter deals with the benign skin tumors and premalignant skin conditions. They account for 1.98%

of the skin conditions in Kerala. Benign skin tumors can arise from the epidermis, dermis or skin appendages. They commonly present with asymptomatic papules or nodules. The common benign skin tumors are given below.

Benign skin tumors

- Seborrheic keratoses
- Acrochordon
- Keratoacanthoma
- Trichoepithelioma
- Syringoma
- Cylindroma

Seborrheic Keratoses

This is a pigmented benign skin tumor composed of epidermal keratinocytes. This presents with single or multiple hyperpigmented flat papules or plaques on the face, neck and upper trunk with a 'stuck-on' appearance (Fig. 233.1). Dermatosis papulosa nigra is a clinical variant presenting with tiny pin head sized hyperpigmented

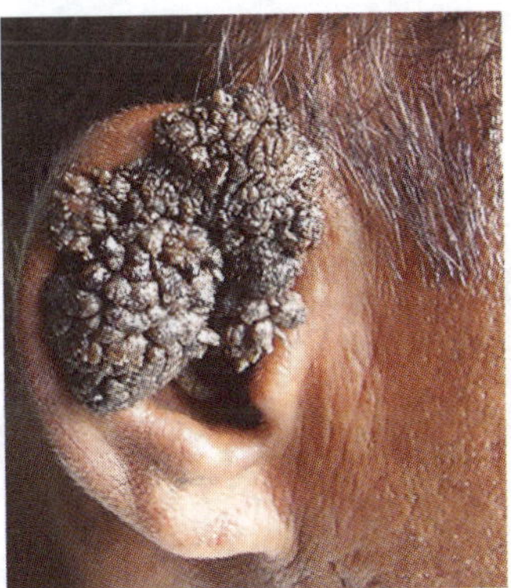

Fig. 233.1: Seborrheic keratoses on external ear

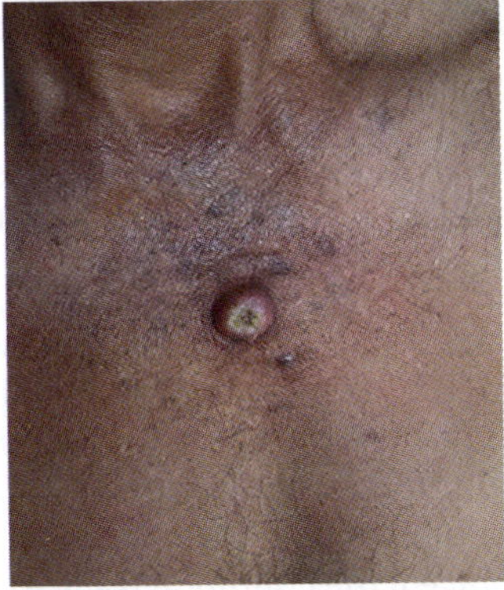

Fig. 233.2: Keratoacanthoma on the front of the chest

papules on the face and neck. Electrosurgery and cryotherapy are the treatment modalities.

Acrochordon

They are also known as skin tags or Templeton's tags and are soft skin-colored pedunculated papules usually seen on the neck, axilla, back and chest. Histologically, they are soft fibromas. *Treatment* is by electrosurgery or cryotherapy.

Keratoacanthoma

This is a benign tumor originating from the pilosebaceous unit containing keratinized squamous cells. It presents as skin-colored, dome-shaped, firm papules or nodules with a central crater filled with a keratin plug usually seen on the central part of the face or upper trunk (Fig. 233.2). This has to be differentiated from squamous cell carcinoma. Spontaneous resolution may occur. Surgical excision, electrocautery or topical 5-fluorouracil are the treatment modalities.

Trichoepithelioma

This is a benign skin tumor arising from hair structures. These may be solitary or multiple. Multiple trichoepithelioma may be an autosomal dominant disorder. It presents with skin-colored papules distributed on the face, specially on the eyelids, cheeks and nasolabial folds (Fig. 233.3). *Treatment* is by excision.

Syringoma

This is a tumor arising from the ductal part of the eccrine sweat glands. It presents with skin-colored papules with a crenated edge on the upper and lower eyelids and cheeks. *Treatment* is by electrosurgery.

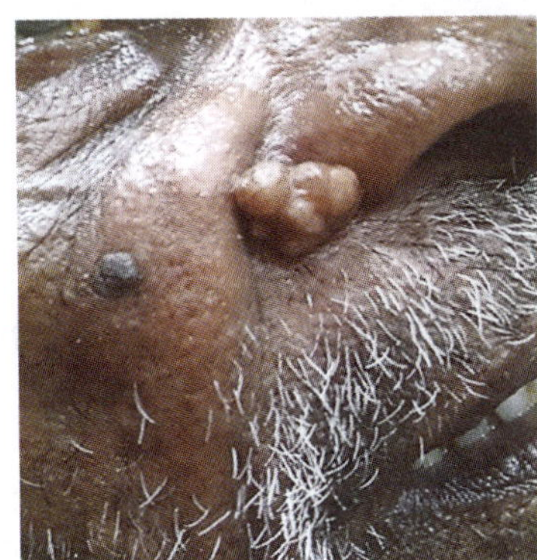

Fig. 233.3: Trichoepithelioma on the nasolabial fold

Cylindroma

It is a benign tumor of the apocrine glands usually presenting on the scalp as reddish tumors and histologically has islands of tumor cells arranged like a 'jigsaw puzzle'. Surgical excision is the treatment of choice.

Miscellaneous

Granuloma pyogenicum is a benign angiomatous tumor of the skin, which is a lobulated capillary hemangioma (Fig. 233.4). Excision, liquid nitrogen cryotherapy and laser therapy are the treatment modalities.

PREMALIGNANT SKIN CONDITIONS

Some common premalignant skin conditions are given in below. They usually lead to squamous cell carcinoma.

Premalignant conditions
• Actinic keratoses
• Arsenical keratoses
• Bowen's disease
• Bowenoid papulosis
• Cutaneous horn
• Erythroplasia of Queyrat

Actinic Keratoses

This occurs due to chronic exposure to sunlight. It is rare in India, but common in white races. It is characterized by skin-colored or hyperpigmented hyperkeratotic papules and plaques on the sun-exposed areas like the face and dorsum of hands. They may lead to squamous cell carcinoma. Small and superficial lesions can be treated with liquid nitrogen cryotherapy and topical 5-fluorouracil. Large indurated lesions must be excised and sent for biopsy. *Prevention* consists of avoidance of

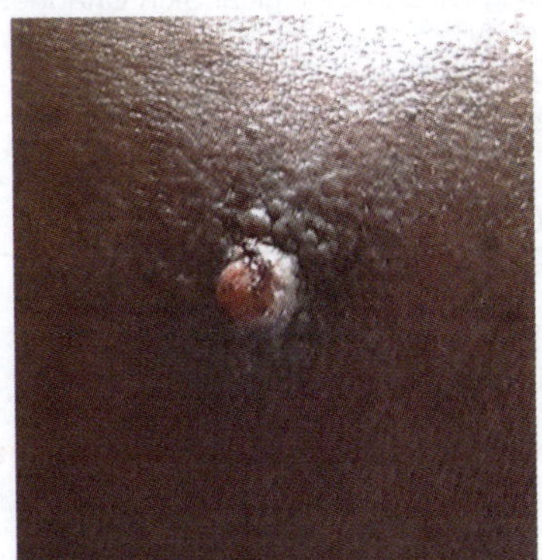

Fig. 233.4: Granuloma pyogenicum on the shoulder

direct sunlight and regular use of sunscreens containing avobenzones, oxybenzones and cinnamates.

Arsenical Keratoses

This occurs in individuals who are exposed to chronic arsenic poisoning. It presents as multiple discrete punctate keratotic papules and plaques on the palms and soles. It may be associated with lung carcinoma. *Treatment* is difficult, but keratolytic agents can be tried.

Bowen's Disease

It is a form of intraepidermal squamous cell carcinoma. Exposure to ultraviolet (UV) radiation is an important cause. It starts as an asymptomatic scaly erythematous macule, which enlarges irregularly. Scales are easily detached giving a moist red and granular appearance. The lesions are slightly raised with a well-demarcated margin (Fig. 233.5). It can occur anywhere on the skin or mucous membrane. Ulceration is a sign of invasive carcinoma. Cryotherapy, electrosurgery, surgical excision and topical 5-fluorouracil are the treatment options.

Bowenoid Papulosis

This is caused by human papilloma virus (HPV), HPV-16 and 18, presentings with multiple discrete lichenoid papules usually on the shaft of the penis. They may progress to squamous cell carcinoma. *Treatment* is by electrosurgery, cryotherapy and topical 5-fluorouracil. Topical immune response modifier, *imiquimod* is also effective.

Cutaneous Horn

This presents as hard yellowish brown horny plugs or outgrowths on the upper part of the face and ears.

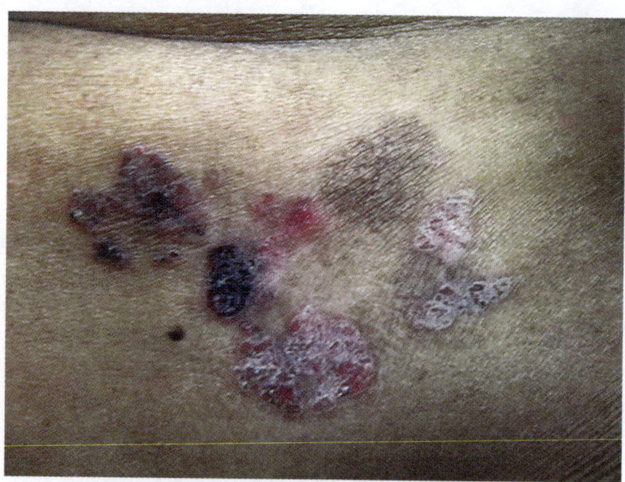

Fig. 233.5: Bowen's disease

Treatment consists of excision. Underlying squamous cell carcinoma should be excluded by histopathology.

Erythroplasia of Queyrat

This presents as red velvety plaques with a moist appearance on the glans penis in people with intact prepuce. It is considered to be a form of squamous cell carcinoma *in situ*. *Treatment* is with topical 5-fluorouracil if there is no submucosal invasion. Mohs surgery is the treatment of choice if the condition is invasive.

RECENT ADVANCES

Immunoenzyme histochemistry studies can be done to distinguish between various appendageal tumors, as arising from eccrine, apocrine or hair structures.

CHAPTER

234

Pregnancy and Skin

Usha Vaidhyanathan

Chapter Summary

- General Considerations
  - Physiological and Biological Skin Changes in Pregnancy
- Specific Dermatoses of Pregnancy
- Disorders Affected during Pregnancy

GENERAL CONSIDERATIONS

Historically, Hebra was the first to introduce the concept of pregnancy dermatoses in 1872. Pregnancy dermatoses can be classified into groups.

Physiological and Biological Skin Changes in Pregnancy

Physiological skin changes occur early in pregnancy and are considered as normal variations. Hence, it is important to avoid unnecessary interventions. The common skin changes are described.

- **Hyperpigmentation** occurs in up to 90% of cases, especially in darker women. Darkening of normally pigmented areas, like areola, nipples and genitalia, occurs commonly. Linea nigra is a brown linear streak of pigmentation along the midline of the abdomen, reaching up to the symphysis pubis. Darkening of freckles, nevi and recent scars can occur.
- **Melasma** or **the mask of pregnancy** is more common in the second half of pregnancy and presents as irregular hyperpigmented patches on centrofacial or malar pattern. Melasma associated with pregnancy usually disappears within a year of delivery and does not require treatment.
- **Hair:** Women usually have a prolonged **anagen phase** and thickening of scalp hair. After delivery, due to

abrupt reduction in estrogen levels, a large proportion of hair enters **telogen phase** and results in increased hair shedding, called telogen effluvium. This usually begins 4–20 weeks postpartum and complete hair regrowth occurs in 15 months.

- **Other changes** include striae gravidarum, vascular and hematological changes like transient thrombocytopenia, varices, gingivitis, epulis gravidarum and dental caries. Palmar erythema, spider angioma and purpura of lower extremities can also occur. Most conditions resolve spontaneously within a few months postpartum.

Specific Dermatoses of Pregnancy

A group of pathological conditions that develop during gestation or shortly after delivery is called the **specific dermatoses of pregnancy**. This includes pruritic urticarial papules and plaques of pregnancy (PUPPP), impetigo herpetiformis and herpes gestationis. Less well-defined conditions are grouped as **prurigo of pregnancy** and include prurigo gestationis of Besnier and papular dermatitis of Spangler.

Pruritic Urticarial Papules and Plaques of Pregnancy

This is most commonly diagnosed benign pruritic dermatosis of pregnancy of unknown etiology. Progesterone has been shown to aggravate inflammatory process at the tissue level and increased progesterone receptor immunoreactivity has been detected in skin lesions. Damage to connective tissue within the striae may also be a trigger.

Clinical features: PUPPP predominantly occurs in the 3rd trimester in first pregnancy. Recurrence in subsequent pregnancies is uncommon. It presents as erythematous papules and urticarial plaques on the abdomen, in the striae, thighs, arms and buttocks. Palms, soles and periumbilical regions are spared. Vesicles, target lesions and polycyclic erythema may also be seen.

Prognosis: It is excellent with no fetal or maternal morbidity or mortality. Spontaneous resolution occurs.

Treatment: Conservative treatment with topical emollients and topical corticosteroids would suffice.

Impetigo Herpetiformis

It is a rare pustular disorder of pregnancy often associated with hypocalcemia. It is considered as a form of generalized pustular psoriasis.

Clinical features: Eruption begins in early 3rd trimester of pregnancy, symmetrically in the flexural areas and then extends centrifugally to become a generalized rash. It presents as erythematous patches with grouped sterile pustules at their margins which erode and crust leaving postinflammatory hyperpigmentation. Mucous membrane may show erosions of tongue, mouth and esophagus. Onycholysis may occur.

Complications: Recurrences with each subsequent pregnancy and occurrence earlier in the pregnancy are common. Placental insufficiency results in an increased risk of fetal abnormalities and stillbirths. Fluid and electrolyte imbalance increases morbidity. It is often associated with hypocalcemia and low serum vitamin D levels.

Histopathology: It is similar to that of generalized pustular psoriasis with spongiform pustules in the epidermis and infiltrates of lymphocytes and neutrophils in the papillary dermis. Direct immunofluorescence is negative.

Treatment: Systemic corticosteroid at a low dose of prednisolone 15–30 mg/day is the treatment of choice. Systemic antibiotics are needed in case of secondary infection. Parenteral calcium and vitamin D are also useful. Treatment is essential as the disease is life-threatening.

Herpes Gestationis (Pemphigoid Gestationis)

It is a rare autoimmune vesiculobullous eruption related to bullous pemphigoid, which develops during the 2nd or 3rd trimester of pregnancy. It is associated with an increased frequency of human leukocyte antigen (HLA) DR-3.

Clinical features: The eruption has an acute onset of severely pruritic urticarial papules, plaques and annular lesions with vesicles around the umbilicus. This rapidly spreads to extremities, abdomen, back and chest. A generalized bullous eruption follows. Mucous membranes, palms, soles and face are spared.

The disease recurs in subsequent pregnancies, usually earlier in gestation and more severe. Histopathology and immunofluorescence are similar to those of bullous pemphigoid.

Treatment: Oral prednisolone in a dose of 0.5 mg/kg/day is the treatment of choice.

Prurigo of Pregnancy

The other less defined pruritic conditions of pregnancy are grouped as prurigo of pregnancy and include prurigo gestationis of Besnier and papular dermatitis of Spangler.

Prurigo gestationis of Besnier: Prurigo gestationis clinically appears as small excoriated erythematous papules grouped over the abdomen and distal extensor extremities and heal with postinflammatory hyperpigmentation. Histopathology is nonspecific and direct immunofluorescence is negative.

Some patients have an atopic background. Intrahepatic cholestasis of pregnancy predisposes to prurigo gestationis.

Symptoms usually disappear after delivery. **Treatment** is symptomatic with topical steroids and antihistamines.

Papular dermatitis of Spangler: Spangler described a more widespread papular eruption associated with a high fetal mortality. **Clinical features** are similar to prurigo, but more widespread, rather than grouping of lesions on extensor surfaces as in prurigo gestationis.

Elevated beta-human chorionic gonadotropin (β-HCG) and decreased cortisol and estrogen levels are also described. The condition responds to high doses of oral steroids and clears rapidly after delivery.

Skin Disorders Influenced by Pregnancy

Certain dermatoses are aggravated and some improve during pregnancy.

- **Psoriasis:** The effects of pregnancy on psoriasis are variable, though often consistent in the same woman. Most patients improve during pregnancy and some can worsen.
- **Atopic dermatitis** worsens in most pregnant women. This is partly due to pruritus of pregnancy.
- **Acne:** It may improve during pregnancy.
- Conditions, like *Hidradenitis suppurativa* and **Fox-Fordyce disease** show clinical improvement during pregnancy as the apocrine activity is decreased during pregnancy. Pregnancy may trigger **erythema multiforme** and **urticaria**.

CHAPTER

235

Basic Concepts

N Krishnan Kutty

Chapter Summary
- General Considerations
- Signs and Symptoms of Mental Disorders
- Clinical Examination of a Psychiatric Patient
- Classification of Mental Disorders

GENERAL CONSIDERATIONS

What is Psychiatry?

A German clinician, Dr Johann Reil originated the term *psychiatry* from the Greek root *psyche* (mind) and *iartos* (treatment). Psychiatry or psychological medicine can be defined as that branch of medicine concerned with the study, diagnosis, treatment and prevention of disorders of the mind. Psychiatric disorders are termed variously as *insanity, mental illness, mental disease, emotional disorders, behavioral disorders, functional disorders* and the like in the past. Psychiatry differs from psychology. *Psychology* deals with scientific study of behavior of normal man and animal.

Evolution of Psychiatry

Though in prehistoric times, physical and psychological illnesses were treated with contempt; with the renaissance movement the attitude toward the victim of illness came to be one of compassion. The *moral treatment* of insane was initiated by Philippe Pinel in France in the 18th century by setting free the lunatics from chains in the mental asylum.

Mental hospitals have a long history of evolution. Originally, these were called *mad houses, lunatic asylums* or *mental asylums*. The mental hospitals are gradually giving way to *general hospital* and *community psychiatry* practice, especially with the advent of modern drugs. The psychiatric patients are seen in general hospital set-up along with the general stream of patients (physically ills) and offered every kind of treatment there, including admission and discharge. The custodial care in the mental hospital is discouraged. The patients are allowed to remain in the community as far as possible. The family and community are given more and more responsibility in their care. Such an approach helps to facilitate early recovery, to minimize psychiatric morbidity and to reduce the social stigma attached to mental disorders. This practice of general hospital and community psychiatry is the modern concept.

SIGNS AND SYMPTOMS OF MENTAL DISORDERS

The symptoms are mostly subjective in nature. Often the patients are mocked at and alleged of simply imitating the symptoms. These symptoms are manifested as disturbances in the basic mental functions. They are best described as disturbances of mood, cognition and conation (psychomotor activity).

Signs and symptoms of mental disorders

Disturbance of mood

Pleasant mood states	Unpleasant mood states	Other mood states
• Euphoria	• Anxiety	• Apathy
• Elation	• Depression	• Anhedonia
• Ecstasy	• Irritability	• Blunting
• Exaltation	• Hatred	• Incongruous

Disturbance of cognition

Disturbance of thinking

Of formal thought	Of abnormal content
• Loosening of association	• Delusions
• Flight of ideas	• Obsessions
• Neologism	• Phobias
• Perseveration	• Suicidal ideas
Of stream	Of possession
• Thought block	• Thought deprivation
• Pressure of talk	• Thought insertion
• Poverty of thinking	• Thought broadcast
• Circumstantiality	

Disturbance of perception

Hallucinations	• Hypnopompic
• Visual	• Extracampine
• Auditory	• Synesthetic
• Olfactory	Illusions
• Tactile	• Macropsia
• Gustatory	• Micropsia
• Lilliputian	Derealization
• Hypnagogic	Depersonalization

Disturbance of memory

Immediate	Amnesia—anterograde and retrograde
Recent	Confabulation
Remote	

Disturbance of consciousness

Clouding	Stupor
Confusion	Coma

Disturbance of orientation

Disorientation to time, place, person

Disturbance of attention and concentration	
Distractibility	Fleeting
Disturbance of conation	
Psychomotor activity	Perseverations
Psychomotor retardation	Echolalia
	Echopraxia
Psychomotor overactivity	Catatonia
	Waxy flexibility
Stereotypy	Posturing
Mannerisms	

Disturbance of Mood

Laughing, crying, anger and the like are expressions of emotion. Emotion is the subjectively experienced feeling tone of mind. It is commonly noted as affect and mood. Though both are used interchangeably in the clinical setting, there are subtle differences. *Affect* is a momentary accentuation of emotion and *mood* is a more sustained emotional state. The normal mood of a person is congruent with the ideas, action and behavior. It is appropriate to situation. It is stable and adequate in intensity.

The common disturbances of mood include incongruity, anxiety, depression, elation, euphoria, ecstasy, flattening (blunting), lability, apathy and anhedonia. When mood is not in harmony or congruent to the ideas or actions it is called *incongruous affect*. For example, the person may start smiling on hearing the tragic news about a dear one. *Anxiety* refers to an unpleasant fearful mood. *Depression* denotes sadness of mood. Anxiety, depression, irritability, hatred and others are *dysphoric (unpleasant) mood states*. *Elation, euphoria* and *ecstasy* are euphoric (pleasant) mood states. Elation is a well-sustained cheerful mood. Euphoria is a happy mood with grandiosity and increased physical well-being. Ecstasy is the extreme degree of pleasure (rapture). In *labile affect*, the mood frequently changes from one state to another without reason *(emotional incontinence)*. In *affective blunting* (flattening), the degree of emotional expression is reduced much (constricted). Loss of emotional expression is called *apathy*. The inability to feel or share pleasure is referred as *anhedonia*.

Typically the mood is sad in depressive disorder, elated in manic disorder, anxious in anxiety disorder, incongruous or blunted in schizophrenia and labile in organic disorders.

Disturbance of Cognition

Cognition refers to an individual's thoughts, knowledge, interpretation, understanding and ideas about himself and his environment.

Thought (thinking) is the goal-directed arousal of symbols, ideas and associations leading to a reality-oriented conclusion. The thought comes to light through verbalization (talk/speech), writing and gestures. Normally, thinking is coherent (fully understandable) and relevant to the context. It follows logic and contains only relevant matters as contents.

Disturbances in thinking may involve in its formation, stream (flow), contents and ownership (possession). Loosening (looseness) of association, flight of ideas, neologism and perseveration, are formal thought dis-orders. In *loosening of association,* the grammatical alliance of talk is lost and no meaningful relation occurs between the ideas. The talk lacks comprehension. Apparently it looks like a flight of ideas. In *flight of ideas,* the talk jumps from topic to topic in quick succession, the ideas are related to each other and they are comprehensible. The logical connection between words or ideas is lost and the words and ideas are linked on the basis of similarities of sound rather than meaning (Clang association). *Neologism* denotes the formation of new words which have no meaning to others (e.g. hirschsprung, heboobi). *Perseveration* is the involuntary repetition of the same thought (talk or activity) given in response to one stimulus when a subsequent stimulus is presented. Thought is said to be *irrelevant* when it is not to the context. It is *incoherent* when it is not meaningful. Thought block, pressure of talk, poverty of thinking, tangential thinking and circumstantiality are disturbances of the stream of talk. When the stream of talk suddenly stops in the midst and fails to proceed further it is termed *thought block*. In *pressure of talk,* ideas continue to rush out of the mind due to its richness. On the other hand, in *poverty of thinking* the talk is scanty and flow is slow. In *circumstantiality,* the talk is prolonged by lengthy narration of unwanted details before coming to the right point finally. In *tangential thinking,* the flow of talk deviates in different directions and a final goal (point) is not reached. The thought may be disturbed by abnormal contents like delusions, obsessions, phobias and suicidal ideas.

A *delusion* is an abnormal belief not shared by other people. It is a false, fixed notion which cannot be corrected even by giving evidence to the contrary. It is not in tune with once cultural and educational background. Delusion can be corrected by treatment. The various kinds of delusions are persecutory, paranoid, grandiose, poverty, guilt, nihilistic, infidelity, control and hypochondriacal or somatic. In persecutory delusion, the patient may have the wrong notion that attempts are being made to harm or kill him. He believes that secret plots are made against him; he is poisoned, he is spied upon and so on. News in the media, a gesture observed, and a conversation he heard may be construed as referring to him only, and that they are deliberately done by his enemies *(delusion of reference)*. *Paranoid delusion* is synonymous with persecutory delusion though it actually includes grandiose delusions as well. In case of *grandiose delusion,* the patient may retain the false notion that he is immensely rich, he is having close contact with people of high caliber, he is very powerful or that he is a big scholar or scientist. In *delusion of poverty,* he holds the wrong notion that he is extremely poor having lost everything and he may even start begging. In *delusion of guilt*, the false belief is that the patient is a sinner who has done sinful deeds in the past or in the previous birth and attributes guilt to himself. The wrong notion held in *nihilistic delusions* is that part of his body, he himself or the world itself is not existing. In *delusion of infidelity* (amorous delusions, jealous husband's or wife's syndrome, pathological jealousy), the wrong notion is that the spouse is having

Table 235.1: Clinical importance of delusions

Types of delusion	Characteristic false belief of paranoid	Typical mental disorder
Persecutory	Persecution to kill or to harm	Schizophrenia depression (when mood congruent)
Reference	Actions of others have special reference/meaning	-do-
Grandiose	One-self being high, big, rich	Mania
Poverty	Poverty or loss	Depression
Guilt	Sinful action	Depression
Nihilistic	Non-existence of part or whole of self or the world itself	Depression
Somatic/ hypochondriasis	Bodily disease	Depression
Jealousy	Illicit sexual relationship	Delusional disorder, alcoholism
Love	Being loved	Delusional disorder
Primary		Schizophrenia
Secondary delusions		Mood disorder or any psychosis

illicit sexual relations. In ***delusions of love (erotomania),*** it is wrongly believed that someone is in sincere love with him or her. In ***delusions of control*** (influence/passivity feeling), the person's belief is that his thoughts, mood and actions are being controlled by people outside. In ***hypochondriacal delusion,*** the patients may think that he suffers from some incurable illness (Table 235.1).

Primary delusion (autochthonous delusion) is the sudden development of delusion without being preceded by any psychological event in the background.

Secondary delusion occurs as a consequence of some psychological events such as mood changes, hallucinations, delusions or others.

Systematized delusions are a complex set of delusions built one upon another around a single theme or an event.

Obsession denotes recurrent intrusion of unwanted thoughts into mind in spite of the efforts made to stop it. ***Phobia*** denotes a kind of fear specific to an object or a situation which are normally harmless. ***Suicidal*** idea is another abnormal content.

The ownership ***(my-ness)*** of thought may be changed. Thought deprivation, thought insertion and thought broadcasting are disturbances in possession of thought. In ***thought deprivation (withdrawal),*** the patient believes that ideas are stolen or taken away from his mind by outside agencies. In ***thought insertion,*** the belief is that ideas are introduced into his mind from outside agencies. In ***thought broadcast,*** the belief is that his thoughts (unexpressed) are known to others as soon as it occurs to him. He may believe that his actions and thought are being controlled.

Formal thought disturbance is frequent in schizophrenia. Cognitive decline is the hallmark of dementia. Sad gloomy thought pervades in depression often with delusion of guilt.

Disturbance of perception: Perception is a cognitive process of becoming aware of the objects and the environ-ment around us by way of the sense organs. The various kinds of perceptions include visual (seeing objects), auditory (hearing sounds), tactile or haptic (feeling touch), olfactory (smelling odors) and gustatory (feeling taste). Hallucinations, illusions, macropsia and micropsia are a common disturbances of perception. ***Hallucination*** is a vivid sensory (perceptive) experience occurring in the absence of the corresponding external object or stimulus. Thus, there can be visual, auditory, tactile, olfactory, and gustatory hallucinations. In ***auditory hallucinations,*** one may hear voices or noises in the absence of the corresponding external stimulus. In ***visual hallucination,*** one may see objects in the absence of such real external objects. In a similar way, the hallucination may be olfactory, tactile or gustatory. In ***olfactory hallucination,*** smells like burning of rubber or rags or foul gases may be experienced. Worms creeping under the skin, radiations touching the skin and the like are perceived in ***tactile hallucinations.*** In ***lilliputian hallucinations,*** the hallucinatory objects especially the people appear much smaller. Auditory and haptic hallucinations are common in schizophrenia. Visual hallucinations are common in organic disorders such as delirium. Visual illusions occur in delirium and auditory illusions are common in depression. The hallucinations experiencing outside the visual field is called ***extracampine hallucination.*** One may have the experience behind the head. One may hear voices speaking at London when the person is in Delhi. In ***synesthetic hallucination,*** the real sensory experience getting in one sensory organ is experienced in another sensory modality. A music heard is experienced as beautiful colors or good taste. This is common with hallucinogens such as lysergic acid diethylamide (LSD), mescaline and cannabis. In dereality feeling the sense of the real world is disturbed. It is an ***as if feeling.*** The environment may appear as if changed in some mysterious way (***derealization***) or the person may appear to him as if changed in some mysterious way (***depersonalization***). Hallucinations and illusions are not always pathological. ***Hypnagogic hallucinations*** occurring as one falls to sleep and ***hypnopompic hallucinations*** occurring as one awakens from sleep are normal phenomena. This may be a normal phenomenon (Table 235.2).

Illusion: This refers to misrecognition of objects. A rope may be misperceived as a snake or a shadow of a tree may be viewed as a ghost. The illusion can be corrected by verifying the truth by closer examination.

Micropsia: In micropsia, the real object or figure appear smaller than what they actually are, and in ***macropsia*** it is the reverse. They are usually found in temporal lobe epilepsy.

Disturbance of memory: The function of memory includes ***registration, retention*** and ***recollection*** of past events and information. Events once registered are retained and stored in the memory centers, and are recalled later according to need. Recollection with the help of a cue is recognition.

The common disturbance of memory is ***amnesia,*** which denotes loss of memory. Amnesia may be global and progressive or selective for certain events only. The memory

Table 235.2: Types of hallucinations and its disorders	
Type of hallucinations	**Typical disorder**
Auditory • Third person—running commentary; discussion, arguing, conversation • Second person—blaming, accusing, prompting suicide • Hearing one's own thought aloud	• Schizophrenia • Major depression • Schizophrenia
Visual • Insects—spiders, snakes and the like • Lilliputian	• Organic-delirium • Temporal lobe epilepsy (TLE)
Olfactory • Aura-burnt smell • Foul odor emanating from the body • Poisonous, foul smelling gas applied from outside	• TLE (uncinate fit) • Major depression • Schizophrenia
Tactile • Cocaine 'bug' • Bizarre sensation such as radiation, electromagnetic waves, cosmic rays all caused by enemies outside	• Cocaine psychosis • Schizophrenia

loss may be for immediate events (loss of retention) or for recent or remote events. The gap in memory may be filled up by fabricated and irrelevant events and information. This phenomenon is called *confabulation.* Anterograde amnesia refers to loss of memory for immediate past followed by an event, usually head trauma. Retrograde amnesia refers to the forward memory loss followed by an event usually head trauma. Amnesia may be for personal events such as date of birth, the school where one studied, the name of the headmaster. The amnesia can also be for impersonal events such as the republic day, the date of worldwar, the first Prime Minister of India and like.

Disturbance of intelligence: Intelligence is a global capacity of an individual to think rationally, to act swiftly and to adjust adequately to the surroundings. Intelligence grows and develops with physical growth and maturation. Intelligence can be measured and expressed in terms of ***intelligence quotient (IQ).*** The average IQ is 100 ± 16. When intelligence is not proportionately grown and developed ***mental retardation*** results. In ***dementia,*** on the other hand, the normally acquired intelligence deteriorates. Dementia is an acquired disorder and mental retardation is developmental disorder.

Disturbance of consciousness: These affect the clarity of the sensorium. The disorder of consciousness includes ***clouding, confusion, stupor*** and ***coma.*** Functional psychiatric symptoms develop in a clear conscious setting. On the other hand, if the symptoms are found to supervene on an impaired state of consciousness, an organic illness has to be considered. In hysterical fainting, there is no real loss of consciousness, and they will be aware of the surroundings.

Disturbance of orientation: Orientation is the appreciations of one's own temporal, personal and spatial relations at a given moment. ***Disorientation*** is the disturbance of orientation. Disorientation may pertain to time, place or persons. These may occur in delirium.

Disturbance of attention and concentration: Distractibility is a disorder in which attention is impaired. Fluctuating levels of attention are found in organic brain syndromes, e.g. delirium. Lack of concentration is seen in depression, schizophrenia, dementia and delirium.

Disturbance of insight: This denotes the abnormalities in the state of awareness of physical or mental health. Psychotic patients believe that they have no illness and so refuse treatment, whereas neurotic patients admit their illness but generally refuse to admit that their illnesses are psychological. They prefer treatment from doctors other than psychiatrists.

Disturbance of Conation (Motor Activity)

Conation represents the will to carry out an activity. It can be expressed as psychomotor or motor activity. It is different from neurological motor function. The disorder of motor activity may include decreased, increased and repetitive activity and disturbance of posture. The condition is called ***psychomotor retardation*** when the rate of motor activity is decreased. In ***psychological stupor***, the motor activity is reduced to a minimum and the patient is fully conscious, unlike in organic stupor (the stupor due to physical causes). When the rate of motor activity is increased it is termed as ***psychomotor overactivity***. Motor activity is increased to a very high degree in states of psychotic excitement. Repetitive motor activity includes stereotypy, mannerism, perseveration, echopraxia and echolalia.

Stereotypy: This term refers to monotonous, purposeless, repetition of an activity. ***Mannerism*** also is a repetitive activity but is not monotonously repeated and often goes with normal personality. The repetition of a previous activity in spite of the patient's effort to move on to a new activity is called ***perseveration of activity***. ***Echopraxia*** denotes involuntary repetition or imitation of an activity just seen. ***Echolalia*** denotes involuntary repetition or imitation of words just heard.

Catatonia: This term refers to widespread rigidity which may manifest as waxy flexibility, posturing, negativism and excitement. In ***waxy flexibility (flexibilitas cerea/ catalepsy),*** the limb can be positioned in any awkward posture for any length of time. ***Posturing*** refers to maintenance of imposed postures, which may be even bizarre and uncomfortable for long periods of time, however, awkward they may be.

Negativism: This term refers to the resistance to perform an activity or doing opposite to what is expected for a given stimulus.

Disturbance of behavior: Behavior is a general term. It is any activity either physical or mental, like walking, crying, speaking, eating, writing and the like. This term may broadly be used to describe mental function in general.

Somatic symptoms: Physical symptoms pertaining to any bodily system may be associated with psychiatric disorders and occasionally be the presenting symptom of such disorders.

CLINICAL EXAMINATION OF A PSYCHIATRIC PATIENT

Examination of a psychiatric patient in general is similar to that of a medical case. The first part consists of history taking and the next consists of the mental state examination. In addition, a full physical examination is required for all cases. An informant to whom the patient is closely known should be selected for eliciting the history, especially in case of psychosis and mental retardation. It is important to establish an understanding relationship (rapport) with the patient. A scheme followed in psychiatric examination is given below:

- **History**
  - Biodata
  - Presenting complaints
  - History of the present illness
  - History of past medical and psychiatric illness
  - Family history
  - Personal history
  - Premorbid personality
- **Mental status examinations**
  - Appearance and general behavior
  - Psychomotor activity
  - Mood (affect)
  - Thinking
  - Perception
  - Consciousness
  - Orientation
  - Attention and concentration
  - Memory
  - Intelligence
  - Judgment
  - Insight
- **Physical examination**
  - General
  - Systemic
- **Provisional diagnosis**
- Investigations biological and psychological
- Final diagnosis.

History

Biodata: The name, address, age, sex, income, education, occupation and marital status are noted.

Presenting complaints: The common presenting complaints include aggression, violence, excessive talk, retarded motor activity, suicidal behavior, insomnia, loss of appetite, bodyaches and pains, paralysis, loss of memory, poor intelligence, habituation to drugs and intoxicants, and sexual disorders. The presenting complaints are recorded in sequential order.

History of present illness: All details of the illness from its onset to the present state should be vividly described. Precipitating/aggravating factors and daily variation of symptoms are enquired into details of treatment have to be recorded. Leading questions may be required to bring out features such as suicidal tendencies, substance abuse, sexual disturbances, obsessions, delusions or hallucinations.

History of past illness: This should include all the past psychiatric problems, medical illness, physical trauma and accidents. Important events from birth including birth injuries and milestones of development have to be obtained.

Family history: All details of the family members, their inter-relationship, family structure, attitude of other family members toward patient and the occurrence of psychiatric illness in family have to be elicited. It is always desirable to construct a family tree.

Personal history: A biographic scheme is to be derived. Intrauterine history; details of delivery, diseases, trauma during childhood, administration of drugs, peer group relations and details of education are taken. All details regarding occupation, work, socioeconomic status, sexual activity, addictions, marriage and martial adjustments and details of the children should be recorded. History of physical torture and sexual assault during childhood should also be elicited if any.

Premorbid personality: This refers to the personality of an individual before developing the illness. This should include the general behavioral pattern, his hobbies, likes and dislikes, character trait, habits, attitude, social relations and others. The patient comes back to premorbid personality, once he recovers from the mental illness.

Mental Status Examination

Appearance and general behavior: The look of the patient, his dressing, hair style, level of co-operation, communication skills and level of activity are noted.

Psychomotor activity: Note whether the activity is normal, decreased or increased and then look for specific disturbances of motor activity such as stereotypy, stupor, mannerism, negativism and others.

Affect and mood: The mood is assessed objectively and subjectively. The patient is asked to tell about his mood state which gives the subjective mood state. Objectively the mood may be assessed by the interviewer. Normally, both subjective and objective mood should be the same (congruent). Abnormalities of mood, if any, are determined.

Thinking: This is brought out by noting the talk, writing and gestures of the patient. Disturbance of thinking manifests as disturbance of the form, stream, content and possession of the thought. Suicidal tendencies, obsessions and sexual matters have to be brought out by specific interrogation. When the patient is mute, gesture or written language is taken for analysis.

Perception: Spontaneous gestures and self-conversation may give clue to hallucinations. Symptoms such as hearing voices or other sensory experiences, in the absence of any real source should suggest hallucinations. In the presence of auditory hallucination, its content, the person (whether first, second or third) and the related mood should be elicited.

Consciousness: The level of consciousness has to be carefully recorded through inspection and interrogation.

Orientation: Orientation in time (day, date, week and year), place and persons should be assessed.

Attention and concentration: Attention can be assessed during interrogation. Normally, attention is prompt and sustained as-long-as the stimulus continues. Attention and concentration can be tested by:

- **Forward and backward counting test:** The patient is made to count 1–20 forwards and then backwards.

- ***Serial deduction test:*** To deduct serially 3s from 40 or 9s from 100. The rate of performance and errors committed will give an idea of the state of attention and concentration. These factors also depend to great deal on the level of his education.
- ***Digit span test:*** In the digit forward, test the patient is asked to repeat digits given by the interviewer containing three, four, five, six, seven or eight digits (e.g. 729, 3194, 27106....). In the backward digit test, the digits given by the examiner have to be repeated in the reverse order (i.e. 8139 as 9318). Seven digits forward and 5 digits backward constitute normal ability. It is lowered when the attention or immediate memory is impaired.

Memory: Immediate memory (power of retention), recent memory and remote memory have to be separately assessed.

How to Elicit Memory?

- ***Immediate memory*** can be assessed by the digit span test. Five objects can be selected and hidden. The patient is taught the hidden place. Distract the attention of patient. After 5 minutes, ask the patient the hidden places. Errors indicate the loss of immediate memory.
- ***Recent memory*** can be assessed by asking the patient the events that happened in the recent past; such as the persons who visited him that day, the items of food taken that day and the previous day and the like. Errors indicate the impairment of recent memory.
- ***Remote memory*** can be tested by asking the personal events like date of birth, the school he has studied, the name of the headmaster and the like, and impersonal events like the independence day, religious festivals days, the time of the worldwar and the like. Incorrect answers indicate the impairment of remote memory.

Intelligence: This can be assessed clinically by knowing his adaptive skills, general knowledge, occupational adjustments, educational achievement, motor skills, management of finance, household and others, during the interview. Intelligence can also be measured by scales of intelligence.

Judgment: This can be assessed by making the patient take decisions when confronted with specific situations. For example, the patient is asked '***What will you do when you see a house on fire?***', '***What will you do when you get a wound on your finger?***' Answers to these types of questions help to reveal impairment in judgment.

Insight: This is the appreciation of one's own physical and mental state. To assess the level of insight the patient is just asked whether he is sick or he needs any treatment. Patients who have no insight often answer that they are not ill and that they do not require any treatment inspite of severe symptoms.

Physical Examination

No mental examination is complete without a thorough physical examination.

At the end of the psychiatric and physical examinations, a provisional diagnosis can be arrived at in most cases. To arrive at a final diagnosis, it is mandatory to undertake the physical and psychological investigations as per indications.

Biochemical, hematological and basic imaging studies, all routine investigations of urine, blood, stool, liver function test (LFT), renal functions, blood-sugar, serum lipids, hematological and other basic investigations such as electrocardiogram (ECG) and chest X-rays.

Psychological Investigations

Psychological testing: Psychometry is the method of measuring psychological processes and states. These tests are ancillary to clinical assessment. They measure specific aspects of intelligence, personality and thinking. Neuropsychological tests help to quantify and localize the brain damage.

The common scales of intelligence are:

- Wechsler Adult Intelligence Scale (WAIS), Wechsler Intelligence Scale for Children (WISC)
- Raven's Progressive Matrices test
- Binet-Simon Intelligence Scale
- Bhatia's Battery of Intelligence Scale

Personality tests: These assess the type of personality, its change or deterioration, if any. The usual tests are:

- Minnesota Multiphasic Personality Inventory (MMPI)
- Rorschach test by Hermann Rorschach
- Bender Visual Motor Gestalt Test (BVMG).

Memory tests: These quantify the loss of memory, e.g.

- Boston Memory scale
- Wechsler Memory scale
- BVMG.

Rating scales: These are questionnaires, interviews and checklists that help to quantify behavior, thought and mood. For example:

- Brief psychiatric rating scale (BPRS)
- Hamilton's rating scales for depression
- Hamilton's rating scales for anxiety
- Abnormal involuntary movements scales (AIMS).

CLASSIFICATION OF MENTAL DISORDERS

The terms ***psychiatric*** and ***mental*** which are used synonymously, denote disorders pertaining to the mind. A major impediment in the classification of mental disorders is the absence of a specific etiological factor. So the term disorder is preferred in place of disease or illness. For the same reason, an etiological classification may not always be possible. The psychiatric disorders are, therefore, categorized into diagnostic entities based on sets of symptom patterns having a separate course (categorical classification). The American Psychiatric Association has made a system of classification known as ***Diagnostic*** and ***Statistical Manual of Mental Disorders*** (DSM). The World Health Organization (WHO) has made its own system known as ***International Classification of Diseases and Related Health Problems (ICD)***. The DSM-5 and ICD-10 are currently in vogue.

ICD-10 are widely followed. The diagnostic categories are given under chapter V (F). Each diagnostic category is given an alphabetic letter code (F) followed by a number code (alpha numerical coding). The disorders range from F-00 to F-99.

A simplified version of the main category of mental disorders followed in ICD-10:

- **F00–F09:** Organic mental disorders
- **F10–F19:** Mental disorders due to psychoactive substance use
- **F20–F29:** Schizophrenia and delusional disorders
- **F30–F39:** Mood (affective) disorders
- **F40–F49:** Neurotic stress-related and somatoform disorders
- **F50–F59:** Behavioral syndromes associated with physiological disturbance
- **F60–F69:** Personality disorders
- **F70–F79:** Mental retardation
- **F80–F89:** Psychological developmental disorders
- **F90–F98:** Childhood emotional disorders
- **F99:** Unspecified mental disorders.

The terms such as *psychosis, neurosis* and *functional* disorders are not in common use at present.

Features of psychoses and neuroses are given in Table 235.3.

Table 235.3: Features of psychoses and neuroses

Psychoses	*Neuroses*
Major psychological disturbance with:	*Minor psychological disturbance with:*
• Loss of contact with reality	• No loss of contact with reality
• Loss of insight	• No loss of insight
• Disintegration of personality	• No disintegration of personality
• Presence of delusions	• No delusions
• Presence of hallucination, e.g. schizophrenia, delirium	• Typically no hallucination, except rarely, e.g. anxiety neurosis, hysterical neurosis

By tradition, a disorder or symptom is said to be functional when there is no demonstrable physical abnormality in any organ system.

Textbook of Medicine

CHAPTER

236

Organic Mental Disorders

N Krishnan Kutty

Chapter Summary

- General Considerations
- Delirium
- Dementia
- Amnestic Disorders

GENERAL CONSIDERATIONS

These are a group of psychiatric disorders resulting from diagnosable structural disease of the brain or dysfunctions of the brain as a result of disease outside the brain. Though there are a large number of physical diseases, the psychiatric manifestations mainly occur as three syndromes.

DELIRIUM

Syn: Acute psycho-organic syndrome, acute brain disorder, toxic metabolic encephalopathy and acute confusional state

It is a syndrome and not a disease.

Clinical features: The clinical features of delirium depend on the degree of severity. It may vary from mild to severe abnormality. Symptoms are rapid in onset, transient in duration and reversible in outcome. These often fluctuate with brief spells of symptom-free intervals (lucidity). Children and old people are more vulnerable. Widespread psychological (cognitive) disturbance is seen. The cardinal feature is impairment of the level of consciousness. The clarity of sensorium is reduced. It leads to clouding, confusion, stupor or even coma. Orientation in time is lost early and later to place and even to person. Attention is fleeting with distractibility. Concentration is poor. Immediate and recent memory is impaired, affecting comprehension and learning. Visual hallucination of insects, reptiles and small objects and visual illusions are characteristic. Disturbed thinking results in irrelevant and incoherent talk and persecutory delusions. Mood becomes irritable, anxious and apprehensive. It may either be perplexed, labile or even depressed. Disturbance in motor function produces severe restlessness, excitement or violent and aggressive behavior. It brings danger to self and to others. Sometimes, underactivity is seen. Insomnia is one of the earliest features of delirium. It is typically associated with daytime somnolence and insomnia at night. Sleep-wake cycle is altered. Insight and judgment are lost. These mental symptoms are accompanied by physical symptoms such as dehydration, tremors, incoordination, aphasia and incontinence. The electroencephalogram (EEG) may show generalized slowing of activity, but in delirium tremens due to alcohol withdrawal, overactivity is more common in the EEG.

Delirium is due to generalized metabolic disturbances. The major neurotransmitter implicated is acetylcholine. Reticular activating system is the main seat of pathogenesis. Delirium occurs in a large number of physical conditions as listed in Table 236.1.

Diagnosis and management: Delirium is an emergency. The diagnosis is made from the clinical features and relevant investigations. The identification of the primary medical condition and its management are the goals. Good supporting environment and nursing care play a key role. Mild delirium may clear up with supportive care. In other cases, appropriate drugs are needed. These include injection of lorazepam and tabs of diazepam (5–10 mg or lorazepam 2 mg oral may help to relieve restlessness and anxiety). Injection of haloperidol 2–5 mg intramuscular

Table 236.1: Common causes of delirium	
Metabolic disturbances	**Vascular causes**
Electrolyte disturbances	**Cerebrovascular disorders**
• Acidosis/alkalosis	• Cardiac failure
• Hypo/hyperglycemia	• Acute myocardial infarction
• Hepatic failure	• Cerebral edema
• Uremia	• Hypertensive encephalopathy
Endocrine disturbances	• Eclampsia
• Hypo/hyperthyroidism	**Drugs:** Consumption/withdrawal
• Hypo/hyperparathyroidism	of:
• Adrenal dysfunction	• Alcohol
• Pituitary dysfunction	• Barbiturates
CNS infections	• Anticholinergics
• Meningitis	• Antipsychotics
• Encephalitis	**Nutritional deficiencies**
• Cerebral abscess	• Thiamine, niacin
Systemic infections	• Vitamin B_{12} and folates
• Pneumonias	**Others**
• Enteric fever	• Epilepsy
• Viral fevers	• Head trauma
• Septicemia	

Abbreviation: CNS = Central nervous system

(IM) reduces psychotic features such as delusions, violence and excitement. The drugs may have to be repeated and later changed to oral route and gradually withdrawn.

DEMENTIA

This is a syndrome, not a particular disease. The word dementia in Latin means general mental deterioration. It is a neuropsychiatric syndrome produced by brain diseases. Dementia is characterized by decline of intellect, memory and personality without impairment of consciousness. Associated symptoms may develop. Dementia is of insidious onset and runs a chronic progressive course. Primary dementia is generally irreversible in nature.

Clinical features of dementia depend on the stage of the disorder. Loss of recent and immediate memory is noted early. It interferes with day-to-day functions. Remote memory is affected only gradually and it leads to disorientation. The gap in memory is filled by irrelevant events and information (confabulation). Other cognitive areas such as thinking, attention, concentration, intelligence, perception and judgment also show decline. Thinking is slow with low word output. Grandiose and persecutory delusions may be seen. Attention and concentration are impaired, but the level of consciousness is unaffected. Visual hallucinations, loss of judgment and loss of insight occur. Personality changes are obvious. Lack of personal care, filthy habits, sexual disinhibition, stealing, lying and drug abuse may be there. Mood deteriorates to one of depression, elation or lability. Changes in the motor activity lead to restlessness and wandering, which predispose to accidents. Suicidal thoughts and attempts are not rare. When the patient fails to cope up with the stress, it produces temper outbursts (catastrophic reaction). The patient follows a rigid, stereotyped routine (organic orderliness). Insomnia is common. Aphasia, agnosia, apraxia, tremors, myoclonus, peripheral neuropathy and other neurological signs may appear. All symptoms worsen as the disease progresses.

Several diseases may give rise to dementia. These are described in.

Reversible Dementia

- Endocrine
- Metabolic
- Nutritional
- Tumor/Trauma
- Infections.

Diagnosis and treatment: The typical clinical features and relevant investigations help to identify the condition and detect the cause. Dementia is to be differentiated from mental retardation, delirium and pseudodementia. Mental retardation is a developmental disorder. Delirium is an acute reversible state. ***Pseudodementia*** is a depressive illness with cognitive impairment and is a reversible condition. The major aim of treatment is to remove the cause whenever possible, in order to reverse dementia or at least to arrest its progress. Attention to general health is important. Regular physical exercise, proper nutrition and prevention of accidents are essential. Counseling to the patient and family is needed. The involvement of community and social agencies can help to reduce the burden of management. Unmanageable cases need institutional care. Any common psychotropic drug can be used symptomatically to reduce restlessness, wandering, insomnia, delusions, hallucination and depression.

Drugs with minimum anticholinergic side effects are preferred and they should be given in minimal effective doses.

Drugs used in dementia
• Lorazepam: 0.5–1 mg (antianxiety and hypnotic)
• Risperidone drops/tablet: 0.5–1 mg (antipsychotic)
• Olanzapine tab: 2.5–5 mg (antipsychotic)
• Quetiapine: 12.5–25 mg (antipsychotic)
• Mirtazapine: 7.5–15 mg (antidepressant)
• Citalopram: 5–10 mg (antidepressant)
• Fluoxetine: 10–20 mg (antidepressant)

Cognitive enhancers: These are newer drugs tried in Alzheimer's diseases, but they are still experimental.

- ***Memantine (5–15 mg):*** This drug is an N-methyl-D-aspartate (NMDA) receptor blocker.
- ***Donepezil (5–15 mg):*** Acetylcholinesterase inhibitor.
- Cortisol, estrogen, vitamin E and plant products like ginkgo biloba are other agents tried from time to time.

Since there is no specific drug for dementia, the emphasis should be on prevention.

AMNESTIC DISORDERS

These disorders are characterized by profound impairment in recent memory with minimal impairment of other cognitive functions. Consciousness is not affected. Ability to learn new information (***anterograde amnesia***) and ability to recall previously learned information are impaired. Orientation to time and place may be lost, but orientation to person is retained. Visuospatial and geographical memory are unaffected. The amnestic gap may be filled by unrelated information (***confabulation***). Full insight is retained. Lesions are demonstrable in the hippocampus, amygdala, fornix and midline structures like the mammillary bodies and dorsomedial thalamus.

Course: The disorder may be of gradual or sudden onset. It may recover fully or run a chronic course.

The common amnestic disorders include transient global amnesia, alcoholic black out, **Korsakoff syndrome**, multiple sclerosis, cerebrovascular diseases (CVD) and such other conditions.

Treatment: Treatment is directed to the cause. In addition to the supportive psychotherapy, drugs can be used to allay the anxiety.

General features of delirium and dementia are discussed in Table 236.2.

Table 236.2: General features of delirium and dementia

Features	Delirium	Dementia
Onset	Rapid within hours to days	Gradual—years
Course	Fluctuating with lucidity	Slow progressive

Contd...

Contd...

Features	Delirium	Dementia
Consciousness	Altered, confused	Clear
Orientation	Usually disoriented in time and place	Disorientation confusion late to occur
Attention	Fluctuating	Intact, shifting or delayed
Sleep	Impaired	Impaired late in the disease
Behavior	Excited, retarded	Excited, wandering in late stages
Talk	Irrelevant, persecutory delusion	Relevant coherent
Mood	Apprehensive	Euthymic
Perception	Hallucination of small insects—illusion	Within normal limits
Insight and judgment	Impaired	Impaired late
Sensorium	Impaired	Not impaired

CHAPTER 237

Schizophrenia and Delusional Disorders

N Krishnan Kutty

Chapter Summary

- Schizophrenia
  - Clinical Features
  - Classification of Schizophrenia
  - Diagnosis
  - Course
  - Schizoaffective Disorder
- Persistent Delusional Disorders

SCHIZOPHRENIA

A precise definition of schizophrenia is lacking. It is a mental disorder characterized by specific psychological symptoms which interfere with the thinking, emotion, conation and motor behavior of the patient. Often the disorder runs a chronic deteriorating course. Whether schizophrenia is a single disorder or a group of many disorders is an unsettled riddle. Schizophrenia is a serious psychiatric disorder. The concept of schizophrenia was initially introduced by **Emil Kraepelin** and termed it **dementia praecox** (dementia = intellectual deterioration, praecox = early onset). To him, it was an illness among adolescents and young adults which gradually lead to intellectual deterioration. Later, **Eugen Bluler** showed that splitting of emotion, thought and behavior among themselves, was the essential feature of schizophrenia. Hence, he coined the term **schizophrenia** (Schizo = split; phrenum = mind).

Etiology

The exact etiology is not clear, but several factors play their roles.

- **Heredity:** Genetic factors play a major role in the etiology. The incidence of schizophrenia is about 1% in the general population. There is higher incidence of the disorder among the family members of schizophrenic patients. About 5% of the parents, 8% of the siblings and 12% of the children of schizophrenics are seen to be affected by the disorder. In twin studies, the concordance rate is 57% in monozygotic twins whereas it is only 12% for dizygotic twins. The mode of transmission may be monogenic or polygenic and the gene may be dominant or recessive. Defects in the long arm of chromosomes 7, 11 and 18 and the short arms of chromosomes 19 and X have been shown in linkage studies.
- **Personality:** Many schizophrenic patients show schizoid personality trait. These individuals are very shy, sensitive and are largely unsocial.
- **Family background:** In many instances, there may be disturbances in family. These include faulty parental attitudes, irrational and incoherent family atmosphere, defects in family communication, broken homes and the like. Emotional instability is found in many families.
- **Social factors:** Schizophrenia is more common in the lower socioeconomic groups. Urbanization and industrialization are other significant contributory factors.
- **Biochemical:** Dopamine hypothesis—is hypothesized that schizophrenia is the result of **dopaminergic hyperactivity** in the central nervous system (CNS), especially of D-2 receptor. Hyperactivity of other amine

receptors for **serotonin (5HT)** and **norepinephrine** are also probable. But these findings are not specific to schizophrenia. The **GABAergic** neuronal loss observed in the hippocampus suggests a role for gamma-aminobutyric acid (GABA). GABA is known to regulate dopaminergic activities. The role of the excitatory amino acid, glutamine has also been implicated.

- **Neuropathology:** Pathological changes are noted in the frontal lobe, hippocampus and basal ganglia. The size of the hippocampus, parahippocampus and amygdala is reduced on postmortem studies. Cell loss is also seen in the putamen and globus pallidus. Neuro-developmental disturbances and neurodegenerative changes have also been attributed.

  In the electroencephalogram (EEG), the evoked potential P300 is found to be relatively smaller and appear with reduced latency. The N100 evoked potential is found to be abnormal.

  The smooth pursuit eye movement is seen to be interrupted.

- **Stress:** Schizophrenia may be precipitated by physical stress like infection, injury, general debility, childbirth or by several forms of psychological stress. Life events too are important factors.

Clinical Features

Schizophrenia is a disease with protean manifestations. The symptoms of the illness include disturbances in thinking, mood, perception and motor behavior. These symptoms occur in a clear conscious setting of the mind.

Common schizophrenic thought disorders

- Loosening of association
- Thought blocking
- Neologism
- Autism
- Loss of abstract thinking
- Primary delusions
- Thought insertion
- Thought withdrawal
- Thought broadcasting
- Passivity feeling

- **Disturbance in thinking:** Thought disorder is a prominent symptom of schizophrenia. There is loss of meaningful connection in the sequential pattern of ideas **(loosening of associations)** which is a formal thought disorder. So the talk becomes incoherent. The stream of thought is affected. The thought becomes suddenly arrested and fails to proceed further (thought block). Circumstantiality, stereotypy and preservation may be observed. New words or phrases may be invented which may not make any sense to others **(neologism)**. The patient may detach from reality and live in his own inner world of phantasy **(autism)**. Occasionally, the patient may be mute. At times, there may be excessive, incoherent and irrelevant talk and activity at a high rate (excitement). They may fail to catch the wider implied meaning of proverbs which are interpreted in a purely literal sense **(concrete thinking)**. This is due to the **loss of abstract** thinking. It may be their experience that the feelings, thoughts or activities are being carried out under external control **(passivity)**.

- **Delusions:** They are common. They may arise without an attributable cause. Such primary delusions are characteristic of schizophrenia. It may be of persecutory, grandiose, somatic or religious themes. Secondary delusions also may exist. The thoughts may be alienated, i.e. the patient experiences that ideas are being taken away from his mind **(thought withdrawal)**; or that thoughts are being introduced into the mind **(thought insertion)**. Another phenomenon is the feeling that thoughts are being known to others as soon as it occurs in the mind **(thought broadcasting)**.

- **Disturbances of affect:** All forms of affective changes may be seen in schizophrenia. In the early stages, loss of emotional feelings **(anhedonia)** may be present. Usually, the patients show an incongruous or blunted affect. In some cases liability, depression, elation, anxiety or exaltation may be the affective changes.

- **Disturbances of perception:** The most common abnormality is auditory hallucination which occurs in a clear, conscious setting. Hallucinatory voices may pass comments or make simple statements about the patient (third person auditory hallucination) or give orders to the patient (second person hallucination). Voices may be threatening, accusatory and obscene. Tactile hallucinations in the form of electromagnetic waves, electricity, vibrations or cosmic rays may be experienced. Visual hallucinations are uncommon and other kinds of hallucinations are rare.

- **Motor disturbances:** The patient lacks energy, initiative and drive. The motor activity may be completely blocked-up at times (catatonic stupor). The patient may carry-out all given instructions without any resistance, even if they are harmful **(automatic obedience)**. The patient's limbs shows spasm and can be passively molded to any awkward posture for any length of time **(waxy flexibility/catalepsy)**. They may actively resist instructions or may do just the opposite of what is excepted normally (negativism). Negativism also causes retention of saliva/urine. Other motor disturbances like repetition of activities such as stereotypy mannerisms, perseveration or echopraxia are also found. At times, they exhibit spells of senseless excitement or states of complete withdrawal from the surroundings. Impulsive, suicidal and homicidal behavior may occur. These may be in response to delusion or hallucination.

- **Cognitive disturbances:** Attention, concentration and vigilance are impaired in schizophrenia. This adversely affects the immediate memory. In chronic cases, intellectual deterioration is also seen.

- **Other clinical features:** Mental functions such as consciousness, orientation, memory and intelligence are usually fully preserved but reasoning, judgment and insight are impaired.

- **Soft neurological signs:** Certain nonlocalizing neurological signs (soft signs) have been reported in schizophrenia. They include tics, stereotypies, grimacing, abnormal motor tone, abnormal movements, dysdiadokokinesis, astereognosis, diminished dexterity and the like.

Box 237.1: Fundamentals symptoms of schizophrenia

The 4 A's are:
- *Autism:* Withdrawal into one's own self into an internal world
- *Association loosening:* Illogical and meaningless connection in talk and thinking
- *Ambivalence:* Simultaneous presence of opposite action or thought, do/dont's
- *Affective blunting/snap prop:* Inappropriate facial expressions of mood.

Table 237.1: Positive and negative symptoms of schizophrenia

Positive symptoms	Negative symptoms
• More acute	• More chronic
• Productive symptoms	• Deficit symptoms
• More in acute disease	• More in chronic disease
• Formal thought disorders	• Anhedonia, lack of initiative and poverty of thinking
• Delusions	• Incongruity and flattened affect
• Hallucinations	• Social withdrawal
• Inappropriate affect	• Impaired attention and concentration
• Disturbance in motor activity	• Decrease in dopamine in prefrontal cortex
• Increase of dopamine in subcortical tissues	

- **Eye signs:** The blink rate may be increased. The patient does not make eye-to-eye contact with others. The smooth pursuit eye movement is seen interrupted.
- **Fundamental symptoms:** *Eugen Bleuler* classified the clinical features into fundamental symptoms and accessory symptoms. *Autism, ambivalence* and disturbances *in affect* and *associations* (4 A's) are the fundamental symptoms (Box 237.1). All the other symptoms like delusions hallucinations, etc. are included under *accessory symptoms*. The fundamental symptoms are diagnostic of schizophrenia.
- **Positive and negative symptoms:** All the symptoms of schizophrenia can be grouped into two sets: (1) positive symptoms and (2) negative symptoms (Table 237.1).

Classification of Schizophrenia

Classically, schizophrenia is divided into four types. These are as follow:

1. In *catatonic* schizophrenia, motor disturbances are very prominent.
2. In the *paranoid* form, delusions and hallucinations are the prominent features.
3. In *hebephrenia*, florid thinking disturbances and marked mood changes are predominant.
4. In *simple* schizophrenia, an insidious onset, lack of interest and initiative and gradual social withdrawal are the characteristic features.

This classification is made on the basis of the dominant clinical features.

Schizophrenia types (Eugen Bleuler)

- Catatonic schizophrenia
- Paranoid schizophrenia
- Hebephrenic schizophrenia
- Simple schizophrenia

In addition to these classic forms, many other special varieties have been described.

Diagnosis

Schizophrenia is diagnosed on the basis of clinical features. Broad diagnostic criteria are set in Diagnostic and Statistical Manual of Mental Disorders (DSM)-IV and International Classification of Diseases and Related Health Problems (ICD) system of classification. Delusion, hallucination, disorganized speech, disorganized or catatonic behavior, negative symptoms, social or occupational dysfunction are the essential criteria. The symptoms should be present at least for a period of one month. Projective tests may be helpful. Schizophrenia has to be differentiated from physical disorders like uremia and other organic mental disorders and also from masked depression, mania, dissociative disorders and others.

Course

Some cases of schizophrenia may recover fully. Others show remissions and exacerbations. A few deteriorate gradually and progressively. The prognosis depends on many factors.

Treatment

Schizophrenia poses the threat of chronic handicap and, therefore, treatment should be instituted early. Mainly three modalities of treatment are at hand. These include antipsychotic drugs (Box 237.2), electroconvulsive therapy (ECT) and psychosocial therapy.

Antipsychotic Drugs

Both conventional antipsychotics such as phenothiazines and haloperidol and newer atypical anti-psychotics such as risperidone, clozapine, olanzapine, quetiapine, ziprasidone and aripiprazole are currently in use (*See* Ch 250).

A suitable drug is to be selected depending upon the efficacy, availability, affordability, side effects, drug compliance and general health of the patient. The starting dose should be small and dose is increased to the effective range and maintained for symptom control. Drug therapy may have to be continued for at least for 24–36 months.

Depot preparations like injections of fluphenazine decanoate 25 mg intramuscular (IM) once in 2–4 weeks and injections of haloperidol decanoate are more advantageous than oral preparations in the maintenance phase in cases of poor drug compliance.

Box 237.2: Common drugs used in schizophrenia

Conventional antipsychotics
- Chlorpromazine
- Trifluoperazine
- Thioridazine
- Haloperidol

Atypical antipsychotics
- Risperidone
- Clozapine
- Olanzapine
- Quetiapine
- Aripiprazole

Depot preparations
- Injection fluphenazine decanoate
- Injection haloperidol decanoate

Electroconvulsive Therapy

It is beneficial in catatonic schizophrenia, acute schizophrenic episodes and in schizophrenic excitement.

Psychosocial Treatment

Steps are taken to keep the patients socialized by means of psychosocial education, close personal contact, group therapy, recreational therapy and occupational therapy so that the patient can readily come back to the social milieu after the treatment. The relatives are counseled regarding the nature of the disorder and role they have to adopt. Chronically handicapped persons need rehabilitation.

Cognitive therapy significantly reduced psychiatric symptoms in patients with schizophrenia spectrum disorders who have decided not to take anti-psychiatric drugs.

Source: Anthony P Morrison et al. The New Eng J Med 2014, 383; 1355.

Schizoaffective Disorder

This term is coined by Jacob Kasanin in 1933 to denote a type of mental disorder characterized by feature of both schizophrenia and affective (mood) disorder. The symptoms fall clearly into neither of these disorders. Psychotic symptoms like delusion and hallucination, affective symptoms of depression like depressive mood, hopelessness and guilt and of mania, such as elated mood, flight of ideas, or grandiosity may be noted. The illness has good prognosis. Anti-depressant mood stabilizers or antipsychotics are indicated, based upon the clinical presentations.

PERSISTENT DELUSIONAL DISORDERS

These are a group of disorders characterized essentially by a single type of long-standing delusion. It was known previously as *paranoid, monomania, paranoid psychosis or paraphrenia*.

The symptoms do not fit into any other type of mental disorders such as schizophrenia, mood disorders or organic psychosis. The delusions may be of different types as:

- Some important person is strongly in love with the person—*delusion of love (Clérambault's syndrome, erotomania)*.
- The spouse has extramarital relationship *(morbid jealousy, jealous husband/wife syndrome, delusion of infidelity, othello syndrome)*. Common in alcoholics.
- Infestation by a parasite or venereal disease or cancer *(parasitophobia/venereophobia, cancerphobia)*.
- Mis-shapening of body parts such as nose or face *(dysmorphophobia)*
- Emanation of foul order from body parts.
- The delusion is treated by antipsychotics and psychosocial therapy.

CHAPTER

238

Mood Disorders: Mania, Depression, Dysthymia

N Krishnan Kutty

> **Chapter Summary**
> - General Considerations
> - Mania
> - Depression (Major Depression)
> - Dysthymic Disorders

GENERAL CONSIDERATIONS

A persistent change in the affect or mood is the basic abnormality in mood disorders. What was originally described as *manic depressive psychosis (MDP)* by Emil Kraepelin is presently known as *mood disorders*. A persistent change in mood is the basic abnormality in this disorder. When the mood remains sad (depressed), the resulting clinical condition is called *depression*. It is called *mania* when the mood remains elevated and cheerful. The disorder usually runs an episodic course with recovery and recurrence. In between, lucid intervals occur in which the patient is symptom free. Mood disorders may be unipolar depression, or bipolar mood disorders (BPMD). In unipolar depression, only depressive episodes occur but they occur consecutively at least thrice. In BPMD, both depressive and manic episodes occur. In bipolar-I disorder, both mania and major depression or mania alone occurs. In bipolar-II, instead of mania there occurs hypomania.

MANIA

Etiology

The etiological factors for mood disorders fall under two broad groups—biological and psychosocial. The important biological factors may be genetic, biochemical, endocrine or neuroanatomical.

- *Genetic factors:* The incidence of mood disorders is high among the close relatives of the patients. Children born to affected parents develop the disorders even when the environment is different. In monozygotic twins, the prevalence rate is 69% compared to the general population. Nonbiological children and dizygotic twins have prevalence rates of only 19%.
- *The central monoamines,* residual sodium and melatonin are more important biochemical factors implicated. *Norepinephrine, serotonin* and *dopamine* are the brain neurotransmitters involved. The concen-

tration, turnover and postsynaptic receptor sensitivity of these neurotransmitters are diminished in depression. The converse is true in mania. Reserpine, which depletes serotonin from its stores, causes depression. **The residual sodium,** both intracellular and bone marrow sodium is increased up to 50% in depression and 200% in mania.

- **Endocrine** disorders such as Cushing's syndrome, hypothyroidism and hyperparathyroidism are known to produce depression. The secretion of cortisol is high in depression due to hyperactivity of the hypothalamic-pituitary-adrenal (HPA) axis. This secretion is not suppressed by exogenous dexamethasone unlike as in normal persons. This is the basis of **dexamethasone suppression test**.

- **Organic disorders** like cerebral atherosclerosis, neurosyphilis, acquired immunodeficiency syndrome (AIDS), Parkinson's disease and frontal lobe lesions may produce depression. Positron emission tomography (PET) and single-photon emission computed tomography (SPECT) studies have demonstrated reduced cerebral blood flow and reduced oxygen and glucose consumption in the frontal cortex among such patients **(hypofrontality)**. The hypothalamus, basal ganglia and limbic cortex are probably the anatomical sites affected in depression.

Psychological and social factors are closely linked. The prominent psychosocial factors are recent stressful life events, obsessive and cyclothymic mood swings, personality traits, loss of maternal affection during childhood, loss of loved objects, loneliness, helplessness, and cognitive distortions. In simple terms, cognition simply means thinking. **The cognitive theory** proposes that depression results primarily due to negative cognition, negative view of the self, of the world and of the future. The mood change is secondary.

Clinical Features

- **Elation of mood** is the characteristic disturbance. It is expansive. Generally, the manic patient appears well-dressed, often in colorful clothing and is cheerful. He is entertaining and often highly interfering. He forms focus of attention by his talk, boosted self-esteem and jocularity. In case of hypomania, the mood is one of euphoria with a generalized feeling of increased well-being. In case of manic excitement, the mood is one of excitement. Occasionally, the mood may be irritable.

- **Thought/talk:** The patient talks excessively and he is rich in ideas. The talk is often coherent, but may not be relevant. Since the rate of talk is high, too many ideas may be crowded into the mind, **giving rise to pressure of talk**. Often, the ideas shift from topic to topic giving rise to **flight of ideas**. The talk may contain typically grandiose delusions or persecutory delusions. The talk is jocular.

- **Disorders of perception** such as illusions may be present during manic excitement. Hallucinations are rare in mania.

- **Motor activity:** Mania is associated with exuberant energy and overactivity. He may get-up very early in the morning and engage himself in various kinds of unwanted activities. The actions are left incomplete. He unnecessarily interferes in the affairs of other people when he is hyperactive and picks up quarrels. In states of excitement, he may turn violent, aggressive, destructive and uncontrollable.

- **Other symptoms:** These include increased sexual urge, extravagance, drug abuse and intoxication. Intelligence is well-preserved. There is apparent impairment of memory on account of rapid flight of attention. Insight and judgment are impaired. Insomnia is a regular feature.

Diagnosis

The diagnosis is based on the clinical features. The Diagnostic and Statistical Manual of Mental Disorders (DSM) and International Classification of Diseases (ICD) prescribe a diagnostic criteria. The symptoms are to be present for one week. Persistently elevated expansive mood, inflated self-esteem, insomnia, flight of ideas, grandiosity, distract ability, marked impairment in social occupational are the core features. In hypomania, mood is elevated with high energy and confidence but without significant impairment of function. Mania is to be differentiated from schizophrenia, general paralysis of the insane, alcoholic excitement and delirium.

Common features of mania
• Elated, expansive mood
• High motor activity
• Richness of ideas
• Flight of ideas
• Jocularity
• Grandiose delusions

Treatment

Pharmacotherapy and electroconvulsive therapy (ECT) are employed in the treatment of mania. Antipsychotics and mood stabilizers are the drugs of choice for acute manic symptoms. Excited and violent patients have to be sedated with parental drugs. In some cases, mechanical restraint and hospitalization may be needed.

ECT may be necessary to bring down violent excitement rapidly.

DEPRESSION (MAJOR DEPRESSION)

Depression may be a symptom, a syndrome or a disease entity (depressive illness). Several terms such as **psychotic depression, endogenous depression, MDP depression, agitated depression, involutional melancholia** or **masked depression** are used to designate depressive disorder. The symptoms of depression are subject to diurnal variation, being worse in the morning. Depressive episodes may be mild, moderate or of severe degree.

Common features of depression
• Sadness of mood
• Retarded motor activity
• Poverty of thinking
• Delusion of guilt
• Hopelessness
• Worthlessness
• Suicidal ideas and attempts

- Loss of appetite
- Loss of weight
- Loss of libido
- Insomnia
- Other somatic symptoms.

Clinical Features

- **Mood:** The symptoms of depression are centered around the disturbance in mood. The mood is sad. The face appears gloomy with wrinkled forehead, drooping of the eyelids and sagging of the angles of the mouth. They show no interest in pleasurable activities *(anhedonia)*. Sometimes, the mood is one of irritability and anxiety.
- **Thought and speech:** The speech is slow and voice is low. Poverty of thinking and loss of self-confidence are prominent symptoms. They are pessimistic. They may retain ideas or delusions of guilt, worthlessness and hopelessness. Out of such thoughts may spring-up suicidal ideas and attempts. Eighty percent of suicides are attributable to depression. In most cases of suicide, the attempts are well-planned and secretly executed. Nihilistic and hypochondriacal delusions are not uncommon. In severe cases, they may become mute *(depressive mutism)*.
- **Disorders of perception:** Auditory hallucinations of accusatory nature may be found.
- **Motor activity:** Motor activity is retarded. The movements are slow. The patient tends to stoop while walking or sitting. Depressed patients become self-centered and prefer to be left undisturbed. The routine work may be avoided due to feeling of general weakness. In the extreme form, the patient may go into a state of *depressive stupor* where all the activities are minimal with least response to external stimuli.
  - *Their attention and concentration* are impaired
  - *The insight and judgment* may be impaired.
- **Pseudodementia:** The sluggishness of mental activity and impairment of attention and concentration may give an apparent impression of dementia.
- **Somatic symptoms:** Loss of appetite, loss of weight, constipation, loss of libido and late insomnia are vital symptoms of depression. Other bodily symptoms such as headache, giddiness, chest pain, backache and amenorrhea are common. Many give history of depressive symptoms preceding MI.

Diagnosis

Diagnosis of depression is made on the basis of clinical features. ICD-10 and DSM specify diagnostic criteria. The essential criteria are—depressed mood, lack of interest, weight loss, insomnia, psychomotor retardation, worthlessness and preoccupation with death. Depression has to be differentiated from organic disorders, schizophrenia, endocrine disorders and substance use disorders.

Course

The symptoms of depression may recover fully, but the risk of recurrence is present either as depression or as mania.

Treatment

Pharmacotherapy, psychotherapy and ECT are effective. Combination therapy brings about more rapid recovery.

- **Inpatient care:** Patients in depressive stupor and those with suicidal ideas require hospitalization.
- **Drugs:** Antidepressants are the drugs of choice. Tricyclic antidepressants, selective serotonin reuptake inhibitors and other atypical antidepressants are in common use. The treatment is initiated with smaller doses and worked up to the optimum level. The drug is maintained for 3–6 months after recovery and then it is gradually tapered off. Hypnotics, antianxiety drugs and other supportive therapy are also indicated.
- **ECT:** It is indicated in cases of depressive stupor, suicidal ideas and suicidal attempts.
- **Psychotherapy:** Cognitive behavior therapy and supportive psychotherapy are beneficial.
- **Rapid cycling:** Mood disorder is an episodic illness. The frequency of episodes varies widely from day to day, to many years. If there are four or more episodes within 12 months period, it is labeled as rapid cycling. The incidence is about 16%.

DYSTHYMIC DISORDERS

This used to be known as neurotic or reactive depression. This is considered as a variant of depression, mild in intensity, chronic in duration and without delusions or hallucinations. Somatic symptoms such as loss of weight, loss of appetite and loss of libido are not marked. Insomnia is early and sleep is fretful. The symptoms are worse in the evenings unlike in the case of mood disorders.

Treatment

This includes counseling, psychosocial therapy and pharmacotherapy with antidepressants.

CHAPTER
239

Anxiety Disorders

N Krishnan Kutty

Chapter Summary
- Generalized Anxiety Disorders (Anxiety Disorders)
- Phobic Anxiety Disorders
- Panic Disorder

INTRODUCTION

Anxiety is a subjective unpleasant feeling of fear, tension, impending danger or panic. In normal persons, fear or anxiety develops as a result of some known external reasons. Anxiety disorders are a group of conditions characterized by severe anxiety. The fear is usually accompanied by autonomic disturbances. There is no obvious external cause, the fear is in the unconscious mind. Three types of anxiety disorders are seen. These are described below.

GENERALIZED ANXIETY DISORDERS (GAD) (ANXIETY NEUROSIS)

In this disorder, the anxiety is free-floating and symptoms are experienced all the time. It was previously known as *anxiety neurosis.*

Etiology

The important causative factors include hereditary predisposition, morbid environment and constitutional defects. Physical factors such as infection, exhaustion and others may precipitate anxiety reaction. According to Sigmund Freud, anxiety develops as a result of the ***conflict*** in the unconscious mind. The conflict occurs when there is rivalry between the reality and needs or wish of the individual, sexual or otherwise. The conflict is unpleasant. So, it gets ***repressed*** into the unconscious part of the mind. When mental energy is diminished, repressed conflict tends to enter into the conscious mind. It is threatening. It is experienced as anxiety. Mental defense mechanisms do not come into play.

Overactivity of the neurotransmitters such as norepinephrine, serotonin and gamma-aminobutyric acid (GABA) are seen in this disorder. Main pathological lesions are seen in the locus coeruleus.

Clinical Features

The symptomatology can be classified as—mental and physical (Box 239.1).

Mental symptoms: Anxiety is the main symptom. It is generalized and present throughout. It hampers the functions of the individual. Anxiety interferes with the functions of attention and concentration and thereby, the memory. Anxiety is the common cause of amnesia in students. The person is preoccupied by ***worries*** and may have many kinds of anxious thoughts and feelings.

Physical symptoms: General features are motor restlessness, fine tremors and generalized muscular tension. This causes aches and pains, especially frontal headache and backache. The pupils are dilated. The mouth is dry due to decreased salivation.

- ***Cardiovascular manifestations:*** Tachycardia, rise in systolic blood pressure, precordial pain and palpitation are common.

- ***Respiratory symptoms:*** Patients with GAD complain of breathlessness and tachypnea. Hyperventilation may lead to alkalotic tetany.

- ***Gastrointestinal (GI) symptoms:*** These include dryness of mouth, dysphagia, diarrhea, constipation, vomiting, abdominal pain, gas and others.

- ***Genitourinary symptoms:*** Anxiety disorder is associated with increased frequency of micturition. Sexual drive (libido) is often diminished. Menstrual irregularities are found in women.

Box 239.1: Symptomatology of anxiety neurons

Mental symptoms (Psychological)
- Severe anxiety
- Irritability
- Lack of attention and concentration
- Worry

Physical symptoms
- Motor
  - Restlessness
  - Tremors
  - Tension
- Central nervous system (CNS)
  - Headache
  - Dizziness
  - Insomnia
- Cardiovascular system (CVS)
  - Palpitation
  - Tachycardia
  - Precordial pain
  - High systolic blood pressure
- Respiratory
  - Tachypnea
  - Breathlessness
  - Hyperventilation
- Gastrointestinal tract (GIT)
  - Dysphagia
  - Dry mouth
  - Diarrhea
- Genitourinary tract
  - Frequency of micturition
  - Menstrual irregularities
  - Sexual dysfunctions
- Skin—cold and clammy

- ***CNS:*** Headache is experienced as a tight band around the head. The patient experiences difficulty in getting into sleep. The sleep is light and fretful.
- The skin is cold and clammy.

Diagnosis

Clinical diagnosis can be made based on the somatic and psychic features. Specific diagnostic criteria are there—the International Classification of Diseases (ICD) and Diagnostic and Statistical Manual of Mental Disorders (DSM) classifications. These included symptoms of autonomous arousal, physical symptoms, mental symptoms and motor symptoms. Not all the symptoms may be there in a case. Persistent anxiety with somatic symptoms is the important feature. Careful search to exclude organic disorders such as endocrine abnormalities, ischemic heart disease (IHD), asthma and malignancy is absolutely essential. Other psychiatric conditions such as delirium, schizophrenia and agitated depression have also to be differentiated.

Treatment

- ***Psychotherapy:*** It is the principal form of treatment. Cases of recent onset may improve with counseling, by giving reassurance and encouragement to make adequate adjustment with the environment. In other cases, relaxation therapy and cognitive therapy may do good.
- ***Drug therapy:*** Antianxiety drugs are needed to give rapid relief. For long-term therapy, any of the antidepressants may be preferred.

Common antianxiety drugs

Benzodiazepines
- Alprazolam
- Diazepam
- Chlordiazepoxide
- Clonazepam

Beta-blockers: Propranolol

Azaspirone: Buspirone

PHOBIC ANXIETY DISORDERS

This disorder is characterized by presence of ***phobia***. Phobia denotes fear which is specific to an object or situation. The fear is unreasonable and out of proportion to the demand of the situation. The subject avoids the object or situation which evokes the phobia.

Clinical features: The symptoms of phobia are very similar to those of GAD but these symptoms occur only in the presence of the stimuli which evoke the phobia, either under imagination or in real situation. The patient is symptom-free at other times.

- In ***simple phobia***, the fear is usually for harmless objects like pen, matchbox, spider, cockroaches, dogs and the like.
- In ***social phobia***, the fear is for social situations such as speaking in public place, eating, writing or voiding urine in comfort stations.
- In ***agoraphobia***, the fear is experienced on getting away from house or being in situations from which escape seems to be difficult. Being in an open space like a *bazaar*, enclosed space like cinema hall or public transport vehicles are such fear-evoking situations.

Diagnosis: It is based on the clinical features in relation to the phobic stimulus. Phobic disorder should be differentiated from GAD, schizophrenia, obsessive compulsive disorder (OCD), epilepsy and depression.

Treatment: The acute symptom can be managed with antianxiety drugs. Behavior therapy, which is intended to desensitize the patient to the phobic stimulus, is the treatment of choice. Systematic desensitization, implosion and flooding are the techniques used (*See* Ch 251).

PANIC DISORDER

The characteristic feature is sudden, unexpected episodes of intense anxiety. It is marked by chest pain, breathlessness, palpitation, sweating and a feeling of imminent death or turning mad. The patient may run for help. Although, a number of general medical conditions such as diabetes may cause panic attacks, some conditions such as mitral valve prolapse, hypoglycemia, anemia, cardiac arrhythmias, carcinoid syndrome, abuse of *Cannabis*, overuse of caffeine, hyperventilation syndrome and temporal lobe epilepsy deserve special mention. Panic disorder may be mistaken for acute myocardial pain. Sometimes, it is associated with agoraphobia. Diagnosis is made from the typical features.

Lactate infusion test: Intravenous (IV) infusion of sodium lactate precipitates panic reaction and this test can be used for the diagnosis.

Treatment: Panic disorder responds well to drugs such as alprazolam, diazepam, selective serotonin reuptake inhibitors, tricyclic antidepressants, sodium valproate, and cognitive and supportive psychotherapies (*See* Ch 251).

CHAPTER 240

Obsessive Compulsive Disorders

N Krishnan Kutty

Chapter Summary

- General Considerations
- Etiology
- Clinical Features
- Diagnosis
- Treatment

GENERAL CONSIDERATIONS

This disorder is characterized by obsessions and compulsions. Obsessions are unwanted thoughts repeatedly intruding into the mind in spite of a strong will to get rid of them. There is the subjective compulsion to act accordingly. Though the patient is fully aware of this absurdity, he is helpless. He is unable to resist this action.

ETIOLOGY

Obsessions usually occur among obsessive personalities. Such individuals are usually very meticulous and methodical and are very particular about cleanliness and orderliness in everything. Many give a family history of obsessive disorder, obsessive trait or mood disorder. Obsession may also result as a sequel of head injury and intracranial infections. Neuroimaging studies have revealed bilateral reduction in the size of the caudate nuclei. There is increased activity in the frontal lobe, basal ganglia and cingulum and dysregulation of central serotonin.

CLINICAL FEATURES (TABLE 240.1)

The obsessions may take the form of ideas, doubts, phobias, impulses, slowness and rumination. The idea may be of any form.

- **Obsessive doubts** may be for an activity that has been just carried out. For example, the patient may go to bed

Table 240.1: Clinical features of obsessions, derealization and delusions

Obsessions	Derealization	Delusions
Doubt	'As if' feeling	Certainty
Minute possibility	No reality	False/bizarre/impossible
Insight	Present	No insight

after bolting the door. He may get up the next moment in doubt whether he had bolted the door or not. This may be continued indefinitely.

- **Obsessive phobia** is the fear that one may do harmful things. For example, a patient may have the fear that poison may be added in the medicine supplied.
- **Obsessive compulsions** are motor activities which are repeated **(obsessive rituals)**. The patient may wash the hand repeatedly, being unsatisfied with the cleanliness. The washing may be continued even to the point of peeling off the skin.
- An impulse may arise to howl or utter obscene words in the church when the mass is on. Obsession may be associated with anxiety or depressive features.

DIAGNOSIS

The premorbid personality, family history and clinical features help to make a diagnosis. The diagnostic criteria included in International Classification of Diseases and Related Health Problems (ICD)-10 are **repetition of thought and actions, compulsion to do it, unpleasantness of repetition, insight for the thought and distress associated with it.** Obsessive compulsive disorder (OCD) has to be differentiated from schizophrenia, psychotic depression and dementia.

Course: In many cases, the illness may recover gradually by itself. In some, the recovery may be sudden even during the early part of the illness. Often willful efforts to suppress the obsession may tend to aggravate the condition.

TREATMENT

Obsessive compulsive disorder responds well to treatment. A combination of pharmacotherapy and behavioral therapy is most suitable. Clomipramine and selective serotonin reuptake inhibitors (SSRIs) are the drugs of choice. They are to be given at the higher dose for 2–3 weeks.

Exposure and *response prevention* are the behavioral therapy techniques employed. This itself may be curative. In addition, supportive therapy and counseling to the family are also indicated.

Psychosurgery like cingulotomy may have to be done in intractable cases.

Conversion Disorders, Dissociative Disorders, Somatoform Disorders, Cultural Bond Syndromes, Reaction to Stress and Adjustment Disorders

N Krishnan Kutty

Chapter Summary

- General Considerations
  - Psychogenesis
- Conversion Disorders
  - Motor Symptoms
  - Sensory Symptoms
  - Special Senses
  - Visceral Symptoms
- Dissociative Disorders
- Somatoform Disorders (SFD)
  - Somatization Disorder
  - Hypochondriacal Disorders
  - Somatoform Pain Disorder
- Culture Bond Syndromes
  - Possession States
  - Dhat Syndrome
- Reaction to Stress and Adjustment Disorders
  - Acute Stress Disorders
  - Post-traumatic Stress Disorder
  - Adjustment Disorders

GENERAL CONSIDERATIONS

For a long time, this disorder was known as *hysteria*, a term coined by *Hippocrates*. Later, it was known as *hysterical neurosis* manifested as a conversion reaction and dissociative reactions based on psychopathology. The disorder is characterized by psychogenic loss or disorder of function. When the symptoms are confined to the sensory, motor or visceral functions, it is called *conversion disorder*. It is called dissociative disorder when the symptoms are psychic in nature. Symptoms are not intentionally produced, but are spontaneous.

Etiology

This disorder develops as a result of environmental stress in subjects who possess defective personalities such as hysterical personality. Such individuals are often emotionally immature. They are defensive, dramatic in behavior, demonstrative and demanding. They show tendency to be untruthful. They are seductive and easily suggestible.

Psychogenesis

- *Sigmund Freud,* the father of psychoanalysis found that hysterical symptom could be produced by suggestion and abolished by persuasion. He stated in his psychodynamic theory that hysterical symptoms develop as a result of psychic (emotional) conflict in the conscious mind. The conflict is repressed into unconscious part of the mind to be forgotten. Later in life, the repressed emotional conflicts try to enter the conscious mind. This produces anxiety which is very unpleasant. The anxiety is made innocuous by the *mental defense mechanisms* of *conversion* into bodily symptoms and *dissociation* into psychic symptoms. The awareness of certain functions gets disintegrated away from the central nervous system (CNS). Actually, there is no organ pathology seen on clinical examinations.

- *Pathophysiology:* Hypometabolism in the dominant hemisphere, hypermetabolism in the nondominant hemisphere and defect in interhemispheric communications have been described.

The relief from anxiety is the *primary gain* in the disorder. The symptoms provide material advantage to the patients. This is the *secondary gain*. The patients are unconcerned about their disability *(La belle indifference)*. In conversion disorders, the emotional abnormality produces physical symptoms pertaining to motor, sensory and visceral systems. It may mimic any disease.

CONVERSION DISORDERS

Syn: Hysterical neurosis

Clinical Features

- *Motor symptoms:* Various types of paresis and paralysis like hemiplegia, monoplegia and paraplegia, bizarre gait, tremors and mutism are common. It is usually a function like movement and not a group of muscles on any nerve distribution that is affected. The proximal parts of the limbs are more affected than the distal parts. The left side is more affected than the right. The paralyzed muscles may be used in one movement, but not in others. Efforts to produce a particular movement in a paralyzed limb may produce spasm in the opposite group of muscles. Examination reveals generalized muscular rigidity with increased tendon reflexes and flexor plantar response. Disuse atrophy may rarely supervene in long-standing cases.
  - *Tremors:* Coarse tremors occurring at rest and exaggerated when attention is drawn to them is suggestive of conversion disorder.
  - *Seizures:* The seizures (fits) occur in emotionally charged situations in the presence of onlookers. Fits do not occur when the patient is alone. Consciousness is not lost during the fits and sequence of events is bizarre. The movements also are bizarre. They may resemble arching or such other acts. Serious injuries do not occur during these episodes. These features help to distinguish hysterical (pseudo) seizures from epileptic (genuine) seizures (Table 241.1).

Table 241.1: Difference between genuine seizures (grand mal fits) and pseudoseizures (hysterical fits)

Genuine seizures (grand mal fits)	Pseudoseizures (hysterical fits)
Prodromal symptoms and aura are common	Absent
Tonic, clonic and relaxation movements are synchronous	No such typical patterns movements are asynchronous. One limb may flex and another may extend
Serious accident or injury when the patient falls down	Minor injuries. No accidents. The patient falls down leaning with support
Bites the tongue	Tongue is not bitten or injured
Incontinence of urine is common	Rare
Fits last for about a minute	Variable, even hours
Confused when awakened	Clear conscious state
No awareness of the events around during the fits	Awareness present
Lethargy may last for about 2–3 days	Active and energetic soon after the fits
Corneal reflex absent and plantar reflex is up going	Corneal reflex present and plantar is down going in the postictal unconscious phase
Postictal raise of prolactin	No raise
EEG abnormalities usual	EEG normal in the ictal period and interictal period

Abbreviation: EEG = Electroencephalogram

- **Sensory symptoms:** These include anesthesia, paresthesia and hyperesthesia. These sensory disturbances do not correspond to any anatomical pattern. Unlike as in neurological lesions, the boundaries are sharply demarcated and extent changes widely with repeated testing. Symmetrical anesthesia affecting the extremities such as gloves and stockings type may occur.
- **Special senses:** Blindness and deafness may occur. The patient can avoid obstacles in the path even when there is **total blindness**. Many patients complain of diplopia as well. Diplopia can be complained of even when one eye is shielded.
- **Visceral symptoms:** Common symptoms are vomiting, retention of urine, constipation, loss of appetite and others.
- All the above disturbances may also be prefixed by **dissociative** as dissociative motor disorders.

DISSOCIATIVE DISORDERS

Clinical Features

In dissociative disorder, the symptoms are confined to the psychic field. Amnesia, fugue, somnambulism, multiple personality and hysterical trance are the common manifestations.

- **Amnesia:** In dissociative amnesia, the loss of memory is confined to a circumscribed event or connected events which are agonizing to the patient. The amnesia occurs in situations of intolerable stress. The intellectual functions are unaffected, unlike in dementia.
- **Fugue:** In dissociated fugue, the person may wander to distant places under loss of identity with complete forgetfulness for the past life. A new identity may be assumed and he may engage in a work quite dissimilar to the previous job. The original identity can be regained under hypnosis, or even spontaneously.
- **Somnambulism:** It is a dissociative state where the individual walks around in sleep. He avoids obstacles on his way. This symptom may also occur in depression and epilepsy.
- **Dual or multiple personality (dissociative identity disorder):** It characterized by the presence of two or more distinct identity of personality that take control of the individual's behavior accompanied by inability to remember important personal information. The patient is possessed by a different personality, usually by a **spirit**—good or evil. In dual personality, the second personality may dominate the activities of the patient and he may not be aware of his real personality.
- **Dissociate trance (twilight state or stupor):** In this disorder, the patient gets detached from reality and may become almost immobile and immersed in his own self or in some other divine power. At times, they may appear possessed by some spirit, ghost and deity temporarily.

Diagnosis

The diagnosis of dissociate disorder (conversion) is made from the clinical picture. Personality tests may be helpful in establishing the diagnosis.

Differential diagnosis: The somatic symptoms may resemble those of physical diseases. The dissociative symptom may be a release phenomenon of CNS pathology. Psychiatric disorders like schizophrenia, depression, dementia and mania have to be differentiated. Coexistence of a physical illness may be there.

Treatment

Reassurance and suggestion are the usual modes of treatment adopted. The success depends on identification and removal of the secondary gain and resolution of the primary emotional conflict. Abreaction, psychotherapy and behavior therapy may be employed. Antianxiety drugs have their role to reduce the internal anxiety. It is not uncommon to find fresh symptoms cropping up when the existing symptom is removed by mere suggestions without resolving the conflict.

SOMATOFORM DISORDERS (SFD)

This includes a set of psychiatric disorders repeatedly presenting with symptoms of a physical illness but with no physical finding either on examination or repeated investigations. The common types of SFDs are:

- In **somatization disorder,** multiple and often changing symptoms are presented. The patient fails to get relief from several doctors. They are eager to get medicines for relief and hunt for drugs.

- In *hypochondriacal disorders,* the patients are preoccupied with presence of physical illness. They demand all kinds of investigations to prove their illness. At the same time, they are afraid to take drugs.
- *Somatoform pain disorder (psychogenic pain disorder):* Chronic pain such as headache, low backache and chest pain of severe nature are common symptoms. The pain is not accounted by physical disorder and is of an emotional nature. The pain may be symbolic of guilt, demand for affection, suppressed aggression or atonement for perceived sin. It may be rewarding to the patients in that they gain attention and care and escape from job or unpleasant task. It may also be the manifestation of other psychiatric disorders such as anxiety, depression or schizophrenia.

Factitious disorder: In this disorder, symptoms of mental or physical illness are purposefully adopted in order to remain in the sick role and avoid specific situations. There is no external gain. Dermatitis artefacta, bruising, brittle diabetes, pyrexia of unknown origin, purgation of unknown origin, chronic wounds and self-medication are examples.

Malingering (feigned insanity): In this condition, symptoms of mental disorder or physical illness may be feigned by the person to get some external gain. The gain may be to get exemption from strenuous work, financial compensation in accident, to get relieved from police action and the like. The symptoms may be vague and they may not suggest any typical disorder. They resist detailed evaluation and give evasive answers. Investigations give negative result. Constant observation and evaluation may bring out the truth. It should be tactfully conveyed to the person.

- The general management principle includes establishing rapport with the patient
- Counseling and supportive psychotherapy
- Antianxiety and antidepressant drugs as indicated.

CULTURE BOND SYNDROMES

These are certain psychiatric syndromes specifically found in certain countries and cultures. A large number of them have been described. For example, Amok, Koro, Latah, Wigo, Voodoo death, *Possession state* and *Dhat* syndrome are just a few examples.

Possession States

Individuals are seen talking and acting, not in their ownself, but in the role of others, being possessed by phenomena such as the spirit of:

- A dead relative or friend or a person who met with an unnatural death
- A god or goddess
- A devil.

They bring out various demands, wishes, orders or warning during the state of possession. These syndromes are more prevalent among young girls especially in rural India. Invocation of the fond deity in trance state is a common religious ritual.

Basically, the syndrome is a dissociative disorder. Major depression, schizophrenia or epilepsy also may appear as possession states. Usually, no treatment is required. Counseling and supportive psychotherapy may help to remove the stress which may precipitate the syndrome. Other cases require appropriate pharmacological agents.

Dhat Syndrome

The syndrome is common among young males mostly prevalent in the northern part of India. They complain of losing semen before and after passing urine. This gives rise to mixed picture of anxiety and depression. Muscular weakness, lack of interest and energy, lack of concentration, palpitation, body aches and visual blurring are complained of. The wrong concept behind this syndrome is that semen (dhatu) is a vital bodily element for vigor and health, and its loss is harmful to health. It is to be treated by counseling and antianxiety drugs.

REACTION TO STRESS AND ADJUSTMENT DISORDERS

Severe stress precipitates many kinds of mental disturbances, but stress reaction (disorder) stands out different from others. An exceptionally severe stress may produce characteristic symptoms known as *stress reaction* or disorder in a person with no previous history of mental illness. Such a stressor may be a major road traffic accident, death caused by lightning, earthquake, flood, bomb explosion, murder, rape, assault and similar situations. If the stressor is of a threatening nature, the symptoms are more like those of an anxiety disorder. When the stressor is one of loss or defeat, the symptoms are more like those of a depressive disorder. Stress disorders may be acute or late post-traumatic.

Acute Stress Disorder

In acute stress disorder, the symptoms follow within minutes or hours of the trauma. It may last for 2–3 days and recover spontaneously. The main symptoms are a dazed feeling, numbness, inability to understand what is said and to answer questions. Autonomic arousal such as anxiety, restlessness, tachycardia, sweating and insomnia may be seen. Symptoms of dissociation, flash back memory of the traumatic event, startle reaction and nightmares are common. Medical help from a general practitioner may be warranted at times. Antianxiety and antidepressant drugs, counseling and other supportive measures offer relief.

Post-traumatic Stress Disorder

In post-traumatic stress disorder (PTSD), the symptoms appear after a latent period ranging from a few weeks to six months. Psychiatric intervention is necessary for relief. The main symptoms are hyperarousal, painful re-experiencing of the traumatic event, emotional numbness, guilt feeling, rejection, humiliation and a pattern of avoidance behavior. Illusions, hallucinations, dissociative state or panic state may manifest. At times aggression, violence and poor impulse control are also seen. The treatment is symptomatic. Counseling, catharsis, direct advice, education to build-up healthy coping skills, cognitive behavior therapy or hypnosis are essential.

Drugs such as tricyclic antidepressants (TCAs), beta-adrenergic blockers and other antianxiety drugs are indicated.

Adjustment Disorders

Syn: Grief reaction

Psychological disturbances may be precipitated by life changes which may turn out to be stressful. Bereavement, migration, divorce, detection of a serious illness, retirement, desertion and financial liabilities are but a few examples. It develops within 1–6 months, usually not later than 6 months. The disturbances would not have developed in the absence of such stress. Worrying, poor concentration, anxiety, depression, irritability, nonspecific aches and pains and palpitation are the usual manifestations. Rarely, aggressive behavior, deliberate self-harm and abuse of drugs and alcohol may occur. In children, it manifests as regressive behavior such as thumb sucking, nail biting, babbling or enuresis.

The **treatment** is directed to resolve the stressful problem. Counseling is the best method to encourage them to talk-out and discuss their problems. Drugs such as antianxiety and antidepressant drugs and hypnotics may also be used.

CHAPTER
242

Torture

N Krishnan Kutty

Chapter Summary

- General Considerations
- Clinical Features
- Treatment
- Prevention

GENERAL CONSIDERATIONS

Torture is the intentional infliction of brutal pain, both physical and mental on a victim with a view to procure information or confession or punishing for committed or suspected crime, or ruining a rival.

Torture is common in several situations in life. It may be present in the family or inflicted by other agencies or persons including governmental establishments, especially during war or postwar situations, for eliciting evidence in crimes and as part of terrorism. Excluded is the pain or suffering arising only inherent in/or incidental to lawful punishment. Torture scenes occur in military setup, police custody, refugee camps, dictator governments, the spread of social violence and also at home (domestic violence). All over the world, intimate partner violence and torture have assumed serious proportions requiring medical and social intervention. The methods of torture involves all sorts of physical violence such as kicking, beating, crushing, burning, mutilating, application of irritant chemicals and mental inflictions such as isolating, humiliating, abusing, accusing, horrifying, guilt-inducing, providing false tragic news of dear persons, giving psychoactive chemicals and forcing to utter slogans opposite to their principles, morals and ethics, and sexual violence, especially against women including unwanted pregnancy. There is no intention to murder. As a result, the torture victim is totally ruined, physically, mentally, morally and spiritually. His/her personality gets disintegrated. Doctors and psychologists are often called in to assist the torturers, especially by governmental agencies in many countries.

CLINICAL FEATURES

The symptoms are related to post-traumatic stress disorder (PTSD). Torture victims present a spectrum of physical and mental symptoms. These may be akin to PTSD but the picture varies depending on the measures used to inflict torture. Prominent ones are the symptoms pertaining to musculoskeletal system, though all systems may be affected. Insomnia, nightmare and lability of mood, lack of concentration, loss of memory, social withdrawal, guilt feeling, insecurity and helplessness are the usual mental symptoms. Other symptoms are fears, apprehension, irritability, anxiety, depression, suicidal ideas and change of personality.

TREATMENT

Torture victims are to be treated and rehabilitated. A holistic approach involving physical, mental, spiritual, legal and cultural measures has to be adopted to give better outcome. The victim is given respect as a human being, his trust and confidence is established. Drugs and psychosocial therapies are given appropriately to relieve symptoms and to rebuild his personality.

PREVENTION

Torture is an inhuman act and unacceptable to democratic principles. The United Nations Convention prohibits the act of torturing and such inhuman acts, since it is a violation of human rights. The International Rehabilitation Council for Torture Victims (IRCT) and many such international organizations are active in its prevention and rehabilitation of the victims. Medical profession is often drawn to assist the torturers. Doctors are forced to stay to prevent death of the victim and they may be forced to issue false medical certificates of tissue damage. They have to treat and rehabilitate the victims, once they are freed. The World Medical Association (WMA) looks down upon torture and makes plea to governments and doctors not to encourage this heinous act.

CHAPTER 243

Disorders of Adult Personality

N Krishnan Kutty

Chapter Summary

- General Considerations
- Etiology
- Primary Ego Defense Mechanisms in Some Personality Disorders
  - Schizoid
  - Obsessive
  - Anxious
  - Histrionic
  - Paranoid
  - Dissocial
- Treatment

GENERAL CONSIDERATIONS

The term, personality is derived from the Greek word **persona = mask.** Personality is the total characteristic of an individual, i.e. everything that a person is made up of. It includes the physical make up, behavior in relation to others, the thinking and feeling. The personality is stable, predictable and measurable. It is in harmony with the sociocultural standards. The characteristic pattern of behavior and mode of thinking that determines a person's adjustment to the environment constitute a normal personality. When the character traits becomes rigid and maladaptable, it results in personality disorders. It produces subjective distress to the person as well as to others in the society.

ETIOLOGY

Genetic factors, constitutional factors and disturbance in family environment during childhood have been implicated. Some psychopaths show an extra 'Y' chromosome (XYY). Some criminal psychopaths may show abnormal electroencephalogram (EEG) patterns.

This disorder develops from early childhood without any clear-cut onset of time. Personality can be assessed by clinical interview and by psychological tests such as Minnesota Multiphasic Personality Inventory (MMPI), Rorschach's test, Thematic Apperception Test (TAT), Personality Assessment Schedule (PAS) and others.

PRIMARY EGO DEFENSE MECHANISMS IN SOME PERSONALITY DISORDERS

Primary ego defense mechanisms in some personality disorders are discussed below.

Disorder	*Defense*
Paranoid personality disorder	Projection
Schizoid personality disorder	Fantasy
Borderline personality disorder	Splitting; acting out
Histrionic personality disorder	Dissociation
Obsessive-compulsive personality disorder	Isolation

Clinical Features

Many types of personality disorders are known. Some common types are given below:

Schizoid Personality Disorder

These individuals are shy, oversensitive and seclusive, often with autistic (fantasy) thinking and poor emotional relationship with others.

Obsessive-Compulsive Personality Disorder (Anankastic Personality Disorder)

These subjects show excessive concern with conformity and adherence to standards of behavior. They are rigid, overinhibited, overcautious and overdutiful and less adaptive. They want perfection and orderliness in everything.

Anxious (Avoidant) Personality Disorder

Persistent feeling of tension and apprehension, avoidance of social interaction and criticism and extreme sensitivity to rejection are the usual features.

Histrionic (Hysterical) Personality Disorder

It is marked by self-suggestibility, attention-seeking behavior, shallow or labile affect, self-dramatization, seductiveness, defensiveness and dependency.

Paranoid Personality Disorder

These individuals are always suspicious and sensitive. They are stubborn and argumentative. They are preoccupied with groundless, conspiratorial explanations of events.

Dissocial (Antisocial) Personality Disorders (Asocial, Psychopathic, Sociopathic Personality)

These personalities are characterized by impulsive behavior, lack of guilt feeling, failure to keep sustained affectionate relationship and failure to learn from past experience. They are labelled as heartless, callous, self-centered persons. They are in the habit of making crimes and offences of all sorts, including substance abuse.

Personality disorder differs from personality changes. **Personality changes** are the deterioration of personality due to brain damage, chronic alcoholism, chronic schizophrenia, chronic distress or chronic epilepsy. On the other hand, personality disorders develop as primary phenomena from early life.

TREATMENT

Since these are life-pattern disturbances, treatment modalities are less effective. Individual and group psychotherapy are the methods of choice. Psychotropic drugs may help during periods of crisis.

CHAPTER 244

Psychoactive Substance-use Disorders and Alcohol-related Disorders

N Krishnan Kutty

Chapter Summary

- General Considerations
- Etiology and Clinical Features
- Treatment
- Prevention
- Alcohol-Related Disorders
- Cannabis-related Disorders
- Opioids-related Disorders
- Nicotine-related Disorders

GENERAL CONSIDERATIONS

These are disorders due to the self-administration of chemical substances for pleasure or to alleviate discomfort. These substances have their effect on the mind. They alter the mood, thought, level of consciousness and behavior. Drug use, drug dependence, drug addiction and habituation were the terms used in the past to denote the same condition. The psychoactive substances (drugs) are of different kinds. The common substances are:

- Alcohol
- Amphetamine and other stimulants
- Barbiturates
- *Cannabis:* Ganja, charas, bhang, hashish
- Cocaine
- *Caffeine:* Coffee and tea
- Hallucinogens like lysergic acid diethylamide (LSD), mescaline
- Volatile solutions such as petroleum, ether, benzene
- Nitrite, nitrous oxide
- Tobacco (nicotine)
- *Opioids:* Morphine, codeine, heroin, pethidine and methadone, pentazocine
- *Sedatives and hypnotics:* Benzodiazepines, e.g. diazepam, lorazepam, alprazolam, librium and others.

All these can be categorized into five groups based on clinical effect as shown below:

1. *Depressants:* Result in behavioral sedation (e.g. alcohol, sedative, anxiolytic drugs)
2. *Stimulants:* Increase alertness and elevates mood (e.g. cocaine, nicotine, caffeine)
3. *Opiates:* Primarily produce analgesia and euphoria (e.g. heroin, morphine, codeine)
4. *Hallucinogens:* Alter sensory perception (e.g. marijuana, LSD)
5. *Other drugs of abuse:* Include inhalants, anabolic steroids and medications.

Administration of or self-medication of these drugs produces several phenomena referable to psychological functions. Most of such drugs lead to dependence on repeated administration. Ultimately they lead to changes in personality and behavior. Several syndromes may be produced by such psychoactive drugs.

ETIOLOGY AND CLINICAL FEATURES

The three major factors involved in substance-use disorders include: (1) personality; (2) substance; (3) environment. They form a closed chain. The personality has to be vulnerable, the drug should be readily available and social environment has to be favorable.

Personality Factors

Family disturbances in early childhood and parental disharmony are important factors. Anxious and depressive personalities get their symptoms apparently relieved by the substance and they continue the abuse. Delinquency and antisocial personality disorders are other common causes. Challenges of day-to-day life and intra and inter personality problems are contributory.

Drug Availability

The drug used may be of medicinal nature such as diazepam, pethidine or mood elevators. Drug trafficking is a major and active menace when there is legal restriction. Substances such as tobacco and alcohol are freely available without restriction.

Social Environment

Many social factors such as unemployment, peer group relationship and social deprivation play a part. Disturbed family circumstances, working environments, marital disharmony, poverty and consumerism are the major social factors.

Physiological Reward Theory

Release of dopamine in large amounts is noted in the nucleus accumbens in drug dependent individuals. The nucleus gets its innervation from the ventral tegmentum. The dopaminergic response is rewarding since it is associated with a sensation of pleasure (positive reinforcement).

Behavior Theory

The pharmacological effect brings on euphoria and relief. This positively reinforces the behavior to repeat the act of substance abuse. When the effect becomes one of flushing, nausea or tachycardia which is unpleasant, it negatively reinforces the behavior and drug consumption is given up. Substance use results in different types of clinical states which are as follows:

- *Acute intoxication:* When the drug use is transient, a picture of acute intoxication results. Abnormal psychic and physical symptoms appear. Symptoms depend upon the drug used. They disappear as the drug is discontinued.

- ***Harmful use (abuse):*** Heavy substance use may lead to damage to physical health (e.g. alcoholic hepatitis), social health (e.g. disapproval and criticism) and mental health (e.g. depression).
- ***Dependence syndrome:*** These are altered physiological and mental states (alteration of mood, behavior and cognition) due to prolonged use of the drug. Withdrawal symptoms occur when the substance is abruptly discontinued. There is overwhelming desire (compulsion) to continue the drug use in order to overcome the unpleasant effects.
- ***Tolerance:*** Tolerance is another feature. Effect of the drug diminishes with repeated use of the same dose. The dose has to be increased progressively to get the same effect. Interest and pleasure in other useful activities diminish.
- ***Withdrawal state:*** This develops once the drug is discontinued after prolonged use. Physical symptoms and psychological symptoms are seen.
- ***Amnesic syndrome:*** Constant impairment in recent memory is the prominent symptom. Events and time sense are confused (confabulation).
- ***Psychiatric conditions:*** Psychiatric conditions like delusions, hallucinations, mood disorders and schizophrenic symptoms may also result.

Diagnosis

Diagnosis is made from the history, physical examination and laboratory findings.

TREATMENT

Principles: Detoxification, psychosocial therapy and ***rehabilitation*** are the methods of treatment.

The treatment of substance abuse is not easy. The first step is the motivation of the patient to accept the treatment. The substance is then totally withdrawn. The withdrawal symptoms which may result are treated medically. Psychotic and mood symptoms require appropriate medications. The abstinence is maintained by psychosocial therapy. Counseling and group therapy may help to resolve personal and interpersonal problems.

Rehabilitation to re-establish their social and economic position is important to prevent relapse. Financial support and social guidance are helpful steps to bring the victim to mainstream lifestyle.

PREVENTION

Substance abuse can be prevented through mass education, banning the production and distribution of drugs, and giving moral education to build-up psychic immunity. Since drug addiction starts early in life, the younger population is at risk; therefore, the college and school students are to be specially targeted.

Among the psychoactive substances, prevalence of alcohol, nicotine (tobacco containing products), cannabis, opioids and LSD use are the most widespread in India.

ALCOHOL-RELATED DISORDERS

See also Section 4, Ch 23

These disorders result from the consumption of ethyl alcohol-containing beverages in quantities large enough to damage the physical, mental and social health of an individual. Brandy, whisky, rum and arrack containing about 30–40% alcohol (referred to as spirits) and toddy, beer and wines which contain alcohol from 5% to 7% to 10% respectively are legally available and they form the bulk of alcoholic drinks consumed in India. In addition, an unknown quantity of illicitly made alcoholic drinks is available in all parts of the country, which are also consumed in large quantities.

Etiology

The role played by genetic factor is important since persons show a genetic and familial predisposition to acquire the habit. Both psychological and environmental factors contribute to the development of alcoholism. Social and family maladjustment, economic factors and vulnerable personality together promote the dependence on alcohol. Anxious and depressed persons find solace in alcohol to get over their symptoms. Antisocial personalities find pleasure in alcohol, especially during periods of crisis.

Alcohol induces euphoria and relief from anxiety. These serve as positive incentives to repeat the consumption. This positive reinforcing effect is associated with a high amount of dopamine release in the ***nucleus accumbens***. In some oriental population such as the Japanese, a variant of the isoenzyme ***aldehyde dehydrogenase*** provides them partial immunity to alcohol. They get negatively reinforced by the production of nausea, flushing and tachycardia on consuming alcohol. Several physical and psychological abnormalities can be caused by alcohol depending upon the amount of consumption, its frequency, type of beverage consumed, co-existent physical and psychiatric illnesses and the nutritional status.

Clinical Features

Alcohol is a cerebral disinhibitant. Acute intoxication causes euphoria or elation, slurred speech, incoordination, polyurea and gait disturbances. During periods of excitement, irrelevant talk, aggressive and violent activity, illusions and persecutory delusions may be observed. In cases of ***chronic alcoholism,*** many other neuropsychiatric complications may be noted. These include continuous auditory hallucinations ***(alcoholic hallucinosis)*** and delirium tremens on withdrawal of alcohol. Other manifestations include delusion of infidelity (***alcoholic paranoia***), loss of recent memory with personality change (***amnestic syndrome/Korsakoff's psychosis),*** intellectual deterioration (alcoholic dementia) and signs of cerebellar degeneration. Depression, schizophrenia and sexual dysfunction may be aggravated by chronic alcoholism. It is a major cause of suicide. Chronic alcoholism causes damage to several organs such as the stomach, liver, peripheral and central nervous system (CNS), heart and others. Consumption of alcohol by drivers is a major contributory factor for road accidents. Alcoholism is a serious major precipitating factor for violence and crimes.

CAGE is a commonly used questionnaire used to diagnose alcoholism. Affirmative answers to any two of the following questions (or to the last question alone) are suggestive of alcohol abuse which:

- Have you ever felt that you should ***Cut*** down your drinking?
- Have you ever felt ***Annoyed*** by others criticizing your drinking?

- Have you ever felt *Guilty* about your drinking?
- Have you ever had a morning drink (*Eye-opener*) after hangover?

Diagnosis of alcoholism is based on the history and clinical features. The severity of intoxication generally correlates with the blood levels of alcohol though there are several exceptions. Blood level can be easily determined by the severity of consumption. It can be rapidly determined by breath tests using breath analyzer.

Treatment

The treatment of alcoholism includes treatment of dependence; psychiatric complications; and *physical complications.* Motivation is absolutely required in all cases. The patient is initially detoxified. Alcohol is withdrawn. The resulting withdrawal reaction, delirium tremens, is medically managed. The patient is quieted with chlordiazepoxide. Electrolyte imbalance and dehydration are corrected. Anticonvulsants and antipsychotics may be needed. After the detoxification process, psychotherapeutic measures are employed. The goal is to improve the environment and personality to maintain sobriety.

Prevention of relapse may be achieved through *behavioral therapy technique* or by *chemical aversion.* For chemical aversion, disulfiram (*antabuse*) is chosen. Initially, a dose of 0.5 g twice daily for the first day, 0.75 g on the second day followed by 0.5 g on the third day and 0.25 g on the fourth day onwards. The patient is advised not to take alcohol containing liquids, since they lead to intense discomfort and even life-threatening consequences when receiving antabuse. Relapse can also be prevented by anti-craving drugs such as *acamprosate* (calcium acetyl homotaurine), a gamma-aminobutyric acid (GABA) analog which inhibits the craving for alcohol. It is given in doses of 333–666 mg thrice daily. Naltrexone is an antagonist of endogenous endorphin. This drug is given in the doses of 50 mg once a day after stopping alcohol for 12 weeks. It helps to maintain abstinence. The neuropsychiatric complications and physical complications are medically managed.

Though many persons get temporary benefit, the motivation for abstinence wanes off and on returning to his home situation the habit returns, often in a more severe form.

CANNABIS-RELATED DISORDERS

Cannabis is widely used as ganja, bhang, charas, hashish, hashish oil, hemp and marijuana for getting its acute intoxicating effect, but unaware of its serious health hazards, on long-term use. The intoxicating effect is produced by its alkaloid content mainly delta 9-tetrahydrocannabinol (delta 9THC). It is a gateway drug as it leads to other type of drug use.

Acute intoxication produces physical and mental alterations. Mood becomes euphoric or elated or intensely anxious. Perception is heightened. Elementary and synesthetic hallucinations, derealization, depersonalization and sense of floating in the air are experienced.

The perceptive changes may be re-experienced at later times in the absence of its use (flashbacks). Headache, tachycardia, tachypnea restlessness and redness of conjunctiva are marked features.

Harmful cannabis use produces more serious symptoms. Anxiety disorders, mood disorders, psychosis with persecutory delusions, (hemp insanity) impairment of cognitive functions are known to be precipitated. The use may be associated with apathy, anergia, loss of interests in personal activities and responsibilities, termed as *Amotivational Syndrome*. Impotency, sterility due to damage of Leydig cells, chromosome damage, cerebral atrophy, coronary heart disease and pulmonary cancer has all been reported.

Cannabis is a drug with reverse tolerance. Physical dependence is disputed but may be mild with short-term anxiety and insomnia. Psychological dependence is there.

Treatment

The cannabis substance is withdrawn. Insomnia, anxiety and mild restlessness that may result is managed with drugs. Psychotherapy and counseling are the ones meant for the maintenance of abstinence.

OPIOIDS-RELATED DISORDERS

The opioids are alkaloid substances contained in the resin opium which is derived from the flower buds of poppy plants. Crude opium, morphine, codeine, heroin (diacetylmorphine—a synthetic derivative) are the commonly abused substances. These are associated with strong physical dependence and severe withdrawal symptoms. Heroin is injected by groups sharing the same syringe and sharing of needle is a potent risk factor for the spread of diseases like acquired immune deficiency syndrome (AIDS), hepatitis and others.

The acute intoxication produces initial euphoria leading to dysphoria, nausea, vomiting, drowsiness, respiratory depression, pupillary constriction and constipation. Psychomotor activity is slowed down. Speech becomes slurred. Attention, concentration and memory are impaired. Anxiety disorders, mood disorders and psychotic disorders may be precipitated. Sexual dysfunctions and impotence may develop. Serious physical problems such as local cellulitis and abscess, human immunodeficiency virus (HIV) and other viral infections are common with unhygienic parenteral administration.

The withdrawal symptoms are characterized by yawning, lacrimation, rhinorrhea, pupillary dilatation, sweating, diarrhea, insomnia, dysphoria, muscle cramps, piloerection, tremors and severe restlessness.

Treatment

Detoxification: The drugs are withdrawn though substitution therapy with methadone a synthetic narcotic.
Clonidine: An adrenergic alpha receptor blocker is in common use; 0.1 mg thrice daily.
Naloxone and naltrexone: These are opioid antagonist with long half-lives. Dose 50–100 mg on alternate days. Naltrexone-clonidine combination is usually preferred. Naltrexone is initially given to produce withdrawal symptoms, when clonidine also is added for relief. After 2–3 weeks the drugs are gradually tapered off.
Buprenorphine: It is another drug that is used in opium withdrawal, dosed at 8–10 mg daily. Detoxification is followed

by counseling psychotherapy and psychosocial rehabilitation including management of physical complications.

Nicotine-related Disorders

See **Section 4, Ch 26**

Nicotine is the causative agent of large number of serious and fatal physical illness including cancer and coronary heart disease. Nicotine is contained in the widely smoked, chewed and snuffed tobacco products. It provides euphoria and mild stimulation. It is an agonist of acetylcholine nicotine receptor. It activates the tegmental dopamine reward system with positive reinforcement. Nicotine enhances secretion of steroids, adrenaline and noradrenaline which contribute to the stimulatory effect.

1571

CHAPTER
245

Behavioral Syndromes Associated with Physiological Disturbances and Physical Factors

N Krishnan Kutty

Chapter Summary

- Eating Disorders
  - Anorexia Nervosa
  - Bulimia Nervosa
- Sleep Disorders
  - Insomnia
  - Hypersomnia
  - Parasomnias
- Sexual Dysfunction
  - Erectile Disorder
  - Premature Ejaculation
  - Abnormalities of Sexual Preference
- Postpartum Psychiatric Disorders (Puerperal Psychosis)

These are a group of disorders where internal medicine as well as psychiatry plays dominant roles both in the causation and management.

EATING DISORDERS

Eating disorders like anorexia nervosa and bulimia nervosa are the most common.

Anorexia Nervosa

This disorder is common among adolescent girls and young women. It is a condition characterized by severe resistance and fear to eat or drink articles of food for prolonged periods leading to severe loss of body weight. There is loss of standard body weight of 15% or more, with the body mass index (BMI) below 17.5. Any attempt to force them to feed may result in vomiting. Vomiting and diarrhea may also be deliberately induced for reducing weight. Though this disorder is more common among prepubertal females, males are not exempt. Body image disturbance is the main cause, but hypothalamic disturbances have also been noted. The fear of becoming obese is the triggering factor. The wish to become a *lean beauty* is also a factor. Amenorrhea, anemia intolerance to cold, growth of lanugo hair, dry skin and cardiac arrhythmias secondary to nutritional deficiencies are also common. Symptoms of depression, obsessive compulsive disorder (OCD) and sexual maladjustment are associated features. In severe cases, cachexia supervenes. The condition is fatal, if untreated.

Treatment

It is mainly supportive. Inpatient care may be required. The patient and family members are educated about the disease. Better interpersonal relationship should be promoted. The patient is encouraged to bring up body weight by eating, helped by counseling and drugs. At least 1,200–1,500 calories should be supplied per day and gradually increased up to 3,000–4,000 calories. Rarely parenteral feeding has to be given. In 6% of cases, *refeeding syndrome* may develop. This may give rise to transient pedal edema. Emergency complications include prolongation of Q-T interval in the electrocardiography (ECG), hypophosphatemia, weakness, confusion and neuromuscular dysfunction.

No drug is specific for anorexia nervosa. Cyproheptadine, chlorpromazine and pimozide are found to be useful. Modified insulin treatment can be used to bring up weight. Some cases may improve with electroconvulsive therapy (ECT).

Bulimia Nervosa

This is characterized by episodes of irresistible urge to overeat (binges). Surprisingly, the body weight remains normal. This is usually achieved by the self-induction of vomiting, use of laxatives or diuretics, or strenuous exercise. It is seen more commonly in women. Amenorrhea is not a feature. Stress encourages overeating. Cognitive behavior therapy and other forms of psychotherapy may help to reduce stress and prevent this disorder. Drugs such as selective serotonin reuptake inhibitors (SSRIs) are helpful adjuncts. Complications may develop on account of repeated vomiting or due to side effects of self-administered drugs which are to be tackled appropriately.

SLEEP DISORDERS

Insomnia, hypersomnia and parasomnias are not uncommon conditions.

Insomnia

Insomnia denotes difficulty in falling asleep or staying asleep or poor quality of the sleep. It is the most common sleep disorder. It may be primary or secondary. The secondary causes are medical and psychiatric. Physical pain, asthma, arthritis, hyperthyroidism, excessive use of caffeine, hunger, use of drugs such as aminophylline and steroids are the common medical causes. Depression, anxiety, mania, OCD, dementia and withdrawal from alcohol or drugs are the common psychiatric causes. The treatment depends on alleviation of the primary cause. Hypnotics can be used temporarily.

In primary insomnia, no specific cause can be found. It is uncommon. There is difficulty in falling asleep or the patient wakes up frequently. The treatment modalities are conditioning of sleep, adoption of sleep hygiene using the bedroom only for sleeping, change of bedroom, and relaxation techniques and use of hypnotic on a short-term basis.

Hypersomnia

In this condition, there is excessive sleep; narcolepsy is the most common condition.

Narcolepsy

It is a hypersomnic condition of unknown etiology characterized by the tetrad of symptoms—sleep attacks, cataplexy, sleep paralysis and hypnagogic and hypnopompic hallucinations. It is an abnormality of rapid eye movement (REM) sleep. REM latency is seen much lowered.

Etiology

The prevalence of narcolepsy is 0.05% in the general population. There is genetic predisposition and is association with human leukocyte antigen (HLA) status. There is deficiency of hipocretin-1, a neuropeptide produced by the hypothalamus.

Clinical features

Sleep attack is the main symptom. There is an irresistible tendency to fall asleep and this may last for 10–15 minutes. The mind is fresh when awake. A less frequently associated symptom is cataplexy, the phenomenon of sudden loss of generalized muscle tone at the peak of intense emotions such as happiness, anger or other emotional outbursts. Sleep paralysis is rare and is manifested as an alarming experience that the person cannot talk nor do any activity when awake. The mind is awake but the body is not. Vivid visual and auditory hallucinations occurring while going to sleep or coming out of sleep are termed hypnagogic and hypnopompic hallucinations, respectively. Other REM sleep abnormalities may also be found.

Diagnosis: Diagnostic criteria are:

- Excessive daytime sleep occurring almost daily for at least 3 months, not attributable to other causes
- Associated cataplexy/sleep paralysis and or hypnagogic and hypnopompic hallucinations
- REM latency reduction in multiple sleep latency test (MSLT)
- Levels of cerebrospinal fluid (CSF) hypocretin-1 below 110 ng/L or less than 30% of normal values are highly suggestive.

Treatment

Narcolepsy has no cure and therefore the management is symptomatic. The medications include:

- Dopamine stimulants to daytime sleepiness and sleep attacks
- Antidepressants (mostly noradrenergic) to control cataplexy and
- Hypnotics for disturbed night-time sleep.

Modafinil, alpha 1-adrenergic receptor antagonist is a wakefulness promoting agent, given in a dose of 100–200 mg in the morning, repeated after lunch if needed. Methylphenidate and amphetamines are commonly used in doses below 60 mg/day. Other stimulants include sodium oxybate, mazindol, pemoline and selegiline. Dose of mazindol is 2–3 mg/day.

Sodium oxybate is the approved drug for cataplexy, given in doses of 3–9 g at night. It reduces day time sleepiness, narcolepsy, sleep paralysis and hypnagogic hallucinations. Adverse side effects include dizziness, headache, nausea and less frequently, pain, depressive mood, enuresis and sleepwalking. Antidepressant drugs (especially SSRIs) are effective in treatment of narcolepsy and cataplexy—especially clomipramine in doses of 10–25 mg.

Parasomnias

These are abnormal events occurring while asleep. They may be nightmares, night terror, somnambulism (sleep walking), somniloquy (sleep talking), bruxism (teeth grinding) and enuresis (bed wetting). These are common in children.

Nightmare

It occurs during REM sleep. The person may get up from sleep with frightening dreams. Sleep may proceed after it. The content of the dream is recollected the next day. It is always nonpathological. But it is common after a stressful experience. Usually no treatment is required. Measures to reduce stress, reassurance, tricyclic antidepressants to reduce REM sleep and diazepam are the modalities of treatment.

Night Terror

The person (often a child) gets up from sleep frightened, terrified, confused, disoriented, screaming aloud, clinging to others around or running for help. Symptoms of autonomous arousal such as sweating palpitation are there. After this episode, the person falls asleep again. The episode is not remembered the next morning. It occurs during non-rapid eye movement (NREM) sleep. It can be a manifestation of temporal lobe epilepsy. Treatment is seldom required. Diazepam or antiepileptic drugs may be required if a seizure disorder is diagnosed (Table 245.1).

Sleep Walking (Somnambulism)

This occurs during NREM sleep. It may be associated with sleep talking. The person may get up while asleep and perform various activities like taking bath, getting dressed up and even going for a walk and returning. He may meet with accidents during this phase. The activity can be terminated by waking him up. The events are not recollected when awake.

Table 245.1: Clinical features and comparison between nightmare and night terror

	Sleeping stage	Characteristics	Treatment
Nightmare (bad dream)	Occurs during REM sleep	• Memory of the events upon awakening • Increases during stress • Reported by 50% of the population	• Tricyclic antidepressant's (TCAs) • Hypnotics • Diazepam • Reassurance
Night terror	Occurs during stages 3 and 4	• Awakened by scream or intense anxiety clinging to another person • No memory of the event • More common in children (boys)	No treatment is necessary or use benzodiazepines

SEXUAL DYSFUNCTIONS

Sexual response is a psychosomatic process. The natural sexual activity in humans is the coital union of man and woman culminating in orgasm in both the partners. Seminal discharge occurs in the male during this state. The causes of sexual disturbances may be physical, psychological or both. The different disorders include:

- Reduction or loss of sexual desire and lack of sexual enjoyment
- Lack of genital response, which includes impotence in men and absence of sexual arousal in women
- Orgasmic dysfunction which includes premature or retarded ejaculation in man and orgasmic failure in women
- Vaginismus and dyspareunia in women and painful ejaculation in men.

Erectile Disorder

Impotence

It is the inability to get or sustain erection sufficient enough for satisfactory coitus. Impotence may be due to physical diseases or may be due to psychological causes. If erection occurs in the presence of another partner or during masturbation, it indicates a psychological cause. Presence of spontaneous early morning erection also points to a psychological cause. Psychological causes leading to impotence include venereophobia, lack of privacy, inertia on the part of the partner, fear of castration, and incestuous feelings.

Diseases such as depression, conversion disorders or anxiety disorder are associated with impotence. Many psychotropic drugs impair erection and delay ejaculation on account of autonomic side effects. Drugs such as bromocriptine, yohimbine and cyproheptadine may be useful in such cases.

Phosphodiesterase type-5 inhibitor such as sildenafil, tadalafil and vardenafil are found very effective. ***Sildenafil*** is very effective to induce strong erection when given in doses of 25–100 mg. SOS to be taken 1 hour before expected intercourse. Only one dose should be taken within 24 hours. Cooperation from the partner is essential for success.

Side effects include vomiting, headache, flushing, dizziness, visual disturbances, raised intraocular pressure, nasal congestion and hypersensitivity reactions. Contraindications include the concurrent use of nitrates, and vasodilators; hypertension, recent stroke, unstable angina, myocardial infarction (MI) and hepatic damage.

Premature Ejaculation

This is the occurrence of ejaculation early during the sexual intercourse before penetration or soon after that. This leads to a sense of frustration in the male and the female partner who does not get orgasm. Physical methods such as the ***stop and start technique*** and ***squeeze technique*** in which the glans penis is squeezed when ejaculation is imminent, may succeed in some cases. Drugs such as fluoxetine and tricyclic antidepressants are helpful to delay ejaculation.

Female orgasmic disorder: Many women may fail to get orgasm or it may be obtained only after undue delay.

Abnormalities of Sexual Preference

Syn: Paraphilias

Fetishism, transvestic fetishism, pedophilia, exhibitionism, sexual sadism, sexual masochism and voyeurism are some of the important disorders.

- ***Fetishism:*** Libido gratification from contact with articles such as dress, hair and others of the opposite sex.
- ***Pedophilia:*** An unnatural urge and desire to have sexual relationship with children of prepubertal age.
- ***Exhibitionism:*** Tendency to exhibit his/her genitals to members of the opposite sex in public for sexual pleasure.
- ***Sexual sadism:*** Sexual pleasure derived from inflicting mental or physical pain on the sexual partner.
- ***Sexual masochism:*** Sexual pleasure derived by being abused or being acted cruelly by the opposite partner.
- ***Voyeurism:*** This is the phenomenon in which a person derives sexual pleasure by observing sexual activity of others.
- ***Scopophilia:*** This is sexual pleasure uptake from visual sources such as nudity in the opposite sex and obscene pictures.

POSTPARTUM PSYCHIATRIC DISORDERS (PUERPERAL PSYCHOSIS)

These are the psychiatric disturbances which are precipitated by the stress of child birth. Two common types are there.

1. ***Postpartum blues*** (Maternity blues) is a mild disturbance of short duration. The main symptoms are irritability, crying spells, labile mood, agitation and confusion immediately following child birth. It may disappear by itself within 2–3 days. To hasten recovery antianxiety drugs may be used.
2. ***Postpartum psychosis*** is a severe kind of disturbance. The symptoms in the majority of cases are those of mood disorders—either of mania or depression with

agitation. Schizophrenia and delirium-like picture do occur at times. The life of the infant is always at risk, because of the delusions involving the baby. So the baby has to be protected. Maternal suicide too is potential risk.

The *diagnosis* has to be made after exclusion of any intracranial pathology. The *treatment* depends upon the clinical presentations. Antidepressants, antipsychotics, antianxiety and anti-hypnotic drugs may be selected according to the clinical presentations.

CHAPTER
246

Psychological Factors Affecting Systemic Medical Disorders

N Krishnan Kutty

Chapter Summary

- Psychosomatic Disorders
- Psychiatric Disorders Caused By General Medical Disorders

PSYCHOSOMATIC DISORDERS

The body and mind interact both in health and illness. The mind plays a major role in many physical illnesses. A physical illness may be precipitated, aggravated or prolonged by psychological factors. This paved the way for the concept of psychosomatic disorders. This term has now been replaced by a new terminology *psychological factors affecting medical conditions*. The psychological factors are many:

- It may be a primary mental disorder which affects the course of a medical disease, e.g. major depression delays recovery from stroke; MI
- It can also be a psychological symptom that adversely affects the disease, e.g. anxiety worsens bronchial asthma. Depressive symptoms delay recovery from surgery
- It may be a personality factor that precipitates a disease, e.g. Type A personality in coronary artery disease (CAD)
- It may be severe stress.

There are many physical disorders where psychological factors play a major role. The common physical disorders which will be affected by psychological stress may affect all systems.

- *Respiratory disorders:* Bronchial asthma, hay fever, vasomotor rhinitis
- *Gastrointestinal (GI) disorders:* Peptic ulcer, irritable bowel syndrome (IBS), ulcerative colitis, anorexia nervosa
- *Cardiovascular disorders:* Hypertension, paroxysmal tachycardia, CAD
- *Nervous system:* Migraine, headaches
- *Endocrine and metabolic disorders:* Hyperthyroidism, diabetes mellitus (DM), menstrual disturbances, obesity
- *Dermatologic disorders:* Eczema, psoriasis, neuro-dermatitis
- *Bones and joints:* Rheumatoid arthritis (RA), backache
- *Maladaptive health behavior affecting a general medical condition*, e.g. treatment is the more important modality, avoidance of physical exercise, overeating, unsafe sex practices and others.

Management

Appropriate medical management which ensures relief relieves the mental tension as well. Antianxiety drugs and mood elevators may be required in some. Other measures include counseling, general behavior therapy techniques such as relaxation, biofeedback, controlled breathing

Table 246.1: Psychiatric symptoms associated with general medical conditions

General medical conditions	Psychiatric symptoms/syndromes
Endocrine disorders	**Psychotic symptoms**
• Hyperthyroidism	Delusions, hallucinations, agitation, insomnia
• Hypothyroidism	**Mood symptoms**
• Hyperparathyroidism	Depression—persistent sadness,
• Cushing's disease	gloomy thought, motor
• Addison's disease	retardation, suicidal intent, ideas
• Pheochromocytoma	and attempts.
Metabolic conditions	Mania-elated, expansive mood,
• Hypoglycemia	hyperactivity, persecutory/
• Hepatic encephalopathy	grandiose delusions, muscular
• Uremia	rigidity, immobility, catatonic
CNS conditions	posturing, negativism, mutism,
Encephalitis sequelae, GPI, poststroke, post-traumatic, Alzheimer's disease, Huntington's chorea, Wilson's disease, tuberous sclerosis, Parkinsonism, frontal and temporal lobe tumors	echolalia and echopraxia
	Anxiety symptoms
	Generalized anxiety, restlessness, panic episodes, obsessive compulsive symptoms, amnesia, dementia
Drugs	
Propranolol, antipsychotics, steroids sympathomimetics, ranitidine, L-dopa, oral contraceptives	**Personality change**
Other conditions	A persistent change in behavior from the previous state and change of character
Vitamin B$_{12}$ deficiency, pellagra, leukemia, systemic lupus erythematosis (SLE)	——Do——

Note: Any psychiatric symptoms may develop in any of the general medical conditions, nonspecifically.

Abbreviations: CNS = Central nervous system; GPI = Genuine progress indicator

Textbook of Medicine

exercises as practiced in yoga and other measures such as hypnosis.

PSYCHIATRIC DISORDERS CAUSED BY GENERAL MEDICAL DISORDERS

Several primary psychiatric disorders are accompanied by somatic manifestations. Similarly, psychiatric symptoms develop in several general medical conditions such as cerebral infarction, encephalitis, drug toxicities and others. These are evident from the history, physical examination and laboratory findings. The psychiatric symptoms are not specific for any particular medical disorder and vice versa. They are not reactions or sequelae of primary medical conditions. There are several medical and surgical conditions which give rise to psychiatric manifestations as part of the disease process. The psychiatric abnormality also clears up when the underlying condition is treated. Though psychotropic drugs too, are needed in the initial phase. These are described along with such disorders in the different sections. Table 246.1 gives a list of important medical conditions which give rise to mental symptoms.

Chapter Summary

- General Considerations
  - Causes of Mental Retardation
- Down's Syndrome (Mongolism)

GENERAL CONSIDERATIONS

(Syn: Mental subnormality/mental handicap/idiocy/ amentia/mentally challenged/oligophrenia/intellectual disability/intellectual development disorder)

Mental retardation is a state of subaverage intellectual functioning resulting in or associated with impairment in adaptive behavior and manifested during the developmental period before the age of 18 years. Normal persons adapt sufficiently to various needs of the society and the environment. Adaptive behavior can be measured using **Vineland Adaptive Behavior Scale (VABS)**. The retardation is graded on the basis of **intelligence quotient (IQ)** into four grades (Table 247.1).

Causes of Mental Retardation

Mental retardation can occur with or without any obvious mental or physical disorder. Several etiological factors are known. A few of them include:

- **Chromosome abnormality**—Down's syndrome, fragile X syndrome, inborn errors of metabolism, e.g. phenylketonuria and the like
- **Congenital brain abnormalities**—microcephaly, hydrocephalus, tuberous sclerosis, cretinism, cerebral palsy
- **Prenatal causes**—maternal rubella, syphilis, lead poisoning, alcohol
- **Perinatal causes**—birth asphyxia, kernicterus
- **Postnatal causes**—hypothyroidism, injury, intoxication with lead and mercury, autism, encephalitis, meningitis.

DOWN'S SYNDROME (MONGOLISM)

See also Section 1, Ch 2

This condition is the most common chromosomal abnormality causing mental retardation. It was described by Langdon Down in 1886. The incidence is 1 in 30 livebirths occurring in children born to mothers aged 45 and above. The risk in the second child is 1 in 100.

Pathology: The 21st chromosome occurs as triple (trisomy) instead of the normal two alleles. About 95% of **trisomy** is due to nondisjunction which happens during meiosis. The rest 5% is due to translocation and **mosaicism**. In mosaicism, the nondisjunction occurs during cell division after fertilization.

Clinical features: Clinical features are characteristic. The face is round with small mouth and pegged teeth, furrowed protruding tongue and high-arched palate. The eyes show oblique palpebral fissures and epicanthic folds. The occiput is flat. The hand is short and broad with a single

Table 247.1: Grades of mental retardation

Grade of mental retardation	IQ range	Mental age	Occurrence rate	Most common cause
Mild/moron or feeble mindedness	50–69	Under 9	85%	Psychosocial
Moderate (Imbecility)	35–49	Under 6	10%	Down's syndrome, fragile X syndrome, phenylketonuria
Severe	20–34	>3 <6	3–4%	Microcephaly, cretinism, cerebral palsy
Profound (Idiocy)	Below 20	Below 3	1–2%	Microcephaly, cretinism, cerebral palsy

Abbreviation: IQ = Intelligence quotient

palmar crease and short curved little finger. Hypotonia and hypermobility of joints may occur. Other less common features are congenital heart disease (CHD), especially septal defects, duodenal obstruction, impaired immune responses, higher incidence of leukemia, hypothyroidism and atlantoaxial dislocation.

Diagnosis: It is done by the clinical findings and IQ measurement. IQ below 70 favors mental retardation. Mental retardation can be predicted during infancy by the presence of clinical features such as microcephaly, mongoloid features, cerebral palsy and others. During early childhood, delay in the developmental milestones, academic backwardness, peer group maladjustment and absconding from school or house may suggest mental retardation. Later in life, such cases present as inability to bear responsibilities and failure in adaptation to life situations, some requiring supervision even in routine work.

Management and care of mental retardation: The main objectives are provision of educational and psychosocial care. It depends on the age of the retarded person and grade of retardation. Fostering, boarding, schooling in special schools and accommodation are their social needs. A team approach, including doctors, nurses, occupational therapists, psychologists, physiotherapists and speech therapists, is most rewarding. Persons with mild handicap can live independently though supervision may be needed in special situations.

Normalization is the modern concept in the management of mental retardation, widely practiced in the USA. The mentally retarded person is made to live in the community and given the chance to experience and participate in social activities. Retarded children are preferably brought up in their own homes. Training and accommodation are provided in the proximity of the family. As in the case of normal persons, the mentally retarded are also prone to develop various psychiatric disorders. Drugs and behavior therapy are given accordingly. (For Down's syndrome *See* Section 1, Ch 2).

CHAPTER 248

Behavioral and Emotional Disorders Occurring in Childhood and Adolescence
(Syn. Psychiatric Disorders in Childhood and Adolescence)

N Krishnan Kutty

Chapter Summary

- Disorders of Psychological Development
- Pervasive Developmental Disorders
  - Childhood Autism (Infantile Autism or Autistic Disorder)
  - Attention Deficit Hyperactivity Disorder (Hyperkinetic Syndrome)
- Conduct Disorders (Juvenile Delinquency)
- Enuresis (Bed-Wetting)

Children too suffer from common psychiatric disorders as other age groups. Some of the disorders are seen exclusively in childhood. The important ones are described here.

DISORDERS OF PSYCHOLOGICAL DEVELOPMENT

Children may lag behind in the development of learning of certain academic skills specifically. Common disorders are:

- Specific reading disorders
- Specific spelling disorders
- Specific mathematics disorders
- Understanding and articulation of spoken language
- Impairment of motor coordination.

Lack of self-esteem and delay in brain maturation may be the cause in many. The disorders may disappear as the child grows. Emotional support and instilling confidence may enhance recovery.

PERVASIVE DEVELOPMENTAL DISORDERS

The symptoms of these disorders are generalized by impairment of social skills, communication skills and general behavior. Childhood autism and attention deficit hyperactivity disorder (ADHD) (hyperkinetic syndrome) are the common disorders accounting for this deficit.

Childhood Autism (Infantile Autism or Autistic Disorder)

The term autism denotes a state of absorption into one's own world of fantasy with loss of contact with the reality. Autistic behavior is the prominent symptom. Reported incidence of childhood autism is 2–5/10,000 livebirths.

Childhood autism was originally described by ***Leo Kanner*** in 1943 as ***Early Infantile Autism. Autistic aloofness, language abnormality and restricted*** and ***compulsive behavior*** are the three main features of this disorder. Boys are more affected than girls. The disorder is unmasked by the third year of life and the child appears normal till then. The child is abnormally quiet, lacks the usual emotional warmth and likes to be left alone. Eye-to-eye contact is avoided. He does not communicate through conversation. Pronouns are reversed. 'You' is used to mean 'I'. Echolalia is common. Words and behavior are stereotypic. The child is fond of sameness in everything. Bizarre behavior such as rocking, whirling the head and flapping of hand may be present. Impulsive violence and destructiveness are common. The arithmetic skill is relatively high. Intelligence quotient (IQ) may be around 70 in most cases. Some have normal IQ. Many cases may be attributable to birth trauma. Autism shows a strong genetic predilection and probably arises from multiple genetic defects. Recurrence within families with one affected child is high.

There is no specific treatment. Antipsychotics are given to control violence and hyperactivity. Behavior therapy may be helpful. Parents are to be counseled regarding management of the child at home. Some may improve spontaneously and may be able to attend normal school. A few may require training in special schools. Some require special residential care.

Attention Deficit Hyperactivity Disorder (Hyperkinetic Syndrome)

This disorder is more common in boys. Persistent inattention, hyperactivity and impulsivity are the cardinal features. These affect their scholastic performance. Impulsive and reckless behavior are common. Brain damage due to birth trauma, allergy to food containing tartrazine, toxicity to lead and overactivity of peripheral adrenergic system are some of the recognized causes.

Treatment

Stimulant drugs such as Dexedrine 2.5–5 mg twice a day, clonidine, tricyclic antidepressants and monoamine oxidase inhibitors are beneficial. Many children become normal as they reach adolescence. Atomoxetine hydrochloride is a recently introduced drug for this condition.

CONDUCT DISORDERS (JUVENILE DELINQUENCY)

These are the most common disorders of childhood. Persistent dissocial, aggressive or defiant behaviors are the presenting features. It is manifested as quarrelsomeness, disobedience, lying, cruelty to people and animals, fighting with people, destructiveness, stealing, absconding from school, fire setting, temper tantrums, running away from home and the like. They may turn into antisocial personalities later in life. The disorder may be the outcome of unsatisfactory family environment, poor academic performance and such other psychosocial adversities.

Treatment

Some may improve spontaneously. Drugs are of little value. Psychosocial therapy is important. The child is given insight-oriented psychotherapy to bring up problem solving skills. Adverse domestic factors are identified and removed. The child's behavior is rectified through rewards, praise and approval (contingency management). The family at risk may be screened and is to be given support and guidance.

Drugs: In selected cases, antipsychotics, selective serotonin reuptake inhibitors (SSRIs), mood stabilizers and anxiolytics may be helpful.

ENURESIS (BED-WETTING)

Almost all children get bladder control by the age of 5. *Nocturnal enuresis is the voiding of urine during sleep persisting after the age of 5 years*. In primary enuresis, the child has never attained bladder control after birth. In secondary enuresis, the child has attained bladder control which is subsequently lost. Delay in brain maturation, emotional factors such as school problems, birth of a younger child, loss of parental affection and other stressful factors may be the underlying causes. Local causes include low volume capacity of the urinary bladder, urinary tract infection (UTI), congenital abnormalities of the lower urinary tract, spina bifida bladder stones and others.

Treatment

Behavior therapy techniques using *mattress alarm (bell or buzzer and pad)*, bladder training exercises and reassurance are the therapeutic modalities. Drugs such as imipramine 25–50 mg at night are useful. Intranasal administration of synthetic antidiuretic hormone spray is effective.

CHAPTER 249

Psychiatric Emergencies

N Krishnan Kutty

Chapter Summary

- Suicide, Attempted Suicide and Deliberate Self-Harm
- Violent and Aggressive Behavior
- Acute Anxiety and Panic Episode
- Stupor
- Acute Psychological Reactions to Physical Disease
- Abnormal Reactions to Psychotropic Drugs

- Suicide and attempted suicide
- Violent or aggressive behavior
- Acute anxiety and panic episode
- Stupor
- Acute psychological reactions to physical illness
- Abnormal reaction to drugs.

SUICIDE, ATTEMPTED SUICIDE AND DELIBERATE SELF-HARM

Suicide is an expression of personal agony. It is a deliberate act or an attempt to kill by oneself (sui = self, cide = murder). Some of these persons may not be actually bent upon causing death but only be trying to seek attention or help, when they are in distress through the self-injurious behavior. Hence, the term *deliberate self-*

INTRODUCTION

A psychiatric emergency can be defined as a sudden disturbance in behavior, thoughts or feelings for which immediate intervention is necessary to avoid danger to the patient, other people, or both. The common psychiatric emergencies are:

harm (DSH) is commonly used at present to denote such self-destructive actions including suicide.

Causes

Suicide can be due to many causes:

- ***Psychiatric disorders:*** Suicide is always the result of mental disorders. Major depression is the most common condition leading to suicide. It can also occur in schizophrenia, dementia, delirium, alcoholism and drug addiction. Less serious suicidal attempts may be made by patients with dissociation/conversion disorders, personality disorders and antisocial personality disorders.
- ***Physical diseases:*** Chronic or serious physical illness like malignancies and degenerative or disfiguring diseases or surgery chronic pain, use of drugs such as steroid, reserpine, antihypertensive like guanethidine and alpha-methyldopa may lead to a feeling of hopelessness and some may attempt or commit suicide.
- ***Social factors:*** Suicidal behavior is high among socially and emotionally isolated individuals as shown by the French Sociologist Émile Durkheim. Persons with broken families, disturbed marriages and stressful occupations are more vulnerable. Though both sexes make suicidal attempts, more serious ones are made by males. Similarly, suicidal behavior is more common among adolescents and elderly subjects.
- ***Psychological factors:*** Acute psychological distress of a severe degree may often lead to suicidal behavior. Loss of job, financial crisis, marital stresses, interpersonal problems in the family, death or serious illness of beloved ones, accidents, failure in examinations, humiliating or painful experiences and other similar factors may predispose to suicidal behavior.

Management

In attempted suicide, emergency medical management is required to prevent deterioration and death. The modalities depend on the type of attempt and substances used as poisons. Once the emergency is tided over, the next step is to identify the predisposing factors and arrange suitable measures to prevent recurrence. In suicidal risk, the first step is to arrange a safe environment where they can be closely observed. The seriousness of suicidal risk is to be evaluated by taking all relevant factors into consideration. The presence of depression, previous history of suicidal attempts, younger age, history of alcohol and drug addiction, presence of serious physical diseases, severe psychological stresses, social isolation and an immature maladjusted personality contribute to increase the suicidal risk. Such patients require psychological support in the form of counseling and psychotherapy. Counseling is directed to solve the interpersonal problem. The family too are given counseling. Drugs are needed to relieve depression, anxiety or psychosis, if they are present. Hospitalization is better when the risk is high.

VIOLENT AND AGGRESSIVE BEHAVIOR

This may result from psychoses like schizophrenia, mania, delirium and intoxication with drugs and alcohol; side effects of drugs such as antipsychotics and sedatives, and systemic drugs like interferons. The patients are briefly evaluated. They should be kept in safe custody to avoid danger to themselves and others. Some of these patients may respond to supportive environment and reassurance. Physical restraints may be necessary in others. Injections of diazepam 10–20 mg IV slowly, lorazepam 2 mg IM or haloperidol 5 mg IM can be given to quieten the patient. The basic disorder is to be identified and managed subsequently.

Note: The doses of these drugs given for psychiatric conditions are higher than the doses used for general medical conditions.

ACUTE ANXIETY AND PANIC EPISODE

This may be secondary to unidentifiable stresses. The patient comes in severe tension, restlessness and with impending feeling of death or disaster accompanied by marked autonomic arousal. After proper evaluation, provision of supportive environment, reassurance and parenteral administration of antianxiety drugs serve to overcome the anxiety. The causative factors need exploration and further management.

STUPOR

Psychiatric stupor is a state of minimal psychomotor activity. The consciousness is not affected in psychological stupor. These patients may refuse to eat and may not cooperate in maintaining proper hygiene. The causes of stupor include catatonic schizophrenia, depressive illness, dissociative disorder and organic conditions. The general management is similar to that of a comatose patient. Further treatment depends on the underlying cause.

ACUTE PSYCHOLOGICAL REACTIONS TO PHYSICAL DISEASE

It is not uncommon to encounter patients in the general wards who present with acute anxiety, tension, depression, fear, agitation or even aggression along with physical disorders such as ischemic heart disease, stroke, accidents, burns, malignancy, postoperative pain and others. These manifestations are a special form of adjustment disorder to serious illness. Denial of the diagnosis and refusal of treatment are not uncommon. It is not rare that such patients may undertake suicidal attempts in this situation.

Such patients need sympathetic consideration, communication, education, reassurance and encouragement. Drugs may be used to control anxiety and depression. The attending physician should extend psychological help as well as appropriate treatment for the basic physical condition. Other situations where acute psychological stress occurs include the following:

- When breaking the news of a serious illness such as AIDS, cancer or leukemia to the patient.
- When giving the first information of death of a close relative.

In such cases, proper empathy from the physician and a supportive attitude toward the persons help to ease the situation.

ABNORMAL REACTIONS TO PSYCHOTROPIC DRUGS

- Dystonia
- Akathisia
- Neuroleptic malignant syndrome (NMS)
- Drug hypersensitivity.

General Principles of Management of Psychiatric Disorders

N Krishnan Kutty

Chapter Summary

- General Considerations
- Physical Methods of Treatment
  - Electroconvulsive Therapy
  - Transmagnetic Stimulation
  - Psychosurgery
- Pharmacological Methods of Treatment
- Antipsychotic Drugs
  - Malignant Neuroleptic Syndrome
- Antidepressant Drugs
- Antianxiety Drugs
- Antiparkinsonism Drugs

GENERAL CONSIDERATIONS

Mental disorders are treatable conditions. Therapeutic modalities in psychiatric medicine fall into three major groups. These methods are:

1. Physical
2. Pharmacological
3. Psychological

Psychiatric cases can be managed in the regular out-patients department (OPD), but inpatient care is needed in cases of violence, stupor, suicidal threat, delirium and feeding problems.

Combination therapies are much better than a single mode.

PHYSICAL METHODS OF TREATMENT

These are electroconvulsive therapy (ECT) and psychosurgery.

Electroconvulsive Therapy (Shock Therapy)

Convulsive therapy was introduced by Von Meduna in 1934 as a treatment for schizophrenia. He observed that schizophrenia and epilepsy seldom occurred together. So his idea was to produce convulsions to drive away schizophrenia. First he used chemical stimulants such as injection of camphor oil, and later, injections of leptazol to induce the convulsions. In 1938, Cerletti and Bini in Italy found that electricity is not fatal and could produce convulsions and so they devised a machine for the same. Thus, electroshock treatment (EST) came into being and later used the terminology, ECT. ECT became very popular because of its efficacy in the management of depression, mania and schizophrenia.

- ***ECT technique:*** In ECT an electric current is applied over the brain in the temporal regions, so as to induce a seizure by the help of an ECT machine. The electrodes are applied on either side of the scalp over the temporofrontal region (bilateral ECT) or one side of the scalp only (unilateral ECT). An electric current of 70/120 V is passed for a period of 0.2–0.6 seconds in order to induce seizure. The seizure so produced, resembles a typical grand mal epilepsy. Two types of techniques are followed: (1) Direct ECT (where no muscle relaxant is used) and (2) modified ECT, at present modified ECT (where muscle relaxant is used) is the method of choice.

- ***Modified ECT:*** ECT is administered after giving a muscle relaxant in order to minimize the muscular convulsion after anesthetizing with thiopentone sodium or propofol. The help of anesthetist is required. For practical purposes, ECT is comparable to a major surgical procedure. Informed consent should be obtained and the procedure should be undertaken by a specialist, only in places with facilities for emergency medical care is available. Injections of atropine just before anesthesia prevent excessive secretion and tachycardia caused by vagal stimulation.

- ***Indications for ECT:*** ECT is still considered as a very effective therapeutic procedure for the following conditions:
  - Major depression with suicidal intent
  - Depressive stupor
  - Resistant depression
  - Catatonic schizophrenia
  - Acute schizophrenic excitement
  - Manic excitement
  - Schizoaffective disorder.

Contraindications: There is no absolute contraindication except for the anesthesia. The contraindications include acute coronary heart disease (CHD), acute febrile illnesses, hypertension, acute respiratory illness and intracranial space occupying lesions. Pregnancy is not a contraindication.

Complications: Mortality is 3–4 per 100,000. It parallels the risk of anesthesia. The other complications include injuries to tongue, skeletal muscles, ligaments and bones, aspiration pneumonia, cardiac arrest, respiratory arrest and postictal anterograde and retrograde amnesia. The amnesia disappears within 1–4 weeks.

Transmagnetic Stimulation

It is a newer technique developed to stimulate the cerebral cortex. A handheld electromagnet is used. Focal areas of the scalp are stimulated. The stimulus may be applied repeatedly and rhythmically repetitive transmagnetic stimulation (rTMS). rTMS is currently found to be more useful in neurology than in psychiatry. The hypofrontality associated with depression is seen rectified with rTMS.

Psychosurgery

It was introduced by Egas-Moniz. These are neurosurgical operations to control intractable mental disorders. Nerve tracts or nuclei concerned with mental functions are severed or destroyed. Proton beams, radioactive implants such as yttrium-90, ultrasonic beams and electrical coagulation are employed for this operation. *Stereotactic tractotomy* severs the connection between the orbital part of the frontal lobe and the limbic area. *Stereotactic limbic leucotomy* interrupts the frontal lobe pathways and cingulate gyrus and amygdala.

Indications for surgery include intractable conditions not responding to medical treatment such as:

- Obsessive compulsive disorders
- Anxiety disorders
- Depression
- Paranoid schizophrenia
- Pain disorders.

The outcome is unpredictable. Some may improve remarkably and others deteriorate, even to the level of vegetative existence.

PHARMACOLOGICAL METHODS OF TREATMENT (DRUG THERAPY)

The discovery of drugs that can rectify disturbed mental function was a major revolution in psychiatry. These drugs which have affinity towards the mind are collectively called *psychotropic drugs*. Such drugs are generally used in the treatment of mental disorders. They can be classified into:

- Antipsychotics
- Antidepressants
- Mood stabilizers
- Antianxiety drugs
- Hypnotics
- Psychostimulants
- Cognitive enhancers
- Antiparkinsonism drugs.

ANTIPSYCHOTIC DRUGS

Neuroleptics or Major Tranquilizers

These drugs are capable of eliminating psychotic symptoms such as delusions, hallucinations, psychomotor excitement and the associated symptoms. Most of these drugs act by blocking dopamine receptors (D_2) or the serotonin (5-HT_2) receptors in the central nervous system (CNS) at the mesocortical and mesolimbic tracts. In addition they also block the histaminic (H_1) cholinergic and adrenergic receptors and these account for their side effects. These drugs are readily absorbed from the gut and are bound to plasma proteins. They are metabolized mostly by hepatic microsomal oxidase system (Table 250.1).

Conventional Versus Atypical Antipsychotics

Phenothiazines are the first group of antipsychotics that came into popular use. Butyrophenone came later. These drugs produced extrapyramidal symptoms (EPS) as side effects, which were very troublesome. The search for EPS-free drugs lead to the discovery of newer antipsychotics. These newer antipsychotics are relatively free of EPS and are called *atypical antipsychotics* (second generation antipsychotics). The original group of drugs, (first generation antipsychotics) are also known as *conventional antipsychotics*.

Table 250.1: List of antipsychotic drugs in common use

Kind of drugs	Starting dose (mg) oral	Max daily dose (mg)	Prominent side effect
Conventional antipsychotics			
Phenothiazines			Common side effect
Chlorpromazine	50–100 tid 50–100	1,500 IM	Sedation Hypotension
Thioridazine Trifluoperazine	50–100 tid 5 tid	800 60	EPS and others
Fluphenazine decanoate	12.5–50 once in 2–4 weeks	IM	EPS
Butyrophenones			
Haloperidol	5–20 mg tid oral 5–10 IM	100	Severe EPS; noncardiotoxic
Haloperidol decanoate	25–250 once in 2–4 weeks	IM	EPS
Diphenylbutylpiperidine			
Pimozide	2–4 mg od	20	EPS
Atypical antipsychotics			
Benzisoxazoles			
Risperidone	1–2 mg bd oral	16	Sedation, EPS
Dibenzodiazepines			
Clozapine	25–50 mg bd	900	Convulsion, leukopenia
Thienobenzodiazepine			Sedation
Olanzapine gain	5–10 mg od hs	20	Sedation weight
Dibenzothiazepine			
Quetiapine	25–50 mg tid	500	Sedation
Others			
Aripiprazole	10–15 od	30	Insomnia
Amisulpride	50–200 mg	1,200	

Abbreviations: EPS = Extrapyramidal symptoms; IM = Intramuscular

drugs, (first generation antipsychotics) are also known as *conventional antipsychotics*.

Indications

These drugs are used to control psychotic behavior in disorders like schizophrenia, mania, delirium, depression with agitation, aggressive and violent behavior, delusions, hallucinations and others in very small doses. It is used to control anxiety symptoms.

Dosage and Administration

Antipsychotics have a wide dosage range with individual variations. Treatment is initiated with small doses. The optimum dose is built up to get symptom control. Maintenance dose is required in disorders like schizophrenia and manic disorders. Drugs which have long half-life need to be administered once daily and those with shorter half-life are given more frequently.

Side Effects of Antipsychotics

- *Extrapyramidal symptoms:* These result from anti-dopaminergic activity at the basal ganglia.
- *Drug-induced parkinsonism:* Tremor, rigidity, akinesia, dysarthria and 'mask-like face'. These respond well

to trimethylphenyl hydrochloride, promethazine, diazepam and other antiparkinsonian agents.

- **Acute dystonia:** Acute spasms of muscles of neck, tongue, face, glottis and other parts. These respond well to antiparkinsonism agents or benzodiazepine, which are to be given parenterally.
- **Akathisia:** Motor restlessness and a drive to move, which is not due to anxiety or agitation. The treatment is by reducing the dose and using drugs, like diazepam or propranolol.
- **Tardive dyskinesia:** Perioral tremors or orofacial dyskinesia or rabbit syndrome, widespread choreoathetosis and dystonia. Prevention is better, since it is not easy to treat. Diazepam, propranolol and antiparkinsonism agents and parenteral benzodiazepine.
- **Anticholinergic (antimuscarinic) symptoms:** Blurred vision, dry mouth, hesitancy of micturation, urinary retention, constipation, precipitation or aggravation of glaucoma.
- **Antihistaminic symptoms:** Sedation and weight gain which are due to H$_1$ receptor blockade.
- **Antiadrenergic symptoms:** Postural hypotension, tachycardia, erectile dysfunction.
- **ECG changes:** Prolongation of Q-T interval and T wave changes.
- **Malignant neuroleptic syndrome (MNS):** It is a rare but very serious side effect mostly seen with high potency antipsychotic drugs like haloperidol. It is characterized by generalized muscular rigidity, hyperpyrexia, unstable blood pressure, tachycardia, excessive sweating, myoglobinuria, urinary incontinence and impaired sensorium. Serum creatine phosphokinase (CPK) is elevated to very high levels. The treatment is symptomatic. The antipsychotic is stopped immediately. Drugs like diazepam, dantrolene, bromocriptine, amantadine and L-dopa help to relieve symptoms. MNS is a medical emergency.

- **Endocrine side effects:** Elevation of prolactin level leading to gynecomastia, galactorrhea, amenorrhea and weight gain.
- **Hematological:** Agranulocytosis.
- **Allergic:** Photosensitivity, skin rashes, itching, exfoliation of skin.
- **Gastrointestinal:** Gastritis, hepatitis and constipation.

ANTIDEPRESSANT DRUGS

Syn: Mood elevators or thymoleptics

These are drugs which elevate the depressed mood by increasing the neurotransmitter levels of norepinephrine and serotonin at CNS synapses. The common antidepressant drugs are given in Table 250.2.

Tricyclic Antidepressants

Tricyclic antidepressants (TCAs) are the first group of antidepressant drugs, which became popular because of their proven efficacy. These are absorbed well from the gastrointestinal tract (GIT) and are highly protein bound. They are metabolized in the liver.

Dosage is 25 mg bd or tds and can be raised to 50 mg tds. This dose is maintained for 3–6 months and gradually tapered off. Weight gain and cardiac toxicity are major

Table 250.2: Common antidepressant drugs				
Name	**Starting dose (mg)**	**Max daily dose (mg)**	**Amine effect**	**Usual side effect (SE)**
Tricyclic antidepressant drugs (TCA)				
Amitriptyline	25 tds od or bd	150	NE 5-HT	Sedation Anticholinergic action, sexual dysfunction, cardiac toxicity, hypotension
Imipramine	25 tds	200	NE, 5-HT	Same as above
Clomipramine	25 tds	300	NE, 5-HT	Same as above
Selective serotonin reuptake inhibitors (SSRIs)				
Fluoxetine	20 od	80	5-HT	GI disturbances, nausea, vomiting, anorexia, delayed orgasm, anorgasmia, insomnia, agitation EPS, mania
Sertraline	25 od	200	5-HT	Dry mouth
Paroxetine	10–20 od	60	5-HT	Sexual dysfunction
Citalopram	10–20 od	60	5-HT	Delayed orgasm, anorgasmia, CNS disturbances
Escitalopram	10–20 od	60	5-HT	Headache, somnolence
Venlafaxine	37.5 bd	375	5-HT, NE	Insomnia, agitation EPS, mania
Monoamine oxidase inhibitors (MAOIs)				
Phenelzine	15	90		Cheese reaction
Tranylcypromine	30	60		CNS—confusion insomnia, headache
Isocarboxazid	10	30		ANS—blurred vision, dry mouth
Moclobemide	150 bd	600		Other side effect—hypotension, sexual disturbance (no cheese reaction with moclobemide)
Atypical antidepressants				
Bupropion	100 bd	450	DA, NE	Agitation, headache insomnia hypotension
Trazodone	50 bd	600	5-HT	Sedation, dry mouth, constipation
Mirtazapine	15 od Bed time	45	5-HT, NE	Increased appetite, sedation, weight gain

Abbreviations: od = Once daily; bd = Twice a day; tds = Thrice a day; CNS = Central nervous system; ANS = Autonomic nervous system; EPS = Extrapyramidal symptoms; NE = Norepinephrine; HT = Hydroxytryptamine; DA = Dopamine; GI = Gastrointestinal

disadvantages. Electrocardiography (ECG) changes include prolongation of P-R and Q-T intervals, ST segment depression, blunting of T wave and arrhythmias.

Selective Serotonin Reuptake Inhibitors (SSRIs)

They have recently become more popular because of their ease of administration and lack of cardiotoxicity. They produce GIT disturbances like nausea, bloating sensations, diarrhea and CNS disturbances like day time sleepiness, headache, agitation, irritability, seizure and some times, extrapyramidal symptoms. Allergic reactions may occur giving rise to skin rashes.

Monoamine Oxidase Inhibitors (MAOIs)

They were the first antidepressants discovered, which led to the discovery of TCAs. These drugs are rarely prescribed because of lack of potency and serious side effects like 'cheese reaction', i.e. a patient on MAOIs goes into a state of fatal hypertensive crisis on consumption of tyramine containing foods like cheese.

Mood Stabilizers

These drugs are primarily meant for the prophylaxis of bipolar mood disorders (BPMDs), but they are also effective in the treatment of acute mania. The common mood stabilizers are lithium, carbamazepine, oxcarbazepine, valproate, lamotrigine, topiramate and gabapentin.

Lithium

The antimanic effect of lithium was discovered by *Cade* in 1949. The carbonate and citrate salts are used.

Dosage: Lithium is given orally. It is absorbed well and excreted through the kidneys. 600–800 mg is given daily in 2–3 divided doses to obtain a serum lithium level of 0.8–1.2 mEq/L for treatment of acute mania. For prophylaxis the level can be 0.4–7 mEq/L and this may be continued for 3–5 years. The level is adjusted by periodic estimation of the level of lithium after a 12-hour lithium fast.

Side effects: Diuresis, tremors, weight gain, hypothyroidism, GIT disturbances, widening of QRS complex in ECG, teratogenicity and others.

Serum levels above 1.4 mEq/L produce toxicity, which includes nausea, vomiting, slurred speech, toxic tremors, seizures and confusion. If, untreated, this may end fatally.

Carbamazepine

It is basically an anticonvulsant.

Dose: 400–1,600 mg given orally in two divided doses. For prophylaxis it is continued for 3–5 years, though in smaller doses. It induces hepatic microsomal enzymes.

Side effects: Diplopia, drowsiness, agranulocytosis, fatal skin reactions such as exfoliative dermatitis, Stevens-Johnson syndrome and toxic epidermal necrolysis. The drug is teratogenic.

Oxcarbazepine

It is an analog of carbamazepine.

Dose: 150–300 mg bd.

Valproate

It is also basically an anticonvulsant.

Dose: This drug is started with a dose of 400–600 mg in divided doses and increased to a maximum of 1–2 g daily.

Serum levels of 50–100 µg/L are optimal. The drug is teratogenic.

Side effects: GIT disturbances, leukopenia and weight gain. Acute pancreatitis and hepatotoxicity are rare serious complications which could be fatal.

Lamotrigine, topiramate and gabapentin are being used recently as adjuncts; but they have not come into common use.

ANTIANXIETY DRUGS (ANXIOLYTICS OR MINOR TRANQUILIZERS)

These are drugs which relieve anxiety symptoms and therefore commonly used in anxiety disorders (Table 250.3). The common antianxiety drugs are the following: The benzodiazepines are the most commonly used drugs. They can be given orally or parenterally, specially intravenous (IV). They bind to the gamma-aminobutyric acid (GABA) receptors and thereby enhance GABA activity. Sedation, ataxia, confusion, drug dependence and withdrawal syndrome are the common adverse effects.

Flumazenil is a beta-2 receptor antagonist which antagonizes the action of benzodiazepine and can be used as an antidote to treat acute toxicity of benzodiazepines.

Hypnotics

These are sleep promoting agents. The drugs in common use are listed in Table 250.4.

Psychostimulant Drugs

These include amphetamine, methylphenidate, cocaine and caffeine. These drugs release dopamine and prevent

Table 250.3: Common antianxiety drugs

Drugs	Dose–oral and parenteral	Remarks
Benzodiazepines		
Lorazepam	1–2 mg once or twice daily 2 mg intramuscular or intravenous (IM or IV)	Short acting
Oxazepam	15–30 bd daily	Short acting
Alprazolam	0.25–0.5 mg 2–3 times daily	Potent drug, long acting
Diazepam	5 mg twice daily 5–10 mg IV	Poorly absorbed when given IM hence IV dose is preferred long acting
Chlordiazepoxide	10–20 mg 2–3 times daily	
Clonazepam	0.5–2 mg once or twice daily	Long acting
Nitrazepam	5–10 mg at bed time	Hypnotic
Flurazepam	5–10 mg at bed time	Hypnotic
β-adrenoreceptor blocker		
Propranolol	10–40 mg twice or thrice daily	Effective against peripheral manifestations of anxiety
Azapirone		
Buspirone	5–10 mg, twice or thrice daily	No sedation No dependence

Table 250.4: Drugs to promote sleep and its oral doses

Benzodiazepines	Oral dose
Nitrazepam	5–30 mg bed time
Clonazepam	2–4 mg bed time
Lorazepam	2 mg bed time
Flurazepam	30–60 mg bed time
Oxazepam	15–30 mg bed time
Nonbenzodiazepines	
Zolpidem	5–20 mg bed time
Zopiclone	3.75–7.5 mg bed time

Table 250.5: Drugs to improve memory and cognitive functions

Drugs	Dosage	Remarks
Cholinesterase inhibitors		
Tacrine Donepezil	30–40 mg qid 5–10 mg qid	Treatment is initiated with small doses and gradually increased to the optimum level
Rivastigmine Galantamine	3–6 mg tid 8–12 mg bid	Gastrointestinal (GI) disturbances may develop
NMDA (N-Methyl-D-aspartate) antagonist		
Memantine	5–10 mg bid	
MAOIs (Monoamine oxidase inhibitors) (beta)		
Selegiline	5–10 mg bd	
Other nonspecific drugs		
Vitamin-E, calcium channel blockers Ginkgo biloba, estrogens		May be useful in some situations, especially as adjuvant drugs

Table 250.6: Antiparkinsonism drugs

Drugs	Dosage
Trihexyphenidyl HCl	1–2 mg bid or tid
Procyclidine HCl	2.5–5 mg bid or tid 2.5–5 mg IM
Promethazine HCl	10–25 mg bid or tid 25–50 mg IM
Diazepam	2–5 mg bid or tid 10–20 mg IV slowly
L-dopa is not recommended as it worsens or induces psychosis	

Abbreviations: HCl = Hydrochloride; IV = Intravenous; IM = Intramuscular

its reuptake. They may lead to drug dependence and development of psychosis.

Amphetamine is used in the treatment of narcolepsy.

Methylphenidate is used in the treatment of attention deficit hyperactivity disorders.

Cocaine is used as a local anesthetic to mucous membranes. Recently it is being tried for therapeutic purposes as well. Being highly habit forming, this drug has to be used with caution.

Cognitive Enhancers

Recently, a few drugs have been introduced to improve memory and other cognitive functions in cases of dementia, specially in Alzheimer's disease. These drugs are mentioned in Table 250.5.

ANTIPARKINSONISM DRUGS

These drugs are very useful in the management of drug-induced EPSs. Commonly used drugs are given in Table 250.6.

CHAPTER 251

Psychological Methods of Treatment (Psychotherapy)

N Krishnan Kutty

Chapter Summary

- Psychoanalytic Psychotherapy
- Principles of Psychoanalysis
  - Narcoanalysis
- Supportive Psychotherapy
- Group Psychotherapy
- Behavior Therapy
- Cognitive Therapy

psychotherapies are in vogue. All of them follow a few fundamental principles.

The therapist should be a trained person. He should establish therapeutic relationship with the patient. Listening and talking takes place between them.

This results in release of pent up emotions in the patient. The patient is given information and explanations of symptoms, guidance, suggestions and advice to restore his lost morale.

PSYCHOANALYTIC PSYCHOTHERAPY

Psychotherapy is also known as **talking cure**. It is based on the communication taking place between therapist and patient. The therapist is a trained person. Removing or modifying symptoms or promoting positive personality growth is the goal of the therapy. Over hundred types of

PRINCIPLES OF PSYCHOANALYSIS

Psychoanalysis is not merely a form of psycho-therapy. It also refers to the process of exploring (analyzing) the mind. Sigmund Freud (1856–1939) is the Father of Psychoanalysis. He was a Viennese Physician. In his classic work, **The Interpretation of Dreams**, he gave a model of the mind called the **Topographical Theory** of the mind. The mind is formed of three regions—the unconscious, preconscious and conscious regions.

1. **The unconscious** part of the mind contains all the repressed (forgotten) ideas and affects. It is the seat of neurotic conflict and influences the conscious mind.
2. **The preconscious** part is the region which is in between the conscious and unconscious regions and it can access both these parts. It contains the events and processes that can be brought to the conscious part, at will.
3. **The conscious** mind is that part which becomes aware of the external and internal world through the senses.

In later years, Freud proposed another model of the mind called the **Structural Theory** of the mind. The mind is formed of three provinces—the id, ego and super ego.

1. **The id:** This is present at birth. It is unconscious and is the reservoir of basic drives and instinct for sex aggression and survival.
2. **The ego:** It is the conscious part. It is the organized portion of the id and includes perception, voluntary movement, memory, judgment and adaptation to reality. It registers sensations from the outside world and internal sources. It is the organ that reconciliates between id and super ego.
3. **The super ego:** It is formed from id and ego. It consists of ethical values and moral principles. It imposes restrictions and prohibitions. It invokes guilt and self-punishment.

The psychotherapy introduced by Sigmund Freud is called **psychoanalytic psychotherapy**. Supportive psychotherapy, group psychotherapy, suggestions, hypnosis, narcoanalysis, abreaction, exposure and response prevention and thought stopping, are some of the other common methodologies of psychotherapy employed.

The classical psychotherapy introduced by Sigmund Freud is psychoanalysis. He devised a technique known as **free association**. The patient is made to rest comfortably on a couch. He is allowed to talk freely, uninhibited, whatever comes to his mind, in sessions lasting for about 45 minutes. Repeated sessions are required. Block in the flow of talk may occur during the sessions. This indicates **resistance**. Resistance is indicative of unconscious painful experiences (conflict). As the psychotherapy proceeds, the patient may develop an emotional relationship (love, liking, hatred) with the therapist. This phenomenon is called **transference**. As a result, neurotic manifestations may develop in the treatment setting. This is known as **transference neurosis**.

The actual neurotic conflict is reflected in this transference neurosis, during the therapeutic sessions. This neurosis is **analyzed and interpreted**. It will help to resolve the neurotic conflict and thereby eliminate the symptoms. The patients also regain insight. The main idea of psychoanalytic psychotherapy is uncovering of the unconscious to resolve the neurotic conflict, the root of neurotic disorder.

Indications

Psychoanalytic psychotherapy is indicated in anxiety disorders, phobic disorders, conversion and dissociative disorders and personality disorders.

Narcoanalysis

The unconscious mind can be reached through the help of narcotic drugs such as short-acting barbiturates like thiopentone sodium and sodium amytal. Usually a 2.5% solution of thiopentone sodium is slowly administered intravenously (IV) to produce a state of cerebral disinhibition. The patient is then allowed to talk freely and uninhibited. Suggestions are given if needed. Narcoanalysis is employed in the following conditions:

- Dissociate and conversion disorders
- Anxiety disorder
- Differential diagnosis of catatonic schizophrenia from depressive and organic stupors. Catatonia improves and the other two worsen.

Abreaction

Abreaction is the secret of religious healing. Abreaction refers to the process of letting out of pent up emotions very freely. It may be done through verbal suggestions or by use of drugs like short-acting barbiturates or stimulant drugs. It is used to bring into conscious mind the unconscious (forgotten) traumatic events and thereby to remove symptoms and disability.

SUPPORTIVE PSYCHOTHERAPY

In this form of therapy, the patient gets support from the therapist, who may be perceived as an authority figure. The patient is given acceptance and he is listened to. The unexpressed emotions are ventilated. It helps to release the inner tensions and strengthens the defense mechanism. The patient is helped to tackle his problem of guilt, shame, anxiety and frustration. The goal is achieved through the process of guidance, persuasion and environmental support. Finally, he may get self-confidence and better outlook of the environment and of himself.

GROUP PSYCHOTHERAPY

In this form of therapy, a group of patients are getting the benefit of psychotherapy simultaneously. A group is formed of 6–10 selected patients and therapists. The group forms a social environment for each patient and that forms the therapeutic agent. Uninhibited free talk is encouraged between members. Each one shares the experiences and problems of others. The group may focus on activities of problem solving and provision of support. Each session may last for 90–120 minutes. The group may meet once or twice a week. Group therapy is indicated in neurotic disorders, psychotic disorders, substance abuse, sexual deviations and personality disorders.

BEHAVIOR THERAPY

Behavior therapy works on the principle of **learning theory**. The neurosis is regarded as a maladaptive behavior learned by the patient and symptoms as conditioned maladaptive pattern of behavior. The patient can be made to unlearn it. Systematic desensitization, implosion (flooding), aversion, exposure and response prevention, and thought stopping are some of the common techniques used in behavior therapy.

COGNITIVE THERAPY

Cognitive Behavior Therapy (CBT)

This therapy is developed by Aron Beck based upon experimental psychology with respect to depression, but later applied to other disorders as well. It is a short-term psychotherapy where the patient and therapist actively participate (collaborate). It is focused on current problems and finding their solutions. CBT is employed in the management of depressive disorder, anxiety disorders, phobic disorders, panic disorder, obsessive compulsive disorder (OCD) and others. The concept is that behavior and emotions are determined by the patient's cognition. Patient's emotions may be the result of *cognitive errors*. Beck found that symptoms of depression were due to disordered ways of thinking *(cognitive distortions)* and not primarily due to downing of the mood. If the errors in thinking are corrected, the rest of the symptoms ought to change and depression should disappear. In the initial stage of cognitive therapy, the cognitive distortions are elicited by repeated interviews and daily monitoring of the thought process. These are analyzed. The patient is made to understand the errors. Correction of the irrational ideas and distortions are then brought out by verbal and behavioral technique.

Systematic desensitization: It is employed in the treatment of phobic disorders. The subject is gradually deconditioned to the phobic stimulus which is thus made innocuous. Initially, the phobic stimulus or object is identified. A graded list (hierarchy) of the anxiety provoking situations is charted out with minimum anxiety at one end and maximum at the other end. The patient is trained to relax. He is then exposed to the phobic stimulus at the minimum end of the hierarchy. Any anxiety that may develop is got over by relaxation. This process is worked upwards serially till the maximum anxiety-arousing situation is got over. This treatment is good for simple phobia.

Implosion (flooding): In this technique, the patient is suddenly exposed to the phobic stimulus. The patient is made to tackle the resulting anxiety manifestations by relaxation and, if necessary, with the help of drugs. He is not allowed to escape from the situation. By a series of such exposures, the patient is deconditioned to the phobic stimulus. This kind of treatment is effective in phobic neurosis. If desensitization is done in real situation, it is called ***flooding*** and if it is done in imagination it is called ***implosion***.

Aversion therapy: This is used in the treatment of alcoholism, drug dependence, sexual deviations, tics, mannerisms and certain dissociative symptoms. The principle is to associate a noxious stimulus with the maladaptive habit and this helps to eliminate the abnormality by negative reinforcement, e.g. in the case of alcohol dependence a strong painful electric shock can be applied on the arm as soon as the patient starts to gulp alcohol in a therapeutic setting. This aversive stimulus may help him to get rid of the habit. The pain produces aversive conditioning.

Exposure and response prevention: It is a good treatment technique for obsessions with ritualistic practice, i.e. when obsessions are accompanied by compulsive rituals. The patient is trained to withdraw from carrying out the act inspite of strong urge to do so. The anxiety may mount up, but lyses gradually within an hour. Slowly the patient gets confidence. His behavior is modified in this way.

Thought stopping: It is a process of distraction of attention from the obsessive thought when it intrudes into the mind by specific techniques, e.g. snapping an elastic band tied around the wrist at the moment.

CHAPTER
252

Principles and Practice of Geriatric Medicine

KV Krishna Das

Chapter Summary

- The Physiology of Aging
  - Life Expectancy and Lifespan
  - Theories of Aging
- Physiological Changes Occurring in the Elderly
- Successful aging
- Frailty

INTRODUCTION

Geriatric medicine is that branch of medicine dealing with the physiological, clinical, psychological and preventive and rehabilitation aspects of illnesses in the elderly. Age above 60 years is included in the geriatric group in India. There are more than 100 million people in this category in India and the number and their proportion in the population are steadily increasing.

Geriatric medicine has been dealt with in the works of Hippocrates and Aristotle (in the late BCs). *Ayurveda* gives description on the illnesses and remedial measures such as rejuvenation therapy, particularly aimed at the elderly population. During the heydays of the *Arabic medicine*, Ibn Sina and others have described this branch of medicine. It was Ignatz Leo Nascher, a Vienna born physician (who migrated to the USA, New York) coined the term *Geriatrics* (1909) from the words *geras* meaning old age and *iatrikos* meaning medical attention.

In India, the specialty of geriatric medicine was established in 1960. Comprehensive treatment facilities for the elderly including geriatric wards in hospitals were started. National Policy on Older Persons (NPOP) was formulated by The Ministry of Social Justice and Empowerment of India in 1999. In 2010, The Ministry of Health and Family Welfare of Government of India promulgated the National Programme for Health Care of the Elderly (NPHCE). This envisaged the creation of specialized regional geriatric care centers in all cities with subsequent extension of the facility to cover all states in the country. Several nongovernmental organizations (NGOs) such as HelpAge International (New Delhi), Alzheimer's and Related Disorders Society of India (ARDSI) at Kochi and many others are creating facilities for the care of the elderly in many parts of India. Several alternate medicine institutions are also active in this direction.

The discipline of geriatrics has become well-established in its own right with its own professional society and postgraduate training programs.

Source: Das T, Chakraborty S. Geriatrics: The great awakening. J Indian Med Assoc. 2014;112(1):12.

Changing demographic pattern worldwide resulted in a steep rise in elderly population both in developed and developing countries. The elderly population in India has risen from 12 million in 1901 to 70 million in 1999 (7% of the total population). India has the second largest elderly population, next only to China in the world. This phenomenal growth of geriatric population is the result of improved life expectancy, better socioeconomic environment, advances in the medical field and prevention and control of communicable diseases and falling birth rates.

Along with this, there is an exponential increase in disability, mental and physical morbidity of the elderly population, needing special health and social services. The manner in which person ages and the capacity to ward off disease are linked to socioeconomic factors, the mental and physical activity patterns and degree of fitness during life. Heredity and lifestyle patterns govern fitness and physiological reserve.

Regulated physical activity protects against obesity, type 2 diabetes mellitus (DM), ischemic heart disease (IHD), hypertension, strokes and orthopedic disabilities. Regular employment protects against depressive illness.

Geriatric medicine is that branch of medicine concerned with preventive, curative and rehabilitative methods of management of medical, psychological and social problems of the aged.

Elderly people behave differently from others in respect to predisposition to disease, general resistance against infections and response to drugs. The discipline of geriatrics deals with the diagnosis and treatment of persons aged 65 years and above. The age of 65 years as the commencement of senescence has been accepted arbitrarily. During senescence, all illnesses are accompanied by a higher mortality than when occurring in younger age groups. A better functional definition of senescence will be as the period when there is commencement of loss of vigor, skin changes of old age, slowed activity of the musculoskeletal system and onset of deterioration of mental functions. The lifespan of man is increasing all over the world. In India, over 7% of the population is above the age of 60 years. The maximum lifespan has not changed despite increase in the average lifespan.

THE PHYSIOLOGY OF AGING

Life Expectancy and Lifespan

Life expectancy refers to the number of years an individual is anticipated to live and this is a parameter common to a socioeconomic group or even a whole nation. This can be calculated at birth of an individual.

Maximum lifespan denotes the number of years an individual lives from birth. The recorded longest living person was a French woman (Jeanne Calment) who lived up to 122 years.

Aging refers to the gradual and progressive decline in cell or tissue structure and function with resulting loss of dynamic equilibrium, reserve function and homeostasis. Aging is associated with physiological decline and accompanying pathology of most of the organ systems with disability and dissatisfaction. Aging changes are universal, decremental and progressive.

Theories of Aging

Several theories are in vogue, although none is completely acceptable. The present views include genetic influences, damage to deoxyribonucleic acid (DNA), mitochondria or telomeres and errors in ribonucleic acid (RNA) and/or DNA synthesis.

Several interventions help to improve the overall health and performance of the elderly. These include:

- Never smoking
- Keeping weight below obese range (BMI < 30)
- Consumption of appropriate calorie diet containing high amounts (at least 500 g) of fruits and fresh vegetables, whole grains, nuts (15–20 g/day), milk and milk products 200 mL/day, fish in sufficient quantities and red meat only in low amounts (< 150 g/day)
- Performing at least 3–5 hours of physical activity (walking, golf, games, swimming and others) per week, regularly
- As far as possible, keeping engaged in activities to which the person is used to.

Special Points to Remember in Aging

- At present, life expectancy is increasing. In India, it is 64 years for men and 67 years for women (WHO data). Many people who die natural deaths live up to 80–90 years or even more. It is also predicted that in many countries (both developed and developing), children born in this century have got a good chance of living up to a century.
- Life expectancy is more in females in humans and also in almost all the mammalian species.
- Chronological age and biological age may not correlate, since the latter depends on comorbidity as well. Pathological changes have to be distinguished from physiological aging.
- Physiological changes of aging produce mild clinical manifestations to which most of the persons adjust, though with discomfort. On the other hand, diseases cause more rapid deterioration and severe disability.
- The elderly may have several concurrent comorbid conditions, some of which may be silent.
- Disease manifestations may be atypical and response to therapeutic modalities may be altered.

Successful aging depends on several factors including genetics, environmental factors and healthy lifestyle.

Physiological Changes Occurring in the Elderly

Gait and Balance

Gait slows 12–16% per decade with age after 30–40 years. The posture becomes stooped and may even resemble that of parkinsonism. The *tandem walking test* may be difficult to perform. Presence of muscle and joint diseases and neurological lesions may add on to the disabilities.

Skin and Hair

There is a decline in the number and functions of several component cells of the skin. These include fibroblasts, mast cells, immune cells (Langerhans cells) melanocytes and sweat and sebaceous glands. All these lead to diminution in their corresponding functions.

Photoaging is the consequence of exposure to ultraviolet (UV) light, environmental pollution and smoking. It is more prominent in fair-skinned persons. Photoaging accounts for more (80%) of the external appearances of aging. *Extrinsic aging* such as wrinkling of the skin, pigmentation, telangiectasia and purpura all are caused by UV light A and B. On the other hand, intrinsic aging is characterized by atrophy, thinness and transparency of the skin, loss of fat, loss of elasticity and wrinkling and dryness of skin leading to pruritus.

Hair and Nails

Hair loss is common with age, hair density drops from the third decade of life. Hair loss starts in the scalp, then may proceed to the eyebrows, axilla and pubis. The nail growth also comes down with age.

Weight and Body Composition

The lean body mass may come down by 30–80% between the third and eighth decade of life.

Age-related sarcopenia (reduction in muscle mass) affects type 2 fibers. Sarcopenia is common in both sexes above the age of 65 years. Hand grip declines with age, but greater loss of muscle strength affects the lower limbs. Bone mass declines in women by 1% and men by 0.7% annually after age of 30 years. During postmenopausal period, 3–5% of bone mass declines rapidly. With further age, the loss of bone mass drops to that of premenopause level and equals that of men. Due to nonenzymatic collagen cross linking, the plasticity of bones diminishes and they become more brittle.

Vital Signs

Age-related changes in vital signs are compounded by pathological processes which are very common.

Stiffening of vasculature gives rise to higher systolic pressure and widening of the pulse pressure.

Autonomic disturbances result in orthostatic and postprandial hypotension.

Thermoregulation is influenced by several factors such as reduced ability to maintain body heat and mount a febrile response. Even infections may not be accompanied by fever and even low-grade fever may indicate serious underlying disease. Hypothermia may occur even in the absence of cold environment and this may herald a poor clinical state and increased mortality.

Vision and Hearing

Delay in adaptation to darkness and light and contrasting colors leads to visual problems. Development of cataracts, rigidity of the iris leading to sluggishness of the pupillary reflexes, presence of floaters in the visual media, reduction of lachrymal secretion and both ectropion and entropion are disturbing problems. Glaucoma, cataracts, macular degeneration and diabetic retinopathy cause serious visual impairment. These predispose to falls.

Hearing impairment is common. The slight dominance of the right ear over the left seen in younger people is magnified further above 80 years of age. Age-related specific hearing defect is presbycusis, i.e. symmetrical bilateral sensorineural hearing loss. The other forms of hearing defects often turn out to be pathological processes. A common easily removable cause of hearing impairment is inspissation of wax in the ears. The hearing impairment in the elderly may be mistaken for cognitive abnormality. This results in withdrawal of social and other activities.

Cardiovascular changes are common as age advances. These include myocardial and vascular stiffening, abnormalities of the electrical activity of the heart, decreased sensitivity of the autonomic nervous system and their consequences. In addition to age-related disease, problems such as ischemia, hypertension and cardiac failure and drug effects are common. Systolic time is prolonged at the expense of diastolic.

By the age of 75 years, almost 90% of the pacemaker cells of the sinoatrial (SA) mode are gone. This leads to reduction in the capacity to increase the heart rate. A simple formula to calculate the acceleratory capacity of the heart is:

> Heart rate maximum = 220 – age in years for males and 190 – age in years for females

Degeneration of conduction system leads to various types of heart block and nonspecific conduction defects. Changes in the autonomic function result in the inability of the cardiovascular system (CVS) to adapt to postural changes. This may manifest as syncope and arrhythmias correctable by pacemakers.

Respiratory System

All components of the respiratory apparatus are affected. These include:

- Reduction of the compliance of the thoracic cage
- Reduction of elastic recoil of the lung
- Increase in pulmonary vascular resistance
- Increase in alveolar size and consequent increase in residual volume
- Decline in strength of the respiratory muscles including the diaphragm.

The breathing pattern and alveolar gas exchange are not significantly altered. These changes tend to stabilize by 70 years.

The formula to calculate the decline in pulmonary arterial oxygen saturation (PaO_2) is given below.

> PaO_2 = 100 – (age in years/3) or 110 – (age in years × 0.4)

The FEV1 decreases. In addition to the mechanical changes, genetic influences have great impact on the aging of the respiratory system.

The immune function of the respiratory mucociliary system declines. Both cellular and humoral immunity are affected. Tobacco smoking-related damage to the lungs is increased in the elderly. Clinically, age-related changes do not result in dyspnea at rest, the latter should suggest added pathological processes. There is increased chance for aspiration, atelectasis, infection and further adverse effects.

The ***renal system*** undergoes structural and functional alterations with age. These include:

- Reduction of renal blood flow at a rate of 10% per decade from 30 to 60 years, the renal cortex being more affected.
- Renal size comes down up to 40% by 80 years of age. Glomerular basement membrane (GBM) undergoes thickening, hyalinization and sclerosis. Functioning tubules comes down and interstitial fibrosis sets in. Glomerular filtration rate (GFR) tends to fall at a rate of 0.8–1% annually after the third decade. This rate is highly variable. Tubular secretions also fall at the rate of 0.7%, annually. The Cockroft-Gault formula is used to calculate the GFR.

Cockroft-Gault Formula

$$\frac{140 - \text{age in years} \times \text{body weight (kg)}}{72 \times \text{serum creatinine (mg/dL)}}$$

Note: For females, multiply by 0.85, because the creatinine clearance is only 85% of this value in females.

Newer formulae have been introduced, e.g. modification of diet in renal disease (MDRD) study and chronic kidney disease-epidemiology collaboration (CKD-EPI) equation (2009).

Source: Levey AS, Stevens LA, Schmid CH, et al. A new equation to estimate glomerular filtration rate. Ann Internal Med. 2009;150(9):604-12.

The ability to conserve water is blunted, sodium homeostasis is commonly deranged, so too is the capacity to eliminate potassium and acid load. Hormonal functions deteriorate. Obstructive uropathy due to prostatomegaly and other causes are frequent. These lead to acceleration of renal dysfunction.

Renal deterioration makes the elderly extremely susceptible to adverse metabolic changes, dietary alterations, electrolyte abnormalities and disturbances in the mineral metabolism. Drug dosages have to be suitably adjusted to avoid toxicity. In general, interventions such as control of blood pressure (BP), blood sugar, weight, diet and calorie intake help to delay renal aging.

The alimentary system: Several age-related changes occur in addition to pathological processes. It is necessary to distinguish the two classes, though at times it may be difficult.

Gastrointestinal Motor Function

Gastrointestinal (GI) motility is altered due to degenerative changes in the submucosal autonomic nervous plexuses. This may present with gastroparesis, loss of motility of segments of the gastrointestinal tract (GIT) leading to discomfort, constipation, stool impaction (fecal incontinence) and postprandial hypotension.

Small intestinal bacteria overgrowth (SIBO) is not uncommon. This may lead to malabsorption. SIBO is predisposed to by decline in gastric acid and with age. Motility disorders with stasis aggravate SIBO. *The gustatory experience* (taste and flavor) is dampened in the elderly. Esophageal function is preserved even in old age and dysphagia, if it occurs, is due to pathological processes. Gastric blood flow comes down and there is slight delay in gastric emptying, specially to liquids and these results in gastric stasis.

In the small intestine, there is reduction in splanchnic blood flow. Calcium absorption is diminished due to resistance to the action of 125-hydroxyvitamin D.

Large intestine shows reduction of rectal wall sensitivity, decrease in anal canal squeeze pressure, delay in colonic transit and higher prevalence of diverticular disease. Constipation is caused by altered gut motility sedentary lifestyle, reduction of fiber in the diet and often the adverse effects of medication.

Pancreas show reduction in insulin secretion but exocrine secretions are preserved.

Liver blood flow declines with age, but liver function is relatively preserved with normal albumin synthesis. Gallbladder stones are more frequent due to lithogenic changes in the bile.

The *gut hormones* show variations. The gut hormones normally regulate motor and sensory activity and cell proliferation, circadian rhythms, nutritional status, energy intake and others. Gut hormones relay signals to the central nervous system (CNS) to coordinate activities. While *ghrelin* stimulates food intake, cholecystokinin, peptide YY (which is a short peptide released by cells in the ileum and colon in response to feeding. It inhibits gastric motility and increases water and electrolyte absorption in the colon). Pancreatic polypeptide and glucagon-like peptide (GLP-1) suppress appetite. Circadian biological rhythms account for food intake, hunger and satiety. Gut hormones such as *motilin* and *ghrelin* help to generate the migrating motor complex (MMC) proceeding downwards. *Gastrin, ghrelin, cholecystokinin* and *serotonin* are involved in the generation of contractions in the small and large intestine. In general, aging changes in gut hormone metabolism do not lead to significant symptoms.

Nervous System

Brain mass decreases with age consistent with decline of cerebral blood flow. Brain atrophy evident in imaging studies is compatible with perfect brain function. In dementia and other diseases, atrophy of selective areas may be prominent. White matter abnormalities detected on imaging are associated with impairment of higher functions (memory, executive function and information processing speed). Presence of intracellular tau protein and extracellular amyloid plaques may indicate damage. While neurofibrillary tangles composed of tau protein and amyloid beta protein may be seen in normal brain tissue, in Alzheimer's disease their extent and distribution are different.

Clinically, normal aging may be associated with diminished vibration sense and position sense and gait abnormalities, even in the absence of demonstrable neurological disease. Mild cognitive decline may be age related but more evident cognitive decline may herald the onset of dementia.

Immune System

Immune system undergoes decline-termed immuno-senescence which affects both innate and adaptive immunity. Thymus involutes by 50 years and the tissue is replaced by fat. Abnormal T and B lymphocyte function leads to decline of both humoral and cellular immunity. Immunosenescence is not accompanied by a total decline in immunity function more often it results in remodeling of the immune processes with selective changes in the different components. Resistance against bacterial and viral disease is reduced. There is upregulation of inflammatory response which may lead to harmful outcome. Death from influenza, pneumonia and septicemia are common in the old. Vaccines may not be optimally effective in them. Increase in the development of malignancies is the result reduction of protective immunity in them.

Sleep disturbances are common. These include phase advance (earlier to bed and earlier to wake up), increase in sleep latency (time taken to fall asleep increases) and fall in sleep efficiency (actual time spent in sleep while in bed). Time spent in deep sleep [nonrapid eye movement (NREM) stages 3 and 4] decline and more time being spent on light sleep (NREM stages 1 and 2). Sleep disturbances contribute to cognitive problems, falls, accidents and impairment of the quality of life. It is important to distinguish physiological sleep changes from pathological sleep abnormalities seen in diseases such as heart failure, respiratory diseases, depression, anxiety, stressful situations, pain, sleep apnea syndrome and others.

Successful aging: This term has been interpreted differently. A practical definition would be 'the state in which an individual makes good use of physiological limitations with a view to achieve a productive and satisfying life keeping his/her dignity as far into life as possible'.

FRAILTY

This term is defined by the concise Oxford English dictionary as *liability to err or yield to temptation, fault, weakness, (weak point)*. In general, the term *frailty* denotes the biological syndrome of reduction of reserves of multiple organ systems, inactivity, stress, poor nutritional intake and altered physiology. Frailty is a term used to describe a subgroup of older adults who experience decreased functional reserve, functional decline and increased vulnerability for morbidity and mortality. When applied to *geriatrics,* it denotes physical weakness, underweight, tiredness and inability to walk easily. Most of frail people are above the age of 80 years, falls and fractures (excluding femoral neck fractures) are common in them. Infections, drug reactions, bereavements, undernutrition, osteoporosis, muscle loss, neuronal loss and overall disability to carry on tasks of day-to-day life are common.

Frailty is defined as the presence of three or more of these conditions. This constitutes the *Frailty Syndrome*. Five key elements form the core of frailty cycle including the following:

1. Unexplained weight loss (> 5% over a year)
2. Poor endurance and energy (self-reported)
3. Poor strength (in lowest 20th percentile)
4. Slow walking speed (Poor **Get up and Go** test)
5. Low physical activity (lowest 20th percentile).

The concept of **homeostenosis** bridges the biologic changes of aging and the increased vulnerability of humans to illness and functional decline in late life, a state commonly referred to as **frailty**. Characterized by multisystem dysregulation that includes:

- Chronic inflammation
- Sacropenia
- Osteoporosis
- Alteration in neuroendocrine function.

Clinical Criteria: 3/5

1. Slow gait speed
2. Low hand grip strength
3. Exhaustion
4. Weight loss
5. Low energy expenditure.

The joint family system which used to be universal in India till 5 decades ago was the best situation for the elderly to enjoy life and maintain their dignity and health. Regular periodic medical check up of the elderly is necessary to detect morbidity and to take preventive steps in time. Age-related changes as per the organ systems are described in Table 252.1.

Source: Pitchumoni CS, Dharmarajan TS. Geriatric Gastro-enterology. Springer 2012.

Table 252.1: Organ systems and age-related changes

Organ system	Age-related change
Cardiovascular	• Impaired contractile function • Decreased conductivity • Decreased ventricular filling • Increased systolic blood pressure • Impaired baroreceptor function

Contd...

Contd...

Organ system	Age-related change
Respiratory	• Decreased lung elasticity • Diminished cough reflex • Decreased maximal breathing capacity • Decreased number of cilia and diminished mucus clearance • Decreased arterial PO_2 • Diminished number of functional alveoli
Gastrointestinal	Decreased esophageal and colonic motility
Renal	• Decreased renal blood flow and glomerular filtration rate (GFR) • Kidney size decreases by 20–30% by age 90 years
Bladder	Decline in bladder capacity from about 500–600 mL to about 250 mL
Immune	• Decreased cell-mediated immunity • Decreased T-cell number • Increased T-suppressor cells • Decreased T-helper cells • Loss of memory cells • Decline in antibody titers to known antigens • Increased autoimmunity
Endocrine	• Decreased hormonal responses to stimulation • Impaired glucose tolerance • Decreased androgens and estrogens • Impaired norepinephrine responses
Autonomic nervous	• Impaired response to fluid deprivation • Decline in baroreceptor reflex • Increased susceptibility to hypothermia
Neurologic	• Decreased vibratory sense • Slowed neuronal transmission • Decreased proprioception
Special senses	• Presbyopia • Lens opacification • Decreased hearing • Decreased taste, smell
Musculoskeletal	Sarcopenia (↓ muscle mass and contractile force)
Integumentary changes	• Decreased skin elasticity: Wrinkling • Increased dryness • Thickened nails • Thinning of hair (baldness) • Decreased subcutaneous fat

CHAPTER

253

Clinical Aspects of Geriatric Diseases

B Krishna Swamy, KV Krishna Das

Chapter Summary

- Aging
- Health Problems in the Elderly
- Disease Pattern in Elderly
- Management Approach to Elderly Patients
- Common Geriatric Symptoms and their Management
- Social Problems in the Elderly
- Development of Geriatric Health Services in India
- Rehabilitation and Physical Therapy of the Aged

AGING

The changes in structure and function occurring in persons after the attainment of sexual maturity constitute **aging**. With advancing age, the adaptability to overcome environmental or internal challenges decreases and the probability of death increases. Tissues differ in their behavior during aging. Visual and auditory functions start deteriorating even in the third decade of life. The rate of deterioration in other organ systems depends to a great deal upon other factors like coexistent diseases, diet, physical exercise and to a great deal on hereditary factors. The present explanations for aging process are not fully satisfactory though many have been put forward.

It is projected that if the present trend of longevity continues through the 21st century, most babies born in developed countries at present (2010–2020) will live for more than 100 years. Low fertility, low immigration rate and long lives make up this situation. Research shows that aging processes are modifiable and that people are living longer without severe disability. Japan has the highest life expectancy. The oldest groups in which elderly who are more than 85 years of the age are the groups that expand most. In general, people are living longer with fewer functional disabilities. Avoidance of smoking has led to longevity. Cancer and chronic respiratory disease are increasing. Cardiovascular mortality is coming down. Hypertension trend is mixed. Prehypertension has increased. Stage 1 hypertension (140–159/90–99) has remained constant and stage 2 hypertension has decreased. Mortality is higher for men compared to women at all ages but women suffer more disabilities.

In dealing with problems in the elderly, it is essential to bear in mind that they may have (1) multiple problems, (2) atypical presentation of diseases and (3) the response to drugs and other therapeutic measures may be unpredictable. Irrespective of the symptom, a full physical examination is absolutely necessary to make a complete diagnosis. Since the aged are very susceptible to adverse drug reactions (ADR), close monitoring is essential. As yet, no drug is available to combat senescence. The aim of therapy is not just to prolong life but to make it useful and enjoyable. General principles of therapeutics in the elderly are given in Chapter 4.

- The term old is used to denote persons aged 75 years and above.
- The term advanced age is used for persons aged above 85 years.

In older persons, compensatory mechanisms are impaired either due to aging or due to disease. Therefore, even minor ailments tip the metabolic equilibrium. From a physiological standpoint, aging may be considered as a progressive diminution of function of each organ system so as to be unable to maintain homeostasis in the presence of a challenge. This graded decline of physiological reserve (homeostenosis) begins in the third decade and occurs in all organs systems independent of each other. This decline may be modified by heredity, environment, diet and personal habits.

Source: Christensen K, Doblhammer G, Rau R, et al. Ageing populations: The challenges ahead. Lancet. 2009;374(9696):1196-208.

Morphological Changes

Cellular changes: The total number of cells comes down in parenchymal organs such as brain, liver and heart. Cell sizes and staining properties become irregular and many binucleate cells appear. The water content of collagen comes down and cross-linkages increase, rendering it increasingly rigid and inflexible. This affects mobility adversely. Elastin also shows degenerative changes. The proportion of body fat in males rises from 19% at 25 years to 35% at 70 years. In females, the change is from 33 to 49%. Serum albumin falls from 4 g/dL in youth to 3.5 g/dL in persons more than 80 years.

Alterations in Organs

Skin: The skin becomes hyperkeratotic, atrophic and wrinkled. Sweat glands and sebaceous glands diminish.

Graying of hair occurs because of the progressively smaller amounts of dopa-oxidase and tyrosinase in hair follicles, both of which are required for the synthesis of melanin. Graying of hair shows a strong genetic predisposition (autosomal dominant) and in the majority of people, 50% of the hairs are gray above the age of 50 irrespective of the sex and hair color.

Heart and blood vessels: Ischemic and hypertensive diseases often supervene as age advances and, therefore, it is difficult to separate these changes from purely aging process. Above the age of 75 years, interstitial fibrosis and fatty infiltration of myocardium develop, even in the absence of any concomitant disease. Lipofuchsin accumulates in the myocardium. Endocardium and valves are thickened. Amyloidosis may develop. Loss of elasticity leads to widening and tortuosity of the aorta. Atherosclerosis accelerates these changes.

Lymphatic organs: The spleen undergoes atrophy. There is increase in the number of plasma cells. Above the age of 70 years, serum globulins are increased and amyloidosis may develop. This form of amyloidosis may affect the heart, islets of Langerhans, peripheral and autonomic nerves, and brain. There is generalized impairment of immune processes and, therefore, infections take a fatal turn.

Cancer: The risk of cancer increases with age and neoplasia accounts for 20% of the total deaths. Atherosclerosis, hypertension and cancer together cause majority of deaths. Invariably, multiple diseases coexist in the elderly patients and diagnosis is often difficult. The symptomatology is atypical.

HEALTH PROBLEMS IN THE ELDERLY

Nutrition: The body weight tends to come down above the age of 70 years. Social neglect, loss of earning capacity and intercurrent illnesses tend to precipitate malnutrition.

Infections: The general resistance against microbes is lowered by malnutrition and impairment of immune mechanisms. The local defense mechanisms of the respiratory, urinary and alimentary tracts, mouth, skin, genitalia and eyes are impaired and, therefore, bacterial infections are common. A common symptom occurring in the elderly subject is alteration in the level of consciousness, delirium and coma, and these must raise suspicion of generalized infection. Fever may not be a prominent symptom in the early stages. Dehydration and electrolyte disturbances are common because of chronic renal impairment and endocrine deficiencies.

Cardiovascular changes: Ischemic heart disease (IHD) is common. Above the age of 80 years, presbycardia results in cardiac failure and arrhythmias. Recurrent thrombo-embolism leads to cerebrovascular occlusion, ischemia

Textbook of Medicine

of limbs and infarction of other vital organs. Varicosity of veins may develop. Dependent edema occurs as a result of exudation of fluid due to loss of elasticity of the skin and fall in tissue tension. Hypoproteinemia, cardiac failure, venous stasis and immobility tend to perpetuate edema.

Respiratory system: Atrophic emphysema, chronic respiratory infection and aspiration pneumonia are disabling problems of old age. Staphylococcal bronchopneumonia may follow influenza and it is a fatal complication. Acute respiratory infection is a common complication of severe illness and this causes death in many cases.

Neurological disorders: Atherosclerosis leads to gradual deterioration of higher functions ending up in dementia. Cerebrovascular accidents (CVA) accelerate this process. Subdural hematomas may develop following minor trauma, or even spontaneously. Cervical spondylosis, lumbodorsal osteoarthritis and ischemia of the spinal cord contribute to pain and dysfunction of the extremities. Peripheral neuropathy occurs frequently. The sensory loss accounts for unsteadiness of gait and clumsiness of movements. Tremor occurring in them aggravates the disability and, therefore, feeding, writing and other activities become difficult or impossible. Parkinsonism is common. This impairs speech and movements further. Cerebellar dysfunction may develop. Herpes zoster is more common in the elderly and postherpetic neuralgia tends to be troublesome.

Autonomic dysfunction: Elderly individuals lose control over the bladder and bowel. There is incontinence of urine and feces. This gives rise to problems of nursing. Postural hypotension may contribute to syncope and falls are common in the elderly. The heat-regulating mechanisms are labile. Accidental hypothermia and hyperthermia may occur due to exposure to external environment.

Special senses: Loss of vision due to cataract, retinal degenerations or chronic iridocyclitis and glaucoma is common. Diabetes and hypertension aggravate the disability. Loss of vision incapacitates them considerably and pastimes like reading, writing and watching television become problematic.

Loss of hearing is common after the age of 50 years and it is a serious handicap. The diminution in hearing may be universal affecting all tones or the higher frequencies may be selectively affected. Deafness impairs their ability to communicate with others and thus makes them isolated. Tinnitus and vertigo may be troublesome. Ageusia or parageusia may occur and these may aggravate their feeding problem.

Alimentary disorders: Loss of teeth makes ingestion of several articles of food difficult. Atrophy of the salivary glands, atrophic gastritis, peptic ulcers, colonic polyps, diverticulosis and cholecystitis are common in the elderly. The poor food intake and immobility lead to constipation. If unattended, this may develop into inspissated feces syndrome in which constipation, alternating spurious diarrhea and fecal incontinence are seen. Malignant lesions in the hepatobiliary system, gallstones and drug-induced hepatotoxicity are more common.

Excretory system: Renal impairment occurs as a result of chronic pyelonephritis and benign nephrosclerosis.

Obstructive uropathy due to enlargement of the prostate is an almost invariable accompaniment above the age of 80 years. The severities of symptoms vary. Several precipitating causes such as urinary infection, prolonged recumbency, instrumentation or sympathomimetic drugs lead to acute obstruction. Elderly women develop senile vaginitis, rectocele, cystocele and uterine prolapse, all predispose to recurrent urinary infections.

Bones and joints: Many weight-bearing joints such as knees, hips and spine, and small joints of the hands and feet develop osteoarthrosis. This tends to make the patient immobile. ***Phlebothrombosis*** and ***embolism*** are common. Accidents and falls are frequent and these initiate the downhill course. Fracture neck of the femur, Colles' fracture and vertebral compression fractures are brought about by osteoporosis. Movements of the shoulder may be restricted by shoulder-hand syndrome.

Muscles: There is generalized atrophy of muscles, myotonia and loss of power. In many areas contractures, cramps or tetany and claudication may develop.

Hematological disorders: Anemia may develop due to poor intake of proteins, iron and vitamins. This is further worsened by loss of blood from hemorrhoids, gastrointestinal (GI) blood losses, diverticulitis and malignancies. Incidence of lymphoma shows a peak in the elderly. Minor trauma in areas such as the dorsum of the hands, wrists lower parts of the legs and feet show senile purpura.

Endocrine system: The gonads, thyroid and adrenal cortex show generalized hypofunction. Myxedema is not uncommon. Since the presentation may be atypical, they may be initially mistaken for primary psychiatric disorders.

Skin: Atrophy of the skin makes it thin and inelastic. There is reduction in subcutaneous fat. These factors make the skin vulnerable to chronic decubitus ulcers. Paresthesia and pruritus are common. The latter may become extremely distressing and intractable, leading to severe distress.

Psychological changes: The elderly become irritable and less adaptable to surroundings. Change in social behavior, emotional instability, loss of self-confidence, mental depression, hallucinations and paranoid, and persecutory fears result in social isolation.

DISEASE PATTERN IN ELDERLY

Aging Changes and Disease States

There is often no clear distinction between changes due to aging and age-associated diseases. Often, medical problems are erroneously considered as aging changes and neglected. Many of the earlier cross-sectional studies on the aging population have created a wrong notion, that aging is always associated with declining function. However, recent longitudinal studies in elderly have clearly shown that physiological functions can be maintained or even improved in the absence of diseases.

The major physiological change associated with aging is the decline in reserve, resulting in a state of ***homeostenosis*** of every organ system. This decline is gradual and often progressive but variable in individuals. However, this decline in function causes no symptoms and possesses few restrictions in the activities of daily living. Loss of adaptability to an acute stress is the key problem in elderly, due to this functional decline.

Unlike in younger age group, multiple diseases are common in elderly. Numerous studies have shown that mean number of diseases per person, for those above the age of 70 years, is around 5. Chronic diseases like hypertension, coronary artery disease (CAD), diabetes mellitus (DM), chronic obstructive pulmonary disease (COPD), degenerative joint diseases, cognitive decline, depressive illness, falls, incontinence and visual and hearing impairment may appear in varying combinations. Multiple symptoms and signs in elderly may be due to different diseases rather than a single disease and unitary disease model approach will lead to wrong diagnosis.

Clinical presentation of diseases also varies in elderly. Some diseases are silent and asymptomatic and many present with atypical symptoms. A disease affecting one organ system can precipitate decompensation in another due to age-related decline in reserve. For example, a respiratory infection can present as acute confusional state, mimicking a central nervous system (CNS) problem. Whatever the underlying acute disease, the weakest areas like cardiovascular, CNS, renal and musculoskeletal systems are often affected and symptoms pertaining to these systems dominate.

A classical presentation of a disease may totally be absent. For example, pneumonia may present often without fever, cough, pleuritic pain and hemoptysis. Myocardial infarction (MI) and intra-abdominal emergency can present as shock or acute confusion.

Because of the decreased reserve, elderly persons develop symptoms at an early stage of the disease and if treated actively, the outcome is much better. Unfortunately, this advantage is set-off by the patients' indifferent attitude toward these early symptoms. The elderly patients seek medical attention at a later stage, when the treatment becomes difficult and the outcome is poor.

At times, coexisting disease may alter the symptoms of another disease, leading to a delay in diagnosis, e.g. disabling old stroke may restrict physical activity, thereby masking an anginal pain of IHD at an early stage. Secondary complications of an acute illness are common in elderly, especially if there is a delay in treatment. For instance, a simple gastroenteritis can lead to dehydration and acute renal failure. However, early diagnosis and prompt therapy result in good outcome.

Though there are no diseases peculiar to elderly, some ailments are more commonly seen in older persons. Sensory deprivation, degenerative joint disease, cardiovascular disorders, vascular and degenerative neurological diseases, DM malignancies and depression are the most common illnesses affecting the elderly. Immobility, unstability (falls), incontinence and intellectual impairment (dementia) constitute the **geriatric giants**, posing management problems.

Tables 253.1 and 253.2 show the diseases patterns in Indian elderly. The main disabilities which afflict the elderly:

Table 253.1: Morbidity pattern in Indian elderly (rural)

Vision problems	88%	Skin problems	13.5%
Locomotor problems	40%	Nutrition problems	11.5%
Cardiovascular system problems	18.7%	Abdominal problems	9.5%
Central nervous system problems	17%	Psychiatric problems	8.5%
Respiratory problems	16%	Hearing problems	8%

Sources:

1. ICMR study—1990, Venkoba Rao
2. VS Natarajan et al.

Table 253.2: Morbidity pattern in Indian elderly (urban)

Cardiovascular system problems	44–48%	Hearing problems	20–24%
Vision problems	40%	Respiratory problems	19–23%
Locomotor problems	36–42%	Psychiatric problems	12%
Central nervous system problems	28–32%	Healthy problems	2%

Sources:

1. Dept of Geriatric Medicine, Govt General Hospital, Chennai
2. Geriatric Clinics, AIIMS, New Delhi
3. KV Krishna Das, Trivandrum.

- Immobility
- Instability and falls
- Incontinence
- Impaired intellect memory
- Frailty
- Depression
- Impaired vision
- Impaired hearing
- Pressure ulcers
- Delirium
- Iatrogenesis and polypharmacy
- Elder abuse and self-neglect
- Caregiver stress and burnout
- Nutritional deficiencies.

These problems impair the quality of life of the elderly and also put great strain on their caretakers who may get exhausted and less caring, thereby adding another dimension to the subjects.

MANAGEMENT APPROACH TO ELDERLY PATIENTS

Multidimensional Geriatric Assessment

Assessment of an elderly patient is always multidimensional and interdisciplinary. It is essential to determine the frail elderly person's medical, psychosocial problems and functional capabilities, with the aim of immediate management, rehabilitation and long-term follow-up. The comprehensive geriatric assessment should include assessment of medical problems and cognitive functions by a physician, assessment of activities of daily living (ADLs) and instrumental activities of daily living (IADLs) by a physiatrist and social problems by a social worker. The aim of initial assessment is to set the realistic goal of improvement and to achieve maximum independence.

The term ADL denotes activities of daily living which includes self-care activities such as eating, bathing, dressing, transferring and toilet, IADL denotes instrumental activities of daily living such as cooking, managing finance, using telephone, driving a car, etc. which demand better functional competence.

Barthel's index of activities of *daily living* is a scoring system which helps to assess the functional capacity of the elderly, specially after a disabling illness.

Several indices have been designed to assess the pathological conditions in the elderly. Hachinski score distinguishes between dementia caused by ischemic brain lesions and nonischemic lesions. The **Barthel's index** is an assessment of functional capacity (Appendix 253.1). It helps to assess the progress in the medical condition of elderly subjects objectively on follow-up:

Appendix 253.1: Hachinski score for ischemic versus nonischemic dementia

Features	Score
Abrupt onset	2
Stepwise course	1
Somatic features	1
Emotional incontinence	1
Systemic hypertension	1
History of strokes	2
Focal neurological symptoms	2
Focal neurological signs	2
Interpretation	
More than 4-Multiinfarct dementia	
Less than 4-Nonvascular dementia	

Barthel's index of activities of daily living

Features	Score
Bowels	
Continence	2
Occasional incontinence	1
Constant incontinence	0
Bladder	
Continent	2
Occasional incontinence	1
Incontinent	0
Feeding	
Independent	2
Needs some help	1
Dependent	0
Combing hair, washing face, cleaning teeth and shaving	
Independent	1
Needs help	0
Dressing	
Independent	2
Can do half	1
Dependent	0

Contd...

Contd...

Features	Score
Transfer (mobility)	
Independent	3
Minor help needed	2
Major help needed	1
Total inability	0
Using the toilet	
Independent	2
Needs some help	1
Dependent	0
Walking	
Independent	3
Walks with one stick	2
Wheel chair	1
Total inability	0
Climbing stairs	
Independent	2
Needs some help	1
Dependent	–
Bathing	
Independent	2
Needs some help	1
Dependent	0

Note: The total score is ascertained immediately after the onset of illness. The total scores are recorded periodically during treatment. Improvement or deterioration can be assessed objectively thereby.

What is Comprehensive Geriatric Assessment?

- A systematic comprehensive problem list focused evaluation of an older person.
- Focus is appropriate medical diagnoses of acute/subacute diseases often superimposed on a background of chronic interacting diseases.
- But focus is also on function, social support, patient and family wishes/expectations and quality of life.

Comprehensive Geriatric Assessments decrease mortality, readmissions to hospital and minimize the impact of *geriatric syndromes* such as cognitive impairment, urinary incontinence and falls.

A geriatric assessment differs from the conventional medical assessment by its attention to many different functional and cognitive domains, as well as its attention to preventative health and their current socioenvironmental situation. Domains covered in an assessment include:

- Medical history
- Medications
- Current living situation and social supports
- Basic activities of daily living and IADLs
- Vision/hearing/mobility/bowels/bladder/diet
- Cognitive status
- Emotional status.

Investigations

Since a coherent history is rarely possible and clinical presentation is often varied and atypical, investigations become essential to arrive at a clinical diagnosis. When an elderly person presents with an acute illness, basic biochemical and radiological tests should be done at the earliest. In asymptomatic patients, safety and usefulness of the test should be considered. In general, noninvasive tests are preferred in elderly although age is not a bar for invasive procedures.

Drug Therapy in the Elderly

The problems associated with drug therapy include alteration in drug metabolism due to changes in body mass and composition, polypharmacy, drug interaction, self-medication, ADR, compliance and cost of therapy. Worldwide data suggest that elderly are the major consumers of the drugs and ADR are more frequent in them. Sedatives, nonsteroidal anti-inflammatory drugs (NSAIDs), diuretics, anticholinergics and antimicrobial drugs lead to adverse side effects frequently. The principle of **start slow and go low** is the practical method of preventing ADR and one has to consider the age-related changes in absorption, distribution and metabolism of a drug before prescribing.

Pharmacotherapy in old age: Adverse drug reactions (ADR) are more common. Most of them are dose-related. Drug distribution changes with the changes in the proportion of fat in the body. Lipid- and water-soluble drugs show corresponding changes in distribution. Drugs such as cimetidine, digoxin and morphine have a smaller volume distribution, hence they show higher blood levels. Fall in the plasma albumin levels results in greater proportion of drugs to be in the free form and this leads to higher side effects, e.g. warfarin, oral antidiabetes drugs, NSAIDs and others. Drugs which depend upon hepatic metabolism may show vagaries in their concentration and actions. Glomerular filtration falls by 35% in the elderly, so too the renal tubular function. Drug dosage has to be adjusted depending upon the creatinine clearance (*See* Section 16, Ch 192).

Changes in hepatic functional impairment, autonomic nervous function and neuromuscular activity influence the actions of drugs. The best method is to individualize the dose on a trial and error basis. A simple prescription with clear instruction of dosage and duration of therapy is mandatory. Periodic review of medication and compliance will be beneficial. In addition to a definitive diagnosis and analysis of risk benefit of therapy, one has to consider the concomitant diseases before choosing a drug.

COMMON GERIATRIC SYMPTOMS AND THEIR MANAGEMENT

There are a few symptoms which are more prevalent in elderly, requiring different approach and management. Pain, dizziness, constipation, dyspepsia, pruritis, memory disturbances, multiple somatic complaints falls and delirium are some of the common symptoms seen in geriatric clinics. A brief review of these symptoms will be useful. Many physicians adopt a syndromic approach while treating geriatric patients. This takes into consideration the functional disabilities such as restriction of movement, diminution of vision, falls and so on, irrespective of the exact pathology. Reduction of the ill effects of age-related phenomena and diseases is the main goal of geriatric medicine.

Constipation

Constipation is defined as less than three bowel movements per week and its prevalence varies from 40 to 60% in elderly. Dietary inadequacy, multiple medications, anorectal problems, reduced gastrointestinal (GI) motility are often contributing factors for constipation. Acute constipation associated with acute medical problems often produce distressing symptoms like abdominal distension, confusion and urinary retention. Laxatives in the form of rectal suppositories and enema are useful and often digital evacuation has to be done. Dietary adjustments in the form of increased fluid and fiber in the diet, regular exercise and a fixed time of bowel evacuation are simple measures of preventing chronic constipation. Bulk and osmotic laxatives are the preferred form of therapy and reassurance that chronic constipation is age-related and benign, is quite useful.

Dyspepsia

Sedentary habits and reduced GI motility often leads to dyspeptic symptoms. Acid peptic disease, reflux eso-phagitis and upper GI malignancy and drugs are the common causes of dyspepsia. Upper GI endoscopy and barium studies are useful and safe in evaluation. Drugs that improve motility like domperidone and H_2 receptor blockers are widely used.

Memory Disturbances

Many elderly patients complain of declining memory function but often perform well during mental status examination. History obtained from the caregiver of declining memory is more reliable and needs evaluation. Age-associated memory impairment (AAMI) has to be differentiated from early Alzheimer's disease. A thorough neurological examination and a regular follow-up can differentiate benign AAMI from progressive dementia. While memory loss is the lone disturbance of the higher function in AAMI, there is a diffuse and progressive alteration of mental functions in dementia. A treatable dementia is always to be considered in any dementing illness and a thorough evaluation is mandatory.

Pain

More than 50% of the elderly patients attending a geriatric clinic will present with pain as the primary complaint. Degenerative joint diseases, osteoporosis, muscular pain, neuritic pain, malignant and somatoform disorders are some of the underlying diseases producing pain. Nondrug method of physical therapy is the first line of management. When medication is required, paracetamol is safe and widely used. NSAIDs should be used with caution in elderly, but should not be withheld when required. Adjuvant pain therapy in the form of antidepressants and anticonvulsants is often useful in chronic and neuritic pain. Opioids should be reserved for intractable pain associated with malignancies. Referral to ***pain clinics***, where multimodel approach is provided, will be beneficial in chronic pain associated with malignancy and depressive illness.

Dizziness and Vertigo

Prevalence of these symptoms vary from 30 to 40% in elderly. Benign positional vertigo, vestibular dysfunction, age-related changes in the sensory system and drugs are some of the common causes of vertigo in the elderly. A thorough ear, nose and throat (ENT) and neurological evaluation is mandatory but often does not contribute in diagnosis or management. The major complication of dizziness includes a fall and fracture in a frail elderly, which should be prevented. Vestibular rehabilitative exercises are the main form of therapy and vestibular sedatives should be used with caution. Walking aids in the form of walking sticks and walking frames are often useful in preventing a fall. The elderly are very prone to develop hyponatremia and this should be looked for in all cases.

Multiple Somatic Complaints

Often multiple complaints are the presenting problems in elderly. A depressive illness is usually the cause of multiple somatic complaints and psychiatric counseling will be useful. A thorough clinical and diagnostic evaluation has to be performed in every case to rule out an organic basis and periodic re-evaluation is ideal.

Falls

Instability and frequent falling may be the presenting symptom in the frail elderly, the prevalence varying from 20 to 30% in the community. Multiple medical illnesses are often the cause for a fall rather than simple aging. Environmental hazards like poor lighting, uneven floor, slippery toilets and stairs without hand rails can lead to falls. Age-related changes in the nervous system, Parkinsonism, cognitive decline, polypharmacy and cardiac arrhythmias are the intrinsic causes of recurrent falls. Physical injuries, fractures and psychological trauma and fear of fall can lead to invalidism. Identifying the basic disease and measures to improve the muscle strength and balance, specially of the lower limbs and physical training can prevent falls.

Delirium

Many a time elderly patients are brought in a state of acute confusion. Delirium involves altered consciousness with impaired attention and diminished arousability. Infection, dehydration, electrolyte disturbances, hypoxia, hypotension and drugs are the frequent causes of acute confusion in elderly. Since delirium is often a clinical manifestation of the underlying serious systemic disease, it has to be identified, evaluated and actively managed. Many times outcome of an acute confusional state is rewarding, provided it is treated early.

SOCIAL PROBLEMS IN THE ELDERLY

Elderly persons have several problems which cause hardship. These include health problems, financial problems, social alienation and possibly others. The elderly person tends to become uncooperative, withdrawn and cynical in behavior. They are not accepted by the younger folk. Many of them are left alone due to death of the near relations or desertion by them. Helplessness is a real medical problem for those above the age of 65 years. Mortality among elderly persons living alone is 3.2% per annum. Mortality is higher in the months of extreme cold and heat. Social rehabilitation measures including living places, hostels, provision of the help at home and device such as emergency alarm for summoning help are available in developed countries. Ideal situation is one in which no elderly person has to live alone and to face death alone.

Socioeconomic problems add and aggravate medical, physical and psychological disabilities in the elderly. The changing demographic pattern has resulted in more number of elderly are joining the *dependent population*. Psychosocial problems are the result of retirement, loss of occupation and income, housing problems and bereavement in the family. The joint family system which is the basic social support in the community is unfortunately disintegrating because of the migration of children for better opportunities. Neglect, loss of respect for elders and elder abuse are increasing in the community. It is vital to promote and protect joint family system to provide basic social and emotional support to the elders. Though old age homes are increasing in number in our country, they can never be a substitute for family care. Developing day care centers, senior citizen clubs and friendly visiting services would help to provide recreation, group activity and emotional outlet for the elders.

DEVELOPMENT OF GERIATRIC HEALTH SERVICES IN INDIA

At present, there are not many geriatric health units available in India. The few available are mostly placed in larger cities. Since most of elderly population lives in the rural area, geriatric health care should be included in the primary health care system. Multipurpose health workers can be trained to identify health problems of the elderly and to provide simple remedies and referral system whenever required. Taluk and headquarters hospitals should provide outpatient and inpatient geriatric services. Teaching hospitals should develop full-fledged geriatric units and provide geriatric training programs for primary care physicians. Many institutions in India are offering postgraduate instructions and training in geriatrics at present. It is also vital to develop nursing homes or long stay hospitals with nursing and rehabilitative services for the elderly with chronic physical disabilities.

REHABILITATION AND PHYSICAL THERAPY OF THE AGED

Interaction with family members and friends, involving in social activities and cultivating a spiritual and philosophical attitude are the most easy and natural way of rehabilitation in old age. Formal groups consisting of physiatrist, occupational and speech therapist, counselor, and appropriate specialist depending upon the major disability can give occupational therapy, with considerable benefits. Rehabilitation includes restoration of the capacity to regain ADL such as bathing, feeding, toileting and transferring and IADL such as cooking, cleaning, shopping and similar functions, along with treatment of underlying morbidities and relief of pain. Wherever available, palliative care services should be provided.

Palliative Care

The center to *Advanced Palliative Care and the American Cancer Society* has defined palliative care as appropriate care at any age and at any stage in a serious illness and can be provided together with curative treatment. This differs from hospice care, in that the former takes care of people who have reasonable lifespan with positive results on therapy.

Source: Sharma OP. Geriatric care. A Textbook of Geriatrics and Gerontology. 3rd Edition. New Delhi: Viva Books; 2008.

Palliative care is not synonymous with ***end-of-life*** care. On the other hand, the ***hospice care*** is care given to patients who are willing to forgo curative treatments and who have a physician-estimated life expectancy of 6 months or less. In case of an individual patient, the physician has to advice the patient and his/her relatives to adopt the appropriate path. Hospice is the facility where a combination of dedicated team consisting of physician, nurse, social worker, counselor including bereavement counseling is available.

The term ***respite care*** denotes the sharing of the care of the elderly by a substitute for varying periods, in order to relieve the stress of the regular caregiver.

Addendum

Editor's Note: With the universal increase in the proportion of the aging population in all countries, comprehensive geriatric assessment (CGA) is a model of healthcare addressed to ensure uniformity.

In principle, it is a thorough multi-domain comprehensive assessment of the patient. There domains include physical health, mental and psychological health, disability normal health and functioning alongside social determinants of health and wellness.

Comprehensive assessment, innovative evaluation, involvement of other service groups in addition to geriatricians and team working in service delivery, are all important to provide appropriate care to prevent disability and treat acute events in this rapidly increasing elderly community.

Index

A

Abadie's sign 1354
Abatacept 736, 789
Abciximab 913, 1185
Abdominal compartment syndrome 520
Abdominal form 383
Abdominal pain 475
Abducent nerve 1321
    palsy 1323
Abetalipoproteinemia 1437
ABO
    hemolytic disease 1078
    system 1097
Abortus fever 243
Abram's pleural biopsy punch 968
Abreaction 1584
Absence seizures 1382
Absolute reticulocyte count 1056
Abstinence 951
Acamprosate 1570
Acanthamoeba 410
Acanthocytes 1056
Acanthosis nigricans 71, 614, 1540
    malignant 1541
Acarbose 592
Accident, management of 123
Accidental hypothermia 108
Accommodation reflex 1319
ACE inhibitors 809
Acetaminophen 140
Acetazolamide 1389
Acetic acid 139
Acetohydroxamic acid 1260
Acetylcholine receptor antibodies 1469
Acetylcholine test 915
Achalasia cardia 486
Achondroplasia 782
Achylia gastrica 1069
Acid maltase deficiency 1479
Acid phosphatase 71
Acid-base
    balance 453
        abnormalities of 452
    disorder 454
        mixed 452, 462
    profile 1484
Acne 1509
    conglobata 1510
    excoriée 1510
    keloidalis nuchae 1536
    occupational 1510
    variants of 1510
    vulgaris 1509
Acneiform eruptions 1530
Acoustic neuromas 1420
Acquired aplastic anemia 1089
Acquired cystic kidney disease 1246
Acquired cysts 1026
Acquired epileptic aphasia 1381
Acquired hemolytic anemias 1075
Acquired hemophilia 1189
Acquired hypertrichosis lanuginosa 1536, 1542
Acquired immune deficiency syndrome 287, 290, 1075
    dementia 293
        complex 293
        encephalopathy 293
Acquired PRCA in adults 1092
Acquired renal cystic disorders 1246
Acquired syphilis 274
Acquired thrombophilia 1204
Acquired von Willebrand disease 1191

Acrochordon 1543
Acrodermatitis
    chronica atrophicans 259
    continua of Hallopeau 1513
Acrokeratosis 71
Acromegaly 650, 651, 786, 936
ACTH 646, 654
    stimulation 692
    testing 687
Actinic keratoses 1543
Actinomyces 382
Actinomycosis 382
Acute attack, management of 775
Acute leukemias, treatment of 1114
Acute malnutrition, moderate 164
Acute myeloid leukemia treatment, high-risk 1121
Acute pharyngitis, microbial causes of 974
Acute poisoning, symptoms of 144
Acute respiratory failure, management of 970
Acute tachycardias, management of 872
Acyanotic congenital heart defects 818, 819
Acyclovir 57, 333, 336
    ointment 336
Acylcarnitine 1487
Acylglycines 1487
Adalimumab 735, 766, 1515
Addison's disease 448, 692, 936
Addisonian pernicious anemia 1069
Adductor reflex, crossed 1291
Adefovir 57
    dipivoxil 348
Adenocarcinomas 1020
Adenoma, bronchial 1019
Adenomatous polyps 509
Adenovirus infections 357
Adie's pupil 1464
Adjustment disorders 1566
Adrenal cortex
    diseases of 688
    disorders of 684
Adrenal cortical
    disorders 687
    hormones 686
        secretory rates of 686
Adrenal crisis 693
Adrenal gland 1145
Adrenal hyperplasia, congenital 691
Adrenal incidentaloma 696
Adrenal medulla, disorders of 684, 694
Adrenergic system, inhibitors of 890
Adrenocortical insufficiency 691
    primary 691
Adrenocortical lesions 690
Adrenocorticotropin hormone 646
Adrenomyeloneuropathy 1430
Adriamycin 1142
Adult personality, disorders of 1567
Adverse drug event 45
Adverse prognostic indicators in stroke 1413
Adverse reactions, management of 100
Aedes aegypti 371
Aerosol
    drug delivery 988
    inhalation 967
    vaccines 330
Aflatoxicosis 145
African river blindness 439
African trypanosomiasis 402
African tumbu fly 90
Agnivesa 1
    tantra 1

Agnogenic myeloid metaplasia 1161
Agonist drugs 40
Agoraphobia 1561
Agranulocytosis 1135
    drug-induced 1135
Air inadvertently during aspiration 1031
Air travel, medical problems of 121
Airway
    clearance 1041
    disease, small 997
    diseases of 1003
        lower 996
    maintenance of 970, 1337
    mechanisms of 955
    resistance 958
        syndrome, upper 1016
    secretion of 954
Akinetic mutism 1337
Alastrim 331
Albendazole 416, 418, 420, 438, 441
Albiglutide 597
Albright's hereditary osteodystrophy 684
Albright's syndrome 705
Albuminocytologic dissociation 1310, 1455
Albuminuria 1214
Alcohol 188, 1349
    acts 1349
    exposure 939
    injection into tumor 561
    intoxication 137
    related disorders 1569
    septal ablation 946
    withdrawal syndrome 137
Alcoholic beverages 951
Alcoholic cirrhosis 533
Alcoholic dementia 1350
Alcoholic hallucinosis 1569
Alcoholic hepatitis 347, 552
Alcoholic hyaline 552
Alcoholic liver disease 552
Alcoholic myopathy 1350
Alcoholic paranoia 1569
Alcoholism 446, 448, 1350, 1438
    chronic 1569
Aldermoniac posture 1474
Aldose reductase inhibitors 785
Aldosterone 687
    antagonists 810
Aldrin 132
Alefacept 1515
Alemtuzumab 1129
Alendronate sodium 771
Aleppo boil 400
Alfa-fetoprotein 560
Alien hand 1291, 1367
Alimentary disorders 476, 1592
    symptoms in 475
Alimentary endoscopy, upper 478
Alimentary manifestations 679
Alimentary pentosuria 618
Alimentary symptoms 176
Alimentary system 666, 1064, 1588
Aliskiren 892
Alkalies 140
Alkalotic tetany 684
Alkaptonuria 628
Alleles 6
Allergen
    identification of 986
    immunotherapy 991
Allergic bronchopulmonary aspergillosis 996

I-ii

Allergic contact dermatitis 1521
Allergic rhinitis 993
   treatment of 973
Allergic to penicillin, treatment of patients 277
Allodynia 1302
Allogenic stem cell transplantation 1157
   in myeloma 1143
Allogenic transplantation 1116
Alopecia 637, 1535
   areata 1535
   totalis 1535
   universalis 1535
Alpha-1 antitrypsin deficiency 1004
Alpha-adrenergic receptor blocking drugs 890
Alpha-fetoprotein 70
Alpha-glucosidase inhibitors 592
Alpha-interferon 57
Alpha-synucleinopathies 1395
ALS-parkinsonism dementia complex 1434
Alternate cover test 1323
Alternative regimen 281, 284
Alveolar hypoventilation, causes of 957
Alveolar membrane 958
Alveolar ventilation 958
Alzheimer's disease 1370, 1371
Amanita muscaria 143
Amanita phalloides 144
Amantadine 57, 324, 1394, 1428
   hydrochloride 56
Amblyomma 94, 267
   americanum 267
Ambrisentan 835
Ambulatory electroencephalogram 1303
Ambulatory peritoneal dialysis, continuous 1280
Ameba rare 1357
Amebiasis 405
   treatment of 408
Amebic dysentery, acute 406, 409
Amebomas 407
Amenorrhea 709
American cutaneous and mucocutaneous
   leishmaniasis 401
American trypanosomiasis 403
Amifostine 77
Amikacin 50
Amino acids 1487
Aminoglutethimide 690
Aminoglycosides 50, 1285
Aminophylline 992
Amiodarone 867, 868
Amlodipine 776, 892
Ammonia 456
Ammonium 456, 1486
   chloride 456
Amnesia 1548, 1564
Amnesic syndrome 1569
Amnestic disorders 1553
Amnestic syndrome 1569
Amebic meningoencephalitis 1357
   primary 409
Amotivational syndrome 1570
Amoxicillin 48
Amphoric breathing 966
Amphotericin B 58, 59, 399, 410
Ampicillin 48
Amplified Mycobacterium tuberculosis detection 303
Amylin 474, 582
   agonists 598
Amylnitrate 144
Amyloid
   A, secondary 1146
   light-chain 1264
   type of 1146
Amyloidosis 448, 938, 1144, 1146, 1264
   localized 1145
   secondary 731
Amyotrophic brachial diplegia 1433
Amyotrophic lateral sclerosis 457, 1431
Anacrotic pulse 848
Anaerobes 268
Anaerobic
   bacteria, role of 61
   food poisoning 143
   infections 268
   organisms 981

Anagen 1535
   phase 1544
Anagrelide 1167
Anakinra 736, 775
Anal canal 476
Anamnestic reaction 231
Anankastic personality disorder 1567
Anaphylactic
   reaction, type I 29
   shock 817
Anaphylactoid purpura 1264
Anaplasma 267
   phagocytophilum 267
Anaplasmataceae 267
Anaplasmosis 263, 267
Anastrozole 78
Anca-associated vasculitis 756
Ancylostoma duodenale 417
Ancylostomiasis 413, 417
Andreas Vesalius 2
Androgen
   excess 708
   functions of 699
Androgenic alopecia 1536
Anemia 1057, 1089
   aplastic 346, 1089, 1091
   based etiopathogenesis, classification of 1058
   correction of 1066
   etiology of 1059
   in rheumatoid arthritis 1070
   in systemic diseases 1070
   management of 1060
   of chronic diseases 1071
   of infections 1071
   severe 389
   treatment of 1241
Anesthesia dolorosa 1302
Anesthetic risk 1018
Anetoderma 1538
Aneuploidy 16
Aneurine 174
Aneurysmectomy 812
Angioedema 1526
Angiofibromas 715
Angiogenesis 72
Angioimmunoblastic
   lymphadenopathy 1159
   lymphoma 1157
Angioplasty, primary 946
Angiosarcomas 944
Angiostrongyliasis 441
Angiostrongylus
   cantonensis 441
   costaricensis 441
Angiotensin converting enzyme 448
   inhibitors 891
Angiotensin receptor blockers 447, 809, 891
Angiotensin-converting enzyme inhibitors 1285, 1286
Angiotensinogen 1211
Angiotensin-receptor blockers 908
Angular chelitis (perleche) 1506
Anhedonia 1555, 1559
Anhidrotic heat exhaustion 104
Anidulafungin 59
Animal rabies 362
Anisakiasis 441
Anisocoria 1319
Anistreplase 906
Ankylosing spondylitis 513, 764, 1027, 1035
Ankyrin 1046
Annual influenza vaccination 1000
Anomalous origin 829
Anomalous pulmonary venous connection 834
Anorectal lesions 282
Anorexia 475
   nervosa 653, 1571
Anosmia 1367
Anosognosia 1297
Anoxic damage to liver, acute 347
Antagonist drugs 40
Anterograde amnesia 1553
Anthracosis 1007
Anthrax 239, 240
Anthropometry 154, 638

Antianginal
   agents 911
   therapy 910, 914
Antianxiety drugs 1582
Antiarrhythmic 811
   drugs 880
Antibacterial
   agents 47, 1500
   drugs 327
   spectrum 50
Antibiotic 61, 76, 271, 539, 970, 983, 1286
   misuse of 61
   regimens, start initial 980
   resistance, future strategies in 61
Antibody 1374
   against viruses 322
   demonstration of 1074
   dependent immunity 29
   response 25
   to clotting factors 1192
Antibody-based therapies 1117
Antibody-detection tests 398
Anticholinergic agents 990, 999
Anticoagulant 811, 908, 913, 1194
   detection of circulating 1174
   indications of 1194
   rodenticides 134
   therapy 174
Anticoagulation, initial 927
Antidepressant 152
   drugs 1581
Anti-diphtheritic serum 224
Antidiuretic hormone 442, 642
Antidotes 127
   to cyanides 134
Antiepileptic drugs 1386
Antifolates 75
Antifungal drugs 58
Anti-GBM disease 1225
Antigen 25
   detection 363
Antiglomerular basement membrane disease 1028
Anti-GPIIB/IIIA antibodies 1185
Antihypertensive
   drug choices 894
   therapy 892
Anti-idiotype therapy 74
Anti-IGE treatment 994
Anti-immunoglobulin E 991
Anti-inflammatory agents 213, 1000, 1499
Anti-ischemia therapy 910
Antimicrobial
   agents 47
   drugs 249
   regimen 232
   resistance 194
   spectrum 51
   therapy 235, 244
Antimicrosomal antibody 661
Antimitochondrial antibody 526, 534
Antimutagens 70
Antimycobacterial drugs 55
Antineutrophil cytoplasmic antibodies 724
Anti-n-methyl-d aspartate syndrome 1377
Antinuclear 526
   antibodies 723, 724, 731, 743, 1262
Antiparkinsonism drugs 1583
Anti-pellagra vitamin 175
Antiphospholipid antibody 724
   syndrome 739, 743, 747
Antiplatelet
   agents 910, 913
   drug 913
     in stroke 1412
     therapy 1185
   therapy 1185
Antipruritic agents 1499
Antipsychotic
   atypical 1580
   conventional 1580
   drugs 1556, 1580
   side effects of 1580
Antipurines 75
Antipyrimidines 75
Antirabic serum 364

Antiretroviral therapy 295
Antirheumatic drugs 736
Anti-snake venom 99
Anti-sterility vitamin 173
Antistreptolysin O titer 723
Antitetanus serum 271
Antithrombin 1172
Antithrombotic mechanisms 1172
Anti-thyroglobulin antibodies 662
Anti-TNF agents, biological 1010
Antitrypsin deficiency 1003
Antituberculous drugs 1286
Antitumor necrosis factor agents 735
Antiviral drugs 56
Antiviral therapy in special population 349
Anti-voltage gated potassium channel syndrome 1376
Anti-β-cell agents 736
Anton's syndrome 1297
Anuria 1212
Anxiety
    acute 1578
    disorders 1560
    neurosis 1560
Anxiolytics 1582
Anxious personality disorder 1567
Aorta
    aneurysms of 930
    diseases of 928
Aortic diseases 928
Aortic incompetence 850
Aortic regurgitation 850
    acute 853
    causes of 850
    signs of 852
Aortic stenosis 847, 848
    congenital 819, 847
    severity of 849
Aortic syndrome, middle 929
Aortic valve, degenerative calcification of 848
Aortoarteritis, type III 929
Aortography 1219
Aphasia
    conduction 1300
    management of 1481
Aphthous ulcers
    major 481
    minor 481
Aplastic anemia
    congenital 1089
    moderate 1090
    severe 1090
    treatment of 1091
    very severe 1090
Aplastic crisis 1084
Apnea test 1338
Apnea-hypopnea index 1016
Apocrine glands 1497
Apoptosis 69
Appendages, infection of 1500
Appetite 475
Apraxic gait 1303
Aprotinin 1194
Aquagenic pruritus 1164
Aquagenic urticaria 1526
Aquaporin channels 465
Arabic medicine 1586
Arbovirus 365, 1360
    group B 370
Arenaviridae 359
Arenavirus 358
    infections 358
Argas persicus 258
Argatroban 1198
    dabigatran 914
Argemone mexicana 145
Argentine 359
Arginine vasopressin 443, 642
    role of 804
Argyll Robertson pupil 1319, 1354, 1367
Armadillo gait 1303
Arnold-Chiari malformation 1450
Arrhythmias 811, 902, 942, 1413
Arrhythmogenic right ventricular
    cardiomyopathy 917
    dysplasia 872

Arsenical keratoses 1544
Artemether 392
Arterial blood
    gases 452, 454, 926
    pressure 792
Arterial embolism 902
Arterial pulse 793
Arterial strokes 1406
Arterial wall, examination of 794
Arteriographic studies 915
Artery
    peripheral 857
    syndrome, basilar 1410
Artery-to-artery embolism 1407
Artesunate 393
Arthralgia 377, 740
Arthritis 210, 377, 513, 767, 740
    inflammatory 727
Arthropod bites 91
Arthroscopy 726, 779
Articular involvement 728
Asbestosis 1007
Ascariasis 413
Ascites 518, 537
    management of 531
    prognosis of 519
Ascitic fluid ultrafiltration 532
Asclepid hippocrates 1
Ascorbic acid 178, 1347
Aseptic meningitis 355
Ashworth scale 1291
Asian opticospinal multiple sclerosis 1428
Asiatic schistosomiasis 431
Aspartate transaminase 901
Aspergillosis 378
Aspergillus 1361, 1362
    flavus 145
Aspermia 706
Aspiration 409, 1031
    elective 1031
    emergency 1030
    pneumonia 979, 981
Aspirin 734, 903, 1185
    in dose 915
Astanga hridaya 1
Astanga sangraha 1
Asterixis 1405
Asthenopia 1297
Asthenospermia 706
Asthma 985, 993, 1042
    acute severe 992
    atopic 985
    bronchial 984
    complications of 994
    controller drugs in 988
    exacerbation, acute 993
    management of 991
    reliever drugs in 988
    severity of 988
    signs to assess severity of 992
Astringents 1499
Astrocytoma 1420
    high-grade 1420
Astrovirus 250
Asymptomatic bacteriuria 1250, 1254, 1273
    in pregnant women 1254
Asymptomatic coronary artery disease 915
Asymptomatic cyst passers 409
Asymptomatic hyperuricemia 776
    treatment of 776
Asymptomatic microscopic hematuria 1220
Asymptomatic non-nephrotic proteinuria 1220
Ataxia 1366, 1437, 1484
    telangiectasia 1438
Ataxic dysarthria 1300
Ataxic gait 1302
Atherosclerosis 896
Atherosclerotic
    complication 885
    renovascular disease 1268
Athetosis 1400
Athletics heart 919
Atlantoaxial dislocation 1449
    types of 1450
Atlantoaxial subluxation 729

Atonic seizures 1382
Atrial fibrillation 843
Atrial flutter 868
Atrial natriuretic peptide, detect 1464
Atrial premature beats 863
Atrial septal defect 823, 947
Atrophic candidiasis, chronic 1506
Atrophic gastritis, chronic 490
Atropine 131
    toxicity 131
Attacks, acute 626
Attention deficit hyperactivity disorder 1577
Atypical pneumonia, primary 319, 320, 979
Auchmeromyia luteola 90
Auditory hallucinations 1548
Auditory nerve 1328
Auscultation 796
Austin flint murmur 851
Autistic disorder 1576
Autoimmune 1425
    diseases 32, 581, 1075
        treatment of 32
    encephalitis 1374, 1376
    encephalopathies 1370, 1375
    hemolytic anemia 1075
    hepatitis 556
    neonatal thrombocytopenia 1180
    polyglandular syndrome 32
    thyroiditis 674
Autoimmunity 581
Autoinfection 419
Autologous
    peripheral stem cell transplantation 1157
    stem cell transplantation 789, 1143
Autonomic function, tests of 1464
Autonomic nervous system
    alterations in 804
    disorders of 1460
Autonomous bladder 1465
Autosomal chromosomes 7
Autosomal disorders 16
Autosomal dominant
    inheritance 12
    polycystic kidney disease 1244
Autosomal recessive
    inheritance 12
    polycystic kidney disease 1245
Autosomes 6
Autosplenectomy 1083
Autotransfusion 1102
Aversion therapy 1585
Avian embryo vaccines 364
Avian flu 325
Avicenna 1
Axon reflex 1463
Ayurveda 1, 1586
Azathioprine 1471
Azidothymidine 57
Azithromycin 51, 235, 266, 281
Azoles 59
Azoospermia 703, 706
Azotemia 810
Aztreonam 49

B

B cell lymphoma, diffuse large 1156
B. novyi 258
B$_{12}$ deficiency, effects of 177
B$_2$-agonists 989
Babinski's reflex 1300
Bacillary angiomatosis 253
Bacillary dysentery, acute 512
Bacillus
    anthracis 240
    cereus 142
Bacitracin 55
Back leak theory 1232
Baclofen 1428
Bacteremia 236, 237, 238, 255
Bacterial endocarditis, subacute 855
Bacterial index 317
Bacterial infection 1075, 1500
    of childhood 223
    secondary 324

Bacterial meningitis 1364
Bacterial nephritis, acute 1243
Bacterial prostatitis
    acute 1254
    chronic 1255
Bacterial vaginosis 284
Bacteriological tests 966
Bacteriuria 1250
    significant 1250
Bacteroides 539
Baghdad boil 400
B-agonists 999
Bainbridge reflex 863
Baker's cysts 729
Balamuthia mandrillaris 410
Balanced diet 161
Balanoposthitis 1506
Balantidiasis 405, 411
Balantidium coli 411
Bald tongue 484
Ballism 1402
Ballistic movements 1400
Balloon
    atrial septostomy 947
    kyphoplasty 1143
    mitral valvotomy 843
    procedures 946
    tamponade 548, 549
Bamboo spine 764
Band forms 1048
Banded krait 96
Banding techniques 19
Bangarus caeruleus 96
Bangarus fasciatus 96
Barbara Wartenberg's sign 1328
Barbiturates 135
Barcelona clinic liver cancer 561
Bariatric surgical techniques 191
Barium
    enema 478, 512
    meal 477, 563
    swallow 477
Barlow's syndrome 846
Barometric pressure 109, 121
    alterations in 109
    increased 109
Barotrauma 109
Barr bodies 18
Barthel's index 1594
Bartonella bacilliformis 253
Bartonella henselae 253
Bartonella quintana 253
Bartonellosis 253
Bartter's syndrome 446, 459, 1249
Basal cell layer 1496
Basal ganglia
    circuits 1398
    physiology of 1391
Basedow's disease 664
Basedow's paraplegia 1493
Basement membrane 1261
Basilar invagination 1448
Basket cells 1128
Basophilic leukemia, chronic 1127
Basophils 1050
Bass player's thumb 721
Batista procedure 812
B-cell origin 1149
BCG vaccination 309
BCP crystal arthropathy 777
Beau's nails 1537
Becker muscular dystrophy 1476
Bedside peak flow meter 987
Bedside testing methods 1299
Bed-wetting 1577
Beef tapeworm 423
Bees 92
Beevor's sign 1441
Behavior theory 1568
Behavior therapy 1584
Behavioral symptoms, adjunctive therapies for 1371
Behavioral syndromes 1571
Behavioral therapy technique 1570
Behçet's disease 759
Behçet's syndrome 759, 760

Bell's palsy 1326
    prognosis of 1327
Belly tendon method 1304
Belt system 1328
Bender visual motor gestalt test 1551
Bentiromide test 566
Benzene 1090
Benzodiazepines poisioning 136
Bereitschafts potential 1289
Bernard-Soulier syndrome 1182
Berry aneurysms 1414
Beta 2-agonists, long-acting 990
    inhaled 994
Beta adrenergic blockers 914
Beta blockers, treatment with 810
Beta interferon 57
Beta thalassemia major 1086
Beta-adrenergic
    blockers 904
    blocking drugs 891
    receptor pathway, alterations in 804
Beta-blockers 668, 809, 910, 915, 1286
    benefits of 809
Betaine 555
Bethlem myopathy 1473, 1474
Bhatia's battery of intelligence scale 1551
Bicarbonate, administration of 606
Biermer's anemia 1069
Biguanides 590
    adverse effects of 591
Bile acid diarrhea 499
Bile culture 230
Bile ducts 563
    major 562
Bilharziasis 430
Biliary cirrhosis 533
    primary 533
    secondary 533
Biliary disorders 499
Biliary obstruction, acute 347
Biliary tract disease 562
Binet-Simon intelligence scale 1551
Binswanger's disease 1373
Bioactive phytochemicals in food 158
Biochemical
    abnormalities 523, 689
    changes 171, 540
    disorders 1383
    feedback 152
    investigation 1234, 1484
    tests 476, 519, 525, 679, 1217, 1464
Biofilm formation 61
Biological agents 734, 736, 788, 789
Biomarkers 926
Biomphalaria 430
Biopsy 201, 479, 1132, 1313
    role of 201
    studies 502, 968
Biosimilars 789
Biosynthesis 580
Biot's breathing 957
Bioterrorism 194
Biotin 176, 1346
    metabolism, defects of 1485
Bipyridyl herbicides 133
Birbeck granules 1497
Birth defects 1347
Bisferiens pulse 794, 851
Bites, local treatment of 364
Bithional 429
Bivalirudin 1198
BK virus 1243
Black fever 397
B-lactam antibiotics 49
B-lactamase resistant penicillin 48
Bladder
    automatic 1440, 1465
    care of 1337
Blalock-Taussig-Thomas shunt 832
Blastic transformation 1124
Blastomyces 1362
Blatchford scores 497
Bleeding 1197
    arrest of 548
    during delivery, serious 1180
    episodes 1188
        acute 1188

esophageal varices 548
from gums 475
into pleural cavity 1031
tendency 1055
time 1173
Blindness 1084
    denial of 1297
Blink reflex 1305
Blistering disorders, classification of 1523
Block vertebrae syndrome 1450
Blood
    bank procedures 1098, 1103
    chemistry 1060
    component 368
        therapy 1112
    counts 1059
    culture 230, 858
    examination 501
    film
        examination, peripheral 1106
        peripheral 1074, 1120
    findings 359
    formation 1044
    gases 958, 1484
    group
        antibodies 1097
        antigens 1046, 1096
        system 1097, 1098
    losses 1063
    pressure 1413, 1463
        control of 1461
        rapid control of 893
        recording 796
        regulation of 1266
    smear 1059
    substitutes 1102
    supply 522, 1289, 1440
    transfusion 368, 497, 1084, 1087, 1096
    urea 1217
        nitrogen 1217
    vessels 1591
        disorders of 1531
B-lymphocytes 25, 1051, 1052
Boas' sign 563
Body buffers 453
Body fluids, metabolites in 640
Body myositis, inclusion 761, 1473, 1479
Body's response to hypoglycemia 603
Bogorad's sign 1327
Bolivian hemorrhagic fevers 359
Bombay blood group 1098
Bombesin 474
Bone 236, 243, 666, 719, 750, 1592
    age 639
    changes 1139
    densitometry 726
    diseases 780
    lesions 275
    marrow 1093, 1120, 1428
        aspiration 201, 1132
        culture 230
        examination of 1056, 1059, 1140
        transplantation 1084, 1110, 1115, 1143
    resorption 77
        inhibiting agents 1143
    tuberculosis 783
Boogards angle 1446
Bornholm's disease 356
Borrelia duttoni 258
Borrelia recurrentis 94, 257
Borrelial infections 257
Bortezomib 78, 1142
Bosentan 752, 835, 1015
Boston memory scale 1551
Bosutinib 1125
Boswellia carteri 258
Botulism 142
Boutonnière or button hole 729
Bovine cough 962, 976
Bowel
    care of 1337
    disease, inflammatory 511, 1490
    enema, small 477
    infarction of 509
Bowen's disease 1544
Bowenoid papulosis 1544

Brachial
neuralgia 1457
plexitis 1457
plexus 1447
Brachytherapy 73
Bradycardiac agents 911
Bradyphrenia 1368
Brain
biopsy 1315
death 1333, 1338
imaging, role of 1475
parts of 1288
stimulation in epilepsy, deep 1390
Brainstem
auditory evoked response 1305
encephalitis 71
lesions 1328, 1332, 1410
Break bone fever 365
Breasts 638
atrophy of 712
Breath
sounds 965
tests 502
Breathing 956
capacity, maximal 961
chemical control of 956
control of 956
techniques, deep 1463
Brittle asthma 993
Brittle bone disease 782
Broad spectrum 1387
penicillins 48
Broca's aphasia 1299
Brock's syndrome 1002
Broken heart syndrome 920
Bromhexine hydrochloride 1000
Bromocriptine 650, 652
Bronchial asthma, management of 988
Bronchial obstruction 977
Bronchial thermoplasty 991
Bronchial tree, divisions of 953
Bronchiectasis 1001, 1043
sicca 1002
Bronchioloalveolitis, types of 994
Bronchitis
acute 996
chronic 997, 1004
emphysema syndrome, chronic 997
Bronchoalveolar lavage 968
Bronchoconstriction 457
Bronchodilator 999
response 1001
Bronchogenic carcinoma 1019, 1025
Bronchography 967, 1005
Bronchophony 966
Bronchopleural fistula 1031
Bronchopneumonia 980
Bronchopulmonary segments 953, 954
Bronchoscopy 968
Brown induration 1013
Brownell-Oppenheimer variant 1374
Brown-Sequard syndrome 1441
Brucella
abortus 243
canis 243
melitensis 243
suis 243
Brucellosis 239, 243, 1354
chronic 244
treatment of complicated 244
Brudzinski's leg sign 220
Brugia malayi 432
Brugia timori 432
Bruxism 475
Bubonic plague 242
Budd-Chiari syndrome 540, 558
Buffer systems 453
Bulbar palsy 1332, 1433
Bulimia nervosa 1571
Bulinus 430
Bull's angle 1449
Bulla spread sign 1524
Bullous disease of childhood, chronic 1525
Bullous emphysema 1004
Bullous impetigo 1501

Bullous pemphigoid 1524
Bumetanide 459
Bundle branch block 877
partial 877
Buprenorphine 1570
Burkholderia pseudomallei 244
Burkitt's lymphoma 1158
Burtonian line 146
Busse-Buschke's disease 380
Busulfan (myleran) 1126
Buthidae 92
Byssinosis 1008
Bythinia species 429

C

C₃ glomerulopathy 1230
Ca-199 71
Cabergoline 650, 652
Cabot's rings 1045, 1068
Cachexia 1026
Cacosmia 1316
Cadaveric position 976
Cafe coronary 976
Calciferol 169
Calcific pancreatitis 615
Calciphylaxis 1239
Calcitonin 450, 659, 677, 682, 771
gene-related peptide 660
Calcitriol 1,25-dihydroxyvitamin 450
Calcium 179
absorption 677
antagonists 911, 915
channel 861
blockers 868, 1014, 1341
blocking drugs 892
free phosphate binding resin 451
homeostasis 442
disorders of 449
oxalate arthropathy 777
receptor agonists 450
stones 1257
Calcium-channel blockers 914
Callitroga 90, 91
Caloric test 1322, 1329, 1335
Calpainopathy 1473
Calymmatobacterium granulomatis 282
Campylobacter jejuni 251
Canakinumab 775
Canals of Lambert 954
Cancer 938, 1591
prognosis in 72
screening programs 78
therapy, adjuvants in 77
Candida 1361, 1362
Candidiasis 378, 1505
Cangrelor 1185
Canities 1536
Cannabis-related disorders 1570
Cannon waves 795
Capillaria philippinensis 441
Caplan's syndrome 730
Capsule endoscope 478
Captopril 891
Caput medusae 546
Carbamazepine 1325, 1582
Carbenicillin 49, 459
Carbimazole 667
Carbohydrate 156, 586
absorption of 473
digestion of 473
intolerance 504
Carboxylase deficiency, multiple 1346, 1437
Carbuncle 214, 1501
Carcino-embryonic antigen 71
Carcinoid syndrome 510
Carcinoid tumors syndrome 510
Carcinomatous polyarthritis 786
Cardiac aneurysm 903
Cardiac arrest 878
management 878
Cardiac arrhythmias 861
Cardiac assist devices 950
Cardiac cachexia 808
Cardiac catheterization 801, 849

Cardiac cirrhosis 559
Cardiac complications 324
Cardiac cycle 791
Cardiac disease 1494
Cardiac electrophysiology, development in 862
Cardiac failure 803
complications of 807
treatment of 843
Cardiac lesions 856
Cardiac lymphomas 944
Cardiac manifestations 259, 942
Cardiac muscle 453
Cardiac output 792
Cardiac pain, control of 904
Cardiac physiology 791
Cardiac resynchronization therapy 947
Cardiac rupture 903
Cardiac surgery 948
Cardiac transplantation 812, 950
Cardiac tumors 942
malignant 944
secondary 944
Cardiac-specific troponins 901
Cardioembolic stroke, causes of 1407
Cardiogenic shock 814-816, 902
compressive 815
intrinsic 815
Cardiology 791
preventive 951
Cardiomyopathy 917, 946, 952
unclassified 917
Cardiopulmonary exercise test 961
Cardiorenal syndrome 937
Cardiospasm 486
Cardiovascular
abnormalities 638
affection 244
changes 1588, 1591
disease 122, 792, 871
drugs in pregnancy 941
lesions 629
manifestations 671, 1238, 1560
system 293, 609, 666, 681, 730, 741, 774
changes in 885
Carditis 211
Carey-Coomb's murmur 211
Carfilzomib 1142
Carney syndrome 936
Carotene, overdosage of 169
Carotenoids 168
Carotid artery stroke syndrome 1409
Carpal tunnel syndrome 671, 1458
Carphology 229
Carrion's disease 253
Carvallo's sign 853
Caspofungin 59
Cassava toxicity, acute 144
Catagen 1535
Catalepsy 1549
Cataract 610
Catastrophic antiphospholipid antibody syndrome 747
Catatonia 1291
Catatonic stupor 1334
Cathepsin 1000
Catheter-based techniques 822, 825, 827, 828, 927
Catheterization 820, 826
Cat-scratch disease 253
Cauda equina 1441
Causalgia 1454
Causative organism 288
Cave disease 379
Cavernous 965
Cefaclor 50
Cefadroxil 49
Cefamandole 50
Cefazolin 49
Cefepime 50
Cefixime 50
Cefoperazone 50
Cefotaxime 50
Cefotetan 50
Cefoxitin 50
Cefpirome 50
Cefradine 49
Cefsulodin 50

Ceftazidime 50
Ceftizoxime 50
Ceftriaxone 50, 1376
Cefuroxime 50
    axetil 50
Celiac disease 502, 1489
Cell
    based treatments 813
    carcinoma, large 1021
    counts 1055
    culture vaccines 364
    large 1156
    lung cancer
        non-small 1021
        small 1021, 1025
        subtypes, non-small 1021
    lung carcinoma, small 1021
    types of 1045
    wall polysaccharide 379
Cell-mediated immunity 26
Cellular casts 1216
Cellular immunity, deficiency of 33
Cellulitis 208, 1501
Centipedes 94
Central anticholinergic agents 1394
Central cord syndrome 1442
Central core disease 1474
Central hypoventilation syndrome, congenital 1335
Central monoamines 1557
Central nervous system 226, 244, 275, 681, 857,
    1026, 1561
    changes in 886
    gumma of 1354
    infection of 238, 1351
    lymphomas, primary 293
    manifestations 1489
        in respiratory disease 1491
        in systemic disorders 1489
    viral infections 1357
Central neurofibromatosis 1459
Central osmotic demyelination 469
Central pontine myelinolysis 445, 464, 469
Central precocious puberty 705
Central scotoma 1320
Central sleep apnea 1016
Centrifugal devices 812
Cephalexin 49
Cephalic tetanus 270
Cephaloridine 49
Cephalosporins 49
Cephalothin 49
Cerbera odollam 138
Cerberin 138
Cercariae daily 430
Cercarial dermatitis 431
Cerebellar ataxias responsive to specific therapy 1437
Cerebellar cortical degeneration, subacute 1438
Cerebellar dysfunction 671
    causes of 1438
Cerebellar hemorrhage 1416
Cerebellar homunculus 1436
Cerebellar nystagmus, classical 1324
Cerebellar tumors 1438
Cerebellopontine angle tumors 1420
Cerebellum
    diseases of 1435
    inflammatory lesions of 1438
Cerebral artery
    stroke, middle 1409
    syndrome
        anterior 1410
        posterior 1410
Cerebral form 111
Cerebral hemorrhage 1176
Cerebral malaria 388, 1356
Cerebral paraplegia 1447
Cerebral thrombosis 1407
Cerebral toxoplasmosis 293
Cerebral vasculitis 1370
Cerebral venous thrombosis 1413
    treatment of 1414
Cerebrospinal fever 220
Cerebrospinal fluid 1307, 1309
    examination 1308
Cerebrotendinous xanthamatosis 1438

Cerebrovascular accidents 122, 1481
Cerebrovascular disease 609, 1406, 1493
Certolizumab 736
Cervical
    cord compression 731
    dysfunction 706
    radiculopathy 1451
    spondylosis 779, 1343, 1451
Cervicofacial form 383
Cestodiasis 423
Chaddock's sign 1301
Chagas disease 403, 936
Chagoma 404
Chamberlain's line 1446
Chancroid 283
Chandipura virus 1361
    encephalitis 361
Charaka samhita 1
Charcoal, activated 126
Charcot's joint 785, 1354, 1446
Charles Bonnet phenomena 1298
Chelated iron 1066
Chemical carcinogens 69
Chemical pleurodesis 1034
Chemokines 26
Chemoprophylaxis 43, 62, 309, 393
Chemotherapy 74, 317, 561, 1025
    adverse effects of 938
Chenodeoxycholic acid 564
Chest
    examination of 796
    syndrome, acute 1083
    wall, diseases of 1034
Cheyne-Stokes
    breathing 957
    respiration 1335
Chiasm 1317
Chickenpox 332
Chiclero's ulcers 401
Chiggers 266
Chigoe flea 95
Chikungunya 370
    virus 1361
Childhood absence epilepsy 1380
Childhood autism 1576
Childhood epilepsy 1380
    benign 1380
Childhood hypopituitarism 654
Chilopoda 94
Chimerism 16
Chinese liver fluke 429
Chipmunk facies 1086
Chlamydia, lifecycle of 280
Chlamydial respiratory infections 319
Chloasma 1533
Chloramphenicol 52, 1089
Chloride
    resistant metabolic alkalosis 459
    responsive metabolic alkalosis 459
Chlorinated diphenyls 132
Chloroquine 408, 1010
    diphosphate 734
Chlorpropamide 645
Cholangiocarcinoma 564
Cholecystitis 563
    acute 563
    chronic 564
Cholecystokinin 471, 474
Choledochoscopy 479 563
Cholera 246
Cholestasis 346, 525
Cholesterol crystal embolism 932
Cholinergic syndrome, acute 130
Cholinergic urticaria 1526
Cholinesterase inhibitors 1470
Chondrocyte transplantation 779
Chordoma 1419
Chorea 1400
    minor 211
Choroidal artery syndrome, anterior 1410
Christmas disease 1189
Chromatin 7
Chromones 994
Chromosomal disorders 15
Chromosomal translocation 68
    syndromes 18

Chromosome 7
    components of 7
Chronic carriers, treatment of 232
Chronic liver disease, systemic complications of 544
Chronic obstructive pulmonary disease
    acute exacerbation of 1001
    infection in 997
Chronic tobacco addiction, therapy of 149
Chronic undernutrition, severe 164
Chronic valvular diseases, surgery for 949
Chrysomya 90, 91
Churg-Strauss syndrome 757, 935
Cicatricial alopecia 1535
Cidofovir 376
Cigarette smoking 952
Ciliospinal reflex 1319
Cilnidipine 892
Ciprofloxacin 54, 235
Circadian rhythm, exaggerated 199
Circle of Willis 1289
Circulating anticoagulants 1193
Circulatory failure, acute 559
Cirrhosis 346, 533, 561
    of liver 528
    patients 349
Cladribine 1129, 1131
Clarithromycin 51, 52
Claviceps purpurea 146
Cleistanthus collinus leaf 138
Climatic bubo 281
Clindamycin 53, 413
Clinico-pathological correlates, causes of 1236
Cloaca 1207
Clobazam 1388
Clofazimine 318
Clonal origin of neoplasms 69
Clonic phase 1382
Clonidine 890, 1464, 1570
Clonorchiasis 429
Clonorchis sinensis 429
Clonus 1291
Clopidogrel 1185
Clostridia, diseases caused by 269
Clostridial myonecrosis 272
Clostridium
    botulinum 142
    difficile 252
    perfringens 142, 143
    tetani 269
Clot retraction 1173
Clotrimazole 58
Clotting cascade 1171
Clotting time 1173
Cloxacillin 48
Clozapine 1395
Clunking sound 729
Clutton's joints 276
Cnidae 95
Coagulase negative staphylococci 214
Coagulation after warfarin 1197
Coagulation defects 1175
Coagulation disorders 1191
    rare 1193
Coagulation vitamin 173
Coal worker's pneumoconiosis 1007
Coarctation of aorta 820, 947
Coarse hair 1539
Coat hanger phenomena 1462
Cobra 96, 97
    bite 98
Coccidioides 1362
Cochlear system 1328
Cochliomyia 91
Cockroft-Gault formula 1588
Cod fish vertebra 770
Codox-M 1159
Coenurus cerebralis 441
Cogan's twitch sign 1467
Cognition, disturbance of 1546, 1547
Cognitive behavior therapy 1585
Cognitive disturbances 1555
Cognitive enhancers 1553, 1583
Cognitive functions 1296, 1583
Cognitive impairment, mild 1372
Cognitive rehabilitation 1481

Cognitive theory 1558
Cognitive therapy 1585
Coin shadow 1023
Coital headache 1342
Colchicine 775
Cold
    agglutinin-positive pneumonia 979
    agglutinins diseases 1075
    areas 801
    injuries to 107
    sore 336, 1503
    urticaria 1526
Colistin 55
Collagen
    diseases 1027
    disorders 1075
    fiber 1538
        disorders of 1537
    major disorders of 629
Collapsing pulse 794
Collaterals, demonstration of 547
Collet-Sicard syndrome 1331
Colon 472
    cancer, genetics of 516
    carcinoma of 512
    diseases of 511
Colonic mucosa 472
Colonic stricture 512
Colonoscopy 478, 512
Color anomia 1298
Color vision 1318
Column disease, lateral 1442
Coma 388, 1333, 1334, 1336
    causes of 1334
    diagnosis of 1336
    grading of 540
Comatose patient 1334
    management of 1337
Combination therapy 399, 1130
Communication system 89
Community acquired pneumonia 320
Community water, fluoridation of 483
Community-acquired pneumonia, causes of 978
Compensatory emphysema 1003
Complement system, deficiency of 34
Complete heart block 876, 877
Complete left bundle branch block 877
Complete right bundle branch block 877
Complete transverse section 1441
Complex partial seizure 1380, 1381
Complex tremor 1405
COMT inhibitors 1394
Conation, disturbance of 1547, 1549
Conchotome biopsy 1312
Condyloma acuminata 286
Condylomata acuminata 1502
Cone shells 95
Congenital aregenerative anemia, chronic 1092
Congenital heart disease, burden of 817
Congenital myasthenia syndromes, treatment of 1471
Congenital syphilis, diagnosis of 277
Congestive heart failure, chronic 559
Congo maggot fly 90
Conidae 95
Conjunctival reflex 1325
Conn's syndrome 459, 936
Connective tissue disease 747, 752
    mixed 752, 1263
Connective tissue disorders 724
Consciousness 1295
    alteration of 537
    disturbance of 1546, 1549
    levels of 1333
Consecutive optic atrophy 1320
Constipation 476, 1595
    predominant 506
Constitutional symptoms 508
Constructional apraxia 537
Consumer Protection Act 3
Contact dermatitis 1521
Contact urticaria 1527
Continend by rhazes 1
Contractile apparatus, changes in 805
Convalescence 225, 372
Conversion disorders 1563

Convulsions, control of 272
Convulsive status 1389
Cooley's anemia 1086
Coomb's test 1074, 1098
Cope's needle 968
Copper 185, 1348
    accumulation of 527
Coprinus species 144
Coral snake 96
Cord blood 1112
    banking 1102
    transfusion 1102
    transplantation 1088
    uses of 1102
Cordylobia anthropophaga 90
Core system 1328
Corkscrew esophagus 488
Corneal reflex 1325
Corneomandibular reflex 1301, 1325
Coronary
    angiography 802, 913, 915
    heart disease 951
    revascularization 906
    stents 945
Coronary artery
    bypass
        graft 900, 907, 914
        surgery 949
    disease, prevention of 915
Coronavirus 250
Corpus callosum 1298
Corrigan's pulse 794
Corrosive acids 138
Cortical arousal 1463
Cortical blindness 1367
Cortical dementia, mixed 1372
Corticobasal degeneration 1373, 1396
Corticosteroid 327, 687, 734, 745, 1110
    therapy, adverse side effects of 65
    withdrawal 66
Corticotropin group 646
Corticotropin-releasing hormone 642
Corynebacterium diphtheriae 223
Coryza 323
Cosmetic effects 710
Co-stimulation blockers 736
Co-trimoxazole 52
Cough
    fracture 962
    reflex 955
    syncope 962
    variant asthma 993
    with expectoration 962
    without expectoration 962
Councilman bodies 342
Cover test 1323
Cowpox 1503
    virus 1503
COX-2 inhibitors 734
Coxa vara 171
Coxiella burnetii 94, 267
Coxsackieviruses infections 355
CPP crystal deposition disease 776
Crab louse 1509
Crab yaws 256
Crackles 965
Cramps 1453
Cranial arteritis 754
Cranial diabetes insipidus 643
Cranial form 355
Cranial nerve 1316, 1330
    eighth 1328
    palsy 1495
    signs 1367
Craniopharyngioma 1419, 1421
Craniotabes 171
Craniovertebral anomalies 1448
    management of 1450
C-reactive protein 722, 897
    high level of 952
Creatine kinase 901
Creatinine clearance 1217
Creatorrhea 500
Crepitations 965
Crest syndrome 748

Cretinism 670
Creutzfeldt-Jakob disease 1373, 1374
Crigler-Najjar syndrome 524
Crimean-congo hemorrhagic fever 360
Crohn's disease 506
    acute exacerbation of 507
Cross reacting antibodies 31
Crotalaria 145, 558
Crotalidae 96
Croup 975
Crunching sounds 966
Crusted scabies 1508
Cryoglobulinemia
    essential mixed 344
    mixed 758, 1264
Cryoglobulinemic vasculitis 758
Cryoprecipitate 1100, 1188
    infusions 1191
Cryptococcal meningitis 293
Cryptococcosis 380
Cryptococcus 1362
    neoformans 1362
Cryptogenic 1380, 1381
    polycythemia 1163
    stroke 1410
Cryptorchidism 703
Cryptorchism 703
Cryptosporidiosis 294, 405, 413
Cryptosporidium parvum 413
Ctenopharyngodon idellus 144
Cubam receptor 1068
Culex tritaeniorhynchus 372
Culicoides 439, 440
Cultural bond syndromes 1563, 1565
Culture negative-neutrocytic ascites 532
Cupids bow sign 1473
Cupping 171
Curb-65 rule 981
Cushing's disease 652, 688, 689
Cushing's syndrome 459, 688, 786, 936
Cushing's vasomotor phenomena 1419
Cutaneous
    amebiasis 407
    anthrax 240
    candidiasis 1506
    diphtheria 224
    drug reactions 1528
    embolism 857
    forms, management of 626
    horn 1544
    larva migrans 422
    leishmaniasis 400
        diffuse 401
    leukoclastic vasculitis 344
    manifestations 291, 749
        of systemic disorders 1539
Cutis laxa 1538
Cyanide
    poisoning 134
    routes of entry of 134
Cyanocobalamin 177, 1347
Cyanosis 793, 964
Cyanotic CHD, management for 836
Cyanotic congenital heart disease 818, 830
Cyanotic heart disease, congenital 836
Cyclical neutropenia 1049
Cylindroma 1543
Cymevene 57
Cyproheptadine 652
Cystathionine beta-synthase deficiency 630
Cystatin 1234
    C 1217
Cystic disease
    congenital 1244
    of kidneys 1244
    of ovary 709
Cystic disorder 1246
Cysticercosis 424, 425, 1355
    eradication of 426
Cysticercus cellulosae 424
Cystine stones 1257, 1258
Cystitis 1250
    in women, acute uncomplicated 1251

Cystourethrography 1219
Cysts 1040
    congenital 1026
    of kidney 1246
Cytisine 152
Cytokines 1052
    role of 804
Cytomegalovirus 374, 1075, 1359, 1377
    infection 376
        reactivation of 293
Cytotoxic hypersensitivity, type II 30
Cytotoxic test 37

D

Da Costa's syndrome 934
Dabigatran 1198
Daclizumab high-yield process 1428
Danazol 1527
Dancing gait 1401
Dandy fever 365
Dandy-Walker malformation 1450
Dapsone 317
    syndrome 318
Daptomycin 53
Darbepoetin-α 1047
Darling's disease 379
Dasatinib 77, 1125
Dawn phenomenon 608
De Motu Cordis 2
De Quervain's thyroiditis 673
Dead hand 120
Death adder 96
Decadron 1142
Decerebrate posture 1336
Decorticate posture 1336
Decubitus ulcers 1413
Deferiprone 1088
Deficiency
    pathology of 174
    states 174
Degenerative joint disease 777
Dehydration, correction of 606
Deliberate self-harm 1577
Delirium 1552, 1596
    tremens 137, 1350
Delivery, timing of 600
Delta sign, empty 1414
Delusion 1547
    primary 1548
Delusional disorders 1554
Demeclocycline 468
Dementia 1377, 1553
    cortical 1368
    drug in 1553
    praecox 1554
    reversible 1369
    subcortical 1368
    with lewy bodies 1373
Demodarans gait 1303
Demyelinating lesions 1425
Dengue 1361
    attacks of 366
    classification 366
    fever 936
    first attack of 366
    shock syndrome 367
Denosumab 682, 772, 789
Dense deposit disease 1230
Dental
    caries 482
    fluorosis 147
    procedures 860
Denture stomatitis 1506
Deoxyribonucleic acid, antidouble standard 1262
Dependence syndrome 1569
Depression 934, 1413, 1557, 1558
    major 1558
Depressive mutism 1559
Depressive stupor 1559
Deprivation dwarfism 656
Depth electrodes recording 1303
Derealization 1548
Dermacentor 94
    marginatus 361
    reticulatus 361

Dermal vasculature, expansion of 1512
Dermatitis
    atopic 1518
    herpetiformis 502, 1524
    management of contact 1522
Dermatobia hominis 90
Dermatome 1439
Dermatomyositis 760, 761, 1479
Dermatophytosis 1504
Dermis 1497
Dermoepidermal junction 1497
Dermographism 1526
Desferrioxamine 1087
Desmopressin 645, 1188
Detemir 595
Detoxification 1570
Detrusor-external sphincter dyssynergia 1465
Developmental anomalies 1438
Devic's disease 1428
Dexamethasone
    high dose 1178
    suppression test 688
Dexrazone 77
Dextrocardia 836, 837
Dextro-transposition of great arteries 833
Dextroversion 836
Dhat syndrome 1565
Di Guglielmo's syndrome 1118
Diabetes 601, 602, 1260
    during pregnancy 599
    in asymptomatic adult, testing for 580
    insipidus 643
    mellitus 577, 604, 784, 935, 1018, 1539
        and pregnancy 1270
        complications of 601, 609
        type 1 577, 599
        type 2 577, 578, 599
        types of 578
    monitoring control of 588
    patients, estimated number of 578
Diabetic cheiroarthropathy 784
Diabetic coma, management of 606
Diabetic complications, pathogenesis of 609
Diabetic dermopathy 1540
Diabetic dyslipidemia 935
Diabetic foot 613
Diabetic ketoacidosis 604, 605
Diabetic lactic acidosis 608
Diabetic nephropathy 611, 1260
Diabetic neuropathy 1456
    classification of 612
Diabetic patient, education of 586
Diabetic retinopathy 609
    classification of 610
    treatment of 610
Diabetic ulcers 1540
Diabetic, acute problems in 608
Diabetology, future prospects in 614
Dialysis 126, 1276
    adequacy 1279
    dementia 1493
    disequilibrium syndrome 1238, 1492
    in acute kidney injury 1278
    monitor 1277
Diamond on quadriceps sign 1474
Diamond-Blackfan anemia 1092
Diaper dermatitis 1506
Diaphragmatic dysfunction, causes of 1037
Diaphragmatic flutter 1039
Diaphragmatic hernia 1037
Diaphragmatic paralysis 1036
    causes of 1037
Diaphragmatic tic 1039
Diarrhea 476
    antibiotic associated 252
    predominant 506
Diarrheal disease 357
    of children, acute 250
    of infective origin 245
Diastolic heart
    dysfunction 805
    failure 805
Diazepam 1428
Diazoxide 891
Dicobalt-acetate 144

Diet 69
    and environmental factors 44
Dietary advice 1259
Dietary iron, metabolism of 181
Dietary management 502, 586
Dietary modification 951
Dietary sources 178
Dietetic management 249
Diethylcarbamazine 437
Diffusion 465, 1277
Difluoromethylornithine 403
Digastric line 1446
DiGeorge syndrome 33, 939
Digestive organs 470
Digestive symptoms 1462
Digestive system, radiological examination of 477
Digital subtraction angiography 86, 802
Digitalis purpurea 810
Digitorum brevis, extensor 1473
Digitoxicity, treatment of 811
Digoxin 810, 811
Dihydroartemisinin 392
Dilated cardiomyopathy 917
Diloxanidefuroate 408
Diltiazem 892
Diminished hematopoiesis 1095
Dipeptidyl peptidase-4 inhibitors 591
Dipetalonema
    perstans 432
    streptocerca 432
Diphtheria 223, 936
    antitoxin 224
Diphyllobothriasis latum 427
Diphyllobothrium latum 427
Diplococcus pneumoniae 216
Diploid cells 6
Diplopia 1323
    crossed 1322
Dipylidium caninum 428
Direct immunofluorescent antibody 363
Direct thrombin inhibitors 1198
Direct toxicity 1284
Directly acting antivirals 350
Directly observed treatment 306
Disaccharidase deficiency 504
Discoid eczema 1520
Discoid lupus 740
Disease modifying therapy 1427
Disease modifying treatments 1435
Disease states 1592
Disease-modifying antirheumatic drugs 734
Disequilibrium syndrome 1279
Disinfection 1101
Disorders, autonomic 1461
Dispermic chimeras 16
Dissecting aneurysms of aorta 931
Disseminated encephalomyelitis, acute 1425, 1443
Disseminated gonococcal infection 279, 280
Disseminated intravascular coagulation 1200
Disseminated morphea 748
Dissocial personality disorders 1567
Dissociated anesthesia 1446
Dissociative disorders 1563, 1564
Dissociative identity disorder 1564
Disturbances, autonomic 614, 1462
Diuretic 531, 810, 813, 889, 1286
    intractable ascites 531
    resistant ascites 531
    therapy 446, 810
    urogram 1219
Diverticulitis 514
Dizziness 1595
DNA polymorphism 19
Dobutamine 816
Dog tapeworm 426
Doll's eye movements 1335
Domiciliary treatment 305
Donepezil 1371, 1395
Donor feces infusion 252
Donor marrow, infusion of 1111
Donor selection 1282
Donovania granulomatis 282
Donovanosis 282
Dopa-agonist responsive dystonia 1399
Dopamine 816
    agonists 539, 652, 1394

Dopa-responsive dystonia 1399
Dornase alpha 1000
Dowager's hump 770
Down's syndrome 16, 939, 1575
Doxazosin 890
Doxycycline 51, 266, 410
Dracontiasis 440
Dragon worm 440
Dressler's syndrome 903
Dropped fingers 729
Drowning 113
Drowsiness 1333
Drug 188, 485, 554, 702, 709, 733, 766, 770,
    775, 910, 1142, 1438, 1512, 1559
    acting against filarial parasite 437
    administration 40, 43
        during pregnancy 44
        in elderly 43
        in special groups 43
        routes of 40
    alternative 66
    and dialysis 1286
    and kidney 1284
    and toxins 461
    availability 1568
    combinations 868, 889
    distribution 42
    dosage of 1402
    elimination of 42
    emergency 893
    eruption, fixed 1530
    first-generation 905
    in renal failure, dosage of 1286
    interaction 46
        prevention of 46
    L-interactions ataxia behavioral 1387
    metabolism 538
    prophylaxis 1341
    related adverse effects 44
    related problem 45
    reserve 306
    resistance 238, 306
        of microbes 59
        primary 306
    therapy 440, 492, 498, 652, 667, 903, 1088,
        1272, 1327, 1403, 1561, 1580
        in elderly 1595
    to improve memory 1583
    toxicity on liver 557
Drug-drug interactions 44
Drug-resistant
    epilepsy, surgery for 1390
    tuberculosis, extensively 307
Dry beriberi 174
Dry drowning 113
Dual personality 1564
Duchenne muscular dystrophy 933, 1476
Duct occluder device 828
Duction movements 1323
Duke's criteria for diagnosis 857
Dulaglutide 597
Duodenal aspirate, cytology of 566
Duodenal biliary drainage 563
Duodenal ulcer 491
Dupilumab 994
Duplex ultrasound 82
Dupuytren's contracture 614
Dura producing, side of 1334
Duration of fever 196
Dwarf tapeworm 427
Dwarfism 647, 655
Dyken criteria for diagnosis 1360
Dynamic cardiomyoplasty 812
Dysbarism 109
Dysesthesias 1302, 1453
Dysfunction, autonomic 1592
Dyskinesias 1405
Dyslipidemia, treatment of 1241
Dysmyelination 1425
Dyspepsia 1595
Dysphagia 475, 485
    causes of 485
    lusoria 485
Dyspnea 792, 963
Dysprosody 1299

Dysreflexia, autonomic 1291
Dysthymia 1557
Dysthymic disorders 1559
Dystonia 1399
    management of 1400
    primary 1399
    with myoclonus 1399
Dystonia-plus syndromes 1399
Dystonic tremors 1404
Dystrophia
    adiposo genitalis 655
    myotonica 1478
Dystrophinopathies 1478
Dystrophy 1472
Dysuria 1212

E

Ear
    infections 238
    middle 120
Eardrum 120
Eating disorders 1571
Eaton agent pneumonia 979
Ebola vaccine 360
Ebola virus
    disease 360
    infections 359
Ebstein anomaly 836
EBV infection, chronic active 375
Ecallantide 1527
Eccrine glands 1498
Echinocandins 59
Echinococcosis 426
Echinococcus granulosus 426
Echinococcus multilocularis 426
Echo Doppler 947
Echocardiography, uses of 800
Echoing 1299
Echolalia 1549
Echopraxia 1549
Echoviruses 355
E-cigarette 152
Eclampsia 1271, 1495
Econazole 58
Ecthyma 214, 1501
Ectopic ACTH secretion 690
Ectopic adrenocorticotropic hormone 71
Ectopic beats 863
Ectopic Cushing's syndrome 713
Ectopic parathyroid hormone 71
Eculizumab 1096
Eczema 1517
    herpeticum 336, 1503
    management of 1518
Edema 792, 793, 1212, 1237
Edmonston B strains of measles virus 330
Edmonston-Zagreb strains 330
Edward's syndrome 17
Efalizumab 1515
Effusion
    complicated 1029
    uncomplicated 1029
Eflornithine 403
Ehlers-Danlos syndrome 629, 1538
Ehrlichia 267
    chaffeensis 267
    ewingii 267
Ehrlichiosis 267
Eight-and-a-half syndrome 1328
Eisenmenger syndrome 828, 835
Elapidae 96
Elastin fiber, disorders of 1537
Elastin fibers 1538
Elastography 82
Electric shock-like sensation 1451
Electrical injuries 116
Electroconvulsive therapy 1557, 1579
Electrocorticography 1303
Electrodiagnostic tests 1469
Electroencephalogram 537, 1303
Electroencephalography 1338
Electrolyte abnormality 938
Electrolyte balance, abnormalities of 442
Electrolyte depletion 810
Electrolyte disturbances 606

Electrolyte imbalance 539
Electromyography 1304
Electron microscopy 1229, 1475
Electrophoretic study 1141
Electrophysiology study 947
Elephantiasis
    treatment of 438
    verrucosa nostra 1532
Eleventh cranial nerve 1331
Elicit memory 1551
Elicit plantar response 1300
ELISA test, capture 371
Ellsworth-Howard test 678
Elsberg pattern 1441
Eltrombopag 1055, 1179
Embolic episodes 856
Embolic phenomenon 857, 942
Embolic stroke 1407
Embolism 1592
Embryo
    damage to 116
    during renal development 1207
Embryology 685
Emergency management 125, 497, 991
Emery-Dreifuss
    muscular dystrophy 934, 1478
    myopathy 1473, 1474
Emollients 1499
Emotional disorders 1576
Emotions 1461
Emphysema 457, 996, 1003, 1004
    atrophic 1004
Emphysematous cystitis 1255
Empirical therapy 859
Empyema 209, 1029, 1031
    necessitans 1031
    of gallbladder 563
Enalapril 891
Enanthems 328
Encephalitic stage, acute 372
Encephalitis 333, 1373
    acute 1360
Encephalomyelitis 329
    ventriculitis 333
Encephalomyelopathy 337
Encephalopathy
    acute 1483
    chronic 1483
Endemic fluorosis 147
    prevention of 149
Endemic gastroenteritis 250
Endemic goiter 663
Endemic typhus 265
Endocardial involvement 294
Endocarditis 221, 238, 267, 1494
    infective 855, 856
    prophylaxis 860
Endocrine 1267, 1558
    abnormalities 770
    causes 709, 1370
    cells 471
    diseases 784
    disorders 636, 786, 935, 1493
        of breast 711
    disturbances 537
    dwarfism 636
    function 566
        of gut 473
    myopathy 1479
    neoplasia, multiple 715
    organ 1211
    syndromes 713, 714
    system 1592
Endocrine-related conditions 711
Endocrinology 631
Endogenous
    benzodiazepines 536
    eczema 1518
    lipids 620
Endorphins 474
Endoscopic interventions 548, 549
Endoscopic management 528
    elective 498
Endoscopic retrograde
cholangiopancreatography 479, 526, 563, 566

Endoscopic sclerotherapy 549
Endoscopy 408
Endothelin
    receptor antagonists 1015
    role of 804
Endotheliomas 1420
Endovascular intervention 1412
Endrin 132
End-stage of Alzheimer's disease 1375
Energy deficient conditions 618
Enkephalins 474
Entacapone, dose of 1394
Entamoeba histolytica 405, 406, 409
Entecavir 57, 348
Enteral feeding 163
Enteric cytopathogenic human orphan viruses 355
Enteroaggregative *Escherichia coli* 236
Enterobacteriaceae group 237
Enterobiasis 420, 477
Enterococci 209
Enterocolitis 233
Enteroglucagon 474
Enteroinsular axis 473
Enterokinase 473
Enteropathic arthritis 766
Enteropathy 718
Enterovirus 352, 355, 1359
    caused diseases 356
    treatment of 357
    type 70 355
Entrapment neuropathy 730, 1456, 1458
Entry inhibitors 295
Enuresis 1577
Enzyme 76, 97
    determination 525
    levels in
        blood 565
        urine 565
    studies 1487
Enzyme-linked
    immunosorbent assay test 32, 231
    immunospot 303
Eosinophilia 1050
    causes of 1050
Eosinophilic
    esophagitis 486
    fasciitis 751
    gastritis 490
    gastroenteritis 1050
    granulomatosis with polyangiitis 757, 1263
    leukemia 1126
    myocarditis 1050
Eosinophils 1049
Epalrestat 785
Ependymomas 1420
Epidemic dropsy 145
Epidemic gastroenteritis 250
Epidemic keratoconjunctivitis 357
Epidemic myalgia 356
Epidemic spastic paraplegia 146
Epidemic typhus 263
Epidermal proliferation 1512
Epidermis 1496
Epidermoid carcinoma 1020
Epigenetics 11
Epilepsy 122, 1379, 1381
    and pregnancy 1383
    management of 1386
        women with 1384
    primary 1380
    sudden death in 1386
    syndrome 1381
        classification of 1380
    with myoclonic 1381
        absences 1381
Epileptic myoclonus 1403
Epileptic seizures, classification of 1380
Epileptic syndrome 1382
    classification of 1380
Episodic apnea 1468
Epistasis 13, 973
    causes of 973
Epitopes 31
Eplerenone 810, 909

Epoprostenol 751
Epratuzumab 1117
Epstein-Barr virus 339, 374, 1359
Eptifibatide 913
Epworth sleepiness scale 1017, 1018
Eratyrus 404
Erectile disorder 1573
Ergonovine test 915
Ergotamine 146, 1340
Ergotism 146
Eruptive xanthomas 1540
Erysipelas 208, 1501
Erythema annulare centrifugum 1541
Erythema gyratum repens 1541
Erythema multiforme 1528
Erythema nodosum 1009, 1542
    causes of 1542
    leprosum 317
Erythematous 1506
Erythremia 1163
Erythrocyte 1044
    count 723
    preparations 1099
    production, defective 1089
    sedimentation rate 722
Erythroderma 1517
Erythrodermic psoriasis 1514
Erythrogenesis imperfecta 1092
Erythrohepatic porphyria 626
Erythroleukemia 1118
Erythromycin 51, 281
Erythroplakia 483
Erythroplasia of Queyrat 1544
Erythropoietic porphyria, congenital 626
Erythropoietin 714, 1046
Escherichia coli 234, 236, 1075
    enterohemorrhagic 236
    enteropathogenic 236
    infections 236
Esmolol 905
Esophageal
    candidiasis 294
    disease, symptoms in 484
    dysphagia 485
    hiatus hernia 488
    pain 484
    spasm, diffuse 488
Esophagitis 486
Esophago-gastroscopy 526
Esophagus 470
    carcinoma of 489
    diseases of 484
Established neuroleukemia, treatment of 1117
Esthiomene 282
Etanercept 736, 766, 1515
Ethacrynic acid 459
Ethanol 135, 460
Ethical committees 3
Ethylene
    dibromide poisoning 132
    glycol 460
Euglobulin lysis time 1174, 1193
Eunuchoid 629
European blastomycosis 380
European Burkitt's lymphoma 1159
Euthyroid Graves' disease 665, 666
Euthyroid sick syndrome 674
Euvolemic hyponatremia 444, 468
Evan's syndrome 1078
Everolimus 510
Evoked responses 1305
Exacerbating factors 1518
Exacerbations
    severity of 999
    treatment of 1427
Exanthems 328
Excessive fibrinolysis, causes of 1193
Exemestane 78
Exenatide 597
    lar 597
Exercise, benefits of 587
Exfoliative dermatitis 1517
Exfoliative drug eruption 1529
Exhibitionism 1573
Exocrine function, tests for 566

Exogenous eczema 1521
Exophthalmos 669
    malignant 669
Expiratory reserve volume 960
Extra-articular
    features 765
    lesions 728
    manifestations 730
Extra-axial tumors 1420
Extracampine hallucination 1548
Extracellular fluid 442
Extracorporeal liver support 542
Extracorporeal membrane oxygenator 812
Extradural hematomas 1422
Extrahepatic manifestations 344, 346
Extrahepatic portal hypertension 550
Extraintestinal amebiasis 406
Extraintestinal infection 236
Extra-intestinal lesions 406
Extraintestinal manifestations 513
Extrapulmonary complications 983
Extrapyramidal disorders 1398
Extrapyramidal dysfunction 1377
Extrapyramidal movement disorders 1484
Extrapyramidal signs 1366
Extrathoracic manifestations 1023
Extreme pica 1064
Extrinsic allergic alveolitis 994
Exudate pleural effusions 1030
Exudative effusion 1030
Eye 730
    movement 1335
        abnormal 1367
        control 1321
    signs 1462, 1556
Eyelids, movement of 1335
Ezogabine 1388

F

Fabry's disease 938
Facial colliculus 1326
Facial nerve 1326
Facial pains 1339
Facial palsy
    bilateral 1328
    chronic 1328
Facioscapulohumeral dystrophy 1473
    muscular 934, 1478
Factitious disorder 1565
Factitious fever 198
Faint 793
Falciparum malaria 347
    treatment of 392
Fallacies of tests 295
Fallopian tubular dysfunction 706
False localizing sign 1419, 1440
Famciclovir 336
Familial colonic polyposis 509
Familial macrophage activation syndrome 737
Familial spastic paraparesis 1430
Fanconi's anemia 1091
Fanconi's syndrome 451
Fannia 90, 91
Fasciculation 1368, 1432, 1453
Fascioliasis 428
Fat 156
    absorption of 472
    digestion of 472
    functions of 156
Fatal insomnia 1376
Fatigue 636, 1435
Fatigue syndrome, chronic 1463
Fat-soluble vitamins 167
Fatty acid
    diarrhea 499
    oxidation, defects of 1479, 1485
Fatty casts 1216
Fatty liver 552
    of pregnancy, acute 1274
Febrile convulsions 1381, 1383
Febrile encephalopathy, nonspecific 1359
Febrile respiratory illness, acute 357
Fecal fat estimation 501
Fecal immunochemical testing 476

Fecal protein loss 501
Feces 565
    culture 230
    examination of 407, 476, 500, 525
Feigned insanity 1565
Felbamate 1388
Felodipine 892
Felty's syndrome 738
Female infertility 706
Female orgasmic disorder 1573
Female pseudohermaphroditism 707
Female purpura over legs 1177
Fenofibrate 776
Ferri reductase enzyme 181
Ferric carboxymaltose 1067
Ferric gluconate 1066
Ferroportin 181, 182
Festinating gait 1303
Fetal alcohol syndrome 1350
Fetal hemoglobin 1088
Fetal life, irradiation in 116
Fetal monitoring techniques 600
Fetishism 1573
Fetor hepaticus 537
Fever 194, 939, 1055, 1413
    blister 336
    in immunocompromised host 35
    of unknown origin 197
    patterns of 196
    undifferentiated 367
    with joint pain 230
Fiber electromyography, single 1305, 1469
Fibrin degradation products, estimation of 1174
Fibrinogen levels, increase in 952
Fibrinolytic system 1172
Fibrocalcific pancreatic diabetes 615
Fibrocalculous pancreatic disease 615
Fibromas 943
Fibromyalgia 763
Fibrothorax 1029
Fibrous pial 1288
Fibrous thyroiditis 674
Fifth cranial nerve 1324
Fighter aircrafts 122
Filarial infections 439
Filariasis 413, 432
    control of 438
    prevention of 438
Filovirus infections 358
Fine-needle aspiration biopsy 661
Finger clubbing 537
Fingolimod 1428
Fire ants 92
First aid 114
    prevention and 131
Fish poisoning 144
Fish tapeworm 427
Fishgold's line 1446
Fissured tongue 484
Flaccid dysarthria 1300
Flail chest 1036
Flapping tremor 537
Flash pulmonary edema 1268
Flea typhus 265
Flexibilitas cerea 1549
Flexural psoriasis 1513
Floppy valve syndrome 846
Flow cytometry 1133
Flucytosine 58, 59
Fludarabine 1129
Fluent aphasia, progressive 1372
Fluid
    transudation, evidence of 841
    treatment of 1240
Fluke infections 428
Flumazenil 539
Fluorescein angiography 610
Fluorescence
    antibody, indirect 398
    in situ hybridization 19, 1107
Fluorine 184
Focal fibrosis 1010, 1011
Focal segmental glomerulosclerosis 1227
Focal signs 1415
Foix-Alajouanine syndrome 1444

Folate deficiency, causes of 178
Folic acid 177, 1346
    deficiency anemia 1071
Follicular impetigo of Bockhart 215
Folliculitis 1501
    decalvans 1536
Fomepizole 135
Fondaparinux 1195, 1196
Food poisoning 142
    chronic 143
    infection type of 143
    type of 142
Food, function of 156, 158
Foot disease 356
Forced acid diuresis 126
Forced alkaline diuresis 126
Forced diuresis 126
Forced expiratory
    flow 961
    time 960
Formal cognitive assessment 1366
Formic acid 139
Forrest classification 497
Forward heart failure 805
Foscarnet 57, 376
Fossa ovalis 823
Foster Kennedy syndrome 1316
Fothergill's disease 1325
Foville's syndrome 1328
Fractional excretion of sodium 1233
Fragile X-associated tremor ataxia 1405
Fragilitas ossium 782
Fragmentation hemolysis 1199
Frailty syndrome 1589
Fraying 171
Freckles 1533
Fredrickson's classification 621
Free living cycle 419
Free radicals and apoptosis, role of 805
Freezing cold injury 107
Frequent respiratory infections 171
Fresh blood in stools 498
Fresh frozen plasma 1100, 1188
Frey's sign 1327
Friedlander's pneumonia 979
Friedreich's ataxia 934, 1436
Fröhlich's syndrome 655
Frontal lobe
    epilepsies 1380
    hemorrhage 1416
Frontotemporal lobar degeneration 1372
    complex 1434
Frozen shoulder 763
Fructosuria 617
Fulminant hepatic failure 540
Fulminant hepatitis 346
Fulminant meningococcemia 221
Fulvestrant 78
Functional residual capacity 960
Fundamental symptoms 1556
Fundus examination 1320
Fungal infections 292, 382, 1361
    superficial 1504
Furosemide 459
Furuncle 214, 1501
Fusidic acid 53
Fusiform bacilli 483
Fusion toxins 74

G

G6PD deficiency, hemolysis in 1080
Gabapentin 1325, 1388, 1428
Gadolinium diethylenetriaminepentaacetic acid 89
Gag reflex 956
Gait cycle 1302
Galactomannan 379
Galactorrhea 637, 712
Galactosemia 617
Galantamine 1371
Gallbladder 563
    carcinoma of 564
    diseases of 562
Gallium nitrate 450
Gallop 797
    rhythm 797

Gallstone disease 347
Gamma glutamyl transpeptidase 525
Gamma interferon 57
Gamma irradiation of blood 1102
Ganciclovir 56, 57, 376
Gander cough 962
Gangrenous cholecystitis, acute 564
Gaol fever 263
Garcin syndrome 1332
Gardnerella vaginalis 284
Gas exchange 958
    in alveoli 958
Gas gangrene 268, 272
Gas mixing within alveoli 961
Gas transfer across alveolar membrane 961
Gas transport down the airways 959
Gasserian ganglion 1324
Gastric
    acid analysis 477
    drainage, continuous 446
    inhibitory polypeptide 471, 474
    juice 471
    lavage 125
    lesions 1060
    outlet obstruction 496
    surgery 1490
Gastrin 471, 474, 1589
Gastrinomas 715
Gastritis 489
    acute 137, 490
    chronic 490
        superficial 490
Gastroenteritis 229, 255
Gastroesophageal reflux disease 488, 993
Gastrointestinal
    anthrax 240
    bleed, upper 1413
    complications 734
    disease 1489
    endoscopy 478
    hormones 473
    infections 238
    manifestations 1238
    motor function 1588
    symptoms 1560
    system 681, 1461
    tract procedures 860
Gatifloxacin 54
Gaze paralysis 1324
Geftinib 77
Gemcitabine 564
Gene 7, 8
    expression profiling 1107
    mapping 19
    therapy 21, 813, 1084, 1088, 1189
        limitations of 22
General paralysis of insane 1353
Genetic
    aspects of cancer 68
    causes, classification of 1430
    changes 1476
    constitution 1475
    counseling 21, 952
    disorders 18, 1267
    effect 31
    epidemiology 22
    factors 188, 495, 727, 739, 764, 1431, 1557
    newer developments in 19
    role of 1475
    syndromes 939
    testing 919
Geniculate bodies 1317
    lateral 1318
Geniospasm 1404
Genital
    atrophic changes in 710
    warts 286, 1502
Genitalia, external 639
Genitourinary
    infection 221
    schistosomiasis 431
    symptoms 1462, 1560
    system 244
    tract procedures 860
    tuberculosis 1255

Genomics, role of 582
Gentamicin 50
Geographical tongue 484
Geriatric 1586
    assessment
        comprehensive 1594
        multidimensional 1593
    diseases 1590
    giants 1593
    health services, development of 1596
    medicine 1586
    symptoms 1595
        management 1595
German measles 336
Gerstmann-Straussler-Scheinker
        syndrome 1373, 1376
Gestational diabetes mellitus 1270
Gestational hypertension 1271
GH estimation 652
GH receptor antagonist 652
Ghrelin 188, 1589
Giant cell 755
    arteritis 754, 935
    thyroiditis 673
Giant platelet syndromes 1182
Giardia intestinalis 410
Giardia lamblia 410
Giardiasis 405, 410
Gigantism 650
Girdle sensation 1302, 1440
Gitelman syndrome 1249
Glabellar tap 1325
Glanders 245
Glargine 595
Glasgow Coma Scale 1336
Glatiramer acetate 1428
Gleevec 1125
Glioblastoma 1420
    multiforme 1420
Gliomas 1420
Global aphasia 1300
Global initiative for asthma 984
Glomerular proteinuria 1221
Glomerulonephritis 1212, 1222, 1225
    acute 230, 1508
    chronic 1223
Glossodynia 484
Glossopharyngeal
    nerve 1330
    neuralgia 1343
Glucagon 471, 474
    like polypeptide-1 474
Glucagonoma 715
Glucocorticoid 65, 213, 682, 686, 1010
    advantages of 64
    in typhoid, role of 232
    resistance 66
        in inflammatory diseases 66
    therapeutics of 63
    therapy 65
Gluconeogenesis, disorders of 1485
Glucose 1310, 1484
    metabolism 522
Glucose-6-phosphate dehydrogenase deficiency 1080
Glulisine 595
Glutamate decarboxylase antibody 1374
Glutaminase 456
Glutamine 456
Gluten-induced enteropathy 502
Glyceryl trinitrate, side effects of 904
Glycogen storage
    disease 938, 1479
    disorders 1485
Glycogenolysis defects 1479
Glycolysis defects 1479
Glycoprotein hormones 646
Glycosylated hemoglobin 588
Glycosylation of proteins 609
Gnathostoma spinigerum 441
GnRH-independent precocious puberty 705
Goalkeeper's fingers 721
Goblet cells 471
Goiter 662
    causes of 662
Goitrous cretinism 184

Golden 's' sign 1023
Goldmann perimetry 1317
Golfer's elbow 763
Golimumab 736
Gonadal disorders
    affecting both sexes 703
    in females 708
    in males 699
Gonadogenesis 696
Gonadotropin 646
    releasing hormone 642
    therapy 654
Gonads disorders 696
Gonda's sign 1301
Gonococcal infection in newborn 279
Gonorrhea 278
    in female 279
    in male 279
Goodpasture's syndrome 1028, 1225
Gopalan's syndrome 1346
Gordon's sign 1301
Gottron's papules 761
Gout 732, 772
    acute 773
    causes of secondary 773
    primary 773
    treatment of chronic 775
Gowers sign 1474
Graded physical activity 951
Graft disease 37
Graft rejection 1283
Graham little syndrome 1515
Graham steell murmur 840
Gram staining 1364
Granular casts 1215
Granular layer 1497
Granulocyte 1048
Granulocyte-macrophage colony-stimulating
        factor 1047
Granulocytic sarcomas 1124
Granuloma
    annulare 1540
    inguinale 282
    pyogenicum 1543
    venereum 282
Granulomatosis
    infantiseptica 255
    with polyangiitis 757, 1263
Granulomatous
    colitis 506
    gastritis 490
    thyroiditis, subacute 673
Graves' disease 664
Green pit viper 96
Green symptoms 153
Gregor Mendel 2, 6
Griseofulvin 58
Groove sign of Greenblatt 282
Group psychotherapy 1584
Growth hormone 646, 714
    releasing
        hormone 642
        inhibiting hormone 642
Growth of baby, regulation of 648
Growth, abnormalities of 636
Guarnieri bodies 330
Guillain-Barre syndrome 374, 457, 933, 1310, 1454
Guinea worm 440
Gustatory experience 1589
Gustatory sweating 1327
Gut flora in health and disease 473
Gut hormones 1589
Guttate psoriasis 1512
Gynecological causes 709
Gynecomastia 637, 707, 712
    causes of 707, 712

H

H$_2$ receptor blocker 492
Habitual hyperthermia 199
Hachinski ischemic score 1417
Hemophilia, complications of 1189
Haemophilus influenzae 1363
    frequently causes pharyngitis 227
    infections 223, 227
    meningitis 227
    type B 227

Haff disease 143
Hair 1498, 1544, 1587
    abnormalities of 636
    disorders of 1534
    loss of 637
    pigmentation, variation in 1535
    shaft abnormalities 1535
Hairy cell leukemia 1130
Hairy tongue 484
Halitosis 475
Hallucination 1548
Hallux valgus 729
Ham acid 1095
Hammer toe 729
Hampton's hump 925
Hand and foot warts 1502
Hand disease 356
Hansen's disease 312
Hantavirus infections 359
Haploid cells 6
Hapten 25, 31
Harmful cannabis 1570
Harmful use 1569
Harrison's sulcus 171
Hartmann's pouch 522
Hartmannella 410
Hartnup disease 1437
Hashimoto's disease 674
Hashimoto's encephalopathy 674, 1377
Hashitoxicosis 674
HBV
    hepatitis, chronic 555
    infection 294, 341, 349
HCV
    hepatitis, chronic 556
    infection 294
        acute 343
        chronic 343
Head louse infestation 1509
Headache 1339, 1342
    chronic daily 1341
    drug-induced 1343
    secondary 1339
    syndromes, primary 1339
Health problems 1551
    in elderly 1591
    occupational 153
Healthcare personnel through counseling 152
Healthcare-associated pneumonia 978
Healthy carrier 192
Hearing 1588
    impairment 1588
    loss, age-related 1347
Heart 114, 210, 1591
    block 874
        etiology of 876
        first degree 876
        second degree 876
        third degree 876
    disease 939, 941
        congenital 817, 837, 947, 948, 952
        critical congenital 838
    failure 803, 808
        acute 805
        backward 805
        chronic 805
        diagnosis of 807
        pathophysiology of 803
        types of 805
    malpositions of 836
    muscle disease, specific 920
    rate related tests 1463
    rate, controlling 842
    sounds 791
Heat cramps 106
Heat hyperpyrexia 102
Heat stroke 102
    first aid for 104
Heat syncope 105
Heat-shock proteins 103
Heavy chain estimation 1140
Hebephrenia 1556
Heberden's nodes 777, 778
Heidenhain variant 1374
Heimlich maneuver 976

Heine-Medin disease 352
Heinz bodies 1074, 1081
Helicobacter heilmannii 491
Helicobacter pylori 491
  diagnosis of 491
  eradication of 493
  infection, treatment of 491
Heliotrope rash 761
Heliotropium 558
Heller's operation 487
HELLP syndrome 1271
Helmet cell 1200
Helminthiasis 413
Helminthic infestations 441
Helper function 26
Helper T-cells 1051
Hemangioma liver 562
Hemaphasalis leachi 267
Hemaphysalis 94
Hematemesis 496
Hematochezia 476, 498
Hematogenous tuberculosis, acute 310
Hematological abnormalities 389
Hematological diseases 122
Hematological disorders 786, 1055, 1154, 1494, 1592
Hematological manifestations 1238
Hematological values, normal 1057
Hematology 743, 1044, 1132, 1139
Hematomyelia 1445
Hematopoietic growth factors 1046
Hematuria 1212
Heme iron 181
Hemidesmosomes 1496
Hemiplegic syndromes, crossed 1410
Hemisphere functions 1296
Hemochromatosis 535, 623, 937
Hemodialysis 1276
  complications of maintenance 1279
Hemodynamic 819, 820, 822, 823, 825, 827, 829, 831, 833
  alterations 803
  changes 845, 857
  of pregnancy 940
  theory 1233
Hemodynamically-mediated renal failure 1284
Hemoglobin 181, 453, 723
  E disease 1085
  estimation 1055
Hemoglobinometry 1059
Hemoglobinopathy 1081, 1088
Hemogram 1234
Hemolytic anemia 1071, 1072, 1095
  secondary 1076
  type of 1075
Hemolytic disease of newborn 1076
Hemolytic jaundice 527
Hemolytic uremic syndrome 1202, 1273
Hemoperfusion 126
Hemophilia
  A 786, 1185
  B 1189
  defects 786
Hemoptysis 962
  in mitral stenosis, causes of 840
  management of 963
Hemopumps 812
Hemorrhage 226
Hemorrhagic conjunctivitis, acute 355
Hemorrhagic disease of newborn 174
Hemorrhagic disorders 1173
Hemorrhagic fever 358, 361
Hemorrhagic thrombocythemia 1166
Hemosiderin 182
Hemosiderosis 1102
Hemostasis 1169, 1192
  normal 1169
Henderson Patterson bodies 1502
Henderson-Hasselbalch's equation 453
Henoch-Schonlein
  purpura 759, 1264
  syndrome 758, 1183
Hepar lobatum 275
Heparin 1194, 1195
  in ischemic stroke 1412
Heparin-induced thrombocytopenia 1195

Hepatic adenoma 562
Hepatic amebiasis 407, 409
Hepatic cirrhosis, management of 530
Hepatic coma, treatment of 539
Hepatic disease 937
Hepatic disorders 551
Hepatic encephalopathy 536, 538, 1490
Hepatic failure 536
  acute 540, 541
  biochemical disturbances in 536
  causes of acute 540
  chronic 536
Hepatic function 1018
Hepatic precoma, treatment of 539
Hepatic transplantation 542
Hepatic veno-occlusive disease 145, 558
Hepatitis 525
  A virus 339
  B 351
    chronic 349
    infection 526
    virus 340
  C 350
    chronic 349
    virus 342
  chronic 346, 555
  delta virus 344
  drug induced 347
  E virus 344
  viruses 345
Hepatobiliary system 521
Hepatocellular
  carcinoma 346
  failure 527
Hepatocyte 453
  transplantation 542
Hepatojugular reflux 795
Hepatolenticular degeneration 535, 624
Hepatorenal syndrome 540, 551
Hepatosplenomegaly 171, 1055
Hepcidin 181, 182
Hephaestin 182
Hereditary angioedema 1527
  treatment of 1527
Hereditary ataxias 1436
Hereditary connective tissue diseases 770
Hereditary coproporphyria 626
Hereditary disorders 1425
Hereditary elliptocytosis 1079
Hereditary hemochromatosis gene product 182
Hereditary hemorrhagic telangiectasia 1184
Hereditary motor sensory neuropathy 1458
Hereditary myelopathies 1444
Hereditary nonspherocytic hemolytic anemias 1080
Hereditary spastic paraplegia 1438, 1444
Hereditary spherocytosis 1078
Hereditary thrombasthenia 1182
Heredity 1554
Heredodegenerative dystonias 1399
Heredofamilial ataxias 1436
Hermaphroditism 706
Herniation 1334, 1419
Herpangina 356
Herpes febrilis 336
Herpes genitalis 285
  in newborn 285
Herpes gestationis 1545
Herpes gladiatorum 336, 1503
Herpes simplex 1503
  virus 336
    encephalitis 336
    type 1 1357
    type 2 1359
Herpes viruse 1357
Herpes zoster 334
Herpesvirus hominis 336
Herpetic whitlow 1503
Hess tourniquet test 1173
Heterophyes heterophyes 429
Heterophyiasis 429
Heteroplasmy 20
Hexachlorobenzene compounds 132
Hexadecylphosphocholine 399
Hiatus hernia 488
HIB infection 227

Hiccough, causes of 1038
Hiccup 1038
High altitude
  disease 113
  pulmonary edema 112
Hippocratic fingers 963
Hippocratic oath 2
Hip-up sign 1474
Hirsutism 1535, 1536
Hirudo medicinalis 95
His bundle electrography 799
Histamine headache 1342
Histopathologic lesions, staging of 554
Histoplasma 1362
Histoplasmosis 379, 1362
Histrionic personality disorder 1567
Hitchhiker's thumb 729
Hockey stick sign 1375
Hodgkin's disease 1148
Hoffman's syndrome 638, 671, 1473, 1474
Holiday heart syndrome 939
Holmgren's wool 1318
Holter monitoring 799
Homeopathic system 2
Homeostenosis 1590
Homme rouge 1128
Homocysteine, total 1070
Homocystinuria 629, 630
Homoplasmy 20
Homunculus 1289
Hormonal abnormalities 1025
Hormonal disorders, indirect indices of 649
Hormonal factors 728
Hormonal interactions 711
Hormonal metabolism 523
Hormonal studies 649
Hormone 76, 687
  actions 633
  estimation of 640
  metabolism 632
  of pituitary 641
  receptors 633
  replacement therapy 772
    in women 710
  secretion of 640
  types of 640
Horn, anterior 1442
Horner's syndrome 1319, 1446, 1464
Horny envelope 1497
Horny layer 1497
Horton's syndrome 1342
Hospital staff, infection control precautions for 325
Hospital treatment 114
Hospital-acquired pneumonia 977
Host disease 37
Host parasite interaction 414
Hot cross bun skull 276
Howell-Jolly bodies 1045, 1068
Hughes syndrome 747
Hughlings Jackson syndrome 1331
Human anaplasmosis 267
Human brain, adult 1288
Human chorionic gonadotropin 714
Human ehrlichiosis 263, 267
Human genome
  mapping project 2
  project 9, 69
Human herpes
  virus-types 6 and 7 1359
  virus-types 7 and 8 1359
Human immunodeficiency virus 278, 287, 936, 1075
  associated cognitive motor complex 293
  co-infection 397
  infection 287, 316, 601
    management of 295
  test 294
Human insulin 594
Human leukocyte antigen
  associations 581
  status, determination of 724
  system in humans 36
Human metapneumovirus 327
Human monocytotropic ehrlichiosis 267
Human placental lactogen 71
Human polymicrobial infections 193

Human rabies 362
immunoglobulin 364
Human T-cell lymphocytotropic virus 1361
Human-to-human transmission 362
Humming bird sign 1396
Humoral hypercalcemia of malignancy 682
Humoral immunity 27
deficiency of 33
Huntington's disease 1401
Huntington's like diseases 1401
Hutchinson's pupillary reaction 1422
Hutchinson's teeth 276
Hyaline casts 1215
Hyalomma 267
Hybrid techniques 87
Hydantoin-linked lymphoma 1159
Hydatid worm 426
Hydralazine 811, 891
Hydrazine derivatives 76
Hydrocele 434
surgery for 438
treatment of 438
Hydrocephalus 1423
developing in infancy, causes of 1423
in adults, causes of 1424
Hydrophidae 96
Hydrophobia 361, 363
Hydropneumothorax 1033
Hydrops fetalis 1077
Hydrostatic pressure gradient 1277
Hydroxy
indole acetic acid 71
proline 71
Hydroxycarbamide 1126
Hydroxychloroquine 734
Hydroxyurea 1084, 1126, 1165, 1167
Hymenolepis diminuta 428
Hymenolepis nana 427
Hyperadrenocorticism 1493
Hyperaldosteronism 446, 936
classification of primary 694
primary 694
Hyperalgesia 1302
Hyperalimentation 504
Hyperamylasemia, causes of 566
Hyperamylasuria, causes of 566
Hyperbaric oxygen 110
Hypercalcemia 180, 442, 450, 679, 680, 714, 938
acute 681
management 681
Hypercapnia 969
manifestations of 970
Hyperchloremic metabolic acidosis 460
Hypercholesterolemia, newer drugs in 622
Hypercortisolism 688
Hypereosinophilia 1050
Hypereosinophilic syndrome, management of 1050
Hyperesthesias 1453
Hyperglycemia 587, 609
Hyperhomocysteinemia 629, 952
causes of 630
Hyperkalemia 442, 448, 938, 1285
management of 448
treatment of 1240
Hyperkalemic distal RTA 460
Hyperkinetic circulation 537
Hyperkinetic movement disorders 1399
Hyperkinetic syndrome 1577
Hyperlipidemias 620
management of primary 621
primary 621
secondary 623
Hypermagnesemia 442, 451, 939
Hypernatremia 442, 445
management of 445
Hyperosmolar
hyperglycemic nonketotic state 607
nonketotic
coma 607
diabetic coma 445
states 464, 466
Hyperparathyroidism 716, 1238, 1493
primary 678
secondary 682
tertiary 682

Hyperpathia 1302, 1453
Hyperphenylalaninemia 627
Hyperphosphatemia 442, 451
Hyperpigmentation 1530, 1544
Hyperpigmented palms 71
Hyperplasia, demonstration of 679
Hyperplastic type 1506
Hyperprolactinemia 649, 708
Hyperpyrexia 195
Hypersensitivity, delayed 27
Hypersomnia 1572
Hypersplenism 1168
causes of 1169
Hypertension 882, 938, 952, 1213, 1238, 1266,
1268, 1269
accelerated 887, 1269
causes of secondary 883, 1267
chronic 1271
classification of 1266
complications of 885
drug in 889
essential 883, 885, 1267, 1269
in children 894
in pregnancy 894, 1272
malignant 887
secondary 883, 885, 1267
causes of 1268
Hypertensive
emergencies 893
encephalopathy 886
nephrosclerosis 1269
urgencies 893
Hyperthermia, malignant 199
Hyperthyroidism 664, 936, 1493
during pregnancy 669
to thyroiditis 669
Hypertransfusion 1087
Hypertrichosis 1535, 1536
Hypertrophic
cardiomyopathy 917, 918
gastritis 490
osteoarthropathy 71, 780
classification of 780
pulmonary osteoarthropathy 780
Hypertrophy of breasts 712
Hyperuricemia 1143
Hyperventilation 957
Hyperviscosity
state, management of 1126
syndrome 1143
Hypervitaminosis D 173, 450
Hypervolemic hyponatremia 444, 468
Hypesthesia 1453
Hypnagogic hallucinations 1548
Hypnic headache 1342
Hypnopompic hallucinations 1548
Hypoadrenocorticism 1493
Hypoaldosteronism 448
Hypocalcemia 180, 442, 450, 938
Hypocomplementemia 1262
Hypofrontality 1558
Hypoglossal nerve 1331
Hypoglycemia 388, 587, 602-604, 1484
management of 603
symptoms of 603
Hypogonadism 699
in women 708
secondary 699
treatment of 701
Hypokalemia 442, 446, 939
antibiotic induced 446
management of 447
Hypomagnesemia 442, 448, 452, 939
Hyponatremia 442, 1413
causes of 467
hypovolemic 444, 468
management of 444
Hypo-osmolar disorders 464, 467
Hypoparathyroidism 682, 1493
treatment of 684
Hypophosphatemia 180, 442, 448, 451
Hypopituitarism 653, 1493
Hypoplastic anemia 1071
congenital 1092
Hypopnea 1016
syndrome 1018

Hyposmia 1316
Hyposplenism 1169
causes of 1169
Hypostatic
congestion 1013
pneumonia 980
Hypotension 810
Hypothalamic
anovulation 708
causes 709
disorders 643
hormones 642
Hypothalamo-pituitary
adrenal axis, suppression of 65
disorders 648
Hypothalamus
defective regulatory control by 649
disorders 641
Hypothermia 108, 939
Hypothyroidism 670, 936, 1493
secondary 672
Hypotonia 1291
Hypotonic duodenography 478, 566
Hypoventilation syndromes 1492
Hypoxanthine-guanine phosphoribosyltransferase 773
Hypoxia 969
correction of 970
manifestations of 969
Hypoxic form 111
Hypsarrhythmia 1382
Hysterical attacks 1384
Hysterical coma 1334
Hysterical fever 199
Hysterical neurosis 1563

I

Iatrogenic Cushing's syndrome 689
Ibandronate 682
Icatibant 1527
Ice-cream headache 1343
Icepack test 1467, 1469
Ice-pick scars 1510
Icroangiopathy hemolytic anemia 1200
Icterus gravis neonatorum 1077
Ideal body
mass index 951
weight 586
Idiopathic hypereosinophilic syndrome 1050
Idiopathic hypogonadotropic hypogonadism 701
Idiopathic inflammatory myositis 761
Idiopathic intracranial hypertension 1424, 1495
Idiopathic polyneuropathy, acute 1454
Idiopathic portal hypertension 551
Idiopathic thrombocytopenic purpura 1175
Idiopathic thrombocytosis, primary 1166
Idiopathic ulcerative colitis 511
Idoxuridine 56, 57
IGF-1, estimation of 652
Ill patients, chronically 122
Illnesses with treatable dementia 1369
Iloprost 751
Imatinib 77, 1125
Imidazole derivatives 54, 76
Imiquimod 286, 1544
Immersion syndrome 113
Immune
complex mediated tissue damage, type III 30
dysfunction 718
reconstitution inflammatory syndrome 308
response 25, 362
secondary 26
system 1589
therapy
long-term 1470
short-term 1470
thrombocytopenic purpura 1175
Immune-mediated damage 1284
Immunity 230, 246
active induced 37
against
infections 26
malaria 387
tuberculosis 300
Immunity-based therapeutic innovations in cancer 74
Immunization, active 350, 351

Immunoblastic lymphadenopathy 1150
Immunochromatographic test 436
Immunocompetent individuals 335, 1359
Immunocompromised individuals 335
Immunoconjugate 1122
Immunocytes 1051
Immunodeficiency states 33
   combined 33
   primary 34
   secondary 34
Immunoglobulin A
   nephropathy 1224
   vasculitis 758
Immunological (immune) tolerance 32
Immunological changes 69
Immunological disorders 747
Immunological disturbances 857
Immunological tests 526
Immunologically-mediated paraneoplastic
   neurological syndromes 1025
Immunology 434, 738
Immunomodulation 1110
Immunomodulatory drugs 1142
Immunopathogenesis 1426, 1511
Immunosuppressant drugs 735, 745
Immunosuppressed hosts 1359
Immunosuppression 1204
Immunotherapy 93
Immunotoxins, therapy with 74
Impetigo contagiosa 1501
Impetigo herpetiformis 1513, 1545
Implantable cardioverter defibrillator 812, 947
Implantable devices 812
Implosion 1585
Impotence 702, 1573
Impulse noise, effects of 120
Inappropriate antidiuretic hormone 71
   secretion 51
Inborn errors of metabolism 618
Incontinentia pigmenti 1533
Incretins 581
Incubation period 362
Indeterminate leprosy 314
Indian Council of Medical Research 1293
Infant botulism 143
Infant hercules 639
Infantile acne 1510
Infantile autism 1576
Infantile B_{12} deficiency 1068
Infantile paralysis 352
Infantile spasms 1381, 1382
Infantilism 637
Infarct, core of 1408
Infection 192, 312, 581, 728, 936, 1075, 1092,
   1370, 1413, 1425, 1443, 1512, 1591
   abdominal 236, 237
   mixed 389, 393
   primary 1503
   secondary 335
   severe 43
   subacute 857
   types of 192
Infection-associated stones 1257
Infectious mononucleosis 374
Infective agent, isolation of 200
Infective endocarditis, acute 855
Infective episodes, treatment of 1000
Infertility 705
Inflammation 1051
Inflammatory
   demyelinating polyneuropathy
      acute 1454
      chronic 1455
   disease
      chronic 770
      nonspecific 481
      of bowel, chronic 767
   myelopathy 1443
   response, inhibitors of 1000
Infliximab 735, 766, 1515
Influenza 323
   A viruses, emergent 325
   virus 1075
      pneumonia, primary 324
Influenzal pneumonia 324

Infusion urogram 1219
Ingested poisons 125
Ingrowing toenail 1537
Inhalation anthrax 240
Inhaled corticosteroids 994
Inhaled glucocorticoids 1000
Inhaled steroids 989
Inheritance pattern 1082
Inheritance, types of 12
Inherited disorders 1185
   of connective tissue 628
   of erythrocytes 1078
Inherited forms of rickets 172
Inhibit neutrophil elastases 1000
Inhibit osteoclast activity 681
Inosine pranobex 58
Insomnia 1572
Inspiratory
   capacity 960
   reserve volume 960
Insulin 474, 606
   action 580
   analogues 594
      long-acting 595
      short-acting 594
   antagonists, role of 582
   combination 591
   degludec 595
   injection 595
      devices 596
   like growth factors 647
   presbyopia 610
   pumps 596
   rapid-acting 594
   release 587
   resistant states 647
   secretion 580
   structure of 580
   synthesis 580
   therapeutics of 595
Insulin-like growth factor 647, 714
   side effects of 648
Insulinomas 715
Insulin-receptor effects 590
Integrase inhibitors 295
Intelligence quotient 1549
Intelligence scale for children 1551
Intelligence, disturbance of 1549
Intensity
   conditioning allografts, reduced 1116
   modulated radiation therapy 1152
Intensive insulin therapy 595
Intention tremors 1404
Intercalated cells 446
Intercritical gout 774
Intercurrent infections 532
Interferon 27, 57, 322, 1110
   alfa 348, 1126
   beta 1b 1427
   gamma release assays 303
Interferon-alpha 76
Interleukin 27, 76, 1000
Intermediate syndrome 130
Intermittent porphyria, acute 353, 626
International Physician for Prevention of
   Nuclear War 118
International prognostic index 1155
Interstitial
   edema 1363
   fibrosis 1010, 1011
   fluid 442
   keratitis 278
   nephritis, acute 1242
Interstitium, diseases of 1242
Interval gout 774
Intervention, type of 825
Interventional cardiology 802, 948
Interventional radiology 87
Intestinal absorption 501
Intestinal amebiasis 406
   chronic 409
Intestinal angina 510
Intestinal blood loss 539
Intestinal capillariasis 441
Intestinal contents 477, 502

Intestinal diseases 499
Intestinal hemorrhage 230, 232
Intestinal myiasis 91
Intestinal nematodes 415
Intestinal pathogenic strains 236
Intestinal perforation 230, 232
Intestinal polyposis 508
Intestinal schistosomiasis 431
Intestinal tuberculosis 508
Intestine
   infective disorders of 767
   large 472, 1060
   small 471, 509
   ulceration of 508
Intolerant to methotrexate 1010
Intoxication 1349
   acute 1568, 1570
Intra-aortic balloon
   counter-pulsation 947
   pump 914
Intra-articular steroids 779
Intracardiac repair 832
Intracellular
   compartment 448
   fluid 442
   to extracellular compartment 448
Intracerebral hemorrhage 1415
Intracranial hematomas 1422
Intracranial hemorrhagic stroke, causes of 1407
Intracranial hypertension, benign 1320, 1424
Intracranial neoplasms 1420
   primary 1420
Intracranial space-occupying lesions 1417
Intracranial structures, traction on 1342
Intractable cardiac failure 813
Intraluminal bacterial proliferation in intestines 504
Intraoral bite wing X-rays 482
Intrasellar cyst 657
Intrasellar-subarachnoid space 657
Intrasplenic pressure 547
Intrathecal drugs 1115
Intravascular
   fluid 442
   hemolysis 1074
   ultrasound 82, 946
Intravenous
   drug users 288
   immunoglobulin 1178, 1455, 1470
   urography 1218
Intrinsic factor deficiency, congenital 1070
Inulin clearance 1234
Invasive tests 491
Involuntary movements 1366
Iodine 183, 667, 1349
   induced hyperthyroidism 184
   nutrition in community 184
Ionizing radiations 118
   injuries to 115
Iothalamate 1234
Ipratropium bromide 992
Ipsilateral hemiparesis 1419
Irbesartan 892
Iron 181, 1348
   chelating agents 1087
   deficiency
      anemia 1063, 1494
      development of 183
      effects of 183
   preparations 1066
   sorbitol citrate 1066
   sucrose 1066
Irritable bowel syndrome 505
Irritable heart syndrome 934
Irritant contact dermatitis 1521
Ischemic cardiomyopathy 915
Ischemic heart disease 895, 1493
Ischemic imbalance 900
Ischemic neurological deficit, reversible 1406
Ischemic penumbra 1408
Ischemic stroke
   in young 1407
   management of 1411
   syndromes 1409
Ischemic syndromes 938
Ishihara pseudoisochromatic plate 1318

Islet cell transplantation 596
Isolated demyelinating syndromes 1425
Isolated joint 513
Isomerism 837
Isometric handgrip test 1463
Isonicotinylhydrazide 1287
Isoprenaline 816
Isoprenaline-B 1464
Isopropyl alcohol 460
Isosexual precocity in boys, incomplete 704
Isosorbide dinitrate 811, 904
Isotope renography 1219
Isotope studies 1060
Isotopic liver scan 526
Isotopic tests 660
Itraconazole 58
Ivabradine 812, 912
Ivermectin 416, 419, 420, 437, 441
Ixodes 94
    scapularis 267

J

Jaccoud's arthritis 210
Jacksonian motor seizures 1381
Jacobson's triad 1316, 1326
Janeway lesions 857
Janus kinase 1161
    inhibitors 736
Japanese encephalitis 372, 1360
Japanese river fever 266
Jarisch-Herxheimer reaction 258, 277
Jaundice 389, 523, 1055
    classification 523
    complications to 526
    management of 528
    types of 524
Jaw jerk 1325
Jellife's syndrome 1345
Jellyfish 95
Jeryl-lynn strain 339
Jigger 95
Jod-Basedow phenomenon 184, 664
Joint 243, 720, 749, 750, 1592
    manifestations, drug-induced 787
    tuberculosis 783
Jones criteria, exceptions to 212
Jugular vein, engorgement of 806
Jugular venous pulse 794
Junctional premature beats 863
Juvenile absence epilepsy 1380
Juvenile delinquency 1577
Juvenile idiopathic arthritis 737
Juvenile myoclonic epilepsy 1382
Juvenile neutrophils 1048
Juvenile Paget's disease 782
Juvenile polyposis 509

K

Kala-azar 397
Kallikrein-kinin system 1211
Kallmann's syndrome 643, 653
Kampavata 1391
Kanamycin 50
Kaposi's sarcoma 292, 1075
Kaposi's varicelliform eruption 336, 1503
Karokampam 1391
Kartagener's syndrome 1002
Karyotyping 8, 19
Kasabach-Merritt syndrome 562, 1201
Katayama disease 431
Katayama syndrome 431
Kawasaki disease 757, 935, 756
Kayser-Fleischer ring 535
Kearns-Sayre syndrome 20
Keloid and hypertrophic scar 1538
Keratinization 1496, 1497
Keratoacanthoma 1543
Keratoderma blennorrhagica 1516
Keratolytic agents 1499
Kerley B lines 841
Kernicterus 1077
Kernig's sign 220
Keshan disease 186, 1349
Kestenbaum's number 1319

Ketoacidosis 452, 461, 606
Ketoconazole 58, 59, 652, 1505
Ketogenic diet 1390
Ketolides 52
Ketones 1485
Ketotifen 994
Kidney 114, 741, 749, 1260, 1266, 1268
    artificial (dialyzers) 1277
    changes in 886
    development of 1207
    disease 1231
        chronic 786, 937, 1236
    disorders 1540
    function of 1207, 1210, 1211
    injury
        acute 1212, 1230
        in pregnancy, acute 1272
        intrinsic acute 1233
    structure of 1207
    transplantation 1282
        immunosuppression in 1283
    vulnerability of 1284
Kiel classification 1153
Killed vaccine 373
Killer cells 1051
Killing function 1049
King cobra 96
Klebsiella granulomatis 282
Klebsiella pneumoniae 234, 979
    infections 237
Klinefelter's syndrome 17, 701, 1445, 1450
Knee syndrome 777
Knidosis 1526
Knock knees 171
Knodell classification 555
Kocher-Debre-Semelaigne syndrome 1473
Koebner's phenomenon 1502, 1512
Koilonychia 1064
Köllner's rule 1318
Koplik's spots 328
Korotkoff's sounds 796
Korsakoff's psychosis 1569
Korsakoff's syndrome 1345, 1554
Krait 96, 97
    bite 98
    venom 99
Kreb's tricarboxylic acid cycle 174
Kupffer's cells 522, 1051
Kuru 1374, 1376
Kussmaul's breathing 460, 957
Kussmaul's respiration 605
Kwashiorkor 163, 166, 1349
Kyasanur forest disease 370, 1360
Kyphoscoliosis 1034

L

LA appendage exclusion 947
Labile diabetes 598
Lacosamide 1390
Lactate dehydrogenase 525, 901
    deficiency 1479
Lactate infusion test 1561
Lactic acidosis 452, 460, 607, 1485
    type A 461
    type B 461
Lactitol 539
Lactose absorption 501
Lactosuria 617
Lactulose 539
Lacunar stroke syndromes 1409
Lacunar syndromes 1410
Laennec's cirrhosis 552
Lafora body disease 1383
Lambert-Eaton myasthenic syndrome 1468
Lamellar granules 1497
Lamina propria 471
Lamivudine 57, 348
Lamotrigine 1387, 1388
Langerhan's cells 1051
Language disorders 1300
Lanreotide 652
Lanthanum carbonate 1241
Laparoscopy 479, 519, 526
Laparoscopy-assisted panendoscopy 478
Larva migrans 422

Larval migration 420
Laryngeal
    diphtheria 224
    obstruction, acute 976
    paralysis 976
Laryngitis
    acute 975
    chronic 975
Laryngysmus stridulus 171
Lasegue's sign 1452
Lassa fever 359
Latent syphilis 274, 277
Latent tuberculosis 299
Late-onset rubella encephalitis 1361
Latex agglutination tests 1311
Lathyrism 146
Latrodectus mactans 91
Lazy leukocyte syndrome 1049
Lead poisoning 146
    acute 146
    chronic 146
Lean nonalcoholic steatohepatitis 553
Leech infestations 95
Leeuwenhoek 2
Leflunomide 735, 1010
Leg raising test 1452
Legionella pneumophila 267
Legionellosis 253, 254
Legionnaires disease 254
Leiomyosarcomas 944
Leishmaniasis 384, 394
    prevention of 401
Lenalidomide 1142
Lenegre's disease 876
Lennox-Gastaut syndrome 1381, 1382
Lentigines 1533
Lepore hemoglobins 1088
Lepra reaction 316
Lepromatous
    borderline 314
    leprosy 313
Lepromin test 314
Leprosy 298, 316
    borderline 314
    reactions in 316
Leptins, role of 188
Leptospirosis 260, 347, 936, 1243
Leptotrombidium deliense 266
Leser-Trélat sign 1541
Lesion 254, 268
    at chiasm 1318
    demonstration of 688
    in optic pathway 1318
    of conus medullaris 1441
    of peritoneum, malignant 520
    of vestibular division 1329
    outside
        brainstem 1332
        cranial cavity 1332
    primary 1498
    produced by staphylococci 214
    secondary 1498
    structural 504
    superficial 214
Letermovir 376
Letrozole 78
Leukapheresis 1100, 1126
Leukemias 786, 1103
    acute 1104, 1113, 116
    chronic 1104, 1122
    classification of 1104
    congenital 1109
    diagnosis of 1106
    drug in 1109
    treatment trials 1122
Leukemic reticuloendotheliosis 1130
Leukemoid reaction 1108
Leukocyte
    alkaline phosphatase score 1123
    count 723
    groups 1098
    patterns 196
Leukoerythroblastic blood picture 1134
Leukomyelitis 1443
Leukonychia 537, 1537

Leukopenia 231
Leukoplakia 483
Leukotriene 27
    modifiers 990, 994
Lev's disease 876
Levamisole 77
Leveen peritoneovenous shunt 532
Levodopa 1393
Levofloxacin 54
Levosalbutamol 992
Levothyroxine sodium 672
Lewis system 1098
Lewy body dementia 1375
    diffuse 1395
Lhermitte's sign 1302, 1354, 1440
Lice 94
Lichen planus 1515
Lichenoid eruptions 1530
Liddle's syndrome 459
Life support measures 874
Life-threatening
    bleeding 1179
    Clostridium difficile infection, chronic 252
    complications 1235
Lightning pains 1354
Limb girdle
    muscular dystrophy 1478
    weakness 1473
Limbic encephalitis 1369, 1377
    common infections 1377
Limbs, temperature of 793
Linagliptin 591
Linamarin 144
Lincomycin 53
Linear immunoglobulin A disease 1525
Linear scleroderma 748
Linezolid 53
    optic neuropathy 53
Lingual dystonia 1300
Lipid
    lowering agents 555
    metabolism 523, 590
    storage-related disorders 1479
Lipid-lowering agents 908, 910
Lipomas 715, 944
Lipoprotein, increase in 952
Liposomal amphotericin B 399
Lipoxygenases 1000
Liquorice ingestion 459
Lispro 594
Listeria monocytogenes 254
Listeriosis 253, 254
    during pregnancy 255
Lithium 935, 1582
    toxicity 1375
Live attenuated
    measles vaccine 330
    varicella zoster virus vaccines 334
Live vaccine 65
Liver 42, 535, 1145, 1540
    abscess, complications of 407
    biopsy 201, 526, 534, 554, 561
    carcinoma of 560
    disease 44
        chronic 1070
        end stage 530, 612
    dysfunction in circulatory impairment 559
    failure
        acute 540, 541, 1491
        chronic 540
    function
        test 525
        zones in 523
    involvement 244
    pyogenic abscess of 559
    structure of 521
    support, artificial 542
    transplantation 535, 542–544
        types of 543
Liver-based metabolic conditions 543
Lixisenatide 597
Loa loa 432
Lobar hemorrhage 1416
Lobar pneumoniae 217
Lobe syndrome, middle 1002

Local radiation injury 116
Local reactions 93, 98
Localized myeloma, treatment of 1143
Locked-in syndrome 1337
Locomotor system 344
    disease of 719
Löfgren's syndrome 1009
Loiasis 438
Lomefloxacin 54
Long-chain fatty acids 1487
Losartan 892
Louse borne
    relapsing fever 257
    typhus 263
Low backache, inflammatory 765
Low birth weight 884
Low grade fever 537
Low tension headache 1343
Lower cranial nerves 1332
Lower GIT bleeding, management of 498
Lower motor neuron 1291
Low-molecular-weight heparin 1195
Lucio leprosy 316
Lucio phenomenon 317
Lues venerea 274
Lugol's iodine 667
Lumbago-Sciatica syndrome 762
Lumbar canal stenosis 1452
Lumbar disc lesions 1452
Lumbar puncture 311, 1415
Lumbosacral plexus 1448
Lumefantrine 392
Lundh test 566
Lung 114
    abscess 981
    allergic disorders of 984
    biopsy 968
    cancer 1541
        classification of 1020
        manifestations of 1022
        signs of 1022
        symptoms of 1022
    capacity 960
        total 960
    circulatory disturbances in 1012
    diseases, occupational 1005
    microbiome 956
    neoplasms of 1019
    perfusion 961
    purpura 1028
    transplantation 1001
    ventilation of 957
    volume 959
        reduction surgery 1000
Lupus erythematosus cell phenomenon 724
Lupus nephritis 1225
Lyme arthritis 32
Lyme borreliosis 253
Lyme disease 936
Lymnaea truncatula 429
Lymph node 508
    biopsy 968
    moderate enlargement of 1055
Lymphangitis 208
    carcinomatosa 1023
Lymphatic drainage 955
Lymphatic filariasis 432, 438
    in children 435
Lymphatic leukemia
    acute 1113
    chronic 1127
Lymphatic organs 1591
Lymphatic structures 1151
Lymphatics, disorders of 1531, 1532
Lymphedema 1532
    treatment of 438
Lymphoblastic leukemia, acute 1113
Lymphocyte 1051
    tumors 1159
Lymphocytic choriomeningitis 359
Lymphocytic lymphoma 1156
Lymphocytic thyroiditis
    chronic 674
    subacute 673
Lymphocytotoxic crossmatch 1282

Lymphogranuloma
    inguinale 281
    venereum 281
Lymphoid cells, malignant disorders of 1147
Lymphoid stem cell 1149
Lymphoid tissue lymphoma, mucosa-associated 738
Lymphokines 26
Lymphoma 450, 1147, 1150, 1157
    in cancer statistics 1148
    malignant 786
    staging of 1151
    types of 1159
Lymphoproliferative malignancies 1494
Lymphorrhage 434
Lymphoscintigraphy 436
Lynch syndrome 495
Lyssa 361

M

Maccallum's patch 210
Macro electromyography 1305
Macroangiopathy 583
Macrocytic anemias 1067
Macrolides 51
Macrophage activation syndrome 737
Macropolycytes 1068
Macroscopic hematuria 1221
Macular atrophy 1538
Macular degeneration, age-related 1347
Macular splitting 1318
Maculopapular 1528
Mad cow disease 1374
Madame-Louis-Bar syndrome 1438
Madura foot 383
Maduramycosis 383
Magnesium 185, 1349
    homeostasis 442
        disorders of 451
    salts 908
    sulfate 992
Magnetic resonance spectroscopy 85, 1306
Magnetic susceptimetry 1087
Maintenance therapy 1115
Major tranquilizers 1580
Malabsorption 527
    causes of 499
    states 499
    syndromes 1489
Malaria 384, 1075
    in pregnancy 390, 393
    treatment of severe 393
    vaccines 394
Malarial hepatopathy 389
Malassezia furfur 1519
Male infertility, causes of 705
Male pseudohermaphroditism 707
Malignant pustule 240
Mallory bodies 552
Mallory-Weiss syndrome 496, 548
Malnutrition 155
    mild acute 164
    severe acute 163, 164
    treatment of 1241
Malt lymphoma 1157
Malta fever 243
Mania 1557
Manioc 144
Mansonella ozzardi 432, 440
Mansonella perstans 439
Mantle cell lymphoma 1157
Mantoux test 200
Mao-B inhibitors 1394
Maple syrup urine disease 1437
Marasmic kwashiorkor 166
Marasmus 166
Marburg virus 359
Marchiafava-Bignami disease 1350
Marcus Gunn pupil 1319
Marfan's syndrome 629, 939
Marginal zone lymphoma 1157
Marie's quadrilateral space 1299
Marie-Bamberger syndrome 780
Marie-Strümpell disease 764
Marine animals, injuries to 95
Marrow cells, ablation of recipient's 1111

Masked hypertension 882
Maternal problems during pregnancy 941
Mature erythrocyte 1046
Maturity-onset diabetes of young 584
Maxillary sinusitis, causative organism in acute 975
Maximal voluntary ventilation 961
May-Hegglin anomaly 1182
McConnell's sign 926
McGregor's line 1446, 1449
MDR-TB, treatment of 307
MDT regimens, alternative 318
Measles 328, 329, 1360
    atypical 329
    inclusion body encephalitis 329, 1360
Measly pork 424
Mebendazole 418, 419
Mechanical ventilation 971
Medial medullary syndrome 1332, 1410
Mediastinal lymphadenopathy 1009
Mediastinal tumors 1039
Mediastinoscopes 968
Mediastinum, diseases of 1039
Medical disorders 1575
Medical errors 45
Medical genetics 5
Medical nutrition therapy 586
Medical Research Council Breathlessness Scale 963
Medical Research Council Modified
        Dyspnea Scale 1001
Medical synovectomy 737
Medical termination of pregnancy 337
Medically active stones 1257
Medication overuse headache 1341
Medicinal iron 1066
Medicine
    computers in 5
    evidence-based 5
    history of 1
Medium vessel vasculitis 755
Medullary cystic kidney disease 1245
Medullary sponge kidney 1246
Medullary syndrome, lateral 1410
Medullary thyroid carcinoma 716
Medulloblastoma 1420
Medulloepithelioma 1419
Mee's nails 1537
Megakaryoblast 1053
Megakaryoblastic leukemia, acute 1118, 1120
Megakaryocyte 1053
Megakaryocytic myelosis 1166
Megaloblastic anemias, congenital 1070
Megaloblasts 1067
Melanonychia, longitudinal 1537
Melarsoprol 403
Melasma 1533, 1544
Melatonin 657
Melioidosis 239, 244
Meliturias, causes of 615, 617
Melkersson-Rosanthal syndrome 1328
Melphalan 1142
Membranoproliferative glomerulonephritis 1229
Membranous nephropathy 1228
Memory
    disturbance of 1546, 1548
    disturbances 1595
    impaired patient, examination of 1365
    testing 1299, 1551
    types of 1365
MEN1 syndrome 715
MEN2 syndrome 715, 716
Mendel-Bekhterev sign 1301
Mendelson's syndrome 1013
Ménétrier's disease 490
Menghini's needle 968
Ménière's disease 1330
Ménière's syndrome 1330
Meningeal
    anthrax 241
    irritation 1343
Meningiomas 1420
Meningitis 255, 333, 338, 1360
    etiology of 1363
Meningococcal infections 219
Meningococcal meningitis 220
Meningococcemia 221
    chronic 221

Meningoencephalitis 255, 374, 1360
Menopause 1384
    medical problems of 710
Mental disorders
    classification of 1551
    signs of 1546
    symptoms of 1546
Mental retardation 1575
    causes of 1575
Mental status examination 1550
Mental stress 934
    ischemia 934
Mental symptoms 1560
Mepolizumab 994
Meralgia paresthetica 1458
Meropenem 49
Mesobuthus tamulus 92
Mesonephros 1207
Metabolic acidosis 388, 452, 460
    treatment of 1240
Metabolic agents 911
Metabolic alkalosis 452, 459
Metabolic arthropathies 769
Metabolic causes 1370
Metabolic disorders 618, 938, 1182
Metabolic disturbance 1438
Metabolic emergencies 602
Metabolic functions, zones in 523
Metabolic muscle diseases 1479
Metabolic syndrome 619, 952
    diagnosis of 619
Metabolism 185
Metanephros 1207
Metastasis 71, 943
Metastatic
    neoplasms 786
    tumors 1421
Metformin 555, 590, 591
    effects of 590
Methacholine test 915
Methanol 460
    poisoning 135
Methisazone 331
Methotrexate 735, 766, 1010, 1514
Methyldopa 890
Methylprednisolone 1178
Methylthiouracil 667
Methylxanthines 990
Metolazone 459
Metrifonate 431
Metronidazole 54, 408
Metyrapone 652, 690
Meyer's loop 1317
Micafungin 59
Miconazole 58
Microalbuminuria 611, 1221, 1261
Microarray analysis 19
Microbial flora 855
    normal 1250, 1500
Microbial virulence factors 1251
Microbiology 1251, 1252, 1253, 1254
Microdermabrasion 1510
Microfilaria detection tests 435
Micropsia 1548
Microscopic polyangiitis 758
Microscopic polyarteritis nodosa 1263
Micturating cystogram 1219
Midnight cortisol 687
Mid-systolic click syndrome 846
Miglitol 592
Migraine 1339-1341
    classic 1340
    drug in 1340
    management of transformed 1341
    with aura 1340
    without aura 1340
Migrating motor complex 471
Migrating thrombophlebitis 1542
Miliary tuberculosis 310
Milk-alkali syndrome 459
Milker's nodule 1503
Millard-Gubler syndrome 1328, 1410
Millennium development goals 3
Miller-Fisher syndrome 1455
Miltefosine 399

Milwaukee shoulder 777
Mimicking coma 1337
    clinical conditions 1337
Mimicking dementia 1368
Minamata disease 143
Mineral bone disease, treatment of 1240
Mineralocorticoid 686, 693
    excess 1267
    hypertension 894
    receptor antagonist 810, 909
Minerals 179
Minimally conscious state 1337
Mini-mental state examination 1296, 1366
Minnesota multiphasic personality inventory 1551
Minocycline 51
Minoxidil 891
Minute sequence pictures 1219
Miracidia 430
Mirodenafil 703
Mirror movements 1450
Miscellaneous infections 294
Mite
    fever 266
    typhus 266
Mitgehen 1291
Mithramycin 450
Mitochondria 20
Mitochondrial diseases 1397, 1473, 1479
Mitochondrial encephalomyopathy 1383
Mitochondrial genetics 20
Mitochondrial inheritance 20
Mitochondrial myopathy 934
Mitotic pool 1048
Mitoxantrone 1428
Mitral annuloplasty 812
Mitral incompetence 844
Mitral regurgitation 844
    acute 845
    cause of 844
    surgery in chronic 846
Mitral restenosis 843
Mitral stenosis 839-941
Mitral valve
    apparatus 839
    prolapse syndrome 846
    repair 812
    replacement 843
Mitral valvotomy, closed 843
Miyoshi myopathy 1474
MMR vaccines 339
Mobile phone radiation 1495
    complications 1495
Mobiliferrin 182
Mobiluncus 284
Mobitz type
    I block 875
    II block 875
Moderately severe patients, treatment of 513
Modern ultrathin fiber-optic bronchoscopes 1024
Modified jones criteria 212
Modified Schober test 765
Molecular characteristics of lymphomas 1158
Molecular genetic
    of epilepsy 1380
    studies 1488
Molecular mimicry 32
Molecular pathogenesis 1123
Molluscum body 287, 1502
Molluscum contagiosum 1502
Mönckeberg's sclerosis 794
Monge's disease 113
Mongolism 1575
Monoamine oxidase inhibitors 935, 1582
Monoclonal antibodies 77, 1130
Monoclonal gammopathy 1143, 1144
Monocytes 1050
Monocytic leukemia, chronic 1127
Monomelic atrophy 1434
Mononeuritis 1456
    multiplex 731, 1454, 1456
Mononeuropathy 1454
Mononuclear phagocytes 1050
Monosomy 16
Montelukast 994
Montenegro skin test 399

Mood
  disorders 1557
  disturbance of 1546, 1547
  elation of 1558
  stabilizers 1582
Morbid anatomy 138
Morphea 748
Morphine 140, 904
Morphology 417, 418, 424, 426, 432, 440
  life cycle 421, 429, 430
  pathogenesis 429
Mosaic wart 1502
Motilin 474, 1589
Motion sickness 121
Motor activity 1558, 1559
Motor denervated bladder 1465
Motor disturbances 1555
Motor functions 1289
Motor impersistence 1400
Motor neuron disease 1430, 1473
Motor polyneuropathy, acute 353
Motor predominant 1454
Motor symptoms 1563
Motor system
  disease 1430
  examination of 1300
Mountain sickness
  acute 111
  chronic 113
Mouth
  disease 356, 480
  dryness of 475
Movement disorders 1350, 1482, 1495
  drug-induced 1405
Moxifloxacin 54
Mucocutaneous lymph node syndrome 756
Mucopolysaccharides 1487
Mucor 1361
Mucormycosis 1362
Mucous membrane lesions 275
Muehrcke's nails 1540
Multiceps multiceps 441
Multicystic dysplastic kidneys 1246
Multifocal atrial tachycardia 865
Multifocal leukoencephalopathy 293, 1361
Multiple personality 1564
Multiple systems atrophy 1395
Mumps 338, 937, 1075, 1361
Munro microabscess 1512
Murine typhus 265
Murmurs 797
Murphy's sign 563
Muscle 749, 1592
  action potential, compound 1304
  biopsy 1311, 1312
  disease 1472
    inflammatory 761, 1479
      tests for 1311
    problems 1482
    stretch reflexes 1301
    training 1041
Muscular atrophy, progressive 1432
Muscular dystrophy 933
  classification of 1476
  congenital 1475, 1477
  diagnosis of 1475
  distal 1478
Musculoskeletal
  system 638
  tissue 860
Mushroom poisoning 143
Myasthenia 1473
  congenital 1468
  gravis 1466, 1468
    diagnosis of 1469
  in pregnancy 1471
Myasthenic crisis 457
  treatment of 1471
Myasthenic reactions 1472
Myasthenic syndrome, congenital 1468
Mycetoma 383
Mycobacterial infections, atypical 294
Mycoplasma 1075
  hominis 284
  pneumonia 979, 1075

Mycosis fungoides 1159
Myelin, role of 1425
Myelitis 333
Myelodysplastic syndrome 1131
Myelofibrosis 1161
  causes of secondary 1163
  primary 1161
Myeloid leukemia
  acute 1117
  chronic 1122
Myeloid metaplasia 1161
Myeloma 450, 1141
  evolution of 1138
  genetics of 1138
  multiple 786, 1075, 1138, 1264, 1494
  staging of 1141
  variant forms of 1143
Myelomatosis 1138
Myelomonocytic leukemia
  acute 1118
  chronic 1127
Myelopathy 731, 1444
  compressive 1441, 1451
Myelophthisic anemia 1071
Myeloproliferative disorders 1160
Myiasis 90
Myoadenylate deficiency 1479
Myocardial disease 938
Myocardial infarction 900, 901
  acute 898
  classification of 900
Myocardial involvement 294
Myocardial ischemia 1413
Myocardial scanning 801
Myocardial stunning 902
Myocarditis 916
  acute 916
  chronic 917
Myocardium, diseases of 916
Myoclonic epilepsy
  progressive 1383
  severe 1381
Myoclonic jerks 1382
Myoclonus 1366, 1377, 1403
Myopathy 933, 1484, 1493
  secondary 761
Myositis 1473
Myotome 1439
Myotonia 1473
  congenta 1478
Myotonic disorders 1478
Myotonic dystrophy 934, 1478
Myxedema 671, 751, 1473
  coma, treatment of 672
  madness 671
Myxomas 943

N

N-acetylcysteine 1000
NADH oxidation, defects of 1485
Naegleria gruberi 1357
Nail 857, 1498, 1587
  changes 1064
  diseases of 1536
  disorders of 1534
  half 1540
  infection 1506
  psoriasis of 1513, 1537
Nailfold capillaroscopy 750
Naja bangarus 96
Naja hanna 96
Naja naja 96
Nakayama yoken strain 373
Nalorphine 539
Naloxone 1570
Naltrexone 1570
Narcoanalysis 1584
Narcolepsy 1572
Narcotics 140
Nasal diphtheria 224
Natalizumab 1428
Nateglinide 590
National Institute of Virology 361
National Leprosy Control Program 319
National Leprosy Eradication Program 319

Natriuretic peptides, role of 804
Natural immunity, active 37
Natural killer cells 25
Nausea 475
Near reflex 1319
Nebulizers 989
Necator americanus 417
Necrobiosis lipoidica diabeticorum 614
Necrolytic migratory erythema 1541
Necrotizing fasciitis 208, 608, 614
Necrotizing myelopathy 1444
Necrotizing ulcerative gingivitis, acute 483
Needle biopsy 1312
Negative phenomena 1453
Neglect syndromes 1296
Negligent adverse event 45
Neisseria gonorrhoeae 278
Neisseria meningitides 219, 1363
Nelson's syndrome 653, 690
Neologism 1547
Neonatal
  alloimmune thrombocytopenia 1180
  diabetes mellitus 601
  gonococcal conjunctivitis 280
  infection 236, 286
  myasthenia gravis 1468
  seizures 1381
  thrombocytopenia 1179, 1180
Neoplasia 1265
Neoplasms 1071
  malignant 1071
Neoplastic cells, characteristics of 70
Neoplastic syndromes 1375
Neorickettsia 267
Neostigmine injection test 1469
Nephritic syndrome 1221
  acute 1212, 1220
Nephrogenic diabetes insipidus 443, 1249
Nephrolithiasis 1213, 1256
Nephron 1208
Nephronophthisis 1245
Nephropathy, contrast-induced 948
Nephrotic syndrome 1212, 1220, 1221, 1285
Nerve
  biopsy 1313
  conduction 1304
  disease, peripheral 1454
  of arnold 1331
  of hering 1330
  peripheral 584
  problems 1482
  roots, diseases of 1439
  stimulation studies 1468
Nervous involvement 1145
Nervous system 344, 730, 742, 1288, 1344,
    1349, 1589
  damage to 527
  in pregnancy 1495
  peripheral 1026
Netilmicin 50, 51
Neural mechanisms 884
Neuralgia 1453
Neuralgic
  amyotrophy 1457
  headache 1343
Neuraminidase inhibitors 57
Neurilemmoma 1420
Neurinoma 1420
Neuritic leprosy, pure 316
Neuro lupus 742
Neuroacanthocytosis 1405
Neurocirculatory asthenia 934
Neurocysticercosis 425
  treatment of 425
Neurodegenerative disorders 1310
Neuroendocrine 1267
Neurofibroma 1420
Neurofibromatosis 1458
  peripheral 1458
Neurogenic
  dysphagia 1482
  pulmonary edema 356
Neurohumoral activation 810
Neurohumoral alterations 804
Neuroleptic malignant syndrome 199

Neuroleptics 1580
Neuroleukemia 1114
Neurologic disorders 933
Neurologic manifestations of liver disease 1490
Neurological causes 1334
Neurological complications 100, 324, 329, 333, 1451, 1492, 1494
Neurological cretins 670
Neurological disorders 1037, 1307, 1381, 1592
Neurological examination 1294
Neurological investigations 1294
Neurological lesions 356
Neurological manifestations 293, 1139
Neurological system 1366
Neuroma 1420
Neurometabolic disorder 1483
Neuromuscular junction, function of 1466
Neuromyelitis optica 1428
    spectrum disorders 1425
Neuromyopathy, critical illness 1493
Neuromyotonia 1453
Neuron specific enolase 71
Neuronal cell 453
Neuronal ceroid lipofuscinosis 1383
Neuronal plasticity 1292
Neuroparalytic syndromes 144
Neuropathic arthritis 785
Neuropathic ulcers 1532
Neuropathology 1347, 1555
Neuropathy
    critical illness 1457
    drug-induced 1456
    peripheral 293, 1368, 1454, 1459, 1493
Neuroprophylaxis 1115, 1117
Neuropsychiatric manifestations 1238
Neurosyphilis 1353
    diagnosis of 1354
    treatment of 1354
Neurotensin 474
Neutralizing antibodies 1188
Neutropenia 1049
    diagnosis of 1136
    idiopathic benign 1049
    severe 1135
Neutropenic patients 62
Neutrophil 1048
    counts, alteration in 1049
    leukocytosis 1049
Neutrophilic leukemia, chronic 1123
Neutrophils
    functional defects of 1049
    functions of 1048
New immune strategies 1117
New therapeutic regimens 1121
Newer antiamyloid treatment studies 1147
Newer antiplatelet drugs 913
Newer drugs 392, 507
Nezelof's syndrome 33
Niacin 175, 1345
Niclosamide 425
Nicorandil 911
Nicotinamide 175
Nicotine replacement therapy 152
Nicotine-related disorders 1571
Nicotinic acid 175, 1345, 1346
Nicotinic receptor partial agonists 152
Nifedipine 892
Night terror 1572
Nightmare 1572
Nikolsky sign 1524
Nilotinib 1125
Nipah virus 327
    encephalitis 1361
Nitazoxanide 250
Nitrates 904, 911, 914
Nitrofurantoin 54
Nitrosoureas 76
Nocardia 382
    brasiliensis 383
Nocardiosis 383
Nocturia 1212
Nocturnal diarrhea 614
Nodular encephalitis 1359
Noise 119
    pollution 120

Nonalcoholic fatty liver disease 553
Nonanticoagulants rodenticides 134
Nonanticytokine BRMs 789
Nonatopic asthma 985
Noncardiogenic pulmonary edema 389
Non-cholera vibrios 250
Noncirrhotic portal fibrosis 551
Non-communicable disease burden, chronic 4
Non-compressive myelopathies 1444
Noncoronary vascular interventions 947
Nondysenteric amebiasis 407
Non-enzyme peptides 97
Nonepileptic seizure 1384
Nonfluent aphasia, progressive 1372
Non-freezing cold injury 107
Nongonococcal genital infections in women 281
Nongonococcal infections in
    children 281
    infants 281
Nongonococcal urethritis 280
Non-heme iron 181
Non-Hodgkin's lymphoma 1153, 1154, 1159
Noninfantile neuronopathic Gaucher's
    disease 1383
Noninflammatory arthritis 727
Noninsulin parenteral therapeutic agents 597
Noninsulin-dependent glucose 587
Noninvasive insulin delivery methods 596
Noninvasive tests 491
Nonisotopic tests 660
Nonlymphocytic leukemia, acute 1117
Nonmetastatic syndrome 1495
Nonmotor manifestations 1392
Nonmyeloablative transplants 1116
Non-nephrotic proteinuria, fixed 1221
Nonobstructive pyelonephritis, acute 1252
Nonparalytic polio 353
Non-polio enteroviruses 1360
Non-Rh hemolytic anemias 1078
Nonsecretory myeloma 1138, 1144
Nonseptic cerebral venous thrombosis 1414
Nonskeletal manifestations 148
Nonsteroidal anti-inflammatory drugs 448, 734, 1284, 1286
    related hematemesis 734
Nonsulfonylurea secretagogues 590
Nontuberculous mycobacteria 298, 312
Non-typhoid Salmonella infections 233
Non-uremic renal osteodystrophy 1239
Non-Wilsonian cerebral degeneration 1491
Noonan's syndrome 939
Normoblasts 1200
Norovirus infections 251
Norwalk viruses 250
Norwalk-like agents 251
Norwegian scabies 1508
Novartis 1125
Novel target visualization 1322
Novel therapeutic approaches 991
Novel therapies 1262
Nuclear angiocardiography 801
Nuclear explosion, dangers of 118
Nuclear imaging 902
Nuclear medicine techniques 86
Nuclear winter 118
Nucleoproteins 7
Nucleus ambiguous, rostral part of 1330
Nummular eczema 1520
Nutraceuticals 779
Nutrient solutions 504
Nutrition 154, 156, 1042, 1591
Nutritional amblyopias 1349
Nutritional anemia, causes of 1070
Nutritional deficiencies 1438
Nutritional disorders 916, 1344
Nutritional inadequacy 1063
Nutritional megaloblastic anemia 1067
Nutritional recovery syndrome 1349
Nutritional science 154
Nutritional status 154
    maintenance of 1235
Nystagmoid movements 1324
Nystagmus 1324
    congenital 1324
Nystatin 58

O

Obesity 186, 457, 582, 636, 884
    hyperventilation syndrome 1016
Obeticholic acid 555
Objective vertigo 1329
Obliterative cardiomyopathy 920
Obsessive compulsive disorders 1562
Obsessive phobia 1562
Obsessive-compulsive personality disorder 1567
Obstruction 1017
    jaundice 527, 528, 937
Obstructive lesions 818, 819
Obstructive lung disease, chronic 997
Obstructive nephropathy 1259
Obstructive pulmonary disease, chronic 937, 996, 1001, 1042
Obstructive shock 814
Obstructive sleep apnea 937, 1017, 1018, 1492
    syndrome 1015
Obstructive uropathy 1273, 1284
Occipital lobe epilepsies 1380
Occipital paroxysms 1380
Ochronosis 628
Octreotide 549, 652
    long-acting release 652
Ocular lesions 629
Ocular manifestations 639
Oculocephalic reflex 1335
Oculomotor nerve palsy 1322
Oculo-orogenital syndrome 175
Odland bodies 1497
Odynophagia 475
    causes of 485
Oestrus 90, 91
Ofatumumab 1130
Offspring, complication in 1383
Ofloxacin 54
Ogilvie's disease 513
Ogilvie's syndrome 367
Oil drop sign 1513
Olfactory nerve 1316
Oligodendrogliomas 1420
Oligosaccharides 1487
Oligosecretory myeloma 1144
Oligospermia 706
Oliguria 1212
Olmesartan candesartan 892
Omalizumab 991, 994
Omega-3 fatty acids 622
Onchocerca volvulus 432
Onchocerciasis 439
Oncogenes 68
Oncogenic osteomalacia 714
Oncogenous osteomalacia 71
Oncology 67
Oncomelania 430
Oncoproteins 68
Onco-suppressor genes 69
Ondine's curse 1335
Onyalai 145
Onychomycosis 1536
Oophoritis 338
Opaque nerve fibers 1320
Open biopsy 1311
Open mitral valvotomy 843
Operative cholangiography 563
Ophthalmic herpes 335
Ophthalmic myiasis 91
Opioids 140
Opioids-related disorders 1570
Oppenheim's sign 1301
Opsoclonus 1324
Optic atrophy 1320, 1354
    secondary 1320
Optic disk pallor 1367
Optic fundus, examination of 1335
Optic nerve 1316, 1317
Optic neuritis 1320
Optical coherence tomography 946
Oral
    antidiabetic drugs 589
        classification of 589
    cancer 484
    cinacalcet 681

corticosteroid therapy, short-course 989
  hairy leukoplakia 483
  mucosa 484
  submucous fibrosis 481
Orally administered drugs 40
Orbital lymphoma, female with 1155
Orchitis 338
Organic acid 1487
  metabolism, defects of 1485
Organic causes 702
Organic disorders 1558
Organic laryngeal paralysis, causes of 976
Organic mental disorders 1552
Organic reflexes 1301
Organism, isolation of 322
Organochlorine insecticides 132
Organophosphorus compounds 130
Ornithodoros lahorensis 258
Ornithodoros tholozoni 258
Orofacial granulomatosis 481
Oropharyngeal
  anthrax 240
  candidiasis 1505
  dysphagia 485
    causes of 485
  infections 279
Oroya fever 253
Orthopnea 792, 964
Orthostatic
  hypotension 894, 1462
  intolerance 895, 1462
  proteinuria 1214, 1221
  tremors, primary 1404
Oseltamivir 57, 324
Osler's disease 1163
Osler's nodes 857
Osmolality, disorders of 466
Osmolar gap 461
Osmole 465
Osmometer 465
Osmoreceptors 442
Osmosis 465
Osmotic demyelination 464
Osmotic equilibrium, disturbances of 464
Osmotic fragility of erythrocytes 1056
Osteitis
  deformans 780
  fibrosa 1239
Osteoarthritis 732, 777
Osteoarthrosis 777
Osteogenesis imperfecta 629, 782
Osteomalacia 172, 1239
Osteomyelitis 215, 221
  variolosa 331
Osteoporosis 648, 769, 770, 789
  localized 770
  primary 770
  secondary 770
Osteosclerotic myeloma 1144
Ostium
  primum defect 823
  secundum 823
Otitic barotrauma 109
Otogenic reflex cough 962
O-toluidine blue 476
Ovarian cancer antigen 71
Ovarian failure 708
  primary 709
  secondary 708, 709
Ovarian function 708
Ovarian hormonal disorders 708
Overlap syndrome 752
Overt nephropathy 612
Ovulatory dysfunction 706
Oxamniquine 431
Oxantel pamoate 419
Oxcarbazepine 1387, 1582
Oxybutinin 1428
Oxygen 904
  therapy 1000
Oxytocin 643
Oxyuriasis 420

P

Pacemaker implantation, temporary 947
Packed cell volume 1059
Paget's disease of bone 780

Pain 78, 1595
  management 78
    chronic 1482
Painful cranial neuropathies 1339
Painful thyroiditis 673
Painless thyroiditis 673
Palatal tremor 1404
Palindromic rheumatism 739
Palinopsia 1298
Palla's sign 925
Palliative care 78, 1596
Pallidotomy 1394
Palmar erythema 537, 1545
Palmomental reflex 1301
Palmoplantar psoriasis 1513
Palmoplantar pustular psoriasis, chronic 1513
Pamidronate 77, 766
Pancoast's syndrome 1022
Pancoast's tumor 1022
Pancreas 579, 582
  artificial 596
  diseases of 565
  isotopic scanning of 566
Pancreatic
  disorders 499
  function tests 565
  polypeptide 474
  transplants 596
Pancreatitis 338, 566
  acute 566
Pancreolauryl test 566
Pancytopenia, congenital 1091
Paneth cells 471
Panhypopituitarism, adult 653
Panic disorder 1561
Panic episode 1578
Pantothenic acid 176, 1346
Papanicolaou's staining 966
Papanicolaou's method 1023
Papillary dermis 1497
Papillary fibroelastomas 944
Papillary muscle dysfunction 903
Papillary necrosis 1285
Papilledema 1320, 1367, 1418
Papular dermatitis of spangler 1545
Papulosquamous disorders 1511
Paracentesis 532
Paracetamol 140
Paracoccidioides 1362
Paradoxical aciduria 447
Paradoxical embolism 828
Paradoxical split 797
Parainfluenza 326
Parakinesia 1400
Paralytic form 363
Paralytic polio 353
Paramyotonia 1478
Paraneoplastic 1375
  limbic encephalitis 1374
  pemphigus 1524
  syndromes 71, 1025
Paranoid 1556
  personality disorder 1567
Paraphilias 1573
Paraplegia in
  extension 1447
  flexion 1447
Paraproteinemias 1182
Paraproteinemic neuropathies 1456
Parasite
  detection 398
  life cycle of 385, 395
  malignancy of 428
Parasitic infections 1354
Parasitology 405
Parasomnias 1572
Parasylvian 1300
Parasympathetic system 1461
Parathormone 450, 676
  actions of 677
Parathyroid 676, 678
  diseases 785
  disorders 676
  function, tests of 677
  hormone 676, 677, 772
    actions of 677
  hyperplasia 715, 716

Paratonia 1291
Paratyphoid fever 233
Parenteral iron 1066
  side effects of 1066
Parenteral nutrition 162, 392, 504
Parenteral routes 40
Paresthesias 1301, 1453
Parietal lobe 1296, 1318
  epilepsies 1380
Parietal pain 476
Parkinson's disease 1391
  disorders 1391
Parkinsonian syndromes 1395
Parkinsonian tremors 1404
Parkinsonism syndromes 1398
Paromomycin 399
Paronychia 1536
  acute 1536
Parosmia 1316
Parotid enlargement, causes of 480
  bilateral 480
Paroxysmal atrial tachycardia 865
Paroxysmal dyskinesia, part of 1399
Paroxysmal hemicranias, chronic 1342
Paroxysmal nocturnal
  dyspnea 792, 964
  hemoglobinuria 1095
Paroxysmal tachycardias 864
Parrot's fever 320
Parrot's nodes 276
Parry's disease 664
Partial pressure of oxygen 121
Partial seizures 1380, 1381
Parvovirus 374
  infection 376, 377
Paschen bodies 330
Passive immunization 350, 351, 364
Passive induced immunity 37
Passive natural immunity 38
Passive smoking 151
Patau's syndrome 17
Patch test 1521
Patent ductus arteriosus 827, 947
Patent foramen ovale 947
Pathological fibrinolysis 1193
Pathological nystagmus 1324
Pathological tremors 1403
Paton's lines 1320
Paul-Bunnell test 375
Peak expiratory flow rate 960
Pectus carinatum 1035
Pectus deformities 1035
Pectus excavatum 1035
Pediatric autoimmune neuropsychiatric disorders 32
Pediculidae 94
Pediculosis 1509
  capitis 1509
  corporis 1509
  pubis 1509
Pediculus humanus
  capitis 94
  corporis 94, 257
Pedophilia 1573
PEEP sign 1467
Pegvisomant 652
Pegylated interferon 58
Peliosis hepatis 558
Pellagra 176, 1345
  sine pellagra 176
Pelvic infection 236
Pemberton's sign 664
Pemphigoid gestationis 1545
Pemphigus
  drug-induced 1524
  erythematosus 1524
  foliaceus 1524
  neonatorum 215
  vegetans 1524
  vulgaris 1523
Pendred syndrome 671
Pendulum breathing 1036
Penicillin 47
  adverse effects of 277
Penicilliosis 294
Pentamidine isothionate 382

Pentavalent antimonials 399
Pentostatin 1129, 1131
Pentosuria 618
Pepper pattern in skull 1239
Peptic esophagitis 488
Peptic ulcer 490, 491
Peptic ulceration
   acute 490
   chronic 490
Perception, disturbances of 1555
Perchlorate discharge tests 662
Percutaneous biopsy 1312
Percutaneous coronary intervention 900, 914
Percutaneous left ventricular assist device 947
Percutaneous transluminal coronary angioplasty 906
Pergolide 650
Pericardial aspiration 923
Pericardial disease 294, 938
Pericardial effusion 922
Pericardiectomy 924
Pericardiocentesis 947
Pericarditis 902
   acute 921
   constrictive 923
Pericardium, diseases of 921
Perineal warts, large 1502
Perinephric abscesses 1255
Periodic alternating nystagmus 1324
Periodic fevers 199
Periodic paralysis 457, 639, 934
Peripheral nervous system, diseases of 1453
Peripheral neuropathy, causes of 1454
Peripheral vesicles 1525
Peritoneal dialysis 1280
   adequacy of 1281
   automated 1281
Peritoneoscopy 479, 526
Peritoneum, diseases of 518
Peritonitis 519
   acute 519
   chronic 519
   in cirrhosis 532
   secondary 532
Permanent pacemaker implantation 946
Pernicious anemia 1069
Persistent delusional disorders 1557
Persistent vegetative state 1337
Personal prophylaxis 249
Personality
   changes 1567
   disorders 1567
   factors 1568
   tests 1551
   type A 934
   type D 934
Pertussis infections 223, 225
Pervasive developmental disorders 1576
Petit mal 1382
Petroleum products 141
Peutz-Jeghers syndrome 495, 509, 1534
Phagocytes, deficiency of 33
Phagocytic function 1168
Phagocytosis, defective 1049
Pharmacotherapy 548
Pharyngeal diphtheria 224
Pharyngitis 974
Pharyngoconjunctival fever, acute 357
Phenformin 460, 591
Phenoxybenzamine 890
Phentolamine 890
Phenylketonuria 627
Pheochromocytoma 694, 716, 936
   multisystem crisis 695
Philadelphia chromosome 1107, 1122
Phlebothrombosis 902, 1592
Phlebotomus papatasi 369
Phobia, simple 1561
Phobic anxiety disorders 1561
Phoma sorghina 145
Phosphate homeostasis 442
   disorders of 451
Phosphide poisoning 132
Phosphodiesterase inhibitors 1000
Phosphonoformate 56
Phosphorus 180

Phosphorylase B deficiency 1479
Photochemotherapy 1514
Photosensitive
   dermatitis 1522
   drug reaction 1530
Photostress test 1317
Phototoxicity 1522
Phrynoderma 1348
Phthirus 94
Physical activity, resumption of 909
Physical examination 495, 507, 638, 793, 806, 910,
   913, 932, 965, 1003, 1022, 1029, 1176, 1551
Physical inactivity 582
Physiological changes 710, 1587
Physiological functions of liver 523
Physiological nystagmus 1324
Physiological proteinuria 1214
Physiological reward theory 1568
Physiological skin changes in pregnancy 1544
Physiological tremor, enhanced 1403
Pickwickian syndrome 1016
Piece meal vision 1298
Pierre marie's three paper test 1299
Pigeon chest 1035
   deformity 171
Pigment casts 1216
Pigment gallstones 528
Pigmentation
   disorders of 1533
   of tongue 484
Pineal body 657
Pineal gland 657
   disorders 657
Pineal tumors 1421
Pinworm 420
Pioglitazone 591
Pipecolic acid 1487
Piperaquine 392
Pironella conica 429
Pit vipers 96
Pitless vipers 96
Pituitary
   anterior 646
   apoplexy 1493
   Cushing's syndrome 689
   disorders 641
   fossa tumors 1421
   gland 641
   hormones, ectopic secretion of 649
   hyperfunction 649
   tumor of 649, 1493
Pityriasis rosea 1516
Pityriasis versicolor 1507
Plague 239, 241
Plantar warts 1502
Plasma
   cell
      dyscrasias 1137
      leukemia 1138, 1143
      proliferative disorders, classification of 1137
   exchange 1203, 1470
   lipids 951
   protein binding 42
Plasmacytoma 1140
Plasmapheresis 1100, 1455
Platelet 1053, 1170
   adhesion, tests for 1173
   aggregometry 1173
   antigenicity of 1170
   count 723, 1202
      even women with 1180
   disorders 1174
   dysfunction 1238
   function 1181
      acquired disorders of 1182
   functional disorders, treatment of 1182
   groups 1098
   plug, formation of 1170
   transfusion 1099, 1100
   ultrastructure of 1170
   vascular diagnosis 1175
Plateletpheresis 1100
Platinum complexes 76
Platybasia 1449
Pleiotropy 13

Pleura 955
   diseases of 1028
   tumor of 1032
Pleural biopsy 968
Pleural effusion 1028
   bilateral 457
   malignant 1022
Pleural friction rub 966
Pleural shock 1031
Pleurisy 1028
   etiology of 1028
Pleuropericardial sounds 966
Pleuropulmonary amebiasis 981, 983
Plexopathy 1454
Plexuses, diseases of 1439
Plumbism 146
Plummer-Vinson syndrome 484
Plus minus sign 1467
Pneumococcal infection 216, 1085
   treatment of 219
Pneumococcal meningitis 218
Pneumococcal peritonitis 219
Pneumococcal pneumonia 217
Pneumoconiosis 1005
   types of 1006
Pneumocystis jirovecii
   infection 381
   pneumonia 290
Pneumomediastinum 1040
Pneumonia 209, 221, 236, 357, 977, 978
   nonspecific 979
Pneumonic plague 242
Pneumothorax 1032
Podoconiosis 437
Podophyllin resin 286
Podophyllotoxin 75, 286
Poems syndrome 1144
Poikilocytosis 1056
Poisoning
   acute 124
   prognosis of 127
Poisonous snakes, identification of 96
Poisons 130
   classification of 124
Polioencephalitis 353
Poliomyelitis 352, 457, 1443
Poliovirus 1359
Poly hill sign 1473
Polyarteritis nodosa 755, 935, 1263
Polycystic kidney disease 1244
Polycystic ovary syndrome 709
Polycythemia 71
   causes of secondary 1164
   rubra vera 1163
   secondary 1165
   vera 1165, 1494
Polydipsia, primary 644
Polyendocrinopathy 718
Polyene antibiotics 55
Polyglandular autoimmune syndrome 717
   type 1 717
   type 2 718
Polymerase chain reaction 19, 231, 322, 1311
Polymicrobial bacterial ascites 532
Polymorphism, restriction site 19
Polymyalgia rheumatica 755
Polymyositis 760, 761, 1479
Polymyxin B 55
Polyneuropathy 337, 1454
Polyopia 1298
Polyostotic fibrous dysplasia of bone 705
Polyphagia 636
Polysomnography 1303
Polyuria 636, 1212
Pomalidomide 1142
Pompholyx 1520
Poncet's disease 732
Poncet's syndrome 302, 787
Pontiac fever 254
Pontine hemorrhage 1416
Porch index of communicative ability 1299
Pores of kohn 954
Porphyria 625
   cutanea tarda 626
Portacaval anastomosis 550

Portal hypertension 545
   in cirrhosis 546
   signs of 546
Portal hypertensive
   colonopathy 548
   enteropathy 550
   gastropathy 548
Portopulmonary syndrome 550
Posaconazole 58, 59
Positive inotropes 812
Post kala-azar dermal leishmaniasis 400
   of brahmachari 400
Postencephalitic parkinsonism 1397
Postexposure prophylaxis 297, 364
Post-gonococcal urethritis 281
Posthepatitis syndrome 346
Postherpetic neuralgia 335, 1343
Posthyperventilation apnea 1335
Postinfectious measles encephalitis, acute 329
Postinfective polyneuropathy 1454
Post-lumbar puncture headache 1343
Postmitotic maturation pool 1048
Postobstructive diuresis 445, 1275
Postpartum blues 1573
Postpartum psychiatric disorders 1573
Postpartum psychosis 1573
Postpartum thyroiditis 661, 674
Postpolio syndrome 354
Postprimary tuberculosis 300
Postrenal failure 1233
Poststreptococcal glomerulonephritis 214, 1223
Post-traumatic stress disorder 1565
Postural drainage 983
Postvaccinal encephalitis 332
Postviral encephalomyelitis 1360
Potassium
   channel antibodies 1369
   homeostasis 442
     disorders of 446
   perchlorate 667
Potential favorable effects 894
Poverty of thinking 1547
Pradhan's sign 1474
Pralidoxime hydrochloride 131
Pramlintide 598
Prasugrel 913, 1185
Praziquantel 425, 429, 431
Prazosin 890, 915
Prebiotics 475
Precancerous lesions 72
Precocious puberty 637, 704
Precordial pain 793
Precordium, examination of 806
Prediabetes, diagnosis of 579
Predisposing to infection 238
Pre-eclampsia 1271, 1495
   management of 1271
Pre-excitation syndrome 867
Pre-exposure immunization 364
Pregnancy 278, 335, 650, 736, 745, 747, 840,
     939-942, 1274, 1544
   associated diseases 1495
   complicating aids 296
   first trimester of 1383
   high-risk 940
   indicators of high-risk 940
   mask of 1544
   plaques of 1545
   specific dermatoses of 1545
Pregnant asthmatic 993
Pregnant patients 277
Pregnant women, active rubella in 337
Prehemorrhagic phase 361
Preherpetic neuralgia 335
Premature ejaculation 1573
Premature ovarian insufficiency 709
Prenatal diagnosis 19
Prenatal management 1077
Prescription of drugs 46
Presinusoidal 546
Pressure hydrocephalus, normal 1370, 1424
Pressure natriuresis 1269
Presystolic gallop 797
Prevention-vaccination 219
Prevotella 284

Priapism 1084
Primary tumor, location of 1022
Primordial T-cells 1051
Principal cells 446
Prinzmetal's angina 914
Prion disease 1373
Prion protein disease 1374
Prion transmitted diseases 1376
Probable tuberculous meningitis 1352
Probenecid 776
Producing stomatocytosis 1080
Prognostic factors, unfavorable 1112
Progressive ataxia, chronic 1437
Prolactin 647
   inhibitory factor 647
Prolactinomas 650
Prolonged fever, causes of 198
Prolymphocytic leukemia 1131
Promyelocytic leukemia, acute 1110, 1118, 1206
Pronephros 1207
Propagation of clot 1171
Propantheline 1428
Prophylactic
   antibiotics 62
   management 1386
   measures 1084
   treatment 280
Prophylaxis 239, 326, 334, 350, 364, 418, 517,
     860, 1026, 1067
   active 228
   antibiotic regimen for 860
   long-term 549
   primary 1188
   secondary 213, 927
   treatment and 285, 556
Propranolol 868, 1341
Propylthiouracil 667
Prosopagnosia 1298
Prostacyclin 1014
Prostaglandin 712, 1211
   clinical uses of 713
Prostate specific antigen 71
Prostatitis, chronic 281
Prosthetic valves 942
Protease inhibitors 295, 1000
Proteasome 77
   inhibitors 1142
Protein 587, 1310
   absorption of 473
   binding 42
   C 1172
   digestion of 473
   energy malnutrition 163, 1349
   metabolism 522
   S 1172
   utilization 157
Proteinuria 1214, 1221
   fixed 1214
   functional 1221
   significant 1221
Proteolytic enzymes 473
Proteomic 11
   account on 11
   finger printing methods 304
Proteus infections 234, 239
Protodiastolic gallop 797
Protozoal diseases 384, 1075
Proximal neuropathy 1456
Prozone effect 649
Prurigo gestationis 1545
Prurigo of pregnancy 1545
Pruritic urticarial papules 1545
Pruritus 1539
   vulvae 614
Prussian blue stain 1093
Pseudobulbar palsy 1332
Pseudocholinesterase in serum 131
Pseudodementia 1368, 1553, 1559
Pseudodystonias 1400
Pseudogout 776
Pseudohemophilia 1190
Pseudohermaphroditism 707
Pseudohyperphosphatemia 181
Pseudohyponatremia 443
Pseudohypoparathyroidism 683, 1493

Pseudolym 1150
Pseudolymphoma 1159
Pseudomembranous colitis 252
Pseudomonas 234
   aeruginosa 238
Pseudomyxoma peritonei 520
Pseudopseudohypoparathyroidism 684
Pseudothrombocytopenia 1175
Pseudotumor cerebri 1424
Pseudoxanthoma elasticum 1538
Psittacosis 319, 320
Psoriasis 1511
   treatment of 1515
   vulgaris 1512
Psoriatic arthritis 732
Psoriatic arthropathy 767
Psychiatric conditions 1569
Psychiatric disorders 934, 1334, 1575, 1576
   in adolescence 1576
   in childhood 1576
   management of 1579
Psychiatric emergencies 1577
Psychiatric patient, clinical examination of 1550
Psychiatric pharmacotherapy 935
Psychiatric problems 1484
Psychiatric symptoms 638
Psychiatry 1546
   evolution of 1546
Psychoanalysis, principles of 1583
Psychoanalytic psychotherapy 1583
Psychogenesis 1563
Psychogenic
   blindness 1321
   causes 702
   dwarfism 656
   fevers 199
   headache 1343
   tremors 1404
Psychological changes 1592
Psychological development, disorders of 1576
Psychological methods of treatment 1583
Psychological testing 1551
Psychometry 1551
Psychosocial treatment 1557
Psychosomatic disorders 1574
Psychosurgery 1580
Psychotherapy 1559, 1561, 1583
Psychotropic drugs, abnormal reactions to 1578
Pteroylglutamic acid 177
PTH resistance syndrome 683
Ptyalism 475
Puberty
   causes of delay in 703
   delayed 637, 703
Puerperal psychosis 1573
Pulfrich phenomena 1317
Pulmonary angiography 967
Pulmonary arterial hypertension 1014
   causes of 1014
Pulmonary arteriovenous fistula 836
Pulmonary artery 829
Pulmonary blood flow
   increased 819
   reduced 818
Pulmonary circulation 955
Pulmonary collapse 1005
Pulmonary compliance 958
Pulmonary complications 982
Pulmonary cysts 1026
Pulmonary diseases 122
Pulmonary edema 1012, 1031
   acute 1012
   chronic 1013
   emergency treatment of acute 813
Pulmonary embolism 857, 902, 924, 1413
Pulmonary eosinophiliosis 995
Pulmonary fibrosis 1010
Pulmonary function 959
   tests 959
Pulmonary hypertension 937, 1084
Pulmonary infections 237
Pulmonary manifestations 1021
Pulmonary mechanics 958
Pulmonary physiology 956
Pulmonary rehabilitation 1000, 1041, 1042

I-xxiv

Textbook of Medicine

Pulmonary response 815
Pulmonary stenosis 822
Pulmonary thromboembolism 1013
Pulmonary tuberculosis, complications of 302
Pulmonary tumors, isotopic localization of 967
Pulmonary valve, acquired lesions of 854
Pulmonary vasculature abnormalities 841
Pulmonary wedge pressure 801
Pulsatile devices 812
Pulsating empyema 1031
Pulse oximetry 838
Pulseless disease 929
Pulsus
   alternans 794
   paradoxus 794
   parvus 794, 848
Pulvinar sign 1375
Pump handle test 765
Pupil 1319, 1335
   abnormal 1320
Pupillary dilatation, relative afferent 1319
Purgatives 126, 539
Purpura over palate 1177
Purpuric disorders 1173
Pursuit system 1322
   abnormalities of 1322
Purulent conjunctivitis 221
Pustular psoriasis 1513
   of pregnancy 1513
Putaminal hemorrhage 1416
Pyelonephritis 1255
   acute 1250, 1273
Pyloric obstruction 496
Pyloric stenosis 446
   congenital 496
Pyoderma 1500
   gangrenosum 1531
   primary 1500, 1501
   secondary 1500
Pyogenic thyroiditis 673
Pyramidal dysfunction 1377
Pyramidal signs 1367
Pyramidal tract syndrome 1442
Pyrantel pamoate 416, 418
Pyrethroid
   exposure, effects of 133
   poisoning 133
Pyrexia 197
Pyridoxine 176, 1346
   dependency, congenital 1346
Pyrimethamine 412
Pyrrolizidine alkaloids 558
Pyruvate kinase deficiency 1081
Pyruvate metabolism, defects of 1485
Pyuria 1250

Q

Q fever 263, 267
   acute 267
   chronic 267
Quantitative sudomotor axon reflex test 1464
Quetiapine 1395
Quinagolide 650
Quincke needle 1308
Quinidine 868
Quinine 393
Quinolones 54
Quinupristin-dalfopristin 53

R

Rabies 361, 1360
   diagnosis, rapid 363
Rachitic rosary 171
Radiation hazards 948
Radiation sickness 74
Radiation syndrome, acute 115
Radiation therapy, adverse effects of 938
Radioactive iodine uptake test 660
Radioactive rain 118
Radiocontrast agents 1285
Radiofrequency ablation 561, 947
   catheter 868
Radioimmunotherapy 74
Radioiodine treatment 668

Radioisotopic investigations 967
Radiosensitivity 73
Raloxifene 772
Ramp movements 1399
Rampant caries 482
Ramsay-Hunt syndrome 1328
Ranolazine 912
Rational therapeutics 45
Raven's progressive matrices test 1551
Raynaud's phenomenon 120, 741, 749
   secondary 749
Rayport clamp 1311
Reactions, treatment of 318
Reactive arthritis 768
Readiness potential 1289
Reaven's syndrome 619
Rebound nystagmus 1324
Recombinant tissue plasminogen activator,
     dose of 1412
Rectum 476
Recurrent acute cystitis 1252
Recurrent aphthous ulcer 480
Recurrent ataxia, acute 1437
Recurrent infection 1254
Recurrent lesions 1503
Recurrent severe hypoglycemia 604
Recurrent vaginitis 614
Red blood cell 1059, 1487
Red cell
   aplasia in children 1092
   aplasia, pure 377, 1092
   enzymopathies 1080
   indices 1056
   membrane 1046
      disorders 1079
   plasmalogens 1487
   production 1044
Red flag signs 506
Red pulp 1168
Reduvid bugs 403
Referred headache 1343
Referred pain 476
Reflex epilepsy 1383
Reflex eye movements 1335
Refractive errors 610
Refractory ascites 531
Refractory cardiac failure 813
Refractory cases, relapse of 1143
Refsum's disease 1438
Regional enteritis 506
Regulatory peptides 473
Regurgitant lesions 818
Rehabilitation 167, 1569
   in neurology 1481
Rehydration therapy 248
Reinfection 1250
Reiter's syndrome 768, 1516
Relapse, treatment of 233, 1117
Relapsing fevers 253, 257
Relapsing-remitting type 1426
Relaxation techniques 1041
Renal abscesses 1255
Renal artery stenosis 937
Renal biopsy 1219, 1234
Renal causes 770
Renal cell carcinoma 1246
Renal changes 98
Renal complications 1143, 1269
Renal cystic neoplasms 1246
Renal damage 774, 1284
   drug-induced 1284
Renal denervation 893
Renal disease 344, 937, 1212, 1213, 1269,
     1272, 1492
   intrinsic 1267
Renal disorders 786
Renal dysfunction
   causes of 1240
   treatment of complications of 1240
Renal failure 101, 389, 527, 1139, 1286
   acute 144, 1070
   chronic 1070, 1212
Renal glycosuria 1247
Renal hormones 884
Renal hypertension 894

Renal indices 1233
Renal infarction 857
Renal involvement 731, 1084, 1270
Renal lesions 583, 1265
   classification of 742
Renal manifestations 679
Renal parenchymal hypertension 1268
Renal replacement therapies, continuous 1279
Renal replacement therapy 1235, 1276
Renal response 815
Renal stones, types of 1257
Renal sympathetic denervation 947
Renal symptoms 540
Renal system 1588
Renal transplantation 1272
   complications of 1283
Renal tubular acidosis 446, 1248
   distal 460
Renal tubules
   diseases of 1242
   functional disorders of 1247
Rendu-Osler-Weber syndrome 1184
Renin angiotensin system, alteration in 804
Renin-angiotensin 1211
   system 1266
Renovascular disease 1267
Repaglinide 590
Reperfusion 909
Repetitive nerve stimulation 1469
Replacement fibrosis 1010
Reproductive system 666
Reserpine 890
Resistant hypertension 893, 1269
   causes of 893
Resistant malaria, new drug for 393
Respiratory
   acidosis 452, 457
   alkalosis 452, 458
   centers 1335
   chain diseases 20
   diseases 937, 962, 966
   distress syndrome 972
      acute 971
   effort related arousal 1016
   failure 968
      acute 1491
      causes of 969
      chronic 971, 1492
      type I 969
      type II 969
      type III 969
      type IV 969
   lesions 356
   manifestations 1239
   physiotherapy 1041
   re-education 1041
   symptoms 1560
   syncytial virus 326
   syndrome
      middle east 327
      severe acute 326
   system 244, 290, 730, 741, 953, 1588, 1592
   tract 323, 1145
      procedures 860
Restarting warfarin after bleeding 1198
Restless leg syndrome 1405
Restrictive cardiomyopathy 917
   classification of 920
Reticular dermis 1497
Reticulocyte count 1055
   corrected 1055
Reticulocyte proliferation index 1056
Retigabine 1388
Retina
   changes in 887
   macula 1320
Retinal lesions 1318
   inner 1318
Retinoids 168
Retinol 168
Retinopathy 583
Retrograde pyelography 1219
Retroperitoneal fibrosis 520
Retroviral syndrome, acute 290
Retroviruses 1361

Rett syndrome 1405
Revascularization procedures 912
Revised National Tuberculosis Control Programme 306
Rexed laminae 1439
Reye's syndrome 332, 562
Rh incompatibility 1076
Rhabdomyomas 944
Rhabdomyosarcomas 944
Rhagades 276
Rhesus system 1098
Rheumatic aortic stenosis 847
Rheumatic chorea 211
Rheumatic fever
    acute 209
    prophylaxis 843
Rheumatic heart diseases 952
Rheumatic manifestations 212
Rheumatic syndromes 762
Rheumatoid arthritis 727, 788, 935, 1262
    variants of 737
Rheumatoid disease, therapy of 736
Rheumatoid disorders 719
Rheumatoid factor 723, 731, 762
Rheumatoid nodules 730
Rheumatological disorders 721, 1075
Rhinitis 973
Rhinocerebral mucormycosis 608
Rhinophyma 1511
Rhinosporidiosis 381
Rhipicephalus 94
    sanguineus 267
Rhodnius 404
Rhonchi 965
Ribavarin 57, 175, 327, 361
Richter's syndrome 1129
Richter's transformation 1129
Rickets 170
Rickettsia akari 267
Rickettsia mooseri 265
Rickettsia prowazekii 263
Rickettsia typhi 265
Rickettsial diseases 263
Rickettsial pox 267
Riedel's thyroiditis 674
Rifabutin 55
Rifampicin 55, 318, 410
Rifapentine 55
Rifaximin 504, 539
Right isomerism 837
Right ventricular
    infarction 909
    physiology 792
Rigid spine syndrome 1474
Rilonacept 775
Rimantadine 57, 324
Rinne's test 1329
Ristocetin cofactor activity 1190
Ritter's disease 215
Rituximab 788, 1130, 1179
Rivaroxaban 914
Rivastigmine 1371, 1395
Road accidents 121, 122
    injuries caused by 123
Rockall scoring system 497
Rocky mountain spotted fever 267
Rodenticides 134
Roflumilast 1000
Rogers sign 1326
Rolandic epilepsy, benign 1382
Romaña sign 404
Romiplostim 1055, 1179
Rorschach Test by Hermann Rorschach 1551
Rosacea 1509, 1511
Rosenbach's sign 1334
Rossolimo's sign 1301
Rotablator 946
Rotavirus 250
Roth's spots 857
Routine blood counts 723
Roxithromycin 51
Rubella 937, 1075, 1361
    congenital 1361
    embryopathy 337
    in adults 337
    in baby, congenital 337
    syndrome, congenital 337

Rufinamide 1388
Rugger jersey spine 1239
Russel's viper 96
    venom 1174
Rusven-clotting time 1174
Ruxolitinib 1163, 1166
Rytand's murmur 851

S

Sabre tibia 276
Saccadic system 1321
Saddle nose 276
Salaam spasm 1382
Salaam seizures 1381
Salazopyrin 52, 735
Salbutamol 992
Salicylate 460
Saline 469
Salivary glands, inflammation of 480
Salmonella 142
    enteritidis 143, 233
    infections 228
        prevention of 233
    typhimurium 143, 233
Salt and water
    intake 884
    retention 1285
Salt balance 1240
Salt depletion heat exhaustion 105
Sarcoglycanopathy 1473
Sarcoidosis 450, 786, 935, 1008
Sarcomas 944
Sarcopenia, age-related 1587
Sarcophaga 90, 91
Saw-scaled viper 96
Saxagliptin 591
Scabies 1507
Scalded skin syndrome 215
Scalene fat pad biopsy 1024
Scalp psoriasis 1513
Scarlet fever 208
Schaefer's sign 1301
Schirmer's test 1464
Schistocytes 1200
Schistosoma haematobium 430, 431
Schistosoma japonicum 430
    infection 431
Schistosoma mansoni 430
    infection 431
Schistosomiasis 413, 430
Schizoaffective disorder 1557
Schizoid personality disorder 1567
Schizophrenia
    classification of 1556
    disorders 1554
Schizophrenic thought disorders 1555
Schmidt's syndrome 1331
Schwabach's test 1329
Schwartzman phenomenon 221
Scleredema Adultorum Buschke 751
Scleredema diabeticorum 614
Scleroderma 748, 935
    localized 748
Scleromalacia perforans 730
Sclerosing cholangitis, primary 534
Sclerosing panencephalitis, subacute 329, 1360
Sclerosis
    multiple 1425, 1427, 1438
    primary lateral 1433
Scopophilia 1573
Scorpion 92
Scrombotoxicity 144
Scrotal tongue 484
Scrub typhus 266
Scurvy 178
Sea snake 97
    bites 99
Seat worm 420
Sebaceous glands 1497
Seborrheic dermatitis 1519
Seborrheic keratoses 1542
Secondary delusion 1548
Secondary drowning 113
Secondary drug resistance 306

Secondary gout 773
Secondary granules 1048
Second-generation drugs 905
Secretin 471, 474
Sedative drug poisoning 136
Segmental bronchi 954
Seizures
    in stroke 1412
    unclassified 1380
Selenium 186, 1349
Sella syndrome, empty 657
Semantic dementia 1372
Semen analysis, normal 706
Senear-Usher syndrome 1524
Senile plaques 1370
Senile purpura 1184
Sensations, abnormal appreciation of 1301
Sensorimotor peripheral neuropathy 1026
Sensory 1454
    assessment 1325
    denervated bladder 1465
    system 1291, 1301
Sentinel headache 1415
Sepsis 62, 236, 1413
    shock 202
Septal defects, atrioventricular 828
Septic cerebral venous thrombosis 1413
Septic shock 202
Septicemic plague 242
Seriously ill patients, treatment of 514
Serologic diagnosis 503
Serological tests 231, 276, 408, 723, 724, 1220, 1234
    frequency of 276
Seronegative spondyloarthritis 789
Seronegative spondyloarthropathy 763, 764
Serotonin reuptake inhibitors 935, 1582
Serpent worm 440
Serum 452, 455
    albumin 526
    alkaline phosphatase 525
    bilirubin 525
    calcium 1218
    cholesterol 525, 1218
    complement levels 724
    cortisol 687
    creatinine 1217
    electrolytes 1217
    gamma glutamyl transpeptidase 534
    late 101
    sickness 33
    uric acid 724
Serum-free light chain estimation 1140
Sevelamer carbonate 1241
Sevelamer hydrochloride 1241
Sex chromosomal disorders 17
Sex chromosome 7
    related disorders 13
    trisomy of 18
Sex hormones 687
    abnormalities of 690
Sexual act 702
Sexual characters, secondary 638
Sexual differentiation, disorders of 711
Sexual dysfunction 1239, 1462, 1573
Sexual function
    abnormalities of 671
    disturbances of 637
Sexual masochism 1573
Sexual maturation, disorders of 637
Sexual medicine 703
Sexual precocity 704
Sexual preference, abnormalities of 1573
Sexual sadism 1573
Sexually transmitted
    diseases 273
    viral diseases 284
Sézary's syndrome 1159, 1160
Shanchol 249
Shank sign 1474
Sheehan's syndrome 653
Sheep liver fluke 428
Sheep-cell agglutination 375
Shigella 143, 234
    boydii 234
    dysenteriae 234

flexneri 234
infections 234
sonnei 234
Shirokampam 1391
Shock 125, 814
classification of 814
distributive 814
hypovolemic 814, 816
therapy 1579
wave lithotripsy 564
Shohl's solution 461, 1248
Short course chemotherapy 304
Short stature, causes of 655
Short wavelength automated test 1317
Shoulder pad sign 1145
Shoulder-hand syndrome 763, 903
Shunt lesions, left-to-right 823
Shy-Drager syndrome 895
SIADH
causes of 645
diagnosis of 468
Sialadenitis 480
Sialidosis 1383
Sialorrhea 1435
Sick sinus syndrome 879
Sickle cell
anemia 786, 1082, 1494
disease 1082
Sickling crises 1083
Sideroblastic anemia 1093
Siderosis 183
Sigmoidoscopy 512
Sildenafil 702, 752, 835, 1015
Silicosis 1006
Silver
beaten appearance 1424
sulfadiazine 52
Sinecatechins 286
Single-chain antibodies 1117
Sinoatrial block 874
Sinus
arrest 874
arrhythmia 862, 1463
bradycardia 863
of Valsalva, aneurysms of 932
tachycardia 863
venosus type of defect 823
Sinusitis 974
complications of 975
Sister-Joseph's nodules 520
Sitagliptin 591
Situation-related seizures 1381
Sixth cranial nerve palsy 1323
Sjögren's syndrome 738, 1262
secondary 739
Sjögren-Larsson syndrome 1444
SK therapy, complications of 905
Skeletal abnormalities-renal osteodystrophy 1238
Skeletal fluorosis 147
Skeletal manifestations 637, 679
Skeletal muscle 453
changes in 666
Skeletal survey 1060
Skeletal symptoms 1084
Skeleton-fusimotor fibers 1290
Skin 730, 749, 1496, 1544, 1587, 1591, 1592
blood vessels 1461
care of 1337
changes 537, 636
in pregnancy, biological 1544
decontamination of 125
functions of 1498
glands of 1497
infected 860
infection of 238, 1500
infestations 1507
involvement purpura above eyelids 1146
lesions 106, 275, 740
snip 231
structure of 860, 1496
tumors 1542
benign 1542
Skull, salt pattern in 1239
Slapping gait 1303
Sleep apnea 457
mild 1016
severe 1016

Sleep disorders 1571
Sleep disturbances 1589
Sleep walking (somnambulism) 1572
Sleeping sickness 402
Slow channel syndrome 1468
Slow-rising pulse 794
Small intestine, diseases of 499
Smallpox 330
Smokeless tobacco 151
Smoking 150, 727
and women 151
cessation of 951, 999
on asthma, effect of 992
Smooth-muscle antibodies 526
Smouldering multiple myeloma 1143
Smudge cells 1128
Snake bite 96
Snake venom, composition of 97
Sneeze 955
Snout 1301
Social phobia 1561
Sodium 442
nitroprusside 891
valproate 1372
Soft chancre 283
Soft neurological signs 1555
Soft sore 283
Soft tissue infections 236
Solar urticaria 1526
Solitary thyroid nodule 675
Somatic complaints, multiple 1596
Somatic symptoms 1559
Somatoform disorders 1563, 1564
Somatomammotropin group of hormones 646
Somatomedin-C 647
Somatosensory evoked
potentials 1338
responses 1305
Somatostatin 474, 549, 642
receptor ligands 652
Somatotropin-mammotropin group 646
Somatotropin-releasing inhibiting hormone 642
Somnambulism 1564
Soothing agents 1499
Sorafenib 77, 561
Soroche, chronic 113
Sotalol 868
South American hemorrhagic fevers 359
Sparfloxacin 54
Sparganosis 441
Sparganum mansoni 441
Sparse hair 1539
Spastic dysarthria 1300
Spastic gait 1302
Special senses 1592
Specific fungal infections, treatment of 59
Spectinomycin 53
Spectrum of disease 553, 1016
Spectrum penicillins, extended 48
Speech
and language 1299
disorders 1300
Spelling dyslexia 1298
Spherocytes 1200
Spider angioma 1545
Spider nevi 537
Spinal accessory nerve 1331
Spinal artery, anterior 1442
Spinal cord
diseases of 1439
injury 457, 1482
parts of 1288
syndromes 1441
Spinal epidural abscess 1444
Spinal muscular atrophy 1434
Spinal shock 1447
Spinal subarachnoid hemorrhage 1415
Spine X-ray 1445
Spinocerebellar ataxia 1436
Spinothalamic tract involvement 1440
Spiramycin 51, 52, 413
Spiroindolone 393
Spironolactone 448
Spleen 857, 1145
disorders 1167
functions of 1167
Splenectomy 1179

Splenic sequestration syndrome 1083
Spondyloarthritis, undifferentiated 769
Spondyloarthropathies 935
Spontaneous bacterial peritonitis 532
Spontaneous hypotension headache 1343
Spontaneous pneumothorax 1032
Spontaneous subarachnoid hemorrhage 1176
Sporadic goiter 664
Sporadic motor system disorders, classification of 1430
Sports injury 783
Spotted fever group 266
Spurious hemoptysis 962
Sputum 962, 966
examination 302, 966, 1023
Squamous cell 1020
carcinoma 487
St. Louis encephalitis virus 1360
Stable angina
chronic 910
pectoris 910
Stamping gait 1302
Standard nutrition tables 158
Staphylococcal bacteremia 215
Staphylococcal food poisoning 142, 215
Staphylococcal infections, diagnosis of 215
Staphylococcal pneumonia 215, 978
Staphylococcus aureus 142, 214
Staphylococcus epidermidis 216
Staphylococcus saprophyticus 216
Stasis eczema 1520
Stasis ulcer 1531
Statin myopathy 1479
Statistical manual of mental disorders 1551
Status epilepticus 457, 1381, 1383, 1389
Steatorrhea 500
Steinert's dystrophy 1478
Stein-Leventhal syndrome 709
Stem cell 1292
transplantation 1088, 1102, 1428, 1143
peripheral 1112
Stent thrombosis 900
Stenting of coarctation 822
Step-down therapy 889
Stereotactic limbic leucotomy 1580
Stereotactic tractotomy 1580
Stereotypy 1405, 1549
Sternberg's cells 1148
Steroid 992, 1470
courses of 1428
hormone secretion 685
synthesis pathway 685
therapy 100
management of 65
striae, female long-term 1181
withdrawal syndrome 65
Steroid-resistant asthma 993
Stevens-Johnson syndrome 1529
Stiff person syndrome 1405
Still's disease 737
Stimulatory hypersensitivity, type V 30
Stinging fishes 95
Stokes-Adams attacks 793
Stomach 470
abnormalities of 499
carcinoma of 495
diseases of 489
Stone disease 1259
Storage pool disease 1181
Strachan's syndrome 1348
Straight back syndrome 1035
Stransky sign 1301
Stratum basale 1496
Stratum corneum 1497
Stratum granulosum 1497
Stratum spinosum 1496
Street virus 361
Streptococcal bacteremia 208
Streptococcal gangrene 208
Streptococcal impetigo 208
Streptococcal infections 207
Streptococcal myositis 208
Streptococcal pharyngitis 208
Streptococcal toxic shock syndrome 209
Streptococcus agalactiae 209
Streptococcus pneumoniae 216, 1363

Streptococcus viridans 209
Streptococcus, group B 209
Streptomycin 50
Stress 1461, 1555
    disorder, acute 1565
        dosing 693
        reaction to 1563
        reticulocytes 1083
        test 799
Stretch reflex 1290
Striae distensae 1538
Striae gravidarum 1545
Strict bed rest 213
String of pearl 1525
Stroke 933, 1084, 1406, 1408
    anterior circulation 1409
    classification of 1406
    diagnosis of 1408
    posterior circulation 1409
    prevention of 1416
    syndromes 1409
Stroke-related complications, treatment of 1412
Strongyloides stercoralis 419
Strongyloidiasis 419
Strontium ranelate 772
Struvite stones 1258
Stupor 1333, 1578
Subarachnoid hemorrhage 1414
Subclinical hypothyroidism 672
Subcortical aphasia 1300
Subcortical dementia 1372
    mixed 1372
Subcutaneous nodules 210, 212
Subdiaphragm cistern 657
Subdural hematoma 1422
    chronic 1369
Subjective vertigo 1329
Sublingual dose 904
Sublingual mucosa 40
Subsultus tendinum 229
Subtle facial palsy 1328
Sucking 1301
Suicide 1577
    attempted 1577
Sulfadoxine 52
Sulfasalazine 735, 766
Sulfinpyrazone 776
Sulfisoxazole 410
Sulfonamides 52
Sulfonylurea compounds 589
Sulkowitch test 678
Sumatriptan 1341
Summation gallop 797
Sunatinib 77
Sunburn 1522
Sunscreens 1500
Sunstroke, first aid for 104
Superior sulcus tumor 1022
Supportive psychotherapy 1584
Suppression tests 678
Suppressive therapy 286
Suppressor cells 1051
Suppressor function 26
Suppurative infections 215
Supranuclear palsy, progressive 1396
Supraventricular tachycardia, management of 867
Sural nerve biopsy 1313
Suramin 439
Surgery, emergency 494, 498
Surgery, timing of 829
Surgical lung biopsy, absence of 1012
Surgically active stone disease 1257
Swan neck deformity 729
Sweat glands 1461
Sweat test 1463
Sweating 1462
Sweet syndrome 1132
Swimmer's itch 431
Swinging flashlight test 1319
Sycosis barbae 214, 1501
Sycosis nuchae 1501
Sydenham's chorea 211, 1401
Sylvian fissure 1299
Symmetrical neuropathy, distal 1456
Symmetrical polyneuropathy 730
Sympathetic nervous system 1266

Sympathetic system 1460
    activation 587
Sympathomimetic drugs 990
Symptomatic hemolytic anemia 1076
Symptomatic hyponatremia, acute 469
Symptomatic iron deficiency anemia 1065
Symptomatic management during attack 627
Symptomatic myoclonus 1403
Symptomatic purpura 1184
Synacthen stimulation 692
Syncope 793
Syndrome X 619
Synesthetic hallucination 1548
Synovial biopsy 726
Synovial fluid 779
    analysis 726
    aspiration 731
    examination 724
Syphilis 274, 278, 936
    clinical types of 274
    congenital 274, 275
    infective endocarditis 1075
    late 275, 277
    secondary stage of 275
    serodiagnosis of 276
    stage of 274
    treatment regimen for 277
Syphilitic deafness 1354
Syphilitic pemphigus 275
Syphilitic pseudoparalysis 276
Syphilitic wig 276
Syringobulbia 1446
Syringoma 1543
Syringomyelia 1446
Systemic corticosteroids 311, 735
Systemic disease 120, 709, 784, 1027, 1260, 1270, 1334, 1456
    cardiac manifestations of 933
Systemic fungal infections 377
Systemic hypertension 881, 883
Systemic illness 1009
Systemic immune complex disease 33
Systemic lupus erythematosus 448, 739, 745, 788, 935, 1274
    symptomatology in 742
Systemic manifestations 750
Systemic medical disorders 1574
Systemic reactions 93
Systemic responses in fever 195
Systemic rheumatologic disorders 935
Systemic sclerosis, progressive 748, 1263
Systemic steroid-sparing therapies 994
Systemic vasculitis 752
Systolic heart failure 805

T

T- and B-cells, interaction between 1053
Tabes dorsalis 1354
Tabes mesenterica 508
Tabetic crises 1354
Tachycardia
    atrioventricular
        junctional 865
        nodal reentrant 865
        reentrant 866
    prevention of 868
Tacrine 1371
Taenia solium 425
Taeniasis saginata 423
Taeniasis solium 424
Tafenoquine 392
Takayasu's arteritis 755, 929, 935, 1264
Takotsubo cardiomyopathy 919, 920
Takotsubo syndrome 939
Tall stature, causes of 651
Tamoxifen 78
Tandem mass spectrometry 1487
Tandem transplantation in myeloma 1143
Tapir's mouth 1473
Taspoglutide 598
Tauopathies 1395
Taxene group 75
T-cell
    function and migration 1052
    origin 1149

T-cell-mediated hypersensitivity reaction, type IV 30
Teardrop heart 936
Tecarfarin 1196
Teicoplanin 53
Telbivudine 57, 348
Teletherapy 73
Telmisartan 892
Telogen 1535
Temporal arteritis 754
Temporal encoding 1482
Temporal lobe 1318
    epilepsies 1380
Temporomandibular arthritis 729
Tenecteplase 906
Tennis elbow 763
Tenofovir 57
    disoproxil fumarate 348
Tensilon test 1469
Tension headaches 1342
Tension pneumothorax 1032
Tenth cranial nerve 1330
Tentorium cerebelli 1435
Teratospermia 706
Terazosin 890
Terbinafine 58, 59
Teriparatide 789
Terlipressin 549
Terry's nails 1540
Testicular failure, adult 699
Testicular leukemia 1114
    treatment of 1117
Tetanus 268, 269
    antitoxin 271
    local 270
    neonatorum 270
Tetany 171, 638
    treatment of 684
Tetracycline 51
Tetralogy of Fallot 831
Thalamic hemorrhage 1416
Thalamotomy 1394
Thalassemia 1085
    facies 1086
    intermedia 1085
    major 1085
    minima 1085
    minor 1085
    pathophysiology of 1085
    syndromes 1081, 1088
Thalidomide 766, 1142
Theophylline 1000
Therapeutic foods 165
Therapeutic index 40
Therapeutic modalities in rheumatology 787
Thermal injury 118
Thermoregulation 1461
Thiabendazole 420, 440
Thiamine 174, 1344
    deficiency, diagnosis of 175
Thiazide 459
    diuretics 645
Thiazolidinediones 555, 591
Thinking, disturbance of 1546
Thiocarbamides 667
Third-generation drugs 905
Thomsen's disease 1478
Thoracic cage, injuries to 1036
Thoracoscopy 968
Thorborn's sign 1441
Thought
    and speech 1559
    block 1547
    broadcast 1548, 1555
    deprivation 1548
    insertion 1548, 1555
    stopping 1585
    withdrawal 1555
Thought/talk 1558
Threadworm 420
Thrombin time 1174
Thrombocythemia, essential 1166
Thrombocytopathy 1181
Thrombocytopenia 231, 332, 337, 1494
    causes of 1175
    secondary 1181

Thrombocytosis 1494
causes of 1166
Thromboembolic pulmonary hypertension, chronic 925, 1013
Thrombolytic agents 906
classification of 905
Thrombolytic therapy 905, 906, 926
Thrombophilia 1204
Thromboplastin time, partial 1174
Thrombopoiesis-stimulating 1179
agents 1179
Thrombopoietin 1054
stimulating protein 1055
Thrombotic thrombocytopenic purpura 1202, 1494
Thunderclap headache 1343
Thyroid 658
acropachy 666
autoantibodies, demonstration of 661
crisis 669
disorders 658, 785, 1539
function 660
tests 660
tests abnormalities 661
hormone
actions of 659
resistance syndrome 673
medullary carcinoma of 676
peroxidase antibody 1374
scintiscanning 661
storm 668
tumor of 675
Thyroid-associated eye disease 665
Thyroiditis 673
acute suppurative 673
chronic 674
drug-induced 673
subacute 673
Thyroid-stimulating hormone 646
Thyrotoxic
crisis 668
ophthalmopathy 1473
Thyrotropin releasing hormone 474, 642
Thyroxine deficiency 1070
Tiagabine 1388
Tic douloureux 1325
Ticagrelor 913, 1185
Tick 94
paralysis 94
Tick-borne
relapsing fever 258
typhus 266
Ticlopidine 1185
Tidal percussion 965
Tidal volume 959
Tigecycline 51
Tiger snake 96
Tinea barbae 1504
Tinea capitis 1504
Tinea corporis 1504
Tinea cruris 1504
Tinea faciale 1504
Tinea manuum 1505
Tinea pedis 1505
Tinea unguium 1505
Tinea versicolor 1507
Tinidazole 55, 408
Tirofiban 913
Tissue
factor pathway inhibitor 1172
invasion 428
myiasis, deep 91
nematodes 432
plasminogen activator 906
alterations in 952
polypeptide specific antigen 71
serrulatus 92
Tizanidine 1428
T-lymphocytes 25, 1052
TNM descriptors 1024
Tobacco
chewing 151
workers 153
Tobacco-related diseases 150
Tobramycin 50, 51
Tocilizumab 736

Tocopherol 1347
Todd's paralysis 1386
Tofacitinib 736
Tolcapone, dose of 1394
Tongue
atrophy of 484
diseases of 480, 483
Tonic-clonic seizures 1381
Tonsillitis
acute 974
chronic 974
Tophaceous gout, chronic 774
Topiramate 1387
Topographagnosia 1298
Toremifene 78
Torsade-de-pointes 872
Torsemide 459
Torture 1566
Torulosis 380
Total dose infusion 1066
Total health value of food 158
Toxic 1456
adenomas 669
chemicals 1090
diffuse goiter 664
effect 1110
epidermal necrolysis 215, 1529
megacolon 512, 513
shock syndrome 215
Toxic/metabolic 1425
Toxicity
acute 169
chronic 169
Toxin 142, 1392
of staphylococci 214
reduce absorption of 125
Toxin-mediated lesions 214
Toxoplasma gondii 411
Toxoplasmosis 405, 411, 1356
congenital 411
in AIDS 412
in pregnancy 412
treatment of 413
Tracheal obstruction 977
Tracheostomy 272
Tractus solitarius 1326
Tranexamic acid 1188, 1193
Tranquilizers, minor 1582
Transarterial chemoembolization 561
Transarterial radioembolization 561
Transbronchial needle aspiration 1009
Transcellular fluid 442
Transcobalamin II, congenital deficiency of 1070
Transcranial Doppler 1306
test 1338
Transcranial magnetic stimulation 1304
Transcriptase inhibitors, reverse 295
Transcriptase polymerase chain reaction, reverse 329
Transesophageal echo 82
Transference neurosis 1584
Transferrin 182
receptor 182
Transformed bladder 1465
Transformed migraine 1341
Transfusion
indications for 1098
therapy, hazards of 1100
transmitted infections 1101
Transient erythroblastopenia of childhood 1093
Transient ischemic attack 1406
Transient myeloid disorder of infancy 1122
Transient proteinuria 1214
Transjugular intrahepatic portosystemic shunt 1490
Translocational hyponatremia 443
Transmagnetic stimulation 1579
Transmission
electron microscopy 1216
mode of 243
prevention of 1375
Transmyocardial laser revascularization 912
Transplacental transfer 42
Transplacental transmission 411
Transretinoic acid 77, 1110
Transthyretin-related amyloidosis 1147
Trans-tubular K$^+$ gradient 446
Transudate, causes of 1030
Transudative effusion 1030

Transverse myelitis 1443
Trasylol 1194
Trazodone 1372
Treatment failure, management of 549
Trematode infections 428
Tremors, essential 1404
Trench fever 254
Treponema pallidum 274
immobilization 276
pertenue 255
Treprostinil 751
Triatoma 404
magista 404
Trichinellosis 421
Trichinosis 421
Trichoepithelioma 1543
Trichomonas vaginalis 283
Trichomoniasis 283
Trichuriasis 418
Triclabendazole 429
Tricuspid atresia 834
Tricuspid regurgitation 854
causes of primary 854
Tricuspid stenosis 853
Tricuspid valve lesions 853
Tricyclic antidepressants 935, 1581
Trifluridine 56, 57
Trigeminal autonomic cephalalgias 1341
Trigeminal nerve 1324
Trigeminal neuralgia 1325, 1343
Trigeminal neuropathy, bilateral 1326
Trimethoprim 52
Triose-phosphate deficiency 1081
Triplet repeat expansion disorders 15
Triradiate pelvis 171
Trisomy 16
13 17
18 17
Trochlear nerve palsy 1323
Trombicula deliensis 266
Trombone tremor 1353
Tropheryma whipplei 503, 767, 1376
Trophic factors 1402
Trophy sign, calf head on 1474
Tropical pancreatitis 615
Tropical pulmonary eosinophilia 995
Tropical pyomyositis 215
Tropical splenomegaly syndrome 390, 1169
Tropical sprue 503, 1490
Trotter's triad 1326
True hermaphroditism 707
True precocious puberty 704
Trypanids 402
Trypanosoma brucei 402
gambiense 402
Trypanosoma gambiense 402
Trypanosomiasis 384
Tryponosomal chancre 402
Trypsin 473
TSH-receptor antibodies 661
Tsutsugamushi fever 266
Tubeless pancreatic function tests 566
Tuberculin skin test 304
Tuberculoid leprosy 313
Tuberculosis 298, 508, 614, 936
abdominal 507
in HIV positive patients, treatment of 308
of mesenteric lymph nodes 508
prevention of 309
primary 300
Tuberculous 1352
disease 1351
exposure 1351
meningitis 310, 1351, 1352
pleural effusion 1031
Tubular necrosis, acute 1273
Tubular obstruction 1232
Tubular proteinuria 1214, 1221
Tubulointerstitial nephritis 1242
chronic 1243
Tumor 72, 658
benign 1019, 1369
cells, destruction of 26
demonstration of 679
in thorax 1022
kinetics 72

localization of 695
lysis syndrome 1265
malignant 1019
markers 70
necrosis factor 1000
primary 1420
secondary 1420
suppressor genes 11
Tumorigenesis 70
Tunga penetrans 95
Turiya avastha 1333
Turner's syndrome 18, 939
Twelfth cranial nerve 1331
Twenty-nail dystrophy 1537
Typhoid
cholecystitis 564
fever 228
nodules 229
state 229
Typhus exanthematicus 263
Tyrosine kinase inhibitors 1117
Tzanck smear 333

U

Udenafil 703
Ulcerohypertrophic forms 508
Ulcers 490
Ulcus molle 283
Ullrich congenital
muscular dystrophy 1474
myopathy 1474
Unarmed tapeworm 423
Undernutrition, types of 164
Underweight 164
mild 164
moderate 164
severe 164
Undulant fever 243
Uninhibited bladder 1465
Universal health coverage 3
Unstable angina pectoris 912
Unstable diabetes 598
Unverricht-lundborg disease 1383
Upper respiratory tract, diseases of 973
Urea cycle disorders 1437
Ureaplasma urealyticum 284
Uremic acidosis 452, 460
Uremic bleeding, treatment of 1241
Uremic encephalopathy 1492
Uremic lung 1239
Uremic renal osteodystrophy 1239
Uremic toxins, circulating 1238
Ureteric bud 1207
Ureterosigmoidostomy 460
Urethra, distal 1250
Urethritis, nonspecific 280
Uric acid 1218
stones 1257
Uricolytic drugs 775
Uricostatic drugs 775
Uricosuric agents 775
Urinary
anion gap 452, 455, 456
bladder, control of 1461
calcium 678
calculi 637
casts 1216
cyclic adenosine-3', 5'-monophosphate 678
hydroxyproline 678, 771
myiasis 91
phosphate 678
system 1207
tract 1207
anatomy of 1250
defense mechanisms of 1250
fungal infections of 1256
infection 236, 612, 1243, 1250, 1273
infection, complicated 1250, 1253
obstruction 1213, 1274
Urinary-free cortisol 687
Urine
avoids stasis, unobstructed flow of 1250
culture 231
role of 1250
examination 1140, 1213

Urokinase 906
Urologic investigations 1220
Ursodeoxycholic acid 564
Urticaria 1526
Urticarial
acute 1526
drug reactions 1530
treatment of 1527
vasculitis 1526
Ustekinumab 1515
Uterine bleeding, dysfunctional 710
Uterine dysfunction 706

V

Vaccination 250, 251, 325, 337, 360, 1187
indications for 351
Vaccine 233, 297, 339
against hepatitis E virus 351
immune globulin 332
Vaccinia gangrenosum 332
Vaccinology 38
Vacuolar myelopathy 293
Vagabond's disease 94
Vagal nerve 1330
stimulation in epilepsy 1390
Vagus nerve 1330
Valganciclovir 376
Valley sign 1473
Valproate 1582
Valsalva test 1463
Valsartan 892
Valvulae conneventes 471
Valvular heart disease 938, 946
causes of chronic 839
chronic 838
Valvular pneumothorax 1032
Vancomycin 53, 252
Vanillyl mandelic acid 71
Vanishing pulmonary tumor 1029
Vaptans 468
Vaquez's disease 1163
Vardenafil 703
Varenicline 152
Variable vessel vasculitis 759
Variant angina 914
Variceal bleeding, management of 548
Varicella 332, 1075, 1377
during pregnancy 333
gangrenosa 333
pneumonia, primary 333
Varicella-zoster
immune globulin 334
virus 1359
Varicose ulcer 1531
Variegate porphyria 626
Varilrix 334
Variola major 330
Variola minor 330, 331
Variola sine eruption 331
Vascular access
for hemodialysis 1277
routes for coronary interventions 945
Vascular changes 583
Vascular cognitive impairment 1416
Vascular dementia 1373, 1416
Vascular disease 294
peripheral 609
Vascular disorders 509, 1174
Vascular endothelial growth factor 1311
Vascular lesions of cerebellum 1438
Vascular phenomena 537
Vascular purpura 1183
drug-induced 1184
Vasculitic disorders, frequency distribution of 753
Vasculitic neuropathy 1456
Vasculitis 749, 935, 1531
causes of secondary 753
Vasoactive intestinal polypeptide 71, 471, 474
Vasodilator 891
drugs 816
Vasogenic cerebral edema 1363
Vasomotor
dysfunction 814
rhinitis 973
symptoms 710, 1462

Vasopressin 549, 1464
analogues 645
excess 645
Vasopressor drugs 816
Vegetable oil increases bioavailability 1348
Vein of Galen 1289
Vein thrombosis, deep 122, 1412
Velcade 1143
Vena cava
filter, inferior 947
obstruction, superior 938
Venezuelan hemorrhagic fever 359
Venom 97
Veno-occlusive disease of Jamaica 145
Venous drainage 1289, 1440
Venous filters 928
Venous pulsation 1320
Venous strokes 1406
Venous thromboembolism 513, 924
Venous thrombosis 938, 1095
Ventilation 327
assistance to 970
imaging 967
imbalance in 958
perfusion abnormalities 958
regulation of 956
Ventilator-associated pneumonia 977
Ventilatory assistance 992
indications for 993
Ventilatory impairment, severe 987
Ventricular assist devices 812
Ventricular asystole 878
Ventricular encephalitis 1359
Ventricular fibrillation 873
Ventricular premature beats 864
Ventricular septal defect 825, 947
Ventricular standstill 878
Ventricular tachycardia 872
Ventriculectomy, partial left 812
Venturi mask 970
VEP abnormalities, basis of 1305
Verapamil 868, 892
Vergence system 1322
Vernet syndrome 1331
Verocytotoxin 236
Verruca 1501
plana 1502
Verruga peruana 253
Vertebral column causing neurological lesions,
diseases of 1448
Vertebrobasilar ischemia 1451
Vertebroplasty 1143
Vertigo 1329, 1595
causes of 1329
Vesiculobullous 1528
disorders 1523
Vessel vasculitides, small 756
Vessel vasculitis, large 754
Vestibular system 1328
Vestibulocochlear nerve 1328
Vibrio fetus 251
Vibrio parahaemolyticus 143
Vidarabine 56, 57
Vigabatrin 1388
Vigorous achalasia 487
Vildagliptin 591
Villus adenoma 509
Vim-Silverman needle 968
Vinca alkaloids 75
Vincent's angina 483
Vincent's spirochetes 483
Vincristine 1142
Viper 96
bites 98
Viperidae 96
Viral
antigens 322
diarrhea, causes of 251
diseases, prevention of 322
hepatitis 339
B in pregnancy 349
B, acute 349
diagnosis of 346
inclusions, demonstration of 322
infections 321, 323, 1075, 1501

morphology 341
multiplication 321
spread 321
Virtual neck exploration 680
Virus 70, 322, 360
fixed 362
isolation 324
Visceral larva migrans 422
Visceral leishmaniasis 397
Visceral pain 475
Visceral syphilis 275
Viscosupplementation 779
Vision 1588
poor 1320
Visual evoked potential 649, 1305
Visual field 1317
defect 1367
Visual illusion 1298
Visual or cerebellar disturbance 1377
Visuospatial function 1366
Vital capacity 960
Vital signs 1334, 1587
Vitamin 473
A 168, 1348
deficiency, causes of 168
toxicity 169
B₁ 174
deficiency 1344
B₁₂ 177, 1347
absorption 501
B₂ 175
B₃ 175, 1345
B₅ 1346
B₆ 1346
B₇ 176, 1346
B₉ 1346
C 1347
adverse effects of 179
deficiency 1070
in health, major roles of 178
D 169, 1348
dependent rickets type i 172
metabolites 170, 1211
resistant rickets 172
E 173, 1347
deficiency 1437
H 176
K 173
antagonists 1196
deficiency 173, 1192
Vitiligo 636, 1534
Vivax malaria, uncomplicated 392
Vocal cord paralysis, causes of 976
Voglibose 592
Voltage gated potassium channel 1374
Voltage-dependent channels 861
Vomiting 475, 485
von Graefe's sign 1328
von Hippel-Lindau syndrome 1438

von Willebrand's disease 1190
genetic transmission of 1190
Voriconazole 58, 59
Voyeurism 1573
Vulpian-Bernhardt syndrome 1433
Vulvovaginal candidiasis 1506

W

Waddling gait 1303
Waldenstrom's macroglobulinemia 71, 1075
Warfarin 1196
administration 1197
effects 1196
reduce 1196
Warthin Finkeldey cells 328
Warts 1501
common 1501
Wasps 92
Water
abnormalities of 442
and electrolytes 473
balance 442
depletion heat exhaustion 105
deprivation test 467, 1214
loading test 1214
Waterhouse-Friderichsen syndrome 220, 221
Watering-can scrotum 279
Water-soluble vitamins 174
Waxy casts 1216
Waxy flexibility/catalepsy 1555
Weakness 636
Weber's syndrome 1410
Weber's test 1329
Wechsler adult intelligence scale 1551
Wechsler memory scale 1551
Wegener's granulomatosis 757, 1027, 1263
Weight and body composition 1587
Weight, loss of 475, 636
Weil-Felix reaction 266
Weingarten's syndrome 995
Wenckebach phenomenon 875
Wernicke's aphasia 1300
Wernicke's encephalopathy 174, 1345
Wernicke's hemianopic pupillary 1297
Wernicke-Korsakoff syndrome 1344, 1345
West Nile encephalitis 1360
West syndrome 1381
Westermark's sign 925
Western blotting 19
Westphal-Strumpell pseudosclerosis 624
Wet beriberi 174
Wet drowning 113
Wet purpura 1176
Whipple's disease 503, 767, 1375, 1376, 1490
Whipworm infection 418
Whispering pectoriloquy 966
White dermographism 1519
White hand 120
White pulp 1167

White-coat 882
Whitmore's disease 244
Whooping cough 225
Wickham's striae 1515
Widal test 231
Widow's hump 770
Wilson's disease 535, 624, 1396, 1438
Winterbottom's sign 402
Wire loop lesions 742
Withdrawal syndromes 1350
Wohlfahrtia 90, 91
Wolbachia 267
in lymphatic filariasis 434
Wolff-Parkinson-White syndrome 867
Woody thyroiditis 674
Woolsorter's disease 240
World Federation of Neurological Surgeons Scale 1415
World Health Organization classification 1133
World Hepatitis Day 339
World Malaria Day 394
Wound, surgical toilet of 271
Wuchereria bancrofti 432

X

Xanthine oxidase 773
inhibitors 912
Xanthochromia 1309
Xanthogranulomatous pyelonephritis 1255
Xeno diagnosis 405
Xenopsylla cheopis 265
Xerophthalmia 738
Xerostomia 738
Xylose absorption test 501

Y

Yawning sign 1467
Yaws 253, 255
Yellow fever 369, 936
Yellow mexican poppy 145
Yersinia enterocolitica 143
Yersinia pestis 241
Y-linked diseases 15
Yoga exercises 588
Young female arteritis 929

Z

Zanamivir 57, 324
Zenker's degeneration 229
Zika virus infections 373
Zinc 185, 1349
Zoledronate 682
Zollinger-Ellison syndrome 715, 494
Zonisamide 1388
Zoom endoscopes 478
Zoonoses 193
Zoster sine herpete 335
Zovirax 57
Zulu Dancer's hip 721
Zygomycetes 1362